Transplantation

Transplantation

Edited by

LEO C. GINNS, MD
Associate Professor of Medicine
Harvard Medical School;
Medical Director
Lung Transplant Program
Massachusetts General Hospital
Boston, Massachusetts

A. BENEDICT COSIMI, MD
Claude E. Welch Professor of Surgery
Harvard Medical School;
Chief, Transplantation Unit
Massachusetts General Hospital
Boston, Massachusetts

PETER J. MORRIS, MB, PhD, FRS
Nuffield Department of Surgery
University of Oxford;
Oxford Radcliffe Hospital
The John Radcliffe
Oxford, England

Blackwell
Science

Editorial Offices:
Commerce Place, 350 Main Street, Malden, Massachusetts 02148, USA
Osney Mead, Oxford OX2 0EL, England
25 John Street, London WC1N 2BL, England
23 Ainslie Place, Edinburgh EH3 6AJ, Scotland
54 University Street, Carlton, Victoria 3053, Australia

Other Editorial Offices:
Blackwell Wissenschafts-Verlag GmbH, Kurfürstendamm 57, 10707 Berlin, Germany
Blackwell Science KK, MG Kodenmacho Building, 7–10 Kodenmacho Nihombashi, Chuo-ku, Tokyo 104, Japan

Distributors:

USA

Blackwell Science, Inc.
Commerce Place
350 Main Street
Malden, Massachusetts 02148
(Telephone orders: 800-215-1000 or 781-388-8250; fax orders: 781-388-8270)

CANADA

Login Brothers Book Company
324 Saulteaux Crescent
Winnipeg, Manitoba, R3J 3T2
(Telephone orders: 204-224-4068)

AUSTRALIA

Blackwell Science Pty, Ltd.
54 University Street
Carlton, Victoria 3053
(Telephone orders: 03-9347-0300; fax orders: 03-9349-3016)

OUTSIDE NORTH AMERICA AND AUSTRALIA

Blackwell Science, Ltd.
c/o Marston Book Services, Ltd.
P.O. Box 269
Abingdon
Oxon OX14 4YN
England
(Telephone orders: 44-01235-465500; fax orders: 44-01235-465555)

Acquisitions: Christopher Davis
Production: Kevin Sullivan
Manufacturing: Lisa Flanagan
Cover design by Leslie Haimes
Typeset by Best-set Typesetter Ltd., Hong Kong
Printed and bound by Braun-Brumfield, Inc.

Printed in the United States of America
00 01 02 5 4 3 2

Library of Congress Cataloging-in-Publication Data

Transplantation / edited by Leo C. Ginns, A. Benedict Cosimi, Peter J. Morris.
p. cm.
ISBN 0-86542-520-5
1. Transplantation of organs, tissues, etc.
2. Transplantation immunology. I. Ginns, Leo C.
II. Cosimi, A. Benedict. III. Morris, Peter J., 1943–
[DNLM: 1. Transplantation. 2. Transplantation Immunology. WO 660 T7692 1998]
RD120.7.T684 1998
617.9′5—dc21
DNLM/DLC
for Library of Congress 98-37281
CIP

To Nancy, Sara, Laura, Rebecca, Mildred

LCG

To my wife and children, Pat, Lisa, Gregg, and Beth, to my parents, and to Cathy for all their support

ABC

To the pioneers who made it happen

PJM

This book is also dedicated to all those transplant patients who have allowed us to gain the knowledge over the years on which this book is based.

CONTENTS

Mary S. Ametani, BS
Department of Surgery
University of Wisconsin Medical School
Madison, Wisconsin

Hugh Auchincloss, MD
Associate Professor of Surgery
Transplant Unit
Harvard Medical School;
Department of Surgery
Massachusetts General Hospital
Boston, Massachusetts

Leonard L. Bailey, MD
Professor and Chairman
Department of Surgery
Loma Linda University Medical Center;
Surgeon-in-Chief
Loma Linda University Children's Hospital
Loma Linda, California

John C. Baldwin, MD
Vice President for Health Affairs
Dartmouth College;
Dean, Dartmouth Medical School
Hanover, New Hampshire

James F. Burdick, MD
Division of Transplantation
Department of Surgery
Johns Hopkins Hospital
Baltimore, Maryland

Sir Roy Y. Calne, FRS
Emeritus Professor of Surgery
Department of Surgery
Cambridge University
Cambridge, United Kingdom

Charles B. Carpenter, MD
Professor of Medicine
Harvard Medical School;
Laboratory of Immunogenetics and Transplantation
Renal Division, Department of Medicine
Brigham and Women's Hospital
Boston, Massachusetts

Lucienne Chatenoud, MD
Department of Clinical Immunology
Hôpital Necker
Paris, France

A. Benedict Cosimi, MD
Claude E. Welch Professor of Surgery
Harvard Medical School;
Chief, Transplantation Unit
Massachusetts General Hospital
Boston, Massachusetts

Margaret J. Dallman, DPhil
Department of Biology
Imperial College of Science, Technology, and Medicine
London, England

G. William Dec, MD
Medical Director, Cardiac Transplantation Program
Massachusetts General Hospital
Boston, Massachusetts

Francis L. Delmonico, MD
Medical Director, New England Organ Bank;
Director, Renal Transplantation
Massachusetts General Hospital
Boston, Massachusetts

Johan DeMeester, MD
Division of Transplantation
Department of Surgery
Johns Hopkins Hospital
Baltimore, Maryland

Michael Donaghy, DPhil, FRCP
Department of Neurology
The Radcliffe Infirmary
Oxford, England

James D. Eason, MD
Department of Surgery
Harvard Medical School;
Transplantation Unit
Massachusetts General Hospital
Boston, Massachusetts

Richard N. Fine, MD
Department of Pediatrics
State University of New York at Stony Brook
School of Medicine;
Children's Medical Center at Stony Brook
Stony Brook, New York

Jay A. Fishman, MD
Associate Professor of Medicine
Harvard Medical School;
Infectious Disease and Transplantation Units
Massachusetts General Hospital
Boston, Massachusetts

Leo C. Ginns, MD
Associate Professor of Medicine
Harvard Medical School;
Medical Director, Lung Transplant Program
Massachusetts General Hospital
Boston, Massachusetts

Douglas A. Hale, MD
Division of Organ Transplantation
Beth Israel Deaconess Medical Center
Boston, Massachusetts

David Hamilton, FRCS
Renal Unit
Western Infirmary
Glasgow, Scotland

Barry D. Kahan, MD, PhD
Division of Immunology and Organ Transplantation
The University of Texas Medical School at Houston
Houston, Texas

Paul A. Keown, MB, CHB
Professor and Director of Immunology
Vancouver Hospital and Health Sciences Center
Vancouver, British Columbia
Canada

Farrukh A. Khan, MD
Department of Surgery
University of Miami School of Medicine
Miami, Florida

Goran B. Klintmalm, MD, PhD, FACS
Department of Transplantation
Baylor University Medical Center
Houston, Texas

Isamu Koyama, MD
Division of Transplantation
Department of Surgery
Johns Hopkins Hospital
Baltimore, Maryland

Erik Langhoff, MD
Hemodialysis and Continuous Ambulatory Peritoneal
Dialysis Units
Massachusetts General Hospital
Boston, Massachusetts

George V. Letsou, MD
Department of Surgery
Baylor College of Medicine
Houston, Texas

Bruce E. Loveland, PhD
Associate Professor
Complement Research Laboratory
The Austin Research Institute
Heidelberg, Australia

Janet Maurer, MD
Cleveland Clinic Foundation
Cleveland, Ohio

Steven L. McAfee, MD
Instructor of Medicine
Harvard Medical School;
Assistant Director, Bone Marrow Transplant Program
Massachusetts General Hospital
Boston, Massachusetts

Sue V. McDiarmid, MD
Director, Pediatric Liver Transplantation
UCLA Medical Center
Los Angeles, California

Ian F. C. McKenzie, MD, PhD
Professor and Director
The Austin Research Institute
Heidelberg, Australia

Anthony P. Monaco, MD
Division of Organ Transplantation
Beth Israel Deaconess Medical Center
Boston, Massachusetts

Peter J. Morris, MB, PhD, FRS
Nuffield Department of Surgery
University of Oxford;
Oxford Radcliffe Hospital
The John Radcliffe
Oxford, England

James M. Neuberger, MD
Consultant Physician
Liver and Hepatobiliary Unit
Queen Elizabeth Hospital
Edgbaston, Birmingham
United Kingdom

Kevin J. O'Connor, PA, CPTC
Director, Donation Services
New England Organ Bank
Newton, Massachusetts

Israel Penn, MD
Professor of Surgery
Department of Surgery
University of Cincinnati Medical Center
Cincinnati, Ohio

John A. Powelson, MD
Department of Surgery
Harvard Medical School;
Transplantation Unit
Massachusetts General Hospital
Boston, Massachusetts

Stephen C. Rayhill, MD
Assistant Professor of Surgery
University of Iowa Hospitals and Clinics
Iowa City, Iowa

Maria A. Rodino, MD
Division of Endocrinology and Metabolism
Columbia-Presbyterian Medical Center
New York, New York

Robert H. Rubin, MD, FACP, FCCP
Director, Center for Experimental Pharmacology and Therapeutics
Division of Health Sciences and Technology
Gordon and Marjorie Osborne Chair in Health Sciences and Technology
Harvard University—Massachusetts Institute of Technology;
Chief, Surgical and Transplant Infectious Disease
Massachusetts General Hospital
Boston, Massachusetts

David H. Sachs, MD
Harvard Medical School;
Transplantation Biology Research Center
Surgical Service
Massachusetts General Hospital
Boston, Massachusetts

Mauro S. Sandrin, PhD
Professor, Transplantation Laboratory
The Austin Research Institute
Heidelberg, Australia

Marc J. Semigran, MD
Harvard Medical School;
Cardiology Division
Massachusetts General Hospital
Boston, Massachusetts

Ferda Senel, MD
Division of Immunology and Organ Transplantation
The University of Texas Medical School at Houston
Houston, Texas

Neil Shachter, MD
Division of Endocrinology and Metabolism
Columbia-Presbyterian Medical Center
New York, New York

David Shaffer, MD
Associate Professor of Surgery
Harvard Medical School;
Division of Organ Transplantation
Beth Israel Deaconess Medical Center
Boston, Massachusetts

Elizabeth Shane, MD
Division of Endocrinology and Metabolism
Columbia-Presbyterian Medical Center
New York, New York

A. G. R. Sheil, MD
Department of Surgery
University of Sydney;
Department of Transplantation Surgery
Royal Prince Alfred Hospital
Sydney, Australia

Philip L. Shields, MD
Liver and Hepatobiliary Unit
Queen Elizabeth Hospital
Edgbaston, Birmingham
United Kingdom

Hans W. Sollinger, MD, PhD
Folkert O. Belzer Professor of Surgery
Chair, Division of Organ Transplantation
University of Wisconsin Medical School
Madison, Wisconsin

James H. Southard, PhD
Department of Surgery
University of Wisconsin Medical School
Madison, Wisconsin

Thomas R. Spitzer, MD
Associate Professor of Medicine
Harvard Medical School;
Director, Bone Marrow Transplant Program
Massachusetts General Hospital
Boston, Massachusetts

Owen S. Surman, MD
Department of Psychiatry
Massachusetts General Hospital
Boston, Massachusetts

Megan Sykes, MD
Associate Professor of Surgery and Medicine (Immunology)
Harvard Medical School;
Immunologist, Departments of Surgery and Medicine
Massachusetts General Hospital
Boston, Massachusetts

Sanjiv Tewari, MD
Northeast Ohio Pulmonary and Critical Care Associates
Akron, Ohio

Nicholas L. Tilney, MD
Harvard Medical School;
Department of Surgery
Brigham and Women's Hospital
Boston, Massachusetts

Nina Tolkoff-Rubin, MD
Associate Professor of Medicine
Harvard Medical School;
Director, Hemodialysis and Continuous Ambulatory
Peritoneal Dialysis Units
Massachusetts General Hospital
Boston, Massachusetts

Andreas G. Tzakis, MD
Department of Surgery
University of Miami School of Medicine
Miami, Florida

Yves F. Ch. Vanrenterghem, MD
Baxter Chair for Renal Transplantation
University of Leuven;
Department of Nephrology
University Hospital Gasthuisberg
Leuven, Belgium

Johan F. Vanwalleghem, MD
Department of Nephrology
University Hospital Gasthuisberg
Leuven, Belgium

Luca A. Vricella, MD
Clinical Research Fellow
Section of Pediatric Cardiac Surgery
Loma Linda University Medical Center
Loma Linda, California
Surgery Resident
The George Washington University Medical Center
Washington, District of Columbia

Mark Waer, MD, PhD
Professor of Nephrology
Director, Laboratory for Experimental Transplantation
University of Leuven
Leuven, Belgium

John C. Wain, MD
Lung Transplant Program
Massachusetts General Hospital
Boston, Massachusetts

Rowan G. Walker, MD, BS, FRACP
Department of Nephrology
Royal Melbourne Hospital
Melbourne, Australia

Kathryn J. Wood, MD
Nuffield Department of Surgery
University of Oxford
Oxford Radcliffe Hospital
Oxford, England

COMMENTATORS

Christina Brattström, MD, PhD
Attending Surgeon
Department of Transplantation Surgery
Karolinska Institute
Huddinge Hospital
Stockholm, Sweden

Michel Broyer, MD
Infants Malades, Néphrologie Pediatrique
Hôpital Necker
Paris, France

Jeremy Chapman, MD, FRACP, FRCP
Director of Renal Medicine
Westmead Hospital
Sydney, Australia

David K. C. Cooper, MD, PhD, FRCS
Harvard Medical School;
Transplantation Biology Research Center
Massachusetts General Hospital
Boston, Massachusetts

Jessica L. Fewkes, MD
Harvard Medical School;
Department of Dermatology
Massachusetts General Hospital
Boston, Massachusetts

John J. Fung, MD
Department of Surgery
Presbyterian University Hospital
Pittsburgh, Pennsylvania

John M. Goldman, DM, FRCP, FRCPath
Professor of Leukaemia Biology
Chairman, Department of Haematology
Imperial College School of Medicine
London, England

David Grant, MD, FRCS
University of Toronto
Toronto, Ontario
Canada

Carl G. Groth, MD, PhD
Professor of Transplantation Surgery
Department of Transplantation Surgery
Karolinska Institute
Huddinge Hospital
Stockholm, Sweden

Ronald D. Guttmann, MD, FRCPC
Professor of Medicine and Director
Centre for Clinical Immunobiology of Transplantation
McGill University Faculty of Medicine
Montreal, Quebec
Canada

Pekka Häyry, MD, PhD
Professor of Transplantation Surgery and Immunology
Transplantation Laboratory
University of Helsinki and Helsinki University Hospital
Helsinki, Finland

Suzanne T. Ildstad, MD
Institute for Cellular Therapeutics
University of Louisville
Louisville, Kentucky

Darlene S. Johnson, MD
Harvard Medical School;
Department of Dermatology
Massachusetts General Hospital
Boston, Massachusetts

Stuart J. Knechtle, MD
Department of Surgery
University of Wisconsin Medical School
Madison, Wisconsin

Gauke Kootstra, MD
Professor and Chairman
Department of Surgery
University Hospital Maastricht
Maastricht, The Netherlands

Henri Kreis, MD
Service de Transplantation
Hôpital Necker
Paris, France

Paul McMaster, MA, MB, ChM, FRCS, FICS
Clinical Director, Liver and Hepatobiliary Unit
Queen Elizabeth Hospital and University of Birmingham
Birmingham, United Kingdom

J. A. Myburgh, MD
Department of Surgery
University of Witwatersand Medical School
Johannesburg, South Africa

Kazuo Ota, MD
Director, Ota Medical Research Institute
Tokyo, Japan

Leendert C. Paul, MD, PhD
Keenan Professor of Medicine
Director, Renal Division
St. Michael's Hospital
Toronto, Ontario
Canada

David Pegg, MD
Medical Cryobiology Unit
Biology Department
University of York
York, United Kingdom
East Anglia Tissue Bank
National Blood Service
Cambridge, United Kingdom

Dale G. Renlund, MD
Medical Director
UTAH Cardiac Transplant Program
Salt Lake City, Utah

Haval Shirwan, PhD
Institute for Cellular Therapeutics
University of Louisville
Louisville, Kentucky

Arthur J. Sober, MD
Harvard Medical School;
Department of Dermatology
Massachusetts General Hospital
Boston, Massachusetts

Jean-Paul Soulillou, MD
Institut National de la Sante et de la Recherche Medicale (INSERM)
C.H.U. Hotel-Dieu
Nantes, France

Thomas E. Starzl, MD, PhD
University of Pittsburgh;
Department of Surgery
Presbyterian University Hospital
Pittsburgh, Pennsylvania

David E. R. Sutherland, MD
Department of Surgery
University of Minnesota Hospital
Minneapolis, Minnesota

Karl Wagner, MD
Leitender Arzt der IV. Medizinischen Abteilung
Nieren—und Hochdruckkrankheiten
Allgemeines Krankenhaus Barmbek
Rübenkamp, Hamburg
Germany

Ken Welsh, MD
Transplant Immunology
Tissue Typing Laboratory
Oxford Transplant Centre
Oxford, England

Lori J. West, MD, DPhil, FRCPC
Assistant Professor of Paediatrics
University of Toronto;
Medical Director, Heart Transplant Service
Divisions of Cardiology and Immunology
The Hospital for Sick Children
Toronto, Ontario
Canada

FOREWORD

Transplantation mobilizes the talent of a selected corps of qualified experts, who have collectively taken on the challenge of imparting the entire subject of living organ transplantation, save only a few particulars such as corneal and bone transplantation. It is still possible to assemble this information in one place even though an immense amount has been learned about this collection of topics in a scant fifty years. Emphasis is placed on clinical aspects. Transplantation is, in some respects, a rather curious medical specialty. It is not defined in anatomical terms, as, for example, cardiology, gastroenterology, and neurology are, and its surgical aspects are not restricted by any narrow technical limits. Why, then, is transplantation a coherent subject at all? The answer lies in the common challenges faced by all efforts to provide functioning, viable organs to a needy individual from an outside source. Thus, a transplanted lung will mobilize a complex immune response very similar to that encountered by a transplanted heart in another recipient. The available methods utilized to quell this response are also similar for different organs. These are well described in the following pages, where it is made clear that the rejection reaction is managed fundamentally in the same way and the systemic complications that may follow rejection treatment (i.e., other than the transplant itself) likewise are similar for all organ transplants. To be sure, when one approaches the problems of individual patients, there are interesting and important precepts and skills that apply only to recipients of the specific organ concerned. Nevertheless, for the present, it is my opinion that in a large, central hospital the teams engaged in transplantation of each of the organs considered in this volume should work in close coordination with one another in order to make full use of new advances that are generally applicable to all and that will continue to appear along the advancing front of the subject. This is what makes *Transplantation* so worthwhile.

One might naturally speculate that, because the features of transplantation that tend to bring its clinical branches together are clustered around the problems of rejection and its management, future discoveries that bring rejection reaction under easy control may lead eventually to fragmentation, with kidney transplantation becoming a part of everyday urology, liver transplantation a part of general surgery, and so on. This form of disciplinary evolution may be welcomed in due course. It remains my belief, however, that moves in this direction would be ill advised at the present time. This statement also extends to the formation of societies and journals focusing on the transplantation of any single organ. Hopefully, surgeons and other clinicians will play a central role in the gradual development of a full understanding of rejection activity. They have done much to get us where we are today. Nevertheless, even a superficial appraisal of the bounding science of immunogenetics should remind us that powerful new weapons are now being forged at some distance from the clinical arena. Thus, close coordination with relevant fundamental science must be contrived in any way possible by those clinicians who would like to contribute to significant core advances.

In the early clinical trials of kidney transplantation in the mid-1950s, pioneer clinicians stepped into the unknown as they performed a few transplants in an effort to find new answers in the face of desperate circumstances in individual patients. Available techniques were adapted from a variety of sources and the seminal events were observed almost in the same way geographic explorers recorded their encounters in the sixteenth century. Although occasionally transplants without immunosuppression to uremic recipients functioned impressively well for a time, the outcome was almost universally poor, with the striking exception of transplants between identical twins. When clinicians began employing immunosuppression, it consisted of selected levels of sublethal, whole body irradiation and variable doses of corticosteroids. That each of these could have a beneficial effect had been learned from laboratory experiments with animals. These regimens were, however, generally inadequate to the task, and one can only conclude that some of the clinicians involved at that time were not completely informed about the systematic findings of laboratory scientists who were pursuing the subject of transplant rejection, largely because of its intrinsic biologic interest, in thorough animal experiments. This was soon remedied, and one of the most stimulating and healthy aspects of the transplantation field that emerged, particularly for a period of about 15 years after the mid-1950s, was an intense feeling that every aspect was to be considered experimental. Laboratory scientists joined clinical investigators at the center of the process. This theme took on a strong international and interdisciplinary flavor, and as the participants were few and most were well known to one another, a feeling of coherence was maintained.

In those years, clinical transplantation meant almost exclusively kidney transplantation. All who were involved were acutely aware that the future of transplantation as a standard form of treatment was far from assured, as it remained uncertain whether transplantation could become clearly superior to chronic dialysis for the long-term management of renal failure. When the rate of success with kidney transplantation gradually improved, mainly with the introduction of improved methods of immunosuppression, this question was settled. Along with this advance and, it must be acknowledged, when payment for the treatment of renal failure was made a responsibility of the United States government, large numbers of patients were identified as potential beneficiaries and a growing number of clinicians of various stripes entered the field. The sense that transplantation was a highly experimental area, in which a close association between clinical efforts and relevant investigation was imperative, inevitably diminished. Treatment plans tended to fall into fixed protocols that were widely copied in newly established clinical transplantation programs.

This was reinforced by the continuing introduction of new chemical and biologic immunosuppressives that made the management of rejection considerably more reliable, the former class of substances coming entirely from the efforts of pharmaceutical companies, and the latter largely from academic sources. In close association with immunosuppressive developments came a rich period of contributions by surgeons, who built on the experience gained from kidney transplantation and branched out into the transplantation of other organs—first the heart, then the liver, and most recently the pancreas, lungs, and intestine. This rise in technical expertise after sufficiently good control of the rejection reaction had been achieved emphasized how closely the management of immunologic variables governs the range of the field. It can be anticipated that even better levels of control will generate possibilities for further technical advances, for the use of structures from both allogeneic and, perhaps, xenogeneic sources.

Although the potentially great value of producing states of specific immunologic tolerance to the foreign antigens presented by a transplanted structure has long been recognized, steadily improving transplant survival rates led many to believe that this objective may not have been very important after all. There has been a recently growing awareness, however, of the fact that continuing immunologic reactivity to foreign antigens is often associated with destructive effects on transplanted organs that can become manifest months or years after placement of the organ. Thus, the imperfections of chemically induced, nonspecific immunosuppression, as it is currently delivered, have reawakened interest in new approaches to the long-term control of rejection activity. I hesitate to use the precisely defined term "immunologic tolerance" in referring to this general subject, as many of the states of unresponsiveness under study do not fulfill the criterion of specific, central failures of the immune response, which is a prerequisite for being so named. Indeed, much information indicates that a rich set of alternative avenues to states of unresponsiveness exists, and that these alternatives must be carefully characterized for what they are (and what they are not) if they are to be tested in properly sophisticated clinical trials.

When viewed by the enlightened observer outside the field of transplantation and, perhaps even more clearly, by people outside medicine altogether, organ transplantation is known especially for certain easily publicized features. It is expensive. Regrettably, organs from human beings are available in numbers too small to benefit all potential recipients. Furthermore, because the transaction of transferring an organ from one individual to another is an intensely human one at every step in the process—calling on all the wisdom we have for the optimal handling and distribution of donated organs and the selection of their recipients—the attention of a wide range of savants extending from economics and the law to humanities, philosophy and even religion has been attracted. To my way of thinking, the clear shortcoming of our own species as a source of structures for the renewal of its own members can be expected to constitute a strong and continuing stimulus for further advances that will release us from this imperfect source. Thus, the ultimate answers to the trying ethical and moral questions we now face will have to be found in solutions that will circumvent them. The possibility of using xenospecific sources of tissues and organs has drawn much attention in recent years. Efforts are also now being directed at the possibility of utilizing human cells derived directly from the needy patient, then expanding these cells in vitro to the desired level for transplantation. The use of small segments of skin from burned patients for interim expansion in culture, before returning resultant skin sheets as autografts to the individual from whom they came, is an example of this method. The same could conceivably be done one day with small bits of liver tissue, even from a diseased organ, although major obstacles of remodeling and differentiation would have to be traversed. The rapid advances now being made in understanding the differentiation of biologic structures, and the availability of increasing numbers of highly active cytokines that can encourage cell growth in vitro, make this effort increasingly realistic. Meanwhile, the search for successful approaches to the use of animal organs continues. The manifold challenges offered by xenotransplantation are not to be taken lightly, but efforts in this direction are clearly far from hopeless and represent a natural field of activity for those who are aware of the pressing need for alternative organ sources.

Even though many interesting challenges confront the field of transplantation, this text also amply records the astounding progress that has already been made. Simply watching a young patient, previously bed-ridden and gasping for oxygen through a tube, breeze into a clinic for a follow-up check of her transplanted lung, take a deep breath with a sigh and a smile, and report miles run and new feats accomplished is enough to leave an indelible impression. Transplantation is a treatment that can succeed spectacularly. This success is still achieved, however, only by the most careful application of skills and experience. These are demanded especially in the early weeks after a new organ has been put in place, when success requires constant vigilance with a high degree of sensitivity to signs that all is not well. This attentiveness cannot be confined entirely to the early postoperative period, however, as all recipients of new organs must remain under heightened surveillance. Complications, both early and late, are not uncommon and are far better managed if dealt with promptly. Nowhere is this more clearly illustrated than in the management of infections in immunocompromised patients. In the early days of transplantation, the lives of patients were often snuffed out by rapidly evolving pulmonary infections attributable to a considerable range of organisms. This outcome is now rather rare, and the improvement, like many advances in bedside clinical medicine, can be credited to several factors. One stems from the recognition that airborne particulate matter can convey a variety of infections from *Aspergillus* to *Legionella*. This hazard has been greatly reduced by constructing nursing units through which passes only air that is under pressure and has been filtered free of even quite small particles. Even more important for patient survival has been the growing awareness of the contribution of the seasoned expert in infectious diseases who can recognize incipient infections early and with increasing assurance. The infections can then be targeted with specific therapy, often using new agents, with impressive success.

The mention, above, of the fact that many fundamental issues in transplantation management are shared by patients receiving any specific organ should not be interpreted as detracting from the importance of detailed advances that have made the successful transplantation of individual organs possible. These advances are amply illustrated in *Transplantation*, and examples are easy to cite. I will choose some from the surgical frontier. Successful transplantation of lungs or pulmonary lobes awaited the advent of reliable and safe techniques for the anastomosis of graft and recipient airways without leakage or stenosis. Likewise, liver transplantation required a new level of familiarity with the vascular anatomy around the liver, especially for joining the donor and recipient suprahepatic vena cava in the cramped quarters available beneath the diaphragm in a surgical field that did not invade the thorax. Experience also had to be applied to determining the optimal provision for biliary drainage from the new liver. Similar technical considerations were applied to transplantation of the pancreas, and some technical points are still not completely settled. Other important aspects of management for each type of transplant recipient have been steadily improved over recent decades and continue to evolve.

Beyond the cautionary comments stemming from its high cost and manifold social and procedural challenges, another, less well-known criticism of this new field led to its being branded as "half-way technology." This epithet, coined by Lewis Thomas, was designed to point out that many transplants are done for end-stage conditions that we are relatively powerless to combat earlier. The idea was that transplantation will surely be superseded by newer methods (technologies that "go all the way") that will halt or prevent the development of glomerulonephritis, myocardiopathies, or sclerosing cholangitis and make organ replacement obsolete. In that sense, the description "half-way technology" seems apt enough. It should not be forgotten, however, that organ failure is very likely to be an accompaniment of the human condition into the distant future, perhaps on the basis of a gradually changing set of causes, and for those individuals with the bad fortune to be facing its consequences, organ replacement will be the only effective technology. For these patients, it will continue to be an "all-the-way technology" of the first order, and the only answer to their needs.

Paul S. Russell, MD
John Homans Professor of Surgery
Harvard Medical School;
Visiting Surgeon
Massachusetts General Hospital
Boston, Massachusetts

PREFACE

Time is that wherein there is opportunity, and opportunity is that wherein there is little time.

—Hippocrates, *Precepts*

The convergence of science and technology has had no more dramatic impact on the practice of medicine than in the field of transplantation. For patients ravaged by a variety of diseases resulting in organ failure, replacement of the exhausted body part offers the opportunity to improve the quality of life and to extend life expectancy. The successful transplantation of each tissue or organ, however, demands that four barriers be overcome: technical issues, rejection, organ availability, and costs. Thus, each expansion of the field has new challenges for society and for those working in this area. We are pleased to have assembled an internationally recognized group of contributors, representing a wide spectrum of expertise, to review the state of the art and to address some of the more important issues associated with organ transplantation.

Transplantation is a comprehensive text in which we have tried to cover all aspects of organ replacement. It represents an effort to explore, in depth, both surgical and medical considerations in the transplantation of all organs. In addition, we have summarized current principles of histocompatibility, immunosuppression, rejection, organ procurement, and surgical techniques, as well as medical evaluation and management. While there are many books devoted to the science and transplantation of individual organs, the purpose of this text is to provide an authoritative overview of the entire field in one book.

Spaced throughout this book are selected commentaries from a variety of experts in the field of transplantation. Our aim is to provide their added perspective in particular areas of interest in transplantation. The diversity of views, we hope, enriches the text, deepens its insight, and broadens its appeal. The array of contributors also underscores the diversity of disciplines involved in this field.

The success of modern transplantation—and its promise for the next century—rests on the talents of multifaceted teams, working together. Transplant physicians and surgeons, nurses, and coordinators combine with specialists in many fields, social workers, nutritionists, and physical therapists, as well as immunologists, pharmacologists, microbiologists, virologists, pharmacists, and administrators to produce a successful transplant program. As transplants become more common, community practitioners also must develop a greater knowledge of the unique aspects of caring for these patients. We hope that *Transplantation* will be a valuable resource for all these individuals (as well as students, residents, and trainees in the field) and for their patients.

The editors could hardly have accomplished the task of preparing this text alone. We are most grateful to our contributors and commentators. We appreciate also the assistance of our Executive Editor, Chris Davis, and his Senior Editorial Assistant, Karin Commeret, from Blackwell Science. Finally, we acknowledge our own patients, from whom we always learn while we strive to help them, and we recognize all of the donor families and individuals on whom so much of transplantation depends.

LCG
ABC
PJM

Notice: The indications and dosages of all drugs in this book have been recommended in the medical literature and conform to the practices of the general medical community. The medications described do not necessarily have specific approval by the U.S. Food and Drug Administration for use in the diseases and dosages for which they are recommended. The package insert for each drug should be consulted for use and dosage as approved by the FDA. Because standards for usage change, it is advisable to keep abreast of revised recommendations, particularly those concerning new drugs.

Chapter 1

Reaching for the Impossible: The Quest for Tissue Replacement

DAVID HAMILTON

The replacement of human tissue with that from other persons or animals has been one of humanity's most ancient goals, but a solution has been reached only within the current generation. The strategies attempted in the past were based on the clinical and physiologic assumptions of their day. There have been times of progress, times of stagnation, and not a few wrong turnings along the way. The periods of rapid progress were associated with better understandings of the basic mechanisms, but surgical empiricism has had its successes as well. Always a solution is found to achieve desirable clinical ends.

Hopes for tissue restoration went through four great phases, each based on the understandings and assumptions regarding disease and repair current at that time. Until medieval times, a firm belief in magical assistance in human medical matters, including transplantation, held sway. In the medieval period, grafts were attempted by simple adhesion of tissues. From the early 1900s onward, researchers experimented with vascularized organ grafting. There then followed a period of high hopes for specific immunologic tolerance, but instead, the routine use of nonspecific immunosuppression emerged. We may now be at the start of a new era of xenografting—breeding immunologically bland animals for the supply of human organs.

ANCIENT TIMES

Seeking tissue replacement is not new, nor is it even limited to recorded history. The legends of all primitive peoples record tales of repair and replacement of lost bits of the human body, with a frequency only rivaled by the legends of successful raising of the dead. Since it was believed that the inflicting of disease and illness and the outcomes of injury were in the hands of the gods, it was also assumed that supernatural forces could lift illnesses, ensure recovery from injury, and in particular replace lost tissue (1). Because early peoples looked to supernatural powers to restore the body, the folklore of all parts of the world has remarkably similar tales of magical replacement of limbs and eyes—and even terrifying stories of the restoration of decapitated heads the wrong way round.

Another tale meeting a receptive hearing was the possible fusion of animals and humans to form hybrid beasts, such as the centaur, mermaid, sphinx, or chimera. Carrying out such unions—or indeed any form of transplantation—required unusual powers of good or evil not given to ordinary persons. Some special attribute might also be required in the recipient—a state of grace or personal worth—to enable the treatment to proceed. In the Christian tradition, for example, these miracles were carried out by Christ and the saints. Christ is said to have replaced a slave's ear that was cut off during Christ's arrest, and Saint Peter also made such tissue restorations (2). The best known legends of all are the miracles involving the twins Saint Cosmas and Saint Damian, who replaced a gangrenous leg (3).

Skin Grafting: Flaps and Other Methods

A limited amount of conventional plastic surgery had been attempted successfully in ancient times. Hindu texts of the 6th century B.C. describe sensible, practical reconstruction procedures, notably for refashioning noses mutilated by punishment or in war. Pedicle grafting was the most common method, and the forehead-to-nose flap also found its uses after such facial injuries (4). Free "split" skin grafts may have been attempted—obtaining a thin graft through cleavage of the skin by trauma and bleeding after flaying the skin of the buttocks.

However, the sensible Indian methods were forgotten when centers of learning arose in Asia Minor and the

Mediterranean, where the practice of surgery declined in status. The Greek medical writers in particular accorded little place to surgery in general, and even less to plastic surgical operations in particular (5).

THE MIDDLE AGES

As a new secular mood appeared in medieval times, belief in magical powers began to decline. Thus, although recourse to holy places and prayer might grant healing to a penitent person, the ability of individuals to achieve miracles, including tissue replacement, was doubted. However, certain assumptions about tissue transplants remained hard to dispel. There were persistent rumors that someone, somewhere, had achieved the replacement of lost parts of the body, and that tissue from another person could be grafted. But those who experimented with surgical tissue replacement and claimed success still had to be careful that they were not accused of calling up the wrong sorts of supernatural help.

Skin Grafting Revisited

The first known revival of restorative surgery came in Italy in the 14th century. The practice and success of surgical empirics in Sicily came to the notice of the trained surgeons of the northern Italian towns and universities, where the authority of the Greek and Roman texts was being challenged by solid personal observation and experimentation. Surgeons and surgery had high status in these towns, and a new tradition of shared learning through publication and teaching replaced the traditional secrecy of the medieval medical men.

Gaspare Tagliacozzi (1545–1599) is remembered for his great text on plastic surgical methods and his careful description of tissue replacement, mainly of the lip, nose, and ear. In addition to the forehead flap, he also used a forearm flap to replace nose or lip defects, and devised special harnesses to achieve approximation of the parts (6). In his text, Tagliacozzi describes no attempts to transplant skin from an unrelated donor. Indeed, he stated that this would be prevented by the "power and force of individuality." Yet after his death, medieval medical lore, gossipy and inattentive to sources, put it about that he did such surgery (7). This story was further extended to say that he even used a slave as a nose donor, and that the grafted nose fell off when the donor died.

The rumors about Tagliacozzi served to support the flirtation at the time with theories of "sympathetic" medicine and action at a distance, which had currency through the advocacy of Kenelm Digby (1603–1665) (Fig. 1.1). These beliefs would lead to a vogue for the treatment of the weapon, not the wound (8). It is perhaps not surprising that the first of the early English surgical texts, James Cooke's *The Marrow of Surgery*, largely ignored the subject of replacement of tissue and had no details of the sensible plastic surgery of Tagliacozzi except to misrepresent him by stating that he had used the biceps muscle, rather than skin, to repair the nose (9).

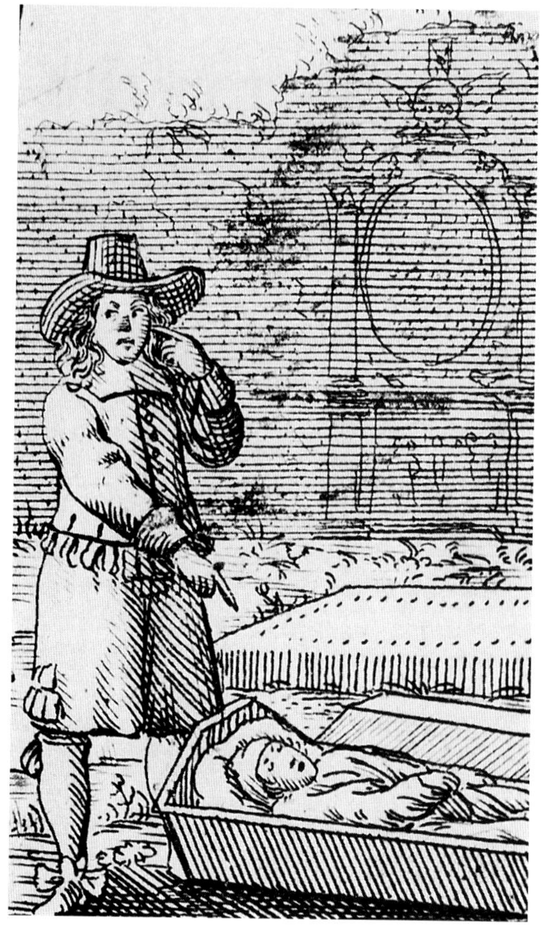

FIGURE 1.1. *The earliest illustration of allograft rejection came from fanciful stories about Tagliacozzi's successful plastic surgical reconstructions in the 1500s. These included false claims that he used slave donors of skin and an embellishment that if the donor died, the distant donor skin died also. This action at a distance is illustrated in Digby's* Powder of Sympathy, *1661.*

More admirable was the mid-17th century London investigation into the matter of grafting by the new pragmatic Royal Society. Members were keen to advance knowledge by experience and experiment and to be free of the hindrance of ancient assumptions. In 1663, they debated the possibility of replacing tissues from other animal sources and proceeded to propose that "an experiment should first be tried . . ." Their plan was to graft skin from one dog to another. However, after much well-meaning muddle, they achieved an inconclusive end—the dog ran away. The matter remained unresolved, and the Royal Society instead turned its attentions to blood transfusion (10).

In spite of the investigative spirit of the age, transplantation and plastic surgery largely were ignored by teachers and writers in surgery. If these areas were mentioned at all, it was in light of the persisting assumption that tissue from one animal would survive in another. This belief was not helped by Trembley's celebrated discovery in the early 18th century that the divided parts of the humble pond polyp would fuse together successfully (11). This new attention to humble life would also reveal the remarkable powers of regeneration of the earthworm.

Thus, until the time of Hunter's experiments, the understanding of the biology of tissue restoration and the reports of success in human transplantation would remain muddled, but the verdict was that tissue regeneration and transplantation might be possible in some circumstances.

THE 19TH CENTURY

John Hunter's Studies

The brothers John and William Hunter came to London from Scotland with little grounding in conventional medical knowledge, ancient or modern, a deficiency that may have been to their advantage. John was to embark on a remarkable range of experimental studies, including transplant work (12). Hunter became skilled at autografting, making the valuable observation that donor tissue must be grafted quickly after removal, otherwise the "life principle" in the graft, as he called it, was lost. He attempted solid fragment grafts of organs such as the testis and ovary, and when months later the lump grossly appeared vascularized and viable, he only claimed tissue survival rather than functional replacement.

At that time, the goal in successful grafting was successful "adhesion"; that is, firm attachment of graft and recipient. The physiologic paradigm of the period held that separated tissues would unite by the blood vessels rejoining in continuity (rather than by ingrowth of new vessels). Understanding this view can help one make sense of the literature of the period: if close and undisturbed adhesion was achieved, then even large solid grafts could survive when the blood vessels rejoined.

This theoretical background, as seen in Hunter's writings, had powerful support from another source. Then, as now, engrafting was common in horticulture, where the tree stems or trunks of one species are routinely merged with stronger or disease-free roots from another. Hunter's era saw no fundamental difference between the plant kingdom and the animal world. All were considered parts of one spectrum of life, known as the "Great Chain of Being." Thus, the mechanisms at work in the animal and plant kingdoms did not differ in principle. Hunter's terminology reveals his horticultural conditioning. He noted that "as the transplanting of teeth is very similar to the ingrafting of trees, I thought the term ['scion' for the graft] might be transferred from gardening to surgery." He would later coin the word "transplant" for his procedure.

Using human donor teeth, Hunter came to obtain a reputation for tooth transplants in his patients (13). It was during this work that he noted, for the first time, the danger of introducing disease from a graft, when he discovered that syphilis had been transferred along with an apparently normal grafted tooth (14).

Hunter's teeth transplants also gave rise to the first ethical concerns with transplantation. In 1806, Joseph Fox noted that servants or soldiers were being coerced into donating teeth to their masters. He complained that this "involved a defect of the moral principle, as one person is injured and disfigured, in order to contribute to the luxury and convenience of another" (15).

Hunter's work showed that tooth and bone transplants could potentially be successful, and he also can be credited with establishing that some exceptional tissue transplants worked—as inert implants for cellular ingrowth. His work is remarkable above all for illustrating that experimentation had a valid role in medical progress.

Rhinoplasty Rediscovered

The expanding British empire of the early 19th century gave its soldiers and travelers many opportunities for scientific studies and observations in novel situations. One of the many discoveries was that in India the ancient art of surgical rhinoplasty was still in use. Skilled empirics offered this service to treat injured noses, ears, or lips, following the same ancient guidelines (16).

Following a report of this surgical procedure and its antiquity in the London *Gentleman's Magazine,* the "Indian method" was given attention in surgical textbooks. It gained approval from the best teachers of the time, including Bell and Thomson in Edinburgh, who would also rediscover, quote, and praise the long-forgotten plastic surgical text by Tagliacozzi.

In London, the first nose reconstruction by a forehead pedicle flap, closely following the Indian methods, was carried out by Carpue in 1812 on a patient whose nose was damaged by syphilis (Fig. 1.2) (17). It was as though the reestablishment of this ancient operation liberated the medical establishment from the dead weight of fanciful myths. Thereafter, replacement surgery made rapid progress. Our modern terminology was to be established by the title of Carl von Graefe's work *Rhinoplastik* of 1818.

Thin, Neovascularized Grafts

The new interest in plastic surgery did have one unfortunate effect: it also revived interest in the old claims for free skin grafting. This was particularly true after Giuseppe Baronio (1758–1811) in Italy had a lucky series of successful full-thickness autografts in sheep (18). The subsequent enthusiasm for free grafting was accompanied by the inevitable dubious claims of success, even for full-thickness skin autografts placed directly on the damaged nose, rather than using a flap (19).

Jacques-Louis Reverdin, a house surgeon in Paris, finally put skin grafting on a sound basis and into regular use with

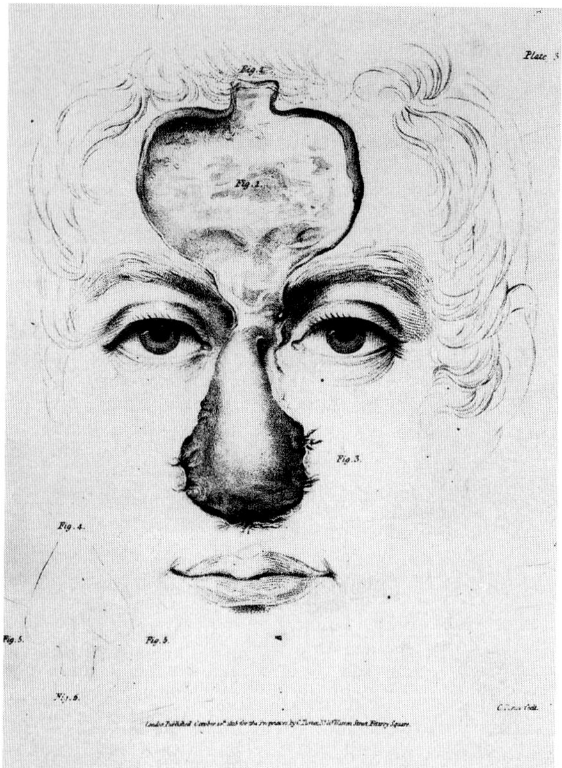

FIGURE 1.2. *Joseph Carpue's forehead flap cases published in 1812 were based on ancient Indian methods and marked the start of modern plastic surgery.*

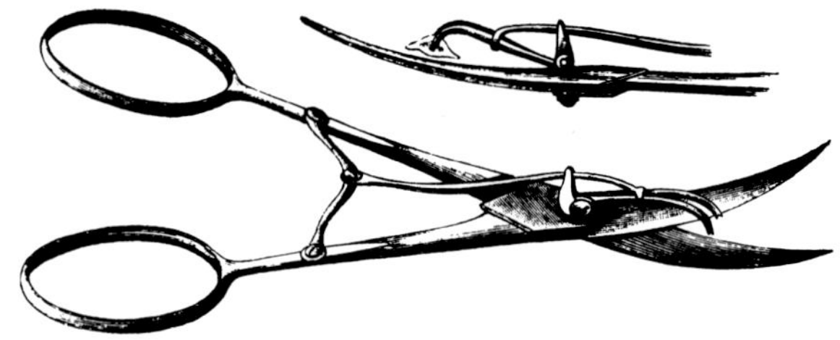

FIGURE 1.3. *Reverdin's demonstration that skin grafts had to be thin to survive made free skin grafting possible. He was aided by his scissors for cutting such thin "pinch" grafts.*

his split-skin pinch grafts, "*lambeaux cutane*" (Fig. 1.3) (20). His discovery that the thin skin would heal in and spread in a way denied to thick skin appears to have been an empirical one (21).

Reverdin may have been aided by the teachings of Paul Bert at the Collège de France, who, shortly after, used the newly evolved microscope to make the crucial observation that any tissue graft was sustained by ingrowth of new vessels. By liberating transplantation from the assumption that the blood vessels of graft and recipient had to adhere, Bert's discovery explained much of the earlier findings, in particular the inability of thick skin grafts to survive. His work not only strongly supported the use of thin split skin, but also showed that for any graft larger than a thin slice to survive, the blood vessels would have to be anastomosed.

Bert is also remembered for his demonstration that animal tissue chemistry is temperature dependent. He made the first demonstration that grafts would survive better if cooled, thus retaining Hunter's "life principle." His perspicacity was less acute, however, when he also claimed that allografts and cross-species transplants survived (22).

The difficulty in judging survival of skin grafts, then as now, is that allografts do survive in the short term, and may survive well on ill patients. The inevitable later immunologic loss could be blamed by an enthusiastic surgeon on either infection or poor management. The additional confusing element of regeneration of host skin beneath and at the edge of defects misled many, including Reverdin, who reported that human donor allografts would survive (a claim that would also be given authority later by Lister in Edinburgh).

The method of split skin grafting spread rapidly from Paris, and enthusiastic reports issued from Pollock in London (23,24) and from Boston (25). These new methods met a need for covering the unhealed ulcers, burns, and wounds of war and the new heavy industry, lesions whose healing was often slowed by malnutrition.

Nor was allografting during this period confined to skin. Human organ allograft slices had uncritical use in uncontrolled circumstances, and there was dreary vogue for their use in diseases known to have a variable clinical prognosis. Ovarian allografting found a role in a variety of complaints, notably infertility, and it was widely used. There even arose a sharp controversy between those who claimed to have invented the procedure (26). The operation was considered respectable enough to start a debate on the legitimacy of the offspring from a mother having received a donor ovary (27).

Because the experimentation during this period of allografting was largely uncritical, it gave confirmation to Hunter's findings that disease, notably syphilis and tuberculosis, could be transferred in apparently normal skin. In particular, the transfer of smallpox in the incubation phase in skin, prior to lesions appearing in the donor, was observed (29). Prudent surgeons also imprudently experimented with skin taken from animals, choosing donor species thought to be disease-free. Once again, skin grafting led to claims for success with skin taken from unrelated humans and even animal donors. These claims were to prove remarkably persistent—in fact, they would continue to be made into the middle of the 20th century.

The popularity of allograft experimentation resulted in the world's first transplant-related litigation. A nurse and doctor in Glasgow Royal Infirmary were fined £5 for removing a patch of skin from a young boy without permission of his parents, to graft it on another patient's wound. Although he had declared them guilty, the sheriff admitted he had no other criticism of the operation (28).

Xenografting

A huge and confusing literature arose in the late 1800s when experiments with skin xenografts were followed by the use of fragments of spleen, pancreas, nerve, thyroid, and ovary taken from animals (30). Respectable scientists made reports of successful organ xenografting. For example, Victor Horsley of London claimed sheep thyroid transplants were of benefit to myxoedema patients. Well into the next century, others would follow in his wake with similar claims for the effects of animal gland-slice grafts.

THE MODERN ERA

Vascular Surgery

The first attempts at vascular surgery came in 1900. Crude suturing with the materials then available gave dismal results in the absence of anticoagulation, but Payr's metal stents allowed occasional restoration of vessel flow when used intravascularly (31). Using this method, progress was made with vascular surgery (32) to the point where organ transplants were attempted experimentally by a number of distinguished surgical scientists in Vienna. Short periods of successful blood flow in organ grafts were recorded by Ullmann (33,34) and Decastello (35).

However, the modern era of vascular surgery truly commenced when members of the Department of Surgery in Lyon, headed by Mathieu Jaboulay (Fig. 1.4), devised better materials and better methods for vascular anastomosis. Jaboulay carried out the first two attempts at human kidney transplant in 1906. Using pig and goat donor kidneys to the arm of patients in chronic renal failure, he reported a 1-hour function of the grafts (36,37). Unger in Berlin also experimented in laboratory transplantation before attempting a monkey-to-human kidney transplant in 1909 (38,39). In 1911, the first human-to-human organ transplant was carried out by Hammond and Sutton in Philadelphia. The operation was a rather improbable vascularized testis allograft, and they claimed function for 3 weeks (40).

Attached to Jaboulay's department in Lyon was the young Alexis Carrel. Carrel's improvements on the departmental vascular surgical methods included use of triangulation and nonpenetrating stitches. His paper in the *Lyon Médicale* is often cited as the start of modern organ transplantation, a claim Carrel did not discourage. When Carrel fell out of favor in France, he emigrated to Chicago, Illinois, where his considerable technical skills and the assistance of the talented Charles Guthrie resulted in a remarkable series of papers on organ transplantation (Fig. 1.5) (41,42). They made many procedural improvements, establishing that cooling of the donor organ was necessary and that the perfusion saline then in use was harmful (43). Carrel later moved to the Rockefeller Institute. There, he found that while he could eventually carry out routine autografting of the dog kidney, there was a barrier to allografting. He realized that "the principles of immunity" might explain this invariable failure.

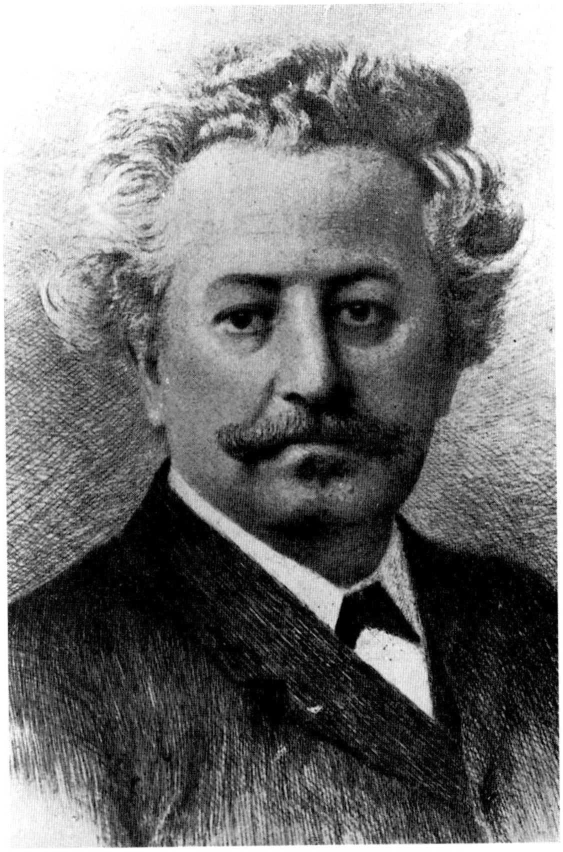

FIGURE 1.4. *One of the early European surgeons interested in organ transplantation was Mathieu Jaboulay in Lyon. He had experience with experimental vascular surgery, and attempted human xenograft kidney transplants in 1906.*

Carrel later ceased his transplant work, in spite of the incentives to continue it. He had become America's first Nobel Prize winner, Rockefeller Institute co-worker James B. Murphy had shown that the reaction against tumor grafts was delayed by radiation or the drug benzol, and Landsteiner was also working in the same building (44,45). After war work on antiseptics, Carrel moved on to study tissue culture, though he did later produce an organ perfusion/storage device with the aviator Charles Lindbergh.

The Immune Response

At the turn of the century, debate had centered on the cellular versus humoral defense of the body. The Metchnikoff view of the central role of the cellular mechanisms began to lose ground, and instead, the humoral theories of Pasteur became dominant (46). But while cell responses were not investigated in transplantation studies, tumor transplantation studies were proceeding, and the loss of tumor grafts was thought to be by an immune response. The prompter rejection of a second tumor graft was established first in 1903 by Jensen in Denmark (47), and then by Bashford in

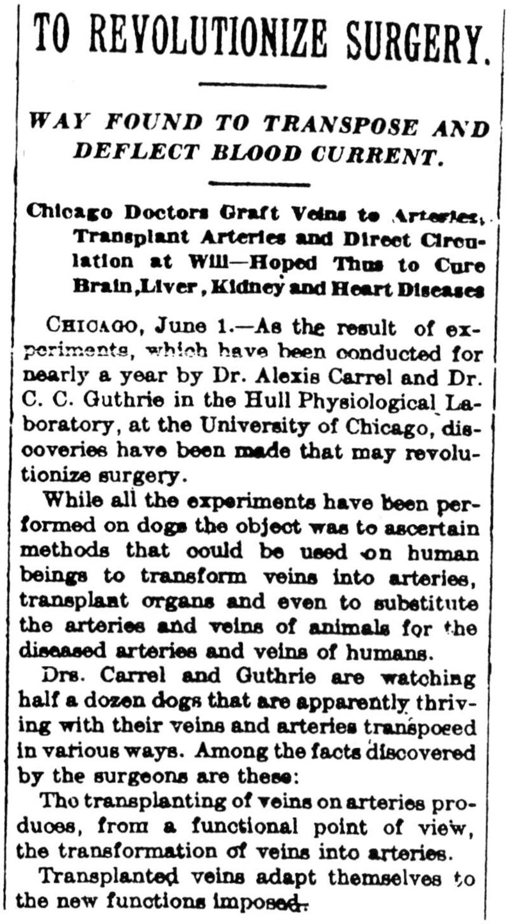

TO REVOLUTIONIZE SURGERY.

WAY FOUND TO TRANSPOSE AND DEFLECT BLOOD CURRENT.

Chicago Doctors Graft Veins to Arteries, Transplant Arteries and Direct Circulation at Will—Hoped Thus to Cure Brain, Liver, Kidney and Heart Diseases

CHICAGO, June 1.—As the result of experiments, which have been conducted for nearly a year by Dr. Alexis Carrel and Dr. C. C. Guthrie in the Hull Physiological Laboratory, at the University of Chicago, discoveries have been made that may revolutionize surgery.

While all the experiments have been performed on dogs the object was to ascertain methods that could be used on human beings to transform veins into arteries, transplant organs and even to substitute the arteries and veins of animals for the diseased arteries and veins of humans.

Drs. Carrel and Guthrie are watching half a dozen dogs that are apparently thriving with their veins and arteries transposed in various ways. Among the facts discovered by the surgeons are these:

The transplanting of veins on arteries produces, from a functional point of view, the transformation of veins into arteries.

Transplanted veins adapt themselves to the new functions imposed.

FIGURE 1.5. *Alexis Carrel pioneered the technical aspect of vascular surgery and organ transplantation, initially in collaboration with C. C. Guthrie in Chicago.* (New York Sun, *June 2, 1906.*)

London, who also noted the lymphocyte infiltrate in the graft (48,49). These findings were thought to be helpful only in the study of cancer progression and regression.

The Inter-War Hiatus

In spite of the promising leads, transplantation progress was hesitant after World War I. The famous European surgical and scientific centers like Vienna never recovered after the war, and British surgery, which was heavily dependent on private practice, had little experimental or research dimension. The discovery of the sulfonamide drugs made the use and development of specific disease vaccines less likely and such research declined, helped by Almroth Wright's high-profile and excessive claims for his vaccine approach. Carrel in New York failed to continue with his organ grafting, and surgical scientists in America were attracted to other rapidly expanding areas.

Practicing surgeons continued to write and teach that allografting of skin could be successful. Occasional critics did appear, such as the American surgeon Holman, who deplored the publicity given to public donations of skin for this purpose: "Grafting is frequently employed to the wondering delight of the credulous laity. That such grafting is most often a failure seems little known" (50). In the middle of the 1920s, gland grafters such as Thorek and Lydston in Chicago and the testis transplanter Voronoff in Paris appeared. These men seem to have been guilty only of self-deception and self-promotion, but Brinkley, the Kansas goat testis transplanter, was definitely a quack (51).

Nor was the inter-war period blessed with any clarity of understanding of rejection mechanisms. The authority of the time, Leo Loeb, made the subject appear impenetrable (52). His use of organ fragment grafts, studied histologically, led to an assumption that a local reaction existed in grafts, thus diverting attention away from consideration of any blood-borne central response. His model concealed that the immune response followed neovascularization.

Histocompatibility

In other specialties and disciplines, notably in tumor transplantation, commendable progress was being made. As Medawar later pointed out, these tumor grafting experiments were carried out without any realization of their significance to the transfer of normal tissue (53). Tumor studies in outbred mice lead to the development of inbred strains of identical mice. The work by C. C. Little and others at Cold Spring Harbor, New York, and later at Bar Harbor, Maine, gave the subject greater precision (54).

Variable survival of grafts was found using transplants between the inbred mice, so it was assumed that a genetic susceptibility to cancer was being studied. Snell, working at Bar Harbor, inverted the thinking and rather than looking at tumor growth, examined tumor loss. He emphasized the genetic control of the strength of the host response, and argued that what was being studied was a normal host reaction. He introduced the term "histocompatibility genes" to explain this phenomenon (55).

J. B. S. Haldane was the first in Britain to obtain inbred mice from Bar Harbor. One of Haldane's pupils, Peter Gorer, was encouraged by his mentor to study tissue transplantation using these new mouse strains. Later, while working on his own in London at Guy's Hospital, Gorer not only detected a powerful controlling antigen in mouse tumor rejection, but also showed that an antibody arose after tumor loss (56). When Snell and Gorer finally met in 1946, they found themselves in broad agreement on their views of histocompatibility: it was clearly a feature of ordinary graft rejection (57).

Other Inter-War Developments

The inter-war period was not without some efforts at kidney transplantation, but these were not followed through. The new availability in the 1920s of the first simple radiological and biochemical kidney function tests seems to have been the stimulus to Williamson and colleagues to study kidney allografting from 1923 to 1926 at the Mayo Clinic. They confirmed Carrel's conclusions on the success of autografts and the failure of allografts (58).

In Russia, Yu Yu Voronoi, a surgeon largely unknown at that time or since, followed his blood transfusion research with the first human cadaveric kidney transplant in 1933. The organ, which was removed 6 hours after the donor's death, was transplanted into an anuric patient with mercury poisoning. Because a blood group difference was present, little function was obtained (59).

Understanding the Rejection Mechanism

A 1942 paper by Gibson and Medawar is considered to mark the beginning of our modern continuous period of interest in tissue transplantation (60). The then-ongoing war in Europe prompted the Medical Research Council in Britain to study burns sustained by aviators, and the Council gave support to young Peter Medawar at Oxford to pursue this work (61). Medawar's grant lead him to the busy Burns Unit at Glasgow's Royal Infirmary (Fig. 1.6), where he would join plastic surgeon Tom Gibson in making a series of classic observations.

Prior to the Medawar and Gibson study, others had suggested that tissue rejection was an almost universal mechanism; however, claims for exceptions and special cases left the matter open, and those who accepted the general rule of rejection of such grafts were far from clear as to what mechanism was involved. An immunologic reaction was not an obvious choice, because responses to one dose of protein antigen were usually feeble, yet graft loss was innate, prompt, and total. In Medawar and Gibson's study, a first set of grafts initially healed in without reaction, but then were destroyed. A second set of grafts was more quickly lost than the first, and the study included histologic evidence of inflammatory cell invasion. These findings, which had only been hinted at by others, firmly showed that rejection was a form of immunologic response.

This was an idea whose time had come. Medawar's later painstaking animal studies further highlighted the serious challenge of tissue rejection. None of the hoped-for exceptions—random matching, blood group matching, young or cultured skin, or superior surgical skill—would be rewarded by increased survival of experimental skin grafts (62). Nor were the "privileged sites" of the brain and anterior chamber of the eye found to be of much practical use, intellectually interesting though they were. Medawar also destroyed the hopes of the gland grafters, showing that endocrine tissue had no special dispensation to survive and revive hormone deficiency states.

John Converse, an American who had been posted in England during World War II, had studied the plastic surgical methods developed by Sir Harold Gillies to treat war injuries. Aware of Medawar's work, he returned to New York with an interest in the field of transplantation. He would advise and help with funding European research during the difficult economic times of the late 1940s (63). In 1954, Converse, in collaboration with Lyndon Peer, Blair Rogers, and Felix Rapaport, helped to organize the first of the international series of conferences by the New York Academy of Science. It was at this meeting that the immunologic term "rejection" found official favor for describing graft loss, supplanting the terms absorption, disintegration, necrosis, or sloughing that were all used up to then. This series of conferences later evolved into the meetings of the international Transplantation Society.

In the 1940s Morten Simonsen (64) of Denmark and William Dempster (Fig. 1.7) (65) in London revived interest in experimental kidney transplantation. They also showed that loss of the organ was apparently an immunologic event, but they were concerned about the absence of any antibody appearing in response to rejection. Simonsen, impressed that the lymphocytes in the graft might be the stimulating antigen, and a mobile one, went on thereafter to study the graft-versus-host reaction in simpler systems. His discovery explained much else later, notably experimental runt disease and the difficulty of bone marrow grafting. In turn, Dempster hypothesized that a subtle antibody responsible for allograft loss would be found, and he tried immune suppression with both radiation and the new drug cortisone. His experiments had but minimal effects on survival in his dog kidney model because, ironically, this animal is insensitive to both agents.

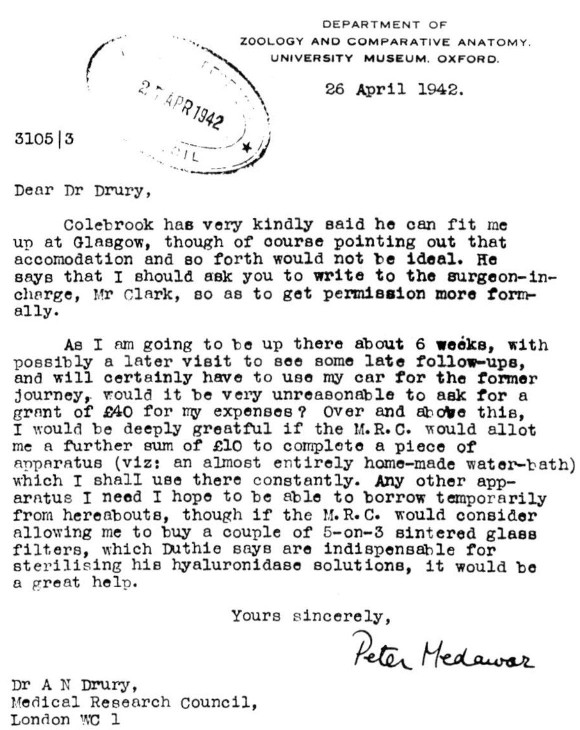
DEPARTMENT OF
ZOOLOGY AND COMPARATIVE ANATOMY.
UNIVERSITY MUSEUM. OXFORD.

26 April 1942.

27 APR 1942

3105|3

Dear Dr Drury,

Colebrook has very kindly said he can fit me up at Glasgow, though of course pointing out that accomodation and so forth would not be ideal. He says that I should ask you to write to the surgeon-in-charge, Mr Clark, so as to get permission more formally.

As I am going to be up there about 6 weeks, with possibly a later visit to see some late follow-ups, and will certainly have to use my car for the former journey, would it be very unreasonable to ask for a grant of £40 for my expenses? Over and above this, I would be deeply greatful if the M.R.C. would allot me a further sum of £10 to complete a piece of apparatus (viz: an almost entirely home-made water-bath) which I shall use there constantly. Any other apparatus I need I hope to be able to borrow temporarily from hereabouts, though if the M.R.C. would consider allowing me to buy a couple of 5-on-3 sintered glass filters, which Duthie says are indispensable for sterilising his hyaluronidase solutions, it would be a great help.

Yours sincerely,

Peter Medawar

Dr A N Drury,
Medical Research Council,
London WC 1

FIGURE 1.6. *Peter Medawar's studies at the Glasgow Royal Infirmary during World War II are considered the beginning of modern transplantation immunology. (Courtesy of the Medical Research Council, United Kingdom.)*

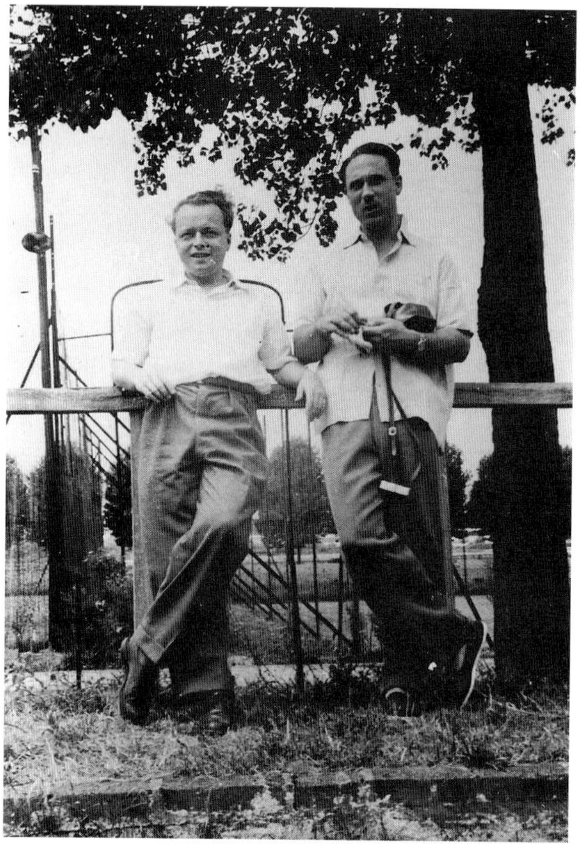

FIGURE 1.7. *The French surgeon Jolibois visiting the pioneer London experimental transplant surgeon William Dempster about 1953 at the Buckston Browne Farm run by the Royal College of Surgeons of England. This laboratory had a distinguished role in supporting experimental surgery, particularly dog kidney transplantation.*

In Britain, Medawar had been almost alone in his interest in the fundamental mechanisms of transplantation, but others joined his group, notably Rupert Billingham and Leslie Brent. The work of Avrion Mitchison, Medawar's pupil, revealed that the powerful rejection mechanism was a cellular one and that the cells involved were the lymphocytes, thus deflecting the call by the critics "to find the antibody" (66). Transplantation biology had not fit into classic immunology—now classic immunology had to accommodate the mechanism of graft rejection. Tissue transplantation study was not the only area liberated from what Medawar called the "tyranny of the antibody." The intense lymphocyte infiltrate in autoimmune disease was now explained and accorded greater importance in the pathogenesis.

Boston and Paris Transplants

In spite of discouraging laboratory findings in skin and kidney transplantation and the feeling that the powerful innate rejection mechanism might never be tamed, a series of human cadaveric kidney transplants were carried out in the early 1950s in Paris and Boston. The Boston surgeons, including David Hume, had the help of pretransplant dialysis with the hospital's pioneer artificial kidney. Also, in these transplants they used small doses of adrenocorticotropic hormone (ACTH) and cortisone (67,68). In Paris, the pioneer nephrologist Hamburger encouraged Küss, Servelle, and Dubost to carry out the surgical procedures, including the first living-related kidney transplant (69,70).

These operations were not without their critics locally and internationally. They were depicted as futile experiments on dying patients. However, they did serve to show that the operation was technically possible, that the pelvic position for the transplanted kidney could be used, and that kidney survival could be greater than predicted from experimental studies. One Boston kidney transplant (to a physician recipient) survived for 5 months without any immunosuppression.

Consequently, similar attempts were made in Chicago, Cleveland, and Toronto, the latter by the gifted surgeon Gordon Murray, who is best known for his introduction of heparin into clinical practice. However, as of 1953 the matter rested, and aside from a brief series of twin transplants (discussed below), kidney allografting would not again be revived on a large scale until 1960.

Corneal Grafting

Corneal grafting was the one transplant service that became established in the 1950s in many parts of the world. The practice of corneal grafting developed through organizations that anticipated many of the structures that were to become necessary later for other types of transplants.

In Britain, corneal scarring from burns was yet another of the legacies of wartime. Benjamin Rycroft of East Grinstead had become interested in corneal grafting as a means of dealing with such eye injuries. Through his work, he improved the technique of corneal grafting; however, he could not meet the demand for such surgery because of the lack of donors. Tissue donation after death was hampered by the legal uncertainties inherent in Britain's Anatomy Act of 1832, which originally had been drafted to thwart grave-robbing for the anatomists.

Rycroft lobbied Parliament to have the restrictive effects of the Act modified. His campaign presaged issues that would be involved much later in organ grafting (71). With the help of interested journalists and television appearances, Rycroft established in the public mind that corneal donation was both noble and respectable. His efforts were rewarded in 1952 by the passage of the Corneal Grafting Act. This act would be copied later in legislation that applied to organs from the rest of the body, in the form of the Human Tissue Act of 1961.

Rycroft's campaign resulted in sufficient donations to meet the then-present needs. Once storage methods were devised, surplus grafts could be transported for some distance and even exported to countries where grafts could not be obtained because of legal or religious obstacles. Rycroft attempted to coax the reluctant Ministry of Health to organize a national scheme for corneal donation, but he was told that this was not the role of government. Such services were to remain voluntary. An organization called "Eye-Will" was formed to organize and publicize the arrangements for donation of corneas after death. The popularity of the program was further established when many celebrities announced their willingness to donate.

Immunologic Tolerance

Although the attempts at human kidney transplantation ceased in 1953, the number of scientists drawn into studying cell-mediated immunity increased (Fig. 1.8). Their research would be rewarded by new insights and some hope of thwarting the immune response.

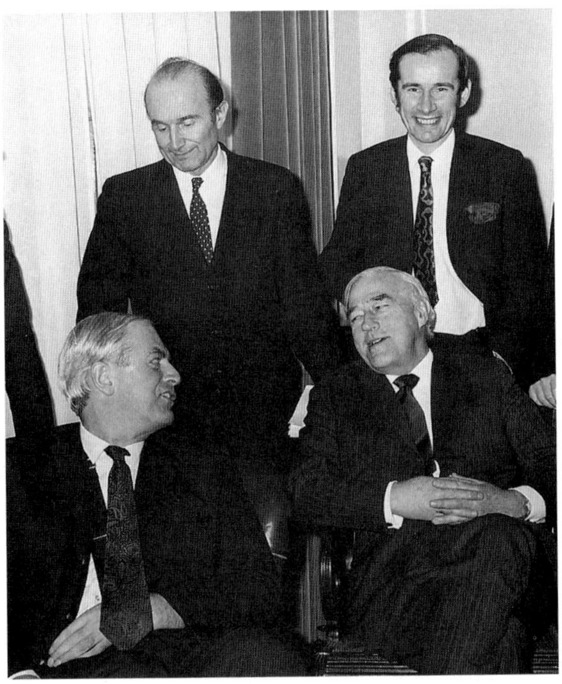

FIGURE 1.8. *Peter Medawar* (bottom left), *shown with the Edinburgh transplant surgeon Michael Woodruff* (bottom right). *Georges Mathé, Parisian pioneer of bone marrow grafting and immunotherapy, is shown top left. (Courtesy of the Ciba Foundation, London.)*

Medawar and Billingham, then in Birmingham, had been working on a major wrong turning, a claim to have found non-Mendelian "plasmagenes" transferred between dendritic cells in the skin. The two reluctantly agreed to help Edinburgh veterinarian Hugh P. Donald use skin grafting to solve the problem of distinguishing between identical and nonidentical cattle twins. The unexpected result of the cattle work was the discovery that nonidentical cattle twins also accepted skin grafts. After initial dismay at this finding, Medawar was reminded of the shared synchorial placenta of such calves. He thus proposed that the animals were "tolerant" as a result of prenatal exchange of blood. This hypothesis was supported by similar suggestions from Hasek, Ray Owen of Wisconsin, and Macfarlane Burnet of Australia that such early exposure to antigen prevented normal adult responses (72).

This proposal was confirmed experimentally by Brent in Medawar's team, with the finding that tolerance could be induced by antigen injection into the fetus and even into newborn mice, a development that simplified the experiments (Fig. 1.9). The use of F_1 hybrid cells prevented "runting." Medawar's work led to a Nobel Prize for himself and Burnet in 1960.

There were high hopes for practical uses of this powerful, specific method of attaining graft survival. It also offered an exciting hypothesis that cell-mediated autoimmunity was a breakdown of self-tolerance. About this time, more of the mysteries about the role of the lymphocyte were solved. For example, its life span was found to be long rather than short, as had been suggested by the huge output from the thoracic duct. That it circulated was demonstrated by Gowans and others in the 1960s (Fig. 1.10) (73). The previously mysterious thymus, usually ignored or thought to be related to prepubertal growth, was found to have the central role in producing the T-cell lymphocyte subset involved in cell-mediated immunity. Above all, the inert lymphocyte lost its bland reputation when it was shown to perform and transform in vitro (74).

Immunosuppression

The Cold War also had affected conventional medical treatments. The study of the effects of radiation became active during the 1950s, and there were hopes of developing a means of protection against lethal exposure. Researchers

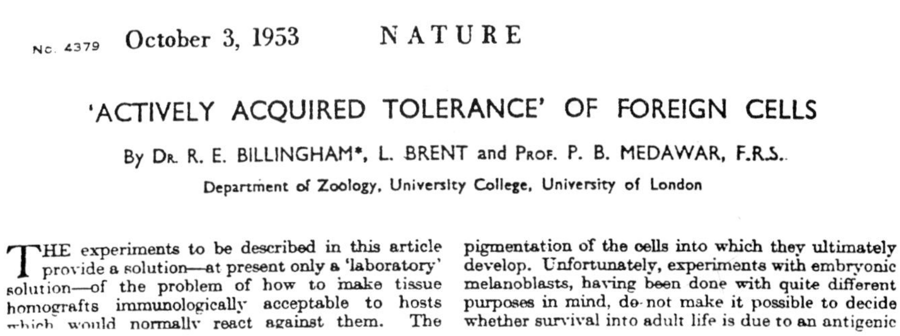

No. 4379 October 3, 1953 NATURE

'ACTIVELY ACQUIRED TOLERANCE' OF FOREIGN CELLS

By Dr. R. E. BILLINGHAM*, L. BRENT and Prof. P. B. MEDAWAR, F.R.S.

Department of Zoology, University College, University of London

THE experiments to be described in this article provide a solution—at present only a 'laboratory' solution—of the problem of how to make tissue homografts immunologically acceptable to hosts which would normally react against them. The pigmentation of the cells into which they ultimately develop. Unfortunately, experiments with embryonic melanoblasts, having been done with quite different purposes in mind, do not make it possible to decide whether survival into adult life is due to an antigenic

FIGURE 1.9. *The demonstration of experimental immunologic "tolerance" in 1953 gave hope that clinical allograft rejection might be eventually overcome.*

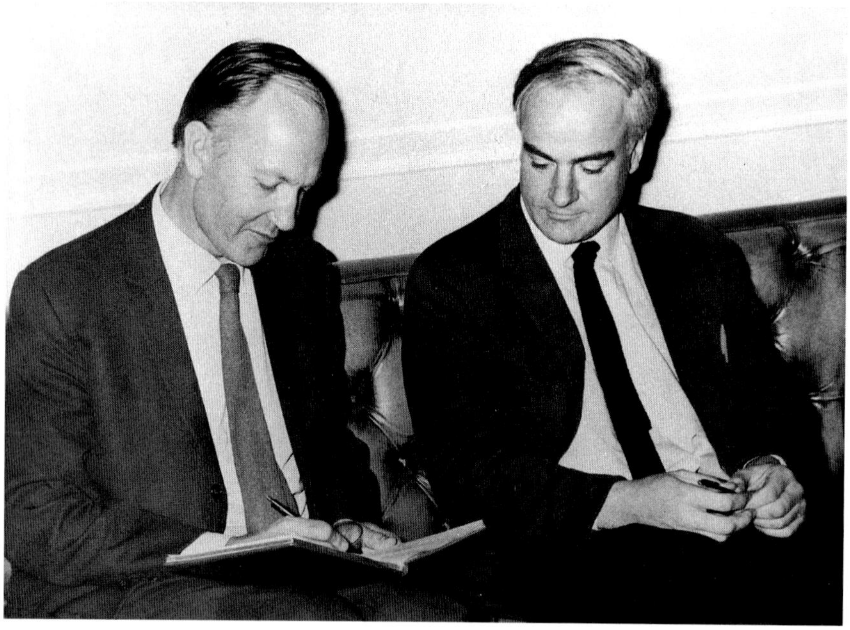

FIGURE 1.10. *Impressive gains in the 1960s clarified the fundamentals of transplantation immunology. James Gowans* (left) *revealed the lymphocyte was an active, recirculating cell, and Avrion Mitchison* (right) *demonstrated the cellular mechanism of allograft rejection. (Courtesy of the Ciba Foundation, London.)*

found that the spleen had such a cellular factor. The protective strategy that thus evolved was to treat fatal radiation damage with bone marrow infusion. This strategy could succeed even when another strain of animal marrow was used, although graft-versus-host disease invariably occurred if hybrid donors were not used. The resulting *chimera* (a classical allusion introduced by Medawar) would accept skin from the donor of the marrow. The persistence of the marrow cellular line was shown by the use of the first cellular marker (76). Main and Prehn and Trentin had also shown this strategy would work, but their experiments were limited by graft-versus-host disease (77).

Practical Application

John Merrill, a Boston nephrologist who had been involved in the earlier Brigham transplants, heard about the new applications for radiation during a visit to John Loutit at the Atomic Energy Research Establishment at Harwell in Britain (Fig. 1.11). Merrill thought that these findings might be useful clinically.

Although kidney allografting had been temporarily halted during this time period (as previously discussed), its earlier technical success allowed that it could be used in the rare situation where one of a set of identical twins had renal failure. From 1954 to 1958, seven kidney transferal operations were carried out on twins with great success (75). These operations provided invaluable nonimmunologic lessons: the kidney would not atrophy, preoperative radiology on the donor was vital, the original disease could return in the transplant, and informed consent had to be taken seriously. In general, the transplanted kidneys worked well, and the donors showed no long-term harm. Thus, the twin transplants kept up researchers' hopes for success, and following Merrill's trip to Britain in 1958, the procedure provided the first chance to attempt transplant immunosuppression.

Radiation and bone marrow were used together only for the first two of the new Boston transplant series. Radiation was then found to be a powerful immunosuppressive agent alone, although it was an unpredictable and uncontrollable one. This approach was used in Boston and Paris from 1958 to 1962 and was also employed at Edinburgh (78). In each center there were one or two long-term survivals of kidneys, measured in years rather than months, but otherwise kidney loss and mortality were high.

Medical Immunosuppression

The effects of the poison nitrogen mustard—which included a capacity to reduce antibody production and kill white cells—had been well known after World War I, but had largely been forgotten over the ensuing years. When the Cold War revived interest in chemical warfare, the U.S. military renewed its study of this alkylating agent by funding cautious, secret human leukemia trials from 1942 onward at Yale University (79).

The hormones of the adrenal cortex were first synthesized in 1948. These hormones quickly proved not only to be curative in Addison's disease, but to have unexpected and remarkable benefits in other diseases, notably rheumatoid arthritis. However, the dangers of the hormone in prolonged or high dosages were soon apparent (80). Tiny amounts of ACTH and cortisone were spared by the manufacturers to use in some of the early Boston kidney transplants.

In 1953, a better derivative was produced, the purine analog 6-mercaptopurine (6-MP). This agent proved particularly successful in treating acute lymphatic leukemia.

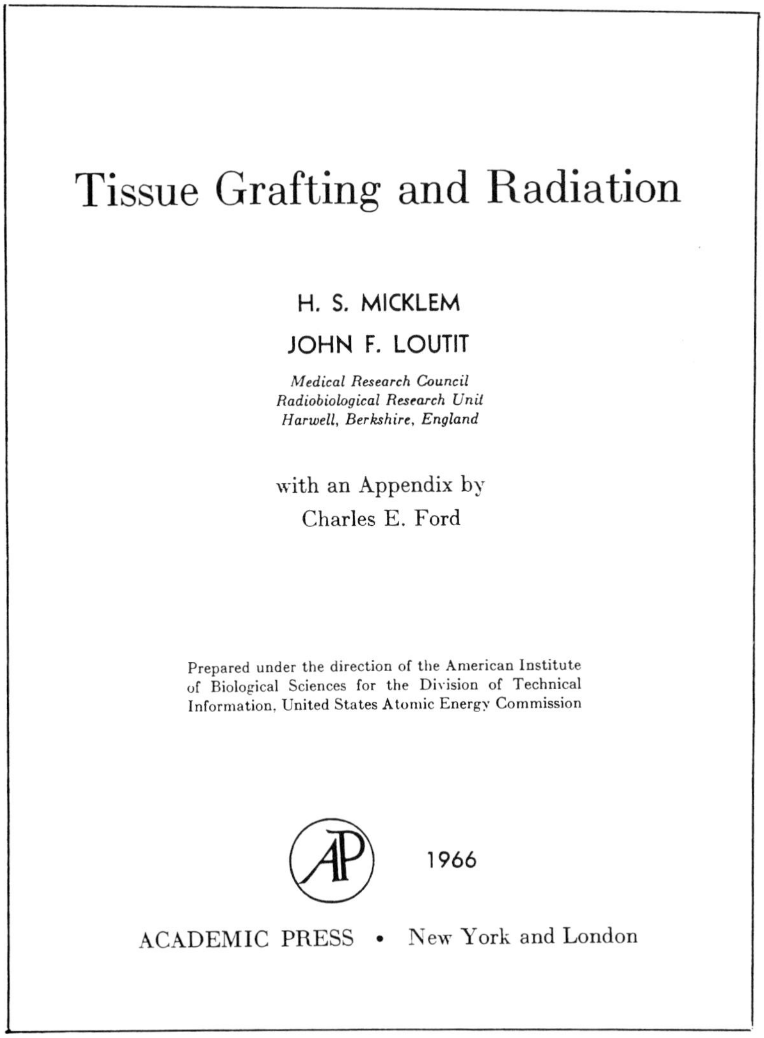

Tissue Grafting and Radiation

H. S. MICKLEM

JOHN F. LOUTIT

Medical Research Council
Radiobiological Research Unit
Harwell, Berkshire, England

with an Appendix by
Charles E. Ford

Prepared under the direction of the American Institute of Biological Sciences for the Division of Technical Information, United States Atomic Energy Commission

1966

ACADEMIC PRESS • New York and London

FIGURE 1.11. *Radiation was the first immunosuppressive agent to be used clinically, starting in Boston, Paris, and Edinburgh. This approach was encouraged by fundamental studies on radiobiology carried out at defense establishments.*

In 1958, Schwartz and Dameshek discovered the immunosuppressive potential of the drugs. Their search for a pharmaceutical alternative to radiation as a bone marrow suppressant led them to experimenting with 6-MP, which they showed was a controllable marrow suppressant in rabbits. After such treatments, they also noted a reduced antibody response; however, the effect was so time dependent that it appeared to have little practical use. Then, in 1960, they investigated this agent's effect on cell-mediated immunity, and found that it also prolonged skin grafts in rabbits (81). Thus, in looking for a pharmacologic bone marrow "space maker" for marrow transplantation, they had found something else—an agent that in limited doses was nontoxic to bone marrow yet immunosuppressive.

Schwartz and Dameshek's work was noticed in London. Roy Calne was at that time working at the Buckston Browne Farm research unit, where the Hammersmith surgeons had carried out their earlier dog kidney work. Calne had noted the uniform failure to prolong kidney survival with a number of regimens, but he quickly obtained modest dog kidney survival with the new agent 6-MP. Charles Zukoski in Richmond made the same observation that same year (82).

Calne followed his work in England with a Boston fellowship, where he proceeded to collect variants on the drug 6-MP from George Hitchings and Gertrude Elion of Burroughs-Wellcome in Tuckahoe (who shared a Nobel Prize in 1988 with James Black). He found that, among the variants, BW57-322 was less toxic and could be used orally. Calne and Murray at Boston found BW57-322 to be effective in dog kidney transplantation, though mortality was high and the surviving kidneys few (83). Murray, who had also been active in the Boston twin transplants, would be awarded a Nobel Prize in 1992.

Using MP-6 and its derivative BW57-322, now called azathioprine (Imuran), human kidney transplants were attempted in London at the Royal Free Hospital by Roy Calne and John Hopewell. Attempts were also made in

Boston and Paris. Uniformly, the results were poor, with high mortality. Conversely, the huge success in basic laboratory studies with induction of tolerance and the discovery of an antibody-mediated "enhancement" seemed to offer greater hope than generalized nonspecific immunosuppression, with all its dangers. Privately, scientific workers and grant-giving bodies urged caution in clinical experiments, and suggested that surgeons instead await elegant solutions from the laboratory.

Attitudes changed in 1963 when a piece of surgical empiricism improved the results of human transplantation. Küss and Hamburger in Paris, Goodwin at UCLA (California), and Starzl in Denver had all noted that steroids reversed rejection episodes when all else had failed (84). Steroids, which had been repeatedly shown to be ineffective immunosuppressants when given alone and had caused severe gastrointestinal problems in dogs, were now combined from the start with azathioprine in the three surgical centers with remarkable results. They found that, fortunately, the dangerous levels of steroids could be reduced in the weeks following grafting as adaptation emerged. In 1963, Starzl's results in 20 of 27 living-related and unrelated kidney transplants were particularly impressive. Optimistically, Reemstma and Hume even attempted monkey kidney transplants in humans and achieved short-term function.

The two-drug regimen of steroids and azathioprine was to become a mainstay for almost 20 years. On occasion there would be temporary enthusiasm for other drugs and modalities: cytotoxic drugs such as cyclophosphamide; biological agents such as antilymphocyte serum; and interventions such as thoracic duct drainage, macrophage blockade, and more targeted radiation. Refinements continued, including improved quality of donor kidneys and the use of better preservation methods.

1960s TO THE PRESENT

During the 1960s, as the results of kidney transplantation slowly improved, the number of units offering the service increased. The clinicians involved grew in number and enthusiasm, and in 1964 the international Transplantation Society assumed the meetings previously organized by the New York Academy of Sciences. The journal *Plastic and Reconstructive Surgery* had, from 1958 to 1962, issued a supplement called the *Transplantation Bulletin*. Reflecting the growing importance of this new discipline, the journal spun off the supplement into the new journal *Transplantation*.

Some pleasant surprises were to accompany the pursuit of this new surgical service. Results simply improved with experience. Belding Scribner's invention of the simple arteriovenous shunt enabled the spreading availability of the artificial kidney and regular dialysis in 1960 (the same year as the introduction of Imuran). This had a revolutionary impact, and made patients fitter than before for surgery. As hemodialysis was available after loss of the kidney, heroic and prolonged antirejection efforts were no longer necessary: the patient's survival was now part of the equation. Both treatments, dialysis and transplantation, had their advocates, and at the time the choice was a difficult one for patients and their advisors—especially when it was discovered that a second transplant might succeed where a first had failed. Each hospital had differing policies according to local experience and facilities.

As kidney transplantations continued, not all of the findings were pleasant. For example, it was demonstrated that pretransplant antibodies might cause immediate rejection of the transplant (85). Prolonged use of steroids was found to give rise to bone disease. Exotic infections were encountered and treated, but the spread of hepatitis B in dialysis and transplant units was occasionally fatal to both staff and patients, casting a cloud over the service for a while. The latter issue was dealt with in the short term by testing the blood used for transfusion; eventually, a vaccine was developed, but initially it was expensive and restricted. The appearance of tumors in allograft recipients raised fundamental questions about tumor origin and surveillance by the immune system, and these de novo malignancies were studied from the first in the Denver Tumor Transplant Registry. Tissue typing labs found that the histocompatibility antigens were associated with disease susceptibility (see below).

The growth in the clinical service sector marched forward in step with the continuing remarkable advances in fundamental immunology at the time. Much of the surgical innovation continued to be empirical, however. The two groups, surgeons and scientists, encouraged each other with their success. The surgeons did not use all of the sophisticated immunology available, but took heart from the vitality and confidence of the laboratories and the strategies they revealed. The scientists not only improved methods of inducing adult tolerance, but even made vital technical innovations, notably the microsurgery methods developed for rat kidney transplantation (86).

For their part, the growing number of immunologists were pleased to know that transplantation success was at hand. They could now show grant-giving bodies that their efforts had practical use. Such was the excitement and intensity of activity in fundamental transplantation studies that it yielded an early case of scientific fraud (87). Later, once the success of organ transplant appeared assured and the methodology became rather routine and unchanging, a number of surgeons and scientists, notably Medawar and Woodruff, turned instead to studies of the relationship of the immune response to cancer.

Tissue Typing

Another product of the optimistic 1960s was tissue typing methods for human organ allografting. Previously, Gorer and Snell had shown the presence of histocompatibility genes in laboratory animals. In 1958, Jean Dausset (later to be awarded a Nobel Prize with George Snell and Baruj Benacerraf) studied the serum of a patient who had multiple blood transfusions and used the anti–white cell antibody he found to identify the MAC antigen (later known as HLA-A2 and A28) found on the rest of the body cells (88,89). Following this, Rose Payne and J. J. van Rood in 1958 realized that mothers who had borne many children were sometimes sensitized against the child's cells, thus enabling them to identify the antigens 4a and 4b (later to be known as HLA-B4 and HLA-B6) (90,91).

The relationship between these tissue antigen types and the results of tissue transplantation was explored via volunteer skin grafting by Rapaport and Dausset. The predictive success rates achieved with matching were supported in human kidney grafting by Terasaki and van Rood in 1966, though the effect was best seen in living-related matches (92). The consequence of the usefulness of matching led naturally to organ-sharing schemes to obtain the best match. These programs developed first locally, then nationally. Eurotransplant, set up in 1969, shared organs over a wider network. Though not everyone agreed that the best match always had to be sought, the sharing schemes were vital in finding suitable kidneys for highly sensitized patients and for obtaining kidneys needed urgently for special cases.

Tissue typing became more sophisticated when the class II HLA antigens, which caused rejection in cadaver kidneys fully matched for the original HLA antigens (later to be known as class I antigens), were identified, leading to DR typing. The in vitro methods were set up initially using cells from the children of first-cousin marriages. Serology advances then led to the introduction of HLA-DR matching in clinical transplantation, and a much greater influence on graft outcome (93). These methods would be of major importance in matching for bone marrow transplantation, where the GvH component was important. Extension of these methods added HLA-DQ and HLA-C to the class II and class I HLA loci, respectively.

In the years since 1992, serologic typing has started to be replaced by DNA typing. These methods have found additional use in medicolegal disputes on parentage.

EVOLUTION OF ORGAN TRANSPLANTATION IN THE 1970s

The evolution of regular transplantation of other organs in human patients followed the pattern set during the pioneer days of kidney transplantation: initial success with experimental studies, then an enthusiastic but difficult start in human cases, followed by a moratorium, and later a cautious reintroduction. A new element had appeared, however: the public was now curious. In the case of the heart transplants, public opinion would play a major role.

The 1970s did not, as expected, see the culmination of transplant success. Rather, it was a time of maturation for the kidney transplant service, with many modest innovations and experience all adding to improved results (Fig. 1.12). Blood transfusion while a patient was on dialysis was found to be favorable, not detrimental, to the results of transplantation. The traditional large steroid dosage could be reduced without risk. At the very end of this decade, a new immunosuppressive agent would appear—cyclosporine was to make transplantation safer and more successful.

Liver Transplantation

In Denver, Tom Starzl, though experienced in both human kidney and animal liver transplants, had shown dismal results in his pioneer attempts at human liver transplantation. In five cases transplanted in 1963 and onward, none survived beyond 23 days (94). Discouraged and acknowledging the formidable technical problems, he ceased such attempts until 1967. In that year, he was joined by Calne at Cambridge in treating a new series of patients. They were encouraged by the availability of human antilymphocyte globulin, a biologic agent that had been studied and refined by Michael Woodruff in Edinburgh and Medawar in London. The technical challenges were overcome with experience and the results improved (95). By 1982, Calne had a 50% 1-year survival. Thus, the service was established, and slowly other centers in North America, Britain, and Europe were set up. By 1998, the European Register could report an 85% 1-year graft survival (see Chapters 19 and 20).

Lung Transplantation

A similar evolution of lung transplantation occurred. Of the first 20 patients, only one was a long-term survivor. However, the technical innovation of the omental patch to prevent bronchial anastomotic leak was helpful in the later success of the procedure (96) (see Chapter 25).

Pancreatic Transplantation

Pancreatic transplantation had a start in 1966 when Kelly and Lillehei carried out the first human vascularized transplant in a diabetic patient, resulting in a 2-month graft function. The serious complications of the surgery were discouraging, and it was not until 1978 that successful strategies using various intra-abdominal positions evolved to deal with the duct system and exocrine part of the gland (97). By the mid-1980s, the international register had about 300 patients, and 50% graft survival was reached in 1985. Eventually, technical success was achieved with combined kidney and pancreas grafting; by 1995 the Registry reported that this procedure comprised 87% of pancreatic transplants, with a 75% 1-year graft survival (98). Pure islet cell transplantation has offered an elegant solution, but, apart from the occasional success, it has proved as difficult as skin allografting to achieve (see Chapter 21).

Heart Transplantation

By the 1960s, experimental heart transplantation was a successful laboratory procedure. Shumway and Lower in

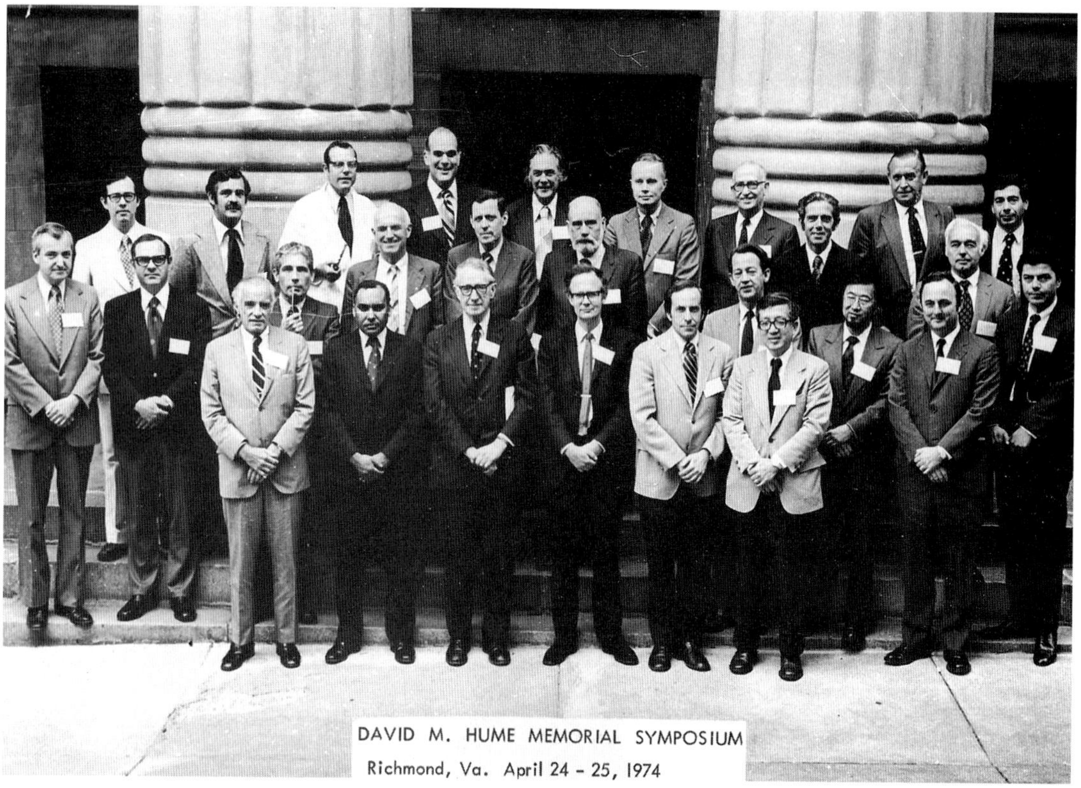

FIGURE 1.12. *The Memorial Meeting for David Hume in 1974 gathered many of the pioneer surgeons, physicians, and transplantation immunologists.*

particular had considerable experience in orthotopic dog heart allografting, as had others (99). South African surgeon Christiaan Barnard would carry out the first human transplant in December 1967 (Fig. 1.13). This case was followed by another, and the second transplant patient was to survive for 2 years (90). The short-term success of Barnard's first case liberated others immediately from any constraints, and six more operations were quickly reported from other centers, though none of the grafts had long-term survival. This initial period of heart transplantation lasted for a little over a year, ceasing in the spring of 1969. Just over 100 heart transplants had been performed in 22 countries, in a rather disorderly and often chauvinistic way. The impetus for the hiatus was, as with the first attempts with other organs, poor results and serious complications.

The public became deeply involved in these heart surgeries. Although they were initially supportive, the media rapidly became intrusive and personalized the events. Public reaction to some aspects of these transplants grew hostile—particularly after the realities of "heart-beating" donor usage were realized. The public ill will, as well as the criticism from the profession itself for the heart procedures, spilled over to other organ programs. The well-established kidney transplant service experienced a fall in donor numbers (100), and even the uncontroversial, low-profile corneal graft service saw a dip in activity. During this time, a Texas patient was being kept alive with the first prototype artificial heart. The controversy over the device's use, combined with a failed heart transplant in this same patient afterward, all added to the general mood against such surgery.

Calls from both outside and inside the profession for a moratorium in heart transplantation followed, and they had to be heeded. US funding for heart transplantation and artificial heart development was cut back. The call was for funding basic immunologic studies rather than clinical experimentation, a view taken not only by immunologists but also by many clinicians. Those advocating prevention of heart disease rather than cure were listened to, as were critics of the costs and the cost-effectiveness of organ transplantation in general. The ethics of transplantation and the methods of allocation of scarce resources became topical and attracted serious study (101). Discussions of formal acknowledgment of "brain death" started in 1968, and successful guidelines became available. The first set of suggestions came from Harvard University, and by the mid-1970s, these or similar guidelines were widely used (102,103).

It was in this climate that Norman Shumway was entrusted with a careful, unostentatious program of human heart transplantation in California. Shumway had had a bad start, with two immediate failures during the enthusiastic "year of the heart." Shumway's results steadily improved after his faltering 1968 start, and by 1972 he had reached a 50%

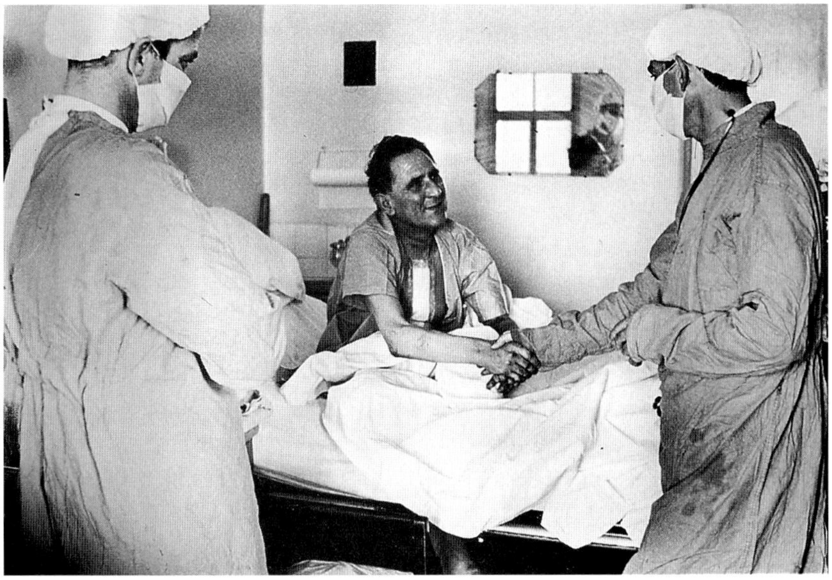

FIGURE 1.13. *Louis Washkansky congratulating the surgeon Christiaan Barnard shortly after the world's first heart transplant operation. (Courtesy of Dr. D. K. C. Cooper, Cape Town, South Africa.)*

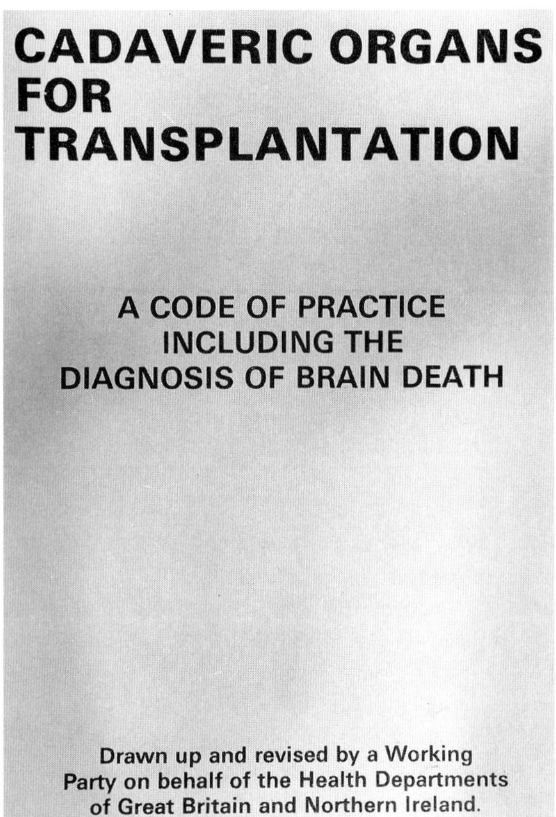

CADAVERIC ORGANS FOR TRANSPLANTATION

A CODE OF PRACTICE INCLUDING THE DIAGNOSIS OF BRAIN DEATH

Drawn up and revised by a Working Party on behalf of the Health Departments of Great Britain and Northern Ireland.

FIGURE 1.14. *Criteria for the diagnosis of death were formalized in Britain in 1979 and greatly aided the emergence of heart and liver transplantation.*

1-year heart allograft survival, aided by regular intracardiac biopsy (104). The sensitive matter of donor organ provision was now studied more calmly, and in 1974 California became the first state to legalize the use of "heart-beating" donors.

The reaction to the controversies of the first period of heart transplantation had been so severe that general attempts were not revived until 12 years after Barnard's first case. In the United Kingdom and elsewhere, not until 1980 were such operations nervously resumed (Fig. 1.14). In Britain, the NHS provided no separate funding for heart transplant research. Instead, the government announced that it would be funding the reintroduction of heart transplants. This novel approach by the government was designed if not to encourage the procedure, then certainly to control it. The expected close public interest did reemerge, but it waned rapidly when the good results allowed an uncontroversial service to emerge in an orderly way (see Chapters 23 and 24).

THE 1980s AND CURRENT ADVANCES

Cyclosporine

In 1979 Calne and White introduced cyclosporine, the first drug to challenge the core regimen of azathioprine and steroids that had persisted in use since the early 1960s (Fig. 1.15) (106). The Sandoz company discovered the agent cyclosporine during routine testing of fungal extracts for biologic activity, notably antibacterial. Cyclosporine's low toxicity and immunosuppressive activity encouraged human use. It was quickly shown to be useful both in experimental grafting and in all forms of human organ transplants (107).

Initially, cyclosporine was a difficult drug to use. With experience, results improved: rejection episodes became less

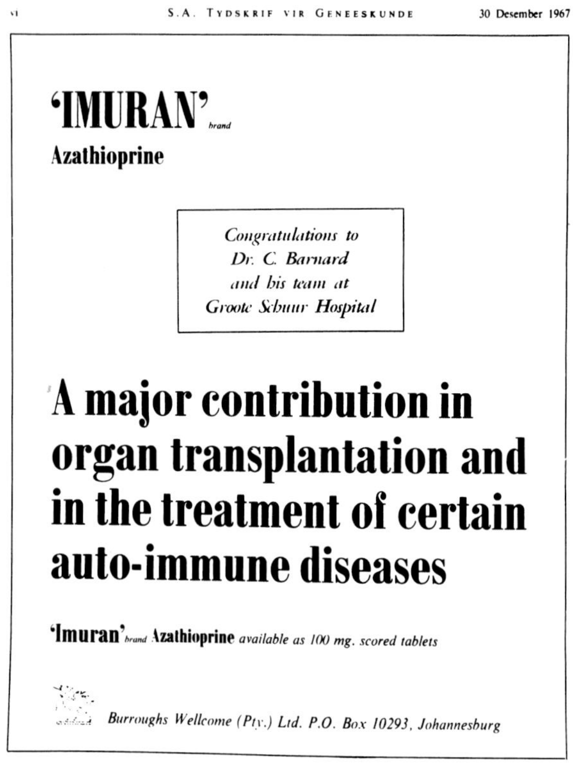

FIGURE 1.15. *Azathioprine and steroids were the unchallenged standard combination of immunosuppressive agents until cyclosporine emerged in the 1980s.*

abrupt, and it partly concealed the effects of tissue typing and blood transfusion. It helped to improve the results of heart and liver transplantation (see Chapter 6).

Service Expansion

Other improvements during this time have given substantial help to the organ transplantation service, such as fine-needle aspiration and cytomegalovirus (CMV) infection detection. New drugs, such as immunoregulatory agents, mycophenolate, and tacrolimus, have found niches. There is also hope for induction of adult tolerance.

But as the service has become successful, need has outstripped the supply of organs. In spite of donor drives run by governments and other agencies, and the sharing schemes of many countries, the donation of organs has risen only slowly. Certainly it cannot meet the need for operations that are now being offered to a wider age range of patients, many of whom are less fit than were previous candidates. The need for organs has led to allegations worldwide of payments to nonrelated donors for kidneys. This practice has been outlawed in many countries. In Britain, for example, stern warnings have been issued by the General Medical Council (108).

Xenografting

As the shortage of donor organs continues, the use of animal donors has returned to the agenda. Until the 1980s, xenograft discussion was based on the assumption that closely related animal organs, notably from monkeys, would be used with powerful immunosuppression plus added measures to thwart the antibody-mediated hyperacute cross-species rejection (109). The emergence in other fields of methods of genetic manipulation and techniques for the modification of the entire histocompatibility mechanism has made closeness of species irrelevant. Thus, modern considerations of xenografting now have centered on the pig—a robust breeder possibly free of any disease threat to humans. The pig has been chosen for possible future human organ provision, with an initial strategy of adding human DNA to the pig in embryo for the rearing of transgenic animals (Fig. 1.16) (see Chapter 40).

RETROSPECT

Historical study of the achievements in tissue transplantation offers unrivaled possibilities for the analysis of the mechanisms of innovation in medicine in general. The usual approach to a history of medicine in a compressed account, as here, makes the progress of any new discipline seem logical and obvious in retrospect. However, during the development of a new discipline the way ahead is not obvious—hindsight reveals that many serious and determined initiatives were pursued in directions that are now not considered to be progress. By merely picking out the line of progress retrospectively, conventional histories not only fail to recreate the mood of the times and its hopes, choices, assumptions, and attitudes, but also can mistakenly attribute the correct insights and goals to contributions now judged to be important. Moreover, future histories may view the straight line of seemingly inevitable progress differently, in the light of developments that are yet to come.

Medical history, if it is to be of use in illuminating present events and aiding our day-to-day choices, must instead attempt to re-create the complexity of the past. Such analysis is of benefit to those with a lively interest in the future—to the scientist who has to choose what to do next and to the grant-giving bodies who are faced with productive allocation of funds.

The demonstration of neonatal tolerance in the mouse, for example, was not regarded by Medawar as directly applicable to specific tolerance of allogeneic tissue in the adult human, even though now we see his work as the initial step toward safe, nonspecific immunosuppression. Should adult human allograft tolerance ever be achieved, we shall revise the core story once again. Should the use of animal organs reach routine use in human medicine, then a new history based on an account of progress toward xenografting will result, and the story of the immunosuppression period will be marginalized and given a less central and final role.

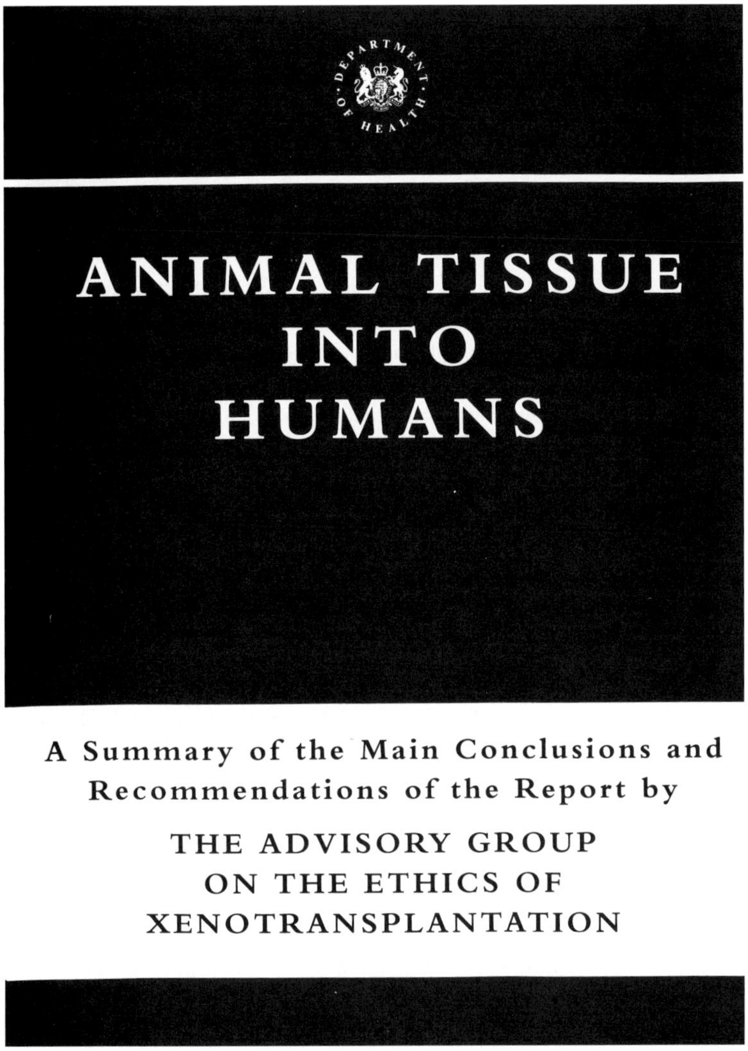
ANIMAL TISSUE INTO HUMANS

A Summary of the Main Conclusions and Recommendations of the Report by

THE ADVISORY GROUP ON THE ETHICS OF XENOTRANSPLANTATION

FIGURE 1.16. *Governments in the mid-1990s cautiously allowed research to proceed into the use of animal organs for human transplantation.*

Other issues emerge from a study of the evolution of tissue transplantation. It is a crucial case study in the relationship between progress in basic science and innovation in the clinical world. Those who advocate that the laboratory should always have first priority for "seed-corn" funding, who see a natural one-way flow of novel findings and methods from the laboratory to the clinic, will not be supported by the detailed history of organ transplantation. In this discipline, empiric clinical and surgical innovation played a more than worthy role. Nor have animal models always been helpful in the development of organ transplantation. In fact, such models sometimes delayed the use of fruitful regimens in humans—the human patient can be the odd mouse out.

Surgical science always benefits from war, and transplantation was no different. World War II and even the Cold War provided transplanters with knowledge of radiation and marrow replacement. We also find examples of the rewards of tedious routine drug testing, from the neutral screening of exotic material that led to the discovery of cyclosporine, to the routine chemical modification of 6-MP that led to azathioprine.

Another matter of historical interest is the role of serendipity. Those looking at susceptibility to tumor transplantation were instead looking at the normal rejection mechanism. The alleged auto-antibody in leukemia was in fact an exciting and useful acquired alloantibody. The hunt for tolerance induction in humans with bone marrow suppression instead showed how useful irradiation and drugs alone could be. Transplantation teaches that those involved in new surgical services will encounter surprises and should be alert for novelties not to be found in the textbooks; the exotic diseases and tumors that developed in immunosuppressed patients are prime examples of the unexpected.

Inspiration in the form of huge successes following the failure of favorite assumptions is a notable part of the history of transplantation. The survival of skin grafts in nonidentical twin cattle, for instance, was a puzzle that hinted at a new immunologic mechanism. The worsening kidney transplant results of the 1970s, which many preferred to ignore as embarrassments, revealed the mysterious benefit of pre-transplant blood transfusions. As transplantation history shows, such paradoxes should not deter researchers, but rather should be regarded as puzzles to solve toward gaining a new understanding of nature and disease.

The rapid emergence of routine organ transplantation illustrates one of the oldest lessons from the history of surgery. At the earliest stages, pioneering surgical methods may be technically baffling and daunting to their originators, who not only may be faced with high mortality among their ill patients, but may also have to confront peer disapproval and public hostility. As we have seen, these methods have often progressed to be carried out with ease in fit patients. Ethical issues have always abounded in the field of organ replacement; although curiously, these concerns have shown a tendency to disappear once a treatment becomes routine and cheaper, with improved results. Thus, desirable goals can be achieved if there is a determination to do so.

REFERENCES

1. Thompson S. Motif-index of folk-literature. Copenhagen: Rosenkilde and Baager, 1955–1958.
2. Tosatti B. Transplantation and reimplantation in the arts. Surgery 1974;75:389–397.
3. de Voragine J. The golden legend. Oxford: The Kelmscott Press, 1900:861–864.
4. Bhishagratna KKL. An English translation of the Sushruta. Calcutta: 1907–1916;1:152–154.
5. Patterson TJS. The Zeis index and history of plastic surgery, 900 B.C.–1863 A.D. Baltimore: Williams & Wilkins, 1977.
6. Tagliacozzi G. De curtorem chirurgia. Venice: Bindoni, 1597.
7. Gnudi MT, Webster JP. The life and times of Gaspare Tagliacozzi. Milan: Hoepli, 1939.
8. Hamilton D, Goodrich JT. An illustration of skin graft rejection and sympathetic medicine from 1661. Bull Hist Med 1986;60:217–221.
9. Freshwater MF. Pre-Baronian tissue transfer. Conn Med 1976;40:613–617.
10. Patterson TJS. Experimental skin grafts in England 1663–64. Brit J Plast Surg 1969;22:384–385.
11. Gibson T. The first homografts: Trembley and the polyps. Brit J Plast Surg 1966;19:301–307.
12. Martin CE. John Hunter and tissue transplantation. Surg Gynecol Obstet 1970;131:306–310.
13. Morse DR. Plantation procedures. J Oral Implant 1977;7:176–192.
14. Hunter J. The natural history of the human teeth. London: J Johnson, 1771.
15. Fox J. The natural history of human teeth. London: 1806:12.
16. Balch CM, Marzoni FA. Skin transplantation during the pre-Reverdin era. Surg Gynecol Obstet 1977;144:767–773.
17. Freshwater MF, Su CT, Hoopes JE. Joseph Constantine Carpue—first military plastic surgeon. Milit Med 1977;142:603–606.
18. Baronio G. On grafting in animals. Joan Bond Sax, trans. Robert Goldwyn, intro. Boston: Boston Medical Library, 1985.
19. Gibson T. Early free grafting. Brit J Plast Surg 1964;17:1–11.
20. Reverdin SL. Greffe épidermique. Bull Soc Imp Chir Paris 1870;10:511–518.
21. Reverdin H. Jaques-Louis Reverdin (1842–1929). Aarau: Sauerländer, 1971.
22. Longacre JJ. Paul Bert and his animal grafts. Plast Reconstr Surg 1984;33:178–186.
23. Pollock GD. Cases of skin grafting. Trans Clin Soc Lond 1871;4:37–54.
24. Freshwater FF. George David Pollock and the development of skin grafting. Ann Plast Surg 1978;1:96–102.
25. Hamilton FH. Healing of ulcers by transplantation. New York Med J 1871; 14:225–232.
26. Simmer HH. Roger Tuttle Morris (1857–1945): a pioneer in ovarian transplants. Obstet Gynecol 1970;35:314–328.
27. Croom JH. A case of heteroplastic ovarian grafting. Trans Edin Obstet Soc 1906;31:194–200.
28. Glasgow Herald, 5 September 1878.
29. Klasen HJ. History of free skin grafting: knowledge or empiricism? Berlin: Springer-Verlag, 1981.
30. Oppenheimer JM. Taking things apart and putting them together again. Bull Hist Med Allied Sci 1980;52:149–161.
31. Payr E. Zur Frage der circulären Vereinigung von Blutgefässen mit resorbirbaren Prosthesen. Arch Klin Chir 1903;72:32–54.
32. Watts SH. The suture of blood vessels. Bull Johns Hopkins Hosp 1907;18:153–178.
33. Ullmann E. Experimentelle Nierentransplantation. Wien Klin Wochenschr 1902;15:281–282.
34. Largiader F. 72 years of organ transplantation: Emerich Ullmann memorial lecture. Eur Surg Res 1974;6:197–208.
35. von Decastello A. Über experimentelle Nierentransplantation. Wein Klin Woch 1902;15:317–318.
36. Jaboulay M. Greffe de reins au pli du conde par soudres artérielles et veineuses. Bull du Lyon Méd 1906;107:575–577.
37. Les biographes médicale de Paris 1936;10:257–272.
38. Unger E. Über Nierentransplantation. Berlin, 1938.
39. Winkler EA. Ernst Unger: a pioneer in modern surgery. J Hist Med Allied Sci 1982;37:269–286.
40. Hammond LJ, Sutton HA. Case of transplantation of testicles. Int Clin (Surgery) 1912;22:150–154.
41. Converse JM. Alexis Carrel: the man, the unknown. Plast Reconstr Surg 1981;68:629–639.
42. Guthrie CC. Blood vessel surgery and its applications. Reprinted with an introduction by Samuel P Harbison and Bernard Fisher. Pittsburgh: University of Pittsburgh Press, 1959.
43. Malinin TI. Surgery and life: the extraordinary career of Alexis Carrel. New York: Harcourt Brace Jovanovitch, 1979.
44. Little CC. James Bumgardner Murphy. Biog Mem Nat Acad Sci 1960;34:183–203.
45. Löwy I. Biomedical research and the constraints of medical practice. James Bumgardner Murphy and the early discovery of the role of lymphocytes in immune reactions. Bull Hist Med 1989;63:356–391.
46. Mazumdar PMH. Immunity in 1890. J Hist Med Allied Sci 1972;29:312–324.
47. Jensen CO. Experimentelle Untersuchungen über Krebs bei Mäusen. Z Bakt Parasit 1903;34:28–122.
48. Bashford EF, Murray JA, Haaland M. Resistance and susceptibility to inoculated cancer. Third Scientific Report of the Cancer Research Fund, 1908:359. (See also the Fifth Report.)
49. Haddow A. Cancer research: its history and prospects. Proc Roy Instit 1959;37:223–240.
50. Holman E. Protein sensitisation in iso-skingrafting: is the latter of practical value? Surg Gynecol Obstet 1924;38:100–106.
51. Hamilton D. The monkey gland affair. London: Chatto, 1986.
52. Hartroft WS. Leo Loeb. Arch Path 1960;70:269–274.
53. Medawar PB. The immunology of transplantation. Harvey Lectures, 1956–57. New York: Academic Press, 144–176.
54. Morse HC. Origins of inbred mice. London: Academic Press, 1978.
55. Snell GD. The genetics of transplantation. J Natl Cancer Inst 1953;14:691–699.
56. Gorer PA. The genetics and antigenic basis of tumour transplantation. J Pathol Bact 1937;44:691–697.
57. Medawar PB. Peter Gorer. Biog Mem Fell Roy Soc 1961;7:95–109.
58. Williamson CS. Further studies on the transplantation of the kidney. J Urol 1926;16:231–252.
59. Hamilton D, Reid WA. Yu Yu Voronoi and the first human kidney allograft. Surg Gynecol Obstet 1984;159:289–294.
60. Gibson T, Medawar PB. The fate of skin homografts in man. J Anat 1942;77:299–310.
61. Medawar PB. Notes on the problem of skin homografts. Bull War Med 1943;4:1–4.
62. Medawar PB. A second study of the behaviour and fate of skin homografts in rabbits. J Anat 1944;79:157–176.
63. Rogers BO. John Marquis Converse 1909–1981. Ann Plast Surg 1982;8:342–358.
64. Simonsen M. Biological incompatibility in kidney transplantation in dogs. II: Serological investigations. Acta Pathol Microbiol Scand 1953;32:1–84.
65. Dempster WJ. Kidney homotransplantation. Brit J Surg 1953;40:447–465.
66. Mitchison NA. Passive transfer of transplantation immunity. Proc R Soc (Biol) 1954;142:72–87.
67. Hume DM, Merrill JP, Miller BF, Thorn GW. Experiences with renal homotransplantation: report of nine cases. J Clin Invest 1955;34:327–382.

68. Hume DM. Early experience in organ homotransplantation in man and the unexpected sequelae thereof. Am J Surg 1979;137:152–161.
69. Küss R, Teinturier J, Milliez P. Quelques essais de greffe de rein chez l'homme. Mem Acad Chir 1951;77:755–764.
70. Starzl TE. France and the early history of organ transplantation. Perspect Biol Med 1993;37:35–47.
71. Rycroft BW. Corneal grafts. London: Butterworth, 1955.
72. Billingham RE, Lampkin GH, Medawar PB, Williams HL. Tolerance of homografts, twin diagnosis and the freemartin condition in cattle. Hereditary 1952;6:201–212.
73. Gowans JL. The effect of the continuous re-infusion of lymph and lymphocytes on the output of lymphocytes from the thoracic duct. Brit J Exp Pathol 1957;38:67–81.
74. Ford WL. The lymphocyte. In: Wintrobe MM, ed. Blood, pure and eloquent. McGraw: New York, 1980:Chapter 14.
75. Murray JE, Merrill JP, Harrison JH. Kidney transplantation between seven pairs of identical twins. Ann Surg 1958;148:343–359.
76. Barnes DWH, Loutit JF. Protective effects of implants of splenic tissue. Proc R Soc Med;46:251.
77. Main JM, Prehn RT. Successful skin homografts after the administration of high dosage X radiation and homologous bone marrow. J Natl Cancer Inst 1955;15:1023–1029.
78. Murray JE, Tilney NE, Wilson RE. Ann Surg 1976;184:565–573.
79. Hektoen L, Corper HJ. The effects of mustard gas (dichlorethylsulphide) on antibody formation. J Infect Dis 1921;28:279–293.
80. Polley HF, Slocumb CH. Behind the scenes with cortisone and ACTH. Mayo Clin Proc 1976;51:471–477.
81. Schwartz R, Dameshek W. Drug-induced immunological tolerance. Nature 1959;189:1682–1683.
82. Calne RY. The rejection of renal homografts: inhibition in dogs by 6-mercaptopurine. Lancet 1960;(i):417–418.
83. Calne RY. The development of immunosuppressive therapy. Transplant Proc 1981;13(suppl 1):44–49.
84. Starzl TE. Personal reflections in transplantation. Surg Clin North Am 1978;58:879–893.
85. Kissmeyer-Nielsen F, Olsen S, Peterson VP, Fjeldborg O. Hyperacute rejection of kidney allografts. Lancet 1966;(ii):662–665.
86. Lee S. Historical significance of rat organ transplantation. Microsurgery 1990;11:115–121.
87. Hixson J. The patchwork mouse. New York: Anchor Press, 1979.
88. Dausset J, Nenna A. Présence d'une leuco-agglutinine dans le sérum d'un cas d'agranulocytose chronique. Compt Rend Soc Biol 1952;146:1534–1541.
89. Dausset J. The birth of MAC. Vox Sang 1984;46:238–242.
90. van Rood JJ, Eernisse JG, van Leeuwen A. Leucocyte antibodies in sera from pregnant women. Nature 1958;181:1735–1736.
91. van Rood JJ. Discovery of 4a and 4b. Vox Sang 1984;46:238–242.
92. Terasaki PI, Vredevoe DL, Porter KA, et al. Serotyping for transplantation. Transplantation 1966;4:688–699.
93. Ting A, Morris PJ. Matching for B-cell antigens of the HLA-DR series in cadaveric renal transplantation. Lancet 1978;(i):575–577.
94. Starzl TE, Marchiori TL, von Kaulla G, Hermann RS, et al. Homotransplantation of the liver in humans. Surg Gynecol Obstet 1963;117:659–676.
95. Starzl T. Experience in hepatic transplantation. Philadelphia: Saunders, 1969.
96. Montefusco CM, Veith FJ. Lung transplantation. Surg Clin North Am 1986;66:503–516.
97. Connolly JE. Pancreatic whole organ transplantation. Surg Clin North Am 1978;58:383–390.
98. Sutherland DER, Gruessner RWG, Gores PF. Pancreas and islet transplantation: an update. Transplant Rev 1994;8:185–206.
99. Cooper DKC. Transplantation of heart and both lungs: 1. Historical review. Thorax 1969;24:383–398.
100. Barnard CN. The operation. A human cardiac transplant: an interim report of a successful operation performed at Groote Schuur Hospital Cape Town. S Afr Med J 1967;41:1271–1274.
101. Letters to editor. BMJ 1968;(i):177, 254, 378, 577.
102. A definition of irreversible coma. Report of the Ad Hoc Committee of the Harvard Medical School to examine the definition of brain death. JAMA 1968;205:337–340.
103. Scarce medical resources. Columbia Law Review 1969;69:620–692.
104. Jamieson SW, Stinson EB, Shumway NE. Cardiac transplantation in 150 patients at Stanford University. BMJ 1979;(i):93–95.
105. Cadaveric organs for transplantation. A code of practice drawn up by a working party on behalf of the Health Departments of Great Britain and Northern Ireland 1979 (revised 1983).
106. Calne RY, White DJG, Thiru S, et al. Cyclosporin A in patients receiving renal allografts from cadaveric donors. Lancet 1978;(ii):1323–1327.
107. Stähelin H. Cyclosporin: historical background. Progr Allergy 1986;38:19–27.
108. The Council of the Transplantation Society. Commercialisation in transplantation: the problems and some guidelines for practice. Lancet 1985;(ii):715–716.
109. Malouin R. Surgeons' quest for life: the history and the future of xenotransplantation. Perspect Biol Med 1994;37:416–428.

GENERAL READING

Patterson TJS, trans, ed. The Zeis index and history of plastic surgery, 900 B.C.–1863 A.D. Baltimore: Williams & Wilkins, 1977.

Marchand P. Der Process der Wundhelung unt Einschluss der Transplantation. Stuttgart: Ferdinand Enke, 1901.

Schöne G. Die Heteroplastiche und Homoöplastische Transplantation. Berlin: Springer, 1912.

Lexer E. Free transplantation. Ann Surg 1914;60:166–195.

Korschelt E. Regeneration und Transplantation. Berlin: Borntraeget, 1931. (Translated and republished in 1990 by Science History Publications, Canton, MA.)

Woodruff MFA. The transplantation of tissues and organs. Springfield, IL: Thomas, 1960.

Moore FD. Give and take: the development of tissue transplantation. Philadelphia: Saunders, 1964.

Medawar PB. Memoir of a thinking radish: an autobiography. New York: Oxford University Press, 1986.

Silverstein AM. A history of immunology. London and New York: Academic Press, 1989.

Starzl TE. The puzzle people: memoirs of a transplant surgeon. Pittsburgh: University of Pittsburgh Press, 1992.

Moore FD. A miracle and a privilege: recounting a half century of surgical advance. Washington, DC: Joseph Henry, 1995.

Brent L. A history of transplantation immunology. London, 1977.

Part I

Immunology

Chapter 2

Immunobiology of Graft Rejection

MARGARET J. DALLMAN

Transplantation of an organ between genetically disparate individuals results in changes in both the host and the graft. Some of these are a consequence of the trauma associated with surgery; others involve specific recognition by the immune system of antigenic differences between donor and recipient. The cumulative effect of these events is a destructive immune response which, if uncontrolled, will lead to immune rejection and loss of the transplant. The outcome following transplantation of material between genetically different individuals has been reiterated by many since it was originally highlighted by workers such as Little and Tyzzer (1). The immunologic nature of tissue rejection was clearly demonstrated over 50 years ago by Gibson and Medawar (2) and by Medawar (3,4) in both human and rodent transplantation, where the rejection process displayed marked specificity and memory for donor tissue and was accompanied by infiltration with leukocytes. Since that time, our understanding of the immune system has developed considerably; consequently, we are now able to describe more fully the molecular and cellular events that result in graft rejection.

An important new tool for our experiments has been mice bearing targeted deletions or mutations in their genome (5). The development of such animals has been made possible through two important technical advances. First, an ability to target pieces of DNA specifically to homologous regions in the genome (gene targeting by homologous recombination) has allowed us to alter the genome in a very specific fashion. Coupling this technique with the second advance—an ability to grow in culture mouse totipotent embryonic stem cells—has allowed the development of "knockout" mice. The first generation of knockout mice that bear deletions from the beginning of development are now being used in transplantation experiments by several groups (6). In theory, these mice allow the investigator to define the activity of a protein by investigating the functioning of the immune system in its absence, a classic approach that has been very valuable in many organisms.

Some interesting and important data have accumulated from experiments with knockout mice, but their use in understanding immunity has been complicated by the hallmark features of the immune system, adaptability and redundancy. As illustrated below, results from transplantation experiments using knockout mice have not always been easy to interpret and are frequently confounded by the elasticity of the immune system and by its resulting ability to circumvent developmental deficiencies using mechanisms that might not normally be employed. Such problems have prompted investigators to develop mice in which the knockout event can be controlled spatially or temporally (7). Although such experiments are still in their infancy, they may prove to be of value in our understanding of immune and transplantation responses.

The aim of this chapter is to review our current understanding of immunity to skin and organ grafts, emphasizing the recent technical and intellectual progress that has advanced knowledge in this area. We assume a basic level of understanding of the cells and molecules involved in immune responses, and refer the reader to other books and reviews for more general descriptions of the immune system (8,9).

TRAUMA AND TRANSPLANTATION

The changes that occur in host and graft following transplantation occur in a series of relatively well-defined stages, as shown in Figure 2.1. The first of these stages involves the rather severe physical assault that the graft undergoes during harvest from the donor and transplantation into the recipient; this is referred to as *ischemia and reperfusion injury.* The result is de novo expression of a variety of genes and infiltration of the graft by inflammatory cells. The induction

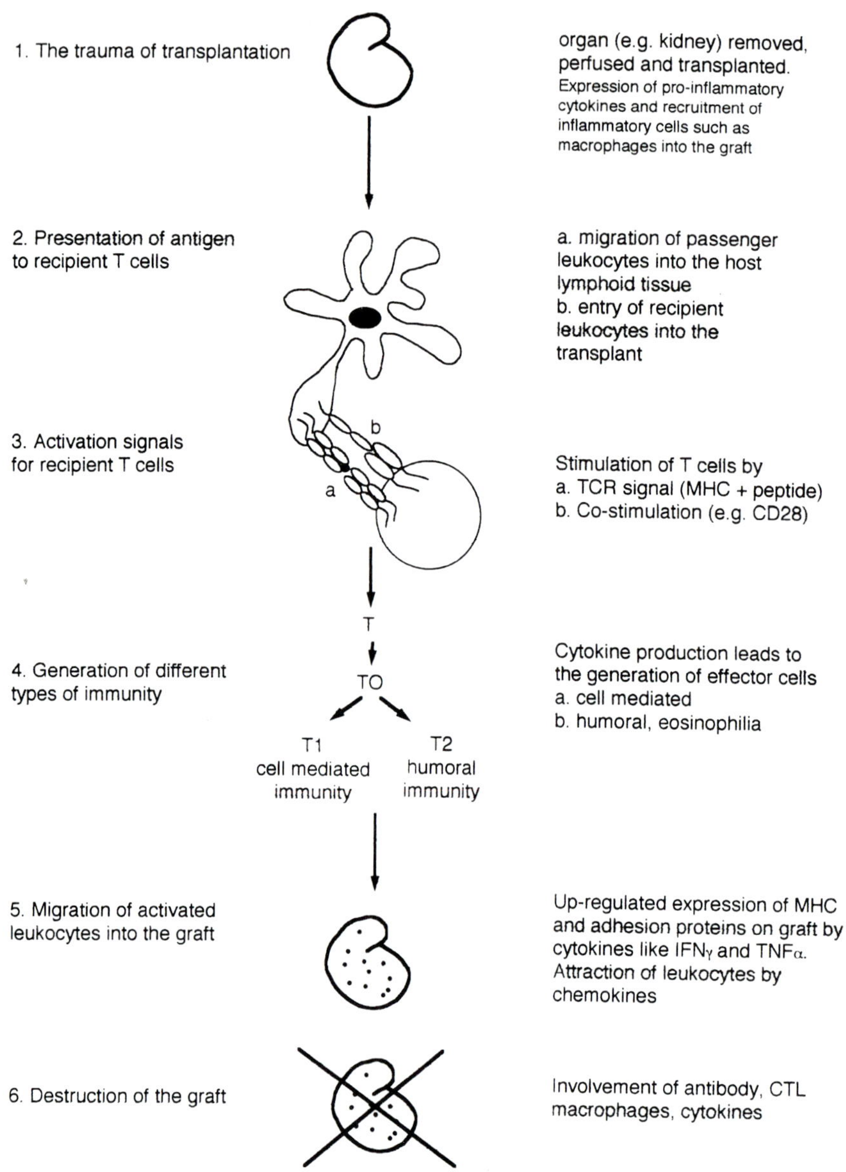

FIGURE 2.1. *The immune response to a graft. The key steps involved in generation of the inflammatory and immune response to an organ transplant. TCR, T-cell receptor; MHC, major histocompatibility complex; IFN, interferon; TNF, tumor necrosis factor; CTL, cytotoxic T lymphocyte.*

Table 2.1. Graft Terminology

Autograft (autologous graft). A graft from one part of the body to another. Examples: skin graft in burn patients, vascular graft.
Isograft (isogenic or syngeneic graft). A graft from one member of a species to a genetically identical member of the same species. Examples: grafts between members of the same inbred mouse or rat strain, grafts between identical twins.
Allograft (allogeneic graft). A graft between nonidentical members of the same species. Examples: grafts between mice or rats of different inbred strains, grafts between unrelated or related but not identical people.
Xenograft (xenogeneic graft). A graft between individuals of different species. Examples: pig or baboon to human, rat to mouse.

of several cytokines (or transcripts of cytokines), including interleukin (IL)-6 and IL-1, has been demonstrated at early time points following transplantation, even in situations in which there is no antigenic difference between donor and recipient and thus no immune response (see Table 2.1 for syngeneic graft terminology) (10,11). This induction of cytokines, together with an increased expression of adhesion proteins on the vascular endothelium of the graft, results in an early infiltration by inflammatory cells, including macrophages (12).

These early events alone do not result in graft rejection, and they are also observed in syngeneic grafts. However, their influence on early graft function and their importance in later rejection when an immune response is stimulated remain unclear.

PRESENTATION OF ANTIGEN TO RECIPIENT T CELLS

Antigens That Stimulate Graft Rejection

Histocompatibility antigens determine the outcome of *allografts*, tissue grafts between different members of the same species. In vertebrate species, histocompatibility antigens can be divided into a single major histocompatibility complex (the MHC) and many minor systems. Incompatibility for either MHC or minor histocompatibility antigens between graft donor and recipient leads to the immune response against the graft. Most vigorous rejection is observed where MHC incompatibilities between donor and recipient are greatest. In a nonsensitized recipient, rejection in the presence of compatibility for the MHC may not occur or may be delayed, except in the case of bone marrow transplantation where minor differences can cause either rapid rejection or graft-versus-host disease (13). However, as has been shown clearly in mice, multiple minor histocompatibility differences may result in skin or cardiac allograft rejection with as rapid a kinetics as that seen for transplantation across the MHC (14).

Major Histocompatibility Complex

There is substantial similarity between the MHC in different species with respect to both immunogenetics and biochemistry, although the order of genes within the complex varies between different species (Fig. 2.2). The genes within the MHC are divided into class I, class II, and class III types (15,16).

Class I proteins are cell surface glycoproteins comprised of two chains: 1) the heavy chain (molecular weight = 45 kd), which is polymorphic and encoded within the MHC by a class I gene; and 2) the nonvariable light chain β_2-microglobulin (molecular weight = 12 kd), which is encoded by a gene at another chromosomal location. Unlike the heavy chain, the β_2-microglobulin is not anchored in the membrane, so it may be exchanged for or stabilized by β_2-microglobulin from the surrounding fluid—an important point when dealing with cells or tissues from β_2-microglobulin knockout mice. MHC class I proteins are expressed on virtually all nucleated cells, albeit at variable levels, and they are, in general, responsible for activating T cells bearing the CD8 surface protein ($CD8^+$ cells; see below).

Class II genes also encode cell surface glycoproteins, which are composed of two chains of similar molecular weight (α chain, molecular weight = 35 kd; β chain, molecular weight = 28 kd), and stimulate T cells bearing the CD4 surface protein ($CD4^+$ cells). The tissue distribution of class II proteins is far more restricted than that of class I, as class II proteins are expressed constitutively only by B lymphocytes, dendritic cells, and some endothelial cells. During an immune response, however, with few exceptions most other cell types may be induced to express MHC class II proteins (17–23).

During the synthesis and transport of MHC class I and class II proteins to the cell surface, they become associated with small peptides. The primary difference between the two MHC classes is in the origin of these peptides: the class I peptides are acquired primarily from intracellularly derived proteins, the class II peptides primarily from extracellularly derived proteins (Fig. 2.3). It is the combination of MHC and peptide that is recognized by the antigen receptor [T-cell receptor (TCR)] on the T cell. During a period of inactivity of the immune system, the peptides contained within the MHC proteins will mainly be self in origin—many

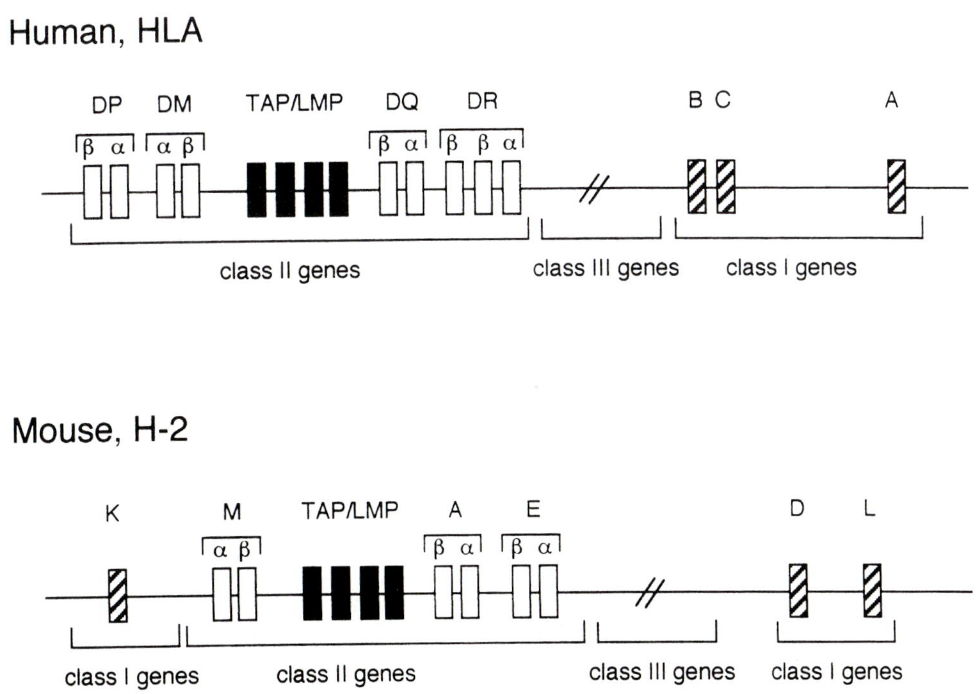

FIGURE 2.2. *MHC loci of human and mouse. The position of MHC class I, II, and III genes within the MHC of human (HLA) and mouse (H-2). Gene positions within the MHC are shown in bars. TAP, transporters associated with antigen processing; LMP, proteosome components.*

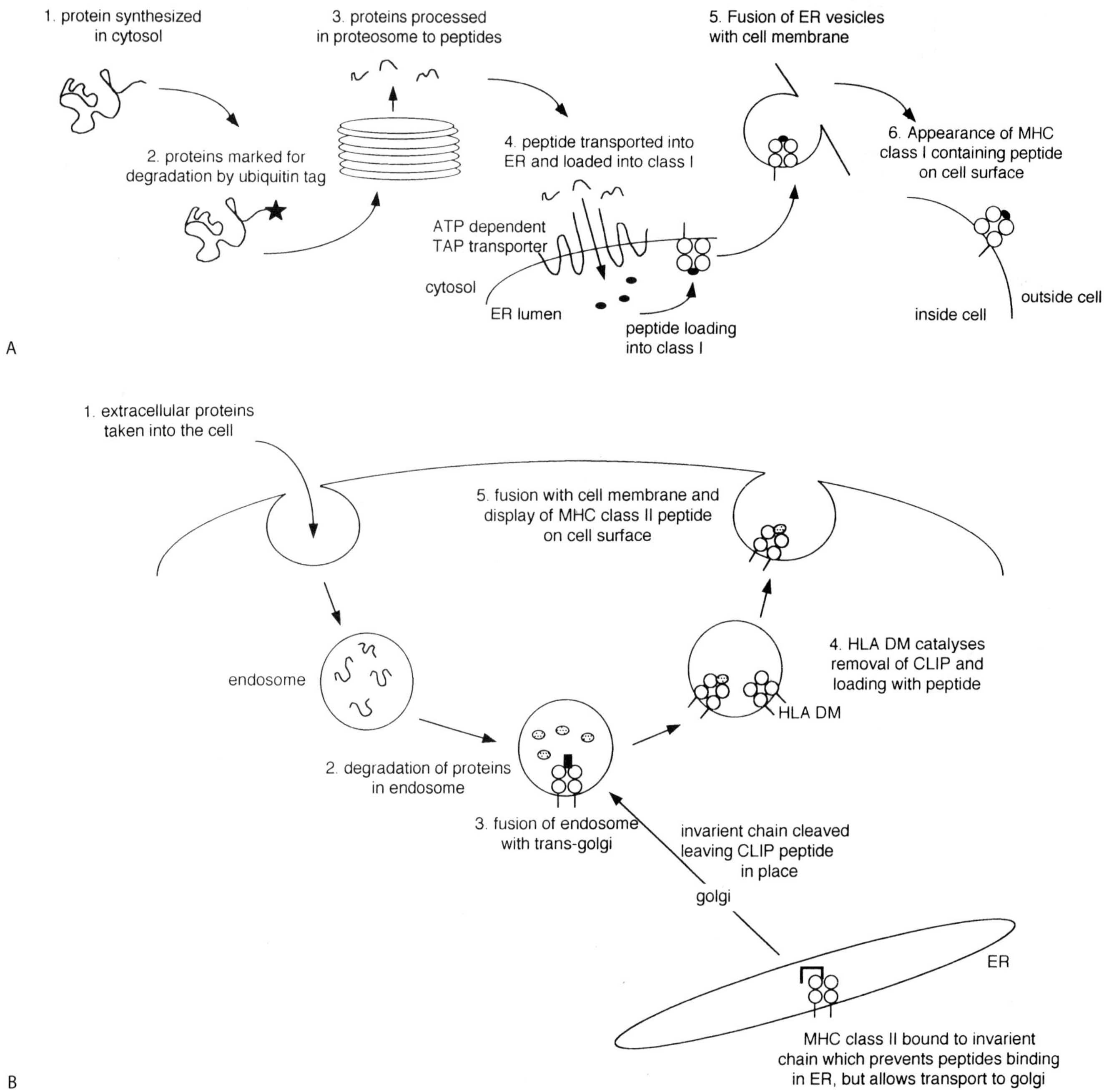

FIGURE 2.3. *Antigen processing and presentation. A simplified version of processing and presentation of proteins in the class I (**A**) and class II (**B**) pathways. TAP, transporters associated with antigen processing; ER, endoplasmic reticulum; MHC, major histocompatibility complex; ATP, adenosine triphosphate; CLIP, class II–associated invariant chain peptide.*

may be derived from the MHC proteins themselves. It is only when a foreign pathogen—or a graft—appears on the scene that the MHC proteins become loaded with foreign peptides. Several proteins encoded within the MHC aid the assembly and loading of class I and II proteins with their peptides.

One type of class II protein, HLA-DM, does not appear on the cell surface but rather plays a role in delivering peptides into other class II proteins before they emigrate to the cell surface (24). The LMP (proteosome components) and TAP (transporters associated with antigen processing) genes also lie within the class II gene region of the MHC. They are involved in the processing (LMP) and loading (TAP) of peptides for class I presentation. Two of the most important advances in immunology over the last decade have been our increased understanding of such antigen processing and presentation pathways (25–31), and our knowledge of the structural resolution of MHC and TCR proteins (32–34).

Mice with disrupted expression of either class II genes (as in class II–/– mice) or β_2-microglobulin (in which surface expression of the whole class I protein is prevented, as in class I–/– mice) have been generated and used as either donor or recipient in transplantation experiments. The literature regarding this work is complex. In many studies, a lack of class I or class II antigens alone on donor tissue had little effect on graft survival (35–39). However other experiments suggested graft survival may be prolonged or permanent when donor tissue lacks either class I (39,40) or class II only (39,41), or lacks both class I and II antigens (35,41,42). Clearly, results vary when different types of grafts are used, probably reflecting a greater or lesser involvement of either $CD4^+$ or $CD8^+$ cells (39,41). However, the interpretation of some of these apparently straightforward experiments is complicated by the suggestion that grafts from class I–/– mice may be reconstituted in their expression of class I by serum β_2-microglobulin in the recipient or may express residual cell surface class I protein in the absence of β_2-microglobulin (36,43).

The class III region of the MHC is large and contains many uncharacterized genes (16). Those genes that have been characterized encode proteins with a variety of different functions. Although they do not stimulate T cells in the same way as do class I and II proteins, many have important activities in generating and influencing immunity. Tumor necrosis factor (TNF)-α and TNF-β, for example, are both encoded in the class III region, and a marker of TNF-α polymorphism associated with high TNF production has been found in heart transplant patients (44).

The very high degree of polymorphism in the class I and II antigens that the MHC encodes is the one notable feature that makes it unlike any other region of the genome, and it is this feature that creates serious problems for the transplant clinician. The extensive polymorphism likely evolved as a product of immune defense mechanisms against infection (15). Species having very limited polymorphism at either class I or class II loci can be devastated by infections that do not present a problem in closely related species with a polymorphic MHC (45). For transplantation purposes, the practical consequence of MHC polymorphism is that MHC-identical donors and recipients are extremely uncommon among unrelated individuals (see Chapter 4). Even when MHC-identical donors are found, the minor histocompatibility antigens are almost undoubtedly different. The only clinically realistic tissue graft involving MHC- and minor histocompatibility–identical antigens is between monozygotic twins. Thus, immunosuppression is routinely needed in clinical transplantation, and acute or chronic rejection still occurs in many patients.

Minor Histocompatibility Antigens

The nature of minor histocompatibility antigens was for many years elusive, although it was clear from genetic studies that many different loci could encode such proteins. Investigators knew T cells could recognize and respond to cells from MHC-identical individuals, but because raising antibodies against the antigens involved was almost impossible, biochemical characterization was very difficult. The knowledge that T cells recognize small peptides from antigens, together with the resourceful application of molecular techniques, has allowed the recent characterization of the prototypic minor histocompatibility antigen, the male antigen or H-Y (46,47). From such work, it is now clear not only that minor histocompatibility antigens are a composite of peptides from low- or non-polymorphic proteins presented in the MHC groove, but also that the so-called H-Y antigen is derived from a group of proteins encoded on the Y chromosome (46–49). The former finding explains why it has been difficult to raise antibodies to minor antigens, because normally antibodies recognize conformational determinants on proteins.

Migration of Passenger Leukocytes from the Organ into Recipient Lymphoid Organs

Isolated MHC proteins or minor histocompatibility antigens can have a surprisingly low level of immunogenicity, but they may be highly immunogenic when found as integrated cell surface proteins. The level of immunogenicity varies considerably with the cell type on which they are found. Researchers have found that cells with the characteristics of bone marrow–derived leukocytes are located throughout the body, in nonlymphoid as well as in lymphoid tissues (50). The nonlymphoid "passenger leukocytes" migrate rapidly out of a tissue following transplantation to the recipient lymphoid organs, where they are able to interact with and stimulate the host immune response (51,52). Such passenger leukocytes have the characteristics of immature dendritic cells (53), which on migration rapidly mature into antigen-presenting cells (APCs) that are particularly potent in their ability to stimulate T cells (54–56). Mature dendritic cells express a high level of both MHC class I and II antigens, and thus are able to stimulate both $CD4^+$ and $CD8^+$ cells. Dendritic cells also have a number of additional features that make them uniquely powerful in stimulating naive (previously unactivated) T cells, earning them the title of "professional" antigen-presenting cells.

Passenger leukocytes certainly can provide an important stimulus for graft rejection. In some instances, their removal from the graft prior to transplantation can prolong the graft's survival (57–59). This is not, however, always the case, which suggests that there is a second route to sensitization of the recipient. It has become clear that dendritic cells can present foreign, graft-derived antigens to the recipient immune system, by either direct or indirect antigen presentation (Fig. 2.4).

Direct Antigen Presentation

Following migration of graft-derived dendritic cells into the recipient lymphoid tissue, they may directly stimulate T cells

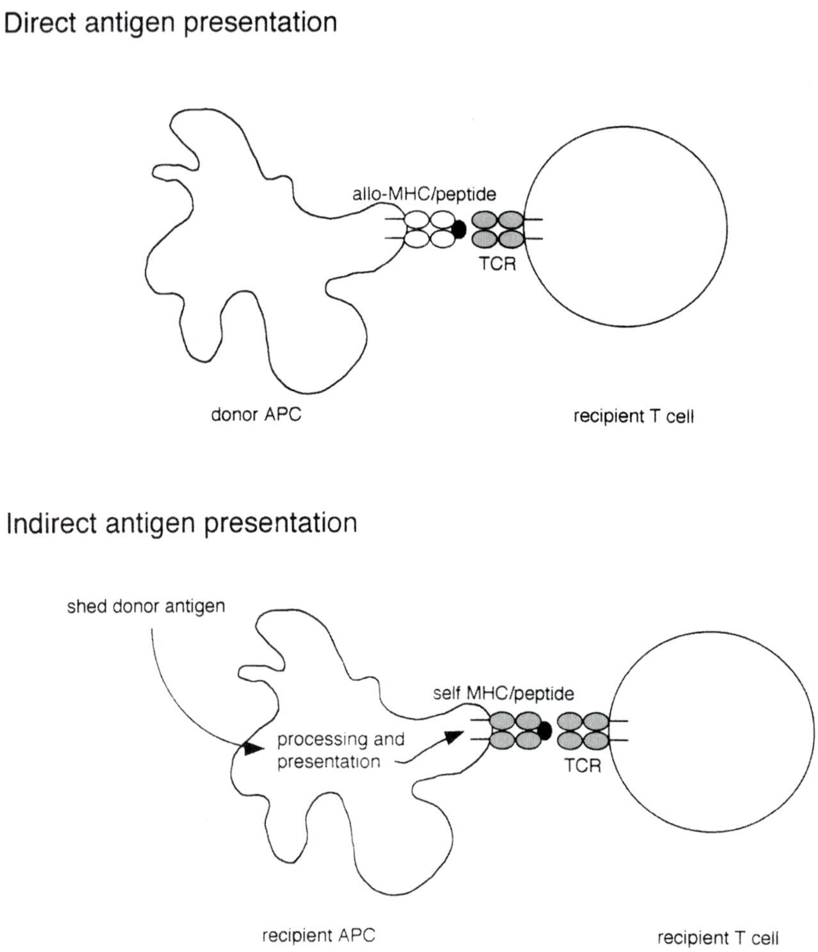

FIGURE 2.4. *Direct and indirect antigen presentation. Methods of sensitization of the recipient by either donor or recipient dendritic cells. APC, antigen-presenting cell; MHC, major histocompatibility complex; TCR, T-cell receptor.*

of the host. This may initially seem surprising if one considers that the T-cell repertoire is skewed toward recognition of peptide in the context of self MHC proteins. However, experiments have shown that allogeneic MHC/peptide complexes provide an extremely strong stimulus to the immune system. A very high frequency of all T cells, up to 1% to 10%, respond to any allogeneic MHC.

As described above, the allogeneic MHC will contain peptides derived from the donor tissue originating mainly from normal nonpolymorphic proteins (60) or the MHC itself (61,62). In the context of self MHC, such peptides would not induce an immune response because the body would be tolerant of them. However, when the MHC is allogeneic (i.e., when a graft is placed into an MHC-disparate recipient) the sum of the MHC + nonpolymorphic peptide may now be recognized as not-self, thus stimulating T cells. The real job of such T cells is obviously not to respond to alloantigen, but to deal with invading organisms. Their ability to respond to alloantigen is thus due to a rather inconvenient cross-reactivity of their receptor for self MHC + foreign peptide with allo-MHC + self peptide. With many T cells that have perfectly respectable reactivity for a foreign peptide + self MHC, cross-reactivity on one or more alloantigens can be demonstrated.

In addition, different peptides may be displayed by the foreign and self MHC proteins due to the different peptide-binding capacities of each MHC groove. Those peptides not normally displayed in self MHC will not have had an opportunity to induce tolerance in the recipient and thus may induce an immune response when presented on allo-MHC proteins. Alloreactive cytotoxic T lymphocytes (CTLs) induced by direct antigen presentation are able to recognize a wide spectrum of different peptide–MHC aggregates and even empty MHC molecules, as elegantly demonstrated by Rotzshe et al (60).

The most likely explanation for the unusually high number of T cells that react to any given allo-MHC is that a very large number of different self peptides are derived from the graft. The combination of these with the allogeneic MHC stimulate a very large number of different T-cell clones in the recipient (63).

Indirect Antigen Presentation

Evidence suggests that allogeneic MHC antigens can be processed in precisely the same way as any other foreign antigen and can be presented in association with self MHC on self antigen–presenting cells (61,64–68). From what we understand about antigen processing and presentation, it seems likely that the majority of allogeneic MHC peptides will be presented in the context of class II MHC antigens, as this is the pathway that deals with proteins exogenous to the cell. There is, however, some crossover between class II and class I pathways such that allogeneic MHC peptides may also be presented in the context of self class I antigens (69,70).

The experiments of Fabre and colleagues (67) suggest that indirect presentation may have a practical significance in transplantation responses. They demonstrated that peptides derived from rat class I antigens are able to immunize animals via the indirect pathway for accelerated rejection of a subsequent skin graft carrying the class I antigens from which the peptides were derived. Further information on this issue was provided by experiments in which skin grafts from class II−/− mice were transplanted to normal mice. APCs from these grafts did not directly stimulate $CD4^+$ cells due to the absence of class II antigen, yet graft rejection still occurred, and importantly was $CD4^+$-cell dependent. In the latter case, the $CD4^+$ cells are presumed to have been stimulated by indirect presentation of donor alloantigens on self MHC (37,43,71).

Despite these compelling data, the actual importance of this pathway in primary acute graft rejection by normal animals remains somewhat obscure. In the view of some researchers, however, indirect antigen presentation not only plays a dominant role in acute rejection (72) but also provides the continued antigenic stimulus required for chronic graft rejection (73).

Entry of Naive Recipient Lymphocytes into Graft Tissue

Dendritic cells can migrate out of a transplant into the local lymphoid tissue to stimulate an immune response, but naive recipient-derived leukocytes can also migrate into the graft. This is particularly obvious following small bowel transplantation, when recipient-derived leukocytes, including T lymphocytes, migrate into the mesenteric lymph nodes and Peyer's patches of the graft, generating a cytokine response within 24 hours of grafting (74–76). Such cells may become activated via direct antigen presentation, as the gut-associated lymphoid tissue will be rich in mature dendritic cells. With other types of transplant, however, the extent to which naive T cells enter and become activated in situ is less clear. Although all tissues contain dendritic cells (as described above), in general they are immature and lack the full stimulatory capacity of lymphoid dendritic cells.

A number of researchers have suggested that the vascular endothelium of the graft may provide another source of stimulation to the host immune system (77,78). Indeed, this is the first part of the donor tissue that the recipient's leukocytes will come in contact with. Studies using cell culture systems have demonstrated that vascular endothelial cells, devoid of dendritic cells, are able to cause marked proliferation of allogeneic lymphocytes and induce the differentiation of cytotoxic effector cells. Human endothelial cells constitutively express MHC class II antigens, whereas rodent endothelium does not, suggesting that the route of recipient sensitization may be more active or important in humans than in rodents. The ability of endothelial cells to stimulate truly naive T cells remains somewhat controversial, particularly because they appear to lack some cell surface proteins that may be critical in T-cell activation (79,80).

Activation of Recipient T Cells

Following the discovery that lymphocytes could be subdivided into two major populations, the T and B cells, it became clear that T cells were required for graft rejection in animals that previously had not been exposed to the donor antigens. Animals deprived of T cells either through genetic mutation or through experimental manipulation are unable to reject grafts (81–83).

Signals Through the T-Cell Receptor

Without an interaction of the TCR with its cognate antigen, T cells remain quiescent and can recirculate through the lymphoid tissues for many months or years (84,85). The majority of T cells bear a TCR comprised of two similar chains: α and β chains. These two chains are complexed with several more proteins of the CD3 complex, the γ, δ, ε, and ζ chains. The TCR binds to the peptide/MHC complex, while the ζ chains of the CD3 complex transduce signals of activation to the T cell (Fig. 2.5). A number of intracellular signaling pathways are activated, resulting in de novo expression of a range of genes, including those encoding cytokines and new cell surface proteins. These signaling pathways have been increasingly well characterized (86), and are now the target of some of our most potent immunosuppressive drugs (87,88) (see Chapter 11).

Second or Costimulatory Signals

Once in receipt of a TCR signal, the destiny of a T cell appears to depend critically on whether it secures other second or costimulatory signals. Without these second signals a T cell may become anergic or unresponsive (89–92), a state that may further enable it to inhibit the growth or activation of neighboring T cells in an antigen-specific fashion (93). Enormous interest has been attracted to studying how depriving the T cell of costimulation results in an unresponsive and even regulatory fate, because harnessing and applying this mechanism could be of major use in preventing graft rejection (see Chapter 13).

Many cell surface proteins on a T cell could potentially contribute to its activation (see Fig. 2.5). The CD4 and CD8 proteins act by binding to class II and class I, respectively, on the APC and are linked to intracellular proteins that are involved in transducing further signals to the T cell. A series of additional proteins on the T-cell surface, such as CD54, CD2, CD11a/CD18, and CD5, act to increase the overall avidity of interaction between the T cell and its APC and may also transduce further signals to the T cell.

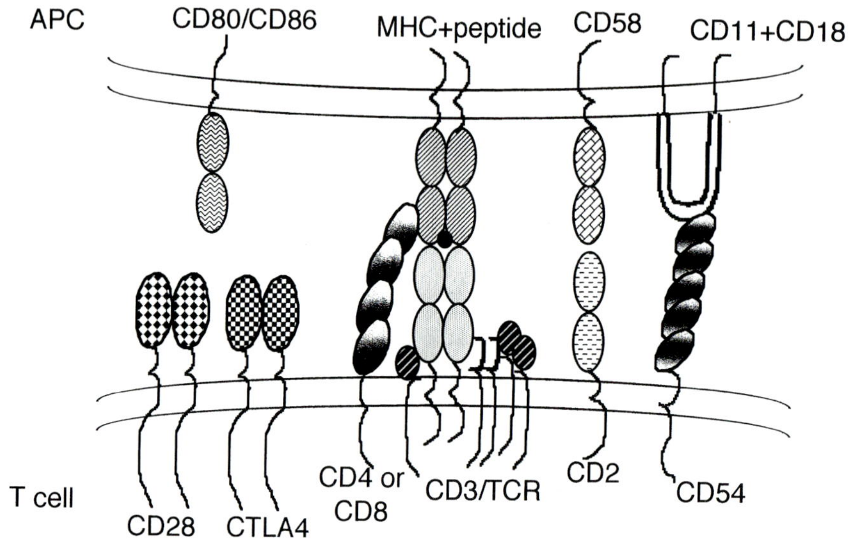

FIGURE 2.5. *Cell surface proteins involved in T-cell activation. Receptors on the T cell are shown with their ligands on the antigen-presenting cell.*

Recently, interest in the area of costimulation for CD4$^+$ T cells has focused on the role of the CD28 pathway (94–97). CD28 is a homodimeric glycoprotein on the surface of T cells that interacts with two counter-receptors, CD80 and CD86, which may be expressed on the surface of APCs. CD80 and CD86 are very similar in structure, although they are not similar at the sequence level. They show different patterns of expression and bind with distinct affinities to CD28 (98–101). CD86, expressed constitutively at a low level by professional APCs (such as dendritic cells) and upregulated rapidly following interaction with the T cell, has a rather low affinity for CD28. CD80 is expressed with slower kinetics and only following interaction of an APC with the T cell. It is expressed at a lower level than CD86, but has a greater binding affinity for CD28 than does CD86. The result of ligation of CD28 by either CD86 or CD80 appears to be increased cytokine synthesis and proliferation following signals through as yet incompletely defined intracellular pathways (102–105). The reason for the apparent redundancy in expression of the costimulatory proteins CD80 and CD86 is as yet unknown, but it is likely (there is some evidence, discussed below) that they may have subtly different roles in the development and resolution of immune responses.

An additional protein, CTLA4 (CD152), is expressed by T cells following activation. Although it is structurally related to CD28, it appears to be critically involved in resolving T-cell responses (106,107). CTLA4 also binds to both CD80 and CD86, not only showing a higher affinity for CD80 than CD86, but also a higher affinity for both than does CD28.

A further complication of this system is that T cells express not only CD28 and CTLA4, but also CD80 and CD86. The role of T-cell CD80 and CD86 is undefined. Clearly, the integration of signals resulting from all of these interactions is complex and as yet poorly understood (97).

The requirement of CD28 signals for CD8$^+$ cells or antigen-primed CD4$^+$ T cells is also unclear. The prevailing view for CD4$^+$ cells is that if they have not recently been stimulated by antigen (i.e., they have developed into memory cells), they will require costimulation for reactivation. Experimentally it has been shown that in certain situations virus-reactive CD8$^+$ cells require neither costimulation through CD28 nor CD28-dependent help (108,109). However, overstimulation of the TCR may occur under these conditions (provided, for instance, by a replicating virus), a situation that may infrequently occur during other immune responses. Even CD4$^+$ cells may lose their requirement for CD28-mediated costimulation in the face of overwhelming TCR signaling. This is suggested by the fact that mice with a disrupted CD28 gene make impaired immune responses, yet can reject skin grafts, albeit in a delayed fashion (110). Nevertheless, blocking this pathway in normal animals may have dramatic effects on the generation of immune responses and may result in prolonged graft survival or even tolerance of grafts (111–113). The potential for blocking this route of immunity in the treatment of transplant patients is as yet unexplored but remains exciting (see also Chapter 13).

Upon activation, T cells express another cell surface protein, gp39 (CD40 ligand). Interaction of this protein with its counter-receptor, CD40, appears to be critical for the activation of B cells, dendritic cells, and monocytes. It may result in the upregulation of CD80 and CD86 on these cells. In an interesting report, Larsen and colleagues (114) showed that blocking the gp39 protein could prolong graft survival in a mouse cardiac transplant model. Even more impressive, however, are more recent data from this group showing that preventing both CD28 and gp39 interactions can induce permanent survival of an allogeneic skin graft in mice with no long-term deterioration of graft integrity (115). Curiously, tolerance to the graft antigens could not be demonstrated in these mice, despite the excellent survival of the transplant itself. This approach has now been extended to nonhuman primate models (116).

In addition to this large number of cell–cell based interactions, T cells receive important signals through the binding of soluble proteins, the cytokines, to specific cell surface cytokine receptors. Through upregulating the expression of receptors for other cytokines, cytokines derived primarily from macrophages, such as IL-1 and IL-12, seem to sensitize T cells to the proliferative and differentiative effects of the (primarily) T-cell–derived cytokines, such as IL-2 and IL-4. A whole cascade of cytokines is produced that amplifies both immune and inflammatory processes following transplantation (reviewed extensively in 117–120; see also below).

GENERATION OF DIFFERENT TYPES OF IMMUNITY

$CD4^+$ and $CD8^+$ Cells

A fundamental aspect of immunity is the initiation of the response by an interaction of the "helper" T cell with an APC. In most cases, such cells bear the CD4 surface protein. However, in certain situations $CD8^+$ cells are able to respond in the absence of $CD4^+$ cells and meet all the requirements of a helper T cell. Once activated, helper T cells recruit and activate other leukocytes, inducing their differentiation into effector cells. That $CD4^+$ cells are frequently required to initiate graft rejection has been shown by many workers in a variety of experimental systems (17,121–124), although depending on the mismatch between donor and recipient, $CD8^+$ cells also may be required or may act independently of $CD4^+$ cells (125–129).

Most recent work on the effects of $CD4^+$ and $CD8^+$ cells in transplantation responses has involved the use of mice deprived of these populations through genetic manipulation. Mice lacking class I or II antigens are severely depleted of $CD8^+$ or $CD4^+$ cells, respectively, as are those mice in which either the CD4 or the CD8 gene has been disrupted (35,38,130–135). The effects on graft rejection of a lack of CD4 or CD8 cells produced in this manner have not been predictable and depend often on the nature of the mismatch between donor and recipient. Further, despite an apparent depletion of $CD8^+$ cells in class I–/– mice, $CD8^+$ CTLs can be generated in large numbers following transplantation and may be involved in the rejection process (71,131,132).

It is probably fair to say that results from the use of knockout mice have not altered our ideas about the roles of these two T-cell subsets in initiating graft rejection. Normally, $CD4^+$ cells seem to play a central part in directing graft rejection, but there are clearly experimental situations (usually when there is a dominant or sole MHC class I mismatch) in which $CD8^+$ cells are also required for rejection to proceed with normal kinetics or act independently of the $CD4^+$ cell.

T1- and T2-Driven Immunity

Following stimulation of the immune system, a response develops in which either humoral or cell-mediated immunity may be seen to dominate (136,137), and cytokines play an important role in determining which type of immunity emerges (138–142; Fig. 2.6). During the early stages of an immune response, T cells will make a wide range of cytokines. Any obvious divergence of cytokine production can be observed only following continued antigenic stimulation. The T1/T2 model is used to describe this phenomenon, although some researchers feel that the T1/T2 paradigm has oversimplified our view of the immune response (143).

The hallmark cytokine of T1 cells is interferon (IFN)-γ. A predominance of this population results in the appearance of cell-mediated immunity involving the generation of both specific CTLs and activated macrophages. T2 cells, on the other hand, make cytokines such as IL-4, IL-5, and IL-6

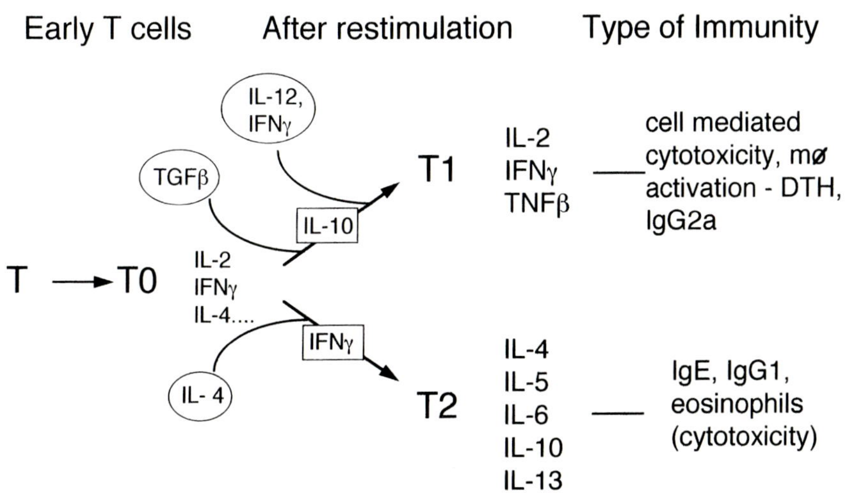

FIGURE 2.6. *T1/T2 cell differentiation and immunity. Cytokines produced at various stages during the evolution of immune responses are shown. Cytokines that positively or negatively influence the divergence of T1 and T2 cells are shown in circles and squares, respectively. DTH, delayed-type hypersensitivity; mø, macrophage.*

that are critical for the induction of humoral immunity (and, in particular, selected immunoglobulin isotypes) and eosinophilia. Recently, it has become apparent that both $CD4^+$ and $CD8^+$ cells can produce these distinct patterns of cytokines.

Exactly how a T1- or T2-dominated response is determined is uncertain, but the local cytokine milieu (144–140), the involvement of APCs other than dendritic cells (150,151), and the type of CD28 signal delivered (i.e., either through CD80 or CD86) (152–155) have been suggested as important factors.

With regard to transplantation responses, particular interest has focused on the possibility that, while a T1-driven response may inevitably be damaging and result in graft rejection, a T2-driven response may not have this effect and may be associated with the induction of tolerance to a graft (118–120,156). A number of studies have found that tolerance or reduced donor-directed reactivity is associated with a decrease in expression of the T1-associated cytokines IL-2 and IFN-γ (157–162). This decrease may be accompanied by (or even due to) the expansion of regulatory T2 cells, and some evidence suggests that the expression of cytokines such as IL-4, IL-5, and IL-10 is preserved during the development of tolerance (161,163,164). However, cells other than T2 cells can produce these cytokines, so their detection does not necessarily infer the presence or action of the T2 population (see also Chapter 5). As discussed in the following sections, an immune response to a transplant is complex. Both humoral and cellular mechanisms can affect graft destruction. Therefore, it is likely that any type of immunity, be it T1 or T2 driven, would result in graft rejection. Rather than prolonged graft survival, a complete shutdown of T-cell cytokine production is frequently observed in models of true tolerance (112,165).

Several groups have tried to assess the role of key cytokines by performing experiments in which the cytokines' overexpression or absence is tested. Using IL-4 knockout mice, two studies have now shown that tolerance can be induced using reagents that block CD28 signaling in the absence of IL-4 (166,167). A very important additional finding from these studies is that tolerance was easier to induce in homozygous −/− mice than in heterozygous IL-4 +/− mice (166). The implication is that the presence of IL-4 itself can be damaging to the graft. Other experiments with knockout mice have shown that neither IL-2 nor IFN-γ is required for rejection (120,168–170). Interpretation of such experiments is complicated because cytokines can often substitute for one another, and therefore whether the phenotype of these mice accurately reflects the importance of these cytokines in normal mice is not clear. For instance, IL-15 can substitute many of the actions of IL-2, and IL-13 can substitute for IL-4. In the experiments described above, IL-15 transcripts were found in grafts put into the IL-2 knockout mice, and IL-13 transcripts were found in those transplanted into IL-4 knockout mice. Thus, the results of these experiments do not address the relative involvement of T1 and T2 cells in rejection and tolerance, but rather look only at the effects of removing single cytokines.

Several experimental studies have tried an alternative approach to this problem: cytokines have been injected or overexpressed in animal transplant models in an attempt to deviate the immune system toward a T1 or T2 response. Injection of IL-2 or IFN-γ can prevent the induction of tolerance (157,159). However, injection or overexpression of IL-4 cannot induce tolerance (171). In fact, while this treatment may marginally prolong graft survival (Dallman et al, unpublished data, 1994), it may actually inhibit tolerance induction (166).

The most plausible conclusion from all of these studies is that immunity driven by either T1 or T2 cells is damaging, although in some cases immunity driven by T2 cells may be less damaging than T1-driven immunity.

MIGRATION OF ACTIVATED LEUKOCYTES INTO THE GRAFT

To enter any site of inflammation or immune response, leukocytes must migrate across the vascular endothelium. This migration process is controlled by the elaboration of cell attractants or chemokines and by cell–cell interactions between the leukocyte and the endothelium.

Cell–Cell Interactions

The adhesion of leukocytes to the endothelium is a complex, multistep process that involves a series of interactions between the surface of the leukocyte and the endothelial cell or its extracellular matrix (85,172). The proteins involved fall into three groups: the selectins, and members of the integrin and immunoglobulin (Ig) superfamilies. Initial interaction and rolling of leukocytes along the endothelium allow the leukocyte to sample the endothelial environment while maintaining its ability to detach and travel somewhere else. This step is largely controlled by the selectins, although α_4 integrins may also play a role at this stage. Under the correct conditions, this interaction will lead to signaling to the leukocyte, thereby slowing down and arresting the rolling process and allowing extravasation. These latter stages are regulated mainly by the integrins and adhesion proteins of the Ig superfamily.

The expression of many adhesion proteins involved in these interactions is upregulated by proinflammatory cytokines. Ischemic damage alone results in increased expression of several cytokines, including IL-1, which upregulates the expression of members of the selectin family (173,174). Other adhesion proteins, such as ICAM 1 and VCAM 1 of the Ig superfamily and E-selectin (endothelial-specific selectin), are known to be upregulated by the type of cytokines induced following the trauma of transplantation. Thus, even before an immune response has been generated, the graft becomes attractive to circulating leukocytes, although naive lymphocytes tend not to home in to nonlymphoid sites. Antigen-activated lymphocytes, however, have an altered recirculation pattern and are perfectly happy to migrate into extra-lymphoid sites (175–177). They may show tissue-selective homing and show preference for sites where they are most likely to reencounter their specific antigen.

In terms of transplantation, one practical aspect of this process is that it may be possible to block the proteins involved in leukocyte extravasation, thereby slowing or preventing the rejection process (see Chapter 13). Blocking these adhesion pathways either by antibodies or by inhibiting their expression has been attempted in both experimental and clinical transplantation (178–181). In general, cocktails of antibodies have a greater beneficial effect than do single antibodies (182,183), although the results are variable and in one case a combination of antibodies to ICAM-1 and LFA-1 was shown to result in accelerated rejection of rat cardiac allografts (184).

Chemokines

A large number of chemokines have been identified, including RANTES, IL-8, and MCP-1 (185,186), which are involved in the attraction of T cells; eosinophils, neutrophils, and basophils; and monocytes, respectively. The initial excitement surrounding the involvement of chemokines in extravasation of leukocytes now has been tempered somewhat by the finding that chemokine receptors are expressed at low levels by resting leukocytes (187). However, in certain situations they appear to play an important role in the development of graft infiltrates (188).

DESTRUCTION OF THE GRAFT

The immune system generates a wide variety of effector mechanisms, depending on the challenge it meets. In certain infections a single mechanism appears to be essential in the clearance of the organism, and the absence of that mechanism renders the host susceptible to disease. For example, in the clearance of lymphatic choriomeningitis (LCMV) infections in mice, cytotoxic cells are absolutely required, so disabling this arm of immunity by disrupting the perforin gene leads to death in infected animals (189). Unfortunately, most of the known effector mechanisms of the immune system seem to be capable of damaging a graft such that the absence of any one effector mechanism has little beneficial effect on graft survival. This is most likely to be the reason that it is so difficult to prevent graft rejection without disabling the central components of the immune system. We will discuss the various effector systems that can damage tissue, along with their role in hyperacute, acute, and chronic rejection.

Antibody

Antibody may cause tissue damage not only through the fixation of complement, but also through the activity of K cells in antibody-dependent cellular cytotoxicity (ADCC). In the latter case, the antibody acts as a bridge between the target tissue and the effector cell, activating the lytic machinery of the K cell and thus damaging the tissue (190). Many different leukocytes appear to be able to express K-cell activity, but although ADCC activity may be recovered from grafts (191), its role in graft rejection is not firmly established.

Patients previously exposed to MHC antigens through transplant, blood transfusions, or pregnancy often develop antibodies reactive with those MHC antigens. Such preformed antibodies can undoubtedly cause hyperacute rejection, where the organ fails immediately following revascularization (192–195). Rejection is accompanied by deposition of antibody and complement and accumulation of polymorphonuclear leukocytes within the graft (193). Hyperacute rejection is now preempted through the use of pretransplant screening by a crossmatch test for antibodies directed toward donor antigens (see Chapter 4). However, the conventional crossmatch test detects not only harmful MHC-directed cytotoxic antibodies, but also harmless autoantibodies (196,197). In most cases it is now possible to distinguish autoreactive from alloreactive antibodies, and thus it has become possible to transplant an increasing number of patients across an apparently positive crossmatch in whom the reactivity is due to autoantibodies.

For some highly sensitized patients, finding a suitable (crossmatch-negative) donor remains quite problematic. Strategies designed to reduce reactivity include intravenous gammaglobulin (IVIG) infusion alone (198) or coupled with cyclophosphamide (199). Therapy with high-dose IVIG after transplantation has also reportedly controlled humoral rejection in renal and cardiac transplant recipients (200).

Of interest is that liver transplantation appears to be an exception to the rules regarding transplantation across a positive crossmatch. Liver transplants are carried out with little regard to the immune system and are performed successfully not only across positive crossmatches but also with little or no attempt at MHC matching the donor and recipient (see Chapter 19). The reasons for the refractoriness to immune rejection displayed by liver grafts are not fully understood. In part, the size and enormous capacity for regeneration displayed by the liver may be responsible. However, the immune response to liver transplants also differs from that to other grafts, with spontaneous tolerance developing in several rat and all mouse strain combinations. An understanding of this phenomenon may help us design new strategies for tolerance induction (201–204).

Many of the changes associated with acute rejection, such as arteriolar thrombosis, interstitial hemorrhage, and fibrinoid necrosis of the arteriolar walls, may result from the deposition of antibody and fixation of complement (205). However, the appearance of donor-specific antibody does not necessarily accompany graft rejection, and its presence may be compatible with unimpaired graft function (206,207). On the other hand, in at least one experimental model in which donor and recipient rats differ only at

MHC class I loci, acute rejection of kidney grafts associates with and can be initiated by donor-specific antibody (208).

Donor-specific antibodies may also be found in the circulation, and immunoglobulin deposits may be seen in vessel walls during chronic rejection (see Chapter 3), but it is not clear whether or how the presence of such antibodies may be causally related to graft dysfunction (209).

An area of increasing interest is *xenotransplantation,* in which the use of animal donors is being considered for human transplantation (see Chapter 40). There are certainly many problems associated with this approach. For example, humans possess circulating antibodies that react with the cells of many animal species including those of the pig, which currently is the animal of choice as a donor in xenotransplantation. These antibodies show a predominant reactivity to sugars on cell surface proteins, which due to the activity of the α-1,3-galactosyltransferase gene are present in pigs (and in many other species) but not in humans (210–214). Such "natural antibodies" result in hyperacute rejection of pig tissue by humans (215,216).

Cellular Mechanisms

The involvement of cell-mediated mechanisms is usually invoked in acute or chronic graft rejection. Although hyperacute rejection has almost always been attributed to antibody, in certain situations a very rapid rejection may occur even when the role of antibody has been excluded. In these situations, a cellular mechanism of rejection has been implicated (217).

Natural Killer Cells

Unlike cytotoxic T cells, described below, the natural killer (NK) cell apparently does not need to interact with antigen to become lytic to target cells, although it is clear that NK activity can be increased by certain cytokines. NK cells may be recovered from the blood or spleen and are able to lyse NK-sensitive targets, which tend to be of tumor origin (218). NK cells are clearly a potent source of cytotoxic activity, but their role in organ graft rejection remains to be established.

Several laboratories, using different experimental models, have found that grafts survive indefinitely in the presence of demonstrable NK effector activity (219–221). On the other hand, NK cells have quite clearly been shown to be involved in the rejection of bone marrow transplants (222,223) (see Chapter 27).

The method of target cell recognition employed by the NK cell is increasingly understood (224–226). Interaction with MHC on a target cell may actually result in the delivery of a negative signal to the NK cell, preventing the activation of its lytic machinery. Conversely, the absence of self class I MHC antigens may trigger the NK cell to attack its target, a finding consistent with the observation that NK cells are capable of rejecting bone marrow cells that express little or no class I antigen (227).

The Specific Cytotoxic T Cell

In cell culture systems, MHC-mismatched lymphocytes proliferate and produce cytokines in response to one another during the so-called mixed lymphocyte reaction (MLR). The resulting cytokine production allows the differentiation of CTLs that lyse target cells bearing the mismatched MHC antigens (228,229). Because a very powerful yet totally antigen-specific response is generated in such MLRs, the CTL has become the prime suspect as the central effector mechanism in graft destruction.

Considerable evidence suggests that CTLs may be involved in graft rejection. First, CTLs may be recovered from allografts that are undergoing rejection, but they are present only at low levels in grafts of animals that have been treated with cyclosporine to prevent rejection (219,220). Second, cloned populations of CTLs are capable of causing the type of tissue damage associated with rejection (230,231). Third, the great majority of class I MHC antigen–directed CTLs express the CD8 protein, and graft rejection may often be delayed in the absence of $CD8^+$ cells (124,125,232–234).

Conversely, graft destruction may occur in the absence of demonstrable CTL activity, and the presence of such cells within a graft may not always lead to graft destruction. The male-specific minor histocompatibility antigen H-Y was first detected in the rejection of male skin grafts by female mice of the same strain. Research using a variety of mouse strains found that although female mice often reject male skin, they do not always mount a detectable cytotoxic T-cell response. Further, in some strains of mice the females are able to generate H-Y–specific cytotoxic cells but do not reject male-derived skin grafts (235,236).

Other experiments have demonstrated the presence of cytotoxic effector cells within a graft that is not rejected (221,237). Rats given a donor-specific preoperative blood transfusion may retain a subsequent renal allograft indefinitely, yet cells extracted from such grafts show high and persistent donor-specific CTL activity. The simple conclusion from these studies is that CTLs cannot always reject grafts. At least two alternate possibilities must be considered: the action of these CTLs may be blocked in the graft itself, only being released to mediate their action on removal from the graft; or the activity of CTLs in cell culture does not accurately reflect their potential in the animal. These results remain intriguing, as they provide direct evidence of cytotoxic effector cells within an organ graft that is not ultimately rejected.

Cytotoxic T cells are able to kill their targets through the elaboration of perforins and granzymes, the activation of the Fas death pathway in the target cell, or the secretion of the cytokine TNF-α. Their involvement in graft rejection has also been questioned by the finding that mice deficient in perforin (perforin knockouts) are able to reject tumor (238), skin (239), and organ (240) grafts, even when the grafts are resistant to Fas-mediated and TNF-α–mediated killing (238). However, in the experiments of Schulz et al

(240), grafts mismatched only at the class I MHC are rejected more slowly in perforin knockout mice, indicating that at least for these grafts, cytotoxic cells play an important role in rejection.

Even if CTLs themselves do not mediate the tissue damage that ultimately results in graft loss, they may still be important in the immune response to the graft. Through the elaboration of high levels of IFN-γ they are able to recruit and activate cells involved in delayed-type hypersensitivity (DTH) lesions, thus initiating acute or chronic rejection.

Macrophages and DTH Reactions

T cells initiate a DTH reaction (241), which involves an essentially nonspecific effector phase [as described by Koch in 1891 in the tuberculin skin reaction (242)] that is characterized by an infiltrate of lymphocytes and cells of the monocyte–macrophage lineage. Damage occurs in a tissue during a DTH reaction due to the elaboration of various noxious substances, including reactive nitrogen, oxygen intermediates, and TNF-α, by the macrophage. Since macrophages themselves do not carry antigen receptors, the specificity of rejection when it is mediated by macrophages must rely on activity of the T cell. This means that the effector step in graft destruction would not itself be antigen-specific—a suggestion difficult to reconcile with data indicating that graft damage may on occasion be incredibly specific (243–245). In other situations, however, tissue destruction can be rather nonspecific, suggesting again that the circumstance of the graft may determine the effector mechanism involved in its destruction.

Support for the role of DTH reactions in graft rejection comes from the studies on rejection of H-Y–disparate grafts. Although cytotoxic cell responses do not always correlate with graft rejection, the generation of DTH reactions to H-Y antigens follows closely the ability of female mice to reject male skin (246). In addition, irradiated rats reconstituted with CD4 cells can reject heart grafts without developing a detectable specific cytotoxic cell response within the transplant (124).

The high level of inflammatory mediators and the type of changes within grafts undergoing chronic rejection suggest a role for activated macrophages in this process (247–250). Cytokines like IL-1, TNF-α, transforming growth factor beta (TGFβ), and platelet-derived growth factor (PDGF) lead to smooth muscle proliferation, and TGFβ and PDGF result in an increased synthesis of extracellular matrix proteins. These cytokines are products of activated macrophages and may result in the atherosclerotic and fibrotic changes associated with chronic graft failure.

In summary, there is evidence for and against the involvement of the specific CTL and DTH effector mechanisms in graft rejection. Several studies have suggested that a specifically activated effector T-cell population, through the elaboration of cytokines like IFN-γ, may recruit cells to mediate tissue destruction through nonspecific or DTH mechanisms (245,251). It seems likely that neither mechanism is unique in its ability to cause acute graft rejection. Frequently both are involved, but in the absence of one mechanism, the other may develop and cause graft rejection.

Cytokines

Undoubtedly, the primary role of cytokines in an immune response to a graft is to initiate the proliferation, differentiation, and homing of leukocytes in the generation of immunity. However, certain cytokines may also directly damage tissue. As described above, TNF-α produced by CTL cells and macrophages may damage a graft. Blocking the effects of TNF by using neutralizing antibodies can prolong organ graft survival (252–254), but the rather minimal effects of these antibodies suggest that TNF may not contribute centrally to graft rejection. Islets appear to be particularly susceptible to damage mediated by proinflammatory cytokines such that these may be a more important component in the rejection of islet transplants (255–258).

Target Cells of Destructive Immunity

Damage to the vascular endothelium, which may express both class I and class II MHC antigens, is likely to result in rapid cell necrosis and graft loss (259). The predominantly vascular changes that occur during rejection of an organ graft suggest that this is the case (260–262). The parenchymal cells may also be targets for tissue destruction, but this is more likely to be secondary to the initial attack on endothelium. The increase in expression of both class I and class II MHC antigens following transplantation might increase the susceptibility of both endothelium and parenchymal cells to destruction. The marked arterial changes seen as a manifestation of both acute and chronic rejection also suggest the importance of the endothelium as the main target of the response. In the case of chronic rejection, the fibrotic changes seen histologically might well be due to ischemia resulting from gradual vascular obliteration (see Chapter 3).

CONCLUSIONS

The immune response to a transplant is complex. Virtually every cell involved in immunity has been implicated in graft rejection, depending on factors such as donor–recipient incompatibility, the type of graft, or the type of immunosuppression. Thus, providing immunosuppression that is adequate to prevent graft rejection without disabling the immune system at a central point is difficult. The unfortunate consequence is that our patients become susceptible to infection and are at increased risk of cancer. The only true solution to our problem is the development of strategies to induce donor-specific tolerance in the recipient. This is straightforward in rodent studies but remains elusive in humans.

COMMENTARY

Leendert C. Paul

Dallman provides an erudite overview on the increasingly complex subject of the immunobiology of graft rejection. Studies of tumor grafts in the early part of the 20th century led Gorer to formulate the concept of graft rejection: "Normal and neoplastic tissue contain isoantigenic factors which are genetically determined. Isoantigenic factors present in the grafted tissue and absent in the host are capable of eliciting a response which results in the destruction of the graft" (1). Subsequent studies by Medawar and colleagues at Oxford confirmed the immunologic basis of graft rejection (2). The availability of congenic lines of rodents differing at a desired polymorphic locus enabled researchers to establish the importance of major histocompatibility complex (MHC)-encoded antigens in acute rejection. We know now that MHC molecules serve as antigen-presenting molecules for various antigens, including foreign MHC peptides.

The classical dogma in immunology states that the immune system recognizes self from non-self and responds to non-self antigens. It has been difficult, however, to unambiguously define self and non-self, and compelling evidence has been presented to suggest that the immune system detects and protects against "danger." It responds to non-self antigens that constitute a threat to the survival of the host, such as invading infectious pathogens (3). According to this hypothesis, genetic disparities between an organ donor and a recipient result in acute rejection if the graft is damaged or "activated." Consistent with this hypothesis are clinical observations from the early 1980s suggesting that ischemic exposure of kidney transplants increases their immunogenicity. Transplants with prolonged ischemic exposure are more likely to experience acute rejection episodes compared with grafts with short ischemic exposure (see also Chapter 17). MHC matching seemed only beneficial in patients who had received a kidney graft exposed to prolonged ischemia (4). Subsequent experimental studies have shown that ischemia enhances the influx of antigen-presenting dendritic cells into the graft (5); enhances or induces the expression of MHC molecules and other cell surface molecules involved in immune reactivity, including cell adhesion molecules (6); and stimulates the release of a myriad of inflammatory mediators, including proinflammatory cytokines such as interleukin (IL)-1.

A large study of living-unrelated, parent-to-child, and cadaveric transplants has demonstrated that the 3-year graft survival rates of the living-unrelated and parent-to-child transplants were equal and were much better than those of cadaveric transplants (7). The superb and equal survival of the living-unrelated and parent-to-child transplants occurred despite the poor MHC matching of the living-unrelated transplants, which is again consistent with the hypothesis that ischemia increases the graft immunogenicity. Moreover, recent work in Tilney's laboratory in Boston has shown that brain death induces widespread expression of various cell adhesion molecules (personal communication). Thus, an organ graft from a brain-dead donor who was exposed to prolonged ischemia is more likely to undergo acute rejection via cytokine and cell adhesion molecule expression. Such a graft initiates a vicious circle in which damage induces a strong immune response, which in turn causes more damage and restimulation of the immune response.

Interaction of the T-cell receptor (TCR) with peptides displayed in the MHC groove of antigen-presenting cells, together with costimulation of the T lymphocyte through one or more costimulatory pathways, results in a tissue-destructive immune response. An absolute requirement for antigen-induced T-cell proliferation is activation of CD45, one of the most abundant leukocyte cell surface glycoproteins (8). CD45 is a phosphatase that acts on the Src family members of protein tyrosine kinases p56*lck* and p59*fyn*. Although the external domain of the molecule does not appear to be required for signal transduction by the TCR, monoclonal antibodies against the CD45RB isoform block signal transduction and prevent rejection in mouse models of acute kidney graft rejection (9).

Dallman discusses the importance of the CD28 and CD40 pathways of costimulation. The CD40L/CD40 pathway appears critical for the activation of B cells, dendritic cells, and monocytes. It has recently become evident, however, that nonhematopoietic cells also express the CD40 receptor, including endothelial cells, fibroblasts, and epithelial cells (10). In the kidney, CD40 is expressed on tubular epithelial cells, and CD40 activation on cultured proximal epithelial cells results in increased production of chemokines like IL-8, MCP-1, and RANTES (11). It is therefore tempting to speculate that tubular CD40/CD40L interactions contribute to the inflammation of acute kidney graft rejection.

The dominant paradigm in the area of T-cell regulation is the notion that cytokine-producing T cells can be classified in two major types: type 1 cells of CD4 or CD8 phenotype synthesize IL-2, interferon (IFN)-γ, and lymphotoxin-α; type 2 cells synthesize IL-4, IL-5, IL-6, IL-10, and IL-13; and both types synthesize IL-3, GM-CSF, and tumor necrosis factor (TNF)-α. The model proposes that signals received from antigen-presenting and bystander cells during T-cell activation direct the development of the T-cell cytokine response to either type 1 or 2 cytokines. The two sets of cytokine genes are reciprocally expressed in either type 1 or type 2 T cells, while within each set they are expressed independently of the others (12). The type 1 and type 2 cytokines in turn differentially regulate a wide variety of antigen-specific and nonspecific immune effector mechanisms.

It is widely accepted that type 1 helper T lymphocytes initiate allograft rejection by promoting the development of alloantigen-specific cytotoxic T lymphocytes (CTLs) and delayed-type hypersensitivity (DTH) responses. Since type 2 helper T cells (T_H2) are antagonistic to type 1 helper T-cell (T_H1) development and function, a popular hypothesis states that preferential induction of allograft-specific T_H2 would downregulate T_H1-driven rejection responses, thereby promoting allograft acceptance. However, many experiments have been presented that show T_H2 may be beneficial, deleterious, and/or irrelevant in the context of transplantation (13). These conflicting observations likely reflect variations in inductive strategies, the type of organ assessed, and whether the graft was immediately vascularized. Clearly, much more work needs to be done to define the role of type 2 cells in rejection.

Finally, various immune mechanisms such as antibodies, CTLs, and cytotoxic cytokines may destroy an allograft. As discussed, cytotoxic T cells may kill their targets through the elaboration of perforins and granzymes, through activation of the Fas death pathway in the target cell, or through the secretion of the cytokine TNF-α. However, the exact mechanisms used in vivo appear to differ under different conditions. More than 90% of cultured proximal tubular epithelial cells express the Fas receptor, suggesting that they are susceptible to Fas-mediated apoptosis. However, Fas ligation on these cells does not result in apoptosis, unless they are incubated with anti-Fas antibodies in combination with cycloheximide (14). Moreover, analysis of cytotoxic T-cell lines derived from renal allograft biopsies obtained at the time of acute rejection showed that such cells bind anti-perforin, anti-granzyme, and anti-FasL antibodies, but the in vitro cytotoxicity of these cells with donor-specific proximal tubular epithelial cells could only be inhibited by preincubation of the cells with concanamycin A, an inhibitor of the perforin/granzyme B pathway; Fas-inhibiting antibodies did not block cytotoxicity or apoptosis. Thus, the perforin/granzyme pathway appears mainly responsible for the cytotoxicity for renal tubular epithelial cells (15). In contrast, studies of pancreas graft biopsies have demonstrated increased numbers of apoptotic cells in biopsies with rejection, as opposed to no increase in granzyme B-positive cells (16), suggesting that apoptosis is the principal cytotoxic pathway in acute pancreas rejection.

Another candidate cell to mediate graft destruction is the eosinophil. Intragraft eosinophilia has been reported during acute and chronic kidney and liver graft rejection (17–19). Studies in a mouse cardiac allograft model have shown that acute rejection episodes in animals depleted of $CD8^+$ cells is characterized by a T_H2-like cytokine pattern and mediated predominantly by eosinophils (20). Eosinophils are extremely caustic cells (21) and are involved in the pathogenesis of asthma and other inflammatory diseases. Although their role as effector cells in allograft rejection remains to be established, eosinophils mediate regression of tumors transfected to produce IL-4 (22).

Along with the recognition that an organ graft transplanted into an allogeneic recipient results in destructive immune responses in the absence of immunosuppressive therapy, it is now increasingly clear that during such a response, immunomodulatory mechanisms are activated that allow long-term graft acceptance despite immunogenetic differences between donor and recipient. These mechanisms are reviewed in Chapter 5.

CHAPTER REFERENCES

1. Little CC, Tyzer EE. Further experimental studies on the inheritance of susceptibility to a transplantable tumour carcinoma (JWA) of the Japanese waltzing mouse. J Med Res 1916;33:393–453.
2. Gibson JM, Medawar PB. The fate of skin homografts in man. J Anat 1943;77:299–310.
3. Medawar PB. Behaviour and fate of skin autografts and skin homografts in rabbits. J Anat 1944;78:176–199.
4. Medawar PB. A second study of the behaviour and fate of skin homografts in rabbits. J Anat 1945;79:157–176.
5. Koller BH, Smithies O. Altering genes in animals by gene targeting. Ann Rev Immunol 1992;10:705–730.
6. Porter ACG, Dallman MJ. Gene targeting: techniques and applications to transplantation. Transplantation 1997;64:1227–1235.
7. Rajewsky K, Gu H, Kuhn R, et al. Conditional gene targeting. J Clin Invest 1996;98:600–603.
8. Janeway CA, Travers P. Immunobiology: the immune system in health and disease. 2nd ed. London/San Francisco: Current Biology, 1996.
9. Halloran PF, Broski AP, Batiuk TD, Madrenas J. The molecular immunology of acute rejection: an overview. Transplant Immunol 1993;1:3–27.
10. Dallman MJ, Larsen CP, Morris CP. Cytokine gene transcription in vascularised organ grafts-analysis using semiquantitative polymerase chain reaction. J Exp Med 1991;174:493–496.
11. Tono T, Moden M, Yoshizaki K, et al. Biliary interleukin 6 levels as indicators of hepatic allograft rejection in rats. Transplantation 1992;53:1195–1201.
12. McLean AG, Hughes D, Welsh KI, et al. Patterns of graft infiltration and cytokine gene expression during the first 10 days of kidney transplantation. Transplantation 1997;63:374–380.
13. Goulmy E. Class I restricted human cytotoxic T lymphocytes directed against minor transplantation antigens and their role in organ transplantation. Prog Allergy 1985;36:44–72.
14. Peugh WN, Superina RA, Wood KJ, Morris PJ. The role of H-2 and non-H-2 antigens and genes in the rejection of murine cardiac allografts. Immunogenetics 1986;23:30–37.
15. Klein J, Juretic A, Baxevanis CN, Nagy ZA. The traditional and a new version of the mouse H-2 complex. Nature 1981;291:455–460.
16. Campbell RD, Trowsdale J. Map of the human major histocompatibility complex. Immunol Today 1993;14:349–352.
17. Dallman MJ, Mason DW, Webb M. Induction of Ia antigens on murine epidermal cells during the rejection of skin allografts. Eur J Immunol 1982;12:511–518.
18. de Waal RMW, Bogman MJJ, Mass CN, et al. Variable expression of Ia antigens on the vascular endothelium of mouse skin allografts. Nature (Lond) 1983;303:426–429.
19. Fellous M, Nir U, Wallach D, et al. Interferon-dependent induction of mRNA for the major histocompatibility antigens in human fibroblasts and lymphoblastoid cells. Proc Natl Acad Sci USA 1982;79:3082–3086.
20. Fuggle S, McWhinnie DL, Chapman JR, et al. Sequential analysis of HLA-Class II antigen expression in human renal allografts. Transplantation 1986;42:144–150.
21. Lampert IA, Suitters AJ, Chisholm PM. Expression of Ia antigen on epidermal keratinocytes in graft-versus-host disease. Nature 1981;293:149–150.
22. Mason DW, Dallman MJ, Barclay AN. Graft-versus-host disease induces expression of Ia antigen in rat epidermal cells and gut epithelium. Nature 1981;293:150–151.

23. Wong GHW, Clark-Lewis I, Harris AW, Schrader JW. Effect of cloned interferon-g on expression of H-2 and Ia antigens on cell lines of hemopoietic, lymphoid, epithelial, fibroblastic and neuronal origin. Eur J Immunol 1984;14:52–56.
24. Roche PA. HLA-DM: an in vivo facilitator of MHC class II peptide loading. Immunity 1995;3:259–262.
25. Belich MP, Trowsdale J. Proteosome and class I antigen processing and presentation. Mol Biol Rep 1995;21:53–56.
26. Cresswell P. Assembly, transport and function of MHC class II molecules. Annu Rev Immunol 1994;12:259–293.
27. Germain RN, Margulies DH. The biochemistry and cell biology of antigen processing and presentation. Annu Rev Immunol 1993;11:403–450.
28. Grey HM, Chestnut R. Antigen processing and presentation to T cells. Immunol Today 1985;6:101–106.
29. Monaco JJ. Major histocompatibility complex-linked transport proteins and antigen processing. Immunol Res 1992;11:125–132.
30. Monaco JJ. Structure and function of genes in the MHC class II region. Curr Opin Immunol 1993;5:17–20.
31. Monaco JJ. Pathways for the processing and presentation of antigens to T cells. J Leukoc Biol 1995;57:543–547.
32. Garcia KC, Degano M, Stanfield RL, et al. An ab T cell receptor structure at 2.5A and its orientation in the TCR-MHC complex. Science 1996; 274:209–219.
33. Bjorkman PJ, Saper MA, Samraoni B, et al. Structure of the human class I histocompatibility antigen, HLA-A2. Nature 1987;329:506–512.
34. Bjorkman PJ. MHC restriction in three dimensions: a view of the T cell receptor/ligand interactions. Cell 1997;89:167–170.
35. Mannon RB, Nataraj C, Kotzin BL, et al. Rejection of kidney allografts by MHC class 1-deficient mice. Transplantation 1995;59:746–755.
36. Li X, Faustman D. Use of donor beta 2-microglobulin-deficient transgenic mouse liver cells for isografts, allografts and xenografts. Transplantation 1993;55:940–946.
37. Auchincloss H, Lee R, Shea S, et al. The role of "indirect" recognition in intiating rejection of skin grafts from major histocompatibility complex class II-deficient mice. Proc Natl Acad Sci (USA) 1993;90:3373–3377.
38. Dierich A, Chan SH, Benoist C, Mathis D. Graft rejection by T cells not restricted by conventional major histocompatibility complex molecules. Eur J Immunol 1993;23:2725–2728.
39. Henretta J, Araneda D, Pittman K, Thomas F. Marked prolongation of incompatible class I deficient heart allografts: paradoxical effects between primarily and secondarily vascularized allografts. Transplant Proc 1995;27:1303–1304.
40. Markmann JF, Bassiri H, Desai NM, et al. Indefinite survival of MHC class I-deficient murine pancreatic islet allografts. Transplantation 1992;54: 1085–1089.
41. Campos L, Naji A, Deli BC, et al. Survival of MHC-deficient mouse heterotopic cardiac allografts. Transplantation 1995;59:187–191.
42. Osorio RW, Ascher NL, Jaenisch R, et al. Major histocompatibility complex class 1 deficiency prolongs islet allograft survival. Diabetes 1993;42:1520–1527.
43. Lee RS, Grusby MJ, Laufer TM, et al. CD8+ effector cells responding to residual class I antigens, with help from CD4+ cells stimulated indirectly cause rejection of "major histocompatibility complex-deficient" skin grafts. Transplantation 1997;63:1123–1133.
44. Turner DM, Grant SC, Lamb WR, et al. A genetic marker of high TNF-alpha production in heart transplant recipients. Transplantation 1995;60: 1113–1117.
45. O'Brien SJ, Roelke ME, Marker L, et al. Genetic basis for species vulnerability in the cheetah. Science 1985;227:1428–1434.
46. Scott DM, Ehrmann IE, Ellis PS, et al. Identification of a mouse male-specific transplantation antigen, H-Y. Nature 1995;376:695–698.
47. Wang W, Meadows LR, den Haan JMM, et al. Human H-Y: a male-specific histocompatibility antigen derived from the SMCY protein. Science 1995;269:1588–1590.
48. Scott DM, Ehrmann IE, Ellis PS, et al. Why do some females reject males? The molecular basis for male-specific graft rejection. J Mol Med 1997;75:103–114.
49. Greenfield A, Scott D, Pennisi D, et al. An H-YDb epitope is encoded by a novel mouse Y chromosome gene. Nat Genet 1996;14:474–478.
50. Hart DN, Fabre JW. Demonstration and characterisation of Ia positive dendritic cells in the interstitial connective tissues of the rat heart and other tissues, but not brain. J Exp Med 1981;154:347–361.
51. Larsen CP, Morris PJ, Austyn JM. Migration of dendritic leucocytes from cardiac allografts into host spleens: a novel pathway for initiation of rejection. J Exp Med 1990;171:307–314.
52. Larsen CP, Steinman RM, Witmer-Pack M, et al. Migration and maturation of Langerhans cells in skin transplants and explants. J Exp Med 1990;172:1483–1493.
53. Reis e Sousa C, Stahl PD, Austyn JM. Phagocytosis of antigens by Langerhans cells in vitro. J Exp Med 1993;178:509–519.
54. Steinman RM, Witmer MD. Lymphoid dendritic cells are potent stimulators of the primary mixed leucocyte reaction in mice. Proc Natl Acad Sci (USA) 1978;75:5132–5136.
55. Steinman RM, Gutchinov B, Witmer MD, Nussenzweig M. Dendritic cells are the peripheral stimulators of the primary mixed leukocyte reaction in mice. J Exp Med 1983;157:613–627.
56. Steinman RM. The dendritic cell system and its role in immunogenicity. Annu Rev Immunol 1991;9:271–296.
57. Billingham RE. The passenger cell concept in transplantation. Cell Immunol 1971;1:1–12.
58. Lafferty KJ, Bootes A, Dart G, Talmage DW. Effect of organ culture on the survival of thyroid allografts in mice. Transplantation 1976;22:138–149.
59. Lechler RI, Batchelor JR. Restoration of immunogenicity to passenger cell-depleted kidney allografts by the addition of donor strain dendritic cells. J Exp Med 1982;155:31–41.
60. Rotzschke O, Falk K, Faath S, Rammensee HG. On the nature of peptides involved in T cell alloreactivity. J Exp Med 1991;174:1059–1071.
61. Golding H, Singer A. Role of accessory cell processing and presentation of shed H-2 alloantigens in allospecific cytotoxic T lymphocyte responses. J Immunol 1984;133:597–605.
62. Parham P, Clayberger C, Zorn SL, et al. Inhibition of alloreactive cytotoxic T lymphocytes by peptides from the OL2 domain of HLA-A2. Nature 1987;325:625–628.
63. Dorling A, Lechler RI. The passenger leucocyte, dendritic cell and antigen-presenting cell (APC). In: Tilney NL, Strom TB, Paul LC, ed. Transplantation biology: cellular and molecular aspects. Philadelphia: Lippincott-Raven, 1996.
64. Butcher GW, Howard JC. Genetic control of transplant rejection. Transplantation 1982;34:161–166.
65. Rock KL, Barnes MC, Germain RN, Benacerraf B. The role of Ia molecules in the activation of T lymphocytes. II Ia-restricted recognition of allo-K/D antigens is required for class I MHC-stimulated mixed lymphocyte responses. J Immunol 1983;130:457–462.
66. Sherwood RA, Brent L, Rayfield LS. Presentation of allo-antigens by host cells. Eur J Immunol 1986;16:569–574.
67. Fangmann J, Dalchau R, Fabre JW. Rejection of skin allografts by indirect allorecognition of donor class I major histocompatibility complex peptides. J Exp Med 1992;175:1521–1529.
68. Liu Z, Braunstein NS, Suciu FN. T cell recognition of allopeptides in context of self MHC. J Immunol 1992;148:35–48.
69. Pfeiffer C, Stein J, Southwood S, et al. Altered peptide ligands can control CD4 T lymphocyte differentiation in vivo. J Exp Med 1995;181:1569–1574.
70. Malaviya R, Twesten NJ, Ross EA, et al. Mast cells process bacterial Ags through a phagocytic route for class I MHC presentation to T cells. J Immunol 1996;156:1490–1496.
71. Lee RS, Grusby MJ, Glimcher LH, et al. Indirect recognition by helper cells can induce donor-specific cytotoxic T lymphocytes in vivo. J Exp Med 1994;179:865–872.
72. Auchincloss H Jr, Sultan H. Antigen processing and presentation in transplantation. Curr Opin Immunol 1996;8:681–687.
73. Cramer DV, Qian S, Harnaha J, et al. Cardiac transplantation in the rat. I. The effect of histocompatibility differences on graft arteriosclerosis. Transplantation 1989;47:414–419.
74. Clark CL, Cunningham AJ, Crane PW, et al. Lymphocyte infiltration patterns in rat small-bowel transplants. Transplant Proc 1990;22:2460.
75. Kim PC, Levy GA, Koh I, Cohen Z. Immunologic basis of small intestinal allograft rejection. Transplant Proc 1991;23:830–832.
76. Toogood GJ, Rankin AM, Tam PKH, et al. The immune response following small bowel transplantation. II. A very early cytokine response in the gut associated lymphoid tissue. Transplantation 1997;63:1118–1123.
77. Hughes CC, Savage CO, Pober JS. The endothelial cell as a regulator of T-cell function. Immunol Rev 1990;117:85–102.
78. Pober JS, Cotran RS. Immunologic interactions of T lymphocytes with vascular endothelium. Adv Immunol 1991;50:261–302.
79. Page CS, Holloway N, Smith H, et al. Alloproliferative responses of purified CD4+ and CD8+ T cells to endothelial cells in the absence of contaminating accessory cells. Transplantation 1994;57:1628–1637.
80. Page CS, Thompson C, Yacoub M, Rose M. Human endothelial stimulation of allogeneic T cells via a CTLA-4 independent pathway. Transplant Immunol 1994;2:342–347.

81. Rygaard J. Skin grafts in nude mice. Acta Path Microbiol Scand 1974;82:93–104.
82. Rolstad B, Ford WL. Immune responses of rats deficient in thymus-derived lymphocytes to strong transplantation antigens. Transplantation 1974;17:405–415.
83. Hall BM, Dorsch S, Roser B. The cellular basis of allograft rejection in vivo. J Exp Med 1978;148:878–889.
84. Gowans JL. The recirculation of lymphocytes from blood to lymph in the rat. J Physiol 1959;146:54–68.
85. Butcher EC, Picker LJ. Lymphocyte homing and homeostasis. Science 1996;272:60–66.
86. Cantrell D. T cell antigen receptor signal transduction pathways. Annu Rev Immunol 1996;14:259–274.
87. Morris RE. Rapamycin: FK506's fraternal twin or distant cousin? Immunol Today 1991;12:137–142.
88. Morris RE. New small molecule immunosuppressants for transplantation: review of essential concepts. J Heart Lung Transplant 1993;12:S275–286.
89. Jenkins MK, Schwartz RH. Antigen presentation by chemically modified splenocytes induces antigen-specific T cell unresponsiveness in vitro and in vivo. J Exp Med 1987;165:302–319.
90. Jenkins MK, Pardoll DM, Mizuguchi J, et al. Molecular events in the induction of a nonresponsive state in interleukin 2-producing helper T-lymphocyte clones. Proc Natl Acad Sci USA 1987;84:5409–5413.
91. Schwartz RH. A cell culture model for T lymphocyte clonal anergy. Science 1990;248:1349–1356.
92. Schwartz RH. T cell clonal anergy. Curr Opin Immunol 1997;9:351–357.
93. Lombardi G, Sidhu S, Batchelor R, Lechler R. Anergic T cells as suppressor cells in vitro. Science 1994;264:1587–1589.
94. June CH, Ledbetter JA, Gillespie MM, et al. T cell proliferation involving the CD28 pathway is associated with cyclosporine-resistant interleukin 2 gene expression. Mol Cell Biol 1987;7:4472–4478.
95. Harding FA, McArthur JG, Gross JA, et al. CD28-mediated signalling co-stimulates T cells and prevents induction of anergy in T-cell clones. Nature 1992;356:607–609.
96. Lenschow DJ, Walunas TL, Bluestone JA. CD28/B7 system of T cell co-stimulation. Annu Rev Immunol 1996;14:233–258.
97. Chambers CA, Allison JP. Co-stimulation in T cell responses. Curr Opin Immunol 1997;9:396–404.
98. Larsen CP, Ritchie SC, Hendrix R, et al. Regulation of immunostimulatory function and costimulatory molecule (B7-1 and B7-2) expression on murine dendritic cells. J Immunol 1994;152:5208–5219.
99. Lenschow DJ, Sperling AI, Cooke MP, et al. Differential up-regulation of the B7-1 and B7-2 costimulatory molecules after Ig receptor engagement by antigen. J Immunol 1994;153(5):1990–1997.
100. Morton PA, Fu X-T, Stewart JA, et al. Differential effects of CTLA-4 substitutions on the binding of human CD80 (B7-1) and CD86 (B7-2). J Immunol 1996;156:1047–1054.
101. Linsley PS, Greene JL, Brady W, et al. Human B7-1 (CD80) and B7-2 (CD86) bind with similar avidities but distinct kinetics to CD28 and CTLA-4 receptors. Immunity 1994;1:793–801.
102. Lindsten T, June CH, Ledbetter JA, et al. Regulation of lymphokine messenger RNA stability by a surface-mediated T cell activation pathway. Science 1989;244:339–343.
103. Thompson CB, Lindsten T, Ledbetter JA, et al. CD28 activation pathway regulates the production of multiple T-cell-derived lymphokines/cytokines. Proc Natl Acad Sci USA 1989;86:1333–1337.
104. Rudd CE, Janssen O, Cai Y-C, et al. Two-step TCR zeta/CD3-CD4 and CD28 signaling in T cells: SH2/SH3 domains, protein-tyrosine and lipid kinases. Immunol Today 1994;15:225–234.
105. Rudd CE. Upstream-downstream: CD28 cosignaling pathways and T cell function. Immunity 1996;4:527–534.
106. Tivol EA, Borriello F, Schweitzer AN, et al. Loss of CTLA-4 leads to massive lymphoproliferation and fatal multiorgan tissue destruction, revealing a critical negative regulatory role of CTLA-4. Immunity 1995;3:541–547.
107. Karandiker N, Vanderlugt CL, Walunas TL, et al. CTLA-4: a negative regulator in autoimmune disease. J Exp Med 1996;184:783–788.
108. Kudig T, Shahinian A, Kawai K, et al. Duration of TCR stimulation determines co-stimulatory requirement of T cells. Immunity 1996;5:41–52.
109. Zimmerman C, Seiler P, Lane P, Zinkernagel RM. Antiviral immune responses in CTLA4 transgenic mice. J Virol 1997;71:1802–1807.
110. Kawai K, Shahinian A, Mak TW, Ohashi PS. Skin allograft rejection in CD28-deficient mice. Transplantation 1996;61:352–355.
111. Lenschow DJ, Zeng Y, Thistlethwaite JR, et al. Long-term survival of xenogeneic panceatic islet grafts induced by CTLA4Ig. Science 1992;257:789–792.
112. Pearson TC, Alexander DZ, Winn KJ, et al. Transplantation tolerance induced by CTLA-4 Ig. Transplantation 1994;57:1701–1706.
113. Turka LA, Linsley PS, Lin H, et al. T-cell activation by the CD28 ligand B7 is required for cardiac allograft rejection in vivo. Proc Natl Acad Sci USA 1992;89:11102–11105.
114. Larsen CP, Alexander DZ, Hollenbaugh D, et al. CD40-gp39 interactions play a critical role during allograft rejection: suppression of allograft rejection by blockade of the CD40-gp39 pathway. Transplantation 1996;61:4–9.
115. Larsen CP, Elwood ET, Alexander DZ, et al. Long term acceptance of skin and cardiac allografts after blocking CD40 and CD28 pathways. Nature 1996;381:434–438.
116. Kirk AD, Harlan DM, Davis TA, et al. CTLA4-Ig and anti-CD40 ligand prevent renal allograft rejection in primates. Proc Natl Acad Sci USA 1997;94:8789–8794.
117. Dallman MJ, Clark GJ. Cytokine and their receptors in transplantation. Curr Opin Immunol 1992;3:729–734.
118. Dallman MJ. Cytokines and transplantation: Th1/Th2 regulation of the immune response to solid organ transplants in the adult. Curr Opin Immunol 1995;7:632–638.
119. Nickerson P, Steurer W, Steiger J, et al. Cytokines and the Th1/Th2 paradigm in transplantation. Curr Opin Immunol 1994;6:757–764.
120. Strom TB, Roy-Chadhury P, Manfro R, et al. The Th1/Th2 paradigm and the allograft response. Curr Opin Immunol 1996;8:688–693.
121. Loveland BE, Hogarth PM, Ceredig R, McKenzie IFC. Delayed type hypersensitivity and allograft rejection in the mouse: correlation of effector cell phenotype. J Exp Med 1981;153:1044–1057.
122. Gurley KE, Lowry RP, Clarke-Forbes RD. Immune mechanisms in organ allograft rejection. II. T helper cells, delayed type hypersensitivity and rejection of renal allografts. Transplantation 1983;36:401–405.
123. Hall BM, DeSaxe I, Dorsch SE. The cellular basis of allograft rejection in vivo: restoration of first set rejection of heart grafts by T helper cells in irradiated rats. Transplantation 1983;36:700–705.
124. Lowry RP, Gurley KE, Clarke-Forbes RD. Immune mechanisms in organ allograft rejection. 1. Delayed type hypersensitivity and lymphocytotoxicity in heart graft rejection. Transplantation 1983;36:391–401.
125. Tilney NL, Kupiec-Weglinski JW, Heidecke CD, et al. Mechanisms of rejection and prolongation of vascularised organ allografts. Immunol Rev 1984;77:185–216.
126. Sprent J, Schaeffer M, Lo D, Korngold R. Properties of purified T cell subsets II. In vivo class I vs class II H-2 differences. J Exp Med 1986;163:998–1011.
127. Rosenberg AS, Mizuochi T, Singer A. Analysis of T cell subsets in rejection of K^b mutant skin allograft differing at class I MHC. Nature 1986;322:829–831.
128. Rosenberg AS, Mizuochi T, Sharrow SO, Singer A. Phenotype, specificity and function of T cell subsets and T cell interactions involved in skin allograft rejection. J Exp Med 1987;165:1296–1315.
129. Rosenberg AS. The T cell populations mediating rejection of MHC class I disparate skin grafts in mice. Transplant Immunol 1993;2:93–99.
130. Lamouse-Smith E, Clements VK, Ostrand-Rosenberg S. Beta 2M −/− knockout mice contain low levels of CD8+ cytotoxic T lymphocyte that mediate specific tumor rejection. J Immunol 1993;151:6283–6290.
131. Schilham MW, Fung-Leung WP, Rahemtulla A, et al. Alloreactive cytotoxic T cells can develop and function in mice lacking both CD4 and CD8. Eur J Immunol 1993;23:1299–1304.
132. Apasov SG, Sitkovsky MV. Development and antigen specificity of CD8+ cytotoxic T lymphocytes in beta 2-microglobulin-negative, MHC class 1-deficient mice in response to immunization with tumor cells. J Immunol 1994;1994:152.
133. Dalloul AH, Chmouzis E, Ngo K, Fung-Leung W-P. Adoptively transferred CD4+ lymphocytes from CD8−/− mice are sufficient to mediate rejection of MHC class II or class I disparate skin grafts. J Immunol 1996;156:411–414.
134. Dalloul AH, Ngo K, Fung-Leing W-P. CD4-negative cytotoxic T cells with a T cell receptor alpha/beta intermediate expression in CD8-deficient mice. Eur J Immunol 1996;26:213–218.
135. Krieger NR, Yin DP, Fathman CG. CD4+ but not CD8+ cells are essential for allorejection. J Exp Med 1996;184:2013–2018.
136. Parish C. The relationship between humoral and cell-mediated immunity. Transplant Rev 1972;13:35–66.
137. Katsura Y. Cell-mediated and humoral immune responses in mice. III. Dynamic balance between delayed-type hypersensitivity and antibody response. Immunology 1977;32:227–235.

138. Mosmann TR, Cherwinski H, Bond MW, et al. Two types of murine helper T cell clone. 1. Definition according to profiles of lymphokine activities and secreted proteins. J Immunol 1986;136:2348–2357.
139. Mosmann TR, Coffman RL. TH1 and TH2 cells: different patterns of lymphokine secretion lead to different functional properties. Annu Rev Immunol 1989;7:145–173.
140. Mosmann TR, Moore KW. The role of IL-10 in crossregulation of TH1 and TH2 responses. Immunoparasitol Today 1991;12:A49–A53.
141. Del Prete GF, De Carli M, Mastromauro C, et al. Purified protein derivative of *Mycobacterium tuberculosis* and excretory-secretory antigen(s) of *Toxocara canis* expand in vitro human T cells with stable and opposite (type 1 T helper or type 2 T helper) profile of cytokine production. J Clin Invest 1991; 88:346–350.
142. McKnight AJ, Barclay AN, Mason DW. Molecular cloning of rat interleukin 4 cDNA and anlaysis of the cytokine repertoire of subsets of CD4+ T cells. Eur J Immunol 1991;21:1187–1194.
143. Kelso A. Th1 and Th2 subsets: paradigms lost? Immunol Today 1995;16:374–379.
144. Gajewski TF, Fitch FW. Anti-proliferative effect of IFN-γ in immune regulation I. IFN-γ inhibits the proliferation of TH2 but not TH1 murine helper T lymphocyte clones. J Immunol 1988;140:4245–4252.
145. Gajewski TF, Schell SR, Nau G, Fitch FW. Regulation of T cell activation: differences among T-cell subsets. Immunol Rev 1989;111:79–110.
146. Swain SL, Weinberg AD, English M, Huston G. IL-4 directs the development of TH2-like helper effectors. J Immunol 1990;145:3796–3806.
147. Swain SL, Huston G, Tonkonogy S, Weinberg AD. Transforming growth factor-β and IL-4 cause helper T cell precursors to develop into distinct effector helper cells that differ in lymphokine secretion pattern and cell surface phenotype. J Immunol 1991;147:2991–3000.
148. Hsieh C-S, Heimberger AB, Gold JS, et al. Differential regulation of T helper phenotype development by interleukins 4 and 10 in an αβ T-cell-receptor transgenic system. Proc Natl Acad Sci USA 1992;89:6065–6069.
149. Hsieh CS, Macatonia SE, Tripp CS, et al. Development of Th1 CD4+ T cells through IL-12 produced by Listeria-induced macrophages. Science 1993;260:547–548.
150. Macatonia SE, Hsieh C-S, O'Garra A, Murphy KM. Dendritic cells and macrophages are required for Th1 development of CD4+ T cells from alpha beta TCR transgenic mice: IL-12 substitution for macrophages to stimulate IFN-gamma production is IFN-gamma-dependent. Int Immunol 1993;5:1119–1128.
151. Macatonia SE, Doherty TM, Knight SC, O'Garra A. Differential effect of IL-10 on dendritic cell-induced T cell proliferation and IFNg production. J Immunol 1993;150:3755–3765.
152. Freeman GJ, Boussiotis VA, Anumanthan A, et al. B7-1 and B7-2 do not deliver identical costimulatory signals, since B7-2 but not B7-1 preferentially costimulates the initial production of IL-4. Immunity 1995;2:523–532.
153. Kuchroo VK, Das MP, Brown JA, et al. B7.1 and B7.2 costimulatory molecules activate differentially the Th1/Th2 developmental pathways: application to autoimmune disease. Cell 1995;80:707–718.
154. Lenschow DJ, Herold KC, Rhee L, et al. CD28/B7 regulation of Th1 and Th2 subsets in the development of autoimmune diabetes. Immunity 1996;5:285–293.
155. Ranger AM, Das MP, Kuchroo VK, Glimcher LH. B7-2 (CD86) is essential for the development of IL-4 producing cells. Int Immunol 1996;8(10): 1549–1560.
156. Dallman MJ. Cytokines as mediators of organ graft rejection and tolerance. Curr Opin Immunol 1993;5:788–793.
157. Dallman MJ, Shiho O, Page TH, et al. Peripheral tolerance to alloantigen results from altered regulation of the interleukin 2 pathway. J Exp Med 1991;173:79–87.
158. Burdick JF, Clow LW. Rejection of primarily vascularized heart grafts. III Depression of the interleukin 2 mechanism early after grafting. Transplantation 1990;50:476–481.
159. Bugeon L, Cuturi M-C, Hallet M-M, et al. Peripheral tolerance of an allograft in adult rats-characterization by low interleukin-2 and interferon-g mRNA levels and by strong accumulation of major histocompatibility complex transcripts in the graft. Transplantation 1992;54:219–225.
160. Mohler KM, Streilein JW. Differential expression of helper versus effector activity in mice rendered neonatally tolerant of class II MHC antigens. Transplantation 1989;47:633–640.
161. Takeuchi T, Lowry RP, Konieczny B. Heart allografts in murine systems. Transplantation 1992;53:1281–1294.
162. Alard P, Lantz O, Perrot JY, et al. A possible role for specific "anergy" in immunologic hyporeactivity to donor stimulation in human kidney allograft recipients. Transplantation 1993;55:277–283.
163. Gorczynski RM. Immunosuppression induced by hepatic portal venous immunization spares reactivity in IL-4 producing T lymphocytes. Immunol Lett 1992;33:67–78.
164. Dallman MJ, Wood KJ, Hamano K, et al. Cytokines and peripheral tolerance to alloantigen. Immunol Rev 1993;133:5–18.
165. Josien R, Pannetier C, Douillard P, et al. Graft infiltrating T helper cells CD45RC phenotype and TH1/TH2-related cytokines in donor specific transfusion-induced tolerance in adult rats. Transplantation 1995;60:1131–1139.
166. Nickerson P, Zheng X-X, Steiger J, et al. Prolonged islet allograft acceptance in the absence of interleukin 4 expression. Transplant Immunol 1996;4:81–85.
167. Lakkis FG, Konieczny BT, Saleem S, et al. Blocking the CD28-B7 T cell costimulation pathway induces long term cardiac allograft acceptance in the absence of IL-4. J Immunol 1997;158:2443–2448.
168. Steiger J, Nickerson PW, Steurer W, et al. IL-2 knockout recipient mice reject islet cell allografts. J Immunol 1995;155:489–498.
169. Konieczny BT, Saleem S, Lowry RP, Lakkis FG. Vigorous cardiac allograft rejection in IFN gamma knockout mice. Proceedings of the 15th Annual Meeting of the American Society of Transplant Physicians 1996:170.
170. Saleem S, Konieczny BT, Lowry RP, et al. Acute rejection of vascularized heart allografts in the absence of IFNg. Transplantation 1996;62:1908–1911.
171. Mueller R, Davies JD, Krahl T, Sarvetnick N. IL-4 expression by grafts from transgenic mice fails to prevent allograft rejection. J Immunol 1997;159:1599–1603.
172. Kirby JA. Function of leucocyte adhesion molecules during allograft rejection. In: Tilney NL, Strom TB, Paul LC, eds. Transplantation biology: cellular and molecular aspects. Philadelphia: Lippincott-Raven, 1996.
173. Pober JS, Gimbrone Jr MA, Lapierre LA, et al. Overlapping patterns of activation of human endothelial cells by interleukin 1, tumour necrosis factor and immune interferon. J Immunol 1986;137:1893–1896.
174. Collins T, Read MA, Neish AS, et al. Transcriptional regulation of endothelial cell adhesion molecules: NF-kappa B and cytokine-inducible enhancers. FASEB J 1995;9:899–909.
175. Butcher EC. The regulation of lymphocyte traffic. Curr Topics Microbiol Immunol 1986;128:85–122.
176. Picker LJ, Butcher EC. Physiological and molecular mechanisms of lymphocyte homing. Annu Rev Immunol 1992;10:561–591.
177. Mackay CR. Immunologic memory. Adv Immunol 1993;53:217–265.
178. Heagy W, Waltenbaugh C, Martz E. Potent ability of anti-LFA-1 monoclonal antibody to prolong allograft survival. Transplantation 1984;37:520–523.
179. Cosimi AB, Conti D, Delmonico FL, et al. In vivo effects of monoclonal antibody to ICAM-1 (CD54) in nonhuman primates with renal allografts. J Immunol 1990;144:4604–4612.
180. Haug CE, Colvin RB, Delmonico FL, et al. A phase I trial of immunosuppression with anti-ICAM-1 (CD54) mAb in renal allograft recipients. Transplantation 1993;55:766–773.
181. Hourmant M, Bedrossian J, Durand D, et al. A randomized multicenter trial comparing leukocyte function-associated antigen-1 monoclonal antibody with rabbit antithymocyte globulin as induction treatment in first kidney transplantations. Transplantation 1996;62:1565–1570.
182. Iwata T, Kamei Y, Esaki S, et al. Immunosuppression by anti-ICAM-1 and anti-LFA-1 monoclonal antibodies of free and vascularized skin allograft rejection. Immunobiology 1996;195:160–171.
183. Yang H, Issekutz TB, Wright JR Jr. Prolongation of rat islet allograft survival by treatment with monoclonal antibodies against VLA-4 and LFA-1. Transplantation 1995;60:71–76.
184. Morikawa M, Tamatani T, Miyasaka M, Uede T. Cardiac allografts in rat recipients with simultaneous use of anti-ICAM-1 and anti-LFA-1 monoclonal antibodies leads to accelerated graft loss. Immunopharmacology 1994;28:171–182.
185. Oppenheim JJ, Wang JM, Chertov O, et al. The role of chemokines in transplantation. In: Tilney NL, Strom TB, Paul LC, eds. Transplantation biology: cellular and molecular aspects. Philadelphia: Lippincott-Raven, 1996:187–200.
186. Oppenheim JJ, Zacharie COC, Mukaida N, Matsushima K. Properties of the proinflammatory supergene "intercrine" cytokine family. Annu Rev Immunol 1991;9:617–648.
187. Bacon KB, Schall TJ. Chemokines as mediators of allergic inflammation. Int Arch Allergy Immunol 1996;109:97–109.
188. Grandaliano G, Gesualdo L, Ranieri E, et al. Monocyte chemotactic peptide-1 expression and monocyte infiltration in acute renal transplant rejection. Transplantation 1997;63:414–420.
189. Kagi D, Seiler P, Pavlovic J, et al. The roles of perforin- and Fas-dependent cytotoxicity in protection against cytopathic and non-cytopathic viruses. Eur J Immunol 1995;25:3256–3262.

190. Perlmann P, Holm G. Cytotoxic effects of lymphoid cells in vitro. Adv Immunol 1969;11:117–193.
191. Tilney NL, Strom TB, MacPherson SG, Carpenter CB. Surface properties and functional characteristics of infiltrating cells harvested from acutely rejecting cardiac allografts in inbred rats. Transplantation 1975;20:323–330.
192. Kissmeyer-Nielsen F, Olsen S, Peterson VP, Fjeldborg O. Hyperacute rejection of kidney allografts associated with pre-existing humoral antibodies against donor cells. Lancet 1966;2:662–665.
193. Williams GM, Hume DM, Hudson RPJ, et al. "Hyperacute" renal homograft rejection in man. New Engl J Med 1968;279:611–618.
194. Morris PJ, Ting A. Studies of HLA-DR with relevance to renal transplantation. Immunol Rev 1982;66:103–131.
195. Patel R, Terasaki PI. Significance of the positive crossmatch test in kidney transplantation. New Engl J Med 1969;280:735–739.
196. Ting A, Morris PJ. Renal transplantation and B cell crossmatches with autoantibodies and alloantibodies. Lancet 1977;2:1095–1097.
197. Ting A, Morris PJ. Positive-crossmatch transplants—safe or not. Transplant Proc 1981;13:1544–1546.
198. Tyan DB, Li VA, Czer L, et al. Intravenous immunoglobulin suppression of HLA alloantibody in highly sensitized transplant candidates and transplantation with a histoincompatible organ. Transplantation 1994;57:553–562.
199. De Marco T, Damon LE, Colombe B, et al. Successful immunomodulation with intravenous gamma globulin and cyclophosphamide in an alloimmunized heart transplant recipient. J Heart Lung Transplant 1997;16:360–365.
200. Jordan SC, Quartel AW, Czer LS, et al. Posttransplant therapy using high-dose human immunoglobulin (intravenous gammaglobulin) to control acute humoral rejection in renal and cardiac allograft recipients and potential mechanism of action. Transplantation 1998;66:800–805.
201. Kamada N, Wight DGD. Antigen-specific immunosuppression induced by liver transplantation in the rat. Transplantation 1984;38:217–222.
202. Kamada N. Experimental liver transplantation. Boca Raton, FL: CRC Press 1988.
203. Farges O, Morris PJ, Dallman MJ. Spontaneous acceptance of liver allografts in the rat: analysis of the immune response. Transplantation 1994;57:171–177.
204. Farges O, Morris PJ, Dallman MJ. Spontaneous acceptance of rat liver allografts is associated with an early down regulation of intragraft IL-4 mRNA expression. Hepatology 1995;21:767–775.
205. Dunnill MS. Histopathology of rejection in renal transplantation. In: Morris PJ, ed. Kidney transplantation: principles and practice. 2nd ed. New York: Grune & Stratton, 1984:355–382.
206. Ting A, Morris PJ. Reactivity of autolymphocytotoxic antibodies from dialysis patients with lymphocytes from chronic lymphocytic leukemia (CLL) patients. Transplantation 1978;25:31–33.
207. Baldwin WMI, Pruitt SK, Sanfilippo F. Alloantibodies: basic and clinical concepts. Transplant Rev 1991;5:100–109.
208. Gracie JA, Bolton EM, Porteous C, Bradley JA. T cell requirements for the rejection of renal allografts bearing an isolated class I disparity. J Exp Med 1990;172:1547–1557.
209. Yilmaz S, Taskninen E, Paavonen T, et al. Chronic rejection of rat renal allograft. I. Histological differentiation between chronic rejection and cyclosporin nephrotoxicity. Transplant Int 1992;5:85–95.
210. Galili U, Rachmilewitz EA, Peleg A, Flechner I. A unique natural human IgG antibody with anti a-galactosyl specificity. J Exp Med 1984;160:1519–1531.
211. Galili U, Macher BA, Buchler J, Shohet SB. Human natural anti-a-galactosyl IgG II. The specific recognition of a (1-3)-linked galactosyl residues. J Exp Med 1985;162:573–582.
212. Sandrin MS, Vaughan HA, Dabkrowski PL, McKenzie IFC. Anti-pig IgM antibodies in human serum react predominantly with Gal(a1-3)Gal epitopes. Proc Natl Acad Sci USA 1993;90:11391–11395.
213. Cooper DKC, Good AH, Koren E, et al. Identification of a-galactosyl and other carbohydrate epitopes that are bound by human anti-pig antibodies: relevance to discordant xenografting in man. Transplant Immunol 1993;1:198–205.
214. Parker W, Bruno D, Holzknecht ZE, Platt JL. Characterization and affinity isolation of xenoreactive human natural antibodies. J Immunol 1994; 153:3791–3803.
215. Platt JL, Fischel RJ, Matas AJ, et al. Immunopathology of hyperacute xenograft rejection in swine-to-human primate model. Transplantation 1991;52:214–220.
216. Platt JL, Bach FH. The barrier to xenotransplantation. Transplantation 1991;52:937–947.
217. Kirkman RL, Colvin RB, Flye MW, Williams GM, Sachs DH. Transplantation in miniature swine. Transplantation 1979;28:24–30.
218. Herberman RB, Djeu JY, Kay HD, et al. Natural killer cells: characteristics and regulation of activity. Immunol Rev 1979;44:43–70.
219. Mason DW, Morris PJ. Inhibition of the accumulation, in rat kidney allografts, of specific-but not nonspecific-cytotoxic cells by cyclosporine. Transplantation 1984;37:46–51.
220. Bradley JA, Mason DW, Morris PJ. Evidence that rat renal allografts are rejected by cytotoxic T cells and not by non-specific effectors. Transplantation 1985;39:169–175.
221. Armstrong HE, Bolton EM, McMillan I, et al. Prolonged survival of actively enhanced rat renal allografts despite accelerated cellular infiltration and rapid induction of both class I and class II MHC antigens. J Exp Med 1987;165:891–907.
222. Murphy WJ, Kumar V, Bennett M. Acute rejection of murine bone marrow allografts by natural killer cells and T cells. Differences in kinetics and target antigens recognized. J Exp Med 1987;166:1499–1509.
223. Murphy WJ, Kumar V, Bennett M. Rejection of bone marrow allografts by mice with severe combined immune deficiency (SCID): evidence that NK cells can mediate the specificity of marrow graft rejection. J Exp Med 1987;165:1212–1217.
224. Colonna M, Brooks EG, Falco M, et al. Generation of allospecific natural killer cells by stimulation across a polymorphism of HLA-C. Science 1993;260:1121–1124.
225. Leibson PJ. MHC-recognising receptors: they're not just for T cells anymore. Immunity 1995;3:5–8.
226. Long EO, Wagtmann N. Natural killer cell receptors. Curr Opin Immunol 1997;9:344–350.
227. Bix M, Liao NS, Zijlstra M, et al. Rejection of class I MHC-deficient haemopoietic cells by irradiated MHC-matched mice. Nature 1991;349:329–331.
228. Hayry P, Defendi V. Mixed lymphocyte cultures produce effector cells: model in vitro for allograft rejection. Science 1970;168:133–135.
229. Hodes RJ, Svedmyr EAJ. Specific cytotoxicity of H-2-incompatible mouse lymphocytes following mixed culture in vitro. Transplantation 1970;9:470–477.
230. Engers HD, Glasebrooke AL, Sorenson GD. Allogeneic tumour rejection induced by the intravenous injection of Lyt-2+ cytolytic T lymphocyte clones. J Exp Med 1982;156:1280–1285.
231. Tyler JD, Galli SJ, Snider ME, et al. Cloned LyT-2+ cytolytic T lymphocytes destroy allogeneic tissue in vivo. J Exp Med 1984;159:234–243.
232. Cobbold SP, Jayasuriya A, Nash A, et al. Therapy with monoclonal antibodies by elimination of T cell subsets in vivo. Nature 1984;312:548–551.
233. Madsen JC, Peugh WN, Wood KJ, Morris PJ. The effect of anti-L3T4 monoclonal antibody treatment on first set rejection of murine cardiac allografts. Transplantation 1987;44:849–852.
234. Madsen JC, Superina RA, Wood KJ, Morris PJ. Induction of immunologic unresponsiveness using recipient cells transfected with donor MHC genes. Nature (Lond) 1988;332:161–164.
235. Hurme M, Chandler PR, Hetherington CM, Simpson E. Cytotoxic T cell responses to H-Y: correlation with the rejection of syngeneic male skin grafts. J Exp Med 1978;147:768–775.
236. Hurme M, Hetherington CM, Chandler PR, Simpson E. Cytotoxic T cell responses to H-Y: mapping of the Ir genes. J Exp Med 1978;147:758–767.
237. Dallman MJ, Wood KJ, Morris PJ. Specific cytotoxic T cells are found in the non-rejected kidneys of blood transfused rats. J Exp Med 1987;165:566–571.
238. Walsh CM, Hayashi F, Saffron DC, et al. Cell-mediated cytotoxicity results from, but may not be critical for, primary allograft rejection. J Immunol 1996;156:1436–1441.
239. Selvaggi G, Ricordi C, Podack ER, Inverardi L. The role of the perforin and Fas pathways of cytotoxicity in skin graft rejection. Transplantation 1996;62:1912–1915.
240. Schulz M, Schuurman H-J, Joergensen J, et al. Acute rejection of vascular heart allografts by perforin-deficient mice. Eur J Immunol 1995;25:474–480.
241. Loveland BE, McKenzie IFC. Cells mediating graft rejection in the mouse. Immunology 1982;46:313–320.
242. Florey HW, Jennings MA. In: Florey HW, ed. General pathology. 4th ed. London: Lloyd-Luke, 1970:124–174.
243. Mintz B, Silvers WK. "Intrinsic" immunologic tolerance in allophenic mice. Science 1967;158:1484–1486.
244. Mintz B, Silvers WK. Histocompatibility antigens on melanoblasts and hair follicle cells. Transplantation 1970;9:497–505.
245. Rosenberg AS, Singer A. Cellular basis of skin allograft rejection: an in vivo model of immune-mediated tissue destruction. Annu Rev Immunol 1992;10:333–358.
246. Liew FY, Simpson E. Delayed type hypersensitivity to H-Y: characterisation and mapping of Ir genes. Immunogenetics 1980;11:255–266.
247. Paul LC, Benediktsson H. Chronic transplant rejection: magnitude of the problem and pathogenetic mechanism. Transplant Rev 1993;7:96–113.

248. Paul LC, Saito K, Davidoff A, Benediktsson H. Growth factor transcripts in rat renal transplants. Am J Kidney Dis 1996;28:441–450.
249. Hayry P, Mennander A, Raisanen-Sokolowski A, et al. Pathophysiology of vascular wall changes in chronic allograft rejection. Transplant Rev 1993;7:1–20.
250. Chen J, Myllarniemi M, Akyurek LM, et al. Identification of differentially expressed genes in rat aortic allograft vasculopathy. Am J Pathol 1996;149:597–611.
251. Snider ME, Steinmuller D. Non-specific tissue destruction as a consequence of cytotoxic T lymphocyte interaction with antigen-specific target cells. Transplant Proc 1987;19:421–423.
252. Imagawa DK, Millis JM, Olthoff KM, et al. The role of tumor necrosis factor in allograft rejection II. Evidence that antibody therapy against tumor necrosis factor-alpha and lymphotoxin enhances cardiac survival in rats. Transplantation 1990;50:189–193.
253. Imagawa DK, Millis JM, Seu P, et al. The role of tumor necrosis factor in allograft rejection. III. Evidence that anti-TNF antibody therapy prolongs allograft survival in rats with acute rejection. Transplantation 1991;51:57–62.
254. Bolling S, Kunkel SL, Lin H. Prolongation of cardiac allograft survival in rats by anti-TNF and cyclosporin combination therapy. Transplantation 1992;53:283–286.
255. Mandrup-Poulsen T, Bendtzen K, Nerup J, et al. Affinity-purified human interleukin I is cytotoxic to isolated islets of Langerhans. Diabetologia 1986;29:63–67.
256. Mandrup-Poulsen T, Helqvist S, Molvig J, et al. Cytokines as immune effector molecules in autoimmune endocrine diseases with special reference to insulin-dependent diabetes mellitus. Autoimmunity 1989;4:191–218.
257. Rabinovitch A, Pukel C, Baquerizo H. Interleukin-1 inhibits glucose-modulated insulin and glucagon secretion in rat islet monolayer cultures. Endocrinology 1988;122:2393–2398.
258. Wolf BA, Hughes JH, Florholmen J, et al. Interleukin-1 inhibits glucose-induced Ca^{2+} uptake by islets of Langerhans. FEBS Lett 1989;248:35.
259. Kauntz SL, Williams MA, Williams PL, et al. Mechanism of rejection of homotransplanted kidneys. Nature 1963;199:257–260.
260. Dvorak HF, Mihm MCJ, Dvorak AM, et al. Rejection of first-set skin allografts in man—the microvasculature is the critical target of the immune response. J Exp Med 1979;150:322–337.
261. Laden AMK, Sinclair RA. Thickening of arterial intima in rat cardiac allografts. Am J Pathol 1971;63:69–84.
262. Porter KA, Calne RY, Zukoski CF. Vascular and other changes in 200 renal homotransplants treated with immunosuppressive drugs. Lab Invest 1964;13:810–824.

COMMENTARY REFERENCES

1. Gorer PA. The antigenic basis of tumour transplantation. J Pathol Bacteriol 1938;47:231–252.
2. Medawar PB. The behaviour and fate of skin autografts and skin homografts in rabbits. J Anat 1944;78:176–199.
3. Matzinger P. Tolerance, danger, and the extended family. Annu Rev Immunol 1994;12:991–1045.
4. Van Es A, Hermans J, Van Bockel JH, et al. Effect of warm ischemia time and HLA (A and B) matching on renal cadaveric graft survival and rejection episodes. Transplantation 1983;36:255–258.
5. Lu CY. Ischemia, injury, and renal allograft rejection. Curr Opin Nephrol Hypertens 1996;5:107–110.
6. Goes N, Urmson J, Ramassar V, Halloran PF. Ischemic acute tubular necrosis induces an extensive local cytokine response. Transplantation 1995;59:565–572.
7. Terasaki PI, Cecka JM, Gjertson DW, Takemoto S. High survival rates of kidney transplants from spousal and living unrelated donors. N Engl J Med 1995;333:333–336.
8. Trowbridge IS, Thomas ML. CD45: an emerging role as a protein tyrosine phosphatase required for lymphocyte activation and development. Ann Rev Immunol 1994;12:85–116.
9. Lazarovits AI, Poppema S, Zhang Z, et al. Prevention and reversal of renal allograft rejection by antibody against CD45RB. Nature 1996;380:717–720.
10. Van Kooten C, Banchereau J. Functions of CD40 on B cells, dendritic cells and other cells. Curr Opin Immunol 1997;9:330–337.
11. Van Kooten C, Gerritsma JSJ, Paape ME, et al. Possible role for CD40-CD40L in the regulation of interstitial infiltration in the kidney. Kidney Int 1997;51:711–721.
12. Fitzpatrick DR, Kelso A. Independent regulation of cytokine genes in T cells. Transplantation 1998;65:1–5.
13. Piccotti JR, Chan SY, VanBuskirk AM, et al. Are Th2 helper T lymphocytes beneficial, deleterious, or irrelevant in promoting allograft survival? Transplantation 1997;63:619–624.
14. Boonstra JG, Van der Woude FJ, Wever PC, et al. Expression and function of Fas (CD95) on human renal tubular epithelial cells. J Am Soc Nephrol 1997;8:1517–1524.
15. Wever PC, Boonstra JG, Laterveer JC, et al. Mechanisms of lymphocyte-mediated cytotoxicity in acute renal allograft rejection. Transplantation 1998;66:259–264.
16. Boonstra JG, Wever PC, Laterveer JC, et al. Apoptosis of acinar cells in pancreas allograft rejection. Transplantation 1997;64:1211–1213.
17. Kormendi F, Amend WJC. The importance of eosinophil cells in kidney allograft rejection. Transplantation 1988;45:537–539.
18. Nolan CR, Saenz KP, Thomas CA, Murphy KD. Role of eosinophils in chronic vascular rejection in renal allografts. Am J Kidney Dis 1995; 26:634–642.
19. Foster P, Sankary HN, Hart M, et al. Blood and graft eosinophilia as predictors of rejection in human liver transplantation. Transplantation 1989;47:72–74.
20. Chan SY, DeBruyne LA, Goodman RE, et al. In vivo depletion of CD8+ T cells results in Th2 cytokine production and alternate mechanisms of allograft rejection. Transplantation 1995;59:1155–1161.
21. Gleich GJ, Frigas E, Loegering DA, et al. Cytotoxic properties of the eosinophil major basic protein. J Immunol 1979;123:2925–2927.
22. Tepper RI, Coffman RL, Leder P. An eosinophil-dependent mechanism for the antitumor effect of interleukin-4. Science 1992;257:548–551.

Chapter 3

Chronic Rejection

NICHOLAS L. TILNEY

Since the first demonstration nearly five decades ago that successful engraftment of a healthy kidney could completely rehabilitate an individual with renal failure, transplantation of several organs has become a unique and exciting chapter in the story of advancement in medicine. In 1993 in the United States alone, about 10,000 kidneys, more than 2500 livers, and over 2000 hearts were transplanted (1). The results, particularly over the short term, have improved progressively, secondary to refinements in tissue typing, better understanding and care of individuals with end-stage organ failure, improved perioperative techniques, and newer and more effective immunosuppressive agents.

Despite these early successes, it has become clear that clinical transplantation has not yet achieved its potential as a long-term or permanent treatment for a life-long disease. In many patients, it provides no more than a short-term amelioration of the existing condition. Thus, regardless of increasingly satisfactory early allograft survival rates, the subsequent rate of graft loss has changed little since the beginning of the experience (Fig. 3.1) (2). Although several factors, including recurrent and de novo disease, drug nephrotoxicity, late acute rejection episodes, and patient death, may contribute to the rate of attrition over time, the inexorable process of chronic rejection is the most important cause of late graft deterioration and failure (3,4). In both United Network for Organ Sharing (UNOS) and Eurotransplant data, the half-life of cadaver donor renal allografts remains at 8 to 9 years, despite more than 80% functioning at the end of the first year (1,2). The rate of decline of other organ grafts is relatively comparable, with the incidence of coronary arteriosclerosis in heart grafts reaching 50% by 5 years (see Chapter 23), leading to a 25% mortality rate (5). The failure of lung transplants, most often from bronchiolitis obliterans (a manifestation of chronic rejection), is as high as 50% within that period (see Chapter 25). The lower occurrence of the condition in liver allografts (50% to 60% functioning at 5 years) has been attributed to several factors (see Chapter 19), including the putatively lower immunogenicity of this organ (6). Thus, *chronic rejection*—which we define as progressive functional deterioration occurring months or years after engraftment, associated with gradual vascular obliteration and other structural changes that lead ultimately to fibrosis—is responsible for most late graft loss, regardless of organ source (7,8).

THE LESION AND ITS PATHOLOGY

The majority of studies of chronic rejection have been limited to descriptions of solid-organ allografts. The common denominator of the process seems to be the development of progressive luminal compromise of hollow structures within the graft, regardless of whether they are vessels, bronchioles, or bile ducts. Whether these and subsequent tissue changes occur secondary to arterial insufficiency and gradual ischemia or develop from unremitting subclinical host immunologic attack or other factors remains undefined. The following sections review the characteristic features that evolve in affected organs.

Kidney

The course of patients experiencing chronic rejection of their kidney grafts is often predictable. Often following a prolonged, satisfactory, stable course, the individual begins to develop progressive proteinuria, hypertension, and deteriorating function, all associated with glomerulosclerosis and nephrosclerosis (Fig. 3.2 and Plate 1). The typical morphologic findings of tubular atrophy, parenchymal fibrosis, and chronic arteritis defects in the elastic fibers of the arterial media were first noted in one of Hume's original (1953) recipients, a nonimmunosuppressed patient sustained by his

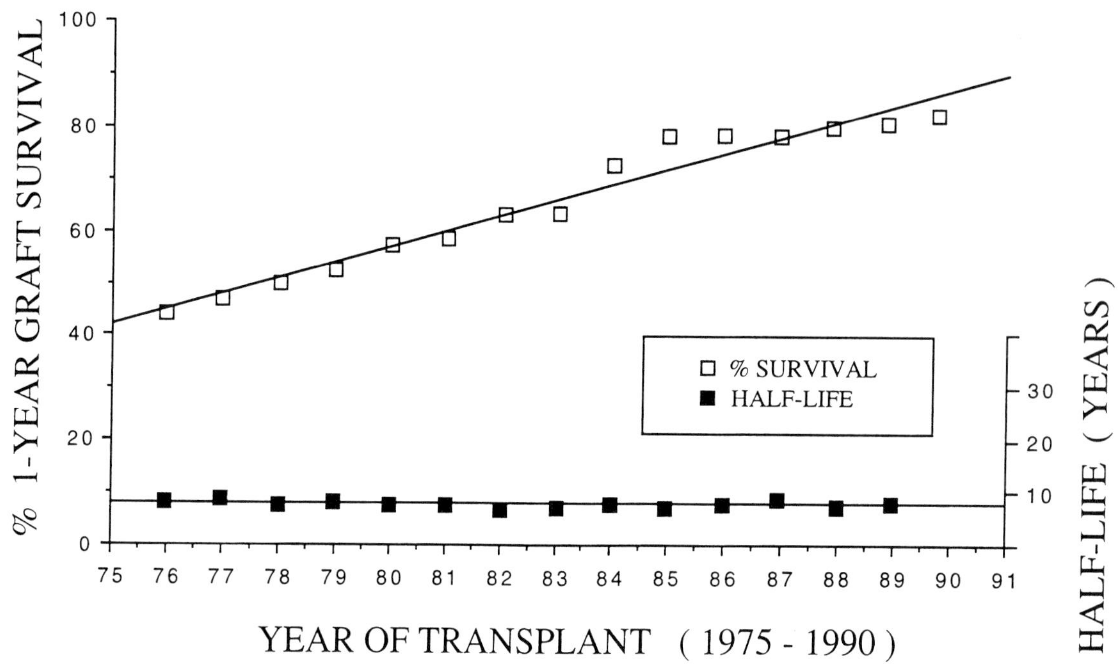

FIGURE 3.1. *The rate of deterioration and failure of organ allografts over the long-term has remained constant despite progressively improving 1-year survival rates. Although grafts fail over time for several reasons, the primary cause is chronic rejection. (Adapted from Giertson DW. Survival trends in long-term first cadaveric donor kidney transplants. In: Terasaki PI, ed. Clinical transplantation 1991. Los Angeles: UCLA Tissue Typing Laboratory, 1992:225.)*

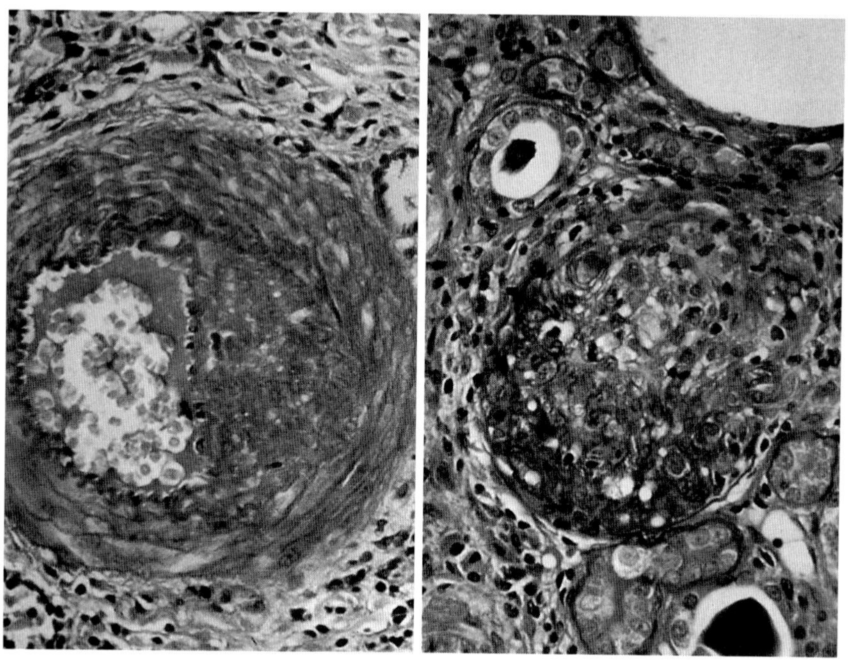

FIGURE 3.2. *The typical lesions of chronic rejection are here demonstrated in a kidney, showing both arterial and glomerular involvement. The arterial lesion is virtually identical to that seen in the coronary vessels of heart allografts. In the glomerulus, there is mesangial proliferation and occlusion of capillary spaces, leading to gradual glomerulosclerosis.*

kidney transplant for 6 months (9). The picture of arterial injury in the graft was similar to that seen in the kidneys of individuals with malignant hypertension or scleroderma, and was described as obliterative endarteritis secondary to proliferation of endothelium and myofibroblasts. Three comparable cases were reported in 1963 among chemically immunosuppressed recipients (10), and several cases were reported in 1964 among drug-treated canine recipients bearing long-standing allografts (11).

Early changes involve enlarged glomeruli with amorphous capillary (nonimmune) deposits beneath the basement membrane. Capillary lumina may narrow. Subsequent gradual functional deterioration occurs coincident with damage to the vascular endothelium, fibro-obliterative arterial lesions, and glomerular and parenchymal fibrosis (12,13). Glomerular changes, less consistent than those evolving in vessels (14–17), include decreased size (probably secondary to ischemia), folding and thickening of the capillary basement membrane, focal hyalinization, and fibrosis (12,18). Fibrinogen, immunoglobulin, and complement may be deposited in peritubular capillaries (12,19). These glomerular alterations evolving over time are probably less associated with major HLA incompatibilities than are the changes that develop during acute rejection; vesicoureteral reflux or hyperfiltration of glomeruli in a single kidney have been also implicated in their etiology (16,18). That such changes may develop on a nonimmunologic basis and not be secondary to recurrent or de novo glomerular disease has been shown in isografted (identical twin) kidneys in which the glomerular lesions of recurrent glomerulonephritis are different from those of chronic rejection, with prominent features including focal mesangial proliferation, increased mesangial matrix formation, and thickening (focal or diffuse) of the basement membranes (20–22). The lack of influence of such intrinsic nephritic processes has also been emphasized by the occurrence of the glomerular alterations of chronic rejection in allograft recipients who did not have glomerulonephritis as their primary renal disease (16,23,24).

Heart

In 1968, coronary artery arteriosclerosis developed in the second heart transplant recipient within a few months of engraftment, causing his death 19 months later (25,44). The donor was only 24 years old, but the recipient's autopsy revealed profound involvement of the coronary arteries. This type of lesion had already been observed in longstanding canine recipients of heart grafts. Because arteriosclerosis normally does not occur in dogs, chronic immune injury was postulated (26). Heart graft recipients afflicted with this condition may experience the sequelae of end-stage coronary artery disease: congestive heart failure, myocardial infarction, ventricular arrhythmias, and sudden death (27). No treatment has been forthcoming.

The lesion is characterized by diffuse fibrous intimal thickening in arteries and arterioles similar to that seen in kidney grafts (28–30). Unlike the type of arteriosclerosis developing in older patients, these abnormalities are usually concentric rather than focal, and often affect the entire coronary tree, including its small branches (Fig. 3.3 and Plate 2). However, proximal intimal plaques do sometimes occur. Histologically, cellular proliferation with variable deposition of collagen, ground substance, and lipid is noted. Varying acute inflammatory changes may be present, especially early in the process (31–33). As similar cell populations have been demonstrated in human arteriosclerotic lesions (34,35), terms such as "transplant arteriosclerosis" or "graft arteriosclerosis" have been used to describe transplant-related changes (36). The consistent finding of T cells and macrophages and the demonstration of immunoglobulin and complement deposition in affected vessel walls have suggested an immunologic basis for this process (28).

In addition, late fibrotic changes may appear throughout the myocardium. The late presence of collagen may be explained in several ways. Deposition of type I collagen in the myocardium of transplanted hearts has been correlated with the length of ischemic time, and type V collagen has been related to cyclosporine (CsA) dose. No correlation has been found with numbers of rejection episodes (37).

Liver

Chronic rejection of liver allografts develops in up to half of the recipients but contributes to only about 20% of graft

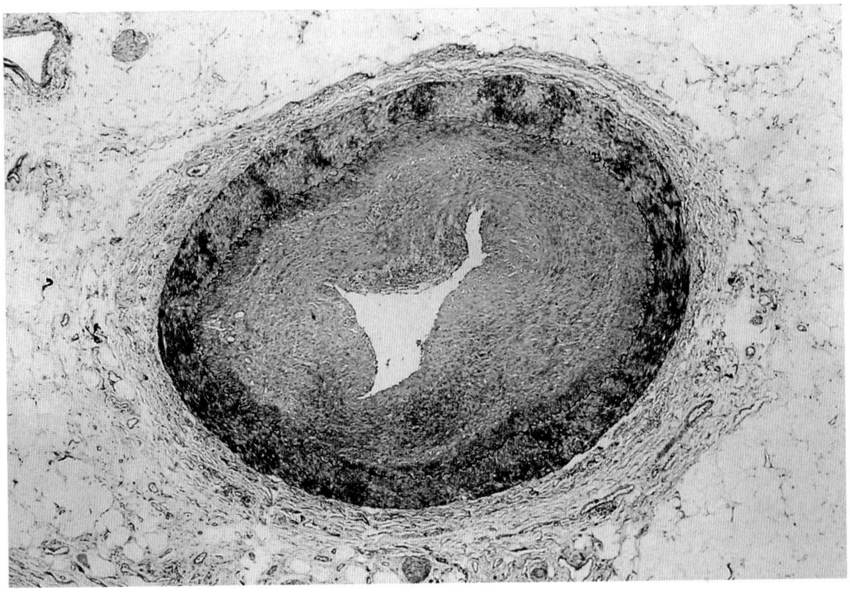

FIGURE 3.3. *Graft arteriosclerosis of cardiac allografts, the primary manifestation of chronic rejection in this organ, involves concentric myointimal proliferation involving the entire coronary arterial tree.*

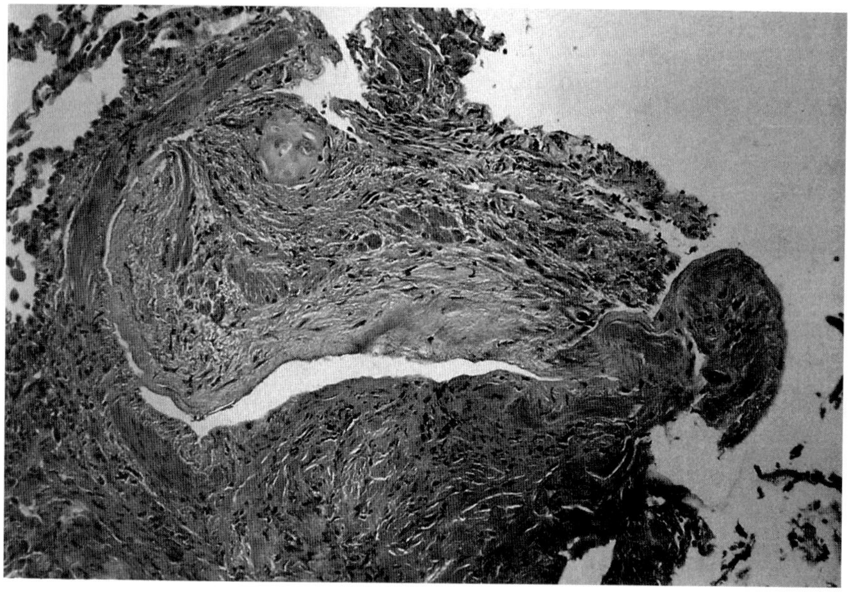

FIGURE 3.4. *Bronchiolitis obliterans is the most common manifestation of chronic rejection of lung allografts. Like graft arteriosclerosis, it involves gradual luminal obliteration of bronchi and bronchioles, with inflammatory cells, granulations, and hypertrophy of smooth muscle.*

failures (38,39). First described in 1981, the process was thought to occur on an immunologic basis because of its resemblance to changes of primary biliary cirrhosis or graft-versus-host disease (40). The lesions have been noted as early as 100 days after engraftment, and have been described as "acute vanishing bile duct syndrome" (6).

Clinically, the gradual development of relatively asymptomatic cholestatic jaundice is followed by increasing levels of serum bilirubin, alkaline phosphatase, and glutamyl transpeptidase. In contrast to acute rejection, where infiltration of inflammatory cells and epithelial cell changes involving both nuclei and organelles distort bile ducts (41), a characteristic of the chronic process is a progressive focal ductal occlusion that particularly involves the smaller interlobular bile ducts (38,40). Arteriosclerotic-like changes of vessels, including the larger branches of the hepatic artery, are closely associated with bile duct narrowing (42). The immunologic nature of this lesion is emphasized by T-cell infiltration of the vessel walls.

Lung

Patients with chronic rejection of lung allografts experience gradually increasing shortness of breath and cough, with decreased exercise tolerance (43,44). The chest roentgenogram is usually negative. Some authors have advocated increased use of steroids; others think that immunosuppression is not helpful (45). The term "bronchiolitis obliterans" was first used to describe the typical diffuse obstruction of terminal bronchioles developing, even after a relatively short time, in up to half of the long-surviving recipients of heart–lung grafts (44). The condition becomes manifest by a peribronchial inflammatory infiltrate, as well as epithelial ulceration with intraluminal plugs of mucus, necrotic cells, and granulation tissue (43). As the process evolves over time, infiltrating macrophages and lymphocytes decrease in number, and the bronchiolar lumina become progressively obliterated by fibrosis (Fig. 3.4 and Plate 3). Arteriosclerotic changes occur in small arteries and veins. Immunoglobulin or complement deposition is rare, although increased class I and class II major histocompatibility complex (MHC) antigens have been described in biopsies of the pulmonary vasculature and bronchiolar epithelium (46).

The phenomenon may be less common in single-lung allografts than after combined heart–lung transplantation, although data are as yet insufficient to establish this point. It remains puzzling that rejection of the heart in a combined heart/lung transplant occurs less frequently than after engraftment of the isolated heart, and that its involvement does not necessarily correlate with rejection of the lung (47).

PATHOPHYSIOLOGY OF CHRONIC REJECTION

The initial development of chronic rejection and associated vascular obliterative lesions has been conceptualized as consisting of three phases:

1. An antibody-mediated phase in which the donor organ is damaged by antibody or antigen–antibody complexes and complement
2. A period of cellular damage mediated first by T lymphocytes and later by macrophages
3. A phase of tissue remodeling dependent primarily on cytokines and growth factors (8,36)

Humoral Activity

The process of chronic rejection has long been thought to develop as a direct result of host humoral activity, since complement, immunoglobulins, and anti–endothelial cell antibodies have been noted in areas of intimal thickening and necrosis of vessel walls. A closer review of the literature, however, reveals that this concept is less clear, as such changes have been well documented in some studies but not in others (48). Although the presence of these humoral mediators may be nonspecific and reflect altered vascular permeability (49), it has recently been shown in heart grafts in severe combined immunodeficiency disease (SCID) mice that transfer of anti-donor antibody may cause graft arteriosclerosis (50). Indeed, it seems likely that an initial wave of antibody deposition after engraftment may produce early injury that may affect later events, as the ultimate progression of anti-donor antibody titers are usually decreased and may be absent thereafter in recipient serum. Peptide-specific anti-endothelial antibodies have been identified by Western blots in heart graft recipients with chronic rejection (51). Anti-HLA antibody immune complexes may be involved. Conversely, anti-idiotypic antibodies or broadly reactive anti-immunoglobulin autoantibodies may prevent chronic changes (52). The immunoglobulin responses of stimulated peripheral blood leukocytes are decreased in recipients of long-term well-functioning grafts. In contrast, T-cell–dependent B-cell responses are normal in patients with chronic rejection (53); the diminished B-cell response noted in those with stable graft function has been explained by increased T-suppressor activity and diminished T-helper effects (54). However, a monocyte defect may be more important, as this population may also be reduced significantly in patients with stable grafts (55).

Initial ischemia/reperfusion injury may influence later processes, with upregulation of inflammatory mediators that themselves may influence the presence of host antibodies. For instance, changes in the endothelial phenotype of ischemic tissues may trigger expression of new antigens that in time may cause immune complex deposition, activation of the classic complement pathway, and loss of membrane complement regulatory proteins (56). Antibodies may be activated by nonspecific stimuli, as in burned patients in whom increased titers produced by stimulated host lymphocytes parallel temporally upregulated complement activation (57,58). These humoral events may provoke a further inflammatory cascade (59).

Cells and Cell Products

During acute rejection episodes, which often occur relatively early following engraftment, an intense mononuclear cell infiltration of the foreign organ becomes evident, reflecting a host cellular immune response against incompatible graft antigens. In addition, the nonspecific ischemic/reperfusion injury may also cause infiltration of similar cell populations, which may act as a trigger for subsequent immune events. The numbers of graft-infiltrating cells then gradually diminish, coincident with the changes of chronic rejection (60). Although numbers of T lymphocytes associated with the earlier acute rejection episodes decline to relatively low levels, they and their products may continue to provide persisting low-grade immunologic responsiveness and ongoing subclinical injury to the graft over time. As noted in experimental models, this population may produce various effector cytokines, including RANTES, a macrophage chemoattractant.

Macrophages seem particularly important in the etiology of chronic rejection and other types of graft dysfunction. In human renal allografts experiencing the process, subendothelial plaques consisting of macrophages in foamy transformation have been described (61). Intimal foam cells, derived mostly from macrophages and to a lesser extent from smooth muscle cells, were prominent in the coronary lumina of heart grafts in cholesterol-fed and immunosuppressed rabbits (62). In a clinically relevant rat kidney allograft model, large numbers of monocyte/macrophages infiltrate the graft substance several weeks after transplantation; in isografts, macrophages increase progressively after a longer time period (Fig. 3.5) (63,64). Macrophage infiltration of both allografts and isografts has been associated with expression of their fibrosis-inducing products, including particularly interleukin (IL)-1, IL-6, tumor necrosis factor (TNF)-α, and macrophage chemoattractant protein (MCP)-1, and growth factors, especially basic fibroblast growth factor (bFGF) and transforming growth factor (TGFβ); expressed strongly both in glomeruli and in and around vessels (65), these products presumably contribute to progressive vascular hypertrophy, glomerulosclerosis, and fibrosis. Platelet-derived growth factor (PDGF) may also be involved. Adhesion molecules, primarily intracellular adhesion molecule (ICAM)-1 and vascular adhesion molecule (VCAM)-1, are present on glomerular capillary endothelium as well as other renal structures. Lymphocyte function–associated antigen (LFA)-1 and very late antigen (VLA)-4, upregulated on infiltrating cells along with other molecules, presumably direct the positioning of infiltrating host cell populations within the graft substance (63,66). Based on studies of experimental glomerulonephritis and of acute immunologic injury of kidney and heart grafts, it appears that chronic graft dysfunction, regardless of etiology, shares features similar to those in other inflammatory responses that involve the cytokine adhesion molecule cascade (67–69).

Graft Components

Individual graft components may respond differently to both initial and late injury. The vascular obliteration associated with chronic rejection, regardless of organ, is thought to derive from a vessel progressing through repetitive episodes of endothelial activation or cell injury, followed by repair, proliferation of smooth muscle cells and fibroblasts, and deposition of extracellular matrix proteins (8). Many of these events are similar to those occurring in atherosclerosis and may lead to concentric narrowing of the arterial lumina (67). Such vascular lesions may arise in response to focal vessel wall damage incurred by alloimmune reactions; however, similar lesions have been described in other con-

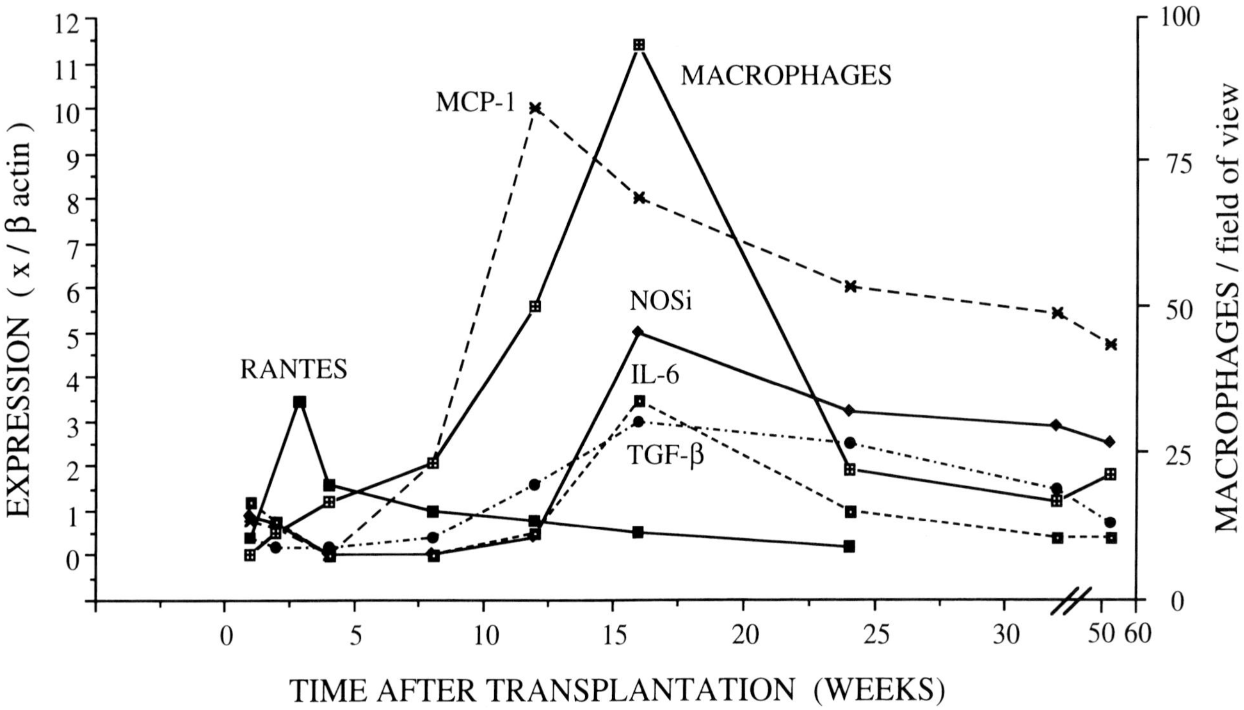

FIGURE 3.5. *The sequence of events of chronic rejection have been defined using a well-established and clinically relevant rat renal allograft model (63,65). The importance of macrophages and their products in the evolution of the process is demonstrated. After a T-cell mediated acute rejection episode at about 1 week, there is a sharp increase in the T-cell factor RANTES, a potent macrophage chemoattractant. This is followed by a sharper peak of MCP-1, another macrophage chemoattractant. There is then a dramatic influx of macrophages into the substance, followed by striking upregulation of fibrosis-inducing macrophage-derived factors, which presumably cause the structural changes of chronic rejection over the long term.*

ditions such as malignant hypertension, scleroderma, radiation nephritis, and hemolytic uremic syndrome (62), as well as in long-surviving isografts (20,70). Early upregulation of complement and adhesion molecules occurs independent of whether the initial stimulus is antigen dependent or independent in origin. Inflammatory products including leukotrienes and oxygen free radicals, elaborated by reperfusion events, probably amplify the insult.

Autoimmune responses against heat shock proteins induced on activated endothelial cells may also be important in the eventual development of graft arteriosclerosis (67). The phenotype of activated endothelial cells may change from those with anticoagulant surfaces to cells with procoagulant characteristics. Exposure of subendothelial collagen to platelets and circulating plasma proteins by endothelial cell denudation may also promote local coagulation and thrombus formation. As in acute rejection of organ allografts, fibrin deposition has been noted around infiltrating macrophages that produce tissue factor–related procoagulant (62); an ischemic insult may produce similar dynamics. Various cytokines, chemoattractants, and mediators are released by injured or activated endothelial cells, including thromboxanes, leukotrienes, growth factors including PDGF and platelet-activating factors, inducible nitric oxide synthase (NOSi), and elastin (59). Circulating leukocyte populations migrate to the area of injury via chemoattractants and adhesion molecules, diapedese into the vessel walls and perivascular spaces, and elaborate a further series of cytokines and growth factors that cause progression of the inflammatory and tissue remodeling processes leading to vascular compromise.

The glomerular lesions of chronic kidney graft rejection are variable and consist of focal or global changes (71). Infiltrating macrophages and their products, particularly IL-6 and various proinflammatory mediators, increase proliferation of mesangial cells and cause overproduction of mesangial matrix; indeed, IL-6 is the most potent mitogen for mesangium known (63). Altered eicosanoid metabolism by glomerular macrophages may accelerate the progression of early glomerular injury toward ultimate sclerosis. Hypertension may activate the glomerular capillary endothelium and increase the activities of cytokines and adhesion molecules (72). Gradual functional deterioration secondary to the development of glomerulosclerosis and vascular obliteration may also produce systemic hypertension, which may itself cause the remaining functioning glomeruli to hyperfilter before they eventually fibrose, establishing a self-sustaining vicious cycle of progressive deterioration (73). Interstitial fibrosis and tubular atrophy are nonspecific and may occur autonomously in the compromised and injured organ.

Thus, transplanted organs receiving an initial injury, regardless of etiology, may experience a gradual but progressive decline in function over months or years despite the continued use of immunosuppressive drugs. These changes seem to be related primarily to structural changes in various anatomic compartments and may have little correlation with host immunologic drive.

RISK FACTORS

Several potential risk factors have been implicated in the presumably multifaceted etiology of the chronic process (Table 3.1). These have been divided into antigen-dependent events such as the influence of HLA matching and early acute rejection, and antigen-independent factors including early ischemia/reperfusion injury, drug nephrotoxicity, viral infection, and other stimuli. The end result of all these forces is thought to be a reduction in the number of functioning nephron units, which may lead to hyperfiltration and gradual fibrosis of the remainder (Fig. 3.6). As a result, function of the graft deteriorates progressively.

Table 3.1. Risk Factors for Chronic Rejection of Kidney Grafts

Antigen Dependent
HLA matching
Acute rejection
Ongoing subclinical immunologic injury
Antigen Independent
Brain death
Ischemia/reperfusion injury
Inadequate renal mass (donor age, gender, race, organ size)
Hypertension and hyperlipidemia
Drug nephrotoxicity
CMV and other infections

Alloantigen-Dependent Events

The relatively prompt development of the characteristic findings of chronic rejection in allografts (both in well-controlled experimental systems and clinically), as compared to the relative lack of such changes in isografts, supports the notion that host immunologic responsiveness is an important factor in the process. In experimental heart transplantation, for instance, graft arteriosclerosis evolves more rapidly in recipients after immunization with donor splenocytes prior to engraftment (74). In human transplantation, antigenic differences between host and donor increase the possibility that chronic rejection will occur; renal allografts from cadavers are more likely to become affected than those from living-related sources (1). Similarly six HLA-antigen–matched cadaver-donor–recipient combinations do better over the long term than those that are less histocompatible (see Chapter 4).

Early acute rejection has been shown in many clinical series to be the critical antigen-driven risk factor for later chronic events (75,76). In one series, for instance, cadaver kidney recipients who had never experienced an early acute rejection episode had a 5-year graft survival of 92%, compared with 45% in recipients who had undergone one or more such crises (77). Two hypotheses have been proffered to explain the influence of ongoing subclinical immunologic rejection on later events. According to one, such activity may persist over time despite putatively sufficient immunosuppression. This continuing immune stimulation may allow indirect presentation of donor MHC peptides to increase

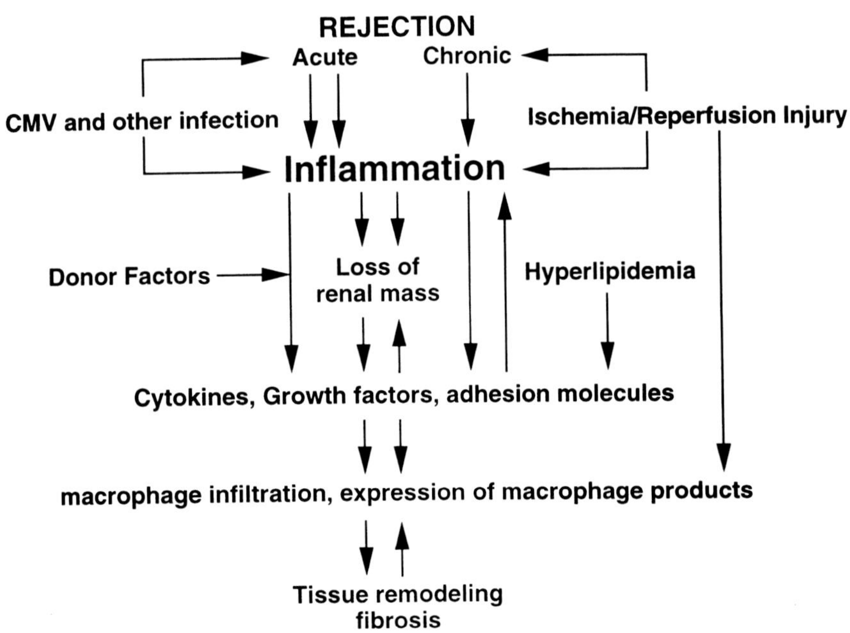

FIGURE 3.6. *The postulated cascade of events of chronic rejection is shown here. The grafted tissue may be injured in several ways within the first days of its placement. These involve both antigen-dependent and antigen-independent factors that may cause loss of renal mass. Various cells and their factors are upregulated, macrophages infiltrate, and their products ultimately produce the typical changes associated with the phenomenon.*

gradually (see Chapter 2). These peptides may be responsible for continuation and/or amplification of long-term host alloresponsiveness (78). Although donor MHC class II+ passenger leukocytes may have been depleted from the grafts, other populations expressing MHC may interact with recipient lymphocytes. A potential role for anti-MHC class I antibody produced by its shedding into the circulation during allograft rejection has been suggested (79).

Alternatively, ongoing immunologic injury from repeated subclinical acute rejection episodes may progressively reduce the amount of functioning nephron units, which may produce gradual organ deterioration over time in an autonomous "alloantigen-independent" fashion. This concept may also explain the later graft compromise secondary to early acute rejection injury.

Antigen-Independent Events

As there have been several suggestions, both experimentally and clinically, that the evolution of chronic rejection can be explained by more than continuing host alloresponsiveness alone, increasing attention is being paid to the influence of alloantigen-independent factors in the etiology of the condition. Indeed, the term "chronic rejection" may itself be a misnomer—"chronic graft dysfunction" may be a more accurate description of the phenomenon, as it is less specific and suggests a multifaceted etiology. Seemingly parallel events occurring in long-surviving renal isografts and allografts and after prolonged periods in kidneys that had experienced initial nonimmunologic injury will be emphasized in this section, because more information is available for kidneys than for other organ systems.

The chronic process appears to develop from various immunologic and nonimmunologic factors that cause the affected tissue to become remodeled in an aberrant and irreversible fashion. As already noted, the lower rate of attrition of grafts from living-related donors supports the notion that immunologic mechanisms related to histoincompatibility are key in the long-term results. It is difficult, however, to maintain this argument completely, because recent data have shown that the success rate of allografts from living-unrelated sources may be comparable to those of living-related origin (80). This unexpected observation suggests that as yet undefined factors associated with kidney procurement from brain-dead cadavers and more expeditious harvesting procedures may affect the eventual outcome (see Chapter 17).

The influence of alloantigen-independent events in chronic graft dysfunction has been emphasized by the observation that isografts may eventually develop functional and structural changes that resemble those of chronically rejecting allografts, albeit less intensely and at a slower tempo (64). A relatively large number (40% at 10 years) of human kidney transplants between identical twins were thought to fail secondary to recurrence of their primary renal disease (20). However, the original investigators also suggested that the late obliterative arterial changes and glomerulosclerosis observed in the deteriorated isografts may have been a consequence of other factors, including transplantation injury per se.

Experimentally, long-surviving kidney isografts in rats developed worsening functional, morphologic, and immunohistologic alterations that included progressive proteinuria associated with macrophage infiltration and upregulation of cytokines and growth factors, all changes similar to those occurring earlier in allografts (64). In related studies, kidney allografts and isografts were retransplanted back into donor strain animals at serial intervals after the original engraftment to determine at what stage the chronic lesions could be reversed by removing the continuing host immunologic drive (81). Structural abnormalities were reversible up to but not following a critical period when they not only did not diminish, but continued to progress. This latter finding emphasized the notion that injury beyond a certain physiologic threshold may become autonomous in the organ itself and worsen over time. Thus, the early stages of chronic rejection seem alloantigen dependent and reversible, whereas the later (presumably antigen-independent) changes are irreversible and progressive.

Finally, the advancing autonomous course of chronic renal transplant rejection may be similar to the changes noted in types of chronic kidney failure of disparate etiologies (82). Such potentially influential nonimmune factors include early injury secondary to prolonged ischemia and reperfusion, the long-term effects of diminished functioning renal mass, disorders of lipoprotein metabolism, cytomegalovirus infection, and the nephrotoxic effects of various immunosuppressive drugs (83).

Early Ischemia/Reperfusion Injury

Prolonged ischemia may influence later functional and morphologic changes in the kidney that resemble those of chronic rejection; indeed, 1-year graft survival is diminished in renal grafts with primary nonfunction (84,85). In addition, initial ischemia correlates with the number of reversible rejection episodes within that period. MHC expression after ischemia, particularly class II, may increase the immunogenicity of the allografted tissues and trigger subsequent host alloresponsiveness (86). MHC upregulation in isografts or in ischemic native kidneys may also lead to increased cellular infiltration and subsequent morphologic changes consistent with chronic rejection in allografts. In experimental models, function deteriorated steadily over time in recipients of kidney allografts subjected to early ischemia (60).

Several mechanisms may lead to organ injury from initial ischemia and reperfusion. Mildly ischemic kidneys perfused with primed neutrophils experience acute renal failure, presumably secondary to the effects of the inflammatory products of these cells (87). Adhesion molecules may play a critical role in the pathogenesis of myocardial reperfusion injury. Leukocytes infiltrate ischemic rat myocardium within 2 hours of reperfusion; ICAM-1 is expressed on capillary and venous endothelial cells (88). Levels of soluble epidermal growth factor (EGF) is considerably higher in ischemic kidneys than in uninjured organs. This factor may act in an autocrine or paracrine fashion to promote cell growth in the injured organ (89).

Clinically, kidney graft survival benefited significantly after administration of recombinant superoxide dismutase, which may inhibit the effects of oxygen free radicals from the anoxic tissues (90). As the incidence of acute rejection and early immunologic graft loss was also diminished, this agent may ameliorate the reperfusion injury and reduce graft immunogenicity by inhibiting upregulation of class II MHC antigen and adhesion molecule expression. In addition, long-term graft survival was markedly increased compared to kidneys in untreated hosts, again suggesting the importance of early injury on later events.

Little information is available on the systemic effects of brain death; however, it is possible that a massive release of inflammatory mediators, cytokines, and adhesion molecules into the circulation of such individuals could occur and potentially influence early and late behavior of donor organs. These factors may play a critical role in altering substantially the character of the vascular endothelium of the organ to be transplanted (91,92). Various growth factors that may influence healing, remodeling, and late changes in the vessel wall may be upregulated. For instance, both PDGF and bFGF induce cell migration and smooth muscle proliferation. Angiotensin II, a growth promoter for vascular smooth muscle cells, may affect myointimal proliferation following an injury, in part by increasing production of TGFβ, which stimulates production of collagens, fibronectin, and proteoglycans. The activities and mRNA levels of angiotensin-converting enzyme (ACE) are increased in the injured vessels, so ACE inhibitors have been suggested for ameliorating the process (93–95).

Fibrogenesis and fibrosis may be the end results of these initial injuries. These normal biologic events are involved physiologically in tissue repair but may occur in excess during progressive fibrosis. Several cytokines have been implicated in the process: TGFβ is critical, although TNF-α and IL-1 also enhance synthesis of extracellular matrix proteins. High concentrations of TGFβ contained in platelets are released at the site of injury or inflammation along with other platelet-derived growth factors. This cytokine is chemotactic for leukocytes and fibroblasts, stimulating these populations to secrete bFGF, another fibrosis-inducing product.

Our understanding of cell growth and extracellular matrix deposition in the kidney's response to insult, regardless of etiology, has also increased (96). Acute glomerular injury involves the activities of both cytokines and growth factors, particularly PDGF and TGFβ. The regeneration of tubules after an acute injury may proceed via EGF; upregulation of receptors for this and other growth factors enhances the growth potential of viable cells despite reduction in overall EGF production by the kidney. Tubular hypertrophy occurs infrequently among nephrons affected by the primary process. In contrast, low-grade ischemic insult may lead to tubular atrophy. Growth factors, elaborated and released by injured tubular cells, may stimulate adjacent fibroblasts to proliferate and deposit matrix proteins. The ensuing fibrotic changes may cause obliteration of peritubular capillaries and aggravate primary glomerular injury by compromising the vascular outflow from the glomerulus. This may account for the long-recognized association between tubulointerstitial injury and the progression of various renal diseases. Such events may contribute to both antigen-dependent and antigen-independent aspects of chronic graft dysfunction.

Hyperlipidemia

The influence of hyperlipidemia on the course of chronic rejection is controversial; indeed, how much is cause and how much is effect of steroids and other post-transplant factors is unknown. Hyperlipidemia, frequently occurring in cardiac transplant recipients, has been thought to be a potential risk factor for accelerated graft arteriosclerosis (97). Dialysis patients may exhibit several linked abnormalities. Hypercholesterolemia causes endothelial injury, increasing lipid accumulation and platelet adhesion. Plasma triglyceride levels may predict graft arteriosclerosis, and total low-density lipoproteins may portend a recurrence of arteriosclerosis in retransplanted heart graft recipients (see Chapter 31).

In chronically rejecting rat cardiac allografts, diffuse proliferative coronary lesions may develop independent of the serum lipid profile. Although lipid deposition in areas of intimal thickening was noted in animals fed a high-cholesterol diet, careful morphometric analysis failed to show a significantly different smooth muscle cell proliferative response compared to control groups (98). Hypercholesterolemia in the absence of hypertriglyceridemia influenced eicosanoid metabolism significantly; minor changes in smooth muscle cell proliferation in the wall of chronically rejecting rat aortic allografts were increased, although the overall extent of arteriosclerosis was not affected (99). A high-cholesterol diet and hyperlipidemia associated with nephrosis acted synergistically to alter macrophage function in this model, leading to secretion of vasoactive substances, cellular proliferation and fibrosis, and further damage to an already injured graft. Hypercholesterolemia has been associated with declining function in some clinical studies of renal transplant recipients, but not invariably (100). Dietary protein restriction may stabilize the function of kidney grafts experiencing chronic rejection, although its influence may be relatively transient.

Immunosuppressive Drugs

Some immunosuppressive agents also affect long-term changes in renal allografts. The nephrotoxic effects of CsA are well known but often have been difficult to differentiate from the chronic process (101). Tacrolimus (FK506) also seems to produce severe nephrotoxicity; for example, several patients who received small bowel transplants were treated with FK506, and they lost renal function and became dialysis dependent.

The development of accelerated graft arteriosclerosis has been linked to the use of these agents, both experimentally and clinically. However, endothelialitis and accelerated changes have been noted in the coronary vessels of failed cardiac transplants in both CsA-treated and untreated recipients, suggesting that hypercholesterolemia and hypertension may represent additional risk factors (102).

CsA-induced nephrotoxicity of the native kidneys, sometimes leading to overt failure, is manifested by focal glomerulosclerosis commensurate with reduced glomerular filtration rate and renal plasma flow (101). Interstitial inflammatory infiltrates of helper but not cytotoxic T cells, B cells, and macrophages are present in such kidneys, though the significance of this is unknown.

Aortic allografts in rats immunosuppressed with CsA develop early subendothelial inflammation followed by proliferation of smooth muscle cells, with intimal thickening and accelerated arteriosclerosis (103). Chronic immunosuppression with azathioprine and steroids does not evoke such morphologic alterations. It is interesting that the attrition rate of kidney allografts in human recipients treated with these latter agents parallels that of CsA-treated hosts (2). Although this may be explained, at least in part, by autonomous changes occurring in kidneys with inadequate functioning renal mass, it may also be that inadequate maintenance immunosuppression, regardless of drug, may allow persistent subclinical immunologic rejections that may adversely influence the chronic process (75).

In addition, side effects of high-dose steroids, including post-transplant diabetes mellitus, lipid abnormalities, and hypercholesterolemia, may develop (see Chapter 8). Glomerular capillary hypertension, exacerbated by steroid treatment in models of renal ablation, may lead to progressive renal failure (104).

Cytomegalovirus

Cytomegalovirus (CMV) is an important cause of increased morbidity and mortality in allograft recipients. It may play a role in chronic rejection by influencing vascular obliterative changes. Studies of endomyocardial biopsy specimens from human heart allografts, for instance, showed that CMV-linked immune activation and typical subendothelial inflammation may contribute to graft arteriosclerosis (105). Acute vascular rejection in CMV-infected heart transplant recipients has also been associated with a subendothelial inflammatory response in large epicardial arteries (106).

The mechanisms involved in the putative relationship between viral and perhaps other infections and rejection have been explained in several ways. A subgroup of kidney recipients with late acute rejection who were unresponsive to treatment showed the presence of large numbers of memory-type CD8 T cells in their peripheral blood associated with asymptomatic CMV infection; antiviral therapy improved graft function in the majority (107). An immediate early gene of the virus able to code for a protein with sequence homology and immunologic cross-reactivity with the HLA-DR β chain may increase the alloimmune response of the host to donor antigens (108). In addition, CMV encodes a glycoprotein homologous to the heavy chain of class I MHC antigen that can bind to its light chain (109). Active infection has been strongly associated with expression of VCAM-1 on capillary endothelium (110). Its effects on leukocyte adhesion and infiltration may contribute to long-term changes in the graft. Cytokines associated with the inflammatory response of CMV infection may also increase endothelial cell damage and vasculopathic changes (see Chapter 36).

The Common Denominator: Functioning Renal Mass

As early or ongoing injury, regardless of type, may decrease the functioning renal mass, the amount remaining may be critical in the eventual outcome of the allograft (111). Donor factors, ischemia and reperfusion, acute rejection, hypertension, and CsA nephrotoxicity have all been implicated in affecting ultimate graft behavior (see Table 3.1). Experimentally, many of the characteristic features of chronic rejection (hypertension, proteinuria, and gradual functional deterioration associated with glomerulosclerosis, tubular atrophy, and interstitial fibrosis) are also typical of those occurring in kidney allografts, kidney isografts, and native kidneys, where all the functional and structural changes associated with chronic rejection evolve at an accelerated rate relatively independent of graft immunogenicity (112). Chronic hyperfiltration by the remaining nephrons initiates a vicious cycle of injury progressing through increasing dysfunction to end-stage renal failure (Fig. 3.7). Conversely, at least experimentally, an intact allograft functioning in the presence of excess renal mass (a retained native kidney or two allografted kidneys) develops few chronic changes over time, the extra nephron mass presumably preventing the autonomous progression of antigen-independent events (113,114). Some early, seemingly beneficial clinical results of transplanting both kidneys from "marginal donors" may emphasize this point (see Chapter 15).

A recent analysis of the effects of the kidney weight–to–body weight ratio in human renal transplantation has confirmed many of these concepts (115). Grafts most at risk for chronic dysfunction over the long term include those from very young (<3 years) or elderly (>60 years) donors. This result may be explained by reduced filtration associated with the small and immature nephrons of pediatric kidneys, which may be unable to tolerate adult levels of renal perfusion, and by age-dependent sclerotic changes in older donors with diminished numbers of functioning nephrons (111). Renal grafts from female donors and from black donors (which have fewer nephrons than those of whites) also have relatively poor results when placed in large male recipients.

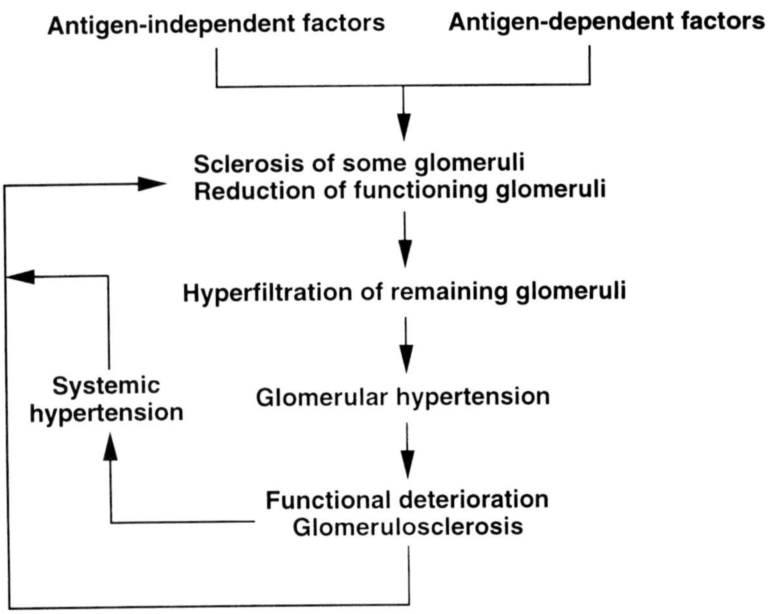

FIGURE 3.7. *During the later course of chronic rejection, remaining functioning nephron units hyperfunction and hyperfilter. Glomerular hypertension is present with gradual functional deterioration of those nephrons, progressive glomerulosclerosis, systemic hypertension, and the vicious cycle of graft deterioration.*

Thus, it may be that not only should donor and host be matched by immunologic criteria, but also that donor kidneys should be distributed on the basis of their predicted physiologic adequacy. The former may improve long-term results based on antigen-dependent criteria, while the latter may reduce antigen-independent variables. In practical terms, such a scheme seems unrealistic in this age of inadequate organ supply. However, if successful xenotransplantation ever becomes a reality, the role of functioning kidney mass may be considered for improving long-term success.

It should be noted in this context, however, that a single uncompromised kidney can continue to function satisfactorily over time. Presumably, there is a critical level of renal mass below which deleterious physiologic and morphologic changes begin to develop. When the behavior of the remaining kidney of living donors was evaluated at >20 years after donation, function was generally unchanged and the frequency of hypertension not higher than that in the general population or amongst sibling controls. A few individuals had developed proteinuria (116). In contrast, although the long-term function of the remaining segment of a solitary kidney that has been partially ablated in patients with bilateral renal cell or transitional cell carcinoma generally remains stable in the short term, some individuals develop increasing proteinuria, glomerulopathy, and progressive renal failure—all changes characteristic of chronic rejection (117).

COMMENTARY

Pekka Häyry

Nicholas Tilney has been a leading expert in the pathophysiology of rejection for nearly 25 years. Upon reading this chapter, I note with admiration how he has been able to cover this difficult topic logically and in detail, yet succinctly. He brings the reader up to date with the pathology of chronic rejection in kidney, heart, liver, and lung transplantation, complete with a description of the pathophysiology of these changes. He dissects the molecular cascades in regard to the host and the graft, emphasizing the role of inflammatory leukocytes (particularly macrophages), cytokines, and growth factors in the development of the pathologic alterations. This discussion is followed by a careful analysis of the risk factors leading to chronic rejection, wherein these risk factors are logically placed in his framework and are analyzed as to how they modulate the cellular and molecular events.

At present it is not possible to describe the molecular cascades in any more detail. We must admit that, even now, the understanding of the pathophysiology of chronic rejection remains primarily descriptive in nature. With time, we will learn to block the various molecules, their ligands, and/or their receptors as expressed in chronically rejecting allografts. We will thereby be able to discover rate-limiting molecules and genes that may be exploited as potential therapeutic targets in the treatment of chronic rejection.

My major comments on Tilney's excellent review will focus on his final interpretation, where I believe that he underestimates the role of acute rejection in allograft arteriosclerosis and overestimates the role of functioning renal mass.

THE TILNEY MODEL

There are two ways for a cell to respond to injury: divide or die. Cell death (via necrosis) is usually followed by fibrotic alterations, and at organ level most of the histologic changes seen in chronically rejecting organ allografts are nonspecific in nature. These changes are rather similar in a variety of other pathologic conditions, regardless of the nature of the original injury.

Of the three types of risk factors—immunologic, extraimmunologic, and infectious—it appears that acute rejection may still be the most important one in kidney transplantation, although geographical variations appear to exist (1). Moreover, it seems that some of the nonimmunologic risk factors, particularly ischemia and reperfusion injury, may not be independent risk factors but rather affect the modifiers via increased immune response. As Tilney clearly states, ischemia/reperfusion injury induces the expression of a whole variety of proinflammatory molecules in rat kidney (2), and these molecules, in turn, induce the transplants to undergo more acute rejection episodes than occur without injury (3).

The major risk factor in heart transplantation is cytomegalovirus (CMV) infection (4). CMV infection is accompanied, in humans (5,6) and in experimental vascular (7) and cardiac (8) transplantation models, with persistent subendothelial "endothelialitis" and perivascular inflammation. The inflamed vessels of CMV-infected recipients seem to express, or overexpress, the same growth factors seen in chronically rejecting transplants without CMV infection (9).

As he is most familiar with renal transplantation, Tilney's final comments have this model primarily in mind. He provides very sound arguments that the size of functioning renal mass is critical and is perhaps the major risk factor determining the eventual outcome of the allograft:

1. Fibrotic vascular glomerular changes are seen also in isografts and in native (aged) kidneys.
2. Several epidemiologic studies have clearly demonstrated that female-to-male transplants, transplants from black donors (who have fewer nephrons than whites), and transplants from very young and elderly donors have relatively poor results (particularly when placed in large male patients).
3. In the rat, functioning recipient kidney protects an allograft from proteinuria (and subsequent chronic rejection), and double transplants do better than single or partial transplants in the F344-to-Lewis renal transplant model.

There are, however, some inconsistencies in the Tilney model, which are discussed below.

Lesions

As I have already stated, fibrotic glomerular changes, as well as vascular sclerosis and interstitial fibrosis (seen also in heart and liver allografts), are nonspecific alterations and common to many different forms of injury. Thus, the fact that the lesions look similar is not proof for or against a similar or dissimilar etiology.

Renal Mass

Without question, the epidemiologic findings are correct: reduced renal mass may contribute to chronic rejection and/or short graft survival. However, in none of the epidemiologic studies regarding (presumed) reduced renal mass have the patients been stratified for acute episodes of rejection. In particular, no such studies are available where the patterns and intensities of acute rejection have been analyzed in the above-mentioned donor-recipient combinations, preferably using protocol core biopsy.

In the few studies where protocol core biopsy has been employed, it appears that the incipient vascular and glomerular changes consistent with chronic rejection histopathology are also frequently seen in stable renal transplants (10–12). Furthermore, the (nonspecific) parenchymal alterations considered characteristic of chronic rejection are virtually always accompanied by low-level inflammation in the vascular periphery, indicating (as suggested also by Tilney), a persistent low-level immunologic insult to the transplant.

A mismatch between the body's metabolic demands and the renal mass available to deal with these demands results in a number of adaptive changes, including glomerular hyperfiltration and hypertension, glomerular hypertrophy, increased glomerular permeability, changes in intrarenal metabolism, and lipoprotein disorders secondary to proteinuria and uremia. These changes may in turn lead to structural damage (13).

Finally, it is hard to believe that insufficient renal mass would be somehow linked to chronic rejection in heart and liver transplants, where strikingly similar vascular and parenchymal changes are seen.

Immune Mechanisms

Several of the adaptive changes associated with insufficient renal mass have been demonstrated by Tilney and others (14) using various forms of renal ablation and transplantation. Thus, both immune and nonimmune mechanisms are involved, but the contribution of each of these factors and their mutual interdependence remain unresolved.

Tilney has been treating recipient rats with a low dose of cyclosporine for a limited time interval, which is not expected to influence immunoresponsiveness. Caution should be exercised in this model—the donor and recipient strains are phenotypically MHC compatible, reciprocal immunizations do not result in hemagglutinating antibodies against class I locus products, and the donor and recipient are nonstimulatory in mixed lymphocyte reactions. A short course of immunosuppression in such combinations may result in profound changes in immunoresponsiveness. While questions regarding the relevance of various experimental models in use to study chronic rejection are beyond the scope of the present discussion, administration of immunosuppressive drugs may erroneously lead to the conclusion that immunologic factors are not important in chronic rejection.

Paul's group (15) used the same donor–recipient combination as used in Tilney's experiments, and the recipient animals were randomized to receive no treatment, antihypertensive drugs that lower the glomerular pressure, or cyclosporine. Whereas antihypertensive drugs, especially drugs that inhibit the formation or action of angiotensin II, inhibited glomerular and to some extent vascular sclerosis, long-term cyclosporine (CsA) in relatively high doses prevented both inflammatory and sclerotic lesions as well as the development of glomerular hypertension. It remains to be established that these rat data are relevant to humans, but the data suggest that immunologic factors are of prime importance in chronic rejection.

Tilney and associates have also demonstrated that their hypothesis is not consistent with experimental findings (16): if a F344-to-Lewis kidney allograft is retransplanted back to the donor strain (prior to a given time point after transplantation), these transplants never develop proteinuria or chronic rejection. Yet, these transplants have undergone a double nonimmune insult (in other words, two transplantations) and they should be particularly prone to chronic rejection.

ALTERNATE MODEL

To overcome what I see as interpretation difficulties in Tilney's excellent review, I would like to propose an alternate model (Fig. 3C.1) for comparison with Tilney's model (Fig. 3C.2).

All forms of injury—immunologic, infectious, and/or mechanical—induce inflammation. Nonimmunologic

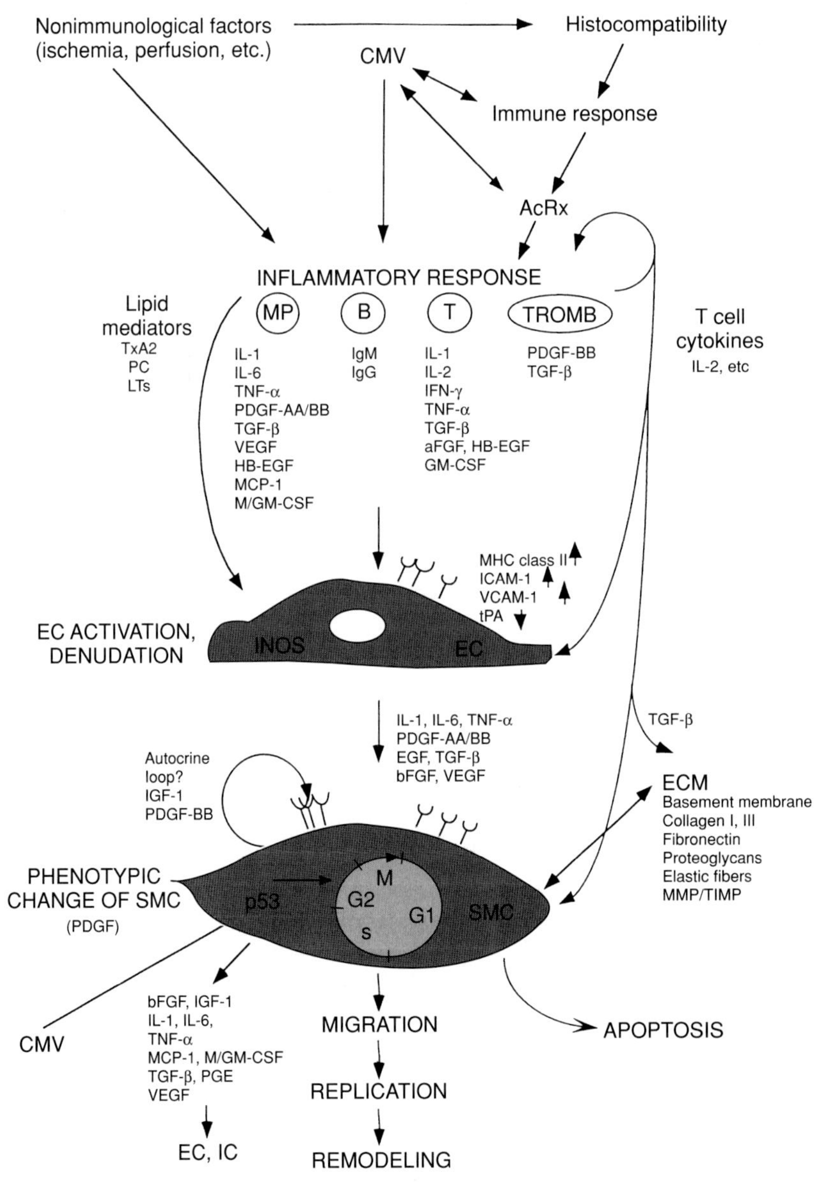

FIGURE 3C.1. *Summary of the major pathways of smooth muscle cell regulation in allograft arteriosclerosis (chronic rejection). The etiology of chronic rejection is most likely multifactorial. We hypothesize that nonimmune and immune inflammation induce persistent low-grade damage to vascular endothelium, which (in concert with inflammatory and smooth muscle cells) begins to secrete growth factors and cytokines to repair the damage. This results in neighboring smooth muscle cell replication in the vascular wall, the influx of myocytes from the media into the intima, and generation of an arteriosclerotic lesion. Within the arterial wall, smooth muscle cells are embedded in and associated with a complex network of noncellular structural elements, called the extracellular matrix (ECM). The ECM is in a steady state of production and degradation. The degradation is mediated by a gene family of proteolytic enzymes called matrix metalloproteinases (MMP), which are secreted as inactive zymogens. They are activated by proteolytic cleavage reactions and their activity is also regulated by a family of specific protein inhibitors, that is, tissue inhibitors of metalloproteinases (TIMP). AcRX, acute rejection; EC, endothelial cells; HB-EGF, heparin-binding epidermal growth factors; iNOS, inducible nitrogenoxide synthetase; LT, leukotrines; MP, macrophages; thromb, thrombocytes; SMC, smooth muscle cells; PC, prostacyclins; TxA2, thromboxane A_2. (Reproduced with permission from Lemström K, Koskinen P, Häyry P. Molecular mechanism of chronic renal allograft rejection. Kidney Int 1995;48:S2–S10.)*

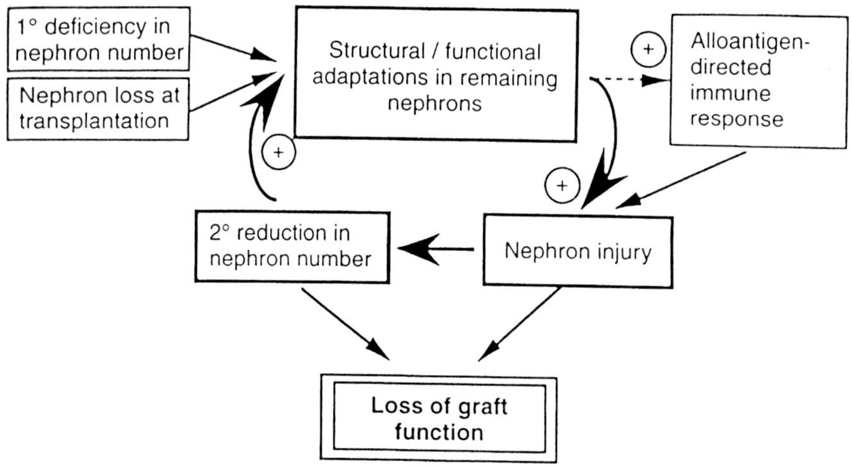

FIGURE 3C.2. *An attempt to integrate injury process initiated by reduced renal mass and the response to alloantigens. Primary deficiency in nephron number may arise through donor factors such as innate deficiency or arteriosclerosis, compounded by losses through ischemic injury and acute rejection and the shortfall already imposed by replacing the workload of two kidneys with a single kidney. The resulting cycle of adaptive changes in surviving nephrons, injuring and ultimately obliterating glomeruli, may amplify the effects of nephron injury through antigen-specific mechanisms. (Source: MacKenzie H, Azuma H, Renneke HG, et al. Renal mass as a determinant of late allograft outcome: insights from experimental studies in rats. Kidney Int 1995;48:S38–S42.)*

etiologies such as ischemia/reperfusion injury also upregulate proinflammatory molecules in graft endothelial cells, leading to increased histoincompatibility and more frequent or severe acute rejection episodes, which contribute again to inflammation. This intragraft inflammation, as shown by Tilney, is T-cell dominated in acute rejection. During chronic rejection, the inflammation localizes more to the vascular periphery or subendothelium. It persists but is lower in intensity, and the level of activation of macrophages predominates over activation of lymphoid cells.

As a consequence of inflammation, regardless of whether it is due to mechanical, immunologic, or infectious injury, the endothelial cells are activated and they express a number of proinflammatory molecules on their surface. To defend themselves against the injury, the endothelial cells (in concert with smooth muscle and inflammatory cells) produce growth factors to repair the lesion. Smooth muscle cells and/or mesangial cells, being in close proximity to endothelial cells, respond to the growth factors by replication, apoptosis, or migration into the subintima in the arterial wall.

The extracellular matrix has an important role in this process, because it must be degraded by smooth muscle cells to provide them access into the intima. Smooth muscle cells express matrix metalloproteinases (17), which may be inhibited or stabilized by tissue inhibitors of matrix metalloproteinases (17,18). The extracellular matrix also provides the heparin-binding growth factors to smooth muscle cells, which may contribute to the induction of their replication and migration.

The final mediators appear to be a (possibly limited) group of smooth muscle cell growth factors, including thrombin, angiotensin II, EGF, platelet-derived growth factor A and B, and insulin-like growth factor 1. The relative importance of these growth factors in the replicatory and migratory process is still incompletely known.

There are two possible angles from which this question can be approached. First, one could modulate the growth factor expression, probably at the messenger RNA level. Second, one could block their receptors either at the level of the receptor (for example, with antibodies or peptides) or at the level of their receptor-specific tyrosine-kinases. According to our current, still-limited information, it appears that the receptors of these growth factors, rather than their ligands, are rate-limiting molecules in the vascular wall (and probably also in the glomerular response) and that the receptors are more likely targets than their ligands in developing new therapies for chronic allograft rejection.

ACKNOWLEDGMENTS

The author is indebted to Drs. Leendert Paul, Karl Lemström, Petri Koskinen, Bengt Fellström, and Eero Taskinen for reading this manuscript and for their valuable contributions.

CHAPTER REFERENCES

1. Cecka JM, Terasaki PI. The UNOS scientific renal transplant registry. In: Terasaki PI, Cecka JM, eds. Clinical transplants 1994. Los Angeles: UCLA Tissue Typing Laboratory:1–18.
2. Giertson DW. Survival trends in long-term first cadaveric donor kidney transplants. In: Terasaki PI, ed. Clinical transplantation 1991. Los Angeles: UCLA Tissue Typing Laboratory, 1992:225.
3. Häyry P, Isonemi H, Yilmaz J, et al. Chronic allograft rejection. Immunol Rev 1993;134:5–19.

4. Paul LC, Benediktsson H. Chronic transplant rejection: magnitude of the problem and pathogenetic mechanisms. Transplant Rev 1993;7:96–113.
5. Hosenpud JD, Norick RT, Preen TJ, et al. The registry of the International Society for Heart and Lung Transplantation: eleventh official report, 1994. J Heart Lung Transplant 1994;13:561.
6. Ludwig J, Wiesner RH, Patts KP, et al. The acute vanishing bile duct syndrome (acute irreversible rejection) after orthotopic liver transplantation. Hepatology 1987;7:476.
7. Tilney NL, Whitley WD, Diamond JR, et al. Chronic rejection—an undefined conundrum. Transplantation 1991;52:389.
8. Fellstrom B, Larsson E, Tufveson G. Strategies in chronic rejection of transplanted organs: a current view on pathogenesis, diagnosis and treatment. Transplant Proc 1991;23:613.
9. Hume DM, Merrill JP, Miller PF, et al. Experiences with renal homotransplantation in the human: report of nine cases. J Clin Invest 1955;34:327.
10. Murray JE, Merrill JP, Harrison JH, et al. Prolonged survival of human kidney homografts by immunosuppressive drug therapy. N Engl J Med 1963;68:1315.
11. Porter KA, Calne RY, Zukoski CF. Vascular and other changes in 200 canine renal homotransplants treated with immunosuppressive drugs. Lab Invest 1964;13:809.
12. Busch GJ, Galvanek E, Reynolds ES Jr. Human renal allografts: analysis of lesions in long-term survivors. Hum Pathol 1971;2:253.
13. Lindquist RR, Guttman RD, Merrill JP, et al. Human renal allografts: interpretation of morphological and immunohistochemical observations. Am J Pathol 1968;53:851.
14. Sibley RK, Payne W. Morphologic findings in the renal allograft biopsy. Semin Nephrol 1985;5:294.
15. Hulme B, Andres GA, Porter KA, et al. Human renal transplants. IV. Glomerular ultrastructure, macromolecular permeability, and hemodynamics. Lab Invest 1972;26:2.
16. Mathew TH, Mathew DC, Hobbs JB, et al. Glomerular lesions after renal transplantation. Am J Med 1975;59:177.
17. Verani RR, Bergman D, Kerman RH. Glomerulopathy in acute and chronic rejection: relationship of ultrastructure to graft survival. Am J Nephrol 1983;3:253.
18. Dunnill MS. Histopathology of rejection in renal transplantation. In: Morris PJ, ed. Kidney transplantation. 2nd ed. London: Grune & Stratton, 1984:355.
19. Porter KA, Andres GA, Calder MW, et al. Human renal transplants. II. Immunofluorescent and immunoferritin studies. Lab Invest 1968;18:159.
20. Glassock RJ, Feldman D, Reynolds ES Jr., et al. Human renal isografts: a clinical and pathologic analysis. Medicine (Baltimore) 1968;47:411.
21. Porter KA, Dossetor JB, Marchioro TL, et al. Human renal transplants. I. Glomerular changes. Lab Invest 1967;16:153.
22. Andres GA, Accinni L, Hsu KC, et al. Human renal transplants. III. Immunopathologic studies. Lab Invest 1979;22:588.
23. Hamburger J, Crosier J, Noel LH. Recurrent glomerulonephritis after renal transplantation. Ann Rev Med 1978;29:67.
24. Peterson VP, Olsen TS, Kissmeyer-Nielson F, et al. Late failure of human renal transplants. Medicine (Baltimore) 1975;54:45.
25. Bernhart GR, Pascoe EA, Mills AS, et al. Accelerated coronary arteriosclerosis in cardiac transplant recipients. Transplant Rev 1987;1:31.
26. Kosek JC, Hurley ET, Lower RR. Histopathology of orthotopic canine cardiac homograft. Lab Invest 1968;19:97.
27. Gao SZ, Shroeder JS, Hunt S, et al. Retransplantation for severe accelerated coronary artery disease in heart transplant recipients. Am J Cardiol 1988;62:876.
28. Palmer DC, Tsai CC, Roodman ST, et al. Heart graft arteriosclerosis. Transplantation 1985;39:385.
29. Billingham ME, Masek MA, Khanna K, et al. Long-term cardiac allograft pathology in human. Lab Invest 1980;42:103.
30. Johnson DE, Shao Zhou G, Schroeder JS, et al. The spectrum of coronary artery pathologic findings in human cardiac allografts. J Heart Transplant 1989;8:349.
31. Oguma S, Banner B, Zerbe T, et al. Participation of dendritic cells in vascular lesions of chronic rejection of human allografts. Lancet 1988;2:933.
32. Hruban RH, Beschorner WE, Baumgartner WA. Accelerated arteriosclerosis in heart transplant recipients is associated with a T-lymphocyte-mediated endothelialitis. Am J Pathol 1990;137:871.
33. Usy CJ, Rose AG. Cardiac transplantation: aspects of the pathology. Pathol Annu 1983;17:147.
34. Jonasson L, Helm J, Skalli O, et al. Regional accumulations of T cells, macrophages, and smooth muscle cells in human atherosclerotic plaque. Arteriosclerosis 1986;6:131.
35. Gown AM, Tsukada T, Ross R. Human atherosclerosis. II. Immunocytochemical analysis of the cellular composition of human atherosclerotic lesions. Am J Pathol 1986;125:191.
36. Feogh ML. Chronic rejection—graft arteriosclerosis. Transplant Proc 1990;22:119.
37. Tazelaar HD, Gay RE, Rowan RA, et al. Collagen profile in the transplanted heart. Hum Pathol 1990;21:424.
38. Snover DC, Sibley RK, Freese DK, et al. Orthotopic liver transplantation: a pathological study of 63 serial liver biopsies from 17 patients with special reference to the diagnostic features and natural history of rejection. Hepatology 1984;4:1212.
39. Jenkins RL. Liver transplantation in the adult. Transplant Rev 1987;1:1.
40. Fennell RH. Ductular damage in liver transplant rejection. Pathol Annu 1981;16:289.
41. Vierling JM, Fennell RH. Histopathology of early and late human hepatic allograft rejection: evidence of progressive destruction of interlobular bile ducts. Hepatology 1985;6:1076.
42. Demetris AJ, Lasky S, Thiel DHV, et al. Pathology of hepatic transplantation. Am J Pathol 1985;118:151.
43. Yousem SA, Burke CM, Billingham ME. Pathologic pulmonary alterations in long-term human heart-lung transplantation. Hum Pathol 1985;16:911.
44. Griffith BP, Paradis IL, Zeevi A, et al. Immunologically mediated disease of the airways after pulmonary transplantation. Ann Surg 1988;208:371.
45. Yacoub MH, Banner NR. Recent developments in living heart-lung transplantation. Transplant Rev 1989;3:1.
46. Taylor TM, Rose ML, Yacoub M. Expression of class I and class II MHC antigens in normal transplanted human lungs. Transplant Proc 1989;21:451.
47. Baldwin JC, Oyer PE, Stenson EB, et al. Comparison of cardiac rejection in heart and heart-lung transplantation. J Heart Transplant 1987;6:352.
48. Taylor DO, Ibrahim HM, Tolman DR, Hess ML. Accelerated coronary arteriosclerosis in cardiac transplantation. Transplant Rev 1991;5:165.
49. Higgy NA, Davidoff AW, Grothman GT, et al. Platelet derived growth factor-receptor expression in rat heart allografts. J Heart Lung Transplant 1991;10:1012–1022.
50. Russel PS, Chase CM, Winn HJ, Colvin RE. Coronary atherosclerosis in transplanted mouse heart. II. The importance of humoral immunity. J Immunol 1994;152:5135–5141.
51. Rose ML. Antibody mediated rejection following cardiac transplantation. Transplant Rev 1993;7:140.
52. Suci-Foca N, Reed E, D'Agati VD, et al. Soluble HLA antigens, anti-HLA antibodies, and anti-idiotypic antibodies in the circulation of renal transplant recipients. Transplantation 1991;51:593–601.
53. Llandsberg DN, Bush LE, Cardella CJ. In vitro immunoglobulin production in long-term renal transplant recipients. Transplantation 1985;39:389.
54. Weimer R, Pomer S, Staehler G, et al. Increased T suppressor activity in renal transplant recipients with long-term stable graft function. Clin Transplant 1990;4:280.
55. Weimer R, Zipperle S, Daniel V, et al. IL-6 independent monocyte/B cell defect in renal transplant recipients with long-term stable graft function. Transplantation 1994;57:54.
56. Väkevä A, Laurila P, Meri S. Regulation of complement membrane attack complex formation in myocardial infarction. Am J Pathol 1993;143:65–75.
57. Moore FD Jr, Davis C, Rodrick M, Mannick JA, Fearon DT. Neutrophil activation in thermal injury as assessed by complement receptor upregulation. N Engl J Med 1986:314:948–952.
58. Davis CF, Moore FD Jr, Rodrick ML, et al. Neutrophil activation after burn injury: contributions of the classic complement pathway and of endotoxin. Surgery 1987;102:477–484.
59. Wiles ME, Hechtman HE, Morel NML, Shepro D. Hypoxia reoxygenation-induced injury of cultured pulmonary microvessel endothelial cells. J Leukocyte Biol 1993;53:490–497.
60. Tullius SG, Heemann UW, Azuma H, Tilney NL. Early ischemic injury leads to long-term functional and morphological deterioration in naive rat kidney and may influence chronic rejection. Transplant Proc 1994;26: 2041.
61. Dimony E, Fellstrom B, Larsson S, et al. Hyperlipoproteinuria in renal transplant recipients: is there a linkage with chronic vascular rejection? Transplant Proc 1993;25:2065.
62. Sasaguri S, Yoshinobu E, Tsakada T, et al. Role of smooth muscle cells and macrophages in cardiac allograft arteriosclerosis in rabbits. J Heart Transplant 1990;9:18.
63. Hancock WW, Whitley DW, Tullius SG, et al. Cytokines, adhesion molecules, and the pathogenesis of chronic rejection of rat renal allografts. Transplant 1993;56:643.

64. Tullius SG, Heemann UW, Hancock WW, et al. Long-term kidney isografts develop functional and morphological changes which mimic those of chronic allograft rejection. Ann Surg 1994;220:425.
65. Nadeau KC, Azuma H, Tilney NL. Sequential cytokine dynamics in chronic rejection of rat renal allografts: Roles for cytokines RANTES and MCP-1. Proc Natl Acad Sci USA 1995;92:8729–8733.
66. Heemann UW, Tullius SG, Azuma A, et al. Infiltration patterns of macrophages and lymphocytes in chronically rejecting rat kidney allografts. Transplant Int 1994;7:349.
67. Ross R. The pathogenesis of atherosclerosis: a perspective for the 1990's. Nature 1993;362:801.
68. Brady HR, Spertini O, Junenez W, et al. Neutrophiles, monocytes and lymphocytes bind to cytokine activated kidney glomerular endothelium all through L-selectin (LAM-I) in vitro. J Immunol 1992;149:2437.
69. Briscoe DM, Schoen FJ, Rice GE, et al. Induced expression of endothelial-leukocyte adhesion molecules in human cardiac allografts. Transplant 1991;51:537.
70. Porter KA. Renal transplantation. In: Heptinstall RH, ed. Pathology of the kidney. 4th ed. Boston: Little, Brown, 1992:1799–1933.
71. Cheigh JS, Mouradian J, Soliman M, et al. Focal segmental glomerulosclerosis in renal transplants. Am J Kidney Dis 1983;2:449–455.
72. Ponticeili C, Montagnino G, Aroldi A, et al. Hypertension after renal transplantation. Am J Kid Dis 1993;21(suppl 2):73.
73. Brenner BM, Milford EL. Nephron underdosing: a programmed cause of chronic renal allograft failure. Am J Kidney Dis 1993;21:66.
74. Cramer DV, Chapman FA, Wu GD, et al. Cardiac transplantation in the rat. II. Alteration of the severity of donor graft arteriosclerosis by modulation of the host immune response. Transplantation 1990;50:554.
75. Almond PS, Matas A, Gillingham K, et al. Risk factors for chronic rejection in renal allograft recipients. Transplantation 1993;55:752.
76. Tesi RJ, Elkhammas EA, Henry ML, et al. Acute rejection episodes—best predictor of long-term primary cadaveric renal survival. Transplant Proc 1993;25:901.
77. Kahan ED. Toward a rational design of clinical trials of immunosuppressive agents in transplantation. Immunol Rev 1993;136:29.
78. Shoskes DA, Wood KJ. Indirect presentation of MHC antigens in transplantation. Immunol Today 1994;15:32.
79. Halloran PF, Schlaut J, Solez K, et al. The significance of the anti-class I response. Transplantation 1992;53:550.
80. Terasaki PI, Cecka JH, Gertson DW, et al. High survival rates of kidney transplants from spousal and living-related donors. N Engl J Med 1995;333:333.
81. Tullius SG, Hancock WW, Heemann UW, et al. Reversibility of chronic renal allograft rejection: critical effect of time after transplantation suggests both host immune dependent and independent phases of progressive injury. Transplantation 1994;58:93.
82. Feehally J, Bennett SE, Harris KPG, Walls J. Is chronic renal transplant rejection a non-immunologic phenomenon? Lancet 1986;i:486.
83. Naumark DMJ, Cole E. Determinants of long-term renal allograft survival. Transplant Rev 1994;8:93.
84. Van Es A, Hermans J, Van Bockel JH, et al. Effect of warm ischemic time and HLA (A and B) matching on renal cadaveric graft survival and rejection episodes. Transplantation 1993;36:255.
85. Cecka JM, Cho YW, Terasaki PI. Analyses of the UNOS scientific renal transplant registry at three years—early events effecting transplant success. Transplant 1992;53:59.
86. Goes N, Urmson J, Ramassar V, Halloran PF. Ischemic acute tubular necrosis induces an extensive local cytokine response. Transplantation 1995;59:565–572.
87. Linas SL, Whittenburg D, Parsons PE, Repine JE. Mild renal ischemia activates primed neutrophiles to cause acute renal failure. Kidney Int 1992;42:610.
88. Yamazaki T, Seko Y, Tamatani T, et al. Expression of inter-cellular adhesion molecule-1 in rat hearts with ischemia/reperfusion and limitation of infarct size by treatment with antibodies against cell adhesion molecules. Am J Pathol 1993;143:410.
89. Schaudies RP, Johnson JP. Increased soluble EGF after ischemia is accompanied by a decrease in membrane-associated precursors. Am J Physiol 1993;264(3 Pt 2):F523.
90. Land W, Schneeberger H, Schleibner S, et al. The beneficial effect of human recombinant superoxide dismutase on acute and chronic rejection events in recipients of cadaveric renal transplants. Transplant 1994;57:211.
91. Dallman M. The cytokine network and regulation of the immune response to organ transplants. Transplant Rev 1992;6:1.
92. Williams TJ, Hellwell PG. Endothelial cell biology. Adhesion molecules involved in the microvascular inflammatory response. Am Rev Resp Dis 1992;146:45.
93. Mii S, Ware JA, Kent KC. Transforming growth factor-beta inhibits human vascular smooth muscle cell growth and migration. Surgery 1993;114:464.
94. Border WA, Nobel NA. Transforming growth factor O in tissue fibrosis. N Engl J Med 1994;331:1286.
95. Ziyadeh FN, Shorma K, Ericksen M, Wolf G. Stimulation of collagen gene expression and protein synthesis in murine mesangial cells by high glucose is mediated by autocrine activation in transforming growth factor B. Lancet 1992;339:213.
96. Fine LG, Norman JT. Renal growth responses to acute and chronic injury: routes to therapeutic intervention. J Am Soc Nephrol 1992;2(suppl 10):S206.
97. Gao SZ, Schroeder JS, Alderman EL, et al. Clinical and laboratory correlation of accelerated coronary artery disease in the cardiac transplant patient. Circulation 1987;76:V-56.
98. Adams DH, Karnovsky MJ. Hypercholesterolemia does not exacerbate arterial intimal thickening in chronically rejecting rat cardiac allografts. Transplant Proc 1989;21:437.
99. Mennander A, Tikkanen MJ, Raisanen-Sokolowski A, et al. Effect of hypercholesterolemia in allograft arteriosclerosis. J Heart Lung Transplant 1993;12:123.
100. Brazy PC, Pirsch JD, Belter FO. Factors affecting renal allograft function in long-term recipients. Am J Kidney Dis 1992;41:123.
101. Myers ED, Poss J, Newton L. Cyclosporine-associated chronic nephropathy. N Engl J Med 1984;311:699.
102. Eich D, Hastillo A, Thompson JA. Hypercholesterolemia in long-term survivors of heart transplantation. J Heart Transplant 1986;5:377.
103. Mennander A, Tiisala S, Paavonen T, et al. Chronic rejection of rat aortic allograft. II. Administration of cyclosporin induces accelerated allograft arteriosclerosis. Transplant Int 1991;4:173.
104. Garcia DL, Rennke HG, Brenner BM, et al. Corticosteroid therapy amplifies glomerular injury in rats with renal obliteration. J Clin Invest 1987;80:867.
105. Hoskinen PK, Krogerus LA, Nieminen MS, et al. Cytomegalovirus infection-associated generalized immune activation in heart allograft recipients: a study of cellular events in peripheral blood and endomyocardial biopsy specimens. Transplant Int 1994;7:163.
106. Norman SJ, Salomon DR, Leelachaikul P, et al. Acute vascular rejection of the coronary arteries in human heart transplantation: pathology and correlations with immunosuppression and cytomegalovirus infection. J Heart Lung Transplant 1991;10:674.
107. Reinke P, Fietze E, Ode-Hakim S, et al. Late acute renal allograft rejection and symptomless cytomegalovirus infection. Lancet 1994;344:1737.
108. Fujinami RS, Nelson JA, Walker L, et al. Sequence homology and immunologic cross reactivity of human cytomegalovirus with HDL-DR beta chain: a means for graft rejection and immunosuppression. J Virol 1988;62:100.
109. Beck S, Barrel BG. Human cytomegalovirus encodes a glycoprotein homologous to MHC class I antigens. Nature 1988;331:269.
110. Koskinen PK. Induction of vascular cell adhesion molecule-1 is associated with cytomegalovirus antigenemia in human heart allograft. Transplant 1993;56:1103.
111. Brenner BM, Cohen RA, Milford EL. In renal transplantation, one size may not fit all. J Am Soc Nephrol 1992;3:162.
112. Heemann UW, Azuma H, Tullius SG, et al. Contribution of reduced functioning kidney mass to chronic renal allograft dysfunction in rats. Transplant 1994;58:1317.
113. Mackenzie HS, Tullius SG, Heemann UW, et al. Nephron supply is a major determinant of long-term renal allograft outcome in rats. J Clin Invest 1994;94:2148.
114. Mackenzie HS, Azuma H, Troy JL, et al. In experimental transplantation, two kidneys are better than one. J Am Soc Nephrol 1994;5:983.
115. Terasaki PI, Koyama H, Cecka JM, et al. The hyperfiltration hypothesis in human renal transplantation. Transplant 1994;57:1450.
116. Najarian JS, Chavers BM, McHugh LE, Matas AJ. 20 years or more of follow-up of living kidney donors. Lancet 1992;340:807.
117. Novick AC, Gephardt G, Gut B, et al. Long-term follow-up after partial removal of a solitary kidney. N Engl J Med 1991;325:1058.

COMMENTARY REFERENCES

1. Isoniemi H, Nurminen M, Tikkanen M, et al. Risk factors predicting chronic rejection of renal allografts. Transplantation 1994;57:68–72.
2. Goes N, Urmson J, Ramarssar V, Halloran PF. Ischemic acute tubular necrosis induces an extensive local cytokine response. Evidence for induction of interferon-γ, transforming growth factor-β1, granulocyte-macrophage colony-

stimulating factor, interleukin-2, and interleucin-10. Transplantation 1995;59:565–572.
3. Yilmaz S, Paavonen T, Häyry P. Chronic rejection of rat renal allograft. II. Impact of prolonged ischemia time on transplant histology. Transplantation 1992;53:823–827.
4. Grattan MT, Moreno-Cabral CE, Starnes VA, et al. Cytomegalovirus infection is associated with cardiac allograft rejection and atherosclerosis. JAMA 1989;261:3561–3566.
5. Hruban RH, Beschorner WE, Baumgartner WA, et al. Accelerated arteriosclerosis in heart transplant recipients is associated with a T-lymphocyte-mediated endothelialitis. Am J Pathol 1990;137:871–882.
6. Koskinen P, Lemström K, Bruggeman C, et al. Acute cytomegalovirus infection induces a subendothelial inflammation (endothelialitis) in the allograft vascular wall; a possible linkage with enhanced allograft arteriosclerosis. Am J Pathol 1994;144:41–50.
7. Lemström KB, Bruning JH, Bruggeman CA, et al. Cytomegalovirus infection enhances smooth muscle cell proliferation and intimal thickening of rat aortic allografts. J Clin Invest 1993;92:549–558.
8. Lemström K, Koskinen P, Krogerus L, et al. Cytomegalovirus antigen expression, endothelial cell proliferation and intimal thickening in rat cardiac allograft after cytomegalovirus infection. Circulation 1995;52:2594–2604.
9. Lemström K, Aho P, Bruggeman CA, et al. Cytomegalovirus infection enhances mRNA expression for platelet-derived growth factor B and transforming growth factor beta 1 of rat aortic allografts; possible mechanism for cytomegalovirus-enhanced graft arteriosclerosis. Arteriosc Thromb 1994;14:2043–2052.
10. Isoniemi H, Taskinen E, Häyry P. Histological chronic allograft damage index (CADI) accurately predicts chronic renal allograft rejection. Transplantation 1994;58:1195–1198.
11. Dimeny E, Wahlberg J, Larsson E, Fellström B. Can histopathological findings in early renal allograft biopsies identify patients at risk for chronic vascular rejection? Clin Transplant 1995;9(2):79–84.
12. Nickerson et al. Sixth International Alexis Carrel Conference; 1996; Banff, Alberta, Canada. Abstract.
13. Hostetter TH, Olson JL, Rennke HG, et al. Hyperfiltration in remnant nephrons: a potentially adverse response to renal ablation. Am J Physiol 1981;241: F85–F93.
14. Kingma I, Chea R, Davidoff A, et al. Glomerular capillary pressures in long-surviving rat renal allografts. Transplantation 1993;56:53–60.
15. Benediktsson H, Chea R, Davidoff A, Paul LC. Antihypertensive drug treatment in chronic renal allograft rejection in the rat. Effect on structure and function. Transplantation 1996;62:1634–1642.
16. Tullius SG, Hancock WW, Heemann U, et al. Reversibility of chronic renal allograft rejection. Critical effect of time after transplantation suggests both host immune dependent and independent phases of progressive injury. Transplantation 1994;58:93–99.
17. Zempo N, Koyama N, Kenagy RD, et al. Regulation of vascular smooth muscle cell migration and proliferation in vitro and in injured rat arteries by a synthetic matrix metalloproteinase inhibitor. Arterioscler Thromb Vasc Biol 1996;16:28–33.
18. Bendeck MP, Irvin C, Reidy MA. Inhibition of matrix metalloproteinase activity inhibits smooth muscle cell migration but not neointimal thickening after arterial injury. Circ Res 1996;78:38–43.

Chapter

4

Histocompatibility Systems

Charles B. Carpenter

The central problem in allografting is the immunogenicity of the grafted organ or tissue, which leads to loss of the graft unless immunosuppressive therapies are applied. Although major strides in clinical transplantation have been made in the past three decades with the increasing application of a variety of immunosuppressive strategies and better management of infectious complications, the need for continuing immunosuppressive drug therapy remains. Furthermore, long-term graft survival rates are not improving in parallel with the improvements in initial (1-year) success. The overall picture is best illustrated with kidney data (Fig. 4.1). It is remarkable that the 1-year graft survival rate for first cadaveric grafts has risen in a linear fashion from 45% to 87% over the past 20 years, while the long-term survival of the same grafts continues to have a half-life ($t_{1/2}$) of 8 to 9 years (1–3). The elements responsible for the improving 1-year success rate are discussed elsewhere (see Chapter 17), as are the problems of long-term, so-called "chronic" rejection, which is refractory to current therapies (see Chapter 3). In both acute and chronic rejection there is evidence of a strong HLA effect, but the role of other "minor" antigen systems has not been investigated systematically as yet because of the lack of sufficient knowledge of non–major histocompatibility complex (MHC) antigens.

The goal of this chapter is to provide current information on histocompatibility systems in humans, regarding not only the immediate issues of HLA matching, but also the background for future developments in the induction and monitoring of unresponsiveness and tolerance.

Inbred congenic mice have provided the firm foundation for the discovery of multiple histocompatibility genes, through the analysis of their rejection responses to tumor and skin grafts by classic genetic studies employing selective backcrossing and intercrossing breeding experiments. The pioneering studies of Snell and colleagues at the Jackson Laboratory (4) revealed a single strong, or major, barrier that they called H-2, as well as a large number of weaker loci (H-1, H-3, H-4, H-5, etc), each linked to different chromosomes, that were as a group called minor H (minor histocompatibility) antigens. The major histocompatibility antigens are encoded by the major histocompatibility complex (MHC) and exist as H-2, HLA, and analogous systems in other species. The MHC is a complex set of linked genes, highly conserved among vertebrate species.

In this chapter, we will first review HLA, the human MHC. We will then discuss recent progress in defining the human minor H system, about which much less is known. Finally, we will consider other non-MHC antigens.

HLA

The term *HLA* is the logo for the human MHC. It comprises several loci on the short arm of chromosome 6 (Fig. 4.2). In humans, antibodies to HLA-encoded antigens are found in sera from multiparous women and from recipients of multiple blood transfusions. Such sera agglutinate or, in the presence of complement, lyse leukocytes from some humans but not others. There are two structural types of MHC molecules: class I and class II (Fig. 4.3). These molecules are involved in recognition of protein antigens and serve to focus immune defenses on the introduction of novel proteins into the body, a process sometimes referred to as distinguishing between "self" and "nonself." MHC molecules act by binding potential antigens in the form of peptide fragments that have been processed in antigen-presenting cells. Clonally determined antigen receptors on T cells then recognize and bind to specific peptide–MHC complexes, setting into motion the appropriate immune response. By comparative analysis of sequences to those of other glycoproteins, portions of MHC molecules show shared ancestry with other molecules of the immune system

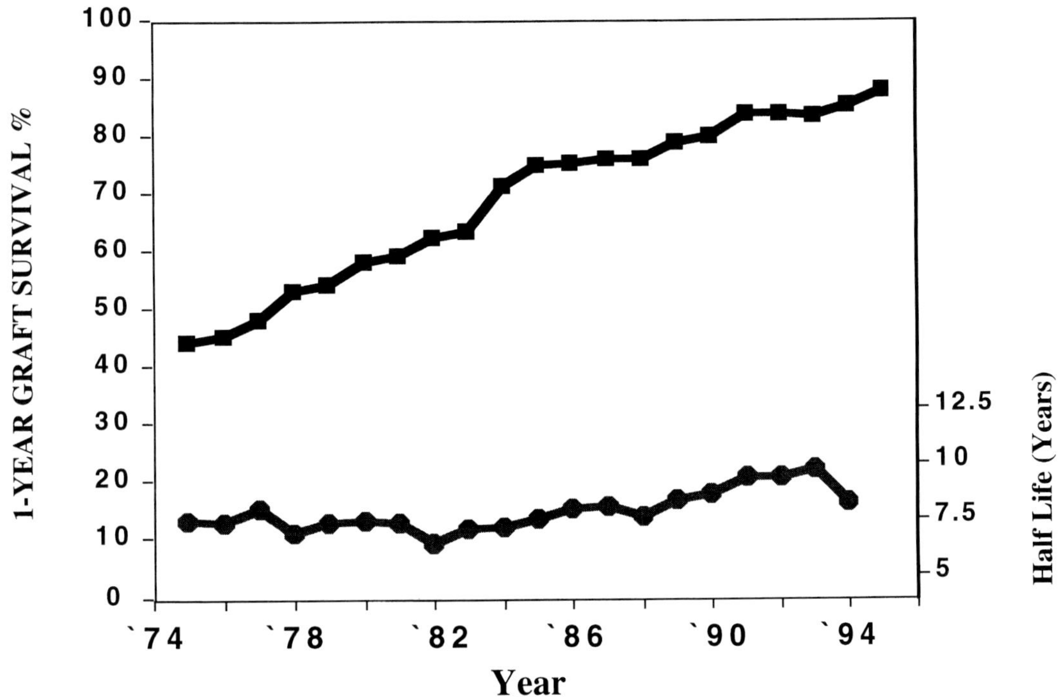

FIGURE 4.1. *Graft survival for first cadaveric kidney transplants from 1975 to 1995. One-year graft survival rates increased linearly over this two-decade period from 45% to 87%, while the subsequent rate of graft loss, expressed as a half-life ($t_{1/2}$) in years, has remained in the 7.5- to 10-year range. The sharper increase in 1-year survival in 1983 is attributable to the general introduction of cyclosporine therapy. However, by 1988 the 1-year rate returned to the new baseline described by the overall slope of 2.5%/year. (Sources: Hata Y, Ozawa M, Takemoto SK, Cecka JM. HLA matching. In: Cecka JM, Terasaki PI, eds. Clinical transplants 1996. Los Angeles: UCLA Tissue Typing Laboratory, 1997:381–396; United Network for Organ Sharing (web site). 1997 update.)*

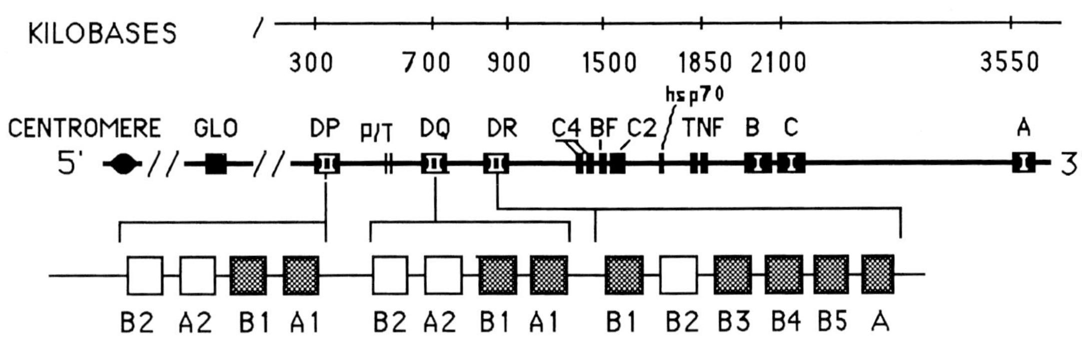

FIGURE 4.2. *Diagram, not to scale, of the HLA region on the short arm of chromosome 6, which encompasses over 3000 kilobases (kb) of nucleotides. Toward the 3′ end are the class I genes, HLA-A, -B, and -C; class II genes are toward the 5′ end of the region. The latter have two genes for each of the components of the heterodimers for HLA-DR, -DQ, and -DP molecules. A and B refer to the genes for the respective α and β chains. Pseudogenes are shown as open boxes. HLA-DR is encoded by a monomorphic A chain and one of four B chains, of which B1 encodes the HLA-DR1 to -DR18 molecules. HLA-DQ and HLA-DP molecules consist of polymorphic A and B chains, although in each case the B chains are more polymorphic. Other loci in the region do not have sequence similarity to HLA, but are of interest: P/T represents two sets of proteosome LMP genes that proteolyze proteins in a controlled manner to make peptides of 8 to 10 amino acids; TAP genes encode chaperone molecules that transport these peptides to MHC class I molecules. The C4, BF, and C2 loci are components of the complement system, and between them and the class I region are heat shock protein gene hsp70 and the tumor necrosis factor (TNF) genes. This diagram omits a large number of other genes, including many class I–like and unknown genes.*

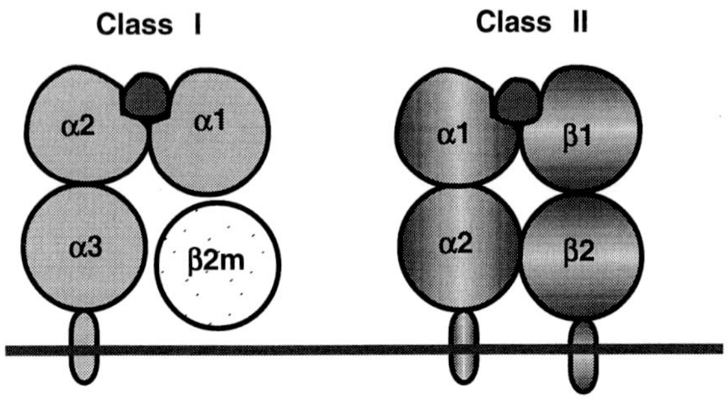

FIGURE 4.3. *The domains of MHC class I and II molecules are schematized to show that class I consists of a three-domain heavy chain (α) inserted into the cell membrane, and is noncovalently associated with a light chain, β_2-microglobulin. The binding groove for peptide is composed of portions of the α_1 and α_2 domains. Class II consists of two chains (α and β), both of which are inserted into the cell membrane. The external domains form a peptide-binding groove very similar to that of class I.*

such as immunoglobulins, T-cell antigen receptors, and T-cell interaction molecules such as CD4 and CD8.

Class I and II MHC Structure

The sequences and structures of molecules bearing MHC antigens have now been extensively elucidated, and it has been determined that the polymorphic, or antigenic, portions of MHC molecules are relatively small in relation to the conserved portions. Such polymorphic epitopes frequently involve as few as one to four amino acid substitutions. The conserved regions of nucleotide sequence and the hypervariable regions are characteristic of each locus (Fig. 4.4).

Class I MHC antigens include HLA-A, HLA-B, and HLA-C, each encoded by a separate genetic locus (see Fig. 4.2). These molecules are identical in general structure and consist of two polypeptide chains, the larger of which traverses the cell membrane (see Fig. 4.3). This heavy chain (44 kd) is divided into three extracellular domains, designated α_1, α_2, and α_3. The other chain is a small protein (11.5 kd) known as β_2-microglobulin, encoded on chromosome 15. It associates noncovalently to support the heavy chain in a stable configuration for peptide binding and T-cell recognition. The surface formed by the α_1 and α_2 domains faces away from the cell surface and is the location of the peptide binding site and the allelic polymorphisms. A large number (>20) of additional class I loci are mapped between HLA-B and HLA-A, and in the region 3′ to HLA-A. These play no defined role as MHC alloantigens.

Each class II antigen consists of two membrane-inserted glycosylated polypeptides, designated α (34 kd) and β (28 kd). These polypeptides are bound together noncovalently (see Fig. 4.3). The extracellular portion of the α chain is divided into two domains, designated α_1 and α_2, and the extracellular portion of the β chain is also divided into two

```
                        β SHEET                                      α    HELIX
        <-------------------------------------------|--------------------------------------------->
DRB1    1        10        20        30        40        50        60        70        80        90
        .        .         .         .         .         .         .         .         .         .
*0101   GDTRPRFLWQLKFECHFFNGTERVRLLERCIYNQEESVRFDSDVGEYRAVTELGRPDAEYWNSQKDLLEQRRAAVDTYCRHNYGVGESFT
*1501   ----------P-R------------F-D-YF---------------F-------------------I---A--------------V----
*1601   ----------P-R------------F-D-YF-----------------------------------F--D--------------------
*03011  --------EYSTS------------Y-D-YFH----N---------F-----------------------K-GR--N--------V----
*0401   --------E-V-H------------F-D-YF-H---Y---------------------------------K-------------------
*0402   --------E-V-H------------F-D-YF-H---Y-----------------------------I--DE--------------V----
*0403   --------E-V-H------------F-D-YF-H---Y------------------------------------E-----------V----
*11011  --------EYSTS------------F-D-YF-----Y---------F----------E--------F--D--------------------
*1201   --------EYSTG--Y-------------HFH----LL--------F---------V--S------I--D--------------AV----
*1301   --------EYSTS------------F-D-YFH----N---------F-------------------I--DE--------------V----
*1401   --------EYSTS------------F-D-YFH----F-------------------A--H---------R---E-----------V----
*0701   ---Q------G-YK----------QF---LF-----F-------------------V--S------I--D--GQ---V------------
*0801   --------EYSTG--Y---------F-D-YF-----Y-------------------S---------F--D---L------------****
*09012  ---Q----K-D--------------Y-H-G------N-------------------V--S------F--R---E---V--------****
*1001   --------EEV------------------RVH----YA-Y-----------------------------R--------------------
```

FIGURE 4.4. *Sequence alignment of the most common alleles of DRB1, from DR1 to DR10. The 90 amino acids comprising the β_1 chain of DRB1 are shown in single letter code from 5′ to 3′, left to right. The first half represents the β-sheet and the second half the α-helix portion. The DR1 (*0101) sequence is the reference for the others. Hypervariable regions are shown by the different amino acids, while identity for the reference sequence is indicated by a dash. The main hypervariable regions are in the vicinity of residues 10, 30, 47, 56–60, and 67–86. Amino acids that are shared with at least one other allele are underlined to show that some regions appear to have been used in several alleles (e.g., EYSTS in *03011, *11011, *1301, *1401, and EYSTG in *1201 and *0801). The first three alleles of DR4 are shown to illustrate how these variants are identical in the β-sheet, but have a few single amino acid differences in the α-helix. Molecular typing is based on methods to discern the patterns of polymorphism at the encoding nucleotide level.*

Table 4.1. Numbers of Defined HLA Alleles

Locus	Serologic/Cellular*	Molecularly Defined
A	28	83
B	60	185
C	10	42
DRB1	21	184
DRB3, 4, 5	3	32
DQA	0	18
DQB	9	31
DPA	0	10
DPB	6	78
Dw	26	

* There have been two biologically significant ways to define HLA antigens: generation of antibodies after pregnancy or transplantation, and the stimulation of MLR proliferation, classified as Dw antigens. A much larger number of DNA sequence–defined alleles exist, and the number continues to grow. The immunologic significance of these new alleles is untested as yet. Some of them may become important immunogens after immunization (already demonstrated for HLA-DP) and become targets for cellular attack (as in graft-versus-host disease or second organ grafts). Others may be important contributors to peptide binding. By definition, there are no additional molecularly defined Dw alleles; however, all the Dw alleles known have been clarified molecularly as determined by class II sequences.

domains, β_1 and β_2. In contrast with class I, the peptide binding and polymorphic external surface of class II is composed of the first domains of each chain, α_1 and β_1. There are three sets of class II molecules having varying degrees of importance to alloimmunity: HLA-DP, HLA-DQ, and HLA-DR (see Fig. 4.2). There are many alleles for each locus, and therefore considerable polymorphism exists (Table 4.1). There are many examples of cellular and serologic correlations with HLA-A, HLA-B, HLA-C, DRB1, DRB3, DRB4, DRB5, DQA1, DQB2, and DPB1 sequences, but not all sequences are definable by classic serologic techniques (see Table 4.1) (22).

Crystallographic studies indicate that MHC class I (5) and class II (6) molecules have similar structures, with the membrane distal domains forming a 2-nm × 1-nm × 1-nm groove for which β-sheets form the base and α-helices form the sides (Fig. 4.5). Although the carbon backbones of class I and II molecules are superimposable, it is the amino acid side chains that provide the different configurations for peptide binding. Indeed, the regions of hypervariability that induce alloimmunization are located primarily along the sides and base of the groove, indicating that they determine various shapes, charges, and hydrophobicity regions for the selection of peptides for presentation to T cells.

Antigen Processing and Presentation

Exogenous and endogenous antigens reach the cell surface by different pathways (7). Cell surface MHC molecules are assembled inside the cell and come to the surface with their peptides already bound (8). Surface MHC molecules lacking peptides are unstable. Exogenous proteins are taken up into endosomes or lysosomes, where they are catabolized into peptides that are usually bound to class II MHC molecules. The class II MHC–peptide complexes are then brought to the surface for presentation to T cells. Peptides from endogenous proteins are complexed in the endoplasmic reticulum to class I MHC molecules, which can be expressed on all cell types except erythrocytes and trophoblasts. Striated muscle cells and liver parenchymal cells are normally negative for class I antigens, but in inflammatory states they can become strongly positive for class I antigens. Viruses replicate inside cells, and their peptides are recognized

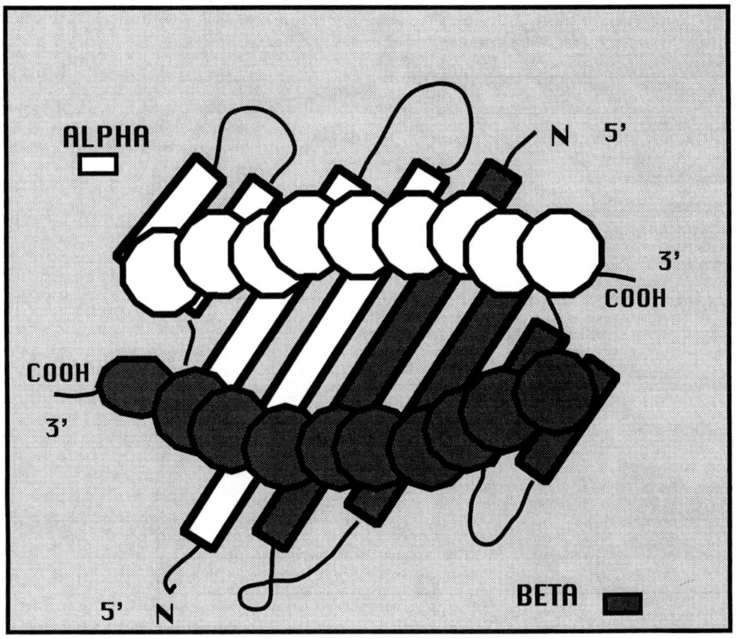

FIGURE 4.5. *A ribbon diagram of the DRB1 molecule, with the two chains shown as white or shaded. This view is looking down on the top of the molecule as it faces away from the cell surface. The α-helices form the sides, and the β-sheets form the floor of a 2-nm × 1-nm × 1-nm groove that binds peptides. The polymorphic regions shown in Figure 4.4 are along the edges and floor of the groove, where their different side chains determine the binding characteristics of a given allele.*

principally by class I–restricted T cells (9). As they are degraded, other intracellular proteins also yield peptides bound to class I molecules (10).

MHC class II antigen expression is limited to B cells, monocytes, macrophages, and dendritic cells. Normally, these cells are the only ones found to bear MHC class II antigens, but, as is the case with class I antigens, inflammatory states cause many other tissues to express class II molecules. Class II–directed T cells are principally concerned with defense against extracellular infectious agents. Class II–expressing antigen-presenting cells degrade molecules from the extracellular space that have been endocytosed or pinocytosed. Because class II–positive cells also carry class I molecules, they may act as antigen-presenting cells for both endogenous and exogenous proteins. The macrophage has the further ability to process exogenous proteins into both class I and II pathways (11).

Selection of Peptides

Genes in the MHC region play a role in the production and transport of peptides for class I binding (see Fig. 4.2). The large multifunctional protease (LMP) proteosome genes encode proteins that are responsible for producing the small peptides required (8 to 10 amino acids long) (12), while the TAP (transporter associated with antigen processing) genes encode chaperones that transport peptides across intracellular membranes (13). There is little evidence that the limited polymorphisms of proteosomes and transporter genes play a role in the patterns of peptide selection for class I presentation. However, study of peptide sequences eluted from MHC crystals do show clearly that certain peptide sequences are MHC allele specific (10,14), confirming the hypothesis that allohypervariability at the margins of the peptide-binding groove defines which peptide sequences will bind.

It is also becoming possible to predict the binding characteristics of class I bound peptides based on four major "supermotifs" found in the sequences of class I HLA-A and HLA-B molecules. Each motif binds peptides of certain characteristics, such as the amino acid at peptide residue 2 and the charge on the C terminal residue (15). Peptides eluted from purified class II HLA-DR molecules are variable in length up to 26 residues and have a minimal length of 13 to 14 amino acids. The elution of a series of class II bound peptides having a common central portion and variable lengths at the 5′ and 3′ ends indicates that proteolysis for class II is a more random process than for class I (16).

T-Cell Recognition

The co-recognition of self-MHC and peptide fragments of an antigen (X) bound in the groove of the class I or II molecules appears to require that the binding surface of the T-cell receptor (TCR) and the binding surface formed by MHC plus peptide be attached at multiple points. The TCR is also composed of an α and β chain, and each variable region (Vα and Vβ) has three hypervariable loops called CDR1, CDR2, and CDR3. CDR3β is more polymorphic than the others, and is likely to have the greatest diversity. Crystallography of the TCR–MHC complex reveals what is likely to be a common orientation for all such interactions. The TCR does not align its α and β chains in parallel with corresponding MHC helices, but it lies at a diagonal, such that CDR3 loops of both Vα and Vβ and CDR1 loops of both Vα and Vβ contact bound peptide. CDR3β also contacts both class I α helices, as does CDR1α. CDR2 loops overlie both helices, but contact only the HLA α_2 helix (17). It is proposed that this study has revealed a common binding mode for all TCR:MHC binding. If so, it identifies the constraints under which direct reactivity to allo-MHC will be explained.

When sufficient costimulation by interactions involving CD4–class II or CD8–class I, CD28:B7, and LFA-1–ICAM-1 has occurred, the T cell becomes activated (see Chapter 2). The need for cross-linking of TCRs is no longer thought to be required; rather, there is evidence that serial engagement of 100 TCRs with each MHC molecule over several minutes (18) is necessary to produce the sustained calcium flux signal required for effective signaling (19).

Selection of the T-Cell Repertoire by Self MHC

There is extensive evidence that the development of the T-cell repertoire in the thymus begins during the fetal period and continues well into adult life, as very large numbers of bone marrow precursor T cells with random TCR gene rearrangements are selected in the thymus (20). The MHC is essential to this process. Many potential clones are destroyed because they have an affinity too high for self MHC, and others with lower affinity are selected to mature and leave to populate the periphery (21). Because the surviving clones have a large variety of TCR rearrangements, a sufficient repertoire of T-cell clones that can recognize self MHC plus peptide remains.

Although the number of MHC polymorphisms increase the likelihood that a particular peptide fragment will be bound so that it can be recognized by T cells, a given individual has a relatively small repertoire of such MHC-binding sites compared with the rich combinatorial possibilities in the TCR gene complex. The inheritance of multiple HLA loci from two parents, however, increases the potential for recognizing a greater number of different self MHC plus peptide complexes, therefore increasing the chances that an individual will survive a given infection.

The presence of polymorphisms for class II on both the α and β chains of HLA-DQ provides an additional increase in the binding repertoire, as it has been shown that HLA-DQ molecules can be composed of α–β combinations from both parental haplotypes. The greater diversity of HLA alleles at the population level should assure survival of at least some portion of the population after exposure to a novel antigen in an epidemic, for example.

Tissue Typing for HLA

For years, the method for defining the expression of HLA antigens in individual humans has been based on serology. Sera from multiparous women has provided the means for defining HLA allelic products. Thus, the development of the field has been dependent on the small number of pregnancy-induced antibody responses that are operationally mono- or duo-specific to single antigen groups and to their subdivisions, known as "splits" (Table 4.2). Miniaturization of the technique by Terasaki, so that only 1 μL of serum is necessary for an assay, made it possible for tens of thousands of typings to be done from a small serum sample, and made sharing of antisera and standardization in worldwide workshops possible.

For the typing procedure, peripheral blood lymphocytes are added to microwells containing antisera predotted in a defined pattern. Rabbit serum is added as a complement source to develop positive cytotoxicity reactions, which are viewed through the microscope. Both T and B cells express class I antigens. Generally, the lymphocyte population is fractionated into T and B cells by nylon wool or magnetic beads coated with T-cell specific monoclonal antibodies, to enrich the B-cell population for use with the class II antisera tray. Anti-class II antibody-containing sera frequently require removal of class I antibodies by adsorption with pooled human platelets, which express class I, but not class II, antigens.

Similar techniques are used for crossmatching, a procedure in which a single patient's serum is tested against potential donor lymphocytes for anti-class I and anti-class II antibodies, as detailed in a later section. Of the class I HLA antigens, products of the HLA-C locus are poorly defined serologically, as are class II HLA-DP antigens (see Table 4.1).

Table 4.2. Splits of Serologically Defined HLA Antigens

Broad Antigen	Splits*
A9	A23, 24
A10	A25, 26
A19	A29, 30, 31, 32, 33, 74
A29	A68, 69
B5	B51, 52
B12	B44, 45
B14	B64, 65
B15	B62, 63, 75, 76, 77
B16	B38, 39
B17	B57, 58
B21	B49, 50
B22	B54, 55
B40	B60, 61
B70	B71, 72
Cw3	Cw9, w10
DR2	DR15, 16
DR3	DR17, 18
DR5	DR11, 12
DR6	DR13, 14
DQ1	DQ5, 6
DQ3	DQ7, 8, 9

* A split can be defined as the offspring of a well-defined "parent" antigen that could be divided by different sets of antisera into two or more closely related alleles. In many cases, the parent is no longer reported after testing, because the offspring are readily identified. Many antigens have no splits. For example, DR4 has more than 20 distinct variants, but these cannot be serologically defined.

Molecular Genetics

The naming of HLA genes is now based on a growing database of DNA nucleotide sequences (22). HLA class I molecules, having a single polymorphic chain, are less structurally complicated than class II heterodimers. The gene encoding the HLA-DR α chain, for example, is called DRA. Similarly, the closely linked genes encoding the β chains have been named DRB1 (encoding the β chains for DR1 through DR18), DRB3 (encoding the β chain for DR52), DRB4 (encoding the β chain for DR53), and DRB5 (encoding the β chain for DR51). DRB2 is a pseudogene that expresses no protein product. Each of the HLA-DR β chains associates with the common nonpolymorphic HLA-DR α chain at the cell surface to form functional class II HLA-DR molecules (see Fig. 4.5). Because there is no variation in DR α chains in the region of the binding groove, the differences in HLA-DR alleles are entirely determined by variations in DR β chains. The HLA-DQ subregion contains the genes DQA1, DQB1, DQA2, and DQB2. DQA2 and DQB2 are pseudogenes, whereas the products of DQA1 and DQB1 are both polymorphic. HLA-DP gene organization is similar to that of HLA-DQ (see Fig. 4.2 and Table 4.1).

Sequence Analysis and HLA Nomenclature

Restriction Fragment Length Polymorphism The first application of molecular techniques to identification of HLA alleles was by restriction fragment length polymorphism (RFLP) analysis, a technique that involves electrophoresis of DNA fragments after the total DNA extracted from a cell sample has been digested by exposure in aliquots to various restriction enzymes. The presence of a known sequence is revealed by Southern blotting with a labeled sequence-specific probe that hybridizes to fragments of appropriate size (23).

Polymerase Chain Reaction The polymerase chain reaction (PCR) technique provides a more convenient and accurate method of typing HLA alleles than RFLP analysis of unamplified DNA, and thus has supplanted it.

One can start with PCR primers that amplify genomic DNA for the α or β chain of a given locus (e.g., DRB1, DQA1), and then hybridize the product, which has been dotted onto a filter, with a series of labeled sequence-specific oligonucleotide probes (SSOPs). Or one can proceed in reverse fashion by previously preparing immobilized probes in microwells or on paper strips and then adding labeled PCR product (PCR-SSOP) (24).

Alternatively, the amplified DNA can be digested in separate aliquots with restriction enzymes, and the allele can be identified by sizing the fragments in gel electrophoresis (PCR-RFLP) (Fig. 4.6).

In a third method, oligonucleotide primers specific for the variable coding regions of specific alleles [sequence-specific primers (SSPs)] can be used in separate aliquots to amplify the DNA for that product. Each aliquot is then electrophoresed and the presence of a band of appropriate size gives a "yes" answer without the use of probes or restriction enzymes (PCR-SSP) (see Fig. 4.6) (25).

The PCR method has the advantage of requiring very small numbers of cells. The PCR-SSP method has been shown to provide results within the same time frame as serology, and is therefore applicable to typing of cadaveric donors (26). Finally, the amplified locus-specific PCR product can be sequenced. This approach has the capability of defining new alleles not revealed by the above methods, but it is generally reserved for that purpose because of cost and time considerations.

Future Techniques Technological advance will continue, and the techniques widely used in clinical laboratories are expected to change and become more rapid and reliable in execution. The application of these techniques for class I and class II typing has already been shown to solve problems of reproducibility in serologic typing (26–28). These problems are based on lack of antibodies for many of the splits in all laboratories, and on subtle differences in technique, including (but not limited to) different lots of complement.

It should also be pointed out that pregnancy-induced antisera are usually quite unique in terms of their content of cross-reacting and additional antibodies. They are not renewable resources, because second bleeds of a donor cannot be expected to be the same. Although monoclonal antibodies might solve some of these problems, they have not provided the power to recognize all required specificities.

Nomenclature Information about DNA sequences is now so extensive that HLA alleles are officially defined by their sequences, rather than by serologic patterns. The sequence information can be used to design new primers and probes for typing. A large number of new alleles, which have not yet been serologically defined, have been identified by sequence analysis (see Table 4.1).

Amino acid differences may occur at several sites, on either the α-helix or the β-sheets (see Fig. 4.4). Although there are three to five areas on an HLA molecule that are most likely to vary by several amino acids, as few as one or two amino acid substitutions may be sufficient to produce a T-cell reactive epitope, or one that is recognized by antibodies. The increased number of alleles identified by molecular techniques (see Table 4.1) is either because of splits of

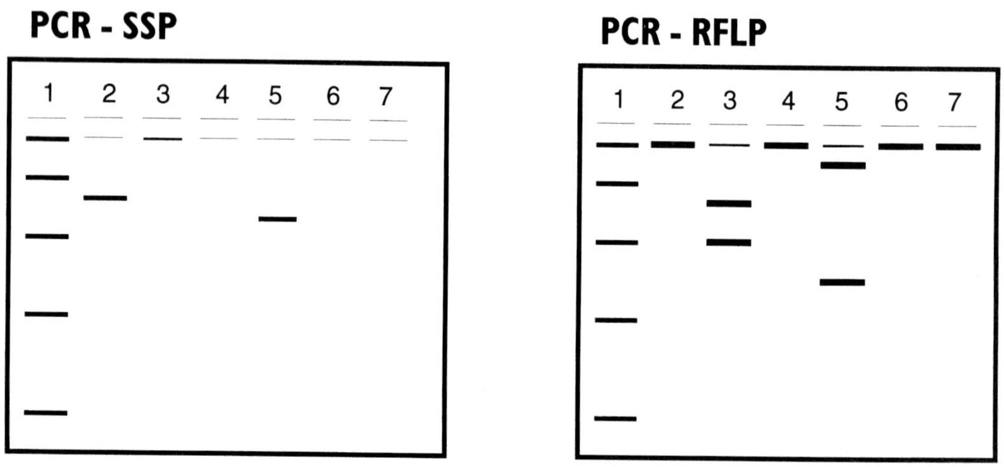

FIGURE 4.6. *Diagrams of the electrophoresis minigel patterns seen when DNA PCR products are displayed in the PCR-SSP and PCR-RFLP techniques. In PCR-SSP, oligonucleotide primers are selected to amplify the β-chain genes of a particular allele, and the result is a "yes/no" answer. In the diagram, lane 1 displays the size standards. The other lanes each contain the amplified sample of a series of primer pairs. In this condensed illustrative example, lanes 2 and 5 show positives. Not only must there be a product, but it must have the expected size for the allele being amplified. For PCR-RFLP, the locus-specific β-chain gene is amplified and subject to the action of restriction enzymes, which have a high degree of specificity to particular nucleotide sequences. Each enzyme is added to a separate aliquot and, after digestion, patterns such as the ones shown will develop. They represent in lanes 3 and 5 different cuts in the sequence that identify the presence of particular sequences.*

broader antigens or because of a unique variant, neither of which can be reproducibly recognized by serology. For example, the comparative sequences of HLA-DRB1 in Figure 4.4 show several motifs that are common to two or more alleles of that locus, suggesting that new alleles have been generated by gene conversion mechanisms (29).

Knowledge of sequences has the possibility of defining apparent differences in cellular (T cell) and antibody epitopes. It has already revealed that several mixed lymphocyte reaction (MLR)-stimulating antigens, termed HLA-Dw, are molecular variants of class II that were poorly appreciated by serologic typing.

Only unique sequences fit within the new nomenclature. The convention is to show first the locus, followed by an asterisk (*), and then a four-digit number. The first two digits are the allele number, and the last two digits indicate a unique sequence for variants. For example, the four most common HLA-A2 variants are now designated as A*0201, A*0202, A*0203, and A*0204. Another example is provided by DR2, which is the parent antigen for the DR15 and DR16 serologic splits (see Table 4.2). It is now known that there are four DRB1 chains for DR2. In the new nomenclature based on nucleotide sequences, DR2 is written as DRB1*1501, DRB1*1502, DRB1*1601, or DRB1*1602. HLA-Dw polymorphisms, which have been classically defined only by reactivity of T cells in the MLR, have been molecularly clarified, with the above four splits of DR2 accounting, respectively, for the previously known HLA-Dw specificities: Dw2, Dw12, Dw21, and Dw22.

Inheritance and Population Frequency of HLA Alleles

Two terms, *haplotype* and *linkage disequilibrium*, describe important associations among MHC genes.

Haplotype

Haplotype refers to the set of genes on any one chromosome. Each individual has two haplotypes of the MHC, one from each parent. Each haplotype has a particular set of antigens determined by the HLA-A, HLA-B, HLA-C, HLA-DR, and other loci, as illustrated in Figure 4.2. Co-expression of DRB3, DRB4, or DRB5 encoded antigens with DRB1 occurs in certain haplotypes, providing DR52, DR53, or DR51, respectively, as additional DRB antigens in serologic typing. HLA antigens are dominantly expressed. There are only rare examples of nonexpression of the products of the major loci, and these defects are usually inherited (30).

When a family is HLA typed, one can usually deduce the haplotypes by observation of the inheritance patterns in children (Fig. 4.7). A crossover event may be observed in the generation being typed at a frequency of 0.8% to 1.5% for each observed inherited haplotype. The probability of distribution of the four possible haplotype combinations in a sibship for the haplotypes ac, ad, bc, and bd is as follows: 25% are HLA-identical sibs (e.g., sharing ac), 25% are HLA-incompatible sibs (e.g., ac vs. bd), and 50% are one-haplotype HLA shared (which is also the case with all parent–child pairs).

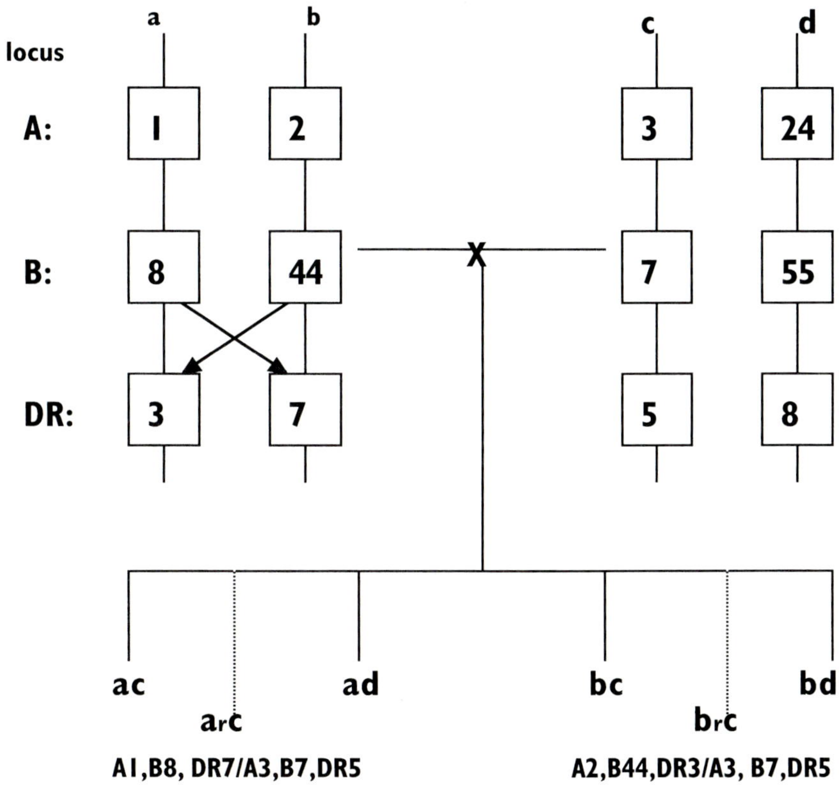

FIGURE 4.7. *Segregation of HLA haplotypes in an illustrative family. Only the HLA-A, -B, and -DR loci are shown, labeled for the allele present. The haplotypes are assigned as a, b, c, and d. The expected combinations found in the children are shown as ac, ad, bc, and bd. For any given child, the chance of having an HLA-identical sib is 25%, the chance of having a totally mismatched sib is 25%, and the chance of having a one-HLA haplotype-matched sib is 50%. Also, either parent to any child is a one-HLA haplotype match. When a recombination has occurred during germline meiosis, illustrated here between B and DR, the recombinant (r) haplotype is evident in that child.*

Linkage Disequilibrium

Linkage disequilibrium refers to the observation that some HLA alleles linked on a single haplotype appear together much more frequently than expected. If HLA genes were distributed independently throughout the population, the frequency at which any two antigens encoded at different linked loci would occur in the general population would simply be the product of their gene frequencies. However, the HLA-A1 antigen and the HLA-B8 antigen are associated six times more often than is predicted.

Recombination, or crossing over, takes place during meiosis and occurs about 1.5% of the time between class I and class II loci (see Figs. 4.2, 4.7). Over many generations, recombination leads to an equilibrium of linked alleles in a population unless selective pressures favor survival of certain haplotypes. A hypothetical example of such selection would be the survival of individuals bearing those HLA haplotypes that may have conferred resistance to epidemics, such as smallpox and plague. Racial differences are reflected in marked variations in the frequencies of certain HLA antigens and haplotypes. Africans show more extensive diversity of alleles than Europeans do, and they also have insignificant degrees of linkage disequilibrium for any HLA haplotypes.

Overall, there are relatively few conserved haplotypes in disequilibrium in the world, with most individuals of all races having almost unique combinations of HLA-A, -B, -C, and -DR (31). This means that identity for HLA among presumably unrelated individuals is at a very low frequency. Within ethnic groups, matching opportunities may be higher. Experience with the large pool of unrelated bone marrow donors is showing that many patients cannot be matched to any donor in a pool size of 100,000 or more (31).

Alloimmunity to HLA

The alloresponse is a special case in immunology, and would not have been encountered in evolution, except during pregnancy. That fetal HLA is immunogenic is clearly demonstrated by pregnancy-induced antibodies used for tissue typing. The allobarrier could have made pregnancy difficult or impossible during evolution except for the presence of several imperfectly understood mechanisms at the placental level that protect the fetus from rejection. The existence of such mechanisms suggests that the need for MHC polymorphisms is primary.

Direct Recognition: The MLR

Alloimmunity employs the same humoral and cellular components of the immune system as are used in body defense against microbes, but there are some important differences. When lymphocytes from one individual are cultured with those from another, the cells are stimulated to divide. This proliferation, which can be measured by following the rate of uptake of ^{3}H-thymidine into the DNA of the cells, is the MLR. By preventing the division of one of the sets of cells by treatment with mitomycin or irradiation, it is possible to study the antigens on the membranes of the treated cells that stimulate this proliferative response. Except for direct activation of T-cell subsets with bacterial superantigens (e.g., staphylococcal exotoxins), the in vitro proliferation of T cells in the MLR is the most vigorous antigen-specific response known because it does not require the priming that is needed to induce proliferation to microbial antigens.

Stimulator cells must be antigen-presenting cells that bear allo-class II, particularly HLA-DR, antigen, and be capable of providing costimulatory signals to T cells. Responding T cells can be cloned, and they are usually CD4^{+} T cells directed to HLA class II. Primed cells are identified by heightened proliferation to any stimulator cell bearing the appropriate target allele. The response can occur in the absence of autologous antigen-presenting cells; hence, the unique feature of this measure of alloimmunity is the direct recognition of intact HLA-disparate molecules on allogeneic cells (32).

The in vitro expansion and differentiation of cytotoxic T cells to HLA class I can also be studied in the MLR, wherein a class II allodifference is generally required in order to induce the CD8^{+} T-cell response to class I, which follows the CD4 response by several hours. The ability to make such cytotoxic cells is termed the cell-mediated lympholysis (CML) assay. Anti-class I CD8^{+} clones also behave as directly reactive effector cells. As with CD4^{+} anti-class II clones, they are not restricted in their response to antigen-presenting cells by self MHC antigens, as is the case for all other T-cell responses to protein antigens.

The ability to respond to allo-MHC antigens in the MLR is a special case in immunology, and has been difficult to explain. One explanation is the high density of alloantigens on cell surfaces, which can be 10 to 50 times the density of a given self MHC plus peptide complex when a microbial antigen has been processed. Also, when T-cell clones raised against nominal antigens are studied for reactivity to allogeneic cells, there are examples of some clones having dual specificity for a self-restricted antigenic peptide and an MHC allele, a finding that strengthens the general assumption that alloreactivity is the result of cross-reactivity with allo-MHC at the level of direct binding to α-helices. There is evidence that changing the self peptides bound to MHC molecules of stimulator cells in the MLR, or in target cells for allocytotoxicity, can alter the strength of response, indicating that direct recognition depends on the conformation of the MHC surface (33–35).

The common mode for TCR binding to MHC, discussed above, provides an ample basis for direct recognition of MHC α-helices. In this regard, it is of interest that the HLA-DR locus, which is the dominant stimulus for the MLR, has a monomorphic α chain, upon which all TCRs are selected in the thymus, thus providing a common baseline level of binding affinity for these clones.

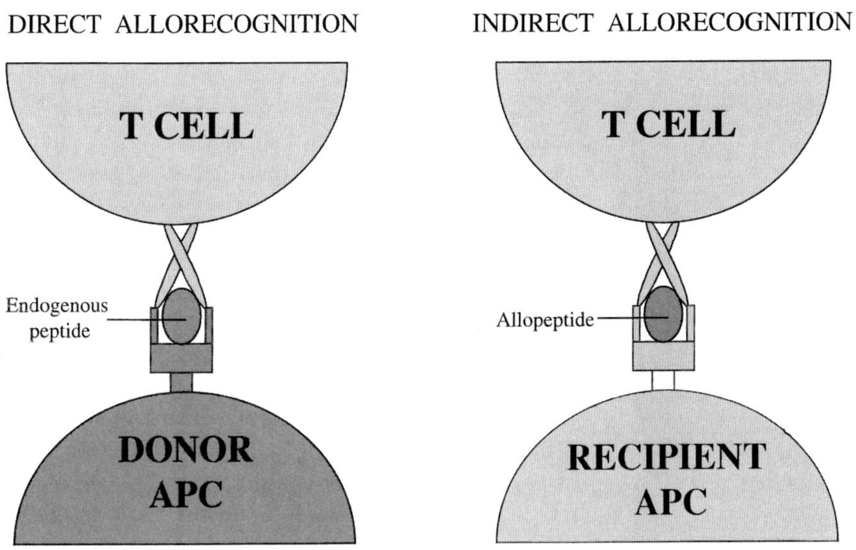

FIGURE 4.8. *Two pathways of allorecognition by T cells. In the direct pathway, which is unique to alloimmunization, the TCR engages the donor APC + peptide configuration, while in the indirect pathway donor alloantigenic peptides are presented by recipient APCs. The indirect pathway is also the mechanism for response to minor H antigens.*

A single locus defined as HLA-D was initially thought to encode the antigenic determinants for the MLR. Subsequently, the HLA-DR (D-related), HLA-DP, and HLA-DQ subregions were serologically defined. HLA-DR antigenic determinants are most influential in evoking a primary MLR, and HLA-DQ antigens play some role. HLA-DP antigens, on the other hand, do not appear to be involved in the primary MLR. However, responding lymphocytes that have been primed by previous exposure to HLA-DR, HLA-DQ, or HLA-DP antigens proliferate early and vigorously when reexposed to the same antigen in a secondary MLR.

Indirect Pathway of Allorecognition

Alloreactive T cells with different TCRs than those reacting directly with intact MHC molecules are known also to perceive allo-MHC as peptides presented on self MHC molecules, termed the "indirect pathway" of alloimmunity (Fig. 4.8) (36–39). The ability to prepare synthetic peptides representing the polymorphisms of MHC has made it possible to study this pathway experimentally. Immunization with synthetic allopeptides alone can cause accelerated graft rejection, whereas administration of such peptides by the oral or intrathymic route can induce hyporesponsiveness or even tolerance to experimental organ transplants (40). Because tolerance to the indirect pathway can prevent the activation of the "firestorm" of acute rejection, in which directly reacting cells can be demonstrated, it has been suggested that the indirect pathway plays a gatekeeper-like initiating role in the CD4-mediated MLR (40). Studies in animals and humans with allopeptides, usually 13 to 20 amino acids in length, have shown that not all potential polymorphic allo-epitopes are immunogenic, and those that are may be from the β-sheets or α-helices of the MHC. The results indicate that in primary responses certain dominant epitopes can be defined that are restricted by the MHC type of the responder (41,42). This opens the possibility of developing tolerance strategies based on the use of dominant epitopes specific to the donor and recipient (see Chapter 5). Monitoring of transplanted patients has shown that acutely or chronically rejecting, but not stable, patients have circulating T cells that proliferate to one or two donor class II MHC peptides (41,42), providing evidence that this pathway is active in vivo. Its role awaits further investigation.

HLA Typing for Transplantation

Crossmatching

There is worldwide variation in the application of HLA testing, both in techniques and in interpretation and application of results. This is particularly true with crossmatching, which at its basic level is the same technique of complement-mediated cytotoxicity used for serologic typing. The avoidance of hyperacute rejection by performance of a crossmatch of recipient serum with donor lymphocytes is well established and highly reliable for kidney transplantation. Sensitization to HLA, as defined by development of antibodies, is the result of prior graft rejections, blood transfusions, or pregnancy. The crossmatch procedures have been principally designed to detect anti-class I antibodies, which are clearly the major player in classic hyperacute rejection (see Chapter 2). There is a general consensus that a negative crossmatch is also desirable for hearts and lungs, but is much less important for livers. The rapidity with which heart and lung transplantation need to proceed can make it difficult to perform complicated crossmatching, and in many centers the absence of antibodies to a panel of cells, defined in advance as PRA (panel reactive antibodies), is considered adequate.

Periodic PRA screening of potential kidney recipients is commonly performed to define low-risk patients who will need only a final crossmatch with the donor, and to provide specificity profiles on patients who have anti-HLA antibodies. Panels for PRA screening are increasingly selected to represent as many HLA class I antigens as possible on the 40 to 50 cells. When antibodies can be defined ("called") in advance, a crossmatch is not necessary with a donor having that antigen. Otherwise, it is common practice to include more than one serum sample in the final crossmatch for patients having PRA, to perform dilutions, and to employ a second more sensitive technique, such as addition of an antiglobulin reagent or the use of flow cytometry (43,44).

It should be noted that the exact protocols vary according to the size of the waiting list being served by the laboratory. In patients who have very weak reactions that can be augmented by a more sensitive technique, the risk is usually considered to be very low for hyperacute rejection, but there is an increased risk for some accelerated rejection activity. Some organ banks have conservative policies to pass over borderline cases in order to avoid any early rejections, while others will give priority to patients with long waiting times willing to accept some increased risk. Recently, enzyme-linked immunosorbent assays (ELISAs) using soluble HLA molecules from well-defined cell lines have been in trial as substitutes for a viable cell panel. The systems do not replace the cell panel, which is superior to the ELISA for defining antibody specificities, but the approach is a promising technical advance and is useful now for general screening (45).

A most important consideration is whether a given patient has rejected a previous graft—particularly whether the rejection was an aggressive one, culminating in graft loss within 3 months or so after transplantation. These patients are likely to have high PRA percentages, and it is in this population that the heightened sensitivity of a positive flow cytometry crossmatch is predictive of poorer graft survival (45,46). It is also considered useful to employ multiple past serum samples in the final crossmatch. Historically positive (>6 months) but currently negative crossmatches are considered to be safe to ignore, and emphasis is currently on the flow cytometer to detect low levels of anti-T cell (class I) antibodies. One should not assume that the antibodies detected are the main effectors in the sensitized response, as these patients are likely to have primed T cells as well. Assay for these is cumbersome and not routinely done.

The significance of having anti-donor B cell antibodies is controversial. First of all, B cells express both class I and class II antigens, and because they express on average a higher density of class I than do T cells, they are more sensitive to lysis by anti-class I antibodies. In sera that have not been absorbed with pooled platelets to remove class I antibodies, the most common cause for a B-cell positive/T-cell negative crossmatch is the presence of anti-class I antibodies. The reports of accelerated, or even hyperacute, rejection from anti-B cell antibodies generally involve relatively high titer reactions (>1 : 4 dilution) in cases having the relevant DR mismatch. There should be some concern for the patient who has high titer anti-class II antibodies (45), and more studies are needed, including screening against a B-cell panel to define class II specificities. It may take more than a high titered anti-class II antibody to cause trouble, since the normal renal vasculature expresses class II antigens relatively weakly. However, with ischemic injury and/or some early rejection activity, class II will be upregulated and the antibodies can then augment the severity of injury.

Some patients have autoreactive antibodies, usually of the IgM class, either anti-B cell or anti-T cell, that are not directed to HLA and can be absorbed out with autologous cells. Alternatively, the reactions can be nullified by incubation of the crossmatch with a reducing substance for IgM such as dithiothreitol (DTT). These antibodies are not deleterious. Flow cytometry can also be used to detect antibodies to B and T cells, and the class of antibody can be defined. Laboratories cannot be expected to perform all possible tests in the middle of a cadaveric donor workup, but patients with high PRA, or who have shown several weakly positive crossmatches, can be worked up electively in the same way that living-related donor cases can be studied—by serum absorptions, titering, and careful B-cell target assays.

HLA Antigen Matching

In the early 1970s it was shown that living-related donor transplantation of kidneys was influenced in a major way by the degree of HLA haplotype matching. The best results were obtained with HLA-identical sib donors, producing a 90% 1-year graft survival rate and half-lives of 20 to 25 years thereafter. Haplo-identical combinations were less successful, with a 70% 1-year survival and a 12-year half-life, while unrelated cadaveric cases attained only a 50% 1-year survival and a half-life of 7 to 8 years (47). At that time the methodology for HLA typing was very limited, but a negative MLR was excellent evidence of HLA identity, and analysis of one haplotype identity was based on parent to child combinations. Since then there has been steady improvement in the 1-year figures in all categories, to the point where currently it takes a large number of cases to discern a difference at 1 year after transplantation among the three levels of compatibility. The half-lives for the three categories, however, have remained close to historical values (Table 4.3).

Definition of the HLA system also has been evolving. For example, in the 1970s there was no knowledge of HLA-DR, and large scale application of mandatory matching criteria did not begin until the early 1980s in Europe and in 1987 in the United States. Analysis of tens of thousands of cadaveric kidney transplants in the past decade shows that the half-life of cadaveric kidney survival after the first year varies in a statistically significant way with the number of incompatibilities for the six antigens of the HLA-A, -B, and -DR loci (see Table 4.3) (2,48). The simple hypothesis in promoting matched transplants had been that full HLA compatibility amongst unrelated donors would equal the results with HLA-identical family donors. The hypothesis has been confirmed only partially, because the extensive

Table 4.3. Effect of HLA Mismatching on Kidney Graft Survival*

Donors	Mismatches	Half-Life (Years)	10-Year Graft Survival (%)
Living-related donor (HLA identical)	0	24.0	74
Cadaveric donor (CAD), 1st graft:			
1992	0	20.3	65
1996	0	14.0	57
Living-related donor (one-HLA haplotype)	3	12.0	54
Living-unrelated donor (spouse)	4	12.0	54
CAD (overall)		9.0	40
CAD	1–2	10.4	45
CAD	3–4	8.4	38
CAD	5–6	7.7	34

* Total number of antigens considered = 6 (2A, 2B, and 2DR).
Sources: Cecka JM and Terasaki PI. The UNOS scientific registry. In: Cecka JM, Terasaki PI, eds. Clinical transplants 1993. Los Angeles: UCLA Tissue Typing Laboratory, 1994:1–18; Hata Y, Ozawa M, Takemoto SK, Cecka JM. HLA matching. In: Cecka JM, Terasaki PI, eds. Clinical transplants 1996. Los Angeles: UCLA Tissue Typing Laboratory, 1997:381–396; Zhou YC, Cecka JM. Effect of HLA matching on renal transplant survival. In Terasaki PI, Cecka JM, eds. Clinical transplants 1993. Los Angeles: UCLA Tissue Typing Laboratory, 1994:499–510.

polymorphism of HLA in the population makes it difficult to duplicate exact matches, as would be found in family members. Furthermore, there are several loci not considered (HLA-C, HLA-DQ, HLA-DP). These would be matched automatically in families because of haplotype inheritance. Finally, the known deleterious effects of ischemia in cadaveric transplants can reduce the rate of overall success. This point is illustrated by living-unrelated donor transplants that have short ischemic times and provide results comparable to those with one-haplotype matched family donors, when they might be expected to be in the less successful range of three antigen-mismatched cadaveric donors (see Table 4.3) (48,49).

First Cadaveric Kidney Grafts

Unrelated cadaveric donors completely matched for HLA-A, -B, and -DR (six antigens) were shown in the first prospective series of 1000 cases distributed through the United Network for Organ Sharing (UNOS) system to have 20-year half-lives and a projected 10-year survival of 65%, versus 7.7-year half-lives and a 10-year survival of 34% for cases with five to six mismatches (see Table 4.3) (50). This study confirmed that A, B, and DR were the most important HLA loci, and added strength to the argument that partial matches for these loci should also be mandated. The difference between the extremes of zero mismatches (best) and six mismatches (worst) is in the range of 17% survival at 3 years, and becomes greater with time (see Table 4.3) (2), but the differences at each level of mismatch are difficult to discern in small numbers of patients. Moreover, the relative strengths of each of these loci are not equal, although the matching protocol in the United States treats them equally. It is interesting that the European transplant results show that the three loci (HLA-A, -B, and -DR) have a time-related influence on graft survival: DR incompatibility is important during the first 6 months, B incompatibility effects last up until 2 years, and A incompatibility first shows its effects after 3 years (51).

From 1990 to 1995, UNOS adopted the addition of a phenotypic match policy to the six-antigen match mandatory protocol. This meant that patients with an unrecognized antigen at a locus—a "blank"—could be considered matched for a donor with the same phenotype. The assumption was made that homozygosity at that locus was most likely; however, as discussed below, this assumption is not supported completely when molecular typing is performed.

Finally, in 1995, UNOS extended the criteria to include a no-mismatch situation in the donor-to-recipient direction when the donor has a blank at a locus but the recipient does not. At present, the short-term (1-year) results are difficult to discern, as the annual overall improvement in all cadaveric grafts (see Fig. 4.1) has continued for all categories of match. The half-lives at 3 years, however, are 13 to 14 years for the no-mismatch cases, considerably better than the concurrent average cadaveric half-life of 8 to 9 years, though less than the 20-year half-life found in the original completely matched cohort.

There is no certain explanation for the fall in half-life at present. With the relatively large numbers of shared kidneys with no mismatches, now at an annual proportion of 20% of all cadaveric transplants in the United States, and the known 15% to 30% error rate in serologic typing (24,25,52), a larger number of patients who are not truly compatible may be included. There are two published studies comparing the survival of first cadaveric kidneys originally transplanted as zero-antigen mismatches, then retyped by DNA molecular techniques for class II and class I antigens. These studies, from Opelz et al in Heidelberg, used submitted data and cell DNA from many centers worldwide. The first study in 1991 assumed that the class I serology was correct (class I molecular typing had not yet been developed), and retyped class II by RFLP. It showed that 53 of 358 transplants (15%) were in fact HLA-DR incompatible. These transplants had a 75% 1-year graft survival rate, compared to 90% for the truly matched (27). The second study in 1997 accepted the submitted class II typings, and retyped class I by PCR-SSOP and PCR-SSP at the level of defining the serologic equivalents. Of 215 cases, 32 (15%) were found to have one or more class I mismatches. These transplants had a 72% 1-year graft survival, compared to 87% for the concurrent truly matched cases (26). The errors were either an inability to recognize an antigen (false-negative blank), or assigning the wrong antigen, most commonly with the splits of A19, B15, B16, B17, B21, and B40 (see Table 4.2).

Although more studies of this nature are needed, the present evidence is sufficient for proceeding with standardization and application of molecular techniques. Better identification of serologically defined HLA antigens can allow truly matched patients to have priority in organ distribution. At the same time, more detailed molecular definition will be needed for bone marrow transplantation and for clinical research into questions of defining permissible mismatches, based on knowledge of immunogenicity as a function of both donor and recipient HLA alleles (53,54).

To provide improved chances for the 80% of patients who cannot be HLA matched, various schemes have been tried to include more patients, particularly those of ethnic/racial groups who do not match well with a majority northern European population. The first scheme was based on the CREG (cross-reactive groups) phenomenon seen with antisera that contain antibodies able to identify "public" antigens common to groupings of the "private" antigens shown in Table 4.2. If CREG groups were used for matching, their lower frequency would make it easier to declare a match. However, it has been impossible to define exact rules for definition of CREGs, as three differing classifications have been proposed (45,55), and it has not yet been possible to fully relate these CREGs to the HLA sequences (i.e., to assign CREGs as expressions of known epitope identities shared among alleles). This approach provides some correlation with graft survival, but not impressively so (55a).

The next step was to analyze graft outcomes in relation to the numbers of amino acids mismatched or to the epitopes of the hypervariable peptide-binding regions (55). More recently, steps have been taken to define "permissible mismatches" by tallying those mismatched epitopes that seem not to matter. There is some indication that the recipient HLA phenotype may influence the results, so more complicated schemes accounting for specific donor–recipient combinations are under study. Because we know that HLA-DR peptide epitopes are immunologically dominant in relation to the recipient HLA-DR type for the indirect pathway of recognition (41), and also that the TCR repertoire for an individual is selected on self-MHC in the thymus, it is reasonable to explore the question of predicting graft survival by avoiding specific donor-epitope/recipient-HLA combinations.

Other Factors

A number of other important issues could impinge on the HLA matching effect. These are variables that, to varying degrees in a very large number of reports, independently are harmful to cadaveric graft survival. It is important to discern whether these variables also affect the overall improvement seen with the zero-HLA-mismatched cases.

Analysis of the UNOS database, which provided the data reviewed above, also provides further information of particular interest regarding first cadaveric grafts (2).

1. The results in HLA-mismatched African-American recipients show a half-life of only 5.5 years, whether the donors were white or black. The small number of zero-mismatched black-to-black transplants also had a 5.5-year half-life, while zero-mismatched cases with white donors had a half-life of 9.2 years.
2. Zero-HLA-mismatched recipients over the age of 60 years had the same early graft survival as younger recipients and a half-life of 15.4 years. When data were adjusted to remove mortality as a cause of graft loss, the >60-year-old HLA-matched group had a half-life of 66.8 years, although the actual patient survival curve had a half-life of 14.3 years. In contrast, the <60-year-old HLA-matched group had a mortality-adjusted half-life of 12.4 years, and an actual patient survival half-life of 24.5 years. With HLA mismatches, these results are lower for all categories except for patients <60 years old, who are not influenced by matching. Clearly, the perception that older recipients are high risk applies only to expected life span. They now do quite well immunologically, especially if HLA matched with their donors.
3. Another contentious subject is the duration of cold ischemia time and its effects on graft survival (see Chapter 16). Assessed at intervals of 3–12, 13–24, 25–36, and >36 hours, there is no ischemia time effect in the zero-HLA-mismatched group. However, for mismatched recipients, there is a 1% to 2% reduction in 1-year graft survival for each 12-hour interval of cold ischemia.

Retransplantation

In general, repeat transplants do not have as much increased risk for rejection-mediated loss as was true in the past, most likely because of improvement in both clinical and cross-matching protocols. Overall, repeat grafts do 8% to 10% less well if the PRA is greater than 50%, but not if the PRA is less than 50% (2). The Collaborative Transplant Study (CTS) database of Opelz shows that the DR-matching effect in first transplants did not require matching for DR splits, but with repeat transplants, matching for DR splits produced a greater than 15% improvement compared to having splits mismatched for both DR alleles. A similar result was found for HLA-DP mismatches; these had no influence in first grafts, but mismatching for both DP alleles produced a 15% detriment in retransplants (56).

Prospectus

All told, the clinical evidence shows that efforts to obtain zero-mismatched cadaveric organs for as many recipients as possible is worthwhile, as results are superior in producing the longest functional survival times. Attempts to make alternative partial-matching schemes work for some portion of the 80% of recipients who will not receive matched organs are in progress, and could be partially successful. Application of molecular typing to the matching problem and development of novel approaches to tolerance induction for those who cannot be matched will be the major effort of the next decade.

MINOR HISTOCOMPATIBILITY ANTIGENS

As single incompatibilities in the mouse, minor histocompatibility antigens (minor H) are characterized by skin graft rejection times of 60 to 100 days, while H-2 incompatibility evokes rejection in 6 to 8 days (4). Multiple minor incompatibilities can be additive, and can equal the strength of H-2, especially when the recipient has been previously immunized to the donor (57). Another general feature of minor H systems is the lack of an antibody response to minor H antigens, in contrast to the strong cytotoxic T lymphocyte (CTL) that develops (58).

The first minor H antigens identified were maternally transmitted in mice, and were shown to be encoded by mitochondrial genes. These are restricted by nonclassic class I MHC antigens, as well as H-2D (59). The Y chromosome of males carries genes for a complex group of minor H antigens, while several other loci are autosomal. Recognition of all of these is restricted by H-2 alleles, which must be present in the responder strain.

Clinically, it has been appreciated for many years that one of the phenomena of severe acute renal allograft rejection in HLA-identical combinations is development of cytotoxic T cells. According to a 1973 report, a nonsensitized female recipient of a female graft started a vigorous rejection a week after transplantation, characterized by a massive cellular infiltrate in the graft (60). This patient had circulating T cells strongly cytotoxic to the donor. In 1976, Goulmy et al (61) reported a case of graft-versus-host disease after bone marrow transplantation in which recipient reactivity was to the donor male H-Y antigen. In 1982, Pfeffer and Thorsby (62) reported a similar case of a nonsensitized female recipient of a male graft who could be shown to kill any cells bearing HLA-A2 or -B7 antigens present in both donor and recipient, but only if the target cells came from a male. Two sets of T cells, one restricted by A2 and the other by B7, were demonstrated. Recently, T cells from HLA-identical bone marrow transplant recipients with graft-versus-host disease have been shown to make HLA class I–restricted cytotoxic T cells directed to Y-chromosome–linked minor H antigens and an autosomal minor H antigen (59).

The major features of minor H systems, as defined in inbred mice and now being confirmed in humans, are:

1. The antigenic moieties are peptides; hence, they are perceived by T cells via the indirect allopathway.
2. They are HLA restricted; that is, they must be presented by class I or II self MHC molecules. Therefore, a given minor H peptide will not be immunogenic if it cannot be presented by the HLA alleles of the recipient.
3. They are mostly (so far) intracellular products presented by class I MHC; therefore, they are recognized by cytotoxic T cells.
4. The sequences so far obtained show no homology to known proteins.
5. They require helper effects from an associated $CD4^+$ response, meaning that there are linked antigenic loci for $CD4^+$ induction, indicating that CD4 effectors are also generated (19,20,25).
6. When multiple minor differences are presented on a skin graft in an H-2 identical combination, the response is frequently to a limited number of immunodominant peptides.

The question of matching for minor H is of particular interest in bone marrow transplantation (see Chapter 27), but many issues need to be addressed. Clearly, the better the HLA match, the more likely it is that minor H restricting elements will be available. However, until genes of minor H are well characterized, all of their restricting elements are known (including class I and II), and their patterns of immunodominance determined, clinical algorithms cannot be developed. A possible future role in organ transplantation would be to assess patients having repeat transplants with good HLA matches for the likelihood of a minor H problem, based on genotyping for minor H incompatibilities and their HLA alleles as restricting elements.

OTHER HISTOCOMPATIBILITY SYSTEMS

Monocyte/Endothelial Antigens

Not all non-MHC antigens are minor H. There are tissue-restricted antigenic systems that may generate antibody responses of potential harm to the graft. HLA-identical sib recipients can generate antibodies that bind to donor endothelium, as well as to monocytes (63) and, in some cases, skin. A high graft failure rate may occur if transplants are done in the face of such a positive crossmatch.

The difficulty has been in defining this system at a molecular and genetic level. This problem is further compounded by a lack of useful typing antisera, and the extreme difficulty in applying crossmatch techniques in tissue typing laboratories, as it appears that only selected cases have antibodies that crossreact with monocytes.

ABH Blood Groups

The blood group polysaccharides are expressed on the endothelium, and any attempt to cross the barrier against natural anti-A and anti-B blood group antibodies has a high risk of hyperacute rejection. As in blood banking, the situation applies in all mismatched combinations except those involving the group O donor. "O" means lacking A or B, but the basic polysaccharide structure (called "H") is still present. Organ procurement organizations have had to restrict such donors to O recipients to avoid disadvantaging O recipients on the list who must receive an O match. The genes controlling ABH expression are not linked to HLA. In working up family members as kidney donors one must be prepared for the disappointment of having individuals with ABH incompatibility in the setting of HLA identity.

In lifesaving emergency transplant situations with heart, lung, or liver recipients, plasmapheresis to reduce the anti-A/anti-B titer has been employed with some success. A state of adaptation in which a rising titer no longer harms the graft can occur if the graft is sustained for several days. A similar phenomenon of adaptation has been reported in some experimental xenograft studies with discordant antibodies.

COMMENTARY

Ken Welsh

Our knowledge of histocompatibility systems is still expanding rapidly, and the chapter by Carpenter is a stimulating read. My commentary on his chapter takes the form of questions that came to mind while I was reading it. I will attempt to answer my questions by drawing on the material in his chapter.

WHY IS DR THE MOST IMPORTANT LOCUS FOR SOLID ORGAN TRANSPLANTATION?

The human major histocompatibility complex (MHC) comprises an approximately 4-megabase stretch of DNA at 6p21.2 (1). Currently, there are a reported 209 genes, pseudogenes, and gene fragments contained therein (2). Within this, the HLA loci encode the most polymorphic system of functional proteins yet detected in humans (there are around 100 HLB-A, 200 HLA-B, 50 HLA-C, 200 HLA-DRBI, 1 HLA-DRA, 30 DQB1, 20 DQA, and 100 DPBI functional alleles).

Within a locus, differential efficacy on transplant outcome is difficult to demonstrate; however, between loci there are major differences for survival and rejection outcomes. For example, in terms of renal allograft survival and rejection after transplant, a HLA-DRB mismatch appears dominant, and HLA-C and HLA-DP appear the least influential. In contrast, for disease, HLA-DQ associations are much more important. It is also well documented that during pregnancy and after blood transfusions or transplants in adults, the most common humoral response is against HLA-class I. Children, on the other hand, commonly produce anti-HLA class II. Because HLA antibodies are generally IgG, such a humoral response also indicates a T-cell response.

It is easy to explain why a HLA class II mismatch is important—a class II difference is necessary to drive cytokine and T-cell responses after transplantation, and such responses then target the class I mismatch of the graft. There are so many different class I alleles that a sequence mismatch is almost guaranteed. It is less easy to explain why HLA-DR is the dominant class II locus. My personal view is that it is the T-cell receptor α (TCRα) that is important here, as the x-ray structure shows that TCRα contacts the polymorphic DRB (3), whereas TCRβ contacts the invariant DRA. Both the α and (more strongly) β chains of the TCR contact peptide, but this specific polymorphic site recognition by the TCRα is restricted to DR because in DQ and DP both chains are polymorphic. The drive against allogeneic DR is thus more directed, in terms of both peptide specificity and DRB polymorphism.

In bone marrow allograft survival, all loci are important, including HLA-C and -DP. However, some studies suggest that certain HLA-DP alleles are more important than others, and it may be that the relative importance of each locus is different for rejection, disease recurrence, and graft-versus-host disease.

WHY CAN WE RETRANSPLANT AFTER PREVIOUS MISMATCHES?

The rules for repeat-mismatch transplants have not changed significantly in 10 years (4). Basically, if the recipient has responded with a humoral response to the mismatch the first time around, then the second graft will most likely fail. Indeed, the same very poor results are obtained if recipients receive a transplant with a mismatch to which they have previously produced an IgG response after transfusion or pregnancy (a nonacceptable mismatch). Nevertheless, if a recipient has not responded to stimulation by a particular antigen (an acceptable mismatch), then it is perfectly safe to retransplant. This all appears clear, but why is it true?

Most of us believe that a T-cell response, not a humoral response, decides the fate of allografts; however, here it appears that the humoral response can accurately predict outcome. One would expect cases where no prior humoral response had been demonstrated would result in rapid rejection due to T-cell memory, but this does not occur. This phenomenon may be immunosuppression related, as higher doses of immunosuppressive drugs are given at transplant, but it is more likely due to the humoral response itself being driven by the T cells that are important in the rejection response. Some centers carrying out pancreas transplants preferentially give mismatches that are shared with functioning renal allografts.

WHY DO HUMANS REQUIRE LONG-TERM IMMUNOSUPPRESSION?

In most rodent models of transplantation, single or limited doses of immunosuppressive drugs are all that are necessary to induce long-term survival. Although some liver transplants can survive in humans without immunosuppression, this only occurs after late withdrawal of immunosuppression (see Chapter 19). Apart from monozygotic identical twins, there are few renal grafts that survive immunosuppression withdrawal. Also, hyperacute rejection is difficult to achieve in experimental rodent models, but in other animals such as dogs and primates hyperacute rejection is common.

The connection between the efficacy of humoral response and differential immunosuppression is difficult to make. Ischemia may play a significant and more obvious role—certainly living-related donor and living-unrelated donor grafts do better with reduced ischemia than would be expected on the basis of HLA match. Part of the answer may also lie in the baseline immunosuppression given to human recipients for ethical reasons; such immunosuppression may interfere with the development of natural tolerance.

SHOULD WE HLA MATCH?

The decision whether to HLA match is easily made for bone marrow transplants: the answer is yes for HLA-A, -B, -C, -DR, -DQ, and if possible -DP. It is not so easy for kidneys, however, and the answer is perhaps best considered separately for first and subsequent grafts.

First Grafts

There is consensus that A-, B-, and DR-compatible grafts do particularly well. There is also no doubt that multicenter studies show the benefits of matching, especially for DR, in renal and cardiac allograft survival. All centers report that DR matching reduces rejection episodes. However, with the advent of the cyclosporine era, many individual centers (including ours at Oxford) do not see a significant influence of matching. In fact, an examination of individual center data reveals that the better a center's results, the less the influence of matching. One explanation for this would be that the better centers are more efficient at treating rejection. Thus, one could potentially obtain a comparable effect simply by using better matched grafts.

This is not to say that good centers must go for the best matches in grafts, but we must recognize that many patients will need retransplantation, which will be more difficult in the face of sensitization. It is much easier to find a second transplant for an individual if the first was well matched. This argument is particularly important for children, because they respond more vigorously and will need more grafts throughout their lives.

In summary, we should use A-, B-, and DR-compatible grafts whenever possible, and this preference should be reflected in national organ exchange programs. However, because fully compatible grafts are so rare, zero-DR-mismatched grafts should be preferred whenever possible, especially in younger recipients.

Second Grafts

In general, the HLA effect for all loci, including DP, is important, and caution is required. A fairly simple audit can be performed: does a center get the same results in sensitized patients and retransplantations as it does for first grafts in unsensitized recipients? Once again, good centers report identical results, but the multicenter studies (described by Carpenter) do show an 8% to 10% difference at 1 year.

While part of the reason for this disparity may be differential immunosuppression, many people, myself included, strongly believe that antibody screening and crossmatching hold the key here. If screening and crossmatching are poor, the results in sensitized patients will also be poor *unless* they are HLA matched.

Unfortunately, no matter how good the screening and crossmatching are technically, they cannot completely overcome the problem of absent samples. If an IgG antibody to a donor MHC was produced but missed, either because the sample was unavailable to screen or because the screening was poor, the result will be the same: an extremely poor prognosis. I predict that as screening improves, the HLA-matching effect for second grafts will decrease and the results will be better than in first grafts.

Hearts, Livers, and Pancreases

Certainly the HLA-matching effect for hearts, livers, and pancreases is less than for other organs, mirroring the lesser importance of antibody. However, there does appear to be a weak DR effect for heart allografts, and certainly a considerable number of heart recipients need additional transplants (mostly kidneys). For livers, any MHC effect appears negligible. For the pancreas, there probably is a significant effect, but the number of pancreatic grafts is as yet too low to establish this with certainty.

SHOULD WE TYPE AT THE MOLECULAR LEVEL?

Figure 4C.1 is an example of a molecular tissue type, a phototype (5), for HLA-A, -B, -C, -DR, and -DQ; HLA-DP is an optional extra. At present, molecular typing has major theoretical problems. For example, nonexpression variants for both HLA class I and HLA class II are known. Additional low-expression variants are also well described. Variants may be one-off mutations, or mutations may occur more often in certain sites that are shared between alleles. Thus, predicting variants is only partially possible by molecular methods, and we must rely on serology to define them. Following their definition, it is relatively easy to incorporate primer sets for their detection.

Another problem with molecular typing is the possible contamination of donor blood with transfused blood. In over 500 transplant donors we have never observed

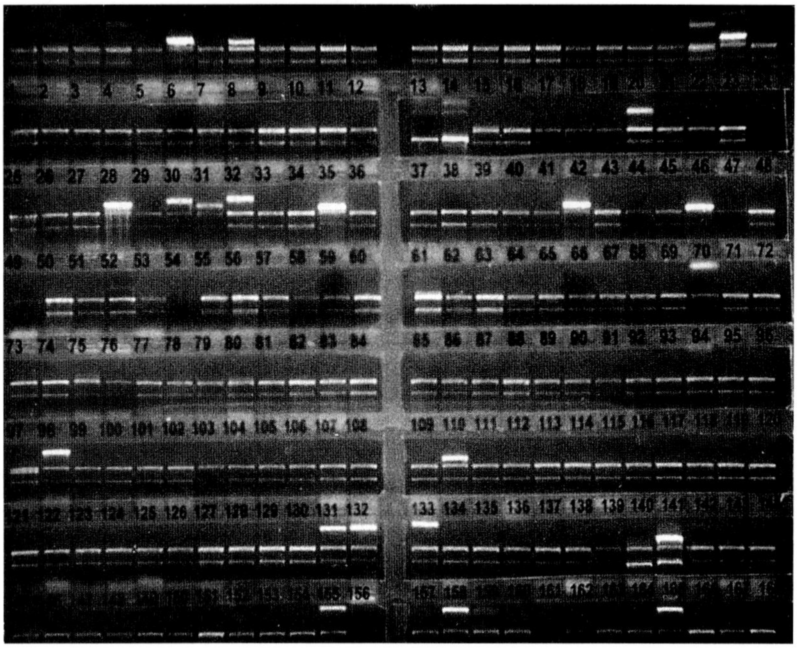

FIGURE 4C.1. *Each well of a 192-well plate is a separate polymerase chain reaction (PCR) containing a control primer pair and a specific primer pair. After reaction, the wells are transferred semi-automatically to a gel. The figure is an actual gel photograph. Control amplification (the constant bands) shows that individual reactions have "worked"—the stronger bands indicate where the specific reactions have worked.*

this, but we still retain the right to retype on spleen or lymph node. Molecular typing for all loci does have major advantages.

1. We can perform bone marrow transplants without recourse to mixed lymphocyte culture (MLC) or precursor frequency assays.
2. Using molecular typing in combination with accurate screening history and peripheral blood crossmatching, we can significantly reduce cold ischemia times for renal transplants.
3. We can define more accurately the contribution of HLA to graft outcome and to incidence of original disease.
4. We can add modules for ABO blood grouping (via transferase polymorphism), cytokine polymorphism, adhesion molecule polymorphism, factor V Leiden mutation, and so on, to our donor–recipient typing without using significant additional resources.

In our laboratory, we stopped serology typing in September 1994, after molecular typing had passed a suitable validation period. In almost 4 years of use on peripheral blood samples from donors, we have found molecular typing to be remarkably trouble free (6). Nevertheless, a well-staffed unit should maintain serology typing alongside molecular typing. A complete switch to molecular typing is not advisable unless resources are restricted. In economic terms, a full HLA-A, -B, -C, -DR, and -DQ type costs around $50, which may seem expensive to those used to free serology reagents but is inexpensive when compared to the cost of commercial plates.

CAN WE PREDICT RESPONSE TO HLA?

Indirect Presentation

It is apparent from the work described on indirect presentation that the number of epitopes that can be defined is restricted and may well be determined by the MHC of the responder. Many T-cell–driven autoantibody responses are IgG and MHC class II restricted. Because self MHC presents and IgG responses are common after indirect presentation, it is likely that the host MHC class II will strongly restrict the specificity observed, just as with autoantibody responses.

Is it then feasible to predict which epitopes will induce indirect presentation? The answer is possibly yes, but other factors will need to be considered. For example, the T-cell repertoire can, in animal models, select on the basis of affinity and chance epitope reactivity. Thus, the jury is still out on how accurate a prediction of indirect presentation for human allografts can be, but the current evidence is hopeful.

Direct Presentation

For direct presentation, the situation is less clear. At present, we can partially predict the specificity of a response. For example, 70% of HLA-A28 individuals in our transplant program have specifically responded to HLA-2–mismatched transplants or transfusions, but no HLA-2 individual has ever responded specifically to HLA-A28.

Unfortunately, the reason for this response lies directly in the sequence. HLA-A2 has several amino acids that are unique to it in the context of all MHC class I. HLA-A28 has no such positions relative to A2. In other words, the positions where A28 differs from A2 are all shared with many other class I antigens. Thus, A2 individuals may have them as part of their own class I, or will respond to them in such a way that the response will not be specific for HLA-A28.

While this response is extremely useful on one level, since it operates for assigning antibody specificity throughout class I, it is not useful for defining total responsiveness. We still cannot define which 70% of A28 individuals will respond.

What Is a Minor Histocompatibility Antigen?

In the light of the description of indirect presentation given by Carpenter, any polymorphism present in the donor tissue could be presented by host MHC and a response will be induced. The requirement for relevance would be the ability to generate a novel peptide in the context of recipient class II and the ability to act as a target in the context of MHC class I or class II of the graft. Although this is a consideration mainly in the context of bone marrow transplants, Carpenter makes the significant point that it may be also important for regrafts. One would certainly expect that, like any protein antigen apart from the MHC, antigen polymorphisms would have a significant immunization factor.

CONCLUSION

Carpenter's chapter prompted me to consider many more questions, but space precludes me from considering them further. I leave one final question: Why do we need rabbit serum in vitro to elicit a positive reaction in the presence of donor-specific antibody in a crossmatch test? Hyperacute rejection of a kidney in the presence of a positive crossmatch occurs without it.

CHAPTER REFERENCES

1. Cecka JM, Terasaki PI. The UNOS scientific registry. In: Cecka JM, Terasaki PI, eds. Clinical transplants 1993. Los Angeles: UCLA Tissue Typing Laboratory, 1994:1–18.
2. Hata Y, Ozawa M, Takemoto SK, Cecka JM. HLA matching. In: Cecka JM, Terasaki PI, eds. Clinical transplants 1996. Los Angeles: UCLA Tissue Typing Laboratory, 1997:381–396.
3. UNOS transplantation data web site. 1997 update.
4. Snell GD. Methods for the study of histocompatibility genes. J Genetics 1948;49:87–98.
5. Bjorkman PJ, Saper MA, Samraoui B, et al. Structure of the human class I histocompatibility antigen, HLA-A2. Nature 1987;329:506.
6. Brown JH, Jardetzky TS, Gorga JC, et al. Three-dimensional structure of the human class II histocompatibility antigen HLA-DR1. Nature 1993;364:33.
7. Harding CV, Unanue ER. Cellular mechanisms of antigen processing and the function of class I and II major histocompatibility complex molecules. Cell Regul 1990;1:499.
8. Germain RN. MHC-dependent antigen processing and peptide presentation: providing ligands for T lymphocyte activation. Cell 1994;76:287.
9. Zinkernagel RM, Doherty PC. Restriction of in vitro T cell-mediated cytotoxicity in lymphocytic choriomeningitis within a syngeneic or semiallogeneic system. Nature 1974;248:701–702.
10. Rotzschke O, Falk K. Naturally occurring peptide antigens derived from the MHC class-I-restricted processing pathway. Immunol Today 1991;12:447.
11. Rock KL, Clark K. Analysis of the role of MHC class II presentation in the stimulation of cytotoxic T lymphocytes by antigens targeted into the exogenous antigen-MHC class I presentation pathway. J Immunol 1996;156:3721–3726.
12. Patel SD, Monaco JJ, McDevitt HO. Delineation of the subunit composition of human proteosomes using antisera against the major histocompatibility complex-encoded LMP-2 and LMP7 subunits. Proc Natl Acad Sci USA 1994;91:296–300.
13. Powis SH, Tonks S, Mockridge I, et al. Alleles and haplotypes of the MHC-encoded ABC transporters TAP1 and TAP2. Immunogenetics 1993;37:373.
14. Hunt DF, Michel H, Dickinson TA, et al. Peptides presented to the immune system by the murine class II major histocompatibility complex molecule I-Ad. Science 1992;256:1817.
15. Sidney J, Grey HM, Kubo RT, Sette A. Practical, biochemical, and evolutionary implications of the discovery of HLA class I supermotifs. Immunol Today 1996;17:261–266.
16. Chicz RM, Urban RG, Gorga JC, et al. Specificity and promiscuity among naturally processed peptides bound to HLA-DR alleles. J Exp Med 1993;178:27.
17. Garboczi DN, Ghosh P, Utz U, et al. Structure of the complex between human T-cell receptor, viral peptide and HLA-A2. Nature 1996;384:134–141.
18. Valitutti S, Lanzavecchia A. Serial triggering of TCRs: a basis for the sensitivity and specificity of antigen recognition. Immunol Today 1997;18: 299–304.
19. Wülfing C, Rabinowitz JD, Beeson C, et al. Kinetics and extent of T cell activation as measured with the calcium signal. J Exp Med 1997;185: 1815–1825.
20. Von Boehmer H. Positive selection of lymphocytes. Cell 1994;76:219.
21. Nossal GJV. Negative selection of lymphocytes. Cell 1994;76:229.
22. Bodmer JG, Marsh SGE, Albert ED, et al. Nomenclature for factors of the HLA system, 1996. In: Charron D, ed. Genetic diversity of HLA: functional and medical implication. Vol 1 Paris: EDK, 1997:505–532.
23. Mytilineos J, Scherer S, Opelz G. Comparison of RFLP-DR beta and serological HLA-DR typing in 1500 individuals. Transplantation 1990;50:870–873.
24. Yu N, Ohashi M, Alosco S, et al. Accurate typing of HLA-A antigens and analysis of serological deficiencies. Tissue Antigens 1997;50:380–386.
25. Lorentzen DF, Iwanaga KK, Meuer KJ, et al. A 25% error rate in serologic typing of HLA-B homozygotes. Tissue Antigens 1997;50:359–365.
26. Mytilineos J, Lempert M, Middleton D, et al. HLA class I typing of 215 "HLA-A,-B,-DR zero mismatched" kidney transplants. Tissue Antigens 1997;50:355–358.
27. Opelz G, Mytilineos J, Scherer S, et al. Survival of DNA HLA-DR typed and matched cadaver kidney transplants. Lancet 1991;383:461–463.
28. Carpenter CB. HLA class I DNA typing in organ transplantation. Tissue Antigens 1997;50:322–325.
29. Erlich HA, Gyllensten UB. Shared epitopes among HLA class II alleles: gene conversion, common ancestry and balancing selection. Immunol Today 1991;12:411–414.
30. Parham P. Filling in the blanks. Tissue Antigens 1997;50:318–321.
31. Mori M, Beatty PG, Graves M, et al. HLA gene and haplotype frequencies in the North American population: the National Marrow Donor Program Donor Registry. Transplantation 1997;64(7):1017–1027.
32. Elliot TJ, Eisen HN. Cytotoxic T lymphocytes recognize a reconstituted class I histocompatibility antigen (HLA-A2) as an allogeneic target molecule. Proc Natl Acad Sci USA 1990;87:5213.
33. Bluestone JA, Kaliyaperumal A, Jameson S, et al. Peptide induced changes in class I heavy chains alter allorecognition. J Immunol 1993;151:3943–3953.
34. Heath WR, Kane KP, Mescher MF, Sherman LA. Alloreactive T cells discriminate among a diverse set of endogenous peptides. Proc Natl Acad Sci USA 1991;88:5101.
35. Molina IJ, Huber BT. The expression of a tissue-specific self-peptide is required for allorecognition. J Immunol 1990;144:2082–2088.
36. Fangmann J, Dalchau R, Fabre JW. Rejection of skin allografts by indirect recognition of donor major histocompatibility complex peptides. J Exp Med 1992;175:1521–1529.
37. Sayegh MH, Khoury SJ, Hancock WW, et al. Induction of immunity and oral tolerance by polymorphic class II major histocompatibility complex allopeptides in the rat. Proc Natl Acad Sci USA 1992;89:7762.

38. Auchincloss H Jr, Lee R, Shea S, et al. The role of "indirect" recognition in initiating rejection of skin grafts from major histocompatibility complex class II-deficient mice. Proc Natl Acad Sci USA 1993;90:3373.
39. Sayegh MH, Watschinger B, Carpenter CB. Mechanisms of T cell recognition of alloantigen: the role of peptides. Transplantation 1994;57:1295.
40. Sayegh MH, Carpenter CB. Role of indirect allorecognition in allograft rejection. Intern Rev Immunol 1996;13:221–229.
41. Liu Z, Colovai AI, Tuguloa S, et al. Indirect recognition of donor HLA-DR peptides in organ allograft rejection. J Clin Invest 1996;98: 1150–1157.
42. Vella JP, Ferreira M, Murphy B, et al. Indirect allorecognition of major histocompatibility complex allopeptides in human renal transplant recipients with chronic graft dysfunction. Transplantation 1997;64(6):795–800.
43. Garovoy MR, Rheinschmidt MA, Bigos M, et al. Flow cytometry analysis: a high technology crossmatch technique facilitating transplantation. Transplant Proc 1983;15:1939–1944.
44. Cook DJ, Terasaki PI, Iwaki Y, et al. An approach to reducing early kidney transplant failure by flow cytometry crossmatching. Clin Transplant 1987;1:253–256.
45. Takemoto SK, Terasaki PI. Evaluation of the transplant recipient and donor: molecular approach to tissue typing, flow cytometry and alternative approaches to distributing organs. Curr Opin Nephrol Hypertens 1997;6:299–303.
46. Mahoney RJ, Norman DJ, Colombe BW, et al. Identification of high- and low-risk second kidney grafts. Transplantation 1996;61:1349–1355.
47. Opelz G, Terasaki PI. Studies on the strength of HLA antigens in related donor kidney transplants. Transplantation 1977;24:106–111.
48. Zhou YC, Cecka JM. Effect of HLA matching on renal transplant survival. In Terasaki PI, Cecka JM, eds. Clinical transplants 1993. Los Angeles: UCLA Tissue Typing Laboratory, 1994:499–510.
49. Carpenter CB. Long-term failure of renal transplants: adding insult to injury. Kidney Int 1995;48(suppl 50):S40–S44.
50. Takemoto S, Terasaki PI, Cecka JM, et al. Survival of nationally shared HLA-matched kidney transplants from cadaveric donors. N Engl J Med 1992;327:834–839.
51. Zantvoort FA, D'Amaro J, Persijn GG, et al. The impact of HLA-A matching on long-term survival of renal allografts. Transplantation 1996:61:841–844.
52. Bozon MV, Delgado JC, Clavijo OP, et al. Error rate for HLA-B antigen assignment by serology: Implications for proficiency testing and utilization of DNA-based typing methods. Tissue Antigens 1997;50:387–394.
53. Doxiadis IIN, Smits JMA, Schreuder GMT, et al. Association between specific HLA combinations and probability of kidney allograft loss: the taboo concept. Lancet 1996;348:850–853.
54. Takemoto S, Terasaki PI. Refinement of permissible HLA mismatches. In: Cecka JM, Terasaki PI, eds. Clinical transplants 1994. Los Angeles: UCLA Tissue Typing Laboratory, 1995:451–466.
55. Takemoto SK. HLA amino residue matching. In: Cecka JM, Terasaki PI, eds. Clinical transplants 1996. Los Angeles: UCLA Tissue Typing Laboratory, 1996:397–424.
56. Starzl TE, Eliasziw M, Gjertson D, et al. HLA and cross-reactive antigen group matching for cadaver kidney allocation. Transplantation 1997;64:983–991.
57. Opelz G. CTS Collaborative Transplant Study Newsletter. 1997:2.
58. Graff RJ, Silvers WK, Billingham RE, et al. The cumulative effect of histocompatibility antigens. Transplantation 1966;4:605–617.
59. Roopenian DC. What are minor histocompatibility loci? A new look at an old question. Immunol Today 1992;13:7–10.
60. Simpson E, Roopenian D. Minor histocompatibility antigens. Curr Opin Immunol 1997;9:655–661.
61. Garovoy MR, Franco V, Zschaeck D, et al. Direct lymphocyte-mediated cytotoxicity as an assay of presensitization. Lancet 1973;1(803):573–576.
62. Goulmy E, Termijtelen A, Bradley BA, Van Rood JJ. Alloimmunity to human H-Y. Lancet 1976;2:1206.
63. Pfeffer PF, Thorsby E. HLA-restricted cytotoxicity against male-specific (H-Y) antigen after acute rejection of an HLA-identical sibling kidney: clonal distribution of the cytotoxic cells. Transplantation 1982;33:52–56.
64. Brasile L, Clarke J, Cerilli J. A probable mechanism for allograft rejection in HLA identical combinations. Transplant Proc 1987;19:894.

COMMENTARY REFERENCES

1. Trowsdale J, Campbell RD. A map of the human MHC. Immunol Today 1993;14(7):349–352.
2. Gruen JR, Nalabolo SR, Chu TW, et al. A transcription map of the major histocompatibility complex (MHC) class I region. Genomics 1996;36:70–85.
3. Fields BA, Ober B, Malchiodi EL, et al. Crystal structure of the V alpha domain of a T cell receptor. Science 1995;270:1821–1824.
4. Welsh KI, van Dam M, Bewick ME, et al. Successful transplantation of kidneys bearing previously mismatched HLA A and B locus antigens. Transplant Int 1988;1:190–195.
5. Bunce M, O'Neill CM, Barnardo MCNM, et al. Phototyping: comprehensive DNA typing for HLA-A, B, C, DRB1, DRB3, DRB4, DRB5, and DQB1 by PCR with 144 primer mixes utilizing sequence specific primers (PCR-SSP). Tissue Antigens 1995;46:355–367.
6. Bunce M, Young NT, Welsh KI. Molecular HLA typing—the brave new world. Transplantation 1997;64:1505–1513.

Chapter 5

Tolerance

MEGAN SYKES DAVID H. SACHS

While improvements in immunosuppressive therapy have dramatically increased the success of clinical organ transplantation, these drugs are associated with life-long risks of infection, malignancy, and graft rejection. Despite improved immunosuppression, chronic rejection is still a major problem and leads to a constant attrition of many types of organ allografts. Induction of donor-specific tolerance with preservation of otherwise normal immune responses is therefore a major goal of research in the field of transplantation. A second impetus for the induction of tolerance arises from the current shortage of allogeneic organs, which has increased interest in the use of other species as xenograft donors. However, immune barriers to xenografts may be even greater than those to allografts (1), and the induction of both B-cell and T-cell tolerance may be essential to the ultimate success of xenotransplantation.

In addition to its potential application for the improvement of organ transplantation, tolerance induction is often considered in relation to bone marrow transplantation (BMT) when used to treat leukemias and other hematologic disorders. Marrow is highly immunogenic, and potent recipient immunosuppression is required to avoid marrow rejection, particularly when major histcompatibility (MHC) barriers are crossed. Furthermore, T cells in the donor marrow have the ability to mount an immune response against the immunosuppressed recipient, leading to graft-versus-host disease (GVHD). Thus, in bone marrow transplant recipients, induction of tolerance in both the host-versus-graft and the graft-versus-host directions might be desirable. However, one exception to this goal is the treatment of leukemia, in which induction of graft-versus-host tolerance may be associated with loss of antileukemic effects from donor T cells. In this situation, the goal should be separation of the graft-versus-leukemia (GVL) response from the graft-versus-normal-host-tissue response. Recently, several approaches to achieving this goal have been attempted. These include efforts to separate graft-versus-host from graft-versus-leukemia activity on the basis of immunologic specificity (i.e., inducing leukemia-specific immune responses) (2), temporal separation of bone marrow transplants from donor T-cell administration (3,4), and functional separation of T-cell responses that induce GVL effects from those that cause GVHD (5). These issues are discussed in more detail elsewhere in this volume. This chapter will focus predominantly on the induction of tolerance in the host-versus-graft direction, which is the major consideration for solid organ transplantation. However, it should be remembered that solid organ transplantation, when accompanied by a significant mass of lymphoid tissue, can lead to clinically significant graft-versus-host reactions. This problem has been observed rarely following liver transplantation and has been a major impediment to small bowel transplantation (6), in which the graft-versus-host response must be balanced against the host-versus-graft response.

MECHANISMS OF TOLERANCE

The thymus is the central organ for T-cell development. Hence, induction of tolerance among developing thymocytes is referred to as "central," as distinguished from the "peripheral" tolerance that may develop among already-mature T cells when they encounter antigen in the peripheral tissues. Peripheral tolerance induction has generally been most successful in animal models involving relatively weak transplantation barriers such as those posed by MHC-matched, minor histocompatibility antigen–disparate grafts (reviewed in reference 7), or by MHC-mismatched cardiac and renal grafts in rodents. However, it is generally more difficult to induce tolerance to vascularized allografts in large animals than in rodents. Unlike central tolerance, peripheral mechanisms alone have not been sufficient to reliably overcome the most stringent transplantation barrier imposed by fully MHC-mismatched primary skin allografts. Thus, central tolerance may prove to be critical to the development of clinical protocols that can ensure the induction of tolerance reliably enough to justify withholding chronic immunosuppressive therapy.

In models involving peripheral tolerance induction, the organ grafts themselves may play an important role in inactivating or deleting preexisting recipient T cells. The role of the graft itself can be illustrated by demonstrating the requirement that the organ graft be present in order for tolerance to be achieved, even if another source of antigen, such as a donor-specific transfusion, is provided (8). Certain types of allografts, such as the murine heart, may be particularly poor in antigen-presenting cells (APCs) and therefore tolerogenic because of their ability to present antigen without adequate costimulation to responding T cells.

The known mechanisms for inducing T- and B-cell tolerance can be grouped into the categories of anergy, suppression, and deletion (and, in the case of B cells, receptor editing). In addition, a graft may simply be ignored by recipient T cells. Each of these mechanisms will be discussed in more detail below.

Lymphocytes Ignoring Graft Alloantigens

Experimental situations in which antigens are ignored by T cells (9) or B cells (10) that can recognize them have been described. This may be due to the presentation of these antigens by "nonprofessional APCs" that are unable to activate T cells, or it may reflect a failure of recipient T cells to migrate to the graft tissue and encounter donor antigens. However, rather than being a true state of systemic tolerance, this may be a more precarious state that can be upset by additional immunologic stimuli provoked by inflammation that may be induced, for example, by infections (9). This state can also be overcome by presentation of antigen on "professional APCs," as has been described for endocrine allografts that are depleted of professional APCs by culturing prior to implantation (11).

Anergy

Another consequence that may occur when T cells encounter peptide/MHC complexes that they recognize without receiving adequate accessory or costimulatory signals is anergy. A lymphocyte is considered "anergic" if it cannot be fully activated by encounter with the antigen that its clonally distributed surface receptor (surface Ig in the case of the B cell, and T-cell receptor in the case of the T cell) specifically recognizes. Frequently in the case of T cells, the anergic state is associated with a lack of interleukin (IL)-2 production and can be overcome by providing exogenous IL-2 (12,13). Numerous methods of inducing T- and B-cell anergy have been described (10,14–17). Anergy of both T and B cells has, in some instances, been associated with T-cell receptor (TCR) and Ig receptor downregulation, respectively (10,18–20). In the case of B-cell tolerance, the ability to induce anergy versus activation may be dependent on antigen concentration (10). In addition to the encounter of antigen without costimulation, T cells may also be anergized by encounter with peptide ligands for which they have low affinity (21,22). Unlike deletional tolerance, however, the anergic state is reversible in vivo and can be overcome by infection (23) or by removal of antigen (24,25).

Several peripheral tolerance models in which the mechanisms are not fully defined may involve anergy (26–28). In the case of rodent vascularized organ allografts, permanent graft acceptance and tolerance are often observed after treatment with a short course of an immunosuppressive agent (29–31). T-cell unresponsiveness to TCR cross-linking has also been described after transplantation of I-E$^+$ islet allografts into I-E$^-$ recipients after anti-CD4 mAb treatment (32). Of course, unresponsiveness to antigenic stimulation does not in itself demonstrate the presence of anergy. T cells with receptors that recognize the donor antigen must still be present in the unresponsive population, and a suppressive mechanism of unresponsiveness must be ruled out.

The presence of donor-reactive TCRs can be demonstrated using mAbs that recognize particular V_β used by T-cell families recognizing superantigens that can be presented by the donor and not the recipient. This approach was used to demonstrate a role for anergy in the induction of tolerance in mice receiving allogeneic BMT after treatment with T-cell–depleting mAbs (27). However, superantigens have not been shown to function as transplantation antigens, so information about mechanisms of tolerance can only be inferred from their analysis. The recent development of TCR-transgenic mice, in which the fate of large numbers of T cells expressing a transgenic receptor recognizing a known transplantation antigen can be followed, has provided a valuable tool for the analysis of anergy and other mechanisms of tolerance (20,33,34).

Other approaches to inducing anergy in transplantation models have involved the administration of "nonprofessional" APCs such as hepatocytes or MHC-transfected fibroblasts intravenously prior to organ transplantation (35,36). It is possible that donor-specific transfusions facilitate tolerance induction (37) because of their B-cell and T-cell contents, both of which can present antigen in a manner that induces anergy (38,39). Another way of inducing anergy by providing antigen in the absence of adequate costimulation involves the use of ultraviolet irradiation to inhibit APC function (40).

Intense interest has recently been focused on inducing tolerance by blocking the B7/CD28 costimulatory pathway. Such blocking can inhibit alloresponses in vitro and induce T-cell anergy (41,42). Induction of peripheral tolerance has indeed been described in animals receiving vascularized allografts (30,43–45) or pancreatic islet xenografts (46) under cover of CTLA4Ig, a synthetic soluble molecule that contains the B7-binding portion of CTLA4, one of the T-cell ligands of B7 (43,46). However, it should be remembered that both islets and vascularized allografts have been shown to have tolerogenic capacity of their own in rodents (47–51). CTLA4Ig blocks CD28 binding to both B7 molecules, B7-1 and B7-2. Recent studies suggest that differential blocking of B7-1 or B7-2 using specific mAbs may have different consequences, depending on the tissue to which tolerance induction is being attempted, and that T_H1-type and T_H2-type T-cell responses may be selectively inhibited by blocking one or the other of these two costimulatory molecules (52). Evidence in a rat renal allograft model suggests that CTLA4Ig may favor the development of T_H2 responses, which may be less acutely destructive than T_H1 responses (see below).

Regarding the induction of tolerance to human islet xenografts under CTLA4Ig cover in mice, the human-to-mouse combination may be so disparate that multiple costimulatory, adhesive, and cytokine-mediated interactions between the two species are defective, resulting in greater ease of tolerance induction when the few functional costimulatory pathways are disrupted. Several known costimulatory pathways and adhesive interactions between human responder T cells and porcine stimulatory cells appear functional (53–55), it is possible that blocking single costimulatory pathways may not be sufficient to reliably ensure induction of tolerance to porcine xenograft donors.

Blocking of the CD28/B7 costimulatory pathway has also been evaluated as an approach to inhibiting GVHD, with limited success (56). However, combined in vitro and in vivo treatment, with exposure to host antigens and a combination of CTLA4Ig and mAb against the β-integrin adhesion molecule LFA-1, can markedly inhibit the capacity of donor T cells to cause GVHD (57). This protocol specifically tolerizes donor T cells to recipient antigens prior to transplant, and does not appear to impair alloengraftment or, importantly, immune reconstitution. However, it remains to be seen whether graft-versus-leukemia responses will be impaired by this treatment.

Recent studies have demonstrated the importance of interactions between CD154 on T cells and its ligand CD40, which is expressed not only on B cells, but on a variety of APCs. Signaling through the interaction of CD40 on APCs with its T-cell ligand is necessary for the conversion of certain nonprofessional APCs, such as B cells, to APCs, in part by upregulating B7 expression. In addition to its important role in providing cognate help for B-cell activation, this interaction probably provides important costimulation leading to T-cell activation. Recent studies suggest that blocking CD154/CD40 interactions can result in graft prolongation or in a state of T-cell tolerance that may be associated with a T_H2-dominant immune response or with a reduction in the production of nitric oxide, an important mediator produced by activated macrophages (58–60). Treatment with anti-CD154 mAb has recently been shown to inhibit GVHD in a parent-to-F1 model and to promote alloengraftment (58). Exposure to recipient alloantigens in the presence of anti-CD154 has also been shown to reduce the GVHD-inducing capacity of donor T cells (61). The role of anergy, if any, in these systems remains to be determined.

Recently, the use of anti-CD154 with or without CTLA4Ig has been shown to have particularly powerful graft-prolonging effects in rodents (62) and in a primate model (63). However, these studies do not show that a state of tolerance is induced by these agents in these stringent models, but rather that the agents serve as potent immunosuppressives. Another model in which anti-CD154 has shown potent graft prolonging effects involves islet (64) or skin (64a) grafting along with donor-specific transfusion. However, systemic tolerance is not induced in this model, and the mechanisms of anti-donor hyporesponsiveness remain to be defined.

T-cell anergy has also been induced in transplantation models by the administration of mAbs that block adhesion molecules (65). Combined treatment with mAbs against lymphocyte function–associated (LFA)-1 and its ligand intracellular adhesion molecule (CAM)-1 has been reported to induce profound tolerance in murine cardiac allograft recipients (66).

Suppression

Graft acceptance may be permitted due to suppressive cell populations that inhibit the responses of donor-reactive T or B cells. Specific suppression of Ig responses by anti-idiotypic antibody was first proposed by Jerne (67). Suppression of T-cell responses has been attributed to T cells, non-T cells, and antibodies, and may be antigen-specific or nonspecific. While functional evidence for the existence of alloantigen-specific suppressor cells of T-cell responses has been obtained in several transplantation models (68–75), such cells have been cloned in only a few instances (76), and it has been difficult to identify suppressor-cell–specific surface markers.

In addition, few mechanisms of specific suppression of alloreactivity have been defined. One such mechanism may involve the cytokine transforming growth factor beta (TGFβ), which has been shown to be involved in the veto cell–mediated inhibition of cytotoxic T lymphocyte (CTL) activity by rhesus monkey bone marrow cells (77). This molecule is also produced by a newly-defined regulatory T-cell type that produces additional cytokines and can inhibit inflammatory bowel disease (78). In a model of antigen-specific T-cell–mediated suppression of responses to a soluble protein antigen, the α chain of the TCR has been implicated as a soluble suppressor factor that confers antigenic specificity of suppression (79).

One additional means of inducing specific tolerance is through a process known as "enhancement," which involves prolongation of graft survival in the presence of donor-specific antibodies. In some cases, enhancement can be passively transferred by these antibodies ("passive enhancement") (80). Enhancement has been most successful in prolonging rodent vascularized allograft transplants in certain strain combinations, and has been much less effective in prolonging skin graft survival. The mechanism of enhancement is incompletely understood. It involves more than the peripheral masking of MHC antigens or antibody-mediated graft APC depletion, as there is clearly a cell-mediated systemic component to the tolerance that results (81).

It seems possible that some suppressive phenomena could be explained by the recently described dichotomy of helper T cell function (82). Many groups have described a shift to the IL-4– and IL-10–producing helper T type 2 (T_H2)-type of response from a proinflammatory [IL-2– and interferon (IFN)-γ–producing] T_H1 response in association with allograft acceptance (31,83–87). Since T_H1 and T_H2 responses mutually downregulate one another, these observations have led to the hypothesis that T_H2 responses are tolerogenic. In a few cases, it has been shown that the use of mAbs that antagonize T_H2 cytokines can impede graft acceptance (84).

T_H2 cytokines may play a role in the induction of "infectious tolerance" observed in mice receiving minor antigen–disparate skin allografts under cover of nondepleting anti-T cell mAbs (7,26). In elegant studies, Waldmann and colleagues demonstrated that CD4 T cells rendered incapable of rejecting the allograft in the original recipients could render naive T cells unresponsive in secondary recipients, and that these tolerant T cells could, in turn, tolerize naive T cells in tertiary recipients (26). T_H2 responses may influence APCs in a manner that prevents them from providing cytokines or costimulation that could cause naive T cells to differentiate into T_H1 cells.

An immune response that is nondestructive and inhibits the development of destructive responses could provide a powerful means of ensuring graft acceptance. However, a T_H1 to T_H2 shift does not appear to fully account for the tolerance in the above model (7). Furthermore, most of the data examining T_H1 and T_H2 cytokines merely demonstrate an association of T_H2-dominant responses with graft acceptance, and only limited data exist to implicate an active role for T_H2 cells in tolerance induction (88).

It seems unlikely that T_H2 responses are benign and nondestructive under all circumstances. Recent studies have demonstrated T_H2 responses in association with allograft rejection (89–91), and others have shown accelerated graft rejection in response to T_H2-type cytokine administration (92). In view of the tendency of T_H2 to provide help for humoral immune responses (82), and of the possible involvement of antibodies in chronic rejection (93), it will be very important to carefully evaluate chronic rejection in models showing T_H2 responses to grafts.

With respect to xenoresponses, it has recently been suggested that xenograft rejection in at least one species combination is associated with a predominant T_H2-type response (94). Thus, the potential of immune deviation to a T_H2 response—or, in fact, any other suppressive phenomenon—to induce xenograft acceptance has yet to be demonstrated.

Recent studies have demonstrated that cytokines whose production was once considered to be regulated as a group of "T_H1-like" or "T_H2-like" molecules are, in fact, regulated independently (95–97). Thus, the T_H1/T_H2 dichotomy is probably an oversimplification, and future studies are likely to better clarify the role of individual cytokines in inducing graft acceptance and rejection.

Deletion

Recent studies have demonstrated that a major mechanism by which self tolerance normally develops among both T and B cells is deletion of developing lymphocyte clones with rearranged receptors that recognize self antigens. Deletion of self-reactive T cells occurs when an immature thymocyte binds with high affinity to a peptide/MHC complex presented in the thymus, hence undergoing apoptotic cell death (21,22). Several marrow-derived cell types, including dendritic cells, B cells, and thymocytes, as well as nonhematopoietic cells of the host thymus (98,99), have the capacity to induce intrathymic tolerance by both deletional and nondeletional mechanisms. Tolerance induced by intrathymic deletion should be very reliable, because the absence of lymphocytes with reactivity to the donor would ensure that a specific response to donor antigens could not be induced under any circumstances.

Deletion may not be unique to immature stages of T-cell development. Peripheral deletion, often following activation, has been described for mature T cells upon exposure to antigen in vivo (20,100). In addition, veto cells (see below) can delete alloreactive CTL precursors.

Because natural antibody (NAb)-producing B cells are a major obstacle to discordant vascularized xenografting, it would be highly beneficial if these cells could be specifically tolerized prior to transplantation. Studies using Ig receptor–transgenic mice suggest that B cells are susceptible to deletion or receptor editing at particular stages of development upon recognition of membrane-bound antigen (10). Antigen expression on radioresistant host cells or a small population of hematopoietic cells appears sufficient to delete immature B cells specific for that antigen (101). To avoid hyperacute rejection, it will be necessary to devise methods of eliminating or tolerizing both preexisting NAb-producing B cells and plasma cells, and of tolerizing B cells that develop subsequent to transplantation.

CHIMERISM AND CENTRAL TOLERANCE

The pioneering work of Owen, Medawar, and others, beginning 50 years ago, led to the observation that hematopoietic chimerism can be associated with a state of donor-specific tolerance (65). Tolerance can most readily be induced by allogeneic hematopoietic cells in animals that are developmentally immunodeficient or in which immunodeficiency has been artificially induced. The capacity of hematopoietic cells to induce tolerance results largely from their ability to induce intrathymic clonal deletion of thymocytes with T-cell receptors that recognize antigens expressed by the hematopoietic cells. The potency of this approach is demonstrated by studies in which preexisting T cells are adequately eliminated and bone marrow engraftment is achieved. In such instances, tolerance to the most immunogenic allografts, such as fully MHC-mismatched skin grafts and small bowel grafts, is reliably attained (102,103).

Obstacles to the Use of Hematopoietic Cell Transplantation for the Induction of Central Tolerance in Man

In view of its potent and reliable ability to induce intrathymic tolerance, it may seem surprising that hematopoietic cell transplantation has not yet been applied to the induction of tolerance in man. However, there are numerous immunologic and physiologic obstacles to the engraftment and function of allogeneic and xenogeneic hematopoietic cells.

Donor cells with long-term multilineage repopulating ability, known as pluripotent hematopoietic stem cells (PHSCs), must survive and function sufficiently to provide a life-long source of donor antigens in the thymus. Furthermore, if the preexisting peripheral alloreactivity is not adequately eliminated, eventual rejection may ensue even if initial intrathymic chimerism is achieved. The barriers to allogeneic and xenogeneic marrow engraftment and hematopoiesis are summarized in Table 5.1.

The simplest and most widely-used approach to overcoming the immunologic and physiologic barriers to marrow engraftment in adult animals has been to pretreat recipients with lethal whole body irradiation (WBI) prior to BMT. While this procedure is well tolerated and reliably induces chimerism and tolerance in rodents, its use is less feasible in humans. Lethal WBI is unduly toxic for use in patients who do not have malignant diseases and who may have a high likelihood of survival without a bone marrow transplant. Furthermore, BMT across HLA barriers is associated with an inordinately high risk of GVHD and engraftment failure (104). Thus, studies in mice showing that sublethal irradiation, with or without cyclophosphamide treatment, is sufficient to allow engraftment of allogeneic marrow given in conventional doses (105,106) are unlikely to be directly applicable to HLA-mismatched allogeneic or xenogeneic transplantation in humans.

Table 5.1. Barriers to Allogeneic and Xenogeneic Hematopoietic Cell Engraftment and Hematopoiesis

Physiologic/Regulatory
Space/physical niches
Cytokines (soluble and stromal cell-bound)*
Adhesion molecules*
Immunologic
T cells (CD4 and CD8; double-negative T cells?*)
Antibodies (from prior sensitization; natural antibodies*)
Natural killer cells*

* May be an especially important barrier to xenogeneic hematopoiesis.

Studies reporting the existence of a novel $CD3^+$, $TCR\alpha\beta^-$, $TCR\gamma\delta^-$, $CD8^+$ bone marrow cell population that facilitates PHSC engraftment (107) have recently received widespread attention. The identity of this unusual cell population and its mechanism of action remain to be determined. While it is well established that conventional $CD8^+$ T cells can enhance marrow engraftment, the ability of a non-T cell expressing CD8 to do so has only been reported by one group and remains to be confirmed by others.

Thus, before the BMT approach to tolerance can be applied clinically it will be necessary to understand the immunologic and physiologic barriers to hematopoiesis in allogeneic and xenogeneic environments, and to develop more specific methods of overcoming these barriers. It would be most desirable to achieve a state of mixed lymphohematopoietic chimerism rather than full donor reconstitution in completely MHC-mismatched combinations. Improved immunocompetence has been observed in mixed chimeras, which contain host-type APCs in the peripheral tissues, presumably because these allow optimal antigen presentation to T cells that have developed in the host thymus and may therefore preferentially recognize peptide antigens presented by host MHC (108,109).

Immunologic Barriers to Allogeneic and Xenogeneic Hematopoietic Cell Engraftment

A model that allows induction of mixed chimerism and donor-specific tolerance across MHC barriers in mice without myeloablative conditioning (102) has helped to define the immunologic barriers to marrow engraftment. This model, which is illustrated in Figure 5.1, involves the use of depleting anti-CD4 and anti-CD8 mAbs followed by a low dose (3 Gy) of WBI and a higher dose (7 Gy) of local irradiation to the thymus. Similar results have recently been achieved using anti-$TCR\alpha\beta$ antibody and 3-Gy WBI (110). These studies (102,111) and others (112) have shown that either $CD4^+$ or $CD8^+$ T cells of the host can readily reject fully MHC-mismatched marrow, and also, as expected, that $CD4^+$ cells reject class II–mismatched marrow and CD8 cells reject class I–disparate marrow. Additionally, CD8 cells play a significant role in rejecting class II–mismatched marrow, and $CD4^+$ host cells pose a weak but detectable barrier to class I–mismatched marrow (111,112). These results are summarized in Table 5.2.

Natural killer (NK) cells, which have long been assumed to resist allogeneic marrow engraftment on the basis of short-term studies of resistance to myeloid progenitor proliferation, actually present only a weak barrier to the engraftment of allogeneic PHSCs (113,114). However, NK cells may play a more significant role in resisting the engraftment of xenogeneic marrow (115).

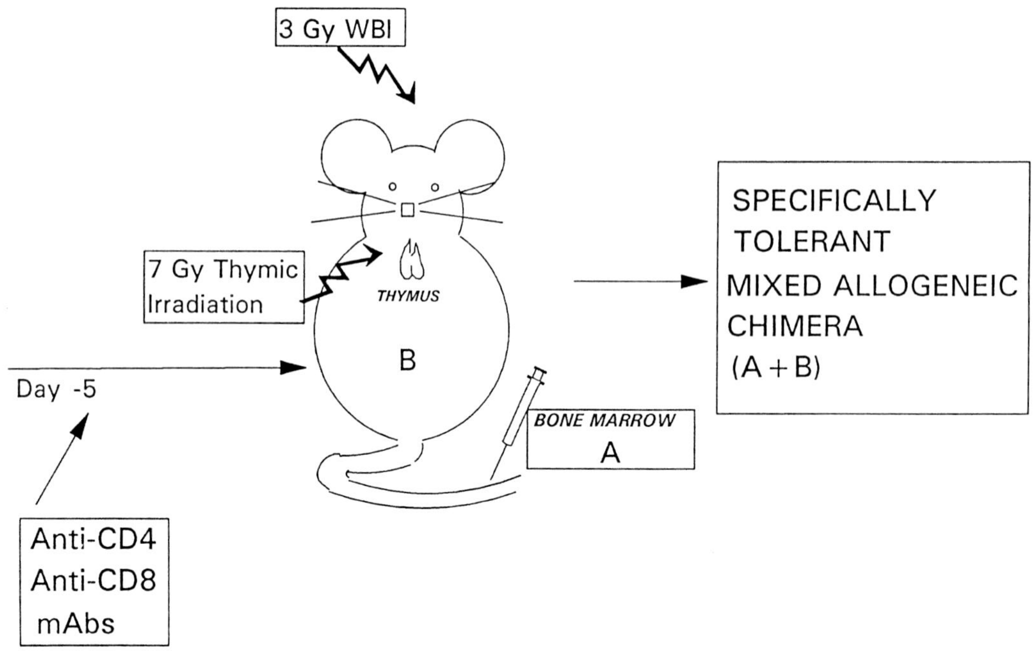

FIGURE 5.1. *Method for producing mixed allogeneic (fully MHC-mismatched) chimeras using a non-myeloablative conditioning regimen. Depleting anti-mouse CD4 mAb is GK1.5 (198), and anti-CD8 mAb is 2.43 (199).*

Table 5.2. Summary of T-Cell Subsets Resisting Allogeneic and Xenogeneic Marrow Engraftment in the Mouse

$CD4^+$ cells resist engraftment of class II–mismatched and, to a lesser extent, class I–mismatched allogeneic marrow.
$CD8^+$ cells resist engraftment of class I–mismatched and class II–mismatched allogeneic marrow.
CD4 and/or CD8 T cells resist engraftment of xenogeneic rat marrow in mice.
$Thy1^+$ (presumably $CD4^-CD8^-$) cells resist rat marrow engraftment in mice.

Physiologic Barriers to Allogeneic and Xenogeneic Hematopoietic Cell Engraftment

The concept that "space" must be created in the hematopoietic compartment to allow donor stem cells to engraft has long been widely accepted. In a syngeneic BMT system in which donors and hosts differed only by nonimmunogenic alleles of the leukocyte common antigen Ly-5, a low dose (1.5 to 3.0 Gy) of WBI was required to make physiologic "space" for engraftment of syngeneic marrow cells, which were given in numbers similar to those which could be obtained from marrow of living human allogeneic marrow donors (116). However, this requirement can be overcome by the administration of very high doses of syngeneic marrow (117,118).The dose of irradiation required to achieve allogeneic marrow engraftment in mice can be reduced by administering increasing numbers of donor marrow cells (119).

Successful engraftment of large numbers of T-cell–depleted HLA-mismatched mobilized peripheral blood and marrow stem cells in humans supports the concept that alloengraftment can also be enhanced by increasing the number of hematopoietic progenitors administered (120).

We have recently demonstrated that engraftment of high doses of allogeneic marrow can be achieved without myelosuppressive treatment in mice that receive T-cell–depleting mAbs (121). However, we have learned from these studies that it is essential to create "space" in the thymus and to achieve high levels of early donor T-cell repopulation in order to achieve permanent skin graft tolerance. Apparently, thymic "space" and peripheral hematopoietic "space" are regulated independently (121).

Using peripheral blood stem cells collected after cytokine mobilization, or using cadaveric donors, it may be possible to transplant large numbers of allogeneic hematopoietic cells to humans. Advances in the ability to propagate primitive hematopoietic cells in vitro using cytokine combinations (122,123), and to reconstitute autologous hematopoiesis in patients with progenitor cells expanded in vitro (124), suggest that ex vivo expansion of allogeneic hematopoietic cells could have clinical utility. The potential to overcome the requirement for host myelosuppression by giving large numbers of hematopoietic cells, which might be available from inbred porcine donors, also deserves exploration in xenotransplantation.

The mechanism by which myelosuppression promotes marrow engraftment is not fully understood, and could include both the creation of physical niches after the destruction of host hematopoietic cells and the upregulation of cytokines that promote hematopoiesis. Homing to the marrow environment depends on interactions between adhesion molecules and their ligands (125), and active

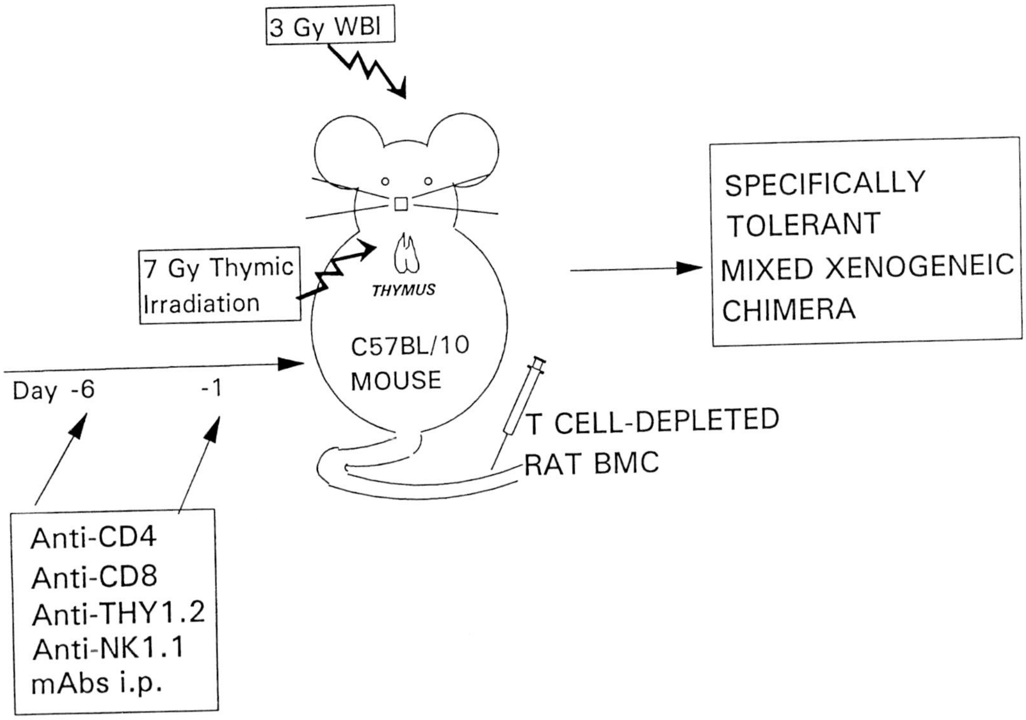

FIGURE 5.2. *Method for producing mixed xenogeneic (rat-to-mouse) chimeras using a non-myeloablative conditioning regimen. Anti-mouse CD4 mAb is GK1.5 (198), anti-mouse CD8 mAb is 2.43 (199), anti-Thy1.2 mAb is 30H-12 (200), and anti-NK1.1 mAb is PK136 (201). Rat marrow was T-cell depleted as described (115).*

hematopoiesis may also depend on specific molecular interactions between the stroma and hematopoietic cells. It is probably the species specificity of some of these interactions (cytokines, adhesion molecules, other cell surface signaling molecules) that accounts for the competitive advantage enjoyed by recipient marrow over xenogeneic donor marrow, as is discussed below.

The mAb-based non-myeloablative approach to host conditioning used in the mouse allogeneic BMT model described above has been extended to the xenogeneic rat-to-mouse combination (Fig. 5.2; see Table 5.2). However, in the xenogeneic model, large numbers of donor bone marrow cells (BMCs) are needed to achieve engraftment, and the level of rat hematopoietic reconstitution gradually declines over time, despite persistent tolerance (115,126). This decline, which can be averted by the late administration of repeated marrow injections (126), is due to a competitive advantage enjoyed by host hematopoietic cells over xenogeneic cells that becomes increasingly evident as recovery of the host from low-dose WBI occurs (127).

Achievement of xenogeneic hematopoietic repopulation has proved to be an even more formidable challenge in more disparate species combinations. Human and pig progenitor cells have been clearly shown to be capable of repopulating murine recipients at low levels (128–130), but the species specificity of critical regulatory molecules may limit the level of donor repopulation. Administration of exogenous donor species-specific cytokines can partially overcome this barrier (129,131).

Tolerance of Natural Antibody-Producing B Cells

Studies in the rat-to-mouse mixed chimerism model described above also demonstrated that mixed chimerism has the capacity to induce tolerance among natural antibody (NAb)-producing B cells, in addition to T cells (132,133). More recently, it has been demonstrated that mixed chimerism can induce tolerance among Nab-producing B cells with the very important anti-α1,3-gal specificity (see below), the major specificity of human Nabs that recognize porcine xenoantigens. These studies (134) were performed in α1,3-gal-deficient mice, which, like humans, produce NAb with this specificity. More recently, similar results have been achieved in α1,3-gal-deficient mice receiving the non-myeloablative conditioning regimen shown in Figure 5.1 (Ohdan H, et al, manuscript submitted).

How Much Intrathymic Chimerism Is Needed to Achieve Full Deletional Tolerance?

In mice receiving allogeneic BMT after conditioning with anti-CD4 and anti-CD8 mAbs, 3-Gy WBI, and 7-Gy thymic irradiation, the first wave of thymocyte recovery (day 10) showed complete deletion of mature host thymocytes recognizing superantigens presented by donor I-E MHC molecules, despite the presence of very small numbers of donor I-E–bearing cells in the thymus at this early time (135). Thymic irradiation can be excluded from this conditioning regimen if a second pretransplant anti-T cell mAb injection is given (136) to overcome residual intrathymic anti-donor alloreactivity (Nikolic B, Sykes M, manuscript in preparation). The second mAb injection reliably permits early intrathymic deletion of donor-reactive host thymocytes (137). However, some animals receiving this regimen (two mAb treatments without thymic irradiation) show gradual decline in chimerism among all lineages and eventual loss of tolerance, as measured by rejection upon repeat donor skin grafting (136).

A low fraction (<20%) of donor cells among T cells that initially repopulate these animals reliably predicts an eventual loss of chimerism in all lineages, even if high levels of engraftment are initially seen in non-T cell lineages (136) (Fig. 5.3). Studies are in progress to determine the reason for this correlation, which might reflect a role for donor thymocytes themselves in the induction of tolerance among residual host thymocytes. Alternatively, it may relate to the fact that thymocytes and intrathymic dendritic cells, which are believed to have strong tolerance-inducing activities, are derived from a common progenitor (138,139).

THE CHIMERISM APPROACH IN LARGE ANIMALS

Tolerance Induction in an Allogeneic Primate BMT Model

Because the non-myeloablative preparative regimen used in mice as described above was far less toxic than the lethal preparative regimen used in previous studies, we have considered it for potential clinical applicability. We have therefore recently developed a similar protocol in cynomolgus monkeys as a preclinical large animal model (140).

Pairs of animals were selected following serologic and mixed lymphocyte reaction (MLR) testing to ensure that they were fully MHC mismatched. Animals were chosen such that at least one mAb was available that reacted with the donor MHC and not with the recipient, for detection of chimerism by flow cytometry (FCM) after transplant.

As illustrated in Figure 5.4, animals received 3-Gy WBI, 7-Gy thymic irradiation, and horse anti-human antithymocyte globulin (ATG) preoperatively. Bilateral nephrectomy,

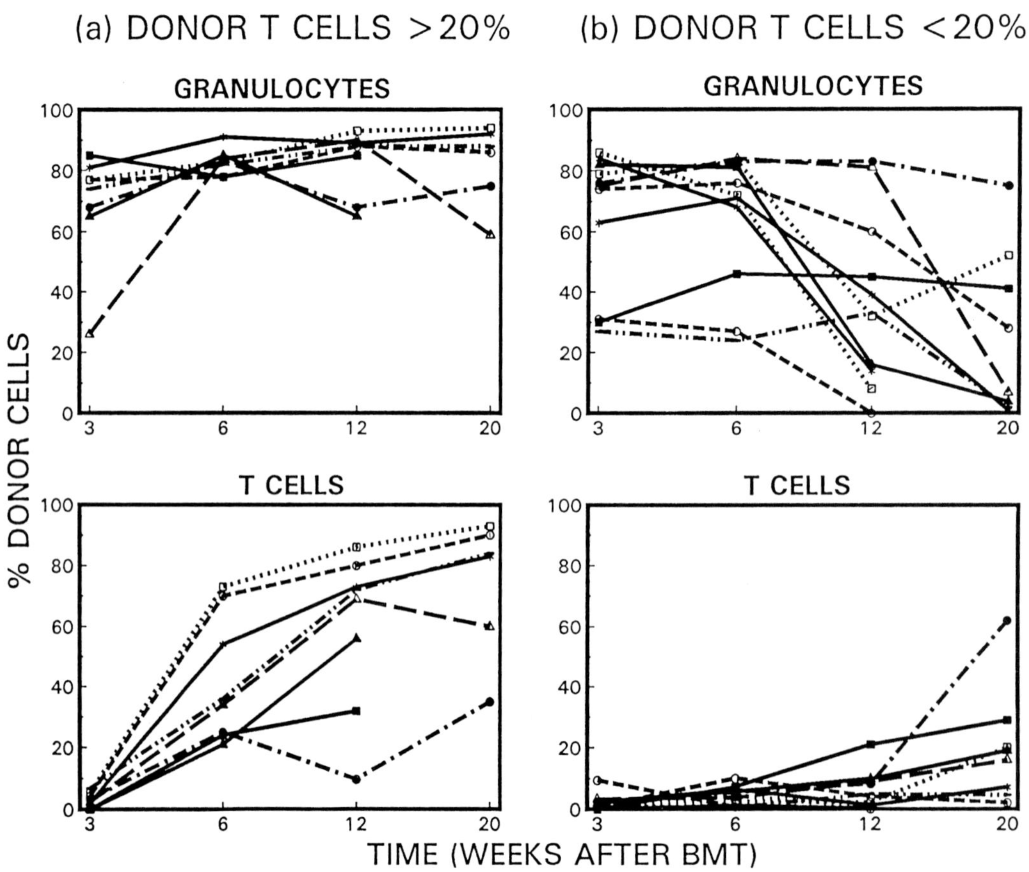

FIGURE 5.3. *Early levels of donor T-cell repopulation predict long-term chimerism in mixed chimeras prepared without thymic irradiation (TI). A relationship is shown between the level of T-cell chimerism at 6 weeks and long-term, stable chimerism in the granulocyte lineage in white blood cells of B10 mice receiving B10.A. BMCs after conditioning with mAbs on days –6 and –1 and 3-Gy WBI on day 0, without TI. Percentages of donor granulocytes and T cells were determined by two-color FCM analysis. Each line represents an individual animal that was studied at each of the indicated time points. (**a**) Mice with >20% donor T cells at 6 weeks showed lasting multilineage chimerism; (**b**) mice with <20% showed a gradual decline in chimerism.*

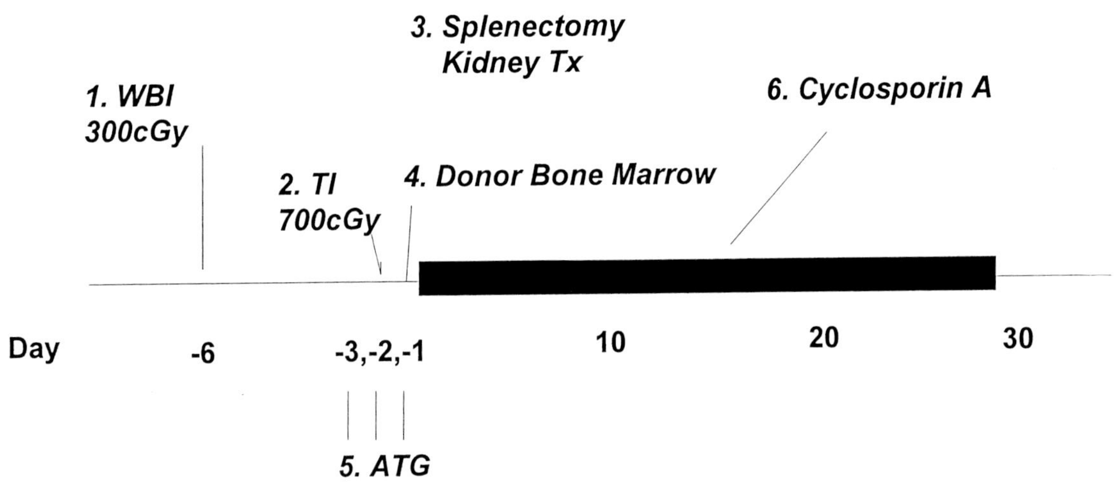

FIGURE 5.4. *Schematic representation of protocol for non-myeloablative preparative regimen to induce tolerance between fully MHC haplotype–mismatched cynomolgus monkeys.*

splenectomy, orthotopic kidney transplantation, and donor bone marrow administration were all performed on day 0 (see below for further details on the preparative regimen). To supplement suppression of mature T cells by ATG, treatment with IM cyclosporine (CsA) was begun on day 1 and continued for 4 weeks. No further immunosuppression was administered after this time. This protocol was thus highly analogous to that used in our previous murine studies (102).

Monkeys treated by this regimen became pancytopenic on day 8 but recovered thereafter, becoming essentially normal hematologically by day 30. Sequential FCM analyses showed clear evidence for chimerism among lymphoid, myeloid, and monocytic subpopulations, generally detected first on about day 8 and persisting until day 30. Thereafter, the levels of detectable chimerism decreased progressively, becoming difficult to distinguish from background staining with isotype control antibodies (i.e., less than 1% to 2%) by FCM. In five of six animals treated by this protocol, transplantation tolerance was induced, as assessed by MLR assays, by monitoring kidney transplant function, and in one case by acceptance of a full thickness graft of frozen skin from the kidney donor (140). In none of these animals was any additional exogenous immunosuppression administered after day 30. We have concluded that specific transplantation tolerance can be induced in primates by this procedure (140).

Mixed Chimerism in a Pig-to-Primate Discordant Xenograft Combination

The Non-myeloablative Protocol

We have recently begun studies attempting to extend the non-myeloablative regimen for production of mixed chimerism to the discordant pig-to-primate (cynomolgus monkey) combination (141). The protocol we have used is illustrated schematically in Figure 5.5. This protocol parallels very closely that which we have previously demonstrated to be effective for inducing long-term graft acceptance in allogeneic mouse combinations (102), in concordant rat-to-mouse xenogeneic combinations (115), and fully MHC-mismatched cynomolgus monkeys (140).

The one main difference from previous protocols is the need to remove natural antibodies from the recipient's circulation to avoid hyperacute rejection. As illustrated in Figure 5.5, this has been accomplished in our model by intraoperative perfusion of the monkey's blood either through an isolated pig liver or through specific antigen-bearing columns via silastic catheters inserted into the aorta and vena cava on day 0, immediately prior to renal transplantation (142). It is interesting to note that a similar procedure using ex vivo pig liver perfusion has been used clinically to treat hepatic coma (143,144). Our use of solid matrix columns bearing appropriate α1,3-galactose sugar linkages is based on reports suggesting that the majority of primate anti-swine natural antibodies are directed to this epitope (145,146), which has been confirmed in our laboratory. Our early results with such columns are encouraging (147).

The preparative regimen we have used is very similar to that used in our monkey allotransplantation model, as described above. Sublethal irradiation consisting of three fractions of WBI (1 Gy each) were administered on days −6 and −5, and 7 Gy of thymic irradiation was administered on day −1. Although it is not clear in either of these large animal models whether thymic irradiation is required, we have retained it in the protocols and are presently testing its necessity in the allogeneic model. Similarly, splenectomy on day 0, although not yet proven to be a necessary part of the preparative regimen, has been included in the protocol because of its apparent usefulness in other transplant models involving preformed antibodies (148,149).

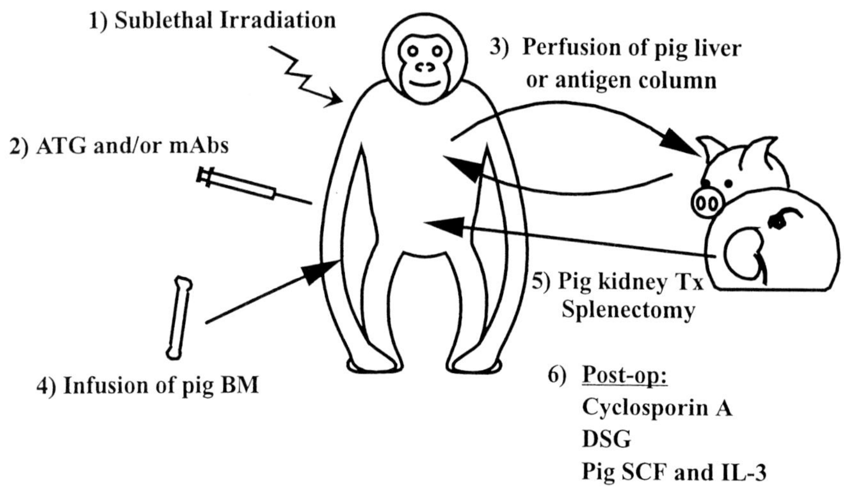

FIGURE 5.5. *Schematic representation of non-myeloablative protocol for attempts to induce transplantation tolerance across the discordant xenogeneic barrier of pig-to-cynomolgus monkey through establishment of mixed chimerism.*

Because no monoclonal antibodies to remove mature T cells from monkeys in vivo are yet available, we have used ATG (Upjohn, Kalamazoo, MI) for this purpose. This reagent was administered on days −2, −1, and 0 (50 mg/kg, IV). As described for our allogeneic primate model (140), examination of lymph nodes indicated that this T-cell depletion was not complete, so we have included a course of CsA (15 mg/kg per day, IV) to further suppress T-cell function in the immediate post-transplant period. Recently, 2 weeks of treatment with 15-desoxyspergualin were also added because of the drug's ability to suppress antibody responses (150).

On day 0, a pig kidney was transplanted into the same large vessels used for the perfusion procedure. Pig bone marrow was harvested and prepared from the same donor, and was infused at approximately 5×10^8 cells/kg perioperatively.

Removal of Natural Antibodies

Removal of NAbs in this combination has been successful in avoiding hyperacute rejection in more than 15 pig-to-monkey xenotransplants performed to date (151). A summary of kidney survivals in this series of animals is shown in Figure 5.6. Following the full preparative regimen, kidney grafts have functioned normally for up to 15 days, achieving normal BUN and creatinine levels. Open biopsies during this time have revealed normal kidneys grossly, and have shown normal kidney histology. However, in all of these animals the kidney subsequently succumbed to a vascular form of rejection, and no long-term kidney survivals were achieved. In addition, with the exception of recent animals in which pig recombinant growth factors were used (see below), there has only been transient evidence for pig cell chimerism, with a low level of pig cells (1% to 5%) in the peripheral blood (151).

The absorption procedure led to an almost complete removal of IgM and IgG anti-pig antibodies, and these antibodies remained at very low levels until shortly before rejection. However, it is possible these low levels were maintained by further in vivo absorption by the kidney itself, as in control animals without kidney grafts these antibodies reappeared rapidly. In animals that rejected the xenografts, IgG antibodies were observed in the serum at the time of rejection, and found by immunofluorescence in large vessels (151).

Preliminary data indicate that this IgG antibody detected additional determinants to those detected by natural antibodies, suggesting that the production of monkey anti-pig IgG represents a T-cell–dependent immune response to the transplant, and that this phenomenon, in addition to the return of natural antibodies, may have contributed to the loss of grafts by vascular rejection during the second week. In recent studies, the use of pig recombinant cytokines after pig bone marrow administration led to absence of sensitization to determinants other than α1,3-gal, suggesting tolerance at the T cell level.

Current Status

Our studies in allogeneic systems have demonstrated that at least initial chimerism is a requirement for achieving lasting transplantation tolerance (87,152,153). Our current efforts have therefore focused on means for increasing reconstitution by pig bone marrow cells in monkey recipients (154). One of the methods being tested involves the use of pig recombinant cytokines (SCF and IL-3) in the postoperative period. Recent results suggest that administration of these cytokines to a monkey receiving the full preparative regimen prolonged survival of pig bone marrow progeny in the monkey's bone marrow for over 6 months (141). In addition, pig cytokines were used postoperatively in the animal with the longest kidney survival, shown in Figure 5.6 (#1094, 15-day survival). Unfortunately, this cynomolgus monkey died from a complication of thrombocytopenia with a functioning kidney transplant (142).

We consider these results to be preliminary, but very encouraging. We are also planning to test the use of fetal pig thymic tissue, which, in the mouse model described below, leads to discordant xenograft tolerance (155). It is our hope that, by combining the approaches being pursued in other laboratories for avoiding hyperacute rejection with

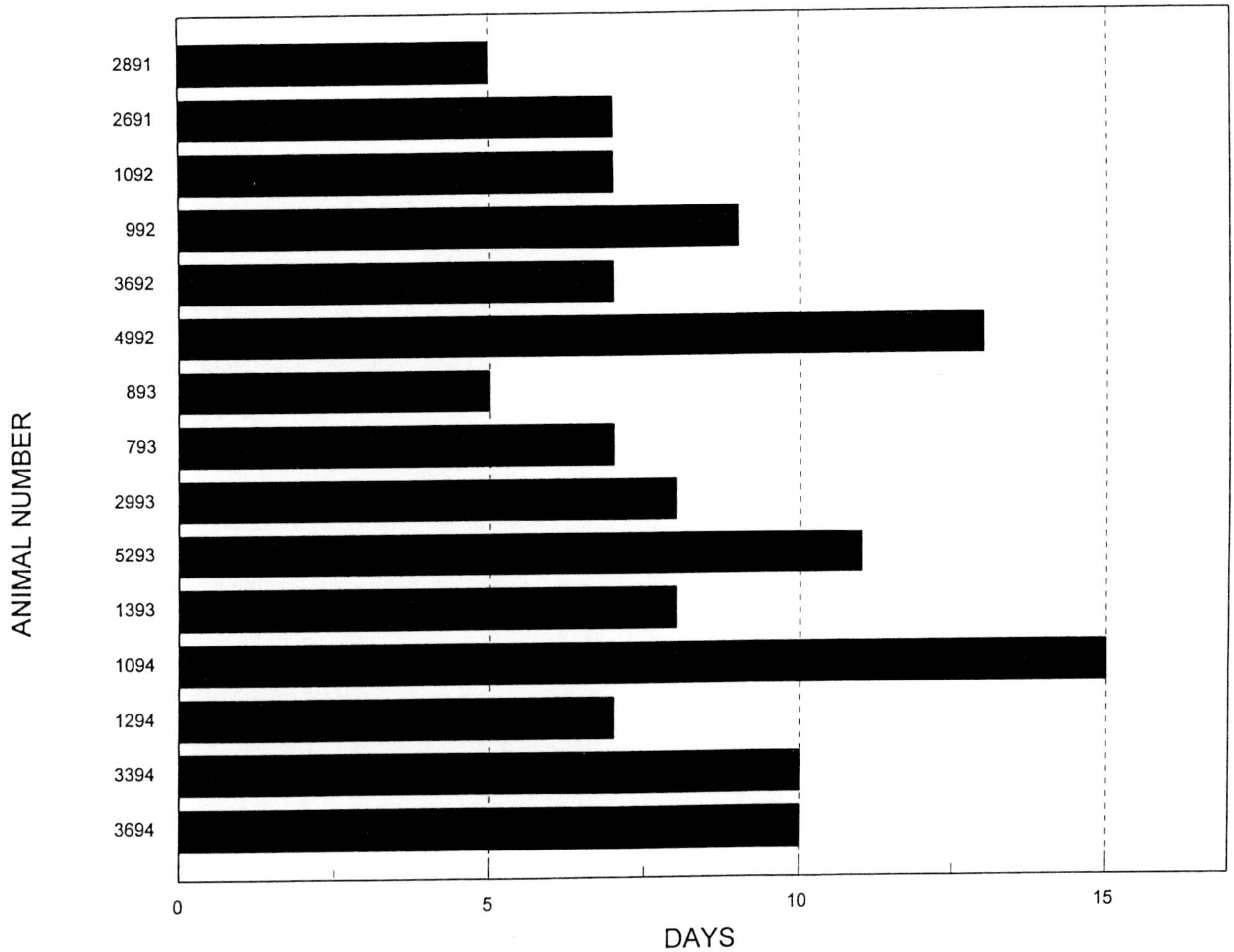

FIGURE 5.6. *Survivals of technically successful pig kidney xenografts in our series of cynomolgus monkeys.*

our own approach to inducing cellular tolerance, long-term acceptance of discordant xenografts will be achieved in the pig-to-primate combination.

DEVELOPMENT OF CHIMERISM AND TOLERANCE WITHOUT T-CELL–DEPLETING OR MYELOSUPPRESSIVE TREATMENT

Based on the recent observation that microchimerism can exist for many years in the tissues of human solid organ allograft recipients (156), it has been hypothesized that microchimerism leads to a state of donor-specific tolerance (51). Since it would be unethical to test this hypothesis by intentionally depleting donor hematopoietic cells from patients, it seems unlikely that the question of whether chimerism induces tolerance or is an epiphenomenon that reflects either tolerance or adequate immunosuppressive pharmacotherapy will be resolved in the near future.

There are a number of mechanisms by which microchimerism, might, in theory, induce peripheral T-cell tolerance. These include nonprofessional APC function of donor-derived B cells (38,157), which can anergize responding T cells. In addition, veto activity of T cells, NK cells, and other cell types eliminates CTLs reactive against antigens expressed on the veto cells (65). T cells can also tolerize other T cells by additional mechanisms (150). Putative veto activity was detected among donor cells isolated from a long-term renal allograft recipient (159), providing the first evidence for a specific mechanism by which incidental chimerism may lead to tolerance in human solid organ allograft recipients.

In addition to the above mechanisms by which chimerism might induce peripheral tolerance, donor leukocytes migrating to recipient thymi might induce central tolerance among T cells that develop subsequent to the time of donor engraftment. Recent evidence suggests that liver grafts may contain self-renewing hematopoietic stem cells (160,161), and dendritic cell progenitors have been detected in the marrow of recipients of spontaneously accepted mouse liver allografts (162).

The observation of lasting microchimerism in long-term human allograft recipients has prompted examination of the role of chimerism in a variety of animal models in which peripheral tolerance is induced. In a mouse model, in which donor-specific transfusions are given with depleting anti-CD4 mAbs prior to cardiac allografting, tolerance has been shown to require the presence of donor antigen in the induction phase, but its maintenance is independent of the lasting presence of donor hematopoietic cells. Antigen presented by the heart allograft, on the other hand, appears to be critical for maintenance of the tolerant state in these mice (163). The presence of microchimerism failed to predict tolerance in a neonatal tolerance model (164) and was not always observed in tolerant rat recipients of cardiac allografts (165). Thus, it has become clear that microchimerism neither predicts tolerance nor is required to maintain tolerance under all circumstances.

Attempts to correlate in vitro measures of donor-specific hyporesponsiveness [MLR, cell-mediated lympholysis assay (CML)] with chimerism and in vivo tolerance (166) have not all showed a correlation (167), and it is not clear that these tests could predict which patients would tolerate withdrawal of immunosuppressive therapy without rejection. Since a fraction of noncompliant long-term allograft recipients who discontinue immunosuppressive therapy do not reject their grafts, and most patients can be maintained on relatively low levels of long-term immunosuppression, it is possible that a state of partial or complete donor-specific tolerance exists in some patients. However, in view of the high rate of chronic graft rejection, it seems unlikely that the level of tolerance in most patients is adequate to allow safe removal of immunosuppressive drugs. Of course, it is possible that immunosuppressive therapy interferes with the induction of tolerance.

Attempts to increase the level of chimerism have been made in human and monkey solid organ transplant recipients by administering donor bone marrow around the time of organ transplantation, without giving specific myelosuppressive therapy (167–169). However, the clinical studies have not demonstrated a reduction in the number of rejection episodes (167,169), even when chimerism has been enhanced (167). These studies did not include intentional peripheral T-cell depletion. In the primate model, which includes recipient pretreatment with antilymphocyte serum (ALS) for T-cell depletion and, for optimal results, total lymphoid irradiation, veto cells in donor bone marrow that inactivate recipient CTLp may promote graft acceptance (77). However, only a fraction of recipients show long-term graft acceptance, with the best results obtained when the donor and recipient share a DR class II MHC allele (168).

Chimerism might contribute to tolerance without the use of myelosuppressive or immunosuppressive conditioning in recipients that are developmentally immunodeficient. In neonatally tolerized animals, several mechanisms have been invoked to explain the observed tolerance. Specific suppressor T cells have been detected (170), and recent studies suggest that a T_H2-type response to the donor may be responsible for the inability to reject donor-specific skin grafts in such animals (87,171). Lasting microchimerism has been detected in some neonatally tolerized mice, and evidence to support an intrathymic deletional mechanism has been obtained in some, but not other, strain combinations (170). Furthermore, the presence of microchimerism does not always predict skin graft tolerance in recipients of allogeneic lymphocytes perinatally, and nontolerant animals can still maintain microchimerism following rejection of donor skin grafts (164,172). Similarly, induction of low levels of chimerism by intrauterine BMT in sheep was not associated with tolerance to donor organ allografts (173). Perhaps the persisting donor cells in these nontolerant animals are T cells that are able to avoid their own destruction through a veto mechanism, but which are insufficient in number to ensure a systemic state of tolerance in the recipient.

Recent studies have challenged the view that neonates are immunoincompetent and hence uniquely permissive for tolerance induction or for induction of a T_H2 response. The tendency of allogeneic cell infusions to result in tolerance and of antigen exposure to result in T_H2 responses in this period may be because of the high ratio of noncostimulatory APCs (T and B cells) in donor inocula to recipient T cells in the neonate, rather than because of any unique susceptibility to tolerance induction.

Neonatal mice can clearly mount T_H1 responses and can be immunized to alloantigens and pathogens (174–176). In fact, the ability of neonates to mount host antigraft responses may be essential for the induction of cell populations that suppress anti-donor responses. When intrathymic deletional tolerance is induced in animals in which the preexisting peripheral T-cell response has been fully ablated, suppressive responses to the donor are notably absent, and tolerance is readily broken by the infusion of nontolerant host-type lymphocytes (153,177). In contrast, tolerance cannot be easily broken by infusion of nontolerant host-type lymphocytes in neonatally tolerized animals (69,170,178).

THE RELATIONSHIP BETWEEN PERIPHERAL T-CELL TOLERANCE AND CENTRAL TOLERANCE

The distinction between central and peripheral tolerance may not always be clear. In a pig "peripheral" tolerance model, in which a class I MHC–mismatched kidney is grafted under cover of a short course of cyclosporine (179), the thymus appears to play a role in the induction of tolerance (180) (Fig. 5.7). Although passenger leukocytes from the graft that enter the thymus might help to tolerize subsequently developing thymocytes, the role of the thymus in tolerizing preexisting T cells in the periphery requires further exploration. Either of these conditions may be possible:

1. T cells that are activated in the periphery by the organ allograft recirculate to the thymus, as has been described (181), and encounter donor antigen there, perhaps on passenger leukocytes, which then inactivates the T cells. This could be a fail-safe

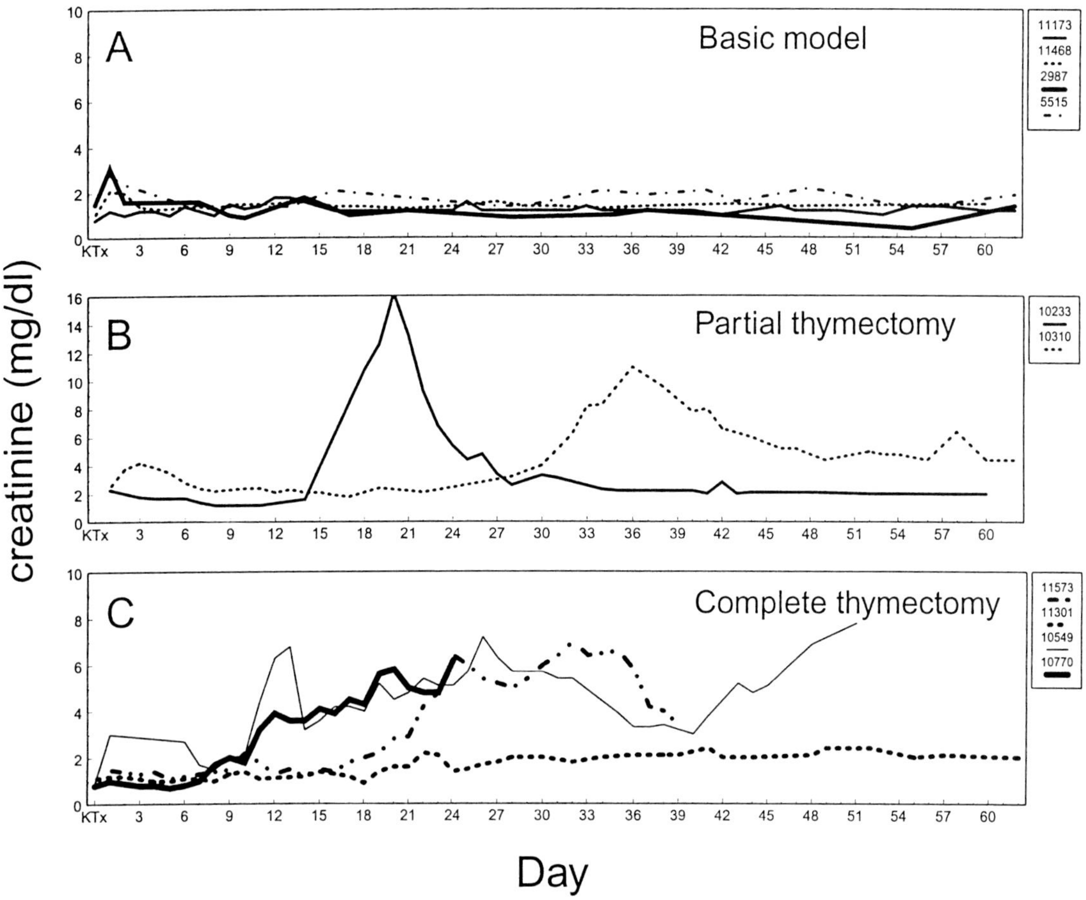

FIGURE 5.7. *Role of the thymus in "peripheral" tolerance induction across a class I barrier in pigs. Pretransplant thymectomy impairs tolerance induced across class I MHC barriers by a short course of high-dose cyclosporine in miniature swine renal allograft recipients. Creatinine levels are shown for individual animals that were thymectomized three weeks prior to kidney transplantation.*

mechanism for ensuring that T cells activated in the periphery of an animal are switched off if the same antigens are present in the thymus.

2. The migration of donor antigen to the thymus may result in the development of T cells that specifically recognize the donor antigen and downregulate the activity of destructive alloreactive T cells, perhaps by secreting T_H2-associated cytokines (68,182).
3. Recent thymic emigrants may be predisposed to becoming suppressive cells when they encounter antigen in the periphery.

A second situation in which the boundary between central and peripheral tolerance is uncertain involves the intrathymic injection of donor antigens. While initial uses of this approach included antibody treatment to deplete peripheral T cells, more recent studies have shown that tolerance to soluble alloantigens can be induced by intrathymic injection without peripheral T-cell depletion (183). Since removal of the thymus before or within the first few days of allografting results in rejection of the allograft (184), the thymus must play an active role in tolerizing preexisting peripheral T cells. This inactivation could be due to recirculation of activated T cells through the thymus or to emigration from the thymus of regulatory T cells. Active regulatory cell populations have been reported in rats receiving intrathymic injections of allogeneic BMCs (185).

The role of the allograft in inducing tolerance in animals receiving intrathymic injection should not be ignored. Transferable tolerance is not induced by intrathymic marrow injection alone without an organ allograft in rats (185), suggesting that the graft itself helps to tolerize the preexisting T-cell repertoire, perhaps by presenting antigen in the absence of costimulation or by activating recipient T cells that then recirculate to the thymus to induce tolerance via the mechanisms described above. In contrast to intrathymic injection, pure intrathymic deletional tolerance is not dependent on the continual presence of antigen in the periphery (153). Donor tissue can be grafted at any time, and tolerance is assured. The intrathymic injection approach has not been successful in "high responder" rat strain combinations and may even induce allosensitization (186,187). Intrathymic injection has not successfully allowed xenotolerance induction, suggesting that its potential may be limited.

THYMIC RECONSTITUTION POTENTIAL IN ADULTS

Depletion or inactivation of preexisting T cells, along with the minimal amount of host conditioning required to allow induction of mixed chimerism, could provide a potent and practical approach to central tolerance induction only if the host thymus is capable of reconstituting the immune system with new T cells. This is likely the case in children. However, the human thymus involutes at puberty, and little is known about its capacity to function when peripheral T-cell depletion provides a physiologic stimulus for thymopoiesis.

Heavily-treated cancer patients demonstrate an age-related delay in recovery of thymically derived CD45RA^{high} naive-type CD4^{+} cells (188,189). Nevertheless, in BMT patients of all ages who do not develop GVHD, the thymic function appears to allow eventual CD4 recovery (189). The potential of the thymus to generate naive T cells after peripheral T-cell depletion in older patients who have not received chemotherapy or radiotherapy remains to be determined. Thus, the age groups for whom peripheral T-cell depletion followed by induction of mixed chimerism and intrathymic tolerance will be practical are currently unknown.

THYMIC TRANSPLANTATION AS AN APPROACH TO CENTRAL TOLERANCE INDUCTION

An alternative approach to inducing central tolerance obviates the requirement for engraftment of donor hematopoietic stem cells that can send progeny to the host thymus and does not depend on a functioning host thymus for the achievement of T-cell recovery. Grafting of thymic tissue to recipients that have been thymectomized (ATX) and depleted of peripheral T cells with mAbs allows host T-cell recovery in the donor thymus. We have recently shown that implantation of fetal pig thymus and liver (THY/LIV) fragments under the kidney capsule of normal C57BL/10 (B10) mice that have been thymectomized (ATX) and treated with the same T- and NK-cell–depleting mAb regimen as that shown in Figure 5.2 can reconstitute immunocompetent CD4^{+} T cells that are specifically tolerant of the discordant xenogeneic donor. Full maturation of mouse $\alpha\beta$TCR^{+} single positive thymocytes from progenitors is seen in these grafts, and CD4^{+} cells repopulate the peripheral lymphoid tissues extensively (155). A state of specific tolerance, which includes the absence of MLR responses to the donor (155) and the acceptance of donor swine leukocyte antigen (SLA)-matched pig skin (190), exists in these animals. To our knowledge, these results provide the first demonstration that donor-specific skin graft tolerance can be induced across widely disparate (discordant) species barriers.

Other studies have demonstrated the capacity of allogeneic or closely related xenogeneic thymic stromal grafts to induce tolerance to antigens expressed by the graft (191,192). In these studies, the grafted thymic stroma was devoid of hematopoietic cells. Donor-specific skin graft tolerance was observed, but in vitro responsiveness to the donor persisted (191,192). Recently, tolerance in this system has been shown to involve an immunoregulatory CD4 cell population (193), and donor-reactive T cells clearly persist (194).

An important difference between those studies and our pig-to-mouse model is that the fetal pig THY grafts used in our model are already seeded with pig hematopoietic cells, including some that express class II MHC, at the time of harvest. Since bone marrow–derived cells may be more efficient than thymic epithelial cells at inducing clonal deletion of developing thymocytes, these pig hematopoietic cells may be responsible for the MLR tolerance to donor pig antigens of mouse T cells that develop in pig thymi. V_β analyses suggest that tolerance to both donor and host develop by an intrathymic deletional mechanism in these animals. Deletion may be induced by both murine and porcine MHC class II^{+} cells with dendritic cell– or macrophage-like morphology, which are both detectable in swine thymus grafts (190).

A surprisingly high level of immunocompetence and host-restricted antigen reactivity has been observed for T cells that develop in pig thymic grafts in these mice. As published studies suggest that thymic epithelial cells determine MHC restriction of CD4^{+} T cells (98), the basis for this immunocompetence and host restriction in thymic xenografts has been investigated. Studies showed that pig MHC mediates positive selection of mouse CD4 cells with no contribution from mouse MHC in these grafts (195). Excellent immunocompetence has been observed in these mice (196) and children with congenital thymic aplasia (DiGeorge anomaly) after grafting with HLA-mismatched allogenic thymi (197). These results suggest that the T-cell repertoire selected by a given MHC may be sufficiently cross-reactive on other MHCs to confer immunocompetence.

CONCLUSIONS

Intrathymic tolerance can be induced by a variety of mechanisms, including deletion, anergy, and suppression, when allogeneic or xenogeneic hematopoietic cells or thymic tissue are successfully engrafted. To rely purely on intrathymic tolerance induction, it is essential to adequately eliminate or inactivate the preexisting peripheral immune system and to ensure a continual supply of tolerance-inducing antigens to the thymus. Advances in the ability to achieve engraftment of hematopoietic and thymic tissue without ablative treatment of the host and the demonstration of efficacy in primate models have brought these approaches closer to clinical application. Furthermore, the development of new approaches to the induction of peripheral tolerance may allow the successful use of methodologies that combine central and peripheral tolerance induction, or perhaps that rely on peripheral tolerance alone.

A deeper understanding of nondeletional mechanisms of tolerance, and of the physiologic mechanisms regulating hematopoietic stem cell engraftment, hematopoietic function, and homing to the thymus should allow the development of minimal host-conditioning regimens that will make reliable allogeneic and xenogeneic tolerance feasible.

ACKNOWLEDGMENTS

We thank Drs. Christine Huang and Andre Simon for helpful review of the manuscript, and Ms. Diane Plemenos for expert secretarial assistance.

COMMENTARY

Kathryn J. Wood

Sykes and Sachs have focused their review of tolerance predominantly on the use of bone marrow as a vehicle for antigen delivery in recipients of solid organ grafts. I enjoyed reading the chapter enormously and was impressed by the amount of work the authors themselves have carried out in developing what is clearly a very elegant and effective approach for the induction of tolerance.

Sykes and Sachs argue very persuasively that a deletional strategy (i.e., one that results in deletion of donor reactive cells centrally in the thymus of the recipient) is likely to be the most effective approach for achieving tolerance in large animal models and ultimately in a clinical situation. While they do not rule out the possibility that other mechanisms such as anergy, suppression, and regulation might also facilitate the induction and maintenance of the tolerant state, my impression is that they feel very strongly that central deletion as a result of the persistence of antigen in the thymus provides the key to achieving long-term tolerance in vivo.

While I would agree that elimination of antigen reactive cells in the thymus via the successful engraftment of allogeneic or xenogeneic hematopoietic cells or thymic tissue into an immunoincompetent host is undoubtedly an effective way of inducing tolerance, I do not think that it is the only approach that can be successful. Moreover, achieving successful long-term engraftment of hematopoietic cells without myeloablation is a challenging objective. As Sykes and Sachs point out, myeloablative strategies are unlikely to be acceptable for the routine treatment of the majority of transplant recipients. The ability to achieve engraftment of hematopoietic tissues without ablative treatment of the host is therefore essential if this approach is to become part of the routine treatment of transplant patients. Sykes and Sachs emphasize this point and describe their strategy for the development of effective nonmyeloablative protocols that result in engraftment without the need for infusion of very large doses of donor bone marrow. With an increased understanding and new insights into stem cell biology, cell migration in vivo and growth requirements for hematopoietic cell engraftment may become easier to achieve without myeloablation in the future.

Another issue that needs consideration is the difficulty of ensuring that deletion of donor reactive leukocytes has been achieved effectively following implementation of a conditioning protocol. Even during the normal development of the immune system only T cells with high avidity for self peptides and MHC are deleted efficiently in the thymus. Cells with a lower avidity have been shown to escape into the periphery where they need to be controlled to ensure that tolerance to self antigens is maintained under all circumstances (1). Very potent mechanisms for regulating immune responses to self antigens in the periphery have been described in recently (2). In my opinion, an alternative mechanism applicable to a wide range of patients waiting for a transplant could be based on a combination approach in which deletion and immunoregulation are used to induce and maintain tolerance. Strategies utilizing this approach would be designed to establish conditions in the host such that any high-avidity donor reactive leukocytes would be deleted and at the same time the potential of natural immunoregulatory mechanisms would be in place to control the reactivity of any low-avidity cells still present in the recipient's repertoire.

Work on novel approaches for developing peripheral tolerance is progressing rapidly as new targets for manipulating immune responses with biologic agents are identified. Blockade of costimulation by targeting the CD28-CD80/86 and/or the CD40-CD40L pathways is producing exciting and impressive results in small and large animal models (3–5). These same agents may also facilitate stem cell engraftment of hematopoietic cells that would lead to deletion of donor reactive cells; work on this has already been initiated in Dr. Sykes' laboratory (6). Clearly, more targets will present themselves as our understanding of the pathways for costimulation and immunoregulation in vivo increases. For example, the role of CTLA4 in downregulating immune responses is intriguing. Further exploration of the molecular mechanisms involved is certain to focus attention on this as a possible way of controlling immune responsiveness in vivo.

New reagents for depleting peripheral leukocytes more effectively are also being developed. Data using an anti-CD3 immunotoxin to manipulate the peripheral T-cell repertoire before transplantation have shown that this can lead to the long-term survival of renal allografts in primates, with tolerance to donor alloantigens developing in some recipients (7,8). The principles highlighted by these experiments have stimulated a number of other studies that may result in the identification of an effective clinical strategy.

The use of biologic agents such as monoclonal antibodies or soluble recombinant ligands at the time of transplantation to facilitate the development of long-term graft survival and ultimately tolerance is not without difficulty and presents challenges of its own. One unresolved issue is how to use biologic agents effectively in combination with conventional immunosuppressive drugs such as cyclosporine, tacrolimus, mycophenolate mofetil, etc. Data from experimental studies suggest that the use of biologic agents and cyclosporine simultaneously at the time of transplantation may inhibit long-term graft survival (3). If this finding is reproducible, the identification of ways in which the biologic agents can be combined effectively with immunosuppressive drugs is essential. Work on this topic is already in progress and new insights into the way the intracellular pathways affected by the drugs and those required for the induction and maintenance of tolerance intersect should emerge before too long.

In the interim, alternative strategies may also be worth considering as short-term approaches to trying to reduce the overall load of immunosuppressive drugs that transplant patients require. As discussed by Sykes and Sachs, although development of immunosuppressive drug therapy has resulted in a dramatic improvement in the success of clinical transplantation, the use of the drugs is associated with many side effects including life-long risks of infection and malignancy. Reducing the total amount of immunosuppression required to maintain the long-term survival of the graft would offer significant benefits by lowering the risks of these side effects.

One strategy that has been shown to be successful for modifying immune responsiveness to alloantigens is the administration of alloantigen before transplantation. Clearly, this approach does not result in true transplantation tolerance (as noted by Sykes and Sachs), but nevertheless it may result in some degree of unresponsiveness to donor antigens becoming established. In the clinical setting pretransplant blood transfusions have been shown to improve renal allograft survival. In the 1970s and early 1980s, pretransplant blood transfusions were used by transplant centers around the world as a means of improving graft survival. For a variety of reasons this practice has fallen into disuse in many centers. However, data from new prospective studies suggest that it may be worth reconsidering as an interim approach (9).

In Oxford we have been developing an approach using pretransplant administration of alloantigen in combination with biologic agents, with the objective of developing specific unresponsiveness to a defined set of alloantigens before transplantation (10,11). In this way we feel that the mechanisms responsible for the development of the unresponsive state will be established before transplantation and, therefore, the administration of immunosuppressive drug therapy. We have recently completed a pilot clinical study investigating such an approach using HLA-typed pretransplant blood transfusions in combination with a nondepleting cdr graft monoclonal antibody targeting the CD4 molecule. The objective of this study was to follow changes in immune responsiveness to the mismatched HLA antigens presented by the blood transfusion. Preliminary analysis of our findings suggests that coadministration of anti-CD4 and alloantigen does result in changes in immune responsiveness—an analysis that is consistent with our results in an experimental model. We feel that such a strategy may facilitate the development of a microenvironment in vivo that, if present at the time of transplantation, will act in concert with the graft itself to promote a degree of unresponsiveness to the graft in the long-term. We have shown not only that the vascularized solid organ grafts are required for the maintenance of operational tolerance (12), but also that they contribute to how unresponsiveness develops.

The ability to switch off or even modify the immune response specifically to the alloantigens expressed by the organ donor without compromising the recipient's ability to respond to other immune challenges after transplantation would represent a major advance in clinical transplantation as we know it. If xenotransplantation is to become a routine clinical procedure, the induction of tolerance may have to become an essential part of any treatment protocol. Thus, if the induction of T- and B-cell tolerance is essential for the ultimate success of xenotransplantation, as Sykes and Sachs suggest, then this area should remain at the forefront of the research effort in transplantation for the foreseeable future.

CHAPTER REFERENCES

1. Auchincloss HA. Why is cell-mediated xenograft rejection so strong? Xeno 1995;3:19–22.
2. Oettel KR, Wesly OH, Albertini MR, et al. Allogeneic T cell clones able to selectively destroy Philadelphia chromosome (Ph1) bearing human leukemia lines can also recognize Ph1 negative cells from the same patient. Blood 1994;83:3390–3402.
3. Sykes M, Sheard MA, Sachs DH. Graft-versus-host-related immunosuppression is induced in mixed chimeras by alloresponses against either host or donor lymphohematopoietic cells. J Exp Med 1988;168:2391–2396.
4. Sykes M, Chester CH, Sachs DH. Protection from graft-versus-host disease in fully allogeneic chimeras by prior administration of T cell-depleted syngeneic bone marrow. Transplantation 1988;46:327–330.
5. Sykes M. Interleukin-2 as graft-vs-host disease prophylaxis. In: Spitzer TR, Mazumder A, eds. Immunotherapy and Bone Marrow Transplantation. Armonk, NY: Futura, 1995:87.
6. Murase N, Starzl TE, Tanabe M, et al. Variable chimerism, graft-versus-host disease, and tolerance after different kinds of cell and whole organ transplantation from Lewis to Brown Norway rats. Transplantation 1995;60:158–171.
7. Cobbold SP, Adams E, Marshall SE, et al. Mechanisms of peripheral tolerance and suppression induced by monoclonal antibodies to CD4 and CD8. Immunol Rev 1996;149:5–34.
8. Pearson TC, Madsen JC, Larsen CP, et al. Induction of transplantation tolerance in adults using donor antigen and anti-CD4 monoclonal antibody. Transplantation 1992;54:475–483.
9. Ohashi PS, Oehen S, Buerki K, et al. Ablation of "tolerance" and induction of diabetes by virus infection in viral antigen transgenic mice. Cell 1991;65:305–317.
10. Goodnow CC. Transgenic mice and analysis of B-cell tolerance. Ann Rev Immunol 1992;10:489–518.
11. Lafferty KJ, Babcock SK, Gill RG. Prevention of rejection by treatment of the graft: an overview. Prog Clin Biol Res 1986;224:87–117.

12. Dallman MJ, Shiho O, Page TH, et al. Peripheral tolerance to alloantigen results from altered regulation of the interleukin 2 pathway. J Exp Med 1991;173:79–87.
13. Schwartz RH. Costimulation of T lymphocytes: the role of CD28, CTLA-4, and B7/BB1 in interleukin-2 production and immunotherapy. Cell 1992;71:1065.
14. Ramsdell F, Fowlkes BJ. Clonal deletion versus clonal anergy: the role of the thymus in inducing self tolerance. Science 1990;248:1342–1348.
15. Schwartz RH. A cell culture model for T lymphocyte clonal anergy. Science 1990;248:1349–1356.
16. Nossal GJV, Pike BL. Clonal anergy: persistence in tolerant mice of antigen-binding B lymphocytes incapable of responding to antigen or mitogen. Proc Natl Acad Sci USA 1980;77:1602–1606.
17. Nossal GJV. Cellular mechanisms of immunologic tolerance. Ann Rev Immunol 1983;1:33–62.
18. Zanders ED, Lamb JR, Feldmann M, et al. Tolerance of T-cell clones is associated with membrane antigen changes. Nature 1983;303:625–627.
19. Schonrich G, Kalinke U, Momburg F, et al. Down-regulation of T cell receptors on self-reactive T cells as a novel mechanism for extrathymic tolerance induction. Cell 1991;65:293–304.
20. Rocha B, Von Boehmer H. Peripheral selection of the T cell repertoire. Science 1991;251:1225–1228.
21. Allen PM. Peptides in positive and negative selection: a delicate balance. Cell 1994;76:593–596.
22. Alam SM, Travers PJ, Wung JL, et al. T-cell-receptor affinity and thymocyte positive selection. Nature 1996;381:616–620.
23. Rocken M, Urban JF, Shevach EM. Infection breaks T cell tolerance. Nature 1992;359:79–82.
24. Rocha B, Tanchot C, Von Boehmer H. Clonal anergy blocks in vivo growth of mature T cells and can be reversed in the absence of antigen. J Exp Med 1993;177:1517–1521.
25. Ramsdell F, Fowlkes BJ. Maintenance of in vivo tolerance by persistence of antigen. Science 1992;257:1130–1134.
26. Qin S, Cobbold SP, Pope H, et al. "Infectious" transplantation tolerance. Science 1993;259:974–977.
27. Waldmann H, Cobbold S. The use of monoclonal antibodies to achieve immunological tolerance. Immunol Today 1993;14:247–251.
28. Alters SE, Song HK, Fathman CG. Evidence that clonal anergy is induced in thymic migrant cells after anti-CD4-mediated transplantation tolerance. Transplantation 1993;56:633–638.
29. Homan WP, Fabre JW, Williams KA, et al. Studies on immunosuppressive properties of cyclosporin A in rats receiving renal allografts. Transplantation 1980;29:361–366.
30. Baliga P, Chavin KD, Qin L, et al. CTLA4Ig prolongs allograft survival while suppressing cell-mediated immunity. Transplantation 1994;58:1082–1090.
31. Mottram PL, Han W-R, Purcell LJ, et al. Increased expression of IL-4 and IL-10 and decreased expression of IL-2 and interferon-gamma in long-surviving mouse heart allografts after brief CD4-monoclonal antibody therapy. Transplantation 1995;59:559–565.
32. Alters SE, Shizuru JA, Ackerman J, et al. Anti-CD4 mediates clonal anergy during transplantation tolerance induction. J Exp Med 1991;173:491–494.
33. Lee NA, Loh DY, Lacy E. CD8 surface levels alter the fate of α/β T cell receptor-expressing thymocytes in transgenic mice. J Exp Med 1992;175:1013–1025.
34. Bertolino P, Heath WR, Hardy CL, et al. Peripheral deletion of autoreactive CD8+ T cells in transgenic mice expressing H-2Kb in the liver. Eur J Immunol 1995;25:1932–1942.
35. Foster S, Cranston D, Wood KJ, Morris PJ. Production of indefinite renal allograft survival in the rat by pretreatment with viable and nonviable hepatocytes or liver membrane extracts. Transplantation 1988;45:228–231.
36. Madsen JC, Superina RA, Wood KJ, Morris PJ. Immunological unresponsiveness induced by recipient cells transfected with donor MHC genes. Nature 1988;332:161–164.
37. Fabre JW, Morris PJ. The effect of donor strain blood pretreatment on renal allograft rejection in rats. Transplantation 1972;14:608–617.
38. Fuchs EJ, Matzinger P. B cells turn off virgin but not memory T cells. Science 1992;258:1156–1159.
39. Lombardi G, Sidhu S, Batchelor R, Lechler R. Anergic T cells as suppressor cells in vitro. Science 1994;264:1587–1589.
40. Kobata T, Ohnishi Y, Urushibara N, et al. UV irradiation can induce in vitro clonal anergy in alloreactive cytotoxic T lymphocytes. Blood 1993;82:176–181.
41. Tan P, Anasetti C, Hansen JA, et al. Induction of alloantigen-specific hyporesponsiveness in human T lymphocytes by blocking interaction of CD28 with its natural ligand B7/BB1. J Exp Med 1993;177:165–173.
42. Gimmi CD, Freeman GJ, Gribben JG, et al. Human T-cell clonal anergy is induced by antigen presentation in the absence of B7 costimulation. Proc Natl Acad Sci USA 1993;90:6586–6590.
43. Pearson TC, Alexander DZ, Winn KJ, et al. Transplantation tolerance induced by CTLA4Ig. Transplantation 1994;57:1701–1706.
44. Sayegh MH, Akalin E, Hancock WW, et al. CD28-B7 blockade after alloantigenic challenge in vivo inhibits Th1 cytokines but spares Th2. J Exp Med 1995;181:1869–1874.
45. Yin D, Fathman CG. Induction of tolerance to heart allografts in high responder rats by combining anti-CD4 with CTLA4Ig. J Immunol 1995; 1655-1659.
46. Lenschow DJ, Zeng Y, Thistlethwaite JR, et al. Long-term survival of xenogeneic pancreatic islets induced by CTLA4Ig. Science 1992;257:789–792.
47. Lafferty KJ, Prowse SJ, Simeonovic CJ, Warren HS. Immunobiology of tissue transplantation: a return to the passenger leukocyte concept. Annu Rev Immunol 1983;1:143–173.
48. Lafferty KJ. A contemporary view of transplantation tolerance: An immunologist's perspective. Clin Transplantation 1994;8:181–187.
49. Calne R, Davies H. Organ graft tolerance: the liver effect. Lancet 1994;343:67–68.
50. Sun J, McCaughan GW, Matsumoto Y, et al. Tolerance to rat liver allografts. I. Differences between tolerance and rejection are more marked in the B cell compared with the T cell or cytokine response. Transplantation 1994;57:1349–1357.
51. Starzl TE, Murase N, Thomson A, Demetris AJ. Liver transplants contribute to their own success. Nature Med 1996;2:163–165.
52. Kuchroo VK, Das MP, Brown JA, et al. B7-1 and B7-2 costimulatory molecules activate differentially the Th1/Th2 developmental pathways: application to autoimmune disease therapy. Cell 1995;80:707–718.
53. Yamada K, Sachs DH, DerSimonian H. Direct and indirect recognition of pig class II antigens by human T cells. Transplant Proc 1995;27(1):258–259.
54. Rollins SA, Kennedy SP, Chodera AJ, et al. Evidence that activation of human T cells by porcine endothelium involves direct recognition of porcine SLA and costimulation by porcine ligands for LFA-1 and CD2. Transplantation 1994;57:1709–1716.
55. Murray AG, Khodadoust MM, Pober JS, Bothwell ALM. Porcine aortic endothelial cells activate human T cells: direct presentation of MHC antigens and costimulation by ligands for human CD2 and CD28. Immunity 1994;1:57–63.
56. Blazar BR, Taylor PA, Linsley PS, Vallera DA. In vivo blockade of CD28/CTLA4:B7/BB1 interaction with CTLA4-Ig reduces lethal murine graft-versus-host disease across the major histocompatibility complex barrier in mice. Blood 1994;83:3815–3825.
57. Blazar BR, Taylor PA, Panoskaltsis-Mortari A, et al. Coblockade of the LFA1:ICAM and CD28/CTLA4:B7 pathways is a highly effective means of preventing acute lethal graft-versus-host disease induced by fully major histocompatibility complex-disparate donor grafts. Blood 1995;85:2607–2618.
58. Durie FH, Foy TM, Masters SR, et al. The role of CD40 in the regulation of humoral and cell-mediated immunity. Immunol Today 1994;15:406–411.
59. Noelle RJ. CD40 and its ligand in host defense. Immunity 1996;4:415–419.
60. Larsen CP, Alexander DZ, Hollenbaugh D, et al. CD40-GP39 interactions play a critical role during allograft rejection: suppression of allograft rejection by blockade of the CD40-gp39 pathway. Transplantation 1996;61:4–9.
61. Blazar BR, Taylor PA, Noelle RJ, Vallera DA. CD4(+) T cells tolerized ex vivo to host alloantigen by anti-CD40 ligand (CD40L : CD154) antibody lose their graft-versus-host disease lethality capacity but retain nominal antigen responses. J Clin Invest 1998;102:473–482.
62. Larsen CP, Elwood EP, Alexander DZ, et al. Long-term acceptance of skin and cardiac allografts after blocking CD40 and CD28 pathways. Nature 1996;381:434–438.
63. Kirk AD, Harlan DM, Armstrong NN, et al. CTLA4-Ig and anti-CD40 ligand prevent renal allograft refection in primates. Proc Natl Acad Sci USA 1997;94:8789–8794.
64. Parker DC, Greiner DL, Phillips NE, et al. Survival of mouse pancreatic islet allografts in recipients treated with allogeneic small lymphocytes and antibody to CD40 ligand. Proc Natl Acad Sci USA 1995;92:9560–9564.
64a. Markees TG, Phillips NE, Noelle RJ, et al. Prolonged survival of mouse skin allografts in recipients treated with donor splenocytes and antibody to CD40 ligand. Transplantation 1997;64:329–335.
65. Charlton B, Auchincloss Jr. H, Fathman CG. Mechanisms of transplantation tolerance. Annu Rev Immunol 1994;12:707–734.

66. Isobe M, Yagita H, Okumura K, Ihara A. Specific acceptance of cardiac allograft after treatment with antibodies to ICAM-1 and LFA-1. Science 1992;255:1125–1127.
67. Jerne NK. Towards a network theory of the immune system. Ann Immunol (Inst Pasteur) 1971;125C:373–389.
68. Pearce NW, Spinelli A, Gurley KE, Hall BM. Specific unresponsiveness in rats with prolonged cardiac allograft survival after treatment with cyclosporine. V. Dependence of CD4+ suppressor cells on the presence of alloantigen and cytokines, including interleukin-2. Transplantation 1993;55:374–379.
69. Roser BJ. Cellular mechanisms in neonatal and adult tolerance. Immunologic Rev 1989;107:179–202.
70. Tomita Y, Mayumi H, Eto M, Nomoto K. Importance of suppressor T cells in cyclophosphamide-induced tolerance to the non-H-2-encoded alloantigens. Is mixed chimerism really required in maintaining a skin allograft tolerance. J Immunol 1990;144:463–473.
71. Tutschka PJ, Ki PF, Beschorner WE, et al. Suppressor cells in transplantation tolerance. II. Maturation of suppressor cells in the bone marrow chimera. Transplantation 1981;32:321–325.
72. Lancaster F, Chui YL, Batchelor JR. Anti-idiotypic T cells suppress rejection of renal allografts in rats. Nature 1985;315(6017):336–337.
73. Maki T, Gottshalk R, Wood ML, Monaco AP. Specific unresponsiveness to skin allografts in anti-lymphocyte serum-treated, marrow-injected mice: participation of donor marrow-derived suppressor T cells. J Immunol 1981;127:1433–1437.
74. Wood ML, Monaco AP. Suppressor cells in specific unresponsiveness to skin allografts in ALS-treated, marrow-injected mice. Transplantation 1980;29:196–200.
75. Wilson DB. Idiotypic regulation of T cells in graft-versus-host disease and autoimmunity. Immunol Rev 1989;107:159–176.
76. Koide J, Engleman EG. Differences in surface phenotype and mechanism of action between alloantigen-specific $CD8^+$ cytotoxic and suppressor T cell clones. J Immunol 1990;144:32–40.
77. Verbanac KM, Carver FM, Haisch CE, Thomas JM. A role for transforming growth factor-beta in the veto mechanism in transplant tolerance. Transplantation 1994;57:893–900.
78. Groux H, O'Garra A, Bigler M, et al. A CD4+ T-cell subset inhibits antigen-specific T-cell responses and prevents colitis. Nature 1997;389:737–742.
79. Byrne MC, O'Hara RM Jr, Kuchroo VK, et al. The role of the T cell receptor alpha chain in antigen-specific immune suppression. Ann N Y Acad Sci 1993;685:611–613.
80. Morris PJ. Suppression of rejection of organ allografts by alloantibody. Immunol Rev 1980;49:93–125.
81. Pearce NW, Spinelli A, Gurley KE, et al. Mechanisms maintaining antibody-induced enhancement of allografts. II. Mediation of specific suppression by short-lived CD4+ T cells. J Immunol 1989;143:499–506.
82. Mosmann TR, Coffman RL. Th1 and Th2 cells: Different patterns of lymphokine secretion lead to different functional properties. Ann Rev Immunol 1989;7:145–173.
83. Kupiec-Weglinski JW, Wasowska B, Papp I, et al. CD4 mAb therapy modulates alloantibody production and intracardiac graft deposition in association with selective inhibition of Th1 lymphokines. J Immunol 1993;151:5053–5061.
84. Gorczynski RM, Wojcik D. A role for nonspecific (cyclosporin A) or specific (monoclonal antibodies to ICAM-1, LFA-1, and IL-10) immunomodulation in the prolongation of skin allografts after antigen-specific pretransplant immunization or transfusion. J Immunol 1994;152:2011–2019.
85. Hancock WW, Sayegh MH, Kwok CA, et al. Oral, but not intravenous, alloantigen prevents accelerated allograft rejection by selective intragraft TH2 activation. Transplantation 1993;55:1112–1118.
86. Takeuchi T, Lowry RP, Konieczny B. Heart allografts in murine systems. The differential activation of Th2-like effector cells in peripheral tolerance. Transplantation 1992;53:1281–1294.
87. Chen N, Field EH. Enhanced type 2 and diminished type 1 cytokines in neonatal tolerance. Transplantation 1995;59:933–941.
88. Bucy RP, Li J, Huang GQ, Honjo K, Xu XY. Allograft tolerance induced by combined anti-LFA-1 and anti-ICAM-1 mAb is associated with shift from Th1 to Th2 cytokine expression in allograft. FASEB J 1995;9:A497.
89. Bishop DK, Chan SY, Eichwald EJ. Th1 and Th2 cytokines promote distinct forms of allograft rejection. FASEB J 1995;9:A497.
90. Martinez OM, Lang T, Villanueva JC, et al. Allograft rejection is associated with a Th2-dominant cytokine profile. FASEB J 1995;9:A497.
91. Alexander DZ, Pearson TC, Ritchie SC, et al. Analysis of the mechanisms of CTLA4-Ig plus bone marrow induced transplantation tolerance. FASEB J 1995;9:A783.
92. Zheng XX, Steele AW, Nickerson PW, et al. Administration of noncytolytic IL-10/Fc in murine models of lipopolysaccharide-induced septic shock and allogeneic islet transplantation. J Immunol 1995;154:5590–5600.
93. Russell PS, Chase CM, Winn HJ, Colvin RB. Coronary atherosclerosis in transplanted mouse hearts. II. Importance of humoral immunity. J Immunol 1994;152:5135–5141.
94. Wren SM, Wang SC, Thai NL, et al. Evidence for early Th2 T cell predominance in xenoreactivity. Transplantation 1993;56:905–911.
95. Szebeni J, Wang M-G, Pearson DA, et al. IL-2 inhibits early increases in serum gamma interferon levels associated with graft-vs-host disease. Transplantation 1994;58:1385–1393.
96. Wang M-G, Szebeni J, Pearson DA, et al. Inhibition of graft-vs-host disease (GVHD) by IL-2 treatment is associated with altered cytokine production by expanded GVH-reactive CD4+ helper cells. Transplantation 1995;60:481–490.
97. Magram J, Connaughton SE, Warrier RR, et al. IL-12-deficient mice are defective in IFN-gamma production and type 1 cytokine responses. Immunity 1996;4:471–481.
98. Matzinger P. Why positive selection? In positive selection in the thymus. Immunol Rev 1993;135:81–117.
99. Matzinger P. Tolerance, danger, and the extended family. Annu Rev Immunol 1994;12:991–1045.
100. Webb SR, Hutchinson J, Hayden K, Sprent J. Expansion/deletion of mature T cells exposed to endogenous superantigens in vivo. J Immunol 1994;152:586–597.
101. Hartley SB, Crosbie J, Brink RA, et al. Elimination from peripheral lymphoid tissues of self-reactive B lymphocytes recognizing membrane-bound antigens. Nature 1991;353:765–769.
102. Sharabi Y, Sachs DH. Mixed chimerism and permanent specific transplantation tolerance induced by a non-lethal preparative regimen. J Exp Med 1989;169:493–502.
103. Orloff MS, Fallon MA, DeMara E, et al. Induction of specific tolerance to small-bowel allografts. Surgery 1994;116:222–228.
104. Martin P. Overview of marrow transplantation immunology. In: Forman SJ, Blume KG, Thomas ED, eds. Bone Marrow Transplantation. Cambridge: Blackwell Scientific, 1994:16.
105. Pierce GE, Watts LM, Clancy J Jr. Sublethal fractionated total-body irradiation and donor bone marrow infusion for induction of allograft tolerance. Transplantation 1985;39:236–241.
106. Colson YL, Wren SM, Schuchert MJ, et al. A nonlethal conditioning approach to achieve durable multilineage mixed chimerism and tolerance across major, minor, and hematopoietic histocompatibility barriers. J Immunol 1995;155:4179–4188.
107. Kaufman CL, Colson YL, Wren SM, et al. Phenotypic characterization of a novel bone marrow-derived cell that facilitates engraftment of allogeneic bone marrow stem cells. Blood 1994;84:2436–2446.
108. Singer A, Hathcock KS, Hodes RJ. Self recognition in allogeneic radiation chimeras. A radiation resistant host element dictates the self specificity and immune response gene phenotype of T-helper cells. J Exp Med 1981;153:1286–1301.
109. Ruedi E, Sykes M, Ildstad ST, et al. Antiviral T cell competence and restriction specificity of mixed allogeneic (P1+P2→P1) irradiation chimeras. Cell Immunol 1989;121:185–195.
110. Nomoto K, Yung-Yun K, Omoto K, et al. Tolerance induction in a fully allogeneic combination using anti-T cell receptor-$\alpha\beta$ monoclonal antibody, low dose irradiation, and donor bone marrow transfusion. Transplantation 1995;59:395–401.
111. Sharabi Y, Sachs DH, Sykes M. T cell subsets resisting induction of mixed chimerism across various histocompatibility barriers. In: Gergely J, Benczur M, Falus A, et al., eds. Progress in Immunology VIII. Proceedings of the Eighth International Congress of Immunology, Budapest, 1992. Proc. 8th Int Cong Immunol 1992:801.
112. Vallera DA, Taylor PA, Sprent J, Blazar BR. The role of host T cell subsets in bone marrow rejection directed to isolated major histocompatibility complex class I versus class II differences of bm1 and bm12 mutant mice. Transplantation 1994;57:249–256.
113. Lee LA, Sergio JJ, Sykes M. Natural killer cells weakly resist engraftment of allogeneic long-term multilineage-repopulating hematopoietic stem cells. Transplantation 1996;61:125–132.
114. Aguila HL, Weissman IL. Hematopoietic stem cells are not direct cytotoxic targets of natural killer cells. Blood 1996;87:1225–1231.
115. Sharabi Y, Aksentijevich I, Sundt TM III, et al. Specific tolerance induction across a xenogeneic barrier: production of mixed rat/mouse lymphohematopoietic chimeras using a nonlethal preparative regimen. J Exp Med 1990;172:195–202.

116. Tomita Y, Sachs DH, Sykes M. Myelosuppressive conditioning is required to achieve engraftment of pluripotent stem cells contained in moderate doses of syngeneic bone marrow. Blood 1994;83:939–948.
117. Ramshaw HS, Crittenden RB, Dooner M, et al. High levels of engraftment with a single infusion of bone marrow cells into normal unprepared mice. Biol Blood Marrow Transplant 1995;1:74–80.
118. Sykes M, Szot GL, Swenson K, et al. Separate regulation of peripheral hematopoietic and thymic engraftment. Exp Hematol 1998;26:457–465.
119. Bachar-Lustig E, Rachamin N, Li H-W, et al. Megadose of T cell-depleted bone marrow overcomes MHC barriers in sublethally irradiated mice. Nature Med 1995;1:1268–1273.
120. Aversa F, Tabilio A, Terenzi A, et al. Successful engraftment of T-cell-depleted haploidentical "three-loci" incompatible transplants in leukemia patients by addition of recombinant human granulocyte colony-stimulating factor-mobilized peripheral blood progenitor cells to bone marrow inoculum. Blood 1994;84:3948–3955.
121. Sykes M, Szot GL, Swenson KA, et al. Induction of high levels of allogeneic hematopoietic reconstitution and donor-specific tolerance without myelosuppressive conditioning. Nat Med 1997;3:783–787.
122. Petzer AL, Hagge DE, Lansdorp PM, et al. Self-renewal of primitive human hematopoietic cells (long-term-culture-initiating cells) in vitro and their expansion in defined medium. Proc Natl Acad Sci USA 1996;93:1470–1474.
123. Emerson SG. Ex vivo expansion of hematopoietic precursors, progenitors, and stem cells: the next generation of cellular therapeutics. Blood 1996;87:3082–3088.
124. Brugger W, Heimfeld S, Berenson RJ, et al. Reconstitution of hematopoiesis after high-dose chemotherapy by autologous progenitor cells generated ex vivo. New Engl J Med 1995;333:283–287.
125. Papayannopoulou T, Craddock C, Nakamoto B, et al. The VLA4/VCAM-1 adhesion pathway defines contrasting mechanisms of lodgement of transplanted murine hemopoietic progenitors between bone marrow and spleen. Proc Natl Acad Sci USA 1995;92:9647–9651.
126. Lee LA, Sergio JJ, Sykes M. Evidence for non-immune mechanisms in the loss of hematopoietic chimerism in rat→mouse mixed xenogeneic chimeras. Xenotransplant 1995;2:57–66.
127. Gritsch HA, Sykes M. Hematopoietic competition limits xenogeneic myeloid reconstitution in SCID mice. Transplant Proc 1996;28:708.
128. Pallavicini M, Flake AW, Bethel C, et al. Creation of human-mouse xenogeneic chimeras by the in utero transplantation of hemopoietic cells. First International Congress on Xenotransplantation 1991:50.
129. Lapidot T, Pflumia F, Doedens M, et al. Cytokine stimulation of multilineage hematopoiesis from immature human cells engrafted in SCID mice. Science 1992;255:1137–1143.
130. Gritsch HA, Glaser RM, Emery DW, et al. The importance of non-immune factors in reconstitution by discordant xenogeneic hematopoietic cells. Transplantation 1994;57:906–917.
131. Yang Y-G, Sergio JJ, Swenson K, et al. Donor-specific growth factors promote swine hematopoiesis in SCID mice. Xenotransplant 1996;3:92–101.
132. Aksentijevich I, Sachs DH, Sykes M. Humoral tolerance in xenogeneic BMT recipients conditioned by a nonmyeloablative regimen. Transplantation 1992;53:1108–1114.
133. Lee LA, Sergio JJ, Sachs DH, Sykes M. Mechanism of tolerance in mixed xenogeneic chimeras prepared with a nonmyeloablative conditioning regimen. Transplant Proc 1994;26:1197–1198.
134. Yang YG, deGoma E, Ohdan H, et al. Tolerization of anti-Galalphal-3Gal natural antibody-forming B cells by induction of mixed chimerism. J Exp Med 1998;187:1335–1342.
135. Tomita Y, Khan A, Sykes M. Role of intrathymic clonal deletion and peripheral anergy in transplantation tolerance induced by bone marrow transplantation in mice conditioned with a non-myeloablative regimen. J Immunol 1994;153:1087–1098.
136. Tomita Y, Sachs DH, Khan A, Sykes M. Additional mAb injections can replace thymic irradiation to allow induction of mixed chimerism and tolerance in mice receiving bone marrow transplantation after conditioning with anti-T cell mAbs and 3 Gy whole body irradiation. Transplantation 1996;61:469–477.
137. Tomita Y, Khan A, Sykes M. Mechanism by which additional monoclonal antibody injections overcome the requirement for thymic irradiation to achieve mixed chimerism in mice receiving bone marrow transplantation after conditioning with anti-T cell mAbs and 3 Gy whole body irradiation. Transplantation 1996;61:477–485.
138. Ardavin C, Wu L, Li C-L, Shortman K. Thymic dendritic cells and T cells develop simultaneously in the thymus from a common precursor population. Nature 1993;362:761–763.
139. Wu L, Vremec D, Ardavin C, et al. Mouse thymus dendritic cells: kinetics of development and changes in surface markers during maturation. Eur J Immunol 1995;25:418–425.
140. Kawai T, Cosimi AB, Colvin RB, et al. Mixed allogeneic chimerism and renal allograft tolerance in cynomologus monkeys. Transplantation 1995;59:256–262.
141. Sablinski T, Sachs DH. Tolerance across discordant xenogeneic barriers. Xenotransplant 1995;2:234–239.
142. Sablinski T, Latinne D, Gianello P, et al. Xenotransplantation of pig kidneys to nonhuman primates: I. Development of the model. Xenotransplant 1995;2:264–270.
143. McDermott WV, Norman JC. Extracorporeal pig liver perfusion in the treatment of hepatic coma. Epatologia 1972;18:265–277.
144. Collins BH, Chari RS, Magee JC, et al. Mechanisms of injury in porcine livers perfused with blood of patients with fulminant hepatic failure. Transplantation 1994;58:1162–1171.
145. Oriol R, Ye Y, Koren E, Cooper DKC. Carbohydrate antigens of pig tissues reacting with human natural antibodies as potential targets for hyperacute vascular rejection in pig-to-man organ xenotransplantation. Transplantation 1993;56:1433–1442.
146. Sandrin MS, McKenzie IF. Gal alpha (1,3)Gal, the major xenoantigen(s) recognized in pigs by human natural antibodies. Immunol Rev 1994;141:169–190.
147. Kozlowski T, Ierenot F, Lambright D, et al. Depletion of anti-Gal(alpha)1-3Gal antibody in baboons by specific alpha-Gal immunoaffinity columns. Xenotransplantation 1998;5:122–131.
148. Alexandre GPJ, Gianello P, Latinne D, et al. Plasmapheresis and splenectomy in experimental renal xenotransplantation. In: Hardy MA, ed. Xenograft 25. New York: Excerpta Medica, 1989:259.
149. Alexandre GP, Squifflet JP, De Bruyere M, et al. Present experiences in a series of 26 ABO-incompatible living donor renal allografts. Transplant Proc 1987;19:4538–4542.
150. Thomas FT, Tepper MA, Thomas JM, Haisch CE. 15-Deoxyspergualin: a novel immunosuppressive drug with clinical potential. Ann NY Acad Sci 1993;685:175–192.
151. Tanaka M, Latinne D, Gianello P, et al. Xenotransplantation from pig to cynomolgus monkey: the potential for overcoming xenograft rejection through induction of chimerism. Transplant Proc 1994;26:1326–1327.
152. Sharabi Y, Abraham VS, Sykes M, Sachs DH. Mixed allogeneic chimeras prepared by a non-myeloablative regimen: requirement for chimerism to maintain tolerance. Bone Marrow Transplant 1992;9:191–197.
153. Khan A, Tomita Y, Sykes M. Thymic dependence of loss of tolerance in mixed allogeneic bone marrow chimeras after depletion of donor antigen. Peripheral mechanisms do not contribute to maintenance of tolerance. Transplantation 1996;62:380–387.
154. Sachs DH, Sykes M, Greenstein JL, Cosimi AB. Tolerance and xenograft survival. Nature Med 1995;1:969.
155. Lee LA, Gritsch HA, Sergio JJ, et al. Specific tolerance across a discordant xenogeneic transplantation barrier. Proc Natl Acad Sci USA 1994;91:10864–10867.
156. Starzl TE, Demetris AJ, Trucco M, et al. Chimerism and donor-specific nonreactivity 27 to 29 years after kidney allotransplantation. Transplantation 1993;55:1272–1277.
157. Eynon EE, Parker DC. Parameters of tolerance induction by antigen targeted to B lymphocytes. J Immunol 1993;151:2958–2964.
158. Lombardi G, Hargreaves R, Sidhu S, et al. Antigen presentation by T cells inhibits IL-2 production and induces IL-4 release due to altered cognate signals. J Immunol 1996;156:2769–2775.
159. Burlingham WJ, Grailer AP, Fechner Jr. JH, et al. Microchimerism linked to cytotoxic T lymphocyte functional unresponsiveness (clonal anergy) in a tolerant renal transplant recipient. Transplantation 1995;59:1147–1155.
160. Murase N, Starzl TE, Ye Q, et al. Multilineage hematopoietic reconstitution of supralethally irradiated rats by syngeneic whole organ transplantation with particular reference to the liver. Transplantation 1996;61:1–4.
161. Taniguchi H, Toyoshima T, Fukao K, Nakauchi H. Presence of hematopoietic stem cells in the adult liver. Nature Med 1996;2:198–203.
162. Lu L, Rudert WA, Qian SG, et al. Growth of donor-derived dendritic cells from the bone marrow of murine liver allograft recipients in response to granulocyte/macrophage colony-stimulating factor. J Exp Med 1995;182:379–387.
163. Bushell A, Pearson TC, Morris PJ, Wood KJ. Donor-recipient microchimerism is not required for tolerance induction following recipient pretreatment with donor-specific transfusion and anti-CD4 antibody. Transplantation 1995;59:1367–1371.

164. Alard P, Matriano JA, Socarras S, et al. Detection of donor-derived cells by polymerase chain reaction in neonatally tolerant mice. Microchimerism fails to predict tolerance. Transplantation 1995;60:1125–1130.
165. Fisher RA, Cohen DS, Ben-Ezra JM, et al. Induction of long-term graft tolerance and donor/recipient chimerism. J Surg Res 1996;60:181–185.
166. Reinsmoen NL, Jackson A, McSherry C, et al. Organ-specific patterns of donor antigen-specific hyporeactivity and peripheral blood allogeneic microchimerism in lung, kidney, and liver transplant recipients. Transplantation 1995;60:1546–1554.
167. Shapiro R, Rao AS, Fontes P, et al. Combined simultaneous kidney/bone marrow transplantation. Transplantation 1995;60:1421–1425.
168. Thomas JM, Verbanac KM, Smith JP, et al. The facilitating effect of one-DR antigen sharing in renal allograft tolerance induced by donor bone marrow in rhesus monkeys. Transplantation 1995;59:245–255.
169. Rolles K, Burroughs AK, Davidson BR, et al. Donor-specific bone marrow infusion after orthotopic liver transplantation. Lancet 1994;343:263–265.
170. Streilein JW. Neonatal tolerance of H-2 alloantigens. Transplantation 1991;52:1–10.
171. Donckier V, Wissing M, Bruyns C, et al. Critical role of interleukin 4 in the induction of neonatal transplantation tolerance. Transplantation 1995;59:1571–1576.
172. Smith JP, Kasten-Jolly J, Field LJ, Thomas JM. Assessment of donor bone marrow cell-derived chimerism in transplantation tolerance using transgenic mice. Transplantation 1994;58:324–329.
173. Hedrick MH, Rice HE, MacGillivray TE, et al. Hematopoietic chimerism achieved by in utero hematopoietic stem cell injection does not induce donor-specific tolerance for renal allografts in sheep. Transplantation 1994;58:110–111.
174. Ridge JP, Fuchs EJ, Matzinger P. Neonatal tolerance revisited: Turning on newborn T cells with dendritic cells. Science 1996;271:1723–1726.
175. Sarzotti M, Robbins DS, Hoffman PM. Induction of protective CTL responses in newborn mice by a murine retrovirus. Science 1996;271:1726–1728.
176. Forsthuber T, Yip HC, Lehmann PV. Induction of Th1 and Th2 immunity in neonatal mice. Science 1996;271:1728–1730.
177. Sykes M, Sheard MA, Sachs DH. Effects of T cell depletion in radiation bone marrow chimeras II. Requirement for allogeneic T cells in the reconstituting bone marrow inoculum for subsequent resistance to breaking of tolerance. J Exp Med 1988;168:661–673.
178. Lubaroff DM, Silvers WK. The importance of chimerism in maintaining tolerance of skin allografts in mice. J Immunol 1973;111:65–71.
179. Gianello PR, Yamada K, Fishbein JM, et al. Long-term acceptance of primarily vascularized renal allografts in miniature swine. Transplantation 1996;61:503–522.
180. Yamada K, Gianello PR, Ierino FL, et al. Role of the thymus in transplantation tolerance in miniature swine I. Requirement of the thymus for rapid and stable induction of tolerance to class I-mismatched renal allografts. J Exp Med 1997;186:497–506.
181. Agus DB, Surh CD, Sprent J. Reentry of T cells to the adult thymus is restricted to activated T cells. J Exp Med 1991;173:1039–1046.
182. Blancho G, Gianello P, Germana S, et al. Molecular identification of porcine interleukin 10: regulation of expression in a kidney allograft model. Proc Natl Acad Sci USA 1995;92:2800–2804.
183. Oluwole SF, Jin M-X, Chowdhury NC, Ohajewkwe OA. Effectiveness of intrathymic inoculation of soluble antigens in the induction of specific unresponsiveness to rat islet allografts without transient recipient immunosuppression. Transplantation 1994;58:1077–1081.
184. Sayegh MH, Perico N, Gallon L, et al. Mechanisms of acquired thymic unresponsiveness to renal allografts. Thymic recognition of immunodominant allo-MHC peptides induces peripheral T cell anergy. Transplantation 1994;58:125–132.
185. Odorico JS, O'Connor T, Campos L, et al. Examination of the mechanisms responsible for tolerance induction after intrathymic inoculation of allogeneic bone marrow. Ann Surg 1993;218:525–531.
186. Debruin RWF, Vanrossum TJ, Scheringa M, et al. Intrathymic injection of alloantigen may lead to hyperacute rejection and prolonged graft survival of heart allografts in the rat. Transplantation 1996;60:1061–1063.
187. Alfrey EJ, Wang X, Lee L, et al. Tolerance induced by direct inoculation of donor antigen into the thymus in low and high responder rodents. Transplantation 1995;59:1171–1176.
188. Mackall CL, Fleisher TA, Brown MR, et al. Age, thymopoiesis, and CD4+ T-lymphocyte regeneration after intensive chemotherapy. New Engl J Med 1995;332:143–149.
189. Weinberg K, Annett G, Kashyap A, et al. The effect of thymic function on immunocompetence following bone marrow transplantation. Biol Blood Marrow Transplant 1995;1:18–23.
190. Zhao Y, Swenson K, Sergio JJ, et al. Skin graft tolerance across a discordant xenogeneic barrier. Nat Med 1996;2:1211–1216.
191. Bonomo A, Matzinger P. Thymus epithelium induces tissue-specific tolerance. J Exp Med 1993;177:1153–1164.
192. Martin C, Ohki-Hamazaki H, Corbel C, et al. Successful xenogeneic transplantation in embryos: induction of tolerance by extrathymic chick tissue grafted into quail. Dev Immunol 1991;1:265–277.
193. Modigliani Y, Tomas-Vaslin V, Bandeira A, et al. Lymphocytes selected in allogeneic thymic epithelium mediate dominant tolerance toward tissue grafts of the thymic epithelium haplotype. Proc Natl Acad Sci USA 1995;92:7555–7559.
194. Modigliani Y, Pereira P, Thomas-Vaslin V, et al. Regulatory T cells in thymic epithelium-induced tolerance. I. Suppression of mature peripheral non-tolerant T cells. Eur J Immunol 1995;25:2563–2571.
195. Zhao Y, Swenson K, Sergio JJ, Sykes M. Pig MHC mediates positive selection of mouse CD4+ T Cells with a mouse MHC-restricted TCR in pig thymus grafts. J Immunol 1998;161:1320–1326.
196. Zhao Y, Fishman JA, Sergio JJ, et al. Immune restoration by fetal pig thymus grafts in T cell-depleted, thymectomized mice. J Immunol 1997;158:1641–1649.
197. Hong R, Moore AL. Organ culture for thymus transplantation. Transplantation 1996;61:444–448.
198. Sharrow SO, Arn JS, Stroynowski I, et al. Epitope clusters of Qa-2 antigens defined by a panel of new monoclonal antibodies. J Immunol 1989;142:3495–3502.
199. Sarmiento M, Glasebrook AL, Fitch FW. IgG or IgM monoclonal antibodies reactive with different determinants on the molecular complex bearing Lyt2 antigen block T cell-mediated cytolysis in the absence of complement. J Immunol 1980;125:2665.
200. Ledbetter JA, Herzenberg LA. Xenogeneic monoclonal antibodies to mouse lymphoid differentiation antigens. Immunologic Rev 1979;47:63–90.
201. Koo GC, Peppard JR. Establishment of monoclonal anti-NK-1.1 antibody. Hybridoma 1984;3:301–303.

COMMENTARY REFERENCES

1. Kawai K, Ohashi P. Immunological function of a defined T-cell population tolerized to low-affinity self antigens. Nature 1995;374:68–69.
2. Heath V, Mason D, Ramirez F, Seddon B. Homeostatic mechanisms in the control of autoimmunity. Semin Immunol 1997;9:375–380.
3. Larsen P, Elwood E, Alexander D, et al. Long-term acceptance of skin and cardiac allografts after blocking CD40 and CD28 pathways. Nature 1996;381:434–438.
4. Larsen C, Alexander D, Hollenbaugh D, et al. CD40-gp39 interactions play a critical role during allograft rejection. Transplantation 1996;61:4–9.
5. Kirk A, Harlan D, Armstrong N, et al. CTLA4-Ig and anti-CD40 ligand prevent renal allograft rejection in primates. Proc Natl Acad Sci USA 1997;94:8789–8794.
6. Wekerle T, Sayegh M, Hill J, et al. Extrathymic T cell deletion and allogeneic stem cell engraftment induced with costimulatory blockade is followed by central T cell tolerance. J Exp Med 1998;187:2037–2044.
7. Knechtle S, Vargo D, Fechner J, et al. FN18-CRM9 immunotaxin promotes tolerance in primal renal allografts. Transplantation 1997;63:1–6.
8. Fechner J, Vargo D, Geissler E, et al. Split tolerance induced by immunotoxin in a rhesus kidney allograft model. Transplantation 1997;63:1339–1345.
9. Opelz G, Vanrenterghem Y, Kirste G, et al. Prospective evaluation of pretransplant blood transfusions in cadaver kidney recipients. Transplantation 1997;63:964–967.
10. Pearson TC, Madsen JC, Larsen C, et al. Induction of transplantation tolerance in the adult using donor antigen and anti-CD4 monoclonal antibody. Transplantation 1992;54:475–483.
11. Bushell A, Morris P, Wood K. Transplantation tolerance induced by antigen pretreatment and depleting anti-CD4 antibody depends on CD4+ T cell regulation during the induction phase of the response. Eur J Immunol 1995;25:2643–2649.
12. Hamano K, Rawsthorne M, Bushell A, Morris P, Wood K. Evidence that the continued presence of the organ graft and not peripheral donor microchimerism is essential for the maintenance of tolerance to alloantigen in anti-CD4 treated recipients. Transplantation 1996;62:856–860.

Part II

Immunosuppression

Chapter

6

Molecular and Clinical Therapeutics of Cyclosporine in Transplantation

PAUL A. KEOWN

MECHANISMS OF ACTION

The cyclosporine family comprises some 25 natural lipophilic cyclic undecapeptides and more than 2000 derivatives originally obtained from the fermentation products of the fungal species *Tolypocladium inflatum Gams* (1). Several analogues exhibit diverse in vitro biologic activities, but only cyclosporin A (CsA) and the natural analogues (Thr^2)-cyclosporin C (CsC), (Val^2)-cyclosporin D (CsD), ($Nval^2$)-cyclosporin G (CsG), and (Nva^2)-cyclosporin M (CsM), produced by substitution of the α-aminobutyric acid at the 2 position, cause selective inhibition of the immune response in vivo.

The unique molecular structure and physiochemical properties of these analogues are integral to their biologic actions and pharmacologic behavior. They consist of 10 known aliphatic amino acids and one novel C9 amino acid [4-butenyl-4-methyl-threonine (MeBmt)] arranged in a cyclic structure, producing a molecular weight of approximately 1200 kd (Fig. 6.1). Solid state x-ray diffraction and nuclear magnetic resonance studies in nonaqueous solution show that the molecule is characterized by two structural motifs (1). Residues MeBmt (AA1) to MeLeu (AA6) comprise an antiparallel β-sheet that is stabilized by three transannular hydrogen bonds (dotted lines in Fig. 6.1), while the residues Ala (AA7) to MeVal (AA11) form a loop in which the 9–10 peptide bond is in the *cis* position. An additional extra-annular hydrogen bond links the NH of DAla (AA8) to the carbonyl oxygen of MeLeu (AA6) (see Fig. 6.1).

The immunosuppressive cyclosporines possess two regulatory domains. Residues 1, 2, 9, 10, and 11 represent the receptor-binding domain, while the antipodean residues 4 to 8 function as the effector domain. Molecular substitution within either of these regions substantially alters the biologic effects of the compound.

CsA binds to several proteins in the eukaryotic cell, the most important of which are the cyclophilins (2). The principal cytoplasmic isoform, cyclophilin A (CyPA), is abundantly expressed in mammalian tissues and binds CsA with high affinity [dissociation constant (K_D) of 6 nmol/L]. This 18-kd enzyme facilitates tertiary protein folding through its peptidyl-prolyl *cis*-trans isomerase function, a function that is abrogated by CsA, although this now appears to be incidental to the immunosuppressive action of the drug and occurs only at much higher concentrations (3).

Several other mammalian cyclophilin isoforms have now been isolated. They contain rotamase domains and exhibit substantial homology with cyclophilin A, but differ in subcellular localization and CsA-binding affinity. The 21-kd protein CyPB (K_D = 9 nmol/L) appears to reside within the endoplasmic reticulum and may mediate translocation into this structure. The 23-kd CyPC (K_D = 6 nmol/L), while also expressed predominantly within the same organelle, shows restricted tissue distribution and is found principally in the kidney (4). Whether this is related to the unique renal toxicity of the cyclosporins is not yet known. A fourth mammalian isoform, CyCD, possesses a signal sequence thought to target it to mitochondria. Finally, a 40-kd cytoplasmic protein termed CyP-40 has recently been identified that is a component of the inactive steroid receptor. This structure contains subunits that can bind with three distinct classes of immunosuppressive agents: glucocorticoids, cyclosporins, and macrolides (tacrolimus and sirolimus). The relevance of this and other binding proteins—such as the 150-kd NK-TR, a component of the putative tumor recognition complex, or the immunophilins expressed in greater concentration in the brain (5)—remains to be determined.

The cyclosporins exert diverse biologic effects that influence many aspects of cell growth and differentiation. For example, selective inhibition of the multiple disease

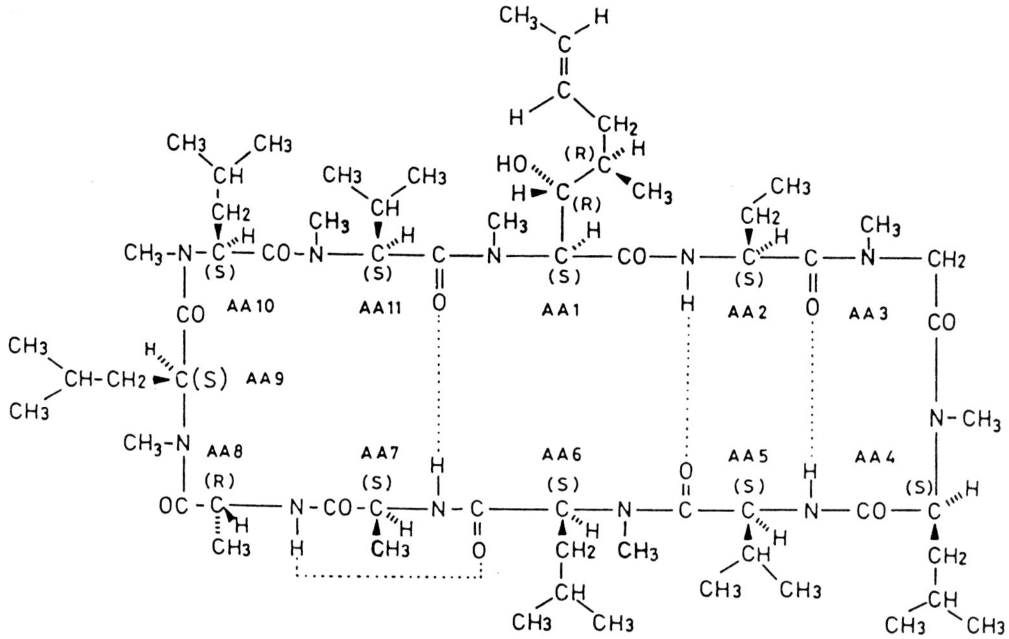

FIGURE 6.1. *Structure of cyclosporine, an 11-amino-acid cyclic peptide. Amino acid residues 1–6 are held together by transannular hydrogen bonds (dotted lines). These, together with the hydrogen bond linking the open loop residues 7–10 to residue 6, contribute to the rigidity of the CsA skeleton.*

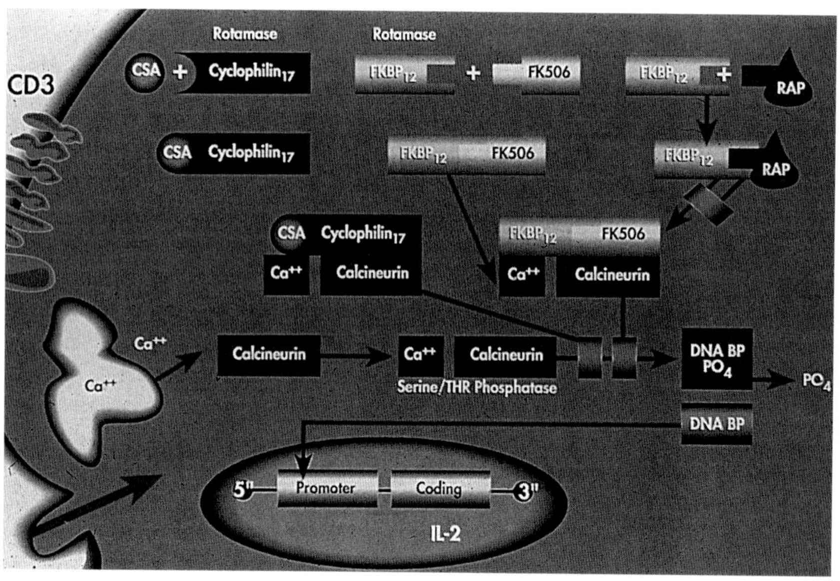

FIGURE 6.2. *Schematic representation of the mechanism of action of CsA, compared with tacrolimus (FK506). CsA bound to cyclophilin (or FK506 to its binding protein, FKBP) complexes with and blocks the enzymatic function of the calcium-activated calcineurin. This prevents dephosphorylation and, therefore, activation of DNA-binding proteins. Thus, IL-2 synthesis is prevented. Sirolimus (RAP) also binds to FKBP (see Chapter 11).*

resistance gene product p-glycoprotein, a leading cause of drug resistance in malignant cells (6), is an action most effectively mediated by [3′-keto-Bmt1]-Val2 cyclosporine, a nonimmunosuppressive cyclosporin D derivative (7). Another recent recognition is that CsA and certain nonimmunosuppressive cyclosporine analogues compete with the Gag polyproteins of the human immunodeficiency virus for binding to cyclophilin A, thereby preventing incorporations of this isomerase into the virions and resulting in a linear reduction of reverse transcription after T-cell infection (8,9).

The most important and extensively studied function, however, is the selective inhibition of lymphocyte signal transduction, a function that appears to be uniquely restricted to those analogues with immunosuppressive potency identified above. The bimolecular complex interacts via the CsA effector domain with the calcium- and calmodulin-dependent serine/threonine phosphatase calcineurin (Fig. 6.2), now recognized as a rate-limiting step in lymphocyte activation (10,11). Blockade of the enzymatic functions of calcineurin prevents dephosphorylation of the

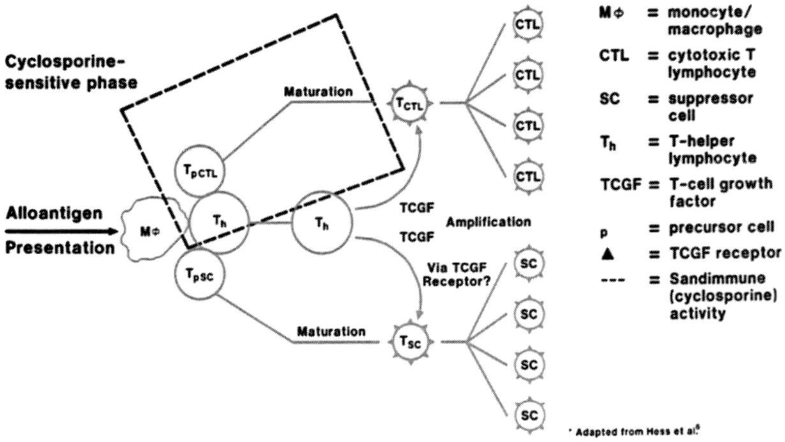

FIGURE 6.3. *Cyclosporine's effect on the immune response. Inhibition of IL-2 and other growth factor synthesis attenuates the maturation from precursor cells to cytotoxic T cells, and possibly favors the development of suppressor cells.*

antigen-inducible transcription factors NFAT1, elk-1, and the cAMP-response element binding protein (CREB) (12,13), also termed DNA-binding proteins (see Fig. 6.2). Translocation to the nucleus is thereby prevented, abrogating transcription of the cytokine gene complex and of the proto-oncogenes *c-myc*, *c-fos*, and n-*ras*. CsA may also directly inhibit the expression of G0/G1 switch genes through an as yet unknown mechanism (14).

As a consequence of these events, entry into the cell cycle is arrested at the G0 or G1 phase, DNA, RNA, and protein synthesis are inhibited, and growth factor production is abrogated. Activation structures are not expressed on the lymphocyte surface, and the generation of specific antibody and cytotoxic T lymphocytes directed against donor antigens is attenuated (Fig. 6.3). CsA also impedes the downstream organization of inflammatory events within the graft by blocking the dynamic upregulation of adhesion molecules and MHC determinants on the high endothelial venule, as occurs under the influence of interferon gamma (IFN-γ), tumor necrosis factor (TNF), and other inflammatory cytokines. Lymphocyte trafficking and accumulation within the graft is attenuated, preventing the T-cell clustering necessary for interaction between graft antigen and the T-cell receptor and the resulting cascade of inflammatory events (15).

CLINICAL PHARMACOLOGY

The intravenous formulation of CsA is stabilized with Cremophor at a concentration of 100 mg/mL, and is administered by either intermittent or continuous infusion over 4 to 24 hours. The oral liquid and gel caplets previously were formulated in corn oil (Sandimmune; Novartis). Advances in pharmaceutical chemistry have now resulted in a new stable microemulsion that combines a lipophilic solvent, a hydrophilic solvent, and a surfactant. This new form is available in both liquid and gel caplet form (Neoral; Novartis) (16). Several generic products are also in the process of clinical evaluation (17).

Absorption

Cyclosporine is absorbed preferentially from the upper intestine via a zero-order process in which the rate of absorption is constant and independent of drug concentration at the absorption site. Presystemic metabolism occurs in the intestinal epithelium under the influence of cytochrome P450-IIIa, reducing the amount of parent drug available for uptake (18). A variable proportion is also recycled into the gut lumen by the multiple drug resistance gene product p-glycoprotein in the epithelial cell membrane (19). The residual unchanged parent compound is absorbed into the portal system (Fig. 6.4); only a small amount is transported via the lymphatics (20).

Absorption following oral administration of Sandimmune is slow, incomplete, and unpredictable, with a lag time of 30 to 60 minutes and an absorption half-life ($t_{1/2}$) of approximately 60 minutes. Peak concentration (C_{max}) in blood or plasma is reached within 3 to 4 hours (mean 2.5 hours), although delayed and secondary peaks are common (21). Uptake is incomplete, with a mean of 30% reaching the systemic circulation (22). Absorption is bidirectionally influenced by food, particularly grapefruit juice (23), and is markedly impaired by reduced bile flow, delayed gastric emptying, intestinal dysmotility, accelerated gastrointestinal transit, or reduced absorptive area, resulting in a high between- and within-subject variability (24–26).

Absorption from Neoral is more rapid, complete, consistent, and dose-linear due to the homogeneous dispersion of uniform particles (<0.15 μ) at the absorptive surface (27–30). The absorption lag is virtually eliminated, and the time to peak concentration (t_{max}) is significantly reduced. C_{max} occurs at 1.5 hours, and delayed or secondary absorption peaks are uncommon (31). While the trough concentration does not differ from that with the oil formulations, C_{max} is increased by more than 60%, and overall bioavailability is increased by 30% to 50% with Neoral (32). Between- and within-patient variability in t_{max}, C_{max}, and exposure throughout the dosing interval (AUC_{0-12}) are also reduced by up to 75% (33,34).

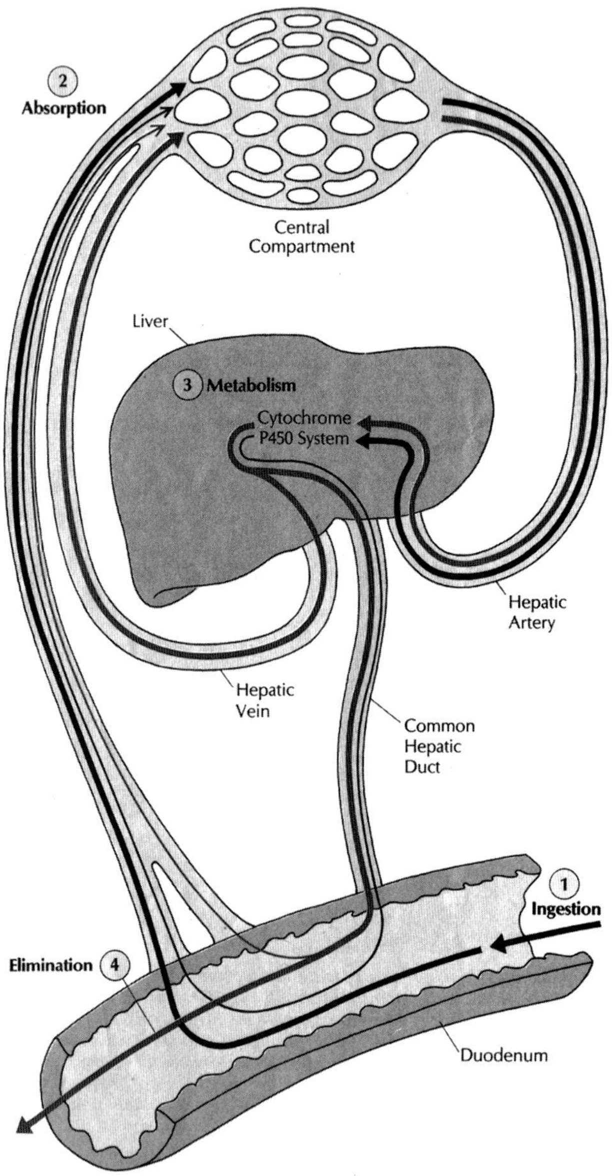

FIGURE 6.4. *Unlike other lipophilic agents, cyclosporine initially bypasses the hepatic portal system. After absorption through intestinal lacteal lymphatics, it goes into the thoracic duct and then to the central blood compartment. From there, cyclosporine enters the liver, where it is metabolized into numerous metabolites (more than 25 have been identified). These metabolites recirculate in the blood, return to the liver, and then move out through the biliary tree into the bowel, where they may be reabsorbed or eliminated. A small amount of the parent compound is probably excreted as well.*

Metabolism

Disposition of CsA is independent of the formulation employed. Partitioning within the blood compartment obeys a temperature-dependent equilibrium in which approximately 50% is bound to erythrocytes, 10% to leukocytes, and 30% to 40% to plasma proteins; only 1% to 6% normally exists in the free state (35). In plasma, 33% to 46% is associated with high-density lipoprotein (HDL), 28% to 35% with low-density lipoprotein (LDL), and 6% to 19% with very-low-density lipoprotein in a ratio inversely reflecting their clearance rates (36). The remaining 11% to 23% of CsA is associated with the nonlipoprotein fraction.

CsA accumulates readily in the body fat, liver, pancreas, heart, lung, kidney, spleen, lymph nodes, and blood. However, it does not readily cross the blood-brain barrier or placenta. Drug concentrations are low in the cerebrospinal fluid, brain, and spinal cord, and the concentration in the fetus represents less than 5% of the maternal drug load (37). Significant concentrations of CsA will accumulate in breast milk, so breast feeding is contraindicated to protect the neonatal immune system (38).

Metabolism of CsA occurs in the liver and bowel under the influence of cytochrome P450-IIIA (39) by demethylation of derivatives on the molecular face opposite the cyclophilin binding site. More than 25 metabolites have been documented in human blood, bile, and urine, all of which retain the cyclic oligopeptide structure (40). The first oxidation products are the primary metabolites M1, M9, and M4N. Further oxidation then produces a second group of metabolites including M19, M49, or M4N9. Other secondary derivatives, such as M4N69 and M69 found in human urine, may represent further oxidation products of M4N9 and M9, respectively. CsA is the major component in plasma, while M1 and M9 are present in high concentration in erythrocytes and other tissues. M1 is the major component in urine, where unchanged CsA represents only 0.1% of the administered dose. An acid derivative of M1 predominates in bile, where CsA is present in only trace amounts. All natural and synthetic metabolites are less immunosuppressive than the parent molecule. CsA is eliminated primarily by biliary excretion, with a median half-life of 6 to 8 hours.

Clearance is higher in children and slower in females (41), reflecting partly the accumulation of the drug in body fat. Alterations in lipid profile modify the distribution and metabolism of CsA; CsA increases lipoprotein concentration, thereby reciprocally modulating its own distribution (36). Clearance of CsA is significantly impaired in patients with liver disease, and the elimination half-life may be prolonged fourfold. Thus, longer dosing intervals or a substantial reduction in dose are necessary in the presence of hepatic dysfunction.

Drug Interactions

Pharmacokinetic interactions (Table 6.1) are commonly due to modulation of cytochrome P450 enzyme activity, which alters the metabolism and clearance of CsA (42). Phenytoin, rifampin, and nafcillin are prototypic of drugs that induce mixed function oxidases—they cause a fall in CsA levels within 72 hours of administration, and may lead to graft rejection unless the interaction is recognized and corrected. Less commonly, drugs such as cholestyramine or the

Table 6.1. Drug Interactions with Cyclosporine

Agent	Pharmacokinetic Action	Consequences
Carbamazepine Nafcillin Phenobarbital Phenytoin Rifampin	Induce cytochrome P450 enzymes	Decrease half-life, blood levels, and immunosuppressive effect
Colchicine Diltiazem Fluconazole Fluoroquinolones Ketoconazole Macrolide antibodies Oral contraceptives Verapamil	Inhibit cytochrome P450 enzymes	Increase half-life, blood levels, and toxicity or immunosuppression
Aminoglycosides Amphotericin B Cimetidine Nonsteroidals Sulfur	Interact at a glomerular or tubular level	Increase nephrotoxicity

somatostatin analogue octreotide influence CsA absorption through direct or indirect means. In contrast, erythromycin, ketoconazole, diltiazem, colchicine, and certain fluoroquinolones inhibit the cytochrome P450 enzyme system. These agents increase CsA exposure within days and may cause acute nephrotoxicity requiring a reduction in CsA dose by 50% or more (43).

Less potent interactions have been reported with the macrolide derivatives josamycin, ponsinomycin, and roxithromycin, and with fluconazole and verapamil. Nifedipine and nitrendipine have no demonstrable influence on CsA pharmacokinetics. Oral contraceptives are weak inhibitors of cytochrome P450 enzymes (44) and may increase CsA concentration in recipients of renal and liver transplants. CsA and prednisolone are metabolized by the same hepatic microsomal enzymes, and human liver microsomal studies show a bidirectional inhibition of CsA and corticosteroid metabolism (45). High-dose intravenous methylprednisolone may transiently increase CsA trough levels (46), but this interaction is of uncertain clinical importance.

Pharmacodynamic drug interactions may also influence the immunosuppression or toxicity of CsA. Median effect analysis in experimental animals shows that immune suppression is additive with azathioprine and mycophenolate, and synergistic with sirolimus (47). In contrast, ciprofloxacin antagonizes CsA in vitro by increasing interleukin (IL)-2 gene transcription, and may increase the risk of acute rejection in vivo (48).

Nonsteroidal anti-inflammatory drugs (NSAIDs) reduce intra-renal blood flow by inhibiting the production of vasodilatory prostaglandins, and may lead to acute renal dysfunction in patients receiving CsA. NSAIDs are generally to be avoided, although short courses may be required for treatment of acute gout or other rheumatologic conditions. Septra, cimetidine, and ranitidine may also elevate serum creatinine, although this occurs by inhibition of tubular secretion rather than by impairment of glomerular filtration (49).

CLINICAL USE OF CYCLOSPORINE

Cyclosporine may be administered intravenously until gastrointestinal function is reestablished. There is little data to determine whether continuous or intermittent infusion is preferable, but in either case the dose should be adjusted to achieve an average concentration ($C_{av} = AUC_{0-t}/t$) above 500 μg/L throughout the dosing interval to minimize the risk of rejection (50). Oral therapy is normally commenced at a dose of 4–5 mg/kg twice daily, although a higher dose or a shorter dosing interval may be required in children and in patients with external bile drainage, gastrointestinal disease, or a decreased elimination half-life (51). Pretransplant pharmacokinetic monitoring may be useful to identify patients with inadequate drug exposure who are at risk of rejection and graft loss, and to predict the dose and dosing interval required (52). Aerosolized CsA has been used in the attempt to reverse acute lung rejection (53); however, demonstration of consistent efficacy awaits larger trials (see Chapter 25).

Prospective, concentration-controlled studies in kidney and liver transplant recipients suggest that Neoral reduces the need for intravenous CsA (54), decreases the risk or severity of acute rejection (55,56), and enables more predictable and cost-effective therapy (57,58). In the international renal study comparing Neoral and Sandimmune, the mean administered CsA dose was 8% lower at 3 months in patients receiving the microemulsion (4.5 versus 4.9 mg/kg/day), although trough levels were comparable at all times. CsA absorption was 49% greater by 2 weeks after transplant (AUC_{0-12h}: 7155 vs. 5221 ng·hr/mL) in these patients, and remained significantly superior throughout the period of follow-up (55). Patient and graft survival were essentially identical for both formulations (98% and 91%, respectively), but acute rejection was significantly less frequent in patients receiving Neoral (42% versus 60%, P = 0.04), without any evidence of increased nephrotoxicity, hepatotoxicity, hypertension, or other adverse effects. The UK multicenter study confirmed these results (56). Target CsA levels were achieved more quickly (2 versus 4 days), while the incidence of both first (35.9% versus 52%) and recurrent rejection (9.7% versus 18.4%) were significantly reduced in patients receiving the microemulsion. Interestingly, the risk of acute rejection was lowest among those who did not receive intravenous cyclosporine (27%, P = 0.026).

Neoral is particularly important in liver transplantation, where external biliary drainage reduces CsA bioavailability from the oil vehicles to less than 5% (59). Absorption is enhanced by two- to sixfold with the new formulation and is closely correlated with age ($r = 0.87$, $P = 0.02$), while total body clearance (12 mL/min/kg) and volume of distribution (Vd_{ss}: 2.2 L/kg) are unchanged (60). Blood levels are comparable to those achieved with intravenous administration within the first 48 hours, and within- (31%) and between-patient variability (17%) are low (61). Intravenous therapy may thus be avoided in 90% of patients (62), while achieving graft survival above 90% and a reduced frequency ($P = 0.02$) and severity ($P = 0.027$) of acute rejection without evidence of incremental toxicity (63,64).

Preliminary studies in pancreas, heart, lung, and heart–lung transplantation confirm these observations, and exposure is increased by approximately twofold and C_{max} by threefold in patients with cystic fibrosis on treatment with Neoral (65–68).

Several large-scale studies have demonstrated that stable patients may be converted safely from Sandimmune to Neoral, offering consistent and predictable immunosuppression at lower cost (69–71). Conversion is normally performed at a 1:1 dose ratio, although the mean dose of CsA must then be reduced by approximately 5% to 12% to maintain constant trough levels. The most extensive pharmacoepidemiologic study encompassed 1097 stable patients randomized 2:1 to receive Neoral or continue on Sandimmune (72). CsA absorption was significantly greater within the first 4 hours after dosing in the Neoral group (3032 ± 1039 versus 1978 ± 934 ng·hr/mL, $P < 0.001$), without any significant change in the trough concentration (203 ± 85 versus 202 ± 95 ng·hr/mL). The magnitude of increase observed was not simply proportional in all patients, but was maximal in the group of patients who experienced the lowest bioavailability from Sandimmune (more than 1 SD below the mean) and were hence at greatest risk of immunologic injury. All of these patients became good or excellent absorbers when converted to Neoral. In contrast, patients who had good bioavailability on Sandimmune saw little incremental improvement in CsA exposure after conversion to Neoral, and thus were not placed at greater risk of toxicity. Apart from a mild and transient increase in serum creatinine in the first month after conversion in the Neoral group, there was no evidence of incremental toxicity throughout the 18 months of follow-up (73). The incidence of acute rejection was similar during the period of observation (5%); the incidence of chronic rejection was slightly lower among patients receiving Neoral (8% versus 11%), but this did not reach statistical significance due to the relatively small cohort size.

Therapeutic monitoring of CsA is widely employed to assist dose adjustment, to detect drug interactions, and to recognize noncompliance with therapy. Adequate bioavailability and consistency of exposure, measured using full pharmacokinetic profiles, have been shown respectively to correlate closely with freedom from acute rejection and chronic rejection (74,75). Because sequential pharmacokinetic profiling is impractical in many settings, the trough (C_0) blood level has been generally accepted for long-term therapeutic monitoring. However, the assumption that this accurately reflects drug exposure has now been shown to be false with Sandimmune ($R^2 = 0.43$) and only marginally superior with Neoral ($R^2 = 0.5$–0.8) (76).

The use of limited sampling strategies to predict exposure throughout the dosing interval, first developed by Johnston et al (77), has now been expanded by other researchers using time points selected from both the absorption and the elimination phases of the dosing interval (78–80). Kahan and colleagues, using a two-point sampling protocol (2 hr and 6 hr post dose) showed a 92% to 99% correlation with full AUC in patients receiving Neoral (82). The Canadian Study Group, for practical purposes of clinical management, has confined the sampling period to the first 4 hours of the dosing interval. In these studies, a four-point protocol with sampling at 0, 1, 2, and 4 hours provided a greater than 97% correlation with the full 12-hour AUC, while selection of just two points at 0 and 2 hours showed a correlation of 94.5% and a mean predictive error of <10% (34). Because of the greater heterogeneity of absorption in the first 2 weeks after transplant, three-point sampling may prove superior during this time, following which two-point sampling using one of several time combinations appears to provide an excellent prediction of drug exposure (83). It is expected that this approach will, for the first time, allow the accurate separation of the transplant population into two groups: those who have excellent and consistent absorption with Neoral and in whom the frequency of monitoring can be markedly reduced or eliminated, and the small but critical population with inadequate or inconsistent exposure who require special attention.

Mycophenolate Mofetil

The use of mycophenolate mofetil (MMF) in combination with CsA has dramatically reduced both the incidence and the severity of acute rejection (84). Initial studies in Canada, Australia, Europe, and the United States were conducted using Sandimmune (85–87), but extensive experience has since been gained with MMF in combination with Neoral. The risk of biopsy-proven acute rejection has declined below 20%, and the frequency of resistant rejection has decreased to almost 5% (84). As a result, this drug is replacing azathioprine as standard therapy for many transplant units.

Apart from an increase in risk of viral infection, largely controlled by routine prophylaxis, there appears to be little cumulative toxicity of these agents. Unfortunately, the rate of chronic graft injury is unaltered, despite the lower incidence of acute rejection episodes following use of this combination. Chronic renal allograft damage remains at 15% to 20% by 3 years, which is in contrast to the early promise of experimental studies (88). Chapter 10 presents a more detailed review of MMF.

Sirolimus (Rapamycin)

Sirolimus (Rapamune, Wyeth-Ayerst) and CsA act at discrete molecular sites (see Fig. 6.2). Sirolimus selectively inhibits a later stage in the immune activation cascade, blocking the downstream effects of the IL-2 receptor signal (89). The two drugs are potently synergistic in experimental animal studies of heart and kidney transplantation, where sirolimus may retard chronic vascular injury (90,91). Phase II studies in human kidney transplantation show that the incidence of acute rejection is reduced to approximately 10% when using optimal combinations of both drugs (92). In addition, sirolimus potentiates the pharmacokinetic exposure to CsA when the two drugs are administered simultaneously (93).

Sirolimus is not nephrotoxic, but may cause thrombocytopenia and hypercholesterolemia, complications also attributed to CsA. Phase III studies now underway will determine the risks and benefits of this combination. A detailed discussion of sirolimus is presented in Chapter 11.

Basiliximab and Daclizumab

Two monoclonal antibodies directed against the IL-2 receptor, basiliximab (Simulect, Novartis) and daclizumab (Zenapax, Hoffman-LaRoche) (94,95), have recently been tested in phase III studies with CsA (see Chapter 13). Both bind to the α-chain of the IL-2 receptor and cause a rapid depletion of cells bearing this structure from the peripheral circulation.

Basiliximab, a chimeric murine monoclonal, is administered on days 0 and 4 post-transplant. The humanized monoclonal daclizumab is given 5 times at 2-week intervals throughout the first 2 months. When combined with CsA microemulsion, both agents produce excellent graft and patient survival (>95% at 6 months). They also provide a significant reduction in the incidence of biopsy-proven acute rejection (basiliximab: 33% versus 51% placebo control, P = 0.001; daclizumab: 28% versus 47% placebo control, P = 0.0001), without any measurable increase in infections, malignancy, or specific toxicity.

Table 6.2. Major Adverse Effects of Cyclosporine Therapy

Effect	Clinical Presentation	Frequency and Severity
Nephrotoxicity*		
Acute	Increased BUN, Cr	Very common (35% to 50%); mild, usually reversible
	Hemolytic uremia	Uncommon; severe, occasionally reversible
Chronic	Increased BUN, Cr Proteinuria, B.P.	Uncommon (7% to 10%); severe, progressive
Cardiovascular	Hypertension*	Very common (70% to 90%)
	Intravascular coagulation	Rare
Neurotoxicity*	Tremor, hyperesthesia	Common (25% to 30%)
	Headache	Usually transient
	Seizures	Uncommon (<5%)
	Severe neurotoxicity (cortical blindness, quadriplegia, seizures, coma, white matter changes on CT or MRI)	Uncommon
Metabolic	Hyperkalemia*	Very common
	Hyperuricemia*	Common
	Hyperglycemia*	Common
	Hyperlipidemia*	Common
	Hypomagnesemia	Uncommon
Gastroenterologic		
GI upset	Nausea, anorexia, cramps, diarrhea	Common; mild, transient
Hepatotoxicity*	Increased SGOT, SGPT, alkaline phosphatase, bilirubin	Uncommon; mild, transient, dose-related
Mucocutaneous	Hirsutism*	Common, often severe
	Gingival hyperplasia*	Common, mild
	Facial dysmorphism	Common (infants)
	Acne, brittle fingernails	Very uncommon
	Decreased scalp hair	Very uncommon
Neoplastic*	PTLD	Uncommon (1% to 8%)
	Epithelial malignancies	Common

* The most commonly cited side effects (often referred to as the "three Ns" and "eight Hs"). Cr, creatinine, B.P., blood pressure.

MAJOR ADVERSE EFFECTS OF CYCLOSPORINE

The side effects of cyclosporine are summarized in Table 6.2.

Renal

Nephrotoxicity is unquestionably the most worrying side effect of CsA and is of particular concern in renal transplant recipients, in whom it has to be distinguished from rejection as a cause of deteriorating renal function. This disadvantage became evident very soon after its initial clinical use. For this reason, investigators have advocated the use of CsA only in patients whose kidneys were diuresing after transplantation (96).

Three clinical types of nephrotoxicity are observed with CsA. The first type occurs immediately after transplantation, usually in a kidney already damaged by ischemia, and is more commonly associated with use of intravenous CsA. The incidence of delayed function after renal transplantation has generally tended to be higher in patients treated with CsA than in those given azathioprine and steroids (97), although there is no general agreement about this (98). The implications of the possible additive effects of CsA nephrotoxicity on an ischemic kidney are important because they suggest that protocols that delay the administration of

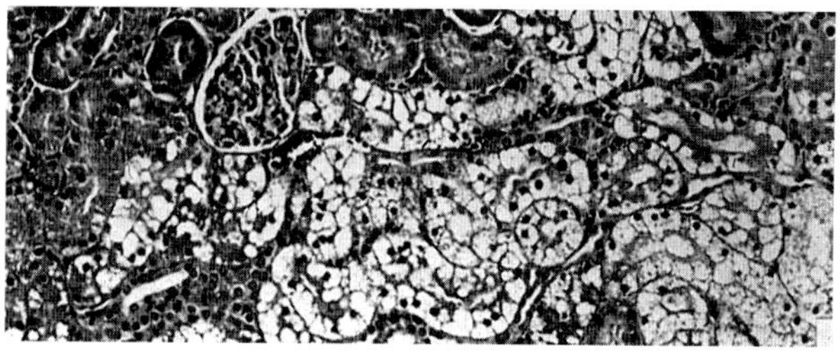

FIGURE 6.5. *Acute CsA nephrotoxicity in a patient with allograft dysfunction 3 weeks after initiation of CsA therapy. Note the extensive proximal tubular vacuolization and sparse cellular infiltrate that are characteristic of CsA nephrotoxicity rather than acute rejection.*

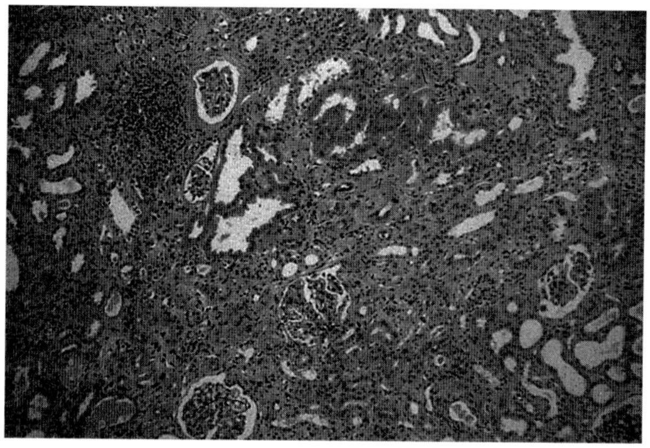

FIGURE 6.6. *Chronic CsA nephrotoxicity. Note the severe ("striped") interstitial fibrosis and diffuse cellular infiltrate. Although intimal proliferation in this biopsy is not dramatic, the histopathologic changes of chronic rejection are often quite similar.*

CsA until adequate renal function is established may be desirable.

The second type of nephrotoxicity is seen any time after the first 2 or 3 weeks and is accompanied by deteriorating renal function, usually but not always associated with high CsA blood levels. This is the type of nephrotoxicity that must be differentiated from an acute rejection episode (see also Chapter 17). Although high serum or blood CsA trough levels are often associated with nephrotoxicity and low levels with rejection, there are numerous exceptions to this. Percutaneous biopsy or fine-needle aspiration of the kidney is essential for making the correct diagnosis. Mild focal infiltrates, tubular vacuolization, and arteriopathy (Fig. 6.5 and Plate 4) are characteristically seen, although differentiation from rejection is frequently difficult. This type of nephrotoxicity recovers rapidly with a CsA dose reduction. Another possible uncommon manifestation of acute CsA nephrotoxicity is a hemolytic-uremia–like syndrome that occurs in the first several weeks after transplantation. Biopsies show striking arteriolopathy and even thrombosis. Despite the striking nature of the histologic findings, a return of renal function has been reported with cessation of CsA or the use of streptokinase and heparin (99).

The third type of nephrotoxicity is a chronic condition in which there is a slow but steady deterioration in renal function. The histology of the kidney typically reveals severe interstitial fibrosis (Fig. 6.6 and Plate 5). This type may show some improvement in renal function with a decrease in the CsA dosage, but it tends to be relatively short lived. It seems likely that many of the changes observed result from chronic rejection, on which is superimposed some element of CsA nephrotoxicity. After cardiac transplantation, this steady deterioration in renal function of patients on CsA has resulted in some patients requiring hemodialysis or renal transplantation (100).

Mechanism

The mechanism of CsA nephrotoxicity has not yet been clarified, but it would seem that a direct toxic action on proximal tubular cells is not a significant factor. Instead, a decrease in renal blood flow with an increased renal vascular resistance at the level of the glomerular afferent arteriole is the primary cause of the nephrotoxicity (101). That acute nephrotoxicity is reversed so rapidly after cessation of CsA is compatible with the concept of renal vasoconstriction as the primary cause of the nephrotoxicity.

Other reports have postulated that the effect of CsA on the production of renal prostaglandin might be responsible for the vasoconstriction as well as the changes in intravascular coagulation (102). The prostaglandins are potent renal vasodilators and are thought to play an important role in modulating the influence of various renal vasoconstrictor factors. There is some evidence that CsA inhibits the production of the prostaglandin metabolites, but CsA may also increase the production of thromboxane, which is a potent vasoconstrictor. Thus, this effect of CsA on the arachidonic acid metabolic pathway within the kidney could explain most of the observed functional and morphologic changes of nephrotoxicity.

Prostaglandins of the E series have immunosuppressive properties and, theoretically, are attractive agents to combine with CsA in order to reduce its nephrotoxicity. Some investigators have shown that misoprostol (a prostaglandin E_1 analogue) improves renal function and safely reduces the incidence of acute rejection in renal transplant recipients treated concurrently with CsA and prednisone (103). However, others have not been able to demonstrate any advantage to the concurrent use of this agent with CsA (104). This strategy has not, therefore, gained universal acceptance.

It has been reported that calcium channel blockers reduce the incidence of primary nonfunction in patients on CsA. Diltiazem has been associated with a marked reduction in CsA dosage with fewer episodes of primary nonfunction and less severe rejection episodes (105). Verapamil resulted in the need for lower CsA doses but equivalent blood levels, but there was no reduction in nephrotoxicity or incidence of rejection (106).

Cardiovascular

Hypertension is commonly associated with the use of CsA and is discussed in detail in Chapter 30. Cyclosporine appears to have complex effects on intravascular coagulation, and there have been reports of an increased incidence of renal artery and vein thrombosis (107,108) and an increase in the incidence of deep venous thrombosis (109). Although it is tempting to attribute these complications, as well as the microangiopathy and hemolytic-uremic syndrome, to CsA's effect on the arachidonic acid metabolic pathway (as discussed earlier), the evidence is too uncertain as yet to draw any firm conclusions.

Neurologic

A variety of neurologic complications have been reported with CsA use, including tremor, headache, convulsions, various paresthesias of the limbs, mania, and depression. These are discussed in detail in Chapter 33. Although the relationship with CsA is not always clear, there is sufficient evidence that such neurologic syndromes can be attributed to CsA toxicity in many instances, because they are typically associated with high blood levels and reverse on lowering the CsA dosage. Evidence suggests that CsA-induced hypomagnesemia may contribute to these neurologic complications, especially the convulsions.

Metabolic

Hyperkalemia is common in patients on CsA and is readily reversible by lowering the dosage or discontinuing the drug. The mechanism is unclear, but the decreased potassium excretion may be a result of decreased serum aldosterone levels or a primary tubular defect (110).

Hyperglycemia may occur in patients on CsA, and is often associated with a raised urine glucose level. The glycosuria is undoubtedly a manifestation of nephrotoxicity, but the hyperglycemia may reflect a toxic effect of CsA on β cells of the pancreas. The condition does appear to be reversible.

Renal handling of uric acid is also affected by the use of CsA, leading to higher serum urate levels even after correction for elevated serum creatinine. These high urate levels slowly return to normal over several weeks after the drug is discontinued. Again, this probably reflects a tubular defect associated with CsA nephrotoxicity. Gout occasionally occurs as a byproduct of the hyperuricemia. Urate levels may need to be lowered with allopurinol, and the leukocyte count needs to be monitored carefully if the patient is also on azathioprine.

Hyperlipidemia is a significant management issue in immunosuppressed allograft recipients. Post-transplant hyperlipidemia has been linked to cardiovascular disease, with its high morbidity and mortality rate (see Chapters 30 and 31). Along with steroid therapy, CsA has been implicated in contributing to hyperlipidemia (111), and conversion from CsA to tacrolimus has been shown to lower cholesterol, LDL, and apolipoprotein B in hyperlipidemic recipients (112).

Hypomagnesemia is due to an increased magnesium clearance in patients on CsA and is usually associated with high blood levels of CsA. This reflects another manifestation of CsA nephrotoxicity. Convulsions, mentioned previously as another possible manifestation of CsA toxicity, have been attributed to hypomagnesemia.

Gastroenterologic

Cyclosporine is unpleasant to take and cannot be adequately disguised, even when taken with flavored drinks such as chocolate milk. Consequently, some patients may experience nausea and anorexia, particularly with large doses. In general, this has been less of a problem with current preparations such as Neoral. The development of the gelatin capsule for CsA has been welcomed by most patients. However, as the capsules are large and difficult to swallow, some patients may prefer to remain with the liquid form.

Hepatotoxicity has been observed in patients on CsA after renal, cardiac, and bone marrow transplantation. Generally this manifests as a temporary elevation of liver function tests that regresses on dosage reduction. No histologic changes have been described in association with these biochemical changes, but high doses of CsA in the rat produce ultrastructural changes and a deterioration in liver function (113). Cyclosporine may be contraindicated in patients with abnormal liver function tests before renal transplantation, because they may be at risk for the development of frank cirrhosis. Furthermore, because CsA is metabolized in the liver, depressed liver function may alter blood levels of the drug.

Mucocutaneous

Mucocutaneous side effects of CsA have been recognized since the drug's introduction. The most common of these side effects are gingival hyperplasia and hypertrichosis. Although plaque control has been shown to be of benefit for gum hypertrophy, gingival surgery has occasionally been necessary. Recently, treatment with azithromycin has been recommended (114), but conversion to tacrolimus is almost always effective in reversing this condition. This approach typically controls hypertrichosis as well.

In children, facial dysmorphism (which was not seen in patients on azathioprine and steroids) can be striking. Again, conversion to tacrolimus, with the admitted increased risk of post-transplant lymphoproliferative disorder (PTLD) (see Chapter 37), is the usual treatment.

Neoplastic

An apparent increased incidence of lymphomas in the early patients treated with CsA caused considerable alarm (115). With time, however, the incidence of lymphoma in renal and cardiac allograft recipients was found to be no greater than expected in recipients treated with conventional immunosuppressive therapy (see Chapter 37). Indeed, most of the patients who have developed lymphomas have received other drugs as well, such as prednisolone and antilymphocyte globulin, suggesting that the occurrence of lymphoma is due to excessive immunosuppression rather than specifically to CsA.

Skin cancer is a major complication after transplantation, particularly in the sun-blessed countries such as Australia. It appears to be just as common among users of CsA as with other types of immunosuppression (described in detail in Chapter 37).

CONCLUSION

Cyclosporine has transformed whole organ transplantation from an experimental procedure with serious morbidity and mortality to a highly successful and economically viable treatment that is universally recognized as the optimal clinical therapy for most patients with end-stage organ failure. Its incorporation into therapeutic protocols has not only improved survival rates for recipients of extra-renal allografts but has also allowed for the reduction of steroid therapy and the accompanying side effects.

European and Canadian clinical trials were among the first to herald this transition (97,116,118), although the highly lipophilic nature of CsA proved a difficult challenge in pharmaceutical chemistry. The formulations initially employed for delivery of CsA resulted in incomplete and erratic absorption, and thus wide variations in exposure occurred within and between individuals. These pharmacokinetic limitations had serious clinical consequences, increasing the risks of both acute and chronic rejection and reducing the value of therapeutic drug monitoring. The introduction of a new microemulsion vehicle has overcome most of these difficulties, cementing the role of CsA as the cornerstone of clinical immunosuppression for renal transplantation.

In the next decade, optimal immunosuppression for organ transplantation must achieve five clinical goals:

1. Patient survival greater than 95%
2. Graft survival exceeding 90%
3. Rejection rate less than 10%
4. Incidence of infection less than 10%
5. Incidence of lymphoma less than 1%

There is now compelling cumulative evidence that the combination of CsA with agents to inhibit nucleotide synthesis, growth factor receptor expression, or growth signal transduction can move renal transplantation over this new threshold of safety and success.

REFERENCES

1. Wenger RM. Structures of cyclosporine and its metabolites. Transplant Proc 1990;22:1104–1109.
2. Fruhman DA, Burakoff SJ, Bierer BE. Immunophilins in protein folding and immunosuppression. FASEB 1994;8:391–400.
3. Bierer BE, Somers PK, Wandless TJ, et al. Probing immunosuppressant action with a non-natural immunophilin ligand. Science 1990;250:556–558.
4. Friedman J, Weissman I. Two cytoplasmic candidates for immunophilin action are revealed by affinity for a new cyclosporine: one in the presence and one in the absence of CsA. Cell 1991;66:799–806.
5. Snyder SH, Sabatini DM, Lai MM, et al. Neural actions of immunophilin ligands. Trends Pharmacol Sci 1998;19:21–26.
6. Demeule M, Beliveau R, Wenger RM. Molecular interactions of cyclosporin A with P-glycoprotein. Photolabeling with cyclosporin derivatives. J Biol Chem 1997;272:6647–6652.
7. Archinal-Mattheis A, Cohen D, Bair KW, et al. Analysis of the interactions of SDZ PSC 83([3′-keto-Bmt1]-Val2]-Cyclosporine), a multidrug resistance modulator, with P-glycoprotein. Oncol Res 1997;7:603–610.
8. Braaten D, Luban J, Phares W, et al. Cyclosporine A-resistant human immunodeficiency virus type 1 mutants demonstrate that Gag encodes the functional target of cyclophilin A. J Virol 1996;70:5170–5176.
9. Bartz SR, Malkovsky M, Rich DH, et al. Inhibition of human immunodeficiency virus replication by nonimmunosuppressive analogs of cyclosporin A. Proc Natl Acad Sci USA 1995;92:5381–5385.
10. Cardenas ME, Muir RS, Breuder T, Heitman J. Targets of immunophilin-immunosuppressant complexes are distinct highly conserved regions of calcineurin A. EMBO J 1995;14:2772–2783.
11. Batiuk TD, Kung L, Halloran PF. Evidence that calcineurin is rate-limiting for primary human lymphocyte activation. J Clin Invest 1997;100:1894–1901.
12. Sugimoto T, Stewart S, Guan KL. The calcium/calmodulin-dependent protein phosphatase calcineurin is the major Elk-1 phosphatase. J Biol Chem 1997;47:29415–29418.
13. Kruger M, Schwaninger M, Blume R, et al. Inhibition of CREB- and cAMP response element-mediated gene transcription by the immunosuppressive drugs cyclosporin A and FK506 in T cells. Naunyn Schmiedebergs Arch Pharmacol 1997;356:433–440.
14. Cristillo AD, Heximer SP, Russell L, Forsdyke DR. Cyclosporin A inhibits early mRNA expression of G0/G1 Switch Gene 2 (G0S2) in cultured human blood mononuclear cells. DNA Cell Biol 1997;16:1449–1458.
15. Borel JF, Baumann G, Chapman I, et al. In vivo pharmacological effects of ciclosporin and some analogues. Adv Pharmacol 1996;35:115–245.
16. Otto MG, Mayer AD, Clarien PA, et al. Randomized trial of cyclosporine microemulsion (Neoral) versus conventional cyclosporine in liver transplantation: MILTON study. Multicentre International Study in Liver Transplantation of Neoral. Transplantation 1998;66:1632–1640.
17. First MR, Alloway R, Schroeder TJ. Development of Sang-35: a cyclosporine formulation bioequivalent to Neoral. Clin Transplant 1988;12:518–524.
18. Kolars JC, Merion RM, Awni WM, Watkins PB. First-pass metabolism of cyclosporin by the gut. Lancet 1991;338:1488–1490.
19. Lown KS, Watkins PB, Benet LZ, et al. Role of intestinal P-glycoprotein (mdr1) in interpatient variation in the oral bioavailability of cyclosporine. Clin Pharmacol Ther 1997;62:48–60.
20. Freeman DJ. Pharmacology and pharmacokinetics of cyclosporine. Clin Biochem 1991;24:9–14.
21. Primmett D, Levine M, Wrishko R, Keown P. A pharmacokinetic study of cyclosporine A: factors affecting the usefulness of trough levels in predicting drug exposure in renal transplant patients. Clin Drug Invest 1997;13:23–36.
22. Kahan BD, Kramer WG, Wideman C, et al. Demographic factors affecting the pharmacokinetics of cyclosporine estimated by radioimmunoassay. Transplantation 1986;41:459–464.
23. Brunner LJ, Munar MY, Vallian J, et al. Interaction between cyclosporine and grapefruit juice requires long-term ingestion in stable renal transplant recipients. Pharmacotherapy 1998;18:23–29.
24. Gupta SK, Manfro RC, Tomlanovich SJ, et al. Effect of food on the pharmacokinetics of cyclosporine in healthy subjects following oral and intravenous administration. J Clin Pharmacol 1990;30:643–653.
25. Lindholm A, Henricsson S, Dahlqvist R. The effect of food and bile acid administration on the relative bioavailability of cyclosporine. Br J Pharmacol 1990;29:541–548.
26. Naoumov NV, Tredger JM, Steward CM, et al. Cyclosporin A pharmacokinetics in liver transplant recipients in relation to biliary T-tube clamping and liver dysfunction. Gut 1989;30:391–396.
27. Mueller EA, Kovarik JM, van Bree JB, et al. Pharmacokinetics and tolerability of a microemulsion formulation of cyclosporine in renal allograft recipients: a concentration-controlled comparison with the commercial formulation. Transplantation 1994;57:1178.

28. Kovarik JM, Mueller EA, van Bree JB, et al. Within day consistency in cyclosporine pharmacokinetics from a microemulsion formulation in renal transplant patients. Ther Drug Monit 1994;16:232–237.
29. Kovarik JM, Mueller EA, van Bree JB, et al. Cyclosporine pharmacokinetics and variability from a microemulsion formulation: multicenter investigation in kidney transplant patients. Transplantation 1994;58:1–5.
30. Mueller EA, Kovarik JM, van Bree JB, et al. Improved dose-linearity of cyclosporine pharmacokinetics from a microemulsion formulation. Pharmacol Res 1994;11:301–304.
31. Keown PA for the National and International Neoral Study Groups. Use of cyclosporine microemulsion (Neoral) in de novo and stable renal transplantation: clinical impact, pharmacokinetic consequences and economic benefits. Transplant Proc 1996;28:2147–2150.
32. Kovarik JM, Mueller EA, Richard F, et al. Evidence for earlier stabilization of cyclosporine pharmacokinetics in de novo renal transplant patients receiving a microemulsion formulation. Transplantation 1996;62:759–763.
33. Kovarik JM, Mueller EA, van Bree JB, et al. Reduced inter- and intraindividual variability in cyclosporine pharmacokinetics from a microemulsion formulation. J Pharmaceut Sci 1994;83:444–446.
34. Keown P, Landsberg D, Halloran P, et al. A randomized, prospective multicenter pharmacoepidemiologic study of cyclosporine microemulsion in stable renal graft recipients. Report of the Canadian Neoral Renal Transplantation Study Group. Transplantation 1996;62:1744–1752.
35. Lindholm A, Henricsson S. Intra- and inter-individual variability in the free fraction of cyclosporine in plasma in recipients of renal transplants. Ther Drug Monitor 1989;11:623–630.
36. Wasan KM, Pritchard PH, Ramaswamy M, et al. Differences in lipoprotein lipid concentration and composition modify the plasma distribution of cyclosporine. Pharmaceutical Res 1997;14:1613–1620.
37. Nandakumaran M, Eldeen AS. Transfer of cyclosporine in the perfused human placenta. Dev Pharmacol Ther 1990;15:101–105.
38. Behrens O, Kohlhaw K, Gunter H, et al. Detection of cyclosporin A in breast milk—is breast feeding contraindicated? Geburtshilfe Fraunenheilkunde 1989;49:207–209.
39. Kronbach T, Fisher V, Meyer UA. Cyclosporine metabolism in human liver: identification of a cytochrome P-450III gene family as the major cyclosporine-metabolizing enzyme explains interactions of cyclosporine with other drugs. Clin Pharmacol Ther 1988;43:630–635.
40. Keown PA. Pharmacokinetics, drug interactions and analytical measurements of cyclosporin. In: Bach J-F. T-cell directed immunointervention. Oxford: Blackwell Scientific, 1993:51–76.
41. Ptachcinski RJ, Venkataramanan R, Burckart GJ. Clinical pharmacokinetics of cyclosporin. Clin Pharmacokinet 1986;11:107–132.
42. Freeman DJ, Laupacis A, Keown PA, et al. Evaluation of cyclosporine-phenytoin interaction with observations on cyclosporin metabolites. Br J Clin Pharmacol 1984;18:887–893.
43. Martell R, Heinrichs D, Stille CR, et al. The effect of erythromycin in patients treated with cyclosporine. Ann Intern Med 1986;104:660–661.
44. Orme ML, Back DJ, Breckenridge AM. Clinical pharmacokinetics of oral contraceptive steroids. Clin Pharmacokinet 1983;8:95–136.
45. Yee GC. Pharmacokinetic interactions between cyclosporine and other drugs. Transplant Proc 1990;22:1203–1207.
46. Klintmalm G, Sawe J. High dose methylprednisolone increases plasma cylosporin levels in renal transplant recipients. Lancet 1984;1:731.
47. Tu Y, Kahan BD, Chou TC, Stepkowski SM. The synergistic effects of cyclosporine, sirolimus, and brequinar on heart allograft survival in mice. Transplantation 1995;59:177–183.
48. Wrishko RE, Levine M, Primmett DRN, et al. Investigation of a possible interaction between ciprofloxacin and cyclosporine in renal transplant patients. Transplantation 1997;64:996–999.
49. Campana C, Molinaro M, Buggia I, Regazzi MB. Clinically significant drug interactions with cyclosporin. An update. Clin Pharmacokinet 1996;30:141–179.
50. Kahan BD, Grevel J. Optimization of cyclosporine therapy in renal transplantation by pharmacokinetic strategy. Transplantation 1988;46:631–644.
51. Cooney GF, Hoppu K, Habucky K. Cyclosporin pharmacokinetics in paediatric transplant recipients. Clin Pharmacokinet 1997;32:481–495.
52. Lindholm A, Kahan BD. Influence of cyclosporine pharmacokinetics, trough concentrations, and AUC monitoring on outcome after kidney transplantation. Clin Pharmacol Ther 1993;54:205–218.
53. Iacono AT, Smaldone GC, Keenan RJ, et al. Dose-related reversal of acute lung rejection by aerosolized cyclosporine. Am J Respir Crit Care Med 1997;155:1690–1698.
54. Levy GA, Neuhaus P, Jamieson NV, et al. Neoral in de novo liver transplantation: adequate immunosuppression without intravenous cyclosporine. Liver Transpl Surg 1997;3:571–577.
55. Keown P, Niese D. Cyclosporine microemulsion increases drug exposure and reduces acute rejection without incremental toxicity in de novo renal transplantation. Kidney Int 1998;54:938–944.
56. Lodge JPA, Pollard SG. Neoral vs. Sandimmune: interim results of a randomized trial of efficacy and safety in preventing acute rejection in new renal transplant recipients. Transplant Proc 1997;29:272–273.
57. Kingma I, Ludwin D, Dandavino R, et al. Economic analysis of Sandimmune Neoral in de novo renal transplant patients in Canada. Clin Transplant 1997;11:42–48.
58. Keown PA, Landsberg D, Lawen J, et al. Economic Analysis of Sandimmune Neoral in Canadian stable renal transplant patients. Transplant Proc 1995;27:1845–1848.
59. Trull AK, Jamieson NV, Alexander GJ, et al. Absorption of cyclosporin from conventional and new microemulsion oral formulations in liver transplant recipients with external biliary diversion. Br J Clin Pharmacol 1995;39:627–631.
60. Dunn SP, Meligeni J, Elder CA, et al. Absorption characteristics of a microemulsion formulation of cyclosporine in de novo pediatric liver transplant recipients. Transplantation 1995;60:1438–1442.
61. Rasmussen A, Kirkegaard P, Heslet L, et al. Induction of immunosuppression by microemulsion cyclosporine in liver transplantation. Transplantation 1996;62:1031–1033.
62. Hemming AW, Levy GA, Aljumah AA, et al. A microemulsion of cyclosporine without intravenous cyclosporine in liver transplantation. Transplantation 1996;62:798–1802.
63. Winkler M, Pichlmayr R, Neuhaus P, et al. A new oral formulation of cyclosporine for early oral immunosuppressive therapy in liver transplant recipients. Transplantation 1996;62:1063–1068.
64. Graziadei IW, Krom RA, Steers JL, et al. Neoral compared to Sandimmune is associated with a decrease in histologic severity of rejection in patients undergoing primary liver transplantation. Transplantation 1997;64:726–731.
65. van der Pijl JW, Cohen AF, van der Woude FJ, et al. Pharmacokinetics of the conventional and microemulsion formulations of cyclosporine in pancreas-kidney transplant recipients with gastroparesis. Transplantation 1996;62:456–462.
66. White M, Carrier M, Jesina C, et al. Pharmacokinetic, hemodynamic, and metabolic effects of cyclosporine Sandimmune versus the microemulsion Neoral in heart transplant recipients. J Heart Lung Transplant 1997;16:787–794.
67. Kesten S, Scavuzzo M, Chaparro C, Szalai JP. Pharmacokinetic profile and variability of cyclosporine versus Neoral in patients with cystic fibrosis after lung transplantation. Pharmacotherapy 1998;18:847–850.
68. Tan KK, Wallwork J, Uttridge JA, Trull AK. Relative bioavailability of cyclosporin from conventional and microemulsion formulations in heart-lung transplant candidates with cystic fibrosis. Eur J Clin Pharmacol 1995;48:285–289.
69. Neumayer HH, Luft FC, Waiser J, et al. Substitution of conventional cyclosporin with a new microemulsion formulation in renal transplant patients: results after 1 year. Nephrol Dial Transplant 1996;11:165–172.
70. Pescovitz MD, Wong RL, Wombolt DG, et al. Safety and tolerability of cyclosporine microemulsion versus cyclosporine: two-year data in primary renal allograft recipients: a report of the Neoral Study Group. Transplantation 1997;63:78–80.
71. Pasha TM, Wiesner RH, Dahlke LM, et al. An open-label study of the safety and tolerability of converting stable liver transplant recipients to Neoral. Liver Transpl Surg 1998;4:410–415.
72. Keown P, Parfrey P, Belitsky P, et al. A randomized, prospective multicenter pharmacoepidemiologic study of cyclosporine microemulsion in stable renal graft recipients. Report of the Canadian Neoral Renal Transplantation Study Group. Transplantation 1996;62:1744–1752.
73. Cole E, Keown P, Landsberg D, et al. Safety and tolerability of cyclosporine and cyclosporine microemulsion during 18 months of follow-up in stable renal transplant recipients: a report of the Canadian Neoral Renal Study Group. Transplantation 1998;65:505–510.
74. Kasiske BL, Heim-Duthoy K, Venkateswara R, Awni WM. The relationship between cyclosporine pharmacokinetic parameters and subsequent acute rejection in renal transplant patients. Transplantation 1998;46:716–722.
75. Kahan BD, Welsh M, Schoenberg L, et al. Variable oral absorption: a biopharmaceutical risk factor for chronic renal allograft rejection. Transplantation 1996;62:599–606.

76. Keown PA, Halloran P, Kahan BD, et al. Optimization of cyclosporine therapy with new therapeutic drug monitoring strategies. Transplant Proc 1998 (in press).
77. Johnston A, Sketris I, Marsden JT, et al. A limited sampling strategy for the measurement of cyclosporine AUC. Transplant Proc 1990;22:1345–1346.
78. Grevel J, Kahan BD. Abbreviated kinetic profiles in area-under-the-curve monitoring of cyclosporine therapy. Clin Chem 1991;37:1905–1908.
79. Cantarovich M, Besner JG, Barkun JS, et al. Two-hour cyclosporine level determination is the appropriate tool to monitor Neoral therapy. Clin Transplant 1998;12:243–249.
80. Melter M, Rodeck B, Kardorff R, Hoyer PF, Brodehl J. Pharmacokinetics of cyclosporine in pediatric long-term liver transplant recipients converted from Sandimmune to Neoral. Transpl Int 1997;10:419–425.
81. Rial M de C, Frias S, Argento J, et al. Convenience of level of cyclosporine-Neoral at time 3 to determine the area under curve in renal transplant. Transplant Proc 1997;29:292–293.
82. Amante AJ, Kahan BD. Abbreviated AUC strategy for monitoring cyclosporine microemulsion therapy in the immediate post-transplant period. Transplant Proc 1996;28:2162–2163.
83. Primmett DRN, Levine M, Kovarik JM, et al. Cyclosporine monitoring in renal transplant patients: two- or three-point methods that estimate area under the curve are superior to trough levels in predicting drug exposure. Ther Drug Monit 1989;20:276–283.
84. Halloran P, Mathew T, Tomlanovich S, et al. Mycophenolate mofetil in renal allograft recipients: a pooled analysis of three randomized double-blind clinical studies in prevention of rejection. Transplantation 1997;63:39–47.
85. The Tricontinental Mycophenolate Mofetil Renal Transplant Study Group. A blinded, randomized clinical trial of mycophenolate mofetil for the prevention of acute rejection in cadaveric renal transplantation. Transplantation 1996;61:1029–1037.
86. Sollinger HW for the US Renal Transplant Mycophenolate Mofetil Study Group. Mycophenolate mofetil for the prevention of acute rejection in primary cadaveric renal allograft recipients. Transplantation 1995;60:225–232.
87. European Mycophenolate Mofetil Cooperative Study Group. Placebo-controlled study of mycophenolate mofetil combined with cyclosporine and corticosteroids for prevention of acute rejection. Lancet 1995;345:1321–1325.
88. The Tricontinental Mycophenolate Mofetil Study Group. A blinded, randomized multicentre study of mycophenolate mofetil (mmf) in cadaveric renal transplantation: results at three years. Transplantation 1989 (in press).
89. Kelly PA, Kahan BD, Behbod F, Gruber SA. Sirolimus, a new, potent immunosuppressive agent. Pharmacotherapy 1997;17:1148–1156.
90. Stepkowski SM, Kahan BD, Chou TC, et al. Synergistic mechanisms by which sirolimus and cyclosporine inhibit rat heart and kidney allograft rejection. Clin Exp Immunol 1997;108:3–68.
91. Morris RE, Berry GJ, Shorthouse R, et al. Studies in experimental models of chronic rejection: use of rapamycin (sirolimus) and isoxazole derivatives (leflunomide and its analogue) for the suppression of graft vascular disease and obliterative bronchiolitis. Transplant Proc 1995;27:2068–2069.
92. Kahan BD. Concentration-controlled immunosuppressive regimens using cyclosporine with sirolimus or brequinar in human renal transplantation. Transplant Proc 1995;27:33–36.
93. Kaplan B, Kahan BD, Napoli KL, Meier-Kriesche HU. The effects of relative timing of sirolimus and cyclosporine microemulsion formulation coadministration on the pharmacokinetics of each agent. Clin Pharmacol Ther 1998;63:48–53.
94. Nashan B, Moore R, Amlot P, et al. Randomized trial of basiliximab versus placebo for control of acute cellular rejection in renal allograft recipients. Lancet 1997;350:1193–1198.
95. Vincenti F, Kirkman R, Light S, et al for the Daclizumab Triple Therapy Study Group. Interleukin-2 receptor blockade with Daclizumab to prevent acute rejection in renal transplantation. N Engl J Med 1998;338:161–165.
96. Calne RY, White DJ. The use of cyclosporin A in clinical organ grafting. Ann Surg 1982;196:330–337.
97. The Canadian Multicentre Transplant Study Group. A randomized trial of cyclosporine in cadaveric renal transplantation. N Engl J Med 1983;309:809–815.
98. Fletchner SM, Payne WD, Van Buren L, et al. The effect of cyclosporine on early graft function in human renal transplantation. Transplantation 1983;36:268–272.
99. Remuzzi G, Bertani T. Renal vascular and thrombotic effects of cyclosporine. Am J Kidney Dis 1989;13:261–272.
100. Goldstein DJ, Zuech N, Sehgal V, et al. Cyclosporine-associated end-stage nephropathy after cardiac transplantation. Transplantation 1997;63:664–668.
101. Remuzzi G, Perico N. Cyclosporine-induced renal dysfunction in experimental animals and humans. Kidney Int Suppl 1995;52:S70–74.
102. Neild GH, Rocchi G, Imberti L, et al. Effect of cyclosporin A on prostacyclin synthesis by vascular tissue. Thromb Res 1983;32:373–379.
103. Moran M, Mozes MF, Maddux MS, et al. Prevention of acute graft rejection by the prostaglandin E1 analogue misoprostol in renal transplant recipients treated with cyclosporine and prednisone. N Engl J Med 1990;322: 1183–1188.
104. Pouteil-Noble C, Chapuis F, Berra N, et al. Misoprostol in renal transplant recipients: a prospective, randomized, controlled study on the prevention of acute rejection episodes and cyclosporin A nephrotoxicity. Nephrol Dial Transplant 1994;9:552–555.
105. Chrysostomon A, Walker RG, Russ GR, et al. Diltiazem in renal allograft recipients receiving cyclosporine. Transplantation 1993;55:300–304.
106. Pirsch JD, D'Alessandro AM, Roecker EB, et al. A controlled, double-blind, randomized trial of verapamil and cyclosporine in cadaver renal transplant patients. Am J Kidney Dis 1993;21:189–195.
107. Canadian Multicentre Transplant Study Group. A randomized clinical trial of cyclosporine in cadaveric renal transplantation. N Engl J Med 1986;314:1219–1225.
108. Rigotti P, Flechner SM, VanBuren CT, et al. Increased incidence of renal allograft thrombosis under cyclosporine immunosuppression. Intern Surg 1986;71:38–41.
109. Vanrenterghem Y, Roels L, Lerut J, et al. Thromboembolic complications and haemostatic changes in cyclosporin-treated cadaveric kidney allograft recipients. Lancet 1985;1:999–1002.
110. Bantle JP, Nath KA, Sutherland DER, et al. Effects of cyclosporine on the renin-angiotensin-aldosterone system and potassium excretion in renal transplant recipients. Arch Intern Med 1985;145:505–508.
111. Satterthwaite R, Aswad S, Sunga V, et al. Incidence of new-onset hypercholesterolemia in renal transplant patients treated with FK506 or cyclosporine. Transplantation 1998;65:446–449.
112. McCune TR, Thacker LR, Peters TG, et al. Effects of tacrolimus on hyperlipidemia after successful renal transplantation. Transplantation 1998;65:87–92.
113. Thomson AW, Whiting PH, Simpson JG. Pathobiology of cyclosporin A in experimental animals. In: Cyclosporin A, White DJ, ed. Amsterdam: Elsevier Biomedical, 1982:177.
114. Nash MM, Zaltzman JS. Efficacy of azithromycin in the treatment of cyclosporine-induced gingival hyperplasia in renal transplant recipients. Transplantation 1998;65:1611–1615.
115. Bird AG, McLachlan SM, Britton S. Cyclosporin A promotes spontaneous outgrowth in vitro of Epstein-Barr virus-induced B cell lines. Nature 1981;289:300–301.
116. Gomez R, Moreno E, Colina F, et al. Steroid withdrawal is safe and beneficial in stable cyclosporine-treated liver transplant patients. J Hepatol 1998;28:150–156.
117. Cyclosporine as sole immunosuppressive agent in recipients of kidney allografts from cadaver donors: preliminary results of a European multicentre trial. Lancet 1982;2:57–69.
118. Beveridge T, Calne RY. Cyclosporine (Sandimmune) in cadaveric renal transplantation. Transplantation 1995;59:1568–1570.

Chapter 7

Azathioprine

Roy Y. Calne

The use of azathioprine as an immunosuppressant for solid organ grafts was a watershed in the development of clinical transplantation. In the Tuckahoe Laboratories of Burroughs-Wellcome, Hitchings and Elion started a program to develop synthetic chemical agents that would be valuable in the treatment of cancer. They deliberately substituted purines and pyrimidines to produce molecules that would act in a fraudulent manner, becoming incorporated in vital biologic processes but then poisoning the cells and preventing their division (1). One of the agents they produced was the thiopurine 6-mercaptopurine (6-MP), which was recognized as valuable in the treatment of certain leukemias.

Schwartz and Damashek (2), working at Tufts Medical School in Boston, used 6-MP in experiments to inhibit the clonal proliferation of lymphocytes that occurs in response to an antigenic stimulus. Rabbits challenged with a foreign protein were treated for 2 weeks with daily doses of 6-MP. This prevented the expected primary and later secondary response to that specific protein, but after the 14-day period of treatment the animals could react against other proteins. The 2-week course of 6-MP appeared to have conferred a specific inhibition of antibody production, determined by the challenging protein at the commencement of the treatment. Of special interest was the observation that this effect lasted for a long time after the 6-MP treatment had stopped. Thus, for a simple foreign protein the drug 6-MP was able to produce tolerance.

At the time, the only clinical success with kidney transplants was between identical twins and very closely matched sibling donors who had been treated with total body irradiation. Many patients within the same irradiation protocol but with less well-matched kidneys developed uncontrollable rejection of the organs or died from the side effects of the irradiation. Infection was a major cause of death. Some clinicians persisted with this treatment, despite the almost universal failure. Developing a safer and more effective form of immunosuppression was essential if organ transplantation was to become established.

Following Schwartz and Damashek's rabbit study, I investigated the effect of this drug in dogs receiving renal allografts, in hope of obtaining similar tolerance to organ grafts. Although tolerance could not be produced, several animals had markedly prolonged survival without rejection of their grafts (3). Similar observations were made independently by Zukoski and Hume, which led to investigations using a variety of antiproliferative drugs, including corticosteroids, for control of the immune process (4).

My quest for a more specific agent than 6-MP led me to a visit to Tuckahoe and discussions with Hitchings and Elion. They gave me a variety of compounds including thiopurines and pyrimidines that they felt were worthy of investigation. I studied these in Joseph Murray's laboratory in Francis Moore's department of surgery at the Peter Bent Brigham Hospital in Boston and found that an imidazole-linked 6-MP, later called azathioprine, was slightly superior to the parent compound (5).

The first use of thiopurines in clinical transplants was in England and France using the parent drug 6-MP (6). Following the observations on azathioprine, however, this agent became part of a new protocol that Murray and his colleagues began to use at the Peter Bent Brigham Hospital in 1962. The early results showed that azathioprine was a superior immunosuppressant to total body irradiation, but alone it did not appear to be sufficiently effective for major clinical development.

In 1960 Goodwin (7) showed that an acute rejection crisis in a clinical renal transplant could be reversed by a large dose of corticosteroids, and that corticosteroids combined with azathioprine was a drug protocol that could give better results in renal allografts than azathioprine alone.

Working in Denver, Starzl and his colleagues performed a series of renal allografts using azathioprine and corticosteroids for immunosuppression. These results were the best that had so far been produced in the clinical setting (8). Rejection crises that continued to occur were treated by higher doses of steroids.

There was a danger that overimmunosuppression would cause infection. Side effects of steroids could be very severe, particularly in children. They caused stunted growth and cushingoid facies, turning the children into monsters who could not socialize in a normal manner. Adults often developed aseptic necrosis of bone from a high steroid dose. The chief side effect of azathioprine was bone marrow suppression, and also some patients had an idiosyncratic hepatotoxic reaction. Long-term treatment with azathioprine may be associated with hypertrophic nodular hepatic adenomata, while macrocytic anemia was another rare complication.

Despite these risks, azathioprine and steroids were used with success throughout the Western world and Australasia. Some of the early patients are still alive, 30 years after renal allografting. This mode of immunosuppression was also used in transplants of the heart, liver, and pancreas. There were some notable good long-term results with grafts of these organs, but the high failure rate did not give confidence to clinicians. We had to await the introduction of cyclosporine to clinical transplantation before transplants of the heart, liver, and pancreas could be considered appropriate therapeutic undertakings (9). Continuing good results have now led to a shortage of organs, which grows more serious every year.

MODE OF ACTION

Azathioprine inhibits both DNA and RNA synthesis, and so interferes with the precursors of purine synthesis and suppresses de novo purine synthesis. It has an effect on both B and T lymphocytes when they are in the process of proliferating. It suppresses both primary T-cell and secondary antibody synthesis, but it does not affect the production of lymphokines. It also has anti-inflammatory action, probably mainly due to its effect on proliferating cells. In addition to marrow suppression and hepatic dysfunction, azathioprine can also cause gastrointestinal disturbance.

The dosage depends on whether azathioprine is being used with other potent agents. Initially, when it is used only with corticosteroids, 3–5 mg/kg/day is given from the time of transplantation. It is usually well tolerated orally, and maintenance doses can often be lowered to 1–3 mg/kg/day. Patients already suffering from liver impairment may require much lower doses or, in some cases, azathioprine may have to be stopped and substituted by another agent such as cyclophosphamide. Azathioprine can also be given intravenously at a similar or slightly lower dose than orally.

When cyclosporine was introduced into clinical organ transplantation, this new agent was used alone or in combination with corticosteroids. Later, it was combined with azathioprine (and corticosteroids) in a triple-drug regimen. In some centers, antilymphocyte antibodies, polyclonal or monoclonal, were given together with the three drugs. To treat a patient with four different immunosuppressive agents requires very careful clinical monitoring, as overimmunosuppression, with accompanying infections and risks of malignancy (particularly B-cell lymphomas), is a hazard. Although the exact immunosuppressive protocol followed by different centers varies in detail, for the past decade triple therapy with cyclosporine, azathioprine, and steroid has been the most common form of treatment.

Currently, the situation is changing. The new powerful purine analogue mycophenolate mofetil (MMF) is thought to have a more specific action on T cells, interfering with their division more than that of other cells. Mycophenolic acid has been used in patients with autoimmune disease, and the MMF derivative has been compared in large multicenter trials with azathioprine. MMF appears to have a better effect in reducing the incidence of acute rejection, although to date there has been no statistically significant improvement in survival of patients or their grafts. Longer follow-up of these studies is now being undertaken.

In summary, for 20 years azathioprine was the lynch-pin of immunosuppression for recipients of solid organ allografts. It was preferred to other antimitotic agents as having a better therapeutic index. Today, however, it may well be replaced by other, more specific agents such as mycophenolate mofetil.

REFERENCES

1. Elion GB, Bieber S, Hitchings GH. The fate of 6-mercaptopurine in mice. Ann NY Acad Sci 1955;60:297–303.
2. Schwartz R, Damashek W. Drug-induced immunologic tolerance. Nature 1959;183:1682–1683.
3. Calne RY. The rejection of renal homografts. Inhibition in dogs by using 6-mercaptopurine. Lancet 1960;1:417.
4. Zukoski CF, Lee HM, Hume DM. The prolongation of functional survival of canine renal homograft by 6-mercaptopurine. Surg Forum 1960;11:470.
5. Calne RY. Inhibition of the rejection of renal homografts in dogs with purine analogues. Transplant Bull 1961;28:445.
6. Hopewell J, Calne RY, Beswick I. Three clinical cases of renal transplantation. Brit Med J 1964;1:411.
7. Goodwin WE, et al. Human renal transplantation: clinical experiences with 6 cases of renal homo-transplantation. J Urol 1963;89:13.
8. Starzl TE, Marchioro TL, Von Kaulla KN, et al. Homotransplantation of the liver in humans. Surg Gynecol Obstet 1963;117:659.
9. Calne RY, White DJG, Thiru S, et al. Cyclosporin A in patients receiving renal allografts from cadaver donors. Lancet 1978;2:323.

Chapter 8

Steroids and Transplantation

ROWAN G. WALKER

From the days of early clinical renal transplantation in the 1960s, steroids (glucocorticoids) provided at least part of the basis of immunosuppressive therapy. For the next 20 to 25 years, steroids would provide the backbone of maintenance immunosuppression, particularly in combination with azathioprine, and virtually stood alone as the treatment for acute rejection. Their major role in maintenance immunosuppression therapy has clearly been lessened by the advent of cyclosporine (early 1980s) and the other calcineurin blockers. Also, to some extent the role of steroids in the treatment of acute rejection episodes has been supplemented, at least in part, by the availability of antilymphocyte serum preparations, particularly the monoclonal anti-T cell antibodies.

Thus, prednisolone, or prednisone in conjunction with azathioprine, has come to be known as "conventional immunosuppression" (1). Although cyclosporine—alone, in combination with steroids, or in triple combination with prednisolone and azathioprine—has probably become the major and most effective form of maintenance immunosuppression, there remains a very significant number of patients for whom steroids are an integral part of the long-term treatment. For these patients, the major problem remains finding the optimal dose and planning for withdrawal of the steroids, with the aim of minimizing the steroids' long-term toxic effects.

HISTORY

As far back as the 1920s, steroids were known to affect the immune system. Their first successful use in renal transplantation was in Boston in 1960, when cortisone was used to reverse a rejection episode in a living-related donor transplant recipient who had been immunosuppressed by whole body irradiation.

In 1961, Elion et al (2) synthesized azathioprine, an imidazole derivative of 6-mercaptopurine (6-MP), which had been found to be less toxic than 6-MP in dogs (3). The development of azathioprine led quite quickly to the undertaking of regular clinical renal transplantation in 1961 (4,5), and steroids were added to azathioprine as maintenance therapy in most centers after 1962 (6). However, following the early observation of successful reversal of acute rejection with large doses of prednisone (7), for many years several centers employed only steroids for the treatment of such episodes (8). Although initially prednisone was the steroid most commonly used, most units replaced it relatively soon with prednisolone.

PHARMACOLOGY

The pharmacology of steroids and their effects on the immune system are known to be extremely complex (9). Steroids affect the immune response in innumerable ways, especially in high doses, and their effects are especially seen on T lymphocytes. Corticosteroids have been shown to block Ca^{2+} ionophore-induced lymphocyte proliferation, which is an in vitro model of postreceptor events occurring after interaction of the T-cell receptor with antigen (10). Although cyclosporine also inhibits Ca^{2+} ionophore-induced proliferation, the mechanism is different (11). The cooperation between monocytes and lymphocytes in the proliferative response is also inhibited by steroids (12).

The block to the activation of T-cell proliferation by steroids has subsequently been shown to be associated with blocking the activation of certain cytokine genes. In particular, steroids block activation of the interleukin 2 (IL-2) gene in T cells (13), and also block activity of IL-1 (14) and IL-6 genes in other cells such as macrophages (15). It has been argued that the ability of steroids to prevent or suppress the fever associated with allograft rejection probably derives from the blocking of the release of these pyrogenic cytokines. As IL-2 is largely dependent on the presence of IL-1 and IL-6, corticosteroids have indirect as well as direct effects on IL-2 production from T cells.

Apart from the inhibition of lymphokines described above, steroids clearly reduce the migration of monocytes toward sites of inflammation. These broad and powerful anti-inflammatory actions of steroids also play an important role in the rejection process. This is particularly evident in the treatment of rejection episodes with high doses of prednisolone (or methylprednisolone) where the clinical effect is most often evident within 1 or 2 hours, which is quite clearly far too rapid to be adequately explained as a true immunosuppressive effect.

MAINTENANCE STEROID REGIMENS

There are virtually no situations where steroids would be used alone as maintenance immunosuppression, except in patients who are intolerant to all other agents or in whom the overall immunosuppression burden needs to be reduced (e.g., a patient developing severe neoplasia where continued use of other agents might hasten the neoplastic disease process). From the early days of clinical renal transplantation, it became increasingly apparent that there was a need to use steroid together with azathioprine; as the pharmacology of these two agents became established, they demonstrated quite different but additive effects (10).

Azathioprine and Steroids

Dual "conventional" immunosuppression maintenance therapy regimens consisting of azathioprine and steroids were used at most centers for the 25 years leading up to the mid-1980s. For the most part, such regimens consisted of:

1. an azathioprine dosage of 2–3 mg/kg/day, given as a single daily dose and reduced only if specifically indicated by complications (mainly leucopenia).
2. a prednisolone dosage, initially quite high (50–100 mg/day) then reduced slowly to a maintenance dose of approximately 10 mg/day over 6 to 7 months, and possibly as low as 5 mg/day over the longer term.

This general type of regimen (with minor variations) was the most common, but a number of exceptions gradually evolved, the most important of which has been the use of low-dose maintenance steroids.

Perioperative Therapy

Virtually all immunosuppressive regimens were established empirically. Whether steroids are given as part of dual (or even triple or quadruple) therapy, a typical perioperative regimen would be preoperative methylprednisolone, 1 gram IV, followed by postoperative hydrocortisone, 100 mg IV every 6 hours until oral therapy could be commenced. There is some evidence to support the approach of administering steroids before antigen exposure, particularly in suppression of humoral immunity. However, in a small controlled clinical trial, Kauffman et al (16) were not able to demonstrate any benefit of perioperative intravenous methylprednisolone. Regardless of the nature of the other immunosuppressive agents in the chosen regimen, many clinicians would continue to use the above approach or something similar.

High-Dose or Low-Dose Steroids

In the late 1970s and early 1980s, McGeown (17,18) consistently achieved excellent graft survival and a low incidence of steroid-related complications with a single daily prednisolone dose of 20 mg/day. The steroid was given from the day of transplantation, with gradual reduction after 6 months. The Necker group deliberately avoided the use of steroids in living donor recipients until the first rejection episode had occurred and discovered that 53% of HLA-identical grafts never developed rejection (19). Although this approach was attempted with cadaveric grafts, nearly all patients developed rejection episodes and subsequently required steroids. These observations strongly suggest that the degree of total immunosuppression, particularly the steroid dosage provided by a typical high-steroid azathioprine regimen, was unnecessary and was associated with an unacceptable rate of complications, especially steroid-related complications.

Eventually, the group at Oxford undertook a prospective trial (20–22). A typical high-dose regimen was compared with a relatively low-dose regimen. The low-dose group received prednisolone, 30 mg/day (as a single morning dose) for the first 60 days with subsequent slow reduction. This was supplemented by methylprednisolone, 1 gram IV on days 6, 7, and 8 after transplantation. Importantly, the study results showed a halving of the rate of steroid-related complications in the low-dose group with preservation of similar patient and graft survival rates to those achieved in patients receiving high-dose steroid. Unfortunately, the number of patients studied (39 on high-dose, 32 on low-dose) was too small to confidently exclude a real difference in graft survival being present in a larger sample. Although other groups (23–25) subsequently reported similar trials and results, there were problems with the relatively small numbers of patients in most of these studies. Nonetheless, the trend of the findings further support the hypothesis that low-dose steroids cause less complications and achieve similar graft survival rates to high-dose steroids (26).

The Influence of Azathioprine Dose

An important Australian multicenter trial (189 patients), showed a significantly worse graft survival in low-dose steroid–treated patients (27). This trial directly compared the original McGeown low-dose steroid regimen with each participating center's standard high-dose steroid therapy—azathioprine dosage was not mandated and each center was at liberty to use its own standard azathioprine dosage protocol.

The results ultimately indicated that the effects of the two steroid regimens could not be considered independently from the azathioprine dosage even after 4 years (28), at which time the apparent differences between the high- and low-steroid regimens demonstrated at 12 months were no longer apparent. It was clear that the combination of low doses of both agents provided inadequate immunosuppression and a poor graft survival, whereas higher doses of azathioprine allowed the use of low-dose steroid without significantly more graft losses than occurred with high-dose steroid. High doses of steroid could compensate to only a variable extent for lower azathioprine doses.

This study (27,28) almost certainly helps to explain the poor results achieved in some units with low-dose steroid regimens. It also indicates that, provided the azathioprine dose is adequate (greater than approximately 2 mg/kg/24 h), it would be possible to exclude any detrimental effect of low-dose steroid on graft survival of 10% or greater with a confidence of 95%.

In patients receiving only the combination of azathioprine and steroids, the important influence of an adequate azathioprine dose can also be demonstrated by analysis of the Australian and New Zealand Dialysis and Transplantation Registry data (Fig. 8.1 and Table 8.1), where the relationship between azathioprine dose and graft survival can be clearly observed irrespective of the steroid dose, even 10 to 15 years after transplantation. Interestingly, the relative importance of azathioprine dose has not been seen subsequently in immunosuppressive regimes that contain cyclosporine (29).

It seems that among "conventional" azathioprine/steroid dual-immunosuppression therapy regimens, the high-azathioprine/low-steroid regimen of the McGeown group is the best option available because it reduces steroid-related complications (28) without risking extra graft losses.

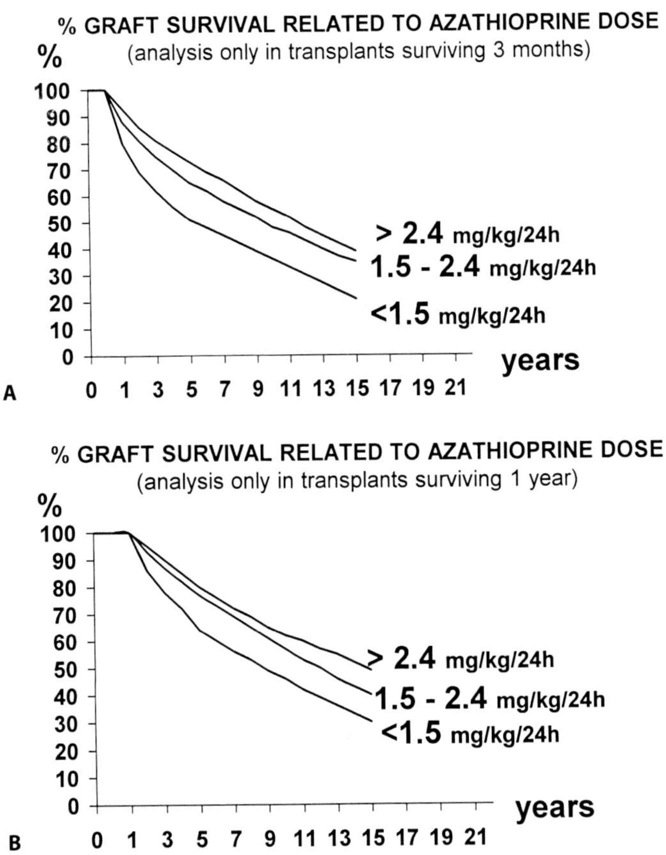

FIGURE 8.1. *Effects of azathioprine (AZA) dose on primary cadaveric graft survival, evaluated at 3 months (**A**) and 12 months (**B**) after transplant. The effect of AZA dose is examined only on grafts that had survived the early post-transplant period. No attempt was made to determine the reason(s) for an AZA dose <1.5 mg/kg/24 h. [Data from the Australian and New Zealand Dialysis and Transplantation Registry (ANZDATA), 1978.]*

Cyclosporine and Steroids Versus Cyclosporine, Azathioprine, and Steroids

Steroids may form part of an immunosuppressive regimen that contains the key immunosuppressive agent cyclosporine (see Chapter 6). Since the introduction of cyclosporine in the late 1970s and early 1980s, it is interesting to reflect that graft outcome (3-year survival) is virtually identical for all

Table 8.1. Effects of Azathioprine (AZA) Dose on Primary Graft Survival (Data Shown in Figure 8.1)

Evaluated 3 Months After Surgery			Evaluated 12 Months After Surgery		
	Number of Patients at Risk			Number of Patients at Risk	
AZA Dose (mg/kg/24 h)	3 Months	10 Years	AZA Dose (mg/kg/24 h)	1 Year	10 Years
<1.5	342	110	<1.5	308	112
1.5–2.4	941	400	1.5–2.4	843	386
>2.4	288	140	>2.4	166	83

Source: Australian and New Zealand Dialysis and Transplantation Registry (ANZDATA), 1978.

regimens, provided that cyclosporine forms one of the components (30). Comparing cyclosporine alone; cyclosporine and steroids; cyclosporine and azathioprine; and cyclosporine, azathioprine, and steroids, the most notable difference is that the relative mean dose of cyclosporine (at 1 year) was lower in the regimen employing all three immunosuppressive agents (so-called "triple" therapy). Of all these regimens, triple therapy is far and away the most popular (31–33), as it allows flexibility in the regimen and a low dose of the potentially nephrotoxic cyclosporine (34,35). Importantly, it also offers the opportunity for tapering the steroid dose to very low maintenance dose levels or even complete withdrawal of steroids (34,35).

It is not yet clear which of the cyclosporine-containing regimens is the optimal maintenance immunosuppressive regimen. One thing that is perhaps clear is the relationship between poor long-term graft outcome (function and survival) and the number and severity of acute rejection events. To what extent a steroid component of the regimen influences these episodes is difficult to determine precisely, particularly in triple-therapy regimens where the dose of cyclosporine is typically reduced compared to monotherapy (cyclosporine alone) or dual therapy (cyclosporine and steroids). The situation has become even more complicated with the introduction of new antiproliferative agents, particularly mycophenolate mofetil (MMF), which in three large multicenter controlled trials (36–38) was shown to reduce the incidence of acute rejection episodes during the early post-transplant months in patients who were simultaneously receiving cyclosporine and steroids (see Chapter 10).

A high proportion of patients receiving monotherapy (cyclosporine alone) require prednisolone (or azathioprine) to be added to the regimen because of immunologic instability. Unfortunately, this approach is not always successful in reversing the rejection process. The alternative approach is to commence with a broader immunosuppression regimen (triple therapy) and consider withdrawing steroids and/or azathioprine sequentially in patients in whom rejection has not proven to be a problem.

Variables Affecting Maintenance Steroid Dose

Patient Size

Children excluded, it is not common for steroid doses to be tailored to body size. Normally, the aim of dose adjustment according to weight would be to give doses in proportion to a patient's metabolic rate. Although surface area most closely reflects metabolic rate, weight is a reasonable guide in adults and is generally easier to measure. However, the correlation between weight and surface area is poor, and it particularly underestimates dosages in children and in small adults (<40 kg) in whom body surface area should be used.

Bioavailability

Prednisone and prednisolone are generally absorbed rapidly from the gastrointestinal tract, with peak plasma concentrations occurring within 1 to 3 hours (39). Prednisone is metabolized by the liver to prednisolone and the efficiency of this conversion is very variable. An average bioavailability of approximately 80% of that achieved by prednisolone (40) is the result of the conversion. Prednisolone is bound partly by the cortisone-binding globulin and also weakly by albumin. Although the binding affinity of albumin is relatively low, it is quantitatively the most important at pharmacologic concentrations of steroids.

Because only free steroid is available to interact with cytosol receptors, conditions that alter the level of plasma binding have marked effects on bioavailability. For example, pregnancy is associated with an increased plasma-binding capacity; consequently, there is reduced bioavailability of steroids in pregnant women. In hypoalbuminemia, the reverse is true—bioavailability is increased, thus explaining the increased incidence of steroid side effects reported in hypoalbuminemic patients (41).

Steroids are almost exclusively inactivated by the liver, so alterations in hepatic functional capacity will influence the half-life. The normal half-life of prednisone is about 60 minutes and that of prednisolone is 200 minutes (42). However, it should be remembered that prednisone is converted to prednisolone, thus the therapeutic effect lasts considerably longer than the half-life would suggest. Chronic liver disease (cirrhosis) can result in a doubling of steroid half-life (41), and certain commonly used drugs such as phenytoin barbiturates and rifampicin shorten the half-life by induction of hepatic enzymes (39).

Renal Function

As steroid metabolism is hepatic, serum activity, and consequently toxicity, is not changed in renal failure.

Timing of Drug Administration

In the era of "conventional" immunosuppression (azathioprine and steroids), it was originally common practice to administer steroids as divided doses (usually twice daily) in adult transplant patients. However, many centers have used a single daily dose, and those particularly concerned with pediatric transplantation have occasionally been inclined to use alternate-day steroids. The aim of single and alternate daily doses of steroid is obviously to reduce the incidence of steroid-related complications, without reducing their effectiveness as antirejection agents.

The logic of using single daily doses is that they be given in the morning to coincide with the cortisol peak, which is subject to diurnal rhythm. Certainly, the suppression of the hypothalamic-pituitary-adrenal axis is less using single morning steroid doses than single evening doses or divided daily doses (43,44). Similarly, there is also less suppression of the axis if steroids are given as a double dose on alternate days (1,45–47). Apart from relative sparing of the adrenal-pituitary axis, it is not clear that other steroid side effects are reduced by single daily doses. The benefits of alternate-day doses are more evident, with less growth retardation, cushingoid characteristics (46), serious infectious complications, and osteonecrosis (48), and these benefits are achievable without detectable loss of anti-inflammatory activity (45,46,49).

There is no appreciable difference in the immunosuppressive efficacy of twice- and once-daily steroids, but alternate-day steroids are definitely less suppressive as judged by their capacity to suppress delayed hypersensitivity skin testing to recall and/or to de novo antigens (49). At a clinical level, although it has not been subjected to trial, single and divided doses seem equally effective; however, many clinicians would argue that compliance is likely to be enhanced with the use of single daily dosing.

In patients receiving azathioprine and steroids, alternate-day prednisolone would predictably be associated with an intensified immune response. Indeed, in more than one study a changeover from daily to alternate-day steroids has been associated with increased rejection events (50–52). However, two prospective trials have not demonstrated a higher incidence of rejection or loss of function (48,53). In trying to interpret this apparent dichotomy, it should perhaps be emphasized that a failure to demonstrate a difference cannot necessarily be extrapolated to the assumption that the two therapies are equally effective, unless the numbers of patients studied are very large.

It has also been suggested that the changeover from daily to alternate-day steroids should be made within a few months of transplantation in children (54). Again, these recommendations were based on experience obtained using a high-dose steroid regimen and cannot be automatically considered to hold true with a low-dose steroid regimen, particularly as the recommended time of changeover is well before the steroid dose is actually down to a "maintenance" level. Growth in pubertal children is particularly sensitive to steroids compared to prepubertal children (55).

One might conclude that, in conventional dual therapy using azathioprine and steroids, in adults low-dose steroid given as a single morning dose would be the optimal regimen, although some would still argue for alternate-day therapy (56). The higher level and the nature of the side effects of daily steroids in children potentially outweigh the possible disadvantages of alternate-day therapy. In regimens containing cyclosporine (and prednisolone) it has been common practice to give the steroid as a single daily dose taken in the morning.

Steroid Withdrawal

Although immunosuppressive therapy including steroids has been discontinued successfully in the long-term in some patients (sometimes inadvertently), it was generally the case that such a practice was often followed by rejection (57). In contrast to complete cessation of immunosuppression in patients on azathioprine and steroids, reduction of the daily dose of azathioprine of stable patients from about 2.0–2.5 mg/kg to 1.5–2.0 mg/kg after 2 years may be relatively safe—the evidence is that azathioprine, rather than the small dose of steroid, contributes to the high risk of malignancy in long-term transplant recipients (see also Chapter 37).

When cyclosporine was first used in clinical transplantation (58) it was suggested that it could be used as sole therapy—thus effectively eliminating the need for maintenance steroid therapy. This view was gradually modified with the recognition that cyclosporine was not only nephrotoxic (59,60), but that the nephrotoxicity was in part dose dependent (61,62). In addition, several studies showed that adding prednisolone and lowering cyclosporine doses reduced toxicity and rejection episodes (63,64). Yet cessation of steroids at 6 or 12 months was likely to be associated with rejection (65,66).

The constant desire to reduce the individual toxicity of the various immunosuppressants eventually led to the development of low-dose "triple therapy" regimens (cyclosporine, azathioprine, and steroids). The synergism between cyclosporine and azathioprine (67) encouraged some clinicians to again consider complete steroid withdrawal. Although this may be achievable in more than 60% of patients (34,68), without rejection and without any adverse effect on graft function or outcome, in the remaining patients rejection episodes still may be observed. As suggested above, incorporation of the newer pharmacologic agents, including MMF (see Chapter 10) and tacrolimus (see Chapter 9), may allow more successful withdrawal of steroids (69). Nevertheless, a steroid-withdrawal approach to immunosuppression is certainly not universally practiced.

Interestingly, the proportion of patients who ultimately require steroids to be introduced into regimens not employing steroids from the outset (70) is strikingly similar to the proportion of patients from whom steroids cannot be successfully withdrawn when steroids are used from the outset.

TREATMENT OF REJECTION EPISODES

Despite the increasing use of antilymphocyte globulin and monoclonal anti-T cell antibodies as antirejection therapy, steroids continue to be the most important first-line treatment of acute rejection. In the treatment of rejection the important issue is not so much the choice of agent but the certainty of the diagnosis. The treatment of rejection is certainly important, but there is no evidence that delaying therapy for 24 hours to make certain of the diagnosis has a detrimental effect on the final outcome. At least 60% of acute rejection episodes can be reversed with oral or intravenous prednisolone (71), although success rates are lower if rejection occurs very early (within the first week) or if the clinical course is complicated by delayed function.

Once the diagnosis of rejection is established, treatment with oral or intravenous "bolus" methylprednisolone (equivalent to 3–15 mg/kg/day) is usually instituted (72). Interestingly, the use of high-dose oral prednisolone (e.g., 200 mg/day for 3 days) as a short course has not been shown to be inferior to intravenous methylprednisolone (0.5–1.0 gram daily for 3 days) in terms of the rate of rejection reversal. The oral regime is simpler, cheaper, and probably better tolerated by patients (73), but intravenous methylprednisolone appears to remain the treatment of choice.

For steroid-resistant rejection, treatment with OKT-3 (71) or antithymocyte globulin (ATG) should be instituted with a high expectation of reversal in the short term (see Chapter 13). For the prednisolone treatments, the incidence of major complications appears to be similar between intravenous and high-dose oral prednisolone therapies. Kauffman et al (74) compared high-dose (30 mg/kg/day) and low-dose (3 mg/kg/day) intravenous methylprednisolone regimens, and established that there was no advantage in high-dose therapy. When high-dose oral prednisolone courses are prolonged, a higher incidence of side effects may be anticipated (75,76).

It is virtually universal practice to repeat a course of high-dose steroid (oral or intravenous) after 3 to 5 days if there is a failure to respond, an incomplete response, or a relapse. The risk of serious complications undoubtedly escalates quite markedly with repeated courses of antirejection therapy. As indicated above, virtually all steroid-resistant rejection episodes respond to polyclonal ATG or a monoclonal T-cell antibody (OKT-3). Common practice is to use OKT-3 or ATG in rejection episodes unresponsive to steroids, and then to repeat the steroid course should the episode either respond and subsequently relapse, or only partially respond. In refractory rejection, an increasing role for other agents such as mycophenolate mofetil or tacrolimus (see Chapter 9) is being progressively established (77,78).

Various forms of in vitro testing of steroid sensitivity have been shown to predict a subsequent response to steroids during acute rejection in the clinical setting. However, the use of such techniques as a guide to immunosuppressive therapy has not gained much acceptance among clinicians (79,80).

COMPLICATIONS AND SIDE EFFECTS

Although it is often possible to ascribe responsibility for particular complications to particular immunosuppressants, many complications are due to the combined immunosuppressive effect of the drug regimen. Because of the nature of those complications, clinicians have always wanted to reduce the steroid burden whenever possible. This desire resulted in enthusiasm for the use of low-dose steroid regimens and steroid-withdrawal protocols when it became clear that the former was probably as effective in preventing graft rejection as conventional high-dose regimens (28), and the latter could be successfully achieved in 60% to 70% of patients taking cyclosporine (34) or in most patients on triple therapy (81).

Complications of Steroids Alone

Growth Retardation

Growth retardation with subsequent failure to reach adult height is one of the most unfortunate features of pediatric renal transplantation (see Chapter 18). Growth rates prior to the availability of recombinant human growth hormone were no better after transplantation than those seen in children on dialysis (82). Many factors potentially influence the final outcome: renal failure itself is a cause of growth retardation owing to impaired somatomedin activity, as are hyperparathyroidism and renal rickets. Similarly, some causes of renal failure, such as cystinosis, are themselves potent causes of growth retardation.

It has been suggested that any improvement in growth velocity occurring after transplantation may be enhanced by the use of alternate-day rather than daily steroids (54). Other important factors include complete normalization of renal function and transplantation prior to the onset of puberty. Puberty is frequently delayed in chronic renal failure, and it may occur soon after transplantation with rapid epiphyseal closure and minimizing of further growth. As stated previously, during puberty, sensitivity of skeletal growth to steroids is marked.

Although the growth velocity after transplantation may reach normal, there is rarely any significant catch-up growth (82). Thus, the degree of growth retardation present before transplantation is some guide to the ultimate best outcome. Immunosuppression regimens containing cyclosporine may offer the best prospects of improved growth (see Chapter 6) after transplantation. The use of recombinant growth hormone before and after transplantation in growth-retarded children (especially prepubertal children) has been so successful that growth retardation is clearly diminishing as a problem in pediatric transplantation. Concerns still remain, however, as to the possible role of recombinant human growth hormone in rejection events (83,84).

Wound Healing

Steroids reduce the rate of wound healing, and this situation is exacerbated by chronic renal failure.

Bone Disease

Steroids are an important predisposing factor in the development of osteoporosis and avascular necrosis (AVN).

Avascular Necrosis The incidence of AVN is as high as 10% to 15% in patients treated with "conventional" high-dose steroid regimens and probably as low as 1% to 2% in patients receiving low-dose steroid. The incidence seems to be more closely related to the level of maintenance steroid than to the short courses ("pulses") of high doses given for rejection. Patients with secondary hyperparathyroidism at the time of transplantation may be at higher risk of developing AVN (85). The AVN lesion most commonly affects the hips and is frequently bilateral (Fig. 8.2). AVN may also affect other joints including the wrists, elbows, knees, ankles, and shoulders (see also Chapter 31).

Pain, often very severe, is the usual presenting symptom. Radiologic changes are typically absent in the early stages. Pain is also the symptom that ultimately is most likely to lead to surgery. Initial treatment is the avoidance of weight-bearing on the affected joint, but compliance with this is difficult to achieve, especially when pain subsides. Contin-

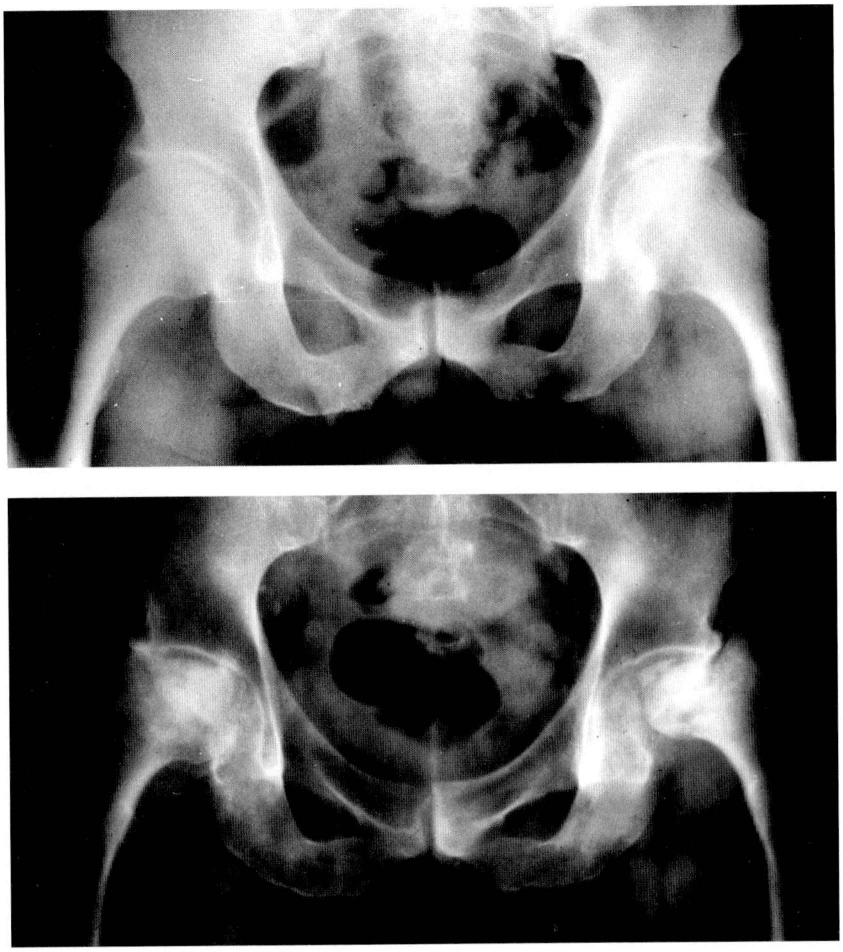

A

B

FIGURE 8.2. *Radiographic appearance of a 24-year-old renal transplant recipient developing the early symptoms of aseptic necrosis, with minimal radiologic changes. The patient's condition 6 months after transplant (**A**) progressed to almost total destruction of both hips (femoral heads) 30 months later (**B**). The patient had received large doses of intravenous corticosteroids for early acute rejection episodes, along with prolonged oral high-dose maintenance prednisolone.*

ued weight-bearing on the joint results in crushing of the femoral head, with a resulting limp. Ultimately, most patients will require surgery (total hip replacement), which is often undertaken relatively early to maximize rehabilitation.

Osteoporosis Osteoporosis associated with steroid use may lead to pathologic fractures. Loss of bone density after transplantation (especially early after transplant) is now well described (86,87) and may be very rapid (88). While glucocorticoids are important (89), the structure of the skeleton is likely to depend on a number of other effects (especially in renal transplant recipients) including exacerbation or remission of hyperparathyroidism, resolution of amenorrhea, increased physical activity, and changes in the renal tubular handling of phosphate (67,90,91).

Cataracts

The incidence of posterior lenticular cataracts is probably as high as 10% in patients receiving high-dose steroid, especially in the peritransplant period (92). The majority of cataracts are small and usually central, and they normally do not cause a very severe handicap. Less frequently (in about 1% to 2% of cases), the cataract is large and necessitates lens removal.

Diabetes

In patients on high-dose steroid regimens, glycosuria in the first 6 months after transplant occurs in about 60% of cases. Most often this is of renal origin, and in only about 20% of patients will hyperglycemia clinically be present. After the first 6 months, when the steroid dose is at maintenance level, glycosuria is much less common (5% of patients). Overall, only 5% to 10% of patients actually require therapy, usually oral hypoglycemic agents, and in many cases this need is transient. One report has suggested that post-transplant glucose intolerance is more likely to be associated with the same HLA-B locus antigens (B8, B18, BW 15, and BW 16) that are associated with juvenile-onset diabetes mellitus (93). There is a clear difference in the incidence of diabetes in patients receiving cyclosporine, where the incidence is low, and those receiving tacrolimus (FK506), where the incidence is high (see Chapter 9). The contribution of prednisolone to the latter is uncertain.

Weight Gain and Obesity

Steroids are frequently associated with a marked increase in appetite, which, coupled with a cessation of dialysis diet restrictions, may result in excessive weight gain (obesity). The problem usually begins to become apparent 2 to 3 months after transplant, and it is most effectively managed using preventative measures rather than by attempts to lose the extra weight. The appetite settles to normal as the steroid dose is reduced. The problem ought to be less marked with a low-dose steroid regimen, but our own experience (28) did not confirm this.

Hyperlipidemia

Hyperlipidemia has been increasingly recognized as a common problem following organ transplantation. Interest particularly centers on hyperlipidemia as a cause of accelerated atherosclerosis and post-transplant coronary and cerebrovascular events (94). In addition, hyperlipidemia may play a role in chronic rejection and late renal graft loss (see Chapter 31).

The precise cause of post-transplant hyperlipidemia is uncertain. In patients treated with prednisolone (and azathioprine), hypertriglyceridemia is the most common finding but is frequently accompanied by hypercholesterolemia. The abnormal lipid profiles are evident early and tend to persist (95). The hypertriglyceridemia probably results from an increased consumption of calories (carbohydrate and fat) following reversal of kidney failure accompanied by glucose intolerance secondary to the steroid administration. In contrast, patients treated with cyclosporine tend to have hypercholesterolemia, which, unlike hyperglycemia, is more severe in cyclosporine- than tacrolimus-treated recipients (see Chapter 9).

The initial therapeutic approach to hyperlipidemia in the transplant recipient is to impose dietary calorie-fat restrictions. The role of pharmacologic lipid-lowering agents in the cyclosporine era is being established (96) (see Chapters 30 and 31).

Cushingoid Features

The characteristic features of Cushing's syndrome, including moon face, acne, altered hair distribution, and truncal obesity with thin extremities, are common with high-dose steroid regimens. The severity of the problem is highly variable. Myopathy can be severe, especially in the elderly and in the early post-transplant months.

Peptic Ulceration

Although there has always been debate about whether steroids cause peptic ulcers, there is clearly an increased incidence and risk in transplant patients, particularly in the early post-graft period when steroid doses are relatively high. Many units use prophylactic H_2 antagonists (e.g., cimetidine) in symptomatic patients or during the period when steroid doses are above 20–30 mg/day. Anecdotal reports suggest that this has been associated with a reduced incidence of peptic ulcers (see also Chapter 29).

Most important for avoiding the potentially fatal complications of peptic ulcers is thorough investigation of all dialysis patients with indigestion prior to transplantation, using elective gastroscopy and/or radiologic studies (barium meal), followed by treatment if any lesions are detected. Silent ulcers are not uncommon in dialysis patients; many patients show minor lesions on gastroscopy, particularly those with hyperparathyroidism. Ulcers detected prior to transplantation should be treated medically first, and then surgically if medical treatment fails.

Colonic Perforation

Colonic perforation is a rare but potentially lethal complication of transplantation. The role of steroids is unclear. In many cases, it is a complication of preexisting diverticulosis, and it may also be seen in overt cytomegalovirus (CMV) infection. Although it is uncommon, its importance lies in the fact that it causes very high mortality in transplant patients. Historically, some units have investigated all potential transplant recipients by barium enema or colonoscopy to exclude diverticular disease. Some units have considered prophylactic surgery, but this is probably not justified in the era of cyclosporine, except perhaps in the occasional patient with a history of recurrent active diverticulitis.

Pancreatitis

Pancreatitis represents another complication in whose etiology the role of steroids is arguable. It is extremely uncommon, and is usually the result of an acute viral infection (e.g., mumps, CMV), preexisting gallstones, or pancreatic disease. Azathioprine should be considered as a possible causative agent in patients receiving the drug as part of the immunosuppression regimen.

Hypertension

Steroids may contribute to the high incidence of post-graft hypertension (at least 50%), but they are rarely the sole cause. The major contributors are the native kidneys, as demonstrated by the low incidence in patients who have been bilaterally nephrectomized; other agents, such as cyclosporine; and transplant arterial disease—either renal artery stenosis or chronic vascular obliteration due to rejection.

Psychiatric Disturbance

Mood changes, most commonly euphoria, are a common side effect of high-dose steroids. Frank psychosis is not rare, but it is almost invariably based on an underlying psychiatric disorder that may not have been readily evident prior to transplantation. Sleep disorders, particularly insomnia, are also a common complaint in the early period; however, such disturbances (particularly involving nightmares) are more often a result of β-blockers for hypertension, rather than steroids (see Chapter 34).

Combined Effects of Steroids and Other Immunosuppression

Infections

Infection in transplant patients remains a relatively common and potentially serious problem (see Chapter 36). The incidence of infections in "conventional" low-dose steroid regimens appears to be less than that found with high-dose regimens (28). Antilymphocyte agents, used either at induction or for the treatment of acute rejection, increase the susceptibility of the patient to infection, especially viral infections such as CMV, herpes simplex, and herpes zoster. Most episodes of acute rejection will have been treated by large bolus doses of prednisolone before the introduction of the antilymphocyte agents.

Malignancy

Malignancy is discussed in detail in Chapter 37. The incidence of virtually all malignancies, especially skin cancer, increases dramatically in immunosuppressed renal transplant recipients (97).

Skin Disorders

The skin is the site of a variety of complications following transplantation. Skin cancers may manifest, but many of the skin problems seen after a transplant are the result of infections (e.g., acne, warts, herpes simplex, and herpes zoster). The etiology is less certain in other skin disorders (98). Steroids induce thinning of the dermis by loss of collagen, a problem most often found in female patients. This common, readily detectable condition creates a risk of shearing injuries from minor trauma, particularly in the skin over the shins.

ACKNOWLEDGMENTS

The author is grateful to the Australian and New Zealand Dialysis and Transplantation Registry for permission to reproduce the data in Figure 8.1 and Table 8.1. The author also wishes to acknowledge the skilled and patient assistance of Miss Christine Whyte, who prepared the manuscript for this chapter.

COMMENTARY

Henri Kreis

Although the majority of transplanters are eager to get rid of steroids, they probably are the only agent for which there is still no surrogate. The chapter by Rowan Walker deals perfectly with the subject of steroids in kidney transplantation, but I do wish to add a few comments on specific points.

Historically, the successful use of steroids in the treatment of acute rejection episodes was first reported in kidney transplantation in 1960 by the Boston group. However, as early as 1951, Jean Hamburger had already used steroids in two of the very first cadaver kidney transplantations performed in the human (1). Unfortunately, the doses used were too small, which led to the erroneous conclusion that steroids were useless in kidney transplantation. For this reason they were subsequently discarded by the Paris group. Were it not for this error, transplantation would have gained about 10 years of positive experience and results.

Today, steroids are widely used, but there is no consensus concerning the innocuousness of steroid withdrawal in post-transplantation protocols. In addition, an increasing number of investigators (2,3) have suggested that steroid withdrawal may increase the risk of chronic allograft rejection. However, in some categories of patients, including recipients of an HLA-identical kidney, steroids can be avoided. In 1973, we reported that this was possible in 53% of such recipients who were on azathioprine alone. However, if an induction therapy of 2 to 4 weeks with a polyclonal, or even better, a monoclonal agent such as OKT-3 is added to the monotherapy, the proportion of patients who will never develop acute rejection episodes despite the lack of steroids can be as high as 70%.

Steroids alone can contribute to the long-term success of kidney grafts when additional immunosuppressive agents have to be discontinued because of cancer. In 1984 we reported the 10-year results for 39 kidney recipients comprising 30 cadaver kidney recipients and 9 living-related recipients on azathioprine/steroid bi-therapy who were withdrawn from azathioprine because they developed cancer (4). Their 10-year graft survival was 56.9% despite the cancer, whereas the graft survival of 79 matched control kidney recipients maintained on bi-therapy was 63.2% at the same end point. Thus, at least in cancer patients, steroids can be successfully used as the only immunosuppressive agent, which is an argument in favor of the efficacy of these drugs.

The fact that mono-agent, bi-agent, or tri-agent cyclosporine-based therapy seems to give identical 3-year graft outcome when analyzing data from the Opelz database may have a number of explanations other than the uselessness of the combination of immunosuppressive agents. It may mean, for example, that the numerous biases present in such a database can cancel out all the very real differences that exist between different groups of patients, and that only results drawn from prospectively randomized series should be considered. But it certainly does not allow the conclusion that steroids combined with cyclosporine are useless (5).

The overall power of the immunosuppressive regimen probably affects graft outcome (i.e., the occurrence of chronic rejection). It is widely accepted today that the number and severity of acute rejection episodes are clearly correlated with the incidence and severity of chronic rejection. Whether steroids help to reduce the number of acute rejection episodes is more difficult to determine precisely. Before the cyclosporine era, our retrospective study compared the incidence of acute rejection episodes in cadaveric-kidney recipients who were on azathioprine only with the incidence among similar patients who had been on azathioprine plus high doses of steroids since the transplantation day (6). We were puzzled by the equal incidence of acute rejection found in both groups. However, transplant biopsies disclosed a higher incidence of inflammatory infiltrates in the transplants of patients who did not receive steroids. It was then suggested that steroids probably act more through their anti-inflammatory mechanisms than through their immunosuppressive properties. For this reason, we further compared patients receiving antithymocyte immunoglobulin (Atgam) induction combined with azathioprine and steroids to patients who received Atgam induction, azathioprine, and the nonsteroidal anti-inflammatory agent Brufen (ibuprofen) (7). The frequency of rejection was higher in the Brufen group (2.18 episodes per patient) than in the steroids group (1.44 episodes per patient).

Since the advent of the cyclosporine era, the role of steroids has become more difficult to assess, as the cyclosporine dose is often lower when it is combined with steroids than when it is used as monotherapy. Nevertheless, three publications reported results observed in controlled studies in which steroids were avoided (8–10). They all showed that the incidence or severity of acute rejection episodes was lower when steroids were used.

Whatever the effect of steroids on acute rejection, they might also play a more direct role in the permanent prevention of chronic rejection by reducing inflammation within the transplant. In fact, studies based on histologic findings suggest that both the rate of sclerosing arteriopathy (11) and that of interstitial fibrosis (12) are higher in patients withdrawn from steroids compared to steroid-treated controls. These findings both correlate closely with chronic rejection. Were this to be confirmed, it would mean that not only the weight of immunosuppression is important for the prevention of chronic rejection but also the presence of other specific agents, including those with anti-inflammatory properties such as steroids.

STEROIDS AND TREATMENT OF REJECTION EPISODES

When used for the prevention of an acute rejection episode, steroids appear more effective in the prevention of the inflammatory changes made of cellular infiltrates and interstitial edema than of the vascular component. Similarly, it is probable that the main target of steroids, when they are used to treat acute rejection, is the inflammatory reaction present in the majority of cases. Their effect on the vascular lesions remains to be proven.

Although steroids continue to be the most important first-line treatment of acute rejection, the way they are used varies greatly from one group to another. Some groups use the intravenous route (with different protocols), while others prefer an oral regime (again, according to different protocols). There is no agreement on the most effective steroid protocol to treat acute rejection. In our group, we have observed a higher number of re-rejection episodes when intravenous boluses were used as compared to high-dose oral administration followed by a slow decrease over weeks.

Because of the variety of approaches used in the treatment of an acute rejection episode, a widely accepted definition of steroid-resistant rejection appears unlikely. Thus, one must be cautious when an immunosuppressive agent is said to be efficient in the treatment of steroid-resistant rejection on the basis of compassionate use. A correct definition of steroid resistance must include the daily dose of steroids, the exact timing of administration, the duration of treatment, and the number of follow-up days required after treatment withdrawal. For multicenter trials, these data must be identical for all the participating centers.

STEROIDS AND AVASCULAR BONE NECROSIS

It is clear that steroids are closely related to the incidence of avascular bone necrosis. In our group, for example, such necrosis has never been observed in recipients of an HLA-identical kidney who did not receive steroids. We have never found an obvious relationship between avascular bone necrosis and the duration or the level of maintenance steroid, but patients who received short courses of high doses for rejection had a higher incidence of bone lesions. This may explain why the incidence of avascular bone necrosis has tremendously decreased today, along with steroid-treated acute rejection episodes.

STEROIDS AND SKIN DISORDERS

That long-term corticosteroid treatment is responsible for atrophy of the skin by loss of collagen is widely accepted today. The deterioration, which is present from the sixth month onward (13), gives the skin an appearance of aging. Up to now, the only way to deal with this complication was for the patient to wear protective apparel or use a protective cosmetic preparation. Seeking a treatment, we studied the effect of topical all-*trans* retinoic acid (0.05%; Galderma Labs) over a 6-month period (14). Clinically, an increase in skin thickness was observed, which was confirmed by noninvasive techniques showing an increase in skin thickness, skin elasticity, skin conductance, and a reduction in the size of the corneocytes. Thus, it appears possible to obtain an improvement in skin atrophy when prevention has not been successful.

CHAPTER REFERENCES

1. Ackerman GL, Nolan CM. Adrenocortical responsiveness after alternate-day corticosteroid therapy. N Engl J Med 1968;278:405–409.
2. Elion GB, Callahan S, Bieber S, et al. A summary of investigations with 6-(1-methyl-4-nitro-r-imidazolyl) thio purine (BW 57-322) Cancer Chemother Rep 1961;14:93–98.
3. Calne RY, Alexandre GPJ, Murray JE. A study of the effects of drugs in prolonging survival of homologous renal transplants in dogs. Ann NY Acad Sci 1962;99:743–761.
4. Murray JE, Merrill JP, Damin GJ, et al. Kidney transplantation in modified recipients. Ann Surg 1962;156:337–355.
5. Murray JE, Merrill JP, Harrison JH, et al. Prolonged survival of human-kidney homograft by immunosuppressive drug therapy. N Engl J Med 1963;268:1315–1323.
6. Starzl TE, Marchioro TL, Waddell WR. The reversal of rejection in human renal homografts with subsequent development of monograft. Surg Gynecol Obstet 1963;117:385–390.
7. Goodwin WE, Mims MM, Kaufman JJ. Human renal transplantation. III. Technical problems encountered in 6 cases of homotransplantation. Trans Am Assoc Genitorin Surg 1985;54:116–125.
8. Kreis H, Lacombe M, Noel LH, et al. Kidney-graft rejection: has the need for steroids to be re-evaluated? Lancet 1978;ii:1169–1172.
9. Cupps TR, Fauci AS. Corticosteroid-mediated immunoregulation in man. Immunol Rev 1982;65:132–155.
10. Dupont E, Schandene L, Denys C, Wybran J. Differential in-vitro actions of cyclosporin, methyl-prednisolone, and 6-metacaptopurine: implications for drugs' influence on lymphocyte activation mechanisms. Clin Immunol Immunopathol 1986;40:422.
11. Metcalfe S. Cyclosporine does not prevent cytoplasmic calcium changes associated with lymphocyte activation. Transplantation 1984;38:161.
12. Gerrard TL, Cupps TR, Jurgensen CH, Fauci AS. Hydrocortisone-mediated inhibition of monocyte antigen presentation: dissociation of inhibitory effect and expression of DR antigens. Cell Immunol 1984;85:330.
13. Crabtree GR. Contingent genetic events in T-cell activation. Science 1989;243:355–363.
14. Knudsen PJ, Dinarello CA, Strom TB. Glucocorticoids inhibit transcription and post-transcriptional expression of interleukin-1. J Immunol 1987;139: 4129–4134.
15. Zanker B, et al. Glucocorticoids block transcription of human interleukin-6 gene by accessory cells. Transplantation 1990;49:183–185.
16. Kauffman HM, Sampson D, Fox PS, Stawicki BS. High-dose (bolus) intravenous methylprednisolone at the time of kidney homotransplantation. Ann Surg 1977;186:631–634.
17. McGeown MG, Kennedy JA, Loughridge WGG, et al. One hundred kidney transplants in the Belfast City Hospital. Lancet 1977;ii:648–651.
18. McGeown MG, Douglas JF, Brown WA, et al. Advantages of low-dose steroid from the day after renal transplantation. Transplantation 1980;29:287–289.
19. Descamps B, Huiglais N, Crosnier J. Renal transplantation between 33 HLA-identical siblings. Transplant Proc 1973;5:231.
20. Chan L, French ME, Beare J, et al. Prospective trial of high-dose versus low-dose prednisolone in renal transplant patients. Transplant Proc 1980;12:323–326.
21. Chan L, French ME, Oliver DO, Morris PJ. High- and low-dose prednisolone. Transplant Proc 1981;13:336–338.
22. Morris PJ, Chan L, French ME, Ting A. Low-dose oral prednisolone in renal transplantation. Lancet 1982;i:525–527.
23. Buckles JAC, Mackintosh P, Barnes AD. Controlled trial of low-versus high-dose oral steroid therapy in 100 cadaveric renal transplants. Proc EDTA 1981;18:394–399.
24. Papadakis JT, Bewick M, Brown CM, et al. Low-dose steroids in renal transplantation (letter). Lancet 1982;i:916–917.
25. Glass NR, Miller DT, Sollinger HW, Belzer FO. A comparative study of steroids and heterologous antiserum in the treatment of renal allograft rejection. Transplant Proc 1983;15:617.
26. Hricik DE, Almawi WY, Strom TB. Trends in the use of glucocorticoids in renal transplantation. Transplantation 1994;57:979–989.
27. d'Apice AJF, Becker GJ, Kincaid-Smith P, et al. A prospective randomized trial of low-dose versus high-dose steroids in cadaveric renal transplantation. Transplantation 1984;37(4):373–377.
28. Walker RG, d'Apice AJF, Mathew TH, et al. Long-term follow-up of a prospective trial of low-dose versus high-dose steroids in renal transplantation. Transplant Proc 1987;19:2825–2828.
29. Walker RG, d'Apice AJF. Non-specific immunosuppression: azathioprine and steroids. In: Morris PJ, ed. Kidney transplantation: principles and practice. 4th ed. Philadelphia: WB Saunders, 1984:202–204.
30. Opelz G. Comparison of immunosuppressive protocols in renal transplantation: a multi-center view. Transplant Proc 1988;20:31–36.
31. Canafax CM, Sutherland DER, Simmons RL, et al. Combination immunosuppression: three drugs (azathioprine, cyclosporine, prednisolone) for mismatched related and four drugs (antilymphocyte globulin, azathioprine, cyclosporine, prednisolone) for cadaver renal allograft recipients. Transplant Proc 1985;17:2671–2672.
32. Hiesse C, Charpentier B, Fries D. Safety of triple immunosuppressive treatment (cyclosporine, azathioprine and prednisolone). Lancet 1985;2:1355.
33. Schareck WD, Hopt UT, Muller GH, et al. Reduction of nephrotoxicity and improvement of immuno-suppression by combination of cyclosporine A and azathioprine. Transplant Proc 1987;19:1937–1939.
34. O'Connell PJ, d'Apice AJF, Walker RG, et al. Results of steroid withdrawal in renal allograft recipients on low dose cyclosporine A, azathioprine and prednisolone. Clin Transplant 1988;2:102–106.
35. Slapak M, Digard N, Wise M, Setakis N. Triple therapy. Transplant Proc 1991;23:2186–2188.
36. Sollinger HW for the US Renal Transplant Mycophenolate Mofetil Study Group. Mycophenolate mofetil for the prevention of acute rejection in primary cadaveric renal allograft recipients. Transplantation 1995;60:225–232.
37. European Mycophenolate Mofetil Cooperative Study Group. Placebo-controlled study of mycophenolate mofetil combined with cyclosporin and corticosteroids for prevention of acute rejection. Lancet 1995;345:1321–1325.
38. Tricontinental Mycophenolate Mofetil Renal Transplantation Study Group. A blinded, randomised clinical trial of mycophenolate mofetil for the prevention of acute rejection in cadaveric renal transplantation. Transplantation 1996;61:1029–1037.
39. Davis M, Williams R, Chakraborty J, et al. Prednisone or prednisolone for the treatment of chronic active hepatitis? a comparison of plasma availability. Brit J Clin Pharmacol 1978;5:501–505.
40. Pickup ME. Clinical pharmacokinetics of prednisone and prednisolone. Clin Pharmacokinet 1979;4:111–128.
41. Lewis GP, Jusko WJ, Burke CW, Graves L. Prednisone side-effects and serum-protein levels. A collaborative study. Lancet 1971;ii:778–780.
42. Baxter JD, Forsham PH. Tissue effects of glucocorticoids. Am J Med 1972;53:573–589.
43. Grant SD, Forsham PH, Di Raimondo VC. Suppression of 17-hydroxycorticosteroids in plasma and urine by single and divided doses of triamcinolone. N Engl J Med 1985;273:1115–1118.
44. Nichols T, Nugent CA, Tyler FH. Diurnal variation in suppression of adrenal function by glucocorticoids. J Clin Endocrinol Metab 1965;25:343–349.
45. Harter JC, Reddy WJ, Thorn GW. Studies on an intermittent corticosteroid dosage regimen. N Engl J Med 1963;269:591–596.
46. Soyka LF, Saxena KM. Alternate-day steroid therapy for nephrotic children. J Am Med Assoc 1965;192:225–230.
47. Fleisher DS. Pituitary-adrenal responsiveness after corticosteroid therapy in children with nephrosis. J Paediatr 1967;70:54–59.
48. Dumler F, Levin NW, Szego G, et al. Long-term alternate day steroid therapy in renal transplantation: a controlled study. Transplantation 1982;34:78–82.
49. MacGregor RR, Sheagren JN, Lipsett MB, Wolff SM. Alternate-day prednisone therapy: evaluation of delayed hypersensitivity responses, control of disease, and steroid side effects. N Engl J Med 1969;280:1427–1431.
50. Diethelm AG, Sterling WA, Hartley MW, Morgan JM. Alternate-day prednisone therapy in recipients of renal allografts. Risk and benefits. Arch Surg 1976;111:867–870.
51. Leb DE. Alternate-day prednisone treatment may increase kidney transplant rejection. Proc Dial Transplant Forum 1979;6:136.
52. Breitenfield RV, Herbert LA, Lemann J Jr, et al. Stability of renal transplant function with alternate-day corticosteroid therapy. J Am Med Assoc 1980;244:151–156.
53. McDonald FD, Horensten ML, Mayor GB, et al. Effect of alternate-day steroids on renal transplant function. A controlled study. Nephron 1976;17:415–429.
54. Potter DE, Holliday MA, Wilson CJ, et al. Alternate-day steroids in children after renal transplantation. Transplant Proc 1975;7:79–82.
55. Van Dieman-Steenvorde R, Donckerwoicke RA, Brack DH, et al. Growth and sexual maturation in children after kidney transplantation. J Pediatr 1987;110:351–356.
56. Briggs JD. A critical review of immunosuppressive therapy. Immunol Lett 1991;29:89–94.
57. Hussey JL. Letter. Discontinuance of immuno-suppression. Arch Surg 1976;111:614.
58. Calne RY, Thiru S, McMaster P, et al. Cyclosporin A in patients receiving renal allografts from cadaver donors. Lancet 1978;2:1323–1327.
59. Kahan BD, Flechner SM, Lorber MI, et al. Complications of cyclosporine-prednisolone immunosuppression in 402 renal allograft recipients exclusively

followed at a single center for from one to five years. Transplantation 1987;43:197–204.
60. Sutherland DER, Fryd DS, Strand MH, et al. Results of the Minnesota randomized prospective trial of cyclosporine versus azathioprine-antilymphocyte globulin for immunosuppression in renal allograft recipients. Am J Kidney Dis 1985;5:318–327.
61. Kupin WL, Venkat KK, Norris C, et al. Effective long-term immunosuppression maintained by low cyclosporine levels in primary cadaveric renal transplant recipients. Transplantation 1987;43:214–218.
62. Wood RFM, Thompson JE, Allen NH, et al. The consequences of conversion from cyclosporine to azathioprine and prednisolone in renal allograft recipients. Transplant Proc 1983;15:2862–2868.
63. Thiel G, Harder F, Loertscher R, et al. Cyclosporine alone or in combination with prednisolone in cadaveric renal transplantation. Transplant Proc 1984;16:1187–1190.
64. Starzl IE, Weil R, Iwatsuki S. The use of cyclosporin A and prednisolone in cadaver kidney transplantation. Surg Gynecol Obstet 1980;151:17–26.
65. Brown MW, Forwell MA. Rejection reaction after stopping prednisolone in kidney-transplant recipients taking cyclosporine. N Engl J Med 1986;314:183.
66. Cristinelli L, Brunori G, Setti G, et al. Withdrawal of methylprednisolone at the sixth month in renal transplant recipients treated with cyclosporine. Transplant Proc 1987;19:2021–2023.
67. Squifflet JP, Sutherland DER, Rynasiewicz JJ, et al. Combined immunosuppressive therapy with cyclosporine A and azathioprine. Transplantation 1982;34:315–318.
68. Chao S-H, Tsai K-S, Chieng P-U, et al. Bone mineral density profile in uremic and renal transplant patients. Transplant Proc 1994;26:2009–2011.
69. Stegall MD, Wachs ME, Everson G, et al. Prednisone withdrawal 14 days after liver transplantation with mycophenolate. Transplantation 1997;64:1755–1760.
70. Russ GR, May S, Jacob CK, et al. Experience with cyclosporine A and azathioprine double therapy in low-risk recipients of first cadaveric renal allografts. Clin Transplant 1990;4:26–31.
71. Thistlethwaite JR Jr, Gaber AO, Haag BW, et al. OKT3 treatment of steroid-resistant renal allograft rejection. Transplantation 1987;43(2):176–184.
72. Barry JM. Immunosuppressive drugs in renal transplantation. Drugs 1992;48(4):554–566.
73. Orta-Sibu N, Chantler C, Bewick M, Haycock G. Comparison of high-dose intravenous methylprednisolone with low-dose oral prednisolone in acute renal allograft rejection in children. BMJ 1982;285:258–260.
74. Kauffman HM Jr, Stromstad SA, Sampson D, Stawicki AT. Randomized steroid therapy of human kidney transplant rejection. Transplant Proc 1979;11:36–38.
75. Gray D, Shepherd H, Daar A, et al. Oral versus intravenous high-dose steroid treatment of renal allograft rejection: the big shot or not? Lancet 1978;i:117–118.
76. Mussche MM, Ringoir SGM, Lamiere NN. High intravenous doses of methylprednisolone for acute cadaveric renal allograft rejection. Nephron 1976;16:289–291.
77. Sollinger HW, Deierho MH, Belzer FO, et al. RS-61443—a phase I clinical trial and pilot rescue study. Transplantation 1992;53:428.
78. Mycophenolate Mofetil Renal Refractory Rejection Study Group. Mycophenolate mofetil for the treatment of refractory, acute, cellular renal transplant rejection. Transplantation 1996;61:722–729.
79. Dumble LJ, Clunie GJA, Macdonald IM, et al. Prediction of renal allograft rejection response to steroids from aDCC response to in vitro steroids. Transplant Proc 1983;15:1145–1147.
80. Francis DMA, Dumble LJ, Bowes LG, et al. Adverse influence of recipient lymphoid resistance to in vitro immunosuppression on the outcome of kidney transplants. Transplantation 1988;46:853–857.
81. Ratcliffe PJ, Dudley CRK, Higgins RM, et al. Randomised controlled trial of steroid withdrawal in renal transplant recipients receiving immunosuppression. Lancet 1996;348:643–648.
82. Rizzoni G, Broyer M, Guest G, et al. Growth retardation in children with chronic renal disease: scope of the problem. Am J Kidney Dis 1986;7:256–261.
83. Watson AR. Safety of growth hormone. Lancet 1991;337:108–109.
84. Fine RN, Yadin O, Nelson PA, et al. Recombinant human growth hormone treatment of children following renal transplantation. Paediatr Nephrol 1991;5:147–151.
85. Woo KT, Junor BJR, Vikraman P, d'Apice AJF. Serum-alkaline-phosphatase as predictor of avascular necrosis of bone in renal-transplant recipients (letter). Lancet 1979;i:620.
86. Horber FF, Casez JP, Steiger U, et al. Changes in bone mass early after kidney transplantation. J Bone Miner Res 1994;9:1–9.
87. Almond MK, Kwan JT, Evans K, Cunningham J. Loss of regional bone mineral density in the first 12 months following renal transplantation. Nephron 1994;66(1):52–57.
88. Julian BA, Laskow DA, Dubovsky J, et al. Rapid loss of vertebral mineral density after renal transplantation. N Engl J Med 1991;325:544–550.
89. Grotz WH, Mundinger FA, Gugel B, et al. Bone mineral density after kidney transplantation. A cross-sectional study in 190 graft recipients up to 20 years after transplantation. Transplantation 1995;59(7):982–986.
90. Wolpaw T, Deal CL, Fleming-Brooks S, et al. Factors influencing vertebral bone density after renal transplantation. Transplantation 1994;58:1186–1189.
91. Grotz WH, Mundinger FA, Gugel B, et al. Bone fracture and osteodensitometry with dual energy X-ray absorptiometry in kidney transplant recipients. Transplantation 1994;58(8):912–915.
92. Shun-Shin GA, Ratcliffe P, Bron AJ, et al. The lens after renal transplantation. Brit J Ophthalmol 1990;74:261–271.
93 d'Apice AJF, Mathews JD, Tait BD, Kincaid-Smith P. Association of HLA antigens with glucose intolerance following renal transplantation. Tissue Antigens 1978;11:423–426.
94. Drueke TB, Abdulmassih Z, Lacour B, et al. Atherosclerosis and lipid disorders after renal transplantation. Kidney Int 1991;39:(suppl 31):S24–S28.
95. Kasiske BL, Umen AJ. Persistent hyerlipidaemia in renal transplant patients. Medicine 1987;66:309–316.
96. Markell MS, Friedman EA. Hyperlipidemia after organ transplantation. Am J Med 1989;87(5N):61N–67N.
97. Sheil AGR, Disney APS, Mathew TH, et al. Cancer development in cadaveric donor renal allograft recipients treated with azathioprine (AZA) or cyclosporine (CyA) or AZA/CyA. Transplant Proc 1991;23:1111–1112.
98. Venning VA. Nonmalignant skin lesion in renal transplant patients. In: Morris PJ, ed. Kidney transplantation: principles and practice. 4th ed. Philadelphia: WB Saunders, 1984:401–411.

COMMENTARY REFERENCES

1. Dubost C, Oeconomos N, Vaysse J, et al. Note préliminaire sur l'étude des fonctions rénales de reins greffés chez l'homme. Bull et Mém Soc Med Hôp de Paris 1951;67:105–106.
2. Almond P, Matas A, Gillingham K. Risk factors for chronic rejection in renal allograft recipients. Transplantation 1993;55:752–757.
3. Basadonna G, Matas A, Gillingham K, et al. Early versus late acute renal allograft rejection: impact on chronic rejection. Transplantation 1993;55(5): 993–995.
4. Campos H, Kreis H, Rioux P, Crosnier J. Azathioprine withdrawal in renal transplant recipients. A long-term follow-up. Transplantation 1984;38(1):29–31.
5. Fries D, Hiesse C, Santelli G, et al. Triple therapy with low-dose cyclosporine, azathioprine, and steroids: long-term results of a randomized study in cadaver donor renal transplantation. Transplant Proc 1988;20(suppl 3):130–135.
6. Kreis H, Lacombe M, Noel L, et al. Kidney-graft rejection: has the need for steroids to be re-evaluated? Lancet 1978;2(8101):1169–1172.
7. Kreis H, Chkoff N, Droz D, et al. Nonsteroid antiinflammatory agents as a substitute treatment for steroids in ATGAM-treated cadaver kidney recipients. Transplantation 1984;37(2):139–145.
8. Johnson R, Mallick N, Bakran A, et al. Cadaver renal transplantation without maintenance steroids. Transplant Proc 1989;21:1581–1582.
9. Salaman J. Cyclosporine mono-drug therapy. Transplant Proc 1988;20(suppl 3):117–120.
10. Tarantino A, Aroldi A, Stucchi L, et al. A randomized prospective trial comparing cyclosporine monotherapy with triple-drug therapy in renal transplantation. Transplantation 1991;52(1):53–57.
11. Offermann G, Schwarz A, Krause P. Long-term effects of steroid withdrawal in kidney transplantation. Transplant Int 1993;6(5):290–292.
12. Isoniemi H, Krogerus L, von Willebrand E, et al. Histopathological findings in well-functioning, long-term renal allografts. Kidney Int 1992;41(1):155–160.
13. Teillac D, Prost Y, Debure A, et al. Clinical and biophysical studies of the skin in renal allograft patients. Clin Transplant 1987;1:1–3.
14. Lacharriere OD, Escoffier C, Gracia A, et al. Reversal effects of topical retinoic acid on the skin of kidney transplant recipients under systemic corticotherapy. J Invest Dermatol 1990;95(5):516–522.

Chapter

9

Tacrolimus

GORAN B. KLINTMALM

HISTORY

Tacrolimus (FK506, Prograf; Fujisawa, Deerfield, IL, USA) is a macrolide compound isolated from *Streptomyces tsukubaensis*, a soil fungus that can be found in Northern Japan (1). Its immunosuppressive properties were first recognized in 1984 during a screening program directed at identifying new immunosuppressive agents. Subsequent in vitro and animal experiments in Japan and at the University of Pittsburgh helped to characterize the mechanism of action of tacrolimus and demonstrated its potent immunosuppressive properties in transplantation (1–6).

IMMUNOLOGY

Most clinically useful immunosuppressive drugs either inhibit the proliferation of T lymphocytes or destroy them. Cyclosporine inhibits cytokine synthesis by binding to cytoplasmic proteins (cyclophylins) in T lymphocytes (see Chapter 6). Tacrolimus functions in a similar fashion, binding to FK-binding proteins (FKBP) in the cytoplasm; however, tacrolimus has a greater binding affinity to FKBP than does cyclosporine to cyclophilin. Rapamycin, which is structurally similar to tacrolimus, does not inhibit cytokine synthesis but rather inhibits the response of T cells to interleukin 2 (IL-2) and other cytokines (see Chapters 6 and 11).

The complex formed by the binding of tacrolimus to FKBP-12 associates with calcium-dependent calcineurin/calmodulin complexes to impede calcium-dependent signal transduction subsequent to stimulation of calcium influx in lymphocytes. Transcription factors that promote cytokine gene activation are direct or indirect substrates for calcineurin, and their activity is reduced by association with the tacrolimus complex. Tacrolimus inhibits the mixed lymphocyte reaction assay, the formation of IL-2 by T lymphocytes, and formation of other soluble mediators including IL-3, IL-4, IL-5, tumor necrosis factor alpha (TNF-α), and granulocyte-macrophage-colony stimulating factor (7). Tacrolimus also inhibits the expression of IL-2 and IL-7 receptors. As an immunosuppressive agent, tacrolimus is approximately 100 times more potent than cyclosporine (8).

PHARMACOKINETICS AND MONITORING

Tacrolimus achieves adequate absorption from the upper small intestine following oral administration, but the extent of absorption is widely variable (range = 5% to 67%) among patients. Administration with food generally does not affect the oral absorption of tacrolimus, although fatty meals may reduce bioavailability (9). Because absorption is bile independent, intravenous administration is not required in most patients (as is often required with cyclosporine [Sandimmune], particularly during the early postoperative period), and dosage changes are not required when clamping a T-tube following liver transplantation (10).

During liver graft failure or hepatic dysfunction, especially with cholestasis, tacrolimus bioavailability increases and clearance decreases owing to its extensive hepatic metabolism. The result is markedly elevated tacrolimus levels with related toxicity necessitating a rapid reduction in dosage (10,11). In contrast, initial dosing reductions usually are not required in patients with renal impairment (10).

Tacrolimus concentrations can be measured either in whole blood or plasma using an enzyme-linked immunosorbent assay (ELISA) (12) or in whole blood with a microparticle enzyme immunoassay (13). Measurement of plasma tacrolimus concentrations may be less desirable both because of the complexity of the methodology and because plasma must be separated at 37°C due to temperature-dependent distribution of tacrolimus into erythrocytes, similar to that of cyclosporine (14). Importantly, plasma levels of tacrolimus measured by ELISA were found to correlate poorly with rejection and toxicity (15), whereas whole blood tacrolimus levels were well correlated with rejection and toxicity (16). Other studies indicated a higher correlation of plasma tacrolimus levels with clinical events (17). As with cyclosporine, plasma level monitoring can be used if samples are handled carefully. However, because of the technical difficulties inherent in plasma level monitoring, whole blood levels are usually considered the standard of care.

During oral therapy with tacrolimus, concentrations should be monitored to maintain 12-hour trough levels in the range of 5 to 15 ng/mL for whole blood or 0.5 to 1.5 ng/mL for plasma to optimize efficacy and minimize toxicity. Clinical experience has shown that high trough tacrolimus levels correlate with a lower incidence of rejection, and high peak levels correlate with increased toxicity (18,19). A definite correlation between tacrolimus levels and nephrotoxicity has not been recognized, but a reduction in serum creatinine levels was reported in liver transplant recipients when tacrolimus levels were reduced (17).

PRECLINICAL EXPERIENCE WITH TACROLIMUS

Numerous animal studies have been conducted demonstrating the in vitro and in vivo effects of tacrolimus (Table 9.1) (20). Although many studies have evaluated the use of tacrolimus in preventing graft rejection, the published literature has also described the effects of tacrolimus on the inhibition of cell-mediated responses, proliferative responses, cytotoxic responses, and humoral responses, as well as its effect on various autoimmune disorders.

An in vitro study evaluated the effect of tacrolimus compared to cyclosporine and prednisolone on the mixed lym-

Table 9.1. Experimental Autoimmune Diseases Suppressed by Tacrolimus

Disease	Species	Tacrolimus Dose (mg/kg/day unless specified)	Reference
Arthritis (Type II collagen-induced)	Rat (Lewis)	0.32[a,b]	Inamura et al, 1988 (21)
	Rat (Outbred)	2.5[c]	Arita et al, 1990 (22)
	Mouse (DBA/1)	2.0	Takagishi et al, 1989 (23)
Type 1 diabetes	NOD mouse	2.0 mg/kg/48 h[a]	Miyagawa et al, 1990 (24)
	Cyclophosphamide-treated NOD mouse	0.2, 1.0, 2.0	Carroll et al, 1991 (25)
	BB rat	1.0[a]	Murase et al, 1990 (26)
	BB rat	25 μg IM[d]	Nicoletti et al, 1991 (27)
Uveoretinitis	Rat (Lewis)	1.0[a,e]	Kawashima et al, 1990 (28)
	Rhesus and cynomolgus monkeys	0.5[f]	Fujino et al, 1990 (29)
Thyroiditis	Rat (PVG)	2.0[g]	Tamura et al, 1992 (30)
Lupus (SLE)	MRL-lpr/lpr mouse	2 mg[h]	Yamamoto et al, 1988 (31)
	NZB/NZW F[1] mouse	2.5 mg/kg/48 h[i]	Takabayashi et al, 1989 (32)
Glomerulonephritis	Rat (Wistar)	0.3 mg[j]	Hara et al, 1990 (33)
(Nephrotoxic antiserum nephritis)	Rat (Wistar)	0.64	Okuba et al, 1990 (34)
Heymann nephritis	Rat (Wistar)	0.64	Okuba et al, 1990 (34)
	Rat (Lewis)	1.0	Matsukawa et al, 1992 (35)
Allergic encephalomyelitis	Rat (Lewis)	1.0	Inamura et al, 1988 (36)
Autoimmune myocarditis	Rat (Lewis)	1.0, 0.32, 1.0	Hanawa et al, 1992 (37)
Experimental allergic contact dermatitis	Farm pig	0.04, 0.4% topical	Meingassner and Stutz, 1992 (38)
Murine (coxsackie B[3]) myocarditis	Mice (C3H/He)	2.5	Hiraoka et al, 1992 (39)

[a] Suppresses induction of disease.
[b] Partially effective during efferent phase of response.
[c] On day of immunization.
[d] Administered daily from 27–120 days of age.
[e] Effective only in induction phase.
[f] Administered from 3 weeks after immunization.
[g] Administered for 3 weeks following induction of disease.
[h] Administered from 8 weeks of age.
[i] From time of immunization.
[j] Administered 5 days per week after immunization.
[k] Administered from day 0–13 or 56–69.

Adapted from Thomson AW, Murase N, Nalesnik MA, Starzl TE. The influence of tacrolimus on experimental autoimmune disease. In: Lieberman R, Mukherjee A, eds. Principles of drug development in transplantation and autoimmunity. Austin, TX: RG Landes, 1996.

phocyte reaction (MLR) (2). Tacrolimus demonstrated dose-dependent suppression of the proliferative response of human lymphocytes to alloantigen stimulation at concentrations higher than 0.1 nmol/L. The IC_{50} values of tacrolimus, cyclosporine, and prednisolone were 0.22, 14.0, and 80.0 nmol/L respectively. Tacrolimus was also shown to inhibit IL-2 production almost completely at concentrations higher than 0.3 nmol/L. With an IC_{50} value of approximately 0.1 nmol/L, tacrolimus was reported to be approximately 100 times more potent than cyclosporine, which had an IC_{50} value of 10 nmol/L. Tacrolimus demonstrated a similar inhibitory effect on interferon (IFN)-γ production.

In a separate study, tacrolimus inhibited the proliferation of murine spleen B lymphocytes induced by anti-mouse IgM by approximately 50% in vitro (40).

In vivo animal studies have investigated the effect of tacrolimus on humoral and cellular immunity. In one study, mice were immunized with sheep erythrocytes and received tacrolimus and cyclosporine orally for 4 days from the day of immunization (1). After 4 days, tacrolimus almost completely suppressed splenic antibody-forming cell (AFC) response at doses of 10 mg/kg or more, whereas cyclosporine almost completely suppressed AFC response at 100 mg/kg. Tacrolimus also suppressed delayed-type hypersensitivity (DTH) responses dose-dependently in mice immunized with methylated bovine serum albumin (MBSA).

The effect of tacrolimus on transplantation of the liver, kidney, heart, islet cells, and abdominal visceral organs has been widely studied in different animal models (41–46). In a liver transplantation study using beagle dogs, 8 of 10 dogs (80%) receiving tacrolimus survived longer than 30 days, providing an early in vivo demonstration that tacrolimus, 1.0 mg/kg, was as potent as cyclosporine, 20 mg/kg (42). Tacrolimus exhibited similar immunosuppressive effects in cynomolgus monkeys undergoing orthotopic liver transplantation (43).

Tacrolimus has also shown promise in animal models of cardiac transplantation. The hearts of F344 rats were heterotopically transplanted into the cervical region of WKA rat recipients receiving either tacrolimus or cyclosporine orally (4). Both agents prolonged acceptance of the cardiac allografts. Tacrolimus significantly prolonged graft survival in rats receiving a heterotopic cardiac transplantation across a strong major histocompatibility complex (MHC) barrier at a dose of 1.28 mg/kg/day (44). When a moderate histoincompatible combination was used, the animal recipients survived indefinitely.

In renal transplantation studies using tacrolimus in unrelated beagle dogs, all the animals in the control group died of renal failure due to graft rejection within 24 days; whereas, animals treated with 1.0 mg/kg/day oral dosage of tacrolimus survived over 140 days after transplantation (3). The effect of tacrolimus in kidney transplantation was also studied in baboons (46). In the tacrolimus groups, 3 of 5 (60%) and 4 of 5 (80%) animals survived longer than 80 days, depending on the dose. All of the animals in the control group died within 14 days of renal failure due to graft rejection. This preclinical trial in subhuman primates suggested that tacrolimus was a promising drug for use in humans.

Preclinical studies of tacrolimus in intestinal transplantation also have been promising (47,48). The efficacy of tacrolimus in several experimental animal models of allotransplantation is summarized in Table 9.2 (49).

EARLY CLINICAL EXPERIENCE IN TRANSPLANTATION

Most early clinical experience with tacrolimus was gained from the pioneering work at the University of Pittsburgh in liver, renal, heart, and small bowel transplantation. Initially, tacrolimus was used as rescue therapy in patients experiencing rejection or toxicity while being treated with cyclosporine. Subsequent trials were expanded to the use of tacrolimus as primary immunosuppression (52–54). This early experience helped to identify the safety and tolerability of tacrolimus as well as its role as primary and rescue therapy following transplantation (Table 9.3).

CLINICAL EXPERIENCE WITH TACROLIMUS FOR SOLID ORGAN TRANSPLANTATION

Liver

Until recently, most clinical experience with tacrolimus had come from its use in liver transplantation as either primary or rescue therapy. Two prospective randomized trials conducted in the United States and Europe found that patient and graft survival were comparable with tacrolimus and cyclosporine but that the incidence of rejection, both acute and steroid refractory, was significantly lower with tacrolimus (55,56).

The US open-label, randomized, multicenter trial compared the efficacy and safety of tacrolimus to a cyclosporine (Sandimmune)-based immunosuppressant regimen in patients undergoing primary liver transplantation (55). Adult and pediatric patients were randomized at the time of transplant to tacrolimus (n = 263) or cyclosporine (n = 266) and followed for 12 months. Study end points were patient and graft survival and the incidence of acute, steroid-resistant, and refractory rejection. Patient and graft survival at 1 year were comparable for the tacrolimus and the cyclosporine groups (Fig. 9.1). Acute and steroid-resistant rejection and treatment failure due to refractory rejection were significantly lower with tacrolimus. Longer-term follow-up of these recipients now suggests a survival benefit for the tacrolimus-treated patients, compared to the Sandimmune-treated group (57). There also appears to be a significant benefit for the tacrolimus-treated liver allograft recipients with hepatitis C. Their 5-year survival rate was 78%, versus only 60% for the Sandimmune-treated HCV-positive patients.

Table 9.2. Tacrolimus in Experimental Allotransplantation

		Strain					
Animal	Organ (Reference)	Donor	Recipient	Dose (mg/kg/day)	Tacrolimus Route	Duration (Days)	Mean Survival (Days)
Rat	Heart (50)	ACI	LEW	0.0	—	—	6.0
				0.6	IM	0–13	39.0
				1.3	IM	0–13	87.0
				1.3	IM	4, 5, 6	91.0
	Liver (41)	ACI	LEW	0.0	—	—	10.0
				1.3	IM	4, 5, 6	>100.0
	Intestine (47)	BN	LEW	0.0	—	—	11.7
				0.6	IM	0–13	>100.0
				1.3	IM	0–13	>100.0
		LEW	BN	0.0	—	—	12.0
				0.6	IM	0–13	27.3
	Multivisceral (51)	BN	LEW	0.0	—	—	10.6
				1.3	IM	0–13	>100.0
Dog	Kidney (5)	Mongrel	Beagle	0.0	—	—	13.0
				0.5	PO	1–90	33.7
				1.0	PO	1–90	31.0
				1.5	PO	1–90	61.0
				2.0	PO	1–90	32.1
				1.0	IM	4, 5, 6	58.0
	Liver (5)	Beagle	Beagle	0.0	—	—	12.4
				1.0	PO	1–90	66.5
				1.0	IM	4, 5, 6	96.6
	Intestine (42)	Mongrel	Mongrel	0.0	—	—	7.8
				0.1	IV	1–90	57.5
				0.2	IV	1–90	23.3
				1.0	IM	3, 4, 5	17.7
Baboon	Kidney (46)	*Papio abunus*	*Papio abunus*	0.0	—	—	9.2
				6.0	PO	1–90	29.5
				12.0	PO	1–90	70.8
				18.0	PO	1–90	74.6
				2.0	IM	4, 5, 6	53.3

LEW = Lewis; BN = Brown-Norway.
Adapted from Todo S and Murase N. Tacrolimus for experimental organ transplantation. In: Lieberman R, Mukherjee A, eds. Principles of drug development in transplantation and autoimmunity. New York: RG Landes, 1996.

Table 9.3. Potential Uses for Tacrolimus

Transplantation
Liver
Kidney
Heart
Intestine
Bone marrow
Lung

Autoimmune Diseases
Psoriasis
Uveitis
Chronic inflammatory diseases of the liver
Nephrotic syndrome

Among pediatric patients, there was a trend toward less rejection and a reduced requirement for steroids with tacrolimus, although patient and graft survival were comparable (58). Major neurologic events and diarrhea were more common with tacrolimus, while hirsutism and higher serum cholesterol levels were reported with cyclosporine.

In a parallel study conducted at eight European transplant centers, 545 patients were randomized to tacrolimus or a conventional cyclosporine (Sandimmune)-based regimen (56). The primary end points were acute, refractory acute, and chronic rejection at 12 months. The rates of rejection were significantly lower with tacrolimus. Patient and graft survival rates were not different between tacrolimus and cyclosporine. The mean corticosteroid dosage

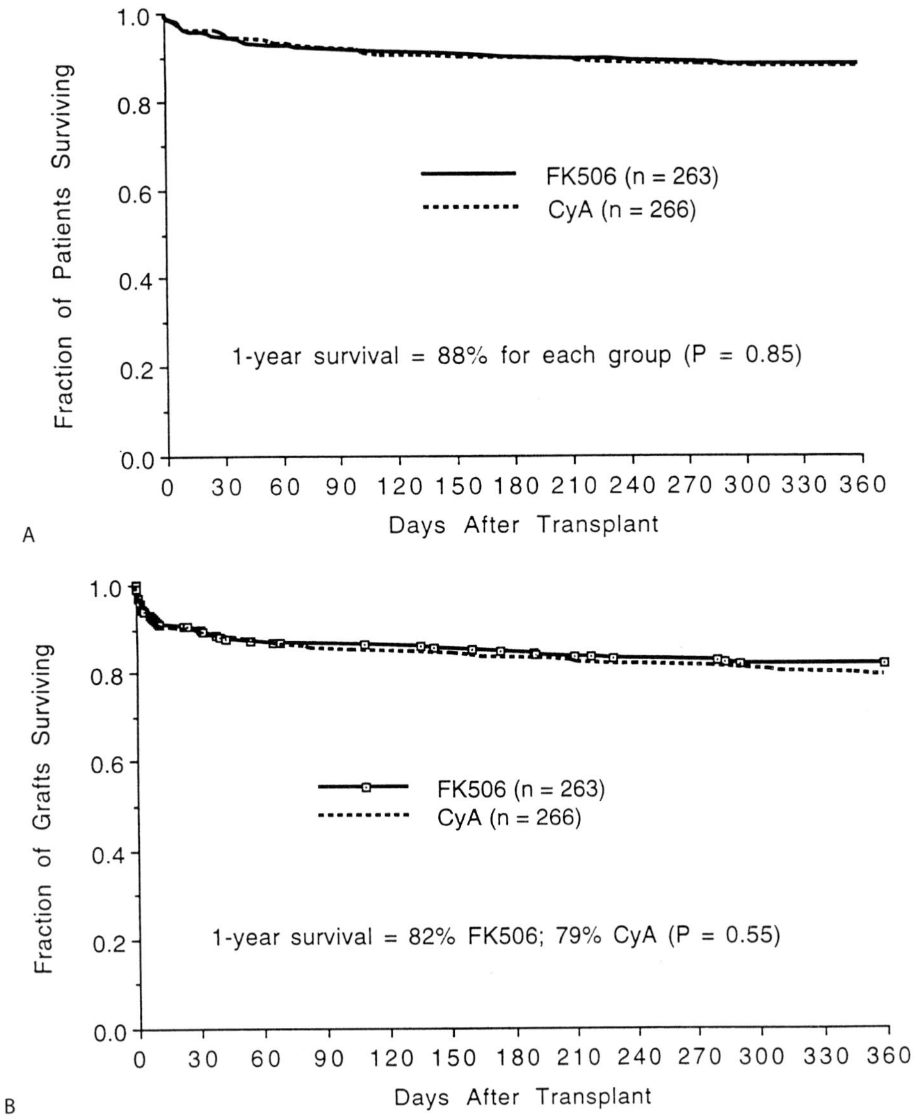

FIGURE 9.1. *Patient survival (**A**) and graft survival (**B**) in patients treated with FK506 or cyclosporine-based (CsA) immunosuppression (55). Kaplan-Meier estimates of 1-year patient and graft survival after liver transplantation were not significantly different between treatment groups.*

was significantly lower and almost no azathioprine or antilymphocyte globulin was required in the tacrolimus group compared with the cyclosporine group.

In the European experience, patients transplanted for fulminant hepatic failure had a particularly impressive response to tacrolimus (59). At 1 week, patient survival was 95.5% with tacrolimus and 82.1% with cyclosporine; by 6 months, survival was 72.7% with tacrolimus and 60.7% with cyclosporine (Fig. 9.2). Similar results were observed for graft survival. Also, the incidence of treated rejection episodes was significantly reduced with tacrolimus. This resulted in a lower mean daily corticosteroid requirement for tacrolimus- versus cyclosporine-treated patients (69 mg/day versus 150 mg/day) and was reflected in a lower incidence of infectious complications with tacrolimus.

A limitation of these studies was the comparison of tacrolimus to Sandimmune, rather than to Neoral therapy (see also Chapter 6). More recent trials suggest a lower incidence of rejection in tacrolimus-treated liver allograft recipients in comparison to those treated with Neoral, but these studies have not yet been completed.

Rescue Therapy Following Liver Transplantation

Tacrolimus in combination with corticosteroids proved to be an effective immunosuppressant regimen for rescue therapy in patients with rejection on a cyclosporine-based regimen after liver transplantation (53). Included were 72 patients with acute rejection, 131 with chronic rejection, and 43 patients with either co-morbid disease or severe cyclosporine-related side effects. At a median follow-up of

240 days, 87% of patients were alive and 79% had functioning grafts. Graft loss was greatest among patients with chronic rejection and a serum bilirubin >2.5 mg/dL (28%) at the start of tacrolimus therapy and among those with viral hepatitis (19%).

An open-label, multicenter study evaluated the safety and efficacy of tacrolimus plus corticosteroids for rescue therapy in 300 adult and 86 pediatric liver transplant recipients experiencing refractory rejection despite conventional immunosuppression (60). All patients were followed for 1 year after conversion to tacrolimus. Of these patients, 260 completed a 1-year follow-up on tacrolimus. Patient survival at 1 year was 74.5% for adults and 79.8% for children, and graft survival at 1 year was 64.7% for adults and 67.9% for children. When outcomes were stratified by baseline total bilirubin levels >6 or <6 mg/dL and by acute versus chronic rejection, patient and graft survival were consistently lower in patients with bilirubin levels >6 mg/dL.

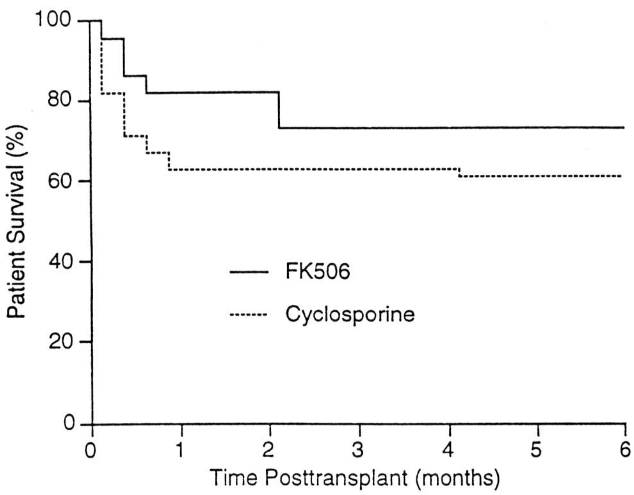

FIGURE 9.2. *Patient survival following liver transplantation for fulminant hepatic failure after treatment with FK506 or cyclosporine (59).*

Kidney

An early multicenter, open-label trial compared various tacrolimus dosages with cyclosporine in 120 patients undergoing primary cadaveric kidney transplant (19). Patients were randomized to a cyclosporine-based regimen or to one of three tacrolimus-based regimens designed to achieve low (5 to 14 ng/mL), medium (15 to 25 ng/mL), or high (26 to 40 ng/mL) trough whole blood levels. This trial revealed that the incidence of neurotoxic and gastrointestinal events was higher among tacrolimus-treated patients during the first month after transplant and correlated with increasing maximum trough tacrolimus concentrations ($P = 0.01$). Also noted was a decreasing rate of rejection with increasing minimum trough tacrolimus concentrations at 1 month ($P = 0.021$) (Fig. 9.3). The range of tacrolimus whole blood levels that optimized efficacy and minimized toxicity was found to be 5 to 15 ng/mL corresponding to an initial oral dose of 0.2 mg/kg/day. At 1 year, patient survival was 98% for all tacrolimus-treated patients and 92% for the cyclosporine group. Graft survival was 93% and 89% in the tacrolimus and cyclosporine groups, respectively (61). The incidence of rejection episodes requiring treatment during the first year was 33% for tacrolimus and 32% for cyclosporine. Until day 42, the incidence of acute rejection was significantly lower (14% tacrolimus, 32% cyclosporine; $P = 0.048$) for the aggregate of all tacrolimus patients versus cyclosporine. In the tacrolimus group, 13 rejection episodes occurred within the first 6 weeks and 17 more were reported at 1 year. In the cyclosporine group, no new rejec-

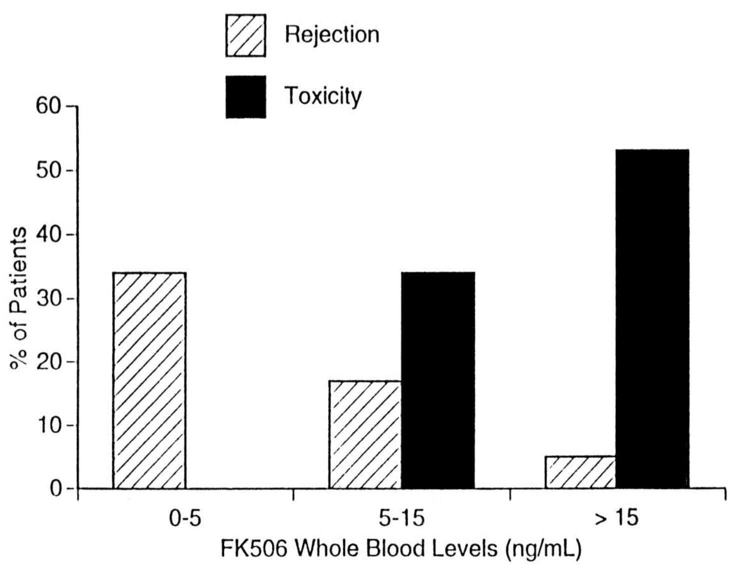

FIGURE 9.3. *Incidence of toxicity and rejection by whole blood FK506 levels (19). A logistic regression analysis was performed to determine the relationship between the occurrence of rejection and toxicity, and the whole blood concentrations of FK506. The occurrence of toxicity requiring a dosage reduction increased significantly with increasing levels of whole blood FK506. Conversely, the likelihood of the occurrence of rejection decreased significantly with increasing whole blood levels of FK506. These data support a recommended target whole blood FK506 level of 5 to 15 ng/mL during the first 42 days of treatment.*

tion episodes were reported beyond 42 days after transplantation. Nephrotoxicity occurred with a similar frequency with tacrolimus and cyclosporine, but the incidence of neurotoxic events and the incidence of new insulin use were higher among tacrolimus-treated patients.

A subsequent randomized, open-label US study compared the efficacy and safety of optimal dosage tacrolimus to cyclosporine (Sandimmune) immunosuppression in patients receiving cadaveric kidney transplants (62,63). A total of 412 renal transplant patients were randomized to tacrolimus (n = 205) or cyclosporine (n = 207). One-year patient survival rates were 95.6% for tacrolimus and 96.6% for cyclosporine (P = 0.576) and 1-year graft survival rates were 91.2% and 87.9%, respectively (P = 0.289). Of note, biopsy-confirmed acute rejection was significantly reduced for tacrolimus patients (30.7%) compared with cyclosporine (46.4%, P = 0.001), and the requirement for antilymphocyte therapy for rejection was also significantly less for tacrolimus (10.7% and 25.1%, respectively; $P < 0.001$). Impaired renal function, gastrointestinal disorders, and neurologic complications, which were rarely treatment limiting, were common in both treatment regimens. Tremor and paresthesia were more frequent for tacrolimus, and the incidence of post-transplant diabetes mellitus was 19.9% for tacrolimus patients versus 4.0% for cyclosporine ($P < 0.001$), but it was reversible in some patients. Hyperlipidemia and hypercholesterolemia were decreased in the tacrolimus group, and hirsutism and gum hypertrophy were rarely seen, resulting in a greater improvement in health-related quality of life for these patients (64).

The results of this study were very similar to those observed in the European multicenter, randomized trial that compared the 12-month efficacy and safety of tacrolimus and cyclosporine (65). In that trial, a total of 448 renal transplant recipients from 15 centers received triple-drug therapy consisting of tacrolimus (n = 303) or cyclosporine (n = 145) in conjunction with azathioprine and low-dose corticosteroids. Twelve months after transplantation, tacrolimus therapy exhibited a significant reduction in the frequency of both acute rejection (tacrolimus 25.9% versus cyclosporine 45.7%; $P < 0.001$) and corticosteroid-resistant rejection (11.3% versus 21.6%, respectively; P = 0.001). Actuarial 1-year patient (tacrolimus 93.0% versus cyclosporine 96.5%; P = 0.140) and graft survival rates (82.5% versus 86.2%, respectively; P = 0.380) did not differ significantly between the two treatment groups. The safety profiles of the tacrolimus- and cyclosporine-based regimens were found to be comparable. No cost comparison results of either of these randomized studies have been reported.

In another randomized, prospective, single center trial of 395 adult patients undergoing renal transplantation, the effect of adding azathioprine to tacrolimus and steroids was evaluated (66). The 2-year actuarial patient and graft survival rates were 95% and 83%, respectively, with tacrolimus-based immunosuppression. There was no significant advantage in either patient or graft survival for patients given azathioprine, but the incidence of acute rejection was significantly higher with double than with triple therapy (54% versus 44%; $P < 0.05$).

Tacrolimus was also evaluated as rescue therapy in 73 patients with biopsy-confirmed renal allograft rejection (67,68). The median time to tacrolimus rescue therapy was 2.5 months (range 18 days to 48 months). At least one course of antilymphocyte therapy had been used in 59 (81%) patients prior to rescue. Responses to tacrolimus therapy included improvement in 78% of patients, stabilization in 11%, and progressive deterioration in 11%. Actuarial patient and graft survival rates were 93% and 75%, respectively, 12 months after initiation of tacrolimus therapy.

In a more recent report, the results of tacrolimus rescue therapy in 169 patients experiencing biopsy-confirmed rejection were summarized (69). The median time to rescue therapy was 2 months (range 2 days to 55 months), and antilymphocyte preparations had been used in 144 (85%) patients prior to rescue. Of the 144 patients unsuccessfully treated with antilymphocyte drugs, 117 (81%) were successfully rescued with tacrolimus. Twenty-eight patients were on dialysis at the time of conversion, and of these 13 (46%) were successfully rescued. In total, 125 (74%) patients were successfully rescued with tacrolimus and had functioning grafts at a mean follow-up of 30 months. Mean prednisone doses decreased from 28.0 ± 9.0 mg/day pre-tacrolimus to 8.5 ± 4.1 mg/day post-tacrolimus.

Of note, successful renal allograft function has been achieved with the addition of tacrolimus therapy even after the patient had been returned to dialysis, sometimes for prolonged periods (70). A review of these and other trials evaluating tacrolimus in renal allograft recipients has been recently published (71).

Kidney–Pancreas

Twenty-three recipients of kidney–pancreas transplants were studied to determine the value of tacrolimus primary immunosuppression in these patients (72). Of the evaluable patients, 10 received cyclosporine and 10 received tacrolimus therapy. The patient survival rate at 1 year was 100% for both the cyclosporine and the tacrolimus group, and the kidney graft survival rate was 90% for both groups. The pancreas graft survival rate was 80% for the tacrolimus group and 100% for the cyclosporine group (not significant). The time to the first rejection episode was significantly longer for tacrolimus compared to cyclosporine (23 versus 12 days, respectively; P = 0.026). There were no significant differences in the incidences of infectious complications or drug-induced nephrotoxicity.

Several other studies, with limited patient populations, have addressed the use of tacrolimus induction and rescue therapy after kidney–pancreas transplantation. In one study, the therapeutic effects of tacrolimus were documented in 61 kidney–pancreas or pancreas-only transplant patients with relapsing and resistant cellular rejection as well as chronic vascular rejection after they had been switched from cyclosporine-based immunosuppression (73). A subsequent follow-up analysis of 166 patients receiving primary tacrolimus therapy revealed a one-year graft survival rate of 88% (74). Similarly, 10 kidney–pancreas transplant patients and 1 pancreas-after-kidney patient were converted to tacrolimus following acute severe cyclosporine nephrotoxicity (75). All 11 patients were alive and 10 combined grafts were still functional 7.7 months after tacrolimus rescue therapy. All of the patients maintained stable renal function and blood glucose levels after the conversion from cyclosporine to tacrolimus. These observations have now encouraged many transplant centers to adopt tacrolimus-based primary immunosuppressive regimens for pancreas–kidney transplant recipients (76) (see also Chapter 21).

Intestinal

Because of the relatively small number of procedures performed, data are more limited on the use of tacrolimus as immunosuppression following intestinal transplantation. Nevertheless, a few reports are available summarizing the results in both adults and children. In an initial report, tacrolimus was used as primary immunosuppression in 12 adults and 11 children who underwent small bowel, small bowel and liver, or multivisceral transplants (77). At a minimum follow-up of 2 months, 19 of 23 patients were alive. In a follow-up that included 15 small bowel recipients from the earlier report, patient and graft survival were 70% and 66%, respectively, at 18 months after transplant (78). This experience, now expanded to 98 consecutive recipients of intestine, liver and intestine, or multivisceral allografts, was recently updated to reveal actuarial 1- and 5-year survival rates of 72% and 48%, respectively (79). As discussed in Chapter 22, these and other reports have concluded that tacrolimus-based immunosuppression provides a higher survival rate following intestinal transplantation than any other currently available regimen.

Heart–Lung

In an open-label study, tacrolimus was evaluated as primary immunosuppression in 62 adult heart transplant recipients and as rescue therapy in an additional 10 patients (80). At a mean follow-up of 1 year, patient survival was 92%. The mean number of rejection episodes was 0.95 per patient during the first 90 days, and recurrent rejection occurred in 28% of patients. Among the 10 patients receiving rescue therapy, 7 remained free from rejection on tacrolimus. In another study of tacrolimus rescue therapy for 16 heart and 15 lung recipients suffering acute or humoral rejection while on cyclosporine, patient survival rates of 100% in the heart recipients and 67% in the lung recipients were achieved (81).

Tacrolimus was used as primary immunosuppression in 26 pediatric heart transplant recipients (82). Patient survival was 82% at 1 and at 3 years, and 60% of patients were rejection-free at 3 and 6 months after transplantation.

Seventy-four adult patients were randomly assigned to tacrolimus or cyclosporine following single or bilateral lung transplant (83). One-year patient survival was similar between groups, but the number of patients free from acute rejection was significantly higher ($P < 0.05$) in the tacrolimus group. One patient (3%) in the cyclosporine group versus 5 of 38 (13%) in the tacrolimus group remained free from acute rejection during the first 120 days after transplant ($P < 0.05$). More patients in the cyclosporine group experienced bacterial infection, which was the major cause of late graft failure in both groups. A follow-up report of 133 patients reported similar 2-year survival rates for tacrolimus and cyclosporine but with a trend toward lower acute rejection rates with tacrolimus (84). Thirteen cyclosporine-treated patients versus 2 tacrolimus-treated patients required crossover to the alternative therapy ($P = 0.02$). The incidence of obliterative bronchiolitis was significantly lower with tacrolimus ($P = 0.025$).

Tacrolimus and cyclosporine were evaluated as primary immunosuppression in 20 pediatric lung transplant patients (85). Eight patients on each drug survived at a mean follow-up of 2 years after transplant. No differences in the incidence of rejection were reported between groups; however, 6 of 7 cyclosporine-treated patients and no tacrolimus-treated patients required antilymphocyte globulin for graft rejection. Furthermore, 4 patients on cyclosporine versus none on tacrolimus developed hypertension.

NONTRANSPLANT USES OF TACROLIMUS

Because of its potent immunosuppressive properties, tacrolimus may have applications in the treatment of autoimmune diseases (see Table 9.3). Clinical experience with tacrolimus has been reported in patients with nephrotic syndrome, psoriasis, chronic inflammatory diseases of the liver, and uveitis (86–90). Seven patients with refractory psoriasis experienced resolution confirmed with skin biopsy following treatment with tacrolimus (87). A marked reduction in proteinuria was observed in 6 of 7 patients with nephrotic syndrome, and the response was sustained for 6 months (86).

Ten patients with primary sclerosing cholangitis were treated with tacrolimus for up to 1 year (84). Serum bilirubin, alkaline phosphatase, and transaminase levels were reduced by 70% to 86%. No adverse effects on serum creatinine or blood urea nitrogen were observed with tacrolimus. In a second trial, 21 patients with autoimmune chronic active hepatitis were treated with tacrolimus for up to 3 months (90). Transaminase levels were reduced by 70% to 80%, with minimal increases in serum creatinine and blood urea nitrogen levels.

Tacrolimus was used to treat 13 patients with refractory uveitis and produced improvement in visual acuity during 6 weeks of follow-up (91).

Tacrolimus also has been investigated for prevention of graft-versus-host disease in patients undergoing bone marrow transplantation (92). In this pilot study, 18 patients were randomized to tacrolimus alone or with methotrexate or methylprednisolone. Eight of 18 patients developed grade II–IV acute graft-versus-host disease, and 1-year disease-free survival was 39%.

SAFETY/TOLERABILITY PROFILE OF TACROLIMUS

Much of the early toxicity reported with tacrolimus was associated with the use of unnecessarily high intravenous doses. The most frequent adverse events with tacrolimus in clinical trials have been renal impairment (highlighting the lack of correlation with blood levels), abnormalities in glucose metabolism, and neurotoxicity (Table 9.4) (55,56). In both of the liver transplant multicenter trials, the incidence of abnormal kidney function in the early post-transplant period was significantly increased with tacrolimus compared with the cyclosporine group. However, serum creatinine concentrations were not significantly different between treatment groups at the 12-month follow-up. The decrease in renal toxicity over time presumably reflected a decrease in the dose of tacrolimus and a more rapid conversion to oral therapy as experience with tacrolimus increased.

A randomized, prospective study on the effects of tacrolimus immunosuppression on lipid profiles in stable cyclosporine-treated renal transplant patients with established hyperlipidemia was undertaken by the Southeastern Organ Procurement Foundation (93). Patients with cholesterol of 240 mg/dL or greater, who were at least 1 year post-transplant with stable renal function, were randomly assigned to remain on cyclosporine (control) or be converted to tacrolimus. Renal function, glucose control, and levels of total cholesterol, triglycerides, total high-density lipoprotein (HDL), low-density lipoprotein (LDL), very-low-density lipoprotein (VLDL), and apoproteins A and B were monitored before conversion to tacrolimus. A total of 53 patients were analyzed (27 in the tacrolimus group and 26 controls) 6 months after conversion. In patients converted to tacrolimus treatment, there was a significant decrease in cholesterol (16%; $P = 0.0031$), LDL cholesterol (25%; $P = 0.0014$), and apolipoprotein B (23%; $P = 0.034$). There was no change in renal function, glycemic control, or incidence of new onset diabetes mellitus in the tacrolimus group. The authors concluded that conversion to tacrolimus from cyclosporine should be considered in the treatment of post-transplant hyperlipidemia.

Table 9.4. Common Adverse Events with Tacrolimus

Gastrointestinal
Anorexia
Diarrhea
Dyspepsia
Nausea
Metabolic
Hyperglycemia
Hyperkalemia
Nephrotoxicity
Neurologic
Confusion
Encephalopathy
Headache
Paresthesia
Psychosis
Seizure
Tremor

New onset diabetes mellitus and hyperglycemia occurred significantly more often with tacrolimus in both the US and the European trial (55,56). Of concern is that many patients developed de novo insulin-dependent diabetes mellitus several months after transplantation, long after high-dose steroid therapy was given. However, later studies combining tacrolimus with mycophenolate mofetil (MMF) suppression indicate the incidence of insulin-dependent diabetes is reduced to 10% or less (94). The incidence of neurologic adverse events, including tremor and paresthesia, was significantly higher with tacrolimus, but the events were generally of mild or moderate severity. However, severe neurologic adverse events—such as convulsions, confusion, psychosis, encephalopathy, and even coma—were also seen, and they responded to a reduction in tacrolimus dosage. In the European trial, a decreased incidence of infection was reported with tacrolimus, while in the US study the incidence of both malignant and nonmalignant neoplasms was lower with tacrolimus. In a 2-year follow-up of the US study, a higher incidence of post-transplant hepatitis C was reported in the tacrolimus group, and the incidence of rejection was higher in this subpopulation of tacrolimus-treated patients. Whether hepatitis C is a more serious problem in those receiving tacrolimus than in those receiving cyclosporine is presently being debated (95,96).

Pediatric patients receiving tacrolimus following liver transplantation have experienced an increased incidence of neurotoxicity, diarrhea, and dyspepsia; however, the incidence of infectious complications was similar to that with cyclosporine (97). In contrast, a higher incidence of viral infections was reported in pediatric patients undergoing kidney transplantation (70). Of particular concern is the high incidence of lymphoproliferative disease, which may approach 10% in the pediatric population (98,99), and the occasional development of red cell aplasia (100) or hemolytic uremia (101). Because a large proportion of children are Epstein-Barr virus (EBV) seronegative and, thus, at risk for primary infection leading to an increased risk of post-transplant lymphoproliferative disease, a role for EBV prophylaxis needs to be clarified (see also Chapter 20).

DOSING AND ADMINISTRATION

Because of good intestinal absorption, intravenous administration of tacrolimus is generally not required in the immediate postoperative period, when tacrolimus can be administered through the nasogastric tube. The initial dose of tacrolimus is 0.05 mg/kg every 12 hours, with subsequent dosage adjustment depending on the measured blood levels. The targeted tacrolimus whole blood level is initially 10 to 20 ng/mL. After 4 weeks the recommended trough level is 5 to 15 ng/mL. The optimal long-term trough level has not yet been well defined. However, in many patients with stable allograft function we see tacrolimus trough levels measuring less that 5 ng/mL, which is below the reliable threshold of the current assay. With improved monitoring techniques, the therapeutic requirements should be better defined in the future.

Pediatric patients have higher clearance and larger volumes of distribution than adult patients and thus require at least two and sometimes three daily full oral doses of tacrolimus to maintain adequate whole blood concentrations (58). Also, pediatric patients are immunologically more active and often require higher drug levels to prevent rejection. Generally, intravenous administration is only required in patients who experience gut complications after transplantation. In those circumstances, the tacrolimus dose is 0.01–0.05 mg/kg per day by continuous infusion. In patients with impaired hepatic function or in patients with stage III–IV encephalopathy, tacrolimus should be initially withheld and an induction protocol using antilymphocyte antibodies considered (see Chapter 13). Also, in patients receiving suboptimal donor organs the tacrolimus starting dose should be reduced.

It should be recognized that the bioavailability of tacrolimus is highly variable, and ordinary doses can quickly make a patient profoundly toxic. Thus, careful monitoring is mandatory in all cases following initiation of therapy. Some patients require an inordinate amount of tacrolimus to produce therapeutic levels (e.g., 0.2–0.3 mg/kg twice daily). In such patients, ketoconazole, itraconazole, or diltiazem have been used effectively to inhibit the metabolism of tacrolimus and allow normalization of the dose requirements. This can be accomplished without any side effects from the antifungal medication.

During initiation of tacrolimus therapy and before stable tissue levels have been achieved, large dosage changes often are necessary. Generally, a 30% to 40% change in dosage achieves the desired results. With stable, well-maintained patients, when fine tuning is desired, small dosage adjustments of 1 mg at a time are appropriate. In patients whose tacrolimus levels are quickly escalating—for example, during periods of sudden deterioration of liver function—the tacrolimus dose should be entirely withheld until nontoxic levels have been restored. This can sometimes take several days, depending on the extent and degree of liver failure. It takes 5 half-lives of any drug before a new steady state has been achieved, and in patients with advanced liver failure, the half-life of tacrolimus could easily reach 60 hours.

The most difficult side effect to manage with tacrolimus is minor neurotoxicity, especially in elderly patients. Minor neurotoxicity can be subtle, and the physician may not notice any abnormal behavior on casual examination. At times, a detailed interview of family and friends may be necessary to identify the cause. This toxicity can occur even with low therapeutic levels of tacrolimus, and its existence may warrant a further dosage decrease, even with blood tacrolimus levels of 5 ng/mL or less. If tacrolimus is not tolerated, one can always switch to cyclosporine. Although cyclosporine also causes neurotoxicity, the signs and symptoms are often different and thus may be relieved by using the alternate drug.

The role of triple therapy in tacrolimus protocols has not been extensively investigated. However, it is clear that the addition of azathioprine and MMF to the immunosuppressive regimen can be beneficial in tacrolimus-treated patients and may limit troublesome toxicity (94). However, with potent drugs such as tacrolimus and mycophenolate mofetil, one of the most common side effects in immunosuppressed patients is overimmunosuppression, which leads to infections and malignancies. Thus, initiation of a triple drug regimen must be done with utmost care.

COMMENTARY

Thomas E. Starzl and John J. Fung

Klintmalm's chapter contains useful information, the exploitation of which requires an understanding of the management principles that have guided organ transplantation since its inception. Only four drugs have been widely used as baseline immunosuppressants: azathioprine, cyclophosphamide, cyclosporine, and tacrolimus. With each agent, the dosage must be determined individually for every patient. The ceilings are imposed by toxicity, and the dose floors are revealed by breakthrough rejection. The amount of azathioprine and cyclophosphamide that can be given is limited by myelotoxicity, which can be monitored conveniently with serial white blood counts. The more complex side effects of cyclosporine and tacrolimus are shown in Table 9C.1.

HISTORICAL PERSPECTIVE

None of the four baseline drugs can reliably prevent post-transplant rejection when used alone. However, it was learned in 1962 to 1963 that organ rejection, which previously had been considered inexorable, could be reversed and that subsequent dose requirements of immunosuppressive agents frequently declined. The same events have been observed with all treatment regimens and with all organs. Delineation of this pattern of convalescence, which was first observed with the combination of azathioprine and prednisone (1), provided the empirical launching pad for the clinical field of organ transplantation, in which dose-maneuverable prednisone has proved to be the indispensable ingredient.

The introduction of each new drug was accompanied by an easily learned trial and potential error determination of the requisite doses of the individual constituents of the cocktail. With increasingly potent baseline agents, survival of all organ grafts rose in three distinct leaps over a 33-year period. The characteristic immunologic confrontation and resolution process did not change—it merely became easier to manage.

Table 9C.1. Nonimmunologic Profile (4+ = Worst), All Dose-Related

	Tacrolimus	Cyclosporine
Nephrotoxicity	++*	++
Neurotoxicity	+	+
Diabetogenicity	+	+
Growth effects		
Hirsutism	0	+++
Gingival hyperplasia	0	++
Facial brutalization	0	+
Hepatotrophic effects	++++	+++
Gynecomastia	0	+
Other metabolic effects		
Cholesterol increase	0	++
Uric acid increase	+?	++

* Less hypertension.
Sources: From Starzl TE, Abu-Elmagd K, Tzakis A, et al. Selected topics on FK 506: with special references to rescue of extrahepatic whole organ grafts, transplantation of "forbidden organs," side effects, mechanisms, and practical pharmacokinetics. Transplant Proc 1991;23:914–919. (Slide presented at the Transplantation Society Congress, San Francisco, in August, 1990.)

What was being accomplished through this process remained enigmatic until it was discovered in 1992 that long-surviving organ recipients had donor leukocyte chimerism in their blood, skin, lymph nodes, and other sites as late as three decades after transplantation. It was then obvious that the prototypic post-transplant phenomena were the product of a double immune reaction: host-versus-graft (rejection) and graft-versus-host (Fig. 9C.1). Potentially tolerogenic "passenger leukocytes" of bone marrow origin, including pluripotent stem cells, had migrated from organs and engrafted peripherally. This was the seminal mechanism of organ allograft acceptance (2).

The Tacrolimus Pilot Trials

The clinical development of tacrolimus bracketed the chimerism discoveries, beginning 3 years before and continuing for 5 years after. In 1989, we first showed that tacrolimus (FK506) could systematically reverse liver allograft rejection that had been intractable in the face of maximal cyclosporine-based conventional immunosuppression (3,4). The "rescued" patients were maintained thereafter on tacrolimus, and manifested no unique or unexpected toxicity (5). Consequently, a nonrandomized trial was begun in which tacrolimus was substituted for cyclosporine from the time of operation.

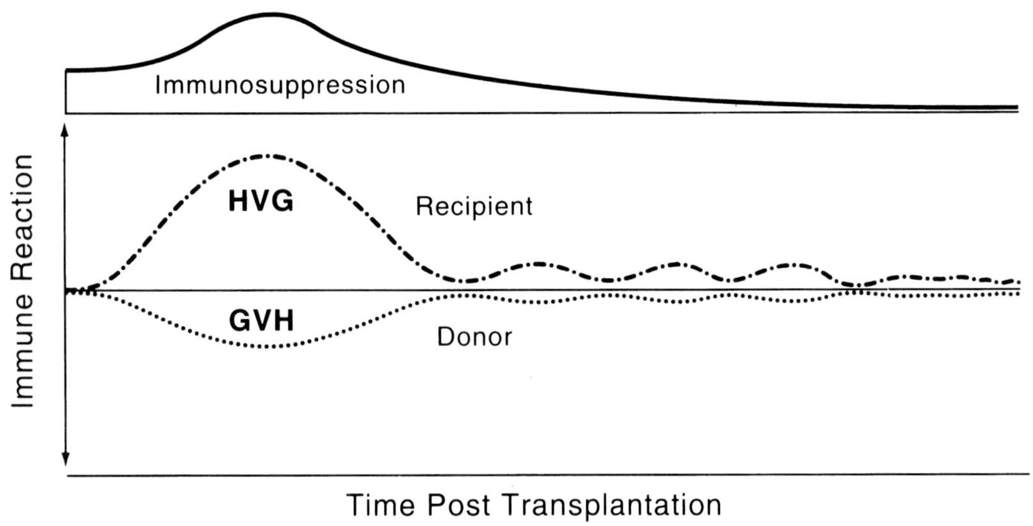

FIGURE 9C.1. *Contemporaneous host-versus-graft (HVG) and graft-versus-host (GVH) reactions in the two-way paradigm of transplantation immunology (2). Following the initial interaction, the evolution of nonreactivity of each leukocyte population to the other is seen as a predominantly low-grade stimulatory state that may wax and wane, rather than as a deletional one.*

By early 1990, nearly 200 liver, kidney, and other-organ recipients who had been entered in the program had superior actuarial survival, lower requirement for prednisone, and better quality of life than we had observed in the past (6–8). Already the upgrading of outlook after liver transplantation was as obvious as it had been a decade before when cyclosporine succeeded azathioprine as the baseline immunosuppressant (Fig. 9C.2). Thus, even as the advent of cyclosporine had elevated transplantation of cadaver kidneys from a previously unacceptable level (9,10), the bar rose for liver and for kidney transplantation with the introduction of tacrolimus (Fig. 9C.3). The same was true for thoracic organs (8).

It was clear by early 1990 that the dose-limiting side effects of cyclosporine and tacrolimus were the same: nephrotoxicity, neurotoxicity, and diabetogenicity (see Table 9C.1). These manifestations could be used from the first day of treatment to determine appropriate doses (6–8,11,12). Invidious toxicity comparisons between cyclosporine and tacrolimus were unwarranted because the scales could be tilted one way or the other by ratcheting the doses up or down. The only adverse effects observed exclusively with one drug but not the other were the dose-related cosmetic changes caused by cyclosporine (see Table 9C.1).

As had been found a decade earlier with cyclosporine (11), it was easy to relate toxic manifestations and rejection to trough plasma and blood concentrations (the plasma/blood ratio of tacrolimus was about 1:10) and promptly endow the laboratory results with clinically relevant meaning (6–8,12,13). Flexibility of dosing was important no matter what the transplanted organ, but it was especially so with the liver because the metabolism of tacrolimus is more dependent than that of cyclosporine on good hepatic function (12,14). By the beginning of 1990, doses and trough levels used for liver, kidney, heart, and lung recipients in Pittsburgh (6,7) were essentially the same as those recommended in

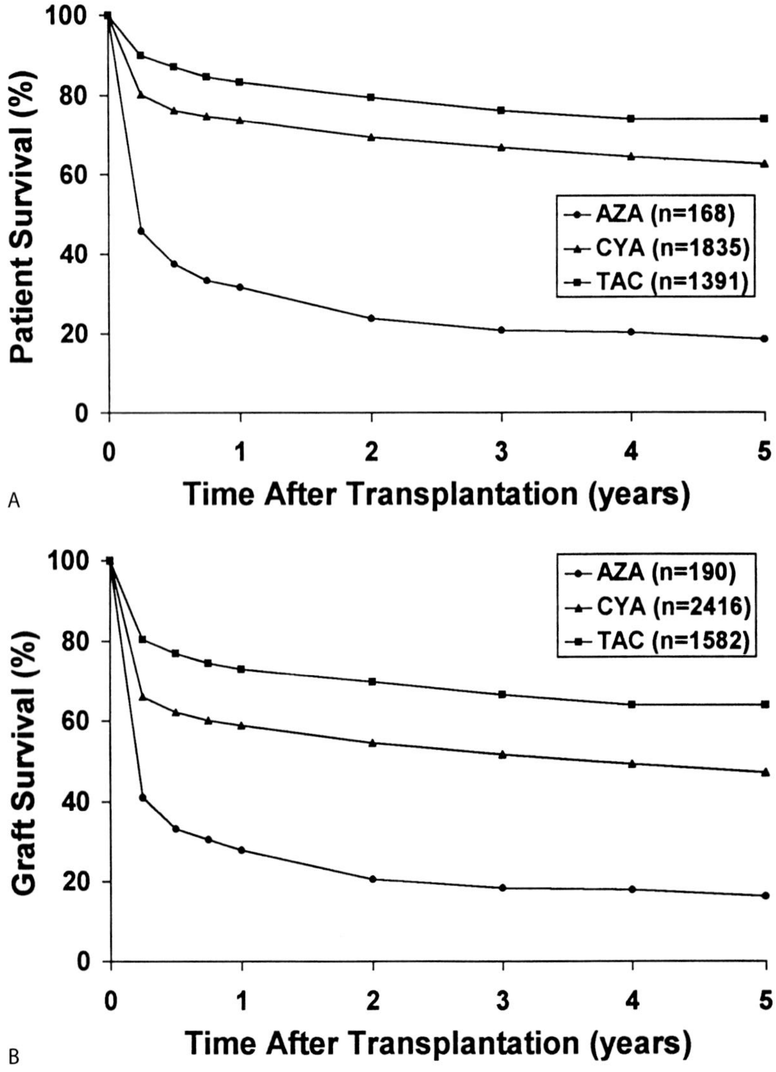

FIGURE 9C.2. *The three eras of orthotopic liver transplantation at the Universities of Colorado (1963–1980) and Pittsburgh (1981–1993), defined by azathioprine, cyclosporine, and tacrolimus (FK 506) immunosuppression.* ***A.*** *Patient survival.* ***B.*** *Graft survival. This was about 10% lower than patient survival in both the cyclosporine era (1980–1989) and the tacrolimus era (1989–1993), whereas patient and graft survival were essentially identical with azathioprine. The difference in later series was explained by effective retransplantation, an option that did not exist previously. AZA, azathioprine; CYA, cyclosporine; TAC, tacrolimus.*

Klintmalm's chapter. The data shown in Figure 9C.4 were presented on April 5, 1990, at the American Surgical Association, and were published 4 months later.

The Randomized Liver Trials

Historically, new immunosuppressive drugs were evaluated in kidney recipients and then applied secondarily to transplantation of unpaired vital organs. This precedent was broken with the development of tacrolimus, largely because liver transplant surgeons demanded that the drug be released for rescue therapy of their patients. Rather than pursuing the question of rescue efficacy, it was decided at meetings with the United States Food and Drug Administration (FDA) during October and November of 1989 to proceed with randomized European and American multicenter trials comparing tacrolimus with cyclosporine as the primary immunosuppressant from the time of liver replacement. By the time these trials started the following autumn, however, a decisive trial that had started in February 1990 in Pittsburgh using the tacrolimus doses shown in Figure 9C.4 was more than half completed.

The Pittsburgh Liver Trial

The Pittsburgh Liver Trial was a single-center, Institutional Review Board (IRB)-mandated trial. Safety and

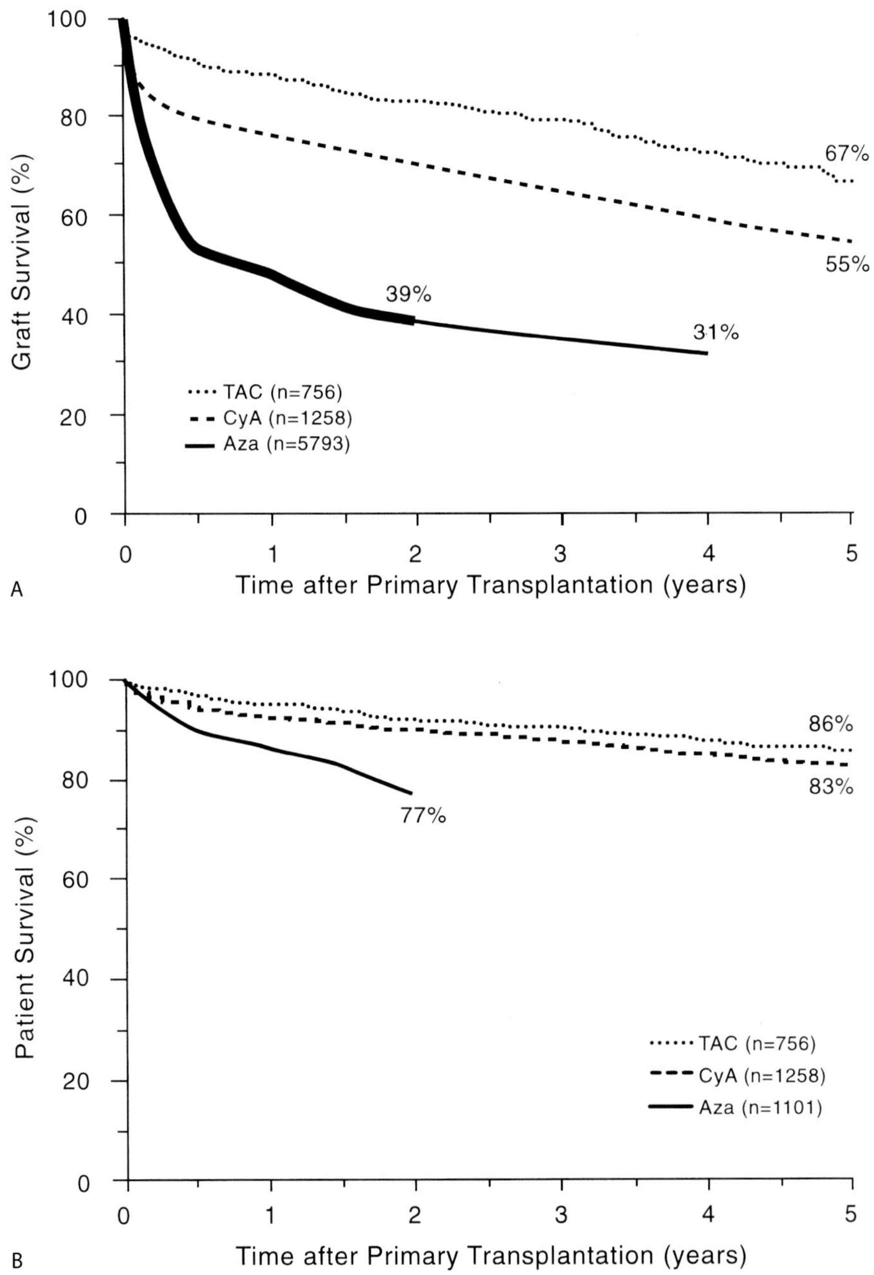

FIGURE 9C.3. *(**A**) Patient survival and (**B**) graft survival after primary cadaveric kidney transplantation at the University of Pittsburgh under cyclosporine (1981–1989) versus tacrolimus-based immunosuppression. These observations suggest the long-term survival of kidney allografts can also be improved by substitution of tacrolimus for cyclosporine. Graft survival curves for azathioprine in **A** are from Terasaki's national register. Early patient survival data are from the Southeastern Organ Procurement Foundation, to which Pittsburgh contributed. TAC, tacrolimus; CyA, cyclosporine; Aza, azathioprine.*

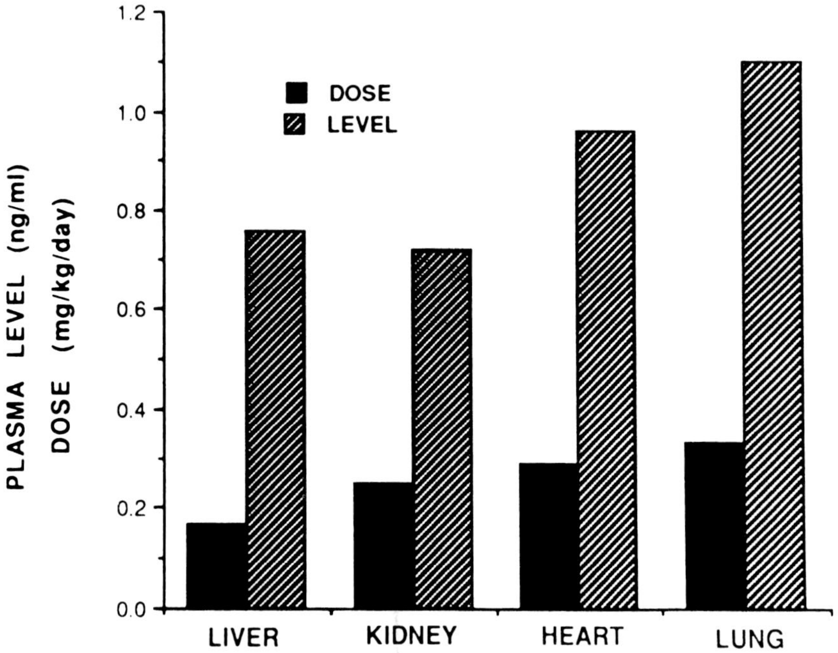

FIGURE 9C.4. *The tacrolimus doses used in the Pittsburgh Liver Trial and initially recommended for recipients of other organs. Because of the dependence on good hepatic function for tacrolimus metabolism, starting doses for liver recipients are slightly lower.*

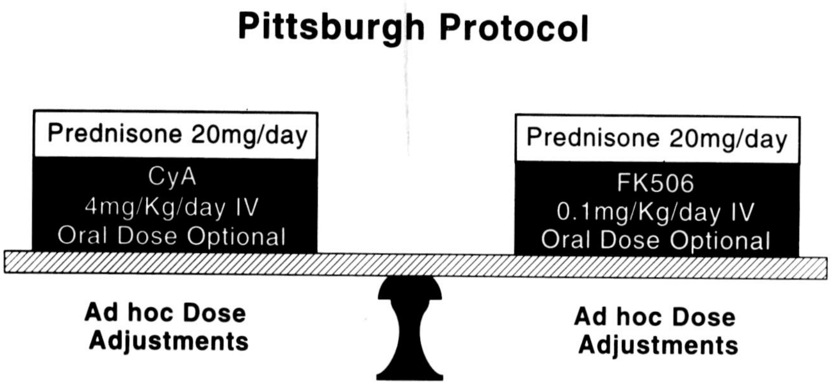

FIGURE 9C.5. *The Pittsburgh Liver Trial protocol, tacrolimus (FK506) versus cyclosporine (CyA). All treatment variables except for the competing drugs were equalized.*

efficacy comparisons were ensured by equalization of all treatment variables except the competing drugs (15,16) (Fig. 9C.5). Definition of end points allowed the liver recipients early access to whichever drug had the better therapeutic margin. The trial was prematurely terminated in 1991 by a multi-institutional oversight committee, which had been insisted upon by the investigators. By the time the trial was stopped, a massive crossover from cyclosporine to tacrolimus had occurred, with only one crossover from tacrolimus to cyclosporine. Throughout the entire 5-year period of subsequent study, tacrolimus enjoyed a statistically significant greater freedom from rejection, either alone or in combination with freedom from graft loss and adverse events (16).

The Multicenter Liver Trials

The design of the subsequent American (17) and European (18) 1iver transplant trials, which involved 20 institutions, was of some concern. In all 20 participating centers, the cyclosporine arm was uploaded with twice (or more) the induction doses of prednisone used for the tacrolimus patients. The cyclosporine-treated recipients also were given a third drug (azathioprine) in 95% of the centers and a fourth agent (polyclonal ALG) in a few (Fig. 9C.6). The tacrolimus doses were set higher than those concurrently used in Pittsburgh, and they remained so until the end of the study (Fig. 9C.7). The combination of excessive dosage and the sometimes delayed response to toxic events on the tacrolimus arm complicated the interpretation of some observations.

The European teams had a 5% better survival of patients on the tacrolimus arm [17% (46/270) versus 22% (61/275) mortality] and a 5% higher graft survival (18). By intent-to-treat analysis, the survival advantage was not statistically significant. However, about 10% of the surviving grafts credited to cyclosporine had been rescued from treatment failure with tacrolimus. The distorting

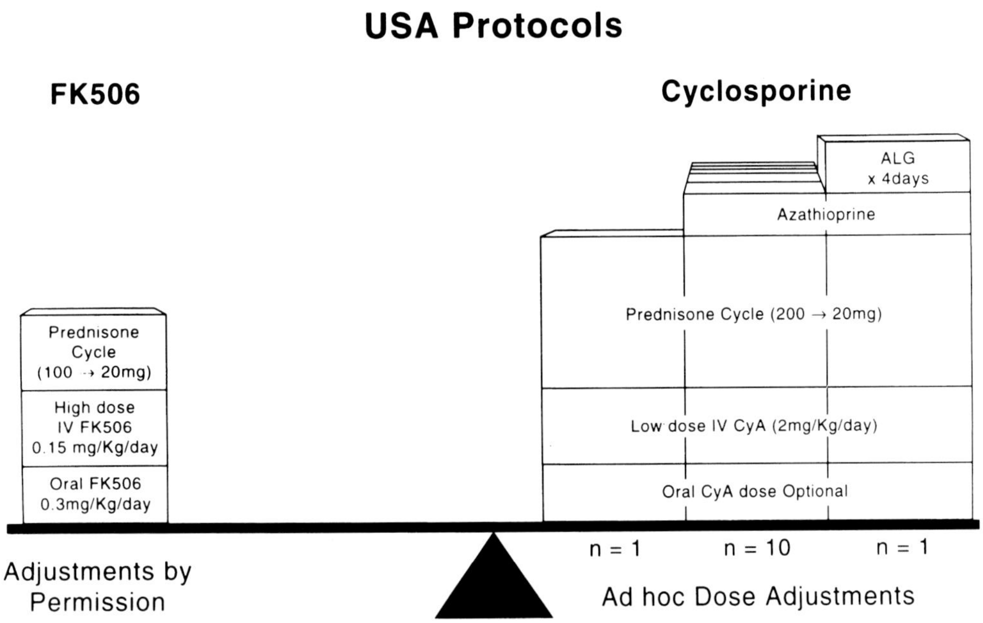

FIGURE 9C.6. *US protocol in the multicenter tacrolimus (FK506) trial. The cyclosporine (CyA) arm was uploaded with twice (or more) the induction doses of prednisone used for the tacrolimus patients. Cyclosporine recipients also were given a third drug (azathioprine) in 95% of the centers; polyclonal ALG was used in a few centers (n, number of centers using the regimen).*

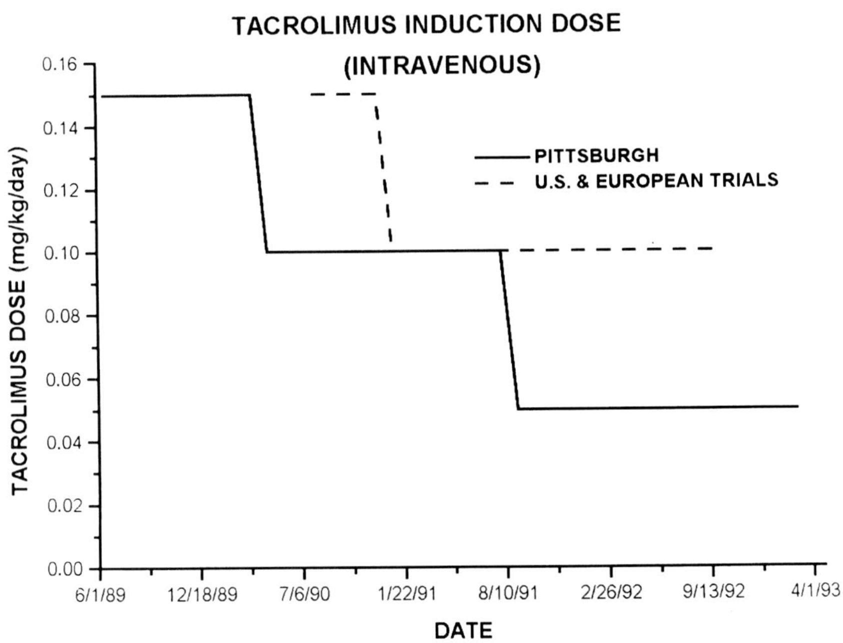

FIGURE 9C.7. *Tacrolimus doses set for the Multicenter Liver Trial. The doses were higher than those used in the Pittsburgh study.*

roles of tacrolimus overdosage and the consequent high rate of toxicity were clarified by separate analyses of the early (high dose) and later (reduced dose) phases of the trial. The statistical analysis, based on the intent-to-treat approach, showed significantly greater freedom from acute rejection, intractable acute rejection, and chronic rejection. The report concluded that tacrolimus had superior therapeutic qualities (18).

In the published American report (17), use of the Kaplan-Meier and intent-to-treat methods created the impression that the better efficacy and greater toxicity of tacrolimus essentially balanced each other. An alternative analysis suggested that freedom from rejection as a single end point was accomplished more frequently with tacrolimus (19). Moreover, the superiority of tacrolimus emerged at all levels, including freedom from adverse events and, most significantly, freedom from refractory rejection. After 1 year of follow-up, 98% of the patients randomized to tacrolimus were not diagnosed with refractory rejection, compared with 87% in the competing arm. The composite freedom at 1 year from the three factors that haunt transplant recipients—refractory rejection, retransplantation, and death—was 80% for tacrolimus and 70% for cyclosporine (19).

Randomized Trialomania

Disquieting scientific and ethical issues were exposed by the events of the 6 years following the placement of tacrolimus on the FDA fast track in November 1989. Neither the new drug's unusual rescue capability (3–5) nor its superiority as a baseline agent (6,7) were in doubt from late 1989 onward. The evidence for this as well as management recommendations had been published by the summer of 1990 (3,6–8,12), although, as with all new therapies, independent confirmation was needed from other centers. The FDA has a range of options for confirmation, as shown in Table 9C.2. However, the agency has increasingly insisted on multicenter, controlled, randomized trials as a prerequisite for marketing new drugs, and tacrolimus would be no different.

The FDA feared that pilot studies might suggest superiority of tacrolimus to potential multicenter participants, making them as reluctant as the Pittsburgh investigators had been to participate in a randomized trial. Therefore, no familiarization cases that used the drug from the time of transplantation were allowed. Also, by the nature of transplantation biology, cocktail regimens can never be applied in exactly the same way to any two recipients. In spite of this, the multicenter trial design insisted on rigidity of therapeutic protocols for tacrolimus (but not for the competing drug).

Although the design and dosing errors of the multicenter liver trials were ascribed to the investigators, the protocols and the trials themselves were efforts to comply with regulatory requirements. The FDA does not ostensibly engage in human experimentation; however, when

Table 9C.2. Spectrum of Most to Least "Adequate" Controls

1. Placebo concurrent control (randomized, double-blinded).
2. Dose-comparison concurrent control (randomized, 2 doses, often with placebo or active treatment arm [competing drug]).
3. No treatment concurrent control (randomized, with no treatment arm).
4. Active treatment concurrent control (randomized versus competing agent).
5. Historical control versus concurrent treatment (special situations, when outcome is self-evident or in absence of equipoise).

Code of Federal Regulations (CFR 314.126). Revised by FDA, April 1, 1994.

the agency imposed a learning curve for tacrolimus on 20 different centers as a condition for the sale of a new drug that was urgently needed for rescue purposes, the agency became the de facto instigator of a human experiment. It is not possible to pull this switch and disavow responsibility for what followed.

Ill-advised or poorly designed randomized trials achieve the opposite objectives of their intent: improved and less expensive patient care. The lack of familiarization studies, together with the inexplicable error in dosing and the disadvantage of no on-site assays for drug monitoring, resulted in the muddled picture of the new drug's potential that emerged in the published literature between 1992 and 1995. Nevertheless, tacrolimus survived the irrational gauntlet not only because it was user friendly, but also because the talented group of multicenter clinical investigators rebelled against the protocol and introduced treatment flexibility. This confirmed our earlier experience, that throughout the entire history of liver transplantation only two key developments have upgraded graft and patient survival: Calne's introduction of cyclosporine in 1979 (21) and its use in combination with prednisone (22), and the arrival of tacrolimus (see Fig. 9C.2).

Other-Organ Uses

Following the uneven literature that came out of the American multicenter liver trials, an avalanche of articles involving organ after organ, and eventually bone marrow transplantation, would confirm essentially every detail of the original Pittsburgh experience (20).

The same developmental leaps were seen in renal transplantation, for example. The 1-year cadaver kidney survival rate in the United States had remained fixed at less than 50% until the advent of cyclosporine, after which it rose to 77% at the University of Pittsburgh. A second abrupt increase to nearly 90% followed the routine use of tacrolimus (see Fig. 9C.3). The maintenance of the gap between cyclosporine and tacrolimus after 1 year was congruent with the report of Gjertson, Cecka, and Terasaki, based on the cadaver kidney half-life projections from 24 American kidney transplant centers with access to tacrolimus. Their suggestion was: "FK 506 (tacrolimus) appears to be the first therapeutic agent to significantly improve long-term kidney graft survival rates" (23). A thorough review of the use of tacrolimus following kidney transplantation has been provided by Laskow et al (24).

POST-TRANSPLANT LYMPHOPROLIFERATIVE DISORDERS

It has not been surprising to observe an incremental increase in post-transplant lymphoproliferative disorders (PTLDs) with the successively more potent baseline immunosuppressants (21,25–27). This risk can be reduced at the outset by avoiding the joint use of the biologic antilymphoid agents (e.g., ALG and OKT-3) in conjunction with cyclosporine and tacrolimus except as a last resort, and then only with extreme caution.

When PTLD is diagnosed early in development, it usually is a trivial problem requiring only drug dose reduction. At the Children's Hospital of Pittsburgh, 9 (13.2%) of 68 recipients (of 69 kidney allografts) treated with tacrolimus-based immunosuppression between 1989 and 1995 developed histopathologically verified PTLD (28). No deaths resulted, nor did any graft losses. All kidneys are still functioning (at the time of this writing) except one that was chronically rejected 3 years later.

At the same institution, histopathologically verified PTLD was diagnosed in 28 (12.1%) of the 232 consecutive primary pediatric liver recipients treated with tacrolimus between 1989 and 1995. Although 5 of the 28 died of potentially PTLD-related complications, the 4-year patient and graft survival rate (82.2%) was essentially the same as in the 204 non-PTLD patients (Table 9C.3) (27). Management was facilitated by the policies of gradual tacrolimus dose reduction with acceptance of lower blood levels as time passes (see Table 9C.3), early discontinuance of prednisone, avoidance of adjunct agents including OKT-3 and azathioprine, and surveillance for Epstein-Barr virus (EBV) infection.

Table 9C.3. Primary Liver Transplantation in Children Under Tacrolimus (n = 232)[a,b]

	Months' Follow-Up				
	3	12	24	36	48
Survival (%)					
Patient	90.2	86	85	84	84
Graft	83	79.2	78.2	77.3	77.3
Tacrolimus (mean)					
Dose (mg/day)	5.6	3.3	2.9	2.9	2.4
Plasma concentration (trough ng/mL)[c]	0.84	0.56	0.43	0.4	0.24
Prednisone (%)					
None	79	82	88	93	91
≤5 mg/day	9	13	7	5	7
>5 mg/day	12	5	5	2	2

[a] September 1989–January 1995. Age 5.0 ± 5.2 (SD) years (medium 2.7). Mean follow-up 44 ± 14.6 months.
[b] 28 patients developed PTLD. Principal sites were the gastrointestinal system (n = 9), lymph nodes (n = 8), liver (n = 6), spleen (n = 2), and tonsils, skin, and blood (leukemia) (n = 1 each).
[c] For approximate whole blood values, multiply by 10.
Data from Dr. Jorge Reyes. Presented at the 2nd International Congress on Pediatric Transplantation, Paris, France, August 23–24, 1996.

Except for their frequent EBV association, human B-cell lymphomas are indistinguishable from those induced by Robert S. Schwartz in a mouse chimerism model (29) 3 years before they were reported in human kidney recipients (30). Schwartz attributed the experimental tumors to an active lymphoproliferative response by the dominant immune apparatus to the persistent subclinical graft-versus-host counterattack of the minority donor leukocyte population. The relevance of his observations to clinical PTLD would only be appreciated 30 years later (27), after the discovery that similar microchimerism was a characteristic feature of successful organ transplantation (2). This fresh insight about PTLD has been used to map treatment strategies of cellular immune modulation as discussed elsewhere (27).

CHAPTER REFERENCES

1. Kino T, Hatanaka H, Miyata S, et al. FK-506, A novel immunosuppressant isolated from a *Streptomyces*. II. Immunosuppressive effect of FK-506 in vitro. J Antibiotics 1987;40:1256–1265.
2. Kino T, Inamura N, Sakai F, et al. Effect of FK506 on human mixed lymphocyte reaction in vitro. Transplant Proc 1987;19:36–39.
3. Ochiai T, Nagata M, Nakajima K, et al. Studies of the effects of FK506 on renal allografting in the beagle dog. Transplantation 1987;44:729–733.
4. Ochiai T, Nakajima K, Nagata M, et al. Studies of the induction and maintenance of long-term graft acceptance by treatment with FK506 in heterotopic cardiac allotransplantation in rats. Transplantation 1987;44:734–738.
5. Todo S, Ueda Y, Demetris JA, et al. Immunosuppression of canine, monkey, and baboon allografts by FK 506: with special reference to synergism with other drugs and to tolerance induction. Surgery 1988;104:239–249.
6. Tsuchimoto S, Kusumoto K, Nakajiwa Y, et al. Orthotopic liver transplantation in rats receiving FK506. Transplant Proc 1989;21:1064–1065.
7. Jiang H, Suguo H, Takahara S, et al. Combined immunosuppressive effect of FK506 and other immunosuppressive agents on PHA- and CD3-stimulated human lymphocyte proliferation in vitro. Transplant Proc 1991;23:2933–2936.
8. Sigal NH, Dumont FJ. Cyclosporin A, FK506, and rapamycin: pharmacologic probes of lymphocyte signal transduction. Ann Rev Immunol 1992;10: 519–560.
9. Mekki Q, Lee C, Carrier S, et al. The effect of food on oral bioavailability of tacrolimus (FK506) in liver transplant patients. Clin Pharmacol Ther 1993;53:229.
10. Lee C, Jusko W, Shaefer M, et al. Pharmacokinetics of tacrolimus (FK506) in liver transplant patients. Clin Pharmacol Ther 1993;53:181–190.
11. Abu-Elmagd K, Fung JJ, Alessiani M, et al. The effect of graft function on FK506 plasma levels, dosages, and renal function, with particular reference to the liver. Transplantation 1991;52:71–77.
12. Jusko WJ, D'Ambrosio R. Monitoring FK 506 concentrations in plasma and whole blood. Transplant Proc 1991;23:2732–2735.
13. Kershner RP, Fitzsimmons WE. Relationship of FK506 whole blood concentrations and efficacy and toxicity after liver and kidney transplantation. Transplantation 1996;62:920–926.
14. Machida M, Takahara S, Ishibashi M, et al. Effect of temperature and hematocrit on plasma concentration of FK 506. Transplant Proc 1991;6:2753–2754.
15. Winkler M, Ringe B, Rodeck B, et al. The use of plasma levels for FK 506 dosing in liver-grafted patients. Transplant Int 1994;7:329–333.
16. Winkler M, Ringe B, Baumann J, et al. Plasma vs whole blood for therapeutic drug monitoring of patients receiving FK 506 for immunosuppression. Clin Chem 1994;40:2247–2253.
17. Backman L, Nicar M, Levy M, et al. FK506 trough levels in whole blood and plasma in liver transplant recipients: correlation to clinical events and side effects. Transplantation 1994;57:519–524.
18. Christians U, Braun F, Schmidt M, et al. Specific and sensitive measurement of FK506 and its metabolites in blood and urine of liver-graft recipients. Clin Chem 1992;38:2025–2032.
19. Laskow DA, Vincenti F, Neylan JF, et al. An open-label, concentration-ranging trial of FK506 in primary kidney transplantation: a report of the United

States Multicenter FK506 Kidney Transplant Group. Transplantation 1996;62: 900–905.
20. Thomson AW, Murase N, Nalesnik MA, Starzl TE. The influence of tacrolimus on experimental autoimmune disease. In: Lieberman R, Mukherjee A, eds. Principles of drug development in transplantation and autoimmunity. Austin, TX: RG Landes, 1996.
21. Inamura N, Hashimoto M, Nakahara K, et al. Immunosuppressive effect of FK506 on collagen-induced arthritis in rats. Clin Immunol Immunopathol 1988;46:82–90.
22. Arita C, Hotokebuchi T, Miyahara H, et al. Inhibition by FK506 of established lesions of collagen-induced arthritis in rats. Clin Exp Immunol 1990;82:456–461.
23. Takagishi K, Yamamoto M, Nishimura A, et al. Effects of FK-506 on collagen arthritis in mice. Transplant Proc 1989;21(pt1):1053–1055.
24. Miyagawa J, Yamamoto K, Hanafusa T, et al. Preventive effect of a new immunosuppressant FK-506 on insulitis and diabetes in non-obese diabetic mice. Diabetologia 1990;33:503–505.
25. Carroll PB, Strasser S, Alejandro R. The effect of FK 506 on cyclophosphamide-induced diabetes in the NOD mouse model. Transplant Proc 1991;23:3348–3350.
26. Murase N, Lieberman I, Nalesnik M, et al. FK-506 prevents spontaneous diabetes in the BB rat. Lancet 1990;ii:373–374.
27. Nicoletti F, Meroni PL, Barcellini W, et al. FK-506 prevents diabetes in diabetes-prone BB/Wor rats. Int J Immunopharmacol 1991;13:1027–1030.
28. Kawashima H, Mochizuki M. Effects of a new immunosuppressive agent, FK 506, on the efferent limb of the immune responses. Exp Eye Res 1990;51:565–572.
29. Fujino Y, Mochizuki M, Raber J, et al. Treatment of S-antigen induced uveitis in primates. Invest Ophthalmol Vis Sci 1990;31:61.
30. Tamura K, Woo J, Murase N, et al. Suppression of autoimmune thyroid disease by FK 506: influence on thyroid-infiltrating cells, adhesion molecule expression and anti-thyroglobulin antibody production. Clin Exp Immunol 1993;91:368–375.
31. Yamamoto K, Mori A, Nakahama T, et al. Experimental treatment of autoimmune MRL-lpr/lpr with immunosuppressive compound FK506. Immunology 1988;69:222–227.
32. Takabayashi K, Koike T, Kurasawa K, et al. Effect of FK-506, a novel immunosuppressive drug on murine systemic lupus erythematosus. Clin Immunol Immunopathol 1989;51:110–117.
33. Hara S, Fukatsu A, Suzuki N, et al. The effects of a new immunosuppressive agent, FK506, on the glomerular injury in rats with accelerated nephrotoxic serum glomerulonephritis. Clin Immunol Immunopathol 1990;57:351–362.
34. Okuba Y, Tsukada Y, Maezawa A, et al. FK-506, a novel immunosuppressive agent, induces antigen-specific immunotolerance in active Heymann's nephritis and in the autologous phase of Masugi nephritis. Clin Exp Immunol 1990;82:450–455.
35. Matsukawa W, Hara S, Yoshida F, et al. Effects of a new immunosuppressive agent, FK506, in rats with active Heymann nephritis. J Lab Clin Med 1992;119:116–123.
36. Inamura N, Hashimoto M, Nakahara K, et al. Immunosuppressive effect of FK506 on experimental allergic encephalomyelitis in rats. Int J Immunopharmacol 1988;10:991–995.
37. Hanawa H, Kodama M, Zhang S, et al. An immunosuppressant compound, FK-506, prevents the progression of autoimmune myocarditis in rats. Clin Immunol Immunopathol 1992;62:321–326.
38. Meingassner JG, Stutz A. Immunosuppressive macrolides of the type FK 506: a novel class of topical agents for treatment of skin diseases? J Invest Dermatol 1992;98:851–855.
39. Hiraoka Y, Kishimoto C, Kurokawa M, et al. The effects of FK-506, a novel and potent immunosuppressant, upon murine Coxsackie virus B3 myocarditis. J Pharmacol Exp Ther 1992;260:1386–1391.
40. Walliser P, et al. Inhibition of murine B lymphocyte proliferation by the novel immunosuppressive drug FK506. Immunology 1989;68:434–435.
41. Murase N, Kim DG, Todo S, et al. Suppression of allograft rejection with FK-506. I. Prolonged cardiac and liver survival in rats following short-course therapy. Transplantation 1990;50:186–189.
42. Todo S, Podesta L, ChapChap P, et al. Orthotopic liver transplantation in dogs receiving FK-506. Transplant Proc 1987;19(suppl 6):64–67.
43. Monden M, Gotoh M, Kanai T, et al. A potent immunosuppressive effect of FK506 in orthotopic liver transplantation in primates. Transplant Proc 1990;22(suppl 1):66.
44. Murase N, Todo S, Lee PH, et al. Heterotopic heart transplantation in the rat receiving FK-506 alone or with cyclosporine. Transplant Proc 1987;5:71–75.
45. Yasunami Y, Ryu S, Kamei T. FK506 as the sole immunosuppressive agent for prolongation of islet allograft survival in the rat. Transplantation 1990;49: 682–686.
46. Todo S, Demetris A, Ueda Y, et al. Renal transplantation in baboons under FK 506. Surgery 1989;106:444–450.
47. Hoffman AL, Makoka L, Banner B, et al. The use of FK506 for small intestine allotransplantation. Transplantation 1990;49:483–490.
48. Yoshimi F, Nakamura K, Zhu Y, et al. Canine total orthotopic small bowel transplantation under FK-506. Transplant Proc 1991;23:3240–3242.
49. Todo S, Murase N. Tacrolimus for experimental organ transplantation. In: Lieberman R, Mukherjee A, eds. Principles of drug development in transplantation and autoimmunity. Austin, TX: RG Landes, 1996.
50. Eiras G, Imventarza O, Murase N, et al. Species differences in sensitivity of T lymphocytes to immunosuppressive effects of FK 506. Transplantation 1990;49:1170–1172.
51. Murase N, Demetris AJ, Matsuzaki T, et al. Long survival in rats after multivisceral versus isolated small-bowel allotransplantation under FK 506. Surgery 1991;110:87–98.
52. Fung J, Abu-Elmagd K, Jain A, et al. A randomized trial of primary liver transplantation under immunosuppression with FK506 vs cyclosporine. Transplant Proc 1991;23:2977–2983.
53. Fung JJ, Todo S, Tzakis A, et al. Conversion of liver allograft recipients from cyclosporine to FK506-based immunosuppression. Benefits and pitfalls. Transplant Proc 1991;23:14–21.
54. Todo S, Fung JJ, Starzl TEA, et al. Liver, kidney, and thoracic organ transplantation under FK506. Ann Surg 1990;212:295–307.
55. U.S. Multicenter FK506 Liver Transplant Study Group. A comparison of tacrolimus (FK506) and cyclosporine for immunosuppression in liver transplantation. N Engl J Med 1994;331:1110–1115.
56. European FK506 Multicentre Liver Study Group. Randomised trial comparing tacrolimus (FK506) and cyclosporin in prevention of liver allograft rejection. Lancet 1994;344:423–428.
57. Wiesner RH. A long-term comparison of tacrolimus versus cyclosporine in liver transplantation: a report of the U.S. FK506 study group. Transplantation 1998;66:493–499.
58. McDiarmid SV, Busuttil RW, Ascher NL, et al. FK506 (tacrolimus) compared with cyclosporine for primary immunosuppression after pediatric liver transplantation. Results from the U.S. Multicenter Trial. Transplantation 1995;59:530–536.
59. Devlin J, Wong P, Williams R, et al. FK506 primary immunosuppression following emergency liver transplantation for fulminant hepatic failure. Transplant International 1994;7:64–69.
60. Klintmalm GB, Goldstein R, Gonwa T, et al. Use of Prograf (FK506) as rescue therapy for refractory rejection after liver transplantation. U.S. Multicenter FK506 Liver Transplant Study Group. Transplant Proc 1993;25:679–688.
61. Vincenti F, Laskow DA, Neylan JF, et al. One-year follow-up of an open-label trial of FK506 for primary kidney transplantation. A report of the U.S. Multicenter FK506 Kidney Transplant Group. Transplantation 1996;61: 1576–1581.
62. Pirsch JD, Miller J, Deierhoi MH, et al. A comparison of tacrolimus (FK506) and cyclosporine for immunosuppression after cadaveric renal transplantation. FK506 Kidney Transplant Study Group. Transplantation 1997;63:977–983.
63. Cavaille-Coll MW, Elashoff MR. Commentary on a comparison of tacrolimus and cyclosporine for immunosuppression after cadaveric renal transplantation. Transplantation 1998;65:142–145.
64. Shield CF, McGrath MM, Goss TF. Assessment of health-related quality of life in kidney transplant patients receiving tacrolimus-based versus cyclosporine-based immunosuppression. Transplantation 1997;64:1738–1743.
65. Mayer AD, Dmitrewski J, Squifflet JP, et al. Multicenter randomized trial comparing tacrolimus (FK506) and cyclosporine in the prevention of renal allograft rejection: a report of the European Tacrolimus Multicenter Renal Study Group. Transplantation 1997;64:436–443.
66. Shapiro R, Jordan ML, Scantlebury VP, et al. A prospective, randomized trial of FK 506/prednisone vs FK506/azathioprine/prednisone in renal transplant patients. Transplant Proc 1995;27:814–817.
67. Woodle SE, Thistlethwaite JR, Gordon JH, et al. A multicenter trial of FK506 (tacrolimus) therapy in refractory acute renal allograft rejection. Transplantation 1996;62:594–599.
68. Woodle SE, Cronin D, Newell KA, et al. Tacrolimus therapy for refractory acute renal allograft rejection. Definition of the histologic response by protocol biopsies. Transplantation 1996;62:906–910.
69. Jordan ML, Naraghi R, Shapiro R, et al. Tacrolimus rescue therapy for renal allograft rejection—five-year experience. Transplantation 1997;63:223–228.

70. Witzke O, Becker G, Erhard J, et al. Tacrolimus rescue therapy in patients with rejection and long-term dialysis after kidney transplantation. Clin Nephrol 1998;49:24–27.
71. Laskow DA, Neylan JF, Shapiro RS, et al. The role of tacrolimus in adult kidney transplantation: a review. Clin Transplantation 1998;12:489–503.
72. Ketel BL, Turton-Weeks S, Reed K, Barone GW. Tacrolimus-based vs cyclosporine-based immunotherapy in combined kidney-pancreas transplantation. Transplant Proc 1996;28:899.
73. Gruessner RWG, Burke GW, Stratta R, et al. A multicenter analysis of the first experience with FK506 for induction and rescue therapy after pancreas transplantation. Transplantation 1996;61:261–273.
74. Gruessner RWG. Tacrolimus in pancreas transplantation: a multi-center analysis. Clin Transplantation 1997;11:299–312.
75. Hariharan S, Munda R, Cavallo T, et al. Rescue therapy with tacrolimus after combined kidney/pancreas and isolated pancreas transplantation in patients with severe cyclosporine nephrotoxicity. Transplantation 1996;61:1161–1165.
76. Gruessner RW, Bartlett ST, Burke GW, Stock PG. Suggested guidelines for the use of tacrolimus in pancreas/kidney transplantation. Clin Transplant 1998;12:260–262.
77. Todo S, Tzakis A, Reyes J, et al. Intestinal transplantation in humans under FK-506. Transplant Proc 1993;25:1198–1199.
78. Todo S, Tzakis A, Reyes J, et al. Small intestinal transplantation in humans with or without the colon. Transplantation 1994;57:840–848.
79. Abu-Elmagd K, Reyes J, Todo S, et al. Clinical intestinal transplantation: new perspectives and immunologic considerations. J Am Coll Surg 1998;186:512–525.
80. Armitage JM, Kormos RL, Morita S, et al. Clinical trial of FK-506 immunosuppression in adult cardiac transplantation. Ann Thorac Surg 1992;54:205–210.
81. Mentzer RM Jr, Jahania MS, Lasley RD. Tacrolimus as a rescue immunosuppressant after heart and lung transplantation. The U.S. Multicenter FK506 Study Group. Transplantation 1998;65:109–113.
82. Armitage JM, Fricker FJ, del Nido P, et al. A decade (1982 to 1992) of pediatric cardiac transplantation and the impact of FK-506 immunosuppression. J Thorac Cardiovasc Surg 1993;105:464–473.
83. Griffith BP, Bando K, Hardesty RL, et al. A prospective randomized trial of FK506 versus cyclosporine after human pulmonary transplantation. Transplantation 1994;57:848–851.
84. Keenan RJ, Konishi H, Kawai A, et al. Clinical trial of tacrolimus versus cyclosporine in lung transplantation. Ann Thorac Surg 1995;60:580–584.
85. Armitage JM, Fricker FJ, Kurland G, et al. Pediatric lung transplantation: the years 1985 to 1992 and the clinical trial of FK506. J Thorac Cardiovasc Surg 1993;105:337–346.
86. McCauley J, Shapiro R, Scantlebury V, et al. FK 506 in the management of transplant-related nephrotic syndrome and steroid-resistant nephrotic syndrome. Transplant Proc 1991;23:3354–3356.
87. Jegasothy BV, Ackerman CD, Todo S, et al. Tacrolimus (FK 506)—a new therapeutic agent for severe recalcitrant psoriasis. Arch Dermatol 1992;128:781–785.
88. Japanese FK 506 Study Group on Refractory Uveitis. A multicenter clinical open trial of FK506 in refractory uveitis, including Behcet's disease. Transplant Proc 1991;23:3343–3346.
89. van Thiel DH, Carroll P, Abu-Elmagd K, et al. Tacrolimus (FK506), a treatment for primary sclerosing cholangitis: results of an open-label preliminary trial. Am J Gastroenterol 1995;90:455–459.
90. van Thiel DH, Wright H, Carroll P, et al. Tacrolimus: a potential new treatment for autoimmune chronic active hepatitis: results of an open-label preliminary trial. Am J Gastroenterol 1995;90:771–776.
91. Ishioka M, Ohno S, Nakamura S, et al. FK506 treatment of noninfectious uveitis. Am J Ophthalmol 1994;118:723–729.
92. Nash RA, Etzioni R, Storb R, et al. Tacrolimus (FK506) alone or in combination with methotrexate or methylprednisolone for the prevention of acute graft-versus-host disease after marrow transplantation from HLA-matched siblings: a single-center study. Blood 1995;85:3746–3753.
93. McCune TR, Thacker LR II, Peters TG, et al. Effects of tacrolimus on hyperlipidemia after successful renal transplantation: a Southeastern Organ Procurement Foundation multicenter clinical study. Transplantation 1998;65:87–92.
94. Eckhoff DE, McGuire BM, Frenette LR, et al. Tacrolimus and mycophenolate mofetil combination therapy versus tacrolimus in adult liver transplantation. Transplantation 1998;65:180–187.
95. Mueller AR, Platz KP, Blumhardt G, et al. The optimal immunosuppressant after liver transplantation according to diagnosis: cyclosporine A or FK506? Clin Transplant 1995;9:176–184.
96. Zervos XA, Weppler D, Fragulidis GP, et al. Comparison of tacrolimus with microemulsion cyclosporine as primary immunosuppression in hepatitis C patients after liver transplantation. Transplantation 1998;65:1044–1046.
97. McDiarmid SV, Colonna JO, Shaked A, et al. Differences in oral FK506 dose requirements between adult and pediatric liver transplant patients. Transplantation 1993;55:1328–1332.
98. Cox KL, Lawrence-Miyasaki LS, Garcia-Kennedy R, et al. An increased incidence of Epstein-Barr virus infection and lymphoproliferative disorder in young children on FK506 after liver transplantation. Transplantation 1995;59:524–529.
99. Cacciarelli TV, Green M, Jaffe R, et al. Management of post-transplant lymphoproliferative disease in pediatric liver transplant recipients receiving primary tacrolimus therapy. Transplantation 1998;66:1047–1052.
100. Misra S, Moore TB, Ament ME, et al. Red cell aplasia in children on tacrolimus after liver transplantation. Transplantation 1998;65:575–577.
101. Walder B, Ricou B, Suter PM. Tacrolimus-induced hemolytic uremic syndrome after heart transplantation. J Heart Lung Transplant 1998;17:1004–1006.

COMMENTARY REFERENCES

1. Starzl TE, Marchioro TL, Waddell WR. The reversal of homografts with subsequent rejection in human renal development of homograft tolerance. Surg Gynecol Obstet 1963;117:385–395.
2. Starzl TE, Demetris AJ, Murase N, et al. The lost chord: microchimerism. Immunol Today 1996;17:577–584.
3. Starzl TE, Todo S, Fung J, et al. FK 506 for human liver, kidney and pancreas transplantation. Lancet 1989;2:1000–1004.
4. Fung JJ, Todo S, Jain A, et al. Conversion of liver allograft recipients with cyclosporine related complications cyclosporine to FK 506. Transplant Proc 1990;22:6–12.
5. Fung JJ, Todo S, Tzakis A, et al. Conversion of liver allograft recipients from cyclosporine to FK506-based immunosuppression: benefits and pitfalls. Transplant Proc 1991;23:14–21.
6. Todo S, Fung JJ, Starzl TE, et al. Liver, kidney, and thoracic organ transplantation under FK 506. Ann Surg 1990;212:295–305.
7. Starzl TE, Fung J, Jordan M, et al. Kidney transplantation under FK 506. JAMA 1990;264:63–67.
8. Armitage JM, Kormos RL, Fung J, et al. Preliminary experience with FK 506 in thoracic transplantation. Transplantation 1991;52:154–167.
9. McDonald JC, Vaughn W, File RS, et al. Cadaver donor renal transplantation by centers of the Southeastern Organ Procurement Foundation. Ann Surg 1981;193:1–8.
10. Opelz G, Mickey MR, Terasaki PI. HLA matching and cadaver kidney transplant survival in North America. Transplantation 1977;23:490–497.
11. Starzl TE, Hakala TR, Rosenthal JT, et al. Variable convalescence and therapy after cadaveric renal transplantation under cyclosporin A and steroids. Surg Gynecol Obstet 1982;154:819–825.
12. Starzl TE, Abu-Elmagd K, Tzakis A, et al. Selected topics on FK 506: with special references to rescue of extrahepatic whole organ grafts, transplantation of "forbidden organs," side effects, mechanisms, and practical pharmacokinetics. Transplant Proc 1991;23:914–919.
13. Starzl TE, Fung JJ. Contempo 90: transplantation. JAMA 1990;263:2686–2687.
14. Abu-Elmagd K, Fung JJ, Alessiani M, et al. The effect of graft function on FK506 plasma levels, doses, and renal function, with particular reference to the liver. Transplantation 1991;52:71–77.
15. Fung J, Abu-Elmagd K, Jain A, et al. A randomized trial of primary liver transplantation under immunosuppression with FK 506 vs cyclosporine. Transplant Proc 1991;23:2977–2983.
16. Starzl TE, Fung JJ, Todo S, et al. The Pittsburgh randomized trial of tacrolimus versus cyclosporine for liver transplantation. J Am Coll Surg 1996;183: 117–125.
17. Klintmalm A for the U.S. Multicenter FK 506 Liver Study Group. A comparison of tacrolimus (FK 506) and cyclosporine for immunosuppression in liver transplantation. N Engl J Med 1994;331:1110–1115.
18. Neuhaus P, Pichlmayr R, Williams R for the European FK 506 Multicentre Liver Study Group. Randomised trial comparing tacrolimus (FK 506) and cyclosporin in prevention of liver allograft rejection. Lancet 1994;344: 423–428.
19. Starzl TE, Donner A, Eliasziw M, et al. Randomised trialomania? The multicenter liver transplant trials. Lancet 1995;346:1346–1350.
20. Transplantation Society in Transplantation Proceedings. Vol. 29. March 1997.

21. Calne RY, Rolles K, White DJG, et al. Cyclosporin A initially as the only immunosuppressant in 34 recipients of cadaveric organs: kidneys, 2 pancreases, and 2 livers. Lancet 1979;2:1033–1036.
22. Starzl TE, Klintmalm GBG, Porter KA, et al. Liver transplantation with use of cyclosporin A and prednisone. N Engl J Med 1981;305:266–269.
23. Gjertson DW, Cecka JM, Terasaki PI. The relative effects of FK 506 and cyclosporine on short- and long-term kidney graft survival. Transplantation 1995;60:1384–1388.
24. Laskow DA, Neylan JF, Shapiro RS, et al. The role of tacrolimus in adult kidney transplantation: a review. Clin Transplantation 1998;12:489–503.
25. Starzl TE, Nalesnik MA, Porter KA, et al. Reversibility of lymphomas and lymphoproliferative lesions developing under cyclosporine-steroid therapy. Lancet 1984;1:583–587.
26. Cox KL, Lawrence-Miyasaki LS, Garcia-Kennedy R, et al. An increased incidence of Epstein-Barr virus infection and lymphoproliferative disorder in young children on FK506 after liver transplantation. Transplantation 1995;59:524–529.
27. Starzl TE. The mother lode of liver transplantation, with particular reference to our new journal. Liver Transpl Surg 1998;4:1–14.
28. Shapiro R, Scantlebury VP, Jordan ML, et al. Tacrolimus in pediatric renal transplantation. Transplantation 1996;62:1752-1758.
29. Schwartz R, Andre-Schwartz J, Armstrong MYK, Beldotti L. Neoplastic sequelae of allogenic disease. Theoretical considerations and experimental design. Ann NY Acad Sci 1966;129:804–821.
30. Penn I, Hammond W, Brettschneider L, Starzl TE. Malignant lymphomas in transplantation patients. Transplant Proc 1969;1:106–112.

Chapter

10

Mycophenolate Mofetil: Experimental and Clinical Experience

STEPHEN C. RAYHILL HANS W. SOLLINGER

The clinical success of solid organ transplantation took a great leap forward in the early 1980s with the development of cyclosporine (see Chapter 6). In synergy with corticosteroids and the antimetabolite azathioprine, cyclosporine significantly reduced cell-mediated graft rejection and allowed for successful organ transplantation. However, despite the improved clinical success produced by this triple drug regimen, enthusiasm was tempered for two reasons: 1) the particular toxicities of the agents; and 2) the nonspecific immunosuppression produced by the regimen, which resulted in opportunistic infections and increased incidence of malignancies. Thus, efforts in developing new immunosuppressive treatments for transplantation have focused on the development of specific immunomodulation and on agents that might additionally produce attenuation of the antibody response, which is felt to be important in the development of chronic rejection (1).

Mycophenolate mofetil (MMF) is the first drug approved for the prevention of allograft rejection in the United States since the development of the calcineurin inhibitors in the 1980s. Like azathioprine, it is an antimetabolite, but it has several advantages. First and foremost, it is more potent and more selective than azathioprine. Because it is a relatively specific inhibitor of lymphocyte proliferation, doses that are strongly inhibitory can be used without major side effects on other proliferating tissues. This represents its major advantage over other antimetabolites. In addition, because it is a strong inhibitor of lymphocyte proliferation, it inhibits both cell-mediated immunity and humoral immunity. As noted, the inhibition of B cells is felt to be important in the attenuation of the development of chronic rejection (see Chapter 3). Thus, the development of MMF to replace azathioprine in the triple immunosuppression regimen is a major advance in immunosuppressive therapy.

MMF was developed by Nelson, Allison, and Eugui of Roche Laboratories (previously Syntex Research) (1). It is a more orally bioavailable prodrug of mycophenolic acid (MPA), its active form, to which it is converted in the gastrointestinal tract. Its development was based on the observation that a deficiency in de novo purine synthesis in lymphocytes results in a general state of immunosuppression. Specifically, they noted that a genetic deficiency in the production of adenine deaminase, an enzyme critical to de novo purine synthesis, resulted in reduced numbers and reduced function of B and T lymphocytes, while producing no other clinical abnormalities (2). In contrast, children with a defect in the salvage pathway for purine synthesis maintain normal lymphocyte responses, despite being unable to recycle purines, a defect that produces significant abnormalities in other systems (3). Thus, they reasoned that human lymphocytes depend almost exclusively on the de novo pathway of purine synthesis, while other cells can fall back on the salvage pathway in the absence of effective de novo purine synthesis. With this in mind, they sought to develop a vector to block de novo purine synthesis and thereby produce a selective inhibitor of lymphocytes.

The purines guanosine and adenosine are produced from inosine via the de novo pathway (Fig. 10.1). Adenosine deaminase converts inosine to adenosine, while inosine monophosphate dehydrogenase (IMPDH) affects the conversion of inosine to guanosine. Inhibition of either enzyme results in decreased production of these nucleotides, and therefore, cell proliferation as the cell becomes deficient in these substrates. In addition, because guanosine nucleotides are important regulatory stimulators of the rate-limiting enzymes catalyzing inosine synthesis, the reduction in intracellular concentration of guanosine has an indirect inhibitory effect. This is in contrast to the adenosine nucleotides, which allosterically inhibit inosine synthesis. Thus, an inhibitor of de novo guanosine synthesis is a particularly effective inhibitor of de novo purine synthesis—both directly, by depleting the levels of guanosine, and

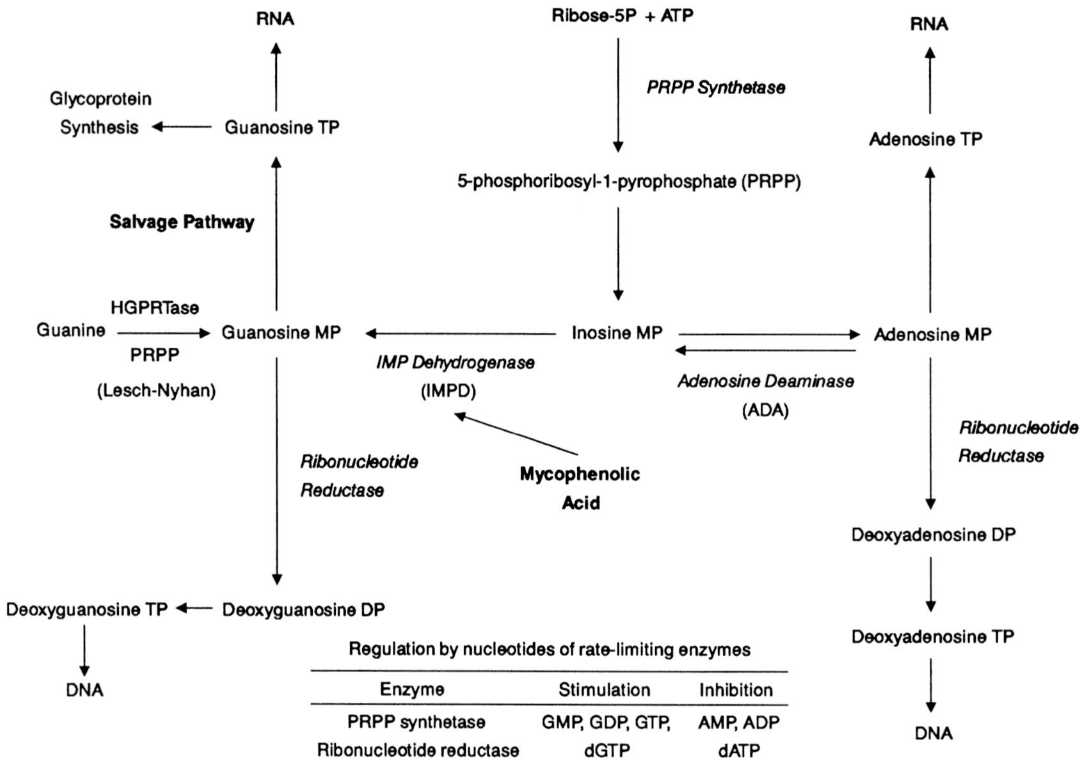

FIGURE 10.1. *The de novo pathway of purine biosynthesis, showing the central position of IMP. MPA inhibits IMP dehydrogenase, thereby depleting GMP, GTP, and dGTP. Two rate-limiting enzymes in the purine synthesis pathway are activated by guanosine ribonucleotides and dGTP, and inhibited by adenosine ribonucleotides and dATP.*

indirectly, by downregulation of enzymes critical to synthesis. Allison, Eugui, and Nelson sought a specific inhibitor of guanosine production. Of the several possible inhibitors of IMPDH available, they selected mycophenolic acid, a fermentation product of several *Penicillium* species, because it is a specific, potent, noncompetitive, and reversible inhibitor of eukaryotic inosine monophosphate dehydrogenases (4,5). It has the additional benefit of not being a nucleoside analog, which, although also inhibitory, could produce undesirable mutagenic effects such as inhibition of DNA repair enzymes and production of chromosomal breaks, which can lead to lymphomas (6). Thus, by defining a specific biochemical pathway critical for the proliferation of human T and B lymphocytes, the development of an organ-specific immunosuppressive was begun.

MECHANISMS OF ACTION

The major advantage of MPA over other antimetabolite immunosuppressants is its relatively selective effect on lymphocyte activation. This is due to two aspects of the drug's mechanism of action. The first is inhibition of purine synthesis. Guanosine and adenosine, the two purine nucleosides, are synthesized via the de novo pathway (see Fig. 10.1). The initial step is the conversion of ribose-5-phosphate and ATP into the amino sugar phosphate 5-phosphoribosyl-amine by 5-phosphoribosyl-1-pyrophosphate synthetase. This step, in which the amide amino group of glutamine replaces the pyrophosphate group of PRPP, is the rate-controlling process of purine synthesis. The 5-phosphoribosyl-1-pyrophosphate synthetase is allosterically inhibited by adeninal nucleotides, and is stimulated by guanosine nucleotides. Via a subsequent series of steps, including the addition of an entire glycene molecule, the pentose sugar is converted into an imidazole ring and then a purine ring, resulting in inosine monophosphate. Inosine monophosphate is the precursor for both adenosine monophosphate and guanosine monophosphate. Inosine monophosphate is converted to adenosine monophosphate by adenosine deaminase and into guanosine monophosphate via inosine monophosphate dehydrogenase. It is the conversion of inosine monophosphate into guanosine monophosphate by IMPDH that is blocked by mycophenolic acid. This competitive inhibition of IMPDH results in the reduction of guanosine monophosphate via decreased synthesis of the molecule and, indirectly, by the loss of its stimulatory effect on the inosine monophosphate synthesis pathway. Thus, the synthesis of both adenosine monophosphate and guanosine monophosphate is inhibited. With these vital DNA substrates depleted, lymphocytes are unable to proliferate. In contrast, cells other than lymphocytes can use the salvage pathway to produce adequate quantities of guanosine monophosphate and adenosine monophosphate by recycling guanine and adenine already present in the cell.

The second mechanism for the selective inhibition of lymphocytes by MPA is based on the unique isoforms of IMPDH employed by lymphocytes. Natsumeda et al have isolated two cDNA clones for two distinct isoforms of IMPDH (7,8). A constitutive form, type I, is the predominant structure expressed in resting human lymphocytes. An inducible form, type II, is found in lymphocytes when they are stimulated by phytohemagglutinin (T cells) or transformed by Epstein-Barr virus (B cells). When stimulated, the type II gene is strongly expressed. The type II isoform of IMPDH is five times more sensitive to MPA than is the type I isoform (1). Thus, rapidly dividing lymphocytes are most susceptible to mycophenolic acid (i.e., the relative susceptibility of lymphocytes to mycophenolic acid is enhanced by their dependence on the type II isoform of IMPDH when activated).

In Vitro Effects of Mycophenolic Acid

Mycophenolic acid, by strongly inhibiting IMPDH, depletes GTP, the precursor for RNA synthesis, and deoxy-GTP (dGTP), the precursor for DNA synthesis in activated peripheral blood lymphocytes and human T- and B-lymphocytic cell lines, locking them in S phase (9). Guanosine monophosphate and adenosine monophosphate must be reduced to deoxydiphosphates and then converted to deoxytriphosphates to be substrates for DNA synthesis. In cells lacking the salvage pathway (those lacking hypoxanthine guanine phosphoribosyl transferase) the addition of deoxyguanosine results in restoration of deoxy-guanosine triphosphate, but not guanosine triphosphate. The restoration of the deoxy version allows DNA synthesis and cellular proliferation. This demonstrates that the depletion of deoxyguanosine triphosphate, the key substrate for DNA polymerase, and therefore for DNA synthesis, is the principal reason that proliferation is inhibited by MPA. In addition to its specific targeting of lymphocytes, MPA also decreases pools of deoxyguanosine triphosphate in human peripheral blood monocytes; however, it does not decrease deoxy-GTP in neutrophils (1). Physiologic concentrations of MPA inhibit the in vitro proliferative responses of human peripheral blood mononuclear cells to phytohemagglutinin, a T-cell mitogen; pokeweed mitogen, a T-cell–dependent B-cell mitogen; and *Staphylococcus* protein A sepharose, a B-cell mitogen (Fig. 10.2) (10). Mycophenolic acid also inhibits the mixed lymphocyte response. Importantly, the

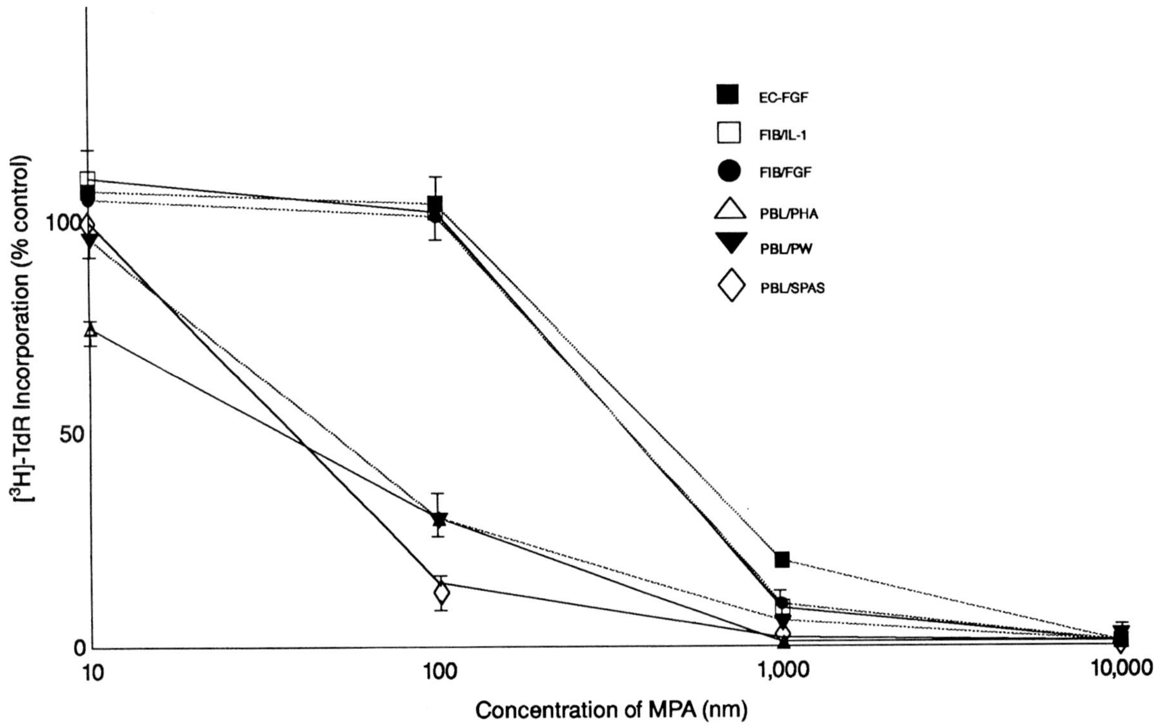

FIGURE 10.2. *Inhibition by MPA of human peripheral blood lymphocyte (PBL) proliferation in response to stimulation by PHA, PWM, and a B-cell mitogen (staphylococcal protein A sepharose). Higher concentrations of MPA are required to inhibit the proliferation of human dermal fibroblasts (FIB) responding to IL-1β and human umbilical vein endothelial cells (EC) responding to basic fibroblast growth factor.*

inhibiting concentration 50% (IC_{50}) is always less than 100 nmol/L, a concentration shown to have no antiproliferative effect on fibroblasts, endothelial cells, and most other cell types studied. Unlike the calcineurin inhibitors, MPA has no effect on IL-2 production by activated lymphocytes (10,11). However, when it is added to a mixed lymphocyte reaction 72 hours after initiation, it is still strongly inhibitory, implying that MPA works at a late stage in T-cell activation. Indeed, consistent with its inhibitory effect on DNA synthesis, cells treated with MPA are blocked at the G_1 to S transition stage (9).

An important secondary effect of purine nucleoside inhibition by MPA may be the disruption of the synthesis of adhesion molecules. Adhesion molecules such as the integrins and selectins are critical in the recruitment of leukocytes to sites of inflammation or rejection (see Chapter 2). They mediate the attachment of these cells to appropriate substrate cells. Both the recruitment of lymphocytes and their activation are decreased in the absence, or with reduced concentrations, of appropriate cell-adhesion molecules such as ICAM-1 and its complementary ligand, LFA-1 (12,13). Glycosylation of proteins and lipids, a required step in the creation of these molecules occurs through nucleotide intermediates. Thus, it follows that MPA, by depleting the purine nucleotide pools in the cells, could inhibit the transfer of the appropriate sugars to nascent membrane glycoproteins. This effect has been confirmed experimentally by measuring the transfer of labeled sugars to glycoproteins and assaying the density of glycoproteins via flow cytometric analysis (14). Thus, MPA may inhibit rejection by attenuating the recruitment of mononuclear cells to rejection sites and by reducing the ability of the lymphocytes to interact with endothelial cells once at the proper location.

In vitro antibody formation by polyclonally activated human B lymphocytes is almost completely inhibited by 100 μmol/L of MPA (10). In contrast to cyclosporine treatment, human spleen cells exposed to tetanus toxoid in the presence of MPA were found to produce no secondary response or subsequent antibody production (15). This may be important in the attenuation of chronic graft rejection.

A second possible mechanism through which MMF may reduce the potential for chronic rejection is through its ability to inhibit human arterial smooth muscle proliferation (Fig. 10.3) (1). Clinically attainable concentrations of MPA inhibit the proliferation of human arterial smooth muscle cells in culture. This has obvious implications for a possible therapeutic benefit with respect to the cellular intimal thickening found in chronic rejection.

The cellular effects of MPA are summarized in Table 10.1.

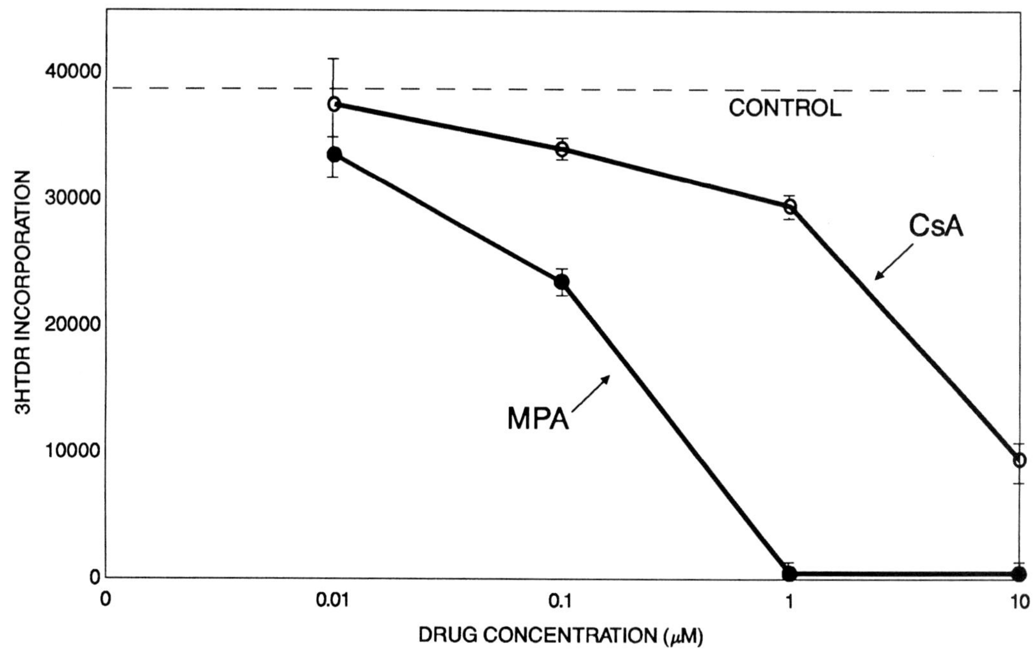

FIGURE 10.3. *The effect of MPA and cyclosporine on the proliferation of human arterial smooth muscle cells in culture. MPA attenuated the proliferative response of human arterial smooth muscle cells grown in culture. This effect occurred at clinically attainable concentrations of MPA (1 to 10 μmol/L) and therefore, might be expected to contribute to a reduction in the arterial wall proliferative response in chronic rejection. Note that the inhibitory concentration for human smooth muscle cells, 10 times greater than that required for inhibition of lymphocytes in culture, was similar to that required for endothelial cells and fibroblasts (see Fig 10.2).*

Table 10.1. The Cellular Effects of Mycophenolic Acid

1. Blocks the proliferative response of both T and B cells.
2. Inhibits adhesion molecule production by inhibiting glycosylation.
3. Inhibits antibody production.
4. Inhibits medial smooth muscle proliferation.

In Vivo Studies

That MPA is lymphocyte selective in vivo was first demonstrated by Eugui et al (16). Mice were given subcutaneous injections of the antigen ovalbumin, which is known to stimulate DNA synthesis in lymph nodes draining the site of injection by stimulating a secondary response. The mice were then given intraperitoneal [^{3}H]-TdR to illuminate the sites of active DNA synthesis. Two groups were evaluated: a control group, which was given the vehicle only, and a treatment group, which was given 100 mg/kg/day of oral MPA. Incorporation of tritiated thymidine into DNA was measured in the appropriate lymph nodes, the spleen, and the testes. MPA strongly inhibited DNA synthesis in the lymph nodes, but had no detectable effect on DNA synthesis in the testes or small intestinal epithelial cells. The spleen was affected, as expected, but there was no effect noted on neutrophils or platelets. Next, mice were challenged with allogeneic tumor cells placed intraperitoneally. The mice treated with MPA had a dose-dependent reduction in the generation of cytotoxic T lymphocytes, and in contrast to untreated mice, they were unable to eliminate tumor cells from their peritoneum.

The effects of MPA on lymphocytes are rapidly and fully reversible (1). Peripheral blood mononuclear cells separated from the plasma of patients treated with MMF respond normally to mitogenic stimulation, whereas that response is strongly attenuated in the presence of the patient's plasma.

Modification of the in vivo antibody response by MMF has been evaluated in rats and mice. Mycophenolate mofetil given orally to mice inhibited the formation of antibodies in a dose-dependent manner (16). When given to rats, it nearly abolished the formation of xenoantibodies, and suppressed resynthesis after plasmapheresis (16,17). Antibody formation from human B cells cultured from the spleen was also inhibited by MMF (15,18).

The effect of MMF on cytokines has been studied by Nagy et al, who demonstrated that in contrast to cyclosporine, which inhibited all cytokines studied at all time points, MMF produced no early (6 to 24 hours) inhibition of cytokine production (19). It did, however, inhibit superantigen-induced cytokine production after 48 hours (only IL-3). This finding was seen in preparations induced with either superantigen or mitogen stimulation. That MPA does not affect IL-2 production was corroborated in a study of mitogen-activated human peripheral lymphocytes (10,11).

STUDIES OF THE EFFECTS OF MYCOPHENOLATE MOFETIL ON ANIMAL ALLOGRAFTS

Studies in Animal Models of Heart Transplantation

The first published reports on the use of MMF in a transplantation model were produced by Morris and co-workers, who studied the effect of MMF on the survival of rat cardiac allografts (20,21). Initially, they found that treatment with MMF prolonged median cardiac allograft survival from 8 to 60 days, and then with an increased dose in a subsequent study to 200 days. In addition, the authors showed that MMF could halt even rejection that was advanced at the onset of treatment (22). Indeed, there was no difference in rats who were treated with MMF from day 1 after transplant versus those begun on day 4 after transplant. When a lower dose of MMF was combined with cyclosporine, the drugs acted additively, further prolonging allograft survival. Rat cardiac allograft recipients surviving 200 days or more after the discontinuation of MMF were given two additional transplants: donor strain and third-party strain atrial allografts. The donor strain allografts were accepted and continued to beat for more than 100 days (suggesting that a state of tolerance may have been achieved). In stark contrast, the third-party atrial grafts were rejected within 14 days. An important additional observation was that graft coronary disease was diminished in the MMF-treated allograft recipients (23). MMF and sirolimus (rapamycin) were found to be synergistic in preventing heart, pancreas, and kidney allograft rejection and in reversing ongoing heart allograft rejection in a rat model (24).

To determine whether MMF might be useful in preventing hyperacute (antibody-mediated) or accelerated acute (T-cell–mediated) rejection, Knechtle et al studied its use in a rat model of sensitized cardiac allograft rejection (25). As shown in Table 10.2, untreated control Lewis recipients were found to have a median survival time of 6 days. Other Lewis rats sensitized with skin grafts from ACI rats were given ACI heart transplants. When untreated, allografts in sensitized rats survived for a median period of 2 days, whereas posttransplant MMF treatment prolonged median survival to 5 days. When given in combination with cyclosporine, MMF prolonged median survival to 14 days. Thus, hyperacute and accelerated acute rejection were prevented; however, acute cellular rejection could not be overcome with MMF alone or in combination with cyclosporine in these sensitized rats.

Investigators from Kobe University and from Syntex Research evaluated combination therapy consisting of MMF and brequinar in the heterotopic rat allograft model (26). Compared to controls, which survived an average of 7 days, animals treated with either MMF or brequinar had a median survival of 15 days. Combination therapy, however, increased median survival to 133 days with no toxic side effects noted. The effect of combination therapy with MMF and brequinar was also evaluated in the setting of rejection rescue

Table 10.2. Allograft Survival in Previously Sensitized Recipients

Group No.	Treatment	Graft Survival Time (Days)	Median Survival Time	*P*	Correlation Between Graft Survival Time and Cytotoxic Antibody Titer (*P*)
1	None	1,1,1,1,1,1,2,2,3,4,4,4,4,4	2	—	0.99
2	MMF (20 mg/kg/d)	1,1,2,5,5,5,5,5,5,5[a],6,6[a],6	5	0.0002 vs. Group 1	0.15
3	CsA (10 mg/kg/d)	1,1,3,7,8,8,8,9,10,14,14,15[a]	8	0.004 vs. Group 1 0.0016 vs. Group 2	0.61
4	MMF + CsA	1,3[a],5[a],11,12[a],13,17[a],18[a],20,24,35,37[b]	15	<0.01 vs. Groups 1, 2, 3	0.45
5	14 days MMF preoperatively, +MMP + CsA postoperatively	1,3[a],3,5[a],9,13,14,14,15,16[a],22[a],33,35	14	0.05 vs. Group 3 0.39 vs. Group 4	0.92

Note: Last two columns represent long-rank tests comparing survival times and the correlation between graft survival and cytotoxic antibody titer.
[a] Rat died.
[b] Rat killed before rejection.
CsA = cyclosporine.

therapy (26). In this experiment, immunosuppressive therapy was withheld until the fifth postoperative day, after the establishment of acute rejection. At this point, treatment with MMF, brequinar, or both was begun. Recipients were evaluated on day 21, when it was noted that either drug by itself, and both in combination, significantly decreased the extent of rejection compared to control animals.

The effect of MMF in a combination therapy regimen was further evaluated in several subsequent studies, including one corroborating Morris' early results, demonstrating that combination therapy with cyclosporine and MMF prolongs rat cardiac allograft survival (27). Another study, in a strongly MHC-incompatible rat cardiac allograft model, evaluated the effect of MMF in combination with leflunomide or tacrolimus (28). It demonstrated that MMF alone or in combination with leflunomide significantly increased allograft survival. Morris et al subsequently demonstrated that MMF treatment significantly prolonged cardiac allograft survival in cynomolgus monkeys, futher supporting its clinical use (23).

The Effect of Mycophenolate Mofetil on Renal Allografts in the Canine Model

The effect of MMF on kidney allograft survival in dogs was evaluated in several studies (29–31). Dogs that received either no treatment or treatment with subtherapeutic doses of cyclosporine and methylprednisolone had median allograft survivals of 8 days. In contrast, MMF prolonged mean survival to 36 days. The strongest effect was noted when MMF was combined with cyclosporine and methylprednisolone, which prolonged median allograft survival to 122 days. Gastrointestinal side effects, which had been seen in dogs receiving MMF alone, were significantly reduced with the lower doses employed in this combination therapy regimen.

A model of rescue therapy for acute renal allograft rejection in dogs was also evaluated (30). A subtherapeutic regimen of MMF, cyclosporine, and methylprednisolone, known from previous experiments to be inadequate for preventing acute allograft rejection, was given. As expected, severe allograft rejection occurred in all dogs within 5 to 10 days of transplantation. Methylprednisolone bolus therapy for 3 days only temporarily reversed this acute rejection, with no dog in this group surviving longer than 20 days after the diagnosis of acute rejection. In contrast, 14 of 16 dogs receiving high doses of MMF for 3 days and then returned to the scheduled combination therapy had complete reversal of rejection. The other two had partial reversal, and all had prolonged survival. Thus, high-dose MMF successfully reversed acute rejection in this canine renal allograft model.

The Effect of MMF on Hepatic Allografts in the Canine Model

The effect of MMF on liver allograft rejection in dogs was also studied (32). As shown in Table 10.3, when used in combination with prednisone and cyclosporine, MMF significantly prolonged canine liver allograft survival. Specifically, this combination therapy, begun on day 1 and continued for up to two weeks, prolonged median survival from 7 days in untreated controls to 70 days in the treatment group. Again, the MMF was well tolerated.

The Effect of MMF on Acute Rejection of Intestinal Allografts in the Animal Model

The effect of MMF on canine intestinal allograft survival was investigated by D'Alessandro et al (33). With no immunosuppressive therapy, median recipient survival was no longer than 10 days; however, triple therapy with MMF,

Table 10.3. Experimental Groups and Survival Following Allogeneic Liver Transplantation in Dogs

Experimental Group	Survival Time (Days)	Mean ± SD	Median	*P* vs. Control
Control Group	6,6,7,8,8	7 ± 1	7	—
Prednisone 0.1 mg/kg	6,8,9,11,11	9 ± 2	9	NS
MMF 20 mg/kg	9,9,10,11,24	13 ± 6	10	<0.05
CsA 5 mg/kg	7,17,22,35,105,120	51 ± 49	29	<0.05
CsA 5 mg/kg, MMF 20 mg/kg	27,36,68,90,110	66 ± 35	68	<0.05
CsA 10 mg/kg	8,22,44,119,126	64 ± 55	44	<0.05
CsA 10 mg/kg, MMF 20 mg/kg (6 wks, then MMF 10 mg/kg)	52,57,65,70,110,125,126	86 ± 33	70	<0.01

NS = not significant; CsA = cyclosporine.

prednisone, and cyclosporine increased median survival to 136 days. In fact, no dog treated with this regimen died due to rejection of the intestinal allograft. This encouraging result was corroborated by a subsequent study of canine small bowel transplantation, which achieved excellent results using combination chemotherapy with prednisone, tacrolimus (FK506), and MMF (34). However, studies using rat models of intestinal transplantation failed to demonstrate increased survival with MMF (35,36).

The Effect of Mycophenolate Mofetil on Animal Hind Limb Allograft Survival

Cyclosporine and MMF combination therapy also prolonged survival of rat hind limb allografts (37). Compared to controls, where the allografts were completely rejected within 10 to 12 days, five of six rats treated with cyclosporine had prolonged allograft survival; however, they demonstrated mild to moderate rejection on biopsy within six months. In contrast, five of six recipients receiving MMF had no rejection at 32 weeks' follow-up, while the remaining recipient demonstrated only slight rejection. Even better results were seen with combination immunosuppressive therapy using both MMF and cyclosporine, where no rejection was observed at all, and full sensation and partial function were observed in all animals. This work, suggesting that MMF was highly effective for immunosuppression in limb transplantation, was corroborated by a study of its efficacy in a rescue model of acute rat hind limb rejection. After being postponed for 7 to 9 days following transplantation, MMF treatment completely reversed rejection in all animals studied (38). A subsequent study using MHC-mismatched rat hind limb allografts—a highly antigenic model—corroborated this finding (39). MMF, along with cyclosporine and prednisone, has permitted successful transplantation of radial forelimb osteomyocutaneous flaps in a porcine model (40). Compared to untreated controls, where all the grafts were completely rejected by day 7, 3 of 10 pigs treated with cyclosporine (CsA), MMF, and prednisone were free of rejection at 90 days, while 3 others developed stable mild-to-moderate rejection. Two pigs died and 2 flaps were lost (by day 29) from severe rejection.

The Effect of MMF in Animal Models of Pancreatic Islet Cell Transplantation

The efficacy of MMF treatment on murine pancreatic islet cell allografts was studied by Howe and co-workers, who observed prolongation of islet survival with treatment (41–43). Allografted islets were transplanted under the kidney capsules of recipients that received either vehicle or 30 daily oral treatments with MMF. As documented by serial blood glucose levels, the authors noted that 9 of the 10 vehicle-treated controls rejected their grafts within 14 to 20 days, whereas 7 of the 11 MMF-treated mice had functioning grafts longer than 100 days after transplantation. No obvious toxic effects were observed. The recipients who maintained a functional allograft for at least 100 days were subsequently challenged with an intraperitoneal injection of donor spleen cells. Only one of the seven recipients then rejected the islet graft. Two weeks later, these recipients were simultaneously transplanted with donor strain and with third-party thyroid tissues. After 30 days, thyroid allograft function was assayed by measuring radioiodine uptake. The donor strain thyroid allografts continued to function, whereas third-party allografts did not, suggesting that not only had MMF reduced rejection of the original islet grafts, but that it had permitted the development of a state of donor-specific tolerance. MMF has also been shown to increase whole pancreas allograft survival in a rat model (44); in combination with IL-2 toxin, it was found to significantly prolong mouse thyroid allograft survival (45). The effects of MMF in animal models of allotransplantation are summarized in Table 10.4.

Table 10.4. A Summary of the Effects of Mycophenolate Mofetil in Animal Models of Allotransplantation

Transplanted Organ	Model	Findings
Heart	Rat and monkey	Prolongs graft survival Reverses ongoing rejection (rescue therapy) Inhibits hyperacute and accelerated acute rejection Protection enhanced when used in combination with cyclosporine, tacrolimus, brequinar, and leflunomide Reduces antibody production Decreases graft coronary artery disease
Kidney	Dog	Prolongs graft survival Reverses ongoing rejection (rescue therapy)
Liver	Dog	Prolongs graft survival
Intestinal	Dog	Prolongs graft survival
Hind limb	Rat	Prolongs graft survival Reverses ongoing rejection (rescue therapy)
Islet cell	Mouse and rat	Prolongs graft survival
Thyroid	Mouse	Prolongs graft survival
Aorta	Rat	Decreases intimal proliferation

The Effects of MMF on Animal Xenograft Models

Several studies have evaluated the efficacy of MMF in combination with cyclosporine in hamster-to-rat heart xenograft models (46,47). In untreated recipients and those treated with cyclosporine alone, rejection occurred on average at 4 days following transplantation. The combination of MMF and cyclosporine increased median survival to 6 days. When cyclosporine, MMF, and brequinar were used as a triple-therapy regimen, median survival was prolonged to 33 days.

MMF has been shown to be effective in increasing the survival of cynomolgus monkey cardiac xenografts transplanted into baboons (48,49). With no treatment, severe humoral and cellular rejection occurred, resulting in a mean graft survival of 9 days. In contrast, treatment with cyclosporine and prednisone increased graft survival to 77 days, while triple therapy with cyclosporine, prednisone, and azathioprine resulted in a mean graft survival of 94 days. However, baboons receiving daily cyclosporine, prednisone, and MMF (70 mg/kg/day) fared best, with a mean graft survival of 296 days. Significantly diminished xenograft vascular disease was also observed in the baboons receiving MMF. Thus, rejection in the MMF-treated baboons occurred with less frequency, less severity, and with less development of vascular disease.

Table 10.5. A Summary of the Effects of Mycophenolate Mofetil in Animal Models of Xenotransplantation

Organ	Combination	Effect
Heart	Hamster-to-rat	Prolongs graft survival
	Monkey-to-baboon	Prolongs graft survival and decreases graft coronary artery disease
Islet	Rat-to-hamster Pig-to-rat	Prolongs graft survival

The effect of MMF on rejection of pancreatic islet cell xenografts has also been studied in a model where rat pancreatic islet cells were transplanted into hamsters (50). Treatment with MMF prevented rejection and maintained islet capillary perfusion, while the untreated islets suffered irreversible failure of capillary perfusion and died. Furthermore, in a pig islet-to-rat model, MMF in combination with cyclosporine and leflunomide prevented islet xenograft rejection (51). The effects of MMF in xenotransplantation are summarized in Table 10.5 (see also Chapter 40).

THE EFFECT OF MYCOPHENOLATE ON ANTIBODY PRODUCTION IN ANIMAL ALLOGRAFTS

To study the effect of MMF on humoral rejection, Knechtle et al placed three successive skin grafts from ACI rats to Lewis recipients at 14-day intervals (25). Assaying antibody production by the chromium-51 release assay, the authors noted significantly higher titers of complement-fixing antibodies in the untreated group. Heterotopic rat cardiac allografts were then performed in the sensitized animals. Median survival of untreated cardiac allografts was 2 days. Treatment with MMF alone increased median survival to 5 days. However, the combination of cyclosporine and MMF increased median survival to 14 days.

THE EFFECT OF MYCOPHENOLATE ON CHRONIC REJECTION IN TRANSPLANT VASCULOPATHY IN ANIMAL MODELS

There are three mechanisms through which MMF may decrease chronic rejection and the development of intimal disease in allografts. The first possible mechanism is through a reduction in acute rejection and the consequent reduction in endothelial injury. Endothelial injury results in a cascade of events triggered to effect repair of the defect—when exuberant, this results in ongoing cellular proliferation, fibrosis, and thus luminal compromise (see Chapter 3). A reduction in endothelial injury would attenuate this process. The second means through which MMF might decrease graft vascular disease is through its effect on antibody-mediated rejection. Antibodies attack endothelial antigens directly, resulting in endothelial damage, subsequent exuberant repair, fibrosis, and narrowing of the lumen. The third mechanism through which MMF might decrease proliferative arteriopathy in transplant vessels is through its effect on smooth muscle cells. The endothelial lesions of chronic rejection tend to be concentric atherosclerotic lesions containing both cellular and fibrous elements. The cellular growth is attributed to proliferation of both smooth muscle cells and fibroblasts (1,52). Clinically attainable concentrations of MMF have been shown to inhibit the proliferation of human arterial smooth muscle cells in culture (1). The effect of MMF on chronic rejection was evaluated in the rat heterotopic allograft model; the incidence and severity of proliferative arteriopathy was found to be low in rats treated with mycophenolate compared to those treated with cyclosporine or FK506 (23). This evidence of an antiproliferative effect was corroborated in rats using an aortic allograft model (53). In this experiment, rats were given orthotopic aortic allografts and were treated with either MMF or no immunosuppression. After three months, the allografts were harvested and evaluated using morphometric analysis. Rats treated with MMF showed much less intimal thickening, with significantly decreased cellular proliferation compared to the control group. Syngeneic aortas, used to control for nonimmunologic effects, did not develop proliferative arteriopathy. These findings are supported by data from the cynomolgus monkey heart-to-baboon recipient model described previously (49); the extent of xenograft coronary artery disease was markedly decreased in animals treated with triple therapy including MMF compared to those treated with azathioprine. Furthermore, in a canine model of allogeneic saphenous vein vasculopathy, cyclosporine and MMF reduced the development of intimal disease. In these animals both humoral and cellular responses were inhibited (54). Thus, animal allograft models suggest that MMF may be effective in attenuating chronic rejection.

CLINICAL STUDIES

The first clinical use of MPA was in the treatment of severe psoriasis. Two studies performed in the 1970s demonstrated attenuation of psoriatic lesions following MPA administration (55,56). It was also used at that time as an antiproliferative agent in the treatment of malignancy (57,58). However, absorption of MPA was poor, and the doses used were high and poorly tolerated. Thus, interest in its use waned until the current development of its prodrug, MMF, as an immunosuppressant for use in transplantation.

Kidney Transplantation

Based on the strong evidence from animal and in vitro models suggesting that MMF both protects against rejection and has a mild side-effect profile, clinical trials were begun. The first trial was a phase I trial designed to test the safety of MMF and to determine proper dosing. Escalating doses of MMF (100–3500 mg/day orally) were administered in combination with cyclosporine and prednisone to patients receiving renal allografts (59–61). The efficacy of MMF and its side effect profile were evaluated in eight groups of six patients at eight different dosages. Significant correlations were observed between the MMF dose, the incidence of rejection, and the number of rescue treatments required to treat acute rejection. The most important finding was that the drug was well tolerated, and especially that there was no nephrotoxicity or hepatotoxicity. The most common side effects were gastrointestinal problems, including mild ileus, gastritis, nausea, and vomiting. The only serious side effect observed was a case of hemorrhagic gastritis, which occurred in one patient receiving 1000 mg/day. The study suggested that doses of 2000 mg/day or higher were most efficacious. Dose reduction was required in five patients because of untoward effects, including nausea and vomiting (two patients), diarrhea, myelosuppression (persistent leukopenia), and prolonged elevation in liver function tests (in a patient with hepatitis C infection). Overall, MMF was tolerated at doses of up to 3500 mg/day for up to two years. Thus, this early clinical study demonstrated that MMF could safely replace azathioprine in a triple-drug regimen.

The next investigation was a multicenter study evaluating the effect of MMF as a rescue agent (60). Seventy-five patients who had previously undergone antirejection therapy with high-dose steroids, OKT-3, or both treatments were entered into the study. Treatment consisted of MMF in doses of either 1000 mg or 1500 mg twice daily, begun within 48 hours of a biopsy confirming acute rejection by Banff criteria. During treatment, maintenance doses of cyclosporine and prednisone were maintained. Successful rescue, defined as stabilization or improvement in renal function, was achieved in 52 of the 75 patients (69%). In patients having a serum creatinine of ≤4 mg/dl at initiation of MMF therapy, a success rate of 79% was noted. No significant nephrotoxicity, hepatotoxicity, or myelosuppression were observed. Thus, this study suggested that MMF was effective for treatment of refractory renal allograft rejection.

The effect of MMF on refractory renal allograft rejection was subsequently studied in a larger trial—an open-labeled, multicenter trial in which it was compared to treatment with high-dose intravenous steroids (62). The trial assigned 150 patients randomly to either MMF or intravenous steroid treatment. Six months after enrollment, graft loss or death was 45% lower in the MMF group compared to the high-dose steroid group. This significant reduction was maintained for the subsequent 12 months. Adverse events were gastrointestinal and hematologic, primarily leukopenia. The frequency of opportunistic infections for each group was similar, and at 35% was comparable to that of previous studies.

Heart Transplantation

The first use of MMF to treat mild rejection in cardiac patients was in an eight-week-long phase I trial (64). Oral doses of 500–3000 mg/day of MMF were substituted for azathioprine in a triple therapy regimen. In 20 of the 30 patients with biopsy-proven rejection, rejection resolved within four weeks. The authors concluded that MMF was safe in cardiac patients, and that MMF-based triple therapy was at least as effective as azathioprine triple therapy. In addition, less myelosuppression was noted with MMF than with azathioprine.

Another group also studied the use of MMF to treat recurrent or persistent heart allograft rejection (65). Seventeen patients with biopsy-proven rejection at a mean of 5.4 months following transplantation were given 3000–3500 mg/day of MMF instead of azathioprine in a standard triple therapy regimen. Of the 17 patients, 14 were doing well 10 months from the start of the MMF triple therapy regimen, and the frequency of rejection episodes was decreased following institution of MMF therapy. Gastrointestinal intolerance was the only limiting factor to the use of MMF in this group of patients. These two studies demonstrated that MMF was safe and effective for heart transplant patients.

A randomized, multicontinental trial of the effect of MMF in heart transplant recipients demonstrated that MMF decreased both mortality and rejection within the first year after cardiac transplantation (66). In this study, 650 patients in 28 centers were randomized to receive, in addition to cyclosporine and corticosteroids, 3000 mg/day of MMF or 1.5–3.0 mg/kg/day of azathioprine. The use of MMF resulted in a significant reduction in both mortality at one year (from 11% to 6%, $P = 0.03$) and the requirement for treatment of rejection within the first 6 months after transplantation (from 74% to 66%, $P = 0.03$). More patients in the MMF group were rejection free at 6 months (34% versus 26%, $P = 0.04$). In addition, high-grade rejection (grade 3 or greater) was also reduced (from 53% to 45%, $P = 0.06$). Despite reduced requirements for OKT-3 or ATGAM (from 21% to 15%, $P = 0.06$), patients receiving MMF had a greater incidence of opportunistic infections—mostly herpes simplex (55% versus 44%, $P = 0.02$). No difference between groups in the rate of CMV infection was detected. Significantly more MMF-treated patients had diarrhea (45% versus 34%, $P = 0.008$). Leukopenia, in contrast, was more common in the azathioprine group (39% versus 30%, $P = 0.04$). There was no difference between groups in the risk of lymphoma.

Liver Transplantation

The use of MMF as rescue therapy to treat liver rejection has also been evaluated (67). In this study, patients on a standard immunotherapy regimen of cyclosporine, prednisone, and azathioprine who had biopsy-proven persistent acute rejection after initial treatment with high-dose steroids and OKT-3 were begun on MMF therapy. In 21 of 23 patients there was a significant decrease in the extent of rejection, with complete resolution in 14 of the 23 patients. There was minimal toxicity of MMF noted.

A second study evaluated the treatment of rejection in liver transplant patients with a combination of MMF and prednisone (68). Four patients with established rejection were begun on the MMF and prednisone regimen, with resolution of the rejection in all four cases. Only one patient subsequently developed recurrent rejection, which was treated with OKT-3. It was felt that MMF could be used either to eliminate or to reduce the dose of cyclosporine in patients intolerant of that drug.

Recently, Eckhoff et al (69) published a retrospective analysis of their experience with the use of MMF in liver transplantation in which 130 consecutive liver transplant recipients were studied. The first 80 recipients received tacrolimus and prednisone, while the subsequent 50 recipients received tacrolimus, prednisone, and MMF (1 g orally twice a day, tapered monthly by 250 mg twice a day until discontinuation at 3 months after transplantation). Although there were no differences in 6-month patient and graft survival between groups, the incidence of acute rejection decreased from 61% to 28% ($P = 0.007$). All patients with rejection in the MMF group responded to a steroid bolus, whereas 3 patients in the non-MMF group required the addition of monoclonal antibody therapy (and 2 others required supplemental MMF). In addition, renal function one month after transplantation was better in the MMF-treated group (creatinine = 1.1 versus 1.5, $P = 0.0001$). No difference was observed between groups in the rate of CMV infection. Glucose intolerance after transplantation, however, was greater in the combined therapy group (26% versus 12%, $P = 0.005$).

The use of MMF with tacrolimus in liver transplantation to allow for early steroid withdrawal has been evaluated by Stegall et al (70). Of the 71 patients studied, 35 were randomized to receive tacrolimus and MMF and 36 to receive cyclosporine and MMF. In all patients, prednisone was tapered off by day 15 after transplantation. No immunologic graft loss occurred in either group and biopsy-proven rejection within the first 6 months was similarly low in both groups (46% for the tacrolimus–MMF group, 42% for the cyclosporine–MMF group). Another study comparing tacrolimus to cyclosporine in liver transplant patients receiving MMF also demonstrated excellent results with both regimens. Indeed, rejection within 6 months of transplantation occurred in only 19% of patients for both groups (71).

The use of MMF in liver transplantation does not appear to increase the risk of infection in recipients (72). In a retrospective study from the University of Pittsburgh, 16 patients who received MMF to permit reduction in the doses of tacrolimus (required because of neurotoxicity or nephrotoxicity) were compared to 136 patients who received tacrolimus and prednisone, but no MMF. Despite a decrease in the incidence of rejection within the first 6 months from 30% to 6% with MMF, no significant increase in CMV infection or disease, PCP pneumonia, fungal infection, or recurrence in hepatitis C was observed. There was an increase in bacterial infections noted in the MMF group

(69% versus 36%, *P* = 0.02), but longer intensive care unit stays for patients in this group may have accounted for the difference.

Pancreas Transplantation

MMF has been an extremely important addition to the arsenal of immunosuppression in pancreas transplantation. It has decreased rejection in pancreas transplantation so dramatically that it has allowed the switch from bladder drainage to enteric drainage and is responsible for the recent success with transplantation of the pancreas alone (see Chapter 21). Sollinger et al, summarizing their experience with simultaneous pancreas–kidney (SPK) transplantation, demonstrated marked improvements in allograft survival, with 2-year renal and pancreas graft survival rates increasing from 86% to 95% (*P* = 0.02) and 83% to 95% (*P* = 0.02), respectively, in the MMF era (versus azathioprine) (73,74). Patient survival rates at 2 years also improved, from 95% to 99% (*P* = NS). These increases in survival were largely due to markedly decreased rejection, with renal allograft rejection decreasing from 75% to 31% (*P* = 0.001) with MMF. Steroid refractory rejection was also reduced, from 24% to 7% (*P* = 0.01).

Similar improvements in patient and graft survival in pancreas transplantation were observed by Gruessner et al (75). Evaluating 61 SPK transplants, 44 pancreas-after-kidney (PAK) transplants, and 15 pancreas transplants alone (PTA), they observed that in the SPK population pancreas survival at one year increased from 79% to 86% versus azathioprine (*P* = NS) and kidney survival increased from 86% to 96% (*P* = NS). The incidence of rejection was significantly reduced with the use of MMF (in combination with tacrolimus), from 43% for azathioprine (AZA) to 15% with MMF (*P* = 0.0003). Notably, 50% of recipients in this series developed GI toxicity (toxicity responded to reduction of the dose of MMF or to switching to AZA, which occurred in 14% of patients within 1 year). A third, smaller analysis of the use of MMF in SPK transplantation also demonstrated similar reductions in rejection (76). In this study, patients who received tacrolimus and MMF (18 patients) or cyclosporine and MMF (18 patients) were compared to recipients who received cyclosporine and AZA. Biopsy-proven rejection within the first 6 months of transplantation was reduced from 77% in the AZA group (a historical group) to 11% for both MMF groups (*P* = 0.01).

PHASE III CLINICAL TRIALS OF MMF IN THE PREVENTION OF ACUTE RENAL ALLOGRAFT REJECTION

The large body of experimental and clinical evidence summarized above indicated that MMF is a powerful immunosuppressant with a favorable side-effect profile and led to worldwide evaluation of the drug in renal transplantation. Three international, multicenter, randomized, phase III clinical trials of MMF as an immunosuppressant for renal allograft rejection were initiated. These studies have now been completed, and the success of the drug demonstrated by these studies prompted rapid FDA approval of MMF for the prevention of renal allograft rejection.

The US multicenter study, a prospective, randomized, double-blind study that enrolled 499 patients in 14 states, used standard four-drug therapy (77). All patients received ATGAM for induction therapy, along with a triple-drug immunosuppression regimen consisting of cyclosporine and corticosteroid therapy, accompanied by either 2 mg/kg/day of azathioprine (166 patients), 2 g/day of MMF (167 patients), or 3 g/day of MMF (166 patients). As shown in Table 10.6, biopsy-proven acute rejection episodes or treatment failures were significantly decreased with MMF. MMF-treated patients had a 31% rate of treatment failure or acute rejection for both the 2-g/day and 3-g/day treatment groups. This was in contrast to a 48% failure rate in the azathioprine group. These were statistically significant differences. In addition, patients in the azathioprine group required a significantly greater number of full courses of antirejection therapy compared to both MMF groups. Most important, the rate of biopsy-proven rejection was essentially cut in half with MMF therapy, dropping from 38% in the azathioprine group, to 20% in the 2 g/day MMF group, and 18% in the 3 g/day MMF group. The incidence of leukopenia and tissue-invasive cytomegalovirus (CMV) disease was slightly higher in the MMF groups. Otherwise, the toxicities were similar. A study comparing the cost effectiveness of MMF 2 g/day and AZA in the patients enrolled in the US multicenter study revealed that, despite its greater cost, MMF, by decreasing rejection, dialysis, and graft failure (without changing the cost of treating opportunistic infections), yielded slightly lower first-year costs than AZA (US$29,158 versus US$27,807) (78).

The European Mycophenolate Mofetil Cooperative Study Group evaluated the effect of mycophenolate as a component of triple therapy in 491 patients receiving cadaveric renal allografts (79). This also was a randomized,

Table 10.6. Incidence of Treatment Failure, Early Termination, and Rejection in US MMF Versus Azathioprine Study of Renal Allograft Rejection[a]

	AZA	MMF 2 g/day	MMF 3 g/day
Number of patients	166	167	166
All treatment failures	48%	31%	31%
Biopsy-proven rejection	38%	20%	18%
Biopsy-proven or presumptive rejection	46%	26%	24%
Early termination[b]	6%	10%	13%

[a] Regimen included antithymocyte globulin induction therapy.
[b] Without prior acute rejection; does not include death and graft loss.
AZA = azathioprine; MMF = mycophenolate mofetil.

double-blind, controlled trial. Patients were given standard immunotherapy with corticosteroids, cyclosporine, and either placebo, MMF 2g/day, or MMF 3g/day. Biopsy-proven allograft rejection or treatment failure for any other reason were considered the primary efficacy variables. Acute rejection was treated with high-dose intravenous corticosteroids, and if necessary, with antilymphocyte agents. As shown in Table 10.7, MMF in the setting of triple therapy significantly reduced the incidence of rejection episodes or treatment failures. Indeed, the reduction was greater than 50%. The placebo group had a 56% incidence of treatment failure, in contrast to 30% for the 2g/day MMF group and 39% for the 3g/day MMF group. These were statistically significant differences. The need for treatment of rejection with corticosteroids or antilymphocyte agents dropped as well, from 59% in patients receiving placebo to 29% for those receiving 2g/day of MMF and to 24% for those receiving 3g/day of MMF. With the exception of usually mild gastrointestinal problems, leukopenia, and opportunistic infections, the frequency of adverse events was similar in all treatment groups. These findings corroborated the US study, demonstrating that MMF was effective in the prevention of renal allograft rejection and was well tolerated.

The largest study, a tricontinental study, took place at 21 sites in Australia, Canada, and Europe. The efficacy of MMF as a component of triple therapy was compared to that of azathioprine (80). A total of 503 patients were randomly assigned to one of three treatment groups, receiving corticosteroid and cyclosporine treatment, as well as either 100–150mg/day of azathioprine (166 patients), 2g/day of MMF (173 patients), or 3g/day of MMF (164 patients). Again, biopsy-proven rejection or treatment failure for any reason occurring within the first 6 months of transplantation was the primary determinant of efficacy. As summarized in Table 10.8, patients receiving MMF had significantly fewer treatment failures than did the patients receiving azathioprine therapy; MMF patients also had significantly fewer episodes of rejection. Specifically, 36% of the azathioprine-treated patients had biopsy-proven rejection versus 20% of those in the 2g/day MMF treatment group and 16% of those in the 3g/day MMF treatment group. Although the side-effect profiles of the drugs were similar, the MMF treatment groups did have higher rates of attrition for non-rejection-related events.

The 3-year follow-up to this study (which was not designed for the evaluation of long-term end points) demonstrated continued improved patient and graft survival for the recipients receiving MMF, but the differences were not statistically significant (81). With 50% of the patients remaining in the study at 3 years, by intent to treat, the total rate of graft loss was 20% for the AZA group, 18% for the MMF 2g/day group, and 15% for the MMF 3g/day group. Excluding death as a cause of graft loss, the rates for graft loss were 15% for the AZA group, 15% for the MMF 2g/day group, and 8% for the MMF 3g/day group. There was no difference in creatinine or the incidence of proteinuria between groups at 3 years, suggesting that there was no major difference in the effect on chronic rejection. As had been seen at one year, the MMF groups had slightly greater gastrointestinal toxicity, infection, and malignancy. There were no differences in lymphoproliferative disorders: PTLD occurred in 1 patient (0.6%) in the AZA group, 2 patients (1.2%) in the MMF 2g/day group, and 3 patients (1.8%) in the MMF 3g/day group. Perhaps the most important finding was that there was no change in the adverse event profile of MMF from that observed at 1 year; thus, long-term treatment with MMF appears to be safe.

The data from all three international phase III studies has been pooled and analyzed as a single study (82). This combined analysis revealed no real differences in results from the individual studies, but strengthened their findings. Specifically, 1-year graft survival for the 1493 patients from the three studies was 90% for the MMF 2g/day group, 89% for the MMF 3g/day group, and 88% for the placebo–AZA group (P = NS). There was also no significant difference between groups in patient survival at one year: 95% for the placebo–AZA and MMF 3g/day groups, and 96% for the MMF 2g/day group. Graft loss due to rejection, however, was significantly greater in the placebo–AZA group (6%) than in the MMF groups (3% for MMF 2g/day, 4% for

Table 10.7. Incidence of Rejection, Graft Loss/Death, and Other Treatment Failures at 6 Months for the European MMF Versus Placebo Study of Renal Allograft Rejection

	Placebo	MMF 2 g/day	MMF 3 g/day
Number of patients	166	165	160
All treatment failures (biopsy-proven rejection, graft loss/death, other)	56%	30%	39%
Biopsy-proven rejection	46%	17%	14%
Graft loss/death	2%	2%	3%
Other (any reason)	7%	12%	23%

MMF = mycophenolate mofetil.

Table 10.8. Incidence of Treatment Failure, Early Termination, and Biopsy-Proven Rejection in Tricontinental (Australia, Canada, and Europe) MMF Versus Azathioprine Study of Renal Allograft Rejection

	AZA	MMF 2 g/day	MMF 3 g/day
Number of patients	166	173	164
All treatment failures	50%	38%	35%
Biopsy-proven rejection	36%	20%	16%
Early termination*	10%	14%	15%

* Without prior acute rejection; does not include death and graft loss.
AZA = azathioprine; MMF = mycophenolate mofetil.

MMF 3 g/day, $P = 0.004$). This reflected significantly greater rates of rejection at 6 months in the placebo–AZA group (41%) than in the MMF 2 g/day group (20%) and in the MMF 3 g/day group (16%) ($P < 0.001$). Consequently, the requirement for antilymphocyte therapy to treat steroid-resistant rejection was greatest in the placebo–AZA group at 20%, versus 9% in the MMF 2 g/day group and 5% in the MMF 3 g/day group. Thus, with no increase in mortality compared to AZA, MMF provided better protection from rejection and graft loss due to rejection.

Similar survival rates and rates of rejection were noted in another placebo-controlled, multicenter study performed in Europe (83). The rates of biopsy-proven rejection within the first year dropped from 46% in the placebo group to 18% in the 2 g/day and 14% in the 3 g/day MMF groups ($P < 0.001$). The requirement for antibody therapy for rejection dropped commensurately.

The use of MMF to treat established rejection has also been evaluated (84). In this double-blinded, controlled trial in 221 renal transplant recipients, MMF, in combination with a corticosteroid bolus and taper, was found to be more effective in treating established rejection than a corticosteroid–AZA regimen. The addition of MMF to the regimen significantly reduced the requirement for antilymphocyte therapy compared to the addition of AZA. This suggests that if a patient is not on MMF at the time of rejection, then it should be started to enhance the response to the steroid bolus.

The efficacy of MMF in the African-American population was evaluated in a reexamination of the data from the US Renal Transplant Mycophenolate Mofetil Study Group (85). African-American recipients of renal transplants benefited from MMF, but required a higher dose (3 g/day) than the non-African Americans. Of the 495 patients studied, 117 (24%) were African American. Biopsy-proven rejection (Banff criteria) in African Americans was diminished from 48% for AZA to 32% for MMF 2 g/day and 12% for MMF 3 g/day (P = NS). Similar efficacy was observed in the non-African-American population, but an MMF dose of 2 g/day was adequate. Specifically, 36% of the non-African-American recipients on AZA rejected within the first 6 months, compared to 16% on MMF 2 g/day and 19% on MMF 3 g/day. When rejection and treatment failure (graft loss, death, or withdrawal from the study for any reason without prior rejection) were considered together, the requirement for greater doses of MMF in African Americans became more evident. Fifty-seven percent of African Americans in the AZA group and 32% in the MMF 2 g/day group experienced rejection or treatment failure. In contrast, only 24% in the MMF 3 g/day group experienced such an adverse event ($P = 0.0008$ versus AZA). For the non-African-American patients, 44% in the AZA group, 27% in the MMF 2 g/day group ($P = 0.007$ versus AZA), and 33% in the 3 g/day group ($P = 0.08$ versus AZA) had an adverse event.

The inadequacy of 2 g/day of MMF in African-American recipients of renal transplants was also observed in a single center study that compared MMF 2 g/day to AZA (86). For Caucasians, biopsy-proven rejection at 6 months dropped from 42% to 17% ($P < 0.001$) with MMF. In contrast, for African Americans receiving 2 g/day of MMF, it only decreased from 37% to 31% ($P = 0.4$).

Thus, three large international, multicenter, randomized studies have demonstrated that MMF is significantly more efficacious than azathioprine or placebo in preventing acute kidney allograft rejection. Now the major concern is not the efficacy of the drug, but the gastrointestinal intolerance to MMF. There is also concern that the stronger immunosuppression effected by MMF might result in greater rates of opportunistic infections, such as CMV and other viruses.

The use of MMF in combination with tacrolimus in renal transplant patients has also been studied. Roth et al (87) retrospectively compared 72 patients who received MMF, tacrolimus, and corticosteroids to 98 patients who received only tacrolimus and corticosteroids. They observed significantly reduced rejection in the MMF group (8% versus 21%, $P = 0.003$). This difference persisted when the recipient's race was considered, with rejection declining from 22% to 14% in Caucasians and from 28% to 10% in African Americans. One-year patient and graft survival did not differ between treatment groups. There also was no difference in post-transplant diabetes mellitus (18% in the MMF group versus 21% in the no MMF group). CMV viremia, however, was significantly more common in patients who received MMF (15% versus 2%, $P = 0.0001$).

MMF IN THE TREATMENT OF CHRONIC REJECTION

With the demonstrated in vitro attenuation of B-cell, fibroblast, and smooth muscle cell activity, it has been hypothesized that MMF might also inhibit the development of chronic rejection. No large studies evaluating the effect of MMF on chronic rejection have been published, but early analyses of its long-term efficacy in the phase III studies have not identified a major impact on chronic rejection. Indeed, no significant difference in graft survival or serum creatinine at 3 years was detected in MMF and AZA groups in the Tricontinental Mycophenolate Mofetil Renal Transplantation Study Group (which was not designed for evaluation of the effects of MMF on chronic rejection) (68a). However, encouraging results have been obtained from several small, preliminary studies of the use of MMF as a replacement for, or to permit reduction of the dose of, cyclosporine in patients with chronic cyclosporine-associated nephrotoxicity (88–91).

THE EFFECT OF MMF ON ANTIBODY PRODUCTION IN HUMANS

A study by Kimball et al evaluated the effect of MMF on anti-ATGAM (IgG) antibody formation in renal transplant recipients (63). Forty-seven patients receiving ATGAM and standard therapy with prednisone and cyclosporine were randomized to receive, in addition, either azathioprine or MMF. Anti-ATGAM antibody was detected in 67% of patients receiving azathioprine, in 17% of those receiving MMF at 25 mg/kg/day, and in only 10% of those receiving MMF at 30 mg/kg/day ($P < 0.02$).

Suppression of the humoral immune response by MMF has also been demonstrated by Smith et al (92), who observed a profound (and statistically significant) depression in the response to influenza vaccination in patients immunosuppressed with MMF. Fifty percent of the nonimmunosuppressed controls responded to the vaccination, 33% of the recipients who received AZA responded, but only 10% of the recipients who received MMF responded.

These studies provide further evidence that MMF attenuates the humoral arm of the human immune system.

PHARMACOKINETICS

As noted earlier, mycophenolate mofetil, a prodrug, was developed by researchers at Syntex who were searching for a conjoiner of MPA with increased oral bioavailability. MMF, the morpholinoethyl ester of MPA (Fig. 10.4) was thus developed. It was initially found in primates to have twice the bioavailability of MPA (93,94). MMF is rapidly hydrolyzed by gastrointestinal tract esterases to MPA, its active metabolite. This metabolism is so rapid and complete that no measurable concentrations of MMF in the plasma have been obtained in healthy volunteers or transplant patients after oral administration (95,96). Mycophenolic acid is then converted in the liver (and likely elsewhere) to its glucuronide metabolite, mycophenolic acid glucuronide (MAPG), which is pharmacologically inactive (see Fig. 10.4). The glucuronide moiety is excreted in the urine; in fact, an average of 90% of radiolabeled drug was recovered in the urine after oral administration to healthy volunteers (97). This confirms that MAPG is indeed the primary metabolite of MPA, and that urinary excretion is its primary route of clearance. MAPG undergoes significant enterohepatic circulation, which results in considerable deglucuronidation and reabsorption as MPA. Enterohepatic circulation produces secondary peaks occurring between 6 and 12 hours following ingestion, and again at approximately 24 hours (96,97). Thus, the mean elimination half-life is approximately 16 hours. The pharmacologic activity of MMF is a function of the concentration of free MPA in the plasma (96,97). MPA is extensively bound to serum albumin in humans. Cyclosporine, FK506, and prednisone do not alter this binding (98). As shown in healthy volunteers, MPA reaches its peak plasma concentration at approximately 1 hour following MMF dosing. However, absorption is delayed for approximately 1 hour in the presence of food (96). The area under the plasma concentration time curve (AUC) for MPA increases in a dose-dependent fashion (59). In the phase I trial, it was noted that blood concentrations of MPA were low in the initial post-transplant period; however, they significantly increased over time. In addition, considerable variation in peak and trough concentrations of MPA were seen between individual patients. The long elimination half-life and the extensive protein binding of MPA may be the cause of the variation in blood concentration between that seen early after renal transplantation and that seen later on. Differences in absorption of MMF do not seem to play a role early on, as there is no significant difference in the AUC between oral and intravenous administration immediately after transplantation (oral and IV MMF have equivalent bioavailabilities) (99). Renal impairment has no effect on the pharmacokinetics of MPA, but it does decrease the clearance of MPAG (as a function of glomeru-

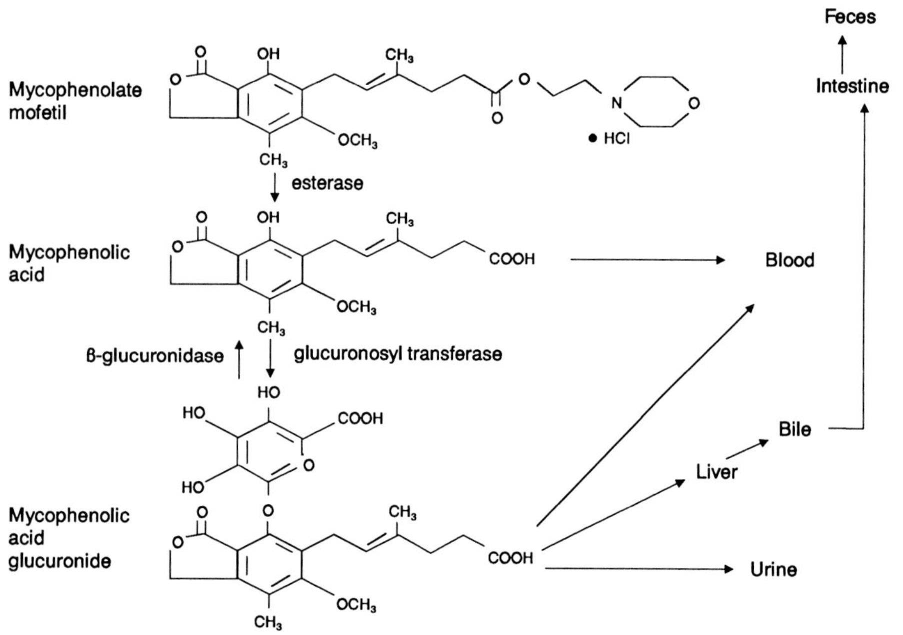

FIGURE 10.4. *The chemical structures of mycophenolate mofetil, mycophenolic acid, and the glucuronide metabolite.*

lar filtration rate). Indeed, the AUCs for MPAG, which is inactive, can increase two to threefold with renal dysfunction after transplantation. Serum levels of the drug are not significantly affected by hemodialysis (96). In addition, the pharmacokinetics of MMF are not changed by coadministration of ganciclovir (100).

THERAPEUTIC DRUG MONITORING

Plasma levels of MPA are measured using high-pressure liquid chromatography. Clinical pharmacokinetic studies suggest a strong correlation between the area under the MPA 24-hour curve and the prevention of rejection (60,97,101). Only free MPA is active (95,97,102). Although direct measurement of MPA is useful, new modes of evaluation to determine the most effective plasma levels for MPA are being developed. Specifically, IMPDH activity in whole blood can be monitored to determine the degree of inhibition of this enzyme by MPA (103,104). Langman et al (105) studied such monitoring in normal patients and in renal transplant recipients. They demonstrated that, in vitro, the maximum inhibition of IMPDH in intact cells in whole blood is 60% to 70%. Fifty percent inhibition occurred at 2–5 mg/L and complete inhibition of IMPDH activity was achieved in lysed cells with 20 mg/L. In vivo, the expected inverse relationship between MPA concentration and IMPDH activity was observed. The maximal inhibition detected, at peak concentrations (occurring 1 hour after dosing), produced 40% inhibition of IMPDH activity. Thus, perhaps only downregulation, not complete inhibition, is required to achieve immunosuppression. Inhibition of IMPDH activity persisted for 8 hours after dosing and little or no inhibition was detected at 12 hours after dosing, suggesting that an 8-hour dosing interval might maintain optimal inhibition of IMPDH. In the 23 normal subjects tested in this study, IMPDH activity followed a gaussian distribution and exhibited considerable variation between subjects (the standard deviation was relatively large with respect to the mean). Such variability might indicate that IMPDH activity in patients should be monitored. To justify widespread monitoring of IMPDH activity, however, the dose–activity relationship must be confirmed in large populations and the minimal activity level required for adequate immunosuppression must also be determined. In practice, drug concentrations or activity measurements may not be needed because interindividual variability in MPA concentrations has been relatively low and the therapeutic, yet tolerable dose range of MMF (2–3 g/day) remains narrow (99). Multicenter trials are required to determine whether MPA levels or IMPDH activity should be routinely monitored.

ADVERSE EFFECTS

The effects of MMF have been studied in over 1500 patients. The major adverse effects of MMF are gastrointestinal and hematologic. Most of the adverse effects are mild, and discontinuation of MMF is seldom required. The most common gastrointestinal side effects are abdominal pain, nausea, diarrhea, gastroenteritis, and gastritis. The most common hematologic disorders are leukopenia and thrombocytopenia, with occasional pancytopenia. As with other immunosuppressive modalities, opportunistic infections, especially with CMV, are somewhat common. Lymphomas have been reported infrequently, and there is reason to believe that the antiproliferative effect of MMF may decrease the rates of lymphoma. The adverse effects observed in the US multicenter study are listed in Table 10.9.

Table 10.9. Infections and Adverse Effects from the US Renal Transplant Mycophenolate Mofetil Study Group

Group	AZA (1–2 mg/kg)	MMF (1 g/BID)	MMF (1.5 g/BID)
Patients enrolled	166	167	166
Patients with 1 or more opportunistic infection	46%	45%	47%
CMV viremia syndrome	15%	15%	13%
Tissue-invasive CMV	6%	9%	11%
Herpes simplex	14%	13%	15%
Herpes zoster	4%	5%	7%
Candida	23%	19%	22%
Diarrhea	24%	32%	37%
Esophagitis	3%	6%	7%
Gastritis	0%	6%	4%
Gastrointestinal hemorrhage	1%	4%	4%
Lymphoma/lymphoproliferative disorder	0%	1%	1%
Neutropenia (absolute neutrophil count <500/μL)	1%	1%	1%
Thrombocytopenia (<50/mL in the first 30 days)	1%	1%	3%
Severe anemia (hemoglobin <6.5 mg/dL)	4%	4%	8%

Mild anemia and hypertension, like diarrhea, were relatively common, but their rates (37% for anemia and 31% for hypertension) did not differ between treatment groups. Leukopenia (1%) and sepsis (1%), which also occurred at similar rates between groups, were the most frequent adverse events leading to discontinuation of the drug.

DRUG INTERACTIONS

The serum concentrations of cyclosporine and tacrolimus are unaltered by MMF. However, tacrolimus appears to increase the immunosuppressive activity of MMF (106). Absorption of MMF is close to 100%, but antacids containing magnesium and aluminum can interfere with absorption, and should not be given concurrently with MMF (96). Cholestyramine decreases enterohepatic recycling, and therefore, decreases the 24-hour AUC for MPA. Thus, bile acid binders should be avoided (95,96).

CONCLUSION

The introduction of MMF into clinical transplantation may be the most important advance since the introduction of the immunophilin binders cyclosporine and tacrolimus. The theoretical considerations of Allison, Nelson, and Eugui have been borne out in the clinical trials of MMF in transplantation. Other than infrequent myelosuppression and gastrointestinal toxicity, which is usually mild, there are minimal untoward effects from treatment with MMF. Because of its greater immunosuppressive activity, however, there does appear to be a higher incidence of tissue-invasive CMV disease.

With the major advances achieved in the treatment of acute allograft rejection, attention is now being focused on chronic rejection. There are several theoretical considerations suggesting that MMF may play a significant role in reducing the severity of chronic rejection. This remains to be seen as long-term data from treatment with MMF become available. Thus, MMF proven safe and efficacious for prevention of rejection in renal allografts, is now being evaluated in the prevention and treatment of rejection in other solid organs. In addition, MMF may have uses outside the realm of transplantation.

COMMENTARY

Carl G. Groth and Christina Brattström

During the past two decades, immunosuppressive protocols have been based on cyclosporine. More recently, tacrolimus has emerged as an interesting alternative. Both of these drugs are characterized by high efficacy but also by dose-limiting, multiorgan toxicity. The goal for the future is to find more specific, less toxic immunosuppressive agents.

Mycophenolate mofetil (MMF) has been introduced as a novel immunosuppressive agent with significant efficacy, high specificity, and low toxicity. Over 3000 patients have by now been enrolled in studies of this drug. Its toxicity differs distinctly from that of cyclosporine and tacrolimus, as the toxic symptoms arise mainly in the gastrointestinal tract and the hematologic system (1). In this commentary, we have elected to focus on the safety of MMF. Also, we have some comments concerning ways of using the drug in clinical practice.

CLINICAL TRIALS

Pioneer studies in animals and humans were performed by Morris (2), Sollinger (3), and their colleagues in the early 1990s. In 1992, three large, prospective, randomized, multicenter studies in renal transplant recipients were launched. One study was located in Europe (4), one covered three continents (5), and the third was done in the United States (6). Each of the studies recruited nearly 500 patients, making this the most ambitious scheme ever employed in evaluating an immunosuppressive agent. The three studies were similar in design, patient population, and timing. All patients received cadaveric renal transplants, and the baseline immunosuppression used was cyclosporine and prednisolone. In the US study the patients were also given antithymocyte globulin (ATG) for induction (6).

In each study the patients were randomized into three groups: 1) control patients, 2) patients given MMF, 2 g/day, and 3) patients given MMF, 3 g/day. In the European study, control patients were given placebo. In the two other studies they received azathioprine. The primary end point of the studies was treatment failure or the occurrence of acute rejection.

Findings in the three studies were remarkably similar, in that the frequency of acute rejection in patients given MMF was approximately half of that in the control groups, whether the latter patients had received azathioprine or placebo (4–6). However, the graft and patient survival figures at 6 and 12 months after transplantation were no better in patients given MMF.

SAFETY OF MMF

The European study, comparing MMF with placebo, was particularly relevant in regards to assessing the toxicity of MMF (4).

In the placebo group, 4% of the patients suffered adverse events that led to discontinuation of the treatment. The corresponding figures were 8.5% in the MMF 2 g/day, and 18% in the MMF 3 g/day groups. Gastrointestinal problems were the most common adverse events. Some symptoms, such as diarrhea, abdominal pain, and dyspepsia, were equally prevalent in all three groups. Stomach and duodenal ulcers, which occurred in a few patients, were also equally distributed between the three groups. Nausea, gastroenteritis, and vomiting, however, were more common in the MMF-treated patients, and these symptoms were most frequently seen in the MMF 3 g/day patients. Life-threatening complications—gastrointestinal hemorrhage, large bowel perforation, and pancreatitis—occurred in a small number of patients treated with MMF, but not in any patient given placebo (Table 10C.1).

Hematologic problems comprised the second largest group of adverse events. Thus, leukopenia had an approximately threefold higher incidence in the MMF-treated patients than in the placebo-treated patients. Anemia was also observed more frequently in the two MMF groups. Thrombocytopenia was equally common in all three groups. Pancytopenia occurred in two MMF 2 g/day patients, and agranulocytosis occurred in two of the MMF 3 g/day patients. All four patients recovered after cessation of MMF (Table 10C.2).

Table 10C.1. Gastrointestinal Adverse Events, European Study

	Placebo (n = 166)	MMF 2 grams (n = 165)	MMF 3 grams (n = 160)
Diarrhea	21 (12.7%)	21 (12.7%)	25 (15.6%)
Abdominal pain	18 (10.8%)	19 (11.5%)	18 (11.3%)
Dyspepsia	9 (5.4%)	5 (3.0%)	8 (5.0%)
Nausea	4 (2.4%)	7 (4.2%)	10 (6.3%)
Gastroenteritis	2 (1.2%)	4 (2.4%)	7 (4.4%)
Vomiting	2 (1.2%)	4 (2.4%)	6 (3.8%)
Stomach ulcer	3 (1.8%)	2 (1.2%)	2 (1.3%)
Duodenal ulcer	1 (0.6%)	2 (1.2%)	1 (0.6%)
Gastrointestinal hemorrhage	0	0	2 (1.3%)
Rectal hemorrhage	0	1 (0.6%)	1 (0.6%)
Duodenal ulcer hemorrhage	0	1 (0.6%)	0
Hemorrhagic pancreatitis and gastritis	0	0	1 (0.6%)
Large intestine perforation	0	2 (1.2%)	2 (1.3%)

Table 10C.2. Hematologic/Lymphatic Adverse Events, European Study

	Placebo (n = 166)	MMF 2 grams (n = 165)	MMF 3 grams (n = 160)
Leukopenia	7 (4.2%)	18 (10.9%)	22 (13.8%)
Anemia	3 (1.8%)	7 (4.2%)	11 (6.8%)
Thrombocytopenia	8 (4.8%)	7 (4.2%)	5 (3.1%)
Pancytopenia	0	3 (1.8%)	0
Agranulocytosis	0	0	2 (1.3%)
Other	8 (4.8%)	17 (10.3%)	8 (5.0%)

Since patients in the MMF arms were given an additional immunosuppressive drug, they ran an obvious risk of developing opportunistic infections. Indeed, herpes zoster and herpes simplex were more common in the MMF-treated patients, and CMV tissue-invasive disease was overrepresented in the MMF 3 g/day group (Table 10C.3). Cytomegalovirus (CMV) viremia/syndrome, however, was equally common in the three groups, as were candidal infections.

In the tricontinental study comparing MMF to azathioprine, gastrointestinal and hematologic symptoms were again the main adverse events (5). Interestingly, the overall incidence of these events was quite similar in all three treatment arms. Diarrhea seemed more common in the MMF-treated patients, whereas thrombocytopenia was perhaps less common (Table 10C.4).

The more severe GI complications in MMF 3 g/day patients included enteric infections (n = 9), colitis (n = 3), and hepatitis (n = 5). These conditions, along with nausea, were the main events leading to discontinuation or interruption of the MMF treatment. With regard to infectious events, CMV tissue-invasive disease occurred more frequently in patients who were given 3 g/day MMF than in those given 2 g/day MMF or azathioprine (Table 10C.5).

Table 10C.3. Opportunistic Infections, European Study

	Placebo (n = 166)	MMF 2 grams (n = 165)	MMF 3 grams (n = 160)
CMV viremia/ syndrome	22 (13.3%)	26 (15.8%)	24 (15.0%)
CMV tissue-invasive disease	4 (2.4%)	5 (3.0%)	11 (6.9%)
Herpes simplex	10 (6.0%)	24 (14.5%)	18 (11.3%)
Herpes zoster	3 (1.8%)	11 (6.7%)	8 (5.0%)
Candida	13 (7.8%)	16 (9.7%)	9 (5.6%)
Pneumocystis carinii pneumonia	4 (2.4%)	0	0
Aspergillus/Mucor	1 (0.6%)	0	0

Table 10C.4. Adverse Events Excluding Infections, Tricontinental Study

	AZA 100–150 mg (n = 162)	MMF 2 grams (n = 171)	MMF 3 grams (n = 164)
Gastrointestinal			
Diarrhea	17%	28%	31%
Abdominal pain	23%	26%	31%
Nausea	20%	14%	20%
Vomiting	6%	12%	16%
Hematologic			
Leukopenia	30%	19%	35%
Anemia	10%	15%	9%
Thrombocytopenia	12%	9%	5%

In the US study, which also made a comparison with azathioprine, the toxicity findings were very similar to those of the tricontinental study (6). However, the incidence of CMV tissue-invasive disease was no higher in the MMF 3 g/day group than in the MMF 2 g/day or azathioprine group.

Data from the placebo-controlled study (4) thus confirmed early findings (1) that MMF may cause significant GI and hematologic toxicity. In most instances these adverse events were mild or moderate, but in some instances life-threatening conditions occurred. As could be expected, adding MMF to cyclosporine and prednisolone caused an increased incidence of viral infections.

Table 10C.5. Infections, Tricontinental Study

	AZA 100–150 mg (n = 162)	MMF 2 grams (n = 171)	MMF 3 grams (n = 164)
Opportunistic infections	44%	46%	46%
CMV viremia/ syndrome	12%	12%	11%
CMV tissue-invasive disease	6%	7%	11%
Herpes simplex	25%	21%	25%
Herpes zoster	7%	7%	8%
Candida	12%	12%	12%
P. carinii pneumonia	2	0	0
Aspergillus/Mucor	<1%	<1%	<1%

Taken together, the tricontinental and the US study included approximately 300 patients who were given azathioprine. The monitoring of these patients has provided an up-to-date database regarding the safety of this classic drug. It is noteworthy that the incidences of leukopenia and anemia were very similar with the azathioprine and MMF treatments. Surprisingly, the incidence of gastrointestinal adverse events was no less in azathioprine-treated patients than in those given MMF—azathioprine is apparently more toxic in this respect than hitherto reported. Regarding viral infections, the findings were very similar in patients given azathioprine and those given MMF.

FUTURE CLINICAL APPLICATIONS OF MMF

Initially, MMF was tried in patients with renal allograft rejection during cyclosporine-based treatment. When these patients had MMF added, more than half of the grafts were rescued (7). More recently, similar results were obtained in a larger study where MMF or steroids were given for refractory rejection (8). Thus, MMF can be used for graft rescue, as has been done with tacrolimus.

The three large multicenter studies have proved that MMF effectively prevents renal graft rejection. A case can therefore be made for employing the drug routinely in all renal transplant recipients. However, some groups have chosen a more restricted use. One reason for this is that the 1-year patient and graft survival figures have not shown significant improvement by MMF treatment. The patients selected for MMF treatment may be immunologically high-risk patients or those who are particularly vulnerable for steroid treatment.

Thus, it may seem rational to limit MMF treatment to the first 6 or perhaps 12 months, as most acute rejection episodes occur within this time. Cost containment could favor such a policy. Such short-term treatment, however, would preclude or reduce the possible gains in regard to chronic rejection.

Because of its ability to suppress B-cell and antibody production, and to inhibit vascular smooth-muscle cell proliferation, MMF has been heralded as a drug that could be effective in chronic rejection. Long-term evaluation of patients in the prevention studies will, hopefully, elucidate this matter. Studies aimed at treatment of chronic rejection are also being contemplated. Patients developing chronic rejection could be randomized to receive MMF or placebo, with renal function and graft histology serving as study parameters. However, no such study has yet been implemented.

On the basis of the findings in the three multicenter studies, the preferred dose of MMF seems to be 2 g/day. This dose was just as effective as 3 g/day in preventing rejection and it has significantly less toxicity. However, MMF at 3 g/day may be used in selected patients. In case of toxicity, a temporary reduction in doses can be made, but prolonged treatment with doses below 2 g/day may not provide adequate immunosuppression. Doses above 3 g/day should not be used, for toxicity reasons.

With the advent of a new immunosuppressive drug, an important question is whether the drug will permit sparing of the old drugs. Indeed, studies in which MMF is given in conjunction with reduced doses of steroids or cyclosporine are in progress. The results are eagerly awaited.

A combination of MMF with other new immunosuppressive drugs offers another highly interesting possibility. Two ongoing studies in renal transplant recipients are exploring such combinations. In a European multicenter phase II study, the efficacy and safety of MMF given in combination with tacrolimus are being assessed. A similar study explores the use of MMF given in conjunction with rapamycin.

CHAPTER REFERENCES

1. Allison AC, Eugui EM, Sollinger HW. Mycophenolate mofetil (RS-61443): mechanisms of action and effects in transplantation. Transplant Rev 1993;7:129–139.
2. Giblett ER, Anderson JE, Cohen F, et al. Adenosine deaminase deficiency in two patients with severely impaired cellular immunity. Lancet 1972;2:1067.
3. Allison AC, Hovi T, Watts RWE, et al. Immunological observations on patients with the Lesch-Nyhan syndrome, and on the role of de novo purine synthesis in lymphocyte transformation. Lancet 1975;2:1179.
4. Franklin TJ, Cook JM. The inhibition of nucleic acid synthesis by mycophenolic acid. Biochem J 1969;113:515.
5. Verham R, Meek TD, Hedstrom L, et al. Purification, characterization and kinetic analysis of inosine-5-monophosphate dehydrogenase of *Trichomonas foetus*. Mol Biochem Parasitol 1987;24:1.
6. Penn I. Tumors of the immunocompromised patient. Annu Rev Med 1988;39:63.
7. Natsumeda Y, Ohno S, Kawasaki H, et al. Two distinct cDNAs for human IMP dehydrogenase. J Biol Chem 1990;265:5292.
8. Konno Y, Natsumeda Y, Nagai M, et al. Expression of IMP dehydrogenase types I and II in *Escherichia coli* and distribution in normal lymphocytes and HL-60 leukemic cells. Cancer Res 1992;52:258.
9. Suthanthiran M, Morris RE, Strom TB. Immunosuppressants: cellular and molecular mechanisms of action. Am J Kidney Dis 1996;28:159–172.

10. Eugui EM, Almquist S, Muller CD, et al. Lymphocyte-selective cytostatic and immunosuppressive effects of mycophenolic acid in vitro: role of deoxyguanosine nucleotide depletion. Scan J Immunol 1991;33:175.
11. Dayton JS, Turka LA, Thompson CB, et al. Comparison of the effect of mizoribine with those of azathioprine 6-mercaptopurine and mycophenolic acid on T-lymphocyte proliferation and purine ribonucleotide metabolism. Mol Pharmacol 1992;41:671.
12. Altmann DM, Hoff N, Trowsdale J, et al. Cotransfection of ICAM-1 and HLA-DR reconstitutes human antigen-presenting mouse L cells. Nature 1989;338:512.
13. Isobe M, Yagita H, Okumura K, et al. Specific acceptance of cardiac allograft after treatment with antibodies to ICAM-1 and LFA-1. Science 1992;225:1125.
14. Allison AC, Kowalski WJ, Muller CJ, et al. Mycophenolic acid and brequinar, inhibitors of purine and pyrimidine synthesis, block the glycosylation of adhesion molecules. Transplant Proc 1993;25(suppl 2):67.
15. Grailer A, Nichols J, Hullet D, et al. Inhibition of human B-cell responses in vitro by RS-61443, cyclosporine A, and FK-506. Transplant Proc 1991;23:314.
16. Eugui EM, Mirkovich A, Allison AC. Lymphocyte-selective antiproliferative and immunosuppressive effects of mycophenolic acid in mice. Scand J Immunol 1991;33:175–183.
17. Kozlowski T, Tibell A, Morpurgo E, et al. Suppression of immunoglobulin resynthesis after plasmapheresis: efficacy of various immunosuppressive drugs—a study in rats. Transplant Proc 1995;27:3545–3546.
18. Burlingham WJ, Grailer AP, Hullett DA, Sollinger HW. Inhibition of both MLC and in vitro IgG memory response to tetanus toxoid by RS-61443. Transplantation 1991;51:545–547.
19. Nagy SE, Andersson JP, Andersson UG. Effect of mycophenolate mofetil (RS-61443) on cytokine production: inhibition of superantigen-induced cytokines. Immunopharmacology 1993;26:11–20.
20. Morris RE, Hoyt EG, Eugui EM, Allison AC. Prolongation of rat heart allograft survival by RS61443. Surg Forum 1989;40:337.
21. Morris RE, Hoyt EG, Murphy MP, Eugui EM. Mycophenolic acid morpholinoethylester (RS-61443) is a new immunosuppressant that prevents and halts cardiac rejection by selective inhibition of T- and B-cell purine synthesis. Transplant Proc 1990;22:1659–1662.
22. Morris RE, Hoyt EG, Eugui EM, Allison AC. Prolongation of rat heart allograft survival by RS-61443. Surg Forum 1989;40:337.
23. Morris RE, Wang J, Blum JR, et al. Immunosuppressive effects of the morpholinoethyl ester of mycophenolic acid (RS-61443) in rat and nonhuman primate recipients in heart allografts. Transplant Proc 1991;23(suppl 2):19–25.
24. Vu MD, Qi S, Xu D, et al. Synergistic effects of mycophenolate mofetil and sirolimus in prevention of acute heart, pancreas, and kidney allograft rejection and in reversal of ongoing heart allograft rejection in the rat. Transplantation 1998;66:1575–1580.
25. Knechtle SJ, Wang J, Burlingham WJ, et al. The influence of RS-61443 on antibody-mediated rejection. Transplantation 1992;53:699–701.
26. Kawamura T, Hullett DA, Suzuki Y, et al. Enhancement of allograft survival by combination RS-61443 and DUP-785 therapy. Transplantation 1993;55:691.
27. Ostraat O, Qi Z, Olausson M, et al. Additive immunosuppressive effect of combined mycophenolate mofetil and cyclosporin A in experimental rat cardiac transplantation. Transplant Proc 1995;27:3540.
28. D'Silva M, Antoniou E, DeRoover A, et al. Immunosuppressive effect of RS-61443 on rat cardiac allograft survival in combination with leflunomide or FK 506. Transplant Proc 1996;28:930–931.
29. Platz KP, Sollinger HW, Hullett DA, et al. RS-61443: a new, potent immunosuppressive agent. Transplantation 1991;51:27.
30. Platz KP, Bechstein WO, Eckhoff DE, et al. RS-61443 reverses acute allograft rejection in dogs. Surgery 1991;110:736.
31. Platz KP, Eckhoff DE, Hullett DA, Sollinger HW. RS-61443 studies: review and proposal. Transplant Proc 1991;23(suppl 2):33.
32. Bechstein WO, Schilling M, Steele DM, et al. RS-61443/cyclosporine combination therapy prolongs canine liver allograft survival. Transplant Proc 1993;25:702.
33. D'Alessandro AM, Rankin M, McVey J, et al. Prolongation of canine intestinal allograft survival with RS-61443, cyclosporine, and prednisone. Transplantation 1993;55:695.
34. Nakajima K, Ochiai T, Nagata M, et al. Effects of triple therapy of cyclosporine, FK 506, and RS-61443 on allogeneic small bowel transplantation in dogs. Transplant Proc 1993;25:595.
35. D'Alessandro AM, Rankin MA. Heterotopic rat intestinal transplantation: effect of cyclosporine and RS-61443 on graft-vs-host disease and rejection. Transplant Proc 1994;26:1611.
36. Shaffer D, Blakely ML, Gottschalk R, Monaco AP. Small bowel transplantation in rats using RS-61443: effect on GVHD and rejection. Transplant Proc 1992;24:1159.
37. Benhaim P, Anthony JP, Lin LY-T, et al. A long-term study of allogeneic rat hindlimb transplants immunosuppressed with RS-61443. Transplantation 1993;56:911.
38. van den Helder TBM, Benhaim P, Anthony JP, et al. Efficacy of RS-61443 in reversing acute rejection in a rat model of hindlimb allotransplantation. Transplantation 1994;57:427.
39. Benhaim P, Anthony JP, Ferreira L, et al. Use of combination of low-dose cyclosporine and RS-61443 in a rat hindlimb model of composite tissue allotransplantation. Transplantation 1996;61:527–532.
40. Ustuner ET, Zdichavsky M, Ren X, et al. Long-term composite tissue allograft survival in a porcine model with cyclosporin/mycophenolate mofetil therapy. Transplantation 1998;66:1581–1587.
41. Hao L, Lafferty KJ, Allison AC, Eugui EM. RS-61443 allows islet allografting and specific tolerance induction in adult mice. Transplant Proc 1990;22:876.
42. Lafferty KJ. Facilitation of specific tolerance induction in adult mice by RS-61443. Transplantation 1992;53:590.
43. Hao L, Wang Y, Chan S-M, Lafferty KJ. Effect of mycophenolate mofetil on islet allografting to chemically induced or spontaneously diabetic animals. Transplant Proc 1992;24:2843.
44. Qi S, Chen H, Xu D, Daloze P. Prolongation of pancreas allograft survival by mycophenolate mofetil in the rat. Transplant Proc 1996;28:932–933.
45. Hullett DA, Landry AS, Eckhoff DE, et al. DAB486-IL-2 (IL-2-toxin) in combination with low-dose RS-61443 (mycophenolate mofetil) prolongs mouse murine thyroid allograft survival. Transplant Proc 1993;25:756.
46. Hullett DA, Kawamura T, Fujino Y, et al. Prolongation of allograft and xenograft survival with mycophenolate mofetil (RS-61443) and brequinar sodium (DUP-785). Transplant Proc 1993;25:700.
47. Fujino Y, Kawamura T, Hullett DA, Sollinger HW. Evaluation of cyclosporine, mycophenolate mofetil, and brequinar sodium combination therapy on hamster-to-rat cardiac xenotransplantation. Transplantation 1994;57:41.
48. McManus RP, O'Hair DP, Komorowski R, Scott JP. Immunosuppressant combinations in primate cardiac xenografts. Ann NY Acad Sci 1993;696:281.
49. O'Hair DP, McManus RP, Komorowski R. Inhibition of chronic vascular rejection in primate cardiac xenografts using mycophenolate mofetil. Ann Thorac Surg 1994;58:1311.
50. Beger C, Vajkoczy P, Menger MD, Messmer K. Effects of RS-61443 on pancreatic islet xenografts. Transplant Proc 1994;26:759.
51. Wennberg L, Wallgren AC, Sundberg B, et al. Immunosuppression with cyclosporin A in combination with leflunomide and mycophenolate mofetil prevents rejection of pig-islets transplanted into rats. Transplant Proc 1996;28:819.
52. Foegh ML. Chronic rejection-graft arteriosclerosis. Transplant Proc 1990;22:119.
53. Steele DM, Hullett DA, Bechstein WO, et al. Effects of immunosuppressive therapy on the rat aortic allograft model. Transplant Proc 1993;25:754.
54. Wagner E, Roy R, Marois Y, et al. Fresh venous allografts in peripheral arterial reconstruction in dogs: effects of histocompatibility and of short-term immunosuppression with cyclosporine A and mycophenolate mofetil. J Thorac Cardiovasc Surg 1995;110:1732–1744.
55. Lynch WS, Roenigk HH Jr. Mycophenolic acid for psoriasis. Arch Dermatol 1977;113:1203–1208.
56. Epinette WW, Parker CM, Jones EL, Greist MC. Mycophenolic acid for psoriasis: a review of pharmacology, long-term efficacy, and safety. J Am Acad Dermatol 1987;17:962–971.
57. Carter SB, Franklin TJ, Jones DF, et al. Mycophenolic acid: an anti-cancer compound with unusual properties. Nature 1969;223:848–850.
58. Williams RH, Lively DH, DeLong DC, et al. Mycophenolic acid: antiviral and antitumor properties. J Antibiot 1968;21:463–464.
59. Sollinger HW, Eugui EM, Allison AC. RS-61443: mechanism of action, experimental and early clinical results. Clin Transplant 1991;5:523–526.
60. Sollinger HW, Deierhoi MH, Belzer FO, et al. RS-61443: phase I clinical trial and pilot rescue study. Transplantation 1992;53:428–432.
61. Deierhoi MH, Sollinger HW, Diethelm AG, et al. One-year follow-up results of phase I trial of mycophenolate mofetil (RS-61443) in cadaveric renal transplantation. Transplant Proc 1993;25:693–694.
62. The Mycophenolate Mofetil Renal Refractory Rejection Study Group. Mycophenolate mofetil for the treatment of refractory, acute cellular renal transplant rejection. Transplantation 1996;61:722–729.
63. Kimball JA, Pescovitz MD, Book BK, Norman DJ. Reduced human IgG anti-ATGAM antibody formation in renal transplant recipients receiving mycophenolate mofetil. Transplantation 1995;60:1379–1383.
64. Ensley RD, Bristow MR, Olsen SL, et al. The use of mycophenolate mofetil (RS-61443) in human heart transplant recipients. Transplantation 1993;56:75–82.

65. Kirklin JK, Bourge RC, Naftel DC, et al. Treatment of recurrent heart rejection with mycophenolate mofetil (RS-61443): initial clinical experience. J Heart Lung Transplant 1994;13:444–450.
66. Kobashigawa J, Miller L, Renlund D, et al. A randomized active-controlled trial of mycophenolate mofetil in heart transplant recipients. Transplantation 1998;66:507–515.
67. Klintmalm GB, Ascher NL, Busuttil RW, et al. RS-61443 for treatment-resistant human liver rejection. Transplant Proc 1993;25:697.
68. Freise CE, Hebert M. Osorio RW, et al. Maintenance immunosuppression with prednisone and RS-61443 alone following liver transplantation. Transplant Proc 1993;25:1758–1759.
69. Eckhoff DE, McGuire BM, Frenette LR, et al. Tacrolimus (FK506) and mycophenolate mofetil combination therapy versus tacrolimus in adult liver transplantation. Transplantation 1998;65:180–187.
70. Stegall MD, Wachs ME, Everson G, et al. Prednisone withdrawal 14 days after liver transplantation with mycophenolate. Transplantation 1997;64:1755–1760.
71. Fisher RA, Ham JM, Marcos A, et al. A prospective randomized trial of mycophenolate mofetil with Neoral or tacrolimus after orthotopic liver transplantation. Transplantation 1998;66:1616–1621.
72. Paterson DL, Singh N, Panebianco A, et al. Infectious complications occurring in liver transplant recipients receiving mycophenolate mofetil. Transplantation 1998;66:593–598.
73. Sollinger HW, Odorico JS, Knechtle SJ, et al. Experience with 500 simultaneous pancreas-kidney transplants. Ann Surg 1998;228:284–296.
74. Odorico JS, Prisch JD, Knechtle SJ, et al. A study comparing mycophenolate mofetil to azathioprine in simultaneous pancreas-kidney transplantation. Transplantation 1998;66:1751–1759.
75. Gruessner RWG, Sutherland DER, Drangstveit MB, et al. Mycophenolate mofetil in pancreas transplantation. Transplantation 1998;66:318–323.
76. Stegall MD, Simon M, Wachs ME, et al. Mycophenolate mofetil decreases rejection in simultaneous pancreas-kidney transplantation when combined with tacrolimus or cyclosporin. Transplantation 1997;64:1695–1700.
77. Sollinger HW, for the U.S. Renal Transplant Mycophenolate Study Group. Mycophenolate mofetil for the prevention of acute rejection in primary cadaveric renal allograft recipients. Transplantation 1995;60:225–232.
78. Sullivan SD, Garrison LP, Best JH, et al. The cost effectiveness of mycophenolate mofetil in the first year after primary cadaveric transplant. J Am Soc Nephrol 1997;8:1592–1598.
79. European Mycophenolate Mofetil Cooperative Study Group. Placebo-controlled study of mycophenolate mofetil combined with cyclosporin and corticosteroids for prevention of acute rejection. Lancet 1995;345:1321–1325.
80. The Tricontinental Mycophenolate Mofetil Renal Transplantation Study Group. A blinded, randomized clinical trial of mycophenolate mofetil for the prevention of acute rejection in cadaveric renal transplantation. Transplantation 1996;61:1029–1037.
81. Mathew TH, for the Tricontinental Mycophenolate Mofetil Renal Transplantation Study Group. A blinded, long-term, randomized multicenter study of mycophenolate mofetil in cadaveric renal transplantation. Transplantation 1998;65:1450–1454.
82. Halloran P, Mathew T, Tomlanovich S, et al. for the International Mycophenolate Mofetil Renal Transplant Study Groups. Mycophenolate mofetil in renal allograft recipients. Transplantation 1997;63:39–47.
83. Weisel M, Carl S, for the European Mycophenolate Mofetil Cooperative Study Group. A placebo controlled study of mycophenolate mofetil used in combination with cyclosporin and corticosteroids for the prevention of acute rejection in renal allograft recipients: 10 year results. J Urol 1998;159:28–33.
84. The Mycophenolate Mofetil Acute Rejection Study Group. Mycophenolate mofetil for the treatment of a first acute renal allograft rejection. Transplantation 1998;65:235–241.
85. Neylan JF, for the U.S. Renal Transplant Mycophenolate Mofetil Study Group. Immunosuppressive therapy in high risk transplant patients. Transplantation 1997;64:1277–1282.
86 Schweitzer EJ, Yoon S, Fink J, et al. Mycophenolate mofetil reduces the risk of acute rejection less in African-American than in Caucasian kidney recipients. Transplantation 1988;65:242–248.
87. Roth D, Colona J, Burke GW, et al. Primary immunosuppression with tacrolimus and mycophenolate for renal allograft recipients. Transplantation 1998;65:248–252.
88. Weir MR, Anderson L, Kink JC, et al. A novel approach to the treatment of chronic allograft nephropathy. Transplantation 1997;64:1706–1710.
89. Ducloux D, Fournier V, Bresson-Vautrin C, et al. Mycophenolate mofetil in renal transplant recipients with cyclosporin-associated nephrotoxicity. Transplantation 1998;65:1504–1506.
90. Zanker B, Schneeberger H, Rothenpieler U, et al. Mycophenolate mofetil-based, cyclosporin-free induction and maintenance immunosuppression. Transplantation 1998;66:44–49.
91. Hueso M, Bover J, Seron D, et al. Low-dose cyclosporin and mycophenolate mofetil in renal allograft recipients with suboptimal renal function. Transplantation 1998;66:1727–1731.
92. Smith KGC, Isbel NM, Catton MG, et al. Suppression of the humoral immune response by mycophenolate mofetil. Nephrol Dial Transplant 1998;13:160–164.
93. Pirsch JD, Sollinger HW. Mycophenolate mofetil—clinical and experimental experience. Ther Drug Monit 1996;18:357–361.
94. Lee WA, Gu L, Miksztal AR, et al. Bioavailability improvement of mycophenolic acid through amino ester derivitization. Pharm Res 1990;7:161–166.
95. Shaw LM, Nowak I. Mycophenolic acid: measurement and relationship to pharmacologic effects. Ther Drug Monit 1995;17:685–689.
96. Bullingham RES, Nicholls A, Hale M. Pharmacokinetics of mycophenolate mofetil (RS-61443): a short review. Transplant Proc 1996;28:925–929.
97. Shaw LM, Sollinger HW, Halloran P, et al. Mycophenolate mofetil: a report of the consensus panel. Ther Drug Monit 1995;17:690–699.
98. Nowak I, Shaw LM. Mycophenolic acid binding to human serum albumin: characterization and relation to pharmacodynamics. Clin Chem 1995;41:1011–1017.
99. Bullingham RES, Nichols AJ, Kamm BR. Clinical pharmacokinetics of mycophenolate mofetil. Clin Pharmacokinet 1998;34:429–455.
100. Wolfe EJ, Mahtur V, Tomlanovich S, et al. Pharmacokinetics of mycophenolate mofetil and intravenous ganciclovir alone and in combination in renal transplantation patients. Pharmacotherapy 1997;17:591–598.
101. Takahashi K, Ochiai T, Uchida K, et al. Pilot study of mycophenolate mofetil (RS-61443) in the prevention of acute rejection following renal transplantation in Japanese patients. Transplant Proc 1995;27:1421–1424.
102. Li S, Yatscoff RW. Improved high-performance liquid chromatographic assay for the measurement of mycophenolic acid in human plasma. Transplant Proc 1996;28:938–940.
103. Langman LJ, LeGatt DF, Yaatscoff RW. Pharmacodynamic assessment of mycophenolic acid-induced immunosuppression by measuring IMP dehydrogenase activity. Clin Chem 1995;41:295–299.
104. Langman LJ, Shapiro AMJ, Lakey JRT, et al. Pharmacodynamic assessment of mycophenolic acid-induced immunosuppression by measurement of inosine monophosphate dehydrogenase activity in a canine model. Transplantation 1996;61:87–92.
105. Langman LJ, LeGatt DF, Halloran PF, et al. Pharmacodynamic assessment of mycophenolic acid induced immunosuppression in renal transplant recipients. Transplantation 1996;62:666–672.
106. Zucker K, Esquenazi V, Rosen A, et al. Unexpected augmentation of MMF pharmacokinetics in renal transplant patients receiving Prograf and CellCept in combination therapy, and analogous in vitro findings. Proceedings of the American Society of Transplant Surgeons 22nd Annual Scientific Meeting 1996:79.

COMMENTARY REFERENCES

1. Sollinger HW, Dierhof MH, Belzer FO, et al. RS-61443—a phase I clinical trial and pilot rescue study. Transplantation 1992;53:428–432.
2. Morris RE, Hoyt EG, Eugui EM, Allison AC. Prolongation of rat heart allograft survival by RS-61443. Surg Forum 1989;40:337.
3. Platz KP, Sollinger HW, Hullett DA, et al. RS-61443, a new, potent immunosuppressive agent. Transplantation 1990;51:27–31.
4. European Mycophenolate Mofetil Cooperative Study Group. Placebo-controlled study of mycophenolate mofetil combined with cyclosporin and corticosteroids for prevention of acute rejection. Lancet 1995;345:1321–1325.
5. The Tricontinental Mycophenolate Mofetil Renal Transplantation Study Group. A blinded, randomized clinical trial of mycophenolate mofetil for the prevention of acute rejection in cadaveric renal transplantation. Transplantation 1996;61:1029–1037.
6. Sollinger HW for the US Renal Transplant Mycophenolate Mofetil Study Group. Mycophenolate mofetil for the prevention of acute rejection in primary cadaveric renal allograft recipients. Transplantation 1995;60:225–232.
7. Sollinger HW, Belter FO, Deierhoi MH, et al. RS-61443 (mycophenolate mofetil). A multicenter study for refractory kidney transplant rejection. Ann Surg 1992;216:513–519.
8. The Mycophenolate Mofetil Renal Refractory Rejection Study Group. Mycophenolate mofetil for the treatment of refractory acute, cellular renal transplant rejection. Transplantation 1996;61:722–729.

Chapter

11

New Small Molecule Immunosuppressive Agents

FERDA SENEL BARRY D. KAHAN

The study of neoplastic agents led to the use of small molecule cytostatic antiproliferative agents, such as 6-mercaptopurine (6-MP), methotrexate (MTX), and cyclophosphamide, as the first immunosuppressive agents. These agents, however, displayed only modest activity when used in the clinical transplant setting, because their nonspecific modes of action caused serious bone marrow suppression with consequent impairment of host resistance and increased infection rates. More recently it was demonstrated that certain agents, namely cyclosporine (CsA), tacrolimus (TRL), and sirolimus (SRL), act selectively on the adaptive host response at different stages of the T- and B-cell cycles and spare nonspecific host resistance (Fig. 11.1). Unfortunately, owing to their significant toxic effects, it has been difficult to optimize the use of individual agents in monotherapy. Therefore, there has been interest in the use of combinations of these immunosuppressants as well as in the introduction of new small molecule agents that specifically alter T-cell function, such as 15-deoxyspergulain (DSG) and FTY720, which offer promising modes of immunosuppression.

NEW NUCLEOSIDE SYNTHESIS INHIBITORS

Mycophenolate Mofetil

Mycophenolate mofetil (MMF; RS-61443, Syntex, San Jose, CA) is the 2-morpholinoethyl ester of mycophenolic acid (MPA; Fig. 11.2), which is produced by several species of *Penicillium* (1). MMF, which is converted primarily in the liver to its active drug, MPA, by ester hydrolysis, was initially used in clinical trials for the treatment of psoriasis and rheumatoid arthritis (2–6) before being applied in experimental animal transplant models and in clinical transplantation by Sollinger et al (7,8). MMF has now been approved by many countries for use in the prophylaxis, but not reversal, of rejection episodes. (See Chapter 10 for a more detailed discussion of mycophenolate mofetil.)

Molecular Mode of Action

MPA noncompetitively and reversibly inhibits inosine monophosphate dehydrogenase (IMPDH) activity during the synthesis (S phase) of the cell cycle (Table 11.1). Because the salvage pathway of purine synthesis in lymphocytes is somewhat less active than the de novo pathway, lymphocytes depend on the conversion of 5-phosphoribosyl-1-phosphate (PRPP), which is synthesized from ribose-5P and adenosine triphosphate (ATP) by PRPP synthetase to inosine monophosphate (IMP). In turn, IMP is converted to guanosine monophosphate (GMP) by IMPDH. Some GMP, in contrast, is formed by the salvage pathway, in which guanine is converted to GMP by the action of hypoxanthine-guanine phosphoribosyltransferase (HGPRTase). MPA inhibits isozyme 2 (9,10), the primary isoform in human lymphocytes, and is upregulated in other cells upon stimulation. The mechanism of action of MMF is similar to that of mizorbine (MZB; Bredinin, C9H13N306, Tojo Pharma, Tokyo, Japan) (11,12) and is far more selective than that of azathioprine (Aza; Imuran, Burroughs-Wellcome, Research Triangle Park, NC), which exerts inhibitory effects on multiple enzymes in the de novo pathway. Eugi et al (13) found that MPA significantly reduced guanine triphosphate (GTP) levels, an effect that was reversed upon addition of deoxyguanosine ribonucleotides (13,14).

MPA inhibits the proliferation of T and B cells because their generation predominantly depends on de novo purine synthesis. After it was serendipitously discovered that MPA possessed immunosuppressive properties, Allison and Eugi (15) observed that MPA inhibited in vitro proliferative responses even when added 72 hours after stimulation with phytohemagglutinin (PHA) or pokeweed mitogen (PWM)

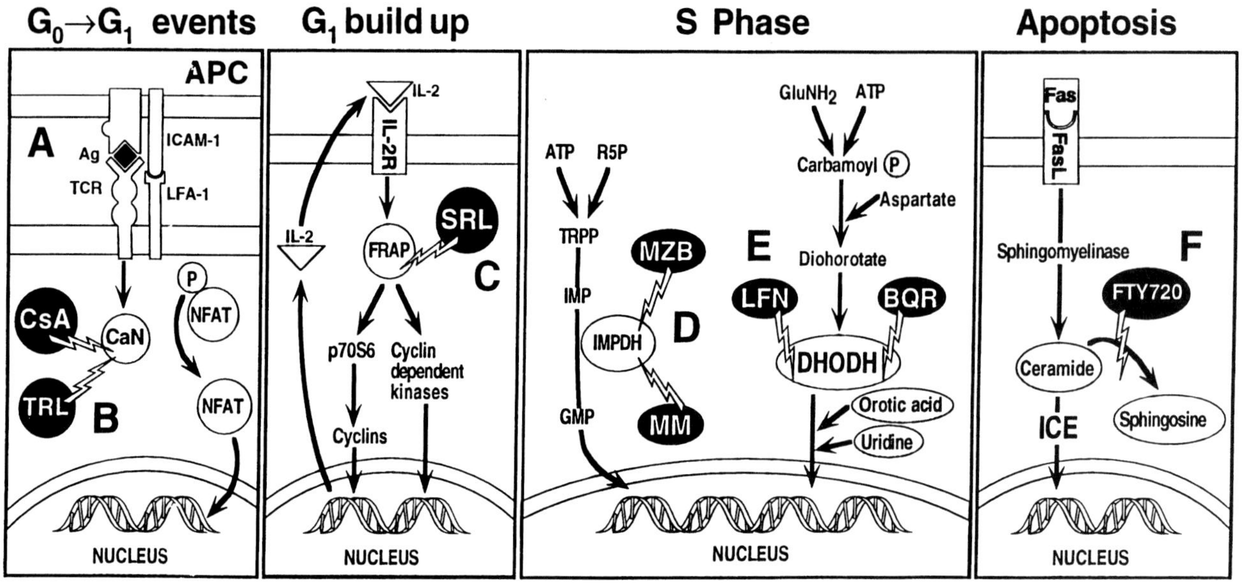

FIGURE 11.1. *Putative sites of T-cell–specific immunosuppressive agents. The sites of action can be classified in the G_0 to G_1 transition, wherein the intercellular adhesion molecule-1 (ICAM-1) antisense phosphorothioate oligonucleotide (PS-Oligo), denoted by A, inhibits the antigen presenting cell function of binding to lymphocyte function antigen-1 (LFA-1) (94). Also, engineered major histocompatibility complex (MHC) antigens act as altered peptide ligands (96). Cyclosporine (CsA) or tacrolimus (TRL) inhibits calcineurin (CaN), denoted by B, in the G_0 to G_1 pathway. During the G_1 buildup, sirolimus (SRL), denoted by C, inhibits the FK-RAPA associated protein (FRAP). In the S phase, mycophenolic acid or its analogue, mycophenolate mofetil (MM), as well as mizorbine (MZB), inhibits purine synthesis (denoted by D), and brequinar (BQR) or leflunomide (LFN) inhibits pyrimidine de novo biosynthesis (denoted by E). FTY720, denoted by F, favors the apoptotic pathway by possibly blocking ceramide degradation, thereby leading to ceramide accumulation and induction of apoptosis.*

Table 11.1. Site of Action of New Small Immunosuppressants During Cell Cycle Progression of Lymphocytes

Phase of Cell Cycle	Inhibitory Drug(s)
G_0	FTY720
$G_0 \rightarrow G_1$	CsA, TRL
G_1	SRL
S	MMF, BQR, LFN

(13). At concentrations of 100 nmol/L, MPA did not inhibit proliferation of nonstimulated fibroblasts or endothelial cells. Unlike CsA and TRL, MPA, at concentrations up to 100 nmol/L, did not affect interleukin (IL)-2 production (16). The depletion of intracellular guanosine-diphosphate intermediates not only affects DNA synthesis but may also inhibit the transfer of mannose and fucose to glycoproteins (17) such as the intercellular adhesion molecules (ICAMs) and very late antigen (VLA)-4 (18), and thereby may impair lymphocyte interactions with target cells (19).

Pharmacokinetics

MMF appears to have a 1.5-fold greater bioavailability than the parent compound MPA (20,21). After single-dose oral administration (20 mg/kg) to cynomolgus monkeys, MMF had a shorter time to peak concentration (t_{max}; 1.3 ± 0.6 hours) and a higher peak concentration (C_{max}) value (34 ± 11 µg/mL) than MPA (13 ± 6.5 hours and 6.9 ± 2.5 µg/mL, respectively) (20). After rapid oral absorption, the prodrug MMF is hydrolyzed in the liver to the active metabolite MPA, which is metabolized principally by hepatic glucuronyl transferase to form an inactive phenolic glucuronide (MPAG), which is secreted into the bile (7). Intestinal glucuronidase converts the inactive compound back into active MPA, which may explain the gastrointestinal toxicity of the drug and enterohepatic recycling (7).

MPA is almost exclusively found in the plasma fraction. Of the MPA in plasma, 7.2% to 16.5% is unbound, less than 10% is bound to lipoproteins, and the rest is primarily bound to nonalbumin proteins (22). Analysis of the pharmacokinetic profiles of cadaveric kidney transplant recipients treated with escalating doses of MMF (1000–1750 mg twice a day) showed that the values for the C_{max} and area under the concentration-time curve over a 24-hour period (AUC_{0-24}) increased in dose-proportionate fashion. For MMF, the C_{max} and AUC_{0-24} values ranged from 1.0 to 3.2 µg/mL and 6.4 to 37.6 µg/hr/mL, respectively. The presence of food lowered the C_{max} by 40% but had no effect on the AUC values. The terminal half-life ranged from 2.3 to 9.6 hours. The AUC_{0-24} values on day 1 after transplant were

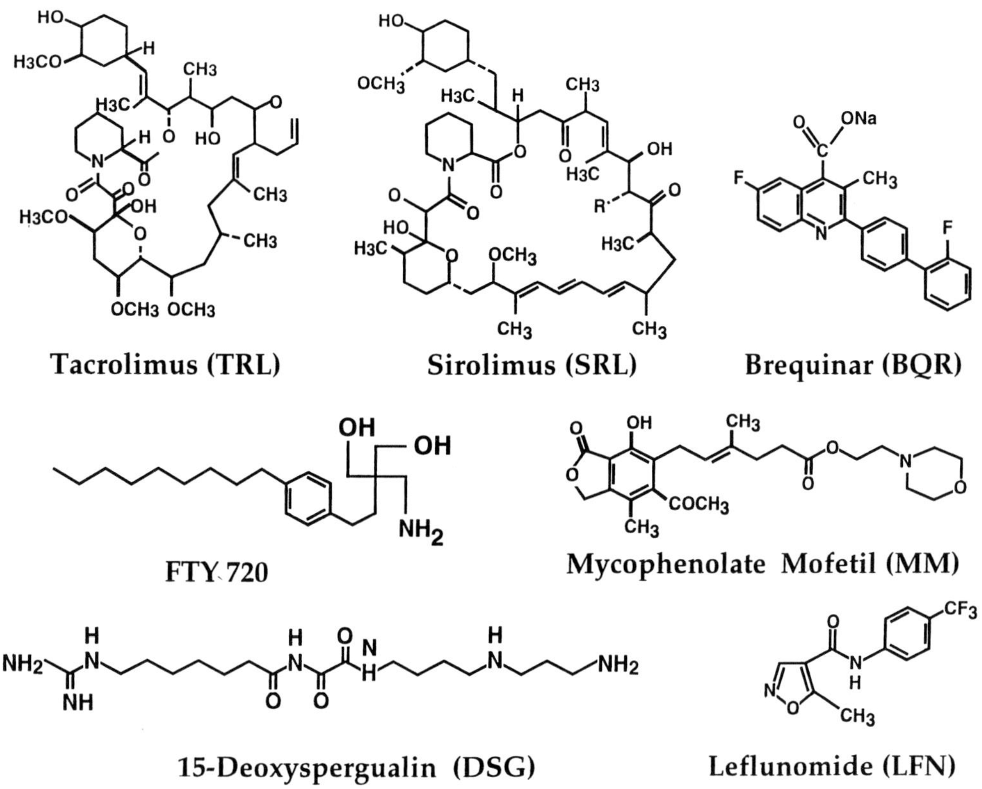

FIGURE 11.2. *Molecular structures of the small molecule immunosuppressants tacrolimus, sirolimus, brequinar, FTY720, mycophenolate mofetil, 15-deoxyspergualin, and leflunomide.*

significantly lower compared to those at day 20, suggesting improved absorption upon resolution of gastrointestinal ileus. In addition, there was also substantial interindividual variation in AUC values (23).

Clinical Applications

Clinical Toxicity in Transplantation and Psoriasis: Phase I Trials Jones et al (4) found that 14 of 29 psoriasis patients showed a clearing of their skin lesions; however, there was a high incidence of gastrointestinal side effects, including nausea, diarrhea, and anorexia. Other studies in psoriasis patients reported an increased incidence of neoplasms (0.08%) (5,6) as well as herpes zoster infections (11.6%) (6,24). Long-term studies in which 1600–7368 mg/day MPA was administered to psoriatic patients revealed that 72.4% of the patients experienced gastric toxicity (6,25), a side effect that was also observed among patients with refractory severe rheumatoid arthritis who were treated with MPA (1.0–1.5 g) twice daily (3,26).

A phase I study that enrolled 48 cadaveric kidney recipients showed that MMF used at doses of 100–3500 mg/day caused a dose-dependent gastrointestinal toxicity (gastritis, mild ileus) with no evidence of bone marrow suppression (23). An open-label single-center trial in which MMF was administered to 21 cadaveric renal transplant recipients at doses ranging from 250–3500 mg/day together with a CsA-prednisone maintenance immunosuppression regimen demonstrated that the limiting side effects of MMF include diarrhea, nausea, elevated liver enzymes, and an increased rate of infections, the most common of which was cytomegalovirus (CMV) (27). In liver transplant recipients, no significant differences were observed in infectious complications between MMF-treated and untreated patients (28).

Prophylaxis of Acute Rejection: Phase II Trials MMF was administered to primary cadaver kidney recipients at doses ranging from 100–3500 mg/day in conjunction with Minnesota Anti-Lymphocyte Globulin (MALG), CsA, and prednisone. A dose-dependent reduction in the incidence of rejection episodes occurred at doses of 2 g/day or more. Moreover, at these doses, there was a less frequent need to use OKT-3 to treat refractory rejection episodes (23). In small cohorts of patients, MMF reduced the incidence of acute rejection episodes among pediatric recipients of cadaveric donor renal allografts and reduced the rate of persistent or recurrent acute rejection episodes among 17 heart transplant patients (29). More recent studies in high-risk renal allograft recipients revealed that acute rejection is best prevented in African Americans (AAs) by an MMF dosage of 3000 mg/day, whereas 2000 mg/day provided a superior benefit/risk ratio for non-AAs (30).

Pilot Studies of Rescue Treatment An open-label study in 20 kidney transplant recipients, who were defined by the investigators as experiencing "refractory allograft rejection," suggested that the episodes were "reversed" in 4 of 5 (80%) living-related donor (LRD) grafts and in 7 of 15 (47%) cadaveric donor grafts (23). A multicenter study (31) of 75 kidney transplant recipients with biopsy-proven rejection episodes that were refractory to at least one course of antilymphocyte globulin (ALG)–OKT-3 revealed that MMF (2000–3500 mg/day) "rescued" the grafts in 52 of 75 (69%) patients, particularly among patients with an entry serum creatinine value below 4 mg/dL (Table 11.2). Another study randomly assigned 150 renal allograft recipients suffering refractory acute cellular rejection to treatment with MMF or steroids. Graft loss or death occurred in 14.3% of the MMF-treated group as compared with 26% of the steroid-treated patients (P = 0.08) (32). Prominent side effects included nausea, diarrhea, and a 40% overall infection rate with drug discontinuation required for patients who experienced pancreatitis, CMV colitis, and severe gastrointestinal complications. Upon review of these and other studies, the United States FDA did not consider the evidence for rejection reversal with MMF compelling.

Prophylaxis of Acute Rejection: Phase III Trials The European, double-blind, placebo-controlled multicenter study (33) enrolled 491 kidney transplant recipients who were randomized to receive placebo (n = 166), 2 g/day MMF (n = 165), or 3 g/day MMF (n = 160) in combination with CsA–prednisone therapy. Biopsy-proven rejection episodes occurred in 17.0% and 13.8% of patients treated with 2 g/day and 3 g/day MMF, respectively, versus a 46.4% rejection episode rate in the placebo group. For all groups, however, no improvement was observed in the six-month graft loss rate, which was 6.7% for 2 g/day MMF, 8.8% for 3 g/day MMF, and 10.2% for placebo. The US double-blind multicenter study (34) included 495 renal transplant recipients who were randomized to receive 2 g/day MMF (n = 167), 3 g/day MMF (n = 166), or 1–2 mg/kg/day Aza (n = 166) together with a CsA–prednisone regimen and antithymocyte globulin (ATG) induction therapy. Compared with a 38.0% rate of rejection episodes among patients in the Aza group, the rates for the 2 g and 3 g MMF groups were 19.8% and 17.5%, respectively, with similar six-month patient and graft survival rates. The time to first biopsy-proven rejection episode or to treatment failure was significantly greater for patients treated with 2 g MMF (P = 0.0036) or 3 g MMF (P = 0.0006) than for those treated with Aza. MMF also appeared to reduce the severity of the rejection episodes. The side effects associated with MMF treatment included diarrhea, leukopenia, tissue-invasive CMV disease, gastrointestinal toxicity, anemia, hypertension, and sepsis.

Potential Effects on Chronic Allograft Vasculopathy MMF has been reported to reduce intimal thickening and graft coronary disease in rats. To four Lewis (LEW; $RT1^l$) recipients of Brown Norway (BN; $RT1^n$) heart allografts, MMF was administered in doses of 30 mg/kg/day from day 1 through day 50, and 20 mg/kg/day from day 51 through day 100. At day 100 one graft had no coronary disease, two grafts had mild intimal proliferation, and one had moderate intimal thickening (35). A subsequent experiment found significantly (P = 0.011) reduced intimal proliferation in ACI aortic allografts transplanted into LEW recipients that received MMF at 40 mg/kg/day for 14 days followed by 30 mg/kg/day thereafter (36). Some researchers, however, failed to document a benefit of MMF in preventing graft vessel disease in a F344-to-LEW heterotopic heart transplant model; similar degrees of arterial intimal thickening in treated versus untreated animals were found (37). Among F344 renal allografts in LEW hosts, administration of MMF (15 mg/kg/day) starting at either day 1 (n = 5) or week 8 after transplant (n = 5) reduced the chronic histologic changes of interstitial fibrosis, tubular atrophy, glomerulosclerosis, and arterial obliteration, and the incidence of proteinuria (38). MMF (40 mg/kg PO for 13 days) also appeared to reduce the degree of arterial intimal thickening in four Sprague-Dawley rats exposed to mechanical injury by balloon dilatation, particularly when combined with sirolimus (1.5 mg/kg). However, there is no evidence that MMF affects the progression of graft vessel disease or chronic rejection in clinical studies.

Table 11.2. Potential Clinical Indications for the Use of Small Molecular Immunosuppressants

	Agent					
Indications	MMF	BQR	TRL	SRL	15DS	FTY720
Presensitized response	0	?	0	0	?	0
Rejection prophylaxis	++[a,b]	++[b]	++[a,c]	+++[b]	0	++[b]
Rejection reversal	0	0	0	+	++[c]	0
Rejection rescue	+	+	+	++	0	0
Chronic rejection	?	?	0	?	0	0

[a] FDA-approved indication for drug use.
[b] Use in combination with CsA.
[c] Use in combination with corticosteroids.

In summary, three randomized clinical studies have shown that MMF decreases the incidence and severity of acute rejection episodes, but fails to improve overall graft or patient survival rates. A recent update failed to show improvement in the three-year graft survival or histopathology among patients treated with CsA–MMF–steroid versus CsA–Aza–steroid or CsA–steroid (39). Nevertheless, MMF is being incorporated into immunosuppressive regimens with increasing frequency for allograft recipients (40). Despite its putatively selective role for T-cell action, clinical experience has documented that MMF inhibits multiple types of rapidly dividing cells, which results in the major side effects of bone marrow suppression and gastrointestinal toxicity, particularly diarrhea. These adverse reactions together with its high cost may limit the long-term application of MMF in future immunosuppressive regimens, unless it can be documented that it reduces the incidence of chronic rejection or permits substantial CsA dose reduction.

Brequinar

Brequinar (BQR; DUP785) was originally developed as an antitumor agent (41), because it inhibits pyrimidine biosynthetic pathways (42). Its high bioavailability and long serum half-life are major advantages, but the drug displays considerable dose-related toxicity.

Molecular Mode of Action

BQR is a synthetic difluoroquinolone carboxylic acid derivative [6-fluoro-2-(2′-fluoro-1,1′biphenyl-4-yl)-3-methyl-4-quinolinecarboxylic acid sodium salt; DuPont-Merck, Wilmington, DE] that inhibits the growth of a wide range of human solid tumors implanted in nude mice (41). BQR displays antitumor effects over a wide range of concentrations, but only displays antilymphocyte effects over a relatively narrow range (22 to 185 nmol/L) (43). In vitro BQR (25 to 75 μM) kills 50% of clone A human colon tumor cells when incubated within 24 hours and 99% after 48 to 72 hours of incubation. Intracellular uridine triphosphate (UTP) and cytidine triphosphate (CTP) pools were depleted to 50% at 3 hours and to undetectable levels (<0.3 pmol) after 24 hours. The addition of exogenous uridine or cytidine to cell cultures reversed the cytotoxic effect.

At concentrations ranging from 15 to 105 nmol/L (44), BQR noncompetitively inhibits dihydro-orotate dehydrogenase (DHO-DH), the enzyme that converts dihydro-orotate into orotic acid. This conversion is a critical step, leading to the formation of uridine- and cytidine-MP. DHO-DH, which blocks the synthesis of DNA and RNA, is the fourth enzyme in the de novo pyrimidine synthesis pathway, located on the outer side of the inner mitochondrial membrane (45). Because lymphocyte pyrimidine pool is limited, activated lymphocytes depend primarily on de novo synthesis, producing a high degree of sensitivity to BQR during the S phase of the immune response (46). In C57Bl/6 mice bearing colon cancer transplants (Colon 38), BQR (50 mg/kg) inhibited plasma and tissue uridine levels to 10% and depleted DHO-DH activity, which persisted for several days, by more than 90% (47).

In Vitro and In Vivo Immunosuppressive Effects

BQR inhibits mixed lymphocyte reaction (MLR) in various species, but most sensitively in human (48). MLR cultures admixing lymphocytes from ACI and LEW rats display a BQR IC_{50} of 0.15 μg/mL (49), and cultures using allogenic human peripheral blood lymphocytes (PBLs), 0.01 μg/mL. Although the IC_{50} concentration is identical to that of CsA, BQR produces 90% inhibition (IC_{90}) at 0.07 μg/mL, a concentration that is considerably lower than that required for CsA (1.2 μg/mL) (50). Just as it inhibited the growth of tumor cells, BQR (10 mg/kg) significantly inhibited the DHO-DH activity in the lymph node cells of antigen-sensitized mice. The delayed-type hypersensitivity response induced by 2,4-dinitrofluorobenzene (DNFB) was 90% inhibited by a BQR dosage of 10 mg/kg, a 10-fold lower dose than that required for CsA. BQR produced dose-dependent inhibition of cytotoxic T-cell proliferation and antibody responses to antigens in C57BL/6 mice. A 50% inhibition of specific lysis was produced by 1.6 mg/kg BQR. There was a strong correlation between drug blood levels and the inhibition of the mitogen-induced lymphocyte proliferation (50). BQR produces synergistic inhibition with CsA toward in vitro human MLR with combination index values ranging from 0.06 to 0.003 at the 95% inhibition level. BQR also displays strong synergism with sirolimus, with CI_{95} values ranging from 0.08 to 0.02. The maximum inhibition degree of lymphocyte proliferation in response to mitogen or MLR-driven stimulation was observed with the triple combination CsA–sirolimus–BQR, with CI values less than 0.0001 over the inhibition range 60% to 95% (51).

BQR inhibits the IgM antibody-mediated xenograft rejection responses in hamster-to-rat heart xenograft models. While the IgM level increased from 218.3 ± 88.4 mg/L to 1631 ± 359.8 mg/L ($n = 6$, $P < 0.01$) in untreated animals, it did not increase in BQR-treated animals (52). At high doses (12 mg/kg, three times a week), BQR prevented both IgM and IgG production in ACI heart allotransplants into skin graft–sensitized LEW rat hosts (53).

The high sensitivity of lymphocytes to the action of BQR compared to comparable purine inhibitors has been attributed to the 100-fold smaller pyrimidine pool than purine pool in these cells (54).

Pharmacokinetics

BQR, a water-soluble compound, is rapidly absorbed from the gastrointestinal tract. The bioavailability is 90%, reaching peak plasma levels between 2 and 4 hours (55). The drug is bound to serum proteins and has a $t_{1/2}$ of 15 hours, a volume of distribution of 15.5 ± 6.0 L/m^2, and a mean plasma clearance of 9.2 ± 7.7 mL/min/m^2. Serum levels of BQR are measured with a reverse phase high-performance liquid chromatography assay (56). After a series of five single daily IV injections of doses ranging from 135 to 300 mg/m^2, the AUC increased linearly as a function of dose (r: 0.85). At higher doses (300 to 2250 mg/kg^2), BQR displayed non-linear pharmacokinetics. BQR is believed to be metabolized in the liver by the P450 cytochrome oxidase system, and excreted primarily in feces (66%) and to a lesser extent in urine (23%) (41). The oral administration of BQR to rats for 1 month did not affect CsA pharmacokinetics (57). Its high bioavailability and long half-life allow BQR to be administered orally on an alternate-day dosing schedule.

Experimental Transplantation

Prevention of Acute and Accelerated Allograft Rejection BQR monotherapy prolongs heart, liver, and kidney allograft survival in rat transplant models. BQR (12 mg/kg, three times a week for 30 days) prolonged cardiac allografts in the ACI-to-LEW rat strain combination from 7.0 ± 0.69 to 45.5 ± 12.26 days. Grafts were rejected approximately 2 weeks after discontinuation of treatment. The same dose of BQR produced graft survivals of more than 230 days for 12 of 26 orthotopic liver transplants and more than 87 days for all kidney transplants. Challenge of long-term liver graft survivors with repeat donor-type (but not with third-party BN cardiac) transplants resulted in permanent survival, demonstrating donor-specific tolerance (49). BQR monotherapy (4 mg/kg orally three times each week) prolonged the survival of heterotopic cardiac allografts in cynomolgus monkeys from 8 ± 0.5 to 20.0 ± 21.5 days (52). BQR (3 mg/kg/day for 90 days) also prolonged mean survival time of hamster heart xenotransplants in LEW recipients from 4.0 ± 0.48 to 24.5 ± 42.2 days. Four animals survived over 90 days (52). BQR administered at a dose of 12.5 mg/kg three times a week from day −10 to day +30 also prevented accelerated rejection of ACI cardiac allograft in LEW recipients that had been presensitized by ACI skin graft placement 7 days prior to transplantation. This regimen prolonged survival from 2.5 ± 0.9 days to 40.0 ± 14.0 days, while CsA (5–15 mg/kg/day for 30 days) was not effective (53).

Combinations with Other Immunosuppressive Drugs In various animal transplant models, the immunosuppressive effect of BQR is potentiated by combination with other agents. The combination of BQR (6 mg/kg) with CsA (1 mg/kg) prolonged liver allograft survival to 220.6 ± 110.3 days, compared with 13.5 ± 83.5 days for BQR alone and 10.0 ± 77.8 days for CsA alone (49). Median effect analysis documented the interaction of CsA and BQR to be synergistic. Administration of BQR (0.25–2.0 mg/kg/day for 14 days) with CsA (0.5 mg/kg) and SRL (0.01 mg/kg) improved the survival of BUF heterotopic heart allografts in Wistar-Furth (WF; RT1^u) recipients from 20.8 ± 2.7 days to 56.6 ± 5.2 days, with a CI value of 0.06 (51). In mice, the addition of BQR (0.125 mg/kg) to the combination of CsA (90.25 mg/kg/day) and sirolimus (SRL) (0.01 mg/kg) prolonged the graft survival from 8.2 ± 1.5 days to 56.6 ± 22.1 days, with a CI of 0.01 (58). In other experiments using a limited array of dose combinations, the addition of MMP to BQR treatment was claimed to prolong significantly the survival of ACI heterotopic heart allografts in LEW recipients (59). In primates, the combination of BQR and CsA also prolonged graft survival. BQR (2 mg/kg three times weekly) and CsA (2 mg/kg) increased graft survival from 8.0 ± 0.5 days in the untreated group and from 22 and 20 ± 21.5 days in both single-drug groups, respectively, to 43 days in the combination group.

Dogs are more sensitive than monkeys or humans to drug-induced myelosuppressive and gastrointestinal (GI) toxic effects, presumably because these tissues undergo rapid cell turnover (47,49). BQR (5 mg/kg) treatment of Sprague-Dawley rats for 1 month caused anemia, leukopenia, bone marrow hypocellularity, GI epithelial growth inhibition, and intestinal mucosal atrophy. The combination of BQR with CsA (10 mg/kg) increased the mortality rate in rats to 69% (22/32) (57), caused hypoplastic changes in the white pulp area of the spleen, and produced mucosal erosive changes in the small intestine and colon in monkeys (60).

Clinical Applications

Phase I Studies Administration of BQR to 45 cancer patients by single daily IV infusion for 5 days over a dose range of 36–300 mg/m^2/day produced dermatitis, mucositis, phlebitis, reversible transaminase elevations, and thrombocytopenia (61). Short-term (10- to 60-minute) IV infusion of BQR repeated every three weeks at doses above 1200 mg/m^2 caused a wide range of dose-dependent side effects, including severe thrombocytopenia, leukopenia, mucositis, nausea, vomiting, and skin rash (56). Phase II studies in cancer using BQR doses of 1800 mg/m^2 failed to reduce the tumor growth (62). There was a strong correlation between the AUC and thrombocytopenia. In a study of 67 cancer patients, 10-minute daily IV infusion of BQR for five consecutive days produced dose-limiting myelosuppression with severe thrombocytopenia; the maximum tolerable doses ranged from 210–350 mg/m^2 (56). BQR was administered at doses ranging from 0.5–4.0 mg/kg to 36 renal (Kahan BD, unpublished data) and 18 orthotopic liver (63) stable adult allograft recipients. The drug was generally tolerated, except for stomatitis, occasional mild diarrhea, and rare viral infections. Concentration-dependent changes occurred in platelet but not in white blood cell counts.

Phase II Studies An initial phase II study in cadaveric kidney recipients failed to document that addition of BQR to a CsA–prednisone regimen reduces the incidence of acute allograft rejection episodes (DuPont-Merck, unpublished data). The study design was flawed, however, and the phase II assessment will need to be repeated in order to draw a firm conclusion about the activity of BQR.

Like other nucleotide synthesis inhibitors, BQR is a potent blocker of the lymphocyte proliferation in vivo and in vitro; however, it also reduces the activity of other dividing cells, such as GI epithelium and bone marrow cells. In animal transplant models, BQR improves graft survival and overcomes accelerated rejection when used alone and acts synergistically with CsA and/or SRL. BQR's unique abilities to suppress antibody responses and to improve the survival of xenotransplants make it likely that the agent will become an important adjunct in clinical immunosuppression. However, the phase I toxicity studies, initially conducted in cancer patients (56,61,62) and then in transplant patients, documented that BQR must play this role only at reduced doses that are subtherapeutic as monotherapy.

Leflunomide

Leflunomide (HWA 486; Hoechst, Basel, SZ), an isoxazol derivative [*N*-(4-trifluoro-methylphenyl)-5-methylisoxazol-4-carboxamide], was initially synthesized to be an agricultural herbicide (see Fig. 11.2). Leflunomide displays immunosuppressive activity in animal models of arthritis, autoimmune diseases, and graft rejection. The parent compound is metabolized quickly to an active metabolite, A771726, which is minimally water soluble. In rodents, A771726 displays a half-life of 10 to 30 hours, which is 10-fold longer in humans. Because the pharmacokinetic characteristics of leflunomide show significant interindividual variability, and because of the agent's severe adverse reaction profile, considerable effort is now underway to produce a less toxic analogue.

Molecular Mode of Action

In vitro A771726 inhibits the proliferation of human PBL upon stimulation with allogeneic PBL in one-way MLR with anti-CD3 MAb plus phorbol myristate acetate (PMA), and with anti-CD28 MAb plus PMA (64,65). Although leflunomide partially inhibits IL-2 production, it does not affect IL-2R expression, and administration of exogenous IL-2 fails to restore T-cell proliferative responses. It has been hypothesized that leflunomide inhibits T-cell activation by inhibiting the lck and fyn families of tyrosine kinases, enzymes that are associated with transduction of many growth factor receptor signals, including IL-2, IL-3, and tumor necrosis factor (TNF)-α, but not IL-1 (66,67). However, leflunomide does not affect the formation of the IL-2/IL-2R complex or initial signal transduction events, such as phosphotyrosine formation and Ca mobilization. These findings were initially interpreted to suggest that the agent principally inhibits the transformation from the G_1 to the S phase of the cell cycle (64–66). However, recent data show that A771726 does not inhibit T-cell receptor (TCR)-mediated signal transduction in Jurkat T cells stimulated by PHA or anti-CD3. Tyrosine kinase–dependent early signal transduction was not affected by A771726. There was no increase in the level of intracellular ionized Ca^{2+}.

Based on the observation that the addition of uridine and cytidine to T cells treated with A771726 restores proliferative responses, an alternate hypothesis has been proposed: A771726 inhibits pyrimidine synthesis (68), in a similar fashion as BQR, by inhibiting dihydro-orotate dehydrogenase (see Table 11.1).

Experimental Animal Models

Leflunomide displays potent immunosuppressive activity against experimental autoimmune disorders, including arthritis (69), systemic lupus erythematosus (70), antibasement membrane antibody–induced glomerulonephritis (71), and tubulointerstitial nephritis (72). It prolongs rat (70) and dog (73) kidney and rat skin graft survival. Kuchle et al (74) demonstrated that treatment with leflunomide (5 and 10 mg/kg/day PO) prolonged BN kidney allograft survival in LEW rats from 8.2 ± 0.3 days to over 60 days. Treatment with 20 mg/kg/day leflunomide significantly prolonged DA skin graft survival in LEW recipients to 29.1 ± 1.8 days from 10.5 ± 1.1 days in untreated controls, and LEW skin graft survival in Fisher rat recipients to 33.8 ± 2.8 days from 16.2 ± 1.0 days in untreated controls. Spleen cells from long-surviving LEW recipients of DA grafts that were treated with leflunomide when transferred prolonged survival of donor-type skin grafts to naive nonirradiated LEW rats (75). Leflunomide monotherapy at daily doses of 0.63–10.0 mg/kg for 7 days significantly prolonged the survival of BN hearts in LEW rats (76). When treatment was extended to 21 days at a leflunomide dose of 5 mg/kg/day, 3 of 6 animals displayed indefinite graft survival. In the hamster-to-LEW rat cardiac xenotransplant model, leflunomide (2.5–20.0 mg/kg/day PO) initiated on day 0 prolonged survival from 3.9 ± 0.3 days to 71.3 ± 17.9 days (10 mg/kg group) (77). The high leflunomide doses (20 mg/kg/day) prolonged survival (MST = 50.9 ± 16.2 days), but caused significant anemia; 4 of 8 animals were lost due to toxicity.

In canine renal transplant models, McChesney et al (73) found that escalating doses of 2–16 mg/kg/day of leflunomide produced dose-dependent effects: 4 mg/kg/day extended survival from 9.0 ± 1.0 days to 15.5 ± 5.0 days with all dogs dying of rejection, and 16 mg/kg/day prolonged survival to 20.7 ± 2.0 days with all dogs dying due to inanition and anemia. The side effects included mild interstitial nephritis and superficial ulcerations of the stomach and jejunal mucosa, as well as anemia and anorexia that were attributed to the generation of an aniline metabolite by hepatic oxidation of the parent compound.

The severe adverse reaction profile of the present compound obviates clinical application of leflunomide. Research is underway to develop less toxic analogues of the A771726 metabolite of leflunomide.

NEW AGENTS THAT SPECIFICALLY ALTER T-CELL FUNCTION

Tacrolimus

During an intensive search to find antibiotics that inhibit IL-2 production in a similar fashion as CsA, the macrolide product of *Streptomyces tsukubaensis* No. 9993 was unearthed from soil samples from Tsukuba, Japan (78). The active compound, tacrolimus (TRL; FK506, Prograf, Fujisawa, Osaka, Japan; molecular weight = 804 daltons molecular weight), is a macrolide lactone with a hemiketal-masked α,βdiketoamide that is functionally incorporated in a 23-member ring (79) (see Fig. 11.2; see Chapter 9 for a more detailed discussion of tacrolimus).

Molecular Mode of Action

TRL forms complexes with FK-binding proteins (FKBPs), which are abundant cytosolic enzymes with intrinsic rotamase activity (80,81), to inhibit the phosphatase activity of calcineurin (82–84), thereby preventing the emigration of the phosphorylated cytoplasmic nuclear factor of activated T cells (NFAT) from the cytoplasm to the nucleus (see Table 11.1). Because NFAT is critical for the upregulation of IL-2 gene transcription, the synthesis of this cytokine is disrupted (85,86) (see Fig. 11.2). Of the four FKBPs characterized to date, it seems most likely that TRL forms a complex with FKBP12, a 12-kd cytosolic protein, which then mediates the immunosuppressive effects of TRL (87).

Pharmacokinetics

Although high-performance liquid chromatography (HPLC) methods unequivocally detect TRL and its metabolites (88), the drug is generally measured in human whole blood samples with an enzyme-linked immunosorbent assay (ELISA) (89). After intravenous administration of TRL, the median half-life is 11.3 hours, with a range of 3.5 to 40.5 hours (90,91). The plasma clearance rate ranges from 5.8 to 103 mL/min/kg. After oral administration, TRL is rapidly absorbed independent of the presence of bile, with a t_{max} of 0.5 to 4.0 hours and a mean oral bioavailability of 25%. The agent is primarily metabolized by the hepatic cytochrome P450-IIIA4 enzyme system (66). Unfortunately, the intraindividual and interindividual variations in TRL pharmacokinetics are as great as those observed with CsA.

Clinical Applications

Prophylaxis of Acute Rejection: Phase III Trials In the phase III open-label, randomized European multicenter trial (92), which enrolled 545 liver transplant recipients, patients in the TRL treatment group displayed an approximately equal incidence of acute rejection episodes compared with those in the CsA treatment group (43.4% versus 53.6%; P = NS). The modest delay in the time to diagnosis ($P = 0.04$) does not seem important, because the trial was unblinded and time to rejection is a subjective measure. The patient and graft survival rates were similar: 82.9% and 77.5%, respectively, for the TRL-treated group, and 77.5% and 72.6%, respectively, for the CsA-treated group. Renal toxicity, altered glucose metabolism, and neurologic complications were more commonly experienced by patients in the TRL group.

The phase III US multicenter trial (93) included 478 adult and 51 pediatric recipients of orthotopic liver transplants. After one year, patients treated with immunosuppressive regimens based on TRL (n = 263) and CsA (n = 266) showed comparable patient and graft survival rates. It was claimed that TRL produced a delay in the onset of all rejection episodes and fewer episodes that were steroid-resistant, but TRL was also associated with substantially more adverse events that required discontinuation of therapy. In renal transplant recipients, acute rejection episodes were significantly reduced in the TRL-treated group and the side effects observed were similar to those in the CsA group (94). As with liver recipients, graft survival rates were not significantly different in the two groups. These findings led to FDA approval of TRL as an alternative to CsA for baseline immunosuppression for transplantation (see Table 11.2).

Rescue Treatment for Acute Refractory Allograft Rejection TRL (0.3–0.15 mg/kg/day) was used by Starzl et al (95) to reverse refractory rejection in 7 of 10 liver allograft patients. The common side effects were nausea and vomiting. A pilot study by Jordan et al (96) found that 20 of 35 renal transplant patients who had been converted to TRL (0.3 mg/kg/day) because of either "uncontrolled" rejection or complications attributed to CsA or steroid therapy showed a return to baseline serum creatinine levels, improvement in histologic features of the allograft on renal biopsy, and/or freedom from chronic dialysis. The observed side effects included CMV or bacterial pneumonia, diabetes, hypertension, cecal perforation, and epistaxis. Another report claimed that with TRL treatment, 57 of 77 patients (74%) experienced "rescue" after refractory rejection episodes of liver, cardiac, and combined pancreas and kidney transplants (97). In a US multicenter trial (98), TRL (0.05–0.075 mg/kg/12 hr IV or 0.15 mg/kg/12 hr PO) was administered to 125 liver transplant recipients with rejection episodes that were refractory to OKT-3. It was reported that 54% of patients experienced beneficial effects after 28 days of treatment. Actuarial graft and patient survival rates were 50% and 72%, respectively, at 12 months after conversion. In 54 of 125 patients, the drug was prematurely discontinued because of treatment failure, severe adverse effects, death, or intercurrent illness.

Armitage et al (99) reported that 5 of 8 rejection episodes in cardiac transplant patients were reversed with TRL (0.2–0.4 mg/kg/day). Although they suggested that TRL therapy permits steroid withdrawal, particularly in pediatric cardiac transplant patients, CsA-based regimens also permit successful withdrawal (100). Based on these equivocal findings the FDA declined to approve TRL for the indication of reversal of refractory rejection.

TRL represents an alternative to CsA that displays greater potency in part due initially to the willingness of physicians to tolerate a greater degree of toxicity than what had been observed with CsA therapy, including hyperglycemia (31.4%), nephrotoxicity (27.1%), cardiac toxicity (18.6%; includes chest pain, chest discomfort, palpitations, abnormal EKG), abdominal distension (18.6%), and tremors (10%) in some reports (101). As further progress helped to clarify optimal dosing regimens for TRL therapy, the drug has become more widely used for recipients of all types of allografs including pancreas (102), kidney (103), and thoracic organs (104).

Sirolimus

Sirolimus (Rapamycin, SRL; Rapamune, Wyeth-Ayerst, Princeton, NJ), a macrocyclic triene antibiotic produced by

Streptomyces hygroscopicus isolated from soil samples collected on Easter Island in 1975 (105,106), was originally developed as an anticandidal and antitumor agent (107,108). SRL is a 31-member macrocyclic lactone (molecular weight = 914.2 kd, C51H79N013) akin in structure to TRL by virtue of an unusual tricarbonyl array (carbons [C] 14–16) consisting of an amide, a ketone, a hemiketal, and a chemically sensitive retroaldol site (C31–C33). Importantly, unlike TRL, SRL also contains a triene segment (C1–C6) (109). The backbone of the macrolide ring is mainly derived from acetates and propionates (110) (see Fig. 11.2).

Molecular Mode of Action

Although SRL binds to FKBP 25, the molecular mechanism of its effect is distinct from the calcineurin-based activity of TRL or even CsA. Sirolimus inhibits a variety of cytokine-mediated, protein kinase C–triggered, and lymphokine-mediated signal transduction pathways, particularly triggered by IL-2 or IL-6 (111). It is thought that SRL inhibits a 282-kd phosphatidylinositol (PI) 3-kinase (FK-Rapamycin Associated Protein, FRAP) (112) that appears necessary for the activation and subsequent protein synthesis of 70-kd S6 kinase ($p70^{S6k}$), a critical enzyme for the activation of the ribosomal protein S6 (113–115). In addition, SRL blocks the phosphorylation (presumably mediated by FRAP) of downstream factors, including: 1) $p34^{cdc2}$ kinase, which forms a heterodimeric complex with cyclin E to produce the maturation-promoting factor, 2) an ill-defined protein that prevents the elimination of $p27^{kip}$, which is a negative regulatory factor for cyclin-dependent kinases, and 3) the eukaryotic initiation factor (eIF-4E)-binding protein necessary for protein translation. The overall effect of these actions is interference with the progression of T cells from the G_1 to the S phase of the cell cycle (116–117).

Pharmacokinetics

The HPLC techniques used to estimate whole blood concentrations of SRL in clinical practice display a detection limit of 2 ng/mL (118). Although liquid chromatography/mass spectrometry (LC/MS) methods are more sensitive, with a detection limit of 80 pg (119), clinical samples generally display concentrations of 5 to 30 ng/mL, and thus LC/MS methods are impractical for use in routine concentration monitoring of SRL. Most of the SRL is found in human red blood and tissue cells, with less than 3% in plasma (120). In contrast to CsA and TRL, the value of the SRL AUC correlates well with the terminal drug concentration (C_{24}; r^2 = 0.9). Because CsA, TRL, and SRL are all metabolized by cytochrome P450-IIIA4 3A/4, drug interactions have been observed in experimental animals (121) and in humans. High SRL trough levels correlate with high CsA average concentration (C_{av}) values (Meier-Kriesche, unpublished observations).

Experimental Animal Models

Prophylaxis of Acute Rejection SRL doses of 3 and 6 mg/kg for 13 days prolong the survival of heart allografts in rats and mice, respectively (122). Single 12-mg/kg doses administered intraperitonealy produced indefinite survival of BN and (LxBN) heart allografts in LEW rats (123). Continuous intravenous infusion of SRL (0.08–0.80 mg/kg/day for 14 days) markedly prolonged transplant survival in rats: kidney graft survival was prolonged from 10 ± 0 to 90.2 ± 62.4 days, and small bowel graft survival from 11.6 ± 1.5 to 26.8 ± 3.7 days (124). In contrast, the pig is more sensitive to SRL: doses of 2 mg/kg SRL extended renal allograft survival from 15.1 to 76 days, although interstitial pneumonitis occurred in 5 of 9 pigs. In dogs, even subtherapeutic doses of 2 mg/kg SRL produced the toxic effects of thrombocytopenia and necrotizing fibrinoid vasculitis in the GI tract (125), a finding that was also observed in baboons (126,127). Interestingly, in all these animal models there was no pathohistologic change in kidney grafts associated with SRL therapy in situations where an equally immunosuppressive dose of CsA was nephrotoxic (128,129).

Passive transfer experiments from hosts demonstrating long-term graft survival to isogeneic virgin hosts demonstrated a unique mechanism of drug-induced unresponsiveness. In both rats and mice, SRL treatment induces the production of IgG-blocking antibodies (130). Serum passively transferred from SRL-treated WF recipients significantly prolonged Buffalo (BUF; $RT1^b$) heart allograft survival from 9.8 ± 1.2 days in controls to 74.4 ± 31.1 days ($P = 0.002$). The sera were directed toward donor foreign histocompatibility antigens rather than specific T-cell receptors.

Rescue Treatment When SRL treatment (0.8 mg/kg/day) for 14 days was initiated on day 3 or 4, but not day 5, the rejection process of BUF heart allografts in WF recipients that had been treated with a subtherapeutic dose of CsA was reversed and the transplants enjoyed prolonged survival (131). The same SRL dose prevented accelerated cardiac allograft rejection in presensitized WF recipients, an effect that was also associated with significantly lower levels of donor-specific IgG compared with sensitized, untreated hosts (132).

Prevention of Chronic Allograft Vasculopathy Treatment with SRL reduced intimal thickening and prevented development of experimental chronic allograft vasculopathy in two cardiac transplant models—LEW-to-F344 and BN-to-LEW rats (133,134). In untreated mice, at 30 and 50 days after cardiac transplantation, the incidences of intimal thickening were 55% and 60%, respectively. These rates improved with SRL treatment (135). In addition, the intimal thickening and endothelial proliferation observed in the carotid artery after mechanical balloon injury in rats were reduced by 85% after SRL therapy (136). Presumably these results are related to the immunosuppressive actions of SRL, as well as to its blockade of the proliferative effects of epidermal- and fibroblast-derived growth factors and/or of other cytokines that induce endothelial proliferation.

Combination Therapy with Other Immunosuppressive Agents SRL acts synergistically with CsA in vivo and in vitro. The SRL–CsA combination displays a strong synergistic effect on the order of a 10- to 1000-fold augmentation of the potency of the individual agents to inhibit proliferative responses (137) and reduce the generation of cytotoxic cells (138). The beneficial synergistic interactions noted by Meiser et al (139) and by Ochiai et al (140) in dogs were also documented in the rat by application of the rigorous median effect analysis (138). In contrast to the strong synergistic interaction of the combination of SRL (0.01 mg/kg/day) and CsA (0.05 mg/kg/day) to prolong rat cardiac allograft survival (157), the combination of SRL and TRL showed antagonism, perhaps due to mutual competition for FKBPs (82,141). SRL has been found to act synergistically with MMF in preventing heart, kidney, and pancreas allograft rejection in rat models (142).

Clinical Applications

Clinical Toxicity in Transplantation: Phase I Trial In a double-blinded randomized phase I study, Murgia et al (143) administered SRL or placebo for 14 days as twice daily doses to renal transplant recipients who had remained stable for at least 6 months on a CsA–steroid regimen. Thirty patients were divided into three groups: low-dose (1–3 mg/m^2/day), medium-dose (5–6 mg/m^2/day), and high-dose (7–13 mg/m^2/day); 10 patients received placebo. The major toxic effect of SRL was hypertriglyceridemia. In addition, SRL produced a dose-dependent decrease in platelet counts and to a lesser extent in white blood cell counts. These effects were more pronounced in patients with initially low cell counts. However, SRL treatment did not affect the CsA AUC, blood pressure values, or kidney or liver function tests.

A phase I trial of ascending doses of SRL (0.5–7.0 mg/m^2) administered de novo together with CsA and prednisone showed a reduction in the incidence of acute rejection within the first 6 months to 6.7% (2 of 30) in SRL-treated patients from 36.9% for a historical cohort of 65 patients who were treated with CsA–prednisone alone ($P = 0.02$) (144).

Prophylaxis of Acute Rejection: Phase II Trial A multicenter trial of SRL (1, 3, or 5 mg/m^2/day) in combination with CsA and prednisone confirmed that SRL treatment reduced the incidence of acute rejection episodes among 149 renal transplant recipients. Within 6 months the CsA–prednisone–placebo group showed a 40% incidence of rejection episodes, whereas the groups of patients treated adjunctively with 1 and 3 mg/m^2/day SRL experienced a 10% and 7% rejection incidence, respectively. The one-year graft survival was 96% and 87% in patients given placebo and SRL, respectively. A significant racial difference was observed in the incidence of rejection episodes when CsA doses were halved. Nonblack patients treated with a reduced-dose CsA regimen and 1, 3, or 5 mg/m^2 SRL experienced approximately a 10% incidence of rejection episodes, whereas black patients treated with a reduced-dose CsA regimen and the same doses of SRL experienced rejection rates comparable to patients treated with a full-dose CsA regimen without SRL (145).

In a subsequent phase II multicenter study, SRL with azathioprine and steroids was compared to CsA with azathioprine and steroids in cadaver donor renal transplant recipients (145). The incidence of rejection and graft survival rates at one year were similar in both patient groups. SRL had a favorable safety profile compared to CsA with regard to tremor, hirsutism, and renal function but produced more significant abnormalities in triglyceride and cholesterol levels.

More recently, SRL has been combined with CsA in phase II/III global multicenter dose-escalation trial for mismatched cadaveric or living-donor renal allograft recipients (146). The investigators noted a reduction in the incidence of acute rejection episodes to 11% from 29% in patients previously treated with CsA and prednisone (Fig. 11.3). The SRL-treated patients had more severe hyperlipidemia, thrombocytopenia, and leukopenia but could be withdrawn more successfully from adjunctive corticosteroid treatment. Additional clinical trials with this agent are underway.

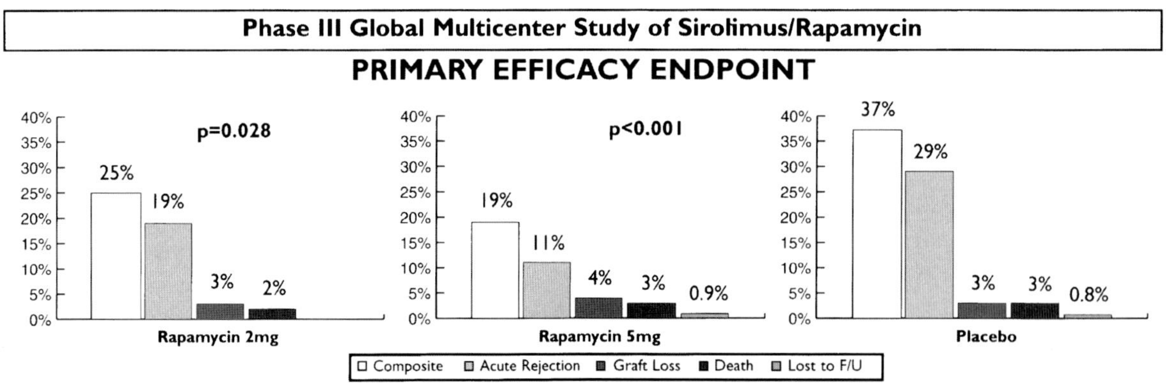

FIGURE 11.3. *Data from 576 recipients of cadaveric or mismatched living-donor renal allografts randomized to receive Rapamycin (2 mg/day or 5 mg/day), or placebo together with CsA and steroids. (Adapted from Highlights of the Transplantation Society XVII World Congress. Montreal, 1998;1:1–2.)*

15-Deoxyspergualin

Spergualin (1-amino-19-guanitido-11,15-dihydroxy-4,9,12-triazanonadecane-10,13-dione), a water soluble peptide (molecular weight = 496 d) (147) fermentation product of *Bacillus laterosporus*, was synthetically dehydroxylated to produce 15-deoxyspergualin (DSG; Behringwerke, Marburg, Germany) (148), an agent with antibacterial, antitumor (148–150), and immunosuppressive properties (151–155). The DSG derivative, a racemic mixture of positive and negative enantiomers, has a broader range of activity and greater potency than DSG, but a similar toxicity profile to spergualin.

Molecular Mode of Action

DSG only moderately inhibits Con-A-, LPS- or MLR-stimulated blastogenesis, as well as cytotoxic T-cell activity (154,156–158), without affecting IL-2 production. DSG is active even when added to cell cultures 3 or 4 days after stimulation (156), suggesting that DSG acts at a later stage during the cell cycle than CsA, perhaps during generation and/or differentiation of antigen-specific cytotoxic T lymphocytes. These immunosuppressive effects are antagonized by supplementation of the lymphocyte medium with IFN-γ, but not IL-2 (156,157,159–161). DSG (5 mg/kg) also dampens antibody production in immunotoxin-treated mice (162) and surface IgM expression after lipopolysaccharide or IFN-γ induction by a murine pre-B-cell line (163). Although the molecular mode of action of DSG is unknown, the compound specifically binds to Hsp70, a member of the heat shock protein family, which may represent a class of immunophilins distinct from the cis-trans proline isomerase immunophilins, cyclophilins, and FKBPs (164). In addition, DSG inhibits the monocyte/macrophage functions of liposomal enzyme release, superoxide production, class II antigen upregulation, and IL-1 production (165,166).

Pharmacokinetics

DSG must be delivered parenterally because it is a highly polar molecule with poor (3% to 6%) oral bioavailability (167). After intravenous infusion (80–2160 mg/m^2/day), DSG and its major (among 6) metabolite, desaminopropyl-DSG, reach steady-state concentration within 2 hours and show no accumulation over 5 days (168–171). The AUC of DSG correlates well with the administered dose ($r^2 = 0.97$). The drug is cleared in a biexponential manner. The α-phase half-life ranges from 5 to 30 minutes, the β-phase half-life ranges from 44 to 160 minutes, and the total body clearance rate ranges from 258 to 451 mL/min/m^2 (mean 364 ± 78 mL/min/m^2) (168). The drug is primarily eliminated by the kidney, with 4% to 14% of the administered dose excreted unchanged in the urine (168,172).

Experimental Animal Models

Prophylaxis of Acute Rejection DSG modestly prolongs the survival of rat skin (154) or islet (151) allografts and mouse heart pinnal implants (173), as well as liver, pancreas, thyroid, and pancreaticoduodenal transplants in rats and mice (153,174). In canine models, DSG caused significant gastrointestinal toxicity, and in baboons 4 mg/kg/day DSG improved cardiac, but not renal, allograft survival (175). Furthermore, DSG modestly inhibited accelerated rejection responses in skin graft–sensitized rats, prolonging survival from 4.2 ± 0.5 days to 7.2 ± 0.5 days ($P < 0.01$).

Rescue Treatment for Acute Allograft Rejection Because it was observed in rats that DSG was more effective if administered 10 days after skin transplantation rather than perioperatively (155,176), canine experiments were conducted and showed that DSG treatment (2.4 mg/kg/day for 12 days) reversed acute rejection episodes, although the dogs experienced severe gastrointestinal toxicity (177).

Combination Therapy with Other Immunosuppressive Agents Although DSG adds little benefit to CsA immunoprophylaxis, there was no additive interaction between CsA and DSG (3–4 mg/kg/day) to improve the survival of monkey heart xenotransplants into chacme baboons (178). DSG showed a stronger interaction with the antirat T-cell receptor MAb R73 than with CsA. In a multimodality protocol, the combination of low doses of DSG (0.5 mg/kg/day), CsA (20 mg/kg/day), Aza (2.5 mg/kg/day), and ALG (2.5 mg/kg/day) treatment during a 14-day induction period showed an additive interaction to prolong canine islet graft survival in chacme baboons, which unfortunately suffered gastrointestinal toxicity.

Clinical Applications

Toxicity in Cancer Patients: Phase I Trials Administration of DSG (20–600 mg/m^2) as a 3-hour infusion for 5 consecutive days to 28 cancer patients produced dose-dependent gastrointestinal toxicity (nausea/vomiting, anorexia), alopecia, tongue and perioral numbness, hypotension, and bone marrow suppression (granulocytopenia, leukopenia, and anemia) (169). There was extensive formation of the drug metabolite desaminopropyl-DSG, with less than 10% of the administered dose excreted unchanged in the urine (168).

Prophylaxis of Rejection: Phase II Trials In a de novo treatment protocol in 10 patients, Koyama et al (179) administered the combination of DSG (2–5 mg/kg/day for 5 to 14 days), prednisone, CsA (4–6 mg/kg/day), and mizorbine (2–3 mg/kg/day) or Aza (1–2 mg/kg/day). They observed that facial numbness was the most common side effect, and bone marrow suppression was the most serious, albeit reversible, side effect. The most striking clinical result in phase II studies was that two patients with type I diabetes mellitus were insulin-independent at 9 months after simultaneous single donor islet and kidney transplants when treated with DSG, prednisone, MALG, and CsA (180).

Rescue Treatment for Acute Allograft Rejection: Phase II Trials An initial study reported that DSG (40–220 mg/m^2) produced remissions in 27 of 34 acute rejection episodes after renal transplantation (181), particularly when combined with methylprednisone (MP) (182). DSG (3–5 mg/kg) administered as seven daily 3-hour infusions produced a 76% rate of reversal of 260 acute rejection episodes within the first six months after transplantation. Among 30 rejection episodes graded by Banff criteria, DSG was more effective in reversing grade I (20 of 22; 88%) compared with grade IIa (3 of 8; 38%) episodes (183). In addition, DSG reversed 70% of steroid-resistant rejection episodes. However, the combination of DSG and MP produced the highest rate of rejection reversal (87.5%). The adverse effects observed in patients treated for allograft rejection included numbness of the face, lips, and limbs (14%), gastrointestinal toxicity (9%), bone marrow suppression (26 to 54%), and the occurrence of infection (9%). These results led to approval of DSG in Japan in 1994 for the treatment of acute rejection episodes in kidney transplant recipients (184).

Inhibition of Preformed Antibody Synthesis: Phase II Trials The combination of DSG (5 mg/kg/day for 5 days) with other agents (CsA, MP, and ALG) appears to inhibit secondary synthesis of preformed antibodies in ABO-incompatible or HLA-presensitized kidney transplant recipients. Combination therapy beginning de novo on postoperative day 1 was used with pretransplant plasmapheresis in 14 renal transplant patients. Five subjects did not experience rejection episodes, one lost his graft, and two died (one from a B-cell lymphoma and the other from cerebral hemorrhage) (185). Administration of DSG (4 mg/kg for 5 days) in three xenografted patients appeared to facilitate pig islet cell survival for several weeks to months, as manifested by urinary excretion of small amounts of porcine C-peptide (186).

Thus, although DSG seems to reverse allograft rejection episodes effectively, it displays a lower efficacy for prophylaxis of allograft rejection episodes than CsA. However, the clinical trials to date do not document the agent's therapeutic efficacy, but rather show its limitations, such as low oral bioavailability and severe gastrointestinal toxicity. Because of these characteristics, DSG must be administered systemically and for only limited periods of time.

FTY720

Myriocin (ISP-1) is an immunosuppressive compound that was isolated from the culture broth of *Isaria sinclairii* (ATCC 24400) (187). Its semisynthetic derivative FTY720 (188), a phenyl ring inserted into the side chain (2-octadecyl-2-amino-1,3-propanediol) is less toxic than ISP-1 (189).

Molecular Mode of Action

The parent compound ISP-1 inhibits the proliferation of lymphocytes in allogenic mouse MLR 5- to 10-fold more potently than CsA, but fails to dampen human leukemia cell proliferation. In vivo, ISP-1 inhibits T-cell–dependent antibody formation 10-fold and alloreactive CTL production 100-fold more effectively than CsA (187). In contrast, even at high (1000 nmol/L) concentrations, FTY720 does not inhibit the production of IL-2 or IL-3 (190), and therefore must act on a distinctive activation pathway. ISP-1, but not FTY720, inhibits serine palmitoyl transferase activity in IL-2–dependent CTLL-2 cells (191). One hypothesis advocated by Suzuki et al (192) suggests that antigen-induced apoptosis, as evidenced by the formation of apoptotic bodies and the presence of DNA ladders on agarose gel analysis of rat spleen cells, is produced by a three-hour in vitro incubation with drug. A second hypothesis is based on the observation that administration of FTY720 (10 mg/kg) to rats causes peripheral lymphocytopenia within three hours, seemingly due to a reduced expression of α_4-integrin. In contrast, FTY720 does not reduce the numbers of circulating polymorphonuclear leukocytes, peripheral B cells, bone marrow cells, or thymocytes, or the splenic content of B cells. Conversely, the numbers of T and B cells in mesenteric and peripheral lymph nodes increase, suggesting acceleration of lymphocyte homing, producing sequestration from the allograft. The effect may be mediated by upregulated expression $\alpha4/\beta7$-integrin on lymphocytes that bind Gly CAM-1 and Mad CAM-1, both of which are expressed on the cell surface of high endothelial venules (HEV) in lymph nodes and Peyer's patches (193).

Experimental Animal Models

Prophylaxis of Acute Rejection Administration of ISP-1 at doses of 0.03–0.30 mg/kg intraperitoneally prolonged the survival of rat skin allografts in dose-dependent fashion, but with severe toxicity. FTY720 (0.1–10.0 mg/kg IV) prolonged LEW skin allograft survival in F344 rats (188). Administration of low doses (0.5 mg/kg) of FTY720 for 14 days prolonged ACI liver allograft survival in LEW rats from 11.5 to 27.5 days. A two-day course of FTY720 (5 mg/kg/day) initiated either one day before and on the day of transplant, or on days 3 and 4 after transplant, prolonged graft survival from 11.5 to 28.5 or 23 days, respectively. The former two-dose regimen of FTY720 administration prolonged the median survival time of canine kidney grafts from 9 to 21 days, a result that was not inferior to that obtained by administering a daily regimen of FTY720 (192).

Combination Therapy with Cyclosporine FTY720 (0.1 mg/kg) potentiated the immunosuppressive effects of CsA to prolong the survival of rat skin allografts (194). Subtherapeutic daily CsA doses (10 mg/kg PO) starting on day 1 in combination with 1 or 5 mg/kg/day doses of FTY720 starting on day 1 produced 36.5- or 74-day mean allograft survivals, respectively (192). Further studies showed that even lower FTY720 doses of 0.1 to 1.0 mg/kg/day in combination with CsA significantly prolonged canine renal graft survival compared with CsA alone (195). Median effect analysis of rat heart allograft survivals documented that combinations of FTY720 with CsA displayed a greater degree of synergism than did FTY720 with SRL (Kahan et al, unpublished observations). Phase I clinical trials studying an FTY720–CsA combination were begun in December of 1998.

SUMMARY

During the past two decades, since the cyclosporine revolution, there has been an explosion of interest in the discovery and development of small molecule immunosuppressants that reduce the rate of acute allograft rejection episodes and increase graft and patient survival rates. The nonspecific cytostatic immunosuppressive chemicals are now being superseded by agents that act specifically on T-cell function. As a result, there has been a trend to eliminate azathioprine and corticosteroids, the primary components of the immunosuppressive regimens used from 1962 to 1982, from the regimens because of their adverse effects on elements of nonspecific host resistance. Although some physicians contend that the more selective purine synthesis inhibitor mycophenolate mofetil significantly reduces the incidence of acute allograft rejection episodes, others are concerned about the agent's well-documented side-effect profile. Although leflunomide and brequinar specifically inhibit de novo pyrimidine synthesis, their adverse effect of marked myelodepression results in a narrow therapeutic window and consequently little advantage over the purine synthesis inhibitors mycophenolate mofetil and mizorbine. In contrast, two new agents introduced since the advent of the cyclosporine era, tacrolimus and sirolimus, specifically disrupt cytokine generation by acting on T lymphocytes, and therefore may serve to improve graft survival in clinical transplantation. Although tacrolimus seems to be little more than an alternative to cyclosporine, sirolimus, particularly when combined with CsA, produces a synergistic interaction that reduces the incidence of acute rejection episodes, permits early steroid withdrawal, and/or allows marked CsA dose reduction. Among the other new agents, 15-deoxyspergualin, which has been used primarily by Japanese physicians to treat refractory renal allograft rejection, is not presently under clinical development, although it might play a future role in the treatment of allo-presensitized recipients or in xenotransplantation. In contrast, there is considerable excitement about the new agent FTY720, which may cause antigen-induced apoptosis and certainly interacts synergistically with CsA both in rodents and in dogs. The drug is currently being prepared to begin clinical trials.

As the enormous number of new small molecule compounds that display in vitro antilymphocyte activity are evaluated as immunosuppressants in rodent, canine, and primate models, we are likely to witness an evolution in immunosuppressive therapy. Soon, highly selective drug therapy may be based on our knowledge of the molecular events that lead to acute or chronic allograft rejection.

COMMENTARY

Karl Wagner

The evolution of immunosuppressive therapy has reached the point where basic questions must be addressed. The development of cyclosporine (CsA) and its subsequent widespread use in highly differentiated protocols in combination with steroids resulted in a marked increase in short-term survival among transplant patients. Following renal transplantation, one-year patient and graft survival figures in excess of 95% and 85%, respectively, became achievable. Such an accomplishment is even more impressive when we consider the relative expansion of indications for transplantation, the waiving of various contraindications for transplantation (including coronary heart disease), and the adoption of a more liberal use of organs from elderly donors during the past two decades. The questions raised now, therefore, include: What one-year survival rates can be achieved by using conventional immunosuppressive therapy in multimorbid patients? Can we further improve upon these results without inducing donor-specific tolerance? As we approach the magical limit of 100% one-year survival rates, the size of study groups that would be required to demonstrate the statistical superiority of a new immunosuppressive compound has become extraordinarily large. Since these numbers are seldom achievable, the efficacy of any new agent must compete at least with the results achieved using the "gold standard" CsA. Secondary end points including the occurrence of "immunologic catastrophes" (e.g., steroid-resistant rejection, life-threatening septicemias), changes in vascular risk (hypertension, lipid metabolism) profiles, the severity and clinical relevance of other complications, and economic analyses must, therefore, also be taken into consideration.

Despite the improvement of one-year survival rates with CsA, the subsequent rate of graft loss has not changed considerably over the past decade. This may be the consequence of chronic rejection that might have additional causes other than immunologic imbalance between donor and recipient. As there may be numerous mechanisms involved in the development of chronic rejection, further questions are: What potential role can new immunosuppressive agents play in preventing chronic rejection? Do immunosuppressive agents currently under evaluation exert their effects by any supplementary mechanisms that might be relevant for chronic rejection? Although clinical observations that can answer these questions will only be available from long-term investigations, we should certainly consider these points when evaluating new immunosuppressive agents.

The molecules discussed in this chapter can be divided into three groups: those with proven clinical relevance [mycophenolate mofetil (MMF) and tacrolimus (TRL, FK506)], a second group consisting of agents entering clinical investigation [sirolimus (SRL) and 15-desoxyspergualin (DSG)], and a final group where data are only available from animal experiments (leflunomide and the myriocin derivative, FTY720). With respect to the latter group and specifically leflunomide, the adverse reaction profile of the active compound A771726 obviates clinical application. Whether less toxic analogues can be developed remains to be evaluated. Clinical use of DSG may be limited because of the associated gastrointestinal toxicity; but perhaps more importantly, based on its very low oral bioavailability, it will need to be administered systemically. Although DSG has a proven efficacy in the reversal of ongoing rejection episodes (including steroid-resistant rejection), the assessment of Senel and Kahan that DSG is less efficacious than CsA in the prophylaxis of allograft rejection is supported by the fact that DSG has received formal approval only for the treatment of acute renal allograft rejection.

Thus, of the six compounds discussed in this chapter, only MMF, TRL, and SRL seem to be of current clinical relevance. Besides the different mechanisms of action, there is an additional major distinguishing point that must be recognized: Only TRL has, to date, been considered a primary immunosuppressant capable of replacing CsA, whereas MMF and SRL have been investigated mostly for use in conjunction with CsA.

Conclusions concerning SRL must reflect the fact that patient and graft survival from prospective randomized renal transplant trials are just becoming available. Survival and toxicity observations from the multi-institutional European trial will be of particular interest since this trial will evaluate SRL as primary therapy in place of CsA. Available data from the Sirolimus Multi-Center Study Group phase I/II trials indicate a dramatic reduction in the occurrence of rejection from 40% for the control group (CsA and steroids) to 10% and 7%, respectively, in patients treated with the addition of 1 and 3 mg/m^2/day of SRL. Combination therapy with SRL and CsA appears to exert, at least experimentally, a synergistic immunosuppressive effect. This implies, as shown by the Sirolimus Multi-Center Study Group, the possibility, at least in Caucasians, of reducing the CsA dose in conjunction with SRL with no detrimental effect on rejection rates. The experimental observation that SRL prevents chronic allograft vasculopathy by blockade of the proliferative effects of growth factors might have implications for its effect on chronic rejection. SRL, in conclusion, appears to be a promising substance. However, the data currently available do not yet enable us to answer whether patient and graft survival are comparable to those achieved with conventional CsA-based therapy.

MMF has undergone extensive investigations for the prophylaxis of rejection in prospectively randomized renal transplant recipients (see also Chapter 10). Over 1400 recipients were included in three different trials. One observation from these trials was the finding that conventional triple therapy (CsA, steroids, and azathioprine) offers only a 2% reduction in the incidence of rejection compared with dual therapy (CsA and steroids). The addition of MMF in doses of 2 or 3 g/day to dual therapy resulted in similar patient and graft survival but a significant reduction in rejection episodes (to below 20%). This was accompanied by a reduction in the severity of the rejection as assessed according to the Banff classification. This was paralleled by a reduction in the rate of steroid-resistant rejection and a lower use of OKT-3. The incidence of leukopenia was significantly reduced in patients receiving MMF compared with those treated with azathioprine. These positive effects were somewhat counter-balanced by the frequent occurrence of abdominal discomfort and a slightly higher incidence of viral infections. Since MMF has been shown experimentally to reduce the formation of adhesion molecules, the MMF-treated patients in the above trials have been enrolled in continuing studies investigating the possible role of MMF in limiting the development of biopsy-proven chronic rejection.

It may be concluded that whenever the indication for an augmentation of immunosuppression with the addition of azathioprine is present, it is reasonable to consider incorporating MMF in its place. Whether this may have any impact on the development of chronic rejection can only be determined in further trials. Unfortunately, a misguiding pricing policy, which established the daily cost of MMF to be comparable to that of CsA and therefore far above that of azathioprine, may in the long run prevent the long-term use of MMF.

TRL differs markedly from the molecules discussed above (see also Chapter 9). First, it is the only new molecule thus far established to be effective as baseline immunosuppression in place of CsA. Second, initial clinical experience was gained in liver transplantation. Its mechanism of action, at least in part, seems to be similar to that of CsA. However, TRL complexes with a different intracellular binding protein and its immunosuppressive potency seems to be far higher than that of CsA. In phase III liver transplant studies comparing CsA-based triple therapy and TRL-based dual therapy, patient and graft survival were numerically higher in the TRL treatment groups, although these differences failed to reach statistical significance. In addition, TRL was associated with significant reductions in the incidence of acute and steroid-resistant rejection episodes and a consequent lower usage of OKT-3. In some trials, a reduced incidence of hypertension and smaller disturbances in lipoprotein metabolism were also noted. Subsequent renal transplant studies have now yielded similar results: comparable patient and graft survival in the TRL and CsA treatment groups, but significant reductions in the incidence of rejection and less frequent OKT-3 usage in TRL-treated patients. However, changes in the vascular risk profile (hypertension and lipoprotein metabolism) appeared to be somewhat less prominent. Adverse reactions associated with TRL are similar to those seen with CsA, although some differences are apparent. Nephrotoxicity is comparable, but both gingival hyperplasia and hirsutism are far less prevalent with TRL. A major difference in some trials is the higher diabetogenic effect of TRL, which may be controlled by steroid reduction.

TRL possesses a unique property not as evident with CsA. In numerous trials in both liver and renal transplant recipients, TRL has shown the capacity to reverse refractory allograft rejection. This effect appears to be independent of the preceding administration of antilymphocyte antibodies, and the use of TRL is therefore warranted even in the presence of steroid-resistant graft rejection or when treatment with antilymphocyte antibodies is ineffective or contraindicated. Based on experience with TRL in previous studies of primary immunosuppressive treatment and on the compelling evidence that the drug is effective in rescue therapy, its use in a primary immunosuppressive regimen for immunologic high responders should be considered.

In conclusion, with respect to the emerging clinical role of small molecule immunosuppressive agents, the short-term results appear similar to those achieved with CsA immunosuppression. However, as a result of their distinct properties, they may offer a more flexible individualization of immunosuppression and hopefully, in the long run, for improvement in long-term graft survival.

REFERENCES

1. Gosio B. Ricerche bacteriologiche e chimiche sulle alterazioni del mais. Riv Igiene e Sanita Publica Ann 1896;7:825.
2. Platz KP, Sollinger HW, Hullett DA, et al. RS-61443—a new potent immunosuppressive agent. Transplantation 1991;51:27–31.
3. Schiff MH, Goldblum R, Rees MMC. 2-Morpholino-ethyl mycophenolic acid in the treatment of refractory rheumatoid arthritis. Arthritis Rheum 1990;33s:155.
4. Jones EL, Epinette WW, Hackney VC, et al. Treatment of psoriasis with oral mycophenolic acid. J Invest Dermatol 1975;65:537–542.
5. Lynch WS, Roesnigk HH Jr. Mycophenolic acid for psoriasis. Arch Dermatol 1977;113:1203–1208.
6. Epinette WW, Parker CM, Jones EL, Greist MC. Mycophenolic acid for psoriasis. J Am Acad Dermatol 1987;17:962–971.
7. Sollinger HW, Eugi EM, Allison AC. RS-61443: mechanism of action, experimental and early clinical results. Clin Transplant 1991;5s:523–526.
8. Giblett ER, Anderson JE, Cohen F, Meuwissen HJ. Adenosine deaminase deficiency of two patients with severely impaired cellular immunity. Lancet 1972;2:1067–1069.
9. Natsumeda Y, Carr SF. Human type I and II IMPDH as drug targets. Ann NY Acad Sci 1993;696:88.
10. Franklin TJ, Cook JM. The inhibition of nucleic acid synthesis by mycophenolic acid. Biochem J 1969;113:515–524.
11. Mizuno K, Miyazaki T. Synthesis and cytotoxicity of bredinine 5-monophosphate. Chem Pharm Bull 1976;24:2248–2250.
12. Mita A, Akiyama N, Nagao T, et al. Advantages of mizorbine over azathioprine in combination therapy with cyclosporine for renal transplantation. Transplant Proc 1990;22:1679–1681.
13. Eugi EM, Almquist S, Muller CD, Allison AC. Lymphocyte selective cytostatic and immunosuppressive effects of mycophenolic acid in vitro: role of deoxyguanosine nucleotide depletion. Scan J Immunol 1991;33:161–173.
14. Allison AC, Kowalski WJ, Muller CD, Eugi EM. Mechanisms of action of mycophenolic acid. Ann NY Acad Sci 1993;696:63.
15. Allison AC, Eugi EM. Inhibitors of de novo purine and pyrimidine synthesis as immunosuppressive drugs. Transplant Proc 1993; 25(Suppl 2):8–18.
16. Dayton JS, Turka LA, Thompson CB, et al. Comparison of the effects of mizoribine with those of azathioprine, 6-mercaptopurine or mycophenolic acid on T lymphocyte proliferation and purine metabolism. Molec Pharmacol 1992;141:671.
17. Laurent AF, Dumont S, Poindron P, Muller CD. Mycophenolic acid suppresses protein N-linked glycosylation in human monocytes and their adhesion to endothelial cells and to some substratcs. Exp Hematol 1996;24:59–67.
18. Alices M, Osborne L, Takada Y, Carause C. VCAM-1 on activated endothelium interacts with the lymphocytes integrin VLA-4 at a site distinct from the fiber nectin binding site. Cell 1990;60:577–584.
19. Allison AC, Kowalski WJ, Muller CJ, et al. Mycophenolic acid and brequinar, inhibitors of purine and pyrimidine synthesis, block the glycosylation of adhesion molecules. Transplant Proc 1993;25(3;Suppl 2):67–70.
20. Lee WA, Gu L, Miksztal AR, et al. Bioavailability improvement of mycophenolic acid through amino ester derivatization. Pharmaceut Res 1990;7:161–166.
21. Allison AC, Eugi EM. Immunosuppressive and long-acting anti-inflammatory effect of mycophenolic acid and derivatives, RS-61433. Br J Rheum 1991;30(Suppl 2):57–61.
22. Propper DJ, Woo J, Macleod AM, et al. The effects of rapamycin on humoral immunity in vivo: suppression of primary responses but not of ongoing alloantibody synthesis or memory responses. Transplantation 1992;54:1058.
23. Sollinger HW, Deierhoi MH, Belzer FO, et al. RS-61443: a phase I clinical trial and pilot rescue study. Transplantation 1992;53:428–432.
24. Marinairi R, Fleischmajer R, Schragger AH, Rosenthal AL. Mycophenolic acid in treatment of psoriasis: long term administration. Arch Dermatol 1977;113:930–932.
25. Jones EL, Frost P, Epinette WW, Gomez E. Mycophenolic acid: an evaluation of long-term safety. In: Faber M, ed. Psoriasis: Proceedings of the Second International Symposium. New York: Yorke, 1977:442–443.
26. Goldblum R, McHugh D, Schiff M, et al. 2-morpholino-ethyl mycophenolic acid (ME-MPA) inhibits lymphocyte mitogen responses in rheumatoid arthritis. J Clin Pharm Ther 1990;47:193.
27. Deierhoi MH, Kauffman RS, Hudson SL, et al. Experience with mycophenolate mofetil (RS61443) in renal transplantation at a single center. Ann Surg 1993;217:476–484.
28. Paterson DL, Singh W, Panebianco A, et al. Infectious complications occurring in liver transplant recipients receiving mycophenolate mofetil. Transplantation 1998;66:593–598.
29. Kirklin JK, Bouge RC, Naftel DC, et al. Treatment of recurrent heart rejection with mycophenolate mofetil: initial clinical experience. J Heart Lung Transplantation 1994;13:444–450.
30. Neylan JF for the U.S. Renal Transplant Mycophenolate Mofetil Study Group. Immunosuppressive therapy in high-risk transplant patients. Transplantation 1997;64:1277–1282.
31. Sollinger HW, Belzer FO, Deierhoi MH, et al. RS-61443: a multicenter study for refractory kidney transplant rejection. Ann Surg 1992;216:513–519.
32. The Mycophenolate Mofetil Renal Refractory Rejection Study Group. Mycophenolate mofetil for the treatment of refractory acute cellular renal transplant rejection. Transplantation 1996;61:722–729.
33. European Mycophenolate Mofetil Cooperative Study Group. Placebo-controlled study of mycophenolate mofetil combined with cyclosporin and corticosteroids for prevention of acute rejection. Lancet 1995;345:1321–1325.
34. Sollinger HW, for the US Renal Transplant Mycophenolate Mofetil Study Group. Mycophenolate mofetil for the prevention of acute rejection in primary cadaveric renal allograft recipients. Transplantation 1995;60:225–232.
35. Morris RE, Wang J, Blum JR, et al. Immunosuppressive effects of the morpholinoethyl ester of mycophenolic acid (RS-61443) in rat and nonhuman primate recipients of heart allografts. Transplant Proc 1991;23(Suppl 2):19–25.
36. Steele DM, Hullett DA, Bechtein WO, et al. The effects of immunosuppressive therapy on rat aortic allograft model. Transplant Proc 1993;25:754.
37. Schmid C, Heemann U, Azuma H, Tilney NL. Comparison of rapamycin, RS-61443, cyclosporine, and low-dose heparin as treatment for transplant vasculopathy in rat model of chronic allograft rejection. Transplant Proc 1995;27:438–439.
38. Azuma H, Binder J, Heeman U, et al. Effects of RS61443 on functional and morphological changes in chronically rejecting rat kidney allografts. Transplant Proc 1995;27(1):436–437.
39. Mathew TH for the Tricontinental Mycophenolate Mofetil Renal Transplantation Study Group. A blinded, long-term, randomized multicenter study of mycophenolate mofetil in cadaveric renal transplantation. Transplantation 1998;65:1450–1454.
40. Gruessner RWG, Sutherland DER, Drangstveit MB, et al. Mycophenolate mofetil in pancreas transplantation. Transplantation 1998;66:318–323.
41. Dexter DL, Hesson DP, Ardecky RJ, et al. Activity of a novel 4-quinolinecarboxylic acid, NSC368390 [6-fluoro-2-(2′fluoro-1,1′biphenyl-4-yl)-3-methyl-4-quinolinecarboxylic acid sodium salt], against experimental tumors. Cancer Res 1985;45:5563–5568.
42. Chen SF, Ruben R, Dexter D. Mechanism of action of the novel anti-cancer agent 6-fluoro-2-(2′-fluoro-1,1 byphenyl 4-yl)-3 methyl-4 quinolone carboxylic acid sodium salt. Inhibition of de novo pyrimidine nucleotide biosynthesis. Cancer Res 1986;46:5014.
43. Simon P, Townsend RM, Harris RR, et al. Brequinar sodium: inhibition of dihydro-orotic acid dehydrogenase, depletion of pyrimidine pools and consequent inhibition of immune function in vitro. Transplant Proc 1993;25(Suppl 2):77–80.
44. Chen SF, Papp LM, Ardecky RJ, et al. Structure-activity relationship of quinoline carboxylic acids: a new class of inhibitors of dihydro-orotate dehydrogenase. Biochem Pharmacol 1990;40:709–714.
45. Chen JJ, Jones ME. The ceullar location of dihydro-orotate dehydrogenase: relation to de novo biosynthesis of pyrimidines. Arch Biochem Biophys 1976;176:82–90.

46. Makowka L, Chapman F, Cramer DV. Historical development of brequinar sodium as a new immunosuppressive drug for transplantation. Transplant Proc 1993;25(Suppl 2):2–7.
47. Peters GJ, Nadal JC, Laurensse EJ, et al. Retention of in vitro antipyrimidine effects of brequinar sodium (DUP-785; NSC 368390) in murine liver, bone marrow, and colon cancer. Biochem Pharmacol 1990;39:134–144.
48. Makowka L, Sher LS, Cramer DV. The development of brequinar as an immunosuppressive drug for transplantation. Immunol Rev 1993;136:51.
49. Cramer DV, Chapman FA, Jafee BD, et al. The effects of a new immunosuppressive drug: brequinar sodium on heart, liver and kidney allograft rejection in the rat. Transplantation 1992;53:303–308.
50. Jaffee BD, Jones EA, Loveless SE, Chen SF. The unique immunosuppressive activity of brequinar sodium. Transplant Proc 1993;25(Suppl 2):19.
51. Kahan BD, Tejpal N, Gibbons S, et al. The synergistic interactions in vivo and in vitro of brequinar sodium with cyclosporine or rapamycin alone and in triple combination. Transplantation 1993;55:894.
52. Cramer DV, Chapman FA, Jaffee BD, et al. The prolongation of concordant cardiac hamster-to-rat xenograft by brequinar sodium. Transplantation 1993;54:403–408.
53. Yasunaga C, Cramer DV, Chapman FA, et al. The prevention of accelerated cardiac allograft rejection in sensitized recipients following treatment with brequinar sodium. Transplantation 1993;56:898.
54. Eiras-Hreha G, Cramer DV, Cosenza C, et al. Brequinar sodium: monitoring immunosuppressive activity. Transplant Proc 1993;25(3;Suppl 2):32–36.
55. Shen HS, Chen SF, Behrens C, et al. Distribution of the novel anticancer drug candidate brequinar sodium (Du 785, NSC 36890) into normal and tumor tissues of nude mice bearing human colon carcinoma xenografts. Cancer Chemother Pharmacol 1988;22:183–186.
56. Schwartzmann G, Dodion P, Vermorken JB, et al. Phase I study with brequinar sodium (NSC 368390) in patients with solid malignancies. Cancer Chemother Pharmacol 1990;25:345–351.
57. Barnes TB, Campbell P, Zajac I, Gayda D. Toxicological and pharmacokinetic effects following coadministration of brequinar sodium and cyclosporine to Sprague-Dawley rats. Transplant Proc 1993;25(Suppl 2):71–74.
58. Stepkowski SM, Tu Y, Chou TC, Kahan BD. Synergistic interactions of cyclosporine, rapamycin, and brequinar on heart allograft survival in mice. Transplant Proc 1994;26:3025–3027.
59. Kawamura T, Hullet DA, Suzuki Y, et al. Enhancement of allograft survival by combination RS-61443 and DUP-785 therapy. Transplantation 1993;55: 691–695.
60. Makowka L, Tixier D, Chaux A, et al. The use of brequinar sodium for preventing cardiac allograft rejection in primates. Transplant Proc 1993;25(Suppl 2):48–53.
61. Artega CL, Brown TD, Khun JG, et al. Phase I clinical and pharmacokinetic trial of brequinar sodium. Cancer Res 1989;49:4648.
62. Maorun J, Ruckdeschel J, Natale R, et al. Multicenter phase II study of brequinar sodium in patients with advanced lung cancer. Cancer Chemother Pharmacol 1993;32:64.
63. Sher LS, Eiras-Hreha G, Kornhauser DM, et al. Safety and pharmacokinetics of brequinar sodium in liver allograft recipients on cyclosporine and steroids. Hepatology 1993;18:746.
64. Chong AS-F, Gebel H, Finnegan A, et al. Leflunomide, a novel immunomodulatory agent: in vitro analyses of the mechanism of immunosuppression. Transplant Proc 1993;25(1):747–749.
65. Chong AS-F, Finnegan A, Jiang XL, et al. Leflunomide, a novel immunosuppressive agent: the mechanism of inhibition of T cell proliferation. Transplantation 1993;55:1361–1366.
66. Chong AS, Xiao F, Xu XL, Williams JW. In vivo and in vitro immunosuppression with leflunomide. New immunosuppressive drugs. Glenview, IL: Physicians and Scientists, 1995:163–176.
67. Bartlett RR, Dimitrijevic M, Mattar T, et al. Leflunomide (HWA 486), a novel immunomodulating compound for the treatment of autoimmune disorders and reactions leading to transplantation rejection. Agents Actions 1991;32:10–21.
68. Cao WW, Kao PN, Choa AC, et al. Mechanism of antiproliferative action of leflunomide. A77 1726, the active metabolite of leflunomide, does not block T-cell receptor-mediated signal transduction but its antiproliferative effects are antagonized by pyrimidine nucleosides. J Heart Lung Transplant 1995;14:1016–1030.
69. Bartlett RR, Schleyerbach R. Immunopharmacological profile of novel isoxazol derivative HWA 486, with potential antirheumatic activity-I. Disease modifying action on arthritis of the rat. Int J Immunopharmacol 1985;7:7–18.
70. Popovic S, Bartlett RR. The use of the murine chronic graft vs. host disease, a model for systemic lupus erythematosis, for drug discovery. Agents Actions 1987;21:284.
71. Ogawa T, Inazu M, Gotoh K, Hayashi S. Effects of leflunomide on glomerulonephritis induced by antibasement membrane antibody in rats. Agents and Actions 1990;31:321–328.
72. Thoenes GH, Sitter T, Langer KH, et al. Leflunomide (HWA 486) inhibits experimental autoimmune tubulointerstitial nephritis in rats. Int J Immunopharmac 1989;11:921–929.
73. McChesney L, Xiao F, Sankary H, et al. Evaluation of leflunomide in the canine renal transplantation model. Transplantation 1994;57:1717–1722.
74. Kuchle CCA, Thoenes GH, Langer KH, et al. Prevention of kidney and skin graft rejection in rats by leflunomide, a new immunomodulating agent. Transplant Proc 1991;23:1083–1086.
75. Schorlemmer HU, Seiler FR, Bartlett RR. Prolongation of allogeneic transplanted skin grafts and induction of tolerance by leflunomide, a new immunosuppressive isoxazol derivative. Transplant Proc 1993;25:763–767.
76. Williams JW, Xiao F, Foster P, et al. Leflunomide in experimental transplantation. Transplantation 1994;57:1223–1231.
77. Xiao F, Chong A, Foster P, et al. Effect of leflunomide in control of acute rejection in hamster-to-rat cardiac xenografts. Transplant Proc 1993;26:1263–1265.
78. Kino T, Hatanaka H, Hoshimata M, et al. FK 506, a novel immunosuppressant isolated from a streptomyces. I. Fermentation, isolation, and physicochemical and biological characteristics. J Antibiotics 1987;40:1249–1255.
79. Tanaka H, Kurado A, Marusawa H, et al. Structure of FK 506: a novel immunosuppressant isolated from a streptomyces. J Am Chem Soc 1987;109:5031–5033.
80. Harding MW, Galat A, Uehling DE, Schreiber SL. A receptor for immunosuppressant FK506 is a peptidyl prolyl cis-trans isomerase. Nature 1989;341:758–760.
81. Siekierka JJ, Hung SHY, Poe M, et al. A cytosolic binding protein for the immunosuppressive FK506 has peptidyl prolyl isomerase activity but is distinct from cyclophilin. Nature 1989;341:755–757.
82. Liu J. FK506 and cyclosporine, molecular probes for studying intracellular signal transduction. Immunol Today 1993;14(6):290–295.
83. Klee CB, Draetta GF, Hubbard MJ. Advances in enzymology and related areas of molecular biology. Vol. 61. New York: Wiley, 1988:49–209.
84. Fruman DA, Klee CB, Bierer BE, Burakoff SJ. Calcineurin phosphatase activity in T lymphocytes is inhibited by FK506 and cyclosporin A. Proc Natl Acad Sci 1992;89:3686–3690.
85. O'Keefe SJ, Tamura J, Kincaid RL, et al. FK-506 and CsA-sensitive activation of the interleukin-2 promoter by calcineurin. Nature 1992;357:692–694.
86. Tocci MJ, Matkovich DA, Collier KA, et al. The immunosuppressant FK506 selectively inhibits expression of early T cell activation genes. J Immunol 1989;143:718–726.
87. Bram RJ, Hung DT, Martin PK, et al. Identification of the immunophilins capable of mediating inhibition of signal transduction by cyclosporin A and FK506. Roles of calcineurin binding and cellular localization. Mol Cell Biol 1993;13:4760–4769.
88. Takada K, Oh-hashi M, Yoshikawa H, et al. Determination of a novel potent immunosuppressant (FK506) in rat serum and lymph by high-performance liquid chromotography with chemiluminescence detection. J Chromatography 1990;530:212–228.
89. Warty V, Zuckerman S, Venkataramanan R, et al. FK506 measurement: comparison of different analytical methods. Ther Drug Monit 1993;15:204–208.
90. Venkataramanan R, Jain A, Warty VW, et al. Pharmacokinetics of FK506 following oral administration: a comparison of FK506 and cyclosporine. Transplant Proc 1991;23:931–933.
91. Venkataramanan R, Jain A, Cadoff E, et al. Pharmacokinetics of FK506: preclinical and clinical studies. Transplant Proc 1990;22(Suppl 1):52.
92. European FK 506 Multicenter Liver Study Group. Randomised trial comparing tacrolimus (FK506) and cyclosporin in prevention of liver allograft rejection. Lancet 1994;344:423–428.
93. The U.S. Multicenter FK506 Liver Study Group. A comparison of tacrolimus (FK506) and cyclosporine for immunosuppression in liver transplantation. N Eng J Med 1994;331(17):1110–1115.
94. FK506 Kidney Transplant Study Group. A comparison of tacrolimus (FK506) and cyclosporine for immunosuppression after cadaveric kidney transplantation. Transplantation 1997;63:977–983.
95. Starzl TE, Todo S, Fung J, et al. FK 506 for liver, kidney and pancreas transplantation. Lancet 1989;2:1000–1004.

96. Jordan ML, Shapiro R, Jensen CWB, et al. FK 506 conversion of renal allografts failing cyclosporine immunosuppression. Transplant Proc 1991;23:3078–3081.
97. Jordan ML, Shapiro R, Vivas CA, et al. FK 506 "rescue" for resistant rejection of renal allografts under primary cyclosporine immunosuppression. Transplantation 1994;57:860–865.
98. The U.S. Multicenter FK506 Liver Study Group. Use of prograf (FK506) as rescue therapy for refractory rejection after liver transplantation. Transplant Proc 1993;25:679–688.
99. Armitage JM, Kormos RL, Griffith BP. A clinical trial of FK 506 as primary and rescue immunosuppression in cardiac transplantation. Transplant Proc 1991;23:1149.
100. McMaster P, Dousset B. The improved results of liver transplantation. Transplant Int 1992;5:125.
101. Japanese FK 506 Study Group. Japanese study of FK 506 on kidney transplantation: results of phase II study. Transplant Proc 1993;25:649–654.
102. Tacrolimus Pancreas Transplant Study Group. Tacrolimus in pancreas transplantation: a multicenter analysis. Clin Transplant 1997;11:299–312.
103. Laskow DA, Neylan JF, Shapiro RS, et al. The role of tacrolimus in adult kidney transplantation: a review. Clin Transplant 1998;12:489–503.
104. Keck BM, Bennett LE, Fiol BS, et al. Worldwide thoracic organ transplantation: a report from the UNOS/ISHLT International Registry for Thoracic Organ Transplantation. In: Terasaki PI, Cecka JM, eds. Clinical transplants 1997. Los Angeles: UCLA Tissue Typing Laboratory, 1998:29–43.
105. Vezina C, Kudelski A, Sehgal SN. Rapamycin (AY-22,989), a new antifungal antibiotic: I. Taxonomy of the producing streptomycete and isolation of the active principle. J Antibiot (Tokyo) 1975;28:721–732.
106. Sehgal SN, Baker H, Vezina C. Rapamycin (AY-22,989), a new antifungal antibiotic: II. Fermentation, isolation and characterization. J Antibiot (Tokyo) 1975;28:727–732.
107. Douros J, Suffness M. New antitumor substances of natural origin. Cancer Treatment Rev 1981;8:63.
108. Eng CP, Sehgal SN, Vezina C. Activity of rapamycin (AY-22,989) against transplanted tumors. J Antibiot 1984;37:2131.
109. Findlay JA, Radics L. On the chemistry and high field nuclear magnetic resonance spectroscopy of rapamycin. Can J Chem 1980;58:579–584.
110. Paiva NL, Demain AL, Roberts MF. Incorporation of acetate, proprionate, and methionine into rapamycin by *Streptomyces hygroscopicus*. J Nat Prod 1991;54:167.
111. Kahan BD. Immunosuppressive agents acting upon lymphokine synthesis and signal transduction. Clin Transplantation 1993;7:113–125.
112. Kunz J, Henriquez R, Schneider U, et al. Target of rapamycin in yeast, TOR2, is essential phosphatidylinositol kinase homolog required for G1 progression. Cell 1993;73:585–596.
113. Kahan BD, Ghobrial R. Immunosuppressive agents. In: Kahan BD, ed. Surgical clinics of North America: transplantation. Philadelphia: WB Saunders, 1994:1029–1054.
114. Sehgal SN, Molnar-Kimber, Ocain TD, Weichman BM. Rapamycin: a novel immunosuppressive macrolide. Medicinal Res Rev 1994;14(1):1–22.
115. Kuo CJ, Chung J, Fiorentino DF, et al. Rapamycin selectively inhibits interleukin-2 activation of p70S6 kinase. Nature 1992;358(6381):70–73.
116. Morris RE. Rapamycin: antifungal, antitumor, antiproliferative, and immunosuppressive macrolides. Transplantation Rev 1992;6(1):39–87.
117. Morice WG, Brunn GJ, Wiederrecht G, et al. Rapamycin induced inhibition of p34cdc2 kinase activation is associated with G1/S-phase growth arrest in T lymphocytes. J Biochem 1993;268:3734–3738.
118. Streit F, Christians U, Schiebel HM, et al. Sensitive and specific quantification of sirolimus (rapamycin) and its metabolites in blood and urine of kidney graft recipients using HPLC/electrospray-mass spectrometry. Clin Chem 1996;42:1417–1425.
119. Napoli KL, Kahan BD. Routine clinical monitoring of sirolimus whole-blood concentrations by HPLC with ultraviolet detection. Clin Chem 1996;42:1943–1948.
120. Zimmerman J, Kahan BD. The pharmacokinetics of sirolimus in stable renal transplant patients after multiple oral dose administration. J Clin Pharmacol 1997;37:405–415.
121. Stepkowski SM, Napoli KL, Wang ME, et al. The effects of the pharmacokinetic interaction between orally administered sirolimus and cyclosporine on the synergistic prolongation of heart allograft survival in rats. Transplantation 1996;62:986–994.
122. Morris RE, Meiser BM. Identification of a new pharmacologic action for an old compound. Med Sci Res 1989;17:877.
123. Morris RE, Meiser BM, Wu J, et al. Use of rapamycin for the suppression of the alloimmune reactions in vivo: schedule-dependence, tolerance induction, synergy with cyclosporine and FK 506 and effect on host-versus-graft and graft-versus-host reactions. Transplant Proc 1991;23:521–524.
124. Stepkowski SM, Chen H, Dalazo P, Kahan BD. Rapamycin, a potent immunosuppressive drug for vascularized heart, kidney, small bowel transplantation in rat. Transplantation 1991;51:22–26.
125. Calne RY, Collier DS, Lim S, et al. Rapamycin for immunosuppression in organ allografting. Lancet 1989;2:227.
126. Collier DS, Calne R, Thiru S, et al. Rapamycin in experimental renal allografts in dogs and pigs. Transplant Proc 1990;22:1674.
127. Collier DS, Calne RY, Pollard SG, et al. Rapamycin in experimental renal allografts in primates. Transplant Proc 1991;23:2246.
128. Whiting PH, Adam J, Woo J, et al. The effect of rapamycin on renal function in the rat: a comparative study with cyclosporine. Toxicol Lett 1991;58:169–179.
129. Di Joseph JF, Sehgal SN. Functional and histopathologic effects of rapamycin on mouse kidney. Immunopharmacol Immunotoxicol 1993;15:45–99.
130. Ferraresso M, Ghobrial R, Stepkowski S, Kahan BD. Mechanism of unresponsiveness to allografts induced by rapamycin and rapamycin/cyclosporine treatment in rats. Transplantation 1993;55:888–894.
131. Wang M, Stepkowski SM, Ferraresso M, et al. Rapamycin rescue therapy delays rejection of heart allografts in rats. Transplantation 1993;54:704.
132. Chen H, Wu J, Xu D, et al. Reversal of ongoing heart, kidney and pancreas allograft rejection and suppression of accelerated heart allograft rejection in the rat by rapamycin. Transplantation 1993;56:661–666.
133. Adams DH, Wyner LR, Karnovsky MJ. Cardiac graft arteriosclerosis in the rat. Transplant Proc 1993;25(2):2071–2073.
134. Meiser B, Reichart B. Graft vessel disease: the impact of immunosuppression and possible treatment strategies. Immunol Rev 1993;134:99–116.
135. Ardehali A, Billingsley A, Laks H, et al. Experimental cardiac allograft vasculopathy in mice. J Heart Lung Transplant 1993;12:730–735.
136. Gregory CR, Huang X, Pratt RE, et al. Treatment with rapamycin and mycophenolic acid reduces arterial intimal thickening produced by mechanical injury and allows endothelial replacement. Transplantation 1995;59:655–661.
137. Kimball PM, Kerman RH, Kahan BD. Rapamycin and cyclosporine produce synergistic but nonidentical mechanism of immunosuppression. Transplant Proc 1991;23(1):1027–1028.
138. Kahan BD, Gibbons S, Tejpal N, et al. Synergistic interactions of cyclosporine and rapamycin to inhibit immune performances of normal human peripheral blood lymphocytes in vitro. Transplantation 1991;51:232–239.
139. Meiser BM, Wang J, Morris RE. Rapamycin: a new highly active immunosuppressive macrolide with an efficacy superior to cyclosporine. Prog Immunol 1989;7:1195–1198.
140. Ochiai T, Gunji Y, Nagata M, et al. Effects of rapamycin in experimental organ allografting. Transplant 1993;56:15–19.
141. Bierer BE, Somers PK, Wandless TJ, et al. Probing immunosuppressant action with a nonnatural immunophilin ligand. Science 1990;250:556–559.
142. Vu MD, Qi S, Xu D, et al. Synergistic effects of mycophenolate mofetil and sirolimus in prevention of acute heart, pancreas, and kidney allograft rejection in the rat. Transplantation 1998;66:1575–1580.
143. Murgia MG, Jordan S, Kahan BD. The side effect profile of sirolimus: a phase I study in quiescent cyclosporine-prednisone-treated renal transplant patients. Kidney Int 1996;49:209–216.
144. Kahan BD. Sirolimus: a new agent for clinical renal transplantation. Transplant Proc 1997;29:48–50.
145. Groth CG, Brattström C, Claesson K, et al. New trials in transplantation: how to exploit the potential of sirolimus in clinical transplantation. Transplant Proc 1998;30:4064–4065.
146. Kahan BD, Podbielski J, Napoli KL, et al. Immunosuppressive effects and safety of a sirolimus/cyclosporine combination regimen for renal transplantation. Transplantation 1998;66:1040–1046.
147. Falf W, Ulrichs K, Muller-Ruchholtz W. 15-deoxyspergualin (a new guanidine-like drug) blocks T lymphocyte proliferation. Transplant Proc 1991;23:864–865.
148. Takeuchi T, Iinuma H, Kunimoto S, et al. A new antitumor antibiotic, spergualin: isolation and antitumor activity. Antibiotics 1981;34:1619–1621.
149. Hibashami H, Tsukada T, Suzuki R, et al. Deoxyspergualin, an antiproliferative agent, shows inhibitory effects on synthetic pathway of polyamines. Anticancer Res 1991;11:325–330.
150. Umeda Y, Moriguchi M, Kurond H, et al. Synthesis and antitumor activity of spergualin analogues: I. Chemical modification of 7-guanidine-3-hydroxyacyl moiety. J Antibiot 1985;38:886–898.

151. Walter P, Feifel G, Shorlemmer H, et al. A new immunosuppressive active antitumoral drug 15-deoxyspergualin prevents rejection of allogeneic transplanted islets. Transplant Proc 1986;18:1860–1861.
152. Ochiai T, Hori S, Nakajima K, et al. Prolongation of rat heart allograft survival by 15-deoxyspergualin. J Antibiot 1987;40:249–250.
153. Thies JC, Walter PK, Zimmermann FA, et al. Prolongation of graft survival in allogeneic pancreas and liver transplantation by 15-deoxyspergualin. Eur Surg Res 1987;19:129–134.
154. Umezawa H, Ishizuka M, Takeuchi K, et al. Suppression of tissue graft rejection by spergualin. J Antibiot 1985;38:283–284.
155. Masuda T, Mizutani S, Iijima M, et al. Immunosuppressive activity of 15-deoxyspergualin and its effect on skin allografts in rats. J Antibiot 1987;40:1612–1618.
156. Takahara S, Jiang H, Takano Y, et al. The in vitro immunosuppressive effects of deoxyspergualin in man compared with FK 506 and cyclosporine. Transplantation 1992;53:914–918.
157. Tepper MA, Nadler S, Mazzucco C, et al. 15-deoxyspergualin: a novel immunosuppressive drug: studies of the mechanism of action. Ann New York Acad Sci 1993;685:136–147.
158. Kerr PG, Atkins RC. The effects of deoxyspergualin on human cytotoxic T lymphocytes, NK cells, and LAK cells. Kidney Int 1990;38:557–558.
159. Nishimura K, Tokunaga T. Mechanism of action of 15-deoxyspergualin: suppressive effects on the induction of alloreactive secondary cytotoxic T lymphocytes in vivo and in vitro. Immunology 1989;68:66–71.
160. Nishimura K, Tokunaga T. Mode of action of 15-deoxyspergualin: effects on induction and effector function of cytotoxic T lymphocytes (CTL). Int J Immunopharmacol 1988;10:75.
161. Kerr PG, Atkins RC. The effects of deoxyspergualin on lymphocytes and monocytes in vivo and in vitro. Transplantation 1989;48:1048–1052.
162. Pai LH, FitzGerald DJ, Tepper MA, et al. Inhibition of antibody response to *Pseudomonas exotoxin* and an immunotoxin containing *Pseudomonas exotoxin* by 15-deoxyspergualin in mice. Cancer Res 1990;50:7750–7753.
163. Sterbenz KG, Tepper MA. Effects of 15-deoxyspergualin on the expression of surface immunoglobulin in 70Z/3.12 murine pre-B cell line. Ann New York Acad Sci 1993;685:205–207.
164. Nadler SG, Tepper M, Schacter B, Mazzucco CE. Interaction of the immunosuppressant deoxyspergualin with a member of the Hsp 70 family of heat shock proteins. Science 1992;258:484–486.
165. Waaga AM, Ulrichs K, Krzymanski M, et al. The immunosuppressive agent 15-deoxyspergualin induces tolerance and modulates MHC-antigen expression and interleukin-1 production in the early phase of rat allograft responses. Transplant Proc 1990;22:1613–1614.
166. Dickneite G, Shorlemmer HU, Sedlacek HH. Decrease of mononuclear phagocyte cell functions and prolongation of graft survival in experimental transplantation by 15-deoxyspergualin. Int J Immunopharmacol 1987;9:559–565.
167. Thomas FT, Tepper MA, Thomas JM, Haisch CE. 15-deoxyspergualin: a novel immunosuppressive drug with clinical potential. Ann New York Acad Sci 1993;685:175–192.
168. Muindi J, Lee S, Baltzer L, et al. Clinical pharmacology of deoxyspergualin in patients with advanced cancer. Cancer Res 1991;51:3096–3101.
169. Tamura K, Niitaji H, Ogawa M, Kimura K. Phase I and pharmacokinetic study of deoxyspergualin given by 3-hour infusion for 5 days. Proceedings of ASCO 1989;8:74.
170. Sprancmanis LA, Riley CM, Stobaugh JF. Determination of the anticancer drug, 15-deoxyspergualin, in plasma ultrafiltrate by liquid chromatography and precolumn derivatization with naphthalene-2,3-dicarboxyaldehyde/cyanide. J Pharmacol Biomed Anal 1990;8:165–175.
171. Hibasami H, Tsukada T, Suzuki R, et al. Deoxyspergualin, an antiproliferative agents, shows inhibitory effects on the synthetic pathway on polyamines. Anticancer Res 1991;11:325–330.
172. Morris RE. 15-deoxyspergualin: a mystery wrapped within an enigma. Clin Transplant 1991;5:530–533.
173. Yuh DY, Morris RE. The immunopharmacology of immunosuppression by 15-deoxyspergualin. Transplantation 1993;55:578–591.
174. Kamata K, Okubo M, Masaki Y, et al. Effect of 15-deoxyspergualin on the survival of thyroid allografts in mice. Transplant Proc 1989;21:1099–1103.
175. Reichenspeurner H, Hidebrandt A, Human P. 15-deoxyspergualin after cardiac and kidney allotransplantation in primates. Transplant Proc 1990;22:1618–1619.
176. Shorlemmer H, Dickneite G, Seiler F. Treatment of acute rejection episodes and induction tolerance in rat skin allotransplantation by 15-deoxyspergualin. Transplant Proc 1990;22:1626–1630.
177. Amemiya H, Suzuki S, Niya S, et al. A new immunosuppressive agent, 15-deoxyspergualin in dog renal allografting. Transplant Proc 1989;21: 3468–3470.
178. Reichenspeurner H, Human P, Boehm DH, et al. Optimisation of immunosuppression after xenogeneic heart transplantation in primates. J Heart Transplant 1989;8:200–208.
179. Koyama I, Amamiya H, Taguchi Y, et al. Prophylactic use of deoxyspergualin in a quadruple immunosuppressive protocol in renal transplantation. Transplant Proc 1991;23:1096–1098.
180. Gores PF, Najarian JS, Stephanian E, et al. Insulin independence in type I diabetes after transplantation of unpurified islet from single donor with 15-deoxyspergualin. Lancet 1993;341:19.
181. Amemiya H, Suzuki S, Ota K, et al. A novel rescue drug, 15-deoxyspergualin. Transplantation 1990;49:337–343.
182. Amemiya H. Deoxyspergualin: clinical trials in renal graft rejection. Ann NY Acad Sci 1993;685:196–201.
183. Kyo M, Ichikawa Y, Fukunishi Y, et al. Histopathologic classification and clinical effects of kidney transplant rejection treated with 15-deoxyspergualin. Transplant Proc 1995;27:1012.
184. Amemiya and Japanese Collaborative Transplant Study Group of NKT-01. Immunosuppressive mechanism and action of deoxyspergualin in experimental and clinical studies. Transplant Proc 1995;27:31.
185. Takahashi K, Tanabe K, Ooba S, et al. Prophylactic use of a new immunosuppressive agent, deoxyspergualin, in patients with kidney transplantation from ABO incompatible or preformed antibody-positive donors. Transplant Proc 1991;23:1078–1082.
186. Groth CG. Deoxyspergualin in allogeneic kidney and xenogeneic islet transplantation: early clinical trial. Ann New York Acad Sci 1993;685: 193–195.
187. Fujita T, Inoue K, Yamamoto S, et al. Fungal metabolites. Part 11. A potent immunosuppressive activity found in *Isaria sinclairii* metabolite. J Antibiot 1994;47:208.
188. Adachi K, Kohara T, Nakao N, et al. Design, synthesis, and structure-activity relationship of 2-substituted-2-amino-1,3-propanediols: discovery of a novel immunosuppressant, FTY720. Bioorganic & Medicinal Chemistry Letters 1995;5:853–856.
189. Fujita T, Yoneta M, Hirose R, et al. Simple compounds, 2-alkyl-2-amino-1,3-propanediols have potent immunosuppressive activity. Bioorg Med Chem 1995;5:847.
190. Chiba K, Teshima A, Fujii A, et al. FTY720, a novel immunosuppressant, possessing unique mechanism. I. Relationship between immunosuppressive effects and selective decrease of peripheral mature T cells. San Francisco: 9th International Congress of Immunology, 1995:864.
191. Miyake Y, Kozutsumi Y, Nakamura S, et al. Abstracts of the 16th Symposium on the interaction between biological membranes and drugs. Kyoto, 1994:21.
192. Suzuki S, Enosawa S, Kakefuda T, et al. A novel immunosuppressant, FTY720, with a unique mechanism of action, induces long-term graft acceptance in rat and dog allotransplantation. Transplantation 1996;61:200–205.
193. Chiba K, Adachi K. FTY720. Drugs of the Future 1997;22:18.
194. Hoshino Y, Chiba F, Rahman F, et al. FTY720, a novel immunosuppressant, possessing unique mechanism. II. Synergistic prolongation of allograft survival in combination with cyclosporin in rat and dog. San Francisco: 9th International Congress of Immunology, 1995:864.
195. Suzuki S, Kakefuda T, Amemiya H, et al. An immunosuppressive regimen using FTY720 combined with cyclosporine in canine kidney transplantation. Transplant Int 1998;11:95–101.
196. Stepkowski SM, Tu Y, Condon TP, Bennett CF. Blocking of heart allograft rejection by intracellular adhesion molecule 1 antisense oligonucleotides alone or in combination with other immunosuppressive modalities. J Immunol 1994;153:5336.

Chapter

12

Principles of Action of Biologic Immunosuppressants

Lucienne Chatenoud

Polyclonal antilymphocyte sera (ALS) were the first biologic immunosuppressants to be introduced in clinical transplantation for both the prevention and the treatment of acute allograft rejection. This represented, in the late 1960s, a major advance. Prior to that time, prolonged survival of functioning allografts was difficult to achieve using corticosteroids and azathioprine exclusively (1). The introduction of ALS was, in addition, the first step toward the use of drugs having, as opposed to conventional chemical immunosuppressants, a selective activity on immunocompetent cells.

The advent of hybridoma technology in 1975 led to the development of potentially therapeutic monoclonal antibodies directed against T-lymphocyte receptors. This major technologic breakthrough made feasible the characterization of biologic agents that could selectively target functionally distinct cell subsets of immunocompetent cells (Fig. 12.1) (2). Monoclonal antibodies represent, in addition, an excellent alternative to polyclonal antisera, which are laborious to produce, screen, and standardize (see also Chapter 13, Table 13.8). They allow the use of small doses of an homogeneous antibody preparation with predefined specificity for a single cell surface or soluble molecule. More recently, by means of molecular engineering, a new generation of promising biologic agents has emerged in the form of "humanized" monoclonal antibodies and recombinant proteins—immunoadhesins targeting distinct immune cell receptors or products (i.e., cytokines) (Fig. 12.2) (3).

Experimental and clinical experience with biologic agents both in transplantation and in autoimmune disorders has clearly demonstrated that they may exhibit unique therapeutic properties not shared by conventional chemical immunosuppressants (e.g., corticosteroids, azathioprine, cyclosporine). They can, under some circumstances, promote immune tolerance defined operationally as an acquired state of antigen-specific immunologic unresponsiveness that is durable in the absence of generalized chronic immunosuppression (4). The work of Monaco and his group in the early 1970s was seminal in pointing to the ability of ALS to induce tolerance to allografts in rodent skin transplant models (5). Since then, in several models it has been shown that anti-T-cell monoclonal antibodies can induce tolerance to foreign soluble antigens and to tissue alloantigens and autoantigens (6–16).

Understanding the cellular and molecular basis by which biologic agents control deleterious immune responses to allografts requires a discussion of the principal targets.

MAIN TARGETS OF THERAPEUTIC BIOLOGIC AGENTS: IMMUNE CELL RECEPTORS AND SOLUBLE MEDIATORS

Effective immune responses ensue from cooperation between functionally distinct cell types that are antigen-presenting cells (APC), B and T lymphocytes that communicate through an intricate network of cell receptors, and soluble mediators, namely, cytokines. Cell-to-cell cooperation involves a number of surface receptors interacting with their specific ligands as well as with a variety of cytokines (Fig. 12.3). Depending on the context, the stimuli elicited trigger the transduction of intracellular signals leading to immune cell activation, differentiation, functional inactivation (anergy), or programmed cell death (apoptosis).

The allogeneic response of acute rejection is essentially a T-cell mediated immune reaction. In theory, each of the cell actors implicated in this response—namely, the APCs, the $CD4^+$ helper cytokine producers, and $CD8^+$ cytotoxic effectors—and each of their membrane receptors or derived cytokines represent equally good targets for therapeutically relevant immunosuppressants (see Fig. 12.3). In practice,

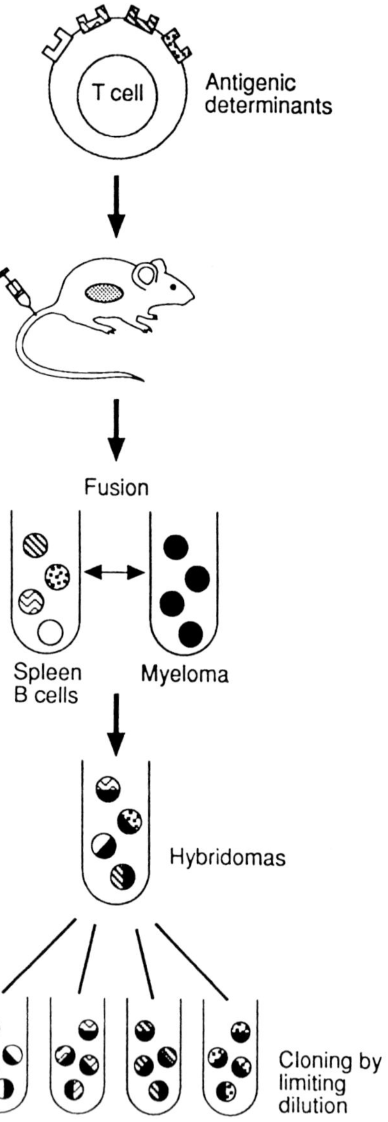

FIGURE 12.1. *Production of monoclonal antibodies according to the technique described by Kohler and Milstein (2). Splenocytes from immunized mice are fused with myeloma cells. The hybridomas obtained are cultured by limiting dilution in individual wells. The supernatants are screened for the desired specificity. Large-scale production of selected hybridomas may then be performed either in vitro or in vivo (i.e., ascites).*

however, this is not the case. As a consequence of the very restricted specificity of monoclonal antibodies, it soon became apparent that the in vivo therapeutic capacity of a given antibody was directly correlated with the functional relevance of its molecular target. For instance, all CD3 antibodies used in vivo so far have proved to be excellent immunosuppressants (17). In contrast, this was not the case for most of the CD2 antibodies tested, despite the fact that both specificities are expressed on all mature T cells (18).

Receptors and Coreceptors Involved in Antigen Recognition

T-cell antigen recognition involves a molecular triad including specialized membrane receptors, some of which are privileged targets for therapeutic biologic agents (see Fig. 12.3). T cells bind peptides presented in the context of major histocompatibility complex (MHC) molecules via specialized dimeric receptors: the T-cell receptor (TCR) α and β chains. The variable regions of the TCR α and β chains dictate antigen specificity. The CD3 molecular complex consists of at least five invariant membrane proteins designated γ, δ, ε, ζ, and η (19). The γ, δ, and ε subunits are expressed as noncovalently linked γ–δ and γ–ε dimers; the ζ and η subunits form disulfide-linked homo-$\zeta\zeta$ and heterodimers $\zeta\eta$. CD3 regulates the assembly and expression of TCR and is responsible for transducing TCR $\alpha\beta$ signals.

The CD4 and CD8 receptors were initially considered to be simple adhesion molecules interacting with their specific ligands: the MHC class II and I products, respectively. It soon became apparent, however, that upon antigen binding the cross-linking of CD4 and CD3/TCR significantly improved T-cell signaling (20). According to recent data CD4, through its noncovalently associated lymphocyte-specific tyrosine kinase $p56^{lck}$, associates to the "activated" form of the CD3 ζ–ζ chains (tyrosine phosphorylated ζ associated to tyrosine phosphorylated cytoplasmic ZAP-70), thereby stabilizing the CD3/TCR–antigen–MHC interaction and amplifying the signaling process. CD4 thus represents an important "coreceptor" of CD3/TCR that actively participates in the delivery of activation signals (Fig. 12.4) (21).

Receptors Delivering "Costimulatory" Signals and Adhesion Molecules

T-cell activation is initiated through the CD3/TCR complex, but this signal is not sufficient to sustain full activation of naive T cells. In contrast, a state of unresponsiveness or anergy may result on rechallenge. In order for sustained T-cell activation to occur, CD3/TCR costimulatory signals derived from specialized receptors must be delivered. In the case of naive T cells, CD28 is one important receptor mediating costimulation on interaction with the B7 family (B7.1, B7.2) of ligands expressed on antigen-presenting cells (22–24) (see Fig. 12.3).

The term *adhesin* encompasses a variety of cell receptors that enhance cell contacts and represent interesting targets for immunosuppressive agents (25–27). Two major systems have been investigated: ICAM-1–LFA-1 and CD2–LFA-3 (25–27). There is increasing evidence that, under certain circumstances, several adhesion receptor–ligand pairs can modulate an immune response not simply by enhancing adhesion, but by providing additional activation signals (28). Thus, in the case of memory T cells that possess a lower

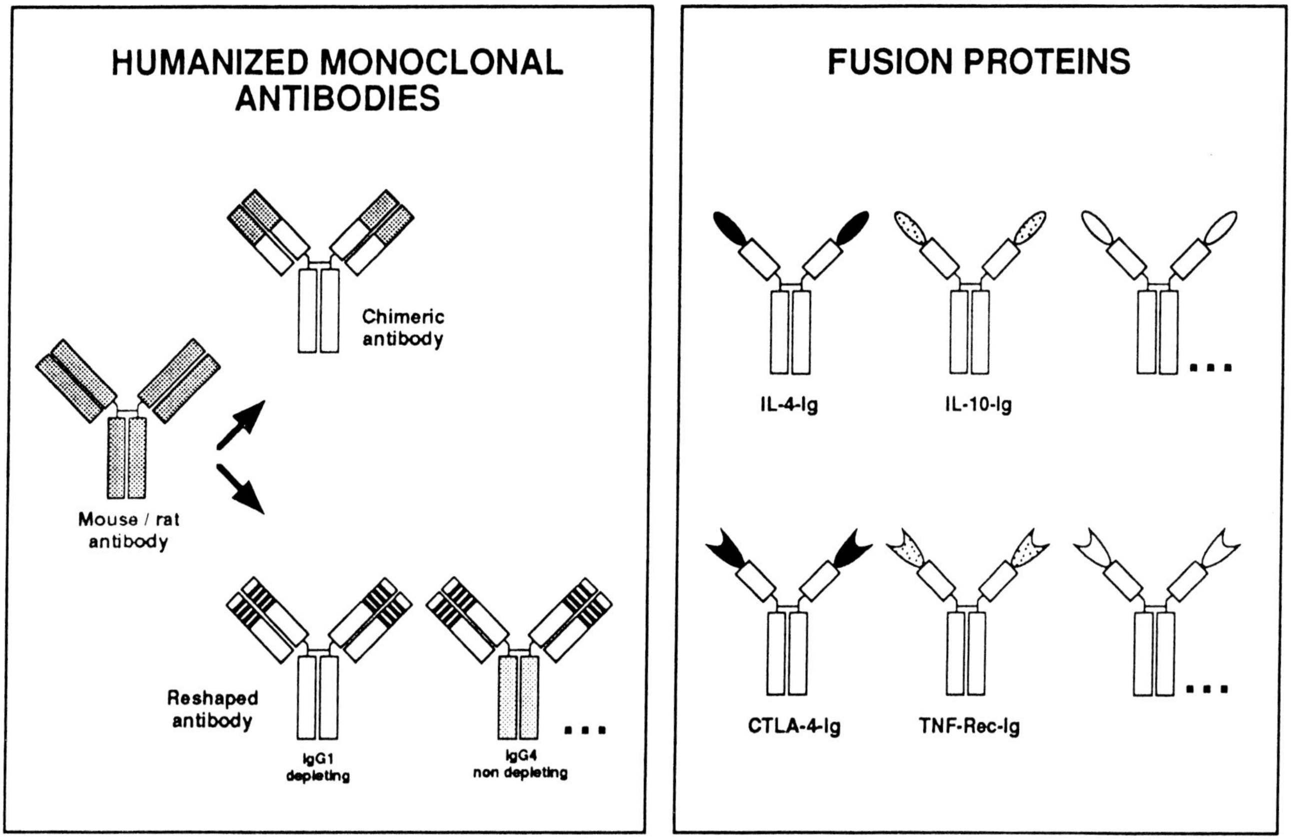

FIGURE 12.2. *Scheme describing the structural characteristics of molecularly engineered monoclonal antibodies and immunoadhesins (3).*

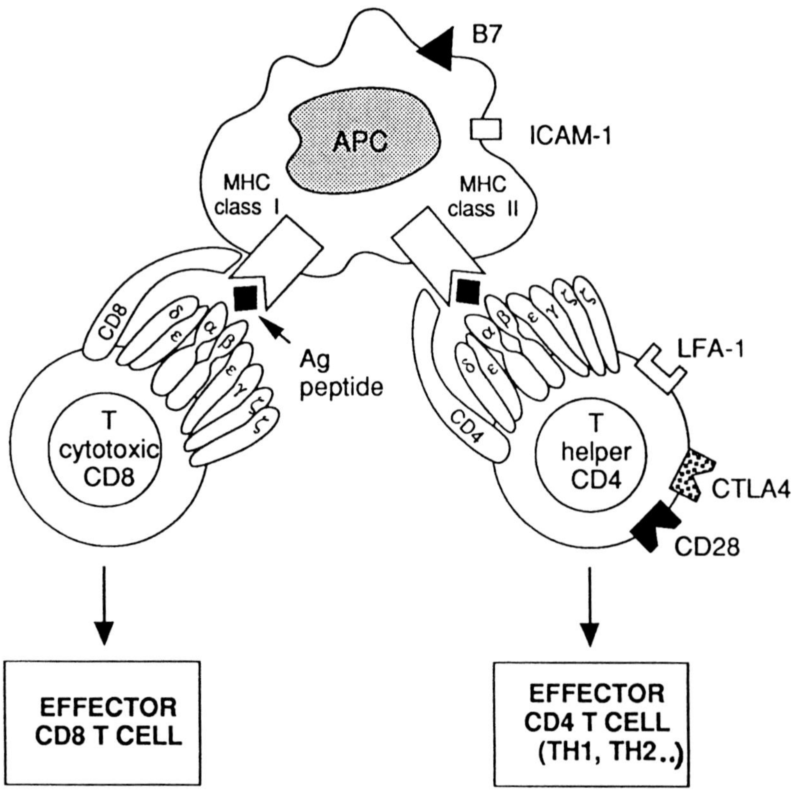

FIGURE 12.3. *Principal targets of therapeutic biologic immunosuppressants expressed at the surface of functionally distinct immune cells.*

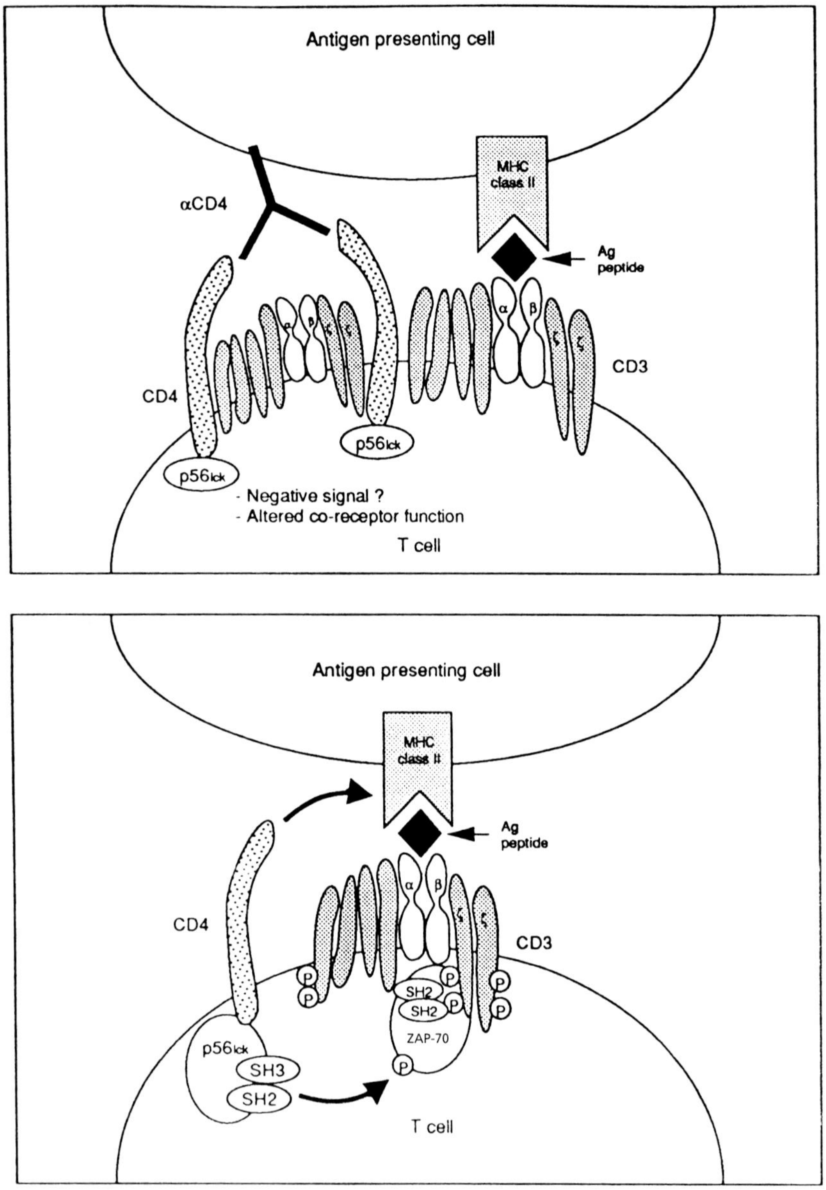

FIGURE 12.4. *The intracellular pathways of T-cell activation: the interaction of CD3 and CD4 molecules (20,21). In addition, the top panel illustrates the hypothesis proposed to explain the mode of action of anti-CD4 monoclonal antibodies. (Adapted from Thome M, Duplay P, Guttinger M, et al. Syk and ZAP-70 mediate recruitment of p561ck/CD4 to the activated T-cell receptor/CD3/zeta complex. J Exp Med 1995;181:1997–2006.)*

activation threshold compared to naive T cells, adhesins may enter into play to deliver effective costimulatory signals.

Receptors Selectively Expressed by Activated Cells

Cytokine receptors probably illustrate the best example of membrane molecules selectively expressed by activated immune cells and used as targets of therapeutic monoclonal antibodies. In transplantation, efforts have been devoted predominantly to the targeting of the interleukin (IL)-2 receptor. Both murine and humanized antibodies directed at the α chain of IL-2 receptor (CD25) have been applied (29). Humanized antibodies to CD25 especially seem to express a potent therapeutic capacity when used for prophylaxis of allograft rejection (29).

Soluble Mediators of Immunity: Cytokines

Cytokines are essential mediators of immunity and inflammation, two processes that operate to variable extents during each of the three essential phases of the alloimmune response: 1) antigen recognition, 2) proliferation and differentiation of committed cells, and 3) target destruction.

A major concept emerged in the mid 1980s from the work of Mosmann et al (30), who proposed that CD4+ T lymphocytes providing help for humoral (B-cell–dependent) or cellular (T-cell–dependent) responses were in fact distinct and could be differentiated on the basis of the cytokines they produced. Thus, two lymphokine patterns termed T_H1 (type 1 helper T cell) and T_H2 (type 2 helper T cell) were identified. Activation of the T_H1 cells [IL-2 and interferon gamma (IFNγ) producers] supports macrophage activation and cell-mediated delayed-type hypersensitivity responses.

Activation of T_H2 cells (IL-4, IL-5, IL-6, IL-10, and IL-13 producers) provides efficient B-cell help, thus favoring humoral responses. Fully differentiated T_H1 and T_H2 subsets do not preexist in the naive immunologically unprimed host. Among the various factors that direct a naive T helper precursor to differentiate upon antigen encounter into a T_H1 or a T_H2 cell are the type of antigen and its dose, the nature of the APC, the genetic background (both MHC and non-MHC genes), and, interestingly enough, the environmental cytokines by themselves. IFNγ, produced by T_H1 cells, inhibits the proliferation of T_H2 cells; conversely, IL-10, produced by T_H2 cells, inhibits the synthesis of cytokines by T_H1 cells by acting at least in part on APCs (31,32). IL-12, an APC-derived cytokine, is a key factor driving the differentiation of T_H1 cells, at least in part through its capacity to induce IFNγ. Conversely, IL-4 strongly directs the development of T_H2 cells and together with IL-10 shows a strong inhibitory capacity on T_H1-type response development (31).

Enormous efforts to delineate the role of a polarization toward a preferential T_H1 or T_H2 helper T-cell phenotype in the establishment and the control of allogeneic responses have paved the way to developing new therapeutic strategies (31,32). In particular, specific, long-term tolerance to alloantigens and autoantigens in rodent models has been interpreted as resulting from a favoring of a T_H2 versus a T_H1 response. Depending on the situation considered—transplantation or autoimmunity—this may be achieved by treatment with antibodies to given cytokines (anti-IFNγ) (33), antibodies to T-cell receptors (CD4, CD4+CD8, CD3, CD28) (34), or with the cytokines themselves (IL-4) (35).

The Particular Case of Polyclonal Antilymphocyte Sera

Polyclonal antilymphocyte globulins (ALG), which are widely used in transplantation, represent a mixture of a wide spectrum of antibody specificities that probably include, in variable proportions, a large number (if not all) of the cell-related specificities mentioned above. It is the variability in the concentration of each given specificity, to which can be added the isotype and the affinity of antibodies, that probably explains the differences in the batch-to-batch therapeutic potencies (36). Among the various in vitro properties ascribed to ALS preparations, only two are relevant to predicting immunosuppressive capacity in vivo. These are inhibition of the mixed lymphocyte reaction, which correlates, albeit moderately, with in vivo immunosuppression, and inhibition of E-rosette formation resulting from the interaction between the adhesion molecules CD2 (on T cells) and LFA-3 (on sheep erythrocytes) (27).

CELLULAR MECHANISMS

Although they are not mutually exclusive, three principal mechanisms have been identified through which biologic therapeutic agents affect the immune response: 1) the physical elimination of the target cells, which raises the issue of the turnover of the removed cell population, 2) the inhibition or blockade of the functional capacity of the target cells, and 3) the triggering of cell-mediated immunoregulatory circuits that redirect a destructive alloreactive effector response toward a nondestructive type of alloreactivity (Fig. 12.5). The latter unique capacity is considered at present as one major mechanism underlying the tolerogenic properties of biologic agents in general and anti-T–cell antibodies in particular. This clearly distinguishes biologic agents from chemical immunosuppressants that exclusively act through mechanisms involving the removal and/or the functional inhibition of their targets.

Cellular Depletion

From the biochemical point of view, the effector functions of an antibody molecule, such as the capacity to interact with Fc receptors and to activate the complement cascade, rely on the structure of the constant region. Cell lysis can occur following direct complement-dependent lysis in the circulation or by means of cell opsonization and removal in the liver and the spleen by reticuloendothelial cells. Trapping in these organs of lymphoid cells preincubated in vitro with polyclonal antilymphocyte antibodies or following their in vivo injection has been shown in both murine and clinical studies (37,38). Only C1, C4, C2, and C3 complement components are needed for effective opsonization. Some data suggest that only C1 and C4 would be sufficient (39).

In contrast, with cell-directed monoclonal antibodies the mechanisms involved in antibody-mediated cell destruction in vivo are more variable and complex. Actually, not only the antibody isotype but also its fine specificity can influence the lytic capacity. Thus, it is not sufficient to select for the adequate antibody isotype to achieve a desired in vivo depleting or nondepleting effect (40,41). When injected into humans, mouse and rat monoclonal antibodies to cell determinants mostly show a rather poor lytic capacity in the presence of human complement. This is due to the now well-characterized membrane-bound factors that inhibit complement activation in a species-restricted manner. Despite this, some antibody specificities, for reasons that are not fully understood, are highly depleting. This was the case for the CAMPATH-1 antibody (CD52) directed to a small GPI-linked protein abundantly expressed on B cells, T cells, and monocytes and extensively used to purge T cells from allogeneic bone marrow prior to transplant for prevention of graft-versus-host disease (GVHD) (40). Using molecular engineering, sets of recombinant antibodies with identical specificities but different constant regions were analyzed and probed for the sequences that determine antibody function (41). These have been used to rank the antibodies with regard to efficiencies in human complement-mediated lysis and also in antibody-dependent cell-mediated cytotoxicity (ADCC) by activated FcγRIII

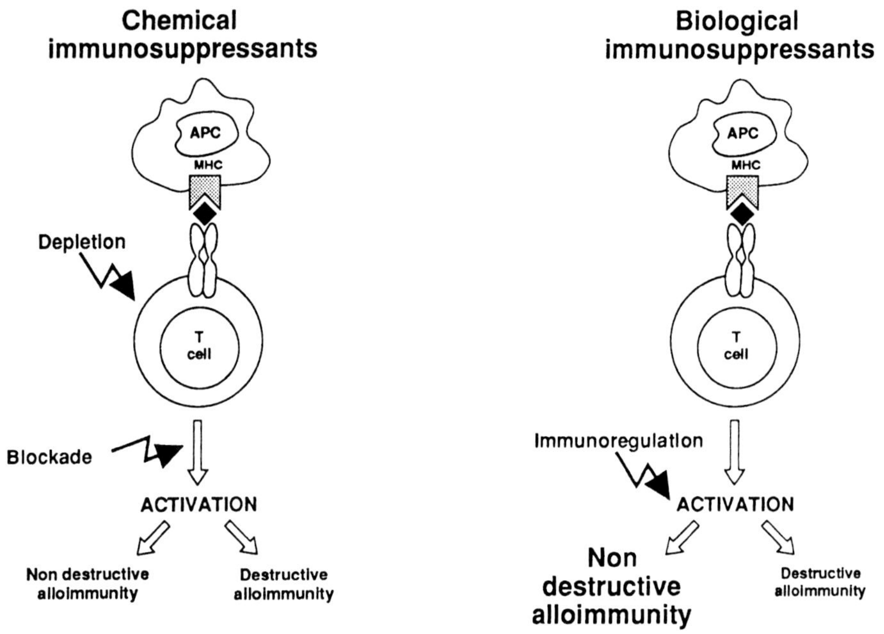

FIGURE 12.5. *Schematic representation of the mechanisms involved in the mode of action of immunosuppressants. The figure highlights the distinct points within an immune response that are the targets for chemical or biologic agents.*

(CD16) expressing effector cells. These studies showed that the lytic capacity of antibodies is greatly influenced by the antibody specificity as well as by the density and the distribution of the antigen on the target cell surface. However, among a given set of monoclonal antibodies sharing the same variable region, a hierarchy in terms of lytic capacity can be established that in the case of human immunoglobulins, for instance, is as follows (from highest to lowest): IgG1, IgG2, IgG3, IgG4.

An antigen may be a poor target for lysis when it easily undergoes antigenic modulation—namely, the disappearance from the cell surface upon binding by a specific ligand (in this case the monoclonal antibody). This is the case for B-cell (surface Ig) and T-cell antigen receptors (CD3/TCR) (see below for more details).

Among the other mechanisms studied and potentially involved in antibody-mediated depletion are redirected T-cell lysis consequent to bridging of cytotoxic T cells to the target (42) and, particularly for antibodies to CD3 and CD4, induction of apoptosis or programmed cell death. Apoptosis is a signal-dependent suicidal process associated with the activation of an endogenous endonuclease that leads to genomic DNA fragmentation. The delivery of apoptotic signals is elicited by the interaction between membrane receptors preferentially expressed at the surface of activated cells, namely, Fas/Fas ligand, TNF/TNF receptor. Apoptosis mediated via CD3/TCR signaling was initially demonstrated in immature thymocytes but it is also triggered in activated mature peripheral T cells (43–45).

To be complete, one may add here immunotoxins that consist of conjugates of a toxin (diphtheria toxin or ricin) coupled to an antibody or to a cytokine (46,47). The immunotoxin is delivered to the target cell by the antibody or the cytokine, whereupon the toxin kills the target cell after being internalized (46,47).

The immunologic effects of cell depletion will depend on the cellular selectivity of the immunosuppressive agent and on the renewal rate of the target cell population. Depletion may globally affect leukocytes (CD52), T cells (CD3), or T-cell subsets (CD4, CD8). In other cases, only activated T cells may be hit, as is the case for IL-2 receptor (CD25)-specific agents. The renewal rate varies considerably with cellular subsets. Pools of B cells and short-lived T cells will rapidly reappear after initial depletion. Conversely, recirculating long-lived T cells will take several weeks in the mouse and several months in humans to replenish initial cell pools. This very slow turnover of circulating T cells explains the T-cell selectivity of polyclonal ALS (48). The case of depleting monoclonal antibodies to CD4 is intriguing and deserves a word of clinical caution. This is best illustrated by the case of the humanized antibody to CD4 MT-412 (human IgG1) that was used in both transplanted and autoimmune patients. Especially at high doses (700 mg of cumulated dosage), peripheral CD4+ cell counts remained very low for several consecutive months (49).

Functional Inhibition

Several nonmutually exclusive mechanisms may account for antibody-mediated inhibition of cell function, including: 1) antibody-mediated cell coating that interferes with physiologic cell-to-cell interactions, 2) the antigenic modulation of the target cell receptor, and 3) the induction of cell anergy.

The relevance of antibody-mediated cell coating was initially discussed with polyclonal antilymphocyte antibodies since absolute lymphocytopenia did not appear to be essential for their therapeutic effect. In fact, T cells that reappeared after treatment were functionally impaired both in vitro and in vivo. It was, however, difficult to identify among the various specificities present in polyclonal ALS preparations which targets were the most relevant for cell inactivation.

Several monoclonal antibodies to human, mouse, and rat CD4 have been described that express immunosuppressive and tolerogenic effects but are nondepleting (9,12,34,50,51). It is likely that CD4 coating, given the contribution of CD4 to TCR/CD3-mediated signaling, not only interferes with lymphocyte binding to MHC class II–bearing cells but also triggers therapeutically relevant but still elusive negative "signals" (52). Thus, upon independent ligation of CD3 and CD4, as may occur with the injection of antibodies to CD4, the physiologic stimulation of resting T cells is significantly inhibited (see Fig. 12.4). In addition, a decrease in induced proliferative responses and lymphokine production response to various stimuli, including soluble antigens, alloantigens, lectins, and antibodies to TCR/CD3, is observed but cannot be accounted for by simple blockade of adhesion to MHC class II (53).

Cell-directed antibodies can also induce antigenic modulation, which is the redistribution of the molecules that they bind on the cell surface (54) (Fig. 12.6). The antigen–antibody complex will ultimately cap at a pole of the cell and disappear upon internalization or shedding. If the molecule is central to the cell function, the loss of the membrane receptor expression will render the cell incompetent. This has been well documented in the case of antibodies to CD3 (54–56). In both mice and humans, therapeutic doses produce only partial depletion (in lymphoid organs 30% to 40% of CD3+ cells). Remaining cells

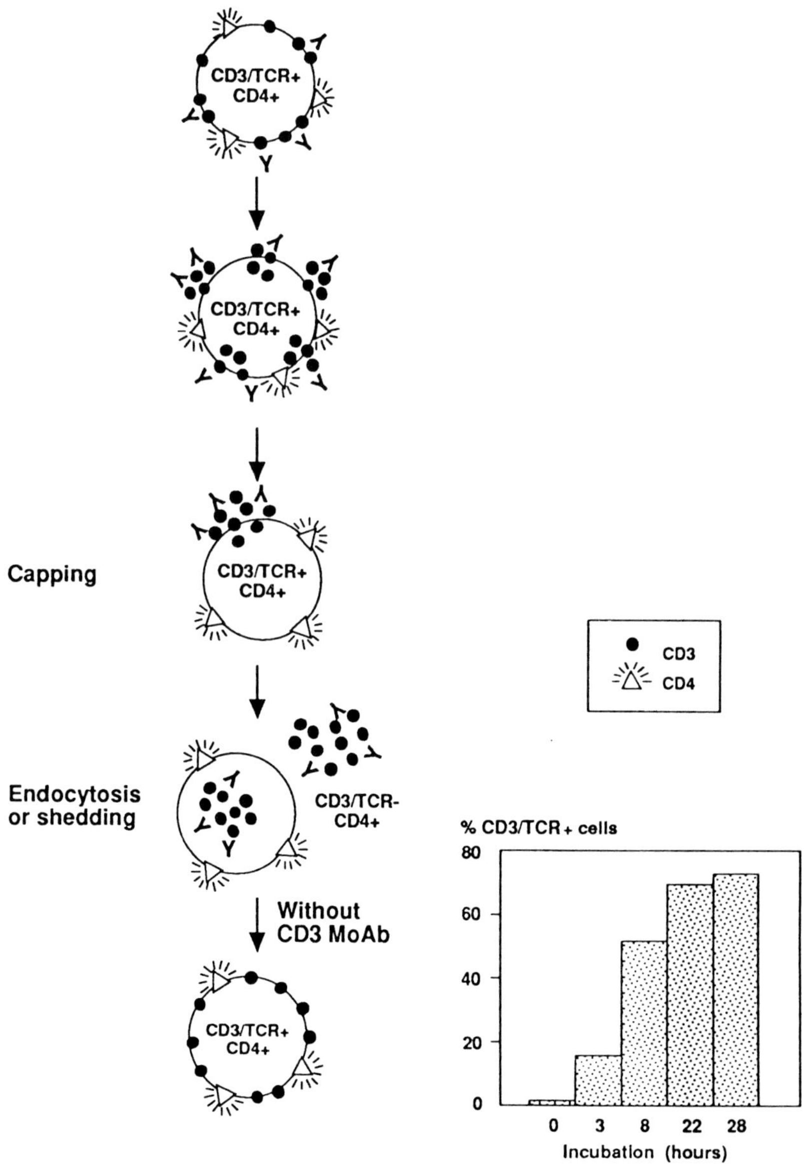

FIGURE 12.6. *Antigenic modulation of the CD3/TCR complex from peripheral blood cells in transplant patients treated with a CD3 antibody. During treatment, cells modulate the CD3/TCR receptor, but within a few hours of in vitro incubation in the absence of the antibody the receptor is re-expressed (54,56).*

undergoing antigenic modulation express a particular phenotype; they are CD3-TCR-CD4+ or CD3-TCR-CD8+ (54,56). The phenomenon is reversible within a few hours (in vitro, 8 to 12 hours) when the antibody is cleared from the surrounding medium. Cells undergoing CD3 antibody-mediated antigenic modulation are completely unresponsive to antigen-specific or mitogen stimulation (54,56). This correlates with the profound in vivo immunosuppression exhibited by these patients, in whom allograft rejection is seldom observed when T cells in the circulation do not express CD3 (17,57).

As mentioned above, sustained T-cell activation upon engagement of CD3/TCR requires the simultaneous delivery of costimulatory signals through specialized receptors, such as CD28 interacting with B7 ligands at the surface of APCs (see Fig. 12.3). Several in vitro models using both murine and human clones showed that occupancy of the TCR alone, in the absence of adequate costimulation, induced a state of unresponsiveness termed *anergy* (58,59). Depending on the system, anergy in vitro is reversible by adding IL-2 either alone or in association with CD2 antibodies (59). The role of anergic cells in physiologic or induced immune tolerance is still debated. At present, only through the injection of superantigens or by using adoptive transfer of TCR transgenic cells can anergic cells be demonstrated in vivo (59).

It is important to mention at this point the very interesting results of using antibodies or fusion proteins that interfere with costimulatory signals in experimental transplantation (11,60,61). Thus, in a mouse heart and skin allograft model, the simultaneous (but not the independent) blockade of the CD28 and CD40 costimulatory pathways promoted long-term allograft survival. Importantly, the technique also inhibited the development of chronic vascular rejection in the grafted hearts (61). Chronic vascular rejection remains a major cause of long-term graft failure for which no effective therapy is available. If confirmed, these data point to selective inhibitors of costimulation as major immunosuppressive tools capable of interfering simultaneously with acute and chronic rejection.

Acquired Transplant Peripheral Tolerance: The Way to "Nonaggressive" Alloreactivity

Achieving donor-specific tolerance while preserving normal immune responsiveness to other foreign antigens is a major goal in clinical transplantation (see Chapter 5). A previously long-held tenet was that physiologic immune tolerance could only result from intrathymic, clonal deletion of immunoreactive cells, a concept supported by the direct demonstration of intrathymic negative selection (4). However, it is now extensively documented that, in normal individuals, although deletion mechanisms ensure the elimination of most autoreactive T and B lymphocytes, this purging is far from complete. Thus, autoreactive T and B cells can be found in all normal subjects. In most cases, however, they do not give rise to clinically evident autoimmune diseases (4). This is because extremely potent, extrathymic nondeletional active mechanisms—cytokine-mediated immune deviation, anergy, suppression, and vetoing—are operative and prevent potentially destructive immunoreactivity (4).

Although transplantation tolerance can be induced through intrathymic deletion of alloreactive T cells (e.g., stable lymphohematopoietic mixed chimerism follows the infusion of allogeneic bone marrow in adequately conditioned recipients), this approach is difficult to apply clinically. Application is limited by its aggressive nature (62,63) as well as by the fact that a loss of functional thymus occurs after puberty.

Peripheral tolerance can be successfully induced and maintained over a long term in adult recipients, even after thymectomy, if the alloantigen is delivered appropriately. Whether antigen presentation is via bone marrow, whole blood, or the allograft itself, the development of tolerance also requires particular biologic agents. As already mentioned, it appears that biologic agents (i.e., natural or biotechnologically engineered antigens, antibodies, receptors, and cytokines) are particularly capable of providing the positive signals required for the reorientation of the immune response leading to peripheral immune tolerance induction.

The groundbreaking experiments by Monaco and Wood in the 1960s (5,64) used a combination of ALS and post-transplantation donor bone marrow infusion to induce specific unresponsiveness to skin allografts (5,64,65). This approach, with modifications, has been successfully used to transplant mismatched renal allografts in nonhuman primates. Prolonged survival of histoincompatible kidney transplants has been achieved in rhesus monkeys with a combination of rabbit ALG plus low-dose lymphoid irradiation and a post-transplantation donor bone marrow (depleted of bright CD3+/DR+ cells) infusion (66–69).

Importantly, monoclonal antibodies can afford the same effect. In the monkey model, a CD3 immunotoxin can also provide the allograft tolerance induced by the ALG + TLI conditioning regimen (70). A nondepleting antibody to CD4 has also been successfully used in this setting.

The unique tolerogenic capacity of antibodies to CD4 has long been known. The first important finding was that rat antibodies to CD4 injected into mice did not trigger an antiglobulin response as was the case with the majority of rodent monoclonal antibodies against other T-cell antigens (6,7). Moreover, specific tolerance to soluble antigens could be induced by delivering them to normal adult euthymic animals under the cover of depleting or nondepleting antibodies to CD4 (6,34,71). Importantly, all that was needed to maintain this immune tolerance was the antigen alone, delivered at regular time intervals, in the absence of any further monoclonal antibody treatment. These findings were rapidly extended to tissue antigens and in particular alloantigens. This protocol has been recently adapted by Wood's group using as a source of antigen donor-type whole blood in association with depleting or nondepleting antibodies to CD4 (12,14). Thus, specific tolerance to completely mismatched fully vascularized cardiac allografts is achieved. Importantly, through the exclusive administration at regular intervals of donor blood, the time of allograft implantation can be delayed for several months (12,14).

In adult euthymic mice, combinations of antibodies to CD4 and CD8, even if nondepleting, can induce classic transplantation tolerance to skin grafts across partial and fully mismatched combinations (72). This antibody-induced tolerance can also be induced and maintained in thymectomized animals, clearly showing that it is a peripheral event. Not unexpectedly, no evidence for clonal deletion of specific alloreactive T cells was found (9,34).

Antibodies to specificities other than CD4 are also of interest. For instance, antibodies to CD3, to LFA-1 and ICAM-1, and to CD25 (especially in rat transplant models), and agents interfering with costimulatory pathways such as CTLA4Ig have been shown to be effective. Combined administration of LFA-1 and ICAM-1 to mice resulted in permanent engraftment of fully mismatched vascularized heart allografts but also specific tolerance to donor-type skin allografts (10). Similarly, antibodies to CD3 can promote long-term specific unresponsiveness to both alloantigens and autoantigens. In the rat, CD3 antibody induces permanent engraftment of histoincompatible vascularized heart grafts and permanent tolerance (i.e., skin graft acceptance) (73). Moreover, in NOD mice, who develop a spontaneous form of T-cell–mediated autoimmune, insulin-dependent diabetes mellitus, low-dose CD3 treatment applied at the stage of overt disease induces permanent remission and restores self tolerance (16). Finally, in both xenogeneic and allogeneic transplant models, CTLA4Ig was shown to have great potential (74,75).

Apart from their potential therapeutic interest, all these models support the fundamental notion that the organ allograft itself may provide an effective presentation of antigen for induction of transplantation tolerance. Moreover, the major features characterizing these models of monoclonal antibody–induced peripheral immune tolerance are their active (dominant) nature and their strict antigen dependence. This is well illustrated by the fact that tolerant animals resist the transfer of immunocompetent naive and sensitized effectors that could reverse or "break" the tolerant state by eliminating or functionally blocking immune cell subsets—mainly regulatory CD4+ cells—that are known to mediate suppression if adoptively transferred into naive recipients (9,34).

Can all this be explained by an exclusive immune deviation from a T_H1 allodestructive response to a T_H2 nondestructive or even protective response? Supporting this hypothesis are the data showing dominant T_H2 responses in neonatal tolerance models in which establishment is completely blocked by the administration of a monoclonal antibody to IL-4 (76). Moreover, although it is more controversial, in some models of CD4 antibody–induced tolerance, the presence of a dominant T_H2 response has been reported (31). However, when it comes to the phenomenon of transferable suppression, the available data show only a partial blockade upon treatment with anti-IL-4 (34). Another important unresolved question concerns the cellular source of IL-4. Although the assumption is that tolerant or suppressor cells would produce it, there is no firm evidence to show their T_H2 origin. Taken together, the present data suggest that diverting to an IL-4–producing phenotype could be but one of the critical factors involved in the tolerance induction phase; whether it is also relevant during the long-term maintenance phase is still unresolved.

An alternate possibility is that tolerant cells might be to some extent anergic, that is, capable of providing no help while competing for APC binding with potentially reactive effectors. There is interesting in vitro and in vivo evidence to support this hypothesis. In vitro, anergic human T-cell clones could suppress the proliferation of potentially reactive cells by nonanergic cells, provided the same APC was presenting the peptides specific for both partners (77). Competition for the APC surface and locally produced IL-2 has been proposed as the mechanism for this effect while excluding a role for "inhibitory" cytokines (i.e., IL-4, IL-10) secreted by the anergic cells (77). Similarly, in vivo, tolerance to a given alloantigen may "spread" to third-party allografts, provided the initially "tolerated" and the third-party alloantigen are presented by the same APC (i.e., usage of organ allografts from F1 donors) (34). This very interesting phenomenon is termed *linked suppression*. Once again, the molecular basis for this "competition" remains obscure and could in principle involve a low cytokine-producing ability (i.e., anergy), the production of cytokines modulating T-cell or APC function (i.e., IL-4, IL-10, TGFβ, etc.), and competition for costimulatory molecules on the APC (34).

In conclusion, although the molecular mechanisms remain to be clarified, T-cell–mediated suppression represents a field that can no longer be ignored by groups attempting to achieve successful clinical immunomodulation.

CELL ACTIVATION AS A PREREQUISITE FOR ANTI-T-CELL ANTIBODY–INDUCED TOLERANCE

Some recent data emphasize the role of T-cell activation in the induction of immune tolerance by means of biologic agents. Of particular relevance are the studies showing that cyclosporine abrogates the tolerogenic properties of antibodies to CD3 or of agents blocking CD28 and CD40 (61). This is particularly evident when cyclosporine is used with biologic agents at the inception of treatment. It is well established that cyclosporine selectively interferes with TCR/CD3 T-cell activation pathways, leading to the transcription of both T_H1 and T_H2 cytokine genes. Thus it inhibits the transcription not only of IL-2 and IFNγ mRNA but also of IL-4 and IL-10 mRNA (78,79). The effect of cyclosporine on IL-10 production depends on the cell source of the cytokine; the inhibition is exclusively noted on stimulation with CD3 antibodies and not with bacterial lipopolysaccharide (79).

This may be of relevance for future clinical strategies of tolerance induction in transplant patients. In fact, in clinical protocols, for obvious reasons, drug association is indispensable. However, it is important to develop the best combinations in order to avoid deleterious, potentially antagonistic effects, for example by preventing the induction of antigen-specific long-term hyporesponsiveness. For instance, a recent report from the Collaborative Transplant Study Group shows that the kidney allograft survival in patients who received OKT-3 as part of their prophylactic regimen was significantly lower if cyclosporine was given from the beginning of OKT-3 treatment, as compared to patients in whom the administration of cyclosporine was delayed (80).

CONCLUSIONS

Most chemical immunosuppressive agents act by promoting cell depletion and/or blockade of cell activation. These therapeutic approaches are nonantigen specific and their major drawback is their relatively long-term ineffectiveness typically resulting in recurrence of the pathogenic immune process at drug cessation. The need to reduce chronic immunosuppression, with its potential for infectious and tumorigenic complications, seems achievable through the use of nontoxic biologic agents.

Moreover, from a more fundamental point of view, an understanding of the molecular basis of the tolerogenic properties of monoclonal antibodies would clear the way for development of more readily applicable therapeutic strategies—simple chemicals or recombinant receptor agonist and/or antagonist ligands that would mimic the desired therapeutic effect. Dissecting the intimate molecular and cellular mechanisms through which antibodies express these subtle modulatory effects certainly promises future exciting challenges for immunopharmacologists.

REFERENCES

1. Starzl TE. Heterologous antilymphocyte globulin. N Engl J Med 1968;279:700–705.
2. Kohler G, Milstein C. Continuous cultures of fused cells secreting antibody of predefined specificity. Nature 1975;256:495–497.
3. Winter G, Milstein C. Man-made antibodies. Nature 1991;349:293–299.
4. Schwartz RH. Immunological tolerance. In: Paul WE, ed. Fundamental immunology. New York: Raven, 1993:677–731.
5. Monaco AP, Wood ML, Russell PS. Studies on heterologous antilymphocyte serum in mice. III. Immunological tolerance and chimerism produced across the H2-locus with adult thymectomy and antilymphocyte serum. Ann NY Acad Sci 1966;129:190–209.
6. Benjamin RJ, Waldmann H. Induction of tolerance by monoclonal antibody therapy. Nature 1986;320:449–451.
7. Gutstein NL, Seaman WE, Scott JH, Wofsy D. Induction of immune tolerance by administration of monoclonal antibody to L3T4. J Immunol 1986;137:1127–1132.
8. Cobbold SP, Qin S, Leong LY, Martin G, Waldmann H. Reprogramming the immune system for peripheral tolerance with CD4 and CD8 monoclonal antibodies. Immunol Rev 1992;129:165–201.
9. Qin S, Cobbold SP, Pope H, et al. "Infectious" transplantation tolerance. Science 1993;259:974–977.
10. Isobe M, Yagita H, Okumura K, Ihara A. Specific acceptance of cardiac allograft after treatment with antibodies to ICAM-1 and LFA-1. Science 1992;255:1125–1127.
11. Lin H, Bolling SF, Linsley PS, et al. Long-term acceptance of major histocompatibility complex mismatched cardiac allografts induced by CTLA4Ig plus donor-specific transfusion. J Exp Med 1993;178:1801–1806.
12. Pearson TC, Madsen JC, Larsen CP, et al. Induction of transplantation tolerance in adults using donor antigen and anti-CD4 monoclonal antibody. Transplantation 1992;54:475–483.
13. Wofsy D, Seaman WE. Reversal of advanced murine lupus in NZB/NZW F1 mice by treatment with monoclonal antibody to L3T4. J Immunol 1987;138:3247–3253.
14. Wood KJ. Transplantation tolerance with monoclonal antibodies. Semin Immunol 1990;2:389–399.
15. Shizuru JA, Taylor-Edwards C, Banks BA, et al. Immunotherapy of the nonobese diabetic mouse: treatment with an antibody to T-helper lymphocytes. Science 1988;240:659–662.
16. Chatenoud L, Thervet E, Primo J, Bach JF. Anti-CD3 antibody induces long-term remission of overt autoimmunity in nonobese diabetic mice. Proc Natl Acad Sci USA 1994;91:123–127.
17. Cosimi AB, Colvin RB, Burton RC, et al. Use of monoclonal antibodies to T-cell subsets for immunologic monitoring and treatment in recipients of renal allografts. N Engl J Med 1981;305:308–314.
18. Jonker M, Goldstein G, Balner H. Effects of in vivo administration of monoclonal antibodies specific for human T cell subpopulations on the immune system in a rhesus monkey model. Transplantation 1983;35:521–526.
19. Clevers H, Alarcon B, Wileman T, Terhorst C. The T cell receptor/CD3 complex: a dynamic protein ensemble. Annu Rev Immunol 1988;6:629–662.
20. Rudd CE. CD4, CD8 and the TCR-CD3 complex: a novel class of protein-tyrosine kinase receptor. Immunol Today 1990;11:400–406.
21. Thome M, Duplay P, Guttinger M, et al. Syk and ZAP-70 mediate recruitment of p56lck/CD4 to the activated T cell receptor/CD3/zeta complex. J Exp Med 1995;181:1997–2006.
22. Linsley PS, Brady W, Urnes M, et al. CTLA-4 is a second receptor for the B cell activation antigen B7. J Exp Med 1991;174:561–569.
23. Van Den Eertwegh AJ, Noelle RJ, Roy M, et al. In vivo CD40-gp39 interactions are essential for thymus-dependent humoral immunity. I. In vivo expression of CD40 ligand, cytokines, and antibody production delineates sites of cognate T-B cell interactions. J Exp Med 1993;178:1555–1565.
24. Boise LH, Noel PJ, Thompson CB. CD28 and apoptosis. Curr Opin Immunol 1995;7:620–625.
25. Springer TA. Adhesion receptors of the immune system. Nature 1990;346:425–434.
26. Makgoba MW, Sanders ME, Shaw S. The CD2-LFA-3 and LFA-1-ICAM pathways: relevance to T-cell recognition. Immunol Today 1989;10:417–422.
27. Springer TA, Dustin ML, Kishimoto TK, Marlin SD. The lymphocyte function-associated LFA-1, CD2, and LFA-3 molecules: cell adhesion receptors of the immune system. Annu Rev Immunol 1987;5:223–252.
28. Clark EA, Ledbetter JA. How B and T cells talk to each other. Nature 1994;367:425–428.
29. Waldmann TA, O'Shea J. The use of antibodies against the IL-2 receptor in transplantation. Curr Opin Immunol 1998;10:507–512.
30. Mosmann TR, Coffman RL. TH1 and TH2 cells: different patterns of lymphokine secretion lead to different functional properties. Annu Rev Immunol 1989;7:145–173.
31. Nickerson P, Steurer W, Steiger J, et al. Cytokines and the Th1/Th2 paradigm in transplantation. Curr Opin Immunol 1994;6:757–764.
32. Bromberg JS. IL-10 immunosuppression in transplantation. Curr Opin Immunol 1995;7:639–643.
33. Bach JF. Anti-gamma interferon (IFN-gamma) monoclonal antibodies. In: Bach JF, ed. Monoclonal antibodies and peptide therapy in autoimmune diseases. New York: Marcel Dekker, 1993:319–391.
34. Cobbold SP, Adams E, Marshall SE, et al. Mechanisms of peripheral tolerance and suppression induced by monoclonal antibodies to CD4 and CD8. Immunol Rev 1996;149:5–33.
35. Rapoport MJ, Jaramillo A, Zipris D, et al. Interleukin 4 reverses T cell proliferative unresponsiveness and prevents the onset of diabetes in nonobese diabetic mice. J Exp Med 1993;178:87–99.
36. Balner H, Eysvoogel VP, Cleton FJ. Testing of anti-human lymphocyte sera in chimpanzees and lower primates. Lancet 1968;1:19–22.
37. Greaves MF, Tursi A, Playfair JH, et al. Immunosuppressive potency and in vitro activity of antilymphocyte globulin. Lancet 1969;1:68–72.

38. Martin WJ, Miller JF. Cell to cell interaction in the immune response. IV. Site of action of antilymphocyte globulin. J Exp Med 1968;128:855–874.
39. Bach JF, Gigli I, Dardenne M, Dormont J. Mechanism of complement action in rosette inhibition and lymphocytotoxicity of antilymphocyte serum. Immunology 1972;22:625–635.
40. Bindon CI, Hale G, Waldmann H. Importance of antigen specificity for complement-mediated lysis by monoclonal antibodies. Eur J Immunol 1988;18:1507–1514.
41. Isaacs JD, Clark MR, Greenwood J, Waldmann H. Therapy with monoclonal antibodies. An in vivo model for the assessment of therapeutic potential. J Immunol 1992;148:3062–3071.
42. Wong JT, Colvin RB. Selective reduction and proliferation of the CD4+ and CD8+ T cell subsets with bispecific monoclonal antibodies: evidence for inter-T cell-mediated cytolysis. Clin Immunol Immunopathol 1991;58:236–250.
43. Smith CA, Williams GT, Kingston R, et al. Antibodies to CD3/T-cell receptor complex induce death by apoptosis in immature T cells in thymic cultures. Nature 1989;337:181–184.
44. Wesselborg S, Janssen O, Kabelitz D. Induction of activation-driven death (apoptosis) in activated but not resting peripheral blood T cells. J Immunol 1993;150:4338–4345.
45. Choy EH, Adjaye J, Forrest L, et al. Chimaeric anti-CD4 monoclonal antibody cross-linked by monocyte Fc gamma receptor mediates apoptosis of human CD4 lymphocytes. Eur J Immunol 1993;23:2676–2681.
46. Kronke M, Schlick E, Waldmann TA, et al. Selective killing of human T-lymphotropic virus-I infected leukemic T-cells by monoclonal anti-interleukin 2 receptor antibody-ricin A chain conjugates: potentiation by ammonium chloride and monensin. Cancer Res 1986;46:3295–3298.
47. Walz G, Zanker B, Brand K, et al. Sequential effects of interleukin 2-diphtheria toxin fusion protein on T-cell activation. Proc Natl Acad Sci USA 1989;86:9485–9488.
48. Lance EM. The selective action of antilymphocyte serum on recirculating lymphocytes: a review of the evidence and alternatives. Clin Exp Immunol 1970;6:789–802.
49. Moreland LW, Pratt PW, Bucy RP, et al. Treatment of refractory rheumatoid arthritis with a chimeric anti-CD4 monoclonal antibody. Long-term followup of CD4+ T cell counts. Arthritis Rheum 1994;37:834–838.
50. Powelson JA, Knowles RW, Delmonico FL, et al. CDR-grafted OKT4A monoclonal antibody in cynomolgus renal allograft recipients. Transplantation 1994;57:788–793.
51. Darby CR, Bushell A, Morris PJ, Wood KJ. Nondepleting anti-CD4 antibodies in transplantation. Evidence that modulation is far less effective than prolonged CD4 blockade. Transplantation 1994;57:1419–1426.
52. Bank I, Chess L. Perturbation of the T4 molecule transmits a negative signal to T cells. J Exp Med 1985;162:1294–1303.
53. Emmrich F, Kanz L, Eichmann K. Cross-linking of the T cell receptor complex with the subset-specific differentiation antigen stimulates interleukin 2 receptor expression in human CD4 and CD8 T cells. Eur J Immunol 1987;17:529–534.
54. Chatenoud L, Bach JF. Antigenic modulation: a major mechanism of antibody action. Immunol Today 1984;5:20–25.
55. Hirsch R, Eckhaus M, Auchincloss H Jr, et al. Effects of in vivo administration of anti-T3 monoclonal antibody on T cell function in mice. I. Immunosuppression of transplantation responses. J Immunol 1988;140:3766–3772.
56. Chatenoud L, Baudrihaye MF, Kreis H, et al. Human in vivo antigenic modulation induced by the anti-T cell OKT3 monoclonal antibody. Eur J Immunol 1982;12:979–982.
57. Vigeral P, Chkoff N, Chatenoud L, et al. Prophylactic use of OKT3 monoclonal antibody in cadaver kidney recipients. Utilization of OKT3 as the sole immunosuppressive agent. Transplantation 1986;41:730–733.
58. Schwartz RH. A cell culture model for T lymphocyte clonal anergy. Science 1990;248:1349–1356.
59. Schwartz RH. Models of T cell anergy: is there a common molecular mechanism? Comment. J Exp Med 1996;184:1–8.
60. Lenschow DJ, Zeng Y, Thistlethwaite JR, et al. Long-term survival of xenogeneic pancreatic islet grafts induced by CTLA4Ig. Science 1992;257:789–792.
61. Larsen CP, Elwood ET, Alexander DZ, et al. Long-term acceptance of skin and cardiac allografts after blocking CD40 and CD28 pathways. Nature 1996;381:434–438.
62. Sykes M, Sheard M, Sachs DH. Effects of T cell depletion in radiation bone marrow chimeras. I. Evidence for a donor cell population which increases allogeneic chimerism but which lacks the potential to produce GVHD. J Immunol 1988;141:2282–2288.
63. Sykes M, Sachs DH. Bone marrow transplantation as a means of inducing tolerance. Semin Immunol 1990;2:401–417.
64. Wood ML, Monaco AP, Gozzo JJ, Liegeois A. Use of homozygous allogeneic bone marrow for induction of tolerance with antilymphocyte serum: dose and timing. Transplant Proc 1971;3:676–679.
65. Maki T, Gottschalk R, Wood ML, Monaco AP. Specific unresponsiveness to skin allografts in anti-lymphocyte serum-treated, marrow-injected mice: participation of donor marrow-derived suppressor T cells. J Immunol 1981;127:1433–1438.
66. Thomas JM, Carver FM, Foil MB, et al. Renal allograft tolerance induced with ATG and donor bone marrow in outbred rhesus monkeys. Transplantation 1983;36:104–106.
67. Thomas J, Carver M, Cunningham P, et al. Promotion of incompatible allograft acceptance in rhesus monkeys given posttransplant antithymocyte globulin and donor bone marrow. I. In vivo parameters and immuno-histologic evidence suggesting microchimerism. Transplantation 1987;43:332–338.
68. Thomas JM, Carver FM, Cunningham PR, et al. Kidney allograft tolerance in primates without chronic immunosuppression—the role of veto cells. Transplantation 1991;51:198–207.
69. Thomas J, Alqaisi M, Cunningham P, et al. The development of a posttransplant TLI treatment strategy that promotes organ allograft acceptance without chronic immunosuppression. Transplantation 1992;53:247–258.
70. Harawy MM, Knechtle SJ. Strategies for tolerance induction in nonhuman primates. Curr Opin Immunol 1998;10:513–517.
71. Wofsy D, Mayes DC, Woodcock J, Seaman WE. Inhibition of humoral immunity in vivo by monoclonal antibody to L3T4: studies with soluble antigens in intact mice. J Immunol 1985;135:1698–1701.
72. Qin SX, Cobbold S, Benjamin R, Waldmann H. Induction of classical transplantation tolerance in the adult. J Exp Med 1989;169:779–794.
73. Nicolls MR, Aversa GG, Pearce NW, et al. Induction of long-term specific tolerance to allografts in rats by therapy with an anti-CD3-like monoclonal antibody. Transplantation 1993;55:459–468.
74. Lenschow DJ, Zeng Y, Thistlethwaite JR, et al. Long-term survival of xenogeneic pancreatic islet grafts induced by CTLA4Ig. Science 1992;257:789–792.
75. Lin H, Bolling SF, Linsley PS, et al. Long term acceptance of major histocompatibility complex mismathed cardiac allografts induced by CTLA4Ig plus donor-specific transfusion. J Exp Med 1993;178:1801–1806.
76. Schurmans S, Heusser CH, Qin HY, et al. In vivo effects of anti-IL-4 monoclonal antibody on neonatal induction of tolerance and on an associated autoimmune syndrome. J Immunol 1990;145:2465–2473.
77. Lombardi G, Sidhu S, Batchelor R, Lechler R. Anergic T cells as suppressor cells in vitro. Science 1994;264:1587–1589.
78. Granelli-Piperno A, Keane M, Steinman RM. Evidence that cyclosporine inhibits cell-mediated immunity primarily at the level of the T lymphocyte rather than the accessory cell. Transplantation 1988;46:53S–60S.
79. Durez P, Abramowicz D, Gerard C, et al. In vivo induction of interleukin 10 by anti-CD3 monoclonal antibody or bacterial lipopolysaccharide: differential modulation by cyclosporin A. J Exp Med 1993;177:551–555.
80. Opelz G. Efficacy of rejection prophylaxis with OKT3 in renal transplantation. Collaborative Transplant Study. Transplantation 1995;60:1220–1224.

Chapter

13

Biologic Immunosuppressive Agents

JAMES D. EASON A. BENEDICT COSIMI

Organ transplantation has become the treatment of choice for many patients with end-stage kidney, liver, heart, or lung disease. Much of the clinical success that has been achieved has relied on life-long administration of pharmacologic agents that rather nonselectively block immune responsiveness. Since the cellular interactions involved in the recipient's reaction to an allograft are mediated through T-cell subsets bearing distinctive cell surface molecules, one approach to providing a more selective immunosuppressive strategy might be through the use of antibodies targeted to specific sites involved in the immune response.

The initial effort to achieve this goal was through the use of polyclonal antilymphocyte sera (ALS). These preparations were designed to attack principally the infiltrating mononuclear cells observed in allograft biopsies coincident with allograft rejection. Such suppression conceptually could retain much of the host's response to bacterial infection, since this is more dependent on B-cell–mediated humoral processes. Following the introduction of antilymphocyte globulin (ALG) by Starzl et al in 1967 (1), extensive clinical studies established the efficacy of these polyclonal preparations for both prophylaxis and treatment of rejection and they continue to be used today in many clinical situations (2–5). However, with the use of classic techniques to immunize animals that generate these polyclonal products, a heterogeneous group of antibodies is produced not only to most T-cell populations, but also to B cells and even nonlymphoid cells. Thus, global suppression can result from the administration of polyclonal antilymphocyte antibodies, not infrequently resulting in opportunistic infections. Hence, the search for even more specific agents has continued.

Another milestone toward this goal occurred when cell hybridization techniques were developed that could yield monoclonal antibodies (MAbs) to single-cell membrane determinants (6). This Nobel Prize–winning technology provided reagents that are reactive only with T cells or, even more importantly, with specific T-cell subsets or other molecular targets. Monoclonal antibody therapy was introduced into clinical protocols in 1981, when Cosimi reported the rapid reversal of acute rejection in renal allograft recipients treated with OKT-3 MAb without the use of increased steroid dosages (7). This MAb has since become the treatment of choice for steroid-resistant rejection in recipients of all types of allografts. As detailed below, its role in induction therapy has been less well established.

With the addition of OKT-3 to therapeutic protocols, it seemed a new clinical era had been entered in which monoclonal ALS would be extensively used to manipulate selected T-cell populations while leaving intact most of the host's other immune competence. Like the polyclonal antilymphocyte preparations, OKT-3 is a pan-T-cell antibody and therefore affects all aspects of cell-mediated immunity. The successful clinical application of this MAb, however, emphasized that this technology could provide further designer proteins targeting less broadly expressed cell surface markers that are important components of the effector pathways of rejection. Unfortunately, progress in defining clinically effective MAbs that provide more selective suppression of immunologic responses than OKT-3 has been frustratingly limited. Undoubtedly, this is due to the complexity of the rejection reaction, which must include alternate pathways that can be utilized to mount an effective response following highly selective blocking of known mechanisms.

Some of the most promising agents currently under investigation are directed toward the integrins or adhesion molecules, the costimulatory pathways, and the cytokine receptors. In addition to the use of MAbs to inhibit the function of these molecules, the use of soluble receptors [e.g., tumor necrosis factor receptor (TNFR), interleukin 2 receptor (IL-2R)] as immunosuppressive agents is being explored. The constantly expanding identification of new molecules involved in the rejection process promotes continuing opportunities for targeting specific components of the immune system. This chapter traces the evolution of antilymphocyte antibodies (both polyclonal and monoclonal) in the context of their preparation, their prophylactic administration, and their abolition of the rejection reaction as well as the possible future role some of these agents may play in the development of conditioning regimens that may even induce donor-specific tolerance.

POLYCLONAL ANTILYMPHOCYTE SERA

ALS, ALG, and antithymocyte globulin (ATG) are xenotypic polyclonal antibody preparations with differing degrees of immunoglobulin purity produced by immunizing animals with different source lymphocytes (see below).

Production of ALS Preparations

Polyclonal antibodies are produced by immunizing animals with human lymphoid cells. The immunized animal produces numerous antibodies, each from an individual cell clone, in response to the various antigens contained on the immunogen. Cultured lymphoblasts (producing ALG) or human thymocytes (producing ATG) are the most commonly employed immunogens. Cultured lymphoblasts have the advantage of being free of contaminants such as erythrocytes, platelets, or stromal elements that induce unwanted antibodies. However, stable cultured clones are typically B cells, so thymocytes remain the immunogen of choice for many commercial preparations (Table 13.1). Thymocytes are obtained from cadaver donors or patients undergoing open heart surgery. The selection of specific animals for immunization is based on practical considerations including cost, animal size, and availability (8). The most commonly used preparations are of equine or rabbit origin. These two species have been demonstrated to produce large volumes of potent antilymphocyte antibodies. Sera from multiple animals are usually pooled in the attempt to achieve batch-to-batch consistency.

Following immunization of the selected animals, sera are harvested and processed to obtain purified globulin. This generally involves extensive absorption with nonlymphoid cells in order to remove contaminating antibodies (e.g., hemolysins) and fractionation, thus obtaining the IgG portion of the serum that contains the immunosuppressive component. Nevertheless, over 95% of the final product is made up of irrelevant equine or rabbit globulin, and it is estimated that only about 2% of the administered antibodies are specifically reactive with human T lymphocytes (9). The steps involved in the production of a typical polyclonal ALS are summarized in Figure 13.1.

Administration

The initial reports of antilymphocyte antibody use involved intramuscular or subcutaneous administration. However, local inflammatory reactions and the increased immunogenicity associated with these approaches plus the need for relatively large volumes of polyclonal agents make intravenous administration the preferred approach. A painful chemical phlebitis can be associated with peripheral administration through low-flow veins, and so antilymphocyte antibodies are sometimes given via central venous access lines or an arteriovenous fistula. Central venous administration also allows for more concentrated individual doses in patients unable to tolerate large volume infusions. The currently available commercial preparations include ATG-Fresenius and Thymoglobulin (Pasteur Merieux; in the

Table 13.1. Comparison of Polyclonal Antilymphocyte Preparations

	ATGAM (Upjohn)	Lymphoglobuline (Merieux)	Thymoglobuline (Merieux)	ATG (Fresenius)	MALG (U. Minn)	RATG (12)
Immunogen	Thymus	Thymus	Thymus	Jurkat Cell Line	Cultured Lymphoblasts	Thymus
Species	Equine	Equine	Rabbit	Rabbit	Equine	Rabbit
Dosage (mg/kg/d)	10–30	10	1.25–2.5	1–5	15–20	1–5
Reactivity Against*:						
CD2	++	++++	+	±	+	+
CD3	++	+	+	0	+	±
CD4	+++	+	±	0	+	+
CD8	++	+++	++	0	+	+
CD11a	++	+	±	0	+	+
CD18	++	++	+	0	++	++++
CD28	+	++	±	±	++	++++
TCR	++	+	+	0	+	N/A

* Comparative in vitro reactivity to specific CD antigens (11–13).

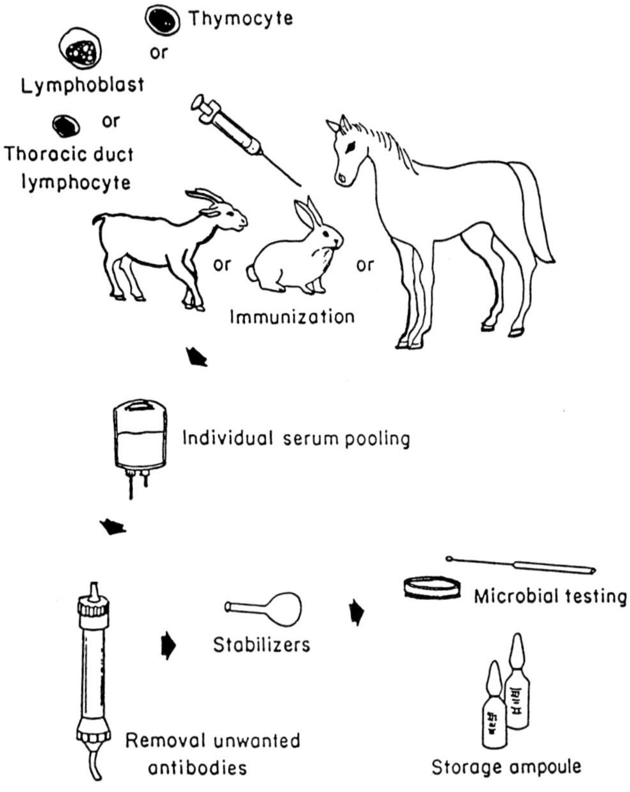

FIGURE 13.1. *Production of polyclonal ALS preparations for human use. Selected animals are immunized with human thymocytes, thoracic duct lymphocytes, or cultured lymphoblasts. Harvested sera are pooled, extensively absorbed to remove unwanted antibodies, and processed to obtain the IgG portion.*

U.S.A., Sangstat Medical Corp.), which are of rabbit origin and are given in doses of 1.25–5.0 mg/kg/day, and ATGAM (Upjohn) and Lymphoglobuline (Pasteur Merieux), which are of equine origin and are given at doses of 10–30 mg/kg/day. Minnesota ALG (MALG), which is currently not available (10), has been administered at a dose of 15–20 mg/kg/day. In addition, some transplant centers continue to produce their own individual products. Since no single agent has been defined as most efficacious, ALS, ATG, and ALG preparations can be considered under the single heading of ALS.

Mechanisms of Action

Polyclonal ALS contain antibodies reactive with multiple common T-cell surface molecules (see Table 13.1). Probably most relevant are antibodies targeting the cluster designation (CD) determinants CD2, CD3, CD4, CD8, CD11a, CD25, CD40, and CD54 (11–13). There appear to be at least three mechanisms of action by which polyclonal antibodies exert their effects. In vivo administration of ALS often results in profound lymphopenia. One mechanism for this lymphopenia appears to be classic complement-mediated cell lysis. Another likely mechanism for the lymphopenia and its resultant immunosuppressive effect is uptake of opsonized T cells by the reticuloendothelial system. ALS-coated T cells can be found sequestered in the reticuloendothelial system of the spleen, liver, lungs, thymus, and lymph nodes of treated animals. A third mechanism by which ALS could exert its immunosuppressive properties is through masking or modulation of essential surface receptors on lymphocytes that remain in the circulation but whose function is blocked. After cessation of ALS therapy, repopulation of peripheral blood lymphocytes usually occurs within 3 to 10 days. However, the proliferative response of these lymphocytes often remains impaired. This phenomenon may result from the development of nonspecific suppressor cells (14).

CLINICAL APPLICATIONS OF POLYCLONAL ANTIBODIES

Polyclonal ALS preparations for intravenous administration are typically diluted in isotonic saline to concentrations not exceeding 4 mg/cc. Dextrose- or heparin-containing solutions are generally avoided because they may result in protein aggregation. Infusion is by slow intravenous administration over approximately four hours in order to minimize toxicity. An in-line filter is recommended to prevent infusion of precipitates that may develop during storage. Corticosteroids along with acetaminophen and antihistamines are often given prior to administration of ALS to limit the side effects resulting from the rapid release of cytokines that is associated with initial infusions (see below). A skin test or a slowly infused test dose has been recommended for exclusion of preexisting type I sensitivity to equine or rabbit serum. Most clinicians, however, have discontinued skin testing since little correlation with allergic reactions has been demonstrated (15). The duration of ALS therapy is generally 5 to 14 days, depending on the specific indication for treatment as well as center preferences.

ALS Rejection Prophylaxis (Induction Therapy)

While there is little disagreement about the efficacy of polyclonal preparations in rejection reversal, the role of these agents for induction therapy is more controversial. Early studies demonstrated a significant delay in the onset of first rejection episodes in renal allograft recipients treated with ALS in conjunction with azathioprine and steroids compared to patients on azathioprine and steroids alone. After cessation of ALS therapy, however, a high incidence of rejection episodes occurred and significant improvement in long-term allograft or patient survival was difficult to demonstrate (16,17). Many of these early studies suggested an improvement in graft survival of approximately 10%, but the low numbers of patients in individual reports, the nonstandardized products being used, and the multiple other variables involved in such clinical trials made it difficult to provide statistically significant conclusions.

The subsequent addition of cyclosporine (CsA) to immunosuppressive protocols clearly improved survival for recipients of all types of allografts, suggesting induction ALS therapy might no longer be a consideration (see also Chapter 6). However, the apparent nephrotoxic synergism between CsA and the physiologic factors associated with acute tubular necrosis (ATN), which are frequently encountered in the early postoperative period especially after renal transplantation, has raised concerns that irreversible renal damage may occur if CsA is being administered when the kidney is in the initial recovery phase. This has prompted many centers to replace CsA with an antilymphocyte preparation until satisfactory renal function is restored (18–22). Observations in patients treated with such protocols have been encouraging, including a lower incidence of delayed graft function, minimally increased risks of viral infections, and a rejection-free early course in the majority of recipients. Improved long-term allograft survival has been achieved only in some individual center reports (23,24). Retrospective analyses of large databases (Table 13.2), however, have documented an advantage of induction antilymphocyte therapy in conjunction with delayed CsA therapy, particularly for recipients of older donor kidneys, highly sensitized patients, retransplant recipients, and those with delayed graft function (25,26). Concerns regarding the costs and potential risks of ALS immunosuppression have led many centers to recommend ALS induction therapy only for these high-risk recipients (27) or to reduce the dosage administered based on T-cell monitoring of individual patients (28). The continuing lack of consensus regarding the most cost-effective approach for induction therapy is emphasized by a recent survey of US transplant programs (29) (Table 13.3).

While most of the early studies using ALS involved renal transplantation, polyclonal antibody induction therapy has more recently been evaluated in recipients of extrarenal allografts. Sequential ALS-CsA induction therapy in hepatic transplant recipients has been reported from some centers to limit renal dysfunction, improve allograft survival and thus require fewer retransplants, and reduce the incidence of rejection. These benefits were achieved without an increased incidence of infectious complications or malignancy. Survival rates of over 90% have been reported using this approach (30,31). A recent study comparing ATG–CsA quadruple immunosuppression to tacrolimus and prednisone showed improved graft and patient survival in the ATG–CsA group with similar rejection rates (32). ALS induction has also been reported to increase survival rates in pediatric recipients of major blood group (ABO)-incompatible liver allografts (33). Some centers, however, caution that ATG therapy is an increased risk factor for subsequent cytomegalovirus (CMV) infection and recommend such induction only in selected high-risk hepatic allograft recipients (34) (see also Chapter 36).

ALS has also been considered an important induction agent in pancreatic transplantation (35). A lower incidence of rejection episodes, along with a delay in onset to first rejection, and pancreatic graft survival rates of over 80% have been reported using sequential ALS–CsA quadruple induction therapy in combined kidney–pancreas transplantation.

ALS was used almost universally in cardiac transplantation prior to the introduction of CsA. In contrast to the observations in recipients of renal allografts, the efficacy of ALS had been felt to be conclusive for cardiac transplantation (36,37). With the addition of CsA to

Table 13.2. The Effect of Induction Therapy with ALS or OKT-3 on CD Renal Allograft Survival

	No Antibody		ALG/OKT-3		
	% 1-Yr Survival	Recipients (*n*)	% 1-Yr Survival	Recipients (*n*)	*P* value
Primary Transplant	78	14,450	80	4820	<0.001
Donor age >55	68	92	76	350	0.006
DGF	64	3690	70	1185	<0.0001
PRA >50%	72	1345	77	550	0.02
Diabetic	76	2830	80	1025	0.004
Retransplant	70	2680	74	1050	0.006
Donor age >55	52	160	65	65	0.04
DGF	53	965	60	390	0.01
PRA >50%	63	770	72	415	0.002
Diabetic	69	310	77	100	NS

NS = not stated.
Source: Adapted from Cecka JM, Terasaki PI. The UNOS Scientific Renal Transplant Registry. In: Teraski PI, Cecka JM, eds. Clinical transplants 1991. Los Angeles: UCLA Tissue Typing Laboratory, 1992:6.

Table 13.3. Preferred Immunosuppressive Approaches of US Transplant Programs

	Kidney		Heart		Liver		Pancreas	
	I[a]	II[b]	I[a]	II[b]	I[a]	II[b]	I[a]	II[b]
Induction Therapy								
Polyclonal Ab	54%	25%	54%	28%	37%	42%	76%	12%
Monoclonal Ab	51%	26%	55%	28%	35%	40%	72%	8%
Rejection Therapy								
Monoclonal Ab	94%	2%	92%	3%	95%	0%	92%	0%
IV Steroids	90%	4%	97%	0%	91%	5%	80%	0%
Polyclonal Ab	73%	12%	82%	5%	67%	7%	68%	4%

[a] Proportion of programs regarding the approach as important or essential to successful patient outcome.
[b] Proportion of programs regarding the approach as unnecessary or undesirable.
Adapted from Evans RW, Manninen DL, Dong FB, et al. Immunosuppressive therapy as a determinant of transplantation outcomes. Transplantation 1993;55:1297–1305.

immunosuppressive protocols, many centers discontinued the use of ALS induction. As in renal transplant recipients, however, the severe nephrotoxic effects of CsA that became apparent following heart transplantation have led some centers to replace CsA with ALS during the immediate post-transplant period (38,39). This approach is reported to reduce the incidence and severity of rejection and improve long-term outcome and renal function in cardiac transplant recipients (40–42). Again, however, this practice is far from universal (see Table 13.3).

Since steroids have been shown to inhibit bronchial healing in lung transplant recipients (43), ALS in conjunction with CsA and azathioprine induction has been used for induction therapy that withholds steroids for up to three weeks in these patients (44).

ALS Rejection Therapy

The first randomized trial comparing ALS to high-dosage steroids for the treatment of established rejection was conducted in 1979 (45). The patients in that study were living–related donor renal allograft recipients who had received induction immunosuppressive therapy with azathioprine and prednisone. With the onset of biopsy-proven rejection, the patients were randomized to receive either high-dose steroids or ALS. ALS proved to be as effective as high-dosage steroids, with the added benefit of more rapid rejection reversal and fewer subsequent rejection episodes. Long-term follow-up indicated that a one-year allograft survival of over 90% could be achieved in azathioprine-steroid–treated recipients of haploidentical renal allografts if rejection was reversed with ALS, versus a survival of only 74% following rejection treatment with steroids (46). The efficacy of ALS in reversing rejection in CsA-treated patients has also been demonstrated (47,48). ALS has even been used to reverse steroid-resistant rejection in patients who had previously received ALS induction, with no increase in infectious morbidity being observed (3,49). The value of ALS, particularly for treating steroid-resistant rejection in renal transplant recipients, is therefore widely acknowledged (see Table 13.3), although, as discussed below, OKT-3 MAb is now usually preferred. Nevertheless, ALS provides a useful option in rejection therapy, especially for patients who may have been sensitized to murine protein after a previous course of MAb therapy.

ALS has also been used to treat primary or steroid-resistant rejection in liver transplantation (50,51). Again, however, with the availability of tacrolimus and OKT-3, current use of ALS in hepatic transplantation is primarily as an induction agent given to patients with perioperative renal dysfunction. ALS has also been used to treat steroid-resistant rejection in pancreatic, cardiac, and pulmonary transplant recipients. The choice of polyclonal versus MAb therapy in each of these situations remains unresolved and will be discussed further below.

ALS Induction of Transplant Tolerance

The feasibility of inducing allograft tolerance in adult recipients has been established in a number of rodent models (see Chapter 5), many of which, interestingly, have required ALS as part of the T-cell–depleting conditioning protocol (52,53). In murine models, highly specific unresponsiveness to donor antigens can be consistently produced using donor blood or bone marrow infusions and ALS. Long-term allograft survival without the requirement for chronic immunosuppression has been much more difficult to achieve in large animal models, but a similar protocol has been extended to nonhuman primates (54). With a brief course of post-transplant ALS therapy, donor bone marrow infusion, and no further immunosuppression after the fifth day following transplant, indefinite renal allograft survival was observed in about one-third of these recipients (55). On the basis of these observations, a pilot trial in humans was undertaken in which cadaveric renal allograft recipients received ALS followed by the transfusion of donor-specific bone marrow. Control patients received the contralateral kidney without bone marrow transfusion (56). Both groups of patients received CsA, azathioprine, and prednisone. The allograft survival rate for the bone marrow group was significantly improved at 12 months, and it was possible to withdraw steroids completely from a number of these patients. No attempt was made to withdraw all immunosuppression as had been done in the nonhuman primate trials.

Recent data have demonstrated that a state of multilineage mixed chimerism and donor-specific tolerance to renal allografts can be produced in the majority of nonhuman primates that have undergone a brief period of T-cell depletion with a conditioning regimen that also requires ALS (57,58). The mechanism of tolerance in these recipients, in contrast to what has been felt to represent peripherally mediated "anergy" in the previous models, appears to involve clonal deletion (see Chapter 5). Because of the highly durable donor-specific unresponsiveness associated with this type of tolerance, this approach is quite attractive for clinical application, although no trials have yet been undertaken. Nevertheless, these demonstrations of donor-specific hyporesponsiveness in large animal models emphasize that transplant tolerance induction in human recipients should be possible and that initial therapeutic protocols are likely to include ALS.

In Vitro Monitoring of ALS Therapy

Since different ALS preparations, and even the same preparation in different individuals, may produce variable immunosuppressive effects, a number of in vitro assays have been utilized in the attempt to both standardize different batches of ALS and monitor the level of suppression that is being achieved during treatment. For quality control and standardization purposes, the lymphocytotoxicity of each preparation may be determined by adding decreasing concentrations of ALS to lymphocytes in order to determine the lowest concentration at which more than 50% of lymphocytes are killed (59). Preparations are also assayed for their ability to inhibit the formation of rosettes by sheep erythrocytes with human T lymphocytes. Rosette inhibition results from the anti-CD2 antibodies contained in the ALS preparations.

Clinical activity has been evaluated by monitoring T-cell numbers in peripheral blood with the use of MAbs (60). Interestingly, some of the T-cell subset alterations have been documented to persist for periods as long as five years after ALS treatment (61). Depression of CD2- or CD3-positive cells (mature T lymphocytes) to less than 10% of pretreatment values has generally been correlated with rejection control (62,63). In contrast, persistent elevation of this cell population is often associated with unresolved rejection, requiring either increased ALS dosages or the addition of other immunosuppressants. Since most of these preparations are contaminated with antibodies reactive with human erythrocytes and thrombocytes, serial hematocrits and platelet counts must also be monitored during therapy and dosages of the administered product adjusted to prevent unacceptable anemia or thrombocytopenia.

Immunogenicity of Polyclonal Preparations

During or following a course of ALS therapy, serum antibodies reactive with rabbit or equine immunoglobulin can be detected in 10% to 30% of patients (49,64). Such antibodies, if present in sufficient titer during therapy, could neutralize the beneficial effects of the agent and might explain why peripheral blood T cells are not effectively depleted in some patients. However, no consistent correlation has been demonstrated between circulating levels of ALS and allograft survival.

The major immunologic concern associated with infusions of heterologous antibodies is the possibility of producing serum sickness. As noted above, pretreatment skin testing has not proved to be useful for predicting the likelihood of reactions to the foreign protein. Fortunately, anaphylactic reactions and serum sickness have been surprisingly infrequent (65), generally being noted in 1% to 3% of treated patients. Furthermore, many patients have been treated with ALS on repeated occasions without adverse effects. This apparent lack of a clinically relevant immune response to the foreign protein is presumably due to multiple factors, including careful deaggregation of the products prepared for clinical infusion, the intravenous route of administration, and the large dosages employed that should provide a significant antigen excess and favor the development of small and highly soluble complexes. In addition, because these polyclonal antisera react with a variety of lymphocyte populations, the ALS may, in combination with the concomitant pharmacologic immunosuppression being administered, suppress the recipient's response to the foreign protein as well (8). Cessation of ALS therapy and administration of high-dosage steroids has effectively controlled the signs and symptoms of serum sickness in the few patients who have developed this condition.

Side Effects of Polyclonal Preparations

The reported incidence and severity of adverse clinical reactions following ALS administration have varied with the preparation used (Table 13.4). Fever, often in association with significant chills and sometimes diarrhea, develops during the initial infusion in the majority of patients. Intensive evaluation of these "first-dose reactions" following either polyclonal or monoclonal antibody therapy has established that increased serum cytokine levels including TNF,

Table 13.4. Clinical Toxicity of ALS Administration

Reported Incidence >10%		Reported Incidence 5% to 10%		Reported Incidence ≤5%	
Early Reactions					
Chills, Fever (d1)	15–60%	Nausea, diarrhea	1–10%	Hypotension	2–5%
(d2)	4–25%	Neutropenia	1–10%	Dyspnea	2–5%
Thrombocytopenia	1–30%	(<2000/mm^3)		Seizures	0–1%
(<50,000/mm^3)		Serum sickness	1–8%	Anaphylaxis	0–1%
Rash/pruritus	1–20%	Arthralgia	1–7%		
Anemia	5–15%				
Local phlebitis	2–15%				
Late Side Effects					
CMV infection		Herpes simplex reactivation		PTLD	
		EBV reactivation			

IL-1 and IL-6, and interferon gamma (IFN-γ) are highly correlated with the side effects (66,67). To limit the morbidity of this cytokine release, patients are usually premedicated with antipyretics, antihistamines, and intravenous steroids. There is also evidence that anti-TNF antibodies or TNF soluble receptors may limit the cytokine release syndrome (68,69). Such approaches have generally been employed only with MAb therapy where the syndrome has been more severe (see below). During ALS treatment, pruritic skin eruptions (Fig. 13.2 and Plate 6) have been noted in approximately 20% of recipients. Although this presumably represents a type of hypersensitivity to the agent, most patients can complete the therapeutic protocol without the development of more significant problems with only antihistamine administration being required for symptomatic relief.

Thrombocytopenia and/or anemia of varying severity have been reported in up to 30% of patients. This is generally dose-related, occurring in patients who require maximum dosages to depress T-cell levels adequately. A modest reduction in ALS dosage, or further reduction in the concomitantly administered azathioprine or mycophenolate mofetil dose, usually resolves this problem without the need for discontinuing ALS therapy (see also Chapter 10). Although thrombocytopenia primarily results from low levels of contaminating antiplatelet antibodies, reversible platelet aggregation within the pulmonary microcirculation in the absence of antiplatelet antibodies has also been demonstrated (70). These aggregates release vasoactive substances that could induce interstitial pooling and hypotensive reactions, even in the absence of hypersensitivity. Such a sequence of events could explain the observation of occasional hypotensive episodes associated with rapid infusions of ALS.

An increased incidence of infectious complications has been reported in many trials of ALS therapy (see also Chapter 36). Of particular importance was the early observation that CMV infection seemed to be disproportionately more frequent and more severe in allograft recipients treated with ALS (8,51). One group observed the incidence of CMV infection to be twice as high in liver allograft recipients treated with ALS compared to those treated with conventional immunosuppression (34). Similar observations were reported in ALS-treated renal and cardiac allograft recipients. Further experience has established that reducing the dosages of concomitantly administered pharmacologic agents, in conjunction with the steroid-sparing effect

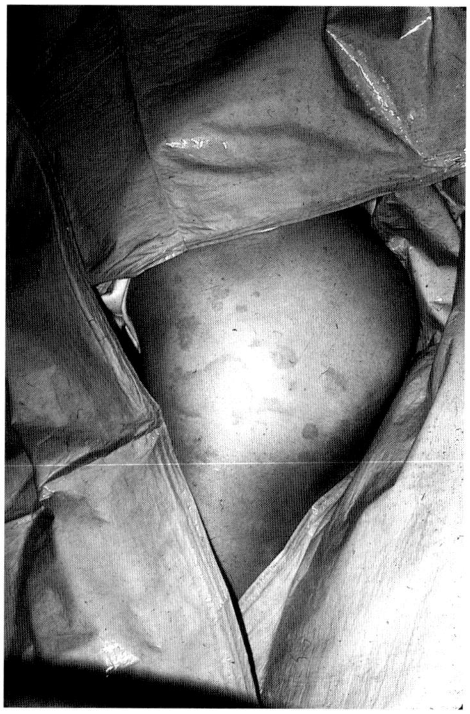

FIGURE 13.2. *Skin rash in an ATG-treated patient. The maculopapular, blotchy eruption developed primarily over the recipient's thighs and buttocks six days after initiating ATG therapy. The 12-day course of treatment, required to reverse the patient's acute rejection episode, was completed without complications following administration of antihistamines for symptomatic relief.*

achieved by ALS, results in infectious complication rates similar to those observed using conventional immunosuppression (17,71). Unfortunately, if concomitantly administered pharmacologic agents are withdrawn completely during ALS therapy, the incidence of sensitization to the heterologous protein is markedly increased. Routine ganciclovir administration during the period of ALS therapy has therefore also been recommended to further limit the incidence of CMV infection (72).

As with any potent immunosuppression (see Chapter 37), administration of ALS is associated with an increased incidence of malignancy (73), particularly post-transplant lymphoproliferative disease (PTLD). This lymphoma-like process results from primary infection (in children) or reactivation (in adults) of Epstein-Barr virus (EBV). This complication is seen most frequently in allograft recipients who have had multiple courses of antirejection therapy, especially if this included ALS.

MONOCLONAL ANTIBODIES

The production of MAbs is based on two well-established observations. First, each B lymphocyte and its expanded clone in an immunized animal produce a single specific antibody but have a very short life span when cultured ex vivo; and second, malignant myeloma cells can be grown permanently in culture but produce antibodies with no predefined specificity. The key breakthrough in MAb technology occurred in 1975 when Kohler and Milstein succeeded in fusing these two cell types, thus combining the essential properties of specific antibody secretion and permanent cell growth (6). Each fusion-derived hybridoma cell line secretes a single antibody of predefined reactivity plus the irrelevant myeloma protein. This methodology allows the production of essentially unlimited quantities of the desired MAb, which can be selected to target virtually any cell surface antigen or circulating molecule. As a result, major advances in both identifying and manipulating cell surface antigens and other immune mediators have occurred.

The previous success of polyclonal ALS in immunosuppressive regimens strongly suggested that MAbs might be even more effectively employed as immunosuppressive agents. This was confirmed when OKT-3, which targets the CD3 complex associated with the T-cell receptor (TCR) expressed on all mature T lymphocytes, was first used clinically (7).

Production of Monoclonal Antibodies

Monoclonal antibody production begins with immunization of mice using human T lymphocytes or selected membrane fragments (Fig. 13.3). After approximately four to six weeks, splenocytes are harvested from the immunized mice. The antibody-producing cells are then mixed with mouse myeloma cells and polyethylene glycol to promote fusion. The hybridomas obtained are assayed and those hybridomas

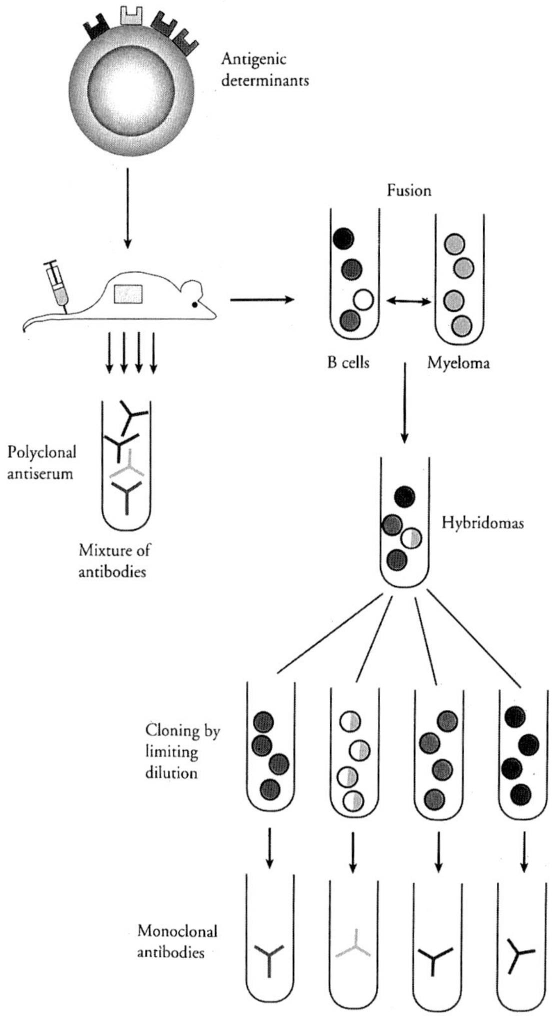

FIGURE 13.3. *Production of monoclonal antibodies for human use. Splenocytes (B cells) from immunized mice are fused with myeloma cells to produce the "immortalized" antibody-producing hybridoma. The desired hybridoma is isolated and expanded by random cloning. (Reprinted with permission. Copyright 1995, Hoffman-La Roche Inc. All rights reserved.)*

demonstrating positive antibody activity are subsequently grown in a hypoxanthine, aminopterin, and thymidine (HAT)-containing medium that kills parental cells but allows the hybridomas to survive. By random cloning, the desired hybridomas are then isolated and expanded. The selected clones are maintained in vitro by mass tissue culture or in vivo by intraperitoneal injection into mice, which results in the formation of an ascites-producing tumor. From these sources, large volumes of tissue culture supernatant or antibody-containing ascites can be sequentially collected for clinical use.

More recent refinements have led to the development of "humanized" monoclonal antibodies (74). Humanized antibodies have been developed in an attempt to overcome the human antimouse antibody (HAMA) response observed in most patients receiving MAbs of murine origin. These HAMAs cause rapid clearance of the murine antibody from the recipient's circulation, thereby reducing the therapeutic efficacy and possibly precluding sequential courses of MAb therapy. As a first step in the production of humanized agents, the mouse variable region is joined to a human constant region (see Chapter 12, Fig. 12.2). Using gene recombinant techniques, the chimeric MAb is further modified so that only the essential antigen-combining sequences of mouse origin are retained (75,76). These segments, termed the *complementary determining regions (CDRs)*, continue to confer antigenic specificity to the antibody. However, since the CDR-grafted antibodies differ from human immunoglobulin only at the epitope-combining site, the HAMA response to these agents is both reduced and predictably anti-idiotypic (77). As a result, the therapeutic course of one humanized MAb should not prevent subsequent treatment with other MAbs bearing different idiotypes. Furthermore, humanized MAbs are less likely to induce the cytokine release syndrome (78,79), and the effective half-life of the administered agent is greatly prolonged in the recipient's circulation (80).

Most recently, MAb immunoconjugates with striking immunosuppressive potency have been developed through fusion technology (81,82). These MAbs allow delivery of drugs or toxins to selected target cells that have surface components reactive with the antibody portion of the conjugate. The immunotoxin portion, which is then internalized by receptor-mediated endocytosis, has proved to be highly efficacious for inducing T-cell depletion in these studies.

Administration

The initial clinical trial using OKT-3 without additional steroids demonstrated the efficacy of this intravenously administered MAb in reversing established renal allograft rejection with dosages as low as 1–2 mg/day (7). However, in some patients, daily T-cell monitoring revealed incomplete depletion or modulation of circulating CD3+ cells. This led to the currently recommended adult dosage of 5 mg/day in order to reduce the need for frequent monitoring. The optimal dosage, however, remains undefined (83) and undoubtedly could be tailored to individual patient requirements by serial monitoring of circulating T lymphocytes (see below). The dosage in children is typically 1.0–2.5 mg/day depending on the size of the child. The duration of therapy may vary depending on whether the drug is being given as an induction agent or as therapy for steroid-resistant rejection. The usual course of OKT3 treatment for rejection is 10 to 14 days, depending on the clinical response, while the course for induction may be shortened depending on the degree of ATN. OKT-3 is injected as a single intravenous bolus and may be given through a peripheral vein. Because OKT-3 may contain particulate protein matter, the drug should be drawn through a 0.22-micron filter prior to infusion. Before initiating therapy, the patient's volume status should be assessed carefully to avoid precipitation of pulmonary edema (see side effects, below).

As with the polyclonal preparations, antihistamines, acetaminophen, and corticosteroids should be given prior to administration of the first one or two OKT-3 doses to alleviate the "first-dose response" (84,85). Concomitant pharmacologic immunosuppression should be reduced to decrease the risks of infection; however, maintenance of at least low-dose CsA may be beneficial to limit the recipient's immune response and prevent recurrent rejection (86). Dosages of other MAbs used in clinical protocols have been widely variable, ranging from as little as 0.5 mg/kg given every two weeks (80) to 1 mg/kg/day (87). As with OKT-3, sequential monitoring of the degree of depletion or modulation of the targeted cell population that is being achieved during therapy has been used to define the appropriate dosage for each preparation.

Mechanisms of Action

Monoclonal antibodies may exert their immunosuppressive effects by several mechanisms (see Chapter 12) including cell depletion (Fig. 13.4), cell coating, and antigenic modulation (88). True T-cell depletion is suggested by a decrease in the number of lymphocytes expressing CD determinants other than the targeted antigen (e.g., absence of cells expressing CD2 following anti-CD3 therapy). Opsonizing antibodies clear T lymphocytes via complement fixation or interaction with Fc receptors that results in reticuloendothelial uptake and lysis in the spleen, liver, and lymph nodes (89). Direct lysis of lymphocytes in the circulation, particularly if a toxin has been conjugated to the MAb, may also contribute to T-cell depletion. Whether opsonization and lymphocyte clearance is more likely from the peripheral circulation or from

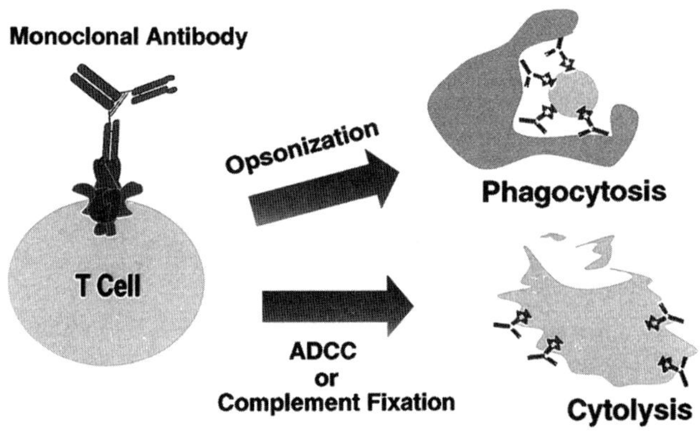

FIGURE 13.4. *T-cell clearance by monoclonal antibodies. Depleting monoclonal antibodies may trigger complement activation through their Fc portion or produce cell cytolysis via antibody-dependent cell cytotoxicity (ADCC). Opsonization and phagocytosis of the antibody-coated cell may contribute to cell clearance in the reticuloendothelial system.*

the transplant itself may be determined by the subclass of administered antibody (90).

Monoclonal antibodies may also exert immunosuppressive activity by coating cell surface antigens. This process may block the function of the cell by interfering with cell-to-cell interactions, by transducing signals that result in inactivation or activation of particular cells, or by cross-linking different cells (91,92). Cells coated with murine MAb can be detected in vitro using antimurine-immunoglobulin–fluoresceinated antibodies. Antigenic coating appears to be the primary mechanism of action for many of the MAbs directed against adhesion molecules (90).

Antigenic modulation (see Chapter 12, Fig. 12.6) is a phenomenon that results in redistribution of antigen–antibody complexes on the cell surface forming a "cap" (88,93). These "caps" of antibody–antigen complexes are then internalized or shed from the cell surface. This process renders the cell unresponsive if the molecule is functionally relevant as in the TCR–CD3 complex, which is targeted by OKT-3 (94). Antigenic modulation may be reversible as demonstrated by reexpression of the molecule if the cells are cultured in vitro or after MAb therapy is withdrawn.

Molecular Targets of Monoclonal Antibodies

While MAbs could be produced against virtually any cell surface or secreted antigen, immunosuppressive activity requires that the antibody be directed against a functionally important molecule. Target antigens for immunosuppressive MAbs are typically expressed on the surface of cells that are known to be involved in the immune response, particularly T cells (see Chapter 2). T cells are equipped with an array of such cell surface molecules (Fig. 13.5) that mediate interactions between nonactivated T cells and antigen-presenting cells (APCs), or between cytotoxic T cells and their targets (e.g., allograft endothelium). Interference with the molecules mediating these interactions therefore represents an attractive approach to selectively interrupting the immune response to an allograft. The important antigens that have been targeted for clinical trials or appear to have significant clinical promise are listed in Table 13.5.

CD2, also known as the E-rosette receptor or lymphocyte function associated antigen-2 (LFA-2), functions as an adhesion and signal transduction molecule. It is expressed on T cells and natural killer (NK) cells. CD2 is physically

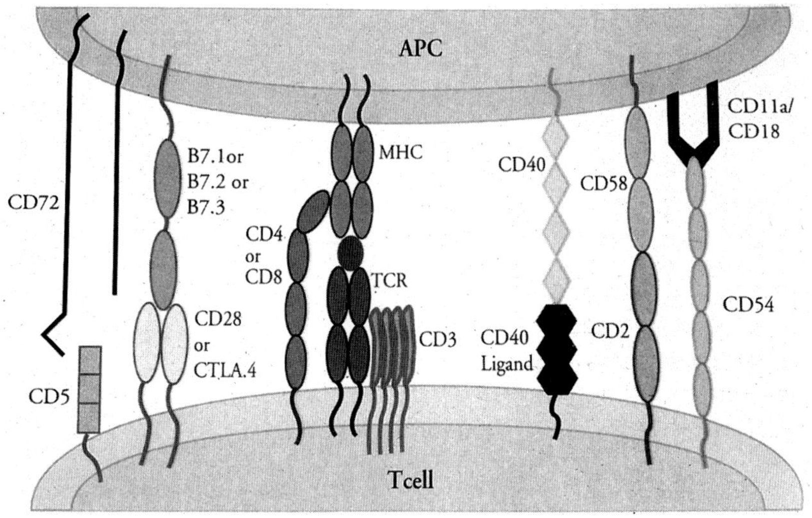

FIGURE 13.5. *Schematic depiction of some of the cell surface molecules involved in T-cell activation. Monoclonal antibodies that are specifically targeted to any one of these determinants can be utilized to selectively interrupt essential intercellular reactions. (Reprinted with permission. Copyright 1995, Hoffman-La Roche Inc. All rights reserved.)*

Table 13.5. Promising Targets for MAb Immunomodulation

Specificity	Distribution	Ligand	Function
CD2 (E-Rosette R)	T cells, NK cells	LFA3	Adhesion with TCR/MHC
CD3	Mature T cells	—	Activation, ↑IL-2
CD4	50–65% T cells	MHC class II	Stabilize TCR/MHC
CD7	T cells, blasts	—	T-cell proliferation
CD8	30–35% T cells	MHC class I	Stabilize TCR/MHC
CD25 (IL-2R)	Activated cells	IL-2	T-cell proliferation
CD28/CTLA4	T cells	B7.1 (CD80), B7.2 (CD86)	Costimulation
CD40L (CD154)	T cells	CD40	APC maturation, ↑IL-12
CD45	BM-derived cells	—	Regulate phosphorylation
CD54 (ICAM)	Endothelium, activated cells	LFA1	Leukocyte adhesion
TCR	T cells	MHC 1 or 2 + peptide	Ag specificity

and functionally linked to TCR and CD3 and enhances their binding to major histocompatibility complex (MHC) antigen. Its ligand is LFA-3 (CD58), found on APCs. Inhibition of CD2 signaling has been shown to result in apoptosis (95) or induction of an anergic state (96). Anti-CD2 MAbs, therefore, could be useful in controlling rejection. Early preclinical studies, however, suggested poor immunosuppressive efficacy of these agents (97). Recently, evaluation of a new anti-CD2 MAb (LO-CD2a) produced from rat ascites has been undertaken in Brussels (98). This agent has been shown to produce prolonged depletion of CD2 reactive cells when administered to chimpanzees and to be minimally mitogenic in vitro. Predictably, therefore, "first dose reactions" should be less severe than those encountered with OKT-3. Initial clinical evaluation of LO-CD2a as treatment for graft-versus-host disease (GVHD) and renal allograft rejection has been encouraging and is continuing.

CD3, a cell-surface immunoglobulin found on mature T cells, is associated with the antigen-recognition site of the T-cell receptor. This molecule is believed to be responsible for T-cell activation and upregulation of IL-2 production along with mitogenesis. OKT-3, which targets this molecule, is the prototype MAb that, to date, has been most widely used for immunosuppression in transplantation (see below).

CD4, a glycoprotein that belongs to the immunoglobulin family, is found on the majority of mature thymocytes and the 55% to 60% of peripheral T cells that bind MHC class II antigens. Historically, these cells were termed *helper/inducer T lymphocytes*. Similarities between human and lower animal CD4 molecules illustrate evolutionary conservation of this component, suggesting its essential role in T-cell function. This molecule is believed to be essential for alloactivation when MHC class II antigen is presented to CD4-bearing T cells. It is an accessory cell adhesion molecule that stabilizes the interaction of the TCR–CD3 complex with the antigen–MHC class II complex. Monoclonal antibodies directed against CD4 block MHC class II–dependent cell proliferation in vitro and block production of IL-2 by T cells in the presence of antigen and thus have been extensively evaluated for clinical use (see below).

CD5, an adhesion molecule found on all T cells and some B cells, apparently plays a role in costimulatory signal transduction. Its importance, however, remains unclear. Xomazyme-65, a ricin-conjugated MAb, is the only preparation directed against CD5 that has been evaluated clinically. Its immunosuppressive efficacy has been difficult to establish (94), and this agent has not been approved for human use.

CD6, an integrin found on all T lymphocytes and some B cells, is apparently involved in costimulatory signal transduction modulating TCR-mediated T-cell activation (99). Monoclonal antibodies directed against CD6 inhibit its interaction with a recently identified ligand, activated leukocyte cell adhesion molecule (ALCAM). Anti-T12, the only anti-CD6 MAb to be evaluated clinically, has not demonstrated consistent efficacy (100).

CD7 is a T-cell surface antigen present on most mature and immature T cells, whose expression is quantitatively increased on T-cell blasts such as those generated by alloactivation. This molecule is an attractive target for selective immunosuppression because of the possibility of removing donor-reactive T-cell blasts without removing resting cells from the circulation (see below).

CD8 is a glycoprotein expressed on the approximately 20% to 40% of peripheral T cells that bind MHC class I antigens. These cells have also been termed *cytotoxic/suppressor T lymphocytes*. CD8 is an important accessory molecule for antigen-dependent T-cell activation and direct adhesion with MHC class I proteins. Leu-2a, an MAb reactive with CD8, has been shown to deplete T cells from the circulation in humans; however, it had limited efficacy as an immunosuppressive agent (101).

CD25, previously known as the IL-2 receptor or Tac, is found on virtually all activated T cells, B cells, and macrophages, plus approximately 15% of resting cells. There are now known to be three IL-2R subunits, α (55 kd), β (75 kd), γ (64 kd). Although the β and γ subunits have been given separate CD designations (CD122 and CD132, respectively), MAbs targeting IL-2R are generally referred to as anti-CD25 reagents. They prevent expansion of CD4 and CD8 cells in mixed lymphocyte reactions (MLRs) and block the generation of cytotoxic T cells in vitro and are thus attractive candidates for selective modulation of immune responses. A number of these MAbs have been evaluated and several have now become available for clinical protocols (see below).

CD40L (CD154), is the T-cell ligand for the CD40 complex on antigen-presenting cells. The CD40/CD40L pathway appears to have a central role in the T-cell helper effector functions governing acute rejection (102). Interaction of CD40 with its ligand leads to APC maturation, increased secretion of the inflammatory cytokine IL-12, and upregulation of other costimulatory pathways including **CD28/B7**. Blocking this pathway with anti-CD40L MAbs results in dramatic prolongation of heart and kidney allograft survival in nonhuman primates (103). No clinical trials have been reported to date. (See further discussion in accompanying Commentary to this chapter.)

CD54, also known as intercellular adhesion molecule (ICAM), is a member of the immunoglobulin supergene family. CD54 is found on endothelial cells, fibroblasts, epithelial cells, and activated lymphocytes. Lymphocyte function associated antigen-1 (LFA-1 or CD11a/CD18), a member of the integrin family, is a ligand for CD54. The interaction of these molecules is involved in the adhesion of leukocytes to blood vessel walls and in their transendothelial migration. The ICAM–LFA-1 interaction is also believed to provide costimulatory signals during antigen presentation and to mediate adhesion between cytotoxic T lymphocytes and target cells (105). Monoclonal antibodies targeting this interaction may be efficacious in limiting reperfusion injury as well as in the prophylaxis and treatment of allograft rejection (see below).

T-cell receptor (TCR) is a heterodimeric polypeptide of the immunoglobulin supergene family closely associated with CD3. The majority (95%) of T cells express the TCR composed of an α and β chain that appear to be responsible for determining the antigen specificity of all cytotoxic and helper T cells. The remaining 5% of T cells express a γ/δ dimer whose function is unknown. The dramatic immunosuppressive efficacy of the anti-CD3 MAb, OKT-3, suggests anti-TCR MAbs could also be useful clinically (see below).

Tumor necrosis factor (TNF) is a cytokine produced by macrophages and activated T lymphocytes. TNF is believed to play a role in the immune response to allografts by stimulating IL-1 production, MHC class I expression on endothelial cells, T-cell proliferation, and initiation of procoagulant activity. TNF is also believed to be one of the primary cytokines responsible for the "first-dose syndrome" observed in recipients of antilymphocyte antibodies. Monoclonal antibodies to TNF and TNF-soluble receptors may be beneficial in limiting the immune response to allografts as well as the cytokine release syndrome (69).

CLINICAL APPLICATIONS OF MONOCLONAL ANTIBODIES

The MAbs that currently have defined clinical efficacy or seem likely to be useful are listed in Table 13.6.

Anti-CD3 Monoclonal Antibodies

OKT-3 is the prototype MAb with demonstrated efficacy particularly for reversal of steroid-resistant rejection in every field of organ transplantation (106). It has been in clinical use for over 15 years and remains the "gold standard" to which newer MAbs are compared for both efficacy and toxicity. While the efficacy of OKT-3 is without question, there are several limitations to its use. Among its limitations are the adverse effects related to the massive cytokine release associated with initial infusions, its immunogenicity, and the not infrequent occurrence of subsequent rejection episodes after discontinuation of OKT-3. Another drawback to OKT-3 is its pan-T-cell suppression that increases the risk of infectious complications and PTLD.

Mechanism of Action

OKT-3, a murine IgG2a MAb, binds the epsilon portion of the human CD3 molecular complex on mature T lymphocytes. Cross-reactivity with other species is limited to the chimpanzee. Consequently, the in vivo evaluation of this MAb has been primarily in humans, where dramatic immunosuppressive effects have been observed (7,107). The CD3 complex is closely associated with the TCR and plays a vital role in T-cell activation and proliferation following presentation of antigen. OKT-3 exerts its effects through opsonization with subsequent complement-mediated cytolysis or reticuloendothelial uptake and destruction of T cells. This initially results in profound T-cell depletion as evidenced by a fall in the total peripheral lymphocyte count, absence of cells expressing other T-cell markers, and a lack of detectable cells coated with mouse immunoglobulin. With continued therapy, antigenic modulation demonstrated by the reappearance of T cells expressing other surface markers (CD4, CD8), but not CD3, occurs. This process involves redistribution of the OKT-3–CD3 complex on the T-cell surface and removal of the complex by internalization or shedding. Since the CD3 antigen is critical for MHC antigen recognition and T-cell–mediated cytotoxicity, the absence of CD3 on the cell surface renders the lymphocytes immunoincompetent (see

Table 13.6. Clinically Useful or [Promising] Monoclonal Antibodies

		Therapeutic Indication		
Specificity	MAb	Induction	Rejection	Other
CD2	[BTI-322]	X	X	GVHD
CD3	OKT-3	X	X	
	[CD3-Immunotoxin]	Preclinical		
CD4	[cMT-412]	X		
CD7	[SDZCHH380]	X		
CD11a/CD18	[Odulimomab]	X		
CD25	BT563	X		
	Zenapax (HAT or daclizumab)	X		
	[33B3.1]	X		
	Simulect (basiliximab)	X		
CD40L	[5C8]	Preclinical		
CD54	[BIRR1]			Autoimmune ?Reperfusion injury
TCR	[T10B9.1A-31]		X	

also Chapter 2). In addition to depletion and antigenic modulation, OKT-3 also causes activation or mitogenesis. While this may seem paradoxical to its immunosuppressive effect, the activated cells are receptorless, as a result of modulation, and do not respond to antigen. It has been suggested that this mechanism of activation may contribute to the induction of suppressor cells (108).

Immunopathologic examination of allograft biopsies following OKT-3 treatment for rejection reveals variable degrees of CD3+ T-cell depletion. A persistent infiltrate, however, has not been reliably correlated with recurrent rejection. Modulation of the CD3 complex, which is observed in circulating lymphocytes, is less pronounced on cells within the allograft. In fact, intragraft T cells appear to be activated as indicated by the expression of IL-2 receptors. The exact mechanism by which OKT-3 reverses rejection at the tissue level therefore remains unclear.

OKT-3 Rejection Prophylaxis (Induction Therapy)

Because OKT-3 inhibits the ability of T cells to recognize antigen, it became a logical choice for prophylaxis in clinical trials. When used as the sole immunosuppressive agent in renal allograft recipients, a vigorous HAMA response was found to rapidly neutralize the effect of OKT-3 (109). Acute rejection occurred in most of these recipients within two weeks of transplantation. A subsequent randomized clinical trial comparing azathioprine and steroids with or without OKT-3 in renal allograft recipients demonstrated a delay in the HAMA response for approximately three weeks (110). Allograft survival of 89% at two years with fewer rejection episodes was observed in the OKT-3 group compared to a 70% graft survival in the control arm. More recently, multicenter trials of renal transplant recipients, comparing induction triple drug therapy including CsA, azathioprine, and steroids with or without OKT-3, demonstrated a significant delay to first rejection, a decreased incidence of rejection, and fewer patients with multiple rejection episodes in the OKT-3–treated group (111,112). As in the previous polyclonal trials, a significant improvement in patient or allograft survival has been difficult to demonstrate in these relatively small studies. Large databases, such as those provided by the Collaborative Transplant Study, however, have demonstrated a survival advantage following OKT-3 induction in conjunction with delayed CsA therapy (113). This approach, in addition to avoiding CsA nephrotoxicity, essentially eliminates the development of early rejection episodes. A disadvantage to the use of OKT-3 as an induction agent is the development of HAMA in some recipients that might preclude later treatment with OKT-3, which could be indicated if severe rejection is encountered. Another concern has been related to the agent's procoagulant activity which has been implicated in cases of graft thrombosis (114).

OKT-3 induction therapy has been evaluated in liver, cardiac, lung, and pancreatic transplant recipients as well. In liver transplantation, the primary rationale for OKT-3 induction is to avoid renal dysfunction associated with CsA or tacrolimus in the immediate post-transplant period, especially since other perioperative factors such as prolonged vena cava clamping, preexisting hepatorenal syndrome, and hemodynamic instability could also enhance the nephrotoxicity of these drugs (see Chapter 19). As in renal transplantation, liver recipients treated prophylactically with OKT-3 have had a lower incidence of rejection, a delay in onset of first rejection, and a decreased incidence of steroid-resistant rejection (115,116).

Attempts to limit the severity of early postoperative renal dysfunction have also been the impetus for OKT-3 induction in cardiac transplantation. Delay in onset of rejection along with fewer rejection episodes have been observed. In addition, some have reported a reduction in late deaths resulting from graft atherosclerosis in patients who had received OKT-3 induction (117). Recent evidence also suggests that these patients may be more easily weaned off of steroids without adverse consequences (see Chapter 23). Some groups, however, have warned of an increased incidence of clinically significant hemodynamic instability associated with early post-heart transplant administration of OKT-3 (118).

OKT-3 has also been used effectively for induction therapy in lung and heart–lung transplant recipients. A recent survey revealed that 52.4% of heart–lung transplant programs favored the use of OKT-3 or other MAb preparations for the prevention of rejection (29). Induction therapy is especially attractive in these patients as an approach that minimizes steroid requirements during the early postoperative period, thereby promoting healing of the bronchial anastomosis (see Chapter 25). The intensity of the suppression provided by OKT-3 must be recognized, and it is clear that concomitant application of carefully designed infection control measures are required in these MAb-treated patients (119).

In the same survey noted earlier (see Table 13.3), 72% of transplant directors suggested that OKT-3 plays an important role in induction therapy for pancreas allograft recipients. A retrospective review of United Network for Organ Sharing (UNOS) data, however, suggested that OKT-3 induction may be associated with a lower graft survival rate than that achieved with ALS induction in pancreas alone and pancreas-after-kidney transplants (120) (see also Chapter 21).

OKT-3 Rejection Therapy

OKT-3 was first evaluated as treatment for established rejection at a time when azathioprine and steroids still constituted the foundation of immunosuppressive induction protocols (7). The initial pilot trial demonstrated that renal allograft rejection could be reversed with as little as 1–2 mg of OKT-3 administered daily. This led to the design of a multi-institutional randomized study in which OKT-3 was compared to conventional therapy for reversal of rejection. In that study, OKT-3 reversed 94% of initial rejection episodes, in contrast to a reversal rate of approximately 70% in conventionally treated patients (121). A number of reports later confirmed the efficacy of OKT-3 in reversing renal allograft rejection that developed in patients on azathioprine and steroids.

A significant limitation in these early trials was the occurrence of subsequent rejection episodes in over 50% of patients, usually within the first eight weeks after OKT-3 had been discontinued. The introduction of CsA partially addressed this limitation. In CsA-based immunosuppressive protocols, about 20% of renal allograft recipients have been found to require OKT-3 therapy if its use is reserved for treatment of acute rejection episodes initially unresponsive to high-dosage steroids (122,123). In 80% to 85% of these patients, a 10- to 14-day course of OKT-3 reverses the steroid-resistant rejection episode, and recurrent rejection has been observed in only 20% of patients receiving maintenance CsA (107,124).

The rather dramatic success of OKT-3 as "rescue" therapy that has been reported even in patients with severe "vascular" rejection (125) has been confirmed in many centers. In a group of nearly 300 patients treated by a number of different investigators, rejection that had failed to respond to CsA, high-dosage steroids, and in many instances ALS, was reversed in 65% of patients. Fifty-six percent of these allografts that were at the point of abandonment under conventional therapy remained functional with a minimum of six months follow-up (122,123).

A meta-analysis of the overall clinical experience published in the English and French literature indicates that OKT-3–treated patients have a threefold higher rate of resolution of the acute episode than do control patients (126). These observations suggest that excessive delay of OKT-3 therapy is probably ill advised. The hazards of prolonged steroid treatment, followed by a course of antilymphocyte antibody therapy, have been well documented. Thus, many clinicians currently recommend limiting the administration of high-dosage methylprednisolone to two or three doses. In those patients with persisting rejection, OKT-3 treatment is then added in preference to more prolonged courses of steroid administration. In fact, some centers advise even earlier institution of OKT-3 as a primary treatment approach for rejection (127), especially in patients with evidence of more severe immunologic injury on histopathologic examination (128).

OKT-3 has also been widely used for steroid-resistant rejection in liver transplantation. Successful allograft rescue can be expected in 75% to 85% of patients treated with OKT-3, with rapid improvement in liver function and resolution of the histologic findings of rejection (129). Failure of OKT-3 treatment in these patients may result from humorally mediated rejection similar to that encountered in ABO-incompatible grafts, which appears to be more resistant to OKT-3 suppression. In a prospective randomized trial, hepatic allograft recipients with first rejection episodes that had failed to respond to one or two boluses of steroids were randomized to receive 10 days of OKT-3 therapy or continued high-dose steroids. This study demonstrated that the results with OKT-3 are significantly better than can be achieved with steroids alone (130). OKT-3 has also been evaluated as first-line therapy for hepatic allograft rejection, where it again proved to be more effective than steroids. However, the incidence of infectious complications was noted to be higher in the patients receiving OKT-3. For this reason, OKT-3 is probably best reserved for patients with steroid-resistant rejection (131).

OKT-3 is typically used to treat steroid-resistant rejection in pancreas transplant recipients as well. In patients who have received simultaneous pancreas and kidney transplants, rejection therapy is usually instituted based on renal dysfunction or biopsy (see Chapter 21). In pancreas alone or pancreas-after-kidney transplantation, pancreatic biopsy may be necessary to differentiate suspected rejection from other causes of pancreatic dysfunction. OKT-3 has been demonstrated to be efficacious even in cases of pancreatic rejection with histopathologic features of chronic rejection (132).

OKT-3 has also proved effective in the treatment of rejection in cardiac and lung transplant recipients. As with other allografts, severe cases of rejection that do not respond to therapy with high-dose steroids or ATG have been effectively reversed with OKT-3 (133,134). The steroid-sparing effect of OKT-3 is of particular benefit in treating rejection in lung transplantation because of concerns of bronchial integrity.

Immunogenicity and Monitoring of OKT-3 Therapy

Because OKT-3 is of murine origin, use of this agent is associated with xenosensitization. The HAMA response occurs in approximately 25% to 30% of patients following initial treatment (135) and in a further similar proportion of patients who were HAMA-negative after initial treatment but then required retreatment (136). The probability of a HAMA response, therefore, appears to be relatively constant per exposure and not strongly influenced by intrinsic differences in the patient's immune responsiveness. However, as suggested above, concomitant immunosuppression does influence the likelihood of HAMA formation that decreased from 36% in patients receiving double drug immunosuppression to 21% in those receiving triple drug suppression (137).

Two classes of anti-OKT-3 antibodies have been identified (138). Anti-isotypic antibodies cross-react with all murine IgG2a immunoglobulins (Fig. 13.6). These HAMA therefore could interfere with subsequent therapy using either OKT-3 or any other IgG2a murine MAb. In contrast, anti-idiotypic antibodies react specifically with the antigen-binding region of OKT-3 and, therefore, may preclude the subsequent administration of OKT-3 but not of other murine MAbs (139). As described above, administration of humanized MAbs has been found to greatly reduce the magnitude of the HAMA response. Clinical trials using a humanized OKT-3 preparation are just being initiated.

In most patients, anti-OKT-3 antibodies first become detectable 7 to 10 days after discontinuing therapy, and

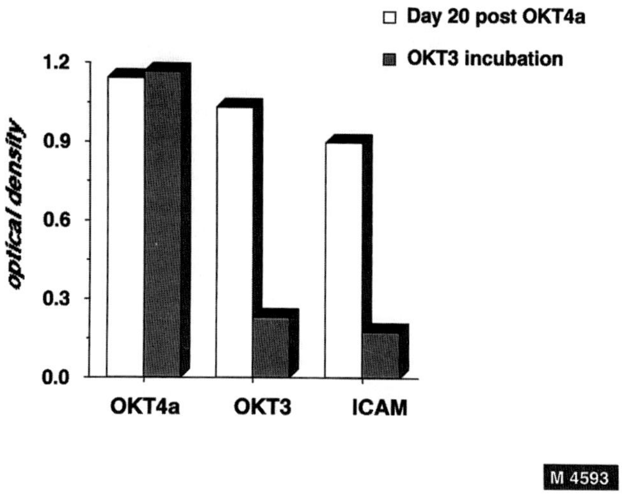

FIGURE 13.6. *Human antibody response to murine monoclonal antibodies. Anti-OKT-4a reactivity [increased optical density in ELISA assay (139)] was detectable in the patient's serum 20 days following initial treatment with this IgG2a MAb. Incubation of the serum sample with OKT-3 resulted in removal of reactivity (anti-isotypic) to OKT-3 and anti-ICAM (both IgG2a), but retention of anti-OKT-4A reactivity (anti-idiotypic).*

therefore do not interfere with the initial therapeutic effect. Occasionally, the antibody response becomes detectable during the course of OKT-3 therapy, resulting in neutralization of the immunosuppressive effect and in resurgence of rejection. Since the development of HAMA is heralded by the reappearance of CD3+ T cells in peripheral blood, flow cytometric monitoring has been recommended every two to three days during OKT-3 administration (136,140). A rise in detectable CD3+ T cells may be overcome by increasing the OKT-3 dose, thereby re-establishing CD3 clearance or modulation and continued control of the rejection episode. It has been suggested that T-cell monitoring may also be useful in predicting the likelihood of rejection after discontinuing OKT-3, since a correlation between early rejection and the rapidity of recovery of CD3+ T-cell counts has been observed (141,142). On the other hand, because of the costs associated with sequential T-cell monitoring, some centers have adopted an escalating dose regimen to ensure adequate OKT-3 serum levels without the need for frequent in vitro monitoring (143).

Retreatment with OKT-3

Since approximately 20% of CsA-treated patients in whom rejection is successfully reversed with OKT-3 subsequently develop further rejection episodes, multiple courses of high-dosage suppression are sometimes required. As with the initial episode, recurrent rejection may be treated with steroids, another antilymphocyte preparation such as ALS, or a second course of OKT-3. Unfortunately, the risks of opportunistic infections or PTLD are greatly increased by sequential courses of antilymphocyte antibody therapy (see Chapter 37). This approach should therefore be used sparingly.

Before re-treating with OKT-3, the patient's HAMA level should be assayed to rule out the presence of high titers of anti-OKT-3 antibody (139). Interestingly, low levels of reactive endogenous antibodies to murine MAbs can be detected in a small proportion of individuals even before initial therapy. However, clinically evident reactions suggesting anaphylaxis have been distinctly unusual in these OKT-3–treated allograft recipients, and the presence of these preexisting antibodies does not seem to alter the efficacy of therapy or predict the likelihood of subsequent rejection episodes (144).

Side Effects of OKT-3

The side effects of OKT-3 therapy can be categorized into direct toxic effects and the consequences of overimmunosuppression. The common side effects of OKT-3 therapy are summarized in Table 13.7. The "cytokine-release syndrome," manifested by fever and chills typically beginning within one to two hours after the initial injection, may also include nausea, vomiting, diarrhea, dyspnea, headaches, arthralgias, and myalgias. Aseptic meningitis and pulmonary edema may occur infrequently. Seizures have been reported, but these are rare. As noted earlier, TNF appears to be the primary cytokine responsible for these adverse events (145), although complement activation has also been implicated recently (146,147). High-dosage corticosteroid administration prior to initiation of OKT-3 therapy has been shown to inhibit the release of the cytokines responsible for this syndrome and decrease the severity of the reactions (67,84). Anti-TNF therapy with MAb or TNF-soluble receptors has also been shown to decrease the severity of this syndrome (68,69). TNF-soluble receptors may also inhibit the frequently observed temporary rise in serum creatinine that presumably results from cytokine-induced nephrotoxicity (148,149). Since respiratory symptoms may be more severe in patients with significant fluid retention, the patient's volume status should be assessed carefully and treated with diuretics or ultrafiltration if volume overload is present prior to initiation of OKT-3 therapy. The use of OKT-3 has also been reported to be associated with arterial thrombosis in renal allografts (114). It has been suggested that this complication could result from the procoagulant (endothelial activation) consequences of increased cytokine levels (see also Chapter 30).

As with any agent, overimmunosuppression can result in opportunistic infections (particularly viral). An increased incidence of Herpes group virus infections including CMV and the EBV-associated PTLD has been reported in recipients of every type of organ allograft following treatment with OKT-3 (150,151). Clinical presentation may range from annoying, but easily controllable, herpes simplex stomatitis to life-threatening lymphoproliferative disease. CMV infections were frequent complications of the early ALS trials, until the need for reducing concomitant immunosup-

Table 13.7. Clinical Toxicity of OKT-3 Administration

Cytokine Release Syndrome		Overimmunosuppression		Immunogenicity	
Reaction	Incidence	Reaction	Incidence	Reaction	Incidence
Chills, fever		CMV infection	20–60%	Rash/Pruritus	0–5%
d1	70–90%	Fungal infection	15–35%	Anaphylaxis	<1%
d2	10–20%	Herpes simplex	5–25%		
Nephrotoxicity	30–40%	PTLD	0–8%		
Vomiting, diarrhea	15–30%				
Dyspnea	10–20%				
Pulmonary edema	0–4%				
Aseptic meningitis	0–3%				
Arterial thrombosis	<1%				

pression and the importance of the serologic status of donor and recipient were recognized (151). The risk for CMV infection has proved to be highest (58%) in seronegative recipients of allografts from a seropositive donor, intermediate in seropositive recipients (36%), and negligible when both donor and recipient are seronegative (3%). Preemptive therapy with ganciclovir, particularly for seronegative recipients (72), has greatly reduced these risks (see Chapter 36).

Latent EBV is reactivated by OKT-3, leading to the outgrowth of virally transformed B cells. These proliferating cells may then evolve from benign EBV-dependent polyclonal B-cell lines to a malignant EBV-independent monoclonal B-cell lymphoma (73), particularly in children previously unexposed to EBV (152). The progression to lymphoma is related to the intensity of the immunosuppression rather than specifically to any particular agent (see Chapter 37). For example, an increased PTLD incidence was noted retrospectively among 154 heart transplant patients after two weeks of OKT-3 prophylaxis was introduced without reduction of the concomitantly administered triple drug therapy (150). In contrast, one month of OKT-3 prophylaxis, in combination with azathioprine and steroids but without CsA, resulted in no lymphomas in 150 renal transplant patients (110). These observations emphasize the importance of decreasing the dosages of concomitant immunosuppressive therapy during the period that any antilymphocyte antibody is being administered. We recommend at least a 50% reduction in the daily CsA and azathioprine dosages during the period of OKT-3 or ALS administration. A further drastic reduction in immunosuppression or even complete elimination, if possible, should be instituted if the diagnosis of PTLD is made (153).

Choice of Polyclonal ALS versus OKT-3 MAb

Both ALS and OKT-3 are directed against T cells, admittedly with a differing degree of selectivity. Nevertheless, the indications for their uses overlap, and the preferred clinical circumstances for one versus the other preparation remain controversial (154–158). A comparison of some of the important features that distinguish these two generations of antilymphocyte preparations is summarized in Table 13.8. OKT-3 administration is simpler but with more pronounced side effects following the initial infusions. This drawback is countered by the general impression that OKT-3 is somewhat more reliable for treatment of severe acute rejection, since it has been successfully used to rescue allografts in recipients who failed to respond to ALS.

Table 13.8. Comparison of Monoclonal Versus Polyclonal Antilymphocyte Antibodies

Characteristic	Monoclonal vs. Polyclonal (Superiority)
Ease of production	Monoclonal
Cost	Monoclonal
Antibody variability	Monoclonal
Specificity	Monoclonal
Ease of administration	Monoclonal
Rejection reversal (early)	Monoclonal
Rejection reversal (overall)	Equal
Viral infection	Equal
PTLD	Equal
Recipient survival	Equal
Side effects	Polyclonal
Immunogenicity	Polyclonal
Retreatment possibility	Polyclonal

When used as induction agents, ALS and OKT-3 have virtually indistinguishable low rates of rejection and delayed graft function. Conflicting observations regarding the incidence of infection have been reported with some studies indicating that ALS is associated with a significantly increased incidence of CMV infections (157) while others found OKT-3 resulted in symptomatic side effects and more infections (158).

How then does a clinician choose between ALS and OKT-3? One approach is to use pharmacologic therapy

(CsA or tacrolimus plus MMF and/or steroids) for initial baseline induction immunosuppression. In kidney recipients with delayed graft function or extrarenal allograft recipients with renal dysfunction, the introduction of CsA or tacrolimus is delayed in favor of ALS prophylaxis. This allows for subsequent rejection treatment with OKT-3 if it is required. For initial acute rejection episodes, two high-dosage steroid boluses are administered. If rejection is not reversed, OKT-3 therapy is usually begun. This approach attempts to take advantage of the relatively equivalent efficacy of either pharmacologic or antilymphocyte antibody induction therapy in patients with adequate renal function, the apparent heightened susceptibility to CsA or tacrolimus nephrotoxicity during periods of ATN, and the greater reliability of OKT-3 for treatment of acute rejection.

Anti-CD4 Monoclonal Antibodies

While OKT-3 has proven to be effective for both induction therapy and treatment of rejection, its nonselective suppression of all T lymphocytes can result in increased risks of infection and malignancy. This has naturally stimulated evaluation of MAbs more specifically targeted to T-cell subsets or other molecules crucial for rejection. One such molecule is the CD4 antigen, which is important during the initial stages of alloactivation, when presentation of MHC class II alloantigen to CD4 results in increased avidity with the TCR and releases cytokines that amplify the rejection process (159). Because CD4+ T cells play an important role in this initial activation and amplification of the alloresponse, anti-CD4 MAbs were predicted to be most effective before effector mechanisms become self-sustaining (160). Multiple studies have confirmed this supposition. For example, rats treated with an anti-CD4 MAb for seven days prior to transplantation have been observed to have marked prolongation of allograft survival in contrast to animals treated with the same protocol beginning on the day of transplantation (161). With this type of early treatment, donor-specific unresponsiveness has been achieved in many experimental models using anti-CD4 MAbs, again suggesting that these MAbs may be more effective when used in induction immunosuppressive regimens than for rejection reversal (159).

Mechanism of Action

Anti-CD4 MAbs may be classified as depleting or nondepleting based on their effect on peripheral blood CD4+ cells. Monoclonal antibodies that are depleting in nature trigger complement activation through the Fc portion of the molecule with resultant target cell lysis (159,162). The depletion of CD4+ cells in peripheral blood and graft infiltrates has correlated in most experimental models with the immunosuppressive activity of these antibodies. Rejection has been observed to occur promptly upon the return of CD4+ cells to the circulation. One disadvantage of depleting antibodies can be the longevity of their effects. CD4+ cells may remain depressed to levels as low as 60% of baseline for up to six months after treatment is discontinued in nonhuman primates (163). Similar results have been reported in patients with depletion persisting for up to two years in one case (164). Precursor lymphocyte depletion could theoretically explain this phenomenon, since immature T cells co-express CD4 and CD8 (165). The clinical consequences of this persistent depletion are unclear.

Nondepleting anti-CD4 MAbs may exert their effect through CD4 modulation or blockade. Modulation presumably removes any contribution of the CD4 molecule to T-cell activation, either as an adhesion molecule or as a signal-transducing molecule. This can lead to significant delay of rejection in rats (166). Similarly, modulation of the CD4 molecule in monkeys was associated with prolonged renal allograft survival. In these animals, intragraft cells were found to be unresponsive to IL-2, suggesting that CD4 modulation prevents T-cell sensitization even in the absence of depletion (167).

CD4 blockade may result from interference with interactions between CD4 and MHC, or between CD4 and the TCR–CD3 complex. Like modulation, this interference might prevent the CD4 molecule from contributing to T-cell activation. Interestingly, CD4 blockade appears even more immunosuppressive than modulation in some models (168). It is possible that CD4 bound by MAb, in contrast to modulation of the CD4 molecule, actually transduces a negative signal to the T cell, thereby suppressing its activation (169).

Since CD4+ T cells are pivotal in the initial activation of the alloresponse, anti-CD4 MAbs have been particularly targeted for their potential to direct the alloresponse toward donor-specific tolerance rather than sensitization. As noted above, striking results have been obtained in rodent models (170–172). Most of these tolerance models have relied on depleting MAbs. Although nondepleting anti-CD4 MAbs may also induce specific tolerance (168), the hyporesponsive state achieved with these agents has usually been to relatively weak antigens or has been confined to limited strain combinations (171). In these models, the CD4+ T cells are presumably rendered anergic when they bind donor antigen without a complete activation signal (173). Interestingly, thymectomy prevents tolerance induction in some anti-CD4 MAb models. It is possible that an intact thymus is necessary for the development of suppressor T cells or that CD4-depleted cells must migrate through the thymus in order to then be rendered anergic when engaging antigen in the periphery (174).

Preclinical Studies

The first anti-CD4 MAb to be evaluated in a nonhuman primate model was OKT-4 in 1980. OKT-4, as the sole immunosuppressive agent, prolonged allograft survival for as long as 42 days, while control animals developed terminal rejection between 8 and 11 days. Multiple epitopes of the CD4 molecule were identified during these initial studies, and population surveys revealed the absence of the OKT-4 reactive site in some human subjects. Subsequently, OKT-4A, a murine IgG2a immunoglobulin, was produced. OKT-4A binds to a universally expressed epitope of the human CD4 antigen that is separate and noncompeting from the epitope recognized by OKT-4. Prolonged renal allograft survival was observed in nonhuman primate preclinical studies of OKT-4A as well (175). Since there was minimal CD4+ T-cell depletion, the mechanism involved appeared to be through antigenic modulation with interference of signal transduction, blocking of the MHC class II–CD4 interaction, or suppressor cell induction.

Despite the efficacy of these murine anti-CD4 MAbs in monkeys, two significant differences from the earlier rodent observations were apparent. First, allograft rejection, though delayed, eventually occurred in all anti-CD4 MAb treated nonhuman primates; and, second, all monkey recipients developed antimouse antibodies. To address these problems, humanized versions of OKT-4A and other murine MAbs were developed. In the modified OKT-4A, only the original murine CDRs were preserved (see Chapter 12). Since these regions bind the target antigen on CD4, the original specificity of OKT-4A was preserved while the remainder of the molecule was completely humanized. To accomplish this, the murine CDRs were grafted onto a human variable region framework, and the resultant structure was then combined with either a human IgG1 or IgG4 constant region (176). These isotypes were selected because of documented differences in their effector functions: human IgG1 antibodies activate complement, with resultant target cell lysis, whereas IgG4 antibodies do not (177). The CDR-grafted OKT-4A preparations retained only 8% of the murine sequence but had comparable binding affinity for the CD4 molecule.

As anticipated, in vivo monkey studies revealed only MAb coating of CD4+ T cells with the IgG4 preparation but consistent and prolonged CD4+ T-cell depletion following IgG1 administration (178). Both MAbs retained the immunosuppressive potency of the parent murine preparation; however, their immunogenicity was reduced and recipient serum levels were maintained for a longer period than following treatment with the murine preparation (179). Moreover, the antibody response was only anti-idiotypic, presumably restricted to the original CDR, and thus would not preclude sequential therapy with MAbs targeting another epitope, such as OKT-3.

Anti-CD4 Rejection Prophylaxis (Induction Therapy)

Based on the encouraging preclinical results, a number of clinical trials have been undertaken mostly in cadaveric renal allograft recipients (159) (Table 13.9). The murine preparation OKT-4A has been well tolerated without first-dose side effects, but the immunosuppressive efficacy has proved inconclusive. A HAMA response occurred in 82% of recipients of this MAb. A subsequent trial evaluating the CDR-grafted OKT-4A was encouraging, with no graft failures; however, the dose used was insufficient to consistently prevent rejection. Two other murine anti-CD4 MAb preparations of the IgG2a isotype, designated BL4 and MT151, have been evaluated in renal allograft recipients. These patients had a discouragingly high incidence of early rejection episodes (180). Recently, B-F5, a murine IgG1 anti-CD4 MAb, was reported to provide significant CD4+ cell depletion in renal allograft recipients and excellent transplant survival. However, one-half of the treated patients experienced an episode of acute rejection within the first three postoperative months (181). The chimeric anti-CD4 MAb, cMT-412, has been evaluated in conjunction with CsA-based triple drug induction therapy in heart and heart–lung recipients (182). This antibody is a combination of the CD4-reactive murine hypervariable regions with human IgG1 constant region. Comparable depletion of CD4+ cells in cMT-412–treated patients and ATG-treated controls was observed. All MAb-treated patients had a benign postoperative course with significantly fewer rejection episodes and fewer infectious complications despite long-lasting T-cell depletion. Despite the partial humanization of the MAb, however, a HAMA response was detected in 64% of patients treated with this agent. Nevertheless, the promising immunosuppressive observations have stimulated continued clinical investigation of this MAb.

Anti-CD4 Rejection Therapy

Since reversal of established rejection would not be predicted to be likely using anti-CD4 MAbs (see above), there have been limited clinical trials for this indication. The anti-CD4 MAb, Max.16H5, which was also initially studied in

Table 13.9. Clinical Trials Using Anti-CD4 Monoclonal Antibodies

Study	MAb	Report	Outcome	Isotype
Kidney Induction	OKT-4A	Delmonico (159)	Variable efficacy	Murine IgG2a
Kidney Induction	OKT-cdr4A	Delmonico (159)	Inconclusive	Humanized IgG4
Kidney Induction	BL4	Land (180)	Ineffective	Murine IgG2a
Kidney Induction	MT151	Land (180)	Ineffective	Murine IgG2a
Kidney Induction	BF5	Dantal (181)	Ineffective	Murine IgG1
Kidney Rejection	Max.16H5	Reinke (183)	Reversed rejection	Murine IgG1
Heart Induction	cMT-412	Meiser (182)	↓Rejection	Humanized IgG1

patients with rheumatoid arthritis, has been administered to renal allograft recipients suffering late-onset rejection (183). This MAb was shown to dramatically deplete CD4+ T cells, improve allograft function, and eliminate the histopathologic features of rejection in the majority of treated patients. In addition, neither anti-isotypic nor anti-idiotypic antibodies to Max.16H5 were detected in any of the recipients. Despite these compelling results, further trials with this MAb have not yet been reported.

Anti-CD7 Monoclonal Antibodies

The anti-CD7 MAb, SDZCHH380, which has been produced through recombinant DNA technology, is composed primarily of human IgG1 with murine hypervariable regions that determine its binding specificity (184). In vitro studies have revealed marked inhibition of T-cell proliferation by this agent. A prospective randomized trial comparing SDZCHH380 to OKT-3 induction in conjunction with CsA-based conventional therapy was performed in cadaveric renal allograft recipients. In this study, the time to first rejection was comparable in both groups of patients; the anti-CD7 MAb was well tolerated with induction of lower levels of TNF and IL-6 than detected in recipients of OKT-3; and no patients produced antibody to SDZCHH380 in contrast to the 70% of OKT-3 recipients with a HAMA response. The investigators concluded that SDZCHH380 could play an important role in induction protocols in renal transplantation. Further trials, however, have not been reported.

Anti-CD25 Monoclonal Antibodies

The interaction between IL-2 and its receptor is required for the proliferation of T cells and the generation of cytotoxic effector T cells. Since IL-2 receptor expression is upregulated on the T-cell surface during lymphocyte activation, the use of anti-CD25 MAbs to block the interaction between IL-2 and its receptor or to eliminate cells expressing CD25 could presumably limit clonal expansion at this critical stage of the immune response (185). The validity of this hypothesis has been established in some murine models where anti-CD25 MAb therapy provided indefinite survival of vascularized allografts (186).

Anti-CD25 Rejection Prophylaxis (Induction Therapy)

A number of randomized trials evaluating the efficacy of anti-CD25 MAb induction therapy have been reported (Table 13.10). Use of the murine anti-Tac MAb in human renal allograft recipients in combination with CsA, azathioprine, and prednisone provided a modest decrease in frequency of rejection episodes and delay in onset of rejection compared to controls, but no improvement in graft or patient survival was achieved (187). Two rat anti-CD25 MAbs have been similarly evaluated. One of these antibodies, 33B3.1, was compared in a randomized trial to ATG as an induction agent in cadaveric renal allograft recipients (188). This trial demonstrated that 33B3.1 was well tolerated but somewhat less effective than ATG in preventing acute rejection. Similar results were observed in renal–pancreas recipients (189). The second rat anti-CD25 MAb, Lo-Tact-1, was compared in liver allograft recipients to two other induction protocols: an OKT-3–treated group and a triple drug (CsA-steroid-azathioprine) control group (190). After two years, patient survival in the Lo-Tact-1 group was significantly higher than in the control group, but not higher than in the OKT-3–treated group. The overall rejection rates in the two MAb-treated groups were similar and both were significantly lower than that observed in the control group.

The most extensively studied anti-CD25 MAb has been the murine agent, BT563, which has been evaluated in randomized trials in kidney (191), liver (192,193), and heart (194) allograft recipients. The incidence of rejection was reduced in the kidney and liver trials, although no significant improvement in allograft or patient survival was achieved. In the heart recipient trial, the frequency of rejection was similar in patients

Table 13.10. Randomized Clinical Trials Evaluating Anti-CD25 Induction Therapy

Allograft	MAb	Control	Report	Efficacy vs. Control
Kidney	Tac	(1)	Kirkman (187)	Equivalent
	33B3.1	ATG + (1)	Soulillou (188)	Equivalent
	BT563	(2)	van Gelder (191)	↓Rejection
	Simulect (basiliximab)	(2)	Nashan (197)	↓Rejection
	Zenapax (HAT or daclizumab)	(1)	Vincenti (198)	↓Rejection, ↑Survival
Liver	Lo-Tact-1	OKT-3 + (1)	Reding (190)	Equivalent
	BT563	ATG + (2)	Nashan (192)	Equivalent
	BT563	ATG + (1)	Langrehr (193)	↓Rejection
Heart	BT563	OKT-3 + (3)	van Gelder (194)	Earlier rejection

(1) CsA-steroids-azathioprine.
(2) CsA-steroids.
(3) CsA (delayed)-steroids-azathioprine.

treated with either BT563 or OKT-3, but rejection occurred earlier in the BT563-treated recipients.

In all of these trials, two major problems were identified that appeared to contribute to the relatively limited effectiveness of the anti-CD25 MAbs in preventing allograft rejection. First, their immunogenicity and short circulating half-life may not have induced adequate periods of immunosuppression. Second, because of their murine or rat structure, the MAbs are less effective than human antibodies in recruiting immune effector functions. To circumvent these limitations, genetic engineering has been used to prepare humanized agents. Initial studies of this approach in nonhuman primates were more promising (195), as was a phase I clinical trial in renal allograft recipients (80). In these patients, the half-life of the humanized agent was extended to over 270 hours in contrast to the 40 hours observed with the parent murine MAb. Similar observations have been made using another humanized anti-CD25 MAb that had a mean half-life in renal allograft recipients of 13.1 days (196). Initial reports of the efficacy and safety of these anti-CD25 MAbs are quite encouraging (197–200). Administration of these agents has been greatly simplified since in vitro monitoring revealed effective depletion of the targeted cell population even with doses given at bi-weekly intervals (201). Both of these agents have recently received FDA approval for clinical use in renal transplant recipients.

Anti-CD25 Rejection Therapy

As with the anti-CD4 agents, there has been limited experience with the use of anti-CD25 MAbs for treatment of ongoing acute rejection. In a report of 33B3.1 MAb treatment for acute renal allograft rejection, only 2 of 10 patients responded immediately to the MAb and 4 others had a delayed response (202). Possible explanations for this limited efficacy might include insufficient MAb reaching the allograft to provide neutralization of the high levels of IL-2 that are undoubtedly present at the rejection site. It is also possible that the immune response that leads to graft destruction is no longer completely under IL-2 control by the time of MAb treatment and that alternative pathways produce continued cytotoxic effects despite IL-2R blockade. Interestingly, anti-CD25 therapy, using the MAbs BT563 or HAT, has been successful in the treatment of steroid-resistant GVHD (203,204).

Anti-CD54 and Other Adhesion Molecule Monoclonal Antibodies

The rapid infiltration by inflammatory cell populations that is characteristic of acute rejection is also the histologic hallmark of ischemic reperfusion injury (205). As a barrier between blood and parenchyma, the endothelium is well positioned to regulate cellular migration from the circulation into tissues (206). The endothelial cell apparently recruits infiltrating cells by expressing adhesion molecules on its surface. These adhesion molecules also play an essential role in providing the accessory signals required for optimal activation of antigen-stimulated cells. Accordingly, disabling these adhesion molecules should limit the inflammatory phenomena associated with cell infiltration, thereby possibly interrupting both the alloresponse and the effects of ischemic injury.

Cell surface adhesion molecules have been grouped into three classes: selectins, integrins, and immunoglobulins. Selectins are small glycoproteins with a lectin domain and an epidermal growth factor (EGF)-like motif. This structure is well adapted for binding surface carbohydrate ligands (207). These molecules are primarily expressed on activated endothelium, platelets, or leukocytes, where they are designated E-, P-, or L-selectin, respectively. In general, selectins mediate the initial weak binding between endothelial cells and leukocytes, setting the stage for stronger binding by other adhesion molecules (208). To date, there has been minimal large animal or clinical evaluation of antiselectin MAbs as immunosuppressive agents.

Integrins are much larger molecules, composed of two noncovalently linked polypeptide chains, each of which has a CD designation. Because they span the cellular membrane, integrins are well adapted to coordinate extracellular contacts with intracellular events (208). As a result, integrins play an important role in regulating the sequential adhesion and deadhesion required for cellular migration into tissues. The integrin LFA-1 (CD11a/CD18), expressed on lymphocytes, granulocytes, and monocytes, is the ligand for CD54. Both of these molecules have been of particular interest as possible targets for MAb therapy.

The immunoglobulin supergene family includes the TCR, MHC classes I and II, CD3, CD4, CD8, and the intercellular adhesion molecules (ICAM-1 or CD54, ICAM-2, and ICAM-3). Resting cells express only limited amounts of these ligands on their surface, but inflammation or early antigen recognition leads to a dramatic upregulation. In general, adhesion molecules in this family bind either integrins or other members of the immunoglobulin supergene family.

Preclinical Studies

Anti-adhesion molecule MAbs have been remarkably effective in some rodent models. For example, MAb combinations targeting T-cell and APC receptor–ligand pairs, such as LFA-1 (CD11a/CD18) and its ligand CD54 (209) or LFA2 (CD2) and its ligand CD48 (210), have induced permanent allograft survival. With such therapy, the TCR presumably interacts with processed antigen within the context of the MHC on the APC, but without concomitant adhesion molecule costimulation. This results in an incomplete activation signal and T-cell hyporesponsiveness rather than activation (211).

The immunosuppressive efficacy of anti-adhesion molecule immunotherapy in the rodent allograft models has prompted further preclinical evaluation of both anti-CD54 and anti-LFA-1 MAbs in monkey allograft recipients. Renal allograft survival in monkeys that were treated with the anti-CD54 MAb, BIRR1, as the sole immunosuppressive agent was prolonged from 9.2 ± 0.6 days in controls to 24 ± 2.4 days (105). Similar prolongation of skin allograft survival was observed in monkeys treated with anti-LFA-1 MAb (212). Recently, an alternative approach to the interruption of adhesion molecule interactions has been reported in which an entirely human fusion protein rather than the MAb was administered to monkey allograft recipients with encouraging prolongation of allograft survival (213). The mechanism of action involved in the anti-CD54–mediated immunosuppression appears to be through inhibition of ICAM-1–mediated functions, including antigen-independent interactions necessary for leukocyte adhesion and recruitment and antigen-dependent functions such as MHC peptide presentation and effector cytotoxicity (214). Of potential relevance for recipients, particularly of cadaver donor organs, has been the observation that reperfusion injury is also attenuated by the MAbs targeting these adhesion molecules (215–217). As noted above, ischemia activates the endothelium, resulting in adhesion molecule upregulation. This causes circulating neutrophils to adhere to vascular endothelium and infiltrate the reperfused ischemic tissues. There, they release toxic proteases and reactive oxygen metabolites resulting in damage to the ischemic organ. Apparently, this process can be inhibited by anti-adhesion molecule therapy.

Anti-CD54 Rejection Prophylaxis (Induction Therapy)

The encouraging observations in nonhuman primates led to a phase I clinical study to evaluate the toxicity, dosage requirements, and potential efficacy of BIRR1 in cadaver donor renal allograft recipients (87). Patients with a high risk of acute graft rejection (because of prolonged allograft preservation time or highly sensitized recipient) were included. At 36 months, 78% of the allografts were functional versus 56% of the contralateral kidneys transplanted in a noncontrolled group that received conventional immunosuppression. Subsequently, over 600 cadaver donor renal allograft recipients were enrolled into three randomized, double-blinded, multi-institution trials conducted in European and North American transplant centers. In one of the studies, there was significantly reduced ($P < 0.05$) severity of rejection and a trend ($P = 0.07$) toward decreased rejection in the MAb-treated group, but neither of the other trials confirmed these observations. As a result, further clinical evaluation of this MAb in renal allograft recipients has been discontinued. A similar protocol using BIRR1 has been conducted in a phase I study in liver transplant recipients (218). Patients who maintained therapeutic levels of BIRR1 had a 40% incidence of rejection compared to a 70% incidence of rejection in conventionally treated liver recipients. All of these trials indicated that relatively large doses of this MAb were necessary to achieve therapeutic levels.

Clinical trials of MAbs targeting LFA-1, the ligand for the CD54 molecule, have also been undertaken. Bone marrow transplant patients were the first recipients of MAb 25.3, which is directed against the CD11a epitope of LFA-1. This agent appeared to improve engraftment in a group of pediatric recipients that was compared to historical controls. However, the same MAb administered to adult leukemic bone marrow recipients was unable to prevent rejection of T-cell–depleted HLA-matched transplants (219). A MAb directed against the CD18 epitope on LFA-1 provided results comparable to those observed in a historical group of renal allograft recipients receiving ATG. A subsequent randomized trial has confirmed this observation (220).

A single report using anti-LFA-1 MAb to treat established rejection in renal allograft recipients noted unsatisfactory reversal of the rejection episode (221).

Anti-TCR Monoclonal Antibodies

The TCR is essential for antigen recognition that, in conjunction with costimulatory signals, leads to T-cell activation. T10B9.1A-31 (T10B9), an antihuman T-cell MAb of murine IgM isotype, is reactive with the α/β chain of the TCR and, thus, is a pan-T-cell antibody with the exception of γ/δ T-cell sparing. Approximately 99% of mature CD3+ cells are lysed by T10B9. This MAb is not mitogenic and therefore does not induce the first-dose reactions associated with cytokine release (222). T10B9 has been evaluated in a prospective randomized trial of renal allograft recipients comparing it to OKT-3 for treatment of acute rejection (148). The trial included 76 evaluable renal allograft recipients treated with conventional immunosuppression until rejection occurred. At this point, therapy with one of the MAbs was initiated. Graft survival was excellent in both groups with a trend toward improved survival at three and four years in the T10B9 group. Recurrent rejection and the requirement for crossover to the other agent were essentially the same in both groups. The incidence and severity of "first-dose" symptoms were decreased in the T10B9-treated patients. The explanation for this difference is the observation that plasma levels of TNF and IFN were much lower following treatment with T10B9 than with OKT-3. In addition, there was no cytokine-induced nephropathy in the T10B9 patients, who therefore had a more rapid reversal of renal dysfunction. There was no statistically significant difference in the incidence of infectious complications between the two groups. The development of a HAMA response was similar in the two groups, but most importantly, there was no cross-reactivity of the HAMA of one MAb with those produced in response to treatment by the other agent. Thus, an alternative therapy would be available should the first MAb fail or if re-rejection occurs.

CONCLUSIONS

Over the last two decades, new and more specific immunosuppressive agents have increased the one-year survival of transplanted organs to the 70% to 90% range. With the current availability of CsA, tacrolimus, mycophenolate mofetil, ALS, and OKT-3, clinicians can devise individualized, multifaceted strategies that provide effective induction therapy and treatment of acute rejection, while limiting the nephrotoxicity of CsA and tacrolimus. A newer pan-T-cell MAb, T10B9.1A-31, could provide even more flexible immunosuppressive strategies, because it could be used in patients who fail to respond to, or have been previously sensitized to, OKT-3. It has not yet been approved for clinical use, however.

Despite these many advances, it remains evident that none of these therapeutic combinations lead reliably to donor-specific tolerance. Thus, the longer-term surviving transplant recipient is continuously threatened by a relentless attrition in allograft survival and continuing morbidity from the chronically administered immunosuppressive agents. The successful clinical application of OKT-3 has emphasized that MAbs could be a potential solution to many of the limitations of conventional immunosuppression. It is now possible to reliably design MAbs to essentially any molecular component essential to the immune response, rather than relying on serendipity for the discovery of new immunosuppressive agents.

There is much current interest in immunotoxin conjugates of MAbs (81,223,224) and in MAbs targeting costimulatory molecules such as CD4, CD25, CD28, and CD40L, since the accessory signals provided by these molecules are essential for immune activation (225,226). Based on the encouraging observations of tolerance induction by such agents in preclinical models, it is hoped that these agents may play an important role in future clinical protocols.

One of the most promising additions to MAb technology is the recombinant DNA technology that is used to "humanize" murine or rat preparations. With these methods, novel antibody molecules that retain only short sequences from the rodent variable region can be consistently constructed. The initial clinical trials using these designer molecules are highly encouraging and have already provided sufficient evidence of immunosuppressive efficacy to justify regulatory approval for several of these agents (197–200). The development of these new molecular agents, more effectively directed to specific cellular targets, should play an increasingly important role in future clinical protocols and perhaps finally provide a means to achieve long-term tolerance in human transplant recipients.

COMMENTARY

Jean-Paul Soulillou

James D. Eason and A. Benedict Cosimi have thoroughly reviewed many of the bioreagents, defined as "biologic immunosuppressive agents," that have entered clinical trials or are expected to be soon available to patients. Although the gap between experiments in test tubes, first clinical trials, and the actual drug registration is extremely long (for instance, 10 years between the first clinical report on the effect of anti-IL-2 receptor in humans and the first double-blind phase II/III trial of modified MAb) (1,2), the high specificity of action and low level of side effects associated with biologic agents (with the exception of the commercial OKT-3) may open new avenues in the treatment of graft recipients and maybe of autoimmune diseases. Moreover, humanized/chimeric forms of these agents may make longer or repeated usage possible and suggest that they could be used for induction therapy during the first months after transplantation, instead of only the first weeks. These agents might thus become popular drugs and the repeated assessment that has restricted them to marginal usage might be a lack of vision for the future!

In this short commentary I would like to elaborate on several issues that could further increase the usefulness of these reagents. However, the number of potentially interesting molecules itself acts as a self limitation, owing to the cost of clinical studies and their rather restricted application as compared to conventional drugs, at least as used currently.

Early phases after grafting are crucial for long-term graft function, principally because of the occurrence of two major events: delayed graft function and acute rejection, both of which are associated with inferior long-term graft function. Therefore, owing to the usual restricted period of time of administration, antilymphocyte antibodies have been mostly devoted to overcoming ongoing rejection and preventing very early rejection and, more recently, reperfusion injuries. The strategy of restricting powerful immunosuppressive treatments to short intervals of time after grafting has recently received some support by the demonstration that—at least for kidney recipients—even "normal" long-term immunosuppression might have overall detrimental effects and, that the current paradigm attributing most overimmunosuppression hazards to induction treatment may be wrong (3). Instead, the intensity of early treatment might be crucial, after which long-term treatment might be reduced. Therefore, the use of bioreagents at the time of transplantation could be the method of choice for treating graft recipients.

TARGETING SECOND SIGNAL MOLECULES

Experimental data, including preliminary results in monkeys (4,5), suggest that inhibiting second signal molecules could be extremely effective. So far, besides recently recognized new targets (CD40L, CD28/B7 interaction, see below), several encouraging reports are already available on the effect of anti-CD2 or anti-LFA-1 (6,7). Interestingly, anti-LFA-1, which is considered to primarily inhibit the interaction between recipient immunocompetent cells and donor endothelial cells, could also act by inhibition of secondary signals (8). This is also suggested—although not well documented yet—by a recent randomized study where anti-LFA-1 administration was associated with the same rate of early rejection as observed in controls, despite no CsA being given during the first 10 days in the anti-LFA-1 arm of the trial (7). This is more suggestive of an action on early rejection than a major effect of ischemia reperfusion (the rate of delayed graft function was not significantly affected). Whether anti-ICAM-1 could be placed on the same level in terms of both efficacy and mechanism of action is still undetermined. The causal events that have been responsible for the interruption of the clinical trials have not yet been released. One can, however, mention the predictable activation on endothelial cells that express high levels of this inducible target molecule after various stimuli such as ischemia and surgical stress.

The use of agents blocking another major second signal, anti-CD40 ligand (CD40L), alone or in association with anti-B7, have produced extremely interesting preliminary results in animals. Long-term allograft acceptance was first observed in rodents, when associated with inhibition of the CD28 pathway (9) [although combined anti-LFA-1 and anti-ICAM-1 were reported to have similar effects (10)]. Similar results were more recently achieved in primates (4). A very promising possibility, which has also been claimed but not confirmed for anti-CD4 and anti-LFA-1, is that agents inhibiting CD40L/CD40 or B7/CD28 pathways might also inhibit help to B cells and the resulting antibody formation, including against their own determinants (4,5). In primates, inhibition of CD40L/CD40 pathway could be even more efficient than that of CD28/B7. The manipulation of CD28/B7 interaction is so far mostly related to the use of CTLA4 Ig fusion molecules or anti-B7 antibody usage. However, this approach might not be optimal and could even be harmful in patients with underlying autoimmune disorders. Indeed, both agents inhibit, without discrimination, the CD28/B7 costimulatory signal *and* the regulatory signal CTLA4/B7. The importance of this negative signal has been—as for CD40L signal in a mirror representation—exemplified by the lethal phenotype due to severe inflammatory processes of the CTLA4 Knock Out (KO) mice (11). The nondiscriminative blocking of these two B7 ligands could also—as for CsA (9)—inhibit the induction of tolerance that appears to require CTLA4 (12). A more adequate option would therefore be to selectively inhibit B7/CD28 interaction that provides a powerful and CsA-insensitive signal for T_H1 cytokine production, without interfering with CTLA4/B7 interaction that is likely to provide regulatory signals after the CTLA4 upregulation that follows TCR ligation. As all described MAbs against CD28 are agonists, such aims would require a more sophisticated design avoiding CD28 cross-linking. Nevertheless, these preliminary results, particularly with combinations of reagents, make imaginable a control of early rejection (without mention of the possibility of tolerance induction). Owing to their well-identified targets, the combination of such reagents is likely to be as efficient as presently available therapies, but with fewer side effects and the opportunity for more precise monitoring.

Interestingly, recent data have also raised the possibility that the inhibition of the CD28/B7 pathway could have some utility in preventing the damage of reperfusion syndrome (13). Indirectly, these data reinforce the hypothesis that anti-LFA-1 (see above) could also act on reperfusion syndrome by an inhibitory effect on T-cell activation rather than through the blockade of leukocyte/endothelial cell interaction only.

TARGETING THE IL-2 RECEPTOR

Although KO mice for various cytokines can develop almost normal rejection, inhibition of a single signal, such as that controlled by the inducibe IL-2R required for T-cell growth, has proven to be highly effective in animals and humans. The possibility of increasing effectiveness by reducing redundancy (such as IL-15, IL-4, IL-7, IL-2 for T-cell growth) is nevertheless suggested by the behavior of KO mice. This could be achieved on the IL-2R target of activated T cells by using a combination of antibodies blocking different epitopes [e.g., IL-2R α-chain for IL-2, IL-2R β chain for IL-15 (14,15)]. Even more efficient would be the possibility of interaction on the γ-chain of the IL-2R involved in multiple cytokine-mediated signals (IL-2, IL-4, IL-7), the mutation of which has been associated with severe immunodeficiencies in humans. This possibility of having both a rather specific effect and a decreased redundancy, drawn from the IL-2/IL-2R pathway, is not the only example. Molecular interactions governing the binding of leukocytes and endothelial cells of various integrins, selectins, and chemokine receptors are also characterized by an extremely high level of redundancy evidenced by both the effect of the corresponding KO gene and the high efficiency of the association of blocking antibodies, suggesting again that multiple interactions also could be strongly beneficial to a "biologic" activity (16). Newly designed antibodies reacting at two epitopes could be useful in the future (17).

BEYOND MONOCLONAL ANTIBODIES

Antibodies or fusion molecules that use parts of immunoglobulins, such as CTLA4 Ig, do not summarize all biologic immunosuppressive agents. There is a diversity of molecules that could be used, including competing soluble receptors (such as soluble TNFR, soluble CR1 complement receptor, or inhibitory cytokines). These agents could be used to inhibit nonspecific inflammation, immune response, or endothelial cell activation in hyperimmunized patients or to prevent reperfusion injury. This field, currently being actively explored in the test tube and in the rodent model, has not yet reached clinical application. Moreover, there is also the possibility to introduce some immunoregulatory cytokines [through recombinant viruses, such as adenoviruses or adenovirus-associated viruses (AAV) for the corresponding molecule] in organs before transplantation. This gene-therapy–derived device for "treating" the organ's microenvironment, rather than the recipient's, may be applicable in the future.

Bioreagents, owing to their property to specifically target functional molecules, used alone or in combination, are also likely to be the tools for inducing tolerance. In this regard, donor MHC expressed by non-APC recipient cells (18) or soluble MHC molecules (19) are interesting. These "biologic agents" might mimic the signals that induce peripheral tolerance following donor blood infusion, a model that has been one of the most efficient in animals.

In conclusion, although long considered to be marginal, bioreagents have gained solid reliability with ATG and OKT-3 and now appear as unique tools as we imagine the future of immunointervention. Interestingly, for instance, two injections (day 0 and day 4 following transplantation) of an antibody directed at the α-chain of IL-2 receptor have been shown to provide about the same level of effect on prevention of early graft rejection, without side effects, as six months of treatment with MMF (20). This example could foreshadow a new paradigm in immunointervention.

CHAPTER REFERENCES

1. Starzl TE, Porter KA, Iwasaki Y, et al. The use of heterologous antilymphocyte globulins in human homotransplantation. In: Wolstenholme GEW, O'Connor M, eds. Antilymphocyte Serum. Boston: Little, Brown, 1967:1.
2. Gantenbein H, Bachmann P, Huynh U, et al. Comparison of two antilymphocyte globulins replacing cyclosporine A after first kidney allotransplantation and prolonged graft ischemia. Clin Transplant 1996;10:384–385.
3. Malinow L, Walker J, Klassen DK, et al. Antilymphocyte induction immunosuppression in the post-Minnesota antilymphocyte globulin era: incidence of renal dysfunction and delayed graft function. A single center experience. Clin Transplant 1996;10:237–242.
4. Guttmann RD, Fleming C. Sequential biological immunosuppression. Induction therapy with rabbit antithymocyte globulin. Clin Transplant 1997;11:185–192.
5. Gaber AO, First MR, Tesi RJ, et al. Results of the double blind randomized multicenter phase III clinical trial of thymoglobulin versus ATGAM in the treatment of acute graft rejection episodes after renal transplantation. Transplantation 1998;66:29–37.
6. Kohler G, Milstein C. Continuous cultures of fused cells secreting antibody of predefined specificity. Nature 1975;256:495.
7. Cosimi AB, Burton RC, Colvin RB, et al. Treatment of acute renal allograft rejection with OKT3 monoclonal antibody. Transplantation 1981;32:535.
8. Cosimi AB, Delmonico FL. Antilymphocyte antibody therapy. In: Burdick JF, Racusen LC, Solez K, eds. Kidney transplant rejection. 2nd ed. New York: Marcel Dekker, 1992:541–565.
9. Simpson MA, Monaco AP. Clinical uses of polyclonal and monoclonal antilymphoid sera. In: Chatenoud L, ed. Monoclonal antibodies in transplantation. Austin, TX: RG Landes, 1995:1–19.
10. Lum CT, Umen AJ, Kasiske B, et al. Clinical impact of replacing Minnesota antilymphocyte globulin with ATGAM. Transplantation 1995;59:371–376.
11. Bonnefoy-Berard N, Vincent C, Revillard JP. Antibodies against functional leukocyte surface molecules in polyclonal antilymphocyte and antithymocyte globulins. Transplantation 1991;51:669–673.
12. Rebellato LM, Gross U, Verbanac KM, et al. A comprehensive definition of the major antibody specificities in polyclonal rabbit antithymocyte globulin. Transplantation 1994;57:685–694.
13. Bourdage JS, Hamlin DM. Comparative polyclonal antithymocyte globulin and antilymphocyte/antilymphoblast globulin anti-CD antigen analysis by flow cytometry. Transplantation 1995;59:1194–1200.
14. Thomas JM, Carver FM, Halsch CE, et al. Suppressor cells in Rhesus monkeys treated with antithymocyte globulin. Transplantation 1982;34:83–89.
15. Brooks CD, Karl KJ, Francom SF. ATGAM Skin Test Standardization: comparison of skin testing techniques in horse-sensitive and unselected human volunteers. Transplantation 1994;58:1135–1137.
16. Wechter WJ, Broodie JA, Morrell RM, et al. Antithymocyte globulin (ATGAM) in renal allograft recipients. Transplantation 1979;28(4):294–307.
17. Cosimi AB. The clinical value of antilymphocyte antibodies. Transplant Proc 1981;13(1):462–468.
18. Novick AC, Ho-Hsieh H, Steinmuller D, et al. Detrimental effect of cyclosporine on initial function of cadaver renal allografts following extended preservation. Transplantation 1986;42:154.
19. Sommer BG, Henry M, Ferguson RM. Sequential antilymphoblast globulin and cyclosporine for renal transplantation. Transplantation 1987;43(1):85–90.
20. Grundmann R, Hesse U, Wienand P, et al. Graft survival and long-term renal function after sequential conventional cyclosporin A therapy in cadaver kidney transplantation—a prospective randomized trial. Klin Wochenschr 1987;65:879–884.
21. Ferguson RM. A multicenter experience with sequential ALG/cyclosporine therapy in renal transplantation. Clin Transplant 1988;2:285–290.
22. Stratta RJ, D'Alessandro AM, Armbrust MJ, et al. Sequential antilymphocyte globulin/cyclosporine immunosuppression in cadaveric renal transplantation. Transplantation 1989;47:96–102.
23. Stratta RJ, Mason B, Lorentzen DF, et al. Cadaveric renal transplantation with quadruple immunosuppression in patients with a positive antiglobulin crossmatch. Transplantation 1989;47(2):282–286.
24. Hariharan S, Alexander JW, Schroeder TJ, First MR. Outcome of cadaveric renal transplantation by induction treatment in the cyclosporine era. Clin Transplant 1996;10:186–190.
25. Cecka JM, Terasaki PI. The UNOS Scientific Renal Transplant Registry. In: Terasaki PI, Cecka JM, eds. Clinical transplants 1991. Los Angeles: UCLA Tissue Typing Laboratory, 1992:6.
26. Shield CF, Edwards EB, Davies DB, Daily OP. Antilymphocyte induction therapy in cadaver renal transplantation. Transplantation 1997;63:1257–1263.
27. Slakey DP, Johnson CP, Callaluce RD, et al. A prospective randomized comparison of quadruple versus triple therapy for first cadaver transplants with immediate function. Transplantation 1993;56:827–831.
28. Abouna GM, Al-Abdullah IH, Kelly-Sullivan D, et al. Randomized clinical trial of antithymocyte globulin induction in renal transplantation comparing a fixed daily dose with dose adjustment according to T cell monitoring. Transplantation 1995;59:1564–1568.
29. Evans RW, Manninen DL, Dong FB, et al. Immunosuppressive therapy as a determinant of transplantation outcomes. Transplantation 1993;55:1297–1305.
30. McVicar JP, Kowdley KV, Emond MJ, et al. Induction immunosuppressive therapy is associated with a low rejection rate after liver transplantation. Clin Transplant 1997;11:328–333.
31. Langrehr JM, Nussler NC, Neumann U, et al. A prospective randomized trial comparing interleukin-2 receptor antibody versus antithymocyte globulin as part of a quadruple immunosuppressive induction therapy following orthotopic liver transplantation. Transplantation 1997;63:1772–1781.
32. Jonas S, Kling N, Bechstein WO, et al. Rejection episodes after liver transplantation during primary immunosuppression with FK506 or a cyclosporin-based regimen: a controlled, prospective randomized trial. Clin Transplant 1995;9:406–414.
33. Renard TH, Andrews WS. An approach to ABO-incompatible liver transplantation in children. Transplantation 1992;53(1):116–121.
34. Stratta RJ, Shaeffer MS, Pharm D, et al. Cytomegalovirus infection and disease after liver transplantation: an overview. Digest Dis Sci 1992;37(5):673–688.

35. Sollinger HW, Stratta RJ, Kalayoglu M, et al. Pancreas transplantation with pancreaticocystostomy and quadruple immunosuppression. Transplantation 1987;102(4):674–679.
36. Griepp RB, Stinson EB, Dong EJ, et al. Use of antithymocyte globulins in human heart transplantation. Circulation Suppl 1972;15:147.
37. English TAH, McGregor C, Wallwork J, et al. Aspects of immunosuppression for cardiac transplantation. Heart Transplant 1981;4:281.
38. Devineni R, McKenzie N, Keown P. Cyclosporine in cardiac transplantation. Transplantation 1984;27:252–254.
39. Deeb MG, Kolff J, McClurken JB, et al. Antithymocyte gamma globulin, low-dose cyclosporine, and tapering steroids as an immunosuppressive regimen to avoid early kidney failure in heart transplantation. J Heart Transplant 1987;6:406–414.
40. Kormos RL, Armitage JM, Stephen AJ, et al. Optimal perioperative immunosuppression in cardiac transplantation using rabbit antithymocyte globulin. Transplantation 1990;49(2):306–311.
41. Menkis AH, Powell AM, Novick RJ, et al. A prospective randomized controlled trial of initial immunosuppression with ALG versus OKT3 in recipients of cardiac allografts. J Heart Lung Transplant 1992;11:569–576.
42. Carrier M, Pelletier G, Cartier R, et al. Induction of immunosuppression with rabbit antithymocyte globulin: five-year experience in cardiac transplantation. Can J Cardiol 1993;9(2):171–176.
43. Cooper JD. Lung Transplantation. Ann Thorac Surg 1989;47:28–44.
44. Stuart S, Griffith B. Single and double lung transplantation. In: Starzl TE, Shapiro R, Simmons RI, eds. Atlas of organ transplantation. New York: Gower Medical, 1992:1–29.
45. Shield III CF, Cosimi AB, Tolkoff-Rubin N, et al. Use of antithymocyte globulin for reversal of acute allograft rejection. Transplantation 1979;28(6):461–464.
46. Nelson PW, Cosimi AB, Delmonico FL, et al. Antithymocyte globulin as the primary treatment for renal allograft rejection. Transplantation 1983;36:587–589.
47. Richardson AJ, Higgins RM, Liddington M, et al. Antithymocyte globulin for steroid resistant rejection in renal transplant recipients immunosuppressed with triple therapy. Transplant Int 1989;2:27–32.
48. Gaber AO, First MR, Tesi RJ, et al. Results of the double-blind randomized multicenter phase III clinical trial of Thymoglobulin versus ATGAM in the treatment of acute graft rejection after renal transplantation. Transplantation 1998;66:29–37.
49. Bock HA, Gallati H, Zurcher RM, et al. A randomized prospective trial of prophylactic immunosuppression with ATG-Fresenius versus OKT3 after renal transplantation. Transplantation 1995;59(6):830–840.
50. Starzl TE, Iwatsuki S, Van Thiel DH, et al. Evolution of liver transplantation. Hepatology 1982;2(5):614–636.
51. Ascher NL, Freese DK, Paradis K, et al. Rejection of the transplanted liver. In: Maddrey WC, ed. Transplantation of the liver. New York: Elsevier, 1988:167–169.
52. Monaco AP, Wood ML. The potential for induction of specific unresponsiveness to organ allografts in clinical transplantation. Heart Transplant 1982;1:257–260.
53. Cosimi AB. Antilymphocyte globulin—a final (?) look..In: Morris PJ, Tilney NL, eds. Progress in transplantation. Vol. 2. Edinburgh: Churchill Livingston, 1986:167–188.
54. Thomas JM, Carver FM, Foil MB, et al. Renal allograft tolerance induced with ATG and donor bone marrow in outbred rhesus monkeys. Transplantation 1983;36:104–106.
55. Thomas JM, Carver FM, Kasten-Jolly J, et al. Further studies of veto activity in rhesus monkey bone marrow in relation to allograft tolerance and chimerism. Transplantation 1994;57:101–115.
56. Barber WH, Mankin IA, Laskow DA, et al. Long-term results of a controlled prospective study with transfusion of donor-specific bone marrow in 57 cadaveric renal allograft recipients. Transplantation 1991;51:70.
57. Kawai T, Cosimi AB, Colvin RB, et al. Mixed allogeneic chimerism and renal allograft tolerance in cynomolgus monkeys. Transplantation 1995;59(2):256–262.
58. Kimikawa M, Sachs DH, Colvin RB, et al. Modifications of the conditioning regimen for achieving mixed chimerism and donor-specific tolerance in cynomolgus monkeys. Transplantation 1997;64:709–716.
59. Terasaki P. Microdroplet assay of human serum cytotoxins. Nature 1964;204:998–1000.
60. Delmonico FL, Auchincloss H, Rubin RH, et al. The selective use of antilymphocyte serum for cyclosporine treated patients with renal allograft dysfunction. Ann Surg 1987;206:649–654.
61. Muller TF, Grebe SO, Neumann MC, et al. Persistent long-term changes in lymphocyte subsets induced by polyclonal antibodies. Transplantation 1997;64:1432–1437.
62. Kreis H, Mansouri R, Descamps J-M, et al. Antithymocyte globulin in cadaver kidney transplantation: a randomized trial based on T-cell monitoring. Kidney Int 1981;19:438–444.
63. Clark K. Monitoring antithymocyte globulin in renal transplantation. Ann Royal College Surgeons Eng 1996;78(6):536–540.
64. Tatum AH, Bollinger RR, Sanfilippo F. Rapid serologic diagnosis of serum sickness from antilymphocyte globulin therapy using enzyme immunoassay. Transplantation 1984;38:582–586.
65. Lawley TJ, Bielovy L, Gascon P, et al. A prospective clinical and immunologic analysis of patients with serum sickness. N Engl J Med 1984;311:1407.
66. Debets JMH, Leunissen KML, van Hooff HJ, et al. Evidence of involvement of tumor necrosis factor in adverse reactions during treatment of kidney allograft rejection with antithymocyte globulin. Transplantation 1989;47:487.
67. Chatenoud L, Ferran C, Legendre C, et al. In vivo cell activation following OKT3 administration. Systemic cytokine release and modulation by corticosteroids. Transplantation 1990;49:697.
68. Charpentier B, Hiesse C, Lantz O, et al. Evidence that antihuman tumor necrosis factor monoclonal antibody prevents OKT3-induced acute syndrome. Transplantation 1993;54:997.
69. Eason JD, Wee SL, Kawai T, et al. Inhibition of the effects of TNF in renal allograft recipients using recombinant human dimeric tumor necrosis factor receptors. Transplantation 1995;59(2):300–305.
70. Henricsson A, Husberg B, Bergentz SE. The mechanism behind the effect of ALG on platelets in vivo. Clin Exp Immunol 1977;29:515–522.
71. Rubin RH, Cosimi AB, Hirsch MS, et al. Effects of antithymocyte globulin on cytomegalovirus infection in renal transplant recipients. Transplantation 1981;31:143.
72. Rubin RH. Preemptive therapy in immunocompromised hosts. N Engl J Med 1991;324:1057.
73. Malatack JF, Gastner JC, Urbach AH, Zitelli BJ. Orthotopic liver transplantation, Epstein Barr virus, cyclosporine, and lymphoproliferative disease: a growing concern. J Pediatr 1991;118:667–673.
74. Winter G, Milstein C. Man-made antibodies. Nature 1991;349:293–299.
75. Boulianne GL, Hozumi N, Shulman MI. Production of functional chimeric mouse-human antibody. Nature 1984;312:643.
76. Heinrich G, Gram H, Kocher HP, et al. Characterization of a human T cell-specific chimeric antibody (CD7) with human constant and mouse variable regions. J Immunol 1989;143:3589.
77. Delmonico FL, Cosimi AB, Kawai T, et al. Nonhuman primate responses to murine and humanized OKT4A. Transplantation 1993;55:722–728.
78. Alegre M-L, Peterson LJ, Xu D, et al. A non-activating "humanized" anti-CD3 monoclonal antibody retains immunosuppressive properties in vivo. Transplantation 1994;57:1537–1543.
79. Alegre ML, Lenschow DJ, Bluestone JA. Immunomodulation of transplant rejection using monoclonal antibodies and soluble receptors. Digest Dis Sci 1995;40(1):58–64.
80. Vincenti F, Lantz M, Birnbaum J, et al. A phase I trial of humanized anti-interleukin 2 receptor antibody in renal transplantation. Transplantation 1997;63:33–38.
81. Knechtle SJ, Vargo D, Fechner J, et al. FN18-CRM9 immunotoxin promotes tolerance in primate renal allografts. Transplantation 1997;63:1–6.
82. Mottram PL, Han W-R, Murray-Segal LJ, et al. Idarubicin-anti-CD3: a new immunoconjugate that induces alloantigen-specific tolerance in mice. Transplantation 1997;64:684–690.
83. Midtvedt K, Tafjord AB, Hartmann A, et al. Half dose of OKT3 is efficient in treatment of steroid-resistant renal allograft rejection. Transplantation 1996;62:38–42.
84. Chatenoud L, Legendre C, Ferran C, et al. Corticosteroid inhibition of the OKT3-induced cytokine-related syndrome-dosage and kinetics prerequisites. Transplantation 1991;51:334–338.
85. Pescovitz MD, Milgrom ML, Leapman SB, Filo RS. Corticosteroid inhibition of the OKT3-induced febrile and nephrotoxic responses during treatment of renal allograft rejection. Clin Transplant 1993;7:529–536.
86. Thistlethwaite JR Jr, Stuart JK, Mayes JT, et al. Complications and monitoring of OKT3 therapy. Am J Kid Dis 1988;11:112–119.
87. Haug CE, Colvin RB, Delmonico FL, et al. A phase I trial of immunosuppression with anti-ICAM-1 (CD54) mAb in renal allograft recipients. Transplantation 1993;55:766–773.
88. Bach JF, Chatenoud L. Immunology of monoclonal antibodies in solid organ transplantation: yesterday, today and tomorrow. Transplant Sci 1992;2(2)suppl:4–8.

89. Janossy G. Purging of bone marrow and immunosuppression. Br Med Bull 1984;40:247.
90. Burdick JF. Biology of immunosuppression mediated by antilymphocyte antibodies. In: Burdick JF, Racusen LC, Solez K, eds. Kidney transplant rejection. 2nd ed. New York: Marcel Dekker, 1992:505–539.
91. Jonker M, Goldstein G, Balner H. Effect of in vivo administration of monoclonal antibodies specific for human T cell subpopulations on the immune system in a rhesus monkey model. Transplantation 1983;35:521–526.
92. Tite JP, Sloan A, Janeway CJ. The role of L3T4 in T cell activation L3T4 may be both an Ia-binding protein and a receptor that transduces a negative signal. J Mol Cell Immunol 1986;2:179.
93. Kerr PG, Atkins RC. The effects of OKT3 therapy on infiltrating lymphocytes in rejecting renal allografts. Transplantation 1989;48:33.
94. Cosimi AB. The future of monoclonal antibody immunosuppression in solid organ transplantation. Transplant Sci 1992;2(2)suppl:28–34.
95. Rouleau M, Mollereau B, Bernard A, et al. Mitogenic monoclonal antibody pairs predispose peripheral T cells to undergo apoptosis on interaction with a third CD2 monoclonal antibody. J Immunol 1994;152:4861–4872.
96. Boussiotis VA, Freeman GJ, Griffin JD, et al. CD2 is involved in maintenance and reversal of human allo antigen-specific clonal anergy. J Exp Med 1994;180:1665–1673.
97. Thurlow PJ, Lovering E, D'Apice AJF, et al. A monoclonal anti-pan-T-cell antibody. Transplantation 1983;36:293–298.
98. Giovino-Barry VC, Latinne D, Xu Y, et al. Perturbation of CD2 can induce alloantigen specific hyporesponsiveness in naive T cells. FASEB 1995;9:A1345.
99. Starling GC, Whitney GS, Siadak AW, et al. Characterization of mouse CD6 with novel mAbs which enhance the allogeneic mixed leukocyte reaction. Eur J Immunol 1996;26(4):738–746.
100. Kirkman RL, Araujo JL, Busch GJ, et al. Treatment of acute renal allograft rejection with monoclonal anti-T12 antibody. Transplantation 1983;36(6):620–626.
101. Wee SL, Phelan JM, Preffer FI, et al. Anti-Leu2a (anti-CD8) monoclonal antibody therapy: antibody-mediated cell clearance in vivo requires Fc-FcRII interaction. Transplant Proc 1989;21:117.
102. Larsen CP, Elwood ET, Alexander DZ, et al. Long-term acceptance of skin and cardiac allografts after blocking CD40 and CD28 pathways. Nature 1996;381:434–438.
103. Kirk AD, Harlan DM, Davis TA, et al. CTLA 4 Ig and anti-CD40 ligand prevent renal allograft rejection in primates. Proc Natl Acad Sci 1997;94:8789–8794.
104. Goldberg LC, Bradley JA, Connolly J, et al. Anti-CD45 monoclonal antibody perfusion of human renal allografts prior to transplantation. Transplantation 1995;59:1285–1293.
105. Cosimi AB, Conti D, Delmonico FL, et al. In vivo effects of monoclonal antibody to ICAM-1 (CD54) in nonhuman primates with renal allografts. J Immunol 1990;144:4604–4612.
106. Kreis H, Legendre C, Chatenoud L. OKT3 in organ transplantation. Transplant Rev 1991;5:181–199.
107. Delmonico FL, Cosimi AB. Monoclonal antibody treatment of human allograft recipients. Surg Gynecol Obstet 1988;166:89–98.
108. Kunicka JE, Platsoucas CD. Induction of suppressor cells to T- and B-cell proliferative responses and immunoglobulin production by monoclonal antibodies recognizing CD3 T-cell differentiation antigen. Cell Immunol 1988;116:195–215.
109. Vigeral P, Chkoff N, Chatenoud L, et al. Prophylactic use of OKT3 monoclonal antibody in cadaver kidney recipients. Transplantation 1986;41:730–733.
110. Debure A, Chkoff N, Chatenoud L, et al. One-month prophylactic use of OKT3 in cadaver kidney transplant recipients. Transplantation 1988;45:546–553.
111. Norman DJ, Kahana L, Stuart FP, et al. A randomized clinical trial of induction therapy with OKT3 in kidney transplantation. Transplantation 1993;55:44–50.
112. Abramowicz D, Goldman M. OKT3 for induction of immunosuppression in renal transplantation. Transplantation 1993;43:91–95.
113. Opelz G, for the Collaborative Transplant Study. Efficacy of rejection prophylaxis with OKT3 in renal transplantation. Transplantation 1995;60:1220–1224.
114. Abramowicz D, Pradier O, Marchant A, et al. Induction of thromboses within renal grafts by high-dose prophylactic OKT3. Lancet 1992;339:777–778.
115. Millis JM, McDiarmid SV, Hiatt JR, et al. Randomized prospective trial of OKT3 for early prophylaxis of rejection after liver transplantation. Transplantation 1989;47:82.
116. Farges O, Ericzon B-G, Bresson-Hadni S, et al. A randomized trial of OKT3-based versus cyclosporine-based immunoprophylaxis after liver transplantation. Transplantation 1994;58:891–898.
117. Robbins RC, Oyer PE, Stinson EB, Starnes VA. The use of monoclonal antibodies after heart transplantation. Transplant Sci 1992;2:22–27.
118. Griffith BP, Kormos RL, Armitage JM, et al. Comparative trial of immunoprophylaxis with RATG versus OKT3. J Heart Transplant 1990;9:301–305.
119. Kramer MR, Stoehr C, Lewiston NJ, et al. Trimethoprim-sulfamethoxazole prophylaxis for *Pneumocystisis carinii* infections in heart-lung and lung transplantation—how effective for how long? Transplantation 1992;53:586–589.
120. Gruessner A, Sutherland DE. Pancreas transplantation in the United States and non-US. In: Terasaki PI, Cecka JM, eds. Clinical transplants 1996. Los Angeles: UCLA Tissue Typing Laboratory, 1996:47–68.
121. Ortho Multicenter Transplant Study Group. A randomized clinical trial of OKT3 monoclonal antibody for acute rejection of cadaveric renal transplants. N Engl J Med 1985;313:337–342.
122. Ponticelli C, Rivolta E, Tarantino A, et al. Treatment of severe rejection of kidney transplants with Orthoclone OKT3. Clin Transplant 1987;1:99–103.
123. Norman DJ, Barry JM, Bennett WM, et al. The use of OKT3 in cadaveric renal transplantation for rejection that is unresponsive to conventional anti-rejection therapy. Am J Kid Dis 1988;11:90–93.
124. First MR, Schroeder TJ, Melvin DB, et al. OKT3 therapy in kidney, liver, heart, and pancreas transplantation. Clin Transplantation 1988;2:185–189.
125. Gaber LW, Gaber AO, Vera SR, et al. Successful reversal of hyperacute renal allograft rejection with the anti-CD3 monoclonal OKT3. Transplantation 1992;54:930–932.
126. Carrier M, Jenicek M, Pelletier LC. Value of monoclonal antibody OKT3 in solid organ transplantation: a meta-analysis. Transplant Proc 1992;24: 2586–2591.
127. Tesi RJ, Elkhammas EA, Henry ML, Ferguson RM. OKT3 for primary therapy of the first rejection episode in kidney transplants. Transplantation 1993;55:1023–1029.
128. Kamath S, Dean D, Peddi VR, et al. Efficacy of OKT3 as primary therapy for histologically confirmed acute renal allograft rejection. Transplantation 1997;64:1428–1432.
129. Woodle ES, Thislethwaite JR, Emond JC, et al. OKT3 therapy for hepatic allograft rejection. Transplantation 1991;51:1207–1212.
130. Cosimi AB, Cho SI, Delmonico FL, et al. A randomized clinical trial comparing OKT3 and steroids for treatment of hepatic allograft rejection. Transplantation 1987;43:91–95.
131. Solomon H, Gonwa TA, Mor E, et al. OKT3 rescue for steroid-resistant rejection in adult liver transplantation. Transplantation 1993;55:87–91.
132. Nakhleh RE, Sutherland DE. Pancreas rejection: significance of histopathologic findings with implications for classification of rejection. Am J Surg Pathol 1992;16:1098–1107.
133. Gilbert EM, DeWitt CW, Eisworth CC, et al. Treatment of refractory cardiac allograft rejection with OKT3 monoclonal antibody. Am J Med 1982;82:202.
134. Shennib H, Massard G, Reynaud M, Noirclerc M. Efficacy of OKT3 therapy for acute rejection in isolated lung transplantation. J Heart Lung Transplant 1994;13:514–519.
135. Carey G, Lisi PJ, Schroeder TJ. The incidence of antibody formation to OKT3 consequent to its use in organ transplantation. Transplantation 1995;60:151–158.
136. Colvin RB, Preffer FI. Laboratory monitoring of therapy with OKT3 and other murine monoclonal antibodies. Clin Lab Med 1991;11:693.
137. Nelson PW, Jaffers GJ, Fuller TC, et al. Reduction of immune response to OKT3 monoclonal antibody. Transplant Proc 1985;17:644–645.
138. Chatenoud L, Jonker M, Villemain F, et al. The human immune response to the OKT3 monoclonal antibody is oligoclonal. Science 1986;232:1406–1408.
139. Legendre CM, Kreis H, Bach J, Chatenoud L. Prediction of successful allograft rejection retreatment with OKT3. Transplantation 1992;53:87–90.
140. Cosimi AB, Colvin RB, Burton RC, et al. Use of monoclonal antibodies to T-cell subsets for immunologic monitoring and treatment in recipients of renal allografts. N Engl J Med 1981;305:308–314.
141. Stephen RN, Munschauer CE, Kohli RK, et al. Post-OKT3 induction therapy CD complex response predicts renal allograft rejection. Transplantation 1997;63:1183–1186.

142. Sheiner PA, Guarrera JV, Grunstein E, et al. Increased risk of early rejection correlates with recovery of CD3 cell count after liver transplant in patients receiving OKT3 induction. Transplantation 1997;64:1212–1216.
143. Woodle ES, Bruse DS, Josephson M, et al. OKT3 escalating dose regimens provide effective therapy for renal allograft rejection. Clin Transplant 1996;10:389–395.
144. Jaffers GJ, Fuller TC, Cosimi AB, et al. Monoclonal antibody therapy: anti-idiotypic and non-anti-idiotypic antibodies to OKT3 arising despite intense immunosuppression. Transplantation 1986;41:572–578.
145. Chatenoud L, Ferran C, Reuter A, et al. Systemic reaction to the monoclonal antibody OKT3 in relation to serum levels of tumor necrosis factor and interferon γ. N Engl J Med 1989;320:1420.
146. Buysmann S, Hack CE, van Diepen FNJ, et al. Administration of OKT3 as a 2-hour infusion attenuates first dose side effects. Transplantation 1997;64:1620–1623.
147. Vallhonrat H, Williams WW, Cosimi AB, et al. In vivo generation of C4d, Bb, iC3b and SC5b-9 after OKT3 administration in kidney and lung transplant recipients. Transplantation 1999 (in press).
148. Waid TH, Lucas BA, Thompson JS, et al. Treatment of renal allograft rejection with T10B9.1A31 or OKT3. Transplantation 1997;64:274–281.
149. Eason JD, Pascual M, Wee S, et al. Evaluation of recombinant human soluble dimeric tumor necrosis factor receptor for prevention of OKT3-associated acute clinical syndrome. Transplantation 1996;61:224–228.
150. Swinnen LJ, Costanzo-Nordin MR, Fisher SG, et al. Increased incidence of lymphoproliferative disorder after immunosuppression with the monoclonal antibody OKT3 in cardiac transplant recipients. N Engl J Med 1990;323:1723–1728.
151. Hibberd PL, Tolkoff-Rubin NE, Cosimi AB, et al. Symptomatic cytomegalovirus disease in the cytomegalovirus antibody seropositive renal transplant recipient treated with OKT3. Transplantation 1992;53:68–72.
152. Andrews W, Sommerauer J, Roden J, et al. 10 years of pediatric liver transplantation. J Pediatr Surg 1996;31:619–624.
153. Chen JM, Barr ML, Chadburn A, et al. Management of lymphoproliferative disorders after cardiac transplantation. Ann Thorac Surg 1993;56:527–538.
154. Steinmuller DR, Hayes JM, Novick AC, et al. Comparison of OKT3 with ALG for prophylaxis for patients with acute renal failure after cadaveric renal transplantation. Transplantation 1991;52:67–71.
155. Frey DJ, Matas AJ, Gillingham KJ, et al. Sequential therapy—a prospective randomized trial of MALG versus OKT3 for prophylactic immunosuppression in cadaver renal allograft recipients. Transplantation 1992;54:50–56.
156. Cole EH, Cattran DC, Farewell VT, et al. A comparison of rabbit antithymocyte serum and OKT3 as prophylaxis against renal allograft rejection. Transplantation 1994;57:60–67.
157. Hanto DW, Jendrisak MD, So SKS, et al. Induction immunosuppression with antilymphocyte globulin or OKT3 in cadaver kidney transplantation. Transplantation 1994;57:377–384.
158. Block HA, Gallati H, Zurcher RM, et al. A randomized prospective trial of prophylactic immunosuppression with ATG-fresenius versus OKT3 after renal transplantation. Transplantation 1995;59:830–840.
159. Delmonico FL, Cosimi AB, et al. Anti-CD4 monoclonal antibody therapy. Clin Transplant 1996;10:397–403.
160. Powelson JA, Cosimi AB. The experimental and clinical use in transplantation of monoclonal antibodies to CD4 and other adhesion molecules. In: Chatenoud L, ed. Monoclonal antibodies in transplantation. Austin, TX: RG Landes, 1995:21–52.
161. Sablinski T, Sayegh MH, Kut JP, et al. The importance of targeting the CD4+ T cell subset at the time of antigenic challenge for induction of prolonged vascularized allograft survival. Transplantation 1992;53:219–221.
162. Sablinski T, Hancock WW, Tilney NL, Kupiec-Weglinski JW. CD4 monoclonal antibodies in organ transplantation—a review of progress. Transplantation 1991;52:579–589.
163. Powelson JA, Knowles RW, Delmonico FL, et al. CDR-grafted OKT4A monoclonal antibody in cynomolgus renal allograft recipients. Transplantation 1994;57:788–793.
164. Horneff G, Emmrich F, Reiter C, et al. Persistent depletion of CD4+ T cells and inversion of the CD4/CD8 T cell ratio induced by anti-CD4 therapy. J Rheumatol 1992;19:1845–1850.
165. Sprent J. T lymphocytes and the thymus. In: Paul WE, ed. Fundamental immunology. 3rd ed. New York: Raven, 1993:75–109.
166. Lehmann M, Sternkopf F, Metz F, et al. Induction of long-term survival of rat skin allografts by a novel, highly efficient anti-CD4 monoclonal antibody. Transplantation 1992;54:959–962.
167. Wee SL, Stroka DM, Preffer FI, et al. The effects of OKT4A monoclonal antibody on cellular immunity of nonhuman primate renal allograft recipients. Transplantation 1992;53:501–507.
168. Darby CR, Morris PJ, Wood KJ. Evidence that long-term cardiac allograft survival induced by anti-CD4 monoclonal antibody does not require depletion of CD4+ T cells. Transplantation 1992;54:483–490.
169. Darby CR, Bushell A, Morris PJ, et al. Nondepleting anti-CD4 antibodies in transplantation. Evidence that modulation is far less effective than prolonged CD4 blockade. Transplantation 1994;57:1419–1426.
170. Shizuru JA, Seydel KB, Flavin TF, et al. Induction of donor-specific unresponsiveness to cardiac allografts in rats by pretransplant anti-CD4 monoclonal antibody therapy. Transplantation 1990;50:366–373.
171. Pearson TC, Madsen JC, Larsen CP, et al. Induction of transplantation tolerance in adults using donor antigen and anti-CD4 monoclonal antibody. Transplantation 1992;54:475–483.
172. Bushell A, Morris PJ, Wood KJ. Induction of operational tolerance by random blood transfusion combined with anti-CD4 antibody therapy. A protocol with significant clinical potential. Transplantation 1994;58:133–139.
173. Bretscher P. The two-signal model of lymphocyte activation twenty-one years later. Immunol Today 1993;13:74–76.
174. Alters SE, Song HK, Fathman CG. Evidence that clonal anergy is induced in thymic migrant cells after anti-CD4-mediated transplantation tolerance. Transplantation 1993;56:633–638.
175. Cosimi AB, Delmonico FL, Wright JK, et al. Prolonged survival of nonhuman primate renal allograft recipients treated only with anti-CD4 monoclonal antibody. Surgery 1990;108:406–413.
176. Riechmann L, Clark M, Waldmann H, et al. Reshaping human antibodies for therapy. Nature 1988;332:323–327.
177. Greenwood J, Clark M, Waldmann H. Structural motifs involved in human IgG antibody effector functions. Eur J Immunol 1993;23:1098–1104.
178. Powelson JA, Knowles RW, Delmonico FL, et al. CDR-grafted OKT4A monoclonal antibody in cynomolgus renal allograft recipients. Transplantation 1994;57:788–793.
179. Delmonico FL, Cosimi AB, Kawai T, et al. Non-human primate responses to murine and humanized OKT4A. Transplantation 1993;55:722–728.
180. Land W. Monoclonal antibodies in 1991: new potential options in clinical immunosuppressive therapy. Clin Transplant 1991;5:493–500.
181. Dantal J, Ninin E, Hourmant M, et al. Anti-CD4 MoAb therapy in kidney transplantation—a pilot study in early prophylaxis of rejection. Transplantation 1996;62:1502–1506.
182. Meiser BM, Reiter C, Reichenspurner H, et al. Chimeric monoclonal CD4 antibody—a novel immunosuppressant for clinical heart transplantation. Transplantation 1994;58:419–423.
183. Reinke P, Kern F, Fietze W, et al. Anti-CD4 monoclonal antibody therapy of late acute rejection in renal allograft recipients—CD4+ T cells play an essential role in the rejection process. Transplant Proc 1995;27:859–862.
184. Lazarovits AI, Rochon J, Banks L, et al. Human mouse chimeric CD7 monoclonal antibody for the prophylaxis of kidney transplant rejection. J Clin Invest 1993;150:5163.
185. Waldmann TA. The IL-2/IL-2 receptor system: a target for rational immune intervention. Immunol Today 1993;14:264–269.
186. Kupiec-Weglinski J, Diamantstein T, Tilney NL. Interleukin-2 receptor-targeted therapy—rationale and applications in organ transplantation. Transplantation 1988;46:785–792.
187. Kirkman RL, Shapiro ME, Carpenter CB, et al. A randomized prospective trial of anti-Tac monoclonal antibody in human renal transplantation. Transplantation 1991;51:107–113.
188. Soulillou JP, Cantarovish D, Le ML, et al. Randomized controlled trial of a monoclonal antibody against the interleukin-2 receptor (33B3.1) as compared with rabbit antithymocyte globulin for prophylaxis against rejection of renal allografts. N Engl J Med 1990;322:1175–1182.
189. Cantarovich D, Le Mauff B, Hourmant M, et al. Prevention of acute rejection episodes with an anti-interleukin-2 receptor monoclonal antibody. Results after combined pancreas and kidney transplantation. Transplantation 1994;57:198–203.
190. Reding R, Feyaerts A, Vraux H, et al. Prophylactic immunosuppression with anti-interleukin-2 receptor monoclonal antibody Lo-Tact-1 versus OKT3 in liver allografting. Transplantation 1996;61:1406–1413.
191. van Gelder T, Zietse R, Mulder AH, et al. A double-blind, placebo-controlled study of monoclonal anti-interleukin-2 receptor antibody (BT563) administration to prevent acute rejection after kidney transplantation. Transplantation 1995;60:248–252.

192. Nashan B, Schlitt HJ, Schwinzer R, et al. Immunoprophylaxis with a monoclonal anti-IL-2 receptor antibody in liver transplant patients. Transplantation 1996;61:546–554.
193. Langrehr JM, Nussler NC, Neumann U, et al. A prospective randomized trial comparing interleukin-2 receptor antibody versus antithymocyte globulin as part of a quadruple immunosuppressive induction therapy following orthotopic liver transplantation. Transplantation 1997;63:1772–1781.
194. van Gelder T, Balk AHMM, Jonkman FAM, et al. A randomized trial comparing safety and efficacy of OKT3 and a monoclonal anti-interleukin-2 receptor antibody (BT563) in the prevention of acute rejection after heart transplantation. Transplantation 1996;62:51–55.
195. Tinubu SA, Hakimi J, Kondas JA, et al. Humanized antibody directed to the IL-2 receptor β-chain prolongs primate cardiac allograft survival. J Immunology 1994;153:4330–4338.
196. Amlot PL, Rawlings E, Fernando ON, et al. Prolonged action of a chimeric interleukin-2 receptor (CD25) monoclonal antibody used in cadaveric renal transplantation. Transplantation 1995;60:748–756.
197. Nashan B, Moore R, Amlot P, et al. Randomized trial of basiliximab versus placebo for control of acute cellular rejection in renal allograft recipients. Lancet 1997;350:1193–1198.
198. Vincenti F, Kirkman R, Light SE, et al. Interleukin 2-receptor blockade with Daclizumab to prevent acute rejection in renal transplantation. N Engl J Med 1998;338:161–165.
199. Kahan BD, Rajagopalan PR, Hall M, et al. Reduction of the occurrence of acute cellular rejection among renal allograft recipients treated with basiliximab, a chimeric anti-interleukin-2-receptor monoclonal antibody. United States Simulect Renal Study Group. Transplantation 1999;67:276–284.
200. Nashan B, Light S, Hardie IR, et al. Reduction of acute renal allograft rejection by daclizumab. Daclizumab Double Therapy Study Group. Transplantation 1999;67:110–115.
201. Kovarik J, Breidenbach T, Gerbeau C, et al. Disposition and immunodynamics of basiliximab in liver allograft recipients. Clin Pharmacol Ther 1998;64:66–72.
202. Cantarovich D, Le Mauff B, Hourmant M, et al. Anti-interleukin 2 receptor monoclonal antibody in the treatment of ongoing acute rejection episodes of human kidney graft—a pilot study. Transplantation 1989;47:454–457.
203. Herbelin C, Stephan JL, Donadieu J, et al. Treatment of steroid-resistant acute graft-versus-host disease with an anti IL-2R monoclonal antibody (BT563) in children who received T-cell depleted, partially matched, related bone marrow transplants. Bone Marrow Transplant 1994;13:563–569.
204. Anasetti C, Hansen JA, Waldmann TA, et al. Treatment of acute graft-versus-host disease with humanized anti-Tac, an antibody that binds to the interleukin-2 receptor. Blood 1994;84:1320–1327.
205. Grisham MB, Hernandez LA, Granger DN. Xanthine oxidase and neutrophil infiltration in intestinal ischemia. Am J Physiol 1986;251:G567–G574.
206. Pober JS, Cotran RS. The role of endothelial cells in inflammation. Transplantation 1990;50:537–544.
207. Lasky LA. Selectins: interpreters of cell-specific carbohydrate information during inflammation. Science 1992;258:964–969.
208. Heemann UW, Tullius SG, Azuma H, et al. Adhesion molecules and transplantation. Ann Surg 1994;219:4–12.
209. Isobe M, Yagita H, Okumura K, et al. Specific acceptance of cardiac allograft after treatment with antibodies to ICAM-1 and LFA-1. Science 1992;255:1125–1127.
210. Qin L, Chavin KD, Lin J, et al. Anti-CD2 receptor and anti-CD2 ligand (CD48) antibodies synergize to prolong allograft survival. J Exp Med 1994;179:341–346.
211. Woodward JE, Qin L, Chavin KD, et al. Blockade of multiple costimulatory receptors induces hyporesponsiveness. Transplantation 1996;62:1011–1018.
212. Berlin PJ, Bacher JD, Sharrow SO, et al. Monoclonal antibodies against human T-cell adhesion molecules—modulation of immune function in nonhuman primates. Transplantation 1992;53:840–849.
213. Kaplon RJ, Hochman PS, Michler RE, et al. Short course single agent therapy with an LFA-3-IgG fusion protein prolongs primate cardiac allograft survival. Transplantation 1996;61:356–363.
214. Adams D. Therapeutic potential of inhibiting the ICAM-1/LFA-1 pathway of leukocyte adhesion. In: Salomon DR, Sollinger H, eds. Recent developments in transplantation medicine: adhesion molecules, fusion proteins, novel peptides and monoclonal antibodies. Glenview, IL: Physicians and Scientists, 1995:27–43.
215. Byrne JG, Smith WJ, Murphy MP, et al. Complete prevention of myocardial stunning, contracture, low-reflex and edema after heart transplantation by blocking neutrophil adhesion molecules during reperfusion. J Thorac Cardiovasc Surg 1992;104:1589–1596.
216. Kelly KJ, Williams WJ, Colvin RB, et al. Antibody to intercellular adhesion molecule 1 protects the kidney. Proc Natl Acad Sci USA 1994;91:812–816.
217. DeMeester SR, Molinari MA, Shiraishi T, et al. Attenuation of rat lung isograft reperfusion injury with a combination of anti-ICAM-1 and anti-β_2 integrin monoclonal antibodies. Transplantation 1996;62:1477–1485.
218. Davies MH, Tregunno GA, Scharschmidt L, Neuberger JM. Monoclonal anti-ICAM-1 antibodies in liver transplantation—preliminary results of a phase I trial. Hepatology 1993;18:75a.
219. Maraninchi D, Mawas C, Stoppa AM, et al. Anti LFA1 monoclonal antibody for the prevention of graft rejection after T cell-depleted HLA-matched bone marrow transplantation for leukemia in adults. Bone Marrow Transplant 1989;4:147–150.
220. Hourmant M, Bedrossian J, Durand D, et al. A randomized multicenter trial comparing leukocyte function-associated antigen-1 monoclonal antibody with rabbit antithymocyte globulin as induction treatment in first kidney transplantations. Transplantation 1996;62:1565–1570.
221. Le Mauff B, Hourmant M, Rougier JP, et al. Effect of anti-LFA-1 (CD11a) monoclonal antibodies in acute rejection in human kidney transplantation. Transplantation 1991;52:297–299.
222. Brown SA, Lucas BA, Waid TH, et al. T10B9 (MEDI-500) mediated immunosuppression: studies on the mechanism of action. Clin Transplantation 1996;10:607–613.
223. Ghetie MA, Vitetta ES. Recent developments in immunotoxin therapy. Curr Opinion Immunol 1994;6:707–714.
224. Thomas JM, Neville DM, Contreras JL, et al. Preclinical studies of allograft tolerance in rhesus monkeys. Transplantation 1997;64:124–135.
225. Lenschow DJ, Zeno Y, Hathcock KS, et al. Inhibition of transplant rejection following treatment with anti-B7-2 and anti-B7-1 antibodies. Transplantation 1995;60:1171–1178.
226. Eck SC, Chang D, Wells AD, Turka LA. Differential down-regulation of CD28 by B7-1 and B7-2 engagement. Transplantation 1997;64:1497–1499.

COMMENTARY REFERENCES

1. Soulillou JP, Peyronnet B, Le Mauff B, et al. Prevention of rejection of kidney transplants by monoclonal antibody directed against interleukin 2 receptor. Lancet 1987;1:1339–1342.
2. Nashan B, Moore R, Amlot P, et al. Randomised trial of basiliximab versus placebo for control of acute cellular rejection in renal allograft recipients. Lancet 1997;350:1193–1198.
3. Dantal J, Hourmant M, Cantarovich D, et al. Effect of long-term immunosuppression in kidney-graft recipients on cancer incidence: randomised comparison of two cyclosporine regimens. Lancet 1998;351:623–628.
4. Kirk A, Harlan D, Armstrong N, et al. CTLA4Ig and anti-CD40 ligand prevent renal allograft rejection in primates. Proc Natl Acad Sci 1997;94:8789–8794.
5. Ossevoort M, Ringers J, Boon L, et al. Blocking of costimulatory pathways using monoclonal antibodies to prevent transplant rejection in a non-human primate model. 3rd International Conference on new trends in clinical and experimental immunosuppression. Geneva: Fevrier, 1998.
6. Qin L, Chavin KD, Lin J, et al. Anti-CD2 receptor and anti-CD2 ligand (CD48) antibodies synergized to prolong allograft survival. J Exp Med 1994;179:341–346.
7. Hourmant M, Bedrossian J, Durand D, et al. A randomized multicenter trial comparing leukocyte function-associated antigen-1 monoclonal antibody with rabbit antithymocyte globulin as induction treatment in first kidney transplantations. Transplantation 1996;62:1565–1570.
8. Rabb H, Martin JG. An emerging paradigm shift on the roll of leukocyte adhesion molecules. J Clin Inv 1997;100:2937–2938.
9. Larsen CP, Elwood ET, Alexander DZ, et al. Long-term acceptance of skin and cardiac allografts after blocking CD40 and CD28 pathways. Nature 1996;381:434–439.
10. Isobe M, Yagita H, Okumura K, Ihara A. Specific acceptance of cardiac allograft after treatment with antibodies to ICAM1 and anti LFA-1. Science 1992;255:1125–1127.
11. Thompson CB, Allison JP. The emerging role of CTLA4 as an immune attenuator. Immunity 1997;7:445–450.

12. Perez VL, Van Parijs L, Blucklans A, et al. Induction of peripheral T cell tolerance in vivo requires CTLA-4 engagement. Immunity 1997;6:411–417.
13. Chandraker M, Takada M, Nadeau K, et al. The role of the B7 costimulatory pathway in experimental cold ischemia/reperfusion injury. Kidney Int 1997;52:1678–1684.
14. François C, Dantal J, Sorel M, et al. Antibodies directed at mouse IL-2-R α and β chains act in synergy to abolish T cell proliferation in vitro and delayed type hypersensitivity reaction in vivo. Transplant Int 1996;9:46–50.
15. Audrain M, Boeffard F, Soulillou JP, Jacques Y. Synergistic action of monoclonal antibodies directed at p55 and p75 chain of the human IL-2-receptor. J Immunol 1991;77:780–786.
16. Hourmant M, Dantal J. Adhesion molecules in rejection and tolerance of allografts. Nephrol Dial Transplant 1996;11:1661–1666.
17. He XY, Xu Z, Melrose A, et al. Humanization and pharmacokinetics of a monoclonal antibody with specificity for both E- and P-selectin. J Immunol 1998;160:1029–1035.
18. Madsen JC, Superina RA, Wood KJ, Morris PJ. Immunological unresponsiveness induced by recipient cells transfected with donor MHC genes. Nature 1988;332:161–164.
19. Zavazova N, Kvonke M. Soluble HLA class I molecules induce apoptosis alloreactive cytotoxic T lymphocytes. Nat Med 1996;2:1005–1010.
20. Pichlmayer P, Cantarovich D, Soulillou JP, et al. European Mycophenolate Mofetil Cooperative Study Group. Placebo-controlled study of mycophenolate mofetil combined with cyclosporin and corticosteroids for prevention of acute rejection. Lancet 1995;345:1321–1325.

Chapter

14

Use of Irradiation and Photopheresis for Immunosuppression in Transplantation

Mark Waer

The basis of the immunosuppressive effects of ionizing radiation is complex and depends on various elements such as the irradiation dose, the dose per fraction, the emitting source used, and the status of the irradiated tissue. The timing of the irradiation is also important to the immunologic response; for example, a primary antibody response is more radiosensitive than a secondary one (1). It has been shown that lymphocytes are extremely sensitive to radiotherapy. In contrast to most other cells that die a mitotic death because of radiation-related damage of DNA structures, lymphocytes die a so-called interphase death. This occurs within one hour of an LD50 dose (2). In contrast to resting T lymphocytes, activated T lymphocytes are relatively radioresistant (3). B lymphocytes are more radiosensitive than T lymphocytes but, similar to T lymphocytes, can become extremely radioresistant when activated (1).

Photopheresis is based on the principle of activating inert 8-methoxypsoralen (8-MOP) by ultraviolet-A (UVA) irradiation. Subsequently, activated 8-MOP provokes a firm linkage of DNA strands in such a way that they cannot be separated, which is needed for cell division. The use of photopheresis after transplantation is based on the hypothesis that donor reactive lymphocytes will expand in the recipient peripheral blood. When peripheral blood is subjected to photopheresis, it is mainly this population of reactive lymphocytes that will be affected. Moreover, giving back inactivated donor reactive lymphocytes may "vaccinate" the recipient with these cells, which eventually may induce downregulatory (e.g., anti-idiotypic), immune circuits.

TOTAL BODY IRRADIATION AND LOCAL GRAFT IRRADIATION

The immunosuppressive effects of ionizing radiation were noted early in the twentieth century (4,5), and total body irradiation has been used since the first days of human kidney transplantation (6). Unfortunately, it was soon learned that sublethal total body irradiation (TBI) was insufficient to provoke long-term survival of allografts and that higher doses would result in irreversible bone marrow aplasia and severe gastrointestinal toxicity (6). Other, more selective radiation techniques included irradiation of the graft implantation site (7), extracorporeal irradiation of the blood lymphocytes (7), and irradiation of thoracic duct lymphocytes (7,8). Still other approaches involved the injection of radioactive substances with high affinity for lymphoid tissues (9) or intravascular implantation of sources of high-energy beta emitters (7,10). However, due to technical difficulties, serious side effects, or lack of efficacy, none of these radiation procedures is routinely used in clinical organ transplantation.

Local graft irradiation has been used in many centers to treat acute rejection crises (11). As a favorable effect could never be substantiated in a controlled trial, this procedure has now been abandoned by most centers. The prophylactic effect of the postoperative administration of local graft irradiation, consisting of 600 Gy given in four fractions, was evaluated in a randomized trial (12). There was no apparent benefit in kidney function or time to first rejection episode in the group receiving local graft irradiation. Cadaver allograft survival was also not significantly different between the two treatment arms.

The most interesting form of irradiation for transplantation is total lymphoid irradiation (TLI). This procedure is still being extensively explored in experimental models and has been used for the past 15 years in transplant patients by several centers. TLI is therefore discussed in more detail in the sections that follow.

TOTAL LYMPHOID IRRADIATION

Discovery of TLI as an Immunosuppressant

TLI has been a standard form of therapy for treating patients with Hodgkin's disease (13). Irradiation is administered through two ports (Fig. 14.1): a thoracic "mantle" field, and an abdominal "inverted Y" encompassing the major lymph node areas, the thymus, and the spleen. In order to increase the hematologic tolerance of the procedure, the spleen is frequently removed before TLI. Usually a total dose of 40–50 Gy (1 Gy = 100 rad or cGy) is administered in daily fractions of 1.5–2.5 Gy. In a study of patients treated with TLI for Hodgkin's disease, it was found that cellular immunity was strikingly impaired for up to 10 years after TLI. The absolute number of T lymphocytes as well as their in vitro reactivity to the mitogens phytohemagglutinin (PHA) and concanavalin A (ConA) or allogeneic stimulator cells in the mixed lymphocyte reaction (MLR) was significantly decreased (14). Interestingly, secondary hematologic tumors (15) or clinically important infections (16) were not increased after TLI. These clinical observations prompted researchers at Stanford to investigate the immunosuppressive potential of TLI in experimental models (17).

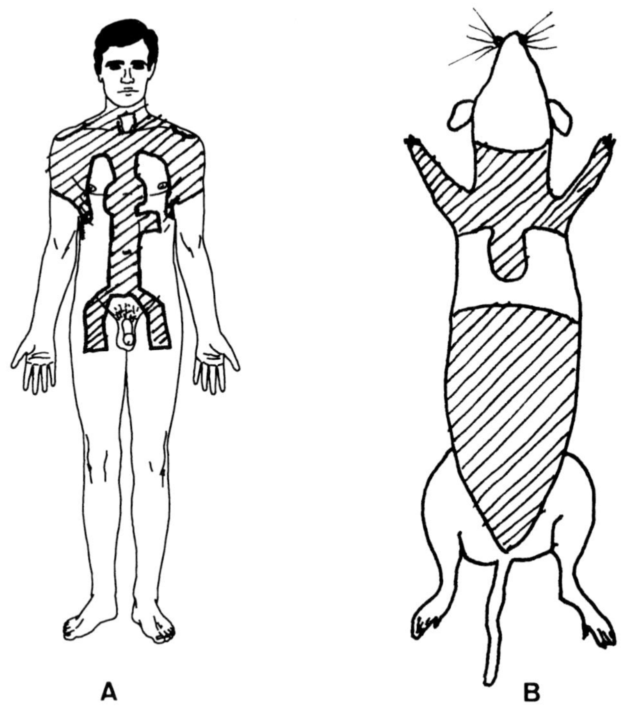

FIGURE 14.1. *TLI irradiation ports as used in patients (**A**) or in experimental studies in rodents (**B**). When no splenectomy is performed, the spleen is usually also included in the irradiation field in patients.*

TLI in Experimental Models

Induction of Specific Transplantation Tolerance in Rodents

A TLI irradiation technique similar to that used in Hodgkin's patients was developed for mice and rats. BALB/c mice were given 17 fractions of 2 Gy daily, delivered to the thoracic and abdominal fields concomitantly. Subsequently, their lymphocyte count as well as PHA, ConA, or MLR reactivity was decreased in a similar fashion as observed in Hodgkin's patients (17). Allogeneic C57BL skin grafts, transplanted one day after TLI, survived five times longer than in unirradiated mice (see Chapter 5). Interestingly, the infusion of 30×10^6 unmanipulated C57BL bone marrow (BM) cells resulted in stable bone marrow chimerism without graft-versus-host disease (GVHD). These chimeras became specifically tolerant to skin grafts originating from the bone marrow donor (17).

The rodent models clearly revealed that several variables determined the success rate of TLI. First, the width of the irradiation field seemed critical. In rats, shielding of even minor parts of the pelvic field prevented the induction of tolerance after TLI (17). Conversely, widening the TLI fields under the form of one or two total body irradiation fractions impressively increased the efficacy of TLI in mice (18). The effect of the total TLI dose was critical (17) and strain related (19). Another important finding with regard to clinical applications was that organ grafts had to be transplanted soon after TLI. Delaying skin graft transplantation to one week after TLI resulted in rapid rejection (17). Presensitization by blood transfusion, even to only minor transplantation antigens, abolished the capacity of TLI to induce stable chimerism (17). The absence of GVHD after TLI was not absolute and depended on the number of T cells present in the bone marrow inoculum (17) or on the level of gut decontamination of the recipient mice (19).

TLI in Large Animal Models

In dogs, although donor bone marrow infusion easily induced chimerism after TLI, it did not appear necessary to obtain long-term heart (20) or kidney allograft (21) survival. Therefore, TLI regimens without bone marrow infusion were further evaluated. A combination of TLI with azathioprine and antithymocyte globulin (ATG) led to an unacceptably high incidence of side effects (22). Addition of continuous high doses (17 mg/kg) of cyclosporine, although very effective, led to lethal lymphomas in 3 of 10 monkeys (22). A combination of 18 fractions of 1 Gy of TLI, followed by a 10-day course of postoperative ATG alone, induced specific transplantation tolerance in 40% of the transplanted dogs (23). A similar regimen was, however, much less effective in a kidney or a pancreas allograft model (24). Hence, from the overall experience in dogs it was not easy to determine which TLI-based regimen would be most suitable for patients.

In splenectomized rhesus monkeys, four to five TLI fractions of 125 cGy each were administered beginning on day 1 after kidney allografting. This was combined with five injections of ATG beginning on day 0. At the time of kidney grafting, recipients received DR– CD3– donor bone marrow cells. An actuarial one-year graft survival without chronic immunosuppression was obtained (25). Microchimerism was documented within skin only. Not depleting the CD3 cells from the donor bone marrow resulted in more generalized microchimerism but, unfortunately, also in subclinical GVHD and inferior one-year graft survival rates (25).

Eight fractions of 1 Gy of TLI delivered over four weeks, but administered through a very wide TLI field, was shown to be very effective in baboons (26). Such a TLI regimen was effective even without administering bone marrow or extra drugs. In two-thirds of the baboons, specific and permanent tolerance toward solid grafts was obtained (26). Altogether, the various experiments performed in monkeys seem to confirm the tolerogenic capacity of TLI as observed in small rodents.

Mechanisms Involved in the Immunomodulatory Action of TLI

Many experiments were performed, mostly in the mouse model, to unravel the mechanisms facilitating tolerance induction after TLI. Suppressor cells were shown to be expanded in the spleen from mice soon after the end of TLI (27). These cells nonspecifically suppressed many immune reactions in vitro. These so-called natural suppressor cells were cloned and shown to express a surface phenotype similar to that of natural killer (NK) cells (i.e., Thy 1+, asialo GM+, Ig–, Lyt 1–, Lyt 2–, Ia–, MAC1–) (28). Nevertheless, these post-TLI suppressor cells did not display NK activity (28). Moreover, they expressed mRNA transcripts for the α, β, and γ T-cell receptor chains, indicating a T-cell–like origin (29). That these nonspecific suppressor cells played a role in the induction of stable BM chimerism after TLI was elaborated from various experiments. First, it was demonstrated that the level of induction of these cells after various TLI regimens correlated well with the relative capacity of these regimens to allow for induction of chimerism after TLI (18,19). Second, coinjection of cloned post-TLI natural suppressor cells was able to prevent the induction of GVHD in cotransfer experiments in mice (30). Third, injection of asialo GM1 antibodies after TLI resulted in the disappearance of post-TLI suppressor cells and concomitantly in the appearance of severe GVHD in a majority of BM transplanted mice (31,32). Whether these nonspecific suppressor cells are also necessary to maintain tolerance after TLI is less clear. Moreover, their persistence or role in inducing specific suppressor cells has been difficult to demonstrate in long-term tolerant TLI-treated mice (33–35). Therefore, other tolerance mechanisms have been suggested to play a role as well.

The presence of clonal anergy in tolerant post-TLI T cells was demonstrated in various models (36,37). These anergized cells were incapable of proliferating, even in the presence of exogenous interleukin 2 (IL-2) (36). In some situations, clonal deletion was demonstrated as well. It was clearly shown that donor- and host-type thymocytes underwent clonal deletion for host and donor antigens, respectively, in the thymus of TLI-treated mice (37). It was also found that TLI-treated rats, developing tolerance for allogeneic antigens, had decreased precursor frequencies of anti-donor cytotoxic T lymphocytes (CTLs) from three months post-TLI (38).

The most recent data suggest that "immunoredirection" may take place after TLI. It is suggested that the post-TLI environment facilitates the preferential development of T_H2-type lymphocytes (secreting IL-4, IL-5, IL-10) at the expense of T_H1 lymphocytes (secreting IL-2 or interferon gamma) (39–41). (See Chapters 5 and 12 for further discussion of T_H1 and T_H2 lymphocytes.) Apparently, alloantigen priming in the immediate post-TLI phase results in a shift of the allospecific cytokine pattern toward T_H2 cytokines by enhancing IL-4–producing CD4 cells and preventing maturation of interferon gamma (IFN-γ)-producing cells. In a study in baboons developing transplantation tolerance toward a kidney allograft, blocking low-affinity IgG antibodies directed at donor antigen presenting cells were demonstrated (42). As the formation of non-Fc binding, noncomplement-fixing IgG antibodies may be the expression of T_H2 activity, this observation may further indicate that TLI facilitates T_H2-type immune reactions.

TLI in Xenotransplantation Experiments

One of the first major hurdles to overcome in xenotransplantation is the occurrence of early humoral rejection, which is mainly provoked by IgM xenoantibodies. These antibodies can be either preexisting, in the case of discordant, phylogenetically distant species combinations, or they can be rapidly induced in the case of closer, concordant combinations (see Chapter 40). Apparently, in most cases these IgM xenoantibodies are T-cell–independent. Although it had been previously shown that TLI was not very active in blocking T-cell–independent antibody formation, it seemed very active in suppressing the antihamster antibody formation in rats. When combined with cyclosporine (CsA) and splenectomy (43), with CsA and anti-CD4 monoclonal antibodies (44), or with deoxyspergualin (45), heart xenograft survival was significantly prolonged and xenoantibody formation was delayed and significantly suppressed. Also in the concordant cynomolgus monkey-to-baboon combination, TLI was exquisitely effective, especially when combined with CsA and methylprednisolone (46–48). Xenograft survival times of more than one year were obtained. Also in these primates, IgM xenoantibody formation was totally suppressed by TLI (46). Nevertheless, the total IgM or IgG blood levels were not altered. These data suggest that TLI may be specifically active on the B-lymphocyte subpopulations that are producing so-called natural xenoantibodies.

Several experiments were performed in order to determine whether TLI could also provoke a decrease of the titer of preexisting IgM xenoantibodies as seen in discordant combinations. In the guinea pig-to-rat combination, a three-week TLI treatment regimen together with azathioprine, cyclosporine, and methylprednisolone resulted in a significant decrease of the preexisting xenoantibody titer. This was unfortunately not accompanied with a prolongation of xenograft survival (49). In the pig islet-into-rat xenograft model, however, TLI was extremely effective when combined with deoxyspergualin (50). Also, in a discordant large animal model involving lamb heart transplantation into pigs, a one-week treatment regimen with TLI, CsA, and azathioprine resulted in a significant decrease of the xenoantibody titer and concomitantly a 30-fold increase of the mean xenograft survival time (51).

In view of the renewed interest in xenotransplantation, the capacity of TLI to influence natural xenoantibodies clearly deserves further exploration.

TLI in Clinical Kidney Transplantation

TLI and Low-Dose Prednisone in Diabetic Renal Allograft Recipients

Between the end of 1981 and the end of 1988, 54 insulin-dependent patients with end-stage renal disease due to diabetic nephropathy were transplanted at the University of Leuven. Twenty-seven of them were given pretransplant TLI followed by low-dose maintenance prednisone after transplantation. The 27 other patients were treated with CsA and a similar low-dose prednisone protocol. The details of the TLI and CsA protocols have been described elsewhere (52–54). TLI patients were given daily fractions of 1 Gy of TLI. In order to be able to irradiate the mantle and inverted Y fields concomitantly, a splenectomy was performed in 18 patients to lower the risk of leukopenia or thrombocytopenia. A minimal total dose of 20 Gy was given to all patients. When a crossmatch-negative donor was not available within two weeks of TLI, extra fractions were administered on a weekly basis, to a maximal cumulative dose of 30 Gy. In all patients, a donor kidney was found within one month after the last TLI fraction. As early transplantation after completion of TLI was considered a priority, only major blood group (ABO) and not histocompatibility matching was taken into account. After transplantation, only 20 to 30 mg of prednisone was given daily and tapered within two weeks to 10 mg per day, which was continued as maintenance therapy. Ten patients in each group were included in a randomized controlled trial. Details and short-term results of this controlled trial have been published elsewhere (54). Here, the long-term results obtained in both groups, also including the patients of the controlled trial, are reported.

As can be seen from Figures 14.2A and 14.2B, patient and graft survival are significantly inferior in the TLI group (Wilcoxon $P < 0.05$ and $P < 0.006$, respectively). Clearly, the TLI regimen as used in this study was unable to provide acceptable graft and patient survival rates. This was also reflected by the fact that TLI-treated patients developed significantly more rejection crises than CsA-treated recipients. Only 4 of the 27 TLI patients did not develop a rejection crisis, and 9 of 27 underwent more than one rejection crisis. In contrast, 14 of 27 CsA patients were rejection free, and only 5 of 27 developed more than one rejection episode. This weak overall immunosuppressive effect of TLI explains why in TLI patients other maintenance immunosuppressants such as azathioprine (4) or CsA (5) had to be introduced. The primary aim of omitting maintenance immunosuppressants in TLI-treated patients was, therefore, not met in the majority of TLI-treated patients.

The major causes of death among the 15 deceased TLI patients were sepsis, which occurred in seven, and cardiovascular accidents, which occurred in five patients. One TLI patient, who was a heavy smoker, died because of lung cancer. In the CsA group, nine patients died of a cardiovascular accident, one of suicide, and three due to sepsis. In all the patients who died as a result of sepsis, high doses of steroids had been given to treat rejection. Hence, the excess mortality due to sepsis that was observed in the TLI patients was indirectly the consequence of the lower capacity of TLI to prevent the occurrence of rejection crises. The overall conclusion of this study is that TLI is insufficient by itself to guarantee good kidney graft survival rates in patients. Clearly, further manipulations such as the infusion of bone marrow cells or the addition of other immunosuppressants than steroids are needed. This experience actually confirms what was observed in most animal models: without the infusion of donor bone marrow or the administration of supplementary immunosuppressants, the induction of transplantation tolerance was rarely achieved with TLI.

TLI with Low-Dose Prednisone and Postoperative ATG

The experience at the University of Leuven clearly showed that a combination of TLI with low-dose prednisone resulted in insufficient immunosuppression in most patients. Based on this preliminary experience and encouraged by the results obtained with TLI combined with ATG in dogs (23), a collaborative program involving preoperative TLI and postoperative ATG and low-dose prednisone (TAP) was initiated at Stanford University and Pacific Medical Center in San Francisco (55,56). Twenty fractions of 1 Gy were administered over a mean period of 12 weeks. A crossmatch-negative cadaver donor was found at a mean interval of nine days after

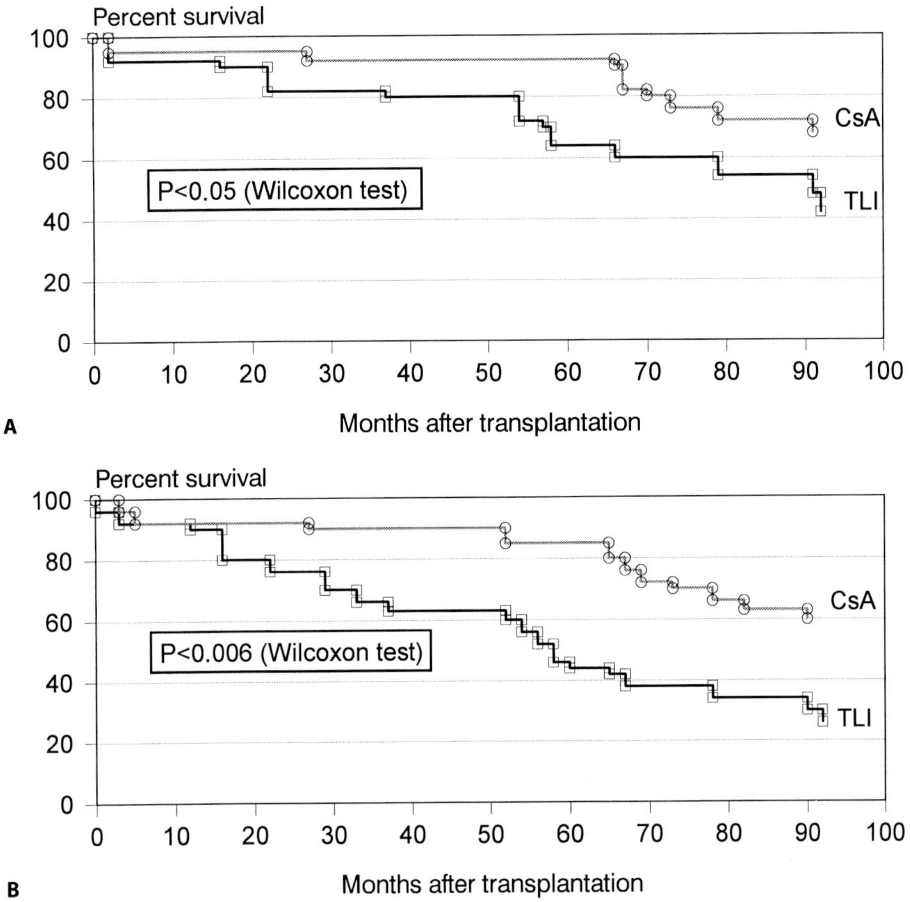

FIGURE 14.2. *Patient survival (**A**) and graft survival (**B**) in patients treated with TLI versus patients receiving CsA immunosuppression.*

the last TLI fraction. After transplantation, six courses of ATG were given and a low-dose prednisone maintenance therapy was initiated. Although the initial short-term results were very favorable (55), a long-term analysis in 52 patients receiving this TAP protocol showed that it was much less effective than a standard protocol of CsA and prednisone (three-year graft survival rates of 50% and 75%, respectively, were observed) (56). All immunosuppressive medication could be stopped in three patients who had remained rejection free for more than one year. Two of these showed specific non-reactivity to their donor cells in MLR (56,57). Unfortunately, two of the patients in whom all drugs were withdrawn developed a rejection six months later.

These results showed that the addition of prednisone and ATG is also not sufficient to increase the efficacy of TLI. Therefore, the same investigators added maintenance therapy with CsA to a similar TAP protocol in six patients. After more than two years, none of these patients underwent rejection crises (56). This protocol, therefore, may hold promise for the future.

Wide-Field TLI with Cyclosporine

A wide-field TLI irradiation protocol was developed at the University of Johannesburg (58,59). The irradiation field involved the entire torso from the base of the skull down to and including the pelvis and proximal end of femora and humeri. Ribs and lungs were shielded. In approximately one-half of baboons receiving this wide-field TLI regimen as eight fractions of 1 Gy over a four-week period, specific allotransplant tolerance without the need for extra drugs was achieved (26).

Fifty-six patients were treated using a similar TLI regimen before allogeneic cadaveric kidney transplantation. After transplantation, CsA and low-dose prednisone were given. The one- and five-year actuarial graft survival was 86% and 60%, respectively (59). In 12 patients, CsA elimination was attempted. However, in nine of them reinstitution of CsA or commencement of azathioprine was necessary.

This illustrates that with this TLI regimen, which was intensively investigated in a relevant baboon preclinical model, the aim of inducing specific tolerance was almost impossible to achieve. The authors suggested that presensitization, which was usually present in their patients, may be responsible for this inferior outcome. Indeed, among their patients, recipients with pretransplantation panel reactive antibodies (PRA) of more than 30% did significantly worse than the other patients (59).

TLI Immunosuppression for Immunologic High-Risk Patients

Twenty patients who previously had rejected a first or second renal allograft were given TLI in a total dose ranging between 10 and 40 Gy at the University of Minnesota (60).

Historically, such patients had a two-year graft survival of less than 40% using an azathioprine-prednisone–based immunosuppression. After TLI, the patients were given post-operative azathioprine and prednisone. The graft survival was significantly increased to 70% at two years and did not change subsequently (61). Later, similarly improved second graft survival rates could be obtained using CsA as well. Because of the ease of the latter regimen, TLI was abandoned (61).

At the University of Rome, two TLI-based regimens were evaluated for treating highly sensitized recipients (62,63). When treated with azathioprine and prednisone, only 10% of similar patients had functioning grafts at one year after transplantation. In a first regimen, 14 patients were given 25–35 Gy of TLI, followed by antilymphocyte globulin (ALG), prednisone, and azathioprine. The one-year graft survival was 64%, and 7 of the 14 patients did not develop any rejection crises (62). A second group of 13 highly immunized patients (four due to blood transfusions and nine due to previous transplantation) was given 20 Gy of TLI, followed by low-dose steroids and CsA. The one-year graft survival in this group was 69%, and 6 patients remained rejection free (62). A follow-up report indicated that the eight-year actuarial graft survival remained at 69% (63).

Post-transplantation TLI for the Treatment of Cardiac Allograft Rejection

Although it is generally accepted that TLI is most effective when administered before the alloantigen challenge, the use of post-transplantation TLI was investigated in a rat model and subsequently successfully explored in cardiac allograft recipients (see Chapter 23). In combination with anti-CD3 monoclonal antibodies, or with ATG together with donor-specific blood transfusions, post-transplantation TLI resulted in long-term specific transplantation tolerance in a strongly immunogenic heart transplant model in rats (64).

After some anecdotal reports of successful clinical use of post-transplantation TLI for the reversal of conventional therapy–resistant cardiac rejection (65,66), the efficacy of 10 fractions of 0.8 Gy of TLI was evaluated in 49 heart transplant patients suffering resistant rejection (n = 44) or early severe vascular rejection (n = 5) at the University of Alabama at Birmingham (67). A significant decrease of the rejection frequency ($P < 0.0001$) was observed in these patients. The reduced post-TLI rejection frequencies were maintained for at least two years. There was no increase in the frequency of infections after TLI, nor were there any deaths during or immediately following TLI (67). These results convinced the investigators that it would be unethical to deny high-risk patients the TLI treatment, despite the lack of appropriate control subjects. Along the same line, based on limited results in six patients, Valentine et al (68) suggested that TLI may be useful for the treatment of intractable acute allograft rejection following heart–lung and lung transplantation.

Discussion

After demonstration of its safety and potential for inducing tolerance in animal models, TLI has been explored in clinical transplantation. The clinical experience reaffirms that TLI is indeed a safe procedure. In nearly all studies, the patient survival rates of the TLI groups were at least as good as in the control groups. Only in the Leuven study in diabetics did TLI-treated patients have significantly lower survival rates. However, as previously mentioned, this excessive mortality was probably related to steroid therapy for rejection crises, which were more common in the TLI group, rather than to intrinsic radiation-related risks.

The major concern when using irradiation in patients is the enhanced risk of tumor development. As could be expected from the experience in Hodgkin's patients, cancers were not more common during the early follow-up of TLI-treated renal transplant recipients. Among the more than 200 such recipients, only five neoplasia-related deaths were documented. Two patients of the Minnesota group developed a lethal lymphoma. As these patients had undergone retransplantation and had previously also received antithymocyte globulins, these deaths are more likely a consequence of overimmunosuppression in general than of TLI in particular. Two other deaths, one due to lung cancer in a heavy smoker in Leuven and one due to pelvic carcinoma in Johannesburg, are also unlikely to be related to irradiation. The only possible irradiation-related death may be the patient dying from myeloid leukemia in Johannesburg. However, in view of a recent report showing a high cumulative incidence of solid tumors in TLI-treated children with Hodgkin's disease starting from 15 years after TLI (69), a close follow-up of TLI-treated transplant patients seems indicated.

As far as the efficacy of TLI is concerned, a distinction must be made between its nonspecific action as an adjunct immunosuppressant and its capacity to induce transplantation tolerance. As an adjunct immunosuppressant added to standard regimens such as azathioprine-prednisone or CsA-prednisone, TLI seems to be extremely efficient. The best example of this comes from the heart transplantation experience. Here, TLI seemed exquisitely effective for the treatment of recurrent or severe vascular rejection. However, as several new immunosuppressive drugs seem able to decrease the incidence of rejection crises when added to CsA-based immunosuppressive schedules, it is unlikely that TLI will find widespread application as an adjunct immunosuppressant for clinical transplantation.

The primary aim of using TLI to achieve transplantation tolerance in a majority of patients has clearly not been achieved. In almost all centers, long-term maintenance immunosuppression was needed. Although the induction of specific transplantation tolerance without maintenance therapy was documented in a few patients, in the majority of other patients, interruption of maintenance immunosuppression was unsuccessful. This weak capacity to induce transplantation tolerance in patients as compared to animals was most striking in the Johannesburg experience. Although these investigators had carefully selected the most efficient TLI-based regimen in a very relevant preclinical model in baboons, a similar TLI schedule was not able to induce tolerance in their patients. Apparently, antigen disparity between donors and recipients is more pronounced in patients than in the less-outbred baboons. Moreover, pre-transplantation sensitization, which was shown in various models to hamper the tolerance-inducing capacity of TLI, is very likely more common in patients.

As multiple TLI regimens have now been explored in the clinic, it seems that a totally new approach is needed in order to achieve clinical tolerance with TLI. From that point of view, the East Carolina University experience in rhesus monkeys involving post-transplant TLI together with the infusion of DR– CD3– donor bone marrow is very appealing, but awaits confirmation in the clinic.

Xenotransplantation is now increasingly considered an achievable option to solve the lack of donor organs for clinical transplantation. Although it was known that the effects of TLI were strongest on T-cell immunity, it is fascinating to observe that TLI is very effective in suppressing or decreasing the formation of T-cell–independent IgM xenoantibodies as well. This suggests that TLI may specifically act on B-lymphocyte subpopulations responsible for the formation of these so-called natural antibodies. A confirmation that TLI suppresses xenoantibody formation will be important if and when xenotransplantation becomes a clinical reality.

THE USE OF PHOTOPHERESIS FOR TRANSPLANTATION

Photopheresis, which includes a combination of leukopheresis and administration of the photosensitive drug 8-MOP followed by extracorporeal photoirradiation with long-wavelength UVA irradiation, was developed by Edelson et al (70) for the treatment of erythrodermic cutaneous T-cell lymphoma. As this treatment achieved remarkable remissions (70) and the proliferating malignant T lymphocytes were primarily of the T helper type, it was hypothesized that a similar treatment regimen may be of use for treating transplant recipients.

Experimental Studies

The potential use of photopheresis was supported by positive experiments in mice (71,72). Spleen cells taken at the time of skin graft rejection were exposed to 8-MOP and UVA irradiation. When reinfused, these cells were able to provoke significant skin graft survival. Studies in a primate cardiac xenotransplantation model showed a synergistic action between CsA, steroids, and photopheresis resulting in extended xenograft survival (73,74).

Clinical Studies

Photopheresis has been used successfully for the treatment of moderately severe heart transplant rejection. In this trial, eight of nine episodes could be reversed with one or two courses (75). However, interstitial T-cell infiltrates persisted longer as compared with steroid-treated control recipients.

Photopheresis was also successfully added to adjunct antibody therapy to prevent rejection of transplants in high-risk patients characterized by the presence of increased levels of lymphocytotoxic antibodies (76). In another study, photopheresis was used for adjunct immunosuppression without concomitant antibody therapy in 15 heart transplant recipients receiving standard triple drug immunosuppression (77). Ten or twenty photopheresis courses were given starting on the first day after heart transplantation. In this study, a new liquid form of 8-MOP was added directly to the buffy coat, resulting in reliable and sufficient drug levels in the cell suspension that is not always achievable after oral application of 8-MOP. Over the total observation time of about 10 months, both photopheresis regimens significantly reduced the number of acute rejection episodes by more than 50% as compared to the control group. Probably as a consequence of the lower need for rejection treatments, photopheresis patients developed significantly fewer infections than control patients. A subsequent multi-institution randomized trial has confirmed that addition of photopheresis to conventional immunosuppression significantly decreases the risk of cardiac rejection; however, survival was not improved in this study (78).

Overall, these first clinical experiences suggest that photopheresis is a safe and effective method of adjunct immunosuppression that should be further explored as an alternative for antibody-based adjunct immunosuppressive regimens.

COMMENTARY

J. A. Myburgh

Experience over some 30 years with experimental organ allotransplantation in the chacma baboon leaves the dominant impression of the uniquely potent tolerogenic effects of a modified regimen of total lymphoid irradiation (TLI), especially when compared with other methods of immune manipulation that are highly effective in rodent models but only modestly so in this primate. Nevertheless, the application of this method to the clinical situation has been rather disappointing, in both our experience and that of a few other centers. The reasons are not wholly clear, but several aspects are probably relevant.

The technique and regimen of TLI used in our baboons was developed from the pioneering work in rodents by Strober and his colleagues at Stanford. One aspect that we have repeatedly emphasized is the *necessity for a wide field of irradiation*. In essence, this includes irradiation of the entire torso from the base of the skull downward, including the pelvis and the upper ends of the humeri and femora (1). In the baboon, shielding to produce fields similar to the mantle and inverted-Y used in the treatment of Hodgkin's disease abolished tolerance production, as was observed in rodents. It is to be emphasized that in nearly all experimental reports from other laboratories and in all clinical series apart from ours, mantle and inverted-Y fields have been used. We believe that the use of the narrower fields is at least partially responsible for the failure of other laboratories to produce tolerance with TLI alone.

In terms of dosage of irradiation, the regimen used in the rodents, namely 17 fractions of 200 cGy each given five days per week, was found to be unacceptably toxic when given to the same wide field in the baboon. An exhaustive series of studies to determine a safe but effective regimen for the baboon resulted in a regimen of a total dose of 800 cGy given in fractions of 80 or 100 cGy twice a week. The dose response curve was parabolic, with lower or higher cumulative doses being less effective in terms of the proportion of recipients made tolerant (1).

The injection of donor bone marrow is certainly not necessary to achieve tolerance in the baboon, and in fact we found it consistently counterproductive whether whole bone marrow, several marrow fractions, or T cell–depleted bone marrow was used. This is in contradistinction to the original rodent experience and is of particular interest in the light of current work on the potential role of microchimerism in tolerance production.

The tolerance produced in baboons by TLI alone is highly specific and durable (2). Skin grafts from the kidney donor are permanently accepted while third-party skin or kidneys are rejected in an unmodified fashion. These baboons have maintained normal graft function for up to 10 years after transplantation, at which time they have been sacrificed for logistic reasons. However, tolerance is attained in only one-third to two-thirds of baboons in different groups and the likelihood of success has not been predictable in individual animals by in vitro tests. Accordingly, over the years we have studied a variety of additive measures in attempts to increase the predictability of tolerance induction and the fraction of tolerant animals obtained. These have included short post-transplant courses of immunosuppressive agents such as both antihuman and antibaboon antithymocyte globulin (ATG), prednisone, cyclosporine, mycophenolate mofetil, and deoxyspergualin; the injection of solubilized donor histocompatibility antigens; and the intrathymic injection of donor lymphoid cells (3). With none of these was there any evidence of a synergistic or even an additive effect to TLI. With all the immunosuppressive agents except ATG, and particularly with cyclosporine, the effect was, in fact, counterproductive in that tolerance was hardly ever obtained. This suggests that these agents were opposing an active tolerogenic mechanism. This is further supported by our finding that the addition of two fractions of TLI after transplantation totally abrogated the tolerogenic effect of the pretransplant course. The addition of intrathymic donor glomeruli had no effect either positive or negative, but intrathymic donor lymphoid cells after pretransplant TLI sensitized the animals and produced accelerated acute rejection. The thymus of most mature adult baboons is atrophic and not encapsulated, and it is not possible to prevent extrathymic extravasation of the injectate. This may be the reason why the results were so different from those obtained in rodents.

It was the unpredictability of tolerance production in individual animals that led us, for obvious ethical reasons, to use conventional immunosuppressive agents following kidney transplantation for patients conditioned with pretransplant TLI. The recognized difference in actuarial survival between patients with panel reactive antibodies of more than 30% and those with less than 30%, and the fact that nearly one-third of our patients were so substantially presensitized (whereas none of our baboons were presensitized), may partially account for the less encouraging results obtained in our clinical trials. We also believe, however, that the results in the baboons showing the counterproductive effects of post-transplant immunosuppressive agents following pretransplant TLI may help to explain the lack of tolerance production in our patients. In addition, attention is drawn again to the fact that other clinical series did not use the wide-field irradiation found to be necessary for tolerance production in both rodents and baboons. While it is clear from the baboon studies that measures in addition to pretransplant TLI, or possibly a modification of the irradiation regimen, will be necessary for more consistent tolerance production, clinical studies without the initial use of additional immunosuppressive drugs after transplantation would appear to be justified and indicated. Attaining tolerance in even one-third of patients, thereby removing the need for post-transplant immunosuppressive drug therapy, would be a very important and most gratifying achievement.

A clearer understanding of the potential mechanisms of tolerance production by TLI should contribute to a more rational search for appropriate additional measures. Our studies in tolerant baboons have shown three patterns of mixed lymphocyte reactions (MLRs): 1) donor specific hypo- or unresponsiveness in 5 of 12 baboons studied up to 4.5 years after transplantation, 2) broad nonspecific hyporesponsiveness to both donor and third-party baboons in another 5 tolerant baboons, and 3) donor responsiveness with a nonspecific suppressor factor in the serum of the other 2 tolerant baboons (5). This suppressor factor was also demonstrated in the serum of three of the baboons with hyporesponsiveness. Nonspecific non-T suppressor cells expressing myeloid-associated antigens CD11b and CD38 were demonstrated by add-in experiments to be involved in most of the MLR suppression (6).

We have also studied this regimen of TLI in chacma baboon–to–vervet monkey kidney xenotransplantation (7,8). The results obtained have approximated those in baboon kidney allotransplantation. With pretransplant TLI alone, 2 of 6 monkeys survived for 364 and 550 days before the grafts were rejected. In a group that received an additional 10 mg/kg of ATG on days −1 and 0, 2 of 4 monkeys survived for 289 and 293 days. However, the additional administration of mycophenolate mofetil was counterproductive in terms of graft survival. As in the baboon allotransplantation studies, the intrathymic injection of donor spleen cells on day 7 abolished the graft-prolonging effect of pretransplant TLI.

Immunologic studies in the two long-surviving monkeys receiving TLI alone revealed the development of low levels of nonspecific cytotoxic antibodies against baboon but not monkey lymphocytes (15% to 29% cell lysis by ^{51}Cr release assays) three weeks after transplantation. These persisted until three months after transplantation. Most of the cytotoxicity was due to IgM. Antibody-dependent cellular cytotoxicity with the use of normal monkey lymphocyte effectors paralleled complement-dependent cytotoxicity, and lymphocyte-mediated cytotoxicity was also present transiently during the antibody-positive period. TLI obliterated the proliferative response of monkey lymphocytes to IL-2, ConA, and PHA. MLR to baboon cells was markedly reduced after TLI, with slow recovery toward pre-TLI levels five months after transplantation. TLI inhibited mitogen-induced IL-2 synthesis to below measurable levels (10 fmol/mL) for two months. Synthesizing ability for IL-2 recovered fully by five months after transplantation without any immediate deterioration of graft function. Sera collected 32 days after transplantation blocked one-way donor-specific and nonspecific MLR using cryopreserved pre-TLI recipient lymphocytes as responders. Open-wedge biopsies of these two grafts three months after transplantation revealed only occasional periglomerular and interstitial foci of chronic inflammatory cells. Immunofluorescence staining revealed focal glomerular deposits of IgM and IgG but no complement.

These findings are of interest and potential relevance to the possibility of baboon-to-human transplantation, although direct extrapolation is clearly not yet possible. The possible impact of species differences is shown by our studies in which the same regimen of TLI was totally ineffective in the reciprocal interprimate combination of monkey-to-baboon kidney transplantation. We feel that TLI should also be studied in discordant combinations such as pig-to-baboon transplantation, in conjunction with measures directed toward the complement and natural antibody components of the immunologic reaction.

CHAPTER REFERENCES

1. Anderson RE, Warner NL. Ionizing radiation and the immune response. Adv Immunol 1976;24:215–335.
2. Kaplan HS. Selective effects of total lymphoid irradiation (TLI) on the immune response. Transplant Proc 1981;13:425–428.
3. Sprent J, Anderson RE, Miller JFAP. Radiosensitivity of T and B lymphocytes. II. Effect of irradiation on response of T cells to alloantigens. Eur J Immunol 1974;4:204–210.
4. Heincke H. Uber die Einwirkung der Röntgenstrahlen auf Tiere. Muenc Med Wochenschr 1903;50:2090–2092.
5. Benjamin E, Sulka E. Antikörperbildung nach experimenteller Schadgung des haematopoietischen Systems durch Röntgenstrahlen. Wien Klin Wochenschr 1908;21:311–314.
6. Hamburger J, Vayse J, Crosnier J, et al. Renal homotransplantation in man after radiation of the recipient. Am J Med 1962;32:854–871.
7. Hume DM, Wolf JS. Abrogation of the immune response: irradiation therapy and lymphocyte depletion. Modification of renal homograft rejection by irradiation. Transplantation 1967;5:1174–1191.
8. Joel DD, Chanana AD, Cronkite EP, Schiffer LM. Modification of skin allograft immunity by extracorporeal irradiation of lymph. Transplantation 1967;5:1192–1197.
9. Hardy MA, Oluwole S, Fawwaz R, et al. Selective lymphoid irradiation. Transplantation 1982;33:237–242.
10. Wolf JS, Hume DM. Transplant immunity in animals with lymphocytopenia induced by indwelling beta irradiation. Surg Forum 1965;16:202–204.
11. Johnson HK, Malcolm A, Al-Abdulla S, et al. The effect of local graft irradiation upon the reversal of cadaveric renal allograft rejection. Transplant Proc 1985;17:2–31.
12. Torrisi JR, Dritschilo A, Harter KW, et al. A randomized study of the efficacy of adjuvant local graft irradiation following renal transplantation. Int J Radiat Oncol Biol Phys 1990;18:1027–1031.
13. Kaplan HS. Hodgkin's disease. 2nd ed. Cambridge, MA: Harvard University, 1980.
14. Fuks Z, Strober S, Bobrove AM, et al. Long term effects of radiation on T and B lymphocytes in peripheral blood of patients with Hodgkin's disease. J Clin Invest 1976;58:803–814.
15. Pedersen-Bjergaard J, Larsen SO. Incidence of acute nonlymphocytic leukemia, preleukemia, and acute myeloproliferative syndrome up to 10 years after treatment of Hodgkin's disease. N Engl J Med 1982;307:965–971.
16. Goffinet DR, Glatstein E, Merigan RD. Herpes zoster-varicella infections and lymphoma. Ann Inter Med 1970;76:235–239.
17. Strober S, Slavin S, Gottlieb M, et al. Allograft tolerance after total lymphoid irradiation (TLI). Immunol Rev 1979;46:87–112.
18. Waer M, Ang KK, van der Schueren E, Vandeputte M. Influence of radiation field and fractionation schedule of total lymphoid irradiation (TLI) on the induction of suppressor cells and stable chimerism after bone marrow transplantation in mice. J Immunol 1984;132:985–990.
19. Waer M, Ang KK, van der Schueren E, Vandeputte M. Allogeneic bone marrow transplantation in mice after total lymphoid irradiation: influence of breeding conditions and strain of recipient mice. J Immunol 1984;132:991–996.
20. Gottlieb M, Strober S, Hoppe RT, et al. Engraftment of allogeneic bone marrow without graft-versus-host disease in mongrel dogs using total lymphoid irradiation. Transplantation 1980;29:487–491.
21. Howard RJ, Sutherland DER, Lum CT, et al. Kidney allograft survival in dogs treated with total lymphoid irradiation. Ann Surg 1981;193:196–200.
22. Pennock JL, Reitz BA, Bieber CP, et al. Survival of primates following orthotopic cardiac transplantation treated with total lymphoid irradiation and chemical immune suppression. Transplantation 1981;32:467–473.
23. Koretz SH, Gottlieb MS, Strober S, et al. Organ transplantation in mongrel dogs using total lymphoid irradiation (TLI). Transplant Proc 1981;13:443–445.
24. Williamson P, Allen RD, Deane SA, et al. Canine pancreas and kidney transplantation following total-lymphoid irradiation. Transplantation 1990;50:576–579.
25. Thomas J, Alqaisi M, Cunningham P, et al. The development of a posttransplant TLI treatment strategy that promotes organ allograft acceptance without chronic immunosuppression. Transplantation 1992;53:247–258.
26. Myburgh JA, Smit JA, Browde S, Stark JH. Current status of total lymphoid irradiation. Transplant Proc 1983;11:659–667.
27. Strober S. Natural suppressor (NS) cells, neonatal tolerance, and total lymphoid irradiation: exploring obscure relationships. Ann Rev Immunol 1984;2:97–115.

28. Schwadron RB, Strober S. Cloned natural suppressor cells derived from the neonatal spleen: in vitro action and lineage. Transplant Proc 1987;19:533.
29. Hertel-Wulff B, Lindsten T, Schwadron R, et al. Rearrangement and expression of T cell receptor genes in cloned murine natural suppressor cell lines. J Exp Med 1987;166:1168.
30. Hertel-Wulff B, Palathumpat V, Schwadron RB, et al. Prevention of GVHD by natural suppressor cells. Transplant Proc 1987;19:536–538.
31. De Ruysscher D, Sobis H, Vandeputte M, Waer M. A subset of asialo GM1+ cells play a protective role in the occurrence of graft-versus-host disease in mice. J Immunol 1991;146:4065–4070.
32. Waer M, Salam A, Vandeputte M. Protective role of asialo GM1+, NK1.1$^-$ cells in the occurrence of graft-versus-host disease after total lymphoid irradiation. Transplantation 1993;56:1049–1050.
33. Okada S, Palathumpat V, Strober S. Identification of donor-derived antigen-specific suppressor cells in murine bone marrow chimeras prepared with total-lymphoid irradiation. Transplantation 1983;36:417.
34. Slavin S, Morecki S, Weigensberg M, et al. Functional clonal depletion versus suppressor cell-induced transplantation tolerance in chimeras prepared with a short course of total-lymphoid irradiation. Transplantation 1986;41:680.
35. Morecki S, Leshem B, Weigensberg M, et al. Functional clonal deletion versus active suppression in transplantation tolerance induced by total-lymphoid irradiation. Transplantation 1985;40:201.
36. Field EH, Steinmuller D. Nondeletional mechanisms of tolerance in total-lymphoid irradiation-induced bone marrow chimeras. Transplantation 1993;56:250–253.
37. Salam A, Vandeputte M, Waer M. Clonal deletion and clonal anergy in allogeneic bone marrow chimeras prepared with TBI or TLI. Transplant Int 1994;7:S457–S461.
38. Florence LS, Jiang GL, Ang KK, et al. In vitro analysis of T cell-mediated cytotoxicity displayed by rat heart allograft recipients rendered unresponsive by total-lymphoid irradiation and extracted donor antigen. Transplantation 1990;49:436–444.
39. Bass H, Strober S. Deficits in T helper cells after total lymphoid irradiation (TLI): reduced IL-2 secretion and normal IL-2 receptor expression in the mixed leucocyte reaction MLR. Cell Immunol 1990;126:129.
40. Bass H, Mosmann T, Strober S. Evidence for mouse TH1 and TH2-like helper T cells in vivo. J Exp Med 1989;170:1495.
41. Field EH, Rouse TM. Alloantigen priming after total lymphoid irradiation alters alloimmune cytokine responses. Transplantation 1995;60:695–702.
42. Stark JH, Smit JA, Myburgh JA. Nonspecific mixed lymphocyte culture inhibitory antibodies in sera of tolerant transplanted baboons conditioned with total lymphoid irradiation. Transplantation 1994;57:1103–1110.
43. Yamaguchi Y, Halperin EC, Harland RC. Significant prolongation of hamster liver transplant survival in Lewis rats by total lymphoid irradiation, cyclosporine and splenectomy. Transplantation 1990;49:13.
44. Steinbrüchel DA, Madsen H, Nielsen B, et al. The effect of combined treatment with TLI, cyclosporine A and anti-CD4 monoclonal antibodies in a hamster-to-rat transplantation model. Transplant Proc 1991;23:579.
45. Marchman W, Araneda D, DeMasi R, et al. Prolongation of xenograft survival after combination therapy with 15-deoxyspergualin and total-lymphoid irradiation in the hamster-to-rat cardiac xenograft model. Transplantation 1993;53:30–34.
46. Roslin MS, Tranbaugh RE, Panza A, et al. One-year monkey heart xenograft survival in cyclosporine-treated baboons. Suppression of the xenoantibody response with total-lymphoid irradiation. Transplantation 1992;54:949–955.
47. Sadeghi AM, Laks H, Drinkwater DC, et al. Heart-lung xenotransplantation in primates. J Heart Lung Transplant 1991;10:442–447.
48. Panza A, Roslin M, Coons M, et al. Successful cardiac xenogeneic transplantation in primates using total lymphoid irradiation. Eur J Cardiothorac Surg 1991;5:161–163.
49. Kaplan E, Dresdale AR, Diehl JT, et al. Total lymphoid irradiation and discordant cardiac xenografts. J Heart Transplant 1990;9:11–13.
50. Thomas F, Pittman K, Ljung T, Cekada E. Deoxyspergualin is a unique immunosuppressive agent with selective utility inducing tolerance to pancreas islet xenografts. Transplant Proc 1995;27:417–419.
51. Tixier D, Levy C, Le Bourgeois JP, et al. Discordant heart xenografts. Experimental study in pigs conditioned by total lymphoid irradiation and cyclosporine A. Presse Med 1992;21:1941–1944.
52. Waer M, Vanrenterghem Y, Ang KK, et al. Comparison of the immunosuppressive effect of fractionated total lymphoid irradiation (TLI) vs conventional immunosuppression (CI) in renal cadaveric allotransplantation. J Immunol 1984;132:1041–1048.
53. Waer M, Vanrenterghem Y, Roels L, et al. Immunological and clinical observations in diabetic kidney graft recipients pretreated with total-lymphoid irradiation. Transplantation 1987;43:371–379.
54. Waer M, Vanrenterghem Y, Roels L, et al. Renal cadaveric transplantation in diabetics using total lymphoid irradiation or cyclosporin A. A controlled randomized study. Transplant Int 1988;1:64–68.
55. Levin B, Collins G, Waer M, et al. Treatment of cadaveric renal transplant recipients with total lymphoid irradiation, antithymocyte globulin, and low-dose prednisone. Lancet 1985;2:1321.
56. Levin B, Bohannon L, Warvariv V, et al. Total lymphoid irradiation (TLI) in the cyclosporine era—use of TLI in resistant cardiac allograft rejection. Transplant Proc 1989;21:1793–1795.
57. Strober S, Dhillon M, Schubert M, et al. Acquired immune tolerance to cadaveric renal allografts: a study of three patients treated with total lymphoid irradiation. N Engl J Med 1989;321:28.
58. Myburgh JA, Meyers AM, Botha JR, et al. Wide field low-dose total lymphoid irradiation in clinical kidney transplantation. Transplant Proc 1987;19: 1974–1977.
59. Myburgh JA, Meyers AM, Margolius L, et al. Total lymphoid irradiation in clinical renal transplantation—results in 73 patients. Transplant Proc 1991;23:2033–2034.
60. Najarian JS, Ferguson RM, Sutherland DER, et al. Fractionated total lymphoid irradiation as preparative immunosuppression in high risk renal transplantation. Ann Surg 1982;196:442–452.
61. Kaufman DB, Kim TH, Slavin S, et al. Long term clinical studies of high-risk renal retransplant recipients given total lymphoid irradiation. Transplant Proc 1989;21:1798.
62. Cortesini R, Molajoni ER, Monari C, et al. Total lymphoid irradiation in clinical transplantation: experience in 30 high-risk patients. Transplant Proc 1985;92:1291–1293.
63. Molajoni ER, Bachetoni A, Cinti P, et al. Eight-year actuarial graft and patient survival of kidney transplants in highly immunized recipients pretreated with total lymphoid irradiation: a single-center experience. Transplant Proc 1993;25:776–777.
64. Woodley SL, Gurley KE, Hoffmann SL, et al. Induction of tolerance to heart allografts in rats using posttransplant total lymphoid irradiation and anti-T cell antibodies. Transplantation 1993;56:1443–1447.
65. Evans MA, Schomberg PJ, Rodeheffer RJ, et al. Total lymphoid irradiation: a novel and successful therapy for resistant cardiac allograft rejection. Mayo Clin Proc 1992;67:785–790.
66. Hunt SA, Strober S, Hoppe RT, Stinson EB. Total lymphoid irradiation for treatment of intractable cardiac allograft rejection. J Heart Lung Transplant 1991;10:211–216.
67. Salter SP, Slater MM, Kirklin JK, et al. Total lymphoid irradiation in the treatment of early or recurrent heart transplant rejection. Int J Radiation Oncol Biol Phys 1995;33:83–88.
68. Valentine VG, Robbins RC, Wehner JH, et al. Total lymphoid irradiation for refractory acute rejection in heart-lung and lung allografts. Chest 1996;109:1184–1189.
69. Bhatia S, Robison L, Oberlin O, et al. Breast cancer and other second neoplasms after childhood Hodgkin's disease. N Engl J Med 1996;334:745–751.
70. Edelson R, Berger C, Gasparro F, et al. Treatment of cutaneous T cell lymphoma by extracorporeal photochemotherapy: preliminary results. N Engl J Med 1987;316:297.
71. Perez M, Edelson R, Lori J, et al. Inhibition of antiskin allograft immunity by infusions with syngeneic photoinactivated effector lymphocytes. J Invest Dermatol 1989;92:669.
72. Perez M, Edelson R, Laroche L. Inhibition of antiskin allograft immunity by infusions with photoinactivated effector T-lymphocytes (PET cells). Yale J Biol Med 1989;62:595.
73. Pepino P, Berger CL, Fuzesi L, et al. Primate cardiac allo- and xenotransplantation: modulation of the immune response with photochemotherapy. Eur Surg Res 1989;21:105.
74. Berger C. Experimental murine and primate models for dissection of the immunosuppressive potential of photochemotherapy in autoimmune disease and transplantation. Yale J Biol Med 1989;62:611.
75. Kraemer KH, Haywood LW, Cohen LF, et al. Effects of 8-methoxypsoralen and ultraviolet radiation on human lymphoid cells in vitro. J Invest Dermatol 1981;76:80.
76. Edelson RL. Light-activated drugs. Sci Am 1988;259:68.
77. Meiser BM, Kur F, Reichenspurner H, et al. Reduction of the incidence of rejection by adjunct immunosuppression with photochemotherapy after heart transplantation. Transplantation 1994;57:563.

78. Barr ML, Meiser BM, Eisen HJ, et al. Photopheresis for the prevention of rejection in cardiac transplantation. Photopheresis Transplantation Study Group. N Engl J Med 1998;339:1744–1751.

COMMENTARY REFERENCES

1. Myburgh JA, Smit JA, Meyers AM, et al. Total lymphoid irradiation in renal transplantation. World J Surg 1986;10:369–380.
2. Myburgh JA, Smit JA. Delineation, durability, predictability and specificity of operational tolerance with total lymphoid irradiation in baboon kidney transplantation. Transplant Proc 1985;17:1442–1445.
3. Smit JA, Stark JH, Myburgh JA. Intrathymic donor antigen in baboon kidney allotransplantation. Afr J Health Sci 1995;2:344–348.
4. Myburgh JA, Meyers AM, Margolius L, et al. Total lymphoid irradiation in clinical renal transplantation—Results in 73 patients. Transplant Proc 1991;23:2033–2034.
5. Stark JH, Smit JA, Myburgh JA. Nonspecific mixed lymphocyte culture inhibitory antibodies in sera of tolerant transplanted baboons conditioned with total lymphoid irradiation. Transplantation 1994;57:1103–1110.
6. Gray CM, Smit JA, Myburgh JA. Identification of non-T suppressor cells with possible contra-interleukin-2 properties in non-human primates tolerant to their renal allografts. Afr J Health Sci 1995;2:354–358.
7. Myburgh JA, Smit JA, Stark JH. Transplantation tolerance following total lymphoid irradiation in baboon-to-monkey kidney xenotransplantation. Transplant Proc 1994;26:1080–1081.
8. Myburgh JA, Smit JA, Stark JH. Experimental concordant kidney xenotransplantation in primates. In Cooper DKC, ed. Xenotransplantation. 2nd ed. Heidelberg, Germany, Pro Edit GmbH 1997:316–322.

Part III

Organ Procurement

Chapter

15

Donor Selection and Management

Kevin J. O'Connor Francis L. Delmonico

The fundamental requirement for transplantation is the organ donor. A comprehensive analysis of the donor is so central to the success of transplantation that a review of the selection and management of organ donors becomes an indispensable measure of the state of the art. The evolution of organ donation, which continues today, has had a profound impact on the practice of transplantation. This practice has interestingly evolved from sole reliance on living-related donors for the initial successful renal transplants, through a period emphasizing mainly the cadaver supply of donor organs, to the present era when living donors have again become an important option for an increasing number of recipients. Reflecting the current approach, this chapter's section on living organ donation is much expanded from previous reviews (1).

The ascendancy of the living donor source is a consequence of the inadequate supply of cadaver organ donors (2). Many transplant physicians have now reluctantly concluded that any significant expansion in the cadaver donor pool may already have been realized (Table 15.1). The number of suitable cadaver donors is not growing as was once anticipated, because of improved trauma care, public awareness of the speeding and drunk-driving penalties, and safer motor vehicle provisions (seat belts, air bags, motorcycle helmets). Moreover, even though public surveys indicate a large majority of society is willing to donate organs at the time of death, the actual consent rate remains at 50% to 60% for most communities, despite an extensive effort in public education over the past decade (3). Therefore, the transplant community is increasingly calling upon an altruistic population of living donors to provide for the huge cadre of patients awaiting not only a renal allograft, but a variety of extrarenal transplants as well (2,4).

As organ replacement is now a well-recognized treatment for end-stage failure, segmental procurement of an unpaired organ from a living donor has broadened the opportunity for lung, liver, and pancreas transplant recipients as well. Furthermore, whereas living donation was once restricted by the degree of human leukocyte antigen (HLA) matching, a genetic relationship is no longer a stipulation. Unrelated spouses and friends of prospective recipients have frequently joined the ranks of organ donors. The observation of comparable success rates for these transplants to those achieved following HLA-matched organ transplantation has fostered a sustained enthusiasm for unrelated-living donation (5). Although living-unrelated donation cannot solve the shortage crisis, this approach will undoubtedly continue to expand until the goal of successful xenotransplantation is clinically attained. Therefore, in this chapter we consider living donation and the ethical concerns and selection criteria that pertain to an unrelated donor.

The shortage of donor organs has catalyzed organ procurement organizations (OPOs) to reconsider also the criteria of cadaver donor suitability. Thus, we review the current criteria for exclusion, including the unacceptable risk of organ recovery from donors with a history of malignancy or HIV, but reconsider historical contraindications related to donor sepsis. The potential transmission of infectious disease via contaminated donor organs is presented in the context of specific bacteriology and by an algorithm of donor serology screening.

Changes in the field of organ donation are nowhere more evident than in a comparison of the current characteristics of the cadaver donor population versus those observed previously. In our experience through the New England Organ Bank (NEOB), we have observed an expansion in the number of cadaver donors now deemed acceptable, especially through the inclusion of those of older age. A review of the NEOB data reveals not only an increase in donors older than 50 years of age, but an increase in donors who have suffered

Table 15.1. US Cadaveric Donors

Year	Donors
1988	4084
1989	4019
1990	4512
1991	4528
1992	4521
1993	4861
1994	5100
1995	5357
1996	5411

Source: Data from the United Network for Organ Sharing, Richmond, VA.

Table 15.2. Cadaveric Organ Donors in the United States by Cause of Death (As Percent of Total)

Year	MVA	CVA
1988	34.3%	27.7%
1989	30.0%	30.6%
1990	27.7%	32.6%
1991	25.8%	34.0%
1992	21.6%	36.2%
1993	21.9%	36.7%
1994	24.5%	41.5%
1995	26.4%	39.2%

MVA = Motor vehicle accident; CVA = cerebral vascular accident.
Source: United Network for Organ Sharing 1996 Annual Report.

brain injury from cerebral vascular accidents. In contrast, the number of "ideal" organ donors dying from traumatic brain injury (motor vehicle accidents or homicide) has fallen sharply. This is not an isolated observation, as the data from the United Network of Organ Sharing (UNOS) are consistent with this trend (Table 15.2) (2). Thus, included in this chapter is a discussion of organ donors who are marginal by previous standards, and also consideration of the renewed interest in the non-heart-beating donor. This is especially relevant today, as adherence to the brain-death definition of death has been questioned (6,7).

Perhaps the most significant obstacle to increasing the number of cadaver organs available for transplantation has been obtaining consent. Separating a family's discussion of the declaration of death with the primary care team from the request for organ donation by an OPO representative permits families to consider donation more favorably. Thus, a suggested OPO practice for maximizing consent is presented in this chapter.

Finally, the prerecovery management of the classic heart-beating donor has been shown to be critically related not only to the immediate function of the transplanted organ but also to the long-term success for the recipient. Thus, our review details the approaches that have been developed to remedy specific organ donor dysfunction after the determination of brain death by current neurologic criteria.

LIVING ORGAN DONATION

Ethical Considerations

As Dr. Joseph Murray prepared for the first successful renal transplant from a living donor in 1954, he was confronted by an ethical dilemma not previously encountered by a physician. He was proposing to operate on a well individual who was to receive no medical benefit from that procedure. Dr. Murray later recalled his experience of consulting members of the medical, legal, and religious communities who were to support this innovative treatment (8). In retrospect, this widespread endorsement was also an important element of the success, notwithstanding Dr. Murray's technical achievement.

Spital has further traced some of the historical process that eventually established the propriety of living organ donation, citing the 1970 report of the Transplantation Society's Committee on Morals and Ethics. The Committee concluded: "Living kidney donors may be used provided the consent is informed, free, and legally acceptable after thorough explanation of the possible consequences has been made" (9).

These fundamental considerations of living donation would appear to be well established and also applicable now to extrarenal donation (10). Nevertheless, the transplant physician today continues to be challenged by ethical issues surrounding living donation. Most of the controversy is related to the continually expanding use of living donors. For example, the "possible consequences" of living donation have been extended to individuals who may have an increased medical risk of undergoing the operative procedure and living the remainder of their lives deficient of the donated organ or resected segment. Moreover, the opportunity for living donation has also been expanded to individuals who may be linked to recipients only by an emotional relationship. Indeed, because of the comparable success from either donor source (11), there would no longer appear to be an ethical distinction between a related and an unrelated living donor (5).

The criteria that allow a living individual to donate must be carefully considered. The importance of an independent psychiatric evaluation of the potential donor cannot be overestimated. The donor should be of legal age and competent; that is, determined not to have major personality disorders or mental retardation. Drug- or alcohol-dependent individuals generally are excluded. Children should be protected from bearing a burden of donation as they are incapable of giving valid consent, especially when there is no "moral imperative" within a family relationship (12).

The volunteerism and altruistic motives of the donor should be carefully assessed. Those donor–recipient dynamics that might introduce the possibility of coercion should be evaluated by psychiatric interview. The psychiatrist can also provide an appropriate escape mechanism for the medically suitable living donor who is afraid to confront the family with a reluctance to donate. In the United States, the psychiatrist must also be alert to the possibility of any remuneration that might be exchanged between the recipient and donor, as the 1984 National Organ Transplant Act has made it illegal to acquire a human organ by monetary compensation. Despite this unequivocal legislation, there are proponents who would establish a brokerage for the purchase of organs, citing two principles of ethics: 1) the respect for autonomous choices (individuals should be at liberty to dispose of their body parts as they see fit), and 2) the principle of utility (sale of organs would be the most effective and efficient way to increase their supply) (13).

Childress (13) has clearly defined the prevailing rationale of a resolute opposition to the sale of human organs: 1) the increased risks of injury to the living donor because the donor is a vendor, 2) such a donor is vulnerable to exploitation and coercion, especially if the donor is destitute, and 3) the sale of organs is an affront to the dignity and value of the human person. With regards to the principle of utility, it is not clear that the sale of organs would increase the supply; moreover, it may adversely influence those who would wish to be altruistic.

These rejoinders have been sufficiently persuasive to limit the sale of organs in most countries, although some countries do permit the commercial traffic of renal allografts (14,15). Thus, the danger of exploitation has clearly been realized. The violation of human rights surrounding organ donation could also develop in societies whose customs forbid the recovery of organs from cadaver and living donors, but sanction the removal of organs from executed prisoners (16). Unfortunately, recipients of organs obtained in desperation from entrepreneurs, under any of these circumstances, have sometimes been subjected to substandard care (17), with a high incidence of surgical complications and human immunodeficiency virus (HIV) infection (18).

As it is an unethical practice to impose the removal of an organ on an individual without consent or for monetary compensation, it may also be unethical for a prospective donor to demand the removal of their organ. Such a scenario has been described. A well-intentioned mother of a child with liver failure was initially rejected as a living donor because of obesity, a smoking history, and use of oral contraceptives. Nevertheless, her insistence to donate led to the performance of the procedure, which, unfortunately, resulted in her death from a pulmonary embolus on the second postoperative day (19). Similarly, family members or friends should be dissuaded from demanding that they be allowed to donate, for example, to a diabetic recipient with advanced coronary and peripheral vascular disease, or to a patient with a high likelihood of recurrent failure in the allograft. These case illustrations emphasize that transplant physicians should not be regarded as mechanics subservient to the dictates of a client. They also reveal a rethinking of the informed consent process particular to living organ donation, which does not neatly fit the classic dogma of *primum non nocere* (20). Moore (20) has suggested that living organ donor ethics should be determined by "the statistical calculation of likelihoods." Thus, as wisdom and experience are applied to the decision of who is a suitable living donor, the transplant physician must exercise the foremost responsibility of *estimating the chance of doing harm*. Unless this risk to the donor is minimal, the circumstances of the donation are medically appropriate, and the prospects for successful transplantation are excellent, living organ donation should not be performed (21).

Medical Suitability

Potential living organ donors should be determined to be ABO blood type compatible with a negative lymphocytotoxic crossmatch (if appropriate) before being subjected to an extensive medical evaluation.

ABO and Lymphocytotoxic Compatibility

Although ABO incompatible donor organs have been transplanted successfully into heart (22), liver (23,24), and kidney allograft recipients (25), ABO-incompatible transplants are usually limited to the following clinical situations: life-threatening emergencies (26), pediatric recipients of liver allografts (27,28), or the special immunologic circumstance in which an A2 blood type donor organ is given to an O (blood group) heart (29) or renal recipient (30). For these transplants to be successful, living donor recipients of ABO-incompatible allografts have usually been treated with additional measures such as splenectomy (31), OKT-3 induction (32), plasmapheresis (33), or immunoadsorption (34), so that the anti-blood group IgM isohemagglutinins do not precipitate a hyperacute rejection of the allograft.

It has also been well established that hyperacute rejection can result from donor-specific lymphocytotoxic antibodies preexisting in the potential heart (35) and renal (36) allograft recipient. This type of immune reactivity remains an absolute contraindication at least to living donor renal (37) and pancreas (38) transplantation. Interestingly, the liver may not predictably suffer the same consequence of hyperacute rejection (39,40). Thus, donor-specific alloantibody in the recipient's serum, a "positive T-cell crossmatch" (see Chapter 4), may not preclude the possibility of successful liver transplantation from a living donor, especially when there are no other donors available.

Donor Age

Although minors (<18 years of age) are considered for organ donation only under special circumstances (41), there is no defined upper age limit of a potential living donor. All donors must be determined to be well and in satisfactory medical condition to undergo the operative procedure. Perhaps surprisingly, a few living kidney donors have been reported at 75 to 80 years of age at the time of their donation (41). Several centers have undertaken a large series of older living renal allograft donors (greater than 55 years of age) whose renal function was normal by creatinine clearance (42,43). However, the renal capacity of these allografts to withstand cyclosporine toxicity or recover from an episode of rejection may not be comparable to that of a renal allograft obtained from a younger donor. Despite the comparable pretransplant creatinine clearances of a younger and older donor kidney, glomerular obsolescence of the elderly allograft may adversely influence the eventual outcome from potentially reversible episodes of renal dysfunction (44). Nevertheless, the outcome following transplantation has been so satisfactory as to permit continued acceptance of medically well elderly donors, even those older than 65 (42).

Other Living Donor Criteria

A history of donor malignancy is nearly always a contraindication to organ donation, as carcinoma (especially renal and colon) has been transmitted to renal allograft recipients from living donors (45). HIV infection is also an absolute contraindication to living donation. Despite the recent improvements in the treatment of HIV, the immunosuppressed recipient should clearly be protected from any identifiable source of life-threatening infection.

All living organ donors should accept HIV screening within two to three months prior to the planned transplant. During the subsequent interval, donors should be instructed to avoid social encounters that might engender an HIV exposure. For example, HIV was transmitted from an asymptomatic living donor of a renal allograft (whose serology was HIV negative eight months prior to the transplant) following homosexual activity between the time of the HIV testing and the transplant (46).

Donors must also be screened by serology for hepatitis and cytomegalovirus (CMV) in proximity to the planned transplant. Previous hepatitis B and C infections are usually considered a contraindication to living donation (37,47). However, a positive donor CMV serology does not preclude living donation, even with the most risky scenario of a CMV-positive donor and a CMV-negative recipient (41) (see Chapter 36).

Screening for diabetes is usually accomplished by a fasting plasma glucose; however, an oral glucose tolerance test is also commonly suggested (37). Some physicians also screen for anti-islet cell antibodies as another risk factor for late onset of donor diabetes in relatives of a diabetic recipient.

Establishing a Genetically Identical Donor

There are rare occasions when the donor may be genetically identical to the recipient, as was the situation of the first successful kidney transplant performed by Dr. Murray. If the donor can be determined to be an identical twin, recipient immunosuppression is not necessary.

We have recently performed kidney transplants into two patients from sibling donors who were thought to be genotypically identical to their respective recipients. Although HLA and red blood cell typing suggested in each instance that the twins were identical, these tests were not felt to be absolutely confirmatory because minor HLA antigens of fraternal twins were possibly undetectable. If the twins were fraternal, then long-term immunosuppression would be advisable. To ensure genotypic identity, we placed a skin graft from the recipient onto the donor's forearm at the time of the kidney transplant. When the skin graft was not rejected at six weeks after transplantation, the renal isograft recipient's immunosuppression was discontinued successfully (in both cases).

Organ-Specific Criteria

Lung The usual screening laboratory data for all living donors are obtained as detailed in Table 15.3. In addition, potential lung donors must have normal pulmonary function and no abnormalities on chest roentgenogram and computed tomography (Table 15.4) (48). There should be no history of a thoracic operation on the side of the intended donation. The size match between the lobe to be

Table 15.3. Living Donor Evaluation

Health history questionnaire:
No significant past medical history
No recent viral infections
Blood pressure (diastolic not >100 mm Hg)
ABO blood type
HLA determination, and lymphocytotoxic crossmatch (if appropriate)
Complete blood count and differential
Coagulation profile (PT, PTT)
Blood urea nitrogen and creatinine, creatinine clearance
Urinalysis, urine for colony count and sensitivity
Electrolytes, glucose, uric acid, Ca, P, Mg, amylase
Liver function tests:
Bilirubin (total and direct)
Alkaline phosphatase
Albumin, (total protein)
SGOT, LDH, CPK
Lipid profile (variable)
CMV antibody
Hepatitis B surface antigen and antibodies
Hepatitis C
Varicella
Toxoplasmosis serology
HIV antibody, antigen
Chest x-ray
Electrocardiogram
RPR

Table 15.4. Evaluation for a Living Lung Donor

Age ≤55 years
High resolution chest CT (no significant pulmonary pathology and completely normal on donor side)
Sputum gram stain, culture, and sensitivity
Cardiac echo with pulse Doppler
Quantitative V/Q scan
Oxygen tension >80 mm Hg on room air
Forced expiratory volume in 1 second and forced vital capacity >85% predicted
No previous thoracic operation on donor side
Skin tests—PPD, mumps, candida

transplanted and the recipient's thoracic cavity is estimated by computed tomographic scans (49). Ventilation/perfusion scans of the right and left lungs are performed to estimate how much of the donor lung function is being removed (49). The recommended room air oxygen tension for a living lung donor is greater than 80 mm Hg, and the forced expiratory volume in one second and forced vital capacity should be greater than 85% of predicted (see also Chapter 25).

Liver Living liver donors undergo essentially the same rigorous assessment as living donors of other organs (see Table 15.3). Because of the space constraint of a child's abdominal cavity, Broelsch also recommends determination of the volume of the left lateral segment of the potential donor liver by volumetric computed tomography and three-dimensional computerized imaging (50). The lateral segment size is generally considered suitable if it is less than 350 mL (19). The hepatic arterial supply is evaluated by selective celiac and mesenteric angiography; a single artery to the left lobe is an absolute requirement (see also Chapter 20).

For children with metabolic disorders, a heterozygous parent may be an acceptable donor, thereby overcoming the homozygous expression of the metabolic defect in the child. An endoscopic retrograde cholangiopancreatography (ERCP) is performed on donors of children with Alagilles syndrome (51).

With such stringent criteria, it is not surprising that at least one-third of potential living liver donor candidates are not accepted because of either increased risk to the donor (including psychosocial instability) or because of liver unsuitability (51).

Pancreas Because of the obvious potential for a pancreas donor to relinquish a vital number of islets of Langerhans (affecting their own genetic predisposition to become diabetic), Gruessner and Sutherland have defined the following inclusion criteria for living pancreas donation: 1) the prospective donor must be at least 10 years older than the age of onset of diabetes in the recipient, 2) if the donor is a sibling, no family member other than the recipient can be diabetic, and 3) the donor's postintravenous glucose stimulation first-phase insulin level must be above the 30th percentile of the normal range (52) (see also Commentary section in Chapter 21).

Kidney The survey of 231 UNOS transplant centers by Bia et al provides an excellent summary of the generally accepted criteria for renal donation (41).

The creatinine clearance should ideally be greater than 80 mL/min/1.73 m^2. Patients with greater than 300 mg/day of proteinuria are excluded, unless the proteinuria is postural and accompanies a normal kidney biopsy. Hematuria (>10 red blood cells per high powered field) is a contraindication, unless a urologic evaluation and kidney biopsy are normal. Most centers exclude a donor with hypertension. However, donors with a history of stone disease are not necessarily rejected. If there are no current stones by intravenous pyelogram and the metabolic studies of calcium, urate, and/or oxalate are normal, then such a patient may be accepted. Some centers do not permit the transplant of a small donor kidney to a relatively large recipient. Brenner et al have suggested that a ratio of donor kidney weight (in grams) to body weight of recipient (in kilograms) of 1.0 or less may pose a risk of glomerular injury by hyperfiltration and, thus, result in a worse outcome (53).

A familial disorder such as polycystic kidney disease is not necessarily a contraindication to donation, if the donor is at least 30 years of age and the computerized tomography of the abdomen is normal. Diabetics, however, are usually excluded from donation.

In addition to a standard profile of renal function, the prospective donor undergoes a renal angiogram prior to nephrectomy, mainly to determine the number of arteries supplying each kidney. The arteriogram also provides further assessment of the renal parenchyma and may reveal the presence of such processes as a renal mass lesion or diseases intrinsic to the renal artery such as fibromuscular dysplasia, arterial stenosis, or aneurysm. These anatomic abnormalities may preclude kidney donation, though we have successfully transplanted kidneys after performing ex vivo renal artery aneurysmorrhaphy.

Living Donor Lung Transplantation

Approximately 80 living donor lung transplants have been reported to the International Registry since 1990. The largest series has been reported by Starnes et al from the University of Southern California Cardiothoracic Center (48). A donor lobectomy was performed from 76 living donors, enabling 37 recipients to undergo bilateral lobar pulmonary transplantation. Seventy-three donors were related to their recipients and three were unrelated.

This group recommends restricting the donated tissue to either the left or right lower lobe (48). The inclusion of a right middle lobectomy has resulted in prolonged air leak from the oversewn middle lobe bronchus. Moreover, the postoperative spirometry of donors who underwent simultaneous lower and middle lobe resection was significantly affected.

The sequence of resection is to first divide the pulmonary artery and then the pulmonary vein (to avoid lobar congestion); the posterior bronchus is transected last (49).

Following lobectomy (Figs. 15.1, 15.2), the lung is immersed in a cold crystalloid solution, with the bronchus intubated and ventilated with 100% oxygen. The pulmonary artery is flushed with cold Collins preservative fluid until the pulmonary vein effluent is clear (48). The donor lobe is

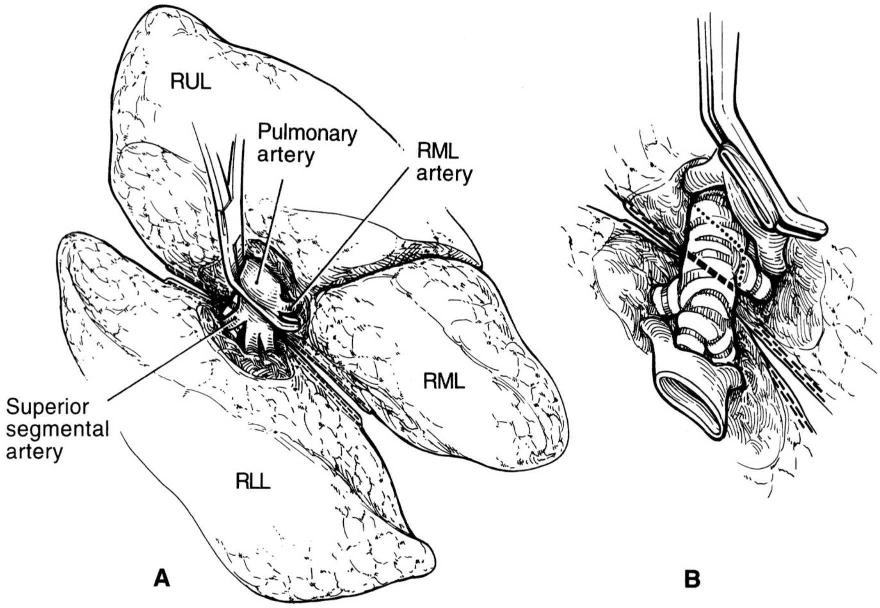

FIGURE 15.1. *Right lower lobe donor lobectomy. **A**. Exposure of the bronchovascular structures is obtained through the major fissure. Following systemic heparinization, a vascular clamp is placed obliquely on the pulmonary artery distal to the origin of the middle lobe branches. The inferior pulmonary vein (not shown) is controlled intrapericardially at its left atrial confluence with a vascular clamp. **B**. Following division of the vascular structures, the lower lobe bronchus is divided obliquely to preserve the superior segmental and basilar segmental orifices (dashed line). In some cases, the close approximation of the superior segmental and middle lobar bronchial orifices makes it necessary to transect the right middle lobe bronchus separately and reimplant it into the distal bronchus intermedius, preserving the function of the middle lobe (dotted lines). (Reproduced by permission from Cohen R, Barr M, Schenkel F, et al. Living-related donor lobectomy for bilateral lobar transplantation in patients with cystic fibrosis. Ann Thoracic Surg 1994;57:1423–1428.)*

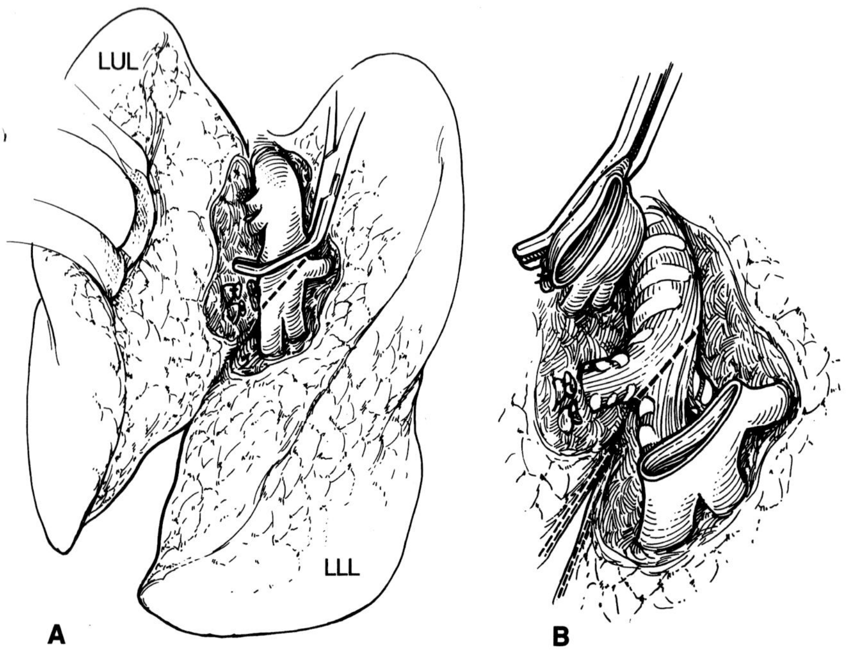

FIGURE 15.2. *Left lower lobe donor lobectomy. **A**. Exposure of the bronchovascular structures is obtained through the major fissure. After systemic heparinization, a vascular clamp is placed obliquely on the pulmonary artery. Ligation and division of the pulmonary artery branches to the lingula of the left upper lobe is frequently required. The inferior pulmonary vein (not shown) is controlled intrapericardially at its left atrial confluence with a vascular clamp. **B**. Following division of the vascular structures, the left lower lobe bronchus is divided obliquely to preserve the superior segmental and basilar segmental orifices (dashed line). Separate division and reimplantation of the lingular bronchus are required infrequently. (Reproduced by permission from Cohen R, Barr M, Schenkel F, et al. Living-related donor lobectomy for bilateral lobar transplantation in patients with cystic fibrosis. Ann Thoracic Surg 1994;57:1423–1428.)*

then transported in cold storage to the recipient operating room for transplantation (see also Chapter 25).

Living Donor Liver Transplantation

As of January 1996, more than 800 liver transplants had been performed from living donors throughout the world (54) following the inception of this approach eight years earlier. This practice has surely been influenced by the high mortality associated with an increased waiting time for an available cadaver donor liver in the United States (55), and by the inability to provide a cadaver donor allograft in certain countries such as Japan (56). As the split-liver approach has become more common, the number of living donor procedures performed appears now to be declining in many countries (see Chapters 19 and 20). Liver transplantation from a living donor is mainly confined to children since a living donor cannot usually provide a sufficient mass of liver tissue for even a small adult recipient (54). Emond et al have suggested that the size of the living donor liver allograft should exceed 25% of the mass expected for an individual recipient (54). Otherwise, recipients may experience poor post-transplant function that may not be capable of sustaining life (see also Chapters 19, 20).

Broelsch and Lloyd perform the donor hepatectomy through a bilateral subcostal incision with an extension to the xiphoid, which is similar to that for a recipient operation (50). A left lateral segmentectomy is usually performed (an anatomic bisegmentectomy of segments 2 and 3), retaining as much length of the left hepatic artery, left portal vein, and left hepatic duct as possible (Fig. 15.3). There may be separate bile ducts emanating from segment 2 and segment 3, each of which requires biliary enteric anastomosis. Interposition donor saphenous vein grafts (versus donor mesenteric veins) are often necessary to extend the donor hepatic artery and portal vein. The left hepatic vein returns the donor hepatic blood to the recipient inferior vena cava. A triangular anastomosis may be created between the donor left hepatic vein and a comparable orifice fashioned in the recipient vena cava by spatulation of the recipient hepatic veins (57); however, alternative methods have been described (58).

Living Donor Kidney Transplantation

The number of living kidney donors is increasing significantly each year. The percentage of living donors in the United States between 1988 and 1995 increased from 20% to 27% of all kidney donors (2).

At the Massachusetts General Hospital, all living kidney donors are admitted on the day of surgery and they are discharged routinely by the fifth day postoperatively. A transcostal, extrapleural incision is usually made across the bed of either the 11th or the 12th rib. If epidural anesthesia is administered, a Foley catheter is placed until the second day following the procedure.

The left kidney is generally preferred for transplantation, as the renal vein is longer and the distance to the origin of

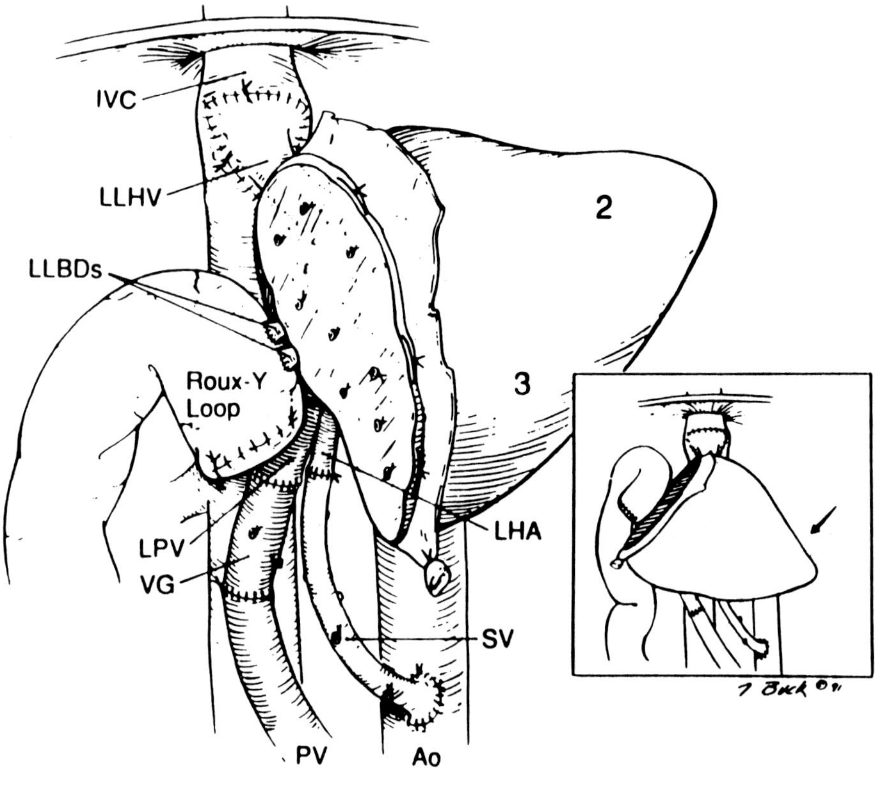

FIGURE 15.3. *Segments 2 and 3 of the donor liver are shown. IVC = inferior vena cava; LLHV = living donor left hepatic vein; LLBDs = living donor left hepatic ducts (with two depicted); LPV = living donor left portal vein; VG = interposition vein graft; LHA = living donor left hepatic artery; SV = recipient saphenous vein graft; PV = recipient portal vein. (Reproduced by permission from Edmon JC, Broelsch C, Lloyd D. Living related donors for liver transplants. In: Cameron J, ed. Advances in surgery. Vol. 26. St. Louis: Mosby-Year Book, 1993:209–221.)*

the renal artery is shorter than on the right (59). Nevertheless, the final selection is made only after a contrast radiographic study reveals the number of renal arteries of each kidney (60). Multiple renal arteries may be found in either kidney in approximately 30% of donors (60). The kidney with a single artery is naturally preferred, but multiple renal arteries may be managed by anastomosis of a polar vessel to the main artery or by anastomosis of the multiple arteries to a teflon patch graft (61).

Ratner and Kavoussi have championed the use of laparoscopic techniques to remove a living donor kidney (62). The implicit advantages of this minimally invasive surgery include less postoperative pain and earlier resumption of lifestyle (including, of course, return to work). Some donors undergoing laparoscopic nephrectomy have suggested that they would have been reluctant to donate if required to do so with a standard flank incision.

Nevertheless, abandoning the open procedure may be premature until the safety and success of a large laparoscopic series is comparatively analyzed over an extended period of time. Some surgeons have already concluded that removal of the right kidney may not be amenable to the laparoscopic method. Technical difficulties related to the short venal vein have resulted in occasional failure of the transplant.

Living-Unrelated Kidney Donors

Nearly 7% of living renal allograft donors in the United States in 1995 were unrelated to their recipients (2). The number of living-unrelated donors doubled between 1994 and 1995 (2). Spouses have become a major source of living donors, the preponderance from wives. Interestingly, the five-year allograft survival of a spousal renal transplant exceeds the likelihood of survival from a cadaver donor by 12% (2). This observation calls into question the emphasis of organ allocation based solely on the degree of HLA matching.

Since the high rate of survival of living-unrelated donor transplants does not appear to be related to HLA matching, other correlates of long-term success such as immediate function assume more importance. Shortening the preservation time of cadaver renal allografts influences initial function; therefore, allocation plans that give local recipients a priority, regardless of the degree of HLA match, may need to be reconsidered in the future.

Nevertheless, the extent of HLA mismatching may be associated with the likelihood of a rejection episode (63). No rejection occurred before hospital discharge in 93% of recipients of spousal allografts with no HLA-DR mismatches, versus 77% of the recipients of grafts with one HLA-DR mismatch and 70% of the recipients of grafts with two HLA-DR mismatches.

There was no difference in survival from allografts transplanted from wives to husbands compared to transplants from husbands to wives, if the wife had not been pregnant. A pregnancy prior to kidney transplantation from a husband donor may adversely affect allograft survival (three-year survival approximately 8% less) (63), as the wife has become sensitized to spousal antigens through the pregnancy and is thus at greater risk for rejection (see also Chapter 17).

Living Donor Pancreas Transplantation

A segmental pancreas was the first extrarenal organ successfully transplanted from a living donor (64). Since 1980, living donor pancreas transplants have been performed alone for diabetics without renal failure; in a sequential manner following cadaver donor kidney transplantation; or recently with a simultaneous kidney transplant (52) (see also Chapter 21). Some diabetics have been preferentially considered for living donor pancreas transplantation following detection of high serum levels of alloantibodies to a potential population of cadaver donors (38). The simultaneous pancreas–kidney procurement is performed through a donor midline abdominal incision (52); however, if a segmental pancreas allograft is to be transplanted alone, the Minnesota group uses a bilateral subcostal incision (65). The tail of the pancreas is mobilized by dividing the distal splenic artery and the splenic vein. The pancreas is transected at its neck (over the course of the portal vein), with the retained pancreatic duct and the pancreatic parenchyma being oversewn. The splenic artery is divided at its celiac axis origin. The proximal splenic vein is divided at the portal vein. The distal pancreatic duct is cannulated, the inferior mesenteric vein is transected, and the preparation is ready for transplantation (65) (Fig. 15.4).

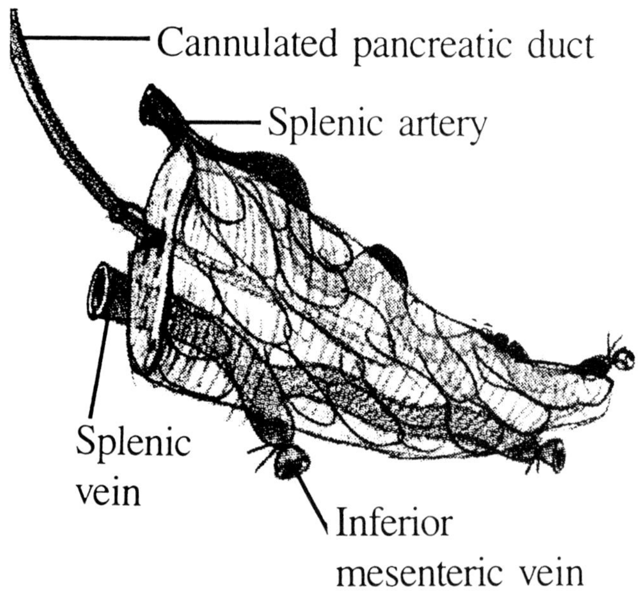

FIGURE 15.4. *Illustration of the segmental living donor pancreatic allograft. (Reproduced by permission from Sutherland D, Ascher N. Distal pancreas donation from a living relative. In: Simmons R, et al, eds. Manual of vascular access, organ donation, and transplantation. New York: Springer, 1984:153–164.)*

Living Donor Risks

Morbidity and Mortality

The perioperative mortality for a living kidney donor is estimated to be 0.03% (37). In the past 30 years, approximately 20 donors have died following renal allograft donation (41,66,67).

As noted earlier, Broelsch et al reported the death of a liver donor due to a pulmonary embolus on the second day following partial hepatectomy (19). A second liver donor death was reported at a conference on split-liver transplantation at the 1997 American Society of Transplant Surgeons meeting. In view of these reported deaths, some prominent transplant surgeons have publicly expressed opposition to the living donation approach (67).

The major postoperative morbidity associated with donor surgery includes pneumonia, wound infection, hematoma, phlebitis, pulmonary embolism, and urinary tract infection. The surgical complication rate for kidney donation is approximately 2% (41).

Starnes et al have reported prolonged air leaks and persistent chest tube drainage in several living lung donors (48). These technical difficulties appear to have been resolved more recently, however, by avoiding removal of the right middle lobe.

Additional risks for living pancreas donors include possible need for splenectomy due to inadvertent injury during dissection of the tail of the pancreas (52).

Some living donors have been reported to experience clinical depression, especially if the transplant is unsuccessful. Usually the disorder is mild and limited (9). Nevertheless, spousal kidney donation may affect marital stability, as a survey of spousal donors has revealed a divorce rate of 3% following transplantation (37).

Organ-Specific Donor Risks

Pulmonary Function Following Lung Donation Although the living lung donors in the study by Starnes et al were noted to have a reduction in their forced vital capacity and their forced expiratory volume, these patients were able to resume their lifestyles without compromise (48).

Diabetes Mellitus Following Pancreas Donation In the University of Minnesota series, none of the living donors who fulfilled the criterion of a normal insulin level following an intravenous glucose tolerance test have become hyperglycemic following hemipancreatectomy (38). However, in the authors' earlier experience, diabetes and several surgical complications had been observed. These included donor small bowel obstruction, a pancreatic pseudocyst, and leakage from the retained pancreatic duct (65).

Renal Failure Following Kidney Donation Partially nephrectomized animals experience progressive proteinuria and glomerulosclerosis as a result of hyperfiltration of the remaining glomeruli (68). Brenner et al have suggested that the reduction in human renal mass resulting from donor nephrectomy could initiate a similar pathophysiology of renal failure in the remaining kidney (53). Uninephrectomy of living donors has been associated with proteinuria and hypertension 6 to 10 years following nephrectomy (69,70). These observations have raised obvious concerns that kidney donors might be at increased risk of developing renal failure. At least 11 living kidney donors have developed end-stage renal failure following their unilateral nephrectomy (37).

However, the long-term outcome of carefully studied kidney donors has not substantiated an increased risk of hypertension or renal failure. Najarian et al have reported the outcome of 57 living renal allograft donors with an average of 23 years of follow-up after donation (66). These donors had no progressive increase in serum creatinine, no greater frequency of hypertension than that of the general population or sibling controls, and no significant rate of proteinuria. Only 4 of the 57 donors had proteinuria greater than 300 mg/24 hr (range 384 to 725 mg).

The US military has studied the consequences of unilateral nephrectomy 45 years after 28 surviving Army personnel had lost their kidneys because of World War II trauma (71). The prevalence of hypertension was not increased, the frequency (4 of 28) and level of proteinuria (377 to 535 mg/24 hr) were not significantly different from expected values, and none of the patients had developed renal failure.

Transplant physicians can also assure women who wish to be donors that they can undergo successful pregnancy after donation without the risk of renal failure (72). In a survey or 33 women with a total of 45 pregnancies after donation of a renal allograft, 75% of the pregnancies were carried to term without complication (73). No increased risk of fetal abnormalities, hypertension, proteinuria, or renal dysfunction was observed.

Living Donor Benefits

The benefit to a living organ donor is mainly psychological. The donor experiences increased self esteem, having contributed greatly to the quality of the recipient's life. Moreover, for parents of a child with end-stage liver failure, hepatic donation provides the satisfaction of having played a personal role in saving the life of their child (50).

Apart from the positive psychological benefits, there are also practical considerations for being a living donor. Of particular importance is the continued ability of the donor to secure an acceptable, low-risk rate of life insurance. Spital and Kokmen conducted a survey of health insurance organizations to inquire whether insurance rates were altered as a result of donor nephrectomy (74). For those already insured, none of the providers responded that they would raise premiums following kidney donation. Furthermore, for those seeking insurance after renal donation, premiums would be maintained at the standard rates considering the extensive evaluation that had been undertaken to determine the medical suitability of a potential living donor. A life insurance company is usually delighted to provide coverage for such a healthy individual.

Recipient Benefit of Living Donation

With more than 50,000 patients awaiting a solid organ transplant from a cadaver donor in the United States alone, the opportunity for a living donor transplant is an obvious advantage. The transplant can be electively scheduled to satisfy the needs of not only the recipient but also the donor (work or school obligations). The alternative is an unpredictable period of waiting for a cadaver organ that may be less than ideal. Moreover, for the extrarenal recipient, this opportunity of transplantation from a living donor may be life-saving. Finally, the potential for less rejection of a living donor allograft, with consequently less maintenance immunosuppression, is also a significant benefit that should foster an aggressive approach by most transplant centers to encourage living donor transplantation.

CADAVER ORGAN DONATION

Although Evans et al have suggested that the supply of cadaver organ donors in the United States could reach a total of 7000 annually, the current number has fallen far short of that expectation (see Table 15.1) (75). Organ procurement efficiency has traditionally been measured by organ donors per million population; however, detailed recent death record reviews by the NEOB now show significant geographic variation in donor potential. This finding may be attributable to the wide variation in homicide and motor vehicle fatality rates between communities. Thus, a better measure of OPO performance should include an objective estimate of the potential for donation in each region as an index to compare the actual rate of organ donation. Notwithstanding these sociodemographic factors, medical exclusion criteria have an additional impact on the opportunity for donation.

Absolute Exclusion Criteria

Age, social and medical history, and specific organ function will determine the suitability of a cadaver organ donor (Table 15.5). There are two well-accepted absolute exclusion criteria for organ donation: 1) a history of malignancy, and 2) HIV infection or AIDS. The risk of these donor diseases to the transplant recipient is the likely transmission of either a donor malignancy or HIV infection through the transplanted organ.

Malignancy

The risk of transplanting a tumor from an organ donor with a known malignancy is significant (approximately 50%) (45). The following cancers have been transplanted to allograft recipients from organ donors: thyroid, bronchial, lung, breast, adenocarcinoma (colorectal and unknown primary), kidney, melanoma, anaplastic, prostatic, and choriocarcinoma (76–80). However, cadaver donors with primary brain tumors, a history of nonmelanoma skin cancers such as basal or squamous cell, or a history of in situ carcinoma of the cervix may be acceptable organ donors. Although none of

Table 15.5. Organ-Specific Evaluation of a Cadaver Donor

	Heart	Lung	Liver	Kidney	Pancreas
Serologies[a]	X	X	X	X	X
ABO	X	X	X	X	X
Creatinine, BUN	—	—	—	X	—
Electrolytes	X	X	X	X	X
LFTs	—	—	X	—	—
PT, PTT	—	—	X	—	—
Serum glucose	—	—	—	—	X
Amylase, lipase	—	—	—	—	X
ABGs	X	X	X	X	X
Bronchoscopy	—	X*	—	—	—
Echocardiography	X	—	—	—	—
Chest x-ray	X	X	—	—	—
Urinalysis	—	—	—	X	—
Blood culture	X	X	X	X	X
Urine culture	—	—	—	X	—
Sputum gram stain and KOH prep	—	X*	—	—	—
Sputum culture	—	X	—	—	—
Cardiac catheterization	X*	—	—	—	—
EKG	X	—	—	—	—

[a] 1997 NEOB serology profile includes anti-HIV, anti-CMV, RPR, anti-HTLV 1/2, anti-HCV, HBSAg, anti-HBs, anti-HBc.
X = test required; X* = test preferred in some cases, but not always required; — = test not required.

these tumors has been transmitted to an allograft recipient in our experience, they warrant additional discussion (see also Chapter 37).

Primary Brain Tumors Although the spontaneous extracranial spread of a primary brain tumor is rare, presumably because of the blood-brain barrier, not all brain malignancies carry the same minimal risk of metastasis (81). Moreover, the possibility of metastasis may be influenced by intracranial operative procedures such as a craniotomy or the insertion of a ventriculo-peritoneal shunt (82). Primary brain tumors have been transmitted from such patients (76). The absence of a shunt, however, does not preclude the possibility of the transmission of a brain tumor to a solid organ allograft recipient (82). If organs are to be recovered from a donor with a primary brain tumor, the thoracic and abdominal cavities must be carefully inspected for metastases.

The diagnosis of a primary brain malignancy must also be differentiated from extracranial malignancies such as melanoma that may have metastasized to the brain (77). Intracerebral hemorrhage may be the presentation of not only a metastatic melanoma but also a renal cell carcinoma or a choriocarcinoma (80,83). Potential female donors with nontraumatic cerebral hemorrhage thought to be secondary to either a primary brain malignancy or a spontaneous subarachnoid hemorrhage should have a blood human chorionic gonadotropin (hCG) level determined (76). If a woman of reproductive age has a measurable blood hCG level, the patient should not be considered an appropriate donor unless there is clear evidence (postmortem) that the patient had either an intrauterine or a tubal pregnancy and the pathology of that gestation does not reveal a choriocarcinoma (Berkowitz R, personal communication, 1997).

In Situ Carcinoma of the Cervix Cervical intraepithelial neoplasia is a dysplastic lesion and a precursor of malignancy that may be suspected by Pap smear but requires a colposcopic biopsy for definitive staging and management (84). A history of absence of invasive cancer permits unrestricted organ donation.

Nonmelanoma Cancers of the Skin Basal cell and squamous cell carcinomas are very frequent in the general population; however, metastasis to the brain, lung, or liver is rare (85). If metastases occur, they are usually detected within six months of initial treatment. Thus, a careful medical history and visceral examination at the time of organ recovery will establish the safety of donation to prospective allograft recipients when a skin cancer history is given by a donor family or by the medical record.

Inadvertently transplanted malignancies may be detected in allograft recipients as early as hours after the procedure (e.g., in allograft nephrectomy or liver allograft biopsy specimens). Otherwise, metastases may become evident within several months following transplantation [choriocarcinoma in the lung of a liver allograft recipient (80)], or they may not become evident until years later [the development of melanoma on the chest, arms, and thighs of a renal allograft recipient (86)].

Interestingly, extrarenal allografts may be the vector of donor-transmitted malignancy even though the organ is typically not a common site of metastasis, for example the heart (79). Presumably the allograft carries the cancer cells that subsequently flourish in the immunosuppressed environment of the recipient. The Penn cancer registry data reveal five heart transplant recipients who developed metastatic malignancy from donors with known cancer (Penn I, personal communication, 1997). Two of these cases in particular emphasize that heart transplant recipients are as vulnerable to the development of donor malignancy as the recipients of other solid organs. First, a 45-year-old cadaver donor with brain hemorrhage underwent a perirecovery liver biopsy that later revealed unsuspected metastatic adenocarcinoma. The heart transplant recipient developed adenocarcinoma metastases to the spine six weeks later. In the second case, four allograft recipients (including a heart recipient who died) developed melanoma following transplantation of organs from a young cadaver donor who died of brain hemorrhage and unsuspected melanoma. This case underscores the risk of melanoma transmission from potential donors with questionable histories, even though they have not suffered metastatic disease. The donor history retrospectively revealed only "benign mole surgery," and there was no evidence of recurrent or metastatic disease at the time of organ donation. A subsequent review by the Armed Forces Institute of Pathology of the previously excised lesion determined the "mole" was most likely a melanoma.

We should note that pathologists may differ regarding the differential diagnosis of a severely dysplastic nevus versus melanoma and that there have been rare instances in which even a thin melanoma (<0.5 mm) has metastasized in a nonimmunosuppressed patient (Mihm M, personal communication, 1998). Thus, a donor history of mole surgery necessitates a careful review of the previous medical records. Any suspicion of melanoma is an absolute contraindication to organ donation, as the risk of transmission of melanoma via either a cadaver or a living donor organ is very high (80%) (77).

Donor Bacteremia

Another contraindication to organ donation, previously considered to be absolute, was the determination of concurrent donor sepsis. However, the increasing shortage of cadaver organs has necessitated a rethinking of this issue, so that organs from every possibly acceptable donor may be recovered.

From an organ bank perspective, sepsis at the time of a patient's death introduces the risk of transmitting infectious disease by donor organs contaminated with pathogens (87). However, before excluding a possibly infected patient as an organ donor, OPOs now routinely evaluate each donor on an individual basis, considering the blood culture bacteriology, the presence and duration of central lines, and the nature of the infection. Transient bacteremia may be the result of an extremity cellulitis (especially adjacent to external orthopedic fixatives), of a repaired intestinal injury, or of other surgery. None of these conditions alone prohibits organ donation.

Similarly, patients with bacterial meningitis may be acceptable for organ donation. *Haemophilus influenzae*, *Streptococcus pneumoniae*, and *Neisseria meningitidis* are the most common bacterial pathogens (88). The administration of at least a broad-spectrum cephalosporin to a potential donor is indicated under these circumstances (88). On the other hand, some bacterial organisms carry a more significant hazard for blood vessel invasion following transplantation. For example, *Staphylococcus aureus* (89), *Bacteroides* species (90), *Klebsiella enterobacter* (91), *Escherichia coli* (91), *Pseudomonas aeruginosa* (92), and fungal infections such as *Candida albicans* (93–95), *Cryptococcus neoformans* (87), and *Histoplasma capsulatum* (90) have been transmitted to allograft recipients from infected donors or preservation fluids and implicated in the subsequent development of recipient mycotic aneurysms and disruption of vascular anastomoses.

In the case of premortem donor bacteremia, if a sufficient course of antibiotic therapy has been administered that minimizes the risk of bacterial transmission, then organ retrieval may be considered. In contrast, fungal contamination is more worrisome because the opportunity for adequate donor treatment is limited. Because *Candida* infections are particularly hazardous to the pancreas transplant recipient (96), many transplant surgeons administer amphotericin B through the nasogastric tube into the donor duodenum during the recovery procedure.

Our NEOB experience with the transplantation of organs from a donor with *Candida* sepsis is informative. Candidemia developed in a 30-year-old trauma victim who became an organ donor eight days following an automobile accident. The donor infection was probably introduced through an indwelling central line that was used for seven days to administer broad-spectrum antibiotics and intravenous hyperalimentation. The donor blood cultures were not found to be positive for *Candida* until hours after the organs had been transplanted. The sensitivity of the *Candida* strain was to amphotericin B and fluconazole. The heart and one of the kidney recipients were treated with amphotericin B for 10 to 14 days following transplantation. During that interval, to minimize the synergistic risks of renal toxicity from cyclosporine and amphotericin, these patients were treated with OKT-3 and steroid immunosuppression. Cyclosporine was begun thereafter. The liver recipient and the other renal allograft recipient were treated with fluconazole and cyclosporine immunosuppression immediately following transplantation. Neither of the renal recipients nor the heart patient has experienced a complication related to the donor *Candida* sepsis. The liver allograft recipient was noted to develop a *Candida* urolithiasis at four months following transplantation. This case illustrates the importance of surveillance donor blood cultures at the time of organ recovery, especially if the donor hospitalization was for longer than seven days' duration or if the donor was treated with intravenous total parenteral nutrition. It also underscores that donor-transmitted infections can be treated successfully in recipients, despite immunosuppression.

The determination of donor tuberculosis is an absolute contraindication to organ donation, as recipient deaths have occurred from disseminated tuberculosis (97). Malaria has been transmitted from bone marrow and solid organs to transplant recipients (98,99). Recipients of allografts from paid organ donors may be at increased risk for the development of this infection (98).

The diagnosis of a herpes simplex virus (HSV) encephalitis is also a contraindication to donation. The HSV may reach the brain through a nasal portal of entry, but biopsy-proven HSV encephalitis infers that viremia has occurred, potentially contaminating visceral organs. Donor HSV infection may be conveyed to an allograft recipient and result in disseminated disease in HSV-seronegative recipients (100). However, unless there is the suspicion of systemic donor HSV disease such as encephalitis, donor HSV testing is not routinely performed.

Serology Testing of the Donor

Most OPOs utilize a panel of "serology" screening to assess donor suitability, including HIV, human T-lymphotropic virus (HTLV), hepatitis B, hepatitis C, cytomegalovirus, toxoplasma, and syphilis. While donor screening for HIV, hepatitis B, and hepatitis C is routinely performed in the United States (101), there are no worldwide standards (102). The practices among OPOs vary widely, as do the interpretation and the reporting of the results (103). The testing laboratories usually employ an enzyme-linked immunosorbent assay (ELISA) to determine the presence of antibodies (with the exception of the hepatitis B surface antigen) in a peripheral blood sample of the prospective donor.

HIV Infection

Human immunodeficiency virus type 1 (HIV) has been transmitted by infected cadaver donors to multiple recipients of organs, resulting in the deaths of the allograft recipients (104,105). UNOS policy states that organs from donors with a positive HIV antibody screening are not suitable, unless subsequent confirmation testing indicates that the screening test was falsely positive. However, a confirmatory Western blot test cannot usually be performed within the time constraints of maximum cadaver organ preservation periods. Therefore, for practical purposes, cadaver donor serum that tests positive for HIV by the preliminary ELISA typically results in the discarding of all donor organs for transplantation. In contrast, there is ample time to perform confirmatory testing on living donors. As noted earlier, all living organ donors should undergo voluntary screening for HIV within two to three months prior to the planned transplant.

The American Red Cross is now screening blood and tissue donors for HIV antigen (p24) by an assay licensed by the Food and Drug Administration (106). This test may be available for organ donor screening in the future and enables HIV antigen detection within 30 days of exposure. The estimated average time between the p24 detection and the development of HIV antibody is approximately seven days; thus, the presumed increased sensitivity of the HIV p24 assay may be limited. However, p24 antigen detection may provide an alternative technique for excluding HIV in rare situations when the organ donor is negative by serology. For example, Simonds et al have reported the transmission of HIV to seven recipients via organs and tissues from a seronegative donor who had HIV p24 antigen retrospectively identified in cultured spleen tissue (107). Presumably p24 antigen could have been detected in a concurrently obtained peripheral blood sample. Five of the seven recipients (including the heart, liver, and kidney recipients) died with HIV infection.

The Center for Disease Control (CDC) has developed guidelines for limiting HIV transmission to organ and tissue recipients (Table 15.6) (108). The OPO staff must obtain a social history of all potential donors that addresses these criteria. When the social or medical history of a potential donor reveals any of the CDC-defined risks, organs may still be offered to potential recipients. The CDC guidelines require, however, that the transplant center inform the recipients of the potential risk of donor HIV infection, even if that risk involves only the donor's behavioral or medical history (109).

Potential donors with a history of incarceration in a correctional institution should be assessed by the usual standards. A negative serology for HIV and hepatitis may be sufficient to permit unrestricted donation if six consecutive months have elapsed since incarceration. Nevertheless, given the hazard of previous intravenous drug use in this population, some former inmates may not be suitable donors because of positive serology screening.

Table 15.6. Center for Disease Control Guidelines for Limiting HIV Transmission

A. *In the preceding 5 years:*
   - Men who have had sex with another man.
   - Persons who report nonmedical intravenous, intramuscular, or subcutaneous injection of drugs.
   - Men and women who have engaged in sex in exchange for money or drugs.

B. Persons with hemophilia or related clotting disorders who have received human-derived clotting factor concentrates.

C. *In the preceding 12 months:*
   - Persons who have had sex with any person described in items A and B above or with a person known or suspected to have HIV infection.
   - Persons who have been exposed to known or suspected HIV-infected blood through percutaneous inoculation or through contact with an open wound, non-intact skin, or mucous membrane.

D. Current inmates of correctional systems.

HTLV I Infection

Although UNOS policy regarding HTLV I screening is the same as it is for HIV (organ donors are not suitable), not all OPOs reject a cadaver donor with a positive anti-HTLV I serology assay (3). The risk of transmission of HTLV I by solid organ transplantation has not been clearly defined. HTLV has been transmitted to recipients of contaminated blood transfusions (110). A patient infected with HTLV I by blood transfusion is at risk for the development of either adult T-cell leukemia or neurologic disorders (111). Thus, HTLV I is considered hazardous, and, consistent with UNOS policy, many regard a positive donor screening for HTLV I to be an absolute contraindication to organ donation. However, depending on the emergent nature and life-threatened status of a particular candidate for transplantation (especially heart or liver), a patient may have little alternative but to accept an organ from a donor whose screening for HTLV I is positive. There is also a possibility that the screening test is falsely positive. The social history may be helpful in discerning whether there is a likelihood of a true positive being confirmed by subsequent testing.

Hepatitis B Infection

There are several serologic profiles for potential organ donors who have been infected with hepatitis B. The implications of donor infectivity vary according to both the serologic profile and the organ to be donated. The following review is categorized by the possible hepatitis B results reported by an OPO to the transplant center.

Hepatitis B Surface Antigen (HBsAg)-Positive HBsAg may be identified in the serum of an infected patient within 30 to 60 days of exposure. Hepatitis B virus (HBV) transmission has been documented to occur through organ transplantation (112,113). Thus, detection of HBsAg in the donor blood sample indicates the donor is at risk for transmitting HBV. The OPO, however, should verify the quality of the serum sample, as a false positive result can arise from a hemolyzed sample of donor blood.

Liver allografts from HBsAg-positive donors have been transplanted successfully to critically ill HBsAg-negative recipients in life-threatening clinical situations (114). Renal allografts from HBsAg-positive donors to HBsAg-negative recipients have also been transplanted without the development of recipient HBV infection; however, the satisfactory clinical course may have been influenced by the presence of previous immunization to HBV (115). Transplant physicians therefore should continue to consider the potential for a poor outcome when organs are transplanted from HBsAg-positive donors (deaths from HBV infection) even for HBsAg-positive recipients.

When the HBsAg-positive result is verified by repeat testing, organ procurement would likely be considered for either heart recipients in a life-threatening emergency status or perhaps those candidates who are anti-HBs-positive (by virtue of immunization or natural immunity).

Anti-HBs-Positive, HBsAg-Negative, HB Core Antibody (Anti-HBc)-Negative This serology profile typically results from previous intentional vaccination of an individual with hepatitis B vaccine; following the administration of HB immune globulin (HBIG); following the transfusion with a blood product from an immunized donor; or following recovery from previous HBV infection.

Antibody to HBsAg, unlike anti-HBc, does not arise during the acute infection but rather during convalescence. Thus, up to six months may elapse following HBV infection before anti-HBs is detected. In contrast, anti-HBc is usually detectable soon after exposure to the HBV, and it will usually persist (see below, the recently recognized importance of detecting anti-HBc).

This potential donor is not likely to transmit HBV because the HBsAg and the anti-HBc are negative. However, serum and liver HBV DNA has been detected by polymerase chain reaction (PCR) technique in patients with idiopathic chronic liver disease whose sera were HBsAg-negative, anti-HBs-positive (116). Moreover, the Mayo Clinic and UCSF groups have reported that a cadaver donor with a serology profile of HBsAg-negative, anti-HBs-positive, and anti-HBc-negative has transmitted HBV to a liver allograft recipient (117). They concluded that the sera from such donors may harbor HBV (as detected by PCR-DNA analysis) despite the negative HBsAg. It should be emphasized that this circumstance appears to occur rarely (<1%). Therefore, a donor serology profile of HBsAg-negative, anti-HBs-positive, and anti-HBc-negative does not appear to present a contraindication to recovery of all organs, especially if the medical history of the donor reveals an HBV vaccination or the administration of HBIG. If no such medical history is elicited, there is the unlikely possibility of HBV transmission from a cadaver donor with this serology profile to a liver allograft recipient (117).

HBsAg-Negative, Anti-HBs-Positive, Anti-HBc-Positive Anti-HBc (IgM) is the earliest antibody detected following HBV infection (10 to 14 days). Anti-HBc (IgG) can persist for the lifetime of a previously infected patient. Although it has been generally accepted that a serology profile of HBsAg-negative, anti-HBs-positive, anti-HBc-positive reveals recovery and immunity to HBV infection, HBV may still reside in the patient's liver. Recent reports are now underscoring the importance of anti-HBc detection regardless of the anti-HBs status (118–120). It is now well established that HBV has been transmitted to liver allograft recipients from cadaver donors whose blood samples revealed a serology profile of HBsAg-negative, anti-HBc-positive, even though the anti-HBs was also positive (120–123). Despite the sera from such donors being HBsAg-negative, the liver clearly continues to harbor HBV. Therefore, following transplantation, HBV can replicate in the newly immunosuppressed environment.

The Pittsburgh database of organ donors has been reviewed to determine the consequence of transplanting a liver allograft from an anti-HBc-positive donor to an HBsAg-negative recipient (119,120). There were 23 evaluable anti-HBc-positive of 982 HBsAg-negative donors. During a mean follow-up of 3.2 years, 19 of 23 (83%) of the patients receiving liver allografts from these donors developed HBV hepatitis (none of the recipients was HBV-positive prior to transplantation). Some of the donors were also anti-HBs-positive, emphasizing the fact that, although anti-HBs positivity may be associated with donor immunity to HBV, it is not necessarily protective against development of HBV hepatitis in the immunosuppressed recipient.

Following a review of their experience with de novo HBV infection transmitted from an organ donor, Douglas et al have suggested that the clinical course may be relatively mild (124). It also appears that the risk of HBV transmission from such HBsAg-negative, anti-HBc-positive donors is mainly for the liver allograft recipient. This serology profile may not carry the same risks for the recipients of other organs (118,125). In the UCSF review, only 1 of 42 kidney and 0 of 7 heart allograft recipients became HBsAg-positive following transplantation of organs from 25 HBsAg-negative, anti-HBc-positive donors, whereas 3 of 6 liver recipients became HBsAg-positive following transplantation. All of these recipients were HBsAg-negative prior to transplantation. Mount Sinai Medical Center and the New York Regional Transplant Program have also recently analyzed the outcome of 52 HBsAg-negative recipients of allografts from 21 anti-HBc-positive donors. Although 4 of 16 liver allograft recipients have become HBsAg-positive, none of the kidney or heart recipients has become positive (126).

Anti-HBc-Positive, HBsAg-Negative, Anti-HBs-Negative A profile of isolated anti-HBc positivity may reflect the window of time in which anti-HBs has yet to become detectable in an HBV-infected individual. Presumably an insufficient period has elapsed for the anti-HBs to become positive. Anti-HBc may be the only marker indicating early recovery from HBV infection, as the HBsAg has decreased in the peripheral blood to undetectable levels and the anti-HBs has yet to increase in sufficient titer to be detectable. It should be noted that the anti-HBc determination is not influenced by exposure to HBV vaccine.

This serology profile is a potential risk for all allograft recipients. HBsAg-negative, anti-HBcAb-positive donors can transmit HBV to renal allograft recipients as noted recently by Satterthwaite et al (127). Miller and his associates have proposed testing donor kidney tissue and serum by PCR analysis on HBsAg-negative, anti-HBcAb-positive donors, further clarifying the risk of HBV transmission for renal allograft recipients (128).

Donor liver function studies may not be helpful because they may be abnormal following premortem hemodynamic instability. A pretransplant liver biopsy should be performed on all HBcAb-positive donors to exclude portal piecemeal necrosis consistent with active hepatitis (118). If the biopsy is positive for hepatitis, the risk of HBV transmission is high.

Finally, there is an association of anti-HBc-positive donors with a positive serology for hepatitis C virus (HCV). A review of the serology profiles of nearly 1000 NEOB donors revealed 44 to be HBsAg-negative, anti-HBc-positive, 10 of whom were concomitantly HCV-positive. Thus, the detection of an HCV-positive serology raises the concern that the anti-HBc-positive result is related to infectious risk behavior.

We should also note that a false-positive anti-HBc result (by the ELISA method) may occur in as many as 30% of the positive results (Dodd R, personal communication, 1997). Turner et al have also evaluated this possibility by screening the sera of 400 HBsAg-negative UK organ donors. Only 5 (25%) of the 20 sera in which anti-HBc was initially detected as positive by the Kodak Amerlite assay were confirmed as anti-HBc-positive with subsequent testing by radioimmunoassay (129). These observations emphasize the need for additional studies to assess true infectivity from potential donors. Such studies include either a positive anti-HBs or HCV serology result, a prerecovery liver biopsy (118), or the PCR analysis of donor kidney tissue (128).

Some OPOs do not routinely assay for anti-HBs in the serologic assessment of a prospective donor (Miller C, personal communication, 1998), but rely only on the anti-HBc determination. If both the HBsAg and the anti-HBc are negative, there are no restrictions to organ recovery. If the serology reveals HBsAg-negative, anti-HBc-positive, the positive anti-HBc result is further defined by testing for IgM versus IgG. IgM-positive donor organs, suggesting recent HBV exposure, would not likely be recovered. However, IgG-positive donor organs may be recovered for life-threatened HBsAg-negative recipients or recipients who are HBsAg-positive. In either of the latter circumstances, Dr. Miller treats his recipients with HBIG following transplantation.

Nevertheless, the determination of an anti-HBs result may be useful in deciding whether extrahepatic organs should be transplanted from a donor with a serology profile of HBsAg-negative and anti-HBc-positive. As noted earlier, a positive anti-HBs determination indicates that the risk of HBV transmission to extrahepatic recipients is minimal.

Caldwell has emphasized the importance of post-transplant treatment of recipients of organs from an anti-HBc-positive donor. Post-transplantation treatment with either HBIG or lamivudine was effective in averting recipient de novo HBV infection (130).

Finally, the presence of anti-HBs in the potential allograft recipient (e.g., following previous HBV vaccination) may also be an important consideration. The risk of HBV infection by transplantation of a liver allograft from a donor who is anti-HBc-positive is reduced for recipients who have preexisting anti-HBs (120). Table 15.7 presents a summary of the risks related to the transmission of HBV infection according to the results of donor serologic testing.

Hepatitis C Virus

The hazard of HCV transmission from a previously infected organ donor is a concern for all allograft recipients. Anti-HCV antibody appears in a peripheral blood sample within two months of HCV exposure. Most OPOs have adopted a policy of screening organ donors for anti-HCV antibody (103); approximately 5% of all organ donors are anti-HCV positive (131). Currently, all organ donors should be tested for anti-HCV antibody using a second-generation enzyme immunoassay that has increased sensitivity and specificity compared to earlier assays (132). Unfortunately, antibody to HCV does not represent donor immunity to HCV. Nevertheless, it is important to emphasize that detecting anti-HCV in the donor serology panel is not predictive of HCV transmission (132).

Approximately 50% of anti-HCV-positive patients have detectable hepatitis C viremia by PCR analysis of peripheral blood (131). All PCR-positive organ donors will transmit HCV to allograft recipients (131); however, the risk of HCV transmission from a PCR-negative (anti-HCV antibody–positive) donor remains unclear (133). Unfortunately, PCR testing (or branched-chain DNA testing) cannot be accomplished within the time constraints necessary for the release of the donor organs. Thus, although exclusion of all

Table 15.7. Summary of the Hepatitis B Serology Risks

Donor Serology Pattern	Presence of HBV DNA in Blood	Risk HBV Transmission to Liver Recipients	Risk of HBV Transmission to Extra-Hepatic Recipients
HBsAg+	Yes	Yes	Yes
HBsAg– Anti-HBs+[a] Anti-HBc–	Unlikely	Yes, but small	Rare
HBsAg– Anti-HBs+/– Anti-HBc+[b]	Possible	Yes, irrespective of anti-HBs+ donor	Yes, but small from anti-HBs+ donor

[a] Check donor history for HBV vaccination.
[b] Clarify whether false positive anti-HBc: check HCV serology result; do prerecovery liver biopsy. Perhaps consider for an anti-HBs+ recipient.

anti-HCV-positive organ donors could eliminate the possibility of HCV transmission, such an indiscriminate policy would unnecessarily discard some organs that are not infected with HCV.

The consequence of receiving an organ from a donor who is anti-HCV-positive can be summarized as follows: approximately 50% of the recipients will develop detectable anti-HCV antibody; 24% will have hepatitis C viremia detectable by PCR analysis; and 35% may develop liver disease (131).

Despite the high risk of transmission of HCV to allograft recipients (134), a positive serologic screening does not necessarily rule out organ donation (133). For example, transplanting an HCV-positive heart allograft when the recipient's life is endangered is an accepted practice even if the recipient is HCV-negative (87,135). More generalized transplantation of organs from HCV-positive donors remains controversial (136). Since effective treatment of HCV infection in an immunosuppressed allograft recipient is typically difficult, some centers regard a positive HCV donor serology as a contraindication to transplantation. Other researchers, such as Fishman et al, have suggested a selective strategy of reserving organs from HCV-positive donors for recipients with previous HCV exposure documented by detectable anti-HCV antibody (133). It must be noted that evidence in both animal models and human studies indicates that "superinfection" with a donor-specific HCV strain can occur even in previously HCV-positive recipients (137,138). Thus, this approach is not without some risk. Nevertheless, liver transplantation from an anti-HCV-positive donor to an anti-HCV-positive recipient does not appear to cause increased morbidity or mortality (139). Similar reasoning has suggested that kidneys from an anti-HCV-positive donor could be targeted for sensitized, diabetic, or elderly recipients who might otherwise have limited opportunity for receiving a donor organ or a relatively limited lifespan during which chronic hepatitis is unlikely to develop (133). This approach seems to be prudent, as the longer-term risk of chronic hepatitis in renal transplant recipients has now been documented (140,141).

Cytomegalovirus

The seminal work of Ho et al (142) established the cadaveric organ donor as an important source of CMV infection in the organ recipient (see also Chapter 36). Thus, all prospective organ donors and recipients should be routinely tested for antibody to CMV. As with HCV, the presence of antibody in either the donor or the recipient indicates the presence of latent viral infection. The specific CMV donor and recipient serologic status has implications for prophylaxis; the highest risk patients are CMV-seronegative recipients of CMV-seropositive donor organs—the so-called primary infection group. Transplantation of an organ from a CMV-positive donor results in reactivation of the latent virus and replication in the immunosuppressed host. In addition, there is molecular evidence that superinfection by the donor strain can occur even in CMV-seropositive recipients (143). However, recent evidence suggests that CMV donor positive–recipient negative mismatches can be successfully overcome by therapeutic strategies incorporating anti-viral prophylaxis (144).

Historically, several studies in kidney, liver, lung, and bowel transplantation had demonstrated decreased survival rates among recipients of CMV-seropositive organs (145,146). In fact, centers performing small bowel transplantation have generally excluded CMV-seropositive donor organs from CMV-seronegative recipients because of the unacceptably high morbidity and mortality (147). The development of post-transplant CMV disease has been associated with increased morbidity and costs (148) as well as other opportunistic infections (149). Recipient CMV infection is also associated with an increased risk of organ rejection, allograft loss, and death (146,150,151). Fortunately for current transplant recipients, the data from many of these studies predates more effective prophylactic strategies for control of CMV infection (152).

The laboratory techniques used for CMV serologic testing of donors include enzyme immunoassay and latex agglutination. These assays have been developed primarily for blood donor screening. As a result, they are very sensitive and generally err toward classifying patients or donors as falsely positive. It is our personal experience that false-positive results may occur in about 10% to 15% of cadaveric donors.

The transplantation of CMV-seropositive donor organs has not been considered an absolute contraindication to transplantation despite the increased risks cited earlier. This is especially pertinent for potential living organ donors (37). The primary reason for accepting such organs for transplantation is the high seroprevalence of the virus in the general population. The prevalence among both organ donors and organ recipients varies from 40% to 80% depending on age, socioeconomic status, and geographic distribution. Fortunately, better control of CMV with refinements in immunosuppression, and the development of effective antiviral agents, has improved the outcome for patients receiving organs from CMV-seropositive donors.

Preferably, testing for CMV should be performed prior to any blood or plasma product transfusion to the organ donor. Testing of organ donors after blood product transfusion presents the additional complexity of assessing the risk of CMV transmission in the transfused blood products, even though this risk should be very small (currently less than 1% risk of acquiring CMV from blood product transfusion). Testing after donor transfusion also introduces the possibility of a false positive CMV assay resulting from the anti-CMV antibody passively transmitted in the blood products.

Use of CMV IgM antibody assays in addition to IgG antibody assays has been advocated by some OPOs. In our experience, IgM anti-CMV is not present in the absence of IgG antibody. Furthermore, the IgM assay lacks sensitivity;

it is not as standardized as the available IgG assays, and false-positive results are not uncommon (153–155). Therefore, from a practical perspective, we do not recommend their use as there is little additional information to be gained by screening for IgM antibody to CMV.

Other Viruses

The transmission of neurotropic viruses such as rabies and Creutzfeldt-Jakob disease from tissue donors has been reported (156). Thus, deaths associated with these diagnoses exclude a potential donor from consideration. Although successful transplantation of renal allografts from donors with Reye's syndrome (encephalopathy and liver failure) has been reported (157,158), some transplant centers may be reluctant to expose their recipients to the risks of an unknown (presumed viral) etiology of donor death.

Over 95% of potential adult donors are seropositive for Epstein-Barr virus (EBV) (IgG antibody); thus, serologic screening of organ donors for EBV has not been routinely performed. Nevertheless, primary EBV infection (i.e., transplantation of an organ from an EBV-seropositive donor to an EBV-seronegative recipient) is associated with an increased risk of post-transplant lymphoproliferative disease (see Chapter 37). Therefore, recognition of this mismatch in a potential allograft recipient known to be EBV-negative may have important prognostic information. Currently there is no effective means of preventing this complication.

Treponemal Antigen (Syphilis)

The detection of antibody to syphilis by the rapid plasma reagin test (RPR) is not a contraindication to organ procurement (90), but it is a contraindication to tissue procurement. The RPR is reactive in more than 90% of patients with primary syphilis, but it may be negative for 6 to 18 months following primary infection. Although syphilis can be transmitted by blood transfusion (159), we are unaware of a recorded infection of a transplant recipient from a syphilitic donor. Moreover, a standard course of penicillin would provide sufficient therapy to prevent syphilitic complications in an allograft recipient (87). This regimen has been reportedly successful in the treatment of two renal allograft recipients intentionally given kidneys from an organ donor whose serology tests for syphilis were positive (159). Thus, a recipient of an allograft from any RPR-positive donor should be treated for 15 days either with penicillin or with doxycycline, tetracycline, or erythromycin for those who are penicillin allergic.

Toxoplasma

The possible transmission of the protozoan *Toxoplasma gondii* is of concern primarily for heart allograft recipients because of the predilection of this parasite for muscle tissue. Organ procurement from seropositive donors is not contraindicated; however, the detection of seropositivity means that the recipient may be placed at higher risk. Fortunately, the use of trimethoprim-sulfamethoxazole typically administered to recipients for *Pneumocystis carinii* prophylaxis also prevents infection by *T. gondii* (160).

Responsibility to Donor Families Regarding Positive Serology Testing

When donor serology screening reveals a positive test, confirmatory testing may be subsequently performed by independent laboratories for each pathogen (including *Treponema*). The practice of the NEOB is to report the confirmed positive findings to the family member who gave consent for donation if there is a hazard that the donor might have transmitted infection to that family member (contact with bodily fluids). This process ensures that any family member who is potentially at risk for having been exposed to HBV, HCV, HIV, HTLV, or syphilis would be appropriately cared for. Such notification would not necessarily apply to estranged family or guardians who consent to donation.

Poison as a Cause of Donor Death

Accidental or suicidal poisonings through inhalation, ingestion, or injection of toxic substances result in several thousand fatalities each year in the United States (161). Barbiturate and benzodiazepine medications are frequently overdosed by suicide victims. Although the majority of these deaths occur in association with cardiopulmonary arrest, some patients are resuscitated for a period of time, only to become brain dead. These patients may be considered for organ donation (Table 15.8).

Each toxic exposure must be evaluated with respect to specific organ injury. Drugs such as acetaminophen may render the liver unsuitable for transplantation because of fulminant hepatic necrosis, but other organs may not be injured. The NEOB has successfully recovered a heart allograft for transplantation from a cadaver donor with fatal acetaminophen-induced liver failure.

Tricyclic antidepressants may cause liver injury and, depending on the tissue concentrations of the tricyclic, adverse effects for recipients of the donor organs (162). The

Table 15.8. Poisons as a Cause of Cadaver Organ Donor Death

Cause of Death	Organs Transplanted	References
Acetaminophen	Heart	169, NEOB
Barbiturates	Kidneys	169
Benzodiazepine	Heart, liver, kidneys	NEOB
Carbon monoxide	Liver, kidneys	164,167,169
Cyanide	Kidneys	166,167,169, NEOB
Imipramine	Liver, kidneys	163, NEOB
Methanol	Heart, liver, kidneys	168, NEOB
Methaqualone	Kidneys	169
Warfarin	Heart, lungs, liver, pancreas, kidneys	NEOB

donor liver may provide tricyclic blood levels in the recipient that produce mental status toxicity and cardiac instability (162). Nevertheless, Fattinger et al have reported successful transplantation of kidneys from a patient who died from a trimipramine overdose, and have suggested that transplantation of the liver might also be feasible from such a donor if the tricyclic level in the donor serum falls to an acceptable level (163).

Carbon monoxide is a common cause of inhalation suicide in the United States (161). Accidental carbon monoxide poisoning can also occur following exposure to solvents in paint removers and by the release of vapors from faulty home heating systems. Death usually occurs from hypoxia prior to arrival in the emergency ward because carbon monoxide rapidly displaces oxygen from the hemoglobin molecule. For those resuscitated patients who subsequently develop anoxic brain death, assessment of renal injury by urine sampling (for myoglobin, protein, and red blood cells) is useful in deciding whether to proceed with kidney procurement, as rhabdomyolysis can affect renal function (164). Depending on liver function and biopsy morphology, liver transplantation should also be considered (165).

Prompt identification of the toxin and treatment to minimize end organ damage can be critical lifesaving measures. These measures can also be consequential to successful organ salvage from patients who cannot be resuscitated from the poison. For example, cyanide causes cellular anoxia within 30 minutes of ingestion or within seconds of inhalation (161). Decreased mitochondrial oxidative metabolism and oxygen utilization leads to lactic acidosis. Unless an antidote regimen of amyl nitrate inhalation, intravenous injection of sodium nitrite, and intravenous injection of sodium thiosulfate is administered promptly, irreversible central nervous system (CNS) damage may ensue (166). Barkoukis et al have reported that use of these cyanide antidotes has resulted in resumption of satisfactory organ function in a patient whose brain injury was beyond resolution following cyanide-mediated suicide, enabling the successful transplantation of the heart and kidneys (166). Liver allografts can also be successfully transplanted from donors with fatal cyanide poisoning, despite initial cyanide toxicity to the liver (166,167).

Hemodialysis and ethanol administration have been used to correct metabolic acidosis and stabilize organ function in a patient who died following methanol ingestion, resulting in the successful transplantation of renal allografts (168). NEOB transplant centers have also successfully transplanted the liver and both kidneys from a donor with fatal methanol toxicity.

Multiple organs have been recovered from an NEOB donor who committed suicide by the ingestion of rat poison. The active ingredient of the poison was sodium brodifacoum. The donor's prothrombin time peaked at 200 seconds but returned to near normal 48 hours later, enabling the successful transplantation of the kidneys, heart, lungs, and liver.

These illustrative cases demonstrate that the toxic organ injury from a fatal poisoning may be reversible. Thus, if the adverse effect of the poison to specific organ function has resolved, recovery and transplantation is appropriate. The function of organs transplanted from donors who have died from poisoning has been satisfactory (169,170).

Donor Consent

As noted earlier, perhaps the most significant obstacle to increasing the number of cadaver organs for transplantation has been obtaining consent. The lack of family consent is the most common reason why potential organ donors are lost, although there are also missed opportunities because the family was never asked to donate (171).

Family consent remains an absolute requirement for organ donation in many communities, irrespective of an individual's previously declared intention as indicated by a donor card. However, the identification of a donor card carried by a deceased person can influence the decision of the family to donate, especially for minority individuals (172). Moreover, there are now statutes that give explicit permission to recover organs with a signed donor card even in the absence of family consent, which makes hospitals legally responsible for referring a potential donor, and mandate that trained personnel introduce the idea of organ donation (Nathan H, personal communication, 1997).

The NEOB has developed an advisory board composed of clergy, media, business leaders, hospital association personnel, legislators, donor families, and transplant recipients—all guided and brought together by the OPO to enhance donation. The goal is to generate new ideas on public education of donation and implementation of new programs geared to promote these ideas.

Although public surveys indicate that a majority of individuals have a positive attitude toward organ donation, there are several misconceptions that can arise at the time of the family permission request and become obstacles to obtaining consent (173). These include confusion about the meaning of brain death, beliefs that transplantation is experimental, concern that there is an underworld market for organs, fear that donor families may face additional medical bills or that the donor's body may be disfigured, and suspicions that the medical profession orchestrating the donation is not trustworthy (174). Thus, to achieve an ideal rate of success the consent process requires structure, consistency, and an experienced person to make the request of a bereaved family.

It is now evident that a discussion of the donation process by the primary care team creates an appearance of conflict of interests that may heighten the family's reluctance to consent. In addition, the primary care team may not be skilled in the request process. In contrast, separating the determination of death by the primary care team from the request for donation made by a representative of the OPO presents a clearer line of responsibility to the family. Family questions regarding the misunderstandings noted above are better answered by a representative of the OPO. Families may subsequently wish to inquire about the outcome of the donation surgery. The OPO coordinator can inform the donor family of the result of their donation without revealing the identity of the organ recipients. This opportunity is an appealing benefit to the donor family.

Thus, the elements included in the best approach to achieve consent for organ donation are: 1) a thorough discussion by the primary care team of the irreversibility of the brain injury that has led to the diagnosis of death, 2) an early referral to the OPO for assessment of donation potential, and 3) after the family accepts the determination of death, introduction of a representative from the OPO to discuss the process of organ donation.

Directed Donation

While it is illegal in the United States to restrict the donation of an organ or organs to a class of individuals (e.g., by gender, race, national origin), directed donation to a specific individual by name may be acceptable. This individual should be known to the family member requesting the directed donation. Since the buying and selling of human organs is also illegal, the primary care physician should not knowingly participate in any directed donation involving monetary exchange or other inducement to directed donation. Thus, the nature of the relationship between the next-of-kin of the donor and the individual to whom the organ is being directed should be ascertained. Unless a relationship is substantiated, the possibility of directed donation is discouraged. The family should also be informed that ABO incompatibility, as well as other medical considerations, may preclude the possibility of directed donation.

Procedure from Donor Referral to Organ Recovery

Stratification of OPO procedures is based on the stage of the clinical situation. The activities noted within each section below are exclusive and they are presented in sequential order. The importance of this paradigm is to illustrate a practice that is both consistent and ethical. There are two cardinal rules that should be emphasized: 1) minimally invasive procedures, such as blood sampling, to determine organ donor suitability may be done after the family gives permission, but prior to declaration of death; 2) no invasive procedure for the purpose of organ donation should be performed unless the patient is declared dead.

Referral for Donation by the Primary Care Team

The initial responsibility of the OPO coordinator is to establish the criteria of donor suitability—age, cause of death, clinical exclusion criteria, and circulatory and ventilator status. The OPO coordinator may consult with the primary care team to discuss the family option for donation and to review the donation procedure.

Verbal Family Interest for Donation

Noninvasive procedures for the sole objective of donor evaluation are indicated. Family consent for donor evaluation should be documented in the patient chart by the primary care team or by the OPO coordinator, independent of consent for donation. Charges for evaluation are the responsibility of the OPO. These include clinical blood sampling, blood type and crossmatch for possible donor transfusion, urinalysis, sputum and urine cultures, chest x-ray, electrocardiogram, and echocardiogram. There should be no written orders by the OPO coordinator until a declaration of death and written family consent are obtained.

Written Family Consent for Donation in Advance of the Diagnosis of Death

HLA typing by peripheral blood samples should be performed if at all possible to expedite the identification of potential recipients. However, this may be contraindicated by red blood cell (RBC) and platelet transfusions given to the donor prior to death. HLA typing is then best accomplished by femoral lymph node procurement after the declaration of death. Serology testing for hepatitis, HIV, HTLV, CMV, and syphilis may now be performed, but not prior to written family consent. Organ placement is now possible, with crossmatching of donor cells with sera from potential recipients as required.

Written Family Consent for Donation Following the Declaration of Death

OPO orders of donor management are now permissible; so too are invasive procedures that include groin node retrieval, bronchoscopy, cardiac catheterization, and placement of infusion lines. Thus, HLA typing and crossmatching by lymph node sampling of the donor is indicated (Figure 15.5). Again, no invasive procedures should be performed until a pronouncement of death has been made. Organ and tissue procurement can now proceed following medical examiner notification if required.

Heart-Beating Cadaver Donor

Brain Death

In 1996, 99% of organ donors in the United States were declared dead by brain death criteria (UNOS, Richmond, VA). Thus, its importance in the process of organ donation cannot be underestimated. The American Academy of Neurology (AAN) defines brain death as "an irreversible loss of the clinical function of the brain, including the brain stem." This understanding of brain death is well accepted in most countries; the major exception until recently was Japan.

In the absence of brain death criteria, deaths are declared by the loss of cardiorespiratory function. However, as a simple and unifying concept, all death occurs when there is permanent loss of the entire brain function.

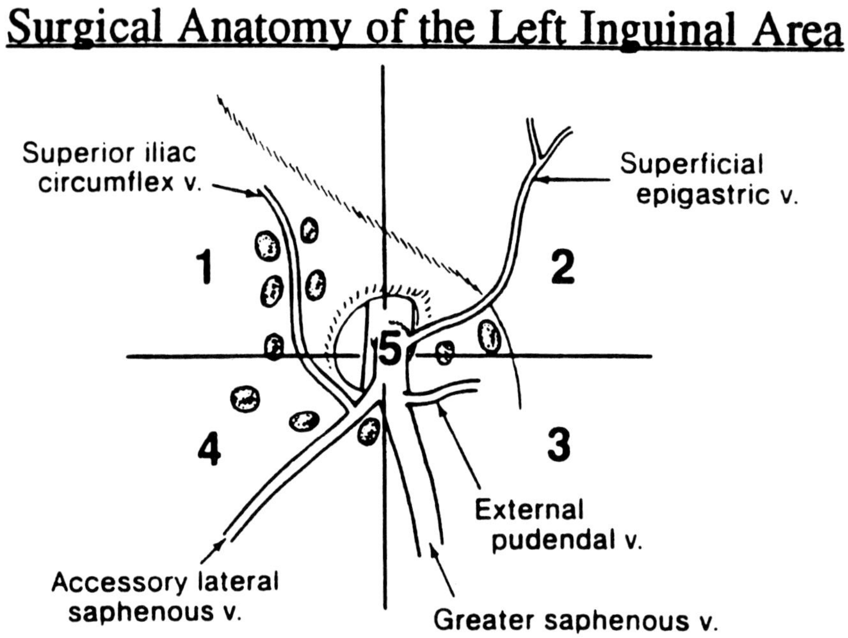

FIGURE 15.5. *Illustration of the groin anatomy of the lymph node recovery. Quadrants 1 and 4 are the location of the best yield of lymph nodes. (Reproduced by permission from Skandalakis JE, Gray SW, Rowe JS Jr. Hernias. In: Anatomical complications in general surgery. New York: McGraw-Hill, 1983:252–281.)*

The identification of brain death as "legal" death is supported widely. However, the criteria that are used to establish brain death may vary. In the United States, the Uniform Brain Death Act approved by the National Conference of Commissioners and Uniform State Laws has declared that "determination of death under this act should be in accordance with reasonable medical standards." Although it is clearly not the responsibility of the transplant physician to diagnose brain death or declare a potential organ donor dead, the transplant physician should be knowledgeable of the criteria that would be "in accordance with reasonable medical standards." The proximate cause for the absence of clinical brain function should be known and demonstrably irreversible. This is especially meaningful today, as the validity of the diagnosis of brain death has been questioned (6).

Guidelines for the clinical diagnosis of brain death promulgated by the AAN are as follows:

A. Prerequisites:
   1. Clinical or neuroimaging evidence of an acute CNS catastrophe that is compatible with the clinical diagnosis of brain death.
   2. Exclusion of complicating medical conditions that may confound clinical assessment (e.g., no severe electrolyte, acid-base, or endocrine disturbance).
   3. No drug intoxication or poisoning.
   4. Core temperature ≥32°C (90°F).

B. Three cardinal findings:
   1. Coma or unresponsiveness.
   2. Absence of brain stem reflexes (pupil, ocular, corneal, pharyngeal, and tracheal).
   3. Apnea.

The brain stem (responsible for spontaneous breathing and vasomotor control) has chemoreceptors that monitor the P_{CO_2} and pH of the cerebrospinal fluid (CSF), which approximate changes in the plasma. An apnea test supports the diagnosis of brain death if the P_{CO_2} is 60 mm Hg or higher and no respiratory movement (abdominal or chest excursion) is detected.

C. Confirmatory laboratory testing (175):
   1. Electroencephalogram.
   2. Contrast or isotope angiography.
   3. Isotope scanning.
   4. Transcranial Doppler ultrasonography.

Although these tests are not mandatory for the diagnosis of brain death in adults, they are recommended for children (176). Specific guidelines for the determination of brain death in children have been published that emphasize the necessity of two clinical examinations, apnea tests, and laboratory confirmation studies 24 to 48 hours apart, depending on the age of the child (176).

Brain Stem Death

In the United Kingdom, Christopher Pallis has concluded that "if there is no functioning brainstem there can be no meaningful or integrated activity of the cerebral hemispheres, no cognitive or effective life, no thoughts or feelings, no social interaction with the environment." Thus, the UK code of brain death focuses on the brain stem reflexes, which include pupillary response to light, corneal (blinking), vestibulo-ocular response to caloric tests, grimacing to painful stimuli, and gagging. If these brain stem functions are absent in a ventilated comatose patient with persistent apnea (in which the cause of the structural brain damage is known and the exclusions of hypothermia and drug toxicity are provided), the patient can be declared dead (177).

Organ-Specific Evaluation

There are few standardized criteria for determining the suitability of specific organs for transplantation. The final decision to use each organ rests with physicians who must judge the capacity of that organ to achieve a life-sustaining function. Poor function of the donor organ can obviously result in the death of the recipient. Thus, the experienced physician, knowing the relative condition of the recipient, determines whether a particular donor organ will be acceptable based mainly on the considerations discussed below.

Cadaver Donor Age Hearts have been transplanted from donors ranging in age from less than 1 week to over 60 years. While many heart transplant centers will consider donors up to age 65, the number of hearts actually transplanted from patients over 50 has been low. Only about 8% of cadaver heart donors in the United States are older than 50 (2). The data are similar for lung donors.

The main concern in using an older heart for transplantation is the likely presence of coronary artery disease (CAD). Cardiac catheterization may be a useful adjunct to assessing the status of the donor coronary circulation. While significant CAD confirmed by coronary angiography usually renders the donor heart unsuitable, there have been reports of ex vivo cardiac surgery (e.g., coronary artery bypass grafting) to repair the donor heart prior to transplantation (178).

In contrast to heart donors, more than 20% of liver donors are older than 50 (2). It is interesting to note that the recent discard rate for liver allografts from donors older than 60 years of age procured by the NEOB was only 28% (18 of 25 transplanted), with an 80.6% rate of recovery of livers from all donors older than 60 (25 of 31) (179). Most centers have now adopted a liberal approach to liver recovery from donors despite their older age (180,181).

Intraoperative liver biopsies appear to be useful for determining hepatic allograft acceptability (182,183). This is best accomplished by a needle biopsy, as wedge biopsies of the liver edge may give a false indication of fibrosis. In our experience, a liver biopsy revealing greater than 50% macrovesicular fat is associated with poor function following transplantation (see also Chapter 19).

The age limits for cadaver donor pancreata are more restrictive than for other vascularized organs; most programs exclude donors under age 10 or over the age of 50. Nevertheless, 7% of UNOS pancreata in 1995 were procured from cadaver donors older than 50 (2).

Kidneys are rarely successfully transplanted from cadavers older than 70. However, an elliptical wedge biopsy of the renal cortex (post-recovery) is useful in deciding whether a kidney from an older-age donor is acceptable. The percent of sclerosed glomeruli is a reliable measure that can be readily determined by frozen section. Generally, donor kidneys with more than 20% glomerulosclerosis are considered unsuitable for conventional transplantation (184). In some cases, these kidneys may be used in "2 for 1" protocols, where both kidneys are implanted into a single recipient (185,186) (see Marginal Donor, below).

Organ-Specific Functional Analysis The preoperative evaluation is based on laboratory tests of organ function, with supplemental imaging studies (echocardiogram) and invasive procedures (cardiac catheterization and bronchoscopy) where appropriate.

Heart Patients with severely depressed cardiac function, significant congenital cardiac anomalies, or significant acquired cardiac disease (such as valvular disease, coronary artery disease, or previous myocardial infarction) are generally deemed unsuitable. Thorough prerecovery evaluation is critical, since current ex vivo cardiac preservation times are limited, and concurrent surgical preparation of the recipient is often required. Laboratory tests should include arterial blood gases (ABG) and creatine phosphokinase (CPK) with myocardial band (MB) fractionation. While the use of donor pulmonary artery pressure monitoring is usually not indicated, serial cardiac indices and calculated systemic vascular resistances should be measured when possible to better assess donor cardiac function and guide donor management.

The donor chest x-rays, 12-lead electrocardiograms, and echocardiogram should be interpreted by an experienced cardiologist. Transesophageal echocardiography can be performed if the transthoracic study is technically limited. Evidence of wall motion abnormalities, global or localized hypokinesis, and estimated left ventricular ejection fraction should be noted as well. Advances in telemedicine (187) may permit routine transmission of these data directly to the transplant center for review prior to the final decision regarding acceptability (see also Chapter 23).

Lung Evidence of chronic lung disease generally precludes donation, although a history of asthma still warrants further consideration.

Careful assessment of pulmonary function necessitates arterial blood gas monitoring. Ideally, the donor should maintain a PO_2 of more than 100 mm Hg on a 0.40 fraction of inspired oxygen (FIO_2). Further testing of lung suitability includes ABG determination on 100% FIO_2, with a goal of PO_2 of more than 300 mm Hg. Serial blood gases help evaluate lung function over time prior to recovery. Chest x-rays at intervals of six to eight hours prior to recovery may be necessary to evaluate evolving pulmonary edema or pneumonia. Bronchoscopy should be performed to exclude gross aspiration or presence of purulent secretions in the bronchial tree. The presence of normal oropharyngeal flora in the sputum culture is not a contraindication (see also Chapter 25).

Liver Liver donor evaluation should include determination of any history of liver disease, liver function tests including coagulation studies, and intraoperative examination of the liver. Mild to moderate elevation of serum transaminases (<6 to 8 × normal) or prothrombin times (<20 seconds) may be acceptable. Blunt force to the right upper quadrant raises the suspicion of traumatic liver injury, but this is best assessed by direct visualization in the operating room. Many liver lacerations do not preclude successful recovery and transplantation (see also Chapter 19).

Kidney Minimum preoperative information to assess donor kidneys includes current blood urea nitrogen (BUN), creatinine, electrolytes, and urinalysis. A history of significant renal disease or injury should be excluded. Evaluation of donor renal function includes serial BUN and creatinine values, quantity and quality (urinalysis) of urine output, history, and physical examination. In general, a terminal creatinine of less than 2.0 mg/dL is desired. For older or borderline donors, a rapid estimate of the creatinine clearance can be obtained using the Cockcroft-Gault formula (188). Ideally, donor urine output should be from 1 to 3 cc/kg/hour, since oliguria in the immediate preoperative interval correlates with poor functional outcomes.

Surgical evaluation includes careful visual inspection of the kidneys. Anatomic variations such as duplicate ureters and multiple renal arteries or veins do not exclude successful transplantation. However, severe mechanical injury such as renal arterial intimal disruption from rapid deceleration trauma or extreme parenchymal injury evidenced by extensive subcapsular hematoma, or evidence of renal malignancy, will usually render the kidneys unsuitable.

Pretransplant inspection of the donor kidney should be carefully performed prior to recipient skin incision to exclude any previously undetected structural problems. Lack of uniform consistency or color may be evidence of perfusion injury and should trigger a diligent search for nonperfused renal arteries. It is critical to identify and reconstruct accessory renal arteries (>1.5 mm diameter), especially lower polar vessels, since ureteral ischemia may lead to necrosis and graft loss (see also Chapter 17).

Pancreas In general, suitability criteria for donor pancreata are more restrictive than for other vascular organs. Since the only indication for pancreas transplantation is insulin-dependent diabetes mellitus, the endocrine function of the donor pancreas must be excellent at the time of donation (see also Chapter 21).

A normal donor serum glucose profile is ideal. Subclinical pancreatitis may be excluded by determination of donor amylase and preferably lipase, since hyperamylasemia may be due to increased salivary amylase release due to facial trauma. When possible, fractionation of the amylase will differentiate between pancreatic and salivary hyperamylasemia. Hyperlipasemia is a more specific finding that generally indicates pancreatic inflammation.

Donor Management

Intensive care unit management of the brain-dead organ donor is a complex and dynamic process directed toward maintenance of end organ function and viability. Commonly encountered clinical problems include hypotension, polyuria, electrolyte imbalances, cardiac dysfunction, and hypothermia (189). Increased blood cytokine levels occur in brain-dead patients. Although interleukin-1 beta (IL-1β) and tumor necrosis factor alpha (TNFα) levels appear to be within normal range, IL-6 levels have been shown to be abnormal (190). The consequence of the IL-6 elevation is not known. However, careful hemodynamic monitoring, anticipation of instability, and rapid treatment are required to maximize the recovery of transplantable organs.

Initial Goals The primary donor management goals include restoration and maintenance of normothermia, normalization of blood pressure, optimization of lung function, restoration of intravascular volume, and correction of acid/base and electrolyte imbalances. Conflicting approaches to ideal management from the various transplant specialties may require the placement of a central line to ensure filling pressures that avoid fluid overload but permit optimal organ perfusion. Without these sophisticated data, the kidney team may prefer aggressive fluid administration and brisk diuresis, the liver and pancreas team may favor adequate but not excessive portal and arterial perfusion pressures, but the thoracic teams may request volume contraction to minimize the development of pulmonary edema. Therefore, preliminary evaluation of organ suitability may be helpful in guiding management when one or more organs are clearly unsuitable. Subsequent management efforts can then be preferentially directed toward those organs that will likely be utilized.

Poikilothermia Loss of thermoregulatory function results from hypothalamic dysfunction in brain-dead patients (191). A capacity for shivering thermogenesis is absent (192). Passive heat loss may lead to progressive hypothermia, which is known to adversely effect cellular metabolism, oxygen release, and cardiac function.

Due to the relatively high body surface area to body mass ratio in neonates and children, core temperatures may fluctuate much more rapidly in these individuals than in adults. In all cases, patient temperature should be carefully monitored and hypothermia should be treated early. It is easier to prevent hypothermia than to reverse it. Effective treatment includes maintenance of room temperature at 75°F or above, keeping the body surfaces well covered at all times, using warming blankets, and heating of intravenous fluids. The use of a warming blanket in the operating room is essential to counter passive heat loss and maintain normothermia. Heating humidified oxygen (to 45°C) via the ventilator may be also of benefit; however, this is not usually necessary. Since oxygen heating may cause thermal injury to the airway, it is not employed unless more routine measures prove ineffective.

Hypertension Severe hypertension [systolic blood pressure (BP) >200 mm Hg] is infrequently encountered in brain-dead patients. However, when hypertension is observed, it is likely related to brain stem herniation and is therefore self-limiting. The reason to treat sustained hypertension is to avoid transient rhythm disturbances. The goal of treatment should be to maintain the diastolic BP below 100 mm Hg.

Sodium nitroprusside (Nipride) infusion is the treatment of choice. Nipride should only be used in cases of severe, persistent hypertension, since prolonged administration may result in cyanide toxicity (193).

Hypotension Alternatively, hypotension (systolic BP <90 mm Hg) is more frequently observed in brain-dead patients, especially at the time of initial referral. Since even brief intervals of prerecovery hypotension can profoundly influence organ function following transplantation, a central venous pressure line and an arterial line are essential in order to manage hypotension appropriately. The most common cause is hypovolemia. If hemodynamic instability persists following volume expansion, a pulmonary artery catheter should be introduced, and serial cardiac outputs and systemic vascular resistance measurements should be determined.

Hypovolemia Excessive intravascular volume loss (hemorrhage, diabetes insipidus) is common in potential organ donors, especially trauma victims. Neurogenic vasodilatation, common in brain-dead individuals, may exacerbate the hemodynamic instability. Intravascular volume deficits should be corrected prior to the use of vasoactive drugs. However, low to moderate dose dopamine hydrochloride (Intropin) infusion (1–5 μg/kg/min) may be required to maintain adequate BP during the initial period of volume repletion. Colloid (albumin, Plasmanate) and blood products (PRBCs) may be necessary for volume expansion in combination with crystalloid solutions. Monitoring of the central venous pressure (ideally 10 to 15 mm Hg) will avoid the development of pulmonary edema, especially in potential lung donors. As the blood volume is restored, vasoactive drugs should be discontinued.

Decreased Vascular Resistance Despite adequate volume restoration, some donors will require additional vasoactive drug therapy because of neurogenic vasodilatation. A dopamine dosage between 5–10 μg/kg/min may be necessary, since the alpha receptors of peripheral blood vessels do not respond with vasoconstriction until this dose range is reached. A dopamine dose that exceeds 10 μg/kg/min usually requires insertion of a pulmonary artery catheter for determination of cardiac filling pressures, cardiac output (CO), and systemic vascular resistance (SVR). The SVR is calculated by thermodilution cardiac output measurements. If the SVR ([(MAP − CVP) × 80]/CO) is less than 400 dynes/sec/cm^{-5}, vasoconstrictor therapy is indicated. Such a scenario suggests the possibility of donor sepsis.

Depressed Cardiac Function Some donors may exhibit depressed cardiac function (not surprising following resuscitation from cardiopulmonary arrest) due to preexisting cardiac disease or secondary to brain stem herniation. Brain death causes a significant loss of both right and left ventricular function. These consequences are greater in the right ventricle and may contribute to early right ventricular failure after transplantation (194). The deterioration of myocardial performance after brain death correlates temporally with desensitization of the myocardial beta-receptor signal transduction system (195). Thus, these patients may be hypotensive despite adequate volume restoration. Donors with depressed cardiac function may require inotropic and chronotropic support to maintain an adequate cardiac output. If the cardiac index (CO/BSA) is less than 2.0 L/min/m^2, inotropic therapy is indicated, preferably with dopamine at a dosage of 3–5 μg/kg/min. The use of vasoconstrictors such as levophed may exacerbate cardiac dysfunction.

Thyroid hormone replacement therapy (triiodothyronine, maximal dose 0.6 μg/kg) has been used to improve myocardial function, allowing the use of donor hearts that might otherwise have been considered unsuitable for transplantation (196,197). However, its usefulness in this setting remains controversial (198).

Mariot et al have extensively analyzed thyroid and cortisol levels in brain-dead donors (199). The free T3 was low in 105 of 120 donors; the TSH was low in 21, but normal in 99; and the cortisol level was low in 19, but normal in 101 patients. These results support the use of either triiodothyronine or cortisol to maintain hemodynamic stability.

Respiratory Insufficiency Brain-dead patients require intensive pulmonary hygiene to prevent atelectasis and to maintain adequate oxygenation. In addition, brain death following head trauma may be associated with an unexplained "neurogenic" pulmonary edema. These patients develop an abnormal capillary permeability, with movement of intravascular fluid into the pulmonary interstitium and eventually into the alveolar space, impairing gas exchange and progressively reducing the volume of ventilated lung tissue. Positive end-expiratory pressure of 5 cm H_2O ("physiologic PEEP") may be helpful to maintain alveolar expansion in these circumstances.

Ventilator settings for brain-dead patients should include a tidal volume of 10 to 15 mL/kg and a respiratory rate sufficient to maintain arterial P_{CO_2} in the 40 to 45 mm Hg range (usually 12 to 16 breaths per minute) (200). The F_{IO_2} should be kept at 40% or less in potential lung donors to prevent pulmonary oxygen toxicity. Levels of PEEP greater than 7.5 cm H_2O may impede venous return and decrease cardiac output.

Hypoxemia Arterial oxygen saturations should be no less than 95%. Hypoxemia should be treated aggressively by adjusting the ventilator F_{IO_2} to maintain P_{O_2} levels greater than 100 mm Hg, which minimizes injury to the transplantable organs other than the lungs, as noted above.

Hypercarbia Apnea testing to confirm the diagnosis of brain death can result in significant hypercarbia leading to respiratory acidosis. Careful attention should be paid to the patient's ventilatory status and ABGs, especially following clinical exams for determination of brain death. The ventilator rate should be increased as needed to normalize P_{CO_2} levels to the 40 to 45 mm Hg range.

Polyuria Polyuria (urine output >500 mL/hr) is frequently seen in brain-dead patients. It may be due to physiologic diuresis, osmotic diuresis (mannitol, hyperglycemia), hypothermia, partial or complete diabetes insipidus (DI), loop diuretics, or a combination of the above. Excessive polyuria due to osmotic diuresis or DI may lead to hypernatremia, hypokalemia, and hyperosmolality. The serum potassium should not fall below 3.5 mEq/L, to avoid arrhythmias. Urine and serum electrolyte levels and osmolality aid in the determination of the cause of polyuria.

Aggressive volume restoration may result in a physiologic diuresis. No treatment is warranted, but intake and output should be monitored carefully. Prior mannitol administration or excessive glucose infusion may result in an osmotic diuresis. Glycosuria and hyperglycemia should be treated with IV insulin therapy (4 units of regular insulin for every 100 dL of blood sugar above 200 dL) to normalize blood glucose levels.

Diabetes Insipidus Once the above mentioned causes for polyuria have been excluded, the diagnosis of DI can be made by evaluating the volume of urine output, urine specific gravity, urine and serum electrolyte levels, and urine and serum osmolality. Three of the following findings noted simultaneously establish the diagnosis of DI:

1. Urine output >500 mL/hr.
2. Serum sodium >155 mEq/L.
3. Urine specific gravity <1.005.
4. Serum osmolality >305 mOsm/L.

Treatment of DI includes intravenous infusion of aqueous pitressin (10 units/250 mL D5W) with an initial dosage of 1.2 units per hour (rate: 30 mL/hr) and subsequent titration to maintain urine output of 150 to 300 mL/hr. Aqueous pitressin should be discontinued for urine output less than 150 mL/hr to minimize the possibility of decreased visceral perfusion (especially in liver and pancreas donors). In addition to pitressin therapy, the free water deficit should be calculated and 50% of the calculated deficit should be infused as rapidly as possible, preferably with hypotonic solutions such as D5W or $^{1}/_{2}$NS. Low-dose arginine vasopressin (AVP) infusion can decrease the plasma hyperosmolality, increase blood pressure, decrease inotrope use, and maintain cardiac output (201).

Disseminated Intravascular Coagulation In addition to the constellation of disorders resulting from brain death (189), many potential organ donors have multiple traumatic injuries that pose further clinical challenges. Disseminated intravascular coagulation (DIC) is often observed following severe head trauma in association with the release of tissue thromboplastin into the peripheral blood circulation (202). DIC presents two problems: 1) the potential for massive blood loss leading to hypovolemic shock, and 2) the possibility of microvascular damage and thrombosis of the end-stage organs. Close attention to the donor coagulation profile in anticipation of DIC, and aggressive treatment with fresh frozen plasma will ameliorate this potentially devastating complication.

Organ Recovery Surgery

Most cadaveric donors are suitable for multiple organ recovery. Therefore, it is now common that three surgical teams may be involved: heart, lung, and abdominal. The donor's arms should be maximally abducted to provide access for intravenous infusion and allow for simultaneous dissection by the thoracic and abdominal teams. A midline incision is made from the suprasternal notch to the pubis. Plasma catecholamines may increase promptly after skin incision of the recovery surgery, and these changes may be associated with an increase in blood pressure and heart rate, even though the patient is brain dead (203). As the thoracic and abdominal cavities are entered, the viscera must be examined for trauma, malignancy, or other pathology.

The operative dissection of the organs has been described previously in several reviews (1,204). However, new surgical approaches to maximize recovery of transplantable organs have been described, including in situ splitting of cadaveric livers (205) and combined liver and whole pancreas procurement in donors with anatomic variations such as a replaced right hepatic artery (206). Because the liver receives a priority of recovery for a life-threatened patient, the pancreas allograft arterial circulation may be reconstructed to allow for the preservation of the celiac axis with the liver. Yang et al have reported the successful use of a Y-graft of the donor common iliac artery, anastomosing the internal iliac to the splenic artery, and the external iliac artery to the superior mesenteric artery (Fig. 15.6) (207).

Perfusion of the intraabdominal organs is accomplished through the portal and aortic cannulas (see Chapter 19). The portal circulation of the donor liver is flushed via the splenic or inferior mesenteric vein. For cardiac perfusion, the cannula is inserted into the ascending aorta just proximal to the innominate artery (see Chapter 23). The cannula for lung perfusion is inserted into the pulmonary artery. With the instillation of the cardioplegia solution, and therefore the cessation of circulation, donor preservation fluid will be compartmentalized to either the chest or the abdomen by cross-clamping the aorta at the diaphragm. Thus, the abdominal organs receive preservation fluid as the thoracic organs are removed. The sequence of abdominal organ removal is usually the liver first, followed by the pancreas and kidneys.

Marginal Donor

The concept of a "marginal" organ donor has emerged as many have attempted to expand the pool of organ donors from individuals dying with less than ideal medical criteria. The shortage of organ donors has demanded such an aggressive approach. The characteristics of a marginal donor are now well established (208–210). These include one or more of the following: a donor age of greater than 60 years; a social history that presents the hazard of infectious disease; a medical history of hypertension or malignancy; or a serology profile that reveals donor viral infection. In contrast, the ideal organ donor is a younger patient, who until suffering a traumatic and irreparable brain injury was otherwise well, with excellent multiorgan function and medical history.

Although a slight increase in the yearly total number of cadaver organ donors has been reported by UNOS, the number of organ donors dying from traumatic brain injury

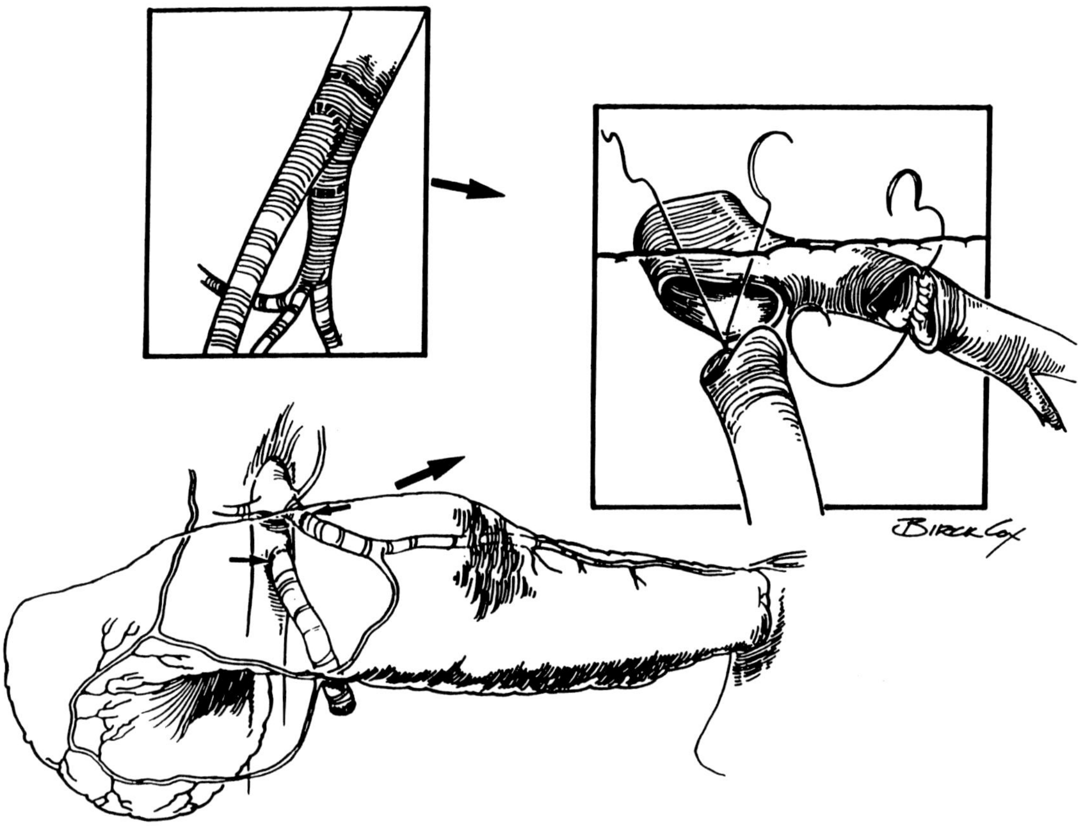

FIGURE 15.6. *Arterial reconstruction of the pancreatic allograft.* Upper left inset: *The donor iliac artery system.* Lower left: *Transection of the allograft splenic and superior mesenteric arteries.* Upper right inset: *The internal iliac artery of the donor Y graft is sewn to the splenic artery, and the orifice of the external iliac artery is sewn to the superior mesenteric artery. (Reproduced by permission from Yang H, Gifford R, Dafoe D, et al. Arterial reconstruction of the pancreatic allograft for transplantation. Am J Surg 1991;162:262–264.)*

(motor vehicle accidents or homicide) has fallen (see Table 15.2). The UNOS data notably reveals an increase in donors older than 50 who have suffered brain injury from cerebral vascular accidents. NEOB data are consistent with this trend. Since 1991, the number of trauma deaths has declined to less than 40% of the NEOB organ donor population. During the same interval, the percentage of NEOB donors over 60 years of age has increased from 8% to 17%. Thus, the percentage of organ donors who are marginal by the criteria detailed above has been rising, and OPOs have been challenged to recover every possible functional organ from a donor population that is markedly changing in profile.

Marginal donor organs are less likely to function satisfactorily following transplantation because of donor hemodynamic instability at the time of death or because of preexisting organ pathology. In a recent review of NEOB data, the rate of dysfunction observed following the transplantation of kidneys from donors older than 60 was high (179). Dialysis was required during the first week following transplantation of kidneys recovered from donors 60 years of age or older in 38.5% of recipients versus 26.4% for donors 60 or younger ($P = 0.01$).

Delayed organ function can obviously present a significant hazard to the allograft recipient. Life-threatened recipients may not survive because a liver or heart allograft functions poorly. It is now evident, however, that preservation injury has more than an immediate consequence for a renal allograft. Halloran et al have presented compelling evidence to suggest that delayed graft function is associated with an increased rate of rejection (211). Consistent with Halloran's experimental data, Cecka and Terasaki have reported significantly more rejection episodes in renal allograft recipients who required dialysis versus those whose allograft functioned well (210). In addition, these allografts have a shorter half-life (212). The risk of failure due to rejection after the first year following transplantation is increased in renal allografts obtained from the expanded donor pool (210,213).

Transplant physicians have also become keenly aware of the impact of delayed graft function on costs, as have insurance providers. Marginal donor kidneys can lengthen the hospital stay, and because of their predilection to rejection, these transplants increase the cost of immunosuppressive treatment and the expense of rehospitalizations (214).

Moreover, as the transplantation of marginal donor allografts influences outcome, it affects the survival data of transplant centers, now widely available for review (215). Health maintenance organizations consider these center-specific data as they determine preferred "centers of excellence." Physicians referring their patients to transplant centers and patient advocate groups also have access to these data. Thus, OPOs are now confronted by economic (216), social, and even ethical disincentives for transplant physicians to accept organs from marginal donors.

In an attempt to resolve this conflict, OPOs have sought to identify prerecovery methods of predicting immediate allograft function following transplantation (184,217,218). In 1993, the NEOB instituted a policy of obtaining a routine biopsy (Bx) on all renal allografts recovered from marginal donors (179). Frozen section Bx evaluation has, in fact, become routine practice for many OPOs because of the transplant center's request to clarify the risk of initial allograft dysfunction.

In the NEOB experience, the results of the Bx study have not been conclusive because of limited data for renal allografts transplanted with a frozen section determination of greater than 20% glomerulosclerosis. Unfortunately, perhaps as a consequence of the routine Bx, there has been an increase in the discard rate of kidneys from donors older than 60 years of age (179). The pressures of a managed-care priority for early discharge, the worsened outcome of older-aged kidneys, the UNOS publication of center-specific data, and the ethical concerns of obtaining informed recipient consent appear to be influencing the center's decision to decline a kidney with less than ideal morphology.

In an effort to reduce the discard rate for renal allografts, innovative approaches are being considered to enable the utilization of these kidneys, even if it requires an experimental protocol. Following the report by Johnson et al (185), the NEOB has devised a prospective study that would permit centers to transplant two potentially discarded kidneys into a single recipient. The donor criteria include: 1) age of greater than 60 years, 2) a Bx finding of at least 20% glomerulosclerosis, and 3) an estimated creatinine clearance of less than 65 mL/min. With these characteristics established, kidneys from such donors would be offered preferentially to a small group of recipients who are older or sensitized or have access problems, and who cannot wait a protracted period for a single ideal kidney.

The OPO responsibility to develop such protocols is underscored by obligations imposed by a society desperate for donor organs. OPOs must contend with a list of candidates that has increased so significantly that it would appear to be beyond resolution (2). Moreover, regulations from government agencies (e.g., the Health Care Financing Administration in the United States) have set standards for not only the number of organ donors but also the number of organs recovered and transplanted. These widely applied rules do not take into account the variability in the cause of patient deaths from one region to another. However, since OPO performance is measured by these criteria, the potential for recovery of every organ from every donor must be considered, even from those who are marginal.

Non-Heart-Beating Donors

A non-heart-beating donor (NHBD) is a donor of organs and/or tissues procured after the donor's death is determined by the absence of heart beat or cardiorespiratory activity. Prior to the establishment of the brain death diagnosis, organs were routinely recovered by this approach. Today, however, few organ donors are NHBD. The UNOS data reveal that only 1% of all organ donors in 1995 were NHBD (2). NHBD are less desirable because the viability of the organs is affected by the cessation of cardiorespiratory function, in contrast to brain-dead donors in whom organ perfusion is interrupted under controlled conditions that minimize ischemia. In the latter situation, the donor's aorta is cross-clamped and blood circulation interrupted as the preservation fluid is infused. Organs procured from NHBD, however, may experience significant periods of warm ischemia prior to the introduction of preservation fluids, while the surgeon awaits cessation of the donor's heart beat. Unless kidneys are recovered from NHBD in carefully controlled situations (219), they may have a high rate of delayed function (220). Ex vivo machine preservation of these allografts may lessen the risk of dysfunction (see Chapter 16) by identifying kidneys that have suffered ischemic injury (221). The release of enzymes such as glutathione s-transferase into the perfusate of the machine-preserved kidneys may be predictive of post-transplant dysfunction (222). Despite these approaches, some of these renal allografts may never function following transplantation and, as a result, the hospital stay of recipients of NHBD donor organs may be significantly extended (220).

Kootstra has reviewed the logistical difficulties entailed with NHBD (223). Perhaps the most significant problem is related to the period of asystole that ensures that the patient is dead. Kootstra has suggested that 10 minutes should elapse before the initiation of organ preservation approaches, so that there is a clear transition from the medical care of a patient to the recovery of organs from a cadaver (223). He acknowledges that the 10-minute period of asystole likely prohibits the recovery of organs other than the kidneys. In contrast, the University of Pittsburgh protocol permits the declaration of death two minutes following the cessation of cardiorespiratory activity, providing at least an opportunity for multiple organ procurement (223).

These variations in approach have fostered public controversy about the validity of the death declaration and other ethical concerns, including the location of the patient at the time of death (intensive care versus the operating room) and the administration of medicines such as heparin and regitine solely to serve the purpose of organ recovery. This controversy resulted in the establishment of a Committee on Medical and Ethical Issues in Maintaining the Viability of

Organs for Transplantation, by the Institute of Medicine (IOM) of the National Academy of Sciences. The Committee was convened in Washington, DC on July 30, 1997, by John T. Potts, MD, of the Massachusetts General Hospital, who served as the Chair. The IOM Committee heard testimony from leaders of the organ procurement and transplant communities, as well as from groups of donor families over a two-day period. The ethical aspects of several NHBD protocols were examined.

The IOM subsequently released its report in December of 1997, fully supportive of the NHBD process. In the report, Dr. Potts noted that "it is critical that all transplant organizations adopt a consistent approach that respects the wishes of patients and families." Thus, there are specific issues that must be addressed at each medical center in developing an acceptable protocol of NHBD. For example, although it might be considered arbitrary, the IOM has recommended that "at least five minutes should elapse after circulation stops before death is pronounced and organ preparation and removal begins" (224).

As the shortage of cadaver organs persists, it is an important time to reconsider fully the NHBD. With the advent of health care proxies, advanced directives, and a public reluctance for extraordinary, life-sustaining measures, there may be an opportunity to increase the number of NHBD. Clinical conditions have become recognized in which irreversible brain injury may be determined without fulfilling the criteria of brain death. With the family's approval, a joint decision with the physician may be given to withdraw life-sustaining support and optimize compassionate care for these patients. Non-heart-beating organ donation may provide these families an important consolation as well as increase the number of organs available for transplantation.

COMMENTARY

Gauke Kootstra

In this chapter, O'Connor and Delmonico note that there is a changing landscape from cadaveric donation to living donor donation. This now really holds only for the kidney because the contribution of living donors in liver, pancreas, and lung allografting is relatively small in number, although especially for children transplantation of a portion of the liver is often crucial for their survival. Obviously, heart donation is impossible when one does not consider the domino heart as being from a living donor. These considerations emphasize that those waiting lists characterized by a high mortality rate, as currently exists for potential liver, lung, and heart recipients, will not be diminished by the expansion of the donor pool with living donors. It is crucial, as the authors note, that in living-related donation the chance of harm for the donor has to be estimated and considered in advance.

Shortage is the crucial item when one writes about donation. There are two points that must be addressed. The first is whether the detection rate is optimal, which is the crucial contribution in the so-called Spanish model. In this approach, donor "detectors" have been placed in every hospital. These detectors are paid by the government and recruited from the hospital staff, and are trained for requesting donation. The second point is to bring down the high refusal rate. It is evident that a reduction in high refusal rates can result in an increase of 15% to 20% in donation. Thus, a combination of improving the detection rate and bringing down the high refusal rate is the first step for increasing postmortem donation.

The authors suggest that the donor shortage may be resolved when xenotransplantation is possible. Is this realistic? What about chronic rejection, which may not be so impressive in liver and heart transplants but which accounts for a 5% loss every year in kidney transplantation? Will xenografts (see Chapter 40) be less subject to chronic rejection?

There are those who continue to believe that we can solve the shortage problem within our own species (1). Stretching the borders of acceptance of donors might help as well. Marginal (2) and non-heart-beating (3) donors are, at least for kidneys, an important source. Horseshoe kidneys (4) should be used, and in living kidney donation kidneys with cysts and some kidneys with fibromuscular disease (5) might be used as well.

The proposal to stretch the criteria to selected donors with sepsis is interesting. Clearly, use of such donors requires extreme caution since donor-transmitted infections may progress rapidly in the immunosuppressed recipient. The potential for mycotic aneurysm development at arterial anastomoses is a deadly risk from donors with bacteremia. These mycotic aneurysms do not present as an aneurysm but rather as a leak, for example, at the anastomosis of the renal artery with the recipient vessel. In such instances, transplantectomy and exclusion of the infected recipient vessel and no local reanastomosis are often crucial for survival. Histology of the resected anastomosis will typically reveal microabscesses in the vessel wall. We have observed fungal infection in two recipients of allografts from a fresh-water drowning victim (6). From this experience, we advise exclusion of fresh-water–drowned patients from donation.

The issue of suspected viral brain infection is sometimes a reason for excluding organ donation. Although no specific virus may be detectable, the analysis of the spinal fluid can be suggestive for it. We lost several potential donors due to this suspected but not detectable viral infection.

Very helpful in this chapter is the serology profile, depicted in Table 15.7, in which the authors stress the results of hepatitis B serology in donors and the potential consequences to transplant recipients.

Blunt trauma to the abdomen should not, as the authors state, always be a reason to exclude organ donation. I always advise exploratory laparotomy to evaluate the macroscopic appearance of the organs. If there is hematoma around the kidney, it is not necessarily a contraindication. The kidneys should be removed and then, on the workbench, be carefully inspected to try to locate the point of bleeding. The same holds for the liver—explore, explant, and decide!

The pretransplant inspection of a shared organ by the recipient team is a crucial step toward a successful transplantation. In every exchange program, one has to reserve time for this important procedure. We tend to do the inspection during the crossmatch in order to confirm the acceptability of the kidney we have received at the very moment the result of the crossmatch is known. This final pretransplant evaluation may reveal the need for ex vivo repair of a damaged organ. An upper polar artery can be left when it has been severed, but lower polar arteries preferably should be repaired.

It is regrettable that on too many occasions in a multiorgan donor the lungs are inspected by the retrieval team and then they are not explanted or are explanted but not used. In Eurotransplant, only 5% of multiorgan donors provide a transplanted lung. One might wonder if the time has come to extend the criteria for acceptance of a lung for transplantation. Most of the patients on the lung waiting list are going to die if an organ does not become available and it might be acceptable to take some risk, especially since experience in lung transplant centers has increased considerably.

There is an interesting discussion in this chapter on the cost increases related to the use of marginal donors. It might be the case for liver, lung, and heart donation that there is a cost increase when the donor organ is not ideal. However, use of marginal kidneys over the long term is nearly always financially profitable. It is alarming that US transplant centers must publish their results through UNOS; centers utilizing more marginal donor organs can be "punished" because the results are worse. This could encourage a very defensive policy on the part of transplant centers with the primary goal being excellent results rather than increasing the number of transplants. Would it be wise to record the results of centers in two categories—those with ideal donors and those with organs from marginal donors? There could be an incentive for centers with relatively good results using large numbers of marginal donors; that is, for those centers that are actively working to reduce the donor shortage. A consensus on the definition of marginal donor would be a prerequisite.

Another approach to enlarging the organ pool is the use of non-heart-beating donors. Such a program has increased our number of available kidneys by 40% (3). In this chapter, attention is mainly focused on the controlled non-heart-beating donor (i.e., category 3 in the so-called Maastricht criteria) (7). These are the "ventilator switch off" cases. We also have achieved reasonable success with the category 2 (unsuccessful resuscitation) donors. Patients in the emergency room are considered potential donors when the resuscitation team decides to discontinue cardiopulmonary resuscitation. Crucial for success of non-heart-beating donation is viability testing of the organs, and this should be developed for the liver as well. Especially with the additional 10 minutes' warm ischemia in the "no-touch" protocol, there is a need for viability testing in the liver. The potential acceptability of these donors for lung transplantation is being evaluated in Leuven, Belgium (8), where lungs of non-heart-beating animals are preserved and tested. Currently in Europe there are enough pancreases available for the need of the pancreas–kidney programs. Thus, there is no immediate need for non-heart-beating pancreas donation.

In conclusion, the donor shortage crisis should be attacked in three ways: a good detection system, extension of donor criteria especially to marginal donors, and a non-heart-beating donor program in every center.

CHAPTER REFERENCES

1. Delmonico F. Organ procurement. In: Morris P, Malt R, eds. Oxford textbook of surgery. Vol. 1. New York: Oxford University, 1994:642–650.
2. UNOS. 1996 annual report of the U.S. scientific registry of transplant recipients and the organ procurement and transplantation network. U.S. Department of Health and Human Services, 1996.
3. Franz H. Public attitudes toward organ donation. J Transplant Coordination 1995;5:50–54.
4. Cohen B, McGrath SMC, DeMeester J, et al. Trends in organ donation. Clin Transplantation 1998;12:525–529.
5. Spital A. Unrelated living kidney donors. Transplantation 1994;57:1722–1726.
6. Shewmon D. Recovery from brain death: a neurologist's apologia. Linacre Q 1997;64:1–96.
7. Truog R. Is it time to abandon brain death? Hastings Cent Rep 1997;27:29–37.
8. Murray J. The first successful organ transplants in man. Nobel Found 1991:201–216.
9. Spital A. Living kidney donation: when is it justified? Am Kid Found Nephrol Lett 1988;5:1–15.
10. Shaw L, Miller J, Slutsky A, et al. Ethics of lung transplantation with live donors. Lancet 1991;338:678–681.
11. Terasaki P, Cecka J, Gjertson D, Takemoto S. High survival rates of kidney transplants from spouse and living unrelated donors. N Engl J Med 1995;333:333–336.
12. Dwyer J, Vig E. Rethinking transplantation between siblings. Hastings Cent Rep 1995;6:7–12.
13. Childress J. The gift of life: ethical issues in organ transplantation. Bull Am Coll Surg 1996;81:8–22.
14. Salahudeen A, Woods HF, Pingle A, et al. High mortality among recipients of bought living-unrelated donor kidneys. Lancet 1990;336:725–728.
15. Frishberg Y, Feinstein S, Drukker A. Living unrelated (commercial) renal transplantation in children. J Am Soc Nephrol 1998;9:1100–1103.
16. Sheil R. Draft report: use of organs from executed prisoners. Transplant Soc Bull 1996;(5):28–31.
17. Qunibi W, Abulrub D, Shaheen R, el-Din A, et al. Attitudes of commercial renal transplant recipients toward renal transplantation in India. Clin Transplant 1995;9:317–321.
18. Lei C, Abdullah K, Morad Z, Suleiman A. Surgical complications of living unrelated kidney transplantations in a third-world country. Transplant Proc 1992;24:1815.
19. Broelsch C, Burdelski M, Rogiers X, et al. Living donor for liver transplantation. Hepatology 1994;20:49S–55S.

20. Moore FD. Three ethical revolutions: ancient assumptions remodeled under pressure of transplantation. Transplant Proc 1988;20:1061–1067.
21. Singer P, Siegler M. Whose kidney is it anyway? Ethical considerations in living kidney donation. Am Kid Found Nephrol Lett 1988;5:16–20.
22. Caruana R, Zumbro G, Hoff R, et al. Successful cardiac transplantation across an ABO blood group barrier. Transplantation 1988;46:472–474.
23. Gugenheim J, Samuel D, Reynes M, Bismuth H. Liver transplantation across ABO blood group barriers. Lancet 1990;336:519–522.
24. Gordon R, Iwatsuki S, Esquivel C, et al. Liver transplantation across ABO blood groups. Surgery 1986;100:342–348.
25. Tanabe K, Takahashi K, Sonda K, et al. Long-term results of ABO-incompatible living kidney transplantation. Transplantation 1998;65:224–228.
26. Farges O, Kalil A, Samuel D, et al. The use of ABO-incompatible grafts in liver transplantation: a life-saving procedure in highly selected patients. Transplantation 1995;59:1124–1133.
27. Yandza T, Lambert T, Alvarez F, et al. Outcome of ABO-incompatible liver transplantation in children with no specific alloantibodies at the time of transplantation. Transplantation 1994;58:46–50.
28. Tanaka A, Tanaka K, Kitai T, et al. Living related liver transplantation across ABO blood groups. Transplantation 1994;58:548–553.
29. Ott G, Norman D, Ratkovec R, et al. ABO-incompatible heart transplantation: a special case for the A2 donor. J Heart Lung Transplant 1993;12:504–507.
30. Nelson P, Landreneau M, Luger A, et al. Ten-year experience in transplantation of A_2 kidneys into B and O recipients. Transplantation 1998;65:256–260.
31. Alexandre G, Latinne D, Carlier M, et al. ABO-incompatibility and organ transplantation. Transplant Rev 1991;5:230–241.
32. Cacciarelli T, So S, Lim J, et al. A reassessment of ABO incompatibility in pediatric liver transplantation. Transplantation 1995;60:757–760.
33. MacDonald A, Belitsky P, Bitter-Suerman H, et al. ABO-incompatible living related donor kidney transplantation: report of two cases. Transplant Proc 1989;21:3362–3363.
34. Mendez R, Sakhrani L, Aswad S, et al. Successful living-related ABO incompatible renal transplant using the BIOSYNSORB immunoadsorption column. Transplant Proc 1992;24:1738–1740.
35. Weil III R, Clarke D, Iwaki Y, et al. Hyperacute rejection of a transplanted human heart. Transplantation 1981;32:71–72.
36. Patel R, Terasaki P. Significance of the positive crossmatch test in kidney transplantation. N Engl J Med 1969;280:735–739.
37. Kasiske B, Ravenscraft M, Ramos E, et al. The evaluation of living renal transplant donors: clinical practice guidelines. J Am Soc Nephrol 1996;7:2288–2313.
38. Sutherland D, Gores P, Farney A, et al. Evolution of kidney, pancreas, and islet transplantation for patients with diabetes at the University of Minnesota. Am J Surg 1993;166:456–491.
39. Iwatsuki S, Iwasaki Y, Kano T, et al. Successful liver transplantation from positive crossmatch donors. Transplant Proceed 1981;13:286–288.
40. Fujita S, Rosen C, Reed A, et al. Significance of preformed anti-donor antibodies in liver transplantation. Transplantation 1997;63:84–88.
41. Bia M, Ramos E, Danovitch G, et al. Evaluation of living renal donors. Transplantation 1995;60:322–327.
42. Kauffman H, Bennett L, McBride M, Ellison M. The expanded donor. Transplant Rev 1997;11:165–190.
43. Fauchald P, Sodal G, Albrechtsen D, et al. The use of elderly living donors in renal transplantation. Transpl Int 1991;4:51–59.
44. Sumrani N, Delaney V, Ding Z, et al. Renal transplantation from elderly living donors. Transplantation 1991;51(2):305–309.
45. Penn I. Malignancies associated with immunosuppressive or cytotoxic therapy. Surgery 1978;83:492–502.
46. Quarto M, Germinario C, Fontana A, Barbuti S. HIV transmission through kidney transplantation from a living related donor. N Engl J Med 1989;320:1754.
47. Fehrman-Ekholm I, Gabel H, Magnusson G. Reasons for not accepting living kidney donors. Transplantation 1996;61:1264–1265.
48. Starnes VA, Barr ML, Cohen RG, et al. Living-donor lobar lung transplantation experience: intermediate results. J Thorac Cardiovasc Surg 1996;112:1284–1291.
49. Starnes V, Barr M, Cohen R. Lobar transplantation; indications, technique, and outcome. J Thorac Cardiovasc Surg 1994;108:403–411.
50. Broelsch C, Lloyd D. Living related donors for liver transplants. In: Cameron J, ed. Advances in surgery. Vol. 26. St. Louis, MO: Mosby-Year Book, 1993:209–221.
51. Sterneck M, Fischer L, Nischwitz U, et al. Selection of the living liver donor. Transplantation 1995;60:667–671.
52. Gruessner R, Sutherland D. Simultaneous kidney and segmental pancreas transplants from living related donors—the first two successful cases. Transplantation 1996;61:1265–1268.
53. Brenner B, Cohen R, Milford E. In renal transplantation, one size may not fit all. J Am Soc Nephrol 1992;3:162–169.
54. Emond J, Renz J, Ferrell L, et al. Functional analysis of grafts from living donors. Ann Surg 1996;224:544–554.
55. Everhart JE, Lombardero M, Detre K, et al. Increased waiting time for liver transplantation results in higher mortality. Transplantation 1997;64:1300–1306.
56. Yamaoka Y, Morimoto T, Inamoto T, et al. Safety of the donor in living related liver transplantation—an analysis of 100 parental donors. Transplantation 1995;59:224–226.
57. Emond J, Heffron T, Whitington P, Broelsch C. Reconstruction of the hepatic vein in reduced size hepatic transplantation. Surg Gynecol Obstet 1993;176:11–17.
58. Egawa H, Inomata Y, Uemoto S, et al. Hepatic vein reconstruction in 152 living-related donor liver transplantation patients. Surgery 1997;121:250–257.
59. Riehle R, Steckler R, Naslund E, et al. Selection criteria for the evaluation of living related renal donors. J Urol 1990;144:845–848.
60. Walker T, Geller S, Delmonico F, et al. Donor renal angiography: its influence on the decision to use the right or left kidney. Am J Radiol 1988;151:1149–1151.
61. Rossi M, Alfani D, Berlocco P, et al. Bench surgery for multiple renal arteries in kidney transplantation from living donor. Transplant Proc 1991;23: 2328–2329.
62. Ratner L, Kavoussi L. Laparoscopic live donor nephrectomy: making live kidney donation easier. Contemp Dialysis Nephrol 1996;11:13.
63. First M. Living unrelated donors. Literature scan. Transplantation 1996;12:22–24.
64. Sutherland D, Goetz F, Elick B, Najarian J. Experience with 49 segmental pancreas transplants in 45 diabetic patients. Transplantation 1982;34:330–336.
65. Sutherland D, Ascher N. Distal pancreas donation from a living relative. In: Simmons R, Finch M, Ascher N, Najarian J, eds. Manual of vascular access, organ donation, and transplantation. New York: Springer-Verlag, 1984:153–164.
66. Najarian J, Chavers B, McHugh L, Matas A. 20 years or more of follow-up of living kidney donors. Lancet 1992;340:807–810.
67. Starzl T. Living donors: con. Transplant Proc 1987;19:174–176.
68. Shimamura T, Morrison A. Progressive glomerulosclerosis in partial five-sixths nephrectomized rats. Am J Pathol 1975;79:95–98.
69. Hakim R, Goldszer R, Breener B. Hypertension and proteinuria: long-term sequelae of uninephrectomy in humans. Kidney Int 1984;25:930–936.
70. Miller I, Suthanthiran M, Riggio R, et al. Impact of renal donation: long-term clinical and biochemical follow-up of living donors in a single center. Am J Med 1985;79:201–208.
71. Narkun-Burgess D, Nolan C, Norman J, et al. Forty-five year follow-up after uninephrectomy. Kidney Int 1993;43:1110–1115.
72. Buszta C, Steinmuller D, Novick A, et al. Pregnancy after donor nephrectomy. Transplantation 1985;40:651.
73. Wrenshall L, McHugh L, Felton P, et al. Pregnancy after donor nephrectomy. Transplantation 1996;62:1934–1945.
74. Spital A, Kokmen T. Health insurance for kidney donors. Transplantation 1996;62:1356–1358.
75. Evans R, Orians C, Ascher N. The potential supply of organ donors. An assessment of the efficacy of organ procurement efforts in the United States. JAMA 1992;267:239–246.
76. Penn I. Transmission of cancer from organ donors. Nefrologia 1995;15: 205–213.
77. Penn I. Malignant melanoma in organ allograft recipients. Transplantation 1996;61:274–278.
78. Baird R, White H, Tribe C. Renal carcinoma in a cadaver graft donor. Br Med J 1975;2:371–374.
79. Loh E, Couch F, Hendricksen C, et al. Development of donor-derived prostate cancer in a recipient following orthotopic heart transplantation. JAMA 1997;277:133–137.
80. Marsh J, Esquivel C, Makowka L, et al. Accidental transplantation of malignant tumor from a donor to multiple recipients. Transplantation 1987;44:449–450.
81. Valerius W. Assessment of potential donors with brain tumors. In: Lewis D, McCoy J, eds. Donor management notes. Vol. 2. 1996:1–15.
82. Colquhoun S, Robert M, Shaked A, et al. Transmission of CNS malignancy by organ transplantation. Transplantation 1994;57:970–978.

83. Meurisse M, Defraigne J, Pirenne J, et al. Organ transplantation from a female cadaver donor with misdiagnosed choriocarcinoma. In: Terasaki P, ed. Clinical transplants. Los Angeles: UCLA, 1989:299.
84. Cannistra S, Niloff J. Cancer of the uterine cervix. N Engl J Med 1996;334:1030–1038.
85. Preston D, Stern R. Nonmelanoma cancers of the skin. N Engl J Med 1992;327:1649–1662.
86. Fairman R, Grossman R, Barker C, Perloff L. Inadvertent transplantation of a melanoma. Transplantation 1980;30:328.
87. Ciancio G, Burke G, Roth D, et al. The significance of infections in donor organs. Transplant Immunol 1996;12:3–14.
88. Quagliarello V, Scheld W. Treatment of bacterial meningitis. N Engl J Med 1997;336:708–716.
89. Doig R, Boyd P, Eykyn S. *Staphylococcus aureus* transmitted in transplanted kidneys. Lancet 1975;2:243–245.
90. Gottesdiener K. Transplanted infections: donor to host transmission with the allograft. Ann Intern Med 1989;110:1001–1016.
91. Weber T, Freier D, Turcotte J. Transplantation of infected kidneys. Transplantation 1979;27:63–65.
92. Nelson P, Delmonico F, Tolkoff-Rubin N, et al. Unsuspected donor pseudomonas infection causing arterial disruption after renal transplantation. Transplantation 1984;37:313–314.
93. Berggren H, Berglin E, Kjellman U, et al. Successful outcome after massive bleeding in a heart transplant recipient with mycotic aortitis. Scand J Thorac Cardiovasc Surg 1994;28:45–47.
94. Benedetti E, Gruessner A, Troppman C, et al. Intra-abdominal fungal infections after pancreatic transplantation: incidence, treatment, and outcome. J Am Coll Surg 1996;183:307–315.
95. Ciancio G, Burke G, Viciana A, et al. Destructive allograft fungal arteritis following simultaneous pancreas-kidney transplantation. Transplantation 1996;61:1172–1175.
96. Bonatti A, Konigsrainer A, Allerberg F, et al. How to treat graft infection after pancreatic transplantation. Transplant Proc 1995;27:3045–3047.
97. Peters T, Reiter C, Boswell R. Transmission of tuberculosis by kidney transplantation. Transplantation 1984;38:514–516.
98. Turkmen A, Sever M, Ecder T, et al. Posttransplant malaria. Transplantation 1996;62:1251–1253.
99. Dharmasena F, Gordon-Smith E. Transmission of malaria by bone marrow transplantation. Transplantation 1986;42:228.
100. Rubin R. Infection in the renal and liver transplant recipient. In: Rubin R, Young L, ed. Clinical approach to infection in the compromised host. 2nd ed. New York: Plenum, 1988:557–621.
101. Novick S, Schrager J, Nelson J, et al. Comparison of two hepatitis B surface antigen and two HIV-1 (p24) antigen EIA test kits with hemolyzed cadaveric blood specimens. Transplant Proc 1996;28:2925–2926.
102. Tjabbes H. Donor screening: an overview of current regulation and practices in Europe. Transplant Proc 1996;28:2950–2952.
103. Domen R, Nelson K. Results of a survey of infectious disease testing practices by organ procurement organizations in the United States. Transplantation 1997;63(12):1790–1794.
104. Center for Disease Control. Human immunodeficiency virus infection transmitted from an organ donor screened for HIV antibody-North Carolina. MMWR 1987;36:306–308.
105. Rubin R, Jenkins R, Shaw B, et al. The acquired immunodeficiency syndrome and transplantation. Transplantation 1987;44:1–4.
106. Center for Disease Control. U.S. Public Health Service guidelines for testing and counseling blood and plasma donors for human immunodeficiency virus type 1 antigen. MMWR 1996;45:1–9.
107. Simonds R, Holmberg S, Hurwitz R, et al. Transmission of human immunodeficiency virus type 1 from a seronegative organ and tissue donor. N Engl J Med 1992;326:726–732.
108. Center for Disease Control. Guidelines for preventing transmission of human immunodeficiency virus through transplantation of human tissue and organs. MMWR 1994:43.
109. Center for Disease Control. Clarification of human immundeficiency virus screening practices for organ donation. Fed Reg 1996;61:56548.
110. Sullivan M, Williams A, Fang C, et al. Transmission of human T-lymphotropic virus types I and II by blood transfusion. Arch Intern Med 1991;151: 2043–2048.
111. Dodd R. The risk of transfusion transmitted infection. N Engl J Med 1992;327:419–429.
112. Lutwick L, Sywassink J, Corry RJ, Shorey J. The transmission of hepatitis B by renal transplantation. Clin Nephrol 1983;19:317–319.
113. Wolf J, Perkins H, Schreeder M, Vincenti F. The transplanted kidney as a source of hepatitis B infection. Ann Intern Med 1979;91:412–413.
114. Gonzalez-Peralta R, Andres J, Tung F, et al. Transplantation of a hepatitis B surface antigen-positive donor liver into a hepatitis B virus-negative recipient. Transplantation 1994;58:114–116.
115. Chan P, Lok A, Cheng I, Chan M. The impact of donor and recipient hepatitis B surface antigen status on liver disease and survival in renal transplant recipients. Transplantation 1992;53:128–131.
116. Liang T, Baruch Y, Ben-Porath E, et al. HBV infection in patients with idiopathic liver disease. Hepatology 1991;13:1044–1051.
117. Douglas D, Rakela J, Marnish D, et al. Transmission of hepatitis B virus (HBV) infection from orthotopic donor livers. Hepatology 1992;16:49A.
118. Wachs M, Amend W, Ascher N, et al. The risk of transmission of hepatitis B from HBsAg(−), HBcAb(+), HBIgM(−) organ donors. Transplantation 1995;59:230–234.
119. Dickson R, Everhart J. Transmission of hepatitis B by transplantation of livers from donors positive for antibody to hepatitis B core antigen. Gastroenterology 1996;110:A1182.
120. Dodson SF, Issa S, Araya V, et al. Infectivity of hepatic allografts with antibodies to hepatitis B virus. Transplantation 1997;64:1582–1584.
121. Donovan J, Schafer D, Goonewardene T, et al. Development of hepatitis B infection after liver transplantation with donor livers from patients with HBcAb. Hepatology 1994;20:129A.
122. Radomski J, Moritz M, Armenti V, et al. Risk of hepatitis B transmission from organ donors who are hepatitis B surface antigen (−) and hepatitis B core antibody (+). Hepatology 1994;20:129A.
123. Radomski J, Moritz M, Armenti V, Munoz S. Hepatitis B transmission from a liver donor who tested negative for hepatitis B surface antigen and positive for hepatitis B core antibody. Liver Transplant Surg 1996;2:130–131.
124. Douglas D, Rakela J, Wright T, et al. The clinical course of transplantation-associated de novo hepatitis B infection in the liver transplant recipient. Liver Transplant Surg 1997;3:105–111.
125. Madayag RM, Johnson LB, Bartlett ST, et al. Use of renal allografts from donors positive for hepatitis B core antibody confers minimal risk for subsequent development of clinical hepatitis B virus disease. Transplantation 1997;64:1781–1786.
126. Paletta L. Organ procurement issues related to viral hepatitis. In: Lewis DD, McCoy J, eds. Donor management notes. Vol. 2. 1996:1–22.
127. Satterthwaite R, Ozgu I, Shidban H, et al. Risks of transplanting kidneys from hepatitis B surface antigen-negative, hepatitis B core antibody-positive donors. Transplantation 1997;64(3):432–435.
128. Cirocco R, Zucker K, Contreras N, et al. The presence of hepatitis B core antibody does not preclude kidney donation. Transplantation 1997;63(11): 1702–1704.
129. Turner D, Zuckerman M, Alexander G, et al. Risk of inappropriate exclusion of organ donors by introduction of hepatitis B core antibody testing. Transplantation 1997;63:775–778.
130. Caldwell S. Hard times and imperfect organs. Liver Transplant Surg 1997;3:181–184.
131. Pereira B, Levey A. Hepatitis C virus infection in dialysis and renal transplantation. Kidney Int 1997;51:981–999.
132. Pereira B, Wright T, Schmid C, et al. Screening and confirmatory testing of cadaver organ donors for hepatitis C virus infection: a U.S. national collaborative study. Kidney Int 1994;46:868–892.
133. Fishman J, Rubin R, Koziel M, Periera B. Hepatitis C virus and organ transplantation. Transplantation 1996;62:147–154.
134. Pereira B, Milford E, Kirkman R, Levey A. Transmission of hepatitis C virus by organ transplantation. N Engl J Med 1991;325:454–460.
135. Lake K, Smith C, LaForest S, et al. Policies regarding the transplantation of hepatitis C-positive candidates and donor organs. J Heart Lung Transplant 1997;16:17–21.
136. Miller J, Roth D, Schiff E. Hepatitis C and organ transplantation. N Engl J Med 1993;328:312.
137. Farci P, Alter H, Govindarajan S, et al. Lack of protective immunity against reinfection with hepatitis C virus. Science 1992;258:135–142.
138. Widell A, Mansson S, Persson T, et al. Hepatitis C superinfection in hepatitis C (HCV) infected patients transplanted with an HCV-infected kidney. Transplantation 1995;60:642–647.
139. Araya V, Rakela J, Wright T. Hepatitis C after orthotopic liver transplantation. Gastroenterology 1997;112:575–582.
140. Kirk A, Heisey D, D'Alessandro A, et al. Clinical hepatitis after transplantation of hepatitis C virus-positive kidneys. Transplantation 1996;62:1758–1762.
141. Kliem V, Van Den Hoff U, Brunkhorst R, et al. The long-term course of hepatitis C after kidney transplantation. Transplantation 1996;62:1417–1421.
142. Ho M, Suwansirikul S, Dowling J, et al. The transplanted kidney as a source of cytomegalovirus infection. N Engl J Med 1975;293:1109–1112.

143. Chou S. Acquisition of donor strains of cytomegalovirus by renal-transplant recipients. N Engl J Med 1996;314:1418–1423.
144. Bueno J, Green M, Kocoshis S, et al. Cytomegalovirus infection after intestinal transplantation in children. Clin Infect Dis 1997;(25):1078–1083.
145. Ettinger N, Bailey T, Trulock E, et al. Cytomegalovirus infection and pneumonitis. Impact after isolated lung transplantation. Washington University Lung Transplant Group. Am Rev Respir Dis 1993;147:1017–1023.
146. Rubin R. Impact of cytomegalovirus infection on organ transplant recipients. Rev Infect Dis 1990;12(suppl 7):S754–S762.
147. Manez R, Kusne S, Green M, et al. Incidence and risk factors associated with the development of cytomegalovirus disease after intestinal transplantation. Transplantation 1995;59:1010–1014.
148. Falagas M, Arbo M, Ruthazer R, et al. Cytomegalovirus disease is associated with increased cost and hospital length of stay among orthotopic liver transplant recipients. Transplantation 1997;63:1595–1601.
149. George M, Snydman D, Werner B, et al. The independent role of cytomegalovirus as a risk factor for invasive fungal disease in orthotopic liver transplant recipients. Am J Med 1997;103:106–113.
150. Grattan M, Moreno-Cabral C, Starnes V, et al. Cytomegalovirus infection is associated with cardiac allograft rejection and atherosclerosis. JAMA 1989;261:3561–3566.
151. Falagas M, Snydman D, Griffith J, Ruthazer R, Werner B. Effect of cytomegalovirus infection status on first-year mortality rates among orthotopic liver transplant recipients. Ann Intern Med 1997;126(4):275–279.
152. Patel R, Snydman D, Rubin R, et al. Cytomegalovirus prophylaxis in solid organ transplant recipients. Transplantation 1996;61(9):1279–1289.
153. Stagno S, Tinker M, Elrod C, et al. Immunoglobulin M antibodies detected by enzyme-linked immunosorbent assay and radioimmunoassay in the diagnosis of cytomegalovirus infections in pregnant women and newborn infants. J Clin Microbiol 1985;21:930–935.
154. Demmler G, Six H, Hurst S, Yow M. Enzyme-linked immunosorbent assay for the detection of IgM-class antibodies to cytomegalovirus. J Infect Dis 1986;153:1152–1155.
155. Chou S, Kim D, Scott K, Sewell D. Immunoglobulin M to cytomegalovirus in primary and reactivation infections in renal transplant recipients. J Clin Microbiol 1987;25:52–55.
156. Center for Disease Control. Update: Creutzfeldt-Jakob disease in a patient receiving a cadaveric dura mater graft. JAMA 1987;258:309–310.
157. Firlit C, Jonasson O, Kahan B, Bergan J. Reye syndrome cadaveric kidneys. Arch Surg 1974;109:797.
158. Richardson C, Warner O, Callender C. Renal transplantation in Reye's syndrome: fate of the recipient—a case report. J Urol 1979;121:497–498.
159. Gibel L, Sterkling W, Hoy W, Harford A. Is serological evidence of infection with syphilis a contraindication to kidney donation? J Urol 1987;138:1226–1227.
160. Podzamczer D, Miro J, Bolao F, et al. Twice-weekly maintenance therapy with sulfadiazine-pyrimethamine to prevent recurrent toxoplasmic encephalitis in patients with AIDS. Ann Intern Med 1995;123:175–180.
161. Lovejoy F, Linden C. Acute poison and drug overdose. In: Isselbacher K, Braunwald E, Wilson J, et al, eds. Harrison's principles of internal medicine. Vol. 2. 13th ed. New York: McGraw-Hill, 1992:2441–2461.
162. Brems J, Merenda G, Hayek M, et al. Orthotopic liver transplantation resulting in amitryptyline toxicity in the recipient. Transplantation 1989;48:159–161.
163. Fattinger K, Rentsch K, Meier P, et al. Safety of liver donation after fatal intoxication with the tricyclic antidepressant trimipramine. Transplantation 1996;62:1259–1262.
164. Hebert M, Boucher A, Beaucage G, et al. Transplantation of kidneys from a donor with carbon monoxide poisoning. N Engl J Med 1992;326:1571.
165. Verran D, Chui A, Painter D, et al. Use of liver allografts from carbon monoxide poisoned cadaveric donors. Transplantation 1996;62:1514–1515.
166. Barkoukis T, Sarbak C, Lewis D. Multiorgan procurement from a victim of cyanide poisoning. Transplantation 1993;55:1434–1435.
167. Snyder J, Unkle D, Nathan H, Yang S. Successful donation and transplantation of multiple organs from a victim of cyanide poisoning. Transplantation 1993;55:425–427.
168. Friedlander M, Rosenmann E, Rubinger D, et al. Successful renal transplantation from two donors with methanol intoxication. Transplantation 1996;61:1549–1552.
169. Hantson P, Mahieu P, Hassoun A, Otte J. Outcome following organ removal from poisoned donors in brain death status: a report of 12 cases and review of the literature. [Review.] J Toxicol Clin Toxicol 1995;33: 709–712.
170. Tenderich G, Koerner MM, Posival H, et al. Hemodynamic follow-up of cardiac allografts from poisoned donors. Transplantation 1998;66:1163–1167.
171. Gortmacher S, Beasely C, Brigham L, et al. Organ donation potential and performance: size and nature of the organ donor shortfall. Crit Care Med 1996;24:432–439.
172. Callender CO, Burston BW, Burton LW, Miles PV. An assessment of the impact of the National Minority Organ Tissue Transplant Education Program. Transplant Proc 1996;28(1):394–397.
173. Franz H, Drachman J, DeJong W, et al. Public attitudes toward organ donation: implications for OPO coordinators. J Transplant Coord 1995;5:50–54.
174. Youngner SJ. Psychological impediments to procurement. Transplant Proc 1992;24(5):2159–2161.
175. Wijdicks EF. Determining brain death in adults. Neurology 1995;45: 1003–1011.
176. Mejia RE, Pollack MM. Variability in brain death determination practices in children. JAMA 1995;274(7):550–553.
177. Pallis C. ABC of brain stem death: from brain death to brain stem death. Br Med J 1982;285:1487–1490.
178. Drinkwater D, Laks H, Blitz A, et al. Outcomes of patients undergoing transplantation with older donor hearts. J Heart Lung Transplant 1996;15:684–691.
179. Delmonico F. Discarding the older age kidney: establishing the need for innovative utilization. Transplant Proc 1997;29:130–131.
180. Wall WJ, Mimeault R, Grant DR, Bloch M. The use of older donor livers for hepatic transplantation. Transplantation 1990;49(2):377–381.
181. Washburn WK, Johnson LB, Lewis WD, Jenkins RL. Graft function and outcome of older (> or = 60 years) donor livers. Transplantation 1996;61(7):1062–1066.
182. Portmann B, Slapak GI, Gane E, Williams R. Pathology and biopsy diagnosis of the transplanted liver. Verh Dtsch Ges Pathol 1995;79:277–290.
183. Ploeg RJ, D'Alessandro AM, Knechtle SJ, et al. Risk factors for primary dysfunction after liver transplantation—a multivariate analysis. Transplantation 1993;55(4):807–813.
184. Gaber L, Moore L, Alloway R, et al. Glomerulosclerosis as a determinant of posttransplant function of older donor renal allografts. Transplantation 1995;60:334–339.
185. Johnson L, Kuo P, Dafoe D, et al. The use of bilateral adult renal allografts—a method to optimize function from donor kidneys with suboptimal nephron mass. Transplantation 1996;61:1261–1277.
186. Lee CM, Scandling JD, Pavlakis M, et al. A review of the kidneys that nobody wanted. Transplantation 1998;65:213–219.
187. Goldberg M. Teleradiology and telemedicine. Radiol Clin North Am 1996;34(3):647–665.
188. Cockcroft DW, Gault MH. Prediction of creatinine clearance from serum creatinine. Nephron 1976;16(1):31–41.
189. Powner D, Jastermski M, Lagler R. Continuing care of multiorgan donor patients. J Intensive Care Med 1989;4:75–83.
190. Amado J, Lopez-Espadas F, Vazquez-Barquero A, et al. Blood levels of cytokines in brain-dead patients: relationship with circulating hormones and acute-phase reactants. Metabolism 1995;44:812–816.
191. Jastremski M, Powner D, Snyder J. Problems in brain death determination. Forensic Sci 1978;11:201–212.
192. Dominguez-Roldan JM, Murillo-Cabezas F, Santamaria-Mifsut JL, et al. Changes in resting energy expenditure after development of brain death. Transplant Proc 1995;27(4):2397–2398.
193. Smith R, Kruszyna H. Nitroprusside produces cyanide poisoning via reaction with hemoglobin. J Pharmacol Exp Ther 1974;191:557–563.
194. Bittner H, Kendall S, Chen E, et al. Myocardial performance after graft preservation and subsequent cardiac transplantation from brain-dead donors. Ann Thorac Surg 1995;60:47–54.
195. D'Amico T, Meyers C, Koutlas T, et al. Desensitization of myocardial beta-adrenergic receptors and deterioration of left ventricular function after brain death. J Thorac Cardiovasc Surg 1995;110:746–751.
196. Jeevanandam V, Todd B, Regillo T, et al. Reversal of donor myocardial dysfunction by triiodothyronine replacement therapy. J Heart Lung Transplant 1994;13:681–687.
197. Novitsky D, Cooper D, Reichart B. Hemodynamic and metabolic responses to hormonal therapy in brain-dead potential organ donors. Transplantation 1987;43:852–854.
198. Howlett T, Keogh A, Perry L. Anterior and posterior pituitary function in brain-stem-dead donors. Transplantation 1989;47:828–834.
199. Mariot J, Sadoune L, Jacob F, et al. Hormone levels, hemodynamics, and metabolism in brain dead organ donors. Transplant Proc 1995;27:793–794.
200. Sethman J, Kappel D. Donor management strategies to maximize lung procurement. J Transplant Coord 1993;3:66–69.

201. Pennefather S, Bullock R, Mantle D, Dark J. Use of low dose arginine vasopressin to support brain-dead organ donors. Transplantation 1995;59:58–62.
202. Bick R. Disseminated intravascular coagulation. Hematol Oncol Clin North Am 1992;6:1259–1285.
203. Fitzgerald R, Dechtyar I, Templ E, et al. Cardiovascular and catecholamine response to surgery in brain-dead organ donors. Anaesthesia 1995;50:388–392.
204. Van Buren CT, Barakat O. Organ donation and retrieval. Surg Clin North Am 1994;74(5):1055–1081.
205. Rogiers X, Malago M, Gawad K, et al. In situ splitting of cadaveric livers. The ultimate expansion of a limited donor pool. Ann Surg 1996;224(3):331–339; discussion 339–341.
206. Shaffer D, Lewis WD, Jenkins RL, Monaco AP. Combined liver and whole pancreas procurement in donors with a replaced right hepatic artery. Surg Gynecol Obstet 1992;175(3):204–207.
207. Yang H, Gifford R, Dafoe D, et al. Arterial reconstruction of the pancreatic allograft for transplantation. Am J Surg 1991;162:262–264.
208. Alexander J, Zola J. Expanding the donor poor: use of marginal donors from solid organ transplantation. Clin Transplant 1996;10:1–19.
209. Ratner L, Kraus E, Magnuson T, Bender J. Transplantation of kidneys from expanded criteria donors. Surgery 1996;119:372–377.
210. Cecka J, Terasaki P. The UNOS scientific renal transplant registry. In: Cecka JM, Terasaki PI, eds. Clinical transplants. Los Angeles: UCLA Tissue Typing Laboratory 1995:1–18.
211. Goes N, Urmson J, Ramassar V, Halloran P. Ischemic acute tubular necrosis induces an extensive local cytokine response. Evidence for induction of interferon-gamma, transforming growth factor-beta 1, granulocyte-macrophage colony-stimulating factor, interleukin-2, and interleukin-10. Transplantation 1995;59:565–572.
212. Shoskes DA, Cecka JM. Deleterious effects of delayed graft function in cadaveric renal transplant recipients independent of acute rejection. Transplantation 1999;66:1697–1701.
213. Cecka JM. The UNOS scientific renal transplant registry. In: Cecka JM, Terasaki PI, eds. Clinical transplants. Los Angeles: UCLA Tissue Typing Laboratory, 1997:1–14.
214. Whiting JF, Golconda M, Smith R, et al. Economic costs of expanded criteria donors in renal transplantation. Transplantation 1998;65:204–207.
215. UNOS. 1994 Center Specific Graft and Patient Survival Rates. Richmond, VA: United Network for Organ Sharing and U.S. Department of Health and Human Services, 1994.
216. Jacobbi L, McBridge V, Etheredge E, et al. The risks, benefits, and costs of expanding donor criteria. Transplantation 1996;60:1491–1496.
217. Seu P, Imagawa D, Olthoff K, et al. A prospective study on the reliability and cost effectiveness of preoperative ultrasound screening of the "marginal" liver donor. Transplantation 1996;62:129–130.
218. Emre S, Schwartz M, Altaca G, et al. Safe use of hepatic allografts from donors older than 70 years. Transplantation 1996;62:62–65.
219. D'Alessandro A, Hoffmann R, Knechtle S, et al. Successful extrarenal transplantation from non-heart-beating donors. Transplantation 1995;59:977–982.
220. Wijnen R, Booster M, Stubenitsy B, et al. Outcome of transplantation of non-heart beating donor kidneys. Lancet 1995;345:1067–1070.
221. Matsuno N, Sakurai E, Tamaki I, et al. The effect of machine perfusion preservation versus cold storage on the function of kidneys from non-heart beating donors. Transplantation 1994;57:293–294.
222. Daemen J, Oomen A, Janssen M, et al. Glutathione s-transferase as predictor of functional outcome in transplantation of machine preserved non-heart-beating donor kidneys. Transplantation 1997;63:89–93.
223. Kootstra G. The asystolic, or non-heart beating donor. Transplantation 1997;63:917–921.
224. Institute of Medicine, National Academy of Sciences. Non-heart beating organ transplantation: medical and ethical issues in procurement. Washington, DC: National Academy, 1997.

COMMENTARY REFERENCES

1. Hoyer J, Kootstra G. Interview. Transplant Int 1997;10:166–168.
2. Abouna GM. Marginal donors: a viable solution for organ shortage. Transplant Proc 1997;29:2759–2764.
3. Kootstra G. The asystolic, or non-heartbeating donor. Transplantation 1997;63:917–921.
4. Vromen M, Kootstra G. The use of horseshoe kidneys for transplantation. Transplant Proc 1988;20:765–766.
5. Linder R, Billing H, Tibell A, et al. Fibromuscular dysplasia in donor kidneys—experience with three cases. Transplant Int 1989;2:228–231.
6. Van der Vliet JA, Tidow G, Kootstra G, et al. Transplantation of contaminated organs. Br J Surg 1980;67:596–598.
7. Kootstra G, Daemen JHC, Oomen APA. Categories of non-heart-beating donors. Transplant Proc 1995;27:2929–2930.
8. Van Raemdonck D, Jannis N, Rega F, et al. Delay of ATP deletion and hypoxanthine formation in rabbit lung after death. Ann Thorac Surg 1996;62:233–241.

Chapter

16

Organ Preservation

JAMES H. SOUTHARD   MARY S. AMETANI

Organ preservation is achieved by rapidly cooling the organ to approximately 4°C using a cold flushout of preservation solution. The organ is then either stored in the cold preservation solution or, in the case of some kidneys, placed on a perfusion device and continuously perfused with cold preservation solution. The length of time an organ can be preserved depends on numerous factors and the particular organ. Experimental methods have been developed for most organs that allow a significantly greater safe preservation time than is needed in most clinical situations. Kidneys can be stored for up to 72 hours by simple cold storage (CS) (1–4) and are routinely stored between 24 to 30 hours in clinical practice. Kidneys can be preserved by machine perfusion (MP) for five (5) to seven (6,7) days and clinically are preserved by this method for 30 hours on average. The liver has been successfully cold-stored for up to 48 hours (8), with clinical preservation times kept between 12 to 20 hours. The pancreas can tolerate 72 hours of preservation (9,10) but clinically is transplanted within 10 to 20 hours of procurement. The heart and lung currently are thought most safely preserved for only about four hours (11,12), although successful transplantations after cold-storage intervals of up to 10 hours have been reported (see Chapter 24). Preservation allows national and international sharing of organs and, in general, organs are not wasted because a safe preservation time is exceeded. Because of the shorter acceptable preservation times, the sharing of hearts and lungs is typically restricted to a smaller geographic region than the intra-abdominal organs. Preservation also allows for the transplant surgery to be performed as a scheduled procedure, which is easier on both the patients and the hospital staff.

For the majority of organs that are transplanted (livers, kidneys, pancreases), the current methods of preservation are very satisfactory and result in good initial function, with only a small percentage of organs never functioning after transplantation. However, a small percentage of organs do develop primary nonfunction (about 6% for livers) and some have delayed function (about 10% for livers and 25% for kidneys). It is unclear what causes primary nonfunction or initial poor function in organs. It is often thought, however, that poor preservation compounded with donor or recipient factors contribute to these problems.

This chapter gives an overview of the current status of clinical organ preservation. This is accomplished by providing first a brief historical account of the developments in organ preservation, then a description of the current status of cold storage and machine perfusion of organs, and finally some comments about the future of organ preservation. There are many good references describing preservation of the various organs used in transplantation. These include descriptions of the fundamental principles of organ preservation (13–15) and assessments of the role of preservation in clinical organ transplantation (16,17).

BRIEF HISTORY OF ORGAN PRESERVATION

In the late 1960s, kidney transplantation between living-related donors was becoming quite successful. There was hope that the recently discovered immunosuppressive drugs (prednisone, azathioprine) would make kidney transplantation possible between unrelated patients and that kidneys could possibly be obtained from cadavers. Because there was at that time no brain death law (see Chapter 15), cadaveric kidneys could only be obtained from non-heart-beating donors. Kidneys from these donors were exposed to a period of no perfusion—warm ischemia (WI)—that was variable but in general lasted for at least 30 minutes. Warm ischemia was known to cause irreversible kidney injury if prolonged beyond one hour. A further complication was the need to transport cadaveric kidneys from the donor hospital to the recipient hospital, and thus a period of preservation of the kidney was necessary.

Folkert Belzer and his colleagues (18) at the University of California at San Francisco had reasoned that preservation could be applied by the use of hypothermia. He believed that the kidney should be continuously perfused for optimal maintenance of viability after WI and prior to transplantation. Belzer, along with Robert Hoffmann, developed a method to perfuse dog kidneys for three days using cryoprecipitated plasma (CPP) (Fig. 16.1). They then developed a portable, battery-operated perfusion machine that could be easily transported (Fig. 16.2). This method was applicable for human kidney preservation and transplantation (19) and thereby had a dramatic effect on the field, increasing the quality and the number of the organs procured.

During this same period, Geoff Collins, working in Paul Terasaki's laboratory, had developed a simpler method of kidney preservation (20). He reported that successful 30-hour dog kidney preservation could be obtained by flushing out the kidney with a phosphate-based glucose solution and storing the organ in a refrigerator at 4°C. Collins solution and Belzer's method of perfusion of kidneys became the standard methods of preservation used throughout the 1970s.

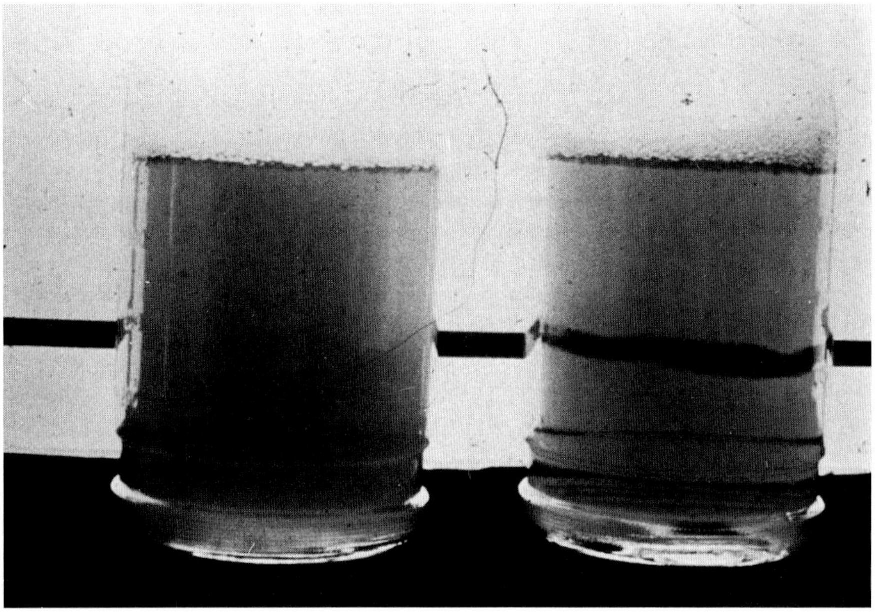

FIGURE 16.1. *In discovering a method to successfully perfuse dog kidneys, Belzer and Hoffmann prepared CPP by freezing autologous dog plasma and thawing the solution. This resulted in aggregation of lipoproteins (bottle on left) that were removed by millipore (0.2 μ) filtration to yield a clear solution of plasma (right). This sterile, lipoprotein-free solution gave successful three-day dog kidney preservation.*

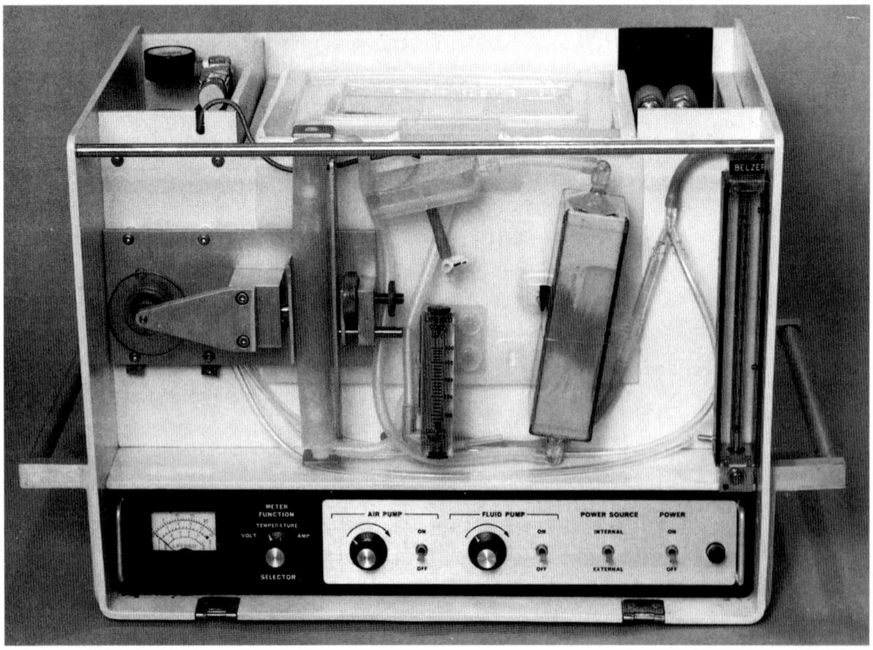

FIGURE 16.2. *The portable Belzer perfusion machine weighed almost 50 pounds and contained a battery. The cassette was cooled by placing ice in the machine. A pulsating pump recirculated CPP, which flowed through a membrane oxygenator. This machine is no longer commercially available.*

These two discoveries had a major impact on the widespread acceptance throughout the world of kidney transplantation for patients with end-stage renal disease. They spawned a flurry of activity in research laboratories to develop even better perfusion methods and cold storage solutions. In Europe, EuroCollins resulted from the modification of Collins solution (21). Magnesium was omitted because it interacted with phosphate to form insoluble crystals that, although not injurious to the kidney, were not a desirable attribute of the preservation solution. Other solutions were also developed including Ross and Marshall's hypertonic citrate solution (2). The composition of these are shown in Table 16.1.

In the 1980s, demonstration of the efficacy of cyclosporine in suppressing graft rejection, especially in liver and pancreas recipients, made transplantation of these organs on a large scale a reality. Preservation of these organs, however, still lagged behind that of the kidney. Collins solution was found not to be particularly effective for these organs. Also, the safe limit of four to eight hours was very constraining on developing a large scale liver or pancreas transplant program.

Belzer, now at the University of Wisconsin at Madison, was working with Southard and colleagues on developing a method to prolong liver and pancreas preservation. Earlier developments included a new synthetic kidney perfusion solution based on sodium gluconate to suppress hypothermically induced cell swelling and hydroxyethyl starch as a colloid to counteract hydrostatic perfusion pressure (22). In 1986, Jan Wahlberg, a visiting transplant surgeon from Sweden, was working on modifying the kidney perfusion solution by replacing gluconate with lactobionic acid. This and a few other minor changes led to the development of the University of Wisconsin (UW) solution, which was first used effectively to extend pancreas preservation in the dog from about 12 hours (with Collins solutions) to 3 days (9). This remarkable discovery had little impact on the transplant community until Jamieson et al (8), working in Belzer's laboratory, showed that the same solution could be safely used to extend liver preservation in the dog from 6 hours to 48 hours. Ploeg et al (1) showed that the UW solution was also capable of excellent dog kidney preservation. These discoveries initiated widespread interest in the UW solution as a means of expanding the donor pool of livers and pancreases. The composition of the UW solution (marketed as ViaSpan) and that of the kidney perfusion solution (marketed as Belzer MPS) are shown in Table 16.2.

Table 16.2. University of Wisconsin Patented Preservation Solutions

ViaSpan		Belzer MPS	
Lactobionic acid	100 mmol/L	Sodium gluconate	80 mmol/L
KOH (5M)	20 mL	Potassium gluconate	10 mmol/L
NaOH (5M)	5 mL	Magnesium gluconate	5 mmol/L
Adenosine	5 mmol/L	KH_2PO_4	15 mmol/L
Allopurinol	3 mmol/L	Adenine	5 mmol/L
KH_2PO_4	25 mmol/L	Ribose	5 mmol/L
$MgSO_4$	5 mmol/L	Glucose	10 mmol/L
Glutathione	3 mmol/L	HEPES	10 mmol/L
Raffinose	30 mmol/L	$CaCl_2$	0.5 mmol/L
Hydroxyethyl starch	5 g%	Hydroxyethyl starch	5 g%
		Glutathione	3 mmol/L
		Allopurinol	1 mmol/L
Insulin	40 U/L	Insulin	40 U/L
Dexamethasone	8 mg/L	Dexamethasone	8 mg/L
Bactrim	2 mL/L	Bactrim	2 mL/L
pH 7.4 Na 25 K 100 mOsm 300		pH 7.4 Na 100 K 25 mOsm 310	

Table 16.1. Composition of Preservation Solutions

Belzer's Early Kidney Perfusion Solution		Collins Solution		EuroCollins Solution		Ross & Marshall's Hypertonic Citrate	
Component	Concentration	Component	Concentration (mmol/L)	Component	Concentration (mmol/L)	Component	Concentration (mmol/L)
Gluconic acid sodium salt	80 mmol/L	Na	10	KH_2PO_4	15	Potassium citrate	28.1
Gluconic acid magnesium salt	5 mmol/L	K	115	K_2HPO_4	42	Sodium citrate	31.8
K_2PO_4	10 mmol/L	Mg	30	KCl	15	Mannitol	188
Glucose	10 mmol/L	Cl	15	$NaHCO_3$	10	$MgSO_4$	83.1
Glutathione reduced	3 mmol/L	HCO_3	10	Glucose	195		
HEPES	20 mmol/L	SO_4	30				
Human serum albumin	37.5 g/L	HPO_4	42.5				
Penicillin	600,000 U/L	H_2PO_4	15				
Phenosulphathelein	12 mg/L	Glucose	195				
Dexamethasone	12 mg/L						
NaCl	10–20 mmol/L						
NaOH (5 M)	To desired pH						
pH 7.5 Na 140 K 10 mOsm 305		pH 7.4		pH 7.4		pH 7.1	

The development of the UW solution inspired other groups to work to develop a better organ preservation solution. Most have been derivatives of the UW solution with addition or subtraction of minor components (23–25). Other solutions are capable of preserving organs by cold storage for 24 to 48 hours with varying degrees of success as compared to the UW solution. Most of the modifications made probably have had little impact on the preservation of organs by simple cold storage.

COLD STORAGE OF ORGANS: HYPOTHERMIA

Simple cold storage of organs is effective because cooling to 4°C slows down the rate of cellular metabolic processes that lead to cell death and organ failure. This may be the most fundamental component of successful organ preservation. Cooling an organ alters many physical and biochemical properties of the organ, such as fluidity of plasma and organelle membranes, activity of enzymes, solubility of substances in the cytosol and membranes, and rates of membrane transport. These alterations do not appear to be particularly harmful, however, and most organs do not show "cold shock" injury common to some biologic materials, such as sperm. Most organs exposed to hypothermia regain function relatively rapidly once reperfused with normothermic blood.

Hypothermia slows down enzyme reactions, alters the physical nature of the cellular membranes, and changes the rate-limiting step in many enzymatic pathways. In general, enzyme activity is slowed approximately twofold for every 10°C drop in temperature. Thus, a temperature decrease from 37°C to a preservation temperature of 4°C would, theoretically, slow metabolism approximately 12-fold. Slowing enzyme activity is critically important because, in cold storage of organs, energy is not put into the organ to help regulate metabolism and, in particular, to stimulate biosynthetic rather than biodegradative reactions. In the absence of a source of energy [adenosine triphosphate (ATP) from oxidative reactions], the degradative reactions become the primary reactions in the cell. These can lead to destruction of important structural elements (phospholipids, cytoskeletal proteins, microtubules, proteins, nucleic acids) that cause not only functional but also structural changes in the cell and in the architecture of the microvascular system of the organ. A summary of some metabolic pathways disrupted by hypothermia is shown in Table 16.3.

Despite the inhibition of enzyme activity by hypothermia, however, these reactions continue. Complete suppression of degradative enzyme activity with specific inhibitors could provide improved preservation. Many attempts have been made to improve organ preservation by treating the organ with enzyme inhibitors that block phospholipases, proteases, eicosanoid metabolism, or other cellular reactions (13–15). Most of these attempts have not warranted clinical trials.

Table 16.3. Metabolic Pathways Disrupted by Hypothermia

Pathway Affected	Consequences
Plasma membrane Na^+–K^+ ATPase	Cell swelling, loss of cytosolic K^+ increases cytosolic Na, Na-Ca^+ exchange, elevates cytosolic Ca^{2+}
Mitochondrial membrane	
Adenine nucleotide translocase inhibited	ATP decreases in cell Activates F_1-ATPase
Ca^{2+} efflux	Elevates cytosolic free Ca^{2+} Destabilizes mitochondrial membrane leading to permeability changes
Endoplasmic reticulum membrane	
Ca^{2+} transport blocked	Cytosolic Ca^{2+} increases
Cytoskeleton	Disruption leading to shape changes, blebbing, endothelial cell dislocation from attachments
Proton metabolism	H^L accumulates due to glycolysis, ATP hydrolysis and loss of sequestration and metabolism

The cold also causes alterations in the physical structure of cellular membranes. Many studies show that at temperatures below the phase transition of the lipid bilayer the membrane undergoes a transition from a liquid crystalline to a gel configuration. In addition, a lateral transition of membrane proteins can occur. These temperature-induced structural changes in cellular membranes, however, appear to be very well tolerated. The effect of cold itself on cells does not appear to be detrimental to organ viability. Normal cellular and organ function are rapidly restored in many organs undergoing cold storage for over 24 hours. In fact, kidneys have been continuously perfused for up to seven days at hypothermic temperatures and then functioned after transplantation (6,7). Other organs (liver, pancreas) will survive exposure to hypothermia for at least two days. Attempts, therefore, to improve organ preservation by utilization of higher temperatures than used currently conceivably would shorten the length of preservation.

Enzymatic reactions continue slowly in the cold, leading to an accumulation of end-products of metabolism. The conditions of organ storage lead to an accumulation of protons with a concomitant decrease in cellular pH, an accumulation of glycolytic intermediates (lactate), increased breakdown products of adenine nucleotides (xanthine, hypoxanthine), and an accumulation of free fatty acids. In addition, there is a decrease in the concentration of important intermediates such as glycogen, glutathione, vitamin E, and some coenzymes. The combination of the accumulation of end-products and the decrease in activity or concentrations of cellular components causes the tissue to become sensitive to reperfusion injury. Also, in the cold, the membrane ion pumps are slow and lack a supply of energy.

Therefore, the cells gain water. This hypothermic-induced cell swelling can exacerbate the injury caused by cold ischemic storage. Thus, suppression of cell swelling is also a key to successful long-term storage of organs. Other complications of cold ischemia may include vasoconstriction induced by exposure of the vascular system to cold solutions, thus restricting optimal flushout of blood from the organ as well as hindering distribution of the protective agents throughout the organ.

Despite the problems associated with hypothermic storage of organs, hypothermia is the key component to successful storage. Managing the complications caused by hypothermia in an effective manner will contribute to improved organ storage.

COLD STORAGE SOLUTIONS

It is reasonably clear that the composition of the cold storage solution is another important factor in successful organ preservation. What is not clear, however, is the precise role of the various components in the different solutions and how these affect viability of the cold-stored organ.

Cold storage solutions have been designed, in principal, to suppress hypothermic-induced cell swelling and to minimize the loss of potassium from the cell (26). This is accomplished with agents that do not readily permeate the cell membrane, because of size and/or charge, and through the use of a cationic composition that resembles the intracellular milieu (high K, low Na) rather than the extracellular environment in order to prevent the loss of cellular potassium. Commonly used impermeants include saccharides such as sucrose, glucose, mannitol, and raffinose; anions such as citrate, phosphate, sulfate, gluconate, or lactobionate; and large molecular mass compounds such as albumin, hydroxyethyl starch (HES), polyethylene glycol, or dextrans. Most of these agents, when mixed in various combinations, will give successful short-term (approximately 24 hours) preservation of organs. The UW solution that contains lactobionate, raffinose, and hydroxyethyl starch is used worldwide for clinical organ preservation. This solution is effective for all organs tested and gives safer, longer-term storage than other solutions. The reasons for this are unclear but may reside in the lactobionate molecule. Lactobionate is impermeable and effectively suppresses hypothermic-induced cell swelling. In addition, lactobionate chelates calcium and lowers the concentration of intracellular calcium in cold-stored tissue. This may be beneficial in suppressing the activities of degradative calcium-dependent enzymes (phospholipases, proteases, etc.) that could lead to cellular disintegration. Lactobionate has also been shown to chelate iron and thus may help to suppress oxidative damage during reperfusion by lowering the concentration of free iron.

The use of a colloid in cold storage solutions is controversial (27,28). Colloids were originally used for successful machine perfusion to counteract the hydrostatic pressure generated by the perfusion pump. Hydroxyethyl starch was found to be the most satisfactory synthetic colloid for long-term (≥72 hours) kidney perfusion (29). Consequently, HES was also included in the UW cold-storage solution. The rationale for using HES was that it would suppress hypothermic-induced cell swelling of endothelial cells, reduce interstitial edema during the initial flushout of organs, and allow for a universal organ preservation solution. In short-term cold storage of the kidney or liver the benefits of a colloid are dubious; however, for successful preservation of the heart and pancreas a colloid may be essential (30,31).

Cold storage solutions often include other agents for their theoretical benefit against potentially injurious processes thought to occur either during storage or on reperfusion. These include such agents as antioxidants, calcium channel blockers, oxidative substrates, energy precursors, and inhibitors of various enzymatic reactions. Studies of experimental models show that solutions including glutathione, allopurinol, nisoldipine, glycine, histidine, chlorpromazine, and trifluoroperazine are beneficial to recovery of function in preserved organs on reperfusion. Many questions about the use of these agents remain, however, and it is not clear how or if these agents are effective clinically. It is unknown how well many of these agents get distributed in the flushed-out organ, whether they penetrate cells during cold static storage, at what concentrations they exist in the cells, and whether they remain in the tissue on reperfusion. Many agents that suppress reperfusion injury in cold or warm ischemic organs are effective only when used in the reperfusion medium and not when incorporated into the cold storage medium. This may be due to the poor uptake of the cytoprotective agents or the rapid dilution of the agent on reperfusion of the organ. The key to the efficacy of cytoprotective agents is their penetration into the cell and the optimization of the concentration at which they should be present during the time when injury can occur. Simple cold flushout of organs followed by static storage may not be sufficient to allow potentially beneficial agents to reach their site of action and remain where needed during the reperfusion period.

WHY THE LIMITS OF SIMPLE COLD STORAGE MAY HAVE BEEN REACHED

The longer an organ is cold-stored the greater the likelihood of injury on reperfusion. This has been amply proven by studies in the laboratory that show increased loss of viability of organs if transplantation is performed after extended preservation times. Dog kidneys can be successfully transplanted after three days of cold storage but not consistently after longer periods of time. Dog livers survive 48 hours' cold storage, rat livers about 40 hours of cold storage, and pig livers about 12 hours of cold storage. Baboon hearts and lungs can tolerate only about 12 hours of cold storage. Clinically, the longer kidneys are preserved the greater the incidence of delayed graft function. There is an increase in

Table 16.4. Agents Used to Suppress Reperfusion Injury

Antioxidants	Calcium Channel Blockers	Anti-inflammatories	Protease Inhibitors	Cytokine Metabolism Inhibitors	Phospholipase Inhibitors
Allopurinol	Nisoldipine	Prostacyclins	Aprotinin	Cyclosporine	Quinicrine
N-Acetylcysteine	Nifedipine	Thromboxane synthetase inhibitors	Pepstatin	Pentoxifillin	Chlorpromazine
Glutathione	Verapamil	Epoprosterol	Leupeptin		Trifluoroperazine
SOD			Glycine		
Catalase					
Lazaroids					
Tocopherols					
Pentoxifillin					

primary nonfunction and initial poor function in livers preserved for greater than 24 hours, and the longer hearts are preserved the greater the incidence of reperfusion injury.

The current limits of safe cold static storage of organs may have been reached and is conservatively about 30 to 40 hours for human organs, with the longest time for pancreases, then kidneys, livers, hearts, and finally lungs. The reason for this may be due to the lack of available energy sources necessary to maintain structural and functional integrity. During storage, lack of continuous perfusion limits oxygen delivery and leads to an accumulation of end products of metabolism and a rate of utilization of ATP that exceeds production. Without energy, the highly organized structural bonds that hold together the cytoskeleton, membranes, proteins, and organelles weaken. Without oxygen and phosphorylation of adenosine diphosphate (ADP) for prolonged periods of time, all organs will lose viability. It appears that at 4°C this takes about two to three days. Evidence that the availability of ATP is a critical determinant to the survival of preserved organs is derived from many studies:

1. A correlation between outcome in human liver transplantation and ATP content of the tissue has been demonstrated (32).
2. In isolated liver cells, the rate of cell death was suppressed by stimulation of glycolytic ATP production with fructose (33).
3. Depletion of liver glycogen and the suppression of glycolytic ATP production increased cell death in the liver (34) and heart (35).
4. Stimulation of a turnover of ATP in kidneys by oxygen persufflation increased tolerance of these organs to both cold and warm ischemia (36).
5. Increased delivery of oxygen to the cold-stored pancreas by a two-layer preservation method increased quality and duration of preservation as tested in a dog transplantation model (37). The benefits of this method were shown to depend on the synthesis of ATP.
6. The inability to cold store hearts for longer than 12 hours has been related to the onset of irreversible ischemic contracture due to loss of ATP. Longer-term preservation was obtained by decreasing the rate of ATP degradation (38).
7. Continuous perfusion of organs maintains ATP concentrations near normal and gives better quality and longer-term preservation of most organs (39).

These studies show that maintaining cellular energy is a critical component to prolonging the tolerance of organs to preservation. This cannot be effectively done for most organs that are cold statically stored; thus most modifications of preservation solutions will have little consequence on the outcome of transplantation unless the changes facilitate an increased supply of energy to the ischemic tissue.

Another limitation to cold storage of organs is the inability of cytoprotective agents to permeate the cell, reach sufficient concentration, and remain present during the initial normothermic reperfusion period when damage to the organ could occur. Most lipophilic compounds have difficulty entering the cell due to their insolubility. Hydrophilic agents may not reach concentrations inside the cell that are sufficient for cytoprotection due to the limited exposure during flushout and poor distribution of the preservative in the tissue. If they do reach equilibrium with the cytosol, it is believed that upon reperfusion these agents may very rapidly be exported from the cell. Therefore, the concentration of these agents is diluted and they may not be effective. The effect of many of these cytoprotective agents may depend more on their presence during reperfusion than in the tissue during the period of cold ischemia.

This is suggested by the fact that there are a large number of agents that have been shown to suppress reperfusion injury in various organs, as shown in Table 16.4. These agents suppressed some forms of reperfusion injury but were effective only if used in pretreatment of the donor or in the reperfusion fluid. Most were not effective when used solely in the preservation solution, unless preservation was by continuous perfusion.

LAZAROIDS AND ORGAN PRESERVATION

The lazaroids represent a class of agents that may be beneficial in improving the outcome of organ transplantation by suppressing tissue damage induced by oxygen free radicals during reperfusion. Studies in diverse organs, including the lung (40), heart (41), kidney (42), and liver (43), have shown a beneficial effect of lazaroids when given to the donor prior to harvesting the organ and when given to the recipient at the time of transplantation. In some of these studies, survival of dogs receiving livers preserved for 48 hours was improved from 0% to 60% (43). Kidneys exposed to WI for 30 minutes prior to 24-hour cold storage also showed an improved survival rate from 0% to 60% (42). The beneficial effects of the lazaroids have been attributed to a decrease in oxygen free-radical damage (lipid peroxidation), decreased neutrophil infiltrations, reduced biosynthesis of adhesion molecules, and suppression of cytokine production. These beneficial effects of lazaroids are not uncommon, and many other types of free-radical scavengers (antioxidants) have shown similar beneficial effects in protecting organs from cold or warm ischemia (44).

The studies showing beneficial effects of lazaroids are often deficient because they do not compare the lazaroid effect to other types of antioxidants such as vitamin E or its analogues, iron chelators, thiol reagents, enzyme inhibitors, or superoxide dismutase (SOD)-catalase mixtures. Another problem in the evaluation of lazaroids for organ preservation (or other agents, for that matter) is related to the deficiencies in the types of models used. The primary goal of organ preservation is related not to extension of the time of preservation but rather to reduction in the incidence of delayed graft function and nonimmunologic-mediated chronic rejection. The models used (dog or rat organ transplantation) do not necessarily represent the actual clinical situation. Thus, it is unclear what impact lazaroids might have in clinical organ preservation and transplantation. Although it is logical that antioxidant therapy should be useful in organ transplantation, because of the evidence showing that after ischemia organs are sensitive to oxidative injury, previous clinical studies using antioxidant therapy in organ transplantation have not shown major beneficial effects. These included trials of SOD as well as allopurinol (45). Thus, enthusiasm for adaptation of antioxidant therapy for use in clinical organ transplantation protocols has not been great. Whether or not such therapy can be demonstrated to affect the long-term outcome of organ transplantation will require the study of a large number of subjects. Because the incidence of delayed graft function is low, the causes are variable and occur at different rates in different centers, and chronic rejection takes three to five years to study, clear evidence of a beneficial effect of these agents will be difficult to establish.

MACHINE PERFUSION

Continuous perfusion preservation is used clinically only for the kidney and then only in a few centers, mostly in the United States. This method has been shown to consistently yield the best quality (lowest delayed graft function rates) and longer successful preservation periods when compared to simple cold storage. Nevertheless, in multicenter comparisons of greater than one-year graft survival results, there is little difference between kidneys preserved by cold storage or machine perfusion. However, there does appear to be a correlation between initial dysfunction of the kidney and loss of the graft long term. It appears that preservation and subsequent reperfusion injury may increase the potential for chronic graft rejection in the kidney and liver (45), although this is controversial (46,47). Even if long-term graft failure is not a factor in influencing the choice of machine perfusion versus cold storage, some would argue that there is evidence suggesting that economic and ethical factors still make machine perfusion more efficacious (48). Since the incidence of delayed graft function from acute tubular necrosis (ATN) is reported to be on average 25% to 35% for cold-stored kidneys but less than 10% for machine-perfused kidneys, a larger number of recipients receiving cold-stored kidneys require dialysis than those receiving kidneys that were machine perfused (49). It has been estimated that the cost to treat a patient with delayed graft function due to ATN is about US$28,000 more than the costs for patients that do not develop ATN (50). Since about 80% of the kidneys currently transplanted are cold stored, this added cost translates into millions of dollars each year that could be saved if all centers used machine perfusion. In addition to the economic aspect, the rewards to a recipient receiving a kidney that functions immediately with no need for continued dialysis is truly the long-awaited gift of life. Again, however, other studies have suggested that simple hypothermic storage is the more cost-effective approach (51).

Machine perfusion has also been studied in a dog liver model in which it allowed safe three-day preservation (52). This method may be the only way to preserve hearts and lungs beyond the current limits of four to six hours. Unlike the liver, kidney, or pancreas, the heart and lung must function normally immediately after transplantation. The abdominal organs, however, can recover from the effects of ischemic injury, and with time and the proper care the tissue can repair itself and become life-supporting. Recipients of intra-abdominal organ transplants are privileged to have methods available that can sustain them during the first few days without a well-functioning organ. No such long-term supports are available for recipients of hearts and lungs. These organs must be preserved extremely well, and machine perfusion may be the only method to accomplish this.

Machine perfusion of organs at hypothermia is effective because a constant supply of nutrients is delivered to the organ and end products of metabolism are removed. At 4°C, metabolism is slowed by nearly 80% to 90%. Even under these conditions it is clear that mitochondria continue to function and can maintain tissue ATP content at or near normal if given the appropriate substrates (adenosine, adenine, ribose, phosphate). Although there is a loss of glutathione during continuous kidney perfusion (53), suggesting the possibility of oxidative stress, glutathione concentrations can be kept near normal with substrate delivery systems such as thioproline. The design of the perfusate, therefore, is critical to successful, long-term machine perfusion. Perfusates with the appropriate pharmacologic agents, nutrients, and substrates could conceivably maintain the viability of organs for prolonged periods of time. The kidney, in fact, has been successfully machine perfused for five to seven days.

Machine perfusion can also advance organ preservation by providing a means of evaluating the viability of organs prior to transplantation. It could also provide a method to salvage organs injured by donor factors, such as hypotension or WI. It seems very plausible that an assessment of some aspect of hypothermic metabolism such as protein synthesis, lipid metabolism, drug metabolism, or nucleic acid uptake could be used as a determinant of how well an organ is preserved. The utility of a reliable "viability" method could be especially important in judging whether to transplant a questionable organ from, for instance, a non-heart-beating cadaver with the potential for prolonged WI injury (54). In fact, the widespread use of non-heart-beating cadavers may be dependent on the use of machine perfusion as a salvage technique, and a "viability" assay for assessment of damage would be of utmost importance here (see also Chapter 15).

VASCULAR EVENTS

During the past six years, evidence supporting injury to the microvascular system as a cause of preservation/reperfusion injury has increased dramatically. It was clear early on in the field of organ transplantation that a hallmark of preservation injury was poor reperfusion of the organ. The events leading to this were unclear and only recently have new insights been gained into the potential mechanisms of vascular injury. This subject has been reviewed in relation to specific organs (55,56) as well as related to the general principles of vascular disease (57).

Cold storage of organs induces a time-dependent change in the structural and functional organization of the components of the vascular system. These events may be closely linked to oxidative stress and the generation of superoxide anions from damaged endothelial lining cells or parenchymal cells. Ischemia leads to a change in the redox state, a loss of naturally occurring antioxidants (glutathione, vitamin E, coenzyme Q, ascorbic acid), activation of oxidases, and the uncoupling of mitochondrial oxidative reactions. Upon exposure to oxygen, there is the opportunity for increased generation of reactive oxygen species such as the superoxide anion or the hydroxyl radical. Reactive oxygen species act as signals for upregulation of the transcription factors for adhesion molecules and cytokine production. These products trigger initiation of the inflammatory response involving the leukocytes, platelets, and complement system. Upon reperfusion, these inflammatory responses injure cells, disrupt the normal flow of blood, and lead to irreversible injury.

Damage to the endothelium impairs vasorelaxation. Vasorelaxation is naturally controlled in part by nitric oxide (NO), which is sensitive to reactive oxygen species. Increased adhesiveness of the endothelial cell lining can also result in vasoconstriction as a result of activated leukocyte infiltration, thrombus formation, and an aggravation of the enzymatic pathways that amplify these processes. Endothelial cell dysfunction predisposes the organ to poor reperfusion and tissue ischemia eventually leading to cell and ultimately organ death. A key component precipitating these events is disruption of the cell-to-cell and cell-to-matrix interactions. The normal structure of the vasculature is maintained by these interactions. Cell-to-cell and cell-to-matrix interactions are integrated by a system of intracellular microtubules and microfilaments composed of contractile proteins. The maintenance of this ultrastructural network is dependent on a supply of energy (ATP) and regulation of the activity of proteases, protein kinases, and calcium-dependent enzymes. Alterations in the supply of energy to the cell or changes in the concentration of cytosolic or total cellular calcium lead to a disruption of the cytoskeletal system. This ultrastructural disruption can lead to the highly injurious inflammatory response seen in cases of primary nonfunction. Furthermore, this type of injury, if not directly responsible for primary nonfunction, may be a contributing factor to later chronic rejection in the kidney, liver, and heart.

FREEZING ORGANS

Freezing organs to liquid nitrogen temperatures would stop nearly all metabolic and molecular reactions and conserve the tissue for long periods of time. The central question is whether this is clinically needed, now or in the distant future, and whether there is evidence that this can be accomplished in a timely and reasonably effective manner.

Freezing would be advantageous only in establishing an organ bank from which organs that exactly match a recipient would be used. This could theoretically reduce immunologic problems, including immunologic-dependent chronic rejection for kidneys. There is currently a shortage of kidneys for transplantation, however, and it is unlikely that any would be available for freezing. Also, the freezing process (use of toxic antifreeze compounds, perfusion, thawing) will undoubtedly cause renal injury (preservation/reperfusion injury) and this could lead to an increased incidence of reperfusion injury–related chronic rejection. It is clear that freezing can be used as a means for preserving single-cell or small multiple-cellular elements (ova); however, it is not clear that large vascularized organs can withstand freezing and thawing. The freezing process inevitably leads to vascular damage, which is a central problem in organ preservation–related injury.

Therefore, the answers to the questions posed above would appear to be that there is no current clinical need for freezing organs for transplantation, no special advantage to be gained, and that the difficulties in accomplishing this appear extremely large and the benefits very small.

FUTURE DIRECTIONS

Because of the large number of variables that can affect the outcome of organ transplantation, it is prudent to try to optimize the ones that can be controlled. The one variable most reasonably and easily controlled relates to preservation. For each organ, preservation conditions should be optimized, and the incidence of preservation-related failures minimized, by using the best methods available and limiting the preservation time to safe limits. Factors unrelated to preservation of the organ can lead to poor recovery of function upon transplantation. Donor age, cause of death, donor management, nutritional status, and organ function at the time of retrieval (discussed in Chapter 15) have been shown to affect initial organ function on transplantation. Recipient factors may also play a role in how readily the organ regains normal function (58). Use of continuous machine perfusion, however, could possibly be the answer to "rescue" some of these organs from less-than-optimal donors, thus achieving better quality and the longer preservation periods that are necessary for the liver, heart, and lung.

Future improvements to cold storage methodologies that affect the current practices of organ preservation and transplantation will be difficult to make. Machine perfusion, however, could be used to develop viability assays to help determine if organs had sustained injury prior to harvest that has made them unsuitable for transplantation. Finally, machine perfusion may significantly lower the number of organs that develop primary nonfunction or initial poor function. This could have a substantial impact on the long-term outlook of the recipient, both by reducing the incidence of chronic rejection and by reducing the cost of organ transplantation.

COMMENTARY

David Pegg

The quality of preserved organs has improved substantially during the past 30 years, as Southard and Ametani so clearly show in this chapter. In the 1960s and early 1970s, experiments in animals had achieved satisfactory renal preservation by vascular flushing followed by refrigeration for 48 hours and by continuous hypothermic perfusion for 96 hours. Livers could be stored for only seven hours. Attempts to store hearts and lungs were even less rewarding. Clinically, primary nonfunction was a common and serious problem, occurring in 30% or more of kidney transplants. Reference to the proceedings of a conference on organ preservation that was held in 1972 (1) shows that the field was dominated by the problems caused by the use of organs that had been damaged by warm ischemia, the need for viability tests to distinguish safe from dangerous transplants, and a fascination with novel, even exotic, perfusion engineering.

The success that has been achieved since then is based on three ideas: that cooling reduces metabolic requirements and thereby prolongs the survival of ischemic organs; that the fluid to which hypothermic organs are exposed should have a typically intracellular balance of solutes; and that vascular perfusion will best provide the residual metabolic support required at low temperatures. These were rational ideas but they proved to be insufficiently precise to stimulate decisive experimentation. As a result, the literature describing empirical organ preservation grew rapidly. Indeed, some of it documented valuable advances—most notably the development of the University of Wisconsin solution in Belzer and Southard's laboratory—but much did not. In particular, attempts to improve on existing preservation solutions by adding assorted metabolites, enzyme and channel blockers, and cofactors have, as Southard and Ametani point out, added little more than confusion.

What then has been responsible for the improvement in the quality of preserved organs that has occurred during the past 30 years? There appear to be two major factors. The first is an improvement in the quality of donated organs before preservation even starts. This has been due to the recognition of brain-death criteria and better medical management of donors (see Chapter 15). The second is the recognition of the importance of preventing cell swelling during storage, which, with the help of a little serendipity, led to the invention of the UW formulation. Research has repeatedly and consistently demonstrated that continuous perfusion is superior to simple hypothermic storage, yet this has failed to have a major impact on clinical practice, no doubt because of increased technical complexity and the perceived cost. As Southard and Ametani show, however, the economic argument is flawed, and scientific, medical, and ethical considerations all argue persuasively for greater use of continuous perfusion methods.

What ideas are there to guide future studies in this field? Southard and Ametani suggest that the limit of simple hypothermic storage time might already have been reached, the crucial factor being exhaustion of chemical energy reserves. If depletion of ATP were the only limiting factor, that would indeed be true, and certainly vascular perfusion is necessary in order to deliver essential metabolites and remove catabolites. Yet if empirical experimentation has demonstrated anything it is that interventions designed solely to maintain ATP levels do not secure greatly prolonged storage; normal reserves of high-energy compounds may be necessary but are not sufficient. The problem is that there are almost certainly several factors, each of which must be satisfied if storage is to be extended. A study published as long ago as 1978

(2) attempted to identify some of these factors including: prevention of cell swelling by the use of impermeant solutes, avoiding the use of excessive potassium concentrations in so-called intracellular perfusates, refining perfusion methods specifically to minimize endothelial damage, removing microvascular obstructions caused by rigid, ATP-depleted erythrocytes, and maintaining cellular ATP reserves. Additional factors might be added to the list today, most importantly perhaps the control of damage caused by oxygen free radicals during reperfusion. It was suggested in that earlier study that the different phases of the preservation process may have different requirements that cannot all be met if a single approach is used throughout. Thus, the first suggested step was to obtain a patent, dilated vascular system free of erythrocytes. The flushing solution should be designed specifically to achieve that end by the inclusion of impermeant solutes in a hypertonic formulation, with red cell disaggregating agents and compounds with anticoagulant, vasodilator, and anti-calcium properties. The second step would be to remove that solution by vascular perfusion with a perfusate designed to maintain metabolism and control cell volume. It would therefore contain metabolites, have a relatively low potassium concentration, and be perfused at a carefully optimized temperature. Selection of the colloid component would be crucial for the avoidance of perfusion-induced endothelial damage. Perfusion might not necessarily be continuous—it might, with advantage, be intermittent. The final stage, when perfusion is discontinued prior to surgical implantation, might call for a different flushing solution, with greater ability to control cell volume by physical means and perhaps to moderate the production or action of oxygen-derived free radicals after reflow. Such a catalogue of objectives invites empirical experiment, but to be effective it really needs to be based on a more extensive knowledge of the physiology and biochemistry of the hypothermic state than we presently possess, and this in turn requires financial support for the research to obtain that knowledge. A willingness to accept greater technical complexity of the process in order to achieve clinical benefits is also required, and most importantly, all the relevant factors must be taken into account when the inevitable cost–benefit analysis is done.

This approach, in agreement with Southard and Ametani, involves a much greater use of perfusion technology, and will inevitably have its own limitations, both practical and theoretical. Is there any prospect of truly indefinite organ storage through cryopreservation approaches? Interestingly, the 1972 conference quoted above (1) included four papers on this topic. The intervening years have taught us much about the problems inherent in this approach. We now know that severe additional problems arise when we attempt to take the cryopreservation techniques developed for cells and apply them to organs. Many of these concern the mechanical effects of ice (3), particularly on the vascular system (4). This has led to a resurgence of interest in the possibility of vitrification—the use of temperatures as low as those used in conventional cryopreservation, but avoiding the formation of ice (5). The greatest progress with this approach has been made by Fahy and his coworkers (6), but two limiting factors remain. The most important is the toxicity of the very high concentrations of vitrifying agents that have to be added. The second is the occurrence of so-called chilling injury, an ill-understood mechanism of damage produced by reduction in temperature, irrespective of freezing. It remains to be shown how these problems will be overcome, but given sufficient resources they will be. The transplant community will then have to decide how best to use these advances—and how to find the resources to pay for them.

CHAPTER REFERENCES

1. Ploeg RJ, Goossens D, McAnulty JM, et al. Successful 72-hour cold storage of dog kidneys with UW solution. Transplantation 1988;46:191–196.
2. Ross H, Marshall VC, Escott ML. 72-hr canine kidney preservation without continuous perfusion. Transplantation 1976;21:498–501.
3. Lam FT, Ubhi CS, Mavor AID, et al. Clinical evaluation of PBS140 solution for cadaveric renal preservation. Transplantation 1989;48:1067–1068.
4. Collins GM, Bravo-Shugarman M, Terasaki PI. Kidney preservation for transportation. Initial perfusion and 30 hours' ice storage. Lancet 1969;2:1219–1222.
5. McAnulty JF, Ploeg RJ, Southard JH, Belze FO. Successful five-day perfusion preservation of the canine kidney. Transplantation 1989;47:37–41.
6. Schilling M, Saunder A, Southard JH, Belzer FO. Five-to-seven day kidney preservation with aspirin and furegrelate. Transplantation 1993;55:955–958.
7. McAnulty JF, Vreugdenhil PK, Southard JH, Belzer FO. Improved survival of kidneys preserved for seven days with a phospholipase inhibitor. Transplant Proc 1991;23:691–692.
8. Jamieson NV, Sundberg R, Lindell S, et al. 24- to 48-hour preservation of canine liver by simple cold storage using UW lactobionate solution. Transplant Proc 1989;21:1292–1293.
9. Wahlberg JA, Love R, Landegaard L, et al. 72-hour preservation of the canine pancreas. Transplantation 1987;43:5–8.
10. Kawamura T, Kuroda Y, Suzuki Y, et al. Seventy-two-hour preservation of the canine pancreas by the two-layer (Euro-Collins' solution/perfluorochemical) cold storage method. Transplantation 1989;47:776–778.
11. Stringham JC, Southard JH, Anderson GM, Belzer FO. Mechanisms of ATP depletion in the cold-stored heart. Transplant Proc 1991;23:2437–2438.
12. Baldwin JC, Frist WH, Starkey TD, et al. Distant graft procurement for combined heart and lung transplantation using pulmonary artery flush and simple topical hypothermia for graft preservation. Ann Thorac Surg 1987;43:670–673.
13. Belzer FO, Southard JH. Principles of solid-organ preservation by cold storage. Transplantation 1988;45:673–676.
14. Clavien P, Harvey PRC, Strasberg SM. Preservation and reperfusion injuries in liver allografts. An overview and synthesis of current studies. Transplantation 1992;53:957–978.
15. Bonventre JV, Weinberg JM. Kidney preservation ex vivo for transplantation. Ann Rev Med 1992;43:523–553.
16. Southard JH, Pienaar H, McAnulty JF, et al. The University of Wisconsin solution for organ preservation. In: Morris PJ, Tilney NL, eds. Transplantation reviews. Philadelphia: WB Saunders, 1990;3:103–130.
17. D'Alessandro AM, Kalayoglu MD, Sollinger HW, et al. Current status of organ preservation with UW solution. Arch Pathol Lab Med 1991;115:306–310.
18. Belzer FO, Ashby BS, Dumphy JE. 24- and 72-hour preservation of canine kidneys. Lancet 1967;2:536–539.
19. Belzer FO, Ashby BS, Gulyassy PF, Powell M. Successful seventeen-hour preservation and transplantation of human-cadaver kidney. N Engl J Med 1968;278(11):608–610.

20. Collins GM, Hartley LC, Clunie GJA. Kidney preservation for transportation. Experimental analysis of optimal perfusate composition. Br J Surg 1972;59:187–189.
21. Dreikorn K, Horsch R. Forty-eight- to 96-hour preservation of canine kidneys by initial perfusion and hypothermic storage using the Euro-Collins solution. In: Marberger M, Dreikorn K, eds. Renal preservation. Baltimore: Williams & Wilkins, 1983:261–275.
22. Hoffmann RM, Southard JH, Lutz MF, et al. Synthetic perfusate for kidney preservation. Its use in 72-hour preservation of dog kidneys. Arch Surg 1983;118:919–921.
23. Roberts RF, Nishanian GP, Carey JN, et al. A comparison of the new preservation solution Celsior to Euro-Collins and University of Wisconsin solutions in lung reperfusion injury. Transplantation 1999;67:152–155.
24. Sumimoto R, Jamieson NV, Wake K, Kamada N. 24-hour rat liver preservation using UW solution and some simplified variants. Transplantation 1989;48:1–5.
25. Roels L, Coosemans W, Donck J, et al. Inferior outcome of cadaveric kidneys preserved for more than 24 hr in histidine-tryptophan-ketoglutarate solution. Leuven Collaborative Group for Transplantation. Transplantation 1998;66:1660–1664.
26. Pegg DE. An approach to hypothermic renal preservation. Cryobiology 1978;15:1–17.
27. Southard JH, van Gulik TM, Ametani MS, et al. Important components of the UW solution. Transplantation 1990;49:251–257.
28. Jamieson NV, Johnston PS, O'Grady JG, et al. Clinical use of UW solution or a simplified liver preservation solution prior to transplantation in 179 human livers, December 1987–July 1989. Transplant Proc 1990;22:2189–2190.
29. Hoffmann RM, Southard JH, Belzer FO. The use of oncotic support agents in perfusion preservation. In: Pegg DE, Jacobsen IA, Halasz NA, eds. Organ preservation: basic and applied aspects. Lancaster, UK: MTP, 1983:261–266.
30. Wicomb WN, Collins GM. 24-hour rabbit heart storage with UW solution: effects of low-flow perfusion, colloid, and shelf storage. Transplantation 1989;48:6–9.
31. Ploeg RJ, Boudjema K, Marsh D, et al. Importance of a colloid in canine pancreas preservation. Transplantation 1992;53:735–741.
32. Kamiike W, Burdelski M, Steinhoff G, et al. Adenine nucleotide metabolism and its relation to organ viability in human liver transplantation. Transplantation 1988;45:138–143.
33. Anundi I, de Groot H. Hypoxic liver cell death: critical PO2 and dependence of viability on glycolysis. Am J Physiol 1989;257:G58–G64.
34. Boudjema K, Lindell SL, Southard JH, Belzer FO. The effects of fasting on the quality of liver preservation by simple cold storage. Transplantation 1990;50:943–948.
35. Wittnich C, Chiu RCJ, McArdle AH. Protection of ischemic myocardium: the roles of nutrition and myocardial glycogen. Can J Surg 1982;25:534–537.
36. Pegg DE, Foreman J, Hunt CJ, Diaper MP. The mechanism of action of retrograde oxygen persufflation in renal preservation. Transplantation 1989;48:210–217.
37. Kuroda Y, Fujino Y, Morita A, et al. Oxygenation of the human pancreas during preservation by a two-layer (University of Wisconsin solution/perfluorochemical) cold storage method. Transplantation 1992;54:561–562.
38. Lagerstrom CF, McElroy DD, Taegtmeyer H, Walker WE. Improved recovery of cardiac function after hypothermic ischemic storage with ouabain. J Thorac Cardiovasc Surg 1988;96:782–788.
39. McAnulty JF, Southard JH, Belzer FO. Comparison of the effects of adenine-ribose with adenosine for maintenance of ATP concentrations in 5-day hypothermically perfused dog kidneys. Cryobiology 1988;25:409–416.
40. Sasaki S, Alessandrini F, Lodi R, et al. Improvement of pulmonary graft after storage for twenty-four hours by in vivo administration of lazaroid U74389G: functional and morphologic analysis. J Heart Lung Transplant 1996;15:35–42.
41. Nishida T, Morita S, Miyamota K, et al. The effect of lazaroid (U74500A), a novel inhibitor of lipid peroxidation, on 24-hour heart preservation. Transplantation 1996;61:194–199.
42. Shackleton CR, Ettinger SL, Scudamore CH, et al. Effect of 21-aminosteroid, U74006F, on lipid peroxidation and glomerotubular function following experimental renal ischemia. J Surg Res 1994;57:433.
43. Todo S, Hamada N, Zhu Y, et al. Lazaroid U-74389G for 48-hour canine liver preservation. Transplantation 1996;61:189–194.
44. Fuller BJ, Gower JD, Green CJ. Free radical damage and organ preservation: fact or fiction? A review of the interrelationship between oxidative stress and physiological ion disbalance. Cryobiology 1988;25:377–393.
45. Land W, Messmer K. The impact of ischemia/reperfusion injury on specific and non-specific, early and late chronic events after organ transplantation. Transplant Rev 1996;10:236–253.
46. Najarian JS, Gillingham KJ, Sutherland DER, et al. The impact of the quality of initial graft function on cadaver kidney transplants. Transplantation 1994;57:812–816.
47. Shackleton CR, Martin R, Melinek J, et al. Lack of correlation between the magnitude of preservation injury and the incidence of acute rejection, need for OKT3, and conversion to FK506 in cyclosporine-treated primary liver allograft recipients. Transplantation 1995;60:554–557.
48. Burdick JF, Rosendale JD, McBride MA, et al. National impact of pulsatile perfusion on cadaveric kidney transplantation. Transplantation 1992;64:1730–1733.
49. Barber WH, Laskow DA, Deierhoi MH, et al. Comparison of simple hypothermic storage, pulsatile perfusion with Belzer's gluconate-albumin solution, and pulsatile perfusion with UW solution for renal allograft preservation. Transplant Proc 1991;23:2394–2395.
50. Rosenthal JT, Danovitch GM, Wilkinson A, Ettenger RB. The high cost of delayed graft function in cadaveric renal transplantation. Transplantation 1991;51:1115–1118.
51. Merion RM, Oh HK, Port FK, et al. A prospective controlled trial of cold storage versus machine-perfusion preservation in cadaveric renal transplantation. Transplantation 1990;50:230–233.
52. Pienaar BH, Lindell SL, van Gulik TM, et al. Seventy-two-hour preservation of the canine liver by machine perfusion. Transplantation 1990;49:258–260.
53. Boudjema K, Lindell S, Southard JH, Belzer FO. Changes in glutathione concentration in hypothermically perfused dog kidneys. J Lab Clin Med 1991;117:131–137.
54. Matsuro N, Sakurai E, Uchiyama M, et al. Role of machine perfusion preservation in kidney transplantation from non-heartbeating donors. Clin Transplantation 1998;12:1–4.
55. Eberl T, Schmid T, Wodlinger R, et al. Which organ preservation solution best protects vascular endothelium. Transplant Proc 1993;25:3019.
56. Satoh S, Stowe NT, Inman SR, et al. Renal vascular response to vasodilators following warm ischemia and cold storage preservation in dog kidneys. J Urol 1993;19:186–189.
57. Gibbons GH, Dzau VJ. Molecular therapies for vascular diseases. Science 1996;272:689–693.
58. Peters TG, Shaver TR, Ames JE, et al. Cold ischemia and outcome in 17,937 cadaveric kidney transplants. Transplantation 1995;59:191–196.

COMMENTARY REFERENCES

1. Pegg DE, ed. Organ preservation. Edinburgh: Churchill Livingstone, 1973.
2. Pegg DE. An approach to hypothermic renal preservation. Cryobiology 1978;15:1–17.
3. Pegg DE. Ice crystals in tissues and organs. In: Pegg DE, Karow AM Jr, eds. The biophysics of organ cryopreservation. NATO ASI Series A: Life Sciences Vol. 147. New York: Plenum, 1987:117–140.
4. Rubinsky B, Pegg DE. A mathematical model for the freezing process in biological tissue. Proc R Soc Lond B Biol Sci 1988;234:343–358.
5. Pegg DE, Diaper MP. Freezing versus vitrification; basic principles. In: Sibinger C, Das PC, Meryman HT, eds. Cryopreservation and low temperature biology in blood transfusion. Boston: Kluwer, Dortrecht, 1990:55–69.
6. Fahy GM, Ali SE. Cryopreservation of the mammalian kidney. II. Demonstration of immediate ex vivo function after introduction and removal of 7.5 molar cryoprotectant. Cryobiology 1997;35:114–131.

Part IV

Organ-Specific Transplantation

Chapter

17

Renal Transplantation

Peter J. Morris

Renal transplantation has become the treatment of choice for most, if not all, causes of end-stage renal disease (ESRD), its application being limited by the availability of kidneys for transplantation. It is remarkable that in the 50 years since Hume and his colleagues performed a series of cadaver kidneys in nonimmunosuppressed recipients at the Peter Bent Brigham Hospital in Boston (1) renal transplantation has become a relatively routine procedure with success rates not dreamed of in the earlier years of transplantation. Indeed, transplantation of the kidney has provided the background in experience and knowledge that has foreshortened the development of transplantation of other organs such as the liver and heart.

The success of renal transplantation has produced its own problems, however, in that there are now far more patients on dialysis waiting for a transplant than there are kidneys available for transplantation, and this discrepancy becomes more marked each year. In the UK, there are nearly 6000 patients waiting for a kidney transplant, but the transplant rate remains relatively stable at around 1600 transplants per year while over 2000 new patients are added to the waiting list each year. This in turn has given rise to widespread discussions concerning the allocation of cadaver kidneys. Should younger patients have priority? Should the time on the waiting list be an overriding factor in allocation? Should nonsensitized patients have preference over sensitized patients? Should patients waiting for a first graft be preferred to those awaiting a regraft? Should diabetic patients be transplanted and to what extent should matching for HLA override these and other factors used for allocation? There is a school of thought that feels, in the presence of a major shortage of such a valuable resource as the cadaver kidney, that only recipients with the best chances of a favorable outcome should be transplanted. The practical effect of such a policy is that patients in whom outcome is likely to be poorer—the diabetic patient, the elderly patient, the highly sensitized patient—would not be transplanted and would remain on dialysis. This is not, of course, compatible with natural justice and is not an approach that receives the support of most of the transplant community. Nevertheless, this is an area that needs widespread discussion not only among the transplant community but also among the public, for the problem of an equitable allocation of cadaver kidneys will only grow over the coming years (2).

INDICATIONS FOR RENAL TRANSPLANTATION

The increasing success of renal transplantation has led to an ever-widening list of indications, and today there is no absolute contraindication to transplantation for ESRD (3). The diseases for which renal transplantation is appropriate management are listed in Table 17.1, which includes virtually all causes of ESRD. Certain of the glomerulonephritides are very likely to recur such as mesangiocapillary glomerulonephritis type 1 and IgA nephropathy, but generally loss of the transplanted kidney as a result of recurrence occurs late, and therefore none of these nephritides represent an absolute contraindication to transplantation (4) (Table 17.2).

The major metabolic disorder causing ESRD is type 1 diabetes mellitus, which in the United States and Scandinavia is the most frequent overall cause of ESRD. The outcome of renal transplantation in diabetics is by no means as good as in the nondiabetic, but as the quality of life for the diabetic is better after transplantation than on dialysis, it remains the treatment of choice for the ESRD diabetic patient. In addition, there is an increasing use of combined kidney and pancreas transplantation in selected patients with end-stage renal failure due to diabetes, and the overall results

Table 17.1. Diseases for Which Renal Transplantation Is Appropriate

Glomerulonephritis
Idiopathic and postinfectious crescentic
Membranous
Mesangiocapillary (type I)
Mesangiocapillary (type II)[a] (dense-deposit disease)
IgA nephropathy[a]
Antiglomerular basement membrane
Focal glomerulosclerosis
Henoch-Schönlein

Chronic pyelonephritis (reflux nephropathy)

Hereditary
Polycystic kidneys
Medullary cystic disease
Nephritis (including Alport's syndrome)
Tuberous sclerosis

Metabolic
Diabetes mellitus
Hyperoxaluria[a]
Cystinosis
Fabry's disease[b]
Amyloid[a]
Gout
Porphyria

Obstructive uropathy

Toxic
Analgesic nephropathy
Opiate abuse

Multisystem diseases
Systemic lupus erythematosus
Vasculitis
Progressive systemic sclerosis

Hemolytic-uremic syndrome

Tumors
Wilms' tumor
Renal cell carcinoma
Incidental carcinoma
Myeloma[b]

Congenital
Hypoplasia
Horseshoe kidney

Irreversible acute renal failure
Cortical necrosis
Acute tubular necrosis

Trauma

[a] Recurrence of the disease is common following transplantation.
[b] Low success rate.
Source: Reproduced by permission from Briggs JD. The recipient of a renal transplant. In: Morris PJ, ed. Kidney transplantation: principles and practice, 4th ed. Philadelphia: WB Saunders, 1994:43–55.

Table 17.2. Some of the Glomerulonephritides and Systemic Diseases Causing End-Stage Renal Disease That May Recur in the Transplanted Kidney

Disease	Approximate Frequency of Recurrence (%)	Loss of Graft Due to Recurrence
Focal segmental glomerulosclerosis	30	Common
Membranous nephropathy	10	Uncommon
Mesangiocapillary type I	20	Common
Mesangiocapillary type II	95	Uncommon
IgA nephropathy	50	Uncommon
Henoch-Schönlein purpura	80	Uncommon
Anti-GBM nephritis	5	Uncommon
SLE	<1	Uncommon
Hemolytic-uremic syndrome	50	Common
Diabetes type I	100	Uncommon
Oxalosis	90	Common
Amyloidosis	30	Uncommon
Cystinosis	5	Uncommon

Source: Adapted from Mathew TH. Recurrent disease after renal transplantation. Transplant Rev 1991;5:31–45.

with careful selection are now very good. Although the outcome of the pancreas grafts are somewhat inferior to that of the kidney grafts, the outcome of the kidney grafts is not jeopardized by the simultaneous pancreas graft.

Other metabolic disorders are relatively rare and present special problems. For example, oxalosis has always had a high recurrence and failure rate although acceptable results can be obtained with immediate and maintained diuresis after transplantation and the addition of pyridoxine, phosphate, and magnesium. Today, however, the ideal management would comprise a combined hepatic and kidney transplant to correct the metabolic defect as well as the ESRD (5).

Hemolytic-uremic syndrome (HUS) is a relatively common cause of ESRD in children (5%) that may recur especially when cyclosporine is used for immunosuppression. There is also a suggestion that HUS is being seen more frequently as a de novo disease in the modern era of immunosuppression.

Tumors of the kidney, Wilms' in children and renal cell carcinoma in adults, are not a contraindication to transplantation, but there should be at least a two-year period free from recurrence before transplantation is performed.

Two other factors that come into consideration in accepting patients for transplantation are age and concurrent disease, especially cardiovascular disease. Neither represents an absolute contraindication in itself and, indeed, most transplant units have no absolute age limit; a decision to transplant is made based on the physiologic status of the patient. Similarly, ischemic heart disease may require angiography with subsequent angioplasty or coronary artery bypass grafting before transplantation. Many units consider that coronary angiography and treatment of significant disease should be mandatory in all diabetic patients before they are accepted on the waiting list for transplantation, and certainly this should be the case before a patient is offered a combined kidney and pancreas transplant.

DONORS

Living Donors

Related

The use of family members as kidney donors is widely practiced and is perhaps increasing in frequency as the shortage of cadaver kidneys becomes more pronounced. The choice of an immediate member of the recipient's family as a donor requires that there is a genuine motivation on the part of the potential donor. This is not always easily established, for often undue pressure can be placed on a potential donor not only by the patient but also by other members of the family. In Oxford, the recipient and potential donor(s) are first seen by a counselor to discuss the advantages and disadvantages of live donation, and at this time the counselor tries to assess the interaction within the family, and especially between donor and recipient. This is particularly helpful in the identification of donors who have doubts about donation and provides them with more time to consider the risks and benefits before they are seen by the transplant surgeons.

The donor must be blood group compatible with the recipient, and there must be a negative serologic crossmatch for HLA antibodies in the serum of the recipient reacting with donor lymphocytes. With respect to matching for HLA, obviously an HLA-identical sibling donor provides the ideal situation for transplantation (apart from the rare identical twin transplant). The donor and recipient sharing one HLA haplotype (e.g., parent to child or 50% of sibling combinations), also provides an excellent outcome. Previously, siblings incompatible for both HLA haplotypes (25%) were generally not considered as donors, but in recent years with modern immunosuppression it has been realized that such transplants do much better than expected and hence are no longer excluded from transplantation on the basis of matching.

The medical evaluation of the donor must be thorough and is preferably done by a physician not immediately involved with the recipient (Table 17.3). Although ideally the potential donor must be completely healthy as well as have normal renal function, the selection criteria may be relaxed a little if the donor is highly motivated, such as is usually the case in parent-to-child transplants, for example. Thus, in such a situation the physician might accept a mild degree of hypertension, especially if labile, provided that any underlying cause was excluded and one could be assured that the donor would comply with subsequent management and follow-up. The last investigation performed is a renal angiogram to establish the anatomy of the arterial blood supply to the kidneys, and this preferably should be a selective renal angiogram. However, magnetic resonance angiography and spiral computerized tomography (CT) scans are also being used effectively to provide this anatomic information about potential donor kidneys.

Table 17.3. Medical Evaluation of a Potential Living Donor of a Kidney

1. Full history and examination
2. HLA typing and crossmatch with recipient sera
3. Full blood count
4. Blood urea nitrogen, serum creatinine, and electrolytes
5. Liver function tests
6. Creatinine clearance and urine analysis
7. Virology serum for hepatitis B and C, HIV, CMV, and EBV
8. Chest x-ray and electrocardiograph
9. Ultrasound examination of kidneys
10. Aortogram

Of interest is the recent report from Sutherland's group of 20 simultaneous kidney and pancreas transplants from living-related donors to diabetic recipients with acceptable results, although not without morbidity in the donor (6). Continuing evaluation of this approach to the management of the diabetic with ESRD is required, as its role remains uncertain because of the inevitable risks to the donor.

Unrelated

In recent years the recognition that transplants between unrelated donors and recipients (but emotionally related, as in transplantation between spouses) do extremely well, presumably because of the lack of any ischemia reperfusion injury, has led to an increasing number of such transplants (7). Although such transplants are acceptable to the profession and the public, it is imperative that the motivation for transplantation is established to be genuinely altruistic without any commercial considerations being involved. In the UK, all unrelated donors and recipients are assessed by an independent committee established by the government—Unrelated Living Transplant Authority (ULTRA)—and no living-unrelated transplants can be performed until this committee has evaluated the proposed donor and recipient and given approval. This legislation was introduced some years ago to guard against the commercial exchange of kidneys and the exploitation of donors from underprivileged classes, either in the UK or from overseas.

Operation

The kidney may be removed from a living donor either via a posterior approach though the bed of the 12th rib (8) or via an anterior transperitoneal approach using a transverse incision. In Oxford, we favor the latter approach as we feel it gives a more controlled view of the vessels and any anatomic anomalies. On the left side the spleen, tail of the pancreas, splenic flexure, and descending colon are reflected to expose the kidney, while on the right side the duodenum, ascending colon, and hepatic flexure are reflected to provide exposure to the vessels and ureter. Usually the left kidney is removed, provided it has a single artery, as a longer length of renal vein can be obtained than on the right side. The dissection of the kidney and its renal artery and vein is carefully completed, and then the ureter is freed down to the brim of the pelvis and ligated and divided. The renal artery is then ligated and divided, followed by the renal vein, and the kidney is removed. The kidney is then immediately placed in ice slush and flushed with an appropriate preservation solution, for example, hypertonic citrate (Marshall's solution), Collins solution, or University of Wisconsin solution. Any remaining dissection is then performed, and if any bench surgery is required, as for example where there is more than one artery requiring anastomosis, then this is carried out at the time.

Recently endoscopic-assisted nephrectomy has been explored in several centers, with encouraging results reported in two quite large series (9,10). Conversion rates to an open procedure were low, as was the complication rate. Furthermore, hospital stay was shorter and, because donors were enthusiastic about the procedure, more living donors were allegedly presenting for evaluation. Nevertheless, these are uncontrolled studies and there is a need for a randomized prospective trial to fully evaluate the true place of endoscopic-assisted live donor nephrectomy.

Cadaveric Donor

Heart-Beating Donor

The conventional cadaver donor is a patient on a ventilator who has been declared brain stem dead (see Chapter 15). The majority of donors have died from irreversible brain damage as a result of trauma or a cerebrovascular accident. In most instances, retrieval of the kidneys is part of a multiorgan retrieval. Again, as pointed out earlier, the potential donor should be maintained in as good a physiologic state as possible in order to diminish the degree of damage occurring in the kidneys before retrieval. There is now evidence, however, that immunologic changes in the kidney are occurring not only after reperfusion following storage but also around the time of death and before removal of the kidneys. These immunologic changes include upregulation of the expression of E selectin, production of P selectin, neutrophil infiltration, and HLA upregulation (11,121).

Non-Heart-Beating Donor

The ever-increasing shortfall between the availability of cadaver donors and the numbers of patients awaiting renal transplantation has led many groups to establish protocols for the emergency perfusion of kidneys in situ and their subsequent removal from patients who have arrested in an emergency room where the cause of death is considered irrecoverable. Undoubtedly this approach has led to a modest increase in donors in centers where this practice has been established, and the outcome of transplantation using such donors has in general been acceptable, although inferior to that using heart-beating donors. On the other hand, there is a group of non-heart-beating donors who were sustained on a ventilator, having been declared brain dead, whose relatives wished the ventilator to be turned off and the heart to have stopped before the kidneys were removed. Such kidneys do as well as heart-beating donor kidneys on the whole, although with a higher rate of delayed graft function. This type of non-heart-beating donor needs to be distinguished from the true non-heart-beating donor referred to above, for the outcome is different and the logistics of organization of retrieval are considerable (12,13).

Operation

If the kidneys are to be removed alone, as in the case of an elderly donor or when permission is refused for other organs, this is performed via a large transverse incision with an en bloc excision of the kidneys after their in situ perfusion (8). The aorta and vena cava are then split to separate the two kidneys, which can then be perfused through the renal artery ostia. Following perfusion with an appropriate perfusate, for example, hypertonic citrate (Marshall's), Collins solution, or University of Wisconsin solution, the kidneys are prepared with a patch of aorta and vena cava on the renal artery and vein, respectively. However, usually kidneys are removed as part of a multiorgan retrieval, in which case they are removed after the heart, liver, and pancreas, all organs being perfused in situ before removal (8). Once removed, the preparation and perfusion of the kidneys is the same as above.

MATCHING AND CROSSMATCHING

This subject has been discussed earlier in the book (see Chapter 4), but the role of antibodies and the crossmatch between the recipient and the donor, both in living-related and in cadaver transplantation, are worthy of further emphasis.

Living-Related Transplants

Serologic typing within a family can be very precise, allowing the members of a family to be genotyped with respect to HLA (see Chapter 4). Twenty-five percent of siblings will be identical for HLA, 50% will share one haplotype (often referred to as haplo-identical), and 25% will share neither haplotype from the parent. Parent-to-child transplants will share one haplotype. The outcome of renal transplants between HLA-identical siblings is excellent and has always provided the evidence that HLA is the major histocompatibility complex in humans. In the azathioprine era, one-haplotype–disparate sibling or parent-to-child transplants did not do as well as HLA-identical siblings, but did do better than two-haplotype–disparate sibling transplants such that most units did not transplant between the latter combination. All this has changed in the cyclosporine era, however. The HLA-identical sibling transplants still have a better outcome but there is no real difference between the other HLA combinations. Today, therefore, most units will use any family member as a donor provided the donor is altruistically motivated to donate a kidney and is in good health.

Cadaver Transplants

The role of matching has always been surrounded by controversy in cadaver transplantation, but today there is little disagreement that transplants between donors and recipients who are identical for the antigens of the A, B, and DR loci (6 antigen match or 000 mismatch) do very well indeed (14,15). Beyond that point there is still disagreement, although the available evidence does probably support the notion that lesser degrees of mismatching do better than badly mismatched pairs provided there is no incompatibility for HLA-DR. However, the influence of HLA-DR matching is not as powerful today in the cyclosporine era as it was in the azathioprine era (16). Certainly the recipient who receives a badly matched kidney that subsequently fails is much more likely to become highly sensitized, making a regraft much more difficult. This by itself suggests that whenever possible a well-matched kidney should be transplanted. What determines a well-matched donor and recipient is not clearly defined, however, other than that matching for HLA-DR remains an important objective. DNA typing is gradually replacing serologic typing (17), and indeed in the Oxford unit DNA typing replaced serologic typing completely in 1996 for both donors and recipients. This allows the donor to be typed before organ retrieval and possible recipients to be selected much earlier than hitherto. Subsequent advances in matching are likely to depend on the definition of the immunogenicity of particular mismatched epitopes on a given HLA background.

Crossmatch

Regular screening of sera from recipients for HLA antibodies, once they have been accepted on a program for transplantation, should be mandatory. This should include the determination of the specificity of the HLA antibodies and also exclude autoantibodies (18). Screening for antibodies has been simplified in recent years using selected pooled lymphocytes or Epstein-Barr virus (EBV)-transformed lymphocytes in a flow cytometry assay, for example. Only with this information about the specificity of antibodies in the recipient can an intelligent interpretation of the crossmatch between recipient sera and donor lymphocytes be made. Traditionally the crossmatch is performed in a serologic complement-dependent cytotoxic assay, but in recent years more units are using flow cytometry for the crossmatch because of its greater sensitivity. If a patient has antibodies, then the crossmatch is the most important part of the tissue typing procedure directed at selecting the appropriate recipient for a given donor. Having said that, it should be possible to dispense with the crossmatch in many, if not most, instances where the antibody specificity in the recipient is clearly defined and none of the relevant antigens detected by those antibodies are present in the donor. This, together with DNA typing of donor and recipient, would allow the appropriate recipient to be selected in advance of organ retrieval, thus decreasing the total cold ischemia time very considerably.

OPERATION

Preparation

When the patient is brought in for transplantation, whether for a living-related or a cadaver transplant, a thorough medical evaluation is made. Depending on the biochemistry, dialysis may be needed before the patient goes into surgery. In addition, a current chest x-ray and electrocardiogram (ECG) are obtained. The first dose of immunosuppressive drugs is usually given some hours before the patient goes to the operating room. An accurate dry weight should be obtained, as this facilitates postoperative management. Prophylactic antibiotics, for example a cephalosporin, should be used and are given with induction of the anesthetic.

Anesthesia

A general anesthetic is used, although renal transplantation under regional anesthesia or a spinal block has been described in the past as an alternative form of anesthesia in high-risk patients. With modern anesthesia and better-prepared patients, however, there would seem to be little indication for these alternative approaches to anesthesia. Effective and safe anesthesia does depend on a knowledge of the effects of uremia on the pharmacokinetics and metabolism of the drugs used (19).

In Oxford, one of the orally administered benzodiazepines is used for premedication, and anesthesia is induced with a sleep dose of thiopental coupled with a loading dose of opioid, for example fentanyl. Neuromuscular blockade is achieved with atracurium or vecuronium. Maintenance of anesthesia is best achieved with inhalation agents, as they are not eliminated by the kidney and may be given with high levels of oxygen in the anemic patient. At the end of surgery, muscular paralysis is reversed with atropine or glycopyrrolate and neostigmine, and anesthesia is discontinued.

A central line is inserted at the time of induction, as this makes monitoring the administration of fluids much easier during the operation and in the postoperative period. Patients who have been on hemodialysis for a long time may be quite dry and require large volumes of fluid to maintain their central venous pressure at a normal level. The central line is most conveniently inserted in the internal jugular vein, as it is only going to be in place for 48 hours. If any technical difficulty is encountered or expected, a

Doppler ultrasound is useful to identify the internal jugular vein before inserting the line.

Transplant

A catheter is inserted with full aseptic technique and connected to a closed drainage system in the operating room. A curved incision is made some 5 cm above the inguinal ligament extending from the midline up toward the costal margin (Fig. 17.1). It is carried down through the oblique muscles to the peritoneum, which is reflected upward and medially to expose the iliac vessels. The lymphatics over the iliac vessels are ligated with silk (diathermy cannot be used as this will lead to a high incidence of lymphoceles; see below) and divided to allow exposure of the external iliac artery or the internal iliac artery if it is to be used for the arterial anastomosis, followed by the external iliac vein. It is our practice commonly to further mobilize the external iliac vein by ligating and dividing the internal iliac vein and any other tributaries. This allows the external and common iliac veins to be brought forward and the venous anastomosis to be performed without any tension, which is particularly useful when there is a short renal vein, as is usually encountered in living donor kidneys.

Following preparation of the kidney, it is biopsied (to provide baseline histology) and then placed within a glove packed with ice to prevent the kidney's warming up during the anastomoses, a small hole being made in the glove over the renal vessels through which they are drawn for the anastomoses. The renal vein is anastomosed end-to-side to the external iliac vein using 5-0 proline, and usually this is the first anastomosis in the case of a cadaver kidney. If a cadaver kidney is to be implanted, it generally will have a cuff of aorta that is trimmed appropriately and then anastomosed end-to-side to the external iliac artery using 6-0 proline. For kidneys removed from live donors, the renal artery is anastomosed end-to-end to the internal iliac artery using a three-point continuous anastomosis with 6-0 proline. Many units also use the internal iliac artery for cadaver kidneys, although the end-to-end anastomosis does require more technical expertise than the end-to-side anastomosis with a cuff of aorta. Where the internal iliac artery is used, it is generally preferable to perform the arterial anastomosis before the venous anastomosis. If the arteries are small it will be necessary to spatulate the ends appropriately as well as perform at least part of the anastomosis with interrupted sutures. On releasing the clamps, one expects to see the kidney perfuse and expand, although in the case of cadaver kidneys it is not uncommon for the kidney to remain rather flabby and even dusky, which is a cause of some concern although not necessarily a predictor of delayed graft function.

The ureter is implanted in the bladder using an antireflux procedure either via a submucosal tunnel into the base of the bladder through an anterior cystotomy (Politano-Leadbetter technique) (20,21) or into the dome of the bladder closing muscle over the ureter to provide an antireflux mechanism (22,23). The latter procedure is not as effective as the former as an antireflux technique (24). Some units routinely insert a double J stent that is removed at six weeks.

The transplanted kidney is then laid in the parapsoas gutter after taking a biopsy. If the common and external iliac vein have been mobilized by ligation and division of the

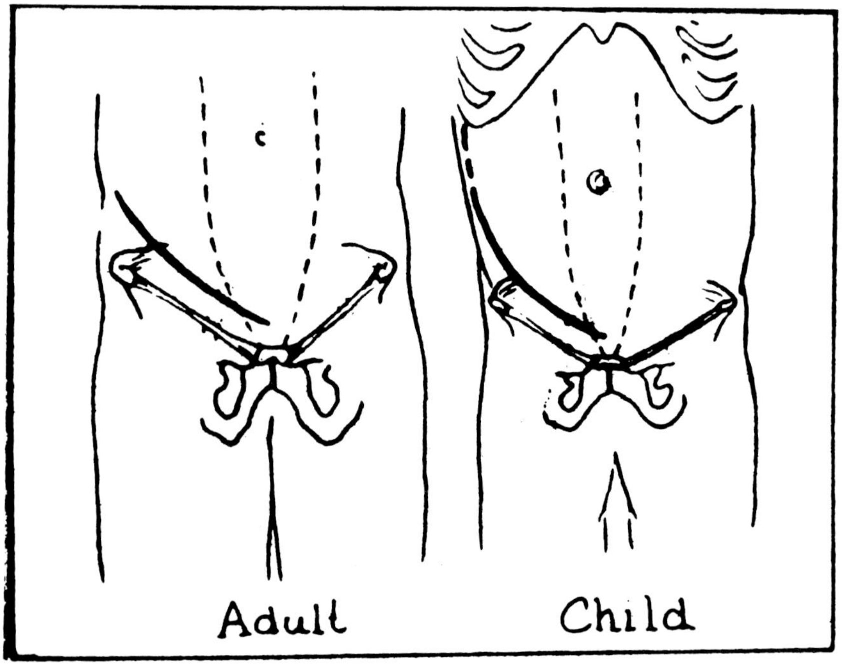

FIGURE 17.1. *Incisions made for implantation of kidney in adult and child. (Reproduced by permission from Morris PJ, ed. Kidney transplantation: principles and practice. 4th ed. Philadelphia: WB Saunders, 1994.)*

internal iliac vein and adjacent tributaries, the kidney will usually lie satisfactorily in the parapsoas gutter without any venous tension, even with a short renal vein. Finally, the wound is closed in layers with nylon and without drainage.

IMMUNOSUPPRESSION

The currently available immunosuppressive agents, both drugs and biologic agents, and those that are about to become available are discussed in detail elsewhere in this book. In this section, the most common approaches to the prevention and treatment of rejection in practice today are discussed, together with the possible uses of some of the newer agents.

Prevention of Rejection

Cyclosporine

Conventional immunosuppressive protocols today are all based on cyclosporine (Table 17.4). Triple therapy (low-dose cyclosporine, azathioprine, and prednisolone) is used by the vast majority of renal transplant units (25); a typical dose regimen used in Oxford is described in Table 17.5. Essentially there is little to choose between these different cyclosporine protocols on the basis of graft survival. However, triple therapy has become popular and is used by some 80% of renal transplant units because it is not only relatively free of side effects but also relatively easy to manage. Recently cyclosporine in a microemulsion (Neoral) has replaced the previous oil-based formulation of cyclosporine (Sandimmune) (26). Although undoubtedly Neoral is better absorbed than Sandimmune, it is not certain that the frequency of rejection is any less. In Oxford, 40% of patients receiving Neoral still experience at least one episode of rejection in the first three months after transplantation, which differs little from the previous frequency of rejection with Sandimmune in our unit. However, for the occasional patient who is a poor absorber of cyclosporine, especially in the first week after transplantation, Neoral is much more effective in that therapeutic blood levels can be achieved quite quickly and maintained more easily.

Table 17.4. Cyclosporine-Based Protocols for Immunosuppression in Clinical Renal Transplantation

Cyclosporine alone (monotherapy)
Cyclosporine + steroids
Cyclosporine + azathioprine
Cyclosporine + azathioprine + steroids (triple therapy)
Cyclosporine ⟶ azathioprine + steroids (conversion therapy)
Cyclosporine + azathioprine + steroids ⟶ azathioprine + steroids (conversion therapy)
ATG/OKT-3 + azathioprine + steroids ⟶ cyclosporine + azathioprine + steroids (sequential therapy)
ATG/OKT-3 + cyclosporine + azathioprine + steroids ⟶ cyclosporine + azathioprine + steroids (quadruple therapy)

Table 17.5. Triple Therapy Immunosuppressive Regimen

Cyclosporine: 8 mg/kg/day given orally in divided doses as Neoral and adjusted according to blood trough levels:
First 6 months: 2–300 ng/mL
After 6 months: 100–200 ng/mL
Azathioprine: 1.5 mg/kg/day
Steroid:
20 mg prednisolone daily in divided doses (if recipient >60 kg)
15 mg prednisolone daily in divided doses (if recipient <60 kg)
At 2 months prednisolone reduced to 10 mg/day over 3 to 5 months
At 12 months prednisolone slowly discontinued

It is not uncommon for units, especially in the United States, to use additional induction therapy with an antilymphocyte agent such as an antithymocyte globulin or OKT-3 (see Chapter 13). The antilymphocyte agent is given over 10 to 14 days or until renal function is established, at which time cyclosporine is introduced (27). This type of therapy does result in less rejection in the early weeks after transplantation and probably results in better graft survival. However, induction therapy with an antilymphocyte agent does increase the incidence of viral infection, especially cytomegalovirus (CMV), and lymphoproliferative disease later on, particularly if additional antilymphocyte therapy has to be given later for steroid-resistant rejection (28). Thus, it is not unreasonable to suggest that except in special circumstances—for example, the highly sensitized patient or the patient with severe acute tubular necrosis (ATN)—antilymphocyte induction therapy should not be used routinely in renal transplantation, either before cyclosporine is introduced or together with cyclosporine.

Although cyclosporine has been commonly used alone or with steroids, this has become a less common practice. In the case of monotherapy with cyclosporine, it appears that a somewhat higher dose of cyclosporine is required with consequently a greater incidence of nephrotoxicity. Some units have nevertheless reported excellent results with cyclosporine monotherapy.

Discontinuation of cyclosporine after a time, ranging from three months to one year after transplantation, and conversion to azathioprine and steroids (conversion protocol) was first described from Oxford (29). This protocol was designed in an attempt to reduce the incidence and degree of nephrotoxicity that was seen in the early days of cyclosporine usage, when larger doses were used than is customary today. A subsequent randomized prospective trial of conversion therapy in Oxford showed that discontinuation of cyclosporine resulted in a dramatic improvement in renal function that was maintained for at least five years (30). However conversion was associated with a 25% incidence of acute rejection within three months of conversion and the need for reintroduction of cyclosporine in a small number of patients. Although graft survival remained very satisfactory (around 70% at five years), this protocol was not widely adopted because of the incidence of acute rejection after conversion, except in developing countries where the cost of cyclosporine prohibited its long-term use. Several other studies later showed very similar results, but all with an incidence of acute rejection after conversion of around 25% to 30%, regardless of the time of conversion (31,32). Nevertheless, graft survival with these conversion protocols remains very satisfactory, as confirmed in a recent meta-analysis (33), and they perhaps deserve further attention.

Cyclosporine (Neoral) is given twice daily as capsules, but an oral solution is available for those patients who are not able to swallow the large capsules. Blood trough levels are monitored regularly (e.g., thrice weekly) in the early weeks after transplantation until stable levels are achieved. They are then monitored approximately once every one to two weeks until a maintenance dose is achieved after three months, when trough levels can be checked relatively infrequently unless drugs that influence liver metabolism are given or there is liver dysfunction. Target trough levels in our triple therapy protocol are 200 to 300 ng/mL during the first six months and 100 to 200 ng/mL thereafter. Although rejection is more likely to be associated with low trough levels and nephrotoxicity with high trough levels of cyclosporine, the correlation is by no means exact. A much better impression of the bioavailability of the drug is given by the area under the curve (AUC), and recent studies suggest that because of the better and more consistent absorption of cyclosporine in its microemulsion formulation (Neoral), the AUC can be accurately calculated from two blood samples at 2 and 6 hours, respectively (34). Cyclosporine is metabolized in the liver by the cytochrome P450 enzyme system, and it is important to be aware of drugs that interact with cyclosporine causing either higher blood levels (e.g., ketoconazole) or lower blood levels (e.g., rifampicin) (Table 17.6), as dose adjustments will be required in the presence of these drugs. Indeed, sometimes cyclosporine has to be discontinued and replaced by another immunosuppressive drug.

Table 17.6. Important Drug Interactions with Cyclosporine

Drugs that increase cyclosporine levels
Ketoconazole
Fluconazole
Erythromycin
Corticosteroids
Diltiazem
Drugs that decrease cyclosporine levels
Isoniazid
Phenobarbitone
Phenytoin
Rifampicin
Drugs that cause additive nephrotoxicity
Aminoglycosides
Amphotericin
Melphalan
Sulfonamides/cotrimoxazole
Trimethoprim

There are a number of side effects associated with cyclosporine, which are listed in Table 17.7. Most of these are to a great extent dose related. The most important side effects are nephrotoxicity, hypertension, and hyperlipidemia. Considerable controversy exists as to whether chronic renal allograft failure is due in many instances to cyclosporine nephrotoxicity or to chronic rejection due to inadequate doses of cyclosporine, which tend to be reduced as renal function deteriorates (35). This is a difficult problem to resolve, but the common occurrence of long-term renal dysfunction of the recipient's own kidneys after cardiac and liver transplantation suggest that cyclosporine nephrotoxicity does persist in many patients. Indeed, it is possible that there is no therapeutic dose of cyclosporine that is not nephrotoxic to some extent.

Tacrolimus

The initial experience with tacrolimus (FK506) was mostly in liver transplantation, but following the demonstration in two large multicenter trials (36,37) that it was at least as effective as cyclosporine in terms of graft survival and resulted in less acute rejection, it was introduced in renal transplantation in place of cyclosporine both as induction therapy and also to rescue grafts undergoing rejection on cyclosporine (see also Chapter 9).

Several randomized prospective trials comparing tacrolimus with cyclosporine have been performed and showed that the incidence of acute rejection episodes in the early months after transplantation is lower in patients receiving tacrolimus, although patient and graft survival are essentially the same (38,39) (Table 17.8). In the European multicenter study, 448 patients were entered into the trial; 303 patients were randomized to receive tacrolimus plus azathioprine and steroids and 145 patients received cyclosporine, azathioprine, and steroids (38). There was not

Table 17.7. Side Effects of Cyclosporine Therapy

Renal	Nephrotoxicity; hemolytic-uremic syndrome
Hepatic	Hepatotoxicity
Neoplastic	Lymphomas; fibroadenoma of breast; squamous cell carcinoma
Dermatologic	Thickening; rashes; hypertrichosis
Gastrointestinal	Anorexia; nausea; failure to gain weight
Metabolic	Hyperkalemia; hyperuricemia; hypomagnesemia; hyperglycemia
Neurologic	Tremor; convulsions; burning sensation in limbs; malaise; depression
Cardiovascular	Fluid retention; hypertension; hypercholesterolemia; Raynaud's phenomenon; intravascular coagulation
Dental	Gingival hypertrophy
Hematologic	Hemolytic anemia

Table 17.8. Patient and Graft Survival and the Incidence of Acute Rejection in Two Large Randomized Prospective Multicenter Trials of Tacrolimus and Cyclosporine in Europe and the U.S.A.

	Tacrolimus (%)	Cyclosporine (%)	*P*
European Trial (n = 448)			
One-year patient survival	93.0	96.5	NS
One-year graft survival	82.5	86.2	NS
Cumulative acute rejection	34.2	57.2	<0.001
Steroid-resistant rejection	11.3	21.6	0.001
US Trial (n = 412)			
One-year patient survival	95.6	96.6	NS
One-year graft survival	91.2	87.9	NS
Cumulative acute rejection	30.7	46.4	<0.001
Use of antilymphocyte agent	10.7	25.1	<0.001

NS = Not stated.
Sources: Data from European Tacrolimus Multicentre Renal Study Group. Multicentre randomised trial comparing tacrolimus (FK506) and cyclosporin in the prevention of renal allograft rejection: a report of the European Tacrolimus Multicentre Renal Study Group. Transplantation 1997;64:436–443; and from Pirsch JD, Miller J, Deierhoi MH, et al. A comparison of tacrolimus (FK506) and cyclosporine for immunosuppression after cadaveric renal transplantation. Transplantation 1997;63:977–983.

only a reduction in the incidence of acute rejection in the tacrolimus group (34.2% versus 57.2%) but also a reduction in the incidence of steroid-resistant rejection (11.3% versus 21.6%). However, patient and graft survival were not different at one year (see Table 17.8). In the US multicenter study, 412 patients were randomized to receive either tacrolimus with azathioprine and steroids or cyclosporine with azathioprine and steroids, and all patients had an induction course of OKT-3 or ATGAM (39). The incidence of acute rejection was reduced in the tacrolimus arm (30.7% versus 46%), as was the use of treatment of acute rejection with an antilymphocyte agent (10.7% versus 25.1%). Furthermore, the incidence of histologic moderate or severe rejection in a blinded independent review of biopsies taken at the time of rejection and graded according to the Banff criteria (see below) was lower in the tacrolimus arm (10.8% versus 26.5%). Once again, however, this was not reflected by improved patient or graft survival at one year in the tacrolimus arm, which were the primary objectives of the trial with respect to efficacy (patient: 95.6% and 96.5%; graft: 91.2% and 87.9% for the tacrolimus and cyclosporine arms, respectively).

Tacrolimus is administered orally in divided doses twice daily at a dose of 0.15–3.0 mg/kg/day initially after transplantation with the aim of achieving trough levels of 10 to 20 ng/mL. Usually the dose can be reduced after the first few weeks while maintaining trough levels at 10 to 15 ng/mL. As tacrolimus is metabolized in the liver by the cytochrome P450 enzyme system, just as cyclosporine, the same potential drug interactions exist as outlined for cyclosporine in Table 17.6. In view of the similar mechanism of action of tacrolimus and cyclosporine, it would be expected that a similar profile of side effects would be evident. This is essentially true, especially with respect to nephrotoxicity, but gum hyperplasia, hirsutism, and facial brutalization do not occur with tacrolimus. On the other hand, there is an increased incidence of insulin-dependent diabetes.

There is a suggestion that tacrolimus may be steroid sparing, although there is no hard evidence that this is so. Nevertheless, a phase I dosage and safety trial of tacrolimus monotherapy involving 28 patients in Manchester (UK) showed a low incidence of rejection (responding to treatment with steroids) and no graft failures at six months, at which time no patients were on steroids (Johnson R, personal communication, 1998).

The use of tacrolimus to salvage grafts where rejection is not being controlled on cyclosporine, by conversion from cyclosporine to tacrolimus, is proving to be of value as judged essentially from an increasing number of anecdotal reports (40,41) and one multicenter trial (42). However, it is of note that the response to conversion is more likely to be favorable if the serum creatinine at the time of conversion is not above 3 mg/dL. This would certainly seem to be a valid use of the drug in renal transplantation. Tacrolimus has also been used to replace cyclosporine in the presence of cyclosporine toxicity, both for nephrotoxicity and for HUS, with some success (43,44).

Tacrolimus may have a place in pediatric transplantation both as primary treatment because of its potential steroid-sparing effect and also for rescue of grafts undergoing rejection on cyclosporine therapy, but data is still rather sparse (45–47). In children, the dose of tacrolimus needs to be one-and-a-half to twice the dose required in adults to achieve the same blood levels. It appeared that the majority of children receiving tacrolimus could be weaned off steroids, with the expected increase in height in those children compared with those remaining on steroids (45,48).

Thus tacrolimus is an effective immunosuppressive agent that may be used in place of cyclosporine. It must be remembered, however, that the prospective trials were not blinded and also that the comparison was with the previous formulation of cyclosporine (Sandimmune) and not the new formulation (Neoral). Thus it might be argued that if Neoral were used there would have been a lower incidence of acute rejection than seen in the comparative trials. Nevertheless, it would seem that tacrolimus is probably as effective as cyclosporine as a primary treatment for the prevention of rejection, and certainly it has a place for the rescue of grafts where rejection is not being controlled on cyclosporine.

Mycophenolate Mofetil

Mycophenolate mofetil (MMF), another antiproliferative agent like azathioprine, has been described in some detail earlier (see Chapter 10). Following the demonstration that it was an effective immunosuppressive agent in animal experiments, phase I studies established dosage profiles that suggested an effective dose in humans of 2–3 g/day in divided doses (49). Although there appears to be an association between the AUC of mycophenolic acid, the active metabolite of MMF, and its immunosuppressive activity, there is not a correlation between dosage, weight, and the AUC. Hence, for the moment, fixed dosages are used—2 g/day in divided doses being the most widely used and recommended dose.

In three large multicenter trials in which two doses of MMF (2 g and 3 g per day) were compared with azathioprine together with cyclosporine and steroids, MMF has been shown to significantly lower the incidence of biopsy-proven acute rejection episodes by 30% to 40% in the first six months after transplantation (50–52). It should also be noted that these three multicenter trials set a new benchmark in clinical trials in transplantation in that they were not only randomized and prospective but also blinded to the participants. Despite the reduction in the incidence of acute rejection episodes in the first six months after transplantation, this has not been reflected by improved graft survival at year 1 or year 3, although it must be said that the numbers in the trials were not powered to show a significant difference in survival, which was a secondary end point of the trials after acute rejection.

MMF has also been used for rescue of grafts undergoing steroid-resistant rejection. The first study was carried out in a number of centers where patients had received steroids and in many instances OKT-3 for acute rejection without response. MMF was added in doses of 1.0 or 1.5 g twice daily in place of azathioprine while continuing cyclosporine and steroids (49). Some 70% of the patients showed an improvement in renal function, and this appeared more likely if their serum creatinines were relatively low (<4 mg/dL) at the time treatment with MMF was commenced. This then led to the establishment of a multicenter study of refractory rejection in which attempts were made to standardize the definition of refractory rejection and patients were randomized to receive further high-dose IV steroids or MMF in place of azathioprine (53). Graft loss or death was significantly lower at six months in the MMF arm of the trial. Studies of refractory rejection are notoriously difficult to plan, however, not the least because of the difficulty in the definition of true refractory rejection. Thus, the results of this trial, although very suggestive that there was an effect, were not able to clearly define the role of MMF as a treatment of true refractory rejection.

MMF has a good safety profile, the major side effects being gastrointestinal and hematologic. The gastroenterologic side effects are nausea, epigastric discomfort, vomiting, and diarrhea; occasional patients may also have a gastrointestinal bleed. The hematologic side effects are similar to azathioprine, namely, leukopenia with occasional patients also displaying thrombocytopenia and anemia. There was no increased incidence of cancer or lymphoma in these trials.

Thus, the results of the multicenter trials would argue strongly in favor of replacing azathioprine with mycophenolate in a triple therapy protocol, although cost is a consideration. It is also possible that the use of mycophenolate with cyclosporine could allow discontinuation of steroids soon after transplantation, but evidence for this still remains to be provided. Furthermore, it may be possible to use MMF with cyclosporine for limited periods of time, for example, 3, 6, or 12 months. Again, there is no evidence for this approach at the present time, although a prospective trial of this type of protocol is in progress.

Sirolimus (Rapamycin)

Sirolimus is a macrolide antibiotic that prevents proliferation of activated T lymphocytes in response to cytokines, especially interleukin (IL)-2, thus acting at an earlier stage of the cell cycle than mycophenolate and azathioprine. It is a potent immunosuppressive agent in experimental animal models (54,55), and its mechanism of action and pharmacokinetics have been discussed in an earlier chapter (see Chapter 11). In experimental models it appears to be synergistic with cyclosporine (56), but as might be expected from the fact that it binds to FKBP 12 at the same part of the molecule as tacrolimus, sirolimus and tacrolimus exhibit competitive antagonism.

As described earlier, phase I studies of dosage and safety established not only a range of doses and potential side effects but also that the addition of cyclosporine and sirolimus had a dramatic effect on the incidence of acute rejection episodes, although thrombocytopenia, leukopenia, and hyperlipidemia were noted (57,58). A multicenter, randomized prospective trial with six arms of 25 patients each has now been completed (Sirolimus Multicenter Study Group—unpublished). The six arms comprised a control group receiving triple therapy with cyclosporine, azathioprine, and steroids and two arms receiving 1 and 3 mg/m^2/day of sirolimus, while the other three arms received half-dose cyclosporine with 1, 3, and 5 mg/m^2/day of sirolimus, respectively. There was a dramatic reduction in the incidence of acute rejection in the two arms receiving full-dose cyclosporine and 1 or 3 mg/m^2/day—10% and 7%, respectively—compared to the control incidence of 40%. This effect was less marked in black patients. A more recent study, again a randomized prospective trial, compared cyclosporine with rapamycin, each group receiving steroids as well; there was no difference in the incidence of acute rejection episodes, which was approximately 40% (59). Side effects are still being defined but hypertriglyceridemia is one major side effect and thrombocytopenia, usually not severe, has been seen not infrequently. In contrast to cyclosporine and tacrolimus, nephrotoxicity has not been observed in either experimental animal models or the initial clinical trials.

Thus, sirolimus is a powerful new immunosuppressive agent that seems likely to have a place in clinical practice, probably used together with cyclosporine, provided side effects are acceptable. A multicenter trial is planned in which patients will receive cyclosporine and sirolimus together with steroids and then at three months be randomized to continue or discontinue cyclosporine. If the discontinuation of cyclosporine proves to be successful, such a strategy might have a significant impact on cyclosporine nephrotoxicity, bearing in mind the improved renal function achieved in the early cyclosporine conversion trials (30). Another property of sirolimus in experimental animal models that may prove to be of value in clinical renal transplantation is its ability to inhibit the vascular changes of chronic rejection (60,61).

Steroid Withdrawal

Because steroids are responsible for many of the medium- and long-term complications of immunosuppression, withdrawal of steroids from immunosuppressive regimens continues to be a desirable objective. Although steroid withdrawal after renal transplantation has undoubted advantages, with reduction in weight, hypertension, and hypercholesterolemia and improved appearance (62–64), there is concern that withdrawal of steroids from cyclosporine-based protocols will be associated with a deterioration in renal function (65). On the other hand, the Collaborative Transplant Study (CTS) registry data suggests that graft survival is superior in those patients in whom steroids are withdrawn (66). A similar recent analysis from the Australian and New Zealand Dialysis and Transplantation Registry also found that patients with a functioning graft at one year who were not on steroids had a better patient and graft survival thereafter compared to patients remaining on steroids (67). However these data have a possible defect in that patients may have remained on steroids because they had a more difficult early course, which might be associated with a poorer long-term graft survival. A meta-analysis of prospective trials of steroid withdrawal in the first 3 months after transplantation suggested an increased incidence of acute rejection after withdrawal (68).

Thus as the medium- and long-term effects of steroid withdrawal on renal function remained uncertain, we began in 1988 a randomized prospective trial in Oxford of steroid withdrawal in patients treated with triple therapy (cyclosporine, azathioprine, and steroids) and with stable renal function at one year or later after renal transplantation (69). This confirmed the benefits of steroid withdrawal, namely an improvement in weight, hypertension, and hypercholesterolemia with a persistent rise in alkaline phosphatase suggesting improved bone mineral metabolism. However, there was an associated 10% decline in renal function, which appeared to be stable at three years (Fig. 17.2). Furthermore, we were not able to define a group of patients (e.g., HLA-matched) in whom steroids could be withdrawn without risk. Thus, an element of caution is required before recommending routine use of steroid withdrawal, even some time after transplantation. It is our practice now in Oxford to withdraw steroids slowly at around one year in patients on triple therapy with stable renal function, provided they have not had rejection episodes after three months from the time of transplantation. The introduction of the newer immunosuppressive drugs such as tacrolimus, MMF, and sirolimus

A

Off	0	47	42	40	41	WG
On	49 (9·7)	2 (6·0)	5 (6·7)	5 (4·5)	3 (5·0)	
Off	0	0	0	17	22	CG
On	51 (9·9)	50 (9·7)	50 (9·5)	31 (7·6)	23 (6·9)	

B

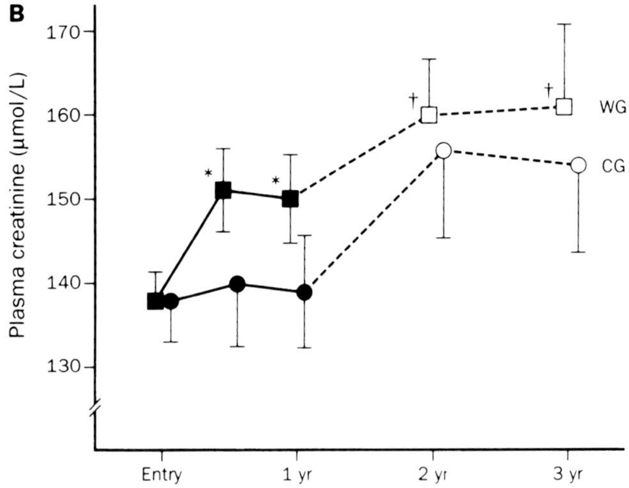

* $P < 0.001$.
† $P < 0.05$.

FIGURE 17.2. *Changes in creatinine during the trial period and after two years of further follow-up.* ***A.*** *Numbers at top are number of patients in each of the original groups who were not taking (off) or taking (on) prednisolone, together with the mean daily dose of prednisolone in those taking steroids.* ***B.*** *Mean plasma creatinine in each group at the trial end points (solid symbols) and subsequent follow-up (open symbols), for each group assigned by intention to treat (squares = withdrawal group; circles = control group). Bars indicate standard errors. Statistical comparison, with entry values by Student's two-tailed paired t-test. (Reproduced with permission from Ratcliff P, Dudley CR, Firth JD, et al. Randomised controlled trial of steroid withdrawal in renal transplant recipients receiving triple immunosuppression. Lancet 1996;348:643-648.)*

may allow steroids to be withdrawn at an earlier stage after transplantation, but this remains to be established in appropriate prospective trials.

Antilymphocyte Agents for Induction

These have been discussed at length in a previous chapter (see Chapter 13), but basically most clinical experience has been with the use of the pan-T-monoclonal antibody, OKT-3, or a polyclonal antilymphocyte antibody, for example, antithymocyte globulin or an antilymphocyte globulin. As already discussed, rejection does not occur during the administration of the antibody but often occurs after cessation of treatment with the antilymphocyte antibody. However, the evidence that graft survival is improved remains uncertain, although a recent meta-analysis of seven randomized controlled trials of induction therapy with an antilymphocyte agent in patients on triple therapy suggested a modest improvement in graft survival in those patients given an antilymphocyte agent (70). Nevertheless, the author does not feel that the routine use of a pan-antilymphocyte antibody for induction is justified in renal transplantation, for there is an increased risk of viral infections and lymphoproliferative disorders. Its use should be restricted to highly sensitized patients and patients with delayed graft function so that commencement of cyclosporine can be delayed until renal function is established.

In more recent years, there has been increasing interest in the use of other monoclonal antilymphocyte agents with specificity against specific molecules such as the IL-2 receptor, CD4, and adhesion molecules. The expectation is that the use of such agents may allow the induction of more specific unresponsiveness (e.g., anti IL-2 receptor antibody) or decrease the ischemia reperfusion injury that occurs in cadaver renal transplantation (e.g., anti-ICAM or anti-LFA-1 antibodies).

Randomized prospective trials of two humanized antibodies against the α chain of the IL-2 receptor have recently shown a significant decrease in the incidence of acute rejection with few or no adverse events accompanying their use (71,72). Furthermore, antibodies against the adhesion molecules may have a role in decreasing ischemia reperfusion injury in the transplanted organ. However, a large multicenter study of induction with an anti-ICAM antibody failed to show any benefit in terms of the incidence of delayed graft function (ICAM Study Group, unpublished data), while a multicenter trial of an anti-LFA-1 antibody only showed a nonsignificant trend in the incidence of delayed graft function in patients at risk (Anti-LFA-1 Study Group, unpublished data).

Other approaches to immunosuppression using antilymphocyte agents in experimental models of organ transplantation that appear exciting are the pretreatment of recipients with donor-specific MHC antigen under an umbrella of anti-CD4 monoclonal antibody (73), and the treatment of recipients with antibodies directed against molecules involved in the delivery of the second signal to the T cell, anti-CD40 ligand, and CTLA4-Ig (74,75). Clinical trials of both these strategies are planned, and undoubtedly the use of monoclonal antibodies in transplantation will be primarily directed at their ability to produce more specific immunosuppression. The major problem of their use in this context is likely to be the need for the concurrent use of conventional immunosuppressive drugs that may interfere with the mechanisms by which the monoclonal antibodies produce specific unresponsiveness in experimental models of organ transplantation.

Treatment of Rejection

The standard therapy for treatment of an acute rejection episode remains high-dose methylprednisolone, given intravenously in doses ranging from 0.5–1.0g daily for three days. In all cases, rejection should be confirmed by biopsy before treatment is started, if at all possible. Some units use oral high-dose methylprednisolone rather than IV administration, but this is no more effective. Furthermore, it usually means the patient is exposed to a greater cumulative dose of steroids and this is (not surprisingly) associated with more complications, as shown some years ago in a randomized prospective trial in Oxford (76).

When there is no response to steroids in terms of renal function or histology, a further course of IV methylprednisolone can be given, unless the initial biopsy showed severe rejection especially with vascular changes, in which case it is preferable to commence treatment with an antilymphocyte agent. Certainly if there is not a response after a second course of steroids, a diagnosis of steroid-resistant rejection can be made and an antilymphocyte agent commenced. Once more, a further biopsy should be performed before commencing an antilymphocyte agent in case the failure to respond to steroids is due to the development of acute tubular necrosis as a response to a severe rejection episode.

The antilymphocyte agents in common use are an antithymocyte globulin (polyclonal) and a monoclonal antibody directed against CD3 on T cells (OKT-3) (27). The administration of OKT-3 is associated with a moderately severe reaction after the first dose due to the release of a host of cytokines such as tumor necrosis factor (cytokine release syndrome). For this reason, most units in Europe use one of the two very effective polyclonal rabbit antithymocyte globulins (ATGs) available, as usually they are associated with relatively little in the way of a reaction with the first dose and appear to be as effective as OKT-3. Around 75% of steroid-resistant rejection episodes respond to treatment with an antilymphocyte agent.

Tacrolimus is also being used increasingly to treat steroid-resistant episodes in patients on cyclosporine, where tacrolimus is substituted for cyclosporine. The available data, which is mostly anecdotal, does suggest that this is a legitimate protocol as previously discussed. Similarly, as already discussed, MMF has been used in steroid-resistant rejection episodes in place of azathioprine in a cyclosporine-based protocol, with reversal of a significant number of such episodes.

EARLY COURSE AFTER TRANSPLANTATION

Immediate Graft Function

In around 60% to 70% of cadaver grafts and virtually all living donor transplants, the graft will function immediately. In recipients of living donor grafts, an initial osmotic diuresis usually occurs, and as much as 25L of urine can be passed in the first 24 hours if the recipient was poorly dialyzed before transplantation. In this situation, accurate fluid balance is essential and sometimes even K+ supplements are required. The sense of well-being in patients with a graft that functions immediately is quite remarkable and will be noted within 24 hours of transplantation. Careful attention to fluid requirements is essential in the first few days, which is greatly facilitated by a central venous pressure line. Fluid intake is initially set at the last hour's urine output plus 50 mL in the form of dextrose saline or normal saline unless otherwise indicated by the central venous pressure. Although a cadaver graft often functions immediately, it rarely achieves normal levels of serum creatinine within the first week in contrast to the living-related graft, which will do so within a few days. Within two to three days, central venous pressure and cardiac monitoring can be discontinued. The urinary catheter is removed on the fifth day in our practice, where we use a Politano-Leadbetter antireflux vesicoureteric anastomosis. The management of the patient with a graft that functions immediately is easier than with a poorly functioning graft, as any complication related to the graft or rejection is usually manifest by a deterioration of renal function.

Delayed Graft Function

Delayed graft function (DGF) is due to ATN and is arbitrarily defined as the need for dialysis in the first week after transplantation. With the use of heart-beating donors, DGF will be seen in about 30% of cadaver transplants. However, most cadaver kidneys do not have optimal function initially, probably due in part to lesser degrees of ATN and ischemia reperfusion injury. Patients with DGF are more difficult to manage, as a deterioration of renal function cannot be used as an indication of a technical complication or early rejection. In our unit, fine-needle aspiration cytology (FNAC) is used to monitor these patients for early signs of rejection; if the cytology is suggestive of rejection, an immediate biopsy is performed (77). Delayed graft function may on occasions last for several weeks and sometimes the graft never functions (primary nonfunction). This phenomenon is seen in patients who receive a badly damaged kidney, as might occur in a kidney removed from a donor who had a prolonged period of hypotension before removal, especially if the donor was elderly.

Deterioration in Renal Function

The causes of a decline in renal function in the early weeks after transplantation are listed in Table 17.9. The two most common causes that need to be distinguished are acute rejection and cyclosporine nephrotoxicity, but the less common causes such as ureteric obstruction and vascular thrombosis must be considered. It should also be remembered that an initial satisfactory urine output in the first few hours that subsequently tails off is compatible with a diagnosis of ATN.

In the presence of early renal dysfunction, the clinician should follow a regular protocol of investigation. First, a whole blood trough level of cyclosporine should be obtained if not available, together with an ultrasound examination of the kidney and its surrounds. A cyclosporine trough level that is elevated (>400 ng/mL) would suggest the presence of nephrotoxicity; one that is low (<150 ng/mL) or within the normal range would be compatible with rejection or a mechanical cause of the renal dysfunction, respectively. The ultrasound scan will allow a diagnosis of ureteric obstruction or a urinary leak to be made, but in addition it will allow the detection of a lymphocele or a hematoma adjacent to the kidney, both of which may obstruct the ureter. If the ultrasound does not detect any obstruction, the next investigation is a needle core biopsy of the kidney, usually performed today with a mechanical needle, such as a Biopty gun. This will allow a diagnosis of rejection to be made and also the severity of the rejection to be assessed.

Table 17.9. Causes of a Deterioration in Renal Function in Early Weeks After Renal Transplantation

Acute tubular necrosis
Vascular
Renal artery thrombosis
Renal vein thrombosis
Bleeding
Lymphatic
Lymphocele
Rejection
Accelerated or acute
Cyclosporine nephrotoxicity
Urologic
Urine leak
Ureteric obstruction

Although renal arterial or venous thrombosis is a cause of acute renal dysfunction in the early days after transplantation, the diagnosis is not a true differential diagnosis in cases of renal dysfunction in that the presentation is acute, with the sudden onset of anuria and, in the case of renal vein thrombosis, the presence of a painful swollen kidney. Indeed, today in the cyclosporine era, the common cause of rupture of a transplanted kidney is renal vein thrombosis, in contrast to the azathioprine era when it was acute rejection. In addition, duplex scanning can be used to confirm that perfusion of the kidney is satisfactory, and this has now replaced isotope scans previously used for this purpose. In our unit, this is performed routinely on day 2 after operation and is particularly reassuring in cases where the graft is oliguric or anuric as a result of ATN.

TECHNICAL COMPLICATIONS AND THEIR MANAGEMENT

Renal Artery

Thrombosis of the renal artery is relatively rare and usually results in loss of the kidney even if it is recognized quickly. It may be recognized at the time of transplantation as a result of an intimal flap caused by damage of the artery during removal of the kidney. When this occurs, it usually is possible to repair the damage. This may be easier if the kidney is removed and reperfused, allowing repair to be performed on the bench, after which the kidney is reimplanted. It more commonly occurs in the first 48 hours after surgery with the sudden onset of anuria. A duplex scan or an isotope renogram will confirm the diagnosis; however, if the kidney is to be saved, it is preferable to take the patient straight back to surgery for exploration.

Renal artery stenosis usually presents with hypertension and deterioration of renal function, especially after the introduction of an angiotensin-converting enzyme inhibitor for better control of blood pressure (78,79). Presentation is most commonly between 3 and 24 months after transplantation but may occur years after transplantation. The frequency of renal artery stenosis is around 5%, but the true frequency is almost certainly higher than that (80). Early occurrence of renal artery stenosis tends to be at the anastomosis and is probably technical in origin. Later stenoses occur distal to the anastomosis and may be related to rejection, turbulence, or undetected damage to the artery at the time of retrieval (Fig. 17.3). In the patient with poorly controlled hypertension and declining renal function, a biopsy should be performed to exclude acute or chronic rejection followed by an angiogram, which remains the gold standard for diagnosis. Treatment in the first instance should be angioplasty, with surgery reserved for recurrent stenoses after angioplasty (80). There may be a place for repeat angioplasty and insertion of a stent, but the long-term outcome of stenting is unknown and it would certainly make any subsequent surgery on the artery very difficult.

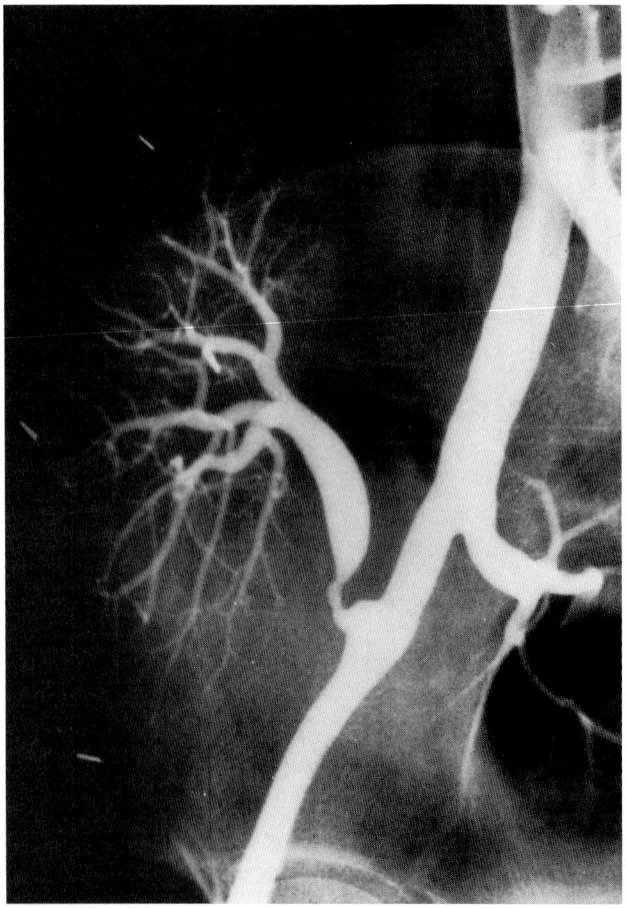

FIGURE 17.3. *A stenosis in the transplant renal artery distal to the end-to-side anastomosis of the renal artery with a cuff of aorta to the external iliac artery.*

Renal Vein

Thrombosis of the renal vein has become relatively common in the cyclosporine era and may be related to the procoagulant properties of cyclosporine (81,82). It also occurs more commonly in diabetics. Typically it occurs around five to seven days after transplantation with the sudden onset of oliguria and a painful swollen kidney. The patient should be explored immediately, as renal vein thrombosis is often associated with a rupture of the kidney; sometimes it is possible to successfully perform a thrombectomy of the renal vein. Prevention of renal vein thrombosis requires attention to the position of the renal vein and avoiding tension and twisting at the time of surgery. However, most renal vein thromboses are not technical, and prophylactic use of aspirin may be appropriate, assuming there is a significant platelet defect induced by cyclosporine. Since we introduced 75 mg of aspirin daily for one month after transplantation some years ago, renal vein thrombosis has virtually been eradicated in our unit.

Lymphatic

A lymphocele is a large collection of lymph that collects retroperitoneally around the kidney and arises from the recipient lymphatics around the iliac artery. The incidence is around 5%, although in the past it was much higher before it was realized that during the dissection of the iliac vessels, lymphatics must be ligated with a nonabsorbable ligature such as silk before division (80,83). A lymphocele produces clinical symptoms and signs by pressure on the iliac vein with swelling of the leg, obstruction of the ureter to produce deterioration of renal function, and pressure on the bladder or rectum with resultant strangury or tenesmus. The diagnosis is clearly made by ultrasound examination. Aspiration may be performed on two or three occasions, but if it still recurs then the lymphocele should be fenestrated into the peritoneal cavity via a transperitoneal approach. Recently it has been possible to do this endoscopically provided the lymphocele is immediately adjacent to the peritoneum (80).

Urologic

The two major urologic complications are ureteric obstruction and urine leakage (84,85). When obstruction occurs early in the post-transplant period, it is generally due to technical reasons at the site of implantation of the ureter into the bladder or twisting of the ureter. Oliguria or anuria in the immediate post-transplant period should make one suspect such problems. The diagnosis is confirmed by ultrasonography in the first instance, followed by antegrade pyelography to define the exact site of obstruction. Early surgical revision is required. Ureteric obstruction by hematoma after a percutaneous needle biopsy is occasionally encountered, but this outcome usually resolves spontaneously over a few days without active intervention. At times remote from the transplant operation, ureteric obstruction is often due to ureteric stricture formation that is presumed to reflect previous ischemic damage to the ureter. Again, ultrasonography and an antegrade pyelogram or an intravenous urogram will confirm the diagnosis, which should always be considered when a gradual deterioration in renal function is seen, especially without evidence of significant chronic rejection. Ureteric strictures may be treated by balloon catheter dilatation and insertion of a double J stent, although formal surgical reconstruction is often necessary.

Urine leakage usually occurs from the lower end of the ureter due to ischemia of this structure, perhaps as a result of skeletonization of the ureter during donor nephrectomy. Leakage from the cystostomy made at the time of ureteric implantation as part of the Politano-Leadbetter technique is relatively uncommon nowadays. Urine leakage is often not evident until at least one week after transplantation, and often several weeks pass before the diagnosis becomes obvious. Oliguria is noted in association with fever, local tenderness, and swelling. Ultrasonography followed by antegrade pyelography or intravenous urography allows a definitive diagnosis. Surgery should be undertaken as soon as possible, since a delay will undoubtedly result in infection, making the inevitable surgery more difficult and hazardous.

There has been a marked reduction in the incidence of urologic complications, both obstruction and leakage, in recent years in the Oxford Transplant Unit. This dates from the change to low-dose steroids in 1979, such that the overall complication rate is around 4.5% (85). Urologic complications can be avoided to some extent by careful attention to the removal of the donor kidney and its implantation.

Management of complications has been revolutionized by the development of minimally invasive techniques such as antegrade and retrograde insertion of stents and balloon dilatation of stenoses, all of which have reduced the need for operative intervention. However, it is important not to persist too long with these less invasive techniques if early correction of the defect is not achieved.

Other urologic complications, such as vesicoureteric reflux in the transplant kidney associated with repeated infection, may require reimplantation of the donor ureter with a more effective antireflux procedure. In an increasingly elderly male population with a renal transplant, bladder outflow obstruction requiring transuretheral resection of the prostate is seen with increasing frequency.

LATE COURSE AFTER RENAL TRANSPLANTATION

Chronic Renal Allograft Failure

This term describes the steady decline in renal function usually occurring any time after three months in a kidney with either relatively early normal renal function or with suboptimal function from the time of transplant. The causes of chronic allograft failure are listed in Table 17.10. Although it has been customary to attribute most instances of chronic allograft failure to a chronic immunologic reaction, so-called chronic rejection, it is now recognized that there are many other causes of a continuing deterioration of renal function after transplantation. It is important to establish a diagnosis because some of the causes of chronic allograft failure, for example, urinary tract obstruction and renal artery stenosis, are amenable to treatment.

Investigation of a patient with a late deterioration of renal function should include ultrasound of the renal tract to exclude obstruction and a renal biopsy to identify either recurrent nephritis, which would be suggested if the original disease was a glomerulonephritis with a high recurrence rate (e.g., focal sclerosing glomerulonephritis or mesangiocapillary glomerulonephritis type 2), or changes compatible with chronic rejection. It should be remembered, however, that occasionally a glomerulonephritis can occur de novo in a transplanted kidney where the original disease was not a nephritis. If the patient has hypertension, especially if receiving an angiotensin-converting enzyme (ACE) inhibitor, then an angiogram should be performed to exclude a renal artery stenosis.

Late Complications of Renal Transplantation

These are dealt with later in the book in considerable detail in descriptions of complications of organ transplantation in general, but some of the more important late complications of renal transplantation (Table 17.11) will be briefly discussed in the context of this overview of renal transplantation. Many of these complications are related to long-term immunosuppression and the nonspecific nature of its effect on the immune response.

Table 17.10. Causes of Chronic Renal Allograft Failure

Causes
Recurrent nephritis
Ischemia reperfusion injury
Cyclosporine nephrotoxicity
Chronic rejection
Renal artery stenosis
Hypertension
Previous acute rejection episodes
Urinary tract obstruction

Table 17.11. Late Complications of Renal Transplantation

Chronic allograft failure
Cardiovascular disease
Infection
Cancer
Osteopenia
Liver dysfunction
Benign skin lesions

Cardiovascular Disease

Cardiovascular disease is a major problem in transplant recipients, and death from myocardial infarction is now the most common cause of death after renal transplantation (78). The high incidence of hypertension and hyperlipidemia, both major risk factors for cardiovascular disease, in renal transplant patients can be attributed to both steroids and cyclosporine (78,86–88). Both diseases are common—some 70% of renal transplant patients are on antihypertensive treatment after one year, and some 30% of patients require treatment for hypercholesterolemia.

Persisting hypertension after renal transplantation may be due to several causes, and it is important to define the cause in case it is correctable. These causes include chronic rejection, diseased native kidneys with a high renin output, the immunosuppressive drugs, and transplant renal artery stenosis. To elucidate the cause, biopsy of the transplanted kidney and a renal angiogram will usually be required. In some patients, selective catheterization of the renal veins of the transplanted kidney and the native kidneys to obtain samples for renin estimations will be helpful in reaching a diagnosis. A significant renal artery stenosis will generally be associated with a deterioration of renal function in addition to hypertension, particularly if an ACE inhibitor has been introduced for the management of the hypertension.

A significant renal artery stenosis is generally treated by angioplasty, provided the transplant renal artery is accessible to the vascular radiologist. This now has quite a high success rate in good hands, but there is a relatively high recurrence rate that may be treated by a repeat angioplasty and perhaps insertion of a stent or surgical reconstruction. Stents should probably be reserved for a further recurrence, as there is insufficient information about the long-term behavior of stents in this situation, and certainly any subsequent surgery on the renal artery would be made extremely difficult in the presence of a stent. It needs to be borne in mind that surgical reconstruction of a transplant renal artery stenosis is often a difficult procedure because of the fibrous reaction around the kidney, and hence the attraction of angioplasty as a primary treatment. In the face of recurrent stenoses after successful angioplasty, however, our practice is to favor surgery over stenting.

Where the native kidneys are thought to be the major cause of the hypertension, bilateral nephrectomy may be indicated (78,89). If the kidneys are small, this can be achieved by embolization of the renal arteries (90), and of the open procedures the translumbar approach is associated with a relatively low morbidity. It is also possible that endoscopic-assisted nephrectomy may have a place in bilateral nephrectomy after renal transplantation.

After renal transplantation, hypertriglyceridemia persists and hypercholesterolemia develops. In at least 30% of patients on cyclosporine, there will be a significant degree of hypercholesterolemia with a lesser number with hypertriglyceridemia (87,88), but steroids undoubtedly play a role in both elevated cholesterol and triglyceride levels.

The aggressive treatment of risk factors for cardiovascular disease in recipients of renal transplants is imperative, remembering the high incidence of death from myocardial infarction in this population. This treatment should include dietary management, cessation of smoking, tight control of hypertension, and if necessary correction of a coexisting transplant renal artery stenosis or bilateral native nephrectomy. The use of one of the statins for correction of hypercholesterolemia not controlled by diet should also be mandatory.

Infection

Infections are a greater problem in the early months after transplantation, as discussed in detail later in this book (see Chapter 36). Cytomegalovirus infection is the biggest problem at this time, particularly in the CMV-seronegative recipient of a seropositive kidney, as the virus is generally transferred in the transplanted kidney (91,92). Although some units advocate routine prophylaxis with ganciclovir in this situation, our practice is a more conservative one in that prophylactic treatment is reserved for patients receiving additional therapy with an antilymphocyte agent, but the patients are monitored for evidence of infection with regular CMV antigen and polymerase chain reaction (PCR) assays. Transplant patients are more susceptible to infection and one must always be suspicious of the possibility of more exotic infections—cryptococcosis, tuberculosis, *Pneumocystis carinii*—in the long-term immunosuppressed recipient with evidence of infection (93). Liver dysfunction is likely to be due to hepatitis A, B, or C, but many cases remain undiagnosed and may be due to drug toxicity, for example with azathioprine or cyclosporine (94,95). Transmission of hepatitis C virus (HCV) with a kidney from a donor with anti-hepatitis C antibody results in a high rate of HCV infection in the recipient with non-A, non-B hepatitis (96), and therefore transplantation should not be performed even in recipients with anti-HCV antibodies.

Cancer

The increased incidence of cancer can be attributed in part to the nonspecific nature of the long-term immunosuppression and the strength of the immunosuppression (see Chapter 37). The latter point was illustrated in a randomized trial of low-dose versus high-dose cyclosporine commencing one year after transplant. There was a significantly lower incidence of cancer in the low-dose cyclosporine group (97). Admittedly, the cancers with the greatest increase in frequency are those with a putative viral etiology such as non-Hodgkin's lymphoma, squamous cell carcinoma of the skin, Kaposi's sarcoma, and cervical cancer in women, but in fact virtually all cancers show an increased frequency in transplant patients (98,99). The data from the Australian and New Zealand Dialysis and Transplant Registry (ANZDATA) provide the most comprehensive registry of cancer after renal transplantation. It is a prospective record of all cancers occurring after renal transplantation since 1963, and records the total number of transplants performed together with the immunosuppression used. The latest report shows that by 30 years after renal transplantation some 80% of patients have developed at least one type of cancer. Most of these cancers are skin cancers, but in addition over 30% of patients have developed a nonskin cancer (100). This contrasts with the risk of developing a cancer in an age-matched general population of around 5%. Some of the risk ratios from ANZDATA for the more commonly occurring cancers are illustrated in Table 17.12.

Osteopenia

Osteopenia is a common problem in long-term transplant patients and may present as osteomalacia, osteoporosis, or osteitis fibrosa cystica (101). Steroids are an important factor in the etiology of post-transplant osteopenia, as are cyclosporine and secondary hyperparathyroidism. Serious consideration should be given to placing all postmenopausal women who have a transplant on hormone replacement therapy unless there are contraindications, as the potential benefits especially as related to the prevention of osteoporosis and cardiac disease outweigh the very small risks of breast cancer, which is not one of the cancers that so far appears to have an increased incidence after renal transplantation (see also Chapter 31).

Table 17.12. The Risk of Development of Some Nonskin Cancers After Cadaveric Renal Transplantation

Site of Cancer	Risk Ratio (O/E)	95% Confidence
Esophagus	5.04	2.49–8.00
Rectum and anus	1.43	0.90–2.16
Lung	2.10	1.61–2.71
Breast (female)	0.96	0.69–1.30
Cervix—in situ	13.51	10.03–17.82
Cervix—invasive	3.78	2.11–6.23
Vulva and vagina	43.43	30.14–57.95
Penis	24.14	9.70–49.73
Bladder	7.19	5.40–9.39
Kidney	6.90	5.18–9.00
Ureter	250.00	119.88–459.75
Lymphoma CNS	>1000	939.00–>10.000
Non-Hodgkin's disease	7.4	5.90–9.18
Kaposi's sarcoma	85.71	50.80–135.47

The data reported here have been supplied by the Australia and New Zealand Dialysis and Transplant Registry. The interpretation and reporting of these data are the responsibility of the editors and in no way should be seen as an official policy or interpretation of the Australia and New Zealand Dialysis and Transplant Registry.

Benign Skin Lesions

Benign skin lesions are also common and include warts, acne, hirsutism, candida and dermatophyte infections, pityriasis versicolor, and nonmalignant skin tumors such as solar keratoses, keratoacanthoma, and Bowen's disease (102). All of these skin lesions are related directly or indirectly to the long-term use of immunosuppression.

Neurologic Complications

These are discussed in detail elsewhere in this book (see Chapter 33) and may be regarded as belonging to one of four broad syndromes: diffuse encephalopathy (e.g., cyclosporine toxicity); focal central nervous system abnormalities (e.g., cerebral lymphoma); seizures (e.g., cyclosporine toxicity); and peripheral nervous system syndromes (e.g., Guillain-Barré syndrome) (103).

REJECTION

The immunologic reaction to the renal allograft is known as rejection. A rejection episode is defined by clinical and biochemical parameters and confirmed wherever possible by a biopsy of the transplanted kidney. This is generally done today with a mechanical needle such as the Biopty gun and is a relatively safe procedure particularly if done with ultrasound guidance. Rejection is classified under several headings according to the timing and histologic parameters (Table 17.13) (104).

Hyperacute Rejection

Hyperacute rejection occurs in the presence of donor-specific antibodies in the recipient, who may have been sensitized by previous transfusions, pregnancy, or transplantation. It will also be seen if a blood group–incompatible transplant is performed in error; for example, a blood group A or B kidney is transplanted to a blood group O recipient. However, it should be noted that transplantation of blood group A2 kidney to O recipients may be successful in the presence of low anti-A titers (105). With the regular screening for HLA antibodies of patients on dialysis await-

Table 17.13. Types of Rejection

Hyperacute rejection
Accelerated rejection
Acute rejection
Chronic rejection

ing a transplant and the use of sensitive assays (e.g., flow cytometry) for the crossmatch between recipient serum and the proposed donor lymphocytes, hyperacute rejection is a rare event and where it does occur may be due to an immediate cellular anamnestic response. In the classic phenomenon, the transplanted kidney will initially perfuse well and become firm and pink, but after 20 minutes or so it will begin to become flabby and blue and a biopsy at that stage will show a massive infiltration of polymorphonuclear leukocytes (106). Some hours later, widespread thrombosis in glomerular capillaries and arterioles together with hyalin necrosis of arteriolar walls will be seen. No treatment will reverse this phenomenon once it has commenced.

Accelerated Rejection

An accelerated rejection occurs within the first five days of transplantation and is assumed to be due to an anamnestic cellular response against donor HLA antigens, as it may occur in the absence of any sensitization as determined by the presence of HLA antibodies before transplantation; in theory it could be related to sensitization against minor histocompatibility antigens in the donor, especially in the presence of HLA compatibility. It is associated with a sudden deterioration of renal function and histologically may be associated with a marked cellular infiltrate with or without vascular changes. In the absence of vascular changes, the response to high-dose intravenous methylprednisolone is usually rapid, whereas in the presence of vascular changes, which are a poor prognostic feature, treatment with antilymphocyte agents often will be necessary, and indeed antilymphocyte agents might be appropriate as the first line of treatment of this type of rejection.

Acute Rejection

Classically, acute rejection occurs between one and three weeks after transplantation. With current cyclosporine-based immunosuppression, it is not usually associated with clinical features such as swelling and tenderness of the kidney or a fever (which were typical features in the pre-cyclosporine era). Acute rejection episodes occur in about 40% to 50% of patients on triple therapy (cyclosporine, azathioprine, and steroids). However, as already noted, a reduction in this incidence has been seen with the use of some of the newer immunosuppressive agents, for example, MMF, sirolimus, and monoclonal antibodies against the IL-2 receptor. Histologically it is characterized by edema, mononuclear cell infiltrate, endothelial cell activation, and in more severe cases interstitial hemorrhage and arterial wall hyalinization. The presence of the latter two changes, so-called vascular rejection, is a bad prognostic sign (104,107,108) and is an indication for aggressive treatment usually with an antilymphocyte agent and possibly intravenous immunoglobulin (109). There has been a major effort in recent years to standardize the histologic assessment of acute and accelerated rejection, using the so-called Banff criteria (Table 17.14) (108). This has been extremely helpful, although further modifications are being introduced as the early grades of Banff have not proved to be predictive of outcome (107).

Table 17.14. System for Grading Acute Rejection in Allograft Biopsies Based on the Banff Schema

Biopsy Finding	Grade
Normal or with minor interstitial lymphoplasmacytic infiltration	Normal
Minor interstitial lymphoplasmacytic infiltration with occasional penetration of tubular epithelium	Borderline
Widespread focal interstitial lymphoplasmacytic infiltration with mild tubulitis; normal glomeruli and arterial vessels	Grade I
Extensive interstitial lymphoplasmacytic infiltration with definite tubulitis and intimal cell prominence with subintimal vacuolation in arterial vessels	Grade II
Extensive interstitial lymphoplasmacytic infiltration with tubulitis and lymphoplasmacytic infiltration of arterial walls sometimes accompanied by fibrinoid change or medial smooth muscle necrosis	Grade III

Usually, most acute rejection episodes respond satisfactorily to treatment with methylprednisolone, but some will be steroid resistant and require treatment with an antilymphocyte agent. Another biopsy should be undertaken to confirm that a rejection episode is persisting in the presence of steroid therapy before embarking on further therapy, as it is not uncommon for a degree of ATN to be produced by an acute rejection insult to the kidney.

Chronic Rejection

This is one cause of chronic renal allograft failure as previously discussed, and classically occurs anytime from three months after transplantation. However, within the various causes of chronic allograft failure are a cohort of patients with probably true chronic rejection where no other cause of failure can be identified (110–112). This is characterized histologically by the appearance of arterial myointimal hypertrophy, interstitial fibrosis, and glomerular sclerosis. The steady deterioration of renal function in general does not respond to treatment with increased steroids or changing to other immunosuppressive agents unless there is some superadded acute rejection on top of the chronic rejection changes. In a recent study in Oxford of a cohort of patients with carefully defined chronic rejection—steady deterioration in renal function, exclusion of other causes of chronic allograft failure, and histologic changes typical of chronic rejection—a number of risk factors were identified in a multivariate analysis. The significant factors were acute rejection either early or late, proteinuria and hypertriglyceridemia at one year, male sex, and serum creatinine at six months. Other factors such as cold ischemia time, donor age and sex, transfusions, and matching for HLA were not found to be significant (113).

RESULTS OF RENAL TRANSPLANTATION

Living Donors

Living-Related Donors

Transplantation within the immediate family of the recipient can produce excellent results, especially between HLA-identical siblings, as both the medium-term and the long-term results are superior to cadaver transplantation (Fig. 17.4). Furthermore, it is often possible to use lower doses of immunosuppression with the attendant benefits that this provides. Occasionally a recipient will have an identical twin, and obviously that is a perfect combination for transplantation in that no immunosuppression is required; although, if the original disease in the recipient was a glomerulonephritis with a high risk of recurrence, most clinicians would feel that some immunosuppression is advisable to decrease the risk of recurrence (114,115).

Living-Unrelated Donors

The inadequate supply of cadaver kidneys has led not only to an increase of living-related donors, especially in Europe, but also to far greater consideration of the use of living-unrelated donors, particularly spouses. Surprisingly, bearing in mind that spouses are usually quite incompatible for HLA, the results of transplantation have proven to be extremely good, equivalent to those of one-haplotype-disparate parent-to-child transplants, for example (Fig. 17.5) (7,116,117). Among spouse transplants, however, more recently it has been demonstrated that there is also an influence of the degree of fortuitous HLA matching between donor and recipient on graft outcome (118). The good results of spouse transplants in the presence of often major HLA incompatibility between donor and recipient underlines the importance of ischemia reperfusion injury in determining the outcome of cadaver kidneys. This has provided a major impetus for the investigation of mechanisms and causes of this phenomenon with a view to developing strategies for its prevention (119).

Cadaver Donors

Many factors may influence the outcome of cadaveric renal transplantation (Table 17.15), but there is now fairly general agreement as to the more important factors between the major registries—UNOS, Eurotransplant, CTS, and the United Kingdom Transplant Service Support Authority (UKTSSA). A recent multivariate analysis from UKTSSA

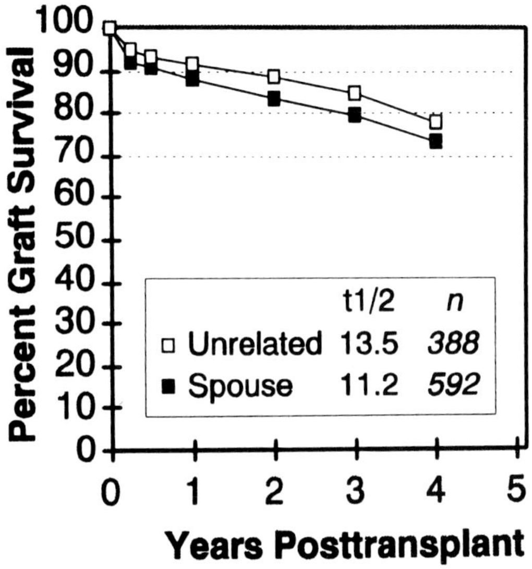

FIGURE 17.5. *Results of genetically unrelated living donor transplants (1991–1995). (Reproduced by permission from Cecka JM. The UNOS Scientific Renal Transplant Registry. In: Cecka JM, Terasaki PI, eds. Clinical Transplants 1996. Los Angeles: UCLA Tissue Typing Laboratory, 1997:1–14.)*

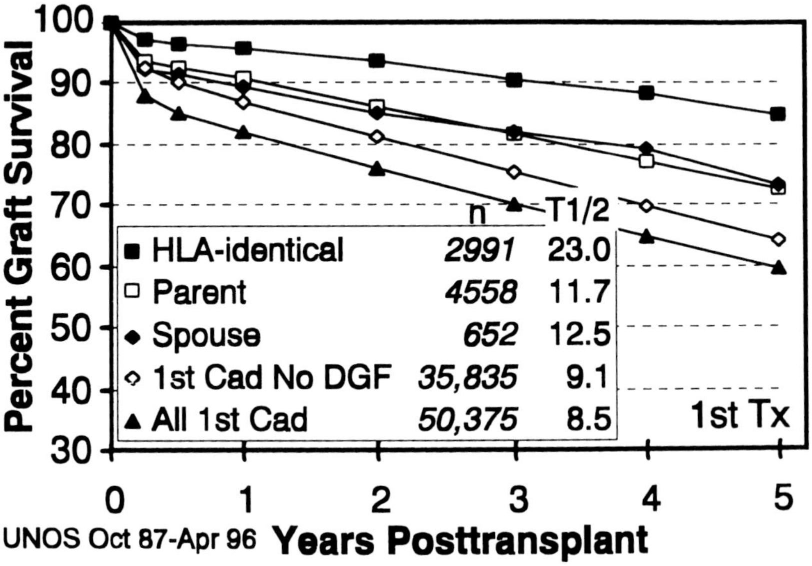

FIGURE 17.4. *Renal graft survival in living-related (HLA-identical and parent-to-child), spouse, and cadaver grafts as recorded by UNOS. Cadaver graft survival is given for grafts with no delayed graft function (DGF) as well as for all first cadaver grafts. (Reproduced by permission from Cecka JM. In: Sickness and health—high success rates of kidney transplants between spouses. Transplant Rev 1996;10:216–224.)*

Table 17.15. Factors Influencing the Outcome of Cadaveric Renal Transplantation

Immunologic
Immunosuppression
Matching for HLA
Sensitization
Rejection

In part immunologic
Recipient age
Bilateral nephrectomy
Ischemia times
Delayed graft function
Race
Original disease

Nonimmunologic
Compliance
Cardiovascular disease
Center effect
Donor and recipient sex
Clinical care

(14) of over 6000 first cadaver grafts with a 99.6% and 97.8% follow-up at one and five years, respectively, identified a number of highly significant factors (points 1 to 5, below) influencing the outcome of such grafts. In addition, other factors influencing graft outcome not addressed in the UK analysis are also described below (points 6 to 12).

1. *Donor age.* The older the donor the poorer the outcome—a finding no doubt related to the often marked reduction in nephron mass in the older kidney (Fig. 17.6). Similarly, the kidney from a very young donor has a poorer outcome due to a higher incidence of vascular thromboses, which are seen both in adult and pediatric kidneys.
2. *Recipient age.* Graft survival is poorer in the older recipient, but here the reason is that more of the older patients are dying with a functioning graft, often of cardiovascular disease (Fig. 17.7). However, it should be noted that the older patient is immunologically less reactive than the younger patient and immunosuppressive therapy should be tailored accordingly. A further analysis showed that the influence of donor and recipient age are

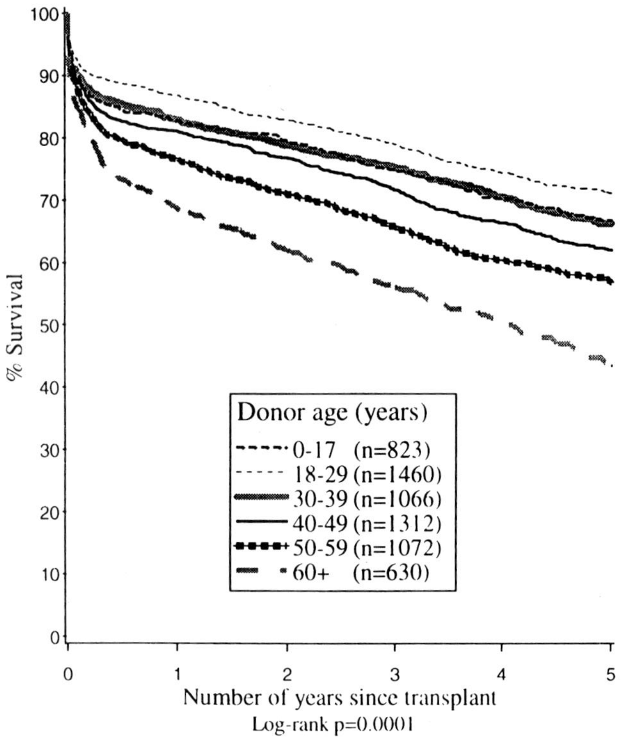

FIGURE 17.6. *The effect of donor age on first cadaveric graft outcome in UKTSSA analysis. (Reproduced by permission from Morris PJ, Fuggle S, Briggs D. Factors influencing outcome of primary cadaveric renal transplantation in the UK. Submitted for publication, 1998.)*

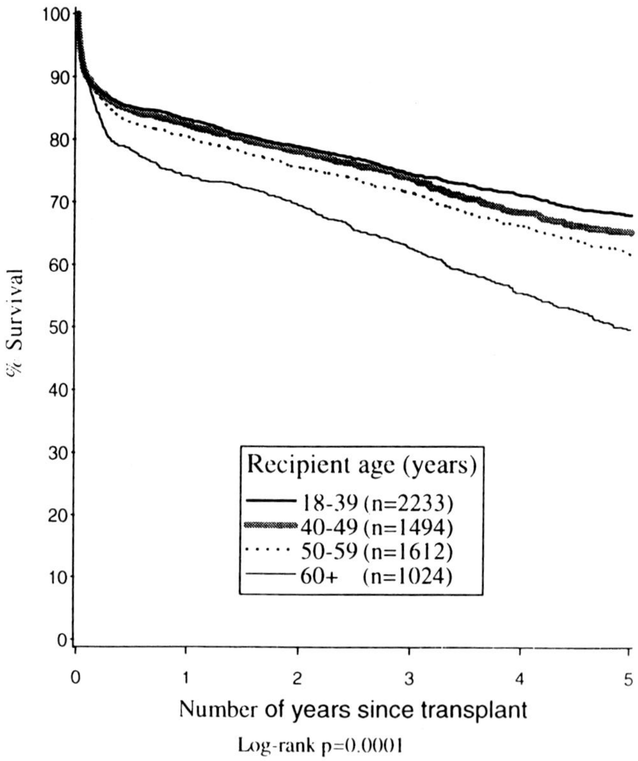

FIGURE 17.7. *The effect of recipient age on first cadaveric graft outcome in UKTSSA analysis. (Reproduced by permission from Morris PJ, Fuggle S, Briggs D. Factors influencing outcome of primary cadaveric renal transplantation in the UK. Submitted for publication, 1998.)*

quite independent, a point that should be borne in mind with the current practice of age-matching donor and recipient.

3. *HLA matching.* It is now generally accepted that well-matched cadaver kidneys have a better outcome than poorly matched cadaver kidneys (14,15,18). This was confirmed in the UK study, where the outcome of transplants between a donor and recipient with 0 mismatches at the HLA-A, B, and DR loci had far superior results to those with other degrees of mismatch (Fig. 17.8) (14). However, there was also a better outcome in transplants with what is defined as a favorable match, namely 100, 010, and 110 mismatches at the HLA-A, B, and DR loci. Thus the exchange of kidneys in the UK continues to be based on matching along the above lines, with the exchange of 000 mismatched kidneys receiving top priority in the national scheme, followed by the so-called favorable matches. However, the new allocation system also uses points based on some of the other factors determining graft outcome to separate equally well-matched donors and recipients on the national matching scheme.

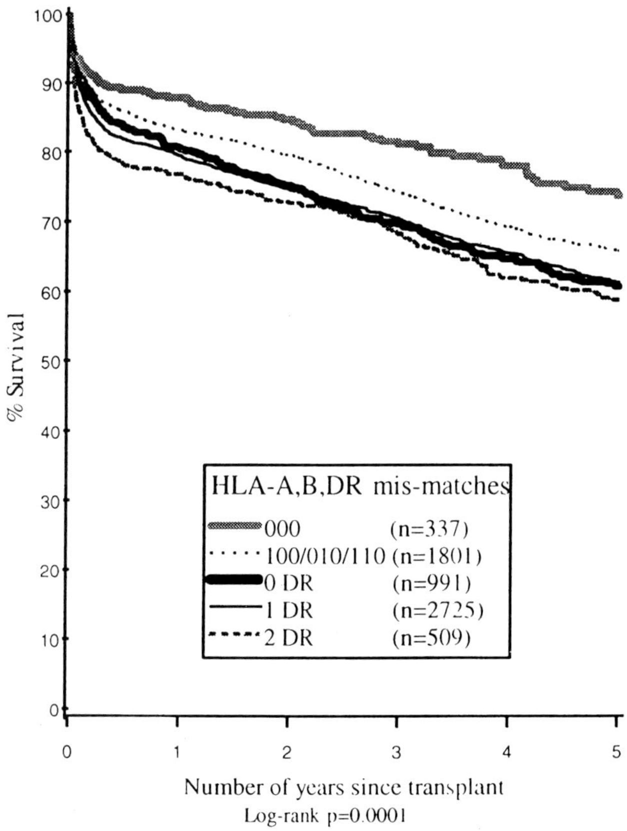

FIGURE 17.8. *The effect of matching for HLA-A, B, and DR on first cadaveric graft outcome in UKTSSA analysis (14). Triple 0 (000) mismatches had significantly better outcome than favorable mismatches (100, 010, 110), which in turn were significantly better than other degrees of mismatch (e.g., 210, 111, etc.).*

4. *Diabetes.* Graft outcome is poorer in the diabetic recipient primarily because of the presence of comorbid disease, especially cardiovascular disease. Stringent screening of potential diabetic recipients for cardiac disease and either their exclusion from further consideration or correction of the cardiac disease with coronary artery bypass grafting can produce results similar to those obtained in a nondiabetic patient (120). Furthermore, there is increasing evidence that a combined kidney and pancreas transplant can enhance the quality of life in the diabetic patient with ESRD, although it is unlikely to influence to any extent the progress of most of the secondary complications of diabetes (121), probably because the correction of the diabetes by a successful pancreatic transplant is too late in the course of the disease. However, the secondary complications do not continue to progress.

5. *Ischemia times.* Prolonged ischemia times do influence graft outcome, and in the UK data this became significant at times over 30 hours. This has been used as an argument not to transport kidneys on the basis of HLA matching. It should be noted, however, that in the UK multivariate analysis the marked influence of HLA matching was after allowing for the deleterious effect of prolonged ischemia times, as well as other potentially deleterious factors such as age of donor and recipient. Nevertheless, every effort should be made to keep ischemia times as short as possible. With the advent of DNA typing, it will be much easier to type a potential donor before organ retrieval, thus expediting the selection of possible recipients (17).

Over recent years there has been increasing recognition of changes that occur in the kidney both around the time of death and after storage and reperfusion, the so-called ischemia reperfusion injury. For example, in a longitudinal study of both cadaver and living-related kidneys in Oxford, upregulation of the adhesion molecule E selectin has been observed in endothelium of kidneys immediately after retrieval, while 30 minutes after reperfusion some 50% of kidneys show a marked expression of P selectin on activated platelets in glomeruli associated with a neutrophil infiltrate (122). Thus, some very significant changes occur in cadaver kidneys related both to the death of the donor and to ischemia times and reperfusion, providing a ripe environment for any subsequent specific inflammatory alloreaction. Hence there are now cogent reasons for reducing ischemia times as much as possible, while still retaining the beneficial effects of matching.

6. *Delayed graft function.* The outcome of grafts with delayed function (DGF), defined as the need for dialysis in the first week after transplantation, is much poorer than in grafts with initial function in most reports. The reasons for this are several and include ATN in association with ischemia reperfusion injury leading to a reduced nephron mass. Furthermore, the combination of DGF and acute rejection is a particularly bad prognostic

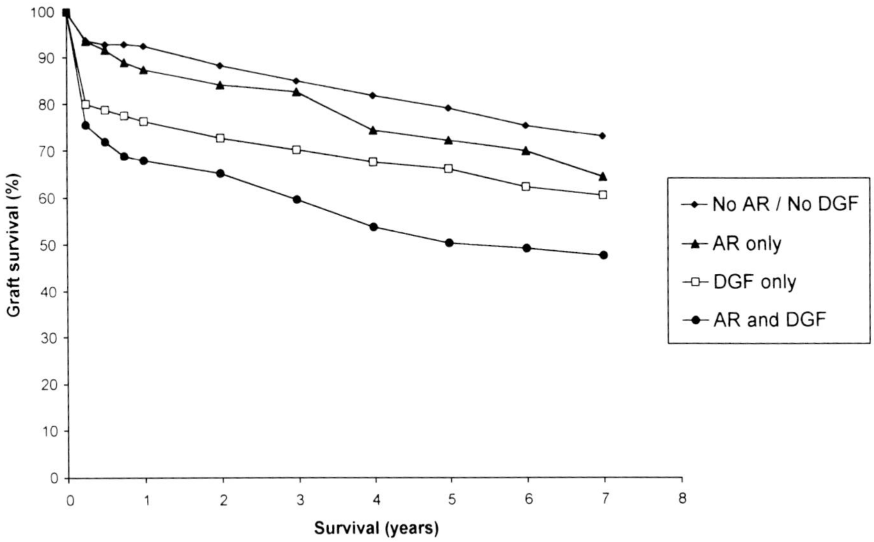

FIGURE 17.9. *Graft outcome in the Oxford Transplant Centre of cadaveric grafts based on the occurrence of acute rejection (AR) in the first six months after transplantation and/or delayed graft function (DGF). All patients received triple immunosuppression (cyclosporine, azathioprine, and steroids) and early technical failures were excluded. (Reproduced by permission from McClaren AJ, Jassem W, Gray DWR, et al. Delayed graft function: risk factors and the relative effects of early function on long-term survival in cadaveric renal transplantation. Clinical Transplantation 1999. In press.)*

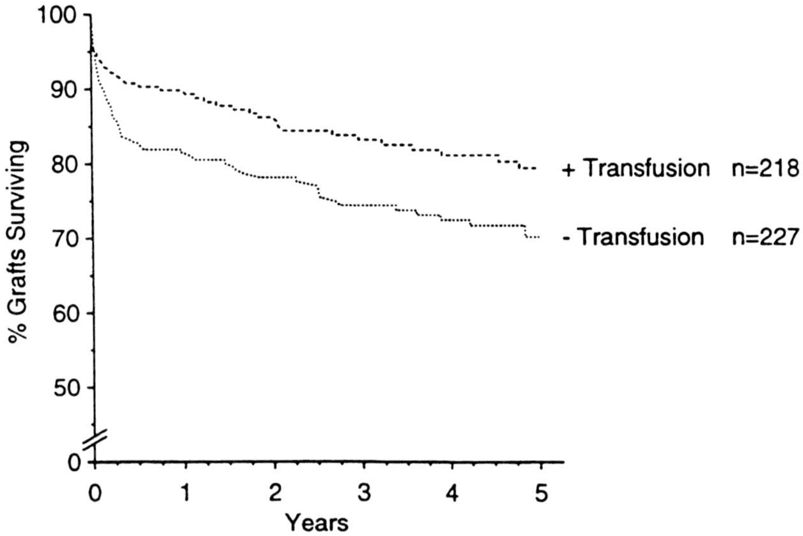

FIGURE 17.10. *Outcome of first cadaveric grafts in a randomized prospective trial of blood transfusion before transplantation. (Reproduced by permission from Opelz G, Vanrenterghem Y, Kirste G, et al. Prospective evaluation of pretransplant blood transfusions in cadaver kidney recipients. Transplantation 1997;63:964–967.)*

indicator, as recently confirmed in an analysis from Oxford (Fig. 17.9) (123).

7. *Center effect.* All registry data show that there is a difference in outcome between centers that can be explained in part by patient selection, but also must be influenced by the expertise of the transplant unit with respect to patient management. A center effect was also evident in the UK analysis.

8. *Blood transfusions.* Although in the azathioprine era the beneficial effects of transfusions before transplantation were clearly evident in subsequent graft survival, this transfusion effect seemed to disappear in the cyclosporine era. However, there are suggestions that if the recipient received blood from a donor sharing HLA-DR with the recipient then a better graft outcome was obtained, and in vitro data have been presented showing a decrease in cytotoxic T-cell precursors, for example, in such situations (124,125). Subsequent studies have not confirmed these observations (126–128). Nevertheless, an important randomized trial of deliberate transfusion of nontransfused recipients before transplantation, where cyclosporine-based protocols were used, has demonstrated a clear benefit of transfusion in the nontransfused recipient (Fig. 17.10) (129). Thus, the transfusion effect probably does still exist, but is not so marked in the cyclosporine era. The mechanism of this effect in humans remains unclear, although it is now well documented in the rodent as being due to downregulation of the T_H1 pathway (130,131).

9. *Sensitization and regrafts.* In the past, the outcome of transplants in patients with preexisting HLA antibodies was poorer than in nonsensitized recipients, as was the outcome of patients receiving a regraft, and this difference still exists in many units. However, in the cyclosporine era this difference has tended to disappear, but due only in small part to the availability of more powerful immunosuppression. Probably the most important developments in these improved results have been the

adoption of more sensitive crossmatch assays, the regular screening of recipients before transplantation for HLA antibodies, and the definition of the specificity of these antibodies.

10. *Sex of the donor and recipient.* As the female kidney is smaller than the male kidney and therefore has a smaller nephron mass, it might be expected that transplantation of a female kidney into a male recipient might have a poorer outcome than a male into male or a male into female, and indeed there is evidence to support this hypothesis (132). On the other hand, there is no data suggesting that incompatibility for the minor histocompatibility antigen, H-Y, influences graft outcome.

11. *Compliance.* In recent years, failure of compliance with immunosuppressive drugs has been recognized increasingly as an important cause of graft loss (133). This is often due to loss of body image in the young person or to financial problems in paying for immunosuppressive drugs.

12. *Associated disease.* The presence of associated disease such as cardiac ischemia or obstructive airways disease will influence graft outcome by the diseases' influence on patient survival. Of the diseases causing ESRD, only diabetes influences graft outcome to any great extent, essentially because of the poorer patient survival in diabetic patients. Graft outcome in patients with systemic lupus erythematosus does appear to be somewhat lower than in patients with other causes of ESRD (134). However, neither condition represents a contraindication to transplantation, as the quality of life with a transplant is preferable to that on dialysis.

REHABILITATION AND QUALITY OF LIFE

A number of studies in the United States and Europe have shown that renal transplantation provides a superior quality of life to that on dialysis, and that a majority of successfully transplanted patients are fully rehabilitated in the sense of returning to their previous occupation (135). It should be remembered, however, that many of these studies were performed before the widespread use of erythropoietin to correct the anemia of ESRD and this has undoubtedly improved the quality of life for patients on dialysis. Indeed, a more recent study of work disability, functional limitations, and health status of transplant recipients suggested that transplantation is not a panacea and that many patients report defects in their well-being and health status (136). Nevertheless, most patients do feel that release from the tyranny of dialysis definitely makes transplantation the preferred option for the treatment of ESRD.

One of the benefits of transplantation is the restoration of fertility to both male and female patients. Pregnancy in female patients is common and, although the incidence of spontaneous abortion is higher, there is no evidence of an increased incidence of fetal abnormalities in pregnancies successfully carried to term (137). There is a risk of rejection associated with pregnancy in about 10% of patients and an impairment of function in about 15% of patients, although this usually occurs in patients with impaired renal function at the time of conception.

CONCLUSIONS

Renal transplantation is undoubtedly the treatment of choice for most if not all cases of ESRD, and there are no definite contraindications to renal transplantation. Both dialysis and transplantation are expensive, although transplantation is the much more affordable option over several years. It must be remembered that many patients will pass from one treatment to another, perhaps several times in the course of their lifetime, and it is therefore important that there be an integrated program of dialysis and transplantation for the management of ESRD so the most appropriate option for therapy can be provided for these patients.

COMMENTARY

Kazuo Ota

The chapter on renal transplantation written by Peter Morris is well organized and covers all the essential and related topics. There are, however, several points in his presentation that differ from our practice in Japan, where more than 70% of the kidneys are donated from living-related donors. Furthermore, nearly all the cadaveric kidneys are retrieved from non-heart-beating donors.

As of the end of 1997, 175,988 patients were being treated with dialysis in Japan, and the annual increase of the patients on dialysis was approximately 13,000. On the other hand, the total number of the kidney transplantations in 1998 was 688, including 509 living donors and 149 non-heart-beating cadaver donors. There were approximately 13,400 patients on the wait-list.

Despite the shortage of donors, we have performed 1046 kidney transplantations in 1029 recipients at Tokyo Women's Medical College between February 1983 and December 1995 using cyclosporine-based protocols. These included 813 (87.3%) living and 133 (12.7%) cadaveric donor transplantations. The patient survival rates were 94.0% and 90.8% at 5 and 10 years, respectively, in the recipients from living donors, and 89.6% and 86.7% in recipients from cadaveric donors. The graft survival rates at 5 and 10 years were 82.6% and 70.0%, respectively, in the living donor recipients, and 76.0% and 59.4% in the cadaveric donor patients.

The survival rates of kidney transplant recipients should be compared with those of age-matched dialysis patients. From the Japanese registry of dialysis therapy, the survival rates of patients as a whole (n = 266,016) at 5 and 10 years were 60.0% and 42.5%, respectively. For an age-matched cohort of 36,930 dialysis patients who started dialysis between the ages of 30 and 44, the rates of 5- and 10-year survival were 86.8% and 76.5%, respectively. In any case, the survival of kidney transplant recipients is longer than dialysis patients, with a better quality of life.

Regarding the relative contraindication in the recipients, as is described in the chapter, IgA nephropathy is a type of glomerulonephritis with a propensity to recur. It is also one of the leading causes of chronic renal failure in Japan. Our study showed that the recurrence rate after kidney transplantation is high (40% to 50%) in this group of patients, which was confirmed in a histologic study. However, excluding those complicated by chronic rejection and/or microangiopathy caused by the nephrotoxicity of cyclosporine, deterioration of renal function was observed in a limited number of cases. Also, focal segmental glomerulosclerosis (FSGS) has a propensity to recur. In our series of 20 patients, 9 lost their grafts by recurrence. Plasmapheresis is effective in removing toxic factors before operation, and it is also effectively used to treat recurrence after transplantation. Among 14 patients thus treated, 12 grafts are functioning.

As regards oxalosis, we have performed successfully sequential living donor liver and kidney transplantations in a patient suffering from type I oxalosis, using her father, who showed a 50% reduction of alanine glyoxylate aminotransferase activity, as a donor. The partial liver was transplanted 54 days prior to the kidney transplantation. During the interval an augmented continuous ultrafiltration using hemofilter was carried out to remove as much oxalate as possible.

Because of the shortage of cadaver donors, we have performed ABO-incompatible kidney transplantation after removing anti-A and/or anti-B antibodies by plasmapheresis or plasma adsorption using Biosynsorb (Chembiomed Ltd., Edmonton, Alberta). Except for the early graft loss caused by humoral rejection occurring in the initial six months, ABO-incompatible kidneys functioned well and similar to ABO-compatible cases. Long-term follow-up study of our 67 cases revealed that the graft survival rates after one year were 79%; after five years, 75%; and after eight years, 73%. There was no significant difference from ABO-compatible cases in terms of the graft survival after five years. The A and B antigens in the transplant were followed histologically. Both of the antigens gradually decreased with time, although they were still observed after eight months.

It is my opinion that the recent improvement in patient and graft survival after kidney transplantations is based on the discovery and evolution of new drugs and medical technologies. First, there has been the introduction of new drugs such as cyclosporine, tacrolimus, gusperimus (15-deoxyspergualin), and antilymphocytic agents including OKT-3. Second, we have witnessed the development of new drugs that are useful to prevent some of the side effects of immunosuppressive drugs, such as H_2 blockers for gastroduodenal ulcers. Third, new technologies for diagnostic imaging such as computerized tomography (CT), magnetic resonance imaging (MRI), and ultrasound, applicable to any parts of the body of the recipients and donors including the grafts, have been developed. The contribution of ultrasound, flow cytometry, and aspiration cytology to diagnose rejection and of assays using the antigenemia method to detect cytomegalovirus (CMV) infection should be emphasized.

A fourth important advance is the invention of new technologies to make surgical intervention less invasive. Stenosis of renal arteries and the ureter can be treated by catheteral intervention. Endoscopic surgery is used effectively to treat surgical complications that otherwise necessitate open surgery.

Finally, there is the improvement of tissue typing, including flow cytometric crossmatch and DNA typing, and the improvement of various modern intensive care technologies.

However, despite the efforts we have made, among 1046 kidneys transplanted in our center and immunosuppressed mainly with cyclosporine, 230 were lost for various reasons. The leading cause of graft loss was chronic rejection, accounting for 121 cases (52.6%), followed by recurrence of de novo nephritis in 37 cases (16.1%). Graft loss by acute rejection, a leading cause of graft failure in the azathioprine era, decreased to 24 cases (10.4%) in this series.

Another important cause of graft loss is the death of the recipients, which occurred in 83 of our patients. The major causes of patient death were infections in 21 patients (25.3%), apoplexy in 13 (15.7%), liver failure in 11 (13.3%), and cardiac failure in 9 (10.8%). Other than these, 26 cases of malignant tumors were found, including 8 cases of renal cell carcinoma, followed by 6 cases of gastrointestinal cancer and 4 cases of malignant lymphomas. Eight of these patients have died.

Skin cancer, which is frequently found among the Caucasian transplant population, is rare among Japanese. Only one case was found among 1029 cases. The difference in the variety of malignant tumors may be related to the race of the recipient and the very long duration of maintenance dialysis prior to transplantation.

From these observations, it has become clear that the most important way to improve the rate of graft survival is to develop a method to avoid or at least to treat the chronic rejection without endangering the lives of the recipients. Induction of tolerance may one day solve the problem.

REFERENCES

1. Hume DM, Merrill JP, Miller BF, Thorn GW. Experiences with renal homotransplantation in the human: report of nine cases. J Clin Invest 1955;34:327.

2. Tilney NL. A crisis in transplantation: too much demand for too few organs. Transplant Rev 1998;12:1–9.
3. Briggs JD. The recipient of a renal transplant. In: Morris PJ, ed. Kidney transplantation: principles and practice. 4th ed. Philadelphia: WB Saunders, 1994:43–55.
4. Mathew TH. Recurrent disease after renal transplantation. Transplant Rev 1991;5:31–45.
5. Watts RW, Dunpure CJ, De Pauw L, et al. Combined liver-kidney and isolated liver transplantation for primary hyperoxaluria type 1: the European experience. Nephrol Dial Transplant 1991;6:502–511.
6. Gruessner RW, Kendall DM, Drangstveit MB, et al. Simultaneous pancreas-kidney transplantation from live donors. Ann Surg 1997;226:471–482.
7. Terasaki PI, Cecka JM, Gjertson DW, Takemoto S. High survival rates of kidney transplants from spousal and living unrelated donors. N Engl J Med 1995;333:333–336.
8. Cosimi AB. The donor and donor nephrectomy. In: Morris PJ, ed. Kidney transplantation: principles and practice. 4th ed. Philadelphia: WB Saunders, 1994:56–70.
9. Flowers JL, Jacobs S, Cho E, et al. Comparison of open and laparoscopic live donor nephrectomy. Ann Surg 1997;226:483–490.
10. Ratner LE, Kouvoussi LR, Sroka M, et al. Laparoscopic assisted live donor nephrectomy—a comparison with the open approach. Transplantation 1997;63:229–233.
11. Fuggle SV, Sanderson JB, Gray DWR, et al. Variation in expression of endothelial adhesion molecules in pretransplant and transplanted kidneys—correlation with intragraft events. Transplantation 1993;55:117–123.
12. Kootstra G. The asystolic, or non-heartbeating, donor. Transplantation 1997;63:917–921.
13. Cho YW, Terasaki PI, Cecka M, Gjertson DW. Transplantation of kidneys from donors whose hearts have stopped beating. N Engl J Med 1998;338:221–225.
14. Morris PJ, Fuggle S, Briggs D. Factors influencing outcome of primary cadaveric renal transplantation in the UK. (Submitted for publication, 1998).
15. Terasaki PI, Cho Y, Takemoto S, et al. Twenty-year follow-up on the effect of HLA matching on kidney transplant survival and prediction of future twenty-year survival. Transplant Proc 1996;28:1144–1145.
16. Ting A, Morris PJ. Matching for B-cell antigens of the HLA-DR (D-related) series in cadaver renal transplantation. Lancet 1978;1:575.
17. Bunce M, O'Neill CM, Barnard MC, et al. Phototyping: comprehensive DNA typing for HLA-A, B, C, DRB1, DRB3, DRB4, DRB5 & DQB1 by PCR with 144 primer mixes utilizing sequence-specific primers (PCR-SSP). Tissue Antigens 1995;46:355–367.
18. Ting A, Welsh K. HLA matching and crossmatching in renal transplantation. In: Morris PJ, ed. Kidney transplantation: principles and practice. 4th ed. Philadelphia: WB Saunders, 1994:109–126.
19. Sear J. Anesthesia in renal transplantation. In: Morris PJ, ed. Kidney transplantation: principles and practice. 4th ed. Philadelphia: WB Saunders, 1994:149–166.
20. Lee HM. Surgical techniques of renal transplantation. In: Morris PJ, ed. Kidney transplantation: principles and practice. 4th ed. Philadelphia: WB Saunders, 1994:127–137.
21. Prout GR, Hume DM, Lee HM, Williams GM. Some urological aspects of 93 consecutive renal homotransplants in modified recipients. J Urol 1967;97:409–425.
22. Campos Freiese G, Goes GM, Campos Freise JG. Extravesical ureteral implantation in kidney transplantation. Urology 1974;3:304–308.
23. Briand O, Nussaume O, Cohen G, et al. Ureterovesical reimplantation: a technique derived from Lich and Gregoir's procedure. N Presse 1982;11:2779–2780.
24. Yadav RV, Johnson W, Morris PJ, et al. Vesico-ureteric reflux following renal transplantation. Br J Surg 1972;59:33–35.
25. Morris PJ. Cyclosporine. In: Morris PJ, ed. Kidney transplantation: principles and practice. 4th ed. Philadelphia: WB Saunders, 1994:179–201.
26. Mueller EA, Kovarik JM, van Bree JB, et al. Pharmacokinetics and tolerability of a microemulsion formulation of cyclosporine in renal allograft recipients —a concentration-controlled comparison with the commercial formulation. Transplantation 1994;57(8):1178–1182.
27. Powelson JA, Cosimi AB. Anti-lymphocyte globulin and monoclonal antibodies. In: Morris PJ, ed. Kidney transplantation: principles and practice. 4th ed. Philadelphia: WB Saunders, 1994:215–230.
28. Opelz G, Henderson R. Incidence of non-Hodgkin lymphoma in kidney and heart transplant recipients. Lancet 1993;342:1514.
29. Morris PJ, French ME, Ting A, et al. A controlled trial of cyclosporin A in renal transplantation. In: White DJ, ed. Cyclosporin A. Amsterdam: Elsevier, 1982:355.
30. Morris PJ, Chapman JR, Allen RD, et al. Cyclosporin conversion versus conventional immunosuppression: long-term follow up and histological evaluation. Lancet 1987;2:286.
31. Hoitsma AJ, Wetzels JF, von Lier HJ, et al. Cyclosporin treatment with conversion after three months versus conventional immunosuppression in renal allograft recipients. Lancet 1987;2:584.
32. Hall BM, Tiller DJ, Hardie I, et al. Comparison of three immunosuppressive regimens in cadaver renal transplantation: long-term cyclosporine, short-term cyclosporine followed by azathioprine and prednisolone, and azathioprine and prednisolone without cyclosporine. N Engl J Med 1988;318:1499.
33. Kasiske BL, Heim-Duthoy K, Ma JZ. Elective cyclosporine withdrawal after renal transplantation. A meta-analysis. JAMA 1993;269:395–400.
34. Amante AJ, Kahan BD. Abbreviated AUC strategy for monitoring cyclosporine microemulsion therapy in the immediate post-transplant period. Transplant Proc 1996;28:2162–2163.
35. Salomon DR. An alternative view minimizing the significance of cyclosporine nephrotoxicity and in favor of enhanced immunosuppression for long-term kidney transplant recipients. Transplant Proc 1991;23:2115–2118.
36. McMaster P. Patient and graft survival in the European Multicentre Liver Study—FK506 vs cyclosporin A. Transplant Int 1994;7:S32–S36.
37. The US Multicenter FK506 Liver Study Group. A comparison of tacrolimus (FK506) and cyclosporine for immunosuppression in liver transplantation. N Engl J Med 1994;331:1110–1115.
38. European Tacrolimus Multicentre Renal Study Group. Multicentre randomised trial comparing tacrolimus (FK506) and cyclosporin in the prevention of renal allograft rejection: a report of the European Tacrolimus Multicentre Renal Study Group. Transplantation 1997;64:436–443.
39. Pirsch JD, Miller J, Deierhoi MH, et al. A comparison of tacrolimus (FK506) and cyclosporine for immunosuppression after cadaveric renal transplantation. Transplantation 1997;63:977–983.
40. Jordan ML, Shapiro R, Vivas CA, et al. FK506 rescue for resistant rejection of renal allografts under primary cyclosporine immunosuppression. Transplantation 1994;57:860–865.
41. Ochiai T, Ishibashi M, Kukao K, et al. Japanese multi-centre studies of FK506 in renal transplantation. Transplant Proc 1995;27:50–53.
42. Woodle ES, Thistlethwaite JR, Gordon JH, et al. A multicenter trial of FK506 (tacrolimus) therapy in refractory acute renal allograft rejection: a report of the Tacrolimus Kidney Transplantation Rescue Study Group. Transplantation 1996;62:594–599.
43. Kitamura M, Hiraga S, Kobayashi T, et al. Clinical experience of FK506 for renal allograft transplantation. Transplant Proc 1994;26:1924–1926.
44. Abdalla AH, Al-Sulaiman MH, Al-Khader AA. FK506 as an alternative in cyclosporin-induced hemolytic uremic syndrome in a kidney transplant recipient. Transplant Int 1994;7:382–384.
45. Ellis D, Shapiro R, Jordan ML, et al. Comparison of FK-506 and cyclosporine regimens in pediatric renal transplantation. Pediatr Nephrol 1994;8:193–200.
46. Shapiro R, Scantlebury VP, Jordan M, et al. FK506 in pediatric kidney transplantation—primary and rescue experience. Pediatr Nephrol 1995;9:3–48.
47. Corey HE, Tellis V, Schechner R. Improved renal allograft survival in children treated with FK506 (tacrolimus) rescue therapy. Pediatr Nephrol 1996;10:720–722.
48. Shapiro R, Scantlebury VP, Jordan ML, et al. Tacrolimus in pediatric renal transplantation. Transplantation 1996;62:1752–1758.
49. Sollinger HW, Deierhoi MH, Belzer FO, et al. RS-6143: a phase I clinical trial and pilot rescue study. Transplantation 1992;53:428.
50. The Tricontinental Mycophenolate Mofetil Renal Transplantation Study Group. A blinded, randomized clinical trial of mycophenolate mofetil for the prevention of acute rejection in cadaveric renal transplantation. Transplantation 1996;61(7):1029–1037.
51. European Mycophenolate Mofetil Cooperative Study Group. Placebo-controlled study of mycophenolate mofetil combined with cyclosporin and corticosteroids for prevention of acute rejection. Lancet 1995;345:1321–1325.
52. The U.S. Mycophenolate Mofetil Study Group. Mycophenolate mofetil for the prevention of acute rejection of primary cadaveric kidney transplants: status of the MYC 1866 study at 1 year. Transplant Proc 1997;29:348–349.
53. The Mycophenolate Mofetil Renal Refractory Rejection Study Group. Mycophenolate mofetil for the treatment of refractory, acute, cellular renal transplant rejection. Transplantation 1996;61:722–729.
54. Camardo JS, Scarola JA, Maida BT. Rapamycin (sirolimus, rapamune). Curr Opin Nephrol Hypertens 1995;4:482–487.
55. Sehgal SN. Rapamune (sirolimus, rapamycin): an overview and mechanism of action. J Therap Drug Monitoring 1995;17:660–665.
56. Kahan BD. Is there a rationale to combine cyclosporin and sirolimus? Nephrol Dial Transplant 1996;11:21–23.

57. Murgia MG, Jordan S, Kahan BD. The side effect profile of sirolimus: a phase I study in quiescent cyclosporine—prednisone—treated renal transplant patients. Kidney Int 1996;49:209–216.
58. Kelly PA, Gruber SA, Behbod F, Kahan BD. Sirolimus, a new, potent immunosuppressive agent. Pharmacotherapy 1997;17:1148–1156.
59. Groth CG, Backman L, Morales JM, et al. Sirolimus (rapamycin) based therapy in human renal transplantation: similar efficacy and different toxicity compared with cyclosporin. Transplantation 1999 (in press).
60. Ardehali A, Billingsley A, et al. Experimental cardiac allograft vasculopathy in mice. J Heart Lung Transplant 1993;12:730–735.
61. Gregory CR, Huang X, Pratt RE, et al. Treatment with rapamycin and mycophenolic acid reduces arterial intimal thickening produced by mechanical injury and allows endothelial replacement. Transplant Proc 1991;23(1): 1027–1028.
62. Pirsch JD, Armbrust MJ, Knechtle SJ, et al. Effect of steroid withdrawal on hypertension and cholesterol levels in living related recipients. Transplant Proc 1991;23:1363–1364.
63. Hricik DE, Bartucci MR, Mayers JT, Schulak JA. The effects of steroid withdrawal on the lipoprotein profiles of cyclosporine-treated kidney and kidney-pancreas transplant recipients. Transplantation 1992;54:868–871.
64. Hricik DE, Lautman J, Bartucci MR, et al. Variable effects of steroid withdrawal on blood pressure reduction in cyclopsorine-treated renal transplant recipients. Transplantation 1992;53:1232–1235.
65. Sinclair WRS, for the Canadian Multicentre Study Group. Low-dose steroid therapy in cyclosporine-treated renal transplant recipients with well functioning grafts. Can Med Assoc J 1992;147:645–657.
66. Opelz G. Effect of maintenance immunosuppressive drug regimen on kidney transplant outcome. Transplantation 1994;58:443–446.
67. Disney APS, Russ GR, Walker R, Sheil AGR, eds. Australian and New Zealand Dialysis and Transplant Registry Report 1997:119.
68. Hricik DE, O'Toole MA, Schulak JA, Herson J. Steroid-free immunosuppression in cyclosporine-treated renal transplant recipients: a meta-analysis. J Am Soc Nephrol 1993;4:1300–1305.
69. Ratcliffe P, Dudley CR, Firth JD, et al. Randomised controlled trial of steroid withdrawal in renal transplant recipients receiving triple immunosuppression. Lancet 1996;348:643–648.
70. Szczech LA, Berlin JA, Aradhye S, et al. Effect of anti-lymphocyte induction therapy on renal allograft survival: a meta-analysis. J Am Soc Nephrol 1997;8:1771–1777.
71. Vincenti F, Kirkman R, Light S, et al. Interleukin-2-receptor blockade with Daclizumab to prevent acute rejection in renal transplantation. N Engl J Med 1998;338:161–165.
72. Nashan B, Moore R, Amlot P, et al. Randomised trial of basiliximab versus placebo for control of acute cellular rejection in renal allograft recipients. Lancet 1997;350:1193–1198.
73. Pearson TC, Madsen JC, Larsen CP, et al. Induction of transplantation tolerance in adults using donor antigen and anti-CD4 monoclonal antibody. Transplantation 1992;54(3):475–483.
74. Larsen CP, Elwood ET, Alexander DZ, et al. Long-term acceptance of skin and cardiac allografts after blocking CD40 and CD28 pathways. Nature 1996;381:434–438.
75. Kirk AD, Harlan DM, Armstrong NN, et al. CTLA4-Ig and anti-CD40 ligand prevent renal allograft rejection in primates. Proc Natl Acad Sci USA 1997;94(16):8789–8794.
76. Gray D, Shepherd H, Daar A, et al. Oral versus intravenous high-dose steroid treatment of renal allograft rejection: the big shot or not? Lancet 1978;1:117–118.
77. Von Willebrand E, Hughes D. Fine needle aspiration cytology of the transplanted kidney. In: Morris PJ, ed. Kidney transplantation: principles and practice. 4th ed. Philadelphia: WB Saunders, 1994:301–313.
78. Raine AEG. Cardiovascular complications after renal transplantation. In: Morris PJ, ed. Kidney transplantation: principles and practice. 4th ed. Philadelphia: WB Saunders, 1994:339–355.
79. Curtis JJ, Luke RG, Whelchel JD, et al. Inhibition of angiotensin-converting enzyme in renal-transplant recipients with hypertension. N Engl J Med 1983;308:377–381.
80. Gray DW. Vascular and lymphatic complications after renal transplantation. In: Morris PJ, ed. Kidney transplantation: principles and practice. 4th ed. Philadelphia: WB Saunders, 1994:314–329.
81. Jones RM, Murie JA, Ting A, et al. Renal vascular thrombosis of cadaveric renal allografts in patients receiving cyclosporin, azathioprine and prednisolone triple therapy. Clin Transplant 1988;2:122–126.
82. Vanrenterghem Y, Roels L, Lerut T, et al. Thromboembolic complications and haemostatic changes in cyclosporin-treated cadaveric kidney allograft recipients. Lancet 1985;1:999–1002.
83. Griffiths AB, Fletcher EW, Morris PJ. Lymphocele after renal transplantation. Aust NZJ Surg 1979;49:626–628.
84. Loughlin KR, Tilney NL, Richie JP. Urological complications in 718 renal transplant patients. Surgery 1984;95:297–302.
85. Cranston D. Urological complications after renal transplantation. In: PJ Morris, ed. Kidney transplantation: principles and practice. 4th ed. WB Saunders, 1994:330–338.
86. Kasiski BL. Possible causes and consequences of hypertension in stable renal transplant patients. Transplantation 1987;44:639–643.
87. Vathsala A, Weinberg RB, Schoenberg L, et al. Lipid abnormalities in cyclosporine-prednisolone treated renal transplant recipients. Transplantation 1989;48:37–43.
88. Bittar AE, Ratcliffe PJ, Richardson AJ, et al. The prevalence of hyperlipidaemia in renal transplant recipients: associations with immunosuppressive and antihypertensive therapy. Transplantation 1990;50:987–992.
89. Curtis JJ, Luke RG, Diethelm AG, et al. Benefits of removal of native kidneys in hypertension after renal transplantation. Lancet 1985;2:729–745.
90. Taylor HM, Benjamin IS, Morris PJ. Control of hypertension after renal transplantation by embolisation of host kidneys. Lancet 1984;2:424–427.
91. Rubin RH, Wolfson JS, Cosimi AB, Tolkoff-Rubin NE. Infections in the renal transplant recipient. Am J Med 1981;70:405–411.
92. Warrell MJ, Chinn I, Morris PJ, Tobin JO. The effects of viral infection on renal transplants and their recipients. QJM 1980;49:219–231.
93. Cohen J, Hopkin J, Kurtz J. Infectious complications after renal transplantation. In: Morris PJ, ed. Kidney transplantation: principles and practice. 4th ed. Philadelphia: WB Saunders, 1994:364–389.
94. Pol S, Cavalcanti R, Carnot F, et al. Azathioprine hepatitis in kidney transplant recipients. A predisposing role of chronic viral hepatitis. Transplantation 1996;61:1774–1776.
95. Martin P, Friedman LS. Chronic viral hepatitis and the management of chronic renal failure. Kidney Int 1995;47:1231–1241.
96. Pereira BJG, Wright TL, Schmid CH, Levey AS. A controlled study of hepatitis C transmission by organ transplantation. Lancet 1995;345:484–487.
97. Dantal J, Hourmant M, Cantarovich D, et al. Effect of long-term immunosuppression in kidney-graft recipients on cancer incidence: randomised comparison of two cyclosporin regimens. Lancet 1998;351:623–628.
98. Sheil AGR. Cancer in dialysis and transplant patients. In: PJ Morris, ed. Kidney transplantation: principles and practice. 4th ed. Philadelphia: WB Saunders, 1994:390–400.
99. McGregor JM, Proby CM, Leigh IM. Virus infection and cancer risk in transplant recipients. Trends Microbiol 1996;4:2–3.
100. Cancer report. In: Disney APS, Russ GR, Walker R, Sheil AGR, eds. Australia and New Zealand Dialysis and Transplantation Registry Report 1997:138–146.
101. Julian BA, Benfield M, Quarles LD. Bone loss after organ transplantation. Transplant Rev 1993;7:82–95.
102. Venning VA. Non-malignant skin lesions in renal transplant recipients. In: Morris PJ, ed. Kidney transplantation: principles and practice. 4th ed. Philadelphia: WB Saunders, 1994:401–411.
103. Donaghy M. Neurological complications. In: Morris PJ, ed. Kidney transplantation: principles and practice. 4th ed. Philadelphia: WB Saunders, 1994:357–363.
104. Dunnill MS. Histopathology of renal allograft rejection. In: Morris PJ, ed. Kidney transplantation: principles and practice. 4th ed. Philadelphia: WB Saunders, 1994:266–285.
105. Nelson PW, Landreneau MD, Luger AM, et al. Ten-year experience in transplantation of A2 kidneys into B and O recipients. Transplantation 1998;65:256–260.
106. Williams GM, Hume DM, Hudson RP, et al. Hyperacute renal-homograft rejection in man. N Engl J Med 1968;279:611–618.
107. Bates WD, Davies DR, Welsh K, et al. An evaluation of the Banff classification of early renal allograft biopsies and correlation with outcome. Nephrol Dial Transplant 1998. In press.
108. Solez K. International standardization of nomenclature for the histological diagnosis of renal allograft rejection: the Banff working classification of kidney transplant pathology. Kidney Int 1993;44:411–422.
109. Jordan SC, Quartel AW, Czer LSC, et al. Posttransplant therapy using high-dose human immunoglobulin to control acute humoral rejection in renal and cardiac allograft recipients and potential mechanism of action. Transplantation 1998;66:800–805.
110. Waagu AM, Rocha AM, Tilney N. Early risk factors contributing to evolution of long-term allograft dysfunction. Transplant Rev 1997;11:208–216.
111. Hayry P. Aspects of allograft rejection, 1: molecular pathology of acute and chronic rejection. Transplant Rev 1995;9:113–120.

112. Paul LC. Aspects of allograft rejection, III: clinical assessment of renal allograft rejection. Transplant Rev 1995;9:138–146.
113. McLaren AJ, Fuggle SV, Welsh KI, et al. Chronic allograft failure in human renal transplantation. A multivariate risk factor analysis. (Submitted for publication).
114. Tilney NL. Renal transplantation between identical twins: a review. World J Surg 1986;10:381–388.
115. Kramer P, Broyer M, Brunner FP, et al. Combined report on regular dialysis and transplantation in Europe, XII. Proc Eur Dial Transplant Assoc 1982;19:1.
116. Cecka JM. In: Sickness and health—high success rates of kidney transplants between spouses. Transplant Rev 1996;10:216–224.
117. Belzer FO, Kalayoghi M, Sollinger H. Donor-specific transfusion in living-unrelated renal donor-recipient combination. Transplant Proc 1987;19:1514.
118. Opelz G. Impact of HLA compatibility on survival of kidney transplants from unrelated live donors. Transplantation 1997;64:1473–1475.
119. Land W, Messmer K. The impact of ischemia/reperfusion injury on specific and non-specific early and late chronic events after organ transplantation. Transplant Rev 1996;10:108–127 and 236–253.
120. Friedman EA, Sommer BG. Renal transplantation for diabetic nephropathy. In: Morris PJ, ed. Kidney transplantation: principles and practice. 4th ed. Philadelphia: WB Saunders, 1994:460–477.
121. Pirsch JD, Andrews C, Hricik DE, et al. Pancreas transplantation for diabetes mellitus. Am J Kidney Dis 1996;27:444–450.
122. Koo DH, Welsh KI, Roake JR, et al. Ischemia/reperfusion injury in human kidney transplantation: an immunohistochemical analysis of changes after reperfusion. Am J Pathol 1998;153:557–566.
123. McClaren AJ, Jassem W, Gray DWR, et al. Delayed graft function: risk factors and the relative effects of early function on longterm survival in cadaveric renal transplantation. Clinical Transplantation 1999 (in press).
124. Lagaaij EL, Henneman IPH, Ruigrok M, et al. Effect of one HLA-DR antigen matched and completely HLA-DR mismatched blood transfusions on survival of heart and kidney allografts. N Engl J Med 1989;321:701.
125. Middleton D, Martin J, Douglas J. Transfusion of one HLA-DR antigen matched blood to potential recipients of a renal allograft. Transplantation 1994;58:545.
126. Van der Mast B, Vietor HE, van der Meer-Prins EMW, et al. Modulation of the T cell compartment by blood transfusion. Transplantation 1997;63: 1145–1154.
127. Baudouin V, de Vitry N, Hiesse C, et al. Cytotoxic T lymphocyte changes after HLA-DR match and HLA DR mismatch blood transfusions. Transplantation 1997;63:1155–1160.
128. Young NT, Roelen DL, Iggo N, et al. Effect of one-HLA-haplotype matched and HLA-mismatched blood transfusions on recipient T lymphocyte allorepertoires. Transplantation 1997;63:1160–1165.
129. Opelz G, Vanrenterghem Y, Kirste G, et al. Prospective evaluation of pretransplant blood transfusions in cadaver kidney recipients. Transplantation 1997;63:964–967.
130. Dallman M, Shiho O, Page TH, et al. Peripheral tolerance to alloantigen results from altered regulation of the interleukin 2 pathway. J Exp Med 1991;173:79–97.
131. Bugeon L, Cuturi MC, Hallet MM, et al. Peripheral tolerance of an allograft in adult rats—characterization by low interleukin-2 and interferon-gamma mRNA levels and by strong accumulation of major histocompatibility complex transcripts in the graft. Transplantation 1992;54:219–225.
132. Terasaki PI, Cecka JM, Gjertson DW, et al. A ten-year prediction for kidney transplant survival. In: Terasaki PI, Cecka JM, eds. Clinical transplant 1992. Los Angeles: UCLA Tissue Typing Laboratory, 1993:50.
133. Colon EA, Popkin MK, Matas AJ, Collies AL. Overview of noncompliance in renal transplantation. Transplant Rev 1991;5:175–180.
134. Mitsuishi Y, Cecka JM. Disease effects and associations. In: Terasaki PI, Cecka JM, eds. Clinical transplant 1992. Los Angeles: UCLA Tissue Typing Laboratory, 1993:371.
135. Evans RW. Quality of life assessment and the treatment of end-stage renal disease. Transplant Rev 1990;4:28.
136. Manninen DL, Evans RW, Dugan MK. Work disability, functional limitations and the health status of kidney transplant recipients post transplant. In: Terasaki PI, Cecka JM, eds. Clinical transplant 1992. Los Angeles: UCLA Tissue Typing Laboratory, 1993:193.
137. Bumgardner GL, Matas AJ. Transplantation and pregnancy. Transplant Rev 1992;6:139–162.

Chapter

18

Renal Transplantation in Children: Current Practices

RICHARD N. FINE

The initial impression of renal transplantation as a treatment modality for children afflicted with end-stage renal disease (ESRD) was not overwhelmingly enthusiastic. Riley (1), in an editorial in the *Journal of Pediatrics* in 1962, reflected on his observations of the pioneering efforts in Denver with the concern that "continued growth retardation would lead to the kidney being based in a healthy dwarf." About a decade later in the same journal, Reinhardt (2) questioned the utility of ESRD care "because of the cost to the child of physical and emotional discomfort."

Fortunately, these concerns did not deter the burgeoning use of renal transplantation as an optimal therapeutic modality for ESRD in infants, children, and adolescents. During the past three decades there have been substantial changes in the clinical management of children requiring renal transplantation. The result has been continued improvement in the patient and graft survival rates and significant advances in minimizing the myriad of adverse consequences accompanying renal transplantation in children.

This chapter describes the latest outcome results of renal transplantation and details the issues that currently adversely affect uniform long-term success.

The North American Pediatric Renal Transplant Cooperative Study (NAPRTCS) was initiated in 1987. The goal of NAPRTCS was to enroll at least 80% of the renal transplants performed in North America in infants, children, and adolescents younger than 18 at transplantation. Serial follow-up data were analyzed and published in an annual report (3–6). Special analyses were performed to address questions that could not be answered with existing data in the registry and special studies were initiated to answer questions that required additional information not routinely collected by the registry. As of December 31, 1995, 4715 renal transplants were enrolled in NAPRTCS. Since analysis of this large database provides the most updated cross-sectional information regarding the status of renal transplantation in children, I will rely heavily on the NAPRTCS data to address the current status of renal transplantation in children.

PATIENT AND GRAFT SURVIVAL

In 1993 Stablein and Tejani (7) analyzed the five-year patient and graft survival rates of the initial 2231 children enrolled in NAPRTCS; 47% were recipients of living-related donor (LRD) grafts and 53% were recipients of cadaver donor (CD) grafts. During the five-year period, 42 (4%) LRD and 82 (7%) CD graft recipients died. The five-year patient survival estimate was 97% and 94% for the LRD and CD recipients, respectively.

Tejani et al in 1995 (8) demonstrated steady improvement in the one- and two-year CD graft survival rates for the five-year period 1987 to 1994. For the 1987 cohort, the one- and two-year graft survival rates were 72% and 65%, respectively, and for the 1991 cohort they were 83% and 78%, respectively ($P = 0.02$). Analysis of practice patterns for the 1258 index (first) transplants performed during the five-year period indicated the following changes associated with the improved CD graft survival rates: increased use of T-cell antibody induction; increased use of cyclosporine (CsA); a higher mean daily dose of CsA at 12 months after transplant; the decreased use of random blood transfusions; and the decreased use of younger CD grafts. The percent graft survival rates for LRD and CD grafts from the 1996 NAPRTCS report are shown in Figure 18.1. The risk factors for graft failure are discussed in detail below.

The shortage of available CD kidneys compared to the increasing demand for CD organs has led to the increased use of living-unrelated donors (LURD) in adult recipients. Limited experience with the use of the LURD has been reported in pediatric recipients. Recently Al-Uzri et al (9) have detailed the experience with 35 LURD reported to

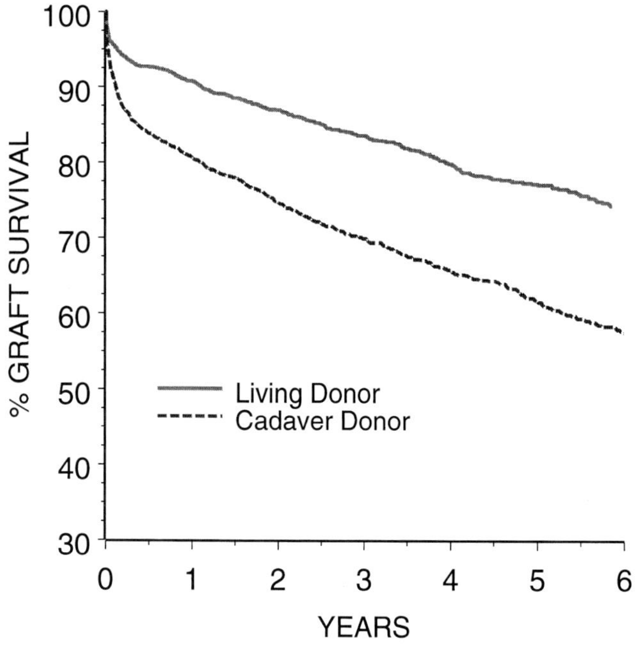

FIGURE 18.1. *Percent graft survival, by allograft source.*

NAPRTCS since 1987. The one- and two-year graft survival rates of 82% and 67%, respectively, for the LURD recipients are inferior to LRD graft survival rates but comparable to the CD graft survival rates performed during the same time period. During the first post-transplant year, the incidence of a first rejection episode was higher in the LURD group (75%) compared to either the LRD (48%) or the CD (63%) group of recipients. Ten grafts failed: one due to vascular thrombosis, two to acute rejection, two to recurrence of disease, one to infection, and four to patient death. The high incidence of graft loss following LURD transplants suggests caution when considering such donor grafts in pediatric recipients. It is possible that patient selection of more clinically compromised patients may have accounted for the inferior outcome of LURD grafts reported.

Preemptive transplantation (PET) has been utilized to avoid clinical deterioration as well as to avoid the need to initiate dialysis in pediatric patients with progressive chronic renal insufficiency (CRI). Fine et al (10) reviewed 2212 primary transplants reported to NAPRTCS between January 1987 and October 1992. Transplantation without prior dialysis was performed in 581 (26.3%). The 1996 annual report of NAPRTCS indicates a current incidence of PET of 24.7% (11). The primary motivation for utilizing renal transplantation as a primary ESRD modality without prior dialysis was found to be the patient's desire to avoid dialysis and the recommendation of the nephrologist/surgeon primarily involved in the child's care.

An LRD graft was utilized twice as often as a CD graft for PET, and the incidence of PET was higher in younger (<6 years of age) recipients. Graft survival rate following PET for either LRD or CD grafts was significantly better compared to recipients receiving prior dialysis. Therefore, PET can be recommended in those potential recipients who want to avoid dialysis and especially in those areas of the world where children have limited access to dialysis facilities but have an available kidney donor.

PATIENT DEATH AFTER TRANSPLANT

In 1994 Tejani et al (12) detailed the 136 patient deaths out of 2457 recipients included in NAPRTCS for an annual mortality rate in pediatric recipients of 24.5 per 1000 patient years. The primary categories of death were infection (40%), cardiovascular disease (21%), hemorrhage (12%), and malignancies (7%). Multiple factors were identified that were associated with an increased risk of patient death. Cadaver donor recipients had a higher mortality rate (6.7%) than LRD recipients (4.0%). Recipient age was a significant factor with mortality rates of 17.5%, 8.0%, 3.6%, and 4.5% in recipients aged 0 to 1, 2 to 5, 6 to 12, and 13 to 17 years, respectively. The combination of young donor and recipient ages was particularly vulnerable.

The underlying renal disease also affected mortality rates, with oxalosis (33%), congenital nephrotic syndrome (15%), pyelonephritis/intestinal nephritis (11.1%), and Denys/Drash syndrome (21.4%) at increased risk. Interestingly, acute tubular necrosis (ATN) and graft failure within the first 30 days after transplant were also identified as being associated with increased patient mortality.

The results of this analysis led to the suggestion that CD grafts should be used with caution in young recipients, especially those aged 0 to 1 year of age, and that assiduous efforts should be made to reduce the incidence of ATN. Kidneys from young donors that are being utilized for young recipients should have as short cold ischemia times as possible in order to limit the occurrence of ATN and early graft failure with their associated risks.

The 1996 report of NAPRTCS confirms the information in the special analysis of Tejani et al (12), with infection remaining the primary cause in the 214 recipient deaths and with younger recipients being more vulnerable. Interestingly, children younger than 2 receiving their index transplant in 1987 through 1993 had a substantial reduction in mortality, with only 1 of 32 in 1992 and 0 of 36 in 1993. Perhaps reduction in the previously identified risk factors from NAPRTCS data has accounted for the reduction in mortality in the youngest recipients. The percent patient survival rates for LRD and CD grafts from the 1996 NAPRTCS report are shown in Figure 18.2.

IMMUNOSUPPRESSION

The use of sequential quadruple immunosuppression has increased over the past decade. Preoperative immunotherapy is utilized currently by 58% of LD recipients (11); however, this frequency has decreased from 71% over the past de-

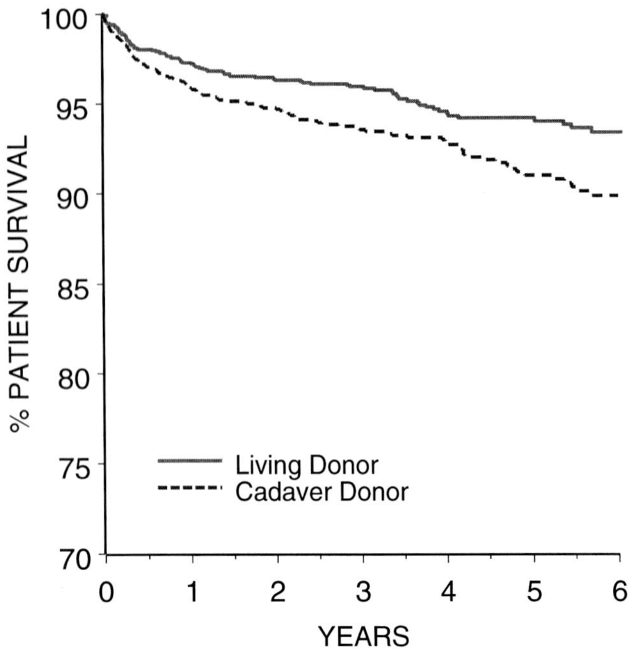

FIGURE 18.2. *Percent patient survival, by allograft source.*

cade (13). During the first 30 days, antilymphocyte globulin/antithymocyte globulin (ALG/ATG) or OKT-3 is used prophylactically until the serum creatinine level is ±2.0 mg/dL, at which time CsA is introduced. Azathioprine and prednisone treatment is initiated in the perioperative period.

The median dose of CsA administered at 30 days is 9.89 mg/kg/day, which is reduced to a median dose of 6.9 mg/kg/day at 6 months with subsequent reduction to a maintenance dose of 5.8 mg/kg/day at 36 months (11).

Harmon and Sullivan (14) reviewed the relationship between CsA dose and graft outcome. They noted that between 6 and 36 months after transplant, recipients who had a first rejection episode or lost their graft had a lower median CsA level than those who did not. Tejani and Sullivan (15) verified that higher maintenance doses of CsA decreased the risk of graft failure in pediatric recipients. They noted that younger recipients were receiving higher doses of CsA and that between 1987 and 1992 the maintenance dose of CsA in both LRD and CD graft recipients increased from 6.4 mg/kg/day to 7.9 mg/kg/day. It appears that dissemination of NAPRTCS data has been effective in altering treatment patterns.

The importance of CsA dosage as reflected by CsA trough levels was recently emphasized by Matas et al (16). The authors demonstrated that the CsA trough level of less than 100 ng/mL was a critical factor for biopsy-proven rejection in pediatric recipients during the first six post-transplant months. In addition, the frequency of CsA administration is increased in pediatric recipients in order to maintain adequate immunosuppression. Because of variable absorption, CsA is usually administered twice daily in pediatric recipients, and in younger recipients it is frequently administered thrice daily (17).

The 1996 NAPRTCS annual report (11) indicates that 43% of the recipients are receiving ATG/ALG in a median initial dose of 15.6 mg/kg/day and 15% are receiving OKT-3 at a median initial dose of 0.11 mg/kg/day as induction therapy. Therefore, 58% of pediatric recipients are currently receiving induction therapy. The incidence of induction therapy is higher for CD than LRD recipients (48% versus 38% with ATG/ALG; 18% versus 11% for OKT-3, respectively). The median initial dose of prednisone is 1.8 mg/kg/day, which is reduced to 0.63 mg/kg/day at 30 days. Gradual reduction continues to a median dose of 0.21 mg/kg/day at 12 months and 0.15 mg/kg/day at 60 months. At four years, 29% of LRD recipients and 23% of CD recipients are receiving alternate-day therapy (ADT) (11). Approximately 88% of the pediatric recipients receive azathioprine at an initial median dose of 2.2 mg/kg/day. At 60 months, the percentage receiving azathioprine is similar, with a median dose of 1.63 mg/kg/day. There is minimal difference in the dosage of azathioprine between LRD and CD recipients. Cyclosporine is initiated on day 1 in LRD recipients and on day 3 in CD recipients at a median initial dose of 8.2 mg/kg/day, which is increased to 9.8 mg/kg/day at 30 days. At 60 months the median dose is 4.6 mg/kg/day. The median dose of CsA is minimally higher in CD recipients.

Three new immunosuppressive drugs have been introduced recently to replace one or more of the drugs in the previously standard regimen. Tacrolimus (FK506) has had limited use in pediatric recipients in lieu of CsA. Shapiro et al (18) reported the use of tacrolimus as primary immunosuppression in 69 pediatric recipients between 1989 and 1995. The mean tacrolimus dose was 0.22 ± 0.14 mg/kg/day and the mean trough tacrolimus level was 9.5 ± 4.8 mg/dL. With 57% of the grafts from CD donors, the four-year overall graft survival rate was 85% with no statistical difference between the outcome of LRD and CD grafts.

In addition to the salutary affect on graft outcome, the use of tacrolimus facilitated discontinuation of prednisone in 73% of the recipients, although it ultimately had to be restarted in 10% of those recipients. The major complications of tacrolimus were new-onset diabetes in 10% (6 of 7 recipients were ultimately weaned off insulin), cytomegalovirus infection in 13%, and post-transplant lymphoproliferative disorder (PTLD) in 10%. The incidence of PTLD decreased in the latter part of the study, and all recipients with PTLD were alive with a functioning graft. Certainly these encouraging data with the use of tacrolimus in pediatric recipients justify a controlled trial in pediatric allograft recipients.

Ettenger et al (19) have reported preliminary data with the use of mycophenolate mofetil (MMF) in lieu of azathioprine in pediatric recipients. Between March 1994 and May 1996, 37 pediatric recipients (16 LRD and 21 CD) received MMF (600 mg/mm^2 twice a day) along with CsA and prednisone. The incidence of clinical acute rejection episodes was 13% and increased to 19% with inclusion of data from routine one-year surveillance biopsies. Only one graft was lost at 5 days consequent to vascular thrombosis. Potentially related infectious complications were cytomegalovirus (CMV) infection in seven patients, bacterial infections in three, urinary tract infection in two, pneumonia in one, oral thrush in two, and herpes stomatitis in two. The most frequent side effects necessitating dosage reduction were neutropenia in three patients and diarrhea/nausea in six.

The increased infection rate especially with CMV indicates a need to increase CMV prophylaxis with MMF. Before MMF is used routinely in pediatric recipients, a controlled trial indicating improved allograft survival rates is required.

Lastly, Ferraris et al (20) have replaced prednisone and/or methylprednisone with deflazacort. Deflazacort was substituted for oral methylprednisone, with 1.5 mg of deflazacort replacing 1.0 mg of methylprednisone. Deflazacort is an oxazoline analogue of prednisone that purportedly has equivalent immunosuppressive potency but reduced side effects. The authors switched 14 pediatric recipients from methylprednisone to deflazacort following at least one year of stable graft function. All recipients received LRD grafts. Growth velocity improved and no patient experienced a rejection episode. The authors also evaluated various immunologic parameters prior to and six months following introduction of deflazacort and found an improvement in the degree of immunosuppression as indicated by changes in the immunologic parameter evaluated. These data are promising and should be verified with appropriate controlled studies.

FACTORS AFFECTING ALLOGRAFT SURVIVAL RATES IN CHILDREN

Donor Age

Harmon et al (21) analyzed the impact of donor age on graft survival in 787 CD renal transplant recipients less than 18 years of age reported to NAPRTCS. The ideal donor was 20 to 25 years of age; increased rates of graft loss were found in both younger and older donors. A neonatal donor had a 2.7-fold increased risk, and a 50-year-old donor a 1.8-fold increased risk, compared to the ideal donor. One-year graft survival rates for donors less than 5 years, 6 to 9 years, 10 to 39 years, and older than 40 years were 62%, 74%, 79%, and 71%, respectively. Analysis of the etiology of graft failure indicated that 10% of the grafts performed from donors younger than 5 years of age resulted from vascular thrombosis, primary nonfunction, and other technical complications. These data led to the decreased preferential utilization of kidneys from young pediatric donors especially for young pediatric recipients. Between 1987 and 1991, 3.2% of CD grafts reported to NAPRTCS were from pediatric donors younger than 2 years of age. Since 1991, only 1% of CD grafts were from pediatric donors of that age group. The latest report of NAPRTCS (11) demonstrates the continued adverse impact of young (<5 years) CD age on graft survival rates at five years (Fig. 18.3). This effect is independent of recipient age.

Because of the shortfall of availability of CD kidneys, there have been continued efforts to maximally utilize kidneys from young pediatric cadaver donors. Recently Bretan et al (22) described their experience with en bloc pediatric kidneys from donors younger than 60 months of age into adult recipients. The graft survival rate at 12 and 24 months was 100% and 85%, respectively. All grafts were said to function immediately and there were no technical losses. All the grafts were primary and were placed in nonsensitized recipients utilizing quadruple immunosuppression with OKT-3 induction. The authors suggest that excellent results with minimal complications can be obtained with young infant donor kidneys if quadruple immunosuppression is used in recipients with decreased immune reactivity.

Since maximal utilization of all potential CD organs is mandatory with the current limited availability, it is likely that further investigative efforts will be undertaken to circumvent the previously identified difficulties with the use of kidneys from young donors for pediatric recipients.

Recipient Age

Young recipients have been identified by NAPRTCS as being at increased risk for graft failure. When comparing four age groups (0 to 1 years, 2 to 5 years, 6 to 12 years,

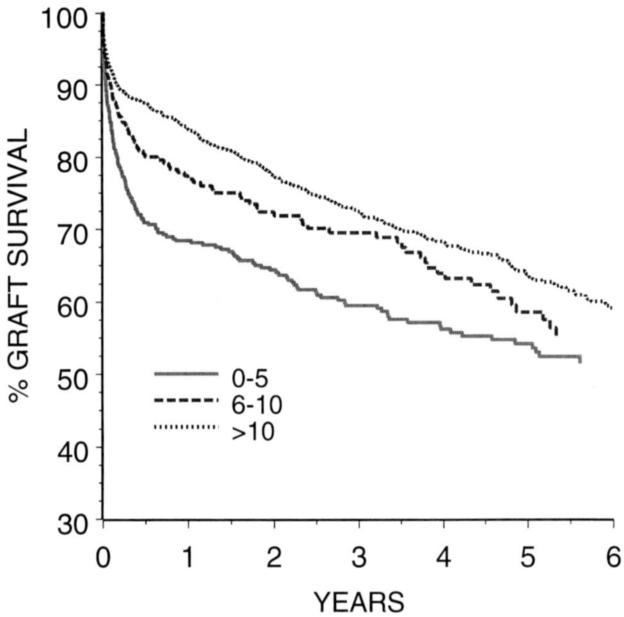

FIGURE 18.3. *Percent graft survival for cadaver donor grafts: donor age.*

and 13 to 20 years), the four-year percent function was similar for the four age groups when an LRD graft was used; however, there was a significant decrease in the 0- to 1-year-old age group (45%) compared to the other three age groups (61% to 68%) when transplanting a CD graft. Such data have led to a recommendation accepted by many that transplantation be deferred until the recipient is at least two years of age with a weight of 10 kg unless an LRD kidney is available.

Primary Diagnosis

Kashtan et al (23) utilized the NAPRTCS database to examine the effect of the primary diagnosis on outcome of renal transplantation in children. In recipients of LRD kidneys, the lowest graft failure rates were associated with cystinosis, familial nephritis, and hemolytic-uremic syndrome (HUS), while the highest failure rates were observed with congenital nephrotic syndrome (CNS) or focal glomerulosclerosis (FGS). In CD graft recipients, the lowest failure rates were associated with glomerulonephritis, congenital/structural diseases, and cystinosis, while recipients with FGS, HUS, and CNS had the highest failure rates. The data from this special analysis suggest that a primary diagnosis of cystinosis has a superior outcome whereas FGS and CNS carry the highest risk of graft failure.

Human Lymphocyte Antigen Matching

McEnery and Stablein (24) in 1992 utilized the NAPRTCS database to address the question "Does human lymphocyte antigen matching improve the outcome in pediatric renal transplants?" Their analysis of four years of registry data concluded that DR matching was associated with improved CD graft outcome. In addition, the analysis demonstrated that no antigen matching clearly had a poorer outcome than those with one or more antigen matches at each loci. An insufficient number of six antigen matches were available for analysis in pediatric recipients to corroborate the beneficial effect noted in adult recipients (25).

Second Transplants

Tejani and Sullivan (26) analyzed 3290 primary and 573 first repeat transplants reported to NAPRTCS between 1987 and 1994. Grafts from LRD accounted for 52% of the primary grafts and only 23% of second transplants. There was a higher percentage of two DR mismatches in the second transplants (40%) compared to primary grafts (27%). The five-year graft survival rates were significantly lower for CD second grafts (47%) compared to primary grafts (62%); however, no significant difference was noted in grafts from LRD. A kidney from a CD less than 6 years of age was the only identified factor predictive of graft failure. These data have contributed to the less than enthusiastic use of CD kidneys from donors younger than 6 years of age into pediatric recipients requiring repeat transplantation.

Induction Therapy

The absence of induction therapy has been identified as a risk factor for the development of acute rejection episodes in pediatric recipients as well as having an adverse impact on graft survival rates. The 1996 report of NAPRTCS (11) revealed a 19.6% failure rate and a 77% four-year graft function rate for recipients of LRD transplants who did *not* receive ATG/ALG or OKT-3 induction therapy compared to 14.2% and 82%, respectively, for those recipients receiving induction therapy (Fig. 18.4). The impact was greater in recipients of CD transplants, with a 36% failure rate and a 60% four-year function rate in those recipients who did *not* receive ATG/ALG or OKT-3 induction therapy compared to 26.8% and 68%, respectively, for those receiving induction therapy (Fig. 18.5). The use of ATG/ALG or OKT-3 as induction therapy did not negatively influence the efficacy of reversing subsequent rejection episodes. For CD recipients, the overall rate of ATN was 19.2%; however, it was slightly increased to 22.4% in those recipients *not* receiving induction therapy.

Therefore, retrospective analysis indicates that the use of induction therapy has a positive impact on graft survival rates in recipients of both LRD and CD grafts, with an apparent greater affect in CD recipients. The use of induction therapy does not adversely affect the subsequent use of ATG/ALG or OKT-3 to treat rejection episodes. Since

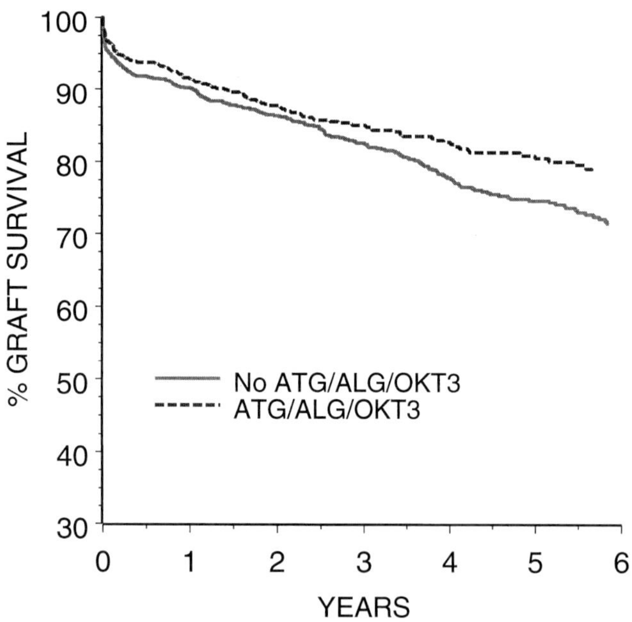

FIGURE 18.4. *Percent graft survival for living donor grafts: early ATG/ALG/OKT-3 therapy.*

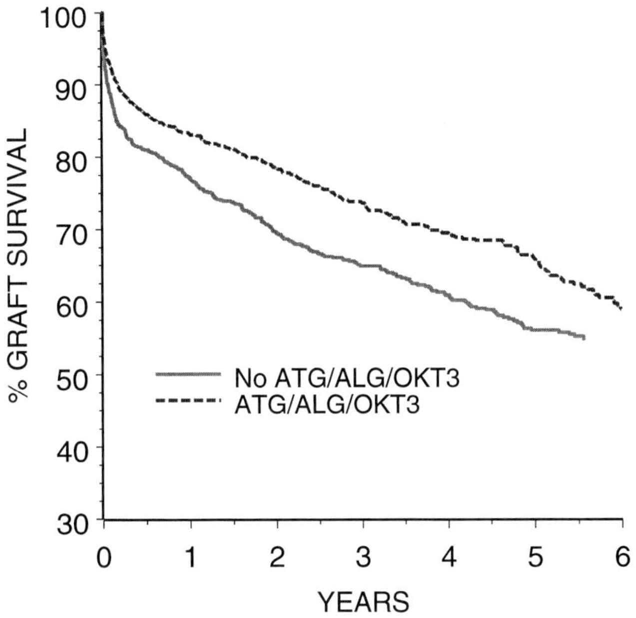

FIGURE 18.5. *Percent graft survival for cadaver donor grafts: early ATG/ALG/OKT-3 therapy.*

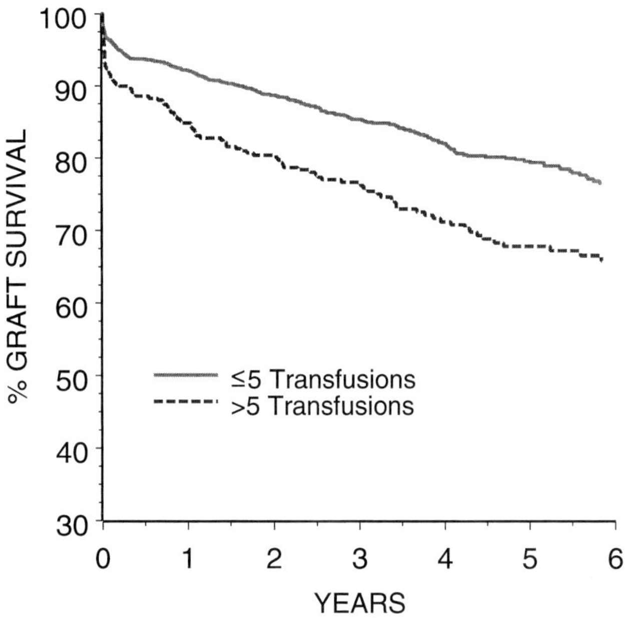

FIGURE 18.6. *Percent graft survival for living donor grafts: transfusion history.*

induction therapy may potentiate infectious complications and the development of de novo malignancy, however, a prospective multicenter controlled study under the auspices of NAPRTCS to definitely determine the efficacy of induction therapy in pediatric recipients is currently in progress.

Pretransplant Blood Transfusion

The availability of recombinant human erythropoietin (rHuEpo) and the improved graft survival rates with the introduction of newer immunosuppressive agents such as CsA in pediatric recipients has led to both a substantial reduction in the therapeutic need for blood transfusions and the elective use of blood transfusions to improve graft outcome. Chavers et al (27) evaluated the impact of pretransplant blood transfusion on graft outcome between 1987 and 1995. Multiple (more than five) pretransplant blood transfusions were a significant risk factor for graft failure in pediatric allograft recipients and should be avoided. However, limited (one to five) pretransplant blood transfusions were associated with a decreased incidence of acute rejection episodes. These data were different from those of adult recipients and suggest that the number of blood transfusions are an important factor in transplant outcome in pediatric recipients.

Current NAPRTCS data (11) indicate that the graft failure and four-year graft function rate are superior in recipients of LRD or CD grafts who received no or one to five pretransplant lifetime transfusions compared to those

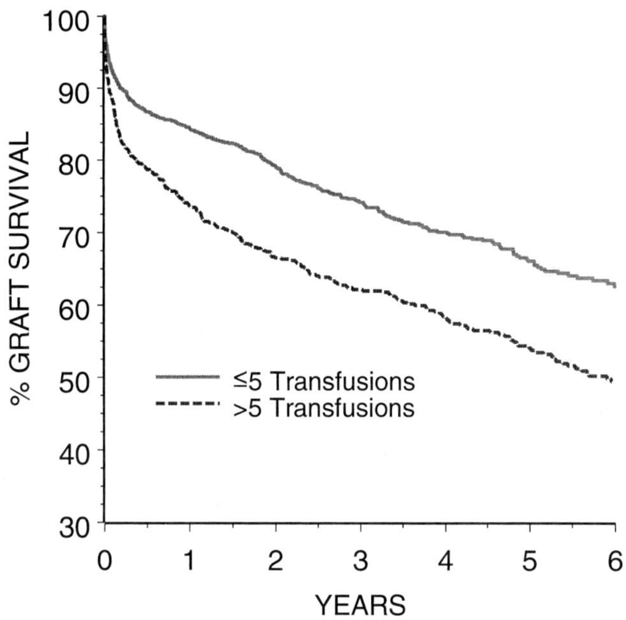

FIGURE 18.7. *Percent graft survival for cadaver donor grafts: transfusion history.*

recipients receiving more than five blood transfusions (Figs. 18.6, 18.7). These data have led to the abandonment of purposeful blood transfusions as a prerequisite for proceeding with renal transplantation in pediatric recipients.

CAUSES OF ALLOGRAFT FAILURE IN CHILDREN

Of the 1170 graft failures reported to NAPRTCS, the most common causes of graft failure were chronic rejection (28.2%), acute rejection (17.9%), vascular thrombosis (12.7%), patient death (10.7%), and recurrence of original disease (6.8%). Tejani et al (28) utilized the NAPRTCS database to determine the clinical correlates of chronic rejection in pediatric renal transplants, as chronic rejection was the most common cause of graft failure. The authors demonstrated that an acute rejection episode, more than two acute rejection episodes, and late (>365 days after transplant) acute rejection episodes were the most common correlates for the development of chronic rejection. Since acute rejection was the most critical element in the genesis of chronic rejection, it is imperative that maximal effort be made to prevent the first rejection episode in pediatric recipients.

Tejani et al (29) analyzed the role of rejection in graft outcome and noted that the index rejection episode more frequently led to graft failure in infants and young children compared to older age groups. This phenomenon probably accounts for acute rejections being the second most common cause of graft failure in the pediatric recipient. Various factors may account for this high incidence of graft failure following an index acute rejection episode.

Infants and young children may have heightened immune response (30) that is inadequately suppressed with current immunosuppressive protocols. Consequently, enhanced dosage with resultant higher immunosuppressive drug blood levels may be indicated to prevent the index rejection episode. Alternately, the failure to reverse the index acute rejection episode may be attributable to a delay in diagnosis because the serum creatinine level is a poor indication of rejection when a large kidney is placed in a small child (31). Other diagnostic indicators such as molecular markers of acute rejection may need to be utilized in infants and young children to indicate the presence of rejection if the diagnosis is to be made before extensive damage to the graft has occurred.

Harmon et al (32) in 1991 utilized the NAPRTCS database to identify vascular thrombosis as an important cause of graft failure in pediatric recipients. Among LRD recipients, vascular thrombosis occurred almost exclusively in recipients less than 6 years of age and had an increased incidence in recipients of preemptive transplants. In CD recipients, vascular thrombosis was not limited to young recipients; however, young donor age and prolonged cold ischemia times were associated with an increased incidence of vascular thrombosis. Identification of young donors and prolonged cold ischemia times as significant risk factors for vascular thrombosis in pediatric CD recipients has contributed to the overall disenchantment with the use of young (<5 years of age) pediatric cadaver donors for transplantation into pediatric (especially young) recipients.

Recurrence of the original native kidney disease in the graft accounts for a substantial number of graft failures in pediatric recipients. The principal disease that recurs in pediatric recipients is focal glomerulosclerosis (FGS). Tejani and Stablein (33) analyzed the outcome of 132 recipients whose original disease was FGS. Twenty-seven (20.5%) of the 132 recipients had biopsy-proven recurrence of FGS. The median time interval to recurrence after transplant was 14 days. Interestingly, the incidence of recurrence was similar in white (23%) and Hispanic (20%) recipients, but was much lower in black recipients (9%). The time from onset of FGS to ESRD was short in those with recurrence (33 versus 52 months). In addition, 18% of CD recipients manifested recurrence compared to 24% in LRD recipients. Fifty percent of the LRD grafts failed as a consequence of recurrence as compared to 25% of the CD recipients.

A special study is currently being undertaken by NAPRTCS to determine the impact of the presence of the recently described permeability factor (34) on the incidence of recurrence following transplantation in patients with FGS. If such a correlation is identified, pretransplant removal of the permeability factor could potentially prevent recurrence.

INFECTIOUS COMPLICATIONS

Varicella/Zoster

Varicella infection following renal transplantation in pediatric recipients can be associated with significant morbidity and occasional mortality. A report (35) spanning the years 1968 to 1979 from the University of Minnesota documented varicella in 19 of 160 recipients. The infection was clinically severe in eight patients, and one patient died from overwhelming varicella. More recently, eight recipients at the Boston Children's Hospital developed varicella, and despite varicella/zoster immunoglobulin and acyclovir therapy, four patients manifested severe disease and two died (36).

Furth et al (37), utilizing the NAPRTCS database, documented varicella infection in 44 of 2320 recipients who enrolled between 1987 and 1994 and who required hospitalization during the first post-transplant year. Recipients in the 6- to 12-year-old age group were at increased risk to develop varicella. When compared to the cohort of 2276 recipients that did not develop varicella, there was no significant difference in the immunosuppressive regimen or number of rejection episodes. Interestingly, graft survival was better in those recipients who developed varicella. No patient lost their graft or died consequent to the varicella infection.

Despite the report of Furth et al (37), the potential for substantial morbidity and possible mortality from overwhelming disease consequent to varicella infection in pediatric recipients does exist. Substantial reduction in the immunosuppressive regimen and administration of varicella/zoster immunoglobulin and acyclovir are advocated with clinical varicella/zoster infection. However, prevention of varicella infection is the optimal approach.

Broyer et al (38) recently reported their experience with varicella vaccination in children with ESRD prior to transplantation. The incidence of varicella was significantly lower (26 of 212, 12%) in those patients who received immunization compared to those recipients who did not and had no history of prior varicella infection (22 of 49, 45%). Clinically the disease was less severe in the immunized recipients, with three deaths among naive recipients and none among the vaccinees. Herpes zoster occurred in 76 of 704 recipients included in the study. The prevalence was 13% in recipients with a history of varicella, 7% in vaccinees, and 38% in naive recipients who developed varicella following transplantation.

Acute rejection episodes occurred in association with varicella in three recipients and with zoster in four recipients; however, neither group had any significant impact of the infection on graft function. These data would argue for a policy that mandates varicella vaccination in naive recipients prior to transplantation. A potential dilemma in the future involves the criteria for a varicella vaccine booster for those recipients who received the vaccine prior to developing ESRD as a primary immunization. The presence of adequate anti-VZ antibody titers prior to transplantation may dictate the appropriate approach in such patients.

Cytomegalovirus Infection

Human cytomegalovirus (CMV) frequently causes opportunistic infection in renal allograft recipients. CMV infection is usually clinically manifest during the initial two to six months after transplant, with multiorgan involvement producing significant morbidity and potential mortality. Graft function may be adversely affected by CMV infection.

Bock et al (39) undertook a special study involving the participating NAPRTCS centers to evaluate the incidence and clinical characteristics of CMV disease in the current immunosuppressive era, and to assess the impact of the various forms of prophylactic therapy on disease outcome. Between 1987 and 1993, 142 of 2517 recipients were identified who required hospitalization for CMV-associated disease during the first 12 months after transplant, for an incidence of 5.6%. The most significant risk factor for hospitalization was receipt of a kidney from a CMV-positive donor.

The prophylactic use of antiviral agents was associated with a decreased risk of major organ involvement during CMV infection, with prophylaxes with enriched anti-CMV IgG significantly reducing the risk of hospitalization associated with CMV infection. Any form of prophylaxis (acyclovir, ganciclovir, pooled IgG, or enriched anti-CMV IgG) was associated with significantly improved three-year graft survival rates. A discouraging observation was the increasing incidence of hospitalization consequent to CMV infection. During 1987 through 1989 the incidence was 4%, whereas from 1990 through 1992 it was 7.7%. The increasing use of anti-T-cell antibody induction therapy was identified as a potential contributor to this increasing incidence.

This study suggested a role for combined enriched anti-CMV IgG and antiviral agent prophylaxis in diminishing the clinical consequences of CMV disease.

Other Immunization

Epidemic influenza infection may produce morbidity in pediatric recipients. Recently, Edvardsson et al (40) evaluated the immunogenicity of the commercially available influenza vaccine in pediatric renal allograft recipients. Influenza vaccination produced equivalent humoral immunity in the transplant recipients compared to normal subjects, and there was no increase in the frequency of acute rejection episodes.

Furth et al (41) assessed the efficacy of pneumococcal vaccine in children with chronic renal insufficiency (CRI), those undergoing dialysis, and in post-transplant recipients. Antibody response was adequate in the majority of the patients in each group compared to published data in normal subjects of similar age. No information was provided regarding the frequency of acute rejection episodes in association with vaccination.

Enke et al (42) have reported that diphtheria and tetanus vaccination can be performed effectively and safely in pediatric recipients.

GROWTH

In 1993, Tejani et al (43) analyzed growth during the first two post-transplant years in 300 recipients entered into NAPRTCS between 1987 and 1990. The mean (±SEM) baseline height z score was −2.41 ± 0.09 and the Δ (change) z score after 2 years was 0.18 ± 0.06 ($P < 0.01$). The Δz score was 1 SD for recipients 0 to 1 years of age and 0.5 SD for recipients 2 to 5 years of age, whereas no improvement was noted during two years in recipients 6 to 17 years of age at transplantation. Renal function had a profound impact of z score, with a −0.17 decrease for every 1 mg/dL increase in the serum creatinine concentration. The special analysis confirmed previous reports from NAPRTCS that increase in growth rate following successful transplantation occurs primarily in recipients younger than 6 years of age.

A further analysis by Tejani and Sullivan (44) in 1993 on 412 recipients with a functioning graft for at least three years indicated a mean height deficit of −2.46 with a Δz score at three years of 0.16 ($P < 0.01$). The age of transplant was again identified as the most important factor contributing to post-transplant growth. Additionally, growth deficit at transplant was identified as a significant factor. The authors concluded that most growth-retarded children over 6 years of age at transplantation are unlikely to exhibit accelerated post-transplant growth.

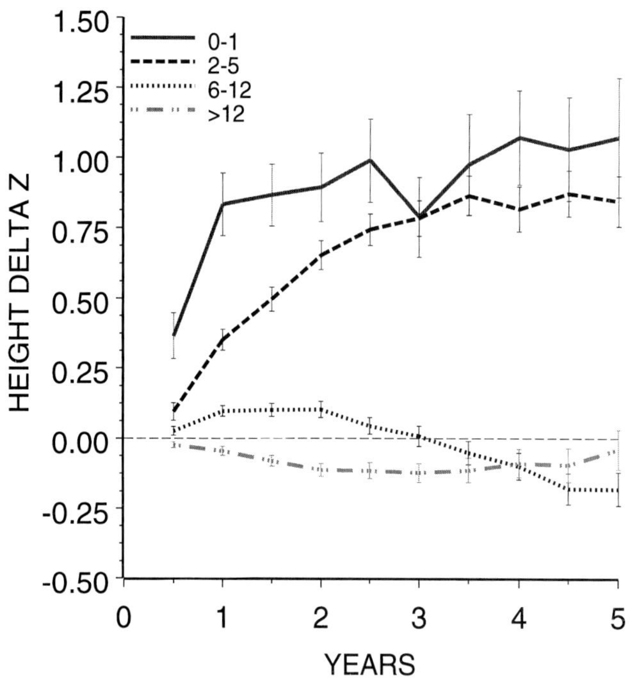

FIGURE 18.8. *Mean change from baseline (with SE) in height standard deviation scores for patients with functioning grafts at each post-transplant time.*

Table 18.1. Mean and SE Height Standard Deviation Scores for Patients with Functioning Grafts at Each Post-transplant Time

	Baseline (n = 4730)		Month 24 (n = 2347)		Month 60 (n = 779)	
	Mean	SE	Mean	SE	Mean	SE
Total	−2.05	0.02	−2.01	0.03	−2.21	0.05
Gender						
Male	−2.13	0.03	−2.08	0.04	−2.23	0.06
Female	−1.94	0.04	−1.90	0.05	−2.18	0.08
Age at transplant						
0–1	−2.57	0.10	−1.93	0.11	−1.69	0.18
2–5	−2.58	0.05	−1.98	0.07	−1.76	0.09
6–12	−2.17	0.04	−2.09	0.04	−2.49	0.06
>12	−1.70	0.04	−1.96	0.06	−2.19	0.11
Prior transplant						
No	−1.94	0.02	−1.90	0.03	−2.13	0.05
Yes	−3.16	0.08	−3.07	0.11	−2.86	0.15

Recently, Tejani et al (45) evaluated growth in 587 recipients with a functioning graft for longer than 54 months and compared the results to the previous studies at two and three years after transplant. Improvement in Δz scores decreased from +0.18 at two years to +0.16 at three years and +0.11 at the end of the 54-month period. Recipient age and magnitude of growth deficit at transplantation were again confirmed as the major factors associated with accelerated growth after transplant. Again, little catch-up growth was observed in recipients older than 6 years of age. The mean change from baseline in height standard deviation scores (SDS) for patients with functioning grafts at each time after transplant as indicated by the 1996 NAPRTCS report are shown in Figure 18.8. The mean height SDS according to gender, age at transplant, and prior transplant at baseline, 24 months, and 60 months as indicated by the NAPRTCS report are shown in Table 18.1. Interestingly, race emerged as a significant factor in this longer-term analysis. Caucasian children had steady improvement in Δz score to +0.18 during the longer period of analysis, whereas African-American and Hispanic children had a deceleration in growth at the end of the longer observation period. The authors suggested that alternative strategies were necessary to improve the quality of life with respect to growth in the majority of pediatric recipients.

A potential alternative strategy is the use of alternate-day steroid dosing. Jabs et al (46) analyzed the impact of alternate-day steroid (ADT) dosing in recipients with a functioning graft for longer than 12 months enrolled in NAPRTCS. The mean change in z score at 24 months was +0.5 ± 0.06 in recipients receiving ADT compared to +0.1 ± 0.03 in recipients receiving daily steroids. Graft survival did not differ on the basis of the steroid dosing pattern, and the decline in graft function did not differ between the daily and ADT groups. The data would indicate improved growth without compromised graft function or survival with use of ADT.

Another potential strategy is the use of recombinant human growth hormone (rhGH) after transplant. Both phase I (47) and phase III (48,49) studies with rhGH in renal allograft recipients have demonstrated consistent improvement in growth velocity. The major concern is the impact of rhGH on allograft function. Specifically, instances of acute rejection in recipients receiving rhGH have been reported as well as accelerated decline of allograft function in recipients manifesting chronic rejection. Despite two controlled studies (48,49), the impact of rhGH on allograft function remains equivocal. Therefore, NAPRTCS is currently undertaking a multicenter study involving 200 pediatric allograft recipients that is designed to address the issue of safety of rhGH after transplant.

NONCOMPLIANCE

Although noncompliance is reported to account for less than 2% of the graft failures reported to NAPRTCS, it is possible that intermittent and permanent discontinuation of immunosuppressive medications contributes to the incidence of chronic rejection as the primary cause of graft failure (11,50). Despite the fact that noncompliance was identified as a significant contributor to decreased graft function and graft loss in pediatric renal allograft recipients almost 20 years ago (51), no specific methodology has yet been developed to identify the at-risk individual or to inter-

cede to prevent the aberrant behavior. Indeed, recidivism has been noted following a subsequent transplant (52) in 50% of recipients who lost an initial graft consequent to noncompliance.

Meyers et al (53) recently detailed their experience from South Africa with noncompliance in 12 of 56 pediatric recipients. The authors identified missing clinic visits; occasional failure to take medications; taking additional medications; failure to know the names of their medications; and decreased knowledge of their disease, their graft function, and their immunosuppressive regimen as risk factors for noncompliance. About 40% of the noncompliant patients were concerned about the side effects of their medications. Although the authors suggest that ongoing education concerning transplantation and consequences is desirable, they conclude that "There are few practical suggestions for improving compliance in children who have had renal transplants."

MALIGNANCY

The 1995 NAPRTCS annual report (54) summarized the 50 malignancies reported to NAPRTCS since its inception in 1987. Twelve of the fifty were reported during 1994. Of the 50 malignancies, 30 were lymphoproliferative malignancies of which 18 were classified as PTLD, 18 were non-lymphoproliferative, and 2 were unknown. In 7 cases, the malignancy occurred in recipients who had received multiple renal allografts. Twenty-three of the 50 recipients have died, 7 within a month of diagnosis. Three malignancies were observed at autopsy and 9 recipients had a functioning graft at the time of death.

Although a detailed analysis of malignancy was not included in the 1996 annual report (11), it was somewhat alarming that 13 additional malignancies were reported during 1995. Critical evaluation of the potential factors contributing to the increased emergence of malignancy in pediatric allograft recipients is warranted. The most likely culprit is the increasing use of newer immunosuppressive agents and the tendency to utilize higher doses of some agents for maintenance immunosuppression. A special study has been undertaken by NAPRTCS to address the factors predictive of malignancy development and is currently being compiled for publication. Hopefully, results of this analysis will pinpoint specific areas requiring modification in order to curtail the increasing development of malignancy in pediatric recipients.

COMMENTARY

Michel Broyer

In this chapter, Richard Fine presents an overview of renal transplantation in children based mainly on data from the North American Pediatric Renal Transplant Cooperative Study (NAPRTCS), and perhaps the title of the chapter should have reflected the source of the data. For example, survival of both patients and grafts among children are often higher in single-center studies than is illustrated by the NAPRTCS data, and perhaps it would have been interesting to cite one or two examples of such data. In his discussion of immunosuppression, Dr. Fine describes the proportion of patients receiving various immunosuppressive drugs and the mean dose of these drugs prescribed in North America.

The NAPRTCS data on induction therapy with an antilymphocyte agent suggest that graft survival is better with induction therapy in both living-related and cadaver transplant in children. However, the statistical significance of these differences is not given and must be marginal, for Dr. Fine suggests that, bearing in mind the risks of antilymphocyte agents in potentiating infectious complications and the development of de novo malignancies, a prospective multicenter controlled study is in progress to examine the overall benefits, or otherwise, of induction therapy in pediatric recipients.

In the section on blood transfusions, the NAPRTCS data suggest that the graft survival was better, both in recipients of living-related transplants and in recipients of cadaver transplants, if they received none or up to five blood transfusions at any time before transplantation compared to graft survival in patients who received more than five blood transfusions. His conclusion that this data have led to the cessation of deliberate blood transfusions in pediatric recipients before transplantation by most centers does not seem entirely rational, and indeed there is no universal consensus for abandoning a limited number of blood transfusions in nontransfused pediatric recipients.

Regarding the discussion about vascular thrombosis in pediatric recipients as an important cause for graft failure mostly occurring in the recipients less than 6 years of age, which admittedly is a generalized observation throughout the world, it is possible that this may be avoided, or certainly its incidence reduced, by the use of low-molecular-weight heparin in those children who are at risk of thrombosis after transplantation.

Recurrence of FSGS was said to be higher in LRD recipients, but is this statistically significant? It might also be noted that some success has been reported by treating a recurrence with immunoabsorption on protein A or with high-dose cyclosporine.

In the section on cytomegalovirus (CMV) infection, it perhaps might have been noted that the availability now of methods of early diagnosis—antigenemia or polymerase chain reaction (PCR)—do allow therapy with ganciclovir to be withheld as routine prophylaxis but commenced when there is early evidence of infection.

In Dr. Fine's discussion on growth, I did not find expressing the mean growth of graft recipients to be particularly useful in describing this phenomenon and

would have been interested in the proportion of patients who underwent catch-up growth in the NAPRTCS data. Furthermore, there is evidence in at least one controlled study to show better growth rate with alternate-day steroids without an increased risk of rejection, as indeed suggested by Dr. Fine. However, the comment that recombinant human growth hormone (rhGH) given after transplant to improve growth velocity may have an impact on allograft function has been challenged by one study showing that rhGH administration was safe in patients who did not develop more than one acute rejection crisis before the onset of treatment for at least one year after transplantation (1).

CHAPTER REFERENCES

1. Riley CM. Thoughts about kidney hemotransplantation in children. J Pediatr 1964;65:797.
2. Reinhart JB. The doctor's dilemma. J Pediatr 1970;77:505–507.
3. Alexander SR, Arbus GS, Butt KMH, et al. The 1989 report of the North American Pediatric Renal Transplant Cooperative Study. Pediatr Nephrol 1990;4:542–553.
4. McEnery PT, Alexander SR, Sullivan K, Tejani A. Renal transplantation in children and adolescents: the 1992 Annual Report of the North American Pediatric Renal Transplant Cooperative Study. Pediatr Nephrol 1993;7:711–720.
5. Avner ED, Chavers B, Sullivan EK, Tejani A. Renal transplantation and chronic dialysis in children and adolescents: the 1993 Annual Report of the North American Pediatric Renal Transplant Cooperative Study. Pediatr Nephrol 1995;9:61–73.
6. Kohaut EC, Tejani A. The 1994 Annual Report of the North American Pediatric Renal Transplant Cooperative Study. Pediatr Nephrol 1996;10:422–434.
7. Stablein DM, Tejani A. Five-year patient and graft survival in North American children: a report of the North American Pediatric Renal Transplant Cooperative Study. Kidney Int 1993;44(suppl 43):S16–S21.
8. Tejani A, Sullivan EK, Fine RN, et al. Steady improvement in renal allograft survival among North American children: a five year appraisal by the North American Pediatric Renal Transplant Cooperative Study. Kidney Int 1995;48:551–553.
9. Al-Uzri A, Sullivan EK, Harmon WE, Fine RN. Living Unrelated Renal Transplantation in Children: a report of the North American Pediatric Renal Transplant Cooperative Study. Presented at the Sixteenth Annual Scientific Meeting American Society of Transplant Physicians, Chicago, May 10–14, 1997.
10. Fine RN, Tejani A, Sullivan EK. Pre-emptive renal transplantation in children: report of the North American Pediatric Renal Transplant Cooperative Study. Clin Transplant 1994;8:474–478.
11. Stablein DM, Sullivan EK. Renal transplantation, dialysis, chronic renal insufficiency: the 1996 Annual Report of the North American Pediatric Renal Transplant Cooperative Study.
12. Tejani A, Sullivan EK, Alexander S, et al. Posttransplant deaths and factors that influence the mortality rate in North American children. Transplantation 1994;57:547–553.
13. Stablein DM. The 1988 Annual Report of the North American Renal Transplant Cooperative Study.
14. Harmon WE, Sullivan EK. Cyclosporine dosing and its relationship to outcome in pediatric renal transplantation. Kidney Int 1993;44(suppl 43):S50–S55.
15. Tejani A, Sullivan EK. Higher maintenance cyclosporine dose decreases the risk of graft failure in North American children: a report of the North American Pediatric Renal Transplant Cooperative Study. J Am Soc Nephrol 1996;7: 550–555.
16. Matas AJ, Gillingham KJ, Chavers BM, et al. The importance of early cyclosporine levels in pediatric kidney transplantation. Clin Transplant 1996;10:482–486.
17. Neiberger R, Weiss R, Gomez M, et al. Elimination kinetics of cyclosporine following oral administration to children with renal transplant. Transplant Proc 1987;19:1525.
18. Shapiro R, Scantlebury VP, Jordan ML, et al. Tacrolimus in pediatric renal transplantation. Transplantation 1996;62:1752–1758.
19. Ettenger R, Cohen A, Nast C, et al. Mycophenolate mofetil as maintenance immunosuppression in pediatric renal transplantation. Transplant Proc 1997;29:340–341.
20. Ferraris JR, Tambutti ML, Redal M, et al. Immunosuppressive activity of deflazacort in pediatric renal transplantation. Transplantation 1996;62:417–420.
21. Harmon WE, Alexander SR, Tejani A, Stablein D. The effect of donor age on graft survival in pediatric cadaver renal transplant recipients—a report of the North American Pediatric Renal Transplant Cooperative Study. Transplantation 1992;54:232–237.
22. Bretan PN, Friese C, Goldstein RB, et al. Immunologic and patient selection strategies for successful utilization of less than 15 kg pediatric donor kidneys—long term experiences with 40 transplants. Transplantation 1997;63:233–237.
23. Kashtan CE, McEnery PT, Tejani A, Stablein DM. Renal allograft survival according to primary diagnosis: a report of the North American Pediatric Renal Transplant Cooperative Study. Pediatr Nephrol 1995;9:679–684.
24. McEnery PT, Stablein DM. Does human lymphocyte antigen matching improve the outcome in pediatric renal transplants? J Am Soc Nephrol 1992;2(suppl 3):S234–S237.
25. Takemoto S, Carnahan E, Terasaki PI. Report on 604 six-antigen-matched transplants. In: Terasaki P, ed. Clinical transplants 1990. Los Angeles: UCLA Tissue Typing Laboratory, 1991:485–495.
26. Tejani A, Sullivan EK. Factors that impact on the outcome of second renal transplants in children. Transplantation 1996;62:606–611.
27. Chavers B, Sullivan K, Tejani A, Harmon W. Pre-transplant (Tx) blood transfusion (BT) and renal allograft outcome: a report of the North American Pediatric Renal Transplant Cooperative Study. Presented at the Fifteenth Annual Scientific Meeting American Society of Transplant Physicians, Dallas, May 26–29, 1996.
28. Tejani A, Cortes L, Stablein D. Clinical correlates of chronic rejection in pediatric renal transplantation. Transplantation 1996;61:1054–1058.
29. Tejani A, Stablein D, Alexander S, et al. Analysis of rejection outcomes and implications—a report of the North American Pediatric Renal Transplant Cooperative Study. Transplantation 1995;59:500–504.
30. Ettenger RB, Blifeld C, Prince H, et al. The pediatric nephrologist's dilemma: growth after renal transplantation and its interaction with age as a possible immunologic variable. J Pediatr 1987;111:1102.
31. Bunchman TE, Fryd DS, Sibley RK, Mauer SM. Manifestations of renal allograft rejection in small children receiving adult kidneys. Pediatr Nephrol 1990;4(3):255–258.
32. Harmon WE, Stablein D, Alexander SR, Tejani A. Graft thrombosis in pediatric renal transplant recipients—a report of the North American Pediatric Renal Transplant Cooperative Study. Transplantation 1991;51:406–412.
33. Tejani A, Stablein DH. Recurrence of focal segmental glomerulosclerois posttransplantation: a special report of the North American Pediatric Renal Transplant Cooperative Study. J Am Soc Nephrol 1992;2:S258–S263.
34. Savin VJ, Sharma R, Sharma M, et al. Circulating factor associated with increased glomerular permeability to albumin in recurrent focal segmental glomerulosclerosis. N Engl J Med 1996;334:878–883.
35. Feldoff CM, Balfour HH, Simmon RL, et al. Varicella in children with renal transplants. J Pediatr 1981;98:25–31.
36. Lynfield R, Herrin JT, Rubin RH. Varicella in pediatric renal transplant recipients. Pediatrics 1992;90:216–220.
37. Furth SL, Neu AM, Sullivan EK, et al. Immunization practices in children with renal disease: a report of the North American Pediatric Renal Transplant Cooperative Study. Pediatr Nephrol 1997;11:443–446.
38. Broyer M, Tete MJ, Guest G, et al. Varicella and zoster in children after kidney transplantation: long-term results of vaccination. Pediatrics 1997;99:35–39.
39. Bock GH, Sullivan EK, Miller D, et al. Cytomegalovirus infections following renal transplantation—effects of antiviral prophylaxis. Pediatr Nephrol 1997;11:665–671.
40. Edvardsson VO, Flynn JT, Deforest A, et al. Effective immunization against influenza in pediatric renal transplant recipients. Clin Transplant 1996;10:556–560.
41. Furth SL, Neu AM, Case B, et al. Pneumococcal polysaccharide vaccine in children with chronic renal disease: a prospective study of antibody response and duration. J Pediatr 1996;128:99–101.
42. Enke BU, Bokenkamp A, Offner G, et al. Response to diphtheria and tetanus booster vaccination in pediatric renal transplant recipients. Transplantation 1997;64:237–241.
43. Tejani A, Fine R, Alexander S, et al. Factors predictive of sustained growth in children after renal transplantation. J Pediatr 1993;122:397–402.
44. Tejani A, Sullivan K. Long-term follow-up of growth in children post-transplantation. Kidney Int 1993;44(suppl 43):S56–S58.
45. Tejani A, Cortes L, Sullivan EK. A longitudinal study of the natural history of growth post-transplantation. Kidney Int 1996;49(suppl 53):S103–S108.

46. Jabs K, Sullivan EK, Avner ED, Harmon WE. Alternate-day steroid dosing improves growth without adverselty affecting graft survival or long-term graft function. Transplantation 1996;61:31–36.
47. Fine RN, Yadin O, Moulten L, et al. Extended recombinant human growth hormone treatment after renal transplantation in children. J Am Soc Nephrol 1992;2(suppl 3):S274–S283.
48. Hokken-Koelega ACS, Stijnen T, deJong MCJW, et al. A placebo-controlled double-blind trial of growth hormone treatment in prepubertal children with renal allografts. Vorden, The Netherlands: Grafitel-Veldwijk, 1994:125–140.
49. Broyer M, Guest G, Crosnier H, et al. A multicenter open randomized controlled study of rhGH therapy in short children after kidney transplantation. J Am Soc Nephrol 1995;6:1075.
50. Cecka JM, Gjertson PW, Terasaki PI. Pediatric renal transplantation: a review of the UNOS data. Pediatr Transplantation 1997;1:55–64.
51. Korsch BM, Fine RN, Negrete VF. Noncompliance in children with renal transplants. Pediatrics 1978;61:872–876.
52. Korsch BM, Negrete VF, Fine RN. Non-compliance with immunosuppressive medications in renal transplants. Arzt und Patient, Jan. 20–23, 1980.
53. Meyers KEC, Thomson PD, Weiland H. Noncompliance in children and adolescents after renal transplantation. Transplantation 1996;62:186–189.
54. Stablein DM, Sullivan EK. The 1995 Annual Report of the North American Pediatric Renal Transplant Cooperative Study.

COMMENTARY REFERENCE

1. Broyer M. Results and side-effects of treating children with growth hormone after kidney transplantation—a preliminary report. Acta Paediatr 1996; 417(suppl):76–79.

Chapter

19

Liver Transplantation

JOHN A. POWELSON A. BENEDICT COSIMI

INTRODUCTION

Despite its remarkable ability for regeneration and healing, the liver can sometimes be irreversibly damaged by chronic disease or by an overwhelming acute illness. In those cases, bleeding, infection, coma, and finally death can be reliably anticipated. Currently, the only lifesaving option is to replace the diseased liver with a healthy human organ. During the three decades since the first successful clinical procedure, liver transplantation has provided a therapeutic option for over 20,000 patients who would have otherwise died from irreversible liver failure (1). The operation has evolved from a risky, experimental procedure, with discouragingly few successes, to the widely accepted therapy of choice for patients with end-stage disease, and is now routinely performed in major hospitals throughout the world.

Because of the numerous perioperative complications encountered during the early development of liver transplantation, the procedure was initially considered only as a last resort that was attempted in patients who were already on life support. Subsequently, clarification of appropriate indications and timing of the transplant, technical refinements, and better immunosuppression (Table 19.1) have improved survival rates, and hepatic replacement has gradually shifted from a heroic salvage operation to the preferred therapeutic option for earlier stages of liver disease. Because of the improvement in long-term survival (Fig. 19.1) and rehabilitation following liver transplantation, the number of candidates for this procedure has rapidly grown. As a result, there may be over a one-year delay from the time the patient is placed on the wait-list to the actual transplantation (Fig. 19.2) (1). Unfortunately, this has led to increasing numbers of candidates dying before a suitable allograft is identified (2). Thus, candidates for hepatic replacement must now be identified and placed on the wait-list at progressively earlier stages of their liver disease. Hepatologists and liver transplant teams, therefore, must now place new emphasis on predicting the rate of progression of various diseases and on accurate timing of potential transplantation, both of which require considerable experience and judgment.

The evolution and development of liver transplantation has also transformed many applications of previously utilized surgical approaches; technical innovations that were originally developed for liver transplantation are now applied to conventional types of liver surgery, such as those for cancer and trauma (3–9). Even more importantly, operative procedures that previously might have been appropriate for patients with early stages of liver disease must now be considered from the perspective that future liver transplantation could be required. For example, because technically feasible but purely palliative operations in the portal area, such as portacaval shunts and complex biliary reconstructions, can limit the success of subsequent transplantation, they should be avoided whenever possible in the potential candidate for liver replacement (10,11). Finally, patients who have previously been considered high-risk candidates for conventional surgery (for instance those with resectable hepatocellular neoplasms but in the presence of significant cirrhosis) may now be offered liver transplantation as a more efficacious approach (12,13). Thus, it has become increasingly important for hepatobiliary surgeons in general to become familiar with the indications for and technical approaches involved with liver transplantation.

HISTORY OF LIVER TRANSPLANTATION

The first reference in the scientific literature to hepatic replacement was by Welch in 1955 (14). Those initial experimental efforts were directed to the transplantation of an extra, or auxiliary, liver into an ectopic site in the abdomen,

Table 19.1. Important Advances in Liver Transplantation

Definition of indications
Appropriate patient selection
Improved timing
New strategies in immunosuppression
CsA, tacrolimus
Monoclonal antibodies
? Rapamycin, mycophenolate mofetil
? Tolerance
Operative refinements
Autotransfusion
Selected use of veno-venous bypass
Organ procurement
Better donor management
UW solution (longer-term preservation)
Retransplantation

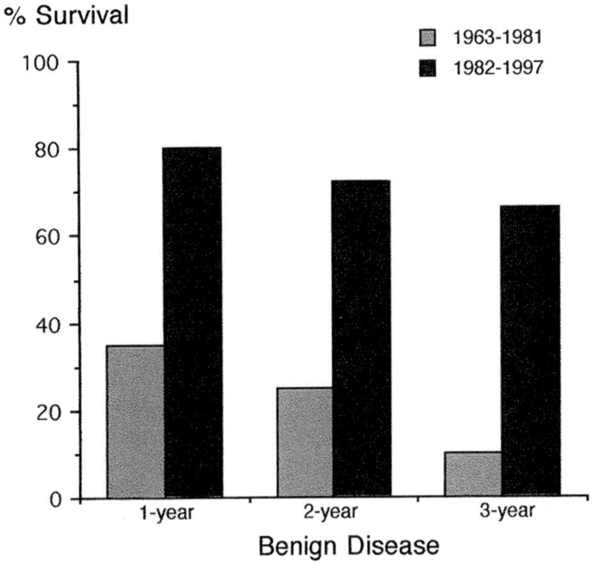

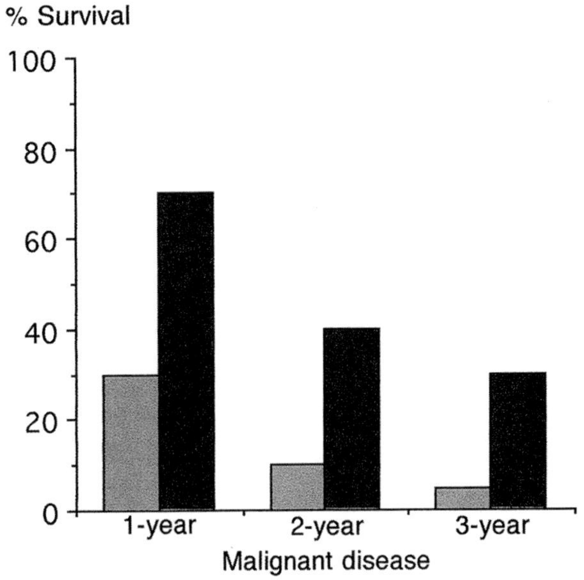

FIGURE 19.1. *Recipient survival following liver transplantation. During its early development, liver transplantation was considered only as a last resort. With current improved survival rates, hepatic replacement has become the preferred therapeutic option for earlier stages of liver disease.*

typically with systemic venous inflow to the portal system. The earliest canine auxiliary allografts were rapidly rejected, making observations beyond a few days impossible. The subsequent more prolonged survival, provided by the introduction of azathioprine immunosuppression, revealed a rapid diminution in the hepatic allograft mass, beginning within two weeks after heterotopic implantation (15). What was missing? The answer came with the definition of hepatotrophic substances, including insulin, in the splanchnic blood (16,17) (see section on auxiliary transplantation). This definition of the requirement for portal inflow to sustain a liver graft provided the impetus for orthotopic liver transplantation.

The techniques of orthotopic liver transplantation were first studied in canine experiments in 1956. Over the next seven years, separate teams led by Moore (18) in Boston and by Starzl (19), first in Chicago and then Denver, independently identified the operation's exacting technical requirements. Based on these extensive studies, the first clinical attempt at liver replacement was undertaken at the University of Colorado in March, 1963 (20). Despite the experience of the operative team, the procedure could not be completed due to massive hemorrhage. Over the next four years, isolated efforts to accomplish this formidable procedure at several institutions worldwide yielded no long-term successes. Ischemic damage and poorly controlled rejection inevitably led to hepatic failure or sepsis. It had become clear that the successful clinical application of the technical skills already available would have to await the development of more effective immunosuppression.

Initial progress in this area occurred in 1966, when antilymphocyte serum (ALS) was added to clinical protocols. Improved results were first reported in renal allograft recipients receiving triple drug therapy including azathioprine, steroids, and ALS. Soon thereafter, in July of 1967, the first human recipient to achieve prolonged survival after hepatectomy and orthotopic liver transplantation was reported from Denver, Colorado. This young patient, who was treated for extensive hepatoma, lived with normal allograft function for more than a year before dying of recurrent cancer (21). Despite such occasional successes and the satisfactory outcomes routinely achieved following kidney transplantation, infectious complications continued to plague liver allograft recipients. An early death rate of at least 70% was encountered. Most centers concluded that the immunosuppressive approaches then available were still too nonselective for successful hepatic replacement: the complex operation was so extensive that recipients were rendered unacceptably vulnerable to infection, even with the use of ALS. More selective immunosuppressive protocols, targeting rejection and not antimicrobial defenses, were required. Over the next 15 years, therefore, a virtual moratorium was imposed on clinical liver transplantation, except for continued efforts by the teams in Colorado and Cambridge, England.

Immunosuppressive agents with greater specificity eventually arrived on the scene. Initially, there was the almost simultaneous clinical introduction of cyclosporine (see Chapter 6) and OKT-3 monoclonal antibody in the early 1980s. This momentous advance, after two decades of disappointments and tragic failures, finally provided the effective balance between therapeutic and toxic effects of immunosuppression that had been needed to demonstrate the clinical feasibility of liver transplantation, which rapidly went from an experimental procedure to one that could be routinely performed with predictable clinical benefits. More recent improvements in the management of rejection, including the addition of tacrolimus (FK506) and mycophenolate mofetil to clinical protocols and the promise of other agents in development (see Chapters 9 through 13), continue to reduce the morbidity faced by all allograft recipients and will undoubtedly further extend the indications for liver replacement. Finally, it is hoped that the ever widening imbalance between the potential candidate pool and the number of available allografts will eventually be addressed by successful approaches to xenogeneic transplantation (see Chapter 40).

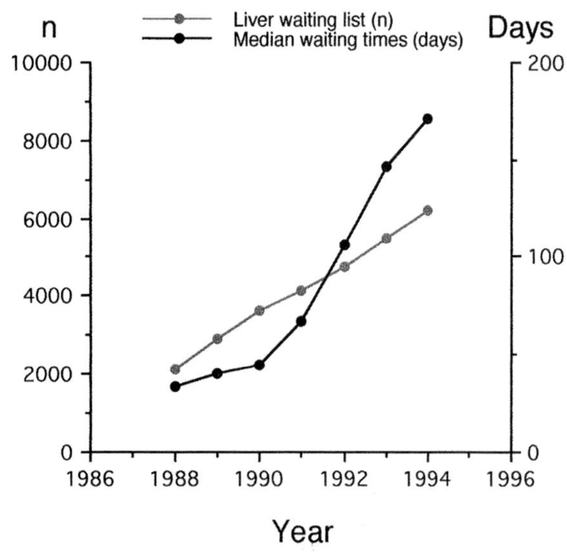

FIGURE 19.2. *Donor organ shortage. The number of patients waiting for a liver transplant is increasing faster than the organ supply. The resultant increased waiting times have led to increasing numbers of candidates dying before a suitable allograft is identified.*

INDICATIONS FOR LIVER TRANSPLANTATION

General Indications

Discernible throughout the indications for liver transplantation are two themes that apply to virtually any patient with progressive, irreversible liver disease (Table 19.2):

1. Liver transplantation is the only currently available treatment for hepatocyte failure. Although complications of liver disease that are not associated with severe hepatocyte dysfunction can often be palliated by conventional surgery, the metabolic and synthetic functions of the hepatocyte itself are far too diverse and complex to be duplicated, even by the most sophisticated current technologies. In patients with cirrhosis, for example, chronic liver disease has caused injury and scarring. If extensive hepatocyte necrosis has also occurred, liver failure (encephalopathy, fatigue, coagulopathy) develops along with the typical complications of portal hypertension (ascites, bleeding varices) (Table 19.3). Liver transplantation is the only effective treatment for such a patient. In contrast, procedures providing portal-systemic venous

Table 19.2. Indications for Liver Transplantation

Chronic advanced cirrhosis
Primarily parenchymal disease
Postnecrotic cirrhosis (viral, drug-related)
Alcoholic cirrhosis
Cystic fibrosis
Autoimmune disease
Primarily cholestatic disease
Biliary atresia
Primary biliary cirrhosis
Sclerosing cholangitis
Cryptogenic cirrhosis
Primarily vascular disease
Budd-Chiari syndrome
Veno-occlusive disease
Acute fulminant hepatic failure
Viral hepatitis
Drug-induced (e.g., halothane, sulphonamides)
Metabolic liver disease (e.g., Wilson's disease, Reyes' syndrome)
Inborn errors of metabolism
Glycogen storage disease
α_1-Antitrypsin deficiency
Wilson's disease
Primary hepatic malignancies
Hepatoma ± cirrhosis
Cholangiocarcinoma
Unusual sarcomas arising within hepatic parenchyma
Retransplantation

Table 19.3. Liver Failure and Portal Hypertension in Cirrhosis

Liver Failure	Portal Hypertension
History	**History**
Fatigue	Upper GI variceal bleeding
Encephalopathy	
Sleep–wake cycle reversal	
Physical exam	**Physical exam**
Jaundice	Ascites
Ecchymosis	Umbilical caput medusa
Tremor, liver flap	Large hemorrhoids
Gynecomastia, spider angioma	Splenomegaly
Testicular atrophy	Petechiae
Shrunken liver	
Laboratory exam	**Laboratory exam**
Coagulopathy	Thrombocytopenia
Hypoalbuminemia	Mild neutropenia
Elevated bilirubin	
Radiologic exam	**Radiologic exam**
CT: Shrunken lobulated liver (a cirrhotic liver may appear normal)	US: Hepatofugal portal flow
	Portal vein thrombosis
	Splenic vein diameter >13 mm

shunting can often effectively treat portal hypertensive complications in patients with adequately preserved hepatocyte function. Thus, the therapeutic plan for patients with portal hypertension must be defined on an individual basis. We have found the algorithm in Figure 19.3 useful in the management of these patients. Primarily parenchymal liver disorders that lead to hepatocyte failure with or without advanced cirrhosis include fulminant hepatic failure, alcoholic cirrhosis, viral hepatitis, metabolic liver diseases, inborn errors of metabolism, and ischemic injury following transplantation.

2. Liver transplantation may also be the best option for some patients with cirrhosis that is primarily cholestatic disease or is associated with an otherwise resectable tumor. In these individuals, the pathologic process in the biliary tree is either too diffuse or too complex to allow biliary drainage by conventional surgery (even though hepatocyte function is relatively preserved), or the hepatic reserve is too compromised to tolerate even partial liver resection. Diseases in this category include biliary atresia, sclerosing cholangitis, primary biliary cirrhosis, cryptogenic cirrhosis, or hepatoma presenting in a patient with cirrhosis from any cause.

These two principles are central in assessing a patient's candidacy for liver transplantation. Early in the course of the patient's disease, the timing of, or even need for, transplantation is typically least clear. Specific features of each disease

Table 19.4. Diagnostic Tests of Cirrhosis

Test	Disease
Blood tests	
Hepatitis B serology	Hepatitis B
Anti-HCV	Hepatitis C
Antimitochondrial antibodies	Primary biliary cirrhosis
Antineutrophil antibodies	Primary sclerosing cholangitis
ANA, DNA binding, smooth muscle antibody	Autoimmune chronic active hepatitis
Iron, binding capacity, ferritin	Hemochromatosis
Alpha1-antitrypsin	α_1-Antitrypsin deficiency
Ceruloplasmin	Wilson's disease
Mean corpuscular volume	Alcoholic liver disease (often >110 fL)
Alpha-fetoprotein	Hepatoma in cirrhosis of any etiology
Hypercoagulability test	Budd-Chiari syndrome
Radiologic tests	
Cholangiography	Cholestatic cirrhosis (e.g., primary biliary cirrhosis, sclerosing cholangitis)
Doppler US, MRI, angiography	Budd-Chiari syndrome

must be considered, including how quickly to expect end-stage liver failure, the likelihood of survival with or without transplantation, and the likelihood of disease recurrence in the allograft. Precise models predicting the clinical course of patients with some liver diseases provide useful measures of the efficacy of transplantation at various time points (22–27). These considerations help to determine when and whether to list a patient for transplantation and are discussed more fully below for the most frequently encountered liver diseases. Cirrhosis, which results from many causes, leads the discussion because it is the common end point for most disorders of the liver.

Cirrhosis

Diagnosis

Cirrhosis is a histopathologic diagnosis describing the end-stage scarring due to a wide variety of liver diseases. Its hallmark is diffuse hepatic fibrosis and nodule formation (28) (Fig. 19.4 and Plate 7). Alcohol abuse and viral hepatitis are the most common causes in the United States and Europe, but cirrhosis can develop following any process that chronically injures the liver. The most important diagnostic test is the liver biopsy, which will confirm the presence of cirrhosis and may suggest the underlying etiology. In addition, the biopsy may reveal ongoing disease activity (indicated by hepatocyte necrosis, inflammatory infiltrates, bile duct proliferation, or cholestasis). Although morphology and prognosis may not correlate completely, such an active process may be medically treatable. In contrast, findings of extensive fibrosis indicate that the process will be unresponsive to medical management. Besides the liver biopsy, other diagnostic tests may be useful (Table 19.4) (28,29). Surprisingly,

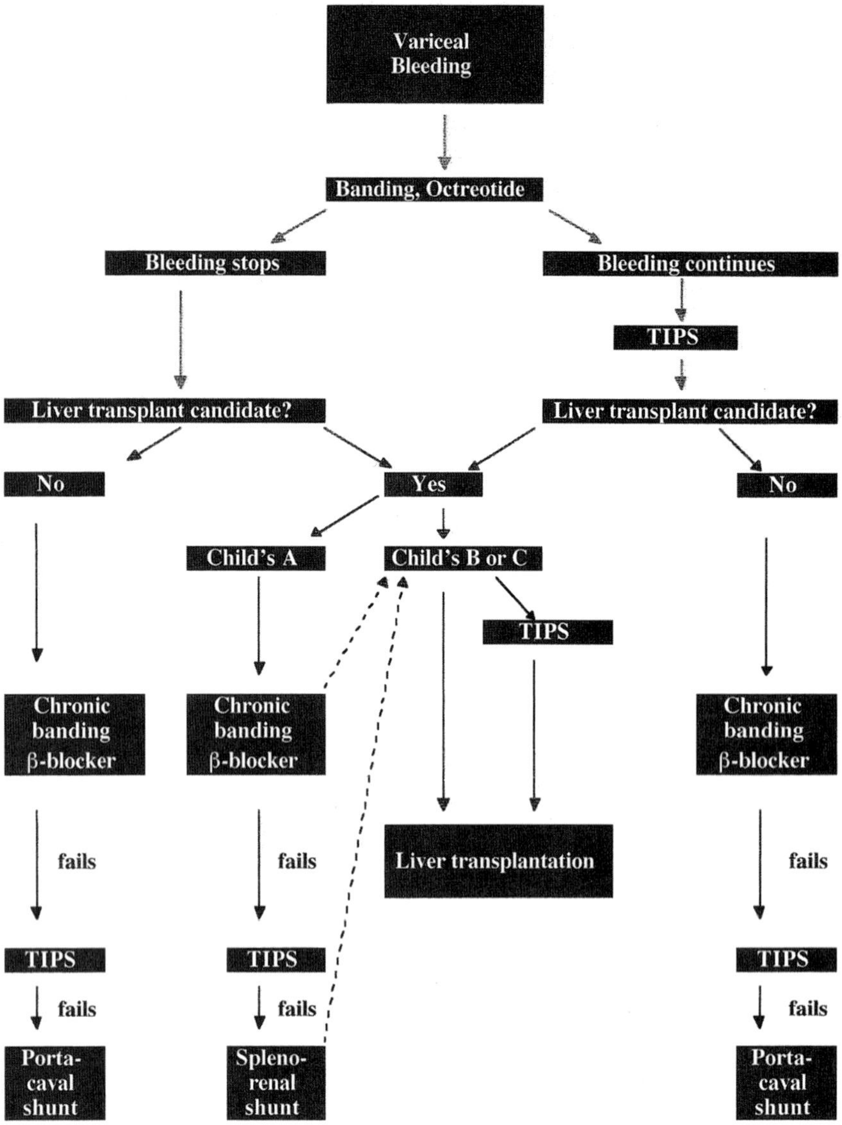

FIGURE 19.3. *Algorithm for the management of portal hypertension in patients with cirrhosis. Portal hypertension (ascites, bleeding varices) with adequately preserved hepatocyte function alone can be treated with systemic portavenous shunting procedures. Liver transplantation is indicated in patients with hepatocyte failure (encephalopathy, fatigue, coagulopathy). The transjugular intrahepatic portasystemic shunt (TIPS) is usually a bridge to transplantation, whereas a surgically constructed shunt is a long-term solution. Since a splenorenal shunt avoids scarring in the portal area, it does not increase the technical difficulty of transplantation. (For CTP classification of hepatocellular function, see Table 19.6.)*

even though bridging fibrosis indicates severe liver injury, the clinical presentation may range from minimal symptoms to incapacitating liver failure. Again, this emphasizes that it is not merely the histopathologic presence of cirrhosis in the biopsy sample that prompts consideration of liver replacement, but the degree of hepatocyte failure.

Hepatocyte Failure in Cirrhosis

Hepatocyte failure occurs when the cirrhotic process has reduced the functional hepatocyte reserve to below that required to maintain the liver's normal synthetic and metabolic functions. For the clinician, the consequences include deranged metabolism, hypoalbuminemia, coagulopathy, and hyperbilirubinemia. For the patient, encephalopathy is usually the most disabling early consequence of liver failure, making driving, working, or even normal sleep patterns impossible (30). As hepatic function progressively deteriorates, encephalopathy typically worsens by stages (Table 19.5) (31), thus helping to define the appropriate time for the transplant. In the earlier stages, a coarse flapping tremor and disturbances in the normal day–night sleep rhythm occur. Although bothersome, these problems alone are usually not severe enough to require immediate transplantation. With further progression, disabling fatigue, periodic amnesia, somnolence, and worsening coagulopathy indicate more advanced liver failure and the need for more urgent liver transplantation. Once hepatic coma develops, the opportunity for optimal treatment has been missed; liver transplantation may still be indicated, but the likelihood of survival is significantly lower in these recipients (Fig. 19.5) (1).

This description of the classic stages of hepatic encephalopathy might suggest that chronic liver failure is predictably incremental and gradual. Why then are clinicians not infrequently faced with a previously stable cirrhotic patient who requires emergency transplantation because of

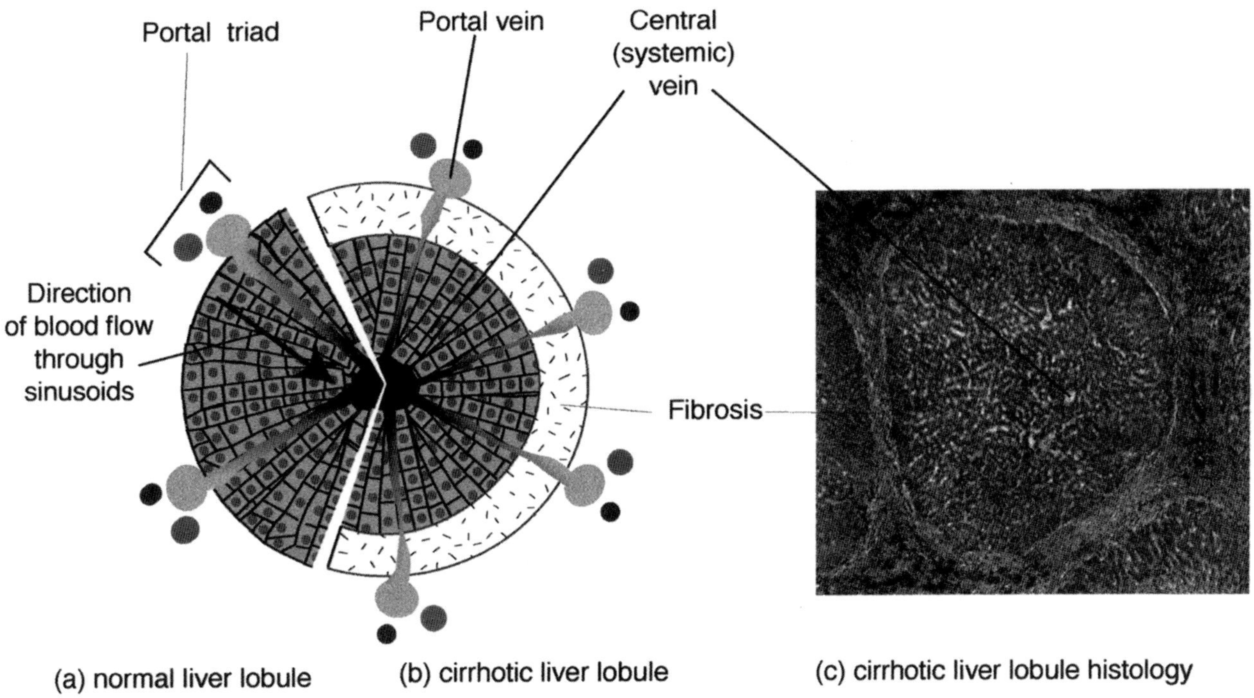

FIGURE 19.4. *Cirrhosis is a histopathologic diagnosis describing the end-stage liver scarring due to a wide variety of liver diseases. Its hallmarks are diffuse hepatic fibrosis and nodule formation. The hepatic fibrosis, by impeding portal venous inflow, results in portal hypertension.*

Table 19.5. Stages of Hepatic Encephalopathy

Stage	Mental Status	Neuromuscular Exam	EEG
I	Mild confusion	Normal	Normal
II	Drowsy but speaking Incontinence Inappropriate	Asterixis Brisk reflexes Increased tone	Generalized slowing
III	Sleeping but arousable Incoherent Confused	Upgoing plantar Clonus Localized or flexion response to pain	Generalized slowing
IV	No response	Sustained clonus Extensor response to pain	Generalized slowing

sudden hepatic decompensation? This circumstance is best explained by considering the liver's central role in response to physiologic stress. Following such challenges as acute trauma, infection, gastrointestinal (GI) bleeding, or surgery, the liver must synthesize crucial proteins, remove toxins from the bloodstream, and provide the energy and metabolic products needed to sustain the entire body. The capacity to satisfy these requirements is available during periods of stress because of the normal liver's functional reserve. Cirrhotic livers, in contrast, may have little reserve. Although the patient may remain stable under ordinary circumstances, there is rapid decompensation when confronted by the increased demands of physiologic stress. Unfortunately, because of their underlying portal hypertension, patients with cirrhosis are particularly susceptible to conditions that may challenge their hepatic reserve. Thus, an episode of variceal bleeding or spontaneously infected ascites may precipitate deepening coma, and even death, before urgent liver transplantation can be accomplished.

Rather than risk the development of such life-threatening complications, the clinician must estimate hepatic reserve by other measures. As a rule, impaired hepatic protein synthesis, indicated by hypoalbuminemia and prolonged prothrombin time, are considered earlier signs of poor hepatic functional reserve, while encephalopathy, as noted above, suggests more advanced liver failure. The Child-Turcotte Pugh classification (Table 19.6), which assesses both neurologic status and synthetic hepatic function, is one useful

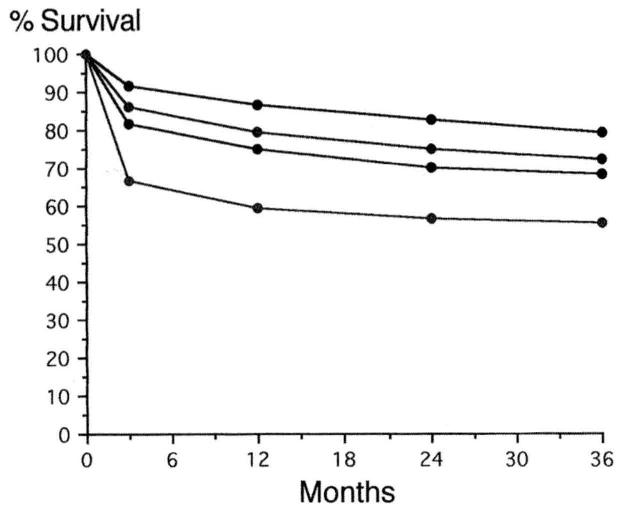

FIGURE 19.5. *Liver transplant recipient survival according to medical status at the time of transplantation (1987 to 1993). The top line represents patients who were not hospitalized (n = 8350); the second line, patients who were hospitalized (n = 3460); the third line, those in intensive care (n = 1585); the bottom line, those on life support (n = 2955). Once terminal stages of liver disease are reached, the opportunity for optimal treatment has been missed; liver transplantation may still be indicated, but the likelihood of survival is significantly lower in these recipients.*

Table 19.6. Child-Turcotte Pugh (CTP) Score to Assess Hepatocellular Function

	Points		
	1	2	3
Albumin (g/dL)	>3.5	2.8–3.5	<2.8
Bilirubin (mg/dL)	<2.0	2.0–3.0	>3.0
Prothrombin (seconds above normal)	<4	4–6	>6
(INR)	<1.7	1.7–2.3	>2.3
Ascites	None	Mild	Moderate
Encephalopathy (grade)	0	I–II	III–IV
Score:	5–6 points	Child's A	
	7–9 points	Child's B	
	9–15 points	Child's C	

Source: Data from Sauerbruch T, Weinzierl M, Kopcke W, Baumgartner G. Prognostic value of Pugh's modification of Child-Turcotte classification in patients with cirrhosis of the liver. Panminerva Med 1992;34(2):65–68; and from Zimmerman H, Reichen J. Assessment of liver function in the surgical patient. In: Blumgart LH, ed. Surgery of the liver and biliary tract. Vol. 2. Edinburgh: Churchill Livingstone, 1994:41.

measure of a patient's degree of hepatocyte failure (23,29). Most class C patients and many class B patients, with complications of portal hypertension such as GI bleeding, are appropriate candidates for immediate liver transplantation, whereas class A patients typically are not.

Portal Hypertension in Cirrhosis

Portal hypertension results in formation of extensive collaterals, including esophageal varices, as alternate channels for return of portal blood to the systemic circulation (Fig. 19.6). Portal hypertension also causes refractory ascites because of the liver and gut engorgement. If high portal pressures persist, varices may rupture, with resultant life-threatening GI hemorrhage (32). Long-term medical efforts to lower portal pressures, for example with nonselective beta-blockers, may reduce the risk of variceal bleeding (33). Not infrequently, however, invasive measures are required to control acute episodes of bleeding. Endoscopic banding is increasingly replacing sclerotherapy as the therapy of choice because it is typically associated with fewer complications. Intravenous octreotide, which decreases portal pressure and collateral flow, has also been found effective in controlling bleeding esophageal varices (34). Combining octreotide with banding or sclerotherapy appears to yield even better results (35). Vasopressin is now used less frequently than in the past because of the ischemic complications associated with its use.

If variceal bleeding recurs despite these measures, three options are typically considered (see Fig. 19.3): a transjugular intrahepatic portasystemic shunt (TIPS) (Fig. 19.7), a surgically constructed portasystemic shunt, or liver transplantation. In Child's C and many Child's B patients with bleeding varices, liver transplantation is more appropriate because it addresses both the hepatocyte failure and the complications of portal hypertension. In many of these individuals, a TIPS is still required to control variceal bleeding during the weeks to months that usually intervene before an appropriate donor organ is identified (36). The TIPS usually controls the variceal bleeding without the need for pretransplant laparotomy and periportal surgery, plus it can be easily removed at transplantation during the native hepatectomy. The TIPS is often an excellent approach for short-term management of intractable ascites as well (37). As with other porta systemic shunts, TIPS may precipitate encephalopathy, but this can generally be controlled with medical measures.

For patients with Class A cirrhosis, liver transplantation is usually not immediately indicated. If these patients develop recurring variceal bleeding, we believe long-term control of portal hypertension is best achieved with a splenorenal shunt (38). This approach avoids dissection and scarring in the portal area that would complicate liver transplantation if it were subsequently required. End-to-side or side-to-side portacaval shunting is generally recommended only for patients with contraindications for transplantation. We have not selected a TIPS procedure for long-term control of portal hypertension because of its reduced patency compared to surgical shunts [currently, TIPS have a 50% one-year patency (39)]. With better stent design and improved patency, it is possible that TIPS could eventually replace the need for most surgically created shunts.

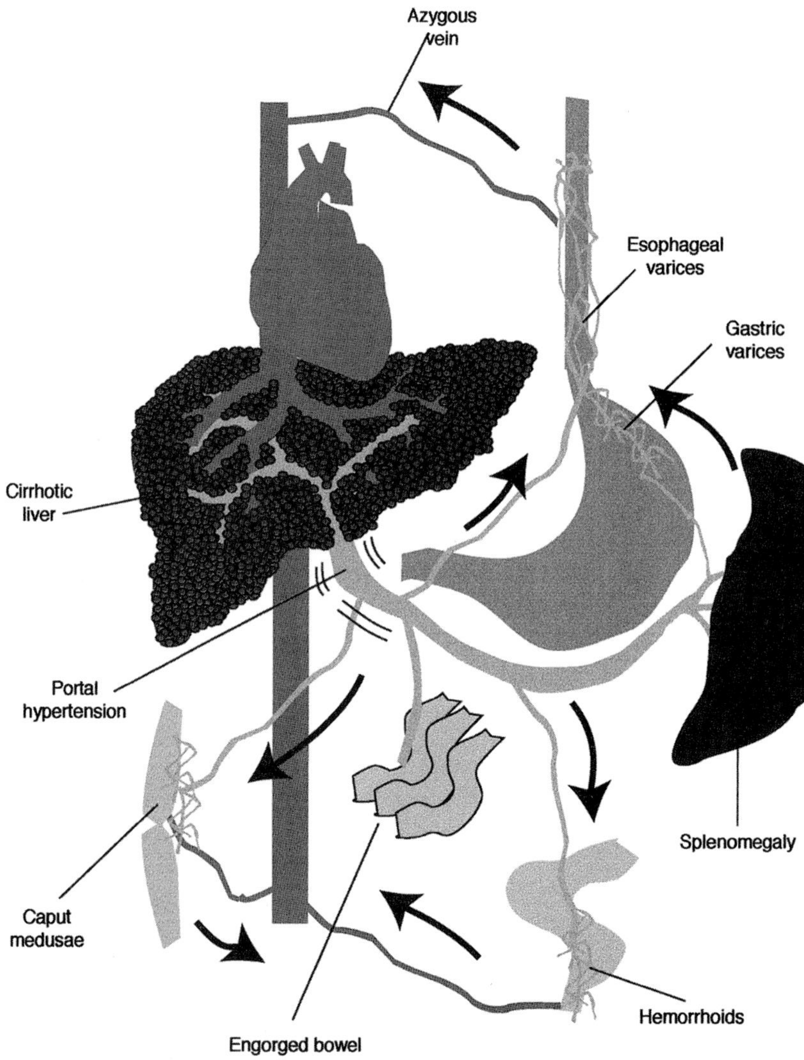

FIGURE 19.6. *Collateral circulation in portal hypertension. Hepatic fibrosis impedes portal venous inflow resulting in elevated portal pressure, which opens collateral veins (esophageal gastric and retroperitoneal varices, anal hemorrhoids, periumbilical caput medusae). Elevated splenic vein pressures produce splenomegaly and associated thrombocytopenia. Elevated splanchnic venous pressures lead to ascites weeping out of peritoneal surfaces.*

Disease-Specific Considerations

Alcoholic Cirrhosis

Alcohol-induced liver injury (Laennec's cirrhosis) is the most common cause of liver failure in North America and Europe (28). Many alcoholics who come to transplantation interestingly have concomitant hepatitis C virus (HCV) infection. A history of amateur tattooing or body piercing is not unusual, but the possible source of the HCV is not apparent in many patients. Because of the association of these two conditions, some have suggested that HCV is an important cofactor for the development of end-stage alcoholic cirrhosis (40). Nevertheless, there are clearly alcoholics who develop end-stage cirrhosis in the absence of HCV. The presence or absence of HCV in the patient with alcoholic cirrhosis does not usually influence the decision regarding the need for transplantation. The risk of HCV reinfection in the allograft does, however, influence the posttransplant course (see below) and is therefore important to the patient's prognosis.

The medical indications for liver transplantation in patients with alcoholic liver disease are similar to those for any cause of cirrhosis. Alcoholics may have other comorbid conditions that would contraindicate transplantation, however, including severe cerebral atrophy and malnutrition. Even more important in these individuals is the assessment of their psychosocial stability and the likelihood of posttransplant noncompliance and recidivism. Consequently, these patients typically undergo more extensive medical, psychosocial, and psychiatric evaluation before liver transplantation (41). Many centers require a measured period of pretransplant abstinence and compliance with a structured alcohol rehabilitation program (42,43). Some recommend signing of an "abstinence contract" as well as random testing of blood alcohol levels during the pretransplant period (44). Unfortunately, even with these measures and extended

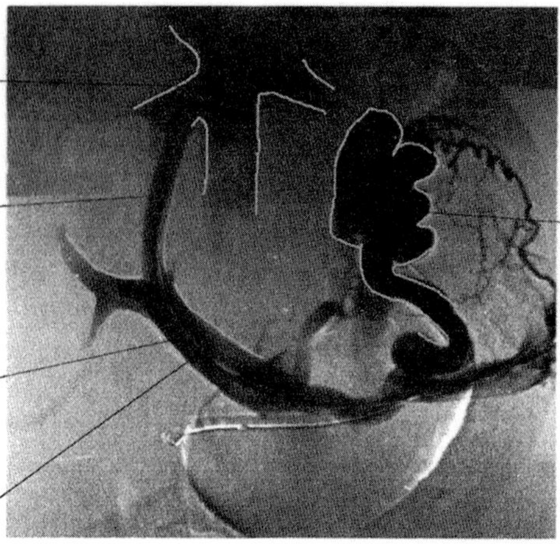

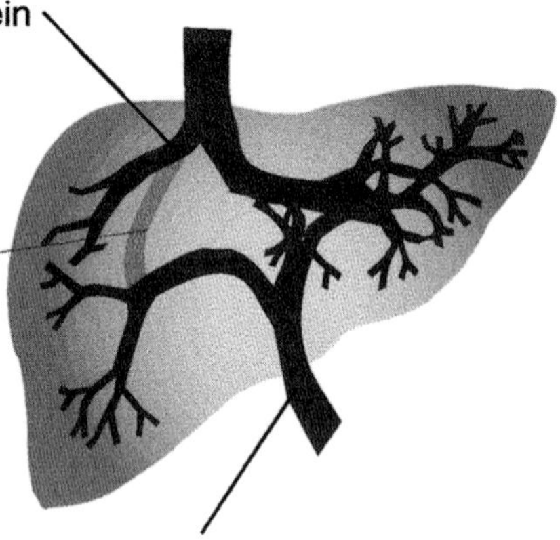

FIGURE 19.7. *Transjugular intrahepatic portasystemic shunt (TIPS). The endoprosthesis is a flexible, self-expanding metal stent connecting the portal and systemic venous systems inside the liver. After the internal jugular vein is accessed percutaneously, a wire is advanced through the right atrium into the hepatic vein. A needle then punctures into the liver parenchyma until blood return indicates penetration of the portal vein. After angiographic verification, the tract between the hepatic and portal veins is dilated and the stent deployed. A stent placed in the liver parenchyma avoids the scarring of a surgical portacaval shunt, and thus does not increase the difficulty of subsequent liver transplantation.*

pretransplant periods of abstinence, post-transplant compliance may not be ensured (45). A previously abstinent alcoholic with a healthy liver allograft may experience a renewed interest in drinking; conversely, an alcoholic who stopped drinking only briefly may find transplantation to be the ultimate sobering experience (45). Accordingly, other measures have been sought to select the most appropriate candidates with Laennec's cirrhosis for transplantation, including the patient's insight into alcoholism, his or her willingness to undergo successful substance abuse therapy, the presence of a supportive family or other associates, and a stable social environment (e.g., not living with an alcoholic spouse or companion). Close post-transplant follow-up and support are also likely to be helpful in maintaining abstinence. Despite all of these efforts, post-transplant recidivism occurs not infrequently (45). Thus, the allocation of such a scarce resource, the allograft, to a patient with a self-inflicted disease and potential for future noncompliance continues to be questioned (46). The basis for the controversy has been founded on both the medical concern regarding the most effective utilization of scarce resources and the moral concern regarding highly costly treatment for consequences of self-inflicted behavior.

Interestingly, despite the significant incidence of alcohol recidivism, most series have not reported that complications of alcohol abuse significantly affect long-term survival rates. With careful pretransplant screening for comorbid conditions and multidisciplinary treatment for substance abuse, transplantation for selected patients with Laennec's cirrhosis has provided results quite comparable to those for other conditions. Thus, a poorly balanced ratio of resource utilization versus benefit has not been apparent in alcoholic transplant recipients. Similarly, the moral objection against committing resources to this specific condition is inconsistent with other widely accepted healthcare policies. These include such practices as treatment for atherosclerotic disease despite continued dietary indiscretion, care for pulmonary disorders despite tobacco abuse, resuscitation following attempted suicide, or care for trauma suffered following substance abuse. Accordingly, most transplant groups have concluded that neither medical nor ethical considerations contraindicate treatment with liver transplantation for at least selected patients with alcoholic cirrhosis. Currently, in fact, Laennec's cirrhosis has become the leading indication for hepatic replacement at many centers.

Hepatitis B

Although the hepatitis B virus (HBV) is known to replicate in hepatocytes, this process itself is apparently not directly damaging to the liver. The host's immune response, however, may cause liver injury and the ensuing clinical illness, presumably as cytotoxic T cells recognize and destroy infected hepatocytes (47). Over 85% of patients recover after a brief illness, and then remain HBV surface antigen free (see Table 19.7 for a description of HBV serologic tests). A small number, however, have such a severe initial response to the virus that hepatocyte function is irreversibly compromised. For these individuals, the only life-saving option is emergent liver transplantation (see section on fulminant hepatic failure). The remaining infected individuals apparently mount an inadequate response to the hepatitis virus, and therefore manifest minimal or no acute illness. These patients remain chronically infected while their immune response to the virus apparently persists and progressively damages the liver. A significant proportion of this group develops either end-stage liver failure or hepatobiliary neoplasia in the cirrhotic liver, and could be considered for liver transplantation.

Table 19.7. Markers of Hepatitis B (HBV) Infection

HBsAg: Hepatitis B surface antigen. A protein on the outer virion coat, and the first detectable marker after HBV infection. *Detectable HBsAg indicates infection, either acute or chronic.*

HBcAg and HBeAg: Hepatitis B core antigen and hepatitis B e antigen. Both are proteins produced by the same genes and become detectable shortly after HBsAg, but HBeAg is secreted into blood and is therefore easily detected, whereas HBcAg is detectable only by histochemical staining. *HBeAg indicates viral replication and the presence of circulating virions.*

HBV DNA: HBV viral DNA. Indicates viral replication and can be detected in serum and in hepatocytes. *HBeAg is a qualitative marker of replication; HBV DNA is a quantitative marker.*

Antibodies (timing of infection)

Anti-HBcAg: The first antibody to appear, usually within two to three weeks of the appearance of HBsAg.

Anti-HBsAg: The antibody to HBsAg emerges after six months and then remains detectable indefinitely, at which time HBsAg becomes undetectable. *There may be a gap between the disappearance of HBsAg and the appearance of anti-HBsAg, during which anti-HBcAg is the only indication of recent infection. However, most cases of isolated anti-HBcAg represent infection in the remote past.*

Anti-HBe: Appears four months after exposure.

Markers of acute versus chronic infection

Acute infection: Typically, the antigens disappear after a few months and the antibodies remain. *Anti-HBsAg protects against reinfection and therefore rules out the presence of chronic infection.*

Chronic infection: HBsAg remains detectable beyond six months. *Chronic infection may exist in two phases:*

1. *Replicative phase:* Detectable HBeAg, HBV DNA, intrahepatic HBcAg, high infectivity, accompanying liver injury.
2. *Nonreplicative phase:* No markers for replication, no intrahepatic HBcAg, low infectivity, minimal liver injury, anti-HBe positive.

Treatment of HBV surface antigen (HBsAg)-positive patients with liver transplantation, like that for Laennec's cirrhosis, has been controversial. Early reports noted a very high incidence of persistent antigenemia in the post-transplant period (48,49) and a rapidly progressive form of cholestatic fibrosis in some allografts (see below) (50,51). With the more recent routine use of long-term HBV immunoglobulin infusions (52–54) and/or nucleoside analogues (55), however, morbidity in these patients has been greatly reduced and many centers now accept these individuals as appropriate candidates for liver replacement.

The evaluation for liver transplantation in the presence of chronic HBV is similar to that for other primarily parenchymal cirrhotic diseases. In contrast to alcoholic liver disease, which may be stabilized and even reversed by abstinence, no effective therapy has traditionally been available for HBV infection. Recent reports do suggest that lamivudine and other nucleoside analogues can effectively inhibit HBV replication in patients both pre- and post-transplantation and that even complete viral suppression may now be possible (55). Thus the number of patients that progress to the need for liver transplantation could be reduced in the future.

Since HBV replicates in extrahepatic sites as well as in hepatocytes, simply removing an infected liver at the time of transplantation will not prevent reinfection of the new liver. Recurrent infection following liver transplantation has been reported in as many as 80% of recipients and depends mainly on the patient's pretransplant infectivity. Not surprisingly, a high level of detectable viral replication (by HBV, DNA, and HBeAg) in the recipient immediately before transplantation is associated with the greatest likelihood of recurrence after transplant (Table 19.8) (54). Conversely, fulminant viral hepatitis, due to a vigorous immune response that destroys both liver and virus, is associated with the lowest likelihood of post-transplant reinfection. Coinfection with the hepatitis D virus also seems to lessen the likelihood of HBV reinfection in the allograft (54,56,57). The reason for this observation is unknown. It has been established that the hepatitis D virus can only replicate in cells infected with HBV (i.e., as a coinfection or superinfection). Nevertheless, recipients infected with both viruses often experience only hepatitis D recurrence in the new liver (58,59). As a result, the post-transplant outcome for patients with chronic hepatitis B and D has proved to be superior to that observed in recipients with chronic HBV alone (see also Chapter 29).

Because of the high likelihood of reinfection following liver transplantation for HBV, some centers continue to exclude these patients from consideration. Particularly disquieting have been the small number of patients that develop a rapidly progressive fibrosing cholestatic disorder

Table 19.8. Recurrence* of Hepatitis B Following Liver Transplantation

Risk of Recurrence by Markers of Hepatitis B Infection Prior to Transplantation		
Hepatitis B cirrhosis (n = 163)	67%	
HBV DNA positive at transplantation	83%	
HBV DNA negative at transplantation	58%	
Hepatitis delta cirrhosis (n = 110)	32%	
Fulminant hepatitis delta (n = 14)	40%	
Fulminant hepatitis B (n = 39)	17%	$P < 0.001$

Lowest recurrence rates occur following fulminant disease and hepatitis delta coinfection.

HBV Recurrence and Survival Following Liver Transplantation	All Patients	Patients with HBV Recurrence
One-year survival	75%	68%
Three-year survival	63%	44%

* HBV recurrence is defined as reappearance of HBV surface antigen in serum.
Source: Data from Samuel D, Muller R, Alexander G, et al. Liver transplantation in European patients with the hepatitis B surface antigen. N Engl J Med 1993;329(25):1842–1847.

Table 19.9. Immune Globulin Prophylaxis in Preventing Post-transplant Recurrence of Hepatitis B

Role of Duration of Prophylaxis in Preventing Recurrence		
No prophylaxis (n = 67)	75% HBV recurrence	
Prophylaxis × 2 months (n = 83)	74%	
Prophylaxis × >6 months (n = 209)	36%	$P < 0.001$

Long-term passive immune prophylaxis is effective in preventing HBV recurrence.

Recurrence Risk at Two Years in Patients Receiving Long-Term Prophylaxis (n = 110)	
Hepatitis B cirrhosis	59%
HBV DNA +ve at transplantation	96%
HBV DNA –ve at transplantation	29%
Hepatitis delta cirrhosis	13%
Fulminant hepatitis B	0%

Long-term passive immune prophylaxis significantly reduced HBV reinfection in patients without evidence of active HBV replication before liver transplantation.

Source: Data from Samuel D, Muller R, Alexander G, et al. Liver transplantation in European patients with the hepatitis B surface antigen. N Engl J Med 1993;329(25):1842–1847; and from Samuel D, Bismuth A, Mathieu D, et al. Passive immunoprophylaxis after liver transplantation in HBsAg-positive patients. Lancet 1991;337(8745):813–815.

(60). Histopathologic examination reveals that allograft hepatocytes are laden with apparently overwhelming quantities of virus, suggesting the infection has flourished without control in the presence of immunosuppression. Retransplantation for this fulminant form of recurrent hepatitis B is associated with a high mortality rate and is probably contraindicated. In most recipients, however, the histopathologic picture of the post-transplant reinfection resembles chronic pretransplant injury and the clinical signs of post-transplant viral hepatitis recurrence are surprisingly benign. Initially reinfection is manifested by asymptomatic HBV antigenemia. The subsequent clinical course is typically complicated by intermittent episodes of low-grade transaminase elevation. Although clinically benign, these episodes are often difficult to interpret, since they can be indistinguishable, even on biopsy, from rejection activity (see below, Post-transplant Viral Hepatitis). The clinical severity of post-transplant disease most likely depends on complex interactions between viral load, subtype of virus [precore mutant being worse (61)], intensity of immunosuppression [lower corticosteroid doses may improve survival (62)], and other unknown factors such as the relationship between allograft and recipient MHC antigens. Despite this complex picture, symptom-free survival rates are only slightly inferior to those achieved for other conditions leading to transplantation (63).

Various forms of therapy have been utilized in the attempt to control recurrent HBV infection following transplantation, but none has proved consistently effective. Interferon-alpha (IFN-α), which leads to a sustained interruption of viral replication in approximately 30% of nontransplant patients (64), has had anecdotal success (65) but generally disappointing results in transplant patients (66). Prostaglandin E may be of benefit, with a response rate in 8 of 12 patients in one series (67). Other agents such as ganciclovir and famciclovir have also been used in small series but with inconclusive results (68).

More recently, HBV immunoglobulin has been administered in the perioperative and postoperative period as passive immunoprophylaxis attempting to reduce both the incidence and severity of reinfection (Table 19.9) (52,54). This experience has shown that immunoglobulin therapy reduces the risk of recurrence to as low as 5% to 30% in those patients at low or intermediate risk of reinfection (patients with acute fulminant hepatitis B, low levels of replicating virus, or hepatitis D coinfection). Some have reported that immunoglobulin therapy fails to affect the risk of reinfection in highly viremic transplant candidates (high DNA levels or HBe antigen positive) (50), although our results in these patients have been more encouraging. Retransplantation for a failing allograft secondary to recurrent hepatitis B has generally led to poor outcomes, but in combination with aggressive immunoprophylaxis to prevent HBV reinfection, it may allow acceptable results (69).

Unfortunately, only long-term anti-HBV immunoglobulin treatment appears effective, and so monthly to bimonthly intravenous infusions are required for indefinite periods. Dosing intervals should be tailored to anti-HBV immunoglobulin titers in the patient's serum. Titers maintained at greater than 500 IU/L for day 0 to day 7 after transplant, greater than 250 IU/L for day 8 to day 90, and greater than 100 IU/L thereafter minimize the risk of HBV recurrence (70). Individualized dosing is particularly important in the first three months following the removal of the infected liver, after which time a steady state of anti-HBV immunoglobulin is reached in most patients, allowing predictable dosing intervals.

Although highly efficacious, the administration of anti-HBV immunoglobulin adds significantly to postoperative costs [in the United States, approximately $10,000 to $15,000 to the immediate perioperative charges and $5000 to $8000 per year for maintenance (70)]. The costs and disadvantages of chronic immunoglobulin therapy have stimulated trials of newer agents such as the nucleoside analogue, lamivudine. In nontransplant patients with hepatitis B, a 12-week course of therapy reduced HBV DNA to undetectable levels in all patients, including those who had not responded to interferon. Moreover, in 19% of patients, HBV DNA did not reappear after stopping therapy (55). Similarly encouraging observations have been made in transplant recipients (71,72), but a significant incidence of viral mutation leading to resistance may limit the long-term efficacy of these agents (73,74). Nevertheless, the availability of lamivudine, ganciclovir (75), and other similar analogues is part of an encouraging wave of new antiviral agents that perhaps, in combination with a brief period of passive immunoprophylaxis, will continue to improve the control of HBV reinfection after transplant (see also Chapter 36).

Hepatitis C

Hepatitis C virus (HCV) is known to be transmitted by occupational exposure to blood, by transfusion of blood products, and by percutaneous contamination from such activity as tattoo placement or intravenous drug use (47). In 40% of patients with HCV, no readily identifiable risk factor can be isolated. Thus, other poorly defined sources, such as sexual or perinatal transmission, may play a role. With the application of serologic and molecular assays for HCV to the blood donor population, the frequency of transfusion-associated transmission has fallen. Nevertheless, the overall prevalence of hepatitis C has remained relatively stable due to increases in other modes of transmission, such as intravenous drug use.

After initial infection with HCV, approximately 50% of patients develop some evidence of chronic disease. Fortunately, the long-term prognosis is relatively benign in the majority of patients, since chronic hepatitis C typically progresses slowly. As noted earlier, the disease progression may be accelerated in patients with other liver disorders, such as Laennec's cirrhosis (40). The indications for liver transplantation in patients with chronically progressive hepatitis C are similar to those cited for other conditions leading to cirrhosis. Survival rates following liver transplantation are also similar to those achieved for these other conditions. In many units, including our own, this is currently the leading indication for liver transplantation.

As with HBV, the post-transplant course in many patients with HCV is complicated by reinfection of the allograft. Unfortunately, as detailed below, no consistently effective medical therapy for recurrent hepatitis C has yet been identified. Anti-hepatitis C is detectable by enzyme immunoassay in over 90% of patients with chronic hepatitis C (47). After transplant, these assays are less reliable and reinfection rates varying between 40% and 60% have been reported (76). The more sensitive viral RNA assays reveal reinfection of the new liver to be nearly universal (77). Most of these recipients will develop histologic evidence of liver disease, and some may even develop a pattern of progressive centrilobular ballooning, bridging fibrosis, and cholestasis, similar to the fibrosing cholestasis seen in transplant recipients with recurrent hepatitis B (78). Some groups have noted that recurrent disease is more common in patients infected with the HCV genotype 1b (79) and following multiple episodes of rejection (80). The immunosuppressive agent administered may also influence the expression of disease. For example, we have observed a higher incidence of post-transplant cirrhosis in patients treated with tacrolimus (31.8%) compared to those treated with cyclosporine (8.9%) (81). Other series, however, have not confirmed such a correlation (82).

Recurrence of hepatitis is heralded by a transaminase elevation (83), which could also indicate rejection or ischemia. Serial biopsies are typically required to differentiate these conditions (see below, Post-transplant Viral Hepatitis) (84). Some groups have suggested the definitive diagnosis can be noninvasively established by polymerase chain reaction (PCR) analysis of RNA (76). However, this test may be too sensitive to differentiate between nonconsequential HCV reinfection and clinically significant hepatitis. Others have suggested that clinically relevant recurrent disease may be best correlated with viral RNA peaks detected on serial PCR analyses (85). Such an approach remains a research tool that may not be generally available; however, we have attempted to establish the diagnosis on the basis of fluctuating, usually low-grade, transaminase elevations associated with mild symptoms of fatigue and histopathologic findings consistent with hepatitis in serial biopsies. The distinction between rejection and recurrent hepatitis, however, is not infrequently unclear, and it is not unusual for these individuals to receive intermittent empiric trials of intensified immunosuppression. Their management, therefore, is often more difficult than that required for patients with hepatitis B.

Therapy for recurrent hepatitis has typically included IFN-α, which has been noted to have an antiviral effect in some patients without a transplant (64). In post-transplant patients, administration of IFN-α will sometimes lead to biochemical improvement or even normalization of liver function (86). Approximately 40% to 60% of these responders, however, will have biochemically detected dysfunction when interferon is stopped. We usually recommend interferon therapy if the transaminase elevation exceeds three times normal and continue a course of 3–5 × 10^6 units three times a week for six months before stopping. If transaminase elevation recurs, therapy is resumed for an indefinite duration. We have observed a trend toward better survival in those patients treated with interferon, but larger sample sizes of randomly treated patients would be required to clearly establish such efficacy. Other groups have reported no efficacy from interferon therapy, and some have warned that the agent's upregulation of the immune system could even precipitate rejection (87). We have not encountered significant complications of rejection during interferon therapy, but this remains a valid theoretical concern.

More recently, the antiviral ribavirin has been evaluated in several series with encouraging results (88,89). Although this agent fails to provide complete viral clearance it appears to be superior to interferon in reducing lobular inflammation. Thus, combination therapy with both agents is now recommended for patients with recurrent HCV following transplantation. Occasional transplant recipients with recurrent disease that progressed to end-stage cirrhosis have been treated with retransplantation (76). Long-term survival in this group has been extremely poor.

Primary Biliary Cirrhosis

Primary biliary cirrhosis (PBC) is a cholestatic disorder characterized by an inflammatory infiltrate in portal tracts that gradually destroys bile ducts (90). The resultant cholestasis leads to symptoms of fatigue, pruritus, and jaundice. In addition, metabolic bone disease may occur, either because of inhibition of bone formation or because of vitamin D malabsorption. As persistent destruction of intrahepatic bile ducts progresses to cirrhosis, symptoms of advanced liver disease, manifested by hyperbilirubinemia and intractable itching in the presence of relatively preserved synthetic function, gradually emerge. Although the etiology of PBC is unknown, an autoimmune process is suggested by the frequent coexistence of other disorders such as thyroiditis or scleroderma (91).

The diagnosis of PBC is established by clinical presentation, positive assays for serum antimitochondrial antibodies, liver biopsy, and the absence of extrahepatic biliary obstruction (Table 19.10). There is no specific treatment, although anti-inflammatory and immunosuppressive agents such as methotrexate alone (92) or in combination with colchicine and ursodiol (93) may sometimes be beneficial. Ursodiol alone can provide symptomatic relief (94) and improved survival (95). Liver transplantation in these individuals is usually required for the intractable symptoms or, more rarely, end-stage cirrhosis. Liver transplantation is extremely effective therapy for the intolerable pruritus, which disappears a few days after surgery (96). Fatigue also disappears after the usual convalescence, and the relentlessly progressive osteodystrophy these recipients had often manifested during the pretransplant period is stabilized and gradually reversed over a period of months. End-stage cirrhosis with the same complications observed in other cirrhotic diseases (e.g., portal hypertension and hepatocellular carcinoma) may also develop in patients with PBC. Prognostic models (97,98),

Table 19.10. Primary Biliary Cirrhosis Versus Sclerosing Cholangitis

	Primary Biliary Cirrhosis	Sclerosing Cholangitis
Site	Intrahepatic portal tracts	Intra- and extrahepatic bile ducts
Symptoms	Pruritus Fatigue Hepatic osteodystrophy	Pruritus Fatigue Hepatic osteodystrophy
Immunoserology	Antimitochondrial antibody (high titer)	Positive polymorph binding test
Cholangiogram	No large duct obstruction No bile duct strictures	Multiple bile duct strictures (beaded bile ducts)
Biopsy (similar in both)	Inflammation progressing to fibrosis	Inflammation progressing to fibrosis Periductal fibrosis ("onion skin")
Associated disease	CRST syndrome Scleroderma Keratoconjunctivitis sicca Inflammatory arthritis Thyroid disease Renal tubular acidosis	Inflammatory bowel disease Cholangiocarcinoma
Biliary anastomosis at transplantation	Choledochocholedochostomy	Roux-en-Y choledochoenterostomy

CRST = calcinosis, Raynaud's phenomenon, sclerodactyly, and telangiectasia.

which include variables such as age, bilirubin level, and presence of cirrhosis, have been devised to more accurately predict patient survival in PBC and are helpful in timing transplantation (99).

In contrast to sclerosing cholangitis, the other major cholestatic disorder presenting in adults, PBC does not affect the extrahepatic biliary tree. Reconstruction of the hepatobiliary tree by choledochocholedochostomy is therefore possible at the time of transplantation. Because of the typically maintained synthetic function and absence of severe portal hypertension in many patients with PBC, their post-transplant recovery is usually less complicated than that experienced by other recipients and reports of one-year survival rates as high as 90% are not unusual. Histologic evidence of recurrent disease (disappearing bile ducts) is difficult to distinguish from chronic rejection but has been suggested in a small number of patients (100).

Sclerosing Cholangitis

Sclerosing cholangitis is also a primarily cholestatic disorder characterized by chronic biliary inflammation that produces diffuse biliary strictures with segmental obliteration (90). Such lesions may, in rare instances, result from prior biliary surgery, recurrent biliary stones, or hepatic artery infusion chemotherapy; however, primary sclerosing cholangitis is the most common underlying disorder that brings patients to transplantation. Like PBC, primary sclerosing cholangitis is usually associated with symptoms and complications of cholestatic disease including pruritus and hepatic osteodystrophy, although either disease can eventually lead to cirrhosis and hepatocellular failure. Indications for transplantation are similar for both diseases and must take into consideration the patient's immediate quality of life during earlier stages as well as the ultimate threat to life by more advanced liver disease (99). Several differences between the two diseases deserve emphasis (see Table 19.10):

- Primary biliary cirrhosis affects only intrahepatic bile ducts whereas sclerosing cholangitis usually involves both intrahepatic and extrahepatic ducts (90). A Roux-en-Y choledochojejunostomy should therefore be used for biliary reconstruction in primary sclerosing cholangitis, in contrast to the choledochocholedochostomy reconstruction typically preferred in PBC.
- Cholangiocarcinoma frequently occurs in association with primary sclerosing cholangitis (101). Unfortunately, it is often difficult to distinguish carcinoma from benign stricturing using routine radiologic studies, surveillance cytologies, or even biopsies. Because of this, most centers recommend resection of the common bile duct and reconstruction by choledochojejunostomy even for patients without obvious extrahepatic stricture at the time of hepatectomy.
- Bile duct strictures are an essential feature for primary sclerosing cholangitis, but not PBC (90). Thus, in sclerosing cholangitis, the cholangiogram shows a diagnostic beaded appearance.
- Over 50% of patients with primary sclerosing cholangitis have concomitant inflammatory bowel disease (102). Surveillance colonoscopy should be performed before transplantation to rule out occult colonic carcinoma and performed yearly after transplant. Most patients will experience improvement in their bowel disease after transplant, possibly because of the immunosuppression required to maintain the allograft.
- Bile duct strictures and resultant bile stasis can cause recurrent episodes of bacterial cholangitis in patients with primary sclerosing cholangitis, especially if prior surgical attempts at biliary reconstruction have been undertaken. Thus, hepatic replacement rather than conventional surgical approaches should be considered for these patients even if advanced liver disease is not present.

Autoimmune Chronic Active Hepatitis

Autoimmune chronic active hepatitis is an inflammatory liver disorder that may progress to hepatocellular necrosis and ultimately fibrosis and liver failure. Its etiology is unclear, but patients typically have circulating antinuclear, DNA-binding, and smooth muscle autoantibodies that are diagnostic markers and suggest a disorder of immune regulation (28). The clinical and biochemical manifestations are often improved by immunosuppressive therapy (103,104), but progression to cirrhosis is observed in a significant proportion of patients. Once cirrhosis is present, the usual indications discussed above lead to the need for liver transplantation (105). Autoimmune chronic active hepatitis is not thought to recur in the allograft, although rare case reports suggest that exceptions may exist.

Hepatocellular Carcinoma

As many as 60% to 90% of primary hepatocellular carcinomas occur in patients with cirrhosis, presumably because the ongoing process of chronic liver injury and repair promotes mutagenesis (106). Thus, newly identified neoplastic lesions are not infrequently detected in patients being serially monitored as part of their management for cirrhosis from any cause. This complication is particularly widespread in Asia and Africa, where chronic HBV and HCV infection are prevalent. The remainder of primary hepatomas, presenting in noncirrhotic livers, are usually not detected, because of their asymptomatic early stages, until bulky disease has developed. At this point, the neoplastic process is often bilobar or involves central structures, making resection for cure possible in only 20% to 30% of these patients. Despite application of other palliative measures, including chemoembolization, cryoablation, or alcohol injection, the median survival for the remaining individuals is only six to eight months. In patients with cirrhosis, the lesions are usually detected much earlier, but the underlying cirrhosis often contraindicates any surgical approach other than a very limited resection.

Since neither of these patient populations can be managed by conventional surgical approaches, they would both appear to be ideal candidates for total hepatectomy and transplantation. Indeed, the presence of a cancer in a cirrhotic liver does not add any particular difficulty to the transplant operation. Consequently, short-term survival in these recipients is often excellent. Unfortunately, long-term survival has been poor due to cancer recurrence. Even patients with no detectable extrahepatic disease at the time of total hepatectomy have had a high risk of recurrence following transplantation. Various disease state characteristics, such as tumor size, number of nodules, and vascular invasion, have been identified as important prognostic variables. Thus, a five-year survival of 68% has been reported for liver transplant recipients whose tumors were less than 5 cm, in contrast to a survival rate of only 25% for patients with tumors greater than 5 cm in diameter (107).

Not unexpectedly, neoplastic disease with more aggressive features is more likely to be associated with occult extrahepatic metastases that progress, sometimes explosively, despite complete removal of the intrahepatic disease (108). It is of interest that the initial site of recurrence of hepatocellular carcinoma following transplantation is not infrequently in the allograft itself. This may indicate that malignant cells are shed into the circulation during the native hepatectomy, after which they preferentially localize in the new liver, or that occult extrahepatic foci metastasize and grow more rapidly in the allograft.

Neoadjuvant therapy could theoretically decrease hepatocellular carcinoma recurrence by eliminating any cancer cells not removed at transplantation. Using peritransplant and post-transplant chemotherapy, one group has reported impressive results in 20 patients (109). Although these patients were at high risk for recurrence (17 had tumors greater than 5 cm, and 11 were stage IVA by TNM classification), overall survival was 63%, and tumor-free survival at three years was 49%. Seventy percent of patients developed leukopenia, but in general, the chemotherapy was well tolerated. The main limitation of this approach is that preoperative chemotherapy cannot be easily timed in relation to transplantation. Thus, many centers have had to rely on intraoperative and postoperative chemotherapy only (110). Whether omitting the preoperative treatment will reduce the apparent beneficial effects previously demonstrated is unknown.

Since the vascular supply of hepatocellular carcinoma is mainly arterial with little portal blood contribution, some centers have recommended chemoembolization prior to transplantation. One group reported their experience with 48 patients who had either a single tumor less than 5 cm, or no more than three nodules, each less than 3 cm in diameter (111). Thirty-three patients with sufficient hepatic function underwent chemoembolization; no postoperative chemotherapy was administered. After four years, the actuarial survival was 75%. As in other experience, tumor size affected survival. Those patients with the smallest tumors in the explanted liver had an actuarial survival of 85%.

Adding some form of cytotoxic therapy thus appears to improve results for transplantation in the treatment of hepatocellular carcinoma. Nevertheless, the literature is replete with conflicting recommendations regarding both the selection of appropriate candidates and the most efficacious pre- and post-transplant adjuvant management (112–115). Most centers currently appear to have accepted, as appropriate candidates, those patients with a single, unresectable tumor no greater than 4 to 5 cm in size or with no more than 2 to 3 nodules, each less than 3 cm in size (12). Portal vein thrombosis in these patients is usually felt to be an absolute contraindication. Many centers advise alcohol injection or chemoembolization of the tumor nodules in the attempt to control the local disease during the 6 to 12 months these potential candidates may have to wait for the actual transplant procedure.

Fulminant Hepatic Failure

Viral infections, drugs, or toxins can cause sudden massive necrosis of a previously healthy liver (Table 19.11) (31,116). This process is termed *fulminant hepatic failure (FHF)*, which is formally defined as hepatic failure leading to encephalopathy within eight weeks of the first symptom of illness (31). This definition embodies the following important concepts

Table 19.11. Causes of Fulminant Hepatic Failure

Infections	Drugs	Toxins	Metabolic Liver Disease
Viral hepatitis (e.g., hepatitis B)	Acetaminophen	Amanita phalloides	Acute fatty liver of pregnancy
Cytomegalovirus	Halothane	Herbal teas	Wilson's disease
Herpes simplex	Isoniazid	Ecstasy (recreational drug)	Galactosemia
Varicella zoster	Ketoconazole		Reye's disease
Epstein-Barr	Antimicrobials, anticonvulsants, anesthetic agents, cardiovascular drugs, and miscellaneous other agents have been reported to cause fulminant hepatic failure		
Adenovirus			

Table 19.12. Fulminant Versus Chronic Hepatic Failure

	Fulminant	Chronic
Duration	Less than 8 weeks	Months to years
Pathology	Cellular necrosis, acute infiltrate (architecture preserved)	Fibrosis, cirrhosis
Prognosis	Reversible	Irreversible
Portal hypertension (ascites, GI bleed)	Rare	Often central feature
Hepatocyte failure (coagulopathy, hypoglycemia)	Central presenting feature	Gradual
Encephalopathy	Can be associated with cerebral edema	Cerebral edema rare

(see also Table 19.12, which compares fulminant to chronic hepatic failure):

- the liver was healthy prior to onset of illness,
- the liver is sufficiently damaged to cause encephalopathy,
- the duration of disease is measured in days to weeks, and
- the liver's basic architecture is preserved.

Survival with medical management alone is often low (<20%) among patients with advanced stages of encephalopathy (117), although etiology clearly influences survival (26). An obvious solution would be to replace the diseased liver with a healthy one.

Appropriate selection of patients with FHF for transplantation, however, poses a difficult dilemma for the clinician. If one waits for progression to the preterminal stages of the disease process, when the need for transplantation is incontrovertible, an allograft may not become available in time, or even if one is available, accumulated complications will greatly compromise post-transplant survival. However, proceeding to transplantation for all patients with FHF early in the disease course will unnecessarily commit the 20% to 30% of patients who spontaneously recover from FHF to transplantation. The wide range of survival rates (58% to 90%) reported from different centers performing liver transplantation in patients with FHF primarily reflects the different philosophies of patient selection (118–120).

Factors that predict irreversible FHF include both static (etiology of fulminant hepatic failure and age) and dynamic (stages of encephalopathy, prothrombin time, factor V levels, serum bilirubin, creatinine, arterial pH, and α-fetoprotein levels) features of the disease (26,31,121). These have been combined in prognostic models (Table 19.13) that are helpful in identifying the most appropriate patients for hepatic replacement before stage IV coma and the sequelae of advanced cerebral edema have become established.

The pretransplant management of patients with FHF is similar to that of patients with decompensated chronic liver failure (see section on pretransplant medical management). The major differentiating feature of the hepatic encephalopathy that develops in fulminant versus chronic liver failure is the typical presence of acute cerebral edema in FHF versus its rare presentation in patients with chronic liver failure (31). This is significant because hepatic encephalopathy, which results from metabolic imbalances, is completely reversible even after prolonged periods if hepatic function is restored. In contrast, the cerebral edema of FHF often progresses rapidly to an irreversible physical condition. Once cerebral-perfusion pressure (the difference between systolic blood pressure and intracranial pressure) falls below 40 mm Hg, cerebral ischemia occurs and is not infrequently followed by fatal brainstem herniation. Thus, although both metabolic encephalopathy and cerebral edema are manifested as coma, only the latter causes irreversible brain damage. Not surprisingly, therefore, cerebral edema is the primary cause of death in patients with FHF and a major determinant of the potential for post-transplant neurologic recovery.

Table 19.13. Indications for Transplantation in Fulminant Hepatic Failure

Paris Criteria
Encephalopathy and age <30 and factor V < 20%
or
Encephalopathy and age > 30 and factor V < 30%
King's College Criteria
Acetaminophen-induced fulminant hepatic failure
Arterial pH < 7.30 (irrespective of encephalopathy grade); *or all of the following:*
Prothrombin time > 100 seconds
Grade III or IV encephalopathy
Creatinine > 300 μmol/L
Nonacetaminophen-induced fulminant hepatic failure
Prothrombin time > 100 seconds (irrespective of encephalopathy grade); *or any three of the following factors:*
Age <10 or >40 years
Etiology: Non-A, non-B, or halothane hepatitis, drug reactions
Jaundice to encephalopathy time >7 days
Prothrombin time >50 seconds
Bilirubin >300 μmol/L

The key aspects of cerebral edema management are summarized in the section on pretransplant medical management and in Table 19.14. Intracranial pressure monitoring with epidural or subdural probes is helpful in guiding management, as well as in permitting more appropriate selection of patients for transplant surgery (Fig. 19.8). Most centers have suggested that refractory cerebral perfusion pressures of less than 40 mm Hg should preclude transplantation.

A number of experimental approaches to the management of FHF have focused on duplicating for liver failure the success of hemodialysis for kidney failure (31). Ex vivo perfusion of the patient's blood through a xenogeneic liver (122) or more recently through an allogeneic organ that was unsuitable for transplantation has occasionally resulted in dramatic, though temporary, reversal of liver failure. Artificial liver biotechnology (123), which is being evaluated in clinical trials, remains investigational but shows considerable promise (124). If technical obstacles could be resolved, auxiliary liver transplants might be the therapy of choice. This approach would provide full liver support while leaving open the possibility of native liver recovery, in which case immunosuppression could be discontinued. This approach has been successful in a small number of patients (125) (see section on auxiliary transplantation).

Table 19.14. Intracranial Hypertension Prevention and Management

Prevention

Treat fever of 100.5°F or more with cooling blankets and alcohol wipes (no Tylenol).
Minimize agitation and arterial hypertension.
Position at 0° to 20°.
Minimize pulmonary suctioning; if needed, squirt lidocaine in endotracheal tube to suppress cough reflex.
Avoid hypoxia and hypercapnia.
Aggressive treatment of low blood pressure (hemodynamic monitoring to guide fluid and pressor administration).

Treatment

Goal:
Maintain CCP >40 to 50 (CCP = MAP − ICP)
If ICP measurements are not available, clinical signs of increased pressure are substituted (tachycardia, increased muscle tone, decreased responsiveness) and an EEG is performed prior to the operation to rule out brain death. CT scan is generally indicated for localizing signs only.
Interventions:
Hyperventilation (P_{CO_2} = 25–35). Useful mainly for short-term treatment (but P_{CO_2} <24 associated with cerebral vasoconstriction).
Diuretics: mannitol until serum osm 310. Furosemide if fluid overloaded.
Drug-induced coma.
Titrate cardiac output/blood pressure to best CCP.

CCP = Cerebral perfusion pressure; ICP = intracranial pressure; MAP = mean arterial pressure.

Budd-Chiari Syndrome

The Budd-Chiari syndrome occurs when hepatic veins are obstructed, usually by thrombosis related to hypercoagulopathy or mechanical obstruction (126). The liver consequently becomes congested and tense, with resultant hepatomegaly and right upper-quadrant pain (Fig. 19.9a). Ascites weeping from the congested liver surface accumulates rapidly. Development of lower extremity edema suggests the venous obstruction has extended into the vena cava. If untreated, the venous hypertension damages the liver parenchyma, resulting initially in patchy fibrosis that then progresses to cirrhosis and end-stage liver failure. In contrast to other parenchymal liver diseases that lead to cirrhosis, portal hypertension in patients with Budd-Chiari syndrome typically precedes the development of cirrhosis. For this reason, the complications of portal hypertension alone are not necessarily an indication for liver transplantation in patients with Budd-Chiari syndrome. Portasystemic shunt procedures, if constructed before significant hepatocellular injury has occurred, can both provide definitive therapy for the portal hypertension and prevent the development of cirrhosis (Fig. 19.9b) (126). However, once histopathologic evidence of fibrosis is detected, the prognosis for patients with Budd-Chiari syndrome becomes much less favorable, even if successful venous decompression can be accomplished. These patients are probably best managed with liver transplantation (127). The operation may be difficult due to distortion by the caudate lobe, which typically undergoes compensatory hypertrophy (Budd-Chiari spares the caudate lobe because its venous drainage is directly into the vena cava, rather than via the hepatic veins). In addition, the suprahepatic vena cava may be encased by inflammatory adhesions or completely obstructed by the thrombotic process. In these patients, the intrapericardial portion of the

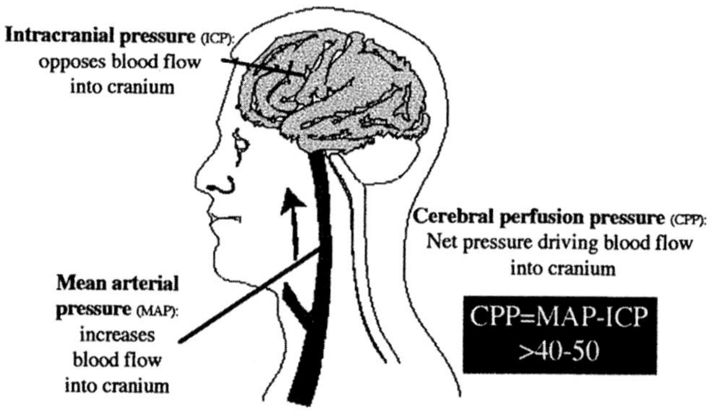

FIGURE 19.8. *Pressures determining blood flow to the brain. Intracranial pressure monitoring with epidural or subdural probes is helpful in guiding management as well as in permitting more appropriate selection of patients for transplant surgery. Most centers have suggested that refractory cerebral perfusion pressures of less than 40 mm Hg should preclude transplantation.*

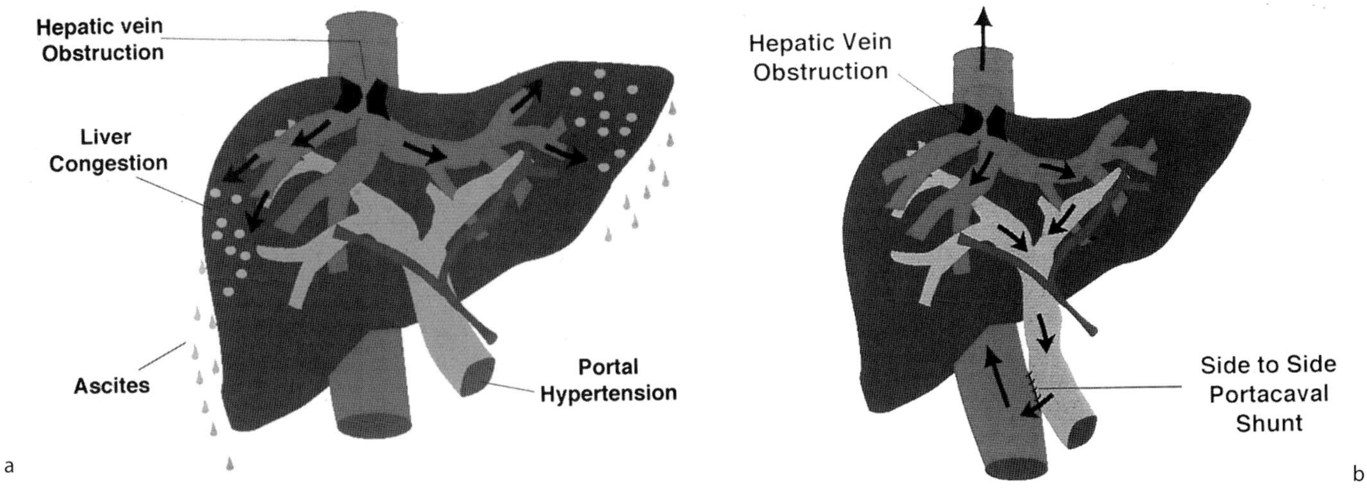

FIGURE 19.9. *Budd-Chiari syndrome. (**a**) Hepatic vein obstruction causes intense hepatic congestion. As a result, the liver becomes tense, swollen, and tender; massive ascites weeps from its surface and portal hypertension results. (**b**) The early treatment of Budd-Chiari syndrome through a portacaval shunt or TIPS procedure may effectively decompress the liver and thus prevent cirrhosis.*

vena cava can be isolated for anastomosis after incising the tendinous portion of the diaphragm. Postoperatively, these recipients are maintained on chronic anticoagulant therapy, since recurrent thrombosis remains an ever-present concern (128).

Retransplantation

Hepatic retransplantation may be indicated for recipients with primary allograft nonfunction resulting from unrecognized irreversible damage sustained in the donor organ either during the agonal prerecovery period or during recovery and preservation; technical complications such as hepatic artery thrombosis; chronic rejection, which is typically manifested by cholestasis and a histologic picture of "vanishing bile ducts"; and, rarely, uncontrolled acute rejection. Retransplantation is contraindicated in conditions known to recur rapidly (e.g., hepatitis and cancer). The reported need for retransplantation has varied between 5% and 25% among different centers, the highest frequency being for pediatric recipients (see Chapter 20).

Overall survival rates following retransplantation are approximately 20% to 30% inferior to those achieved in patients requiring only the primary procedure (129). The likelihood of survival for individual recipients appears to depend on such factors as age, cause of primary graft failure, urgency of retransplantation, and the time interval between primary transplantation and retransplantation (129–131). We found that the one-year actuarial survival rate for retransplantation was 57% if it was performed within three days of transplantation, but dropped to 24% if it was performed between 4 and 30 days after transplantation (130). Thus, an aggressive retransplant policy that attempts to accomplish the procedure within a few days of the primary procedure is more successful than one that pursues protracted periods of supportive care while awaiting improvement in allograft function.

Significant hepatic dysfunction persisting beyond the first few days typically leads to infectious complications and multiple organ failure, which then precludes successful retransplantation. In our experience, late retransplantation (more than one year after the primary transplant) also had an excellent success rate (83%). In these recipients with chronically failing allografts, semielective retransplantation is often possible, thereby providing improved survival when compared to urgent retransplantation.

Pediatric Liver Transplantation

In infants and younger children, biliary atresia has been the most common indication for liver transplantation. Initial management of these patients has almost always included attempts to provide biliary drainage by porticoenterostomy (Kasai procedure) during the neonatal period. Such procedures provide successful biliary diversion and at least temporary stabilization in 50% to 75% of these infants, allowing at least some growth to occur. This greatly increases the likelihood of a size-compatible liver donor becoming available. If the initial Kasai procedure fails, however, most centers now recommend immediate consideration for transplantation, since multiple attempts at revision of biliary drainage greatly compromise the likelihood of success following subsequent hepatectomy and liver replacement.

In later childhood, most candidates for transplantation present with inborn errors of metabolism, postnecrotic cirrhosis, and hepatic neoplasms that are otherwise unresectable. In children with benign conditions, a fall-off from the established growth curve is often the major indication to proceed with transplantation. Thus, if permanent growth retardation is to be avoided, transplantation must be accomplished at a much earlier stage in the evolution of deteriorating hepatic function than what is appropriate in adults.

Pediatric liver transplantation is discussed in detail in Chapter 20.

CONTRAINDICATIONS TO LIVER TRANSPLANTATION

The selection of the most appropriate liver transplantation candidates from those presenting with these many indications primarily depends on the exclusion of coexisting conditions that unacceptably increase the risk of postoperative morbidity and death (Table 19.15). Some contraindications, such as coexisting severe heart or pulmonary disease, are important considerations for any major surgical procedure. Patients with these problems are at high risk because they cannot withstand the hemodynamic and ventilatory demands associated with major surgery. The additional requirement for postoperative immunosuppression in the allograft recipient introduces consideration of comorbidity features that are specifically related to transplantation. For instance, uncontrolled infection or malignancy outside the liver as well as metastatic lesions to the liver almost always precludes successful transplantation because the extrahepatic disease typically progresses with overwhelming rapidity in an immunosuppressed patient. Also, since poor adherence to the post-transplant medical regimen almost inevitably leads to allograft loss or other fatal complications, patients at high risk for noncompliance (e.g., those with active substance abuse, poor mental aptitude, or uncooperative behavior) are generally excluded from receiving scarce organs.

As surgeons have gained increasing experience with liver replacement, a number of factors that were previously felt to preclude transplantation have now been relegated to the relative contraindication category. These include, for example, age over 65 years (a 77-year-old recipient has been reported) or extensive thrombosis of the portal or even mesenteric veins, which has proved to be manageable using vein grafts from the donor. In patients with acute renal failure associated with hepatic decompensation (hepatorenal syndrome), the renal function can be anticipated to rapidly improve following liver replacement. On the other hand, patients with chronic renal failure can be managed with simultaneous liver and kidney transplantation with only moderately increased risks.

Table 19.15. Contraindications to Liver Transplantation

Contraindications
Absolute
Uncontrolled infection outside the hepatobiliary system
Malignancy outside the hepatobiliary system
Secondary hepatic malignancy
Uncorrectable, life-limiting congenital anomalies
Active drug or alcohol abuse
Advanced cardiopulmonary disease
Relative
Age over 65
Portal vein thrombosis
Renal failure not associated with liver disease
Intrahepatic sepsis
Prior extensive hepatobiliary surgery
HIV antibody positivity

RECIPIENT SELECTION AND PRETRANSPLANT MANAGEMENT

As suggested by the discussion above, extensive medical evaluation is required to ensure each patient's suitability for liver transplantation. The transplant coordinator has a central role in this evaluation (see below, Nursing and Paramedical Team), which is to document and summarize the multiple assessments required, including:

- Definition of the cause of liver failure, its irreversibility, and its potential for recurrence in an allograft. Additional studies (e.g., assessment of portal vein patency) may be required.
- Evaluation of comorbid conditions associated with any end-stage liver disease (e.g., hepatorenal or hepatopulmonary syndromes, previous portacaval shunt, etc.) and specific considerations related to individual disease processes (e.g., disease extent in other organs in patients with hemachromatosis, status of colonic pathology associated with sclerosing cholangitis, etc.).
- Screening for coexisting medical conditions (e.g., pulmonary hypertension) (see Chapter 28).
- Assessment of psychosocial suitability for transplantation, particularly in patients with a history of alcohol or drug abuse. In some patients, the excess risk of noncompliance and recidivism may preclude transplantation.
- Identification of significant infectious processes. This includes exclusion of active infection that contraindicates immediate transplantation (e.g., tuberculosis, HIV); treatment of reversible conditions (e.g., poor dentition); and serologic testing for previous infection exposure that could impact post-transplant management [e.g., cytomegalovirus (CMV)].

Liver failure requiring intensive care may necessitate early intubation for airway protection, correction of hypoglycemia and coagulopathy, hemodynamic support, continuous hemofiltration rather than intermittent dialysis, and aggressive prevention and treatment of infection. In fulminant hepatic failure, the management of cerebral edema is critical (see Table 19.14 and Fig. 19.8). As noted above, intracranial pressure monitoring is often helpful for patients with stage III and stage IV encephalopathy, providing continuous assessment of the efficacy of such measures as hyperventilation, diuresis, drug-induced coma, and titration of blood pressure to cerebral perfusion pressure.

DONOR IDENTIFICATION

Wait-List

In order to receive an allograft, a candidate for liver transplantation must be registered on a wait-list maintained by an organ procurement organization (OPO). In the United States, patients are registered with the United Network for Organ Sharing (UNOS), a national network of local OPOs established to allocate organs efficiently and equitably (132). UNOS distributes organs mainly on the basis of the length of time on the wait-list and medical urgency. Organizations with similar goals exist in most countries.

Histocompatibility Testing

Increasing levels of histocompatibility matching between donor and recipient have been correlated with improved allograft survival rates following kidney transplantation (see Chapters 4 and 17). Presumably, a similar survival advantage could be provided by HLA matching in liver transplantation. In fact, class I histocompatibility antigen matching may significantly improve patient and graft survival (133). However, the typical urgency of the recipient operation precludes donor selection based on extensive tissue matching. Histocompatibility testing, therefore, plays little role in selecting an individual recipient for liver transplantation from a particular donor.

Serologic Testing (T-Cell Crossmatch)

Screening for preexisting alloantibody reactive with the potential liver donor also plays little role in selecting recipients for liver transplantation, in contrast to its essential role in kidney transplantation. This observation initially resulted from practical necessity, as the brief duration of ex vivo ischemia tolerated by the liver using early preservation approaches made pretransplant crossmatching impossible. Subsequent retrospective analysis indicated that the survival of transplants performed in the presence of a positive crossmatch had not been adversely affected. A positive crossmatch is, however, associated with a higher likelihood of early rejection episodes (134). Thus, even retrospective knowledge of the crossmatch results may be helpful for identifying high-risk patients who possibly would benefit from more aggressive immunosuppression. Nevertheless, extensive experience has confirmed that numerous other variables are more important determinants of long-term outcome and that a positive cytotoxic crossmatch is not a contraindication for liver transplantation.

One possible explanation for the liver allograft's apparent resistance to the damaging effects of cytotoxic alloantibody is that its large size and functional reserve may allow the allograft to sustain a certain degree of antibody-mediated damage without significant clinical sequelae. Alternatively, the extensive endothelial surfaces in the liver may absorb the donor-reactive antibody, again without clinically evident effects (135). This would explain the observation that a liver allograft appears to prevent hyperacute rejection of a subsequently placed renal transplant despite a positive pretransplant T-cell crossmatch (136).

ABO Blood Grouping

The liver's capacity to withstand antibody-mediated injury also may allow transplantation across the ABO barrier, a circumstance not infrequently encountered when impending death in the candidate precludes waiting for a blood group–compatible organ. Patient survival following ABO-incompatible liver transplantation has been reported in 67% of recipients treated with pretransplant and post-transplant plasmapheresis to lower the isoagglutinin titers (137). The results have been particularly favorable in younger children. Immunoadsorption with synthetic blood group antigens has also been utilized as a more selective alternative to plasmapheresis (137). Unfortunately, transplantation of ABO-incompatible grafts in adults is complicated by a greater incidence of rejection, vascular thrombosis, and biliary complications, making the need for retransplantation more likely (138,139). In one series, biliary complications developed in 82% of ABO-incompatible livers, compared to only a 6% incidence in ABO-matched allografts (140). Presumably, the biliary epithelium, which expresses donor blood group antigen, is highly susceptible to ABO isoagglutinin-mediated injury. Despite this anticipated inferior allograft survival rate, the likelihood of patient salvage is sufficient to justify ABO-incompatible transplantation for some critically ill individuals who have no other available donor. In these patients, it is recognized that the use of an incompatible liver may provide only short-term stabilization until a compatible organ becomes available for retransplantation. Although such an approach has the appeal of rescuing some acutely ill patients, this is accomplished at the price of denying these allografts to other patients with a greater likelihood of success (141). Unfortunately, this difficult choice will persist until the human donor pool expands, artificial liver support devices become available, xenogeneic transplantation becomes a reality, or the humoral response can be better controlled.

For nonemergent procedures, transplantation across ABO-incompatible barriers is generally avoided; however, ABO-unmatched but compatible grafts are not infrequently used (e.g., a blood group O liver into a blood group A, B, or AB recipient). Interestingly, episodes of hemolysis, which are usually self-limiting, occur in approximately one-third of such recipients (142). This apparently results from the continued production of ABO isoagglutinins by donor lymphocytes transplanted with the allograft, that react with the recipient's erythrocytes (142). The resultant clinical syndrome, characterized by anemia and hyperbilirubinemia, is typically benign, lasting for up to two months after transplantation. Treatment with increased steroids is often helpful. If transfusion is required while antirecipient antibodies persist, donor-type red blood cells may be used. In contrast, plasma, if needed, should be recipient ABO identical to avoid infusion of further isoagglutinins and because the plasma may contain soluble ABO antigens that can neutralize ABO alloantibody.

Donor Size

When registering a potential liver allograft recipient, the surgeon specifies the range of acceptable donor size. Reasonable matching for body size between donor and recipient is essential in order to limit the technical difficulties of reimplantation. Preferably, a donor organ should be identified from a person whose weight falls within the range of 25% to 125% of the recipient's. A recipient with a wide costal margin or massive ascites may be able to accommodate a liver from a donor with a much greater weight discrepancy, whereas small individuals have more exacting size constraints. Because of the rarity of potential donors in the pediatric population, one must often consider utilizing larger donors for transplantation into children. In most instances, successful reimplantation of an intact adult allograft into a child is impossible, but this obstacle can be overcome by reducing adult livers to a single lobe or even segment. This approach has been further extended to division of a single cadaver donor liver into two viable grafts for implantation into separate recipients (143,144). This potentially attractive solution to the organ donor shortage has not yet been widely applied due to its exacting techniques and somewhat inferior success rates. Procurement of a single lobe or segment from a living-related donor has also expanded the choices of donors for transplantation into small children (see Chapter 20).

Recipient Allocation

Liver allograft donors in most countries are patients with irreversible cessation of all brain function in the presence of reasonably preserved liver function and sufficient cardiopulmonary stability to maintain hepatic viability (see Chapter 15). Non-heart-beating donors have occasionally provided usable liver allografts, but are not widely used. Once brain death is declared by the patient's attending physician, and the decedent's family agrees to organ donation, the focus of care shifts to correction of the measures that had been instituted while trying to rescue cerebral activity (e.g., dehydration, hypothermia). Potential contraindications to organ donation are carefully evaluated (Table 19.16). If no absolute contraindication is identified, a computerized match-up between donor and potential recipients takes place on the basis of donor size and location, blood group compatibility, waiting time, and medical urgency. The most severely ill patients have priority over less ill patients within each organ-sharing region, regardless of waiting time; for example, a status 1 patient with one-week waiting time has priority over a status 2 patient with one-year waiting time. Using such algorithms, a priority ranking of potential recipients emerges, and the donor liver is offered to the center with the top-ranking patient.

Recipient Team Evaluation

When offered a liver, the recipient team first assesses the quality of the donor organ based on the clinical and biochemical factors that have been correlated with early post-transplant function (Table 19.17). Multiple or prolonged episodes of prerecovery hypoxia and hypotension or marked elevation of transaminases and prothrombin time suggest significant hepatocellular damage with a higher likelihood of early allograft failure. Such an organ is usually not accepted for a stable potential recipient for whom a longer pretransplant waiting time will not represent unacceptable risk. As a general rule, unfavorable donor features tend to be additive. Thus, donor organs from an elderly patient are less likely to tolerate hemodynamic instability than those from an 18-year-old donor. If the potential donor organ is judged to be marginally acceptable, the urgency of the need for liver replacement in the recipient plus the typical waiting times for the region must be considered. While it may be possible to await an ideal donor for a stable liver transplant

Table 19.16. Contraindications to Liver Donation

Absolute contraindications for organ donation	
History of malignancy (excluding primary brain tumors and nonmelanoma skin cancers)	Except for primary brain tumors and nonmelanoma skin cancers, all cancers can be transmitted to allograft recipients through transplantation
HIV positivity	When the social history of a potential donor reveals a high risk for HIV infection, but the serologic test is negative, organs are typically only considered in status 1 patients
Current sepsis	Blood cultures positive for nonskin contaminant bacteria
Hepatitis B surface antigen positivity	Indicates a high risk of transmitting HBV
Relative contraindications for organ donation	
Hepatitis C antibody	Many of these patients will have chronic hepatitis C infection
Hepatitis B core antibody (IgM)	May indicate recent hepatitis B infection and possible infectivity, even in the absence of hepatitis B surface antigen positivity

Table 19.17. Donor Factors That Influence Allograft Function

Donor Factor	Significance
Steatosis	Even if liver function is completely normal, severe macrovesicular steatosis (>50%) (147) has been associated with a high risk of early allograft failure. Steatosis is more common in donors who are old, obese, or diabetic, or have a history of alcoholism.
Oxygen delivery	Multiple episodes of hypotension, requirement for pressors other than dopamine, and poor oxygenation increase the likelihood of organ injury (236).
Donor age	Ideally, less than 60 years. Carefully selected older donors can be used in conjunction with a biopsy (147,237,238). Donors older than 70 years have been used safely.
Transaminase and bilirubin elevation	Abnormal levels in a potential donor may indicate severe organ injury.
Abnormal coagulation profile	If isolated, this may indicate brain injury. Otherwise, abnormal coagulation tests confirm poor hepatic function.
Weight >100 kg	Livers from donors weighing more than 100 kg have a higher likelihood of primary nonfunction (236). Carefully selected heavier donors can be used in conjunction with a biopsy to rule out steatosis.
Length of hospital stay	Prolonged ICU stay (>3 days) has been associated with early allograft damage, though not with early graft survival (236,239).
Malnutrition	Depletion of donor hepatic glycogen reserves may affect the resistance of the graft to ischemic injury (240).
Prior substance or alcohol abuse	A biopsy is required in these donors to rule out steatosis or inflammation.
Cold ischemia time	Keeping cold ischemia time under 12 hours is safe. Livers preserved in University of Wisconsin solution for up to 24 hours have been used, although probably at a higher risk of malfunction (147,154,239).
Warm ischemia time	Ideally, warm ischemia time should be kept under one hour. Over that limit, the longer the ischemia, the higher the likelihood of hepatocyte damage and primary allograft nonfunction.
Donor sex	Livers from female donors have been shown in some series to yield worse graft survival than those from male donors (241). Unknown hormonal factors have been postulated (242).

candidate, the transplant team is compelled to be less selective for those patients who may die before another organ becomes available. As a result, a growing experience with "marginal donors" has been accrued (see Chapter 15). It is now well recognized that the liver from older donors, with unacceptably extensive atherosclerotic disease in other organs, can often be successfully transplanted, possibly because, as first emphasized by Starzl, the atherosclerotic process seems to selectively spare the hepatic arteries. Nevertheless, the graft survival rate from older donors is lower (43% two-year survival for livers from donors older than 60 years versus 71% for younger donors) (145). Again, therefore, liver allografts from older donors are more frequently accepted for the more desperately ill patient who is unlikely to survive a longer wait. Gross and histopathologic examination of the allograft (see below) at the time of donor hepatectomy are crucial final determinants of the organ's suitability for transplantation. Both cold and warm ischemia times should be limited whenever marginal donor livers are used, since these organs have been found to be more susceptible to ischemic injury.

DONOR OPERATION

Preparation

Organ procurement often involves multiple teams traveling to an institution unfamiliar with the procedure. A brief overview of the operation with the local operating room (OR) team will be helpful to avoid confusion. It is critical to enlist anesthesia support to maintain the donor's cardiovascular integrity and normothermia. A frequent misunderstanding involves the use of blood products. Blood products are not wasted in a brain-dead cadaveric donor, and such support should be administered based on the same criteria used for a patient expected to recover (i.e., to maintain oxygen delivery and prevent coagulopathy). Inadequate perfusion of cadaveric organs prior to explantation may have a devastatingly adverse impact on the organ recipients. The procurement teams must recognize that the procedure, while marking a hopeful and technically satisfying beginning for their objectives, usually represents an unpleasant conclusion for the grieving donor hospital. Insensitivity, disrespect, and excessive joviality on the part of the procurement team may leave a lasting negative impression that could result in reluctance to consider future donations. On the other hand, the procurement experience can be positive if features such as its life-saving benefits and the unique anatomic display of the operation are shared with the donor hospital team.

Intraoperative Donor Evaluation

The organs are exposed through a midline incision extending from suprasternal notch to pubis. If the heart is to be procured, it is usually mobilized as the first maneuver so that it can be quickly removed should uncorrectable hemodynamic instability develop during the dissection of other organs. Upon entry into the abdomen, rapid inspection excludes unsuspected sepsis, neoplasia, or other significant pathology. The liver's gross suitability is then confirmed. A normal liver has soft turgor with a smooth, even, sharp-edged surface (146). In contrast, an edematous liver is firm, with rounded edges. If the edema is due to fluid overload, which is typically associated with heart distention and central venous pressure elevation, it should respond to diuresis (146). Otherwise the edema suggests the organ has suffered significant ischemic or toxic injury and probably should not be recovered for transplantation. Other signs of potential organ unsuitability include a yellow hue, heralding significant steatosis, or a firm turgor suggestive of fibrosis. When the common bile duct is transected, the color and quantity of bile can be used as a further measure of the donor liver's quality. Low output of light watery bile indicates significant liver injury (146).

Of major importance during hepatic evaluation is the detection of significant hepatic steatosis, as there is a strong association of this process with post-transplant nonfunction (147). The donors at higher risk for steatosis include elderly or obese individuals, those with a history of diabetes or alcohol intake, and poorly nourished patients with a prolonged premortem hospital course. The precise mechanisms that produce the allograft nonfunction are unknown, since these steatotic livers usually had functioned normally in the donor. Presumably, ischemia and cold preservation irreversibly injure fatty hepatocytes. A steatotic liver may be evident on gross inspection as a large, yellow organ with rounded edges. Once the blood is flushed from the liver, the organ becomes more obviously yellow. A biopsy is essential for determining suitability for transplantation. Organs with severe macrovesicular steatosis (>50%) are generally discarded (Fig. 19.10 and Plate 8). The decision to use organs with less steatosis is based on other donor factors in conjunction with the urgency of the recipient's need for hepatic replacement. Frozen section biopsies of the donor liver are also useful to exclude ischemic necrosis, prominent portal inflammation, periductular fibrosis, granulomatous inflammation, and bridging fibrosis, any of which may influence the final decision to proceed with transplantation (148).

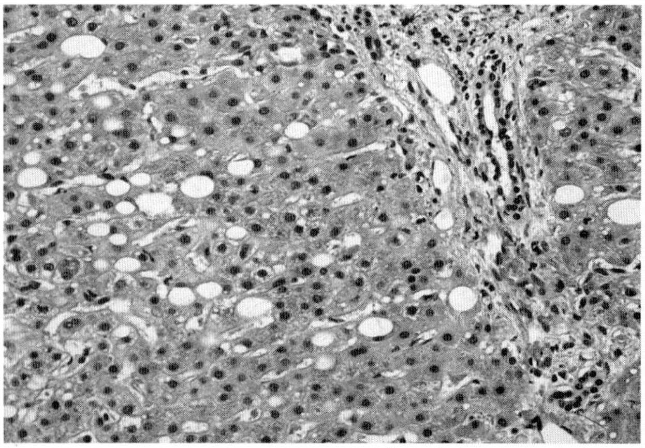

FIGURE 19.10. *Macrovesicular steatosis in the donor liver. Many of the hepatocytes contain one or more vesicles that displace the nucleus and occupy the majority of the cytoplasm.*

Allograft Removal

Although the details will differ depending on the combination of organs removed, certain common principles regarding allograft removal prevail. These include careful coordination among the teams to ensure that there is no compromise in viability of any of the transplanted organs; wide exposure; and removal of the organs in the order of heart and/or lungs, liver, kidney, pancreas, and bowel. Once the supraceliac aorta is clamped, the abdominal organs are flushed and cooled in situ via a cannula in the distal aorta. The liver is usually simultaneously flushed and cooled through its portal system, via a cannula in the splenic or inferior mesenteric vein. The flushed-out blood is collected via a cannula in the inferior vena cava; alternatively, if no thoracic organ is harvested, the right atrium can be incised and the resultant outflow suctioned out of the chest, thus avoiding a caval cannula.

By the end of the isolation procedure, the liver's vasculature is usually completely defined, including the celiac axis down to aorta, any anomalous arterial supply, the portal vein, and the suprahepatic and infrahepatic vena cava. The extent to which this dissection is performed prior to, or after, aortic cross-clamping and allograft cooling will depend on the surgeon's preference as well as the donor's hemodynamic stability. At one extreme is the originally described approach (149), in which a complete dissection of all vessels is performed prior to in situ liver perfusion. This technique has the advantage of completely identifying all structures and allowing rapid removal of the liver following cross-clamping of the aorta; however, the preliminary dissection requires several hours and can be associated with significant blood loss. At the other extreme is the rapid-flush technique, in which cannulation and cold perfusion with minimal prior dissection is performed immediately after initial exploration (150). This technique is ideally suited for hemodynamically unstable patients; however, anomalous structures may not be recognized, and therefore may be injured. Most surgeons use an intermediate combination of these two extremes.

The first step is usually exposure for cannulation of the distal aorta and vena cava, which are approached by elevating the transverse colon and rotating the small bowel to the right. This reveals the ligament of Treitz and the inferior mesenteric vein, which can be encircled at the root of the mesentery and cannulated for portal perfusion (Fig. 19.11 and Plate 9). A slow drip of lactated Ringer's can be instituted through this cannula to keep it open. The soft tissues and lymphatics overlying the aorta and vena cava are then cauterized or controlled with metal clips, and the inferior mesenteric artery is ligated and divided. The aorta and vena cava are then encircled at the iliac bifurcation, paying careful attention to avoiding injury to lumbar vessels or an aberrant renal artery. (As mentioned above, if no thoracic organ is being harvested, encircling the vena cava is not required.) This early dissection allows for rapid cannulation and cold perfusion of the abdominal organs should hemodynamic

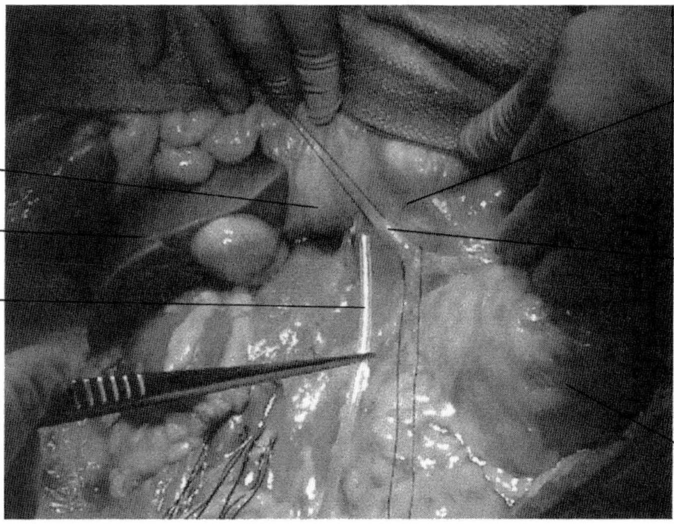

FIGURE 19.11. *The inferior mesenteric vein is found at the base of the distal transverse colon mesentery and can be cannulated to perfuse the portal vein.*

instability develop during the continuing operative procedure.

The next step is to isolate the hepatic blood supply. The round and triangular ligaments are divided and the gastrohepatic ligament is palpated. If an accessory left hepatic artery (18% of donors) (151) is felt, it is freed down to its origin from the left gastric artery, which in turn is followed down to the celiac axis. The remainder of the lesser omentum is divided, and the hepatic hilum encircled by inserting a finger into the foramen of Winslow. The hepatic artery pulse can then be easily palpated. A second pulse detected to the right of the hepatoduodenal ligament and posterior to the portal vein indicates the presence of a replaced right hepatic artery (10% of donors) (146) arising from the superior mesenteric artery. In this circumstance, and if the pancreas is also being recovered for transplantation, a determination of how the vascular structures will be divided must be made. Generally, priority is given to the liver due to its lifesaving function. The common bile duct is then transected near its entrance into the pancreas. The gallbladder is incised and flushed free of bile to prevent autolysis during subsequent cold storage. The right gastric and gastroduodenal arteries are ligated and divided. The pancreas is retracted caudad, and the avascular peritoneum on its superior margin is divided. If the inferior mesenteric vein is not used for portal cannulation, exposure of the splenic and superior mesenteric vein confluence is required. The coronary vein is divided and the portal vein is exposed proximally. If the pancreas is not being retrieved for transplantation, dissection of the portal vein is facilitated by dividing the pancreas through the relatively avascular plane anterior to the mesenteric vessels. The splenic vein is then encircled and cannulated. Preliminary dissection can be interrupted at this point. Alternatively, the celiac axis can be exposed down to the aorta, ligating and dividing the left gastric and splenic arteries (the left gastric artery is left intact in the presence of a replaced left hepatic artery). If a replaced right hepatic artery is present, a Kocher maneuver is required to gain exposure back to its origin from the superior mesenteric artery.

The supraceliac aorta is then encircled after dividing the overlying diaphragmatic crura, in preparation for clamping. (If thoracic organs are not being retrieved, it is often simpler to plan on clamping the easily visible supraceliac aorta in the chest.) The donor is then heparinized, after which cannulae are introduced into the aorta and the vena cava. As the aorta is cross-clamped at the diaphragm, aortic and portal vein perfusion of the liver is begun using University of Wisconsin solution (UW). Ice slush may also be poured into the abdomen to facilitate surface cooling. Concomitant venous decompression via the vena cava cannula prevents hepatic engorgement.

After the cardiectomy, the liver is recovered by dividing the pericaval diaphragm and the distal vena cava just above the renal veins. The arterial dissection is completed by following the hepatic artery down the celiac axis to the aorta. The aorta is divided at an angle to avoid injury to a possibly high-lying renal artery, leaving an aortic patch on the celiac artery. If a replaced right hepatic artery has been identified, the origin of the superior mesenteric artery is included in the aortic patch. The kidney block is then removed, after which segments of donor iliac artery and vein are taken in case vessel grafts are required during hepatic reimplantation.

Cold Preservation

After completion of the donor hepatectomy, the ex vivo allograft is further flushed through the portal vein and hepatic artery. The common bile duct is also flushed with UW solution, which appears to reduce the incidence of post-transplant biliary strictures. The organ is then immersed in a sterile plastic bag containing UW preservation solution for storage on ice until transplantation (Fig. 19.12 and Plate 10). The high potassium concentration, the lactobionate anion, and the raffinose trisaccharide contained in this solution are particularly effective impermeants for limiting hypothermic-induced cellular swelling. The introduction of UW solution into clinical practice has extended the safe period of ex vivo storage to as long as 24 hours. Nevertheless, most centers try to limit the cold ischemia time to no more than 12 to 15 hours (152,153), after which the biliary epithelium appears to sustain worsening degrees of injury (154) manifested in the postoperative period by prolonged periods of severe cholestasis. The relatively prolonged preservation time provided by UW solution increases the opportunity for more distant procurement and also relaxes the logistical constraints of the procedure. The recipient operation can be scheduled on a semielective basis, thus allowing more flexible use of the operation rooms and personnel. Perhaps most importantly, the enhanced margin of safety has made possible the development of new techniques, such as reduced-size liver transplantation, and has further minimized organ wastage by allowing donor hepatectomy to proceed even in circumstances where a recipient is not immediately available.

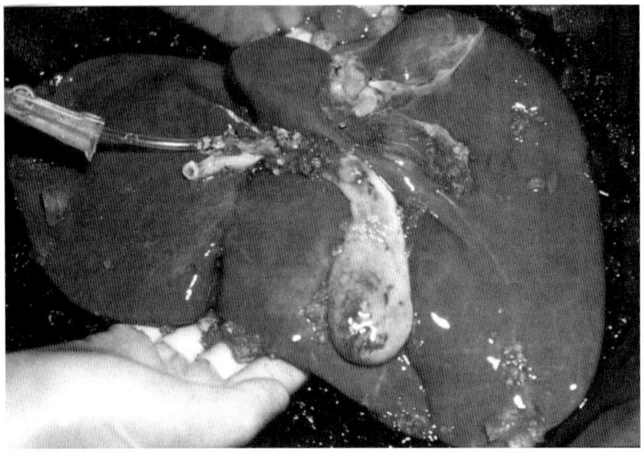

FIGURE 19.12. *A procured liver's inferior surface. The cannula for portal perfusion is still in place. After back-table flushing of the portal vein, hepatic artery, and common bile duct, the liver is packed in preservation fluid and stored in a bag surrounded by ice-cold solution.*

ANESTHETIC CONSIDERATION FOR THE RECIPIENT OPERATION

Preparation

The metabolic and resuscitative management by the anesthesia team is a major determinant of perioperative outcome in liver transplant recipients. The following issues should be kept in mind to minimize complications during, or after, the surgical procedure:

- Because the operation may extend beyond eight hours, all pressure points on the heels, sacrum, elbows, and head must be protected to prevent ischemic ulceration. Focal occipital scalp alopecia that develops during the early post-transplant period is clear evidence of inadequate intraoperative padding.
- Intraoperative rewarming will be required to control the hypothermia that results from prolonged surgery, implantation of an iced allograft, and extracorporeal circulation during veno-venous bypass. Warmed intravenous infusions, a warming blanket, and plastic tents over the head and extremities are commonly used.
- Preparation for major blood loss and hemodynamic instability, particularly during the anhepatic phase, is essential. Specialized equipment must be available, typically including monitoring devices, a rapid blood warming and infusion pump providing transfusion rates as high as 2 L/min, a blood salvage device, an argon beam coagulator, and an extracorporeal pump for veno-venous bypass. In adult recipients, adequate access for infusion and monitoring can be accomplished via a right radial arterial line, a large-bore intravenous catheter in the right arm, and introducers in each internal jugular vein (one for a pulmonary artery catheter and one for the rapid infusion pump). Access sites in the legs are avoided because they would be unreliable during intraoperative vena cava occlusion. The left arm has usually been avoided because the left axillary vein is sometimes used for veno-venous bypass return. Alternatively, many units have begun utilizing a large-bore catheter percutaneously placed into the subclavian vein (155). In small children, a pulmonary artery catheter is neither required nor practical. Instead, a central venous catheter and peripheral venous lines are sufficient.

Anesthetic Approaches

Careful preoxygenation and rapid sequence induction anesthesia are commonly used, because patients with hepatic failure are predisposed to hypoxia from intrapulmonary arteriovenous shunts and from atelectasis due to ascites. The selection of anesthetic agents must take into consideration the high cardiac output and low peripheral vascular resistance typical of end-stage liver disease. A narcotic anesthetic such as Fentanyl and/or morphine is often preferred for hemodynamic stability, but isoflurane inhalational anesthesia, which will reduce systemic resistance, may be used as tolerated. In patients who do not tolerate routine anesthesia administration, a benzodiazepine is often given to block memory (lorazepam is frequently selected because it requires only glucuronidation for excretion).

RECIPIENT OPERATION

Native Hepatectomy

Removal of a diseased liver can be complicated by the severe coagulopathy typically associated with end-stage liver disease, the multiple venous collaterals resulting from portal hypertension, and the dense adhesions from previous operations. Much of the dissection can be performed using electrocautery, reserving suture ligation for large vessels. The argon beam coagulator is useful, especially for control of diffuse bleeding from raw surfaces. Meticulous hemostasis is crucial, since postoperative morbidity and mortality are directly correlated with intraoperative blood loss (156). During this and the anhepatic periods, these patients may develop metabolic acidosis. Interestingly, if this is overcorrected with sodium bicarbonate infusions, severe postoperative metabolic alkalosis, which can delay extubation, may develop. This phenomenon results from the metabolism to bicarbonate, by a functioning allograft, of the significant citrate load that is administered with transfused blood products.

Surgical Exposure

Abdominal exploration in adults is carried out through a bilateral subcostal incision with midline extension (Mercedes incision). The xyphoid is usually excised to maximize the exposure of the suprahepatic vena cava. In children, the midline extension is seldom required. The falciform and round ligaments are divided, often step-wise with ligatures. A mechanical retractor is positioned to spread the costal margin. The suprahepatic dissection is then continued until the anterior surface of the vena cava is defined. The left triangular ligament is divided by cautery to the tip of the left lobe, where its attachments to the diaphragm may be more densely vascularized and require suture ligation. The gastrohepatic ligament (lesser omentum) is similarly divided.

In dissecting the porta hepatis, the recipient common bile duct is divided proximal to the ligated cystic duct, to maximize its length for subsequent choledochocholedochostomy. If the patient had a previous biliary enteric anastomosis, the Roux-loop can be taken down and subsequently used for biliary drainage of the allograft. We attempt to ligate and divide the left and right hepatic arteries individually to avoid possible intimal damage to the more proximal proper and common hepatic arteries, which are often quite fragile. The portal vein is usually skeletonized last, ligating and dividing the coronary vein and any tributaries from the pancreas that may be present. As noted earlier, prior recipient portal vein thrombosis is no longer considered a contraindication to transplantation. If this is encountered, the patency of the portal vein can sometimes be reestablished by thromboendovenectomy. If this is not possible, more proximal dissection beneath the pancreas to the confluence of the recipient's splenic and superior mesenteric veins will sometimes expose a suitable anastomotic site. Occasionally, portal revascularization of the allograft requires approaching the superior mesenteric vein below the pancreas, at the level of the middle colic vein, in order to isolate a site for anastomosis of donor iliac vein graft (Fig. 19.13).

Once the portal dissection has been completed, the infrahepatic vena cava is carefully encircled just above the right renal vein. The right hepatic lobe is elevated and the liver is rotated to the left by the assistant to expose the coronary ligaments. The peritoneal and diaphragmatic attachments are divided with cautery, gradually separating the bare area of the liver from the diaphragm. As the right adrenal vein comes into view posteriorly, it is ligated and divided. Mobilization of the suprahepatic vena cava is accomplished by encircling the cava close to its exit from the liver. By working at this level, the recipient phrenic veins are usually not encountered, remaining with the vena caval cuff

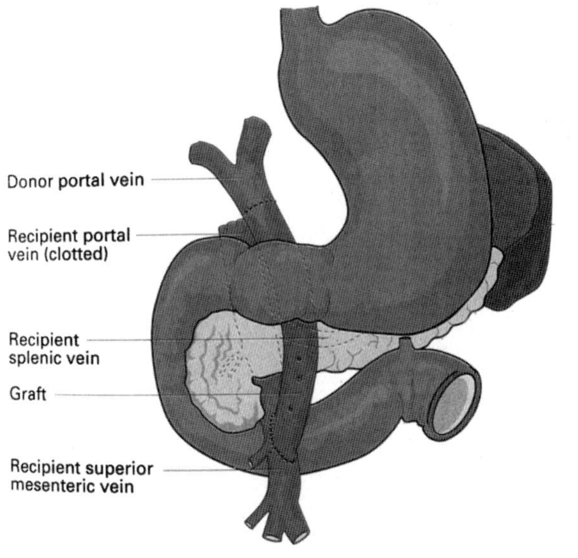

FIGURE 19.13. *Use of donor iliac vein graft to bypass thrombosed recipient portal vein. In patients with extensive thrombosis, the vein graft may have to be placed anterior to the pancreas to extend to a patent superior mesenteric vein. More commonly, a suitable anastomotic site is found behind the pancreas at the confluence of the splenic and superior mesenteric veins.*

above the site where the cava will be divided. Following completion of these maneuvers, the mobilized liver is held in place only by its venous attachments.

An alternative approach utilizes the "piggyback" technique for revascularization of the allograft. With this variant, the retrohepatic cava is preserved and thus not occluded at any time during the surgical procedure (157).

Veno-Venous Bypass

Although venous bypass (158) (Fig. 19.14) during the anhepatic phase is not an essential component of most operations, without it severe splanchnic venous congestion and hemodynamic instability can occur in some patients. Before removing the native liver, therefore, we temporarily cross-clamp the vena cava to assess hemodynamic stability. If hypotension occurs despite adequate volume replacement, a decision is made to either use the piggyback approach or to institute veno-venous bypass. Up to 40% to 50% of the cardiac output can be returned to the heart from the lower body and viscera via this bypass, thereby rapidly stabilizing the patient during the anhepatic period. A significant limitation of bypass is heat loss, estimated at 0.9°C/hr (159). Air emboli can theoretically occur, although we have not observed this, and the risk of clots and platelet plugs appears to be low as long as flow rates exceed 1.5 L/min. Systemic heparinization is not required. The hemodynamic stability provided by this approach allows revascularization of the donor liver in a less urgent fashion, which is a not an insignificant advantage when training inexperienced surgeons in this phase of the operation.

The heparin-bonded veno-venous bypass outflow circuits are placed into the femoral vein, via a cut-down on the left saphenous vein, and the portal vein (after completing the hepatectomy). Both cannulae come together at a Y-connector, which is connected to an in-line centrifugal pump (see Fig. 19.14). The axillary vein is cannulated for return flow via a small incision in the left axilla. Open cannulation of the vessels requires 10 to 20 minutes. Recently, percutaneous femoral and subclavian cannulation with 15F catheters has been recommended in place of open cannulation, thereby simplifying and shortening the procedure without loss of efficacy (155).

Anhepatic Phase

Final resection of the recipient liver is completed by clamping the portal vein and transecting it high in the hilum. Vascular clamps are then placed on the infrahepatic and suprahepatic vena cava. A lengthy suprahepatic caval cuff is developed by incising the liver parenchyma (except in patients with intrahepatic sepsis or neoplasia) and transecting the hepatic veins within the substance of the liver (Fig. 19.15). The infrahepatic cava is severed close to its junction with the caudate lobe. Following removal of the liver from the field, any retroperitoneal bleeding sites are suture-ligated or controlled with cautery. This maneuver typically results in greatly diminished bleeding from the hepatectomy site and allows more complete hemostasis in the exposed hepatic fossa. At this point, the third cannula of the veno-venous bypass can be introduced into the recipient portal vein to decompress the splanchnic venous system.

Allograft Revascularization

Numerous technical approaches have been devised for implanting the new liver. The technique described here emphasizes the important principles involved in the procedure. The suprahepatic vena cava is first tailored by fashioning the recipient hepatic veins into a single caval lumen, thereby providing a lengthy vascular cuff for this difficult anastomosis. The posterior caval wall anastomosis is accom-

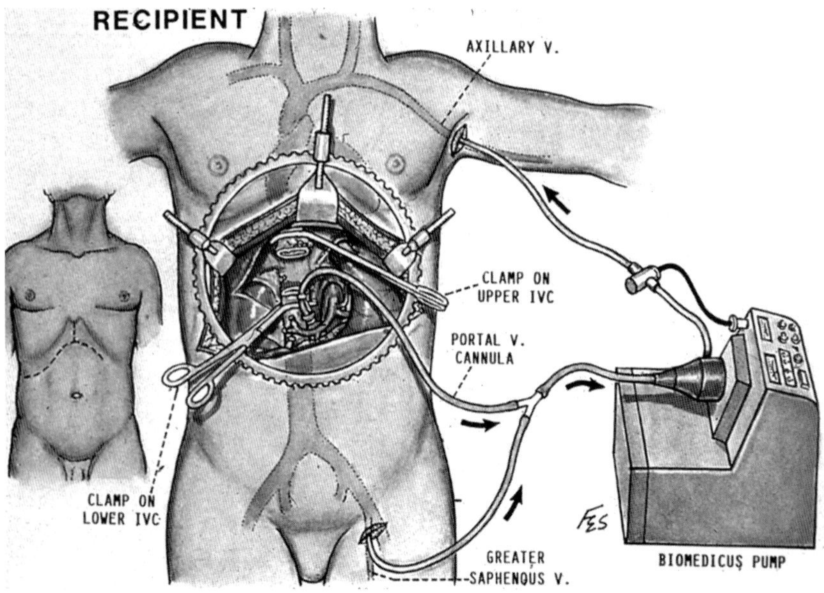

FIGURE 19.14. *Anhepatic stage of the transplant procedure with veno-venous bypass. Lower body systemic venous blood and splanchnic blood are drained via the femoral and portal cannulae, respectively. Blood is returned to the heart by the in-line centrifugal pump via the axillary vein cannula.*

plished using everting mattress sutures placed from within the lumen and the anterior wall by simple over-and-over sutures. Care must be taken not to narrow the lumen of any of the venous anastomoses. Some surgeons address this concern by tying the suture with an "air knot." This "growth factor" allows any purse-stringing of the anastomosis to expand during reperfusion. The infrahepatic cava is reconstructed by usual end-to-end venous anastomotic techniques. Prior to completion of this anastomosis, the allograft is perfused with Ringer's lactate solution via the portal vein in order to flush from the liver the potassium-rich preservation fluid and any air and acidic radicals that have accumulated during cold storage. Some centers prefer leaving a drainage catheter through the infrahepatic caval anastomosis and flushing the allograft with blood following completion of the portal vein anastomosis (160).

If the piggyback approach is used, the donor suprahepatic vena is anastomosed to the common cuff formed by joining the recipient's left and middle hepatic veins. The donor infrahepatic cava is ligated (157).

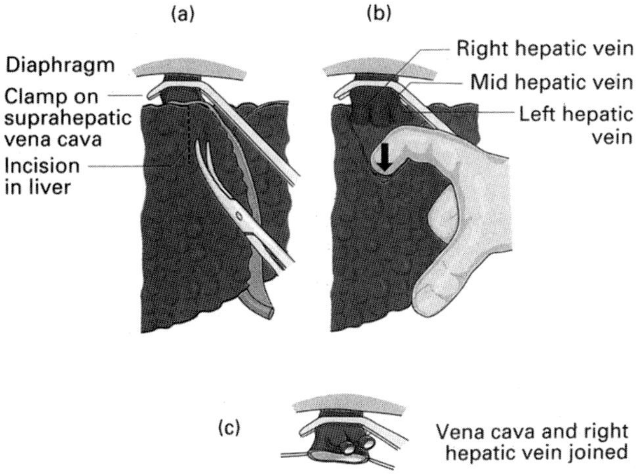

FIGURE 19.15. *Transection of recipient suprahepatic vena cava. (**a,b**) A long cuff is developed by dividing the hepatic veins within the parenchyma of the liver. (**c**) The veins are then opened into the caval lumen to provide the anastomotic site.*

Preparation for the portal vein anastomosis requires removal of the outflow limb of the bypass circuit. As noted earlier, this anastomosis may have to be placed at the confluence of the recipient splenic and superior mesenteric veins or, in some instances, onto a vein graft (161). Following completion of the portal vein anastomosis, we favor immediate reperfusion of the allograft by removing the cava and portal vein vascular clamps. This approach usually limits the warm ischemia interval to less than 60 minutes. The sudden bolus of cold, hyperkalemic, acidotic blood from the lower body and liver may cause pulmonary artery vasoconstriction with resultant hypotension. Prior to unclamping, therefore, the patient's hemodynamic status must be optimized by correcting hypovolemia and acid–base abnormalities and administering calcium chloride to antagonize potential hyperkalemia. As allograft function later improves, potassium supplementation may then be required, because of its uptake into revascularized hepatocytes. Reperfusion of the ischemic liver may also precipitate accelerated fibrinolysis. Aggressive replacement of coagulation factors and antifibrinolytic agent administration may be required to achieve hemostasis at this stage. Once this is accomplished and the patient is stable, the veno-venous bypass circuit is removed to prevent intraluminal clotting.

The hepatic artery reconstruction is then performed. In most patients, we prefer using a Carrell patch of donor aorta for anastomosis to the recipient's common hepatic artery proximal to the gastroduodenal take-off (Fig. 19.16). We usually preserve the recipient's gastroduodenal artery because it may provide collateral inflow in the case of subsequent celiac axis stenosis or compression at the diaphragmatic crural level (median arcuate syndrome) (162). Various donor or recipient arterial anomalies may require modifications for appropriate reconstruction, including the use of an interpositional donor iliac artery as a vascular graft from the recipient's supra celiac or infrarenal aorta (163). If the supraceliac approach is anticipated, we prefer anastomosing the donor iliac graft to the aorta before allograft implantation, which greatly facilitates the exposure of the recipient aorta. The subsequent donor hepatic artery to iliac graft anastomosis can then be easily constructed after the allograft is in place.

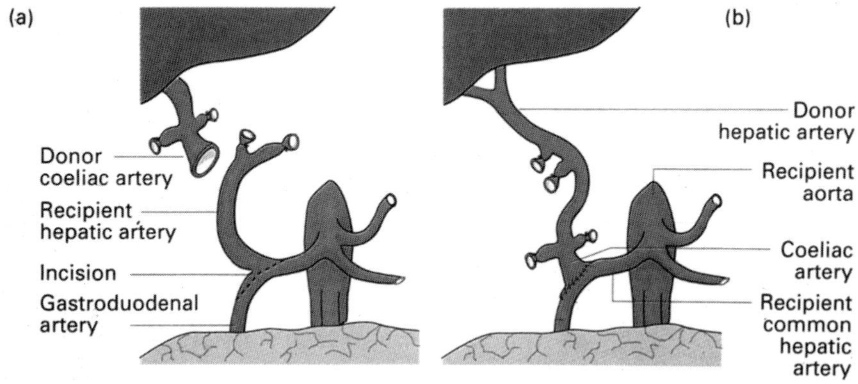

FIGURE 19.16. *(**a**) The arterial anastomosis is between donor celiac axis or Carrel patch of donor aorta to the side of the recipient common hepatic artery at, or proximal to, the origin of the gastroduodenal artery. (**b**) Completed anastomosis.*

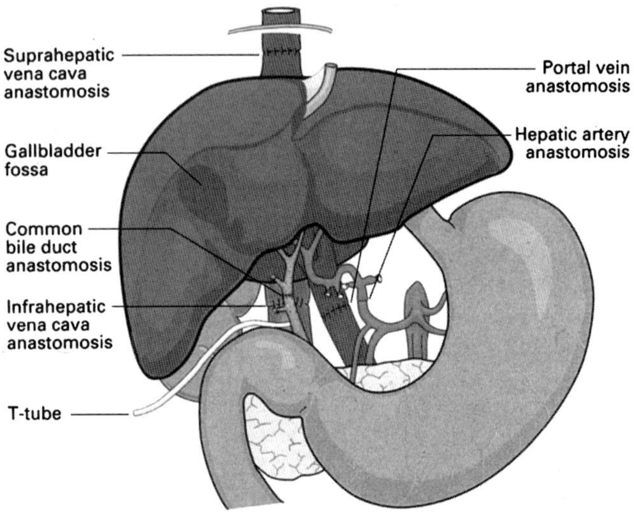

FIGURE 19.17. *Completion of the five anastomoses of orthotopic liver transplantation. The end-to-end suprahepatic vena cava, infrahepatic vena cava, and portal vein anastomoses are performed first to allow early reperfusion of the allograft. Arterial reconstruction may be to the recipient proper hepatic artery as shown here, or, more typically, to the common hepatic artery as in Figure 19.16. The biliary reconstruction is often stented with a T-tube.*

Biliary reconstruction is accomplished as the final step of allograft implantation (Fig. 19.17). End-to-end choledochocholedochostomy using interrupted absorbable suture is preferred for recipients whose native biliary tree is not diseased. In many centers, this anastomosis is routinely stented with an appropriately sized T-tube brought out through the recipient duct. Reconstruction is by choledochoenterostomy into a Roux-en-Y loop of jejunum for patients whose primary hepatic disease involved the biliary tree (e.g. biliary atresia, sclerosing cholangitis, cholangiocarcinoma). We favor stenting this anastomosis as well, using a small feeding tube brought out through the side of the Roux loop. Biliary tree stenting has the advantage of allowing postoperative radiographic studies if any question of obstruction or leak develops. Some centers have concluded that the incidence of complications from these catheters exceeds their benefits and thus recommend not using them (164,165).

Final hemostasis, placement of closed suction drains above and below the liver, and closure of the abdominal, axillary, and groin wounds complete the transplant procedure.

PARTIAL OR SPLIT LIVER TRANSPLANTATION

Because of the limited availability of suitably sized organ donors for the relatively large numbers of infants and small children with end-stage liver disease, a significant proportion of these candidates may die before transplantation can be accomplished. This problem has been addressed by developing reduced-size orthotopic liver transplantation (166). With this approach, livers from cadavers with a weight as great as 10 times that of the recipient can be successfully reduced in size and placed into pediatric recipients. Donor liver procurement is as described above. Anatomic dissection of the graft is then performed ex vivo to provide a right or left lobe or the left lateral lobe for reimplantation into smaller recipients. Growing experience with this technique has more recently progressed to in situ partition of the vascular and biliary structures during donor hepatectomy to obtain two usable allografts for transplantation into separate recipients, the so-called split liver (144). In patients receiving the right lobe (segments 1 and 4–8), recipient hepatectomy and all vascular anastomoses are performed as described above. Biliary reconstruction is via choledochoenterostomy. Recipient hepatectomy in patients receiving the left lobe (segments 2 and 3) involves mobilization of the liver from the retroperitoneum as described, except for preservation of the recipient's inferior vena cava, and suture closure of the right and accessory hepatic vein orifices. The recipient's left hepatic vein is then used for anastomosis to the allograft in piggyback fashion. The shorter lengths of donor left portal vein and hepatic artery may necessitate the use of donor vascular grafts for revascularization in the recipient.

AUXILIARY LIVER TRANSPLANTATION

Transplantation of an auxiliary liver into a heterotopic position has several theoretical advantages for patients with hepatic disorders that do not require removal of the native liver:

- The typically difficult host hepatectomy in the presence of portal hypertension and the instability that may develop during the anhepatic phase are avoided. The procedure may therefore be available for patients with multiple comorbid conditions that might contraindicate the orthotopic approach (167).
- Residual function of the retained native liver can provide temporary support during early postoperative periods of compromised allograft function.
- An auxiliary liver may provide lifesaving hepatic function for patients with acute but potentially reversible liver failure (125,168,169). If satisfactory regeneration of the native liver occurs, immunosuppression can be later withdrawn and the auxiliary graft allowed to reject.
- An auxiliary graft is fully capable of correcting liver-based inborn errors of metabolism that produce extrahepatic manifestations but no other hepatic function abnormalities (e.g., urea cycle deficiencies, Crigler-Najjar syndrome) (170).

As noted in the history of liver transplantation, long-term success rates following earlier clinical attempts at heterotopic liver transplantation were poor. More recent experience with split liver transplantation technology, however, has defined several important principles that have been adopted for more successful auxiliary liver transplantation (166). In one approach, the donor liver is prepared ex vivo by removing the left lobe and reducing the vena cava to a short segment draining the right and middle hepatic veins. Limited recipient dissection is required primarily in the portal area as would be performed for construction of a portacaval shunt. The recipient' s infrarenal aorta is exposed over a length of 3 to 4 cm. The donor's reduced-size right hepatic lobe is oriented in the recipient's right subhepatic region, with the donor vena cava overlying the recipient cava and the allograft hilum facing the aorta (Fig. 19.18). Vascular anastomoses include donor vena cava to side of recipient suprarenal vena cava; donor portal vein to side of recipient portal vein; and Carrell patch of donor aorta to side of recipient aorta. Biliary drainage is into a Roux-en-Y jejunal loop. An alternate approach entails implantation of an auxiliary allograft, consisting of segments 2 and 3, orthotopically into the space provided by resection of the recipient's left lobe (171). Venous revascularization is via donor to recipient left hepatic vein and donor to recipient left portal vein anastomoses. Arterialization is obtained by an interposition graft to the recipient's infrarenal aorta. Biliary drainage is accomplished with a Roux-en-Y jejunal loop.

Despite these improvements, success following auxiliary liver transplantation continues to be inferior to that achieved with orthotopic transplantation (166). Technical complications, particularly venous thromboses resulting from the size constraints imposed by the procedure, have been a major problem. Some patients have recovered after placement of the auxiliary allograft and have been taken off immunosuppression once there was evidence of native liver regeneration. Thus, they were able to be acutely resuscitated without the drawbacks of life-long immunosuppression. Nevertheless, since the results of auxiliary transplantation are less reliable than those for the orthotopic procedure, application of this approach continues to be limited to highly selected patients in a few centers with specialized experience.

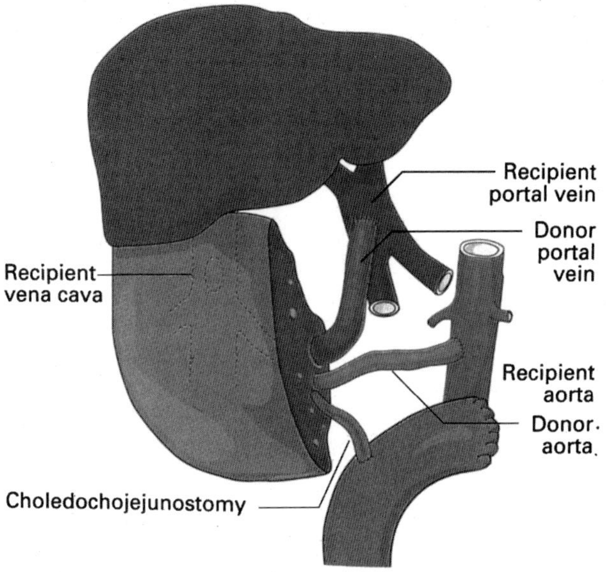

FIGURE 19.18. *Auxiliary partial liver transplantation. The donor right lobe is oriented in the subhepatic region with the hilum facing the recipient aorta. Vascular anastomoses are donor vena cava to side of recipient suprarenal vena cava, donor portal vein to side of recipient portal vein, and Carrel patch of donor aorta to side of recipient aorta. A choledochojejunostomy using a Roux-en-Y loop provides biliary drainage.*

IMMUNOSUPPRESSION FOLLOWING LIVER TRANSPLANTATION

Cyclosporine Induction Protocols

Current conventional immunosuppression for liver transplantation typically includes a combination of either cyclosporine or tacrolimus with azathioprine or mycophenolate mofetil and steroids (172). Since orally administered cyclosporine is largely excreted in the bile, induction therapy using the original Sandimmune preparation (see Chapter 6) requires intravenous cyclosporine administration during the period of external T-tube biliary drainage. Initial doses vary among centers, but a typical protocol includes intravenous (IV) cyclosporine (4–5 mg/kg/day) started on the day of surgery, with Sandimmune (10–12 mg/kg/day) added as soon as it can be tolerated orally in the early postoperative period. The intravenous therapy is discontinued once the T-tube is clamped, after which the oral cyclosporine, divided into twice daily doses, is titrated to maintain trough whole blood levels in the range of 200 to 400 ng/mL. In children, the dosage and frequency of cyclosporine administration required to provide therapeutic plasma levels are usually greater than in adults (173). The new microemulsified formulation of cyclosporine, Neoral (Sandoz Pharmaceutical, Basel, Switzerland) is less dependent on bile salts for absorption and thus obviates some of the variations associated with oral administration of the drug (174). In our experience, treatment with this formulation has provided therapeutic levels without the need for IV cyclosporine even during intervals of external bile drainage.

Steroid dosage recommendations vary tremendously among centers. In our induction protocol, methylprednisolone or prednisone is initiated at a dose of 200 mg/day and then tapered daily by 40-mg decrements to an initial maintenance level of 20 mg/day. Although some centers omit azathioprine, we typically initiate it at a loading dose of 5 mg/kg and then continue it at 1–2 mg/kg/day. Alternatively, mycophenolate mofetil at a dosage of 2 g/day may be used (see Chapter 10). The dosage of azathioprine or mycophenolate mofetil must often be reduced early on because of the neutropenia and thrombocytopenia that are common in patients with portal hypertension and its resultant hypersplenism. Some centers prefer routine initial induction therapy with an antilymphocyte antibody preparation such as antithymocyte globulin (ATG) or OKT-3 (see below and Chapter 13) so that cyclosporine administration can be avoided until stable renal function has been established. We utilize this approach only if significant early renal dysfunction has been encountered, thereby avoiding the need for antilymphocyte antibody therapy in approximately 85% of liver allograft recipients (175–177).

Maintenance

Fortunately, although high levels of immunosuppression are required initially, lower levels with time can be accepted without the risk for rejection (173). Nevertheless, for most patients, it appears to be unwise to completely withdraw cyclosporine, at least during the first several years after the transplant. In a study from the Mayo Clinic, 12 patients who had developed cyclosporine nephrotoxicity a minimum of one year after liver transplantation underwent cyclosporine withdrawal over a period of six months, while also being treated with increased dosages of steroids and a stable dosage of azathioprine (178). A slight transient improvement in renal function was noted, but half of the patients experienced rejection, including two with progressive ductopenia and, eventually, fatal sepsis.

The necessity for continuing cyclosporine therapy in most recipients was further emphasized in a study from Baylor University in which 26 patients who experienced late (more than six months after transplant) acute rejection were all found to have low cyclosporine levels (<150 ng/mL) (179). The interpretation of this report is less clear, however, since noncompliance was the most common reason for the low cyclosporine levels. Prednisone and azathioprine, therefore, may also have been discontinued by these patients. Nevertheless, these two studies, and many anecdotal reports, suggest that long-term rejection-free survival is most commonly observed in cyclosporine-treated patients if maintenance dosages of 3–5 mg/kg/day are targeted during the first several post-transplant years. This usually provides serum levels of approximately 150 ng/mL, which can be allowed to trend down to around 100 ng/mL thereafter. Occasional reports have indicated that cyclosporine, and even all immunosuppression, can be completely withdrawn from some patients 5 to 20 years after transplantation (180). Unfortunately, no reliable measures have been defined that consistently identify individual patients who have achieved such "operational tolerance." Thus, essentially all liver transplant recipients currently receive maintenance immunosuppression indefinitely.

Steroid Withdrawal

Reduction or even discontinuation of steroids, in contrast, is highly desirable in order to avoid the long-term consequences of these agents. Discontinuation of both steroids and azathioprine is possible in children, provided cyclosporine monotherapy is maintained and achieves blood levels of 200 to 250 ng/mL (181). Steroid withdrawal is also possible in adults, albeit at the cost of approximately 7% to 10% of patients experiencing acute or chronic rejection (182). We typically aim for a long-term prednisone maintenance dosage in adults of 5–10 mg/day, with further reduction or conversion to alternate-day therapy in all children and those adult patients who experience significant steroid side-effects.

Tacrolimus Protocols

Tacrolimus (FK506) was introduced clinically in 1989 initially as rescue therapy for cyclosporine-treated liver recipients who had intractable rejection or drug toxicity. The early experience indicated that it compared favorably to cyclosporine-based immunosuppression (183). Two subsequent randomized trials (see Chapter 9) revealed that FK506 provided patient and graft survival equivalent to that achieved with cyclosporine (184,185). FK506 therapy was associated with a significant reduction in acute rejection, steroid-resistant rejection, and chronic rejection. In children, the cumulative corticosteroid dose was less at each time point throughout the first year in the FK506 group (186). FK506, however, was associated with a higher incidence of nephrotoxicity and neurotoxicity. More recent experience suggests that insulin-dependent diabetes may also be more common in FK506-treated patients. On the other hand, hirsutism and gum hypertrophy, which are common complaints of patients receiving cyclosporine, are seldom observed with FK506 (186). Administration of FK506 in the early post-transplant period, like that of Neoral, is simplified by the fact that its oral absorption is reliable, even during external biliary drainage. Thus, IV administration is seldom required.

Based on these observations, many liver transplant programs have replaced cyclosporine with FK506 in their triple-drug induction and maintenance immunosuppressive therapy protocols. The initial dosage of 0.1–0.2 mg/kg/day is administered in two divided doses, aiming for therapeutic levels of 10–20 ng/mL (automated IMX assay; Abbott Diagnostics). Careful monitoring of FK506 blood levels is essential, particularly in patients with delayed liver allograft function, since they require much lower doses to achieve therapeutic whole blood concentrations and severe toxicity can be rapidly induced. Our impression is that FK506-based immunosuppression allows lower long-term steroid doses but requires careful monitoring for management of nephrotoxicity, neurotoxicity, and hyperglycemia. We do not hesitate to convert to cyclosporine if significant complications with FK506 are encountered. Conversely, we have substituted FK506 for cyclosporine in long-term recipients with hirsutism or gum hypertrophy. Thus, although the advent of FK506 has not yielded a dramatic improvement in survival rates, it has simplified early post-liver-transplant management by reducing the incidence of rejection, and it has broadened the choices of immunosuppressive agents to create greater flexibility in designing therapy for individual patients.

Antilymphocyte Induction Protocols

Antilymphocyte agents—OKT-3, ATG, antilymphocyte globulin (ALG)—are highly effective in treating acute rejection (187). Their long-term value in induction therapy has been more controversial, though nearly all studies confirm such therapy significantly delays the onset of first rejection episodes (175–177) (see Chapter 13). For this reason, antilymphocyte agents are sometimes administered to liver allograft recipients instead of cyclosporine or FK506 during the early postoperative period. By withholding these nephrotoxic agents from patients who either have pretransplant renal dysfunction or have developed acute tubular necrosis intraoperatively, the requirement for postoperative renal replacement therapy may be avoided or shortened. In these individuals, therefore, induction with antilymphocyte agents simplifies the early postoperative management. Since the benefits for other liver recipients is less obvious, many centers, including our own, reserve the use of antilymphocyte sera induction therapy for patients with clinical evidence of significant or worsening postoperative renal impairment.

Rejection Therapy

Acute rejection episodes (see section below on diagnosis of rejection) are initially treated with increased steroid dosages. For adults, we usually administer two daily 500-mg pulses of intravenous methylprednisolone. Other centers use even higher dosages. An alternative approach is an oral "steroid recycle," starting with a prednisone dosage of 100 mg twice a day, then reduced to 20 mg daily over the next five days. This avoids the costs as well as a slightly higher incidence of steroid side-effects associated with intravenous steroid therapy. If intensified steroid therapy does not produce satisfactory rejection reversal, OKT-3 monoclonal antibody or other antilymphocyte preparations are added to the regimen. FK506 can also be effective when administered as acute therapy for steroid-resistant rejection (188). Thus, patients who develop mild to moderate rejection while receiving cyclosporine may be converted to FK506 without the need for OKT-3 or additional steroid therapy.

POST-TRANSPLANT MANAGEMENT AND COMPLICATIONS

General Care

Because of their not infrequently precarious pretransplant medical condition, the prolonged operation with its attendant blood loss and fluid shifts, and the coagulopathy and hemodynamic instability that can result if adequate allograft function is delayed, most liver transplant recipients must initially be cared for in a critical care unit. Continuous monitoring is provided by electrocardiography, pulse oximetry, a pulmonary artery or central venous catheter, an arterial pressure line, and a urinary catheter. These evaluations are supplemented with serial physical and laboratory examinations and x-ray studies as indicated. Satisfactory immediate postoperative cardiac output, maintenance of adequate renal function, and correction of abnormal clotting parameters may require aggressive blood and fresh frozen plasma replacement as well as support with vasoactive drug infusions.

Cardiovascular Considerations

The usual hemodynamic profile of patients with end-stage liver disease is one of hyperdynamic circulation with systemic vasodilatation. This may result from a number of factors, including vasodilators released into the systemic circulation from the splanchnic vascular bed as a result of portasystemic shunting and the development of peripheral resistance to vasoconstrictors such as norepinephrine and angiotensin II (189). The high cardiac output and low peripheral resistance commonly persist into the early postoperative period, so that inotropic agents are rarely required in liver transplant recipients (190).

If hypotension occurs, prostaglandin E_1 (PGE_1) infusion (see Renal and Metabolic Considerations below) should be temporarily withheld until the blood pressure is corrected. The usual first therapeutic response is volume administration, which is frequently required because of the massive intraoperative fluid shifts and possible ongoing blood and ascites losses. Replacement should be guided by pulmonary artery or central venous pressures. Excessively high central venous pressures should be avoided, since transmission to the hepatic sinusoids may exacerbate allograft edema already present from reperfusion injury (190). If hypotension persists without detectable hypovolemia or apparent cardiac dysfunction, blood cultures should be drawn and empiric antibiotic therapy initiated. Although early postoperative septic shock is very rare, it may develop in several circumstances.

Perioperative infections that have previously been identified (for instance, the recipient with known liver abscesses) or are unrecognized (for example, intraoperative contamination of ascites by bile or enteric contents) may advance rapidly in an immunosuppressed and debilitated recipient. Alternatively, pathogenic organisms can be transmitted to a previously uninfected recipient from the allograft (see Chapters 15 and 36). Most cadaveric donors have received prolonged, invasive critical care prior to their progressing to brain death and organ donation. Not unexpectedly, this incurs a significant risk for bloodstream infections that may not be detected, because of the time required for the evaluation of the terminal blood cultures, until after the liver transplant procedure has been completed.

Hypertension may also develop in these patients, particularly if they are receiving intravenous cyclosporine. Because of their increased risks of cerebral edema, hemorrhage, and seizures, sustained hypertension requires aggressive treatment. Nitroprusside is often selected in the immediate postoperative period because of the rapid reversibility of its effects. Subsequent therapy may require addition of a calcium channel blocker, and/or diuretics if volume overload is present.

Pulmonary Considerations

Aggressive efforts to prevent pulmonary complications are essential in liver transplant recipients. Intensive chest physiotherapy, postural drainage, and endotracheal suctioning are routine. Flexible fiberoptic bronchoscopy may be required to remove retained secretions that cause segmental atelectasis. Right-sided pleural effusions are common in the early postoperative period. These usually respond to diuretic therapy, but thoracentesis should not be withheld if needed to provide satisfactory lung reexpansion. Even limited episodes of pulmonary dysfunction are poorly tolerated in these nutritionally depleted, debilitated, immunosuppressed patients. Attempted weaning from assisted ventilation is begun as soon as the recipient recovers from anesthesia and demonstrates cough reflexes. If initial oxygenation and ventilation mechanics are satisfactory, successful extubation can be accomplished usually within 12 to 48 hours. Several unusual factors unique to liver allograft recipients may delay weaning. These include right diaphragmatic paralysis, which may result from the intraoperative placement of the suprahepatic vascular clamp, and the development of metabolic alkalosis. Because the latter may contribute to compensatory hypoventilation, correction with potassium chloride, or rarely hydrochloric acid, may be necessary to allow successful early extubation (see also Chapter 28).

Significant hypoxemia resulting from intrapulmonary shunting in patients with chronic liver disease persists to varying degrees into the early postoperative period. Although the prognosis for such patients is somewhat less favorable, such shunting, even advanced to the stage of digital clubbing, has been observed to reverse following successful liver transplantation.

Hepatobiliary Considerations

Satisfactory liver allograft function is manifested by the appearance of deeply pigmented bile in the drainage catheter and early correction of coagulopathy. These recipients will typically have good renal function and will recover rapidly from anesthesia so that successful extubation is possible within 12 to 48 hours. If, in contrast, there is minimal or watery, depigmented biliary output ("white bile"), allograft dysfunction and a complicated early postoperative course can be anticipated (Fig. 19.19). These recipients will require assisted ventilation, intensive infusion of fresh frozen plasma, and other complex resuscitative measures before adequate stabilization is achieved. In 5% to 10% of these

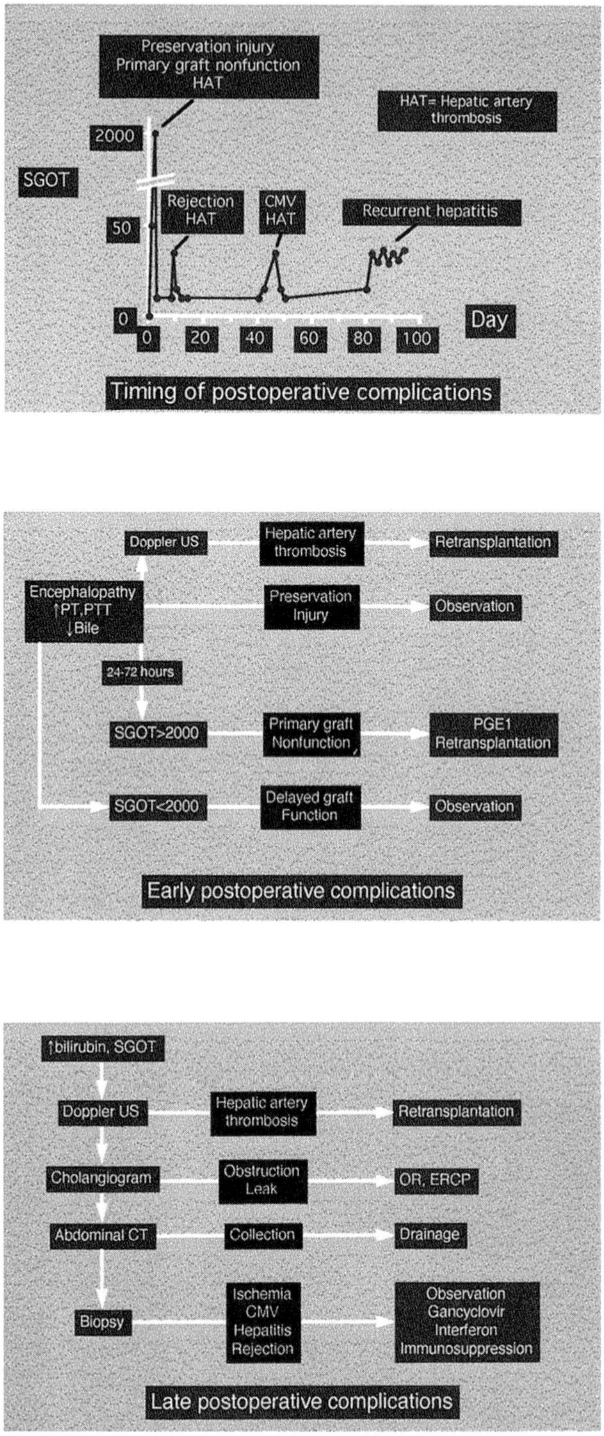

FIGURE 19.19. *Postoperative hepatobiliary complications. Any process that injures allograft hepatocytes will result in an elevated SGOT level* (top)*. The donor allograft quality and subsequent preservation injury dominates the workup of early allograft dysfunction* (middle)*. Hepatic artery thrombosis (HAT), which can present anytime in the postoperative course, can be detected by Doppler ultrasound. Hyperbilirubinemia* (bottom)*, which may indicate bile duct obstruction or leak, possibly resulting from HAT, can be worked up with biliary imaging. If radiographic studies are unremarkable, a biopsy may be required to differentiate between rejection and viral infection.*

recipients, irreversible primary nonfunction is suggested by the protean signs of liver failure (Table 19.18). Primary nonfunction may result from technically inadequate revascularization, but it is most commonly associated with donor characteristics such as obesity, ante mortem hypoxia and hypotension, and hepatic steatosis and with preservation factors such as prolonged warm or cold ischemic times (see Table 19.17). Retransplantation is the only recourse for these patients.

Table 19.18. Indicators of Poor Allograft Function

Mental status	Persistent encephalopathy
Bile production	Clear watery bile, <30 cc /day
Synthetic function	Persistent coagulopathy
Metabolic function	Lactic acidosis, hypoglycemia No bicarbonate production from intraoperative citrate infusion with blood products
Hepatocellular injury	Rising transaminase for >48 hours, peak >2000
Renal function	Low urine output despite rehydration
Thermoregulation	Persistent postoperative hypothermia

Timely identification of the recipients with irreversible allograft ischemic injury is critical if retransplantation is to be successfully accomplished before fatal cerebral edema develops. As in the pretransplant candidate with fulminant hepatic failure, uncorrectable coagulopathy (prothrombin time over 20 seconds), hypoglycemia, acidosis, and new onset of renal failure are ominous. These findings should usually prompt the urgent search for a second allograft.

Postoperative technical complications most commonly include persistent intra-abdominal bleeding, vascular thrombosis, biliary duct problems, or infected fluid collections. The incidence of postoperative bleeding is directly related to the severity of intraoperative bleeding and the quality of immediate allograft function. Despite meticulous surgical technique and apparent hemostasis in the operating room, diffuse capillary oozing may persist until hypothermia and inadequate plasma clotting factor levels have been corrected. If major blood loss persists despite reversal of the coagulopathy, semi-urgent reexploration is indicated to identify a probable surgically correctable cause. In patients whose early bleeding ceases, laparotomy is still usually required 24 to 48 hours after the initial surgery in order to evacuate perihepatic collections that may otherwise become secondarily infected. Such abdominal decompression may also improve renal function by relieving elevated intra-abdominal pressures that impede renal venous outflow typically at pressures greater than 20 to 30 mm Hg (191).

Hepatic artery thrombosis occurs in 2% to 10% of adult liver transplant recipients (162). The key to the pathophysiology of this complication is the biliary tree's unique blood supply (Fig. 19.20). In contrast to the liver parenchyma,

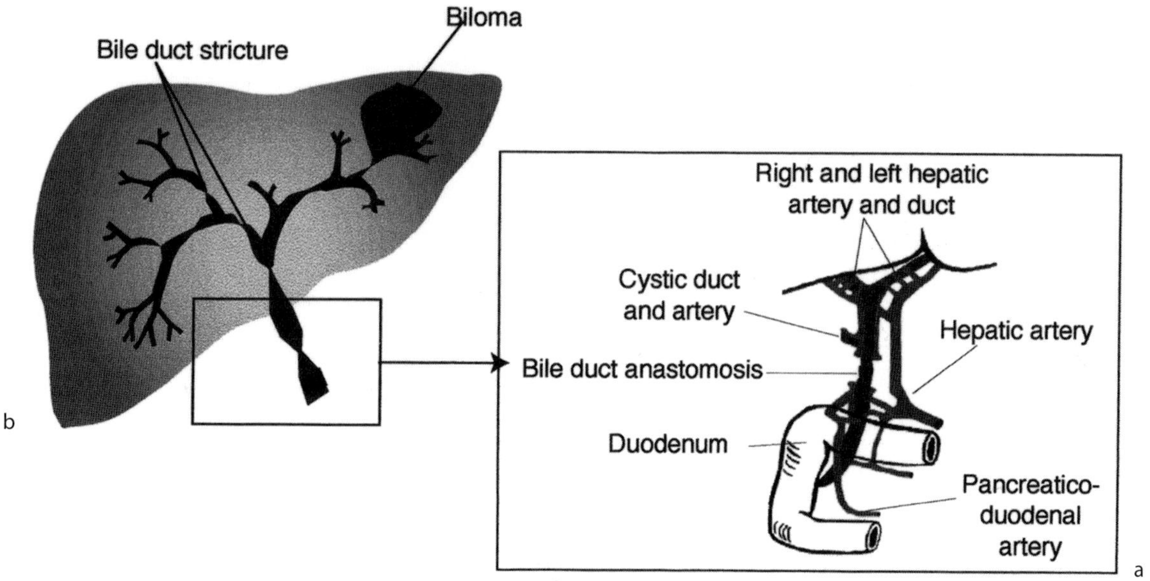

FIGURE 19.20. *Biliary blood supply after transplantation. In contrast to the liver parenchyma, which has a dual portal and arterial blood supply, the biliary tree depends almost entirely on arterial blood. (**a**) Until collateral circulation is reestablished, the allograft bile duct is completely dependent on hepatic artery blood supply. (**b**) This explains the frequent presentation of hepatic artery thrombosis as bile leaks, biliary strictures, or intrahepatic bilomas. Areas of biliary stasis may become infected, resulting in fevers and/or abscesses.*

which has a dual blood supply, the biliary tree depends almost entirely on the hepatic artery (192). This explains the frequent presentation of hepatic artery thrombosis as bile leaks, biliary strictures, or intrahepatic bilomas (193). These biliary abnormalities lead to bile stasis and bacterial overgrowth. Thus, sepsis is common following hepatic artery thrombosis, making this complication a likely diagnosis in liver transplant recipients presenting with relapsing bacteremia or fever of unknown origin. Interestingly, even though some patients present with fulminant hepatic necrosis, hepatic artery thrombosis may be completely asymptomatic in others, presumably because of development of compensatory collateral circulation.

Doppler ultrasound is the first step in establishing the diagnosis of vascular thrombosis, which is then confirmed by angiography. If the clinical presentation is one of fulminant liver failure or relapsing bacteremia, emergent retransplantation is the only viable therapy. The small proportion of patients who develop only mild liver dysfunction without abscess formation or minor biliary leaks, may be conservatively managed while arterial collaterals to the allograft develop. Some groups have successfully rearterialized the allograft either by surgical reconstruction (194) or by percutaneous angiographic techniques. Endoscopic balloon dilatation and placement of metallic stents has also been employed to manage biliary strictures in patients with otherwise satisfactory allograft function despite arterial thrombosis (195).

The presenting symptoms of portal vein thrombosis are usually less devastating. Rarely, in the immediate postoperative period, this complication can produce severe biochemical abnormalities and even hepatic necrosis requiring retransplantation. More commonly, portal vein thrombosis is suggested by recurrent variceal bleeding, new onset ascites, or an unexplained elevation in prothrombin time. Successful management of this complication in patients without severe hepatic dysfunction is usually achieved by operative thrombectomy and correction of any technical abnormality encountered. In the late post-transplant period, a splenorenal shunt may be required.

Vena caval thrombosis is even more rare. If the thrombosis is limited to the infrahepatic cava, the clinical presentation is usually lower extremity edema, and rarely renal dysfunction, which gradually resolves with anticoagulant therapy and development of collateral venous return. If thrombosis extends to the suprahepatic cava, this complication may present as a Budd-Chiari syndrome, which usually requires retransplantation for management.

Bile duct complications, which historically were the Achilles heel of the operation, have greatly decreased in frequency since current reconstructive techniques became standardized. Many centers recommend the use of a feeding or T-tube stent across the anastomosis to provide access for investigation of suspected biliary tract complications and possibly to limit development of late anastomotic strictures. Anastomotic leak, usually manifested by appearance of bile in the abdominal drainage or an unexplained rise in serum bilirubin, occurs during the first several weeks after transplantation. Minimal, well-drained leaks not associated with hepatic artery thrombosis will typically close spontaneously. More extensive bile collections require open drainage to create a controlled fistula or even resection and reanastomosis. Significant leaks secondary to arterial thrombosis must often be managed by retransplantation. Obstruction at the anastomotic site usually occurs in the later postoperative period, since the anastomoses are usually stented for several months following surgery. Short strictures can be dilated via endoscopic or percutaneous approaches (196). Surgical resection of the anastomosis and conversion to choledochojejunostomy may be required for more extensive lesions. Earlier observations of diffuse obstruction by "sludge" within the biliary tree are now seldom encountered. Control of this complication is apparently provided by careful biliary flushing during the donor procedure and improved methods of reconstruction. An interesting and unusual cause of obstruction has been the development of a tension mucocele in a donor cystic duct remnant that shared a common wall with the bile duct, a phenomenon analogous to the Mirizzi syndrome (bile duct obstruction by a cystic duct stone).

Approximately 10% of patients develop bile peritonitis when the T-tube is removed, even as late as six months after transplant. This complication is usually managed with endoscopic placement of an internal stent across the leaking choledochal defect through which the T-tube had exited. Because of this complication, some centers have discontinued the routine use of biliary tree stenting at the time of transplantation (164,165).

Renal and Metabolic Considerations

Most liver allograft recipients develop at least mild postoperative renal dysfunction (197). Contributing to this complication may be preexisting renal insufficiency, intraoperative vena caval occlusion, or significant bleeding and hypotension, postimplantation hepatic allograft dysfunction, and administration of nephrotoxic drugs. In patients whose renal dysfunction progresses to the need for dialysis, mortality rates may be as great as 90% (198,199). Thus, every effort must be made to identify and avoid, whenever possible, those factors that exacerbate post-transplant renal failure.

Preoperative renal function has been found to be one of the most important determinants. Recipients whose pretransplant creatinine was chronically greater than 1.5 mg/dL have an increased likelihood of acute tubular necrosis (ATN) and lower survival rates following liver transplantation. On the other hand, extensive experience has established that, in the presence of satisfactory hepatic allograft function, renal function recovers in patients with pretransplant acute renal failure that resulted from hepatorenal syndrome. These observations suggest that:

- Chronic renal dysfunction is a relative contraindication to liver transplantation.
- High-risk donors should not be considered in patients with marginal preoperative renal function.
- Intraoperative veno-venous bypass or the piggyback approach to vena caval revascularization should probably be used more commonly in patients with marginal renal function, since this may decrease the severity of the postoperative renal failure.

Various medications, including cyclosporine and FK506 (especially when administered parenterally) are major contributors to postoperative renal dysfunction. Both agents cause afferent renal arteriolar constriction, leading to a reduction in cortical perfusion. The exact mechanisms involved are poorly defined, but appear to include a decrease in vasodilatory prostaglandin production (199). This may explain the observation that perioperative PGE_1 infusion led to a significant decrease in renal dysfunction and a trend toward improved survival (200). Based on these considerations, many centers now routinely administer PGE_1 at a dosage of 0.6 μg/kg/hr to liver recipients during the early postoperative period. Some have also advocated low-dose dopamine for its theoretical, though unproved, beneficial effect on renal perfusion (201). Other drugs that increase the nephrotoxic effects of cyclosporine and FK506, for example the aminoglycoside antibiotics, should be avoided, if possible, in these recipients.

If postoperative oliguria persists despite optimized hemodynamics and adequate diuretic trials, we attempt to limit the period of dysfunction by substituting OKT-3 monoclonal antibody for FK506 or cyclosporine. With this approach, dialysis, and its attendant morbidity, is usually avoided, albeit at the cost of using early in the postoperative course a major weapon that could be required later for resistant rejection. If despite these measures dialysis is indicated, we prefer continuous veno-venous hemofiltration, which usually provides greater hemodynamic stability.

Most liver transplant recipients are substantially fluid overloaded (often as much as 10 to 30 kg) above their baseline weight. To help mobilize this excess fluid, diuretics are frequently required during the first postoperative weeks. Early in the postoperative course, priority should be given to maximizing intravascular volume, reserving diuretics for oliguria that does not respond to volume repletion. The role of albumin repletion in hypoalbuminemic, fluid-overloaded liver transplant recipients, though it is widely used, remains controversial. Evidence suggesting that albumin infusions may be beneficial for mobilization of excess body water in patients with borderline renal function includes:

- Patients with uncorrected hypoalbuminemia have a higher mortality (admittedly, the low albumin may be a marker of a high risk, rather than a direct cause, of mortality) (202).
- Albumin is required for the delivery of diuretics to the kidneys.
- Hypoalbuminemia increases bowel edema, which prolongs postoperative ileus and may impair the absorption of immunosuppressive medications.

We therefore favor attempting to keep the serum albumin level above 2.5 g/dL, using either fresh frozen plasma in the presence of a coagulopathy, 5% albumin if additional water is needed, or 25% salt-poor albumin. We do not, however, recommend albumin as a nutritional supplement (see Nutritional Considerations below).

In addition to uremia, other major metabolic derangements that may require correction in the early postoperative period include hypothermia; hyperkalemia, especially in the presence of poor hepatic and renal function; hypocalcemia; metabolic alkalosis; and hypomagnesemia and hypophosphatemia, because of suddenly increased cell metabolism and protein synthesis.

Hematologic Considerations

Leukopenia and thrombocytopenia secondary to hypersplenism typically persist into the postoperative period. The leukopenia is usually of no clinical consequence, although the azathioprine or mycophenolate mofetil dosage may have to be reduced. If the white blood cell count falls below $1500/mm^3$, we favor administering granulocyte colony stimulating factor (GCSF). This may decrease the incidence of postoperative infections. Prolonged thrombocytopenia may require platelet transfusions and similar reductions in drug dosages. These consequences of hypersplenism can be anticipated to gradually resolve over the first few weeks after successful liver transplantation.

We favor maintaining the hematocrit in the range of 25% to 30% during the immediate postoperative period, since higher values may be associated with hepatic artery thrombosis. Hemolysis, at times requiring transfusion, may occur one to two weeks postoperatively. As noted earlier, this most commonly occurs in recipients of an ABO-compatible, but nonidentical, allograft (e.g., blood group O donor to an A recipient) and results from antirecipient isohemagglutinins produced within the graft (142).

Occasionally, patients who received a liver transplant for the treatment of acute non-A, non-B viral hepatitis have developed aplastic anemia. The onset of the aplasia has usually been within one to six months following transplantation and development of subsequent fatal infection has been frequent. Some patients have had recovery of marrow function either spontaneously or following ATG therapy, but the most effective therapeutic approach has not been defined.

Nutritional Considerations

Most liver transplant recipients can be extubated within 12 to 48 hours, tolerate sips by 24 to 72 hours, and can be advanced to a regular diet a few days thereafter (feeding is resumed more cautiously in patients with a Roux-en-Y jejuno-jejunostomy). In these individuals, monitoring caloric and protein intake and adding oral supplements as needed is sufficient to replete preoperative losses and provide for the increased postoperative requirement. The goal in the early postoperative period is to increase the caloric intake to 10% to 20% above baseline requirements and to provide 1.3–2.0 g/kg/day of protein. After the patient recovers, this is reduced back to baseline caloric intake and 1 g/kg/day of protein. Over the longer term, obesity becomes a common nutritional problem [43% of recipients in one study (203)], perhaps because of steroids and the patient's new-found well-being. Careful dietary and exercise counseling, plus medical treatment of hyperlipidemia, then become cornerstones of nutritional management.

More aggressive nutritional repletion may be required in liver transplant recipients who have been chronically malnourished by prolonged preoperative hospitalizations. Little muscle reserve may remain in these patients, who will predictably experience a longer, more complicated, and more expensive postoperative recovery. Although the exact role of malnutrition in these outcomes is unclear, it is likely to increase morbidity by delaying wound healing and reducing resistance to infection. (Conversely, malnourished and debilitated patients probably require lower levels of immunosuppression.) In this subgroup of patients, early postoperative tube feedings, within 12 to 24 hours after transplantation, is an appropriate approach. One group has suggested that this practice may be beneficial for most recipients (204).

As in other critically ill patients, enteric feeding is the preferred route for nutritional support following liver transplantation. Numerous studies have emphasized that enteral nutrition not only has beneficial effects for the gut but also is likely to improve the immune function of distant organs as well, thereby reducing the risks of infection (205). If the need for postoperative tube feedings is anticipated, a nasoenteric tube may be inserted intraoperatively and gently advanced by the surgeon into the distal duodenum or proximal jejunum. Percutaneous jejunostomy or gastrostomy tubes are usually avoided because of their associated high complication rate in immunosuppressed patients.

Patients who have persistent allograft dysfunction present further nutritional challenges, since hepatic failure compromises the metabolism of glucose, fat, and protein. The intolerance to protein is a particular limitation, since protein is essential for hepatic regeneration and tissue repair. To provide sufficient protein without precipitating unacceptable encephalopathy, formulations with low aromatic amino acid and high branched-chain amino acid concentrations have been proposed, although this practice remains controversial (204). Even if only minimal protein loads can be tolerated, caloric needs should be generously supplied, keeping in mind, however, that overfeeding may increase ventilatory needs and produce cholestasis. Hyperglycemia in these patients, which is further exacerbated by FK506 or cyclosporine administration, is generally controlled by insulin administration but may require lowering of the carbohydrate-to-fat calorie ratio.

Neurologic and Psychiatric Considerations

Neuropsychiatric events complicate the postoperative course in 8% to 47% of liver transplant recipients. Identified etiologic factors include preexisting encephalopathy, cerebral edema, electrolyte disturbances, cyclosporine or FK506 toxicity, sleep deprivation, and intraoperative air embolism (now rarely encountered as the importance of flushing the liver prior to reperfusion has been recognized). Persistent postoperative coma most commonly indicates impaired allograft function and the possible need for retransplantation (see Hepatobiliary Considerations above). Persistent obtundation or expressive aphasia, despite good allograft function, is most commonly encountered in patients with Laennec's cirrhosis. This may be due to the cerebral atrophy that results from prolonged alcohol use (206). Rarely, impaired consciousness due to thalamic damage may accompany fluctuations in serum sodium concentrations that produce central pontine myelinolysis. The computerized tomography (CT) scan findings may be unrevealing, but magnetic resonance imaging (MRI) usually reveals the characteristic pontine trident or "bat-wing" shape (206). Management of recipients with neurologic dysfunction presenting as obtundation includes airway protection, correction of identifiable metabolic abnormalities, minimizing cyclosporine or FK506 dosages, and limited use of sedatives and narcotic analgesics. Only small doses of analgesics should be administered initially, preferably using short-acting agents that do not require hepatic metabolism (e.g., Fentanyl). Benzodiazepines are avoided because their long-lasting effects cannot be easily reversed. In contrast, patients with restlessness, irritability, and disordered thinking due to sleep deprivation require appropriate night-time sedation plus limitation of frequent nocturnal nursing interventions to reverse the disorder.

Persistently comatose liver transplant recipients will often blink, move limbs, grimace, smile, and grunt, all without clear evidence of awareness. If brain stem reflexes are absent, the possibility of intraoperative brain death secondary to cerebral edema or intracranial bleeding must be assessed by emergency CT scan and electroencephalogram (EEG). Some patients may appear comatose because motor and reflex activity is absent, but have unmistakable communication through eye movements. This "locked-in syndrome," which may be prolonged, is thought to result from interaction of muscle relaxants with such agents as clindamycin, metronidazole, tetracycline, furosemide, corticosteroids, aminoglycosides, and most antiarrhythmics (206).

Seizure activity is a common neurologic complication following liver transplantation, usually occurring within two weeks of the operation (see also Chapter 33). High blood levels of cyclosporine and FK506 are clearly contributing factors, as are hypocholesterolemia and electrolyte abnormalities such as hyponatremia, hypocalcemia, and hypomagnesemia. Some antibiotics, for example imipenem, also lower the seizure threshold (207). In patients with recurrent seizures, cyclosporine or FK506 may be replaced with an antilymphocyte preparation until the patient stabilizes. Acute treatment for seizures is usually with diazepam or phenobarbitol. Tegretol therapy is generally satisfactory for chronic prophylaxis. We try to avoid the prolonged use of phenobarbitol or dilantin because of the induction of P450 microsomal enzymes that rapidly decrease the blood concentrations of immunosuppressive agents.

Physical Therapy Considerations

Debilitated liver transplant recipients are at high risk for ventilatory insufficiency and postoperative pneumonia. If early ambulation is not possible, continuous lateral rotation beds will decrease respiratory tract infections (208). As soon as the patient is extubated, even if some evidence of confusion persists, aggressive physical therapy is essential to promote early resumption of ambulation and effective pulmonary toilet. Subsequent rehabilitation may require assistive devices for return of complete mobility of limbs that may have become disabled by gout, arthritis, or limb pain (209). Not surprisingly, successfully rehabilitated patients without pain, weakness, or arthritis are 7.8 times more likely to be employed following transplantation (210).

Acute and Chronic Rejection

Despite induction immunosuppressive therapy, 40% to 60% of liver allograft recipients suffer one or more acute rejection episodes, usually first encountered about one week postoperatively. The biochemical and clinical criteria suggesting acute rejection are summarized in Table 19.19. Evidence of rejection presenting between day 5 and day 14 after transplantation is evaluated by radiologic studies to exclude technical complications and usually does not require biopsy confirmation, since this is too early for manifestations of viral hepatitis. Steroid pulse therapy (see Rejection Therapy above) is usually effective. If allograft dysfunction persists and intensified immunosuppression with antilymphocyte therapy is contemplated, we usually recommend biopsy confirmation of the diagnosis.

Histopathologic findings of acute rejection include mononuclear cell infiltrates of portal tracts, subendothelial cells invading portal or central veins, cholestasis, bile duct damage, and variable hepatocellular necrosis (Fig. 19.21 and Plate 11). With more chronic rejection, manifested clinically by cholestatic jaundice, the hepatic artery intima is infiltrated by foamy macrophages that may produce narrowing of the vessel lumen (Fig. 19.22 and Plate 12). Interlobular bile ducts are often reduced in number, and excess fibrosis appears in portal tracts. Unfortunately, many of these biopsy findings can also result from other conditions including cholangitis and viral hepatitis. Thus, the ultimate diagnosis must take into consideration the full constellation of clinical, biochemical, and histopathologic findings, lest overtreatment of multiple suspected but unconfirmed rejection episodes expose the patient to unacceptable risks of infection.

Post-transplant Viral Hepatitis

As with all immunocompromised individuals, cytomegalovirus (CMV) is commonly observed in liver transplant recipients. The severity of the clinical syndrome produced by CMV infection is a function of recipient and donor

Table 19.19. Indicators of Hepatic Allograft Rejection

Clinical
Fever
Right upper quadrant pain, back pain, anorexia, ascites
Decreased bile output and bile pigment
Biochemical
Elevated serum bilirubin
Elevated transaminase
Elevated alkaline phosphatase
Elevated WBC, eosinophilia
Cholangiogram
No leak
No obstruction
Doppler ultrasound
No collection
No ductal dilatation
Patent vessels
Biopsy
Portal inflammation
Hepatocellular necrosis
Endotheliitis

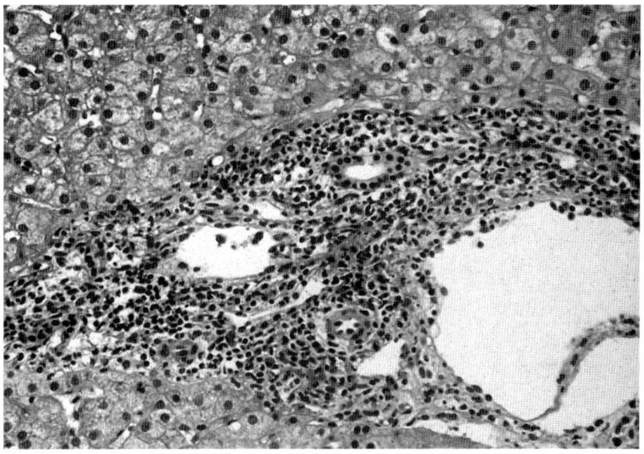

FIGURE 19.21. *Acute cellular rejection. A mixed cellular infiltrate is characteristically seen in the portal tract (portal vein at right of specimen). Such nondestructive lesions are typically reversible.*

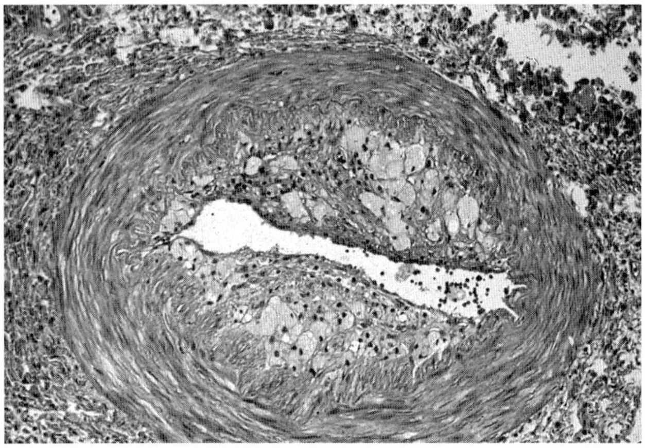

FIGURE 19.22. *Chronic liver allograft rejection. Note artery with severe fibrous intimal thickening and lipid-containing foam cells in the thickened intima.*

serologic status and the amount and type of immunosuppression to which the recipient has been exposed (see Chapter 36). Most CMV infections become evident between the third and eighth postoperative weeks. Disseminated, or extrahepatic, CMV disease is confirmed by positive CMV antigenemia in the presence of typical clinical findings (pneumonia, leukopenia, GI complaints) or histopathologic findings (lung or bowel biopsy). CMV disease in the liver allograft may produce biochemical and clinical findings that resemble those of rejection. Distinguishing between the two is crucial and relies upon blood tests, including CMV antigenemia, to confirm or exclude the presence of active CMV infection. A liver biopsy will almost always be required to exclude coexisting rejection, since active CMV infection may actually precipitate rejection by upregulating MHC receptors on hepatocytes. Typical histopathologic findings of CMV hepatitis are necrotic hepatocytes, with nuclear or cytoplasmic inclusions, scattered throughout the lobule and surrounded by neutrophils (microabscesses) or macrophages and lymphocytes (microgranulomas) (211). The histopathologic presence of CMV can be confirmed with CMV DNA probes. CMV infection, fortunately, is almost always responsive to ganciclovir therapy. Like CMV, other viruses in the herpes family including herpes simplex virus and Epstein-Barr virus may also cause hepatitis, although rarely as an isolated manifestation of the infection.

As discussed previously, many liver allograft recipients whose underlying disease was caused by HBV or HCV experience post-transplant reinfection. Recurrent HBV or HCV hepatitis typically induces biochemical abnormalities that are difficult to distinguish from rejection, so that frequent biopsies are required for these patients as well. Whereas the histopathology of rejection is typically an inflammatory injury involving portal structures, viral hepatitis is more focused on the lobule with resultant spotty hepatocyte necrosis (211). Occasionally, viral hepatitis may also be associated with varying degrees of portal inflammation that can more closely mimic the findings of acute rejection. Again, therefore, the ultimate diagnosis must take into consideration the other clinical findings and may necessitate an empiric trial of rejection therapy.

Long-Term Management

We have found that a flow sheet that details pertinent clinical observations, sequential laboratory values, medication changes, and radiologic and biopsy studies is extremely useful for the long-term management of these complex patients. During their early outpatient course, patients are typically followed with biweekly laboratory checks and weekly visits to the transplant center clinic. Assuming routine recovery, the interclinic visit interval is progressively extended so that by one year, patients are examined only every four months, usually alternating visits with their local physician. We recommend a blood check one or two weeks following any change in the immunosuppressive regimen and more frequent monitoring during attempted steroid withdrawal.

Every outpatient visit must focus on three issues directly related to the liver allograft:

Hepatic function. The significance of any laboratory abnormality must be established by further investigations.

Immunosuppression. Dosage of each agent should be reviewed in terms of routine weaning and current side-effects, particularly progressive renal failure (212).

Nonimmunosuppressive medications. Transplant patients frequently have long lists of medications that should constantly be re-evaluated and simplified. This practice will avoid potentially catastrophic and sometimes unpredictable drug interactions. For example, while H2 blockers and antacids are routinely administered to control gastric hyperactivity, sucralfate is avoided because it inhibits cyclosporine and FK506 absorption by binding these agents in the stomach. Addition of medications, particularly erythromycin or antifungals like fluconazole, increase FK506 or cyclosporine blood levels and may precipitate acute toxicity. Synergistic toxicities should also be considered; a typical example occurs with imipenem, which can lower the seizure threshold in patients receiving FK506 or cyclosporine. While these examples apply to all transplant patients, liver recipients present a further pharmacologic challenge, since the half-life of drugs cleared by the liver may be variably prolonged by delayed allograft function.

In addition to the allograft related issues, a number of common post-transplant conditions, many of which may be addressed by the patient's primary physician, are serially monitored:

Hypertension. Treatment may include calcium channel blockers (e.g., diltiazem), vasodilators (e.g., hydralazine), or reduced dosages of immunosuppressive agents (e.g., cyclosporine, steroids).

Hyperglycemia. Lowering the dosage of FK506, cyclosporine, or steroids; substituting cyclosporine for FK506; diet; and weight loss are all helpful. An oral hypoglycemic agent may be sufficient for glycemic control, but insulin is frequently required.

Weight gain. This common problem requires constant efforts for control with careful education, repeated dietary counseling, and an emphasis on early return to an adequate exercise program.

Hypercholesterolemia. This should be treated aggressively, especially in transplant patients, because of frequent concomitant cardiovascular risk factors.

Gout. Cyclosporine, FK506, and some diuretics such as furosemide all tend to elevate uric acid levels that may precipitate gouty attacks. Treatment includes colchicine and allopurinol, but precautions peculiar to transplant recipients should be kept in mind. For example, since colchicine often causes diarrhea, its administration may impede the absorption of immunosuppressive medications. Additionally, allopurinol has synergistic bone marrow toxicity with azathioprine. Thus, the previously tolerated azathioprine dosage in these patients should be reduced by at least 50% when initiating allopurinol therapy, and the white blood count must be followed carefully.

Routine health maintenance. Mammograms, Pap smears, and careful skin exams, for example, should be carefully monitored (see Chapter 37).

Nursing and Paramedical Team

Most centers have specially trained nurses and paramedical personnel to coordinate each stage of liver transplantation. The initial evaluation of potential candidates for liver transplantation typically involves an extensive diagnostic work-up, multiple referrals to consultants, and general health screening. If the patient is hospitalized for treatment of a complication of hepatic failure, the work-up can be conveniently performed during that visit. Typically, however, cost-containment pressures lead to an outpatient work-up, usually with many of the studies carried out in the patient's local hospital. The pretransplant nurse coordinator is crucial in scheduling these consultations and tests and in following up on their findings. Because this work-up requires frequent communication with the patient, the coordinator becomes the patient's natural source of information and support and often introduces the patient to the complexities of transplantation and immunosuppression with pamphlets and discussions. When the patient's candidacy is confirmed and the patient is placed on the wait-list, the coordinator continues to follow the patient's course, alert to any deterioration that may indicate the need for more urgent transplantation or to developments that would temporarily contraindicate transplantation (e.g., intercurrent infection).

Coordination by specially trained individuals is obviously also required for the complex organ donation process. In hospitals where families of brain-dead patients are routinely approached by trained organ bank coordinators, procurement rates are usually high and grieving families typically report the donation event to be a positive experience despite the obviously tragic circumstance. Once a potential donor is identified, the organ bank coordinator gathers information to allow the transplant surgeon to consider suitability for liver transplantation. Usually, this coordinator also assumes responsibility for bed-side management of the patient after brain death is established, maintaining the hemodynamic stability essential to prevent damage to the potential allografts.

Although liver transplantation is comparable to other major vascular or trauma surgery procedures, the addition of multiple support devices (veno-venous bypass, autotransfusion, rapid infusion, argon beam coagulator, etc.) requires special skills for the operating room team. Many transplant centers, therefore, include specially trained nurses for setting up a compact and functionally efficient operating room and assisting at the surgical procedure.

Postoperatively, liver transplant recipients are typically cared for in specialized units with nurses skilled in both intensive and chronic care. The transplant nurse is often the most accessible caregiver for both the patient and their families, who may be overwhelmed by the complexity of the process (213). A well-informed, sympathetic nurse can help provide information about the transplant procedure, its complications, and immunosuppression with its side-effects. Most centers also have dedicated clinic nurses who coordinate long-term outpatient care. This continuity of care, with a strong emphasis on patient teaching, plays an important role in improving long-term outcome and ensuring compliance with complex medical regimens.

OUTCOME, QUALITY OF LIFE, AND COSTS

Current overall survival rates after liver transplantation are approximately 80% at one year and 73% at three years (1). Thus, the expected long-term survival for these previously untreatable patients now exceeds that provided by modern care for many other commonly encountered conditions, including myocardial infarction and most solid tumors. The majority of deaths occur in the first three months after liver transplantation, with early graft dysfunction or infection being the most common causes of failure. Because of the relatively recent development of liver transplantation, precise survival expectations beyond five years have not yet been established, although death in patients who survived at least five years after transplantation has occurred only rarely. Furthermore, some patients from the earlier experience have now survived for nearly 30 years. This suggests that the prognosis for the approximately two-thirds of recipients currently expected to survive five years is indeed excellent (214).

Nearly complete rehabilitation can be anticipated in the majority of surviving patients, with demonstrable improvements across all health and psychosocial scales (215). Adult recipients are often able to return to a productive place in society. In one study, only 18% of recipients considered themselves not well enough to work (210). Of the remainder, 57% were employed, and the others reported they had taken early retirement (8%), returned to school (3%), could not find work (3%), chose not to work (3%), or were unemployed for family reasons (3%). Not surprisingly, older recipients and those who were continuously out of work for several years before transplantation were the least likely to return to gainful employment after liver transplantation.

Rehabilitation in some patients may be significantly delayed by the complication of osteoporosis, which is common in chronic liver disease (216). Patients at high risk include those with evidence of hypogonadism, overt calcium malabsorption, previous steroid therapy, and cholestatic liver disease (particularly primary biliary cirrhosis). Despite successful transplantation, severe preoperative osteopenia still may progress to compression fractures, back pain, and prolonged disability. Fortunately, this condition generally stabilizes within three to six months following transplantation, again emphasizing the importance of the timely consideration of liver replacement before such secondary complications become too advanced. Other barriers to complete rehabilitation are related to immunosuppression, including nephrotoxicity and hypertension associated with currently used agents, the development of recurrent or de novo malignancies, and chronic rejection requiring retransplantation.

Now that reasonable long-term survival and rehabilitation following liver transplantation have been established, cost-effectiveness issues have engendered increased interest. The average cost of a liver transplant has been estimated to be between US$100,000 and US$200,000. In comparison, the costs of withholding liver transplantation are not insignificant. Chronically ill patients with advanced liver disease incur the costs of income loss, medications, hospitalizations, palliative surgical procedures, and, predictably, terminal care. Interestingly, while expenditures for chronic illness have progressively increased as palliative technology improves, the cost of liver transplantation has actually decreased as improvements in management are defined. For instance, one hospital reduced inpatient organ procurement and physician charges for the transplant hospitalization from $154,000 in 1991–1992 to $103,000 in 1993–1995 (217). These savings were achieved mainly by reducing length of stay, without sacrificing outcome and quality of care. Another group found that the routine use of PGE_1 may save as much as $50,000 for some liver transplants by shortening the duration of intensive care (218). It is also likely that continued improvements in immunosuppression management can result in long-term savings. Thus, although FK506 and cyclosporine-based immunosuppressive regimens provide similar survival rates, FK506 may save an average of $19,290 in the first year because these patients experience fewer rejection episodes (219). In another example, some centers have recommended routine administration of ketoconazole because its effect on cyclosporine metabolism reduces the dosage needed to maintain target levels by 62% at one week and by 80% at one year (220). This can provide savings of $5200 in the first year and $3920 in each subsequent year (inclusive of the cost of ketoconazole).

Nevertheless, the costs of newer medical approaches such as organ transplantation continue to be reviewed in terms of whether the funds being allocated, despite providing life-saving treatment, might not be more justifiably spent in other areas. In a dramatic example, one US state legislature even voted to discontinue payment for all extrarenal transplantation. The not unexpected nationwide reaction to the death of a seven-year-old boy who was denied a bone marrow transplant subsequently led to a review and reversal of the decision. Interestingly, such critical questions are generally asked only of new medical therapies. In part, this is the fault of the medical community, which perhaps should be more active in identifying areas of established therapy that deserve reevaluation. It was rather incongruous, for example, to note that in the same journal issue in which the above state legislature decision was reviewed, a report appeared estimating the cost of treatment for moderate hypertension to be as high as $20,000 to $30,000 per year of life saved. While it is natural for new medical approaches to be the most likely targets for cost containment, scrutiny will probably soon extend to routinely accepted procedures. As has been established in patients with end-stage renal failure (221,222), the new approach (transplantation) may provide not only a better quality of life but may also be a more cost effective long-term option than the alternative (dialysis).

APPLICATION OF TRANSPLANT TECHNOLOGY TO CONVENTIONAL LIVER SURGERY

Retrohepatic Venous Injuries

Trauma to the retrohepatic vena cava or hepatic veins not infrequently results in a lethal injury because of the difficulties encountered trying to gain proximal and distal control of the bleeding site (223). Atriocaval shunts and vascular isolation with sequential clamping have been utilized in patients with these difficult problems; however, results have generally been unsatisfactory (224–227). Occasionally, even extracorporeal bypass and circulatory arrest have been instituted (228), but this approach has the major disadvantage of requiring systemic heparinization that may complicate the management of the patient's other traumatic injuries. Favorable results have been achieved with balloon shunts (229) and with finger fracture resection through liver parenchyma to gain access to the site of venous disruption

(230). Nevertheless, the optimal approach remains to be defined. Since well-defined approaches to retrohepatic control and exposure, veno-venous bypass, and extension of tolerated hepatic ischemic intervals by cold preservation have been developed and reliably applied to liver transplantation, these technologies hold considerable promise for improving the success rates for repair of extensive hepatic and retrohepatic injuries.

Initial experience has already confirmed that veno-venous bypass can be adapted for management of traumatic injuries with minimal modifications. Venous access can be accomplished via either surgical exposure of the saphenous and axillary veins or preferably by percutaneous venous cannulation, using 15F catheters, at groin and subclavian sites (155). We have utilized veno-venous bypass, initiated prior to laparotomy in patients known to have a retrohepatic injury (e.g., involving hemorrhage that was temporarily controlled by packing during earlier laparotomy), with excellent hemodynamic control during the definitive procedure.

Portal vein cannulation can generally be omitted in the trauma setting. If decompression of the splanchnic system is required, for instance to increase venous return or decrease bowel congestion, access can be provided via the inferior mesenteric vein, a technique developed for transplant recipients (231). Cannulation can typically be accomplished at the base of the transverse mesocolon using a 7-mm Gott shunt that is advanced to the confluence of the superior mesenteric and splenic veins (see Fig. 19.11 and Plate 9). The major obstacle to using veno-venous bypass in trauma victims is the requirement for specialized equipment and personnel. If these are not available, the best approach may be temporary packing and transfer to a specialized center.

Other reports have also documented encouraging results using veno-venous bypass for major hepatic and caval trauma (80% survival in five consecutive patients) (3). In this experience, the retrohepatic and perihepatic areas were initially packed to tamponade the active hemorrhage as soon as the presence of major hepatic or retrohepatic injury was established. As the patient was then being stabilized, femoral to axillary veno-venous bypass was established without portal cannulation. Venous bypass flow rates in the range of 2.5 l/min were achieved, after which regional isolation of the bleeding site was provided with the Pringle maneuver and suprahepatic and infrahepatic vena cava clamping. The venous injury could then be repaired in a bloodless fashion.

Extending Hepatic Ischemic Intervals

The in situ human liver can routinely tolerate 20 to 30 minutes of normothermic ischemia (223). In fact, with careful control of volume and cardiac output, ischemic times of 60 to 90 minutes have been tolerated during elective hepatic resections (232). If longer ischemic times are anticipated for performance of complex resections, the techniques of cold preservation developed for transplantation may be applicable.

Ex vivo cold storage times of over 12 hours are routinely tolerated by the liver. Based on this experience, some groups have successfully extended ischemic times, by in situ cold perfusion, to as long as 4 to 5 hours in order to perform difficult resection and reconstructive procedures (233). One group has even reported removal of the liver after cold perfusion in order to perform ex vivo surgery for otherwise unresectable tumors (234). The liver is mobilized and vascular isolation with veno-venous bypass established. The portal vein is then perfused with cold preservation solution and the liver removed for back-table resection. The reconstructed liver is then reimplanted orthotopically. Although theoretically attractive, this method requires a technically challenging reimplantation procedure and would seem rarely indicated.

Either the in situ isolation and cooling approaches already described or ex vivo surgery would appear to provide adequate control and exposure for most procedures. Since the ex vivo surgical approach is limited primarily by potential difficulties with reestablishing continuity of the portal vein, hepatic artery, and common bile duct, preservation of these structures, while mobilizing the cold perfused liver in situ, greatly simplifies the procedure. This approach has been used for extensive centrohepatic resections (5,9), and could also be applicable to liver trauma. Complete vascular exclusion and veno-venous bypass are first established, followed by UW solution hepatic perfusion. Only the suprahepatic and infrahepatic vena cava are divided (Fig. 19.23a). The liver and retrohepatic vena cava can then be elevated out of the hepatic fossa while still tethered by the intact, clamped portal triad (Fig. 19.23b). Alternatively, the vena cava can be left in place and the liver disconnected (Fig. 19.23c). With this exposure, virtually any hepatic resection or injury should be amenable to reconstruction.

Emergency Liver Transplantation for Trauma

For extensive, unreconstructable trauma, liver transplantation has also provided lifesaving treatment (4,7,8,235). A portacaval shunt may be used as a bridging procedure until an allograft becomes available. (Surprisingly, patients can be maintained in the anhepatic state for as long as 30 hours.) Obviously, due to the unreliability of donor organ availability, this approach will rarely be applicable. Future approaches could include support of the anhepatic state until an organ is available by perfusion through an artificial liver device or replacement of the traumatized liver with a xenogeneic organ.

CONCLUSION

Liver transplantation has clearly come of age. The operation is technically difficult and many patients are in poor condition when they are referred for transplantation.

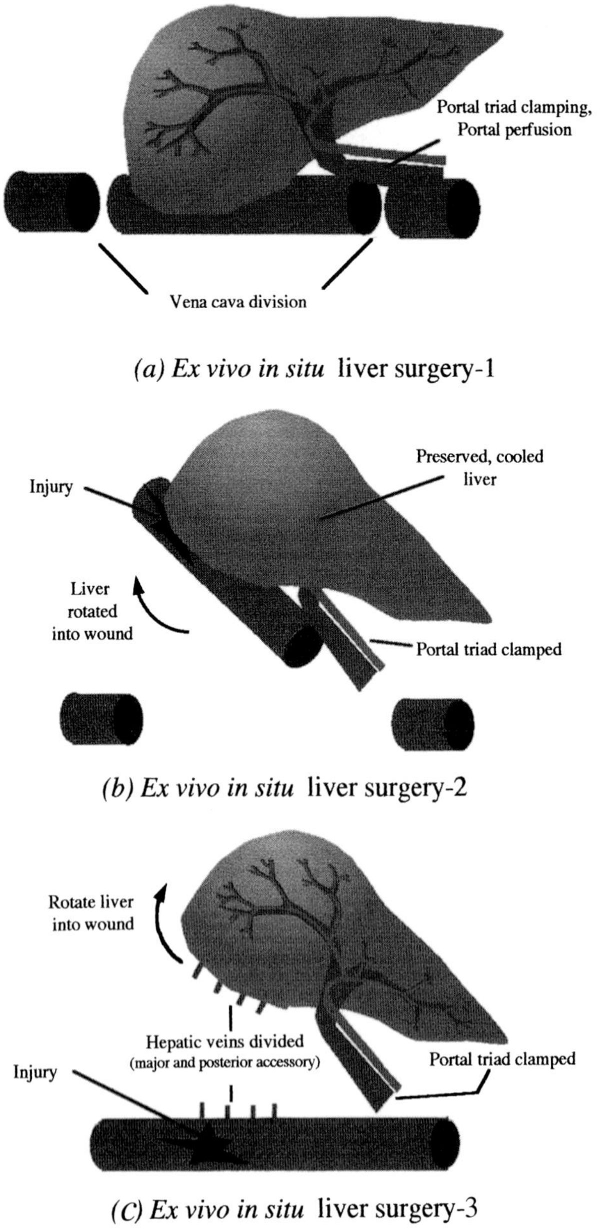

FIGURE 19.23. *Ex vivo in situ liver surgery. Removal of the liver after cold perfusion in order to perform ex vivo surgery for otherwise unresectable tumors is limited primarily by potential difficulties with reestablishing continuity of the portal vein, hepatic artery, and common bile duct. Preservation of portal vein, hepatic artery, and common bile duct while mobilizing the cold perfused liver allows ex vivo but in situ procedures. Complete vascular exclusion and veno-venous bypass are first established, followed by UW solution hepatic perfusion.* ***(a,b)*** *Only the suprahepatic and infrahepatic vena cava are divided.* ***(c)*** *Alternatively, the vena cava can be left in place, and the liver disconnected from the major hepatic veins and the posterior accessory hepatic veins. The liver can then be elevated out of the hepatic fossa while still tethered by the intact, clamped portal triad. With this exposure, virtually any hepatic resection or injury should be amenable to reconstruction. Reimplantation then requires caval anastomoses or use of the "piggyback" technique.*

Nevertheless, the procedure provides the only chance for long-term survival (>5 years) and excellent rehabilitation for two of every three patients whose lifespan would otherwise be measured in terms of months. The identification of more selective and efficacious immunosuppression together with better means to preserve the donor allograft have been two of the most important factors that have made transplantation the preferred therapy for selected patients with end-stage liver cirrhosis or unresectable cancer limited to the liver. Nevertheless, new approaches are needed to lessen, or even completely avoid, the need for long-term administration of immunosuppressive agents.

As for all organ transplants, the major factor currently limiting liver transplantation is the inadequate supply of donor organs. Currently, many patients with hepatic failure or unresectable malignancy are never listed for transplantation and one of every ten patients placed on the waiting list dies before a suitable organ is identified. Yet allografts are successfully transplanted from fewer than one-third of the estimated 12,000 to 18,000 people who die yearly in the United States in circumstances that could make organ donation feasible. Clearly, new approaches are needed to increase the number of allografts available for transplantation and to improve upon the utilization of those organs procured (see Chapter 15).

The extent to which clinical liver transplantation will be applied will be greatly influenced, at least in the short term, by economic and ethical issues. Ultimately, new approaches, possibly including the use of nonhuman donors, more specific immunosuppressive regimens, or even the ability to induce immunologic tolerance to the transplanted liver will undoubtedly make the procedure not only more available but also more effective and economically attractive.

COMMENTARY

Paul McMaster

Remarkable developments in liver transplantation have taken place in the last 25 years and, as the authors of this chapter indicate, it has evolved from a high-risk, complex procedure in the 1970s with little prospect of success to become a major treatment modality for patients with end-stage liver disease. Indeed, there are real signs now that liver transplantation is becoming the "victim" of its own success, with waiting lists growing and organ availability showing no sign of increasing. Between 5% and 10% of adults will die whilst awaiting liver grafting, and the figure for children is perhaps double, with more than 10,000 patients currently listed waiting for liver transplantation in the United States alone.

In many ways we face a classic irony, that application of liver transplantation will be limited because of a shortage of suitable organs at the very time when real success is being achieved. Efforts to ease this growing pressure, however, are being made in a number of areas. There are of course a number of clinicians and scientists who anticipate that the next century will see the successful introduction of xenotransplantation, heralding "a golden era" of clinical transplantation. The recognition that hyperacute rejection is complement activated and might be mitigated by the creation of transgenic animals is an exciting development indeed (see Chapter 40).

Studies by White (1) showed that transgenic pig hearts transplanted into baboons were rarely subjected to hyperacute rejection (2 of 103 transplants), while in nontransgenic donors 65% (17/26) of grafts failed in accelerated fashion. Similar results with kidneys from transgenic pigs suggest the accelerated destruction of grafts may be preventable (2). While this does not mean that acute or indeed chronic rejection is overcome in this setting, it does suggest that important steps are being made in this area. Admittedly, current protocols of immunosuppression in the model using cyclophosphamide have proved to be quite toxic (3). Previous studies in the 1990s in two cases of baboon-to-human liver transplantation showed a remarkable capacity of the liver to function for several months without features of accelerated rejection, although the production of hepatic proteins, coagulation factors, and protein-based bile products suggests the liver may be somewhat late in the order of organs introduced into the clinical practice of xenotransplantation.

In addition to the scientific challenges we face with xenografting, the complex social and economic aspects continue to cause concern. The potential risk of transfer of infection, whether by bacteria or fungi, is an issue that may be overcome by carefully screened breeding pig colonies. Species-specific viruses [pig endogenous retrovirus (PERV)] may, however, in practice be hard to detect. To date, there has been no evidence of porcine retrovirus-mediated disease in humans. Nevertheless, in the era in which Creutzfeld-Jakob disease (CJD) transfer has almost certainly occurred because of prion transmission from animals to humans, it remains uncertain whether this approach would be acceptable to the general community.

A number of recent reports into xenotransplantation in both the United Kingdom and North America have called for more data on safety and efficacy. Calls for a moratorium in clinical experience in xenotransplantation have been made, suggesting that it may be some time before effective clinical xenotransplantation will be a reality.

Alternative approaches to overcome the critical shortage of liver donors have continued to be explored and include the use of living-related transplantation and expanded or so-called "marginal" donors (see Chapter 15). The development of living-related liver transplantation, initially successfully undertaken by Russell Strong in Brisbane, has been fully developed in Japan, where the absence of cadaveric programs has been a potent stimulus. While for a long time living donor kidney grafting has been accepted (UNOS 1990: 2095 living-related kidneys; 1996: 3489 living-related kidneys) outside Japan, increased living donor liver transplantation has been slow to develop (UNOS 1990: 0 living-related livers; 1996: 52 living-related livers).

Living-related liver transplantation has been particularly beneficial in Japan in pediatric transplantation, where segments 2 and 3 from a parent are implanted into a child. Tanaka et al (4) clearly showed that size was crucial: where the ratio between donor graft weight and recipient weight was between 0.8% and 3.0%, two-year survival was 87.8% (140 cases). However, when the ratio between graft weight and recipient weight fell below 0.8%, much less satisfactory results were achieved, with a two-year graft survival of just 58.2% (17 cases). Thus, the critical relationship between the size of the engrafted liver and outcome has been established. The technical skills required to achieve these results should not be underestimated. The introduction of the operating microscope into routine vascular reconstruction in living donor grafts reduced the incidence of hepatic artery thrombosis in these children to under 2% for the first time.

Efforts are now underway to expand the technique of living donor grafting into adults, and early reports from Hong Kong (5) and Japan suggest that for a limited number of small adults, this may prove an appropriate approach. These approaches in adults, however, are still in the developmental phase, and as Lo's pioneering studies of right lobe live donation demonstrated, blood loss can be significant (900 mL median) and hospital stay can be prolonged. In addition, donor reexploration was required in several patients because of biliary leakage. Further experience is needed to resolve these issues.

At this time, therefore, most efforts are being directed to the expansion of cadaveric donor organ use. This can be achieved by the splitting of cadaveric livers so that two recipients can each receive one graft. The left lobe segment 2 and 3 goes to a child, while the right lobe is implanted into an adult; early results have been encouraging. Mirza et al (6), in our own center, reported 27 split livers, creating 40 grafts, with a one-year patient survival of 91% and graft survival of 87.5%. In addition, de Ville et al in a European registry analysis (7) showed that some of the morbidity associated with cadaveric liver splitting could be reduced if the liver was divided prior to removal from the donor, or so-called "in-situ splitting." In a small series of 14 patients from Hanover, Germany, 93% of patients survived the first year with 86% of grafts functioning (8). Further refinement in technique will be needed to reduce the increased morbidity of the right lobe graft, as biliary leakage has occurred in more than 20% of patients.

Cadaveric organ splitting has not been very successful, however, when expanded or marginal donors have been utilized. Personal communication with several centers suggests that they restrict the splitting procedure to the optimal donors, often less than 45 years of age and showing no characteristic of fatty infiltration or instability. Nevertheless, marginal donors increasingly are being utilized. Organs from donors over the age of 55 are now routinely considered as potentially suitable, although extended stays in intensive care unit (ICU), high inotropes, high sodiums, and prolonged hypotension all increase the risk of primary dysfunction or actual failure and nonfunction. In addition, particularly in these marginal donors, extended ischemic and cold preservation times increase risks. Nevertheless, such donors can usually be used, provided recipients are not in a critical or fulminant state, where the delayed function of the graft is insufficient to lead to a rapid recovery of the recipient.

Attempts are being made to evaluate donors on a more rational and consistent basis, including histology to evaluate the degree of macrovesicular fatty infiltrate. A scoring system has been suggested that grades liver function, age, weight, history, and storage on a scale of 100. The presence of adverse factors requires subtracting 20 points from the total, and an overall mean score of less than 45 is associated with primary nonfunction of more than 15%, suggesting that such organs should not be utilized.

The growing interest in the use of non-heart-beating donors for kidney transplantation has also led to a reappraisal of livers harvested from these donors. D'Alessandro was able to harvest 13 pancreases of non-heart-beating cadavers simultaneously with kidneys, and in 12 cases the liver was also used. One-year graft survival of 83.3% is encouraging, although two cases of primary nonfunction in this group suggest it may have a limited place in expanding the potential for liver utilization (9).

Whilst attention to education of both the general public and health care professionals about organ donation may at times seem an unrewarding process, it will in the long term be the mainstay of our efforts to expand organ transplantation over the coming decade. While many still call for legislation to improve the harvesting rates of organs, evidence from Belgium suggests that this may be of limited value. When the Presumed Consent Law was introduced in Belgium nearly a decade ago, organ donation rates doubled in areas where it was widely accepted, but in other parts of the country there was no noticeable change in the rate of organ procurement because of a lack of support from health care professionals and public alike. We must see our program of public education as a medium- to long-term goal, with a particular emphasis on the education of and dissemination of information to young persons, who will form the next generation of potential supporters and donors.

Such a long-term "slog" is perhaps less glamorous and less exciting than the scientific steps that often reach the headlines, but even with success rates in organ transplantation now so high, further improvements in patient survival will be difficult without increased availability of suitable donors to reduce waiting times.

The 1990s have seen five-year survival following liver transplantation improve significantly for many categories of disease. In our own unit, patients with primary biliary cirrhosis (PBC) now have a five-year survival rate of 89%; primary sclerosing cholangitis (PSC), 78%; alcoholic liver disease, 84%; and chronic active hepatitis, 79%. Only in hepatitis B and C, where five-year survival ranges from 70% to 80%, does recurrent disease significantly hinder results of grafting. Transplantation following hepatitis C is almost universally associated with recurrent disease, although severe recurrence occurs in less than 10%, and it remains uncertain what antiviral approach will be beneficial. Although interferon is suggested in several reports to be of help, the morbidity and disruption of the quality of life to the recipient leads many to question its validity. Hepatitis B can be eradicated in some patients with lamivudine, as the authors outline, but there is growing evidence that the viral mutation is most likely in those with the highest viral load at the time of introduction of lamivudine.

Work by Mutimer in Birmingham, England (10) shows that while lamivudine will maintain viral clearance in hepatitis B in a high proportion of patients for at least two years, where high DNA titers of virus are present mutation and graft reinfection will often occur. Current protocols utilize hyperimmune globulin with lamivudine in this particular high-risk group, although medium-term results are still awaited. While steroids and cyclosporine actively stimulate replication of viruses, there is some evidence that rapamycin in vitro inhibits this, and modified protocols of immunosuppression in patients grafted for viral liver disease may require more specific approaches.

As the authors indicate, developments across a whole range of aspects have been required to turn liver transplantation from a high-risk, technically challenging procedure to the success that currently is being achieved. Only by meticulous attention to all aspects of the care—from recipient evaluation to organ procurement and implantation to postoperative care—will this success be further enhanced. More specific protocols of immunosuppression may be required, particularly in the elderly and very young, or in those at risk of recurrent disease. What is not in doubt now is the very high quality of life that can be achieved for many patients undergoing liver transplantation, and the challenge remaining is to make it available to many more individuals.

CHAPTER REFERENCES

1. Seaberg EC, Belle SH, Berringer KC, et al. Long-term patient and retransplantation-free survival: an update from the Pitt-UNOS Liver Transplant Registry. In: Cecka MS, Terasaki PI, eds. Clinical transplants 1997. Los Angeles: UCLA Tissue Typing Laboratory, 1998:15–28.
2. Everhart JE, Lombardero M, Detre KM, et al. Increased waiting time for liver transplantation results in higher mortality. Transplantation 1997;64(9):1300–1306.
3. Baumgartner F, Scudamore C, Nair C, et al. Venovenous bypass for major hepatic and caval trauma. J Trauma 1995;39(4):671–673.

4. Angstadt J, Jarrell B, Moritz M, et al. Surgical management of severe liver trauma: a role for liver transplantation. J Trauma 1989;29(5):606–608.
5. Delriviere L, Hannoun L. In situ and ex situ in vivo procedures for complex major liver resections requiring prolonged hepatic vascular exclusion in normal and diseased livers. J Am Coll Surg 1995;181(3):272–276.
6. Huguet C, Gavelli A, Chieco PA, et al. Liver ischemia for hepatic resection: where is the limit? Surgery 1992;111(3):251–259.
7. Ringe B, Pichlmayr R, Ziegler H, et al. Management of severe hepatic trauma by two-stage total hepatectomy and subsequent liver transplantation. Surgery 1991;109(6):792–795.
8. Ringe B, Pichlmayr R. Total hepatectomy and liver transplantation: a life-saving procedure in patients with severe hepatic trauma. Br J Surg 1995;82(6):837–839.
9. Sauvanet A, Dousset B, Belghiti J. A simplified technique of ex situ hepatic surgical treatment. J Am Coll Surg 1994;178(1):79–82.
10. Terblanche J. Portal hypertension management. Surg Endosc 1993;7(6):472–478.
11. Menegaux F, Keeffe EB, Baker E, et al. Comparison of transjugular and surgical portosystemic shunts on the outcome of liver transplantation. Arch Surg 1994;129(10):1018–1023.
12. Bismuth H, Chiche L, Adam R, et al. Liver resection versus transplantation for hepatocellular carcinoma in cirrhotic patients. Ann Surg 1993;218(2): 145–151.
13. Iwatsuki S, Starzl TE, Sheahan DG, et al. Hepatic resection versus transplantation for hepatocellular carcinoma. Ann Surg 1991;214(3):221–228.
14. Welch CS. A note on transplantation of the whole liver in dogs. Transplant Bull 1955;2:54–55.
15. Starzl TE, Marchiano TL, Porter KA, et al. Factors determining short and long-term survival after orthotopic liver homotransplantation in the dog. Surgery 1965;58:131–155.
16. Starzl TE, Francavilla A, Halgrimson CG. The origin, hormonal nature, and action of hepatotrophic substances in portal venous blood. Surg Gynecol Obstet 1973;137:179–199.
17. Pouyet M, Berard P, Ruckebush Y. Derivation porto-hepatique selective: Origine pancreatique du facteur hepatotrophique portal. Ann Chirg 1969;23:393–398.
18. Moore FD, Wheeler HB, Demissianos HV, et al. Experimental whole-organ transplantation of the liver and of the spleen. Ann Surg 1960;152:374–387.
19. Starzl TE, Kaupp HA, Brock DR, Linman JW. Studies on the rejection of the transplanted homologous dog liver. Surg Gynecol Obstet 1961;112:135–144.
20. Starzl TE, Marchioro TL, Von Kaulla KN. Homotransplantation of the liver in humans. Surg Gynecol Obstet 1963;117:659–676.
21. Starzl TE, Groth CG, Brettschneider L. Orthotopic homotransplantation of the human liver. Ann Surg 1968;168:392–415.
22. Jansen PL. 1-year survey of patients with advanced liver cirrhosis. Prognostic value of clinical and laboratory indexes identified by the Cox regression model. Scand J Gastroenterol 1992;27(10):852–856.
23. Sauerbruch T, Weinzierl M, Kopcke W, Baumgartner G. Prognostic value of Pugh's modification of Child-Turcotte classification in patients with cirrhosis of the liver. Panminerva Med 1992;34(2):65–68.
24. Zoli M, Cordiani MR, Marchesini G, et al. Prognostic indicators in compensated cirrhosis. Am J Gastroenterol 1991;86(10):1508–1513.
25. Murtaugh PA, Dickson ER, Van DG, et al. Primary biliary cirrhosis: prediction of short-term survival based on repeated patient visits. Hepatology 1994;20(1 Pt 1):126–134.
26. O'Grady JG, Alexander GJ, Hayllar KM, Williams R. Early indicators of prognosis in fulminant hepatic failure [see comments]. Gastroenterology 1989;97(2):439–445.
27. Farrant JM, Hayllar KM, Wilkinson ML, et al. Natural history and prognostic variables in primary sclerosing cholangitis. Gastroenterology 1991;100(6):1710–1717.
28. Summerfield JA. Diagnosis of cirrhosis and portal hypertension. In: Blumgart LH, ed. Surgery of the liver and biliary tract. Vol. 2. Edinburgh: Churchill Livingstone, 1994:1602–1611.
29. Zimmerman H, Reichen J. Assessment of liver function in the surgical patient. In: Blumgart LH, ed. Surgery of the liver and biliary tract. Vol. 2. Edinburgh: Churchill Livingstone, 1994:41.
30. Fraser CL, Arieff AI. Hepatic encephalopathy. N Engl J Med 1985;313(14): 865–873.
31. Sussman NL, Lake JR. Treatment of hepatic failure—1996: current concepts and progress toward liver dialysis. Am J Kid Dis 1996;27(5):605–611.
32. Bandoh T, Mitarai Y, Kitano S, et al. Clinical significance of esophageal variceal pressure in patients with esophageal varices. J Hepatol 1994;21(3):326–331.
33. D'Amico G, Pagliaro L, Bosch J. The treatment of portal hypertension: a meta-analytic review. Hepatology 1995;22(1):332–354.
34. Sung JJ, Chung SC, Lai CW, et al. Octreotide infusion or emergency sclerotherapy for variceal haemorrhage [see comments]. Lancet 1993;342(8872):637–641.
35. Besson I, Ingrand P, Person B, et al. Sclerotherapy with or without octreotide for acute variceal bleeding. N Engl J Med 1995;333(9):555–560.
36. Coldwell DM, Ring EJ, Rees CR, et al. Multicenter investigation of the role of transjugular intrahepatic portosystemic shunt in management of portal hypertension [see comments]. Radiology 1995;196(2):335–340.
37. Ferral H, Bjarnason H, Wegryn SA, et al. Refractory ascites: early experience in treatment with transjugular intrahepatic portosystemic shunt. Radiology 1993;189(3):795–801.
38. Orozco H, Mercado MA, Takahashi T, et al. Survival and quality of life after portal blood flow preserving procedures in patients with portal hypertension and liver cirrhosis. Am J Surg 1994;168(1):10–14.
39. Sterling KM, Darcy MD. Stenosis of transjugular intrahepatic portosystemic shunts: presentation and management. AJR Am J Roentgenol 1997;168(1): 239–244.
40. Pares A, Barrera JM, Caballeria J, et al. Hepatitis C virus antibodies in chronic alcoholic patients: association with severity of liver injury [see comments]. Hepatology 1990;12(6):1295–1299.
41. Surman OS, Dienstag JL, Cosimi AB, et al. Liver transplantation: psychiatric considerations. Psychosomatics 1987;28(12):615–618.
42. Bird GL, O'Grady JG, Harvey FA, et al. Liver transplantation in patients with alcoholic cirrhosis: selection criteria and rates of survival and relapse [see comments]. BMJ 1990;301(6742):15–17.
43. Osorio RW, Ascher NL, Avery M, et al. Predicting recidivism after orthotopic liver transplantation for alcoholic liver disease. Hepatology 1994;20(1 Pt 1):105–110.
44. Gish RG, Lee AH, Keeffe EB, et al. Liver transplantation for patients with alcoholism and end-stage liver disease [see comments]. Am J Gastroenterol 1993;88(9):1337–1342.
45. Campbell DA, Lucey MR. Liver transplantation for alcoholic cirrhosis. In: Busutill RW, Klintmalm GB, eds. Transplantation of the liver. Philadelphia: WB Saunders, 1996:145.
46. Moss AH, Siegler M. Should alcoholics compete equally for liver transplantation [see comments]? JAMA 1991;265(10):1295–1298.
47. Dienstag JL. Acute hepatitis. In: Isselbacher KJ, Braunwald E, Wilson JD, et al, eds. Harrison's principles of internal medicine. New York: McGraw-Hill, 1994:1465.
48. Hart J, Busuttil RW, Lewin KJ. Disease recurrence following liver transplantation. Am J Surg Pathol 1990;1(79):79–91.
49. O'Grady JG, Smith HM, Davies SE, et al. Hepatitis B virus reinfection after orthotopic liver transplantation. Serological and clinical implications. J Hepatol 1992;14(1):104–111.
50. Walker N, Apel R, Kerlin P, et al. Hepatitis B virus infection in liver allografts. Am J Surg Pathol 1993;17(7):666–677.
51. Phillips MJ, Cameron R, Flowers MA, et al. Post-transplant recurrent hepatitis B viral liver disease. Viral-burden, steatoviral, and fibroviral hepatitis B. Am J Pathol 1992;140(6):1295–1308.
52. Samuel D, Bismuth A, Mathieu D, et al. Passive immunoprophylaxis after liver transplantation in HBsAg-positive patients. Lancet 1991;337(8745):813–815.
53. Muller R, Gubernatis G, Farle M, et al. Liver transplantation in HBs antigen (HBsAg) carriers. Prevention of hepatitis B virus (HBV) recurrence by passive immunization. J Hepatol 1991;13(1):90–96.
54. Samuel D, Muller R, Alexander G, et al. Liver transplantation in European patients with the hepatitis B surface antigen. N Engl J Med 1993;329(25): 1842–1847.
55. Dienstag JL, Perrillo RP, Schiff ER, et al. A preliminary trial of lamivudine for chronic hepatitis B infection [see comments]. N Engl J Med 1995;333(25):1657–1661.
56. O'Grady JG, Williams R. Liver transplantation for viral hepatitis. Br Med Bull 1990;46(2):481–491.
57. Hopf U, Neuhaus P, Lobeck H, et al. Follow-up of recurrent hepatitis B and delta infection in liver. J Hepatol 1991;13(3):339–346.
58. Konig V, Hopf U, Neuhaus P, et al. Long-term follow-up of hepatitis B virus-infected recipients after orthotopic liver transplantation. Transplantation 1994;58(5):553–559.

59. Ottobrelli A, Marzano A, Smedile A, et al. Patterns of hepatitis delta virus reinfection and disease in liver transplantation [see comments]. Gastroenterology 1991;101(6):1649–1655.
60. Davies SE, Portmann BC, O'Grady JG, et al. Hepatic histological findings after transplantation for chronic hepatitis B virus infection, including a unique pattern of fibrosing cholestatic hepatitis. Hepatology 1991;13(1):150–157.
61. Angus PW, Locarnini SA, McCaughan GW, et al. Hepatitis B virus precore mutant infection is associated with severe recurrent disease after liver transplantation. Hepatology 1995;21(1):14–18.
62. Gish RG, Keeffe EB, Lim J, et al. Survival after liver transplantation for chronic hepatitis B using reduced immunosuppression. J Hepatol 1995;22:257–262.
63. Eason JD, Freeman RJ, Rohrer RJ, et al. Should liver transplantation be performed for patients with hepatitis? Transplantation 1994;57(11):1588–1593.
64. Hoofnagle JH, Peters M, Mullen KD, et al. Randomized, controlled trial of recombinant human alpha-interferon in patients with chronic hepatitis B. Gastroenterology 1988;95(5):1318–1325.
65. Marcellin P, Samuel D, Areias J, et al. Pretransplantation interferon treatment and recurrence of hepatitis B virus infection after liver transplantation for hepatitis B-related end-stage liver disease. Hepatology 1994;19(1):6–12.
66. Lavine JE, Lake JR, Ascher NL, et al. Persistent hepatitis B virus following interferon alfa therapy and liver transplantation. Gastroenterology 1991;100(1):263–267.
67. Flowers M, Sherker A, Sinclair SB, et al. Prostaglandin E in the treatment of recurrent hepatitis B infection after orthotopic liver transplantation. Transplantation 1994;58(2):183–192.
68. Boker KH, Ringe B, Kruger M, et al. Prostaglandin E plus famciclovir—a new concept for the treatment of severe hepatitis B after liver transplantation. Transplantation 1994;57(12):1706–1708.
69. Ishitani M, McGory R, Dickson R, et al. Retransplantation of patients with severe posttransplant hepatitis B in the first allograft. Transplantation 1997;64(3):410–414.
70. Nyman T, Shokouh-Amiri MH, Vera SR, et al. Prevention of hepatitis B recurrence with indefinite hepatitis B immune globulin prophylaxis after liver transplantation. Clin Transplant 1996;10:663–667.
71. Grellier L, Brown D, McPhilips P. Lamivudine prophylaxis: a new strategy for prevention of reinfection in liver transplantation for hepatitis B DNA-positive cirrhosis. Hepatology 1995;22:224A.
72. Ben Ari Z, Shmueli D, Mor E, et al. Beneficial effect of lamivudine in recurrent hepatitis B after liver transplantation. Transplantation 1997; 63(3):393–396.
73. Nery JR, Weppler D, Rodriguez M, et al. Efficacy of lamivudine in controlling hepatitis B virus recurrence after liver transplantation. Transplantation 1998;65:1615–1621.
74. Bartholomew MM, Jansen RW, Jeffers LJ, et al. Hepatitis-B-virus resistance to lamivudine given for recurrent infection afterorthotopic liver transplantation. Lancet 1997;349:20–22.
75. Gish RG, Lau JY, Brooks L, et al. Ganciclovir treatment of hepatitis B virus infection in liver transplant recipients. Hepatology 1996;23(1):1–7.
76. Poterucha J, Rakela J, Lumeng L, et al. Diagnosis of chronic hepatitis C after liver transplantation by the detection of viral sequences with polymerase chain reaction. Hepatology 1992;15:42–45.
77. Gretch DR, Bacchi CE, Corey L, et al. Persistent hepatitis C virus infection after liver transplantation: clinical and virological features. Hepatology 1995;22(1):1–9.
78. Dickson RC, Caldwell SH, Ishitani MB, et al. Clinical and histologic patterns of early graft failure due to recurrnet hepatitis C in four patients after liver transplantation. Transplantation 1996;61(5):701–705.
79. Gane EJ, Portmann BC, Naoumov NV, et al. Long-term outcome of hepatitis C infection after liver transplantation. N Engl J Med 1996; 334(13):815–820.
80. Sheiner PA, Schwartz ME, Mor E, et al. Severe or multiple rejection episodes are associated with early recurrence of hepatitis C after orthotopic liver transplantation. Hepatology 1995;21(1):30–34.
81. Johnson MW, Washburn WK, Freeman RB, et al. Hepatitis C viral infection in liver transplantation. Arch Surg 1996;131:284–290.
82. Zervos XA, Weppler D, Fragulidis GP, et al. Comparison of tacrolimus with microemulsion cyclosporine as primary immunosuppression in hepatitis C patients after liver transplantation. Transplantation 1998;65:1044–1046.
83. Shiffman ML, Contos MJ, Luketic VA, et al. Biochemical and histologic evaluation of recurrent hepatitis C following orthotopic liver transplantation. Transplantation 1994;57(4):526–532.
84. Ferrell LD, Wright TL, Roberts J, et al. Hepatitis C viral infection in liver transplant recipients. Hepatology 1992;16(4):865–876.
85. Duvoux C, Pawlotsky JM, Cherqui D, et al. Serial quantitative determination of hepatitis C virus RNA levels after liver transplantation. A useful test for diagnosis of hepatitis C virus reinfection. Transplantation 1995;60(5):457–461.
86. Wright TL, Combs C, Kim M, et al. Interferon-alpha therapy for hepatitis C virus infection after liver transplantation. Hepatology 1994;20(4 Pt 1):773–779.
87. Feray C, Samuel D, Gigou M, et al. An open trial of interferon alfa recombinant for hepatitis C after liver transplantation: antiviral effects and risk of rejection. Hepatology 1995;22(4 Pt 1):1084–1089.
88. Cattral MS, Krajden M, Wanless IR, et al. A pilot study of Ribavirin therapy for recurrent hepatitis C virus infection after liver transplantation. Transplantation 1996;61(10):1483–1488.
89. Gare EJ, Lo SK, Riordan SM, et al. A randomized study comparing ribavirin and interferon alfa for hepatitis C recurrence after liver transplantation. Hepatology 1998;27:1403–1407.
90. Ryley NG, McGee JO. Cirrhosis and portal hypertension: pathological aspects. In: Blumgart LH, ed. Surgery of the liver and biliary tract. Vol. 2. Edinburgh: Churchill Livingstone, 1994:1589–1602.
91. Locke GR, Dickson ER. Transplantation for primary biliary cirrhosis. In: Busutill RW, Klintmalm GB, eds. Transplantation of the liver. Philadelphia: WB Saunders, 1996:108.
92. Kaplan MM, Knox TA. Treatment of primary biliary cirrhosis with low-dose weekly methotrexate. Gastroenterology 1991;101:1332–1338.
93. Kaplan MM, DeLellis RA, Wolfe HJ. Sustained biochemical and histologic remission of primary biliary cirrhosis in response to medical treatment. Ann Intern Med 1997;126(9):682–688.
94. Poupon RE, Poupon R, Balkau B. Ursodiol for the long-term treatment of primary biliary cirrhosis. The UDCA-PBC Study Group [see comments]. N Engl J Med 1994;330(19):1342–1347.
95. Lindor KD, Therneau TM, Jorgensen RA, et al. Effects of ursodiol considered as a safe, effective, and life-extending treatment in patients with primary biliary cirrhosis. Gastroenterology 1996;110(5):1515–1518.
96. Tzakis AG, Carcassonne C, Todo S, et al. Liver transplantation for primary biliary cirrhosis. Semin Liver Dis 1989;9(2):144–148.
97. Dickson ER, Grambsch PM, Fleming TR, et al. Prognosis in primary biliary cirrhosis: model for decision making [see comments]. Hepatology 1989;10(1):1–7.
98. Grambsch PM, Dickson ER, Kaplan M, et al. Extramural cross-validation of the Mayo primary biliary cirrhosis survival model establishes its generalizability. Hepatology 1989;10(5):846–850.
99. Wiesner RH, Porayko MK, Dickson ER, et al. Selection and timing of liver transplantation in primary biliary cirrhosis and primary sclerosing cholangitis. Hepatology 1992;16(5):1290–1299.
100. Jeyarajah DR, Netto GJ, Lee SP, et al. Recurrent primary sclerosing cholangitis after orthotopic liver transplantation: is chronic rejection part of the disease process? Transplantation 1998;66:1300–1306.
101. Farrant JM, Hayllar KM, Wilkinson ML, et al. Natural history and prognostic variables in primary sclerosing cholangitis. Gastroenterology 1991;100(6): 1710–1717.
102. Martin FM, Rossi RL, Nugent FW, et al. Surgical aspects of sclerosing cholangitis. Results in 178 patients. Ann Surg 1990;212(4):551–556.
103. Jackson LD, Song E. Cyclosporin in the treatment of corticosteroid resistant autoimmune chronic active hepatitis. Gut 1995;36(3):459–461.
104. Stellon AJ, Keating JJ, Johnson PJ, et al. Maintenance of remission in autoimmune chronic active hepatitis with azathioprine after corticosteroid withdrawal. Hepatology 1988;8(4):781–784.
105. Sanchez UL, Czaja AJ, van Hoek B, et al. Prognostic features and role of liver transplantation in severe corticosteroid-treated autoimmune chronic active hepatitis. Hepatology 1992;15(2):215–221.
106. Isselbacher KJ, Dienstag J. Tumors of the liver. In: Isselbacher KJ, Braunwald E, Wilson JD, et al, eds. Harrison's principles of internal medicine. New York: McGraw-Hill, 1994:1495.
107. Yokoyama I, Todo S, Iwatsuki S, Starzl TE. Liver transplantation in the treatment of primary liver cancer. Hepatogastroenterology 1990;37:188–193.
108. Yokoyama I, Carr B, Saitsu H, et al. Accelerated growth rates of recurrent hepatocellular carcinoma after liver transplantation. Cancer 1991;68(10): 2095–2100.
109. Stone MJ, Klintmalm GB, Polter D, et al. Neoadjuvant chemotherapy and liver transplantation for hepatocellular carcinoma: a pilot study in 20 patients [see comments]. Gastroenterology 1993;104(1):196–202.
110. Olthoff KM, Rosove MH, Shackleton CR, et al. Adjuvant chemotherapy improves survival after liver transplantation. Ann Surg 1995;221(6):734–741.

111. Mazzaferro V, Regalia E, Doci R, et al. Liver transplantation for the treatment of small hepatocellular carcinomas in patients with cirrhosis [see comments]. N Engl J Med 1996;334(11):693–699.
112. Schwartz ME, Sung M, Mor E, et al. A multidisciplinary approach to hepatocellular carcinoma in patients with cirrhosis. J Am Coll Surg 1995;180(5):596–603.
113. Cherqui D, Piedbois P, Pierga JY, et al. Multimodal adjuvant treatment and liver transplantation for advanced hepatocellular carcinoma. A pilot study. Cancer 1994;73(11):2721–2726.
114. Chung SW, Toth JL, Rezieg M, et al. Liver transplantation for hepatocellular carcinoma. Am J Surg 1994;167(3):317–321.
115. Castells A, Bruix J, Bru C, et al. Treatment of small hepatocellular carcinoma in cirrhotic patients: a cohort study comparing surgical resection and percutaneous ethanol injection. Hepatology 1993;18(5):1121–1126.
116. Wendon J, Williams R. Transplantation for fulminant hepatic failure. In: Busutill RW, Klintmalm GB, eds. Transplantation of the liver. Philadelphia: WB Saunders, 1996:93.
117. Bernuau J, Rueff B, Benhamou JP. Fulminant and subfulminant liver failure: definition and causes. Semin Liver Dis 1986;6:97–106.
118. Bismuth H, Samuel D, Castaing D, et al. Orthotopic liver transplantation in fulminant and subfulminant hepatitis. The Paul Brousse experience [see comments]. Ann Surg 1995;222(2):109–119.
119. Emond JC, Aran PP, Whitington PF, et al. Liver transplantation in the management of fulminant hepatic failure. Gastroenterology 1989;96: 1583–1588.
120. Asher NL, Lake JR, Emond JC, Roberts JP. Liver transplantation for fulminant hepatic failure. Arch Surg 1993;128:677–684.
121. Bernuau J, Goudeau A, Poynard T, et al. Multivariate analysis of prognostic factors in fulminant hepatitis B. Hepatology 1986;6(4):648–651.
122. Chari RS, Collins BH, Magee JC, et al. Brief report: treatment of hepatic failure with ex vivo pig-liver perfusion followed by liver transplantation [see comments]. N Engl J Med 1994;331(4):234–237.
123. Ellis AJ, Hughes RD, Wendon JA, et al. Pilot-controlled trial of the extracorporeal liver assist device in acute liver failure. Hepatology 1996;24(6):1446–1451.
124. Watanabe FD, Mullon CJ, Hewitt WR, et al. Chemical experience with a bioartificial liver in the treatment of severe liver failure. Ann Surg 1997;225:484–494.
125. Boudjema K, Cherqui D, Jaeck D, et al. Auxiliary liver transplantation for fulminant and subfulminant. Transplantation 1995;59(2):218–223.
126. Orloff MJ, Orloff MS. Budd-Chiari syndrome and veno-occlusive disease. In: Blumgart LH, ed. Surgery of the liver and biliary tract. Vol. 2. Edinburgh: Churchill Livingstone, 1994:1725.
127. Halff G, Todo S, Tzakis AG, et al. Liver transplantation for the Budd-Chiari syndrome. Ann Surg 1990;211(1):43–49.
128. Seltman HJ, Dekker A, Van TD, et al. Budd-Chiari syndrome recurring in a transplanted liver. Gastroenterology 1983;84(3):640–643.
129. Wong T, Devlin J, Rolando N, et al. Clinical characteristics affecting the outcome of liver retransplantation. Transplantation 1997;64(6):878–882.
130. Powelson JA, Cosimi AB, Lewis D, et al. Hepatic retransplantation: a regional experience and survival model. Transplantation 1993;55(4): 802–806.
131. Doyle HR, Morelli F, McMichael J, et al. Hepatic Retransplantation—an analysis of risk factors associated with outcome. Transplantation 1996;61(10): 1499–1505.
132. Lucey MR, Brown KA, Everson GT, et al. Minimal criteria for placement of adults on the liver transplant waiting list. Transplantation 1998;66:956–962.
133. Knechtle SJ, Kalayolu M, D'Alessandro AM, et al. Histocompatibility and liver transplantation. Surgery 1993;114(4):667–671.
134. Doyle HR, Marino IR, Morelli F, et al. Assessing risk in liver transplantation—special reference to the significance of a positive cytotoxic crossmatch. Ann Surg 1996;224(2):168–177.
135. Gugenheim J, Amorosa L, Gigou M, et al. Specific absorption of lymphocytotoxic alloantibodies by the liver in inbred rats. Transplantation 1990;50(2):309–313.
136. Flye MW, Duffy BF, Phelan DL, et al. Protective effects of liver transplantation on a simultaneously transplanted kidney in a highly sensitized patient. Transplantation 1990;50(6):1051–1054.
137. Renard TH, Andrews WS. An approach to ABO-incompatible liver transplantation in children. Transplantation 1992;53(1):116–121.
138. Reding R, de Veyckemans F, et al. ABO-incompatible orthotopic liver allografting in urgent indications. Surg Gynecol Obstet 1992;174(1):59–64.
139. Gugenheim J, Samuel D, Reynes M, Bismuth H. Liver transplantation across ABO blood group barriers. Lancet 1990;336(8714):519–523.
140. Sanchez UL, Batts KP, Gores GJ, et al. Increased bile duct complications in liver transplantation across the ABO barrier. Ann Surg 1993;218(2):152–158.
141. Farges O, Kalil AN, Samuel D, et al. The use of ABO-incompatible grafts in liver transplantation: a life-saving procedure in highly selected patients. Transplantation 1995;59(8):1124–1133.
142. Ramsey G, Cornell FW, Hahn LF, et al. Red cell antibody problems in 1000 liver transplants. Transfusion 1989;29(5):396–400.
143. Emond JC, Whitington PF, Thistlethwaite JR, et al. Transplantation of two patients with one liver. Ann Surg 1990;212:14–22.
144. Goss JA, Shackleton CR, Sev P, et al. In situ splitting of the cadaveric liver for transplantation. Transplantation 1997;64:871–877.
145. Emond JC, Renz JF, Ferrell LD, et al. Functional analysis of grafts from living donors. Implications for the treatment of older recipients. Ann Surg 1996;224(4):544–552.
146. Emre S, Schwartz ME, Miller CM. The donor operation. In: Busutill RW, Klintmalm GB, eds. Transplantation of the liver. Philadelphia: WB Saunders, 1996:392.
147. Strasberg SM, Howard TK, Molmenti EP, Hertl M. Selecting the donor liver: risk factors for poor function after orthotopic liver transplantation. Hepatology 1994;20(4 Pt 1):829–838.
148. Markin RS, Wisecarver JL, Radio SJ, et al. Frozen section evaluation of donor livers before transplantation. Transplantation 1993;56(6):1403–1409.
149. Starzl TE, Hakala TR, Shaw BJ, et al. A flexible procedure for multiple cadaveric organ procurement. Surg Gynecol Obstet 1984;158(3):223–230.
150. Starzl TE, Miller C, Broznick B, Makowka L. An improved technique for multiple organ harvesting. Surg Gynecol Obstet 1987;165(4):343–348.
151. Yanaga K, Podesta LG, Broznick B, et al. Multiple organ recovery for transplantation. In: Starzl TE, Shapiro R, Simmons RL, eds. Atlas of organ transplantation. New York: Gower Medical, 1992:3.1–3.48.
152. Padbury RT, Attard A, Mirza DF, et al. Extended preservation of the liver with UW solution—is it justifiable? Transplantation 1994;57(10):1490–1493.
153. Furukawa H, Todo S, Imventarza O, et al. Effect of cold ischemia time on the early outcome of human hepatic allografts preserved with UW solution. Transplantation 1991;51(5):1000–1004.
154. Carrasco L, Sanchez BF, Sola J, et al. Effects of cold ischemia time on the graft after orthotopic liver transplantation. A bile cytological study. Transplantation 1996;61(3):393–696.
155. Washburn WK, Lewis WD, Jenkins RL. Percutaneous venovenous bypass in orthotopic liver transplantation. Liver Transplant Surg 1995;1(6):377–382.
156. Mor E, Jennings L, Gonwa TA, et al. The impact of operative bleeding on outcome in transplantation of the liver. Surg Gynecol Obstet 1993;176: 219–227.
157. Busque S, Esquivel CO, Concepcion W, So SKS. Experience with the piggyback technique without caval occlusion in adult orthotopic liver transplantation. Transplantation 1998;65:77–82.
158. Griffith BP, Shaw BW, Hardesty RL, et al. Veno-venous bypass without systemic anticoagulation for transplantation of the human liver. Surg Gynecol Obst 1985;160:270–272.
159. Paulsen AW, Whitten CW, Ramsay MAE, Klintmalm GB. Considerations for anesthetic management during veno-venous bypass in adult hepatic transplantation. Anesth Analg 1989;68:489–496.
160. Emre S, Schwartz ME, Mor E, et al. Obviation of prereperfusion rinsing and decrease in preservation/reperfusion injury in liver transplantation by portal blood flushing. Transplantation 1994;57(6):799–803.
161. Kirsh JP, Howard TK, Klintmalm GB, et al. Problematic vascular reconstruction in liver transplantation. Part II. Portovenous conduits. Surgery 1990;107(5):544–548.
162. Imigawa DK, Busuttil RW. Technical problems: vascular. In: Busutill RW, Klintmalm GB, eds. Transplantation of the liver. Philadelphia: WB Saunders, 1996:626–632.
163. Goldstein RM, Secrest CL, Klintmalm GB, Husberg BS. Problematic vascular reconstruction in liver transplantation. Part I. Arterial. Surgery 1990;107(5): 541–543.
164. Rolles K, Dawson K, Novell R, et al. Biliary anastomosis after liver transplantation does not benefit from T tube splintage. Transplantation 1994;57(3):402–404.
165. Randall HB, Wachs ME, Somberg KA, et al. The use of the T tube after orthotopic liver transplantation. Transplantation 1996;61(2):258–261.
166. Broelsch CE, Emond JC, Whitington PF, et al. Application of reduced-size liver transplants as split grafts, auxiliary orthotopic grafts, and living related segmental transplants. Ann Surg 1990;212(3):368–377.
167. Terpstra OT, Schalm SW, Weimar W, et al. Auxiliary partial liver transplantation for end-stage chronic liver disease. N Engl J Med 1988;319(23):1507–1511.

168. Oldhafer KJ, Gubernatis G, Schlitt HJ, et al. Auxiliary partial orthotopic liver transplantation for acute liver failure: the Hannover experience. Clin Transplant 1994:181–187.
169. Chenard NM, Boudjema K, Bernuau J, et al. Auxiliary liver transplantation: regeneration of the native liver and outcome in 30 patients with fulminant hepatic failure—a multicenter European study. Hepatology 1996;23(5):1119–1127.
170. Whitington PF, Emond JC, Heffron T, Thistlethwaite JR. Orthotopic auxiliary liver transplantation for Crigler-Najjar syndrome type 1 [see comments]. Lancet 1993;342(8874):779–780.
171. Gubernatis G, Pichlmayr R, Kemnitz J, Gratz K. Auxiliary partial orthotopic liver transplantation (APOLT) for fulminant hepatic failure: first successful case report. World J Surg 1991;15(5):660–665.
172. Starzl TE, Klintmalm GBG, Poter KA, et al. Liver transplantation with use of cyclosporin A and prednisone. N Engl J Med 1981;305:266–268.
173. Wall WJ, Ghent CN. Immunosuppression in liver transplantation: monitoring, dose adjustment, reduction, and withdrawal. Liver Transplant Surg 1995;1(5):3–10.
174. Winkler M, Haller G, Oldhafer K, et al. A new oral formulation of cyclosporine for early oral immunosupressive therapy in liver transplant recipients. Transplantation 1996;62(8):1063–1068.
175. Cosimi AB, Jenkins RL, Rohrer RJ, et al. A randomized clinical trial of prophylactic OKT3 monoclonal antibody in liver allograft recipients. Arch Surg 1990;125(6):781–784.
176. McDiarmid SV, Millis MJ, Terasaki PI, et al. OKT3 prophylaxis in liver transplantation. Dig Dis Sci 1991;36(10):1418–1426.
177. Millis JM, McDiarmid SV, Hiatt JR, et al. Randomized prospective trial of OKT3 for early prophylaxis of rejection after liver transplantation. Transplantation 1989;47(1):82–88.
178. Sandborn WJ, Hay JE, Porayko MK, et al. Cyclosporine withdrawal for nephrotoxicity in liver transplant recipients does not result in sustained improvement in kidney function and causes cellular and ductopenic rejection. Hepatology 1994:925–931.
179. Mor E, Gonwa TA, Husberg BS, et al. Late-onset acute rejection in orthotopic liver transplantation—associated risk factors and outcome. Transplantation 1992;54(5):821–824.
180. Neuhaus P, Blumhardt G, Bechstein WO, et al. Weaning of immunosuppression in long-term liver transplant recipients. Transplantation 1995;59(2):212–217.
181. Reding R, Wallemacq PE, Lamy ME, et al. Monotherapy with cyclosporine for chronic immunosuppression in pediatric liver transplant recipients. Transplantation 1994;57(4):544–547.
182. Padbury RTA, Gunson BK, Dousset B, et al. Steroid withdrawal from long-term immunosuppression in liver allgraft recipients. Transplantation 1993;55:789–794.
183. Todo S, Fung JJ, Starzl TE, et al. Single-center experience with primary orthotopic liver transplantation with FK 506 immunosuppression. Ann Surg 1994;220(3):297–308.
184. Porayko MK, Textor SC, Krom RA, et al. Randomised trial comparing tacrolimus (FK506) and cyclosporin in prevention of liver allograft rejection. European FK506 Multicentre Liver Study Group [see comments]. Lancet 1994;344(8920):423–428.
185. Wijdicks EF, Wiesner RH, Krom RA. A comparison of tacrolimus (FK 506) and cyclosporine for immunosuppression in liver transplantation. The U.S. Multicenter FK506 Liver Study Group [see comments]. N Engl J Med 1994;331(17):1110–1115.
186. Ramos HC, Reyes J, Abu EK, et al. FK506 (tacrolimus) compared with cyclosporine for primary immunosuppression after pediatric liver transplantation. Results from the U.S. Multicenter Trial. Transplantation 1995;59(4):530–536.
187. Cosimi AB, Cho SI, Delmonico FL, et al. A randomized clinical trial comparing OKT3 and steroids for treatment of hepatic allograft rejection. Transplant Proc 1987;19(1 Pt 3):2431–2433.
188. Jonas S, Kling N, Bechstein WO, et al. FK 506 rescue therapy for hepatic allograft rejection: experience with an aggressive approach. Clin Transplant 1995;9(1):45–52.
189. Wong F, Blendis LM. The patient with renal insufficiency. Liver Transplant Surg 1996;2(5):35–43.
190. Howard TK. Postoperative intensive care management of the adult. In: Busutill RW, Klintmalm GB, eds. Transplantation of the liver. Philadelphia: WB Saunders, 1996:551–563.
191. Diebel LN, Dulchavsky SA, Wilson RF. Effect of increased intra-abdominal pressure on mesenteric arterial and intestinal mucosal blood flow. J Trauma 1992;33:45.
192. Murakami T, Itoshima T, Shimida Y. Peribiliary portal system in the monkey liver as evidenced by the injection replica scanning electron microscope method. Arch Histol Jap 1974;37:245–266.
193. Tzakis AG, Gordon RD, Shaw BW, et al. Clinical presentation of hepatic artery thrombosis after liver transplantation in the cyclosporin era. Transplantation 1985;40:667–671.
194. Langnas AN, Stratta RJ, Wood RP, et al. Hepatic allograft rescue following arterial thrombosis. Transplantation 1991;51:86–90.
195. Sherman S, Jamidar P, Shaked A, et al. Biliary tract complications after orthotopic liver transplantation. Endoscopic approach to diagnosis and therapy. Transplantation 1995;60(5):467–470.
196. Crawford DH, Endre ZH, Axelsen RA. Universal occurrence of glomerular abnormalities in patients receiving liver transplants. Am J Kidney Dis 1992;19:339–344.
197. Ishitani M, Wilkowski M, Stevenson W, Pruett T. Outcome of patients requiring hemodialysis after liver transplantation. Transplant Proc 1993;25:1762–1763.
198. McCauley J, Van Thiel DH, Starzl TE, Puschett JB. Acute and chronic renal failure in liver transplantation. Nephron 1990;55:121–128.
199. Fevery J, Van CE, Nevens F, et al. Reversal of hepatorenal syndrome in four patients by peroral misoprostol (prostaglandin E1 analogue) and albumin administration. J Hepatol 1990;11(2):153–158.
200. Henley KS, Lucey MR, Normolle DP, et al. A double-blind, randomized, placebo-controlled trial of prostaglandin E1 in liver transplantation [see comments]. Hepatology 1995;21(2):366–372.
201. Swygert TH, Roberts LC, Valek TR, et al. Effect of intraoperative low-dose dopamine on renal function in liver transplant recipients. Anesthesiology 1991;75(4):571–576.
202. Kaminski MV, Williams SD. Review of the rapid normalization of serum albumin with modified total parenteral nutrition solutions. Crit Care Med 1990;18:327–335.
203. Munoz SJ, Deems RO, Mortiz MJ. Hyperlipidemia and obesity after orthotopic liver transplantation. Transplant Proc 1991;21:1480–1483.
204. Hasse J. Nutritional aspect of adult liver transplantation. In: Busutill RW, Klintmalm GB, eds. Transplantation of the liver. Philadelphia: WB Saunders, 1996:359–367.
205. Janu P, Li J, Renegar KB, et al. Recovery of gut-associated lymphoid tissue and upper respiratory tract immunity after parenteral nutrition. Ann Surg 1997;225:707–717.
206. Wijdicks EFM. Impaired consciousness after liver transplantation. Liver Transplant Surg 1995;1(5):329–334.
207. Wszolek ZK, Steg RE. Seizures after liver transplantation. Liver Transplant Surg 1995;1(5):334–339.
208. Whiteman K, Nachtmann L, Kramer D, et al. Effects of continuous lateral rotation therapy on pulmonary complications in liver transplant patients. Am J Crit Care 1995;4(2):133–139.
209. Robinson LR, Switala J, Tarter RE, Nicholas JJ. Functional outcome after liver transplantation: a preliminary report. Arch Phys Med Rehabil 1990;71(6):426–427.
210. Adams PC, Ghent CN, Grant DR, Wall WJ. Employment after liver transplantation. Hepatology 1995;21(1):140–144.
211. Demetris AJ, Tsamandas AC, Delaney CP, et al. Pathology of liver transplantation. In: Busutill RW, Klintmalm GB, eds. Transplantation of the liver. Philadelphia: WB Saunders, 1996:681–723.
212. Fisher NC, Nightingale PG, Gunson BK, et al. Chronic renal failure following liver transplantation: a retrospective analysis. Transplantation 1998;66:59–66.
213. Benning CR, Smith A. Psychosocial needs of family members of liver transplant patients [see comments]. Clin Nurse Spec 1994;8(5):280–288.
214. Abbasoglu O, Levy MF, Brkic BB, et al. Ten years of liver transplantation: an evolving understanding of late graft loss. Transplantation 1997;64:1801–1807.
215. Tarter RE, Switala J, Arria A, et al. Quality of life before and after orthotopic hepatic transplantation. Arch Intern Med 1991;151(8):1521–1526.
216. McCaughan GW, Feller RB. Osteoporosis in chronic liver disease: pathogenesis, risk factors, and management. Dig Dis 1994;12(4):223–231.
217. Payne JL, McCarty KR, Drougas JG, et al. Outcomes analysis for 50 liver transplant recipients: the Vanderbilt experience. Am Surg 1996;62(4):320–325.
218. Smith DG, Henley KS, Remmert CS, et al. A cost analysis of alprostadil in liver transplantation. Pharmacoeconomics 1996;9(6):517–524.
219. Lake JR, Gorman KJ, Esquivel CO, et al. The impact of immunosuppressive regimens on the cost of liver transplantation—results from the U.S. FK506 multicenter trial. Transplantation 1995;60(10):1089–1095.
220. Keogh A, Spratt P, McCosker C, et al. Ketoconazole to reduce the need for cyclosporine after cardiac transplantation [see comments]. N Engl J Med 1995;333(10):628–633.

221. Roberts SD, Maxwell DR, Gross TL. Cost-effective care of end-stage renal disease: a billion dollar question. Ann Int Med 1980;92:243–248.
222. Aranzabal JL, Perdigo J, Mijares J, Villar F. Cost analysis of alternative treatments in end-stage renal disease. Transplant Proc 1992;24:335.
223. Feliciano DV, Pachter HL. Hepatic trauma revisited. Curr Probl Surg 1989;26(7):453–524.
224. Yellin AE, Chaffee CB, Donovan AJ. Vascular isolation in treatment of juxtahepatic venous injuries. Arch Surg 1971;102(6):566–573.
225. Krige JE, Worthley CS, Terblanche J. Severe juxtahepatic venous injury: survival after prolonged hepatic vascular isolation without shunting. HPB Surg 1990;3(1):39–43.
226. Cox EF, Flancbaum L, Dauterive AH, Paulson RL. Blunt trauma to the liver. Analysis of management and mortality in 323 consecutive patients. Ann Surg 1988;207(2):126–134.
227. Cogbill TH, Moore EE, Jurkovich GJ, et al. Severe hepatic trauma: a multicenter experience with 1,335 liver injuries. J Trauma 1988;28(10):1433–1438.
228. Launois B, de Chateaubriant P, Rosat P, Kiroff GK. Repair of suprahepatic caval lesions under extracorporeal circulation in major liver trauma. J Trauma 1989;29(1):127–128.
229. McAnena OJ, Moore EE, Moore FA. Insertion of a retrohepatic vena cava balloon shunt through the saphenofemoral junction. Am J Surg 1989;158(5):463–466.
230. Pachter HL, Spencer FC, Hofstetter SR, et al. Significant trends in the treatment of hepatic trauma. Experience with 411 injuries. Ann Surg 1992;215(5):492–500.
231. Ryckman FC, Noseworthy J, Penn I, Alexander JW. The use of mesenteric venous cannulation for portal access during venovenous bypass in orthotopic hepatic transplantation. Clin Transplant 1989;3:331–335.
232. Huguet C, Gavelli A, Bona S. Hepatic resection with ischemia of the liver exceeding one hour. J Am Coll Surg 1994;178(5):454–458.
233. Hannoun L, Panis Y, Balladur P, et al. Ex-situ in-vivo liver surgery [letter]. Lancet 1991;337(8757):1616–1617.
234. Pichlmayr R, Grosse H, Hauss J, et al. Technique and preliminary results of extracorporeal liver surgery (bench procedure) and of surgery on the in situ perfused liver. Br J Surg 1990;77(1):21–26.
235. Esquivel CO, Bernardos A, Makowka L, et al. Liver replacement after massive hepatic trauma. J Trauma 1987;27(7):800–802.
236. Mor E, Klintmalm GB, Gonwa TA, et al. The use of marginal donors for liver transplantation. A retrospective study of 365 liver donors. Transplantation 1992;53(2):383–386.
237. Alexander JW, Vaughn WK. The use of "marginal" donors for organ transplantation. The influence of donor age on outcome. Transplantation 1991;51(1):135–141.
238. Washburn WK, Johnson LB, Lewis WD, Jenkins RL. Graft function and outcome of older (> or = 60 years) donor livers. Transplantation 1996;61(7):1062–1066.
239. Ploeg RJ, D'Alessandro AM, Knechtle SJ, et al. Risk factors for primary dysfunction after liver transplantation—a multivariate analysis. Transplantation 1993;55(4):807–813.
240. Lindell SL, Hansen T, Rankin M, et al. Donor nutritional status—a determinant of liver preservation injury. Transplantation 1996;61(2):239–247.
241. Marino IR, Doyle HR, Aldrighetti L, et al. Effect of donor age and sex on the outcome of liver transplantation. Hepatology 1995;22(6):1754–1762.
242. Kahn D, Gavaler JS, Makowka L, van Thiel DH. Gender of donor influences outcome after orthotopic liver transplantation in adults. Dig Dis Sci 1993;38(8):1485–1488.

COMMENTARY REFERENCES

1. White D. Proceedings of the Novartis Immunosuppression Congress, Florence, Italy, February 1998.
2. Zaidi A, Schmoeckel M, Bhatti F, et al. Life-supporting pig-to-primate renal xenotransplantation using genetically modified donors. Transplantation 1998;65:1584–1890.
3. Schmoeckel M, Bhatti F, Zaidi A, et al. Orthotopic heart transplantation in a transgenic pig-to-primate model. Transplantation 1998;65:1570–1577.
4. Tanaka A, Tanaka K, Shinohara H. Extension of the indication for living related liver transplantation from children to adults based on resolution of graft size mismatch in relation to tissue oxygenation and metabolic load: a case report. Transplant Int 1996;9(suppl I):S174–S177.
5. Lo C-M, Fan ST, Liu C-L, et al. Adult to adult living donor liver transplantation using extended right lobe grafts. Ann Surg 1997;226:261–269.
6. Mirza DF, Achilleos O, Pirenne J, et al. Encouraging results of split liver transplantation. Br J Surg 1998;85:494–497.
7. De Ville de Goyet J, Hausleithner V, Malaise J, et al. Liver procurement without in situ portal perfusion. Transplantation 1993;56:1130–1136.
8. Rogiers X, Malago M, Gawad K, et al. In situ splitting of cadaver livers. Ann Surg 1996;224:331–339.
9. D'Alessandro AM, Kalayoglu M, Sollinger HW, et al. The predictive value of donor liver biopsies on the development of primary non-function after orthoptic liver transplantation. Transplant Proc 1991;23:1536–1537.
10. Multimer D. Proceedings of the International Gastro Congress. Strasbourg, April 1998.

Chapter

20

Liver Transplantation in Children

SUE V. MCDIARMID

The first cases of successful orthotopic liver transplantation (OLT) were in children (1), heralding a new era in pediatric hepatology that offered hope for children dying of liver failure (2). The pediatric liver recipient presents unique challenges to both the transplant surgeon and the physician. The small size of the majority of children who receive liver transplantation (61% are under 5 years of age) (3) incurs a risk of technical complications, the most common of which has been an increased incidence of hepatic artery thrombosis as compared to adult liver recipients (4). However, the small size of pediatric patients awaiting transplant has allowed them more recently to profit from innovative techniques that use partial liver grafts, including living-related grafts, reduced size grafts, and split liver grafts (5–7).

The general principles of immunosuppression in pediatric and adult liver recipients are similar, but children appear to be more immunoresponsive than their adult counterparts (8,9), with the possible exception of young infants in whom rates of rejection were recently noted to be low (10). In spite of children's rejection tendencies, the need to potentiate growth in children after OLT has been the impetus to reducing or withdrawing steroids from maintenance immunosuppressive protocols. As the potency of new immunosuppressive drugs has increased, children receiving organ transplants have experienced fewer rejection episodes, but they have had an associated rising incidence of lymphoproliferative disease, particularly among those children receiving liver transplants (11).

The difference in life expectancy between adults and children after OLT has altered our concept of long-term outcome. The milestones of childhood—growth, development, education, reproductive maturity, and entrance into society as a productive individual—must be achieved in the context of long-term immunosuppression and its possible complications. Because of the relatively short history of successful OLT, our ability to provide the best care over many years to this unique population of children has been hampered by sparse long-term outcome data. However, we now have a new opportunity to evaluate long-term outcomes and devise management strategies that can optimize the care of children in the decades following liver transplantation.

SURGICAL TECHNIQUES, PATIENT AND GRAFT SURVIVALS

The success of pediatric OLT, as reflected in both patient and graft survival, continues to improve. This is in large part due to improved surgical techniques that have decreased the incidence of hepatic artery thrombosis (12–14). Also, the development of reduced size grafts not only decreased the mortality of children waiting, but also shortened the waiting times so that children are in better condition when they receive their transplants (15–17).

The principles of recipient hepatectomy and whole organ transplantation are similar between adult and pediatric recipients (see Chapter 19). The unique surgical aspects of pediatric liver transplantation are the techniques for living-related, reduced, and split liver transplantation (Figs. 20.1, 20.2) (5,18,19). In living donor transplantation, the donor, usually a parent, undergoes a partial hepatectomy, most often of the left lateral segment of the liver. A reduced liver graft uses the left lobe or left lateral segment (less commonly the right lobe) from a whole cadaveric graft, with wastage of the unused portion of the donor organ. In contrast, the split procedure divides the cadaveric organ either in vivo or ex vivo to yield two transplantable segments; the left lateral segment or left lobe is usually placed into a pediatric recipient, and the right lobe is used for an older child or small adult recipient. Although the success of reduced liver trans-

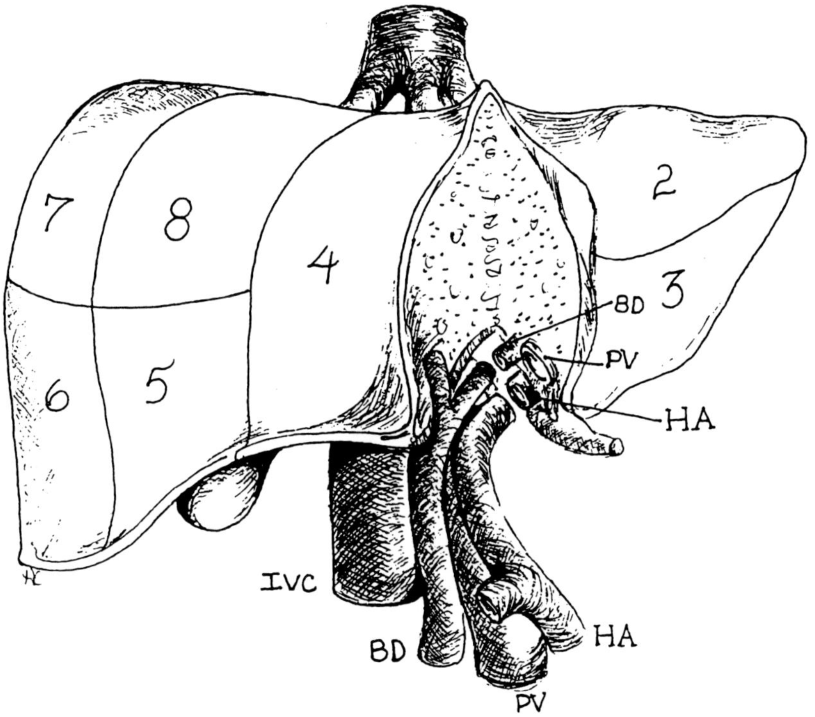

FIGURE 20.1. *The segmental anatomy of the liver is shown. During in situ liver splitting, the dissection is made between segment 4 and segments 2 and 3 after isolating the left hepatic artery, left portal vein, and left hepatic vein in the heart-beating cadaver. BD, bile duct; PV, portal vein; HA, hepatic artery; IVC, inferior vena cava. (Reproduced by permission from Goss JA, Yersiz H, Shackleton CR, et al. In situ splitting of the cadaveric liver for transplantation. Transplantation 1997;64:871–877.)*

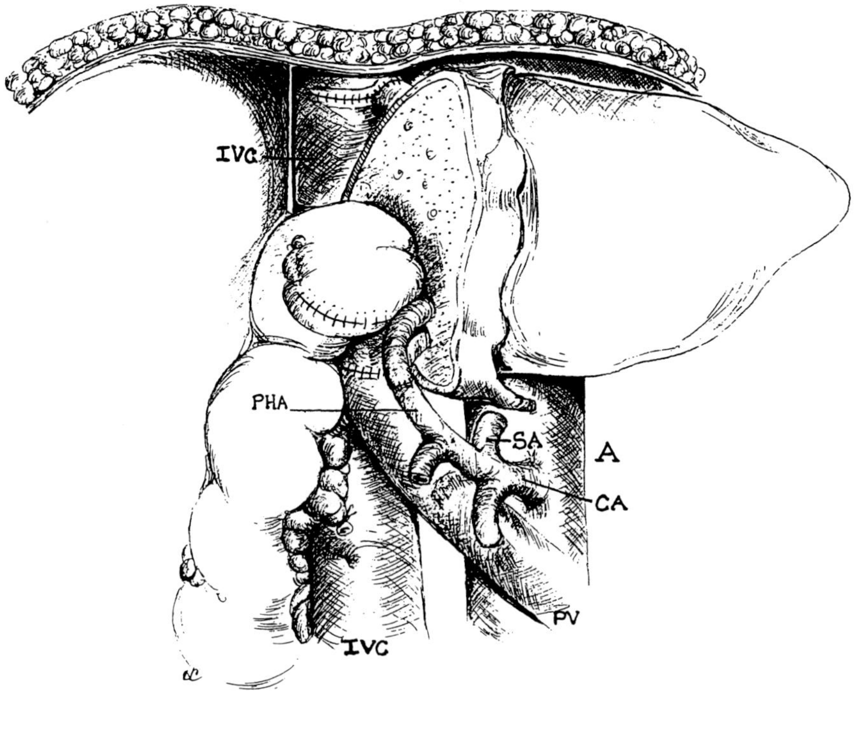

FIGURE 20.2. *A schematic representation of the implanted left lateral segment liver allograft is shown. The patient's inferior vena cava (IVC) is left intact. The following anastomoses are made: donor left hepatic vein to confluence of recipient middle and left hepatic veins; donor left portal vein to recipient portal vein; donor left hepatic artery to recipient common hepatic artery. The biliary reconstruction is a Roux-en-Y hepaticojejunostomy. IVC, inferior vena cava; PHA, proper hepatic artery; SA, splenic artery; A, aorta; CA, celiac axis; PV, portal vein. (Reproduced by permission from Goss JA, Yersiz H, Shackleton CR, et al. In situ splitting of the cadaveric liver for transplantation. Transplantation 1997;64:871–877.)*

plantation made the evolution of both living-related and split transplantation possible, the reduction procedure is now rarely used by programs able to perform the split transplantation. In the face of the increasing deficit in donor organs, the practice of discarding the right lobe should be avoided whenever possible.

The 5-year actuarial patient and graft survival rates after pediatric liver transplantation, as reported in 1996 by the United Network of Organ Sharing (UNOS, the US national database) for the period October 1987 to December 1994, were 75.8% and 59.9%, respectively (3). Tables 20.1 and 20.2 analyze these survival rates by age. Although children less than 1 year of age had a poorer outcome (20,21), recent reports suggest that the reduced waiting time and decreased incidence of hepatic artery thrombosis have removed the survival disadvantage of this group (15,22,23). Several centers have recently emphasized improved results, even in very young infants, following the institution of

Table 20.1. Kaplan Meier Patient Survival: Pediatric OLT Recipients

Age at OLT (Years)	N	3-Month Survival (%)	1-Year Survival (%)	2-Year Survival (%)	3-Year Survival (%)	5-Year Survival (%)
<1	924	80.1	76.8	74.5	72.5	70.2
1–5	1438	82.9	78.3	75.9	74.9	72.7
6–10	504	90.0	85.9	84.2	83.1	82.0
11–17	651	86.9	82.6	82.2	80.8	78.5

October 1987–December 1994. From UNOS 1996 Annual Report.

Table 20.2. Kaplan Meier Graft Survival: Pediatric OLT Recipients

Age at OLT (Years)	N	3-Month Survival (%)	1-Year Survival (%)	2-Year Survival (%)	3-Year Survival (%)	5-Year Survival (%)
<1	924	68.2	62.8	58.4	55.5	53.1
1–5	1438	72.2	65.5	61.1	59.2	56.1
6–10	504	77.3	71.4	62.8	66.5	62.9
11–17	651	77.8	71.0	68.5	65.5	59.8

October 1987–December 1994. From UNOS 1996 Annual Report.

reduced-size grafting and living-related transplantation in their programs (6,22,24–26).

Living-Related Transplantation

Living-related liver transplantation was first described in 1990 (27). It opened up new possibilities for planning transplantation at optimum times for children with chronic liver disease, thus reducing morbidity and mortality from long waiting periods. The success and safety of the procedure are now well documented (22,28). This procedure has gained widespread acceptance in Japan, where cadaveric organs are not generally available. The excellent results attainable are exemplified by the Kyoto experience, where over 300 living-related transplants have been performed. Actual patient and graft survivals are reported at 81.7% and 80.4%, respectively (29). Recently, a more extended application of living-related transplantation in older children and small adults has been described (30).

Other centers that perform both cadaveric and living-related OLT emphasize that living-related transplantation allows children to be transplanted at an optimal time, and thus cadaveric organs can be allocated to very ill children without suitable living donors. One center reported pediatric patient and graft survival for cadaveric grafts of 88% and 74%, respectively, with corresponding patient and graft survival of 94% and 83% for living-related transplantation (6).

Ethical considerations assume critical importance in considering living-related transplant decisions when cadaveric transplants are also available (31,32). Donor safety is paramount and the donor evaluation must include a rigorous psychosocial evaluation as well as a period of intensive education before informed consent is obtained (33–35). The potential donor must also undergo a complete history and physical examination, including careful checking for any transmittable diseases and imaging procedures to evaluate the size of the left lobe and detect any vascular anomalies.

In larger pediatric programs using split liver transplantation techniques, the shortened pediatric waiting time has almost obviated the need for living-related transplantation. The exception is in fulminant liver failure when no suitable donor is available. For ethical reasons some centers will not perform living-related transplantation under such conditions, but several pediatric centers have reported successful outcomes with living-related transplantation (28,36,37).

Split Liver Transplantation

The obvious advantage of the split liver technique is the ability to provide transplants for two recipients using one donor organ (38,39). In the early experience of split OLT, graft survival (particularly of the right lobe graft) was suboptimal (19,38,40), prompting a refinement in the surgical techniques learned from living-related transplantation (41). The European split transplant registry reported a 6-month actual graft survival of elective and urgent OLTs in children of 80% and 61%, respectively, and 72% and 56% in adults (42). These encouraging results prompted more widespread use of the procedure.

The success of split liver transplantation depends on meticulous selection of high quality donors, compatible vascular anatomy, and familiarity with the techniques of reduced or living-related transplantation. Both in vivo and ex vivo splitting (43) have their proponents. The excellent results achievable from in vivo splitting, based on the technique of living-related procurement, are demonstrated by recent reports of patient and graft survivals of 81.2% to 100% and 75% to 80%, respectively (44,45). More widespread use of liver splitting should be an important priority to achieve the benefits of shortened waiting times (particularly for children) and improved use of donor organs. The success of the concept will depend on the ability to place both halves of the donor organ expeditiously, either within the same transplant program or through sharing agreements with other programs.

Auxiliary Liver Transplantation

The auxiliary transplant technique implants a whole or part of an allograft in either the orthotopic or the heterotopic position. All or part of the native liver remains intact (19,46). This technique has been applied most often in fulminant liver failure as a means of temporary restoration of liver function, in hope that the native liver will recover (47). In pediatric patients, the particular application of this technique has been for the treatment of metabolic diseases caused by single enzyme defects in the liver, such as Crigler-Najjar syndrome and urea cycle defects. The mass of a whole liver is apparently not required to restore "normal" metabolism. By leaving a portion of the structurally normal native liver intact, the child is protected from liver failure should the graft fail. Successful application of this concept has been reported in Crigler-Najjar syndrome (48,49), urea cycle defects (19,46), and propionic acidemia (49). However, technical problems, particularly vascular steal syndromes, have limited the more widespread application of the auxiliary transplantation technique.

Factors Affecting Survival

Apart from age, the factors that affect survival after transplantation are the patient's pretransplantation nutritional status, urgency status at time of transplant, the indications for transplant, any previous abdominal surgery or previous liver transplantation, and extrahepatic systemic disease (50).

Children with biliary atresia have traditionally had a worse outcome because of their small size and often malnourished state at the time of transplantation, but more recently improved survivals are being reported (51–53). An 11-year experience of biliary atresia (54) reported actuarial 5-year patient and graft survivals of 78% and 70%, respectively—better than the overall UNOS data. Children with metabolic disease, especially α1-antitrypsin deficiency, have had one of the best prognoses (51,55), perhaps because they are generally older at the time of transplant and usually have not had previous abdominal surgery. Previous abdominal surgery such as a portoenterostomy (the Kasai operation) has been associated with an increased risk of bowel perforation after transplantation. Mortality following this complication has been reported as high as 50% (56). Pediatric liver transplantation for malignancy also carries a poor prognosis, with a reported survival for hepatoblastoma of only 50% at 4 years (57).

As discussed below, malnutrition at the time of OLT has a significant impact on mortality and morbidity after transplantation. Risk scores based on pretransplant bilirubin, body weight, and partial thromboplastin time (PTT) were associated with increased mortality in one study (58).

Retransplantation is associated with a decrease in both patient and graft survival. Hepatic artery thrombosis is still the most common reason for retransplantation, with primary nonfunction (5.3%), initial poor function (2.1%), and chronic rejection (3%) being much less frequent indications (59). In one center's experience, pediatric patient and graft survival were 53.8% and 43.1%, respectively, following retransplantation (60). Whether retransplantation is elective or emergent also affects the outcome: reported patient survival is 82% for elective procedures versus 46% for emergent retransplantation (61). Age less than 3 years also adversely impacted survival after retransplantation (60). It has also been noted that retransplantation at the time of failure of three or more other organ systems is associated with a less than 20% survival (62).

The three most common pretransplant extrahepatic systemic diseases that adversely affect outcome are renal failure, cerebral edema, and hypoxemia. A 47% mortality in children who required pretransplant dialysis has been reported (63). Cerebral edema, seen as a consequence of fulminant liver failure, must be carefully monitored prior to a transplant to avoid a devastating neurologic outcome after a technically successful OLT (64,65). Pretransplant hypoxemia secondary to the poorly understood phenomenon of arteriovenous pulmonary shunts in patients with chronic liver disease (66) may result in an increased risk of posttransplant hepatic artery thrombosis. Although arteriovenous pulmonary shunting was previously considered a relative contraindication to transplant, recent reports suggest these children can be successfully transplanted, with eventual reversal of the shunt (67,68).

INDICATIONS

OLT is performed in children most often for cholestatic or metabolic liver disease (69–72), whereas in adults postnecrotic cirrhosis is the most common indication (73). As listed in Table 20.3, there are six broad categories of indications for OLT: cholestatic liver disease, metabolic liver disease, fulminant liver failure, chronic active hepatitis and cirrhosis, malignancy, and miscellaneous disorders.

Cholestatic Liver Disease

Cholestatic liver disease requiring OLT in children can be divided into two categories: obstructive and nonobstructive processes.

Table 20.3. Categories for OLT Indications

1. Cholestatic Liver Disease
   - Biliary atresia
   - Paucity intrahepatic bile ducts
     - Syndromic (Alagille's)
     - Nonsyndromic
   - Familial cholestasis syndromes
   - Sclerosing cholangitis
   - Caroli's disease
2. Fulminant Liver Failure
   - Viruses (e.g., hepatitis A, B)
   - Toxins (e.g., drugs, mushrooms)
   - Metabolic (e.g., Wilson's disease)
3. Metabolic Liver Disease
   - α1-Antitrypsin deficiency
   - Wilson's disease
   - Tyrosinemia
   - Urea cycle defects
   - Familial hypercholesterolemia
   - Glycogen storage disease (IA and IV)
   - Crigler-Najjar syndrome
   - Neonatal iron storage disease
   - Disorders of bile acid metabolism
   - Hyperoxaluria type 1
   - Selected lipid storage disease
   - Hematologic disorders
     - Hemophilia A, B
     - Protein C deficiency, porphyria
   - Selected organic acidemias
4. Chronic Active Hepatitis/Cirrhosis
   - Autoimmune
   - Neonatal hepatitis
   - Chronic hepatitis C, B
   - Cryptogenic cirrhosis
5. Malignancy
   - Hepatoblastoma
   - Hepatocellular carcinomas
   - Sarcomas
   - Hemangioendothelioma
6. Miscellaneous
   - Budd-Chiari syndrome
   - Trauma
   - Cystic fibrosis
   - Cirrhosis secondary to parenteral nutrition

Obstructive Processes

Of the obstructive processes, biliary atresia is by far the most important diagnosis and is the indication for OLT in more than 50% of children (51). Liver transplantation, however, is not a substitute for a portoenterostomy (the Kasai operation), which should still be performed if the child is diagnosed before 3 months (74–76). However, even with early diagnosis and optimal timing of the portoenterostomy, approximately 75% of children will eventually require OLT—the majority before the age of 5 years (77,78). It is therefore mandatory that children with biliary atresia be assiduously followed so that early referral can be made at the first evidence of liver decompensation.

Other less common obstructive cholestatic disorders for which OLT may be indicated in childhood are sclerosing cholangitis (either primary, or secondary to autoimmune disease), uncorrectable choledochal cyst, and intrahepatic biliary cystic disease (Caroli's syndrome).

Nonobstructive Processes

The nonobstructive cholestatic diseases for which OLT may be required have a variable presentation but are generally characterized histologically by paucity of the intrahepatic ducts (79). The most recognized of these diseases are the syndromic and nonsyndromic forms of Alagille's syndrome (80). The syndromic form, which has variable inheritance, may also be associated with characteristic facies, cardiovascular anomalies (especially pulmonary stenosis), growth retardation, butterfly vertebrae, and posterior embryotoxon in the eye (81). In some rare conditions, disorders of bile acid metabolism have been associated with nonobstructive cholestatic disease (82). However, in several other conditions, such as the familial cholestatic diseases of infancy (83) and Byler's disease, the cause remains unknown. In these conditions, normal γ-glutamyl-transpeptidase activity has been associated with a poor prognosis (84).

Unlike biliary atresia, in which the natural history is usually predictable, the nonobstructive cholestatic diseases may have a variable presentation and clinical course. For example, the cholestasis of Alagille's syndrome may show significant improvement throughout childhood, making liver transplantation unnecessary, or it may follow a course of early liver decompensation requiring transplantation (85,86). Byler's disease frequently causes early liver decompensation for which OLT is lifesaving (87), in contrast to other forms of familial intrahepatic cholestasis which may remain quiescent over time or improve with bile acid therapy (88).

Metabolic Disease

This diagnostic category encompasses a wide spectrum of metabolic diseases, some relatively common with well-established criteria for OLT, others so rare that there are only occasional case reports of successful OLT (89).

The most common of the two metabolic diseases for which OLT is most often performed in childhood is α1-antitrypsin disease (the other is Wilson's disease) (51,90). In general, these children are somewhat older at the time of OLT than are children with biliary atresia, and have an excellent outcome (87.5% 1-year survival in one series) (55). Patients with Wilson's disease typically present in older childhood and adolescence, typically in a setting of previously unrecognized liver disease with portal hypertension and variceal bleeding, or with fulminant liver failure, requiring urgent transplantation (91–93).

The urea cycle defects (94), of which ornithine transcarbamylase deficiency is the most common, are rare metabolic diseases of infancy. Early diagnosis of these conditions in the first days of life, followed by aggressive intervention to control hyperammonemia, is necessary to avoid profound central nervous system damage (95,96). Even with meticulous dietary and medical management, life-threatening hyperammonemic crises can be precipitated by a simple upper respiratory tract infection (97). The outcome with medical therapy alone is dismal: a 79% incidence of neurologic disability with a mean IQ of 43 at 1 year of age (98). Once these children have been identified and stabilized (assuming that central nervous system damage has not occurred), they must undergo transplantation on an urgent basis (99).

OLT is curative for tyrosinemia (100–103), which presents as fulminant liver failure in infancy, as slowly decompensating chronic liver disease in childhood (104), or rarely, with life-threatening neurologic crises (105). The unusual feature of tyrosinemia, and one which influences the timing of OLT, is the likelihood (37% after age 3 years) of the child developing hepatocellular carcinoma (106). Therefore, preemptive OLT before the age of 2 years is advocated by many (107,108). The associated renal disease generally improves after OLT (109,110).

Because of the complexity of metabolic disease in childhood and the frequently associated extrahepatic manifestations, several important principles must be applied to determine whether OLT is indicated (111). The deficient enzyme and its location must be known. If the enzyme is predominantly confined to the liver (as in urea cycle defects or glucuronyl transferase deficiency of Crigler-Najjar syndrome), then liver replacement early in life can be expected to cure the defect (112–114). Careful assessment must be made of possible end-organ damage, such as central nervous system injury in Crigler-Najjar (115) and urea cycle defects, renal failure in hyperoxaluria, and atherosclerosis in familial hypercholesterolemia. Profound central nervous system damage may preclude eligibility for transplantation, but simultaneous liver–kidney replacement for primary hyperoxaluria (116,117) or combined liver–heart transplantation for familial hypercholesterolemia (118,119) may cure end-organ damage as well as replace the missing enzyme. Preemptive liver transplant alone has been used to avoid end-organ damage in hyperoxaluria (120) and familial hypercholesterolemia (121). Wilson's disease provides an example of extrahepatic manifestations (particularly in the central nervous system) that are largely reversible by OLT alone (122).

More widespread expression of the metabolic defect may preclude the possibility that successful OLT will allow long-term disease-free survival. Many storage diseases express the enzyme deficiency in extrahepatic cell lines. Thus, the disease would be expected to progress even after successful OLT. This is especially pertinent to storage diseases that affect the central nervous system and the heart, such as the mucopolysaccharidoses and liposomal storage diseases (e.g., Gaucher's disease and Niemann-Pick disease). OLT alone should not be performed when life-threatening extrahepatic deterioration is predicted.

Fulminant Liver Failure

Age less than 11 years is one of the identified risk factors for poor prognosis in fulminant liver failure (123); prior to the advent of OLT, survival was less than 30% (124). Success rates of 68% without sequelae can be achieved, but early referral to a transplant center is essential to avoid the catastrophe of irreversible cerebral edema (125).

Fulminant liver failure is the indication for OLT in about 8% of children (73). The most common etiologies are hepatitis A, hepatitis B, drug overdose, and Wilson's disease; in many children, however, no cause can be found (125). Potential drug toxicities include acetaminophen, INH (126), halothane, and sodium valproate. Accidental acetaminophen overdoses administered by parents who gave multiple and/or larger-than-recommended doses must always be considered in young children who present with fulminant liver failure (127,128).

Cirrhosis/Hepatitis

In the category of postnecrotic cirrhosis there are relatively few pediatric indications for OLT. The most important indication, autoimmune chronic active hepatitis, usually presents in late childhood, but it is occasionally seen in children before 5 years of age (129).

Malignancy

The most common hepatic malignancy in childhood is hepatoblastoma (130,131). Unlike hepatocellular carcinoma, it is generally locally invasive and relatively slow to metastasize. If the tumor cannot be resected at the time of presentation, chemotherapy will sometimes shrink the tumor and allow successful resection. Should this approach fail, the child should be referred for OLT without delay, particularly when there is tumor in both lobes (132). The key to ultimate tumor-free survival is transplantation before any evidence of distant metastases or large vessel invasion has appeared. Long-term survival of about 50% has been reported after liver transplantation for hepatoblastoma (57).

Hepatocellular carcinoma is rarely seen in children, and it is usually found in the context of preexisting cirrhosis (133), particularly perinatally acquired hepatitis B, or in patients with tyrosinemia. Rare cases have also been reported in the cirrhotic livers of children with biliary atresia and Alagille's syndrome (134,135) or familial cholestatic syndromes (136). The long-term outcome of children following transplantation for hepatocellular carcinoma is unknown, although anecdotal experience suggests a high rate of recurrence.

Miscellaneous Indications

Cystic Fibrosis

Cystic fibrosis with secondary biliary cirrhosis usually presents in older children as portal hypertension (137). The decision regarding OLT is complicated by the anticipated deleterious effect of immunosuppression on existing pulmonary infection. However, children with relatively severe liver disease and more moderate pulmonary disease have been successfully transplanted without inducing major post-OLT pulmonary infectious complications (138–141). Combined lung–liver transplantation has been considered in a few children.

Short Gut Syndrome

Children with short gut syndrome may eventually develop chronic liver failure secondary to the poorly understood effects of long-term parenteral nutrition (142). In recent years, combined liver–small bowel transplantation has had some success in restoring normal liver function and allowing normal enteral nutrition. However, this combined procedure is fraught with major complications, including acute and chronic rejection (particularly of the small bowel allograft), infection, a high incidence of cytomegalovirus (CMV), and post-transplant lymphoproliferative disorder (PTLD). The 1-year actuarial patient and graft survivals in experienced programs are at 51% to 76% and 44% to 61%, respectively (143,144). Careful patient selection and the use of tacrolimus for primary immunosuppression has improved outcome (145) (see also Chapter 22).

LISTING CRITERIA

The appropriate time to list the child with chronic liver disease depends on an understanding of the natural history of the disease as well as knowing the expected waiting times for organ donation. The practice of listing too early (often with the purpose of accumulating waiting-time points) may result in the improper allocation of the scarce donor supply and is to be discouraged. On the other hand, delay in listing children who have indications for OLT can result in significant morbidity and mortality. As the majority of children have cholestatic liver disease, worsening malnutrition, often complicated by recurrent biliary sepsis, becomes an important negative predictor of survival both before and after OLT (146). For this reason, growth failure alone is an important criteria for determining the time of listing in children.

Children should be listed for OLT at the first sign of liver decompensation or if liver decompensation is imminent. However, there are several diseases, including the urea cycle defects and Crigler-Najjar syndrome, in which liver decompensation does not occur but the consequences of the metabolic defect are life-threatening, mandating listing at the highest priority as soon as the disease is identified and the child stabilized. Children with one or more of the criteria shown in Table 20.4 should be placed on the list.

Table 20.4. Conditions That Indicate Listing for Pediatric OLT Is Appropriate

Intractable cholestasis
Portal hypertension with variceal bleeding
Multiple episodes of ascending cholangitis
Failure of synthetic function
Failure to thrive and malnutrition
Intractable ascites
Encephalopathy
Unacceptable quality of life
Metabolic defects for which OLT will reverse life-threatening complications

Very few absolute contraindications remain to transplantation in children. Surgical experience has overcome most of the anatomic obstacles that were previously thought insurmountable (147–149). The improved prognosis of HIV infection has called into question whether even this should remain as an absolute contraindication (150). Relative contraindications are similar to those in adult patients; the most common are life-threatening extrahepatic system failure and sepsis (69). Meticulous assessment and observation of the critically ill child who is a candidate for OLT are essential to determine the time of transplant. This is particularly important in fulminant liver failure, where aggressive management of increased intracranial pressure is necessary to avoid a transplant in a child with irreversible cerebral edema (64).

PRETRANSPLANT CARE

Once the child has been identified for OLT, the major emphasis must be on optimizing nutritional status. Mortality awaiting transplant (151) and morbidity and mortality after transplant are both increased in the malnourished child (146). Malnutrition is particularly common in children awaiting liver transplantation because of the high incidence of cholestatic liver diseases in this group resulting in fat malabsorption, compounded by the catabolic effects of anorexia and intervening sepsis (152). In addition, peripheral insulin resistance in children with end-stage liver disease and increased protein metabolism lead to protein energy malnutrition (153).

Perturbations in the response to growth hormone (GH) and insulin growth factor-1 (IGF-1) are found in children with chronic liver disease (154,155). End-organ resistance is suggested by low IGF-1 levels despite elevated growth hormone concentrations. A study of exogenous GH failed to produce a beneficial response in children with biliary atresia (156).

In the waiting period prior to transplant, inadequate calorie intake should be supplemented either by the enteral route, most often with nocturnal nasogastric feedings (157), or by the parenteral route in children unable to tolerate enteral feedings (158). Parenteral nutrition has the particular advantage of being able to deliver the required calories with the appropriate limitations of sodium and fluid required in children with end-stage liver disease.

Other complications occurring in the pretransplant period such as variceal bleeding, cholangitis, and spontaneous bacterial peritonitis must be quickly identified and aggressively treated to avoid the tragedy of a child too sick to undergo transplantation.

EARLY POSTOPERATIVE COMPLICATIONS

Hepatic Artery Thrombosis

Hepatic artery thrombosis (HAT) remains the most important early postoperative complication distinguishing pediatric and adult recipients (Fig. 20.3). It is the most common reason for retransplantation (59) and one of the most common causes contributing to death in the pediatric population (159). The single most important factor accounting for the increased incidence in children is the technical challenge posed by the very small caliber of the hepatic artery anastomosis.

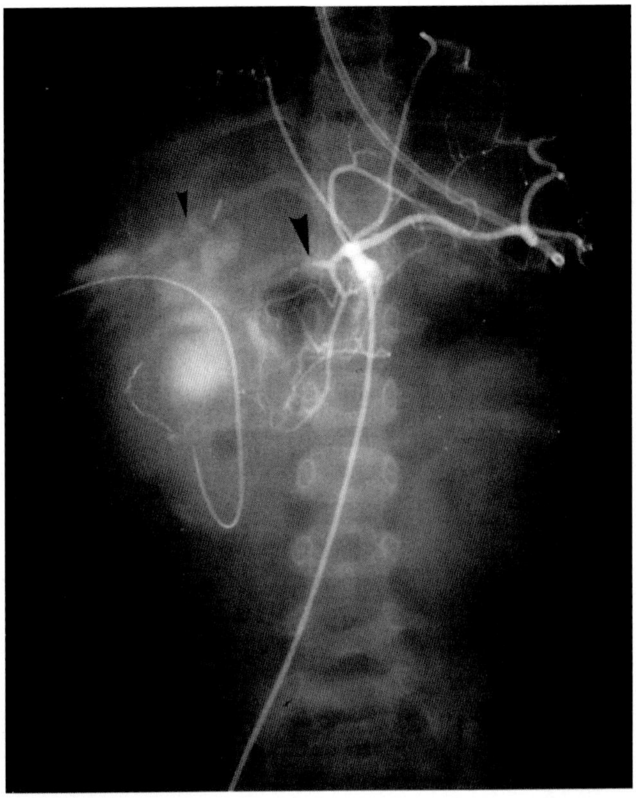

FIGURE 20.3. *Arterial angiography with cannulation of the celiac axis shows complete occlusion of the hepatic artery (*large arrow*). Also shown is the dye from a cholangiogram performed the previous day still pooled in the dilated biliary tree (*small arrows*), indicative of intrahepatic biliary strictures. A biliary stent is in place.*

Previously, the reported incidence was 10% to 15% in children, compared to less than 4% in adults (160). However, recent reports document important progress in reducing the incidence of HAT to as low as 1.7% (12). Meticulous microsurgical techniques and innovative surgical reconstructions are being increasingly used by many pediatric transplant surgeons, with a resultant decrease in the incidence of HAT in many programs (161). In addition, reduced, split, and living-related grafts have a reported lower incidence of HAT (13,14,162).

HAT has four common, but very different presentations (163):

1. In the worst-case scenario, usually occurring within the first days after OLT, HAT causes massive ischemic necrosis resulting in rapid graft failure and the need for immediate retransplantation.
2. Bile leaks and anastomotic breakdown, often with accompanying septicemia, may the first signs of HAT, because the viability of the biliary anastomosis is largely dependent on hepatic artery blood supply.
3. Relapsing bacteremia, usually with multiple enteric organisms but with relatively preserved liver function, can be the only clue to underlying HAT and biliary tract compromise.
4. Later in the postoperative course, HAT may present as biliary strictures, usually intrahepatic and multiple. There may be associated cholangitis and elevation in both bilirubin and transaminases.

Although medical management to decrease the incidence of HAT is of dubious benefit (164), it is still widely used. In general, hyperviscosity should be avoided. Anticoagulation of various types is commonly used. A procoagulant state, particularly associated with low antithrombin III levels, has been described (165,166). Heparinization carries the risk of bleeding and is usually reserved for high-risk patients. Dextran-40 and acetylsalicylic acid are frequently used for their antiplatelet properties (164,166).

Once HAT is suspected, rapid, accurate diagnosis is essential. This may often be easily accomplished, even at the bedside, by duplex ultrasonography. However, beyond the early postoperative period, the ultrasound signal may identify collateral vessels that are falsely interpreted as a patent hepatic artery (167). If clinical suspicion remains, the gold standard is still hepatic artery angiography. Most children with HAT will eventually require retransplantation, although in a few the collateral arterial supply sustains adequate liver graft function indefinitely.

Bowel Perforation

Unlike adults, the majority of children undergoing OLT have had previous major abdominal surgery, usually a portoenterostomy for treatment of biliary atresia. As a consequence, dense adhesions form. Thus, during the transplant operation, these children are predisposed to inadvertent bowel perforation, which carries an associated increase in both morbidity and mortality from septicemia, particularly from fungal infections and peritonitis (168,169). A very grave prognosis is associated with multiple bowel perforations (56). Early suspicion, rapid diagnosis, and exploratory laparotomy combined with broad-based antimicrobial therapy are essential to successful management.

Other Complications

The presentation, diagnosis, and management of the other major postoperative complications—primary nonfunction (PNF), bleeding, sepsis, biliary strictures and leaks, renal failure, and neurologic complications—are essentially the same in children as in adults (see Chapter 19) apart from the following distinguishing points.

Primary Nonfunction

PNF is uncommon in pediatric recipients, occurring in less than 5% of patients (59). The low incidence is most likely due to the relatively better quality of pediatric donors and the use of perfect adult donors for splitting. The exception is livers from neonatal donors, which have an increased risk of PNF (170). An arterial ketone body ratio (a measure of mitochondrial energy production) of less than 0.7 has been used in children to determine which livers are doomed to fail (171).

Bile Duct Complications

The use of reduced sized grafts has not increased the incidence of bile duct complications (172), although partial grafts are associated with more biliary leaks, occurring from the cut surface of the liver. This can often be managed conservatively.

Hepatorenal Syndrome

Dialysis dependence secondary to either hepatorenal syndrome or acute tubular necrosis, whether during the pretransplant or immediate post-transplant period, is uncommon in children. When present it is associated with an increased mortality (63). As in adults, hepatorenal syndrome is usually reversible after successful OLT (173).

Neurologic Complications

Neurologic complications seen in adults during the early post-transplant period, such as pontine myelinolysis syndrome and cerebral vascular accidents, are uncommon in children (174). Seizures, tremors, and relatively mild mental status changes may be seen secondary to either cyclosporine or tacrolimus therapy. These symptoms are generally dose related and reversible.

IMMUNOSUPPRESSION

Immunosuppression regimens for induction, maintenance, and treatment of rejection are generally similar for adult and pediatric recipients. However, there is evidence to suggest children are more immunoresponsive than adults (8,9), so particular attention is required for both adequate induction therapy and the prompt treatment of rejection.

Induction Therapy

Induction therapy is either cyclosporine-based (often combined with azathioprine) or tacrolimus-based (175,176). Both regimens are usually combined with steroids: high-dose intravenous for induction, and low-dose oral for maintenance. Polyclonal or monoclonal antibody induction therapy is not used routinely after pediatric liver transplantation. Although the incidence of early rejection with antibody induction is decreased (177), there has been no proven long-term benefit (178). The rare child with renal failure in the peritransplant period may gain an advantage from antibody induction therapy, so that initiation of cyclosporine or tacrolimus can be delayed until renal function has improved (see also Chapter 13).

Cyclosporine

Neoral, the microemulsion form of oral cyclosporine, is the major recent advance in cyclosporine-based immunosuppression (see Chapter 6). It has particular benefits in pediatric liver recipients (179,180). Neoral's major advantage compared to Sandimmune (the old cyclosporine formulation) is improved absorption with less dependence on bile in the intestinal lumen (181,182). As a result, the time to maximum concentration is shorter, the maximum concentration is higher, and the area under the time versus concentration curve is greater for Neoral compared to Sandimmune (183). These differences are evident even when 12-hour trough levels are held constant between the two formulations.

As young liver recipients are recognized as being relatively poor and erratic absorbers of Sandimmune, frequently needing doses many times in excess of their adult counterparts to achieve similar levels, the Neoral formulation may make cyclosporine management considerably easier (184–186). The effect of an increased total exposure to cyclosporine, assuming target levels remain the same, is still not well understood in children. Whether the rejection incidence will be less, or toxicity increased, remains to be determined (187). A potential advantage of Neoral induction therapy is the avoidance of intravenous cyclosporine and its associated risk of increased toxicity. Trials using Neoral as induction therapy alone indicate that therapeutic cyclosporine levels can be achieved (188).

Tacrolimus

The reduced incidence of rejection reported in the early studies of tacrolimus in pediatric liver recipients (189) prompted the inclusion of pediatric patients in the first large multicenter trial comparing induction and maintenance immunosuppression with tacrolimus versus cyclosporine (Sandimmune) (190). In the adult study there were no differences in patient or graft survival, but in the tacrolimus group there was a statistically significant reduction in overall rejection, steroid resistant rejection, chronic rejection, and cumulative steroid use compared to the cyclosporine group (191,192) (see Chapter 9). The same results were reproduced in the pediatric subgroup, although they did not reach statistical significance because of small numbers (190). However, these encouraging results prompted some centers to change their pediatric liver recipients to induction therapy with tacrolimus. Subsequent reports have confirmed the decreased incidence and severity of rejection and have established guidelines for optimal dosing (29,193–196).

Intravenous tacrolimus is not required to achieve therapeutic levels, thus avoiding some of the previously described toxicity problems (29,197). In addition, successful early steroid withdrawal has been reported (189,198). The toxicity profiles between cyclosporine and tacrolimus are remarkably similar (199,200), with no significant difference in the two most serious adverse events, nephrotoxicity (201,202) and neurotoxicity (203). However, as will be discussed below, tacrolimus may be associated with an increased risk of PTLD in children (204) (see also Chapter 37).

Maintenance Therapy

Maintenance immunosuppression regimens have recently focused on the perils of long-term overimmunosuppression. Reduction of both tacrolimus and cyclosporine levels, as well as steroid withdrawal, is achievable in many patients without precipitating rejection. This is a particularly important consideration in the management of pediatric recipients, in whom the effect of long-term steroid use on growth, or decades of exposure to nephrotoxic drugs, may have far reaching consequences.

Steroid withdrawal has been successfully reported in both cyclosporine (205,206) and tacrolimus regimens (189,198). The incidence of rejection in children is reported to be between 11% (207) and 22% (205). In the few prospective randomized trials of steroid withdrawal, no significant differences in rejection incidence were seen between the withdrawal and control groups (208,209). Caution is required in interpreting these results, as follow-up time is short. The incidence and severity of late rejection after long periods of steroid withdrawal are not yet known.

In stable pediatric liver recipients on Sandimmune, successful conversion to Neoral without significant side effects has been reported (210). However, monitoring of cyclosporine levels is essential in the first month after conversion because dose adjustment, usually reduction, is frequently required (211). A 1 : 1 conversion is generally safe unless the patient malabsorbs Sandimmune (a dose requirement of greater than 10–15 mg/kg/day), in which case the Neoral dose should be reduced to avoid toxic levels.

Rejection Therapy

The incidence of rejection in children after OLT is between 50% to 80%, but it seldom leads to patient death (51,212). First-line treatment for acute rejection in children, as in adults, depends on high-dose intravenous steroids. Steroid resistant rejection, more commonly seen in cyclosporine-based regimens, is treated either by monoclonal antibody therapy with OKT-3 (213) or by conversion to tacrolimus (214). In one report prior to the availability of tacrolimus, OKT-3 was required for 32% of the pediatric liver transplant population, was less efficacious in children compared to adults, and was more likely to induce a human anti-OKT-3 antibody response (215). These findings are consistent with the heightened immune response of children.

The first reports of tacrolimus conversion for steroid-resistant acute rejection in children, usually after failure of OKT-3, described a success rate of up to 80% (176,193,216,217). In addition, chronic rejection, for which no adequate therapy had previously existed, could be resolved in about 50% of cases (216,218).

Important to the success of conversion is switching before the total bilirubin level is higher than about 10 mg/dL (216). The price of this heavy immunosuppressive load, however, was an increased incidence of PTLD, which occurred in 18% to 25% of children (204,216). In an attempt to decrease the overall immunosuppressive burden in children with resistant rejection, several investigators now convert children to tacrolimus without prior OKT-3 therapy (214). The impact of this strategy on the incidence of PTLD is yet to be determined.

Other Agents

Mycophenolate mofetil (MMF) is the other major new immunosuppressant (219) currently available, but unfortunately it has not been well studied in pediatric liver recipients. Extrapolating from their experience in adult OLT recipients, most investigators use MMF in pediatric OLT recipients in conjunction with tacrolimus or cyclosporine, either to control resistant rejection (220) or as a means of lowering the doses of tacrolimus, cyclosporine, or steroids to obviate their side effects (221,222) (see also Chapter 10).

For pediatric liver recipients to receive the potential benefits of new immunosuppressive agents, such as humanized interleukin (IL)-2 receptor monoclonal antibodies, rapamycin, or CTLA4-Ig, they must be included in early trials. As was recently experienced during the early use of tacrolimus, doses (223) and pharmacokinetics (224) may be considerably different in children as compared to adults. Table 20.5 provides guidelines for doses and levels of immunosuppressive drugs used in children after OLT.

Table 20.5. Immunosuppressive Drugs and Doses for Pediatric OLT Guidelines

	Cyclosporine		
	Intravenous (mg/kg/day)	Oral (mg/kg/day)	Therapeutic Range (ng/mL)
Induction			
0–12 months	5–6[a]	10–15[a]	250–400
Maintenance			
1–12 months	0	5–20[b]	200–350
>12 months	0	5–20[b]	100–200
	Tacrolimus		
	Intravenous (mg/kg/day)	**Oral (mg/kg/day)**	**Therapeutic Range (ng/mL)**
Induction			
0–1 months	0	0.1–0.2[a]	12–15
1–3 months	0	0.05–0.30[b]	8–10
>3 months	0	0.05–0.30[b]	5–8
	Steroids		
	Intravenous Methylprednisolone		**Oral Prednisone/Prednisolone**
Induction			
POD 1	10 mg/kg/day		
POD 2	8 mg/kg/day		
POD 3	6 mg/kg/day		
POD 4	4 mg/kg/day		
POD 5	2 mg/kg/day		
Maintenance			0.3 mg/kg/day
Steroid wean, 6–12 months			0.3 mg/kg on alternate days
No rejection			Gradual wean off
Other Immunosuppressants			**Dose**
Azathioprine			1–2 mg/kg/day oral
OKT-3			2.5 mg/day IV (<30 kg) 5.0 mg/day IV (>30 kg)
Mycophenolate mofetil[c]			20–25 mg/kg/dose (given q 12 hours) 600 mg/m^2/dose (given q 12 hours)

[a] Adjust depending on early graft function and renal function.
[b] Adjust to maintain levels in therapeutic range.
[c] Derived from pediatric kidney dosing data (294).
POD = postoperative day.

LONG-TERM COMPLICATIONS

The causes of late graft dysfunction—biliary strictures, acute and chronic rejection, vascular compromise, and infection (225)—are similar in adult and pediatric patients and are described elsewhere. The exception is the low incidence of recurrent disease in the pediatric recipient's allograft, compared to the high incidence of hepatitis C in adult patients. Autoimmune disease and hepatic malignancy both may recur in pediatric liver grafts, but they are unusual indications for transplantation in children (129).

Most of the serious long-term extrahepatic complications after OLT are secondary to immunosuppression, including nephrotoxicity, neurotoxicity, PTLD, and impaired growth and development.

Nephrotoxicity

The majority of children will have some long-term impairment of renal function after liver transplantation (226). The nephrotoxicity of tacrolimus and cyclosporine is of equal magnitude and occurs to some degree almost universally (190,201,227). In the early post-transplant period, the impairment of kidney function is at least partially related to high levels of tacrolimus or cyclosporine, especially if given intravenously (228). This early nephrotoxic stage has a reversible component (229) and reflects the vasoconstrictive effect of tacrolimus and cyclosporine on renal blood flow (230,231). The biggest decrement in glomerular filtration rate (GFR) is seen within 1 month of transplant, and GFR remains relatively constant thereafter (201). By 1 to 2 years after transplant, histologic changes in the kidney may have occurred, making it unlikely that renal impairment will be substantially improved by decreases in tacrolimus or cyclosporine levels (232). Although the nephrotoxic potential of tacrolimus and cyclosporine is similar, hypertension requiring drug management is much less frequent in tacrolimus-treated children (196,201,233).

Few studies have examined true GFR in children after liver transplantation. One center reported that GFR measured by indium DTPA111 was <70 mL/min/1.73 m^2 in 73% of cyclosporine-treated children 1 year after transplant, with a significant further fall-off in mean GFR by 2 years after transplant. In addition, lower GFRs were associated with more hypertension and higher cyclosporine levels (234). Other authors, however, have reported that the loss in GFR can be avoided by cyclosporine dosing 3 times a day (235). The unanswered question is whether there is an inexorable fall in GFR over decades of tacrolimus and cyclosporine use (236).

The renal tubular defects induced by both cyclosporine and tacrolimus are also comparable, with magnesium wasting, metabolic acidosis, and hyperkalemia being the most common (201). The majority of children require long-term magnesium supplementation and may also need exogenous sources of bicarbonate. The correction of acid–base balance is particularly important because prolonged metabolic acidosis may impair growth.

Neurotoxicity

The neurotoxic effects of tacrolimus and cyclosporine are similar (203,237,238). Compared to adults, children appear to be relatively protected from central nervous system neurotoxicity, perhaps because they have less degenerative brain disease. In one study, 23% of adults versus 8% of children had neurologic complications after OLT (239).

Paresthesia and itching (particularly seen with tacrolimus) and tremor are usually dose related and occur most often in the early post-transplant period (199). Cyclosporine and tacrolimus may induce seizures usually in association with another threshold-lowering factor, usually low serum magnesium (240). Low serum cholesterol, by increasing the free drug capable of penetrating the central nervous system, has also been implicated in post-transplant seizures (241,242). Children may also exhibit the diffuse white matter changes described for both tacrolimus and cyclosporine (see Chapter 33), but these are frequently asymptomatic (243). The progression and effects of these gross structural changes in the brain over decades of exposure to these agents are unknown.

Post-transplant Hyperlipidemia

Hyperlipidemia is an important cause of morbidity and mortality in adult transplant recipients (see Chapter 31). Although hyperlipidemia has not yet been well studied in pediatric OLT recipients, one study demonstrated clinically important elevations in both cholesterol and triglycerides in children receiving cyclosporine therapy (Fig. 20.4) (244), which may predispose children to the serious consequences of atherosclerosis later in life. A multivariate analysis was unable to predict cholesterol or triglyceride levels from three predictors: cyclosporine level, prednisone dose, and liver

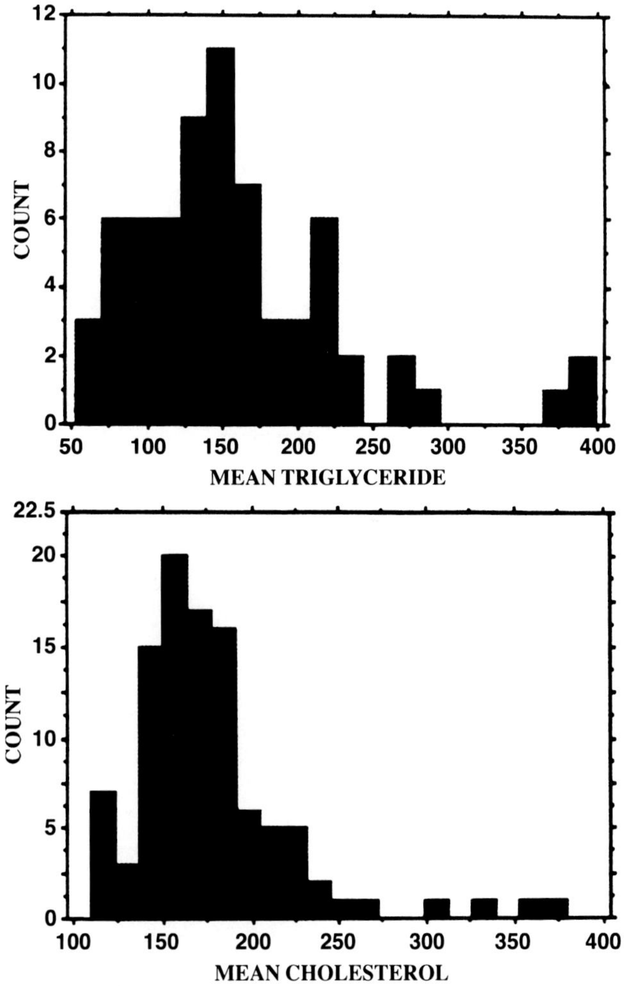

FIGURE 20.4. *The distributions of individual pediatric OLT recipients' mean triglyceride and cholesterol levels are displayed. Note that 47% of children had a mean cholesterol level of >170 mg/dL, and 50% had a mean triglyceride level of >140 mg/dL. (Reproduced by permission from McDiarmid SV, Gornbein JA, Fortunat M, et al. Serum lipid abnormalities in pediatric liver transplant patients. Transplantation 1992;53:109–115.)*

function. Interestingly, tacrolimus does not appear to affect serum lipid levels in children after OLT (190).

Post-transplant Lymphoproliferative Disease (PTLD)

One of the liabilities of the improved potency of new immunosuppressive drugs is an increased incidence of PTLD (11). Eighty-five percent of PTLD is B cell derived and driven by Epstein-Barr virus (EBV), and it may present as a spectrum of disease from a simple mononucleosis-like syndrome to frank lymphoma (245,246). Lymphomas, the most common cause of post-transplant malignancies in pediatric transplant patients, occur more often in nonrenal recipients (247). The three most important risk factors for PTLD are young age, EBV-negative status at transplant, and a primary EBV infection. During the early transplant period, 60% to 80% of seronegative children will contract a primary EBV infection (204). This constellation of risk factors is present in many pediatric liver transplant recipients and makes them a particularly high-risk group (248–250).

An increased incidence and a decreased time to PTLD with each major advance in immunosuppressive potency has been described sequentially with the advent of cyclosporine, then OKT-3 (251,252), and lastly tacrolimus (Figs. 20.5, 20.6; see also Chapter 37) (204,253,254). The liver recipient group with the highest incidence of PTLD (up to 27%) is children with intractable rejections who were converted to tacrolimus, in whom the cumulative immunosuppressive exposure is very high (216,217). Whether the incidence of PTLD is increased in children treated with primary tacrolimus compared to primary cyclosporine immunosuppression is still debated (255). Centers using primary tacrolimus therapy report a PTLD incidence of 6% to 11% (29,189,197,253). Although many centers previously described an incidence of PTLD of 4% or less under cyclosporine therapy (256), these results were often reported before the availability of tacrolimus conversion to treat intractable rejection.

The symptoms, signs, and sites of presentation of PTLD are protean, often making diagnosis difficult (248). A high level of clinical suspicion should be maintained, particularly with post-transplant children who manifest unexplained fever, decreased appetite, weight loss, malaise, and lymphadenopathy. Other common signs and symptoms include diarrhea (particularly associated with protein or blood loss in the stool) (257), stridor, hoarseness, dyspnea, headache, abdominal pain, and mass lesions. The appearance of a monoclonal gammopathy may precede clinical evidence of disease (258). The most common sites of presentation are

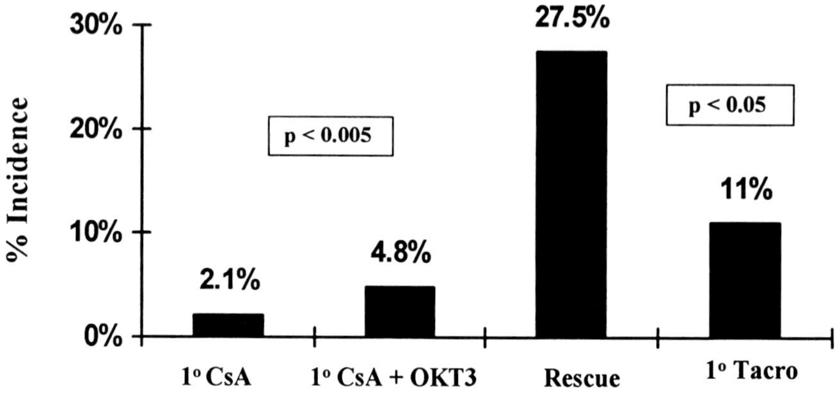

FIGURE 20.5. *The increasing incidence of PTLD as immunosuppressive potency increases in children undergoing OLT at UCLA from 1984 to 1996. There was a significantly lower incidence of PTLD in children receiving primary cyclosporine therapy, OKT-3 rescue therapy, or primary tacrolimus therapy compared to those receiving rescue therapy with tacrolimus.*

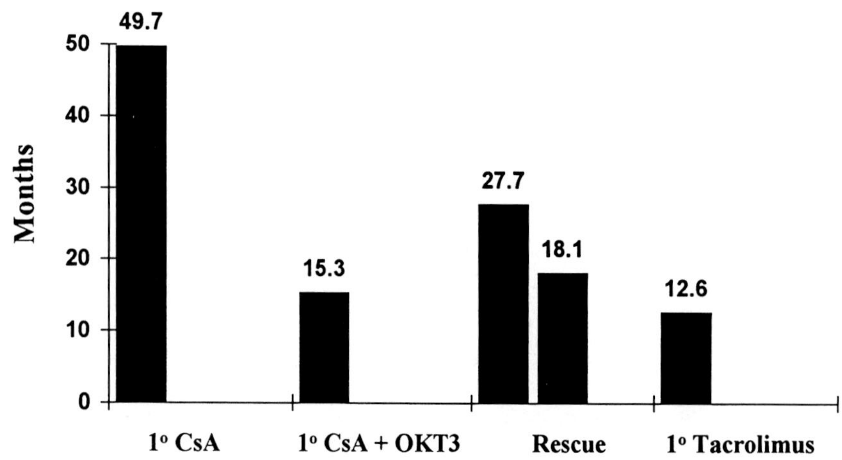

FIGURE 20.6. *The decreasing time to diagnosis of PTLD as immunosuppressive potency increases in children undergoing OLT at UCLA from 1984 to 1996.*

the lymph nodes, the gastrointestinal tract (259), the upper airway, and the liver graft itself (260,261). Histologically, PTLD in the liver graft may present as a lymphocytic infiltrate in the triads, which could be misinterpreted as rejection (Fig. 20.7 and Plate 13). The diagnostic clues for PTLD are atypical lymphocytes, a monotonous uniformity in the appearance of the lymphocytes, and a relative lack of bile duct injury. Unlike other lymphomas, PTLD has a proclivity for the central nervous system, and its first manifestations may be secondary to increased intracranial pressure (262). EBV-associated spindle cell tumors of smooth muscle have been described in children after transplantation (263).

Diagnosis is dependent on a tissue biopsy, which also allows the classification of monoclonal and polyclonal proliferations (264). In general, monoclonal proliferations are associated with a more serious prognosis and a mortality up to 80% (253). Early diagnosis of an asymptomatic primary EBV infection or early PTLD may be aided by polymerase chain reaction (PCR) detection of circulating EBV antigens in the peripheral blood lymphocytes (265), and by in situ hybridization to detect the EBER-1 viral antigen (266).

The ability to easily obtain serial samples to detect a rising viral antigen titer makes peripheral blood monitoring by PCR particularly attractive. Recent reports suggest that serial PCR monitoring of EBV antigens in peripheral blood may allow very early detection of either a primary or a reactivating infection (265). Preemptive therapy with antivirals and decreased immunosuppression can then be initiated to decrease the patient's risk of developing PTLD (267).

Stopping immunosuppression is the most important therapy for PTLD. In many cases, it will allow complete resolution (268). Antiviral therapy with either acyclovir or

A

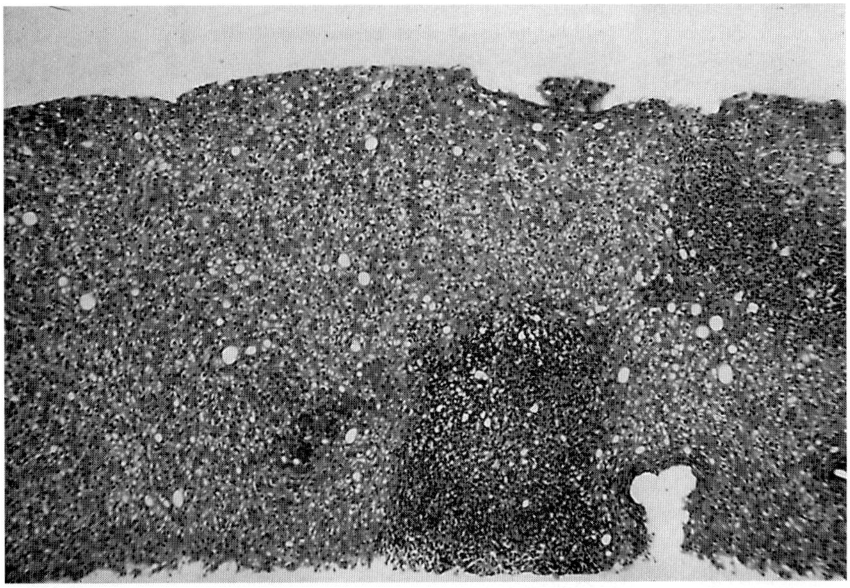

B

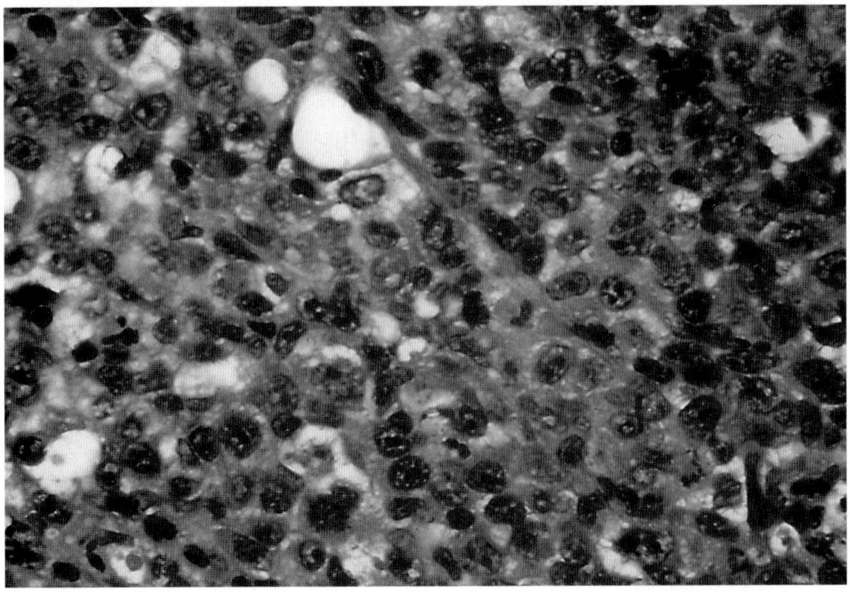

FIGURE 20.7. *The histologic appearance of post-transplant lymphoproliferative disease in the liver allograft is shown.* ***A.*** *Note the infiltrating lymphocytes in the triad, which may be confused with rejection (low-power view).* ***B.*** *A feature of note for distinguishing PTLD from rejection is the monomorphous infiltrate of large immature lymphocytes (high-power view).*

ganciclovir may help control the proliferative stage of acute infection (269). The use of interferon and intravenous γ-globulin to augment the immune response has had some reported benefit (270,271). Recently, CMV hyperimmune globulin, which contains high antibody titers against EBV, has been used. Surgical excision of mass lesions is also advocated. Chemotherapy is seldom warranted. It has a poor response rate and is generally reserved for the more unusual manifestations of EBV malignancy, such as Burkitt's lymphoma or Hodgkin's disease (245). Monoclonal antibody therapy directed against the CD21 and CD24 expressed on the surface of EBV-infected cells has had some success (269).

In addition, infusion of gene-modified, virus-specific autologous T lymphocytes has recently been reported to successfully treat PTLD in patients who were unresponsive to more standard therapy (272).

PTLD is a serious complication with a mortality ranging from 10% to 60% (245) as well as a substantial morbidity. The drastic decreases in immunosuppression required to control the process, as well as the concomitant use of techniques to enhance the immune response, may lead to rejection. At times it may be necessary to sacrifice the graft to allow the remission of life-threatening PTLD. In this circumstance, retransplantation should be delayed as long as possible, and the patient kept off immunosuppression to allow the EBV to become quiescent. Successful retransplantation with reinstitution of immunosuppression has been described, although there is a risk of PTLD recurrence (253).

Growth and Development

One of the unique features differentiating the long-term results of pediatric and adult liver recipients is the child's potential to grow both physically and intellectually. It has been well recognized that despite excellent liver graft function after a transplant, children do not always show normal growth characteristics (273,274).

During the first 18 months after a transplant, weight gain is less affected than is height. Early studies indicated that only 13% to 28% of children showed catch-up growth to greater than the 5th percentile in the first years after a transplant. Normal pretransplant growth was not sustained in the majority of children after transplant, and, of even more concern, some children with previously normal growth lost growth potential after their transplant (275,276). The factors affecting linear growth after pediatric liver transplantation include pretransplant conditions such as age, diagnosis, nutritional status (151), and possibly growth hormone dysregulation (277). Post-transplant factors include nutritional status, graft dysfunction, other intercurrent illness, immunosuppression, and perhaps growth hormone insensitivity (275,278,279).

Most studies find that young age at transplantation allows more potential for catch-up growth (275), although this has been challenged by other studies (280). The indication for transplant may also affect post-transplant growth. Children with biliary atresia appear to have better post-transplant growth (278), but this may be a reflection of their younger age at time of transplant. Poor catch-up growth is a particular problem with Alagille's syndrome, familial cholestasis syndromes, and some metabolic diseases such as tyrosinemia (275,278). Malnutrition in the pretransplant period, which is often associated with cholestatic diseases, may also affect the long-term potential to attain normal predicted growth (146).

In the post-transplant period, the first principle to potentiate growth is provision of adequate nutrition (281). This may be particularly challenging in young infants, or in those children with multiple postoperative complications. Graft dysfunction may affect growth, particularly if long standing and/or associated with increased steroid use for rejection. Chronic rejection and cholestasis have also been associated with poor catch-up growth (275).

The effect of immunosuppression on growth is most obviously related to the use of steroids. Prepubertal children are especially sensitive to steroid-induced growth impairment. Better catch-up growth has been associated with prednisone doses less than 0.1 mg/kg/day, with alternate-day steroids, and with steroid withdrawal (206,207). Successful steroid withdrawal under cyclosporine therapy has been documented by several authors, and in properly selected patients, it does not appear to be associated with more rejection (205–207,282,283). Steroid withdrawal may be attempted more rapidly and perhaps with more success in tacrolimus-treated children (176,198).

In the post-transplant period, growth hormone and its intermediaries appear to return to normal levels, implying that the poor growth noted in many children is secondary to peripheral resistance to growth hormone (279). A pilot study of GH therapy in post-transplant growth-retarded children reported a median increase in growth rate of 7.1 cm/year with an associated increase in IGF-1 and IGF-binding protein-3 levels. No rejection or graft dysfunction was reported (284).

Psychosocial Development

The effect of liver transplantation on the psychosocial development and educational potential of children has not been well studied. Early reports suggested that half of the children were at least 1 year behind the appropriate grade level for their age (285). In a study comparing age-matched children with successful liver transplantation to children with cystic fibrosis, it was noted that the transplanted children had significantly lower nonverbal intelligence, lower academic achievement, and poorer scores for learning and memory (286). Of particular concern are observations that children with the onset of liver disease in the first year of life are more likely to remain delayed in later years (287,288). Although the quality of life is clearly improved for children after pediatric liver transplantation, there is evidence that long-term stress takes an emotional toll on both the child and the family (289,290). Parents have reported greater financial concerns and long-term fears regarding the future of their child (285).

The teenage years are a particular challenge for post-transplant children, their parents, and physicians. One of the most important problems, noncompliance, has been implicated in the increased incidence of both late acute and chronic rejection in teenagers (291). The effect of immunosuppressive drugs on body image, depression, anxiety, and peer pressure associated with the use of drugs and alcohol may become overwhelming problems for teenagers. Although successful pregnancy after liver transplantation has been well described (292), many adolescent boys and girls have serious concerns about their reproductive potential and the effect of immunosuppressive drugs on future children.

In addition, post-transplant teenagers and their parents may fear they will be unable to enter the workforce and become financially independent, particularly if their educational achievement has not been optimal. Many of these patients also lose their childhood insurance policies as they enter adulthood, and finding new insurance coverage can be a major problem.

These major life issues for teenagers often come at a time when they are receiving less frequent follow-up at the transplant center, making intervention more difficult. An increased awareness by both the transplant center and other health professionals is essential during this difficult developmental period.

THE FUTURE

Over the span of only three decades, pediatric OLT has achieved a level of success that could barely have been conceived in the bleak days of the early 1960s when Starzl described the "dismal picture" of liver transplantation in nine patients: "2 of these patients had succumbed within a few hours after operation, and none had lived for longer than 23 days" (293).

Although pediatric patient and graft survival after OLT have improved dramatically as a consequence of improved surgical techniques, advances in immunosuppression, and astute management of early postoperative complications, critical challenges remain for improving outcomes for pediatric liver recipients. These challenges include the donor shortage, access and funding for transplantation, gene therapy for the correction of metabolic disease, protection of growth and development, avoidance of long-term overimmunosuppression, and the eventual goal of achieving donor-specific tolerance.

Although xenotransplantation offers a still-unfilled hope that the donor shortage can eventually be overcome, the technique of split liver transplantation is the first practical advance to date that has expanded the donor supply. Ideally, every suitable donor should be considered for splitting. The development of sharing arrangements between programs could then maximize the use of the right and left liver grafts.

Advances in isolated hepatocyte transplantation and gene therapy targeted to correct metabolic defects may make whole organ transplantation obsolete for single enzyme deficiencies located in the liver. Children suffering from urea cycle defects, Crigler-Najjar syndrome, and familial hypercholesterolemia would be the most likely beneficiaries of the first trials.

Finally, pediatric organ recipients are perhaps the most likely to derive long-lasting advantages from the vigorous research efforts currently underway to avoid long-term overimmunosuppression and eventually achieve donor-specific tolerance. Refinements in the manipulation of the immune response, improved understanding of T-cell signaling, and clarification of the role of chimerism will all contribute to this goal (see Chapter 5). Avoiding several decades of immunosuppression along with its attendant complications may have as yet unmeasured benefits on patients' long-term survival, growth, and quality of life. Providing the resources to achieve these goals—which are a heritage we owe to any child—will require innovative thinking by leaders both in the medical profession and in our society.

ACKNOWLEDGMENT

I would like to gratefully acknowledge Ms. Beatriz Dea's expert preparation of this chapter's manuscript.

REFERENCES

1. Starzl TE, Groth CG, Brettschneider L, et al. Orthotopic homotransplantation of the human liver. Ann Surg 1968;168:392–415.
2. Starzl TE, Koep LJ, Schroter GP, et al. Liver replacement for pediatric patients. Pediatrics 1979;63:825–829.
3. 1996 Annual Report of the US Scientific Registry for Transplant Recipients and the Organ Procurement and Transplantation Network. Transplant Data: 1988–1995. UNOS, Richmond, VA, and the Division of Transplantation, Bureau of Health Resources Development, Health Resources and Services Administration. Rockville, MD: US Department of Health and Human Services, 1996.
4. Todo S, Makowka L, Tzakis AG, et al. Hepatic artery in liver transplantation. Transplant Proc 1987;19:2406–2411.
5. Broelsch CE, Emond JC, Thistlethwaite JR, et al. Liver transplantation, including the concept of reduced-size liver transplants in children. Ann Surg 1988;208:410–420.
6. Emond JC, Heffron TG, Kortz EO, et al. Improved results of living-related liver transplantation with routine application in a pediatric program. Transplantation 1993;55:835–840.
7. Heffron TG, Emond J. Segmental liver transplantation in children: reduced size cadaveric, split and living related. Transplant Sci 1993;2:28–33.
8. Ettenger RB. Age and the immune response in pediatric renal transplantation. Eur J Pediatr 1992;151:S7–S8.
9. Andrews WS, Conlin C. Liver transplantation in children. In: Klintmalm GB, Sollinger H, eds. Liver transplantation. Glenview, IL: Physician and Scientists, 1996:15–27.
10. Murphy MS, Harrison R, Davies P, et al. Risk factors for liver rejection: evidence to suggest enhanced allograft tolerance in infancy. Arch Dis Child 1996;75:502–506.
11. Newell KA, Alonso EM, Whitington PF, et al. Posttransplant lymphoproliferative disease in pediatric liver transplantation. Interplay between primary Epstein-Barr virus infection and immunosuppression. Transplantation 1996;62: 370–375.

12. Inomoto T, Nishizawa F, Sasaki H, et al. Experiences of 120 microsurgical reconstructions of hepatic artery in living related liver transplantation. Surgery 1996;119:20–26.
13. Stevens LH, Emond JC, Piper JB, et al. Hepatic artery thrombosis in infants. A comparison of whole livers, reduced-size grafts, and grafts from living-related donors. Transplantation 1992;53:396–399.
14. Jurim O, Csete M, Gelabert HA, et al. Reduced-size grafts—the solution for hepatic artery thrombosis after pediatric liver transplantation? J Pediatr Surg 1995;30:53–55.
15. Piper J, Whitington PF, Woodle ES, et al. Pediatric liver transplantation at the University of Chicago hospitals. In: Clinical transplants 1992. Terasaki, Cecka, eds. Los Angeles: UCLA Tissue Typing Laboratory, 1992:179–189.
16. Otte JB, de Ville de Goyet J, Sokal E, et al. Size reduction of the donor liver is a safe way to alleviate the shortage of size-matched organs in pediatric liver transplantation. Ann Surg 1990;211:146–157.
17. Goyet JD, Hausleithner V, Reding R, et al. Impact of innovative techniques on the waiting list and results in pediatric liver transplantation. Transplantation 1993;56:1139–1136.
18. Bismuth H, Houssin D. Reduced-sized orthotopic liver graft in hepatic transplantation in children. Surgery 1984;95:367–370.
19. Broelsch CE, Emond JC, Whitington PF, et al. Application of reduced-size liver transplants as split grafts, auxiliary orthotopic grafts, and living related segmental transplants. Ann Surg 1990;212:368–377.
20. Sokal EM, Veyckemans F, de Ville de Goyet J, et al. Liver transplantation in children less than 1 year of age. J Pediatr 1990;117:205–210.
21. Esquivel CO, Koneru B, Karrer F, et al. Liver transplantation before 1 year of age. J Pediatr 1987;110:545–548.
22. Jurim O, Shackleton CR, McDiarmid SV, et al. Living-donor liver transplantation at UCLA. Am J Surg 1995;169:529–532.
23. Cacciarelli TV, Esquirel CO, Moore DH, et al. Factors affecting survival after orthotopic liver transplantation in infants. Transplantation 1997;64:242–248.
24. Emond JC. Clinical application of living-related liver transplantation. Gastroenterol Clin North Am 1993;22:301–315.
25. Bonatti H, Muiesan P, Connelly S, et al. Hepatic transplantation in children under 3 months of age: a single centre's experience. J Pediatr Surg 1997;32:486–488.
26. Woodle ES, Millis JM, So SKS, et al. Liver transplantation in the first three months of life. Transplantation 1998;66:606–609.
27. Broelsch CE, Whitington PF, Emond JC, et al. Liver transplantation in children from living related donors. Surgical techniques and results. Ann Surg 1991;214:428–437;discussion 437–439.
28. Otte JB, de Ville de Goyet J, Reding R, et al. Living related donor liver transplantation in children: the Brussels experience. Transplant Proc 1996;28:2378–2379.
29. Inomata Y, Tanaka K, Egawa H, et al. The evolution of immunosuppression with FK506 in pediatric living-related liver transplantation. Transplantation 1996;61:2:247–252.
30. Emond JC, Renz JF, Ferrell LD, et al. Functional analysis of grafts from living donors. Implications for the treatment of older recipients. Ann Surg 1996;224:544–552;discussion 552–554.
31. Singer PA, Siegler M, Whitington PF, et al. Ethics of liver transplantation with living donors. N Engl J Med 1989;321:620–622.
32. Strong RW, Lynch SV. Ethical issues in living related donor liver transplantation. Transplant Proc 1996;28:2366–2369.
33. Sterneck MR, Fischer L, Nischwitz U, et al. Selection of the living liver donor. Transplantation 1995;60:667–671.
34. Shimahara Y, Awane M, Yamaoka Y, et al. Analyses of the risk and operative stress for donors in living-related partial liver transplantation. Transplantation 1992;54:983–988.
35. Yamaoka Y, Morimoto T, Inamoto T, et al. Safety of the donor in living-related liver transplantation—an analysis of 100 parental donors. Transplantation 1995;59:224–226.
36. Fuchinoue W, Tanaka K, Takasaki K, et al. Living-related liver transplantation for fulminant hepatic failure. Transplant Proc 1997;29:424–427.
37. Cardona J, Houssin D, Gauthier F, et al. Liver transplantation in children with Alagille syndrome—a study of twelve cases. Transplantation 1995;60:339–342.
38. Otte JB, de Ville de Goyet J, Alberti D, et al. The concept and technique of the split liver in clinical transplantation. Surgery 1990;107:605–612.
39. Emond JC, Whitington PF, Thistlethwaite JR, et al. Transplantation of two patients with one liver. Analysis of a preliminary experience with "split-liver" grafting. Ann Surg 1990;212:14–22.
40. McDiarmid SV. Renal dysfunction in pediatric transplant patients. In: Busuttil RW, Klintmalm GB, eds. Transplantation of the liver. Philadelphia: WB Saunders, 1996:596–606.
41. Rogiers X, Otte JB, Malago M, et al. In situ split liver transplantation: a safe way to increase the organ pool. Pediatr Nephrol 1996;10:C56.
42. de Ville de Goyet J. Split liver transplantation in Europe—1988 to 1993. Transplantation 1995;59:1371–1376.
43. Houssin D, Boillot O, Soubrane O, et al. Controlled liver splitting for transplantation in two recipients: technique, results and perspectives. Br J Surg 1993;80:75–80.
44. Rogiers X, Malago M, Gawad KA, et al. One year of experience with extended application and modified techniques of split liver transplantation. Transplantation 1996;61:1059–1061.
45. Goss JA, Yersiz H, Shackleton CR, et al. In situ splitting of the cadaveric liver for transplantation. Transplantation 1997;64:871–877.
46. Terpstra OT, Reuvers CB, Schalm SW. Auxiliary heterotopic liver transplantation. Transplantation 1988;45:1003–1007.
47. Boudjema K, Cherqui D, Jaeck D, et al. Auxiliary liver transplantation for fulminant and subfulminant hepatic failure. Transplantation 1995;59:218–223.
48. Whitington PF, Emond JC, Heffron T, Thistlethwaite JR. Orthotopic auxiliary liver transplantation for Crigler-Najjar syndrome type 1. Lancet 1993;342: 779–780.
49. Rela M, Muiesan P, Andreani P, et al. Auxiliary liver transplantation for metabolic diseases. Transplant Proc 1997;29:444–445.
50. McDiarmid SV. Risk factors and outcomes after pediatric liver transplantation. Liver Transplant Surg 1996;2:5:44–56.
51. Busuttil RW, Seu P, Millis JM, et al. Liver transplantation in children. Ann Surg 1991;213:48–57.
52. Burdelski M, Pichlmayr R, Ringe B, et al. Pediatric liver transplantation—ten years experience in Hanover. Clin Transplant 1987;55–62.
53. Ryckman F, Fisher R, Pedersen S, et al. Improved survival in biliary atresia patients in the present era of liver transplantation. J Pediatr Surg 1993;28:382–385;discussion 386.
54. Goss JA, Shackleton CR, Swenson K, et al. Orthotopic liver transplantation for congenital biliary atresia. An 11-year, single-center experience. Ann Surg 1996;224:276–284;discussion 284–287.
55. Vennarecci G, Gunson BK, Ismail T, et al. Transplantation for end stage liver disease related to alpha 1 antitrypsin. Transplantation 1996;61:1488–1495.
56. Shaked A, Vargas J, Csete ME, et al. Diagnosis and treatment of bowel perforation following pediatric orthotopic liver transplantation. Arch Surg 1994;128:994–999.
57. Koneru B, Flye MW, Busuttil RW, et al. Liver transplantation for hepatoblastoma. The American experience. Ann Surg 1991;213:118–121.
58. Burdelski M, Oellerich M, Duwel J, et al. Pre- and post-transplant assessment of liver function in paediatric liver transplantation. Eur J Pediatr 1992; 151(suppl 1):S39–43.
59. D'Alessandro AM, Ploeg RJ, Knechtle SJ, et al. Retransplantation of the liver—a seven-year experience. Transplantation 1993;55:1083–1087.
60. Newell KA, Alonso EM, Millis JM, et al. Retransplantation for failed hepatic allografts in children. Transplant Proc 1997;29:442–443.
61. Brant de Carvalho F, Reding R, Falchetti D, et al. Analysis of liver graft loss in infants and children below 4 years. Transplant Proc 1991;23:1454–1455.
62. Esquivel CO, Koneru B, Todo S, et al. Is multiple organ failure a contraindication for liver transplantation. Transplant Proc 1987;19:47–48.
63. Ellis D, Avner ED, Starzl TE. Renal failure in children with hepatic failure undergoing liver transplantation. J Pediatr 1986;108:393–398.
64. Lidofsky SD, Bass NM, Prager MC, et al. Intracranial pressure monitoring and liver transplantation for fulminant hepatic failure. Hepatology 1992;16:1–7.
65. Donovan JP, Shaw BWJ, Langnas AN, Sorrell MF. Brain water and acute liver failure: the emerging role of intracranial pressure monitoring [editorial]. Hepatology 1992;16:267–268.
66. Krowka MJ, Cortese DA. Pulmonary aspects of chronic liver disease and liver transplantation. Mayo Clin Proc 1985;60:407–418.
67. McCloskey JJ, Schleien C, Schwarz K, Klein A, Colombani P. Severe hypoxemia and intrapulmonary shunting resulting from cirrhosis reversed by liver transplantation in a pediatric patient. J Pediatr 1991;118:902–904.
68. Hobeika J, Houssin D, Bernard O, et al. Orthotopic liver transplantation in children with chronic liver disease and severe hypoxemia. Transplantation 1994;57:224–228.
69. Shaw B, Wood RP, Kaufman SS, et al. Liver transplantation therapy for children: Part 1. J Pediatr Gastroenterol Nutr 1988;7:157–166.
70. Malatack JJ, Schaid DJ, Urbach AH, et al. Choosing a pediatric recipient for orthotopic liver transplantation. J Pediatr 1987;111:479–489.
71. Whitington PF, Balistreri WF. Liver transplantation in pediatrics: indications, contraindications, and pretransplant management. J Pediatr 1991;118:169–177.
72. Esquivel CO, Iwatsuki S, Gordon R, et al. Indications for pediatric liver transplantation. J Pediatr 1987;111:1039–1045.

73. Starzl TE, Demetris AJ, Van Thiel DH. Liver transplantation. (First of two parts). N Engl J Med 1989;321:1014–1022.
74. Wood RP, Langnas AN, Stratta RJ, et al. Optimal therapy for patients with biliary atresia: portoenterostomy ("Kasai" procedures) versus primary transplantation. J Pediatr Surg 1990;25:153–160;discussion 160–162.
75. Millis JM, Brems JJ, Hiatt JR, et al. Orthotopic liver transplantation for biliary atresia. Evolution of management. Arch Surg 1988;123:1237–1239.
76. Oh M, Hobeldin M, Chen T, et al. The Kasai procedure in the treatment of biliary atresia. J Pediatr Surg 1995;30:1077–1080;discussion 1080–1081.
77. Otte JB, de Ville de Goyet J, Reding R, et al. Sequential treatment of biliary atresia with Kasai portoenterostomy and liver transplantation: a review. Hepatology 1994;20:41S–48S.
78. Karrer FM, Lilly JR, Stewart BA, Hall RJ. Biliary atresia registry, 1976 to 1989. J Pediatr Surg 1990;25:1076–1080;discussion 1081.
79. Alagille D. Liver transplantation in children—indications in cholestatic states. Transplant Proc 1987;19:3242–3248.
80. Alagille D, Odievre M, Gautier M, Dommergues JP. Hepatic ductular hypoplasia associated with characteristic facies, vertebral malformations, retarded physical, mental, and sexual. J Pediatr 1975;86:63–71.
81. Alagille D, Estrada A, Hadchouel M, et al. Syndromic paucity of interlobular bile ducts (Allagille syndrome or arteriohepatic dysplasia): review of 80 cases. J Pediatr 1987;110:195–200.
82. Clayton PT. Inborn errors of bile acid metabolism. J Inherit Metab Dis 1991;14:478–496.
83. Ballow M, Margolis CZ, Schachtel B, Hsia YE. Progressive familial intrahepatic cholestasis. Pediatrics 1973;51:998–1007.
84. Maggiore G, Bernard O, Riely CA, et al. Normal serum gamma-glutamyl-transpeptidase activity identifies groups of infants with idiopathic cholestasis with poor prognosis. J Pediatr 1987;111:251–252.
85. Alagille D. Management of paucity of interlobular bile ducts. J Hepatol 1985;1:561–565.
86. Marino IR, ChapChap P, Esquivel CO, et al. Liver transplantation for arteriohepatic dysplasia (Alagille's syndrome). Transplant Int 1992;5:61–64.
87. Emond JC, Whitington PF. Selective surgical management of progressive familial intrahepatic cholestasis (Byler's disease). J Pediatr Surg 1995;30: 1635–1641.
88. Jacquemin E, Setchell KD, O'Connell NC, et al. A new cause of progressive intrahepatic cholestasis: 3. J Pediatr 1994;125:379–384.
89. Burdelski M, Rodeck B, Latta A, et al. Treatment of inherited metabolic disorders by liver transplantation. Inher Metab Dis 1991;14:604–618.
90. Gartner JC, Zitelli BJ, Malatack JJ, et al. Orthotopic liver transplantation in children: two-year experience with 47 patients. Pediatrics 1984;74:140–145.
91. Riely CA. Wilson's disease. Pediatr Rev 1984;5:217–222.
92. Sternlieb I. Perspectives on Wilson's disease. Hepatology 1980;12:1234–1239.
93. Sokal RJ, Francis PD, Gold SH, et al. Orthotopic liver transplantation for acute fulminant Wilson's disease. J Pediatr 1985;107:549–552.
94. Walser M. Urea cycle enzymopathies. Semin Liver Dis 1982;2:329–339.
95. Batshaw ML, Monahan PS. Treatment of urea cycle disorders. Enzyme 1987;38:242–250.
96. Bachmann C. Diagnosis of urea cycle disorders. Enzyme 1987;38:233–241.
97. Brusilow SW, Danney M, Waber LJ, et al. Treatment of episodic hyperammonemia in children with inborn errors of urea synthesis. N Engl J Med 1984;310:1630–1634.
98. Msall M, Batshaw ML, Suss R, et al. Neurologic outcome in children with inborn errors of urea synthesis. Outcome of urea-cycle enzymopathies. N Engl J Med 1984;310:1500–1505.
99. Todo S, Starzl TE, Tzakis A, et al. Orthotopic liver transplantation for urea cycle enzyme deficiency. Hepatology 1992;15:419–422.
100. Mieles L, Esquivel CO, Van Thiel DH, et al. Liver transplantation for tyrosinemia. A review of 10 cases from the University of Pittsburgh. Dig Dis Sci 1990;35:153–157.
101. Freese D, Tuchman M, Schwarzenberg SJ, et al. Early liver transplantation is indicated for tyrosinemia type I. J Pediatr Gastroenterol Nutr 1991;13:10–15.
102. Flye MW, Riely CA, Hainline BE, et al. The effects of early treatment of hereditary tyrosinemia type I in infancy by orthotopic liver transplantation. Transplantation 1990;49:916–921.
103. Sokal E, Bustos R, Van Hoof F, Otte JB. Liver transplantation for hereditary tyrosinemia—early transplantation following the patient's stabilization. Transplantation 1992;54:937–939.
104. Russo P, O'Regan S. Visceral pathology of hereditary tyrosinemia type I. Am J Human Genet 1990;47:317–324.
105. Mitchell G, Larochelle J, Lambert M, et al. Neurologic crises in hereditary tyrosinemia. N Engl J Med 1990;322:432–437.
106. Weinberg AG, Mize CE, Worthen HG. The occurrence of hepatoma in the chronic form of hereditary tyrosinemia. J Pediatr 1976;88:434–438.
107. Salt A, Barnes ND, Rolles K, et al. Liver transplantation in tyrosinaemia type 1: the dilemma of timing the operation. Acta Paediatr 1992;81:449–452.
108. Starzl TE, Zitelli BJ, Shaw BW, et al. Changing concepts: liver replacement for hereditary tyrosinemia and hepatoma. J Pediatr 1985;106:604–606.
109. Van Thiel DH, Gartner C Jr, Thorp FK, et al. Resolution of the clinical features of tyrosinemia following orthotopic liver transplantation for hepatoma. J Hepatol 1986;3:42–48.
110. Shoemaker LR, Strife CF, Balistreri WF, Ryckman FC. Rapid improvement in the renal tubular dysfunction associated with tyrosinemia following hepatic replacement. Pediatrics 1992;89:251–255.
111. McDiarmid SV. Liver transplantation for metabolic disease. In: Busuttil RW, Klintmalm GB, eds. Transplantation of the liver. Philadelphia: WB Saunders, 1996:198–215.
112. Kaufman SS, Wood RP, Shaw BW, et al. Orthotopic liver transplantation for type I Crigler-Najjar syndrome. Hepatology 1986;6:1259–1262.
113. Shevell MI, Bernard B, Adelson JW, et al. Crigler-Najjar syndrome type I: treatment by home phototherapy followed by orthotopic hepatic transplantation. J Pediatr 1987;110:429–431.
114. Sokal EM, Silva ES, Hermans D, et al. Orthotopic liver transplantation for Crigler-Najjar type I disease in six children. Transplantation 1995;60:1095–1098.
115. van der Veere CN, Sinaasappel M, McDonagh AF, et al. Current therapy for Crigler-Najjar syndrome type 1: report of a world registry. Hepatology 1996;24:311–315.
116. Watts RWE, Calne RY, Rolles K, et al. Successful treatment of primary hyperoxaluria type I by combined hepatic and renal transplantation. Lancet 1987;2:474–475.
117. Schurmann G, Scharer K, Wingen AM, et al. Early liver transplantation for primary hyperoxaluria type I in an infant with chronic renal failure. Nephrol Dial Transplant 1991;5:825–527.
118. Starzl TE, Bilheimer DW, Bahnson HT, et al. Heart-liver transplantation in a patient with familial hypercholesterolaemia. Lancet 1984;1:1382–1383.
119. East C, Grundy SM, Bilheimer DW. Normal cholesterol levels with lovastatin (Mevinolin) therapy in a child with homozygous familial hypercholesterolemia following liver transplantation. JAMA 1986;256:2843–2848.
120. Watts RWE, Danpure CJ, De Pauw L, Toussaint C, European Study Group on Transplantation in Hyperoxaluria Type I. Combined liver-kidney and isolated liver transplantations for primary hyperoxaluria type 1: the European experience. Nephrol Dial Transplant 1991;6:502–511.
121. Sokal E, Ulla L, Harvengt C, Otte JB. Liver transplantation for familial hypercholesterolemia before the onset of cardiovascular complications. Transplantation 1993;55:432–433.
122. Polson RJ, Rolles K, Calne RY, Williams R. Reversal of severe neurological manifestations of Wilson's disease following orthotopic liver transplantation. Q J Med 1987;64:685–691.
123. O'Grady JG, Alexander GJ, Hayllar KM, Williams R. Early indicators of prognosis in fulminant hepatic failure. Gastroenterology 1989;97:439–445.
124. Psacharopoulos HT, Mowat AP, Davies M, et al. Fulminant hepatic failure in childhood: an analysis of 31 cases. Arch Dis Child 1980;55:252–258.
125. Devictor D, Desplanques L, Debray D, et al. Emergency liver transplantation for fulminant liver failure in infants and children. Hepatology 1992;16: 1156–1162.
126. Farrell FJ, Keeffe EB, Man KM, et al. Treatment of hepatic failure secondary to isoniazid hepatitis with liver transplantation. Dig Dis Sci 1994;39:2255–2259.
127. Henretig FM, Selbst SM, Forrest C, et al. Repeated acetaminophen overdosing. Causing hepatotoxicity in children. Clinical reports and literature review. Clin Pediatr (Phila) 1989;28:525–528.
128. Rivera-Penera T, Gugig R, Davis J, et al. Outcome of acetaminophen overdose in pediatric patients and factors contributing to hepatotoxicity [see comments]. J Pediatr 1997;130:300–304.
129. Gregorio GV, Portmann B, Reid F, et al. Autoimmune hepatitis in childhood: a 20-year experience. Hepatology 1997;25:541–547.
130. Newman KD. Hepatic tumors in children. Semin Pediatr Surg 1997;6:38–41.
131. Weinberg AG, Finegold MJ. Primary hepatic tumors of childhood. Hum Pathol 1983;14:512–537.
132. Achilleos OA, Buist LJ, Kelly DA, et al. Unresectable hepatic tumors in childhood and the role of liver transplantation. J Pediatr Surg 1996;31: 1563–1567.
133. Okuyama K. Primary liver cell carcinoma associated with biliary cirrhosis due to congenital bile duct atresia. J Pediatr 1965;67:1:89–93.

134. Kaufman SS, Wood RP, Shaw BW, et al. Hepatocarcinoma in a child with the Alagille syndrome. Am J Dis Child 1987;141:698–700.
135. Adams PC. Hepatocellular carcinoma associated with arteriohepatic dysplasia. Dig Dis Sci 1986;31:438–442.
136. Ugarte N, Gonzalez-Crussi F. Hepatoma in siblings with progressive familial cholestatic cirrhosis of childhood. Am J Clin Pathol 1981;76:172–177.
137. Psarcharopoulos HT, Portman B, Howard ER, et al. Hepatic complications of cystic fibrosis. Lancet 1981;ii:78–80.
138. Cox KL, Ward RE, Furgiuele TL, et al. Orthotopic liver transplantation in patients with cystic fibrosis. Pediatrics 1987;80:571–574.
139. Mieles L, Orenstein D, Teperman L, et al. Liver transplantation in cystic fibrosis. Lancet 1989;1:1073.
140. Cox KL. Liver transplantation in cystic fibrosis. Clin Res 1991;39:6A.
141. Noble-Jamieson G, Valente J, Barnes ND, et al. Liver transplantation for hepatic cirrhosis in cystic fibrosis. Arch Dis Child 1994;71:349–352.
142. Postuma R, Trevenen CL. Liver disease in infants receiving total parenteral nutrition. Pediatrics 1979;63:110–115.
143. Todo S, Reyes J, Furukawa H, et al. Outcome analysis of 71 clinical intestinal transplantations. Ann Surg 1995;222:270–280;discussion 280–282.
144. Langnas AN, Shaw BW, Antonson DL, et al. Preliminary experience with intestinal transplantation in infants and children [see comments]. Pediatrics 1996;97:443–448.
145. Todo S, Tzakis A, Abu-Elmagd K, et al. Cadaveric small bowel and small bowel-liver transplantation in humans. Transplantation 1992;53:369–376.
146. Moukarzel AA, Najm I, Vargas JV, et al. Effect of nutritional status on outcome of orthotopic liver transplantation in pediatric patients. Transplant Proc 1990;22:1560–1563.
147. Woodle ES, Thistlethwaite JR, Emond JC, et al. Successful hepatic transplantation in congenital absence of recipient portal vein. Surgery 1990;107:475–479.
148. Farmer DG, Shaked A, Olthoff KM, et al. Evaluation, operative management, and outcome after liver transplantation in children with biliary atresia and situs inversus. Ann Surg 1995;222:47–50.
149. Busuttil RW, Shaked A, Millis JM, et al. One thousand liver transplants. The lessons learned. Ann Surg 1994;219:490–497;discussion 498–499.
150. Tzakis A, Cooper MH, Dummer JS, et al. Transplantation in HIV+ patients. Transplantation 1990;49:354–358.
151. Shepherd RW, Chin SE, Cleghorn GJ, et al. Malnutrition in children with chronic liver disease accepted for liver transplantation: clinical profile and effect on outcome. J Paediatr Child Health 1991;27:295–299.
152. Kaufman SS, Murray ND, Wood RP, et al. Nutritional support for the infant with extrahepatic biliary atresia. J Pediatr 1987;110:679–686.
153. Balistreri WF, Bucuvalas JC, Ryckman FC. The effect of immunosuppression on growth and development. Liver Transplant Surg 1995;1:5:64–73.
154. Bucuvalas JC, Cutfield W, Horn J, et al. Resistance to the growth-promoting and metabolic effects of growth hormone in children with chronic liver disease. J Pediatr 1990;117:397–402.
155. Bucuvalas JC, Horn JA, Carlsson L, et al. Growth hormone insensitivity associated with elevated circulating growth hormone-binding protein in children with Alagille syndrome and short stature. J Clin Endocrinol Metab 1993;76:1477–1482.
156. Bucuvalas JC, Horn JA, Slusher J, et al. Growth hormone insensitivity in children with biliary atresia. J Pediatr Gastroenterol Nutr 1996;23:135–140.
157. Moreno LA, Gottrand F, Hoden S, et al. Improvement of nutritional status in cholestatic children with supplemental nocturnal enteral nutrition. J Pediatr Gastroenterol Nutr 1991;12:213–216.
158. Handa N, Suita S, Ikeda K, et al. Requirement of parenteral fat in infants with biliary atresia. JPEN J Parenter Enteral Nutr 1985;9:685–690.
159. Kahn D, Esquivel CO, Madrigal-Torres M, et al. An analysis of the causes of death after pediatric liver transplantation. Transplant Proc 1988;20:613–615.
160. Wozney P, Zajko AB, Bron KM, et al. Vascular complications after liver transplantation: a 5-year experience. AJR Am J Roentgenol 1986;147:657–663.
161. Shackleton CR, Goss JA, Swenson K, et al. The impact of microsurgical hepatic arterial reconstruction on the outcome of liver transplantation for congenital biliary atresia. Am J Surg 1997;173:431–435.
162. Rela M, Muiesan P, Bhatnagar V, et al. Hepatic artery thrombosis after liver transplantation in children under 5 years of age. Transplantation 1996;61:1355–1357.
163. Tzakis AG, Gordon RD, Shaw BWJ, et al. Clinical presentation of hepatic artery thrombosis after liver transplantation in the cyclosporine era. Transplantation 1985;40:667–671.
164. Mazzaferro V, Esquivel CO, Makowka L, et al. Hepatic artery thrombosis after pediatric liver transplantation—a medical or surgical event? Transplantation 1989;47:971–977.
165. Jennings I, Calne RY, Baglin TP. Predictive value of Von Willebrand factor to ristocetin cofactor ratio and thrombin-antithrombin complex levels for hepatic vessel thrombosis and graft rejection after liver transplantation. Transplantation 1994;57:1046–1051.
166. Hashikura Y, Kawasaki S, Okumura N, et al. Prevention of hepatic artery thrombosis in pediatric liver transplantation. Transplantation 1995;60: 1109–1112.
167. McDiarmid SV, Hall TR, Grant EG, et al. Failure of duplex sonography to diagnose hepatic artery thrombosis in a high-risk group of pediatric liver transplant recipients. J Pediatr Surg 1991;26:710–713.
168. Cuervas-Mons V, Rimola A, Van Thiel DH, et al. Does previous abdominal surgery alter the outcome of pediatric patients subjected to orthotopic liver transplantation? Gastroenterology 1986;90:853–857.
169. Soubrane O, El Meteini M, Devictor D, et al. Risk and prognostic factors of gut perforation after orthotopic liver transplantation for biliary artesia. Liver Transplant Surg 1995;1:1:2–9.
170. Yokoyama I, Tzakis A, Imventarza O, et al. Pediatric liver transplantation from neonatal donors. Transplant Int 1992;5:205–208.
171. Egawa H, Shaked A, Konishi Y, et al. Arterial ketone body ratio in pediatric liver transplantation. Transplantation 1993;55:522–526.
172. Peclet MH, Ryckman FC, Pedersen SH, et al. The spectrum of bile duct complications in pediatric liver transplantation. J Pediatr Surg 1994;29:214–219;discussion 219–220.
173. Wood RP, Ellis D, Starzl TE. The reversal of the hepatorenal syndrome in four pediatric patients following successful orthotopic liver transplantation. Ann Surg 1987;205:415–419.
174. Martinez AJ, Estol C, Faris AA. Neurologic complications of liver transplantation. Neurol Clin 1988;6:327–348.
175. McDiarmid SV. Special consideration for pediatric immunosuppression after liver transplantation. In: Busuttil RW, Klintmalm GB, eds. Transplantation of the liver. Philadelphia: WB Saunders, 1996:250–261.
176. Tzakis A, Fung JJ, Reyes J, Green M, Starzl TE. Use of FK506 in pediatric patient. Transplant Proc 1991;23:924–927.
177. Ryckman FC, Schroeder TJ, Pedersen SH, et al. Induction therapy with OKT3 in pediatric liver-transplant recipients. Transplant Sci 1994;4(suppl 1):S20–25.
178. McDiarmid SV, Busuttil RW, Levy P, et al. The long-term outcome of OKT3 compared with cyclosporine prophylaxis after liver transplantation. Transplantation 1991;52:91–97.
179. Atkison PR, Grant DR, Williams SE, et al. Sandimmune Neoral in paediatric liver transplant recipients with malabsorption of cyclosporin A. Transplant Proc 1994;26:2953–2954.
180. McDiarmid SV. Uses of Neoral in pediatric liver transplantation. Transplant Proc 1996;28:2264–2266.
181. Holt DW, Mueller EA, Kovarik JM, et al. The pharmacokinetics of Sandimmune Neoral: a new oral formulation of cyclosporine. Transplant Proc 1994;26:2935–2939.
182. Trull AK, Tan KK, Tan L, et al. Enhanced absorption of new oral cyclosporin microemulsion formulation, Neoral, in liver transplant recipients with external biliary diversion. Transplant Proc 1994;26:2977–2978.
183. Dunn SP, Cooney GF, Kulinsky A, et al. Absorption characteristics of a microemulsion formulation of cyclosporine in de novo pediatric liver transplant recipients. Transplantation 1995;60:1438–1442.
184. Superina RA, Strong DK, Acal LA, DeLuca E. Relative bioavailability of Sandimmune and Sandimmune Neoral in pediatric liver recipients. Transplant Proc 1994;26:2979–2980.
185. Whitington PF, Alonso EM, Millis JM. Potential role of Neoral in pediatric liver transplantation. Transplant Proc 1996;28:2267–2269.
186. Hoppu K, Jalanko H, Laine J, Holmberg C. Comparison of conventional oral cyclosporine and cyclosporine microemulsion formulations in children with a liver transplant. Transplantation 1996;62:66–71.
187. Alberti D, Wallemacq P, Falchetti D, et al. Microemulsion formulation of cyclosporine in pediatric liver transplantation. Transplantation 1996;61:512–514.
188. Haller GW, Winkler M, Bechstein WO, et al. Absorption of cyclosporine Neoral early after liver transplantation: is it possible to abandon intravenous cyclosporine A application?. Transplant Proc 1996;28:2239–2240.
189. Tzakis AG, Reyes J, Todo S, et al. Two-year experience with FK 506 in pediatric patients. Transplant Proc 1993;25:1:619–621.
190. McDiarmid SV, Busuttil RW, Ascher NL, et al. FK506 (tacrolimus) compared with cyclosporine for primary immunosuppression after pediatric liver transplantation. Transplantation 1995;59:530–536.
191. The U.S.Multicenter FK506 liver study group. A comparison of tacrolimus (FK 506) and cyclosporine for immunosuppression in liver transplantation. N Engl J Med 1994;331:1110–1115.

192. Randomised trial comparing tacrolimus (FK506) and cyclosporin in prevention of liver allograft rejection. European FK506 Multicentre Liver Study Group. Lancet 1994;344:423–428.
193. Rosh JR, Schwersenz AH, Schwartz M, et al. Therapy with FK 506 in pediatric liver recipients. Transplant Proc 1994;26:152–153.
194. Ueda M, Uemoto S, Inomata Y, et al. A proposal of FK506 optimal dosing in living related liver transplantations. Transplantation 1995;60:258–264.
195. Esquivel CO, So SK, McDiarmid SV, et al. Suggested guidelines for the use of tacrolimus in pediatric liver transplant patients [letter]. Transplantation 1996;61:847–848.
196. McDiarmid SV, Busuttil RW. Primary immunosuppressive therapy with tacrolimus after pediatric liver transplantation. Pediatr Nephrol 1996;10:C41
197. Cacciarelli TV, Esquivel CO, Cox KL, et al. Oral tacrolimus (FK506) induction therapy in pediatric orthotopic liver transplantation. Transplantation 1996;61:8:1188–1192.
198. Uemoto S, Tanaka K, Honda K, et al. Experience with FK506 in living-related liver transplantation. Transplantation 1993;55:288–292.
199. Fung JJ, Alessiani M, Abu-Elmagd K, et al. Adverse effects associated with the use of FK506. Transplant Proc 1991;23:3105–3108.
200. McDiarmid SV, Busuttil RW, Ascher NL, et al. FK506 (tacrolimus) compared with cyclosporine for primary immunosuppression after pediatric liver transplantation. Results from the U.S. Multicenter Trial. Transplantation 1995;59:530–536.
201. McDiarmid SV, Colonna JO, Shaked A, et al. A comparison of renal function in cyclosporine and FK506 treated patients after primary orthotopic liver transplantation. Transplantation 1993;56:847–853.
202. McCauley J, Fung JJ, Todo S, et al. Changes in renal function after liver transplantation under FK506. Transplant Proc 1991;23:3143–3145.
203. Mueller AR, Platz KP, Bechstein WO, et al. Neurotoxicity after orthotopic liver transplantation. A comparison between cyclosporine and FK506. Transplantation 1994;58:155–170.
204. Cox KL, Lawrence-Miyasaki LS, Garcia-Kennedy R, et al. An increased incidence of Epstein-Barr virus infection and lymphoproliferative disorder in young children on FK506 after liver transplantation. Transplantation 1995;59:524–529.
205. Margarit C, Martinez-Ibanez V, Tormo R, et al. Maintenance immunosuppression without steroids in pediatric liver transplantation. Transplant Proc 1989;21:2230–2231.
206. Superina R, Acal L, Bilik R, Zaki A. Growth in children after liver transplantation on cyclosporine alone or in combination with low-dose azathioprine. Transplant Proc 1993;25:2580.
207. Dunn SP, Falkenstein K, Lawrence JP, et al. Monotherapy with cyclosporine for chronic immunosuppression in pediatric liver transplant recipients. Transplantation 1994;57:544–547.
208. De Carlis L, Belli LS, Rondinara GF, et al. Early steroid withdrawal in liver transplant patients: final report of a prospective randomized trial. Transplant Proc 1997;29:539–542.
209. McDiarmid SV, Farmer DA, Goldstein LI, et al. A randomized prospective trial of steroid withdrawal after liver transplantation. Transplantation 1995;60:1443–1450.
210. Hoppu K, Holmberg C, Laine J, Jalanko H. Pharmacokinetic differences between oral cyclosporine (Sandimmune) and cyclosporine microemulsion (Sandimmune Neoral) in children after liver transplantation. European Society of Organ Transplantation, 1995.
211. Holmberg C, Laine J, Jalanko H, et al. Conversion from cyclosporine to Neoral in pediatric recipients for kidney, liver, and heart transplantation. Transplant Proc 1996;28:2262–2263.
212. Dunn SP, Billmire DF, Falkenstein K, et al. Rejection after pediatric liver transplantation is not the limiting factor to survival. J Pediatr Surg 1994;29:1141–1143;discussion 1143–1144.
213. Goldstein G, Kremer AB, Barnes L, Hirsch RL. OKT3 monoclonal antibody reversal of renal and hepatic rejection in pediatric patients. J Pediatr 1987;111:1046–1050.
214. Millis JM, Woodle ES, Piper JB, et al. Tacrolimus for primary treatment of steroid-resistant hepatic allograft rejection. Transplantation 1996;61:1365–1369.
215. McDiarmid SV, Busuttil RW, Terasaki P, Vargas JV, Ament ME. OKT3 treatment of steroid-resistant rejection in pediatric liver transplant recipients. J Pediatr Gastroenterol Nutr 1992;14:86–91.
216. McDiarmid SV, Wallace P, Vargas J, et al. The treatment of intractable rejection with FK506 in pediatric liver transplant recipients. J Pediatr Gastroenterol Nutr 1995;20:291–299.
217. Reding R, Wallemacq PE, Lamy ME, et al. Conversion from cyclosporine to FK506 for salvage of immunocompromised pediatric liver allografts. Transplantation 1994;57:93–100.
218. Egawa H, Esquivel CO, So SK, Cox K, et al. FK506 conversion treatment in pediatric liver transplantation. Transplantation 1994;57:1169–1173.
219. Eugui EM, Almquist SJ, Muller CD, Allison AC. Lymphocyte-selective cytostatic and immunosuppressive effects of mycophenolic acid in vitro: role of deoxyguanosine nucleotide depletion. Scand J Immunol 1991;33:161–173.
220. Klintmalm GB, Ascher NL, Busuttil RW, et al. RS-61443 for treatment-resistant human liver rejection. Transplant Proc 1993;25:697
221. Stegall MD, Wachs ME, Everson G, et al. Prednisone withdrawal 14 days after liver transplantation with mycophenolate: a prospective trial of cyclosporine and tacrolimus. Transplantation 1997;64:1755–1760.
222. Eckhoff DE, McGuire BM, Frenette LR, et al. Tacrolimus (FK506) and mycophenolate mofetil combination therapy versus tacrolimus in adult liver transplantation. Transplantation 1998;65:180–187.
223. McDiarmid SV, Colonna JO, Shaked A, et al. Differences in oral FK506 dose requirements between adult and pediatric liver transplant patients. Transplantation 1993;55:1328–1332.
224. Jain A, Fung JJ, Venkataramanan R, et al. Comparative study of cyclosporine and FK506 dosage requirement in adult and pediatric orthotopic liver transplantation. Transplant Proc 1991;23:2763–2766.
225. George DL, Arnow PM, Fox A, et al. Patterns of infection after pediatric liver transplantation. Am J Dis Child 1992;146:924–929.
226. McDiarmid SV. Renal function in pediatric liver transplant patients. Kidney Int Suppl 1996;53:S77–84.
227. Fung JJ, Abu-Elmagd K, Jain A, et al. A randomized trial of primary liver transplantation under immunosuppression with FK506 vs cyclosporine. Transplant Proc 1991;23:2977–2983.
228. Powell-Jackson PR, Young B, Calne RY, Williams R. Nephrotoxicity of parenterally administered cyclosporin after orthotopic liver transplantation. Transplantation 1983;36:505–508.
229. Chapman JR, Griffiths D, Harding NGL, Morris PJ. Reversibility of cyclosporine nephrotoxicity after three months treatment. Lancet 1985;1:125–130.
230. McCauley J, Studer R, Craven P, Murray S. The effects of cyclosporine A, cyclosporine G, and FK 506 upon prostaglandin production in renal mesangial cells in culture. Transplant Proc 1991;23:3141–3142.
231. Curtis JJ, Laskow DA. Cyclosporine-induced nephrotoxicity: pathophysiology of decreased blood flow. Transplant Proc 1988;20:540–543.
232. Eid A, Perkins JD, Rakela J, Krom RAF. Conversion from standard cyclosporine to low-dose cyclosporine in liver transplant recipients: effect on nephrotoxicity and hypertension beyond one year. Transplant Proc 1989;21:2238–2239.
233. McCauley J, Takaya S, Fung JJ, et al. The question of FK506 nephrotoxicity after liver transplantation. Transplant Proc 1991;23:1444–1447.
234. McDiarmid SV, Ettenger RB, Hawkins RA, et al. The impairment of true glomerular filtration rate in long-term cyclosporine-treated pediatric allograft recipients. Transplantation 1990;49:81–85.
235. Laine J, Krogerus L, Fyhrquist F, et al. Renal function and histopathologic changes in children after liver transplantation. J Pediatr 1994;125:863–869.
236. McDiarmid SV, Ettenger RB, Fine RN, et al. Serial decrease in glomerular filtration rate in long-term pediatric liver transplantation survivors treated with cyclosporine. Transplantation 1989;47:314–318.
237. Eidelman BH, Abu-Elmagd K, Wilson JM, et al. Neurologic complications of FK506. Transplant Proc 1991;23:3175–3178.
238. Lopez OL, Martinez AJ, Torre-Cisneros J. Neuropathologic findings in liver transplantation: a comparative study. Transplant Proc 1991;23:3181–3182.
239. Menegaux F, Keeffe EB, Andrews BT, et al. Neurological complications of liver transplantation in adult versus pediatric patients. Transplantation 1994;58:447–450.
240. Thompson CB, June CH, Sullivan KM, Thomas ED. Association between cyclosporin neurotoxicity and hypomagnesaemia. Lancet 1984;2:1116–1120.
241. de Groen PC. Cyclosporine, low-density lipoprotein, and cholesterol. Mayo Clin Proc 1988;63:1012–1021.
242. de Groen PC, Aksamit AJ, Rakela J, et al. Central nervous system toxicity after liver transplantation. The role of cyclosporine and cholesterol. N Engl J Med 1987;317:861–866.
243. Hall WA, Martinez AJ. Neuropathology of pediatric liver transplantation. Pediatr Neurosci 1989;15:269–275.
244. McDiarmid SV, Gornbein JA, Fortunat M, et al. Serum lipid abnormalities in pediatric liver transplant patients. Transplantation 1992;53:109–115.
245. Rustgi VK. Epstein-Barr viral infection and posttransplantation lymphoproliferative disorders. Liver Transplant Surg 1995;1:5:100–108.
246. Morrison VA, Dunn DL, Manivel JC, et al. Clinical characteristics of post-transplant lymphoproliferative disorders. Am J Med 1994;97:14–24.
247. Penn I. Posttransplant malignancies in pediatric organ transplant recipients. Transplant Proc 1994;26:2763–2765.

248. Ho M, Jaffe R, Miller G, et al. The frequency of Epstein-Barr virus infection and associated lymphoproliferative syndrome after transplantation and its manifestations in children. Transplantation 1988;45:719–727.
249. Lamy M, Favart AM, Cornu C, et al. Epstein-Barr virus infection in 59 orthotopic liver transplant patients. Med Microbiol Immunol 1990;179: 137–144.
250. Sokal EM, Caragiozoglou T, Lamy M, et al. Epstein-Barr virus serology and Epstein-Barr virus associated lymphoproliferative disorders in pediatric liver transplant patients. Transplantation 1993;56:1394–1398.
251. Renard TH, Andrews WS, Foster ME. Relationship between OKT3 administration, EBV seroconversion, and the lymphoproliferative syndrome in pediatric liver transplant recipients. Transplant Proc 1991;23:1473–1476.
252. Penn I. The changing pattern of posttransplant malignancies. Transplant Proc 1991;23:1101–1103.
253. Newell KA, Alonso EM, Whitington PF, et al. Posttransplant lymphoproliferative disease in pediatric liver transplantation. Transplantation 1996;62:3: 370–375.
254. Alfrey EJ, Friedman AL, Grossman RA, et al. A recent decrease in the time to development of monomorphous and polymorphous posttransplant lymphoproliferative disorder. Transplantation 1992;54:250–253.
255. Nalesnik MA, Demetris AJ, Fung JJ, Starzl TE. Lymphoproliferative disorders arising under immunosuppression with FK 506: initial observations in a large transplant population. Transplant Proc 1991;23:1108–1110.
256. Nalesnik MA, Lacker J, Jaffe R, et al. Experience with posttransplant lymphoproliferative disorders in solid organ transplant recipients. Clinical Transplantation 1992;6:249–252.
257. Cao S, Cox K, Esquivel CO, et al. PTLD and gastrointestinal manifestations of EBV infection in children following liver transplantation. Abstract Presented at Am Soc Transplant Phys Dallas, 1996.
258. Badley AD, Portela DF, Patel R, et al. Development of monoclonal gammopathy precedes the development of Epstein-Barr virus-induced posttransplant lymphoproliferative disorder. Liver Transplant Surg 1996;2:5:375–382.
259. Nalesnik MA. Involvement of the gastrointestinal tract by Epstein-Barr virus—associated posttransplant lymphoproliferative disorders. Am J Surg Pathol 1990;14(suppl 1):92–100.
260. Malatack JJ, Iwatsuki S, Gartner JC, et al. Liver transplantation for type I glycogen storage disease. Lancet 1983;1:1073–1074.
261. Markin RS. Manifestations of Epstein-Barr virus-associated disorders in liver. Liver 1994;14:1–13.
262. Penn I, Porat G. Central nervous system lymphomas in organ allograft recipients. Transplantation 1995;59:240–244.
263. Lee ES, Locker J, Nalesnik M, et al. The association of Epstein-Barr virus with smooth-muscle tumors. N Engl J Med 1995;332:19–25.
264. Seiden MV, Sklar J. Molecular genetic analysis of post-transplant lymphoproliferative disorders. Hematol Oncol Clin North Am 1993;7:447–465.
265. Martinez OM, Villanueva JC, Lawrence-Miyasaki LS, et al. Viral and immunologic aspects of Epstein-Barr virus infection in pediatric liver transplant recipients. Transplantation 1995;59:519–524.
266. Randhawa PS, Jaffe R, Demetris AJ, et al. Expression of Epstein-Barr virus-encoded small RNA (by the EBER-1 gene) in liver specimens from transplant recipients with post-transplantation lymphoproliferative disease. N Engl J Med 1992;327:1710–1714.
267. Green M, Reyes J, Jabbour N, et al. Use of quantitative PCR to predict onset of Epstein-Barr viral infection and post-transplant lymphoproliferative disease after intestinal transplantation in children. Transplant Proc 1996;28:5: 2759–2760.
268. Starzl TE, Nalesnik M, Porter KA, et al. Reversibility of lymphomas and lymphoproliferative lesions developing under cyclosporin-steroid therapy. Lancet 1984;1:583–587.
269. Benkerrou M, Durandy A, Fischer A. Therapy for transplant-related lymphoproliferative diseases. Hematol Oncol Clin North Am 1993;7:467–475.
270. Shapiro RS, Chauvenet A, McGuire W, et al. Treatment of B-cell lymphoproliferative disorders with interferon alfa and intravenous gamma globulin [letter]. N Engl J Med 1988;318:1334
271. Taguchi Y, Purtilo DT, Okano M. The effect of intravenous immunoglobulin and interferon-alpha on Epstein-Barr virus-induced lymphoproliferative disorder in a liver transplant recipient. Transplantation 1994;57:1813–1815.
272. Nalesnik MA, Rao AS, Furukawa H, et al. Autologous lymphokine-activated killer cell therapy of Epstein-Barr virus-positive and -negative lymphoproliferative disorders arising in organ transplant recipients. Transplantation 1997;63:1200–1205.
273. Chin SE, Shepherd RW, Cleghorn GJ, et al. Survival, growth and quality of life in children after orthotopic liver transplantation: a 5 year experience. J Paediatr Child Health 1991;27:380–385.
274. Sarna S, Laine J, Sipila I, et al. Differences in linear growth and cortisol production between liver and renal transplant recipients on similar immunosuppression. Transplantation 1995;60:656–661.
275. Moukarzel AA, Najm I, Vargas JV, et al. Prediction of long-term linear growth following liver transplantation. Transplant Proc 1990;22:1558–1559.
276. Urbach AH, Gartner JC, Malatack JJ, et al. Linear growth following pediatric liver transplantation. Am J Dis Child 1987;141:547–549.
277. Sarna S, Sipila I, Vihervuori E, et al. Growth delay after liver transplantation in childhood: studies of underlying mechanisms. Pediatr Res 1995;38:366–372.
278. McDiarmid SV, Gornbein JA, DeSilva PJ, et al. Factors affecting growth after pediatric transplantation. Transplantation 1999;67:404–411.
279. Holt RIG, Jones J, Stone NM, et al. Sequential changes in insulin-like growth factor I (IGF-I) and IGF-binding proteins in children with end-stage liver disease before and after successful orthotopic liver transplantation. J Clin Endocrinol Metabol 1996;81:1:160–168.
280. Codoner-Franch P, Bernard O, Alvarez F. Long-term follow-up of growth in height after successful liver transplantation. J Pediatr 1994;124:368–373.
281. Becht MB, Pedersen SH, Ryckman FC, Balistreri WF. Growth and nutritional management of pediatric patients after orthotopic liver transplantation. Gastroenterol Clin North Am 1993;22:367–380.
282. Andrews WS, Shimaoka S, Sommerauer J, et al. Steroid withdrawal after pediatric liver transplantation. Transplant Proc 1994;26:159–160.
283. Romani F, Belli LS, De Carlis L, et al. Cyclosporin monotherapy (after 3 months) in liver transplant patients: a prospective randomized trial. Transplant Proc 1994;26:2683–2685.
284. Sarna S, Sipila I, Ronnholm K, et al. Recombinant human growth hormone improves growth in children receiving glucocorticoid treatment after liver transplantation. J Clin Endocrinol Metab 1996;81:1476–1482.
285. Zitelli BJ, Miller JW, Gartner C Jr, et al. Changes in life-style after liver transplantation. Pediatrics 1988;82:173–180.
286. Stewart S, Hiltebeitel C, Nici J, et al. Neuropsychological outcome of pediatric liver transplantation. Pediatrics 1991;87:367–376.
287. Stewart S, Uauy R, Waller DA, et al. Mental and motor development, social competence, and growth one year after successful liver transplantation. J Pediatr 1989;114:574–581.
288. Stewart SM, Campbell RA, McCallon D, et al. Cognitive patterns in school-age children with end-stage liver disease. J Devel Behav Pediatr 1992;13: 331–338.
289. Windsorova D, Stewart SM, Lovitt R, et al. Emotional adaptation in children after liver transplantation. J Pediatr 1991;119:880–887.
290. Sokal EM. Quality of life after orthotopic liver transplantation in children. An overview of physical, psychological and social outcome. Eur J Pediatr 1995;154:171–175.
291. Mor E, Gonwa TA, Husberg BS, et al. Late-onset acute rejection in orthotopic liver transplantation—associated risk factors and outcome. Transplantation 1992;54:821–824.
292. Scantlebury V, Gordon R, Tzakis A, et al. Childbearing after liver transplantation. Transplantation 1990;49:317–321.
293. Starzl TE, Groth CG, Brettschneider L, et al. Orthotopic homotransplantation of the human liver. Ann Surg 1968;168:392–415.
294. Ettenger R, Cohen A, Nast C, et al. Mycophenolate mofetil as maintenance immunosuppression in pediatric renal transplantation. Transplant Proc 1997;29:340–341.

Chapter 21

Pancreas Transplantation

HUGH AUCHINCLOSS   DAVID SHAFFER

Pancreas transplantation is performed for the treatment of type 1 diabetes mellitus or occasionally for prevention of diabetes that would result from total pancreatectomy. Rarely, it has been used for patients with type 2 diabetes. Pancreas transplantation is not used to replace the exocrine function of patients with chronic pancreatitis. Thus, unlike most types of organ transplantation described in this textbook, which are performed for organ failure resulting from many different diseases, pancreas transplantation at this time has essentially a single indication.

On the other hand, pancreas transplantation is performed using a wide variety of technical approaches. This reflects the historical difficulty in achieving technically successful transplantation of this organ, partly because the pancreas tolerates surgical manipulation poorly, and partly because its exocrine function is irrelevant therapeutically and the source of many of the complications of the procedure. No universally accepted solutions to these problems have been developed, even after nearly two decades of clinical application.

Pancreas transplantation also differs from many other types of organ transplantation in the greater uncertainty that the procedure is fully justified, medically or economically. Pancreas transplantation is not life-sustaining (as is liver or heart transplantation), so its value must be determined by comparison to the alternative therapy (as also true for kidney transplantation). Because insulin treatment is both relatively inexpensive and extraordinarily effective, even over relatively long periods of time, pancreas transplantation must be justified as a means of providing an improved quality of life for transplant recipients or of preventing the complications of insulin therapy that generally occur over many years.

This chapter on pancreas transplantation covers the standard issues related to any form of organ transplantation, but special attention is devoted to the technical issues and to the justification for the procedure. In addition, because of the strong sense that current approaches to pancreas transplantation are likely to change in the future, more space is devoted to some of the alternatives currently being investigated.

TERMINOLOGY AND CLASSIFICATION

Pancreas transplantation can be performed as a whole organ transplant (often with an accompanying portion of duodenum), as a segmental organ transplant, or as a cellular transplant of islets or of isolated beta (β) cells. Organs for transplantation are almost always obtained from cadaveric donors but have been procured as segments from living donors or as islets from human or animal donors (xenogeneic transplantation). Pancreas transplants are always placed in a heterotopic position, and the recipient does not undergo a native pancreatectomy unless that procedure is itself the indication for pancreas replacement.

Pancreas transplantation is usually performed at the same time as kidney transplantation, using the same donor, in a procedure known as simultaneous pancreas-kidney (SPK) transplantation. Rarely, it has been combined with transplantation of other organs, such as the liver. In nonuremic diabetic patients, pancreas transplantation alone (PTA) can be performed; or pancreas after kidney (PAK) transplantation can be done after a successful cadaveric or living-donor kidney transplant.

Finally, pancreas transplants are often classified according to the manner of handling the exocrine function of the organ. For example, the procedure may involve a duodenocystostomy or a duodenoenterostomy. These terms and the classification of pancreas transplants are summarized in Table 21.1.

Table 21.1. Terminology and Classification for Pancreas Transplantation

Tissue
Pancreas with duodenum
Duodenal button
Duodenal segment
Pancreas
Segmental (distal) pancreas
Islet cells
Unseparated
Highly purified
Beta cells
Donor
Cadaver donor
Living donor
Related
Unrelated
Animal donor (xenogeneic)
Timing
Before other organs: PTA (pancreas transplant alone)
With a kidney: SPK (simultaneous pancreas–kidney)
With other organs: SPL (with a liver)
After kidney transplantation: PAK (pancreas after kidney)
Exocrine Drainage
Duodenocystostomy
Duct-cystostomy
Duodenoenterostomy
Duct ligation
Duct injection

THE RATIONALE FOR PANCREAS TRANSPLANTATION

One obvious rationale for pancreas transplantation is to replace insulin therapy for the recipient. Such therapy is cumbersome and restrictive. It reduces the quality of life for diabetic patients, and it is associated with the risk of life-threatening complications including hyperglycemia and (especially) hypoglycemia.

The other potential benefit from pancreas transplantation is that the maintenance of normal blood glucose levels may prevent the secondary complications of diabetes, including diabetic retinopathy, neuropathy, nephropathy, and accelerated vascular disease. The concept that the complications of diabetes are secondary, stemming from poor control of glucose levels, rather than primary, resulting from a direct effect of the original etiologic agent of the disease, has been referred to as the "glucose hypothesis" (1). Animal studies over many years have supported this hypothesis, but they have usually involved induced forms of insulin-deficiency rather than the idiopathic autoimmune disease of humans. Recently, however, the large Diabetes Control and Complications Trial involving human patients has provided strong evidence supporting the glucose hypothesis (2). In this study, improved (although still imperfect) glucose control was associated with a lower incidence and slower progression of the complications of diabetes. This finding was evident even in patients who had already developed early complications before tight glucose control was instituted (Fig. 21.1). Thus, it is widely believed that secondary complications would not

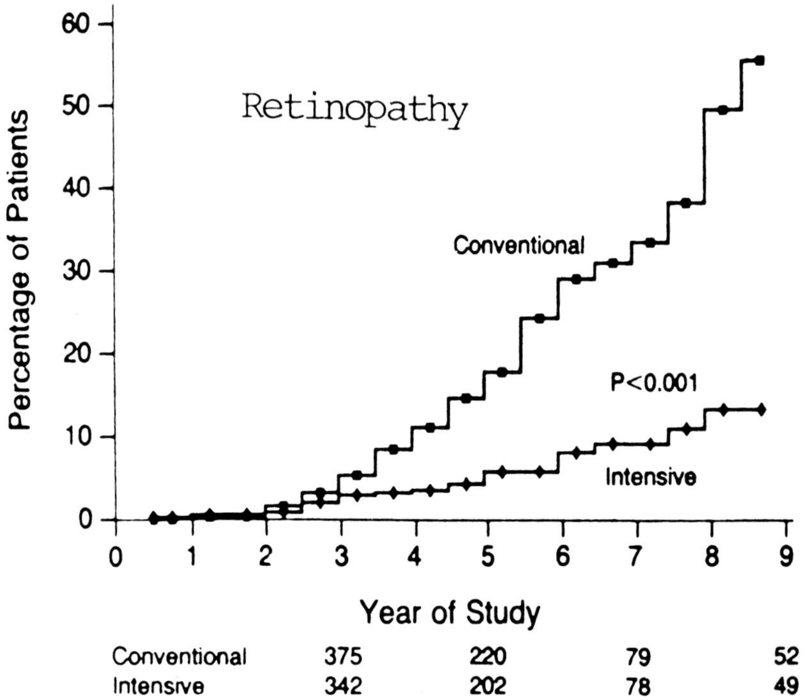

FIGURE 21.1. *Results of the Diabetes Control and Complications Trial show reduced rate of retinopathy with intensive glucose control even in patients with proteinuria at the time of entry into the trial.*

occur if normal glucose homeostasis could be restored shortly after the onset of diabetes (3).

The Diabetes Complications and Control Trial on its own, however, does not prove the value of pancreas transplantation as it is currently performed. Essentially all pancreas transplantation today requires immunosuppressive therapy, and thus pancreas transplantation alone for the treatment of diabetes involves a trade-off of insulin for immunosuppressive drugs. Except in rare cases of exceptionally brittle diabetes with frequent life-threatening complications, insulin therapy is the safer alternative, both in the short and the long term. Therefore, with some notable exceptions, relatively few centers are willing to offer pancreas transplantation until the recipient already requires immunosuppressive therapy for some other indication, usually the transplantation of a kidney for diabetic nephropathy (4). Under these circumstances, the justification for pancreas transplantation based on its ability to control secondary complications presumes that restoration of normal glucose homeostasis will limit the progression of the other secondary complications of the disease, even when at least one severe complication (nephropathy) has already developed. The evidence as to whether pancreas transplantation can achieve this result will be examined later in this chapter.

While the secondary complications of diabetes are familiar to most physicians, those practitioners involved in kidney transplantation may encounter them more forcefully. After it became clear that diabetic patients with renal failure did much better with kidney transplants than on dialysis, the number of diabetic patients receiving kidney transplants increased substantially. As a result, diabetes is now the most common etiology leading to kidney transplantation (see Chapter 17). But while these patients as a group have done remarkably well from the point of view of their kidney transplant, their longer-term survival has allowed the other complications of diabetes to progress relentlessly. Thus, transplant physicians are frequently in the position of watching their patients succumb to the effects of their underlying disease. It is perhaps not surprising, therefore, that the primary impetus for pancreas transplantation has come from transplant surgeons rather than from those who care for diabetic patients in earlier stages of their disease.

THE HISTORY OF PANCREAS TRANSPLANTATION

The history of pancreas transplantation has included four periods. First, between 1890 and 1965, a series of animal experiments demonstrated that total pancreatectomy produced insulin dependence, that transplantation of the pancreas could reverse diabetes, and that surgical techniques could be developed to transplant a vascularized whole organ pancreas.

The second period, from 1966 to about 1980, involved a series of human pancreas transplants that were notable for their remarkably poor survival. The first human attempt, reported by Kelly et al in 1966, involved a young diabetic woman who underwent a segmental pancreas along with a kidney transplant (5). Although she became insulin independent, both organs were subsequently removed because of rejection and complications related to the pancreas transplant. The patient died 2 months after her procedure. Lillehei and associates performed 13 pancreas transplants over the next several years, but only one of them functioned for more than 1 year. Worldwide, by 1977 the overall rate of 1-year graft survival was still only 5% for the 64 pancreas transplants reported to the International Pancreas Transplant Registry.

At the beginning of the third period in the history of pancreas transplantation, the dismal success of the procedure was in striking contrast to the results already being obtained for kidney, heart, and liver transplantation. Efforts to explain this discrepancy suggested at least three major contributing factors:

1. Pancreas transplants had a high rate of early technical failure primarily because of vascular thrombosis.
2. Detecting rejection episodes early enough to reverse them was difficult.
3. There were frequent technical complications related to the management of the exocrine secretions of the organ.

Sollinger, Corry, Starzl, and other investigators addressed these issues in the early 1980s. Their efforts, along with advances in immunosuppressive management, changed the outcome of pancreas transplantation dramatically in a very short period of time (6–8). Some of the key suggestions made during this time are listed in Table 21.2. It is unlikely that all of these ideas were equally important; nonetheless,

Table 21.2. Suggestions During the Early 1980s for Improving the Outcome of Pancreas Transplantation

1. Pancreas transplantation should be done simultaneously with kidney transplantation and from the same donor, thereby allowing assessment of renal function to identify the early onset of rejection episodes.
2. Exocrine drainage of the pancreas should be handled by duodenocystostomy, which is the safest and most reliable anastomosis and one that would also allow monitoring of urinary amylase to determine changes in pancreatic function.
3. Particular attention should be paid to pancreas procurement, since rough handling of the organ will produce graft pancreatitis leading to early thrombosis or peripancreatic collections.
4. The donor spleen should be transplanted with the pancreas to provide a high-flow vascular bed in the early phase of reperfusion. Donor splenectomy should be performed at the completion of the operation.
5. Recipient anticoagulation should be used with low-molecular-weight dextran, aspirin, and/or heparin to avoid early thrombosis.
6. The use of cyclosporine or tacrolimus as a more powerful immunosuppressive agent will lessen the early rejection of pancreas transplants.
7. The pancreas should be preserved with UW solution, which would allow longer preservation times and less ischemic injury.

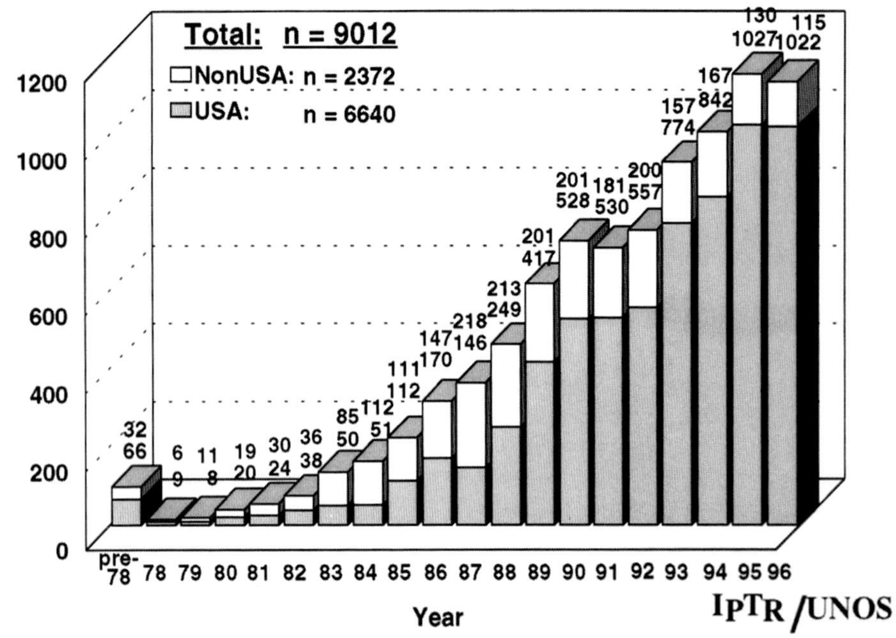

FIGURE 21.2. *Pancreas transplants worldwide show the increasing numbers of pancreas transplants and centers over the years.*

by the end of 1990, 1197 pancreas transplants had been reported in the United States from 60 centers, with an overall 1-year patient survival rate of 92% and a graft survival rate of 72%. Thus, in less than a decade, pancreas transplantation had become a widely practiced procedure (Fig. 21.2) with outcomes that were generally comparable to those for other organs (9–12).

The historical period since 1990 has involved a reassessment of both the techniques for the procedure and its indications. Since this evaluation is ongoing, the results presented in this chapter are certain to be transient. Furthermore, it is not surprising that this period is seeing even greater variations in the approach to pancreas transplantation at different transplant centers. What seems most certain is that both the techniques and the application of pancreas transplantation will continue to evolve, and that we have not yet reached a satisfactory solution to the use of pancreas transplantation in the treatment for diabetes.

SELECTING CANDIDATES FOR PANCREAS TRANSPLANTATION

Currently, no transplant center is willing to offer pancreas transplantation as treatment in the earliest stages of diabetes. A few centers have been willing to perform the procedure for patients who have developed microalbuminuria (a strong predictor of eventual end-stage diabetic nephropathy), especially if the patient has manifested brittle diabetes with frequent and severe hypoglycemic episodes. For the most part, however, pancreas transplantation has been offered only when recipients have at least developed serious proteinuria and diminished glomerular filtration rates (GFRs), and more often when renal failure has progressed to the point where the patient is being evaluated for kidney transplantation. Under these circumstances, pancreas transplantation is offered along with a kidney transplant, as the renal disease is unlikely to be sufficiently reversible and because immunosuppressive therapy usually further damages the already marginal renal function (see Chapter 35).

Clinical experience has indicated that the short-term outcome of SPK transplantation is improved if the procedure is performed early in the course of renal failure (for example, even before the serum creatinine level is above 2 mg/dL) and before the notable manifestation of other secondary diabetic complications. Nonetheless, differences in organ allocation policies of different regions make it impossible to perform early combined organ transplantation in all cases. In some areas, diabetic patients waiting for both pancreas and kidney transplants are listed separately from patients waiting only for kidneys, and the allocation of the two organs is determined by the patient's priority for a pancreas. Since the waiting time for a pancreas is generally much shorter than for a kidney, under this allocation scheme patients can receive both organs early in the course of their renal failure, and almost always sooner than if they had been seeking a kidney transplant alone. At the other end of the spectrum, other regions list candidates for combined organ transplantation together with those waiting for kidneys only; they require that patients be on dialysis before they are listed at all; and they allocate the two organs according to the patient's priority for a kidney. Under these circumstances, combined pancreas and kidney transplantation can rarely be performed until patients have been on dialysis for several years.

These differences in policy reflect the difficulty in balancing the competing interests of different patients. Separate listing for pancreas–kidney recipients allows diabetic patients to receive cadaveric kidney transplants faster than patients with other causes of renal failure. On the other hand, combined listing is likely to make the outcome of pancreas transplantation less favorable; many diabetic patients are no longer suitable candidates for the procedure by the time an organ becomes available. With these competing interests in mind, some regions have adopted intermediate policies that allow combined pancreas–kidney transplantation to occur somewhat earlier than it does for patients waiting only for kidneys, but without putting pancreas–kidney candidates immediately at the top of the list.

Whether early or late in the course of renal failure, diabetic patients are evaluated especially carefully before undergoing combined pancreas–kidney transplantation. In addition to the standard tests used for evaluating any patient considering kidney transplantation, there are several special issues in the combined procedure. First, at those centers using bladder drainage for pancreatic exocrine secretions, the recipient's bladder function should be tested to ensure reasonable emptying. Second, the incidence of asymptomatic cardiac disease is higher in long-term diabetic patients, making it reasonable to include noninvasive testing for ischemic heart disease in these patients. When evaluating the potential benefits of the procedure it is also reasonable to determine the status of other secondary complications of diabetes such as peripheral vascular disease, retinopathy, and peripheral neuropathy. Finally, the potential candidate's difficulty in managing their current insulin therapy may be an important factor in choosing the procedure.

Because of the differences in organ allocation policy described above, the factors determining whether to proceed with pancreas in addition to kidney transplantation are not the same in all cases. When the allocation scheme provides earlier access to kidney transplantation, this becomes a factor in addition to the balance of risks and benefits for pancreas transplantation described later in this chapter. On the other hand, when the allocation policy requires prolonged periods of dialysis before transplantation, potential recipients must recognize that the secondary complications of diabetes are likely to progress during this period, lessening the potential benefits of receiving a pancreas. These candidates may have the option of obtaining a kidney transplant from a living donor, instead of waiting for years on dialysis before receiving both organs from a cadaveric donor. Because the complications of diabetes often progress rapidly while the patient is on dialysis, it is usually preferable to use the living donor for the kidney transplant alone. These patients can then become candidates for a solitary cadaveric pancreas transplant after receiving their kidney from a living donor; however, the outcome of isolated pancreas transplantation is not as good as for the combined procedure (see below).

SELECTING PANCREAS DONORS

With the exception of a small series of living-related segmental pancreas transplants performed at the University of Minnesota (13,14), pancreases are always obtained from cadaveric donors. Selection criteria for a donor include ABO blood group compatibility and documentation of a negative crossmatch with the recipient, just as for kidney donors (see also Chapter 15). Depending on how much cold ischemia time a center is willing to tolerate for a pancreas, crossmatch testing may be required before organ procurement to facilitate pancreas transplantation. Although the outcome of SPK transplantation improves slightly with better HLA matching, the degree of matching is generally considered less important than is waiting time for recipients of both organs, in keeping with the allocation policies for kidney transplants alone. Distribution of combined kidneys and pancreases to HLA-identical recipients on a national basis is usually too cumbersome to accomplish. The degree of HLA matching is a more critical determinant in the outcome of solitary pancreas transplantation and is often used in the allocation of isolated pancreas transplants. Although registry data indicate that cold ischemia times up to 30 hours have no important impact on graft survival, others have found that the occurrence of pancreatic graft thrombosis is related to duration of cold ischemia (15).

There are several organ-specific factors to consider in potential pancreas donors. Evidence of frank pancreatitis or of direct injury to the organ prohibits pancreas procurement. However, mild hyperamylasemia (low levels of serum amylase elevation) is common in cadaveric donors, especially after facial or intracranial trauma, and is not necessarily a contraindication to procurement. A history of heavy alcohol abuse with chronic pancreatitis or a nodular, fibrotic gland noted at the time of procurement precludes donation. Similarly, a history of insulin-dependence or of previous glucose intolerance precludes the use of such donors. However, most cadaveric donors manifest some glucose intolerance in response to the stress of injury and steroid therapy; glucose elevations that have not required insulin therapy are generally not, in themselves, contraindications to organ procurement (16–18). In addition, many centers believe that the age range for acceptable pancreas donors is narrower than for kidneys alone, although little evidence is available to prove this. Cardiac arrest with resuscitation or dependence on vasopressors such as dopamine or Neo-Synephrine does not preclude cadaver pancreas donation, although some evidence suggests that the need for dopamine adversely affects long-term pancreas graft function (16). To avoid post-transplant pancreatitis or ischemic β-cell injury, many centers have stricter criteria for hemodynamic stability for pancreas donors than for liver or kidney donors. Finally, the difficulty of the pancreas procurement procedure is increased considerably if the donor is obese. As with all decisions regarding the suitability of organ donors, the issues to be considered are relative and cannot be quantified with certainty.

SURGICAL PROCEDURES FOR PANCREAS TRANSPLANTATION

Cadaver Donor Pancreatectomy

Pancreas graft procurement is technically the most difficult cadaver organ procurement procedure. It requires familiarity with normal and abnormal anatomy in the upper abdomen and gentle handling of the pancreas and its blood supply. Most pancreases are procured as part of a multi-organ recovery that includes the liver, kidneys, and thoracic organs. Therefore, care must be taken to avoid contaminating the other organs by prematurely opening the bowel. In addition, coordination with the liver procurement effort is essential, especially in cases of abnormal vascular anatomy. In general, the liver, as a life-sustaining organ, is procured with its full vascular supply down to the aorta. Although this requires subsequent vascular reconstruction for the pancreas (see below), experience has shown that both the liver and the pancreas can be obtained from the same donor without adversely affecting either organ (19–21).

Although variations in surgical technique are common between different centers (22–25), the basic elements of the technique for pancreas organ procurement are described briefly as follows. Prior to procurement, amphotericin B solution (50 mL/L) is instilled into the stomach and duodenum via nasogastric tube to reduce the risk of postoperative fungal infections. Povidone-iodine may also be used to reduce bacterial counts. A midline abdominal incision and median sternotomy are performed. Liver dissection is performed first (see Chapter 19). Hepatic arterial anatomy is assessed early in the dissection, the most common anomalies being a replaced right hepatic artery originating from the superior mesenteric artery (SMA), found by palpation in the hepaticoduodenal ligament lateral and inferior to the common bile duct, and a replaced left hepatic artery originating from the left gastric artery in the gastrohepatic ligament. Liver preparation includes mobilization of the right lobe of the liver and isolation of the inferior vena cava (IVC) above the right renal vein, division of the common bile duct and gastroduodenal artery, mobilization of the portal vein in the hepatoduodenal ligament (usually with division of the coronary vein), division of the left triangular ligament and gastrohepatic ligament, and isolation of the supraceliac aorta and identification of the celiac axis, common, and proper hepatic arteries. Following liver preparation, exposure of the pancreas begins.

The origin of the splenic artery from the celiac axis is identified and mobilized for approximately 1 cm. Dissection of the hepatic and splenic arteries is minimized to avoid vasospasm. The gastrocolic ligament and the gastroepiploic and short gastric vessels are divided. The spleen is mobilized by division of its ligamentous attachments and used as a "handle" to allow mobilization of the tail and body of the pancreas. Care is taken not to tear the pancreatic capsule or place excessive traction on the pancreas itself to avoid posttransplant pancreatitis or bleeding. The tail and body of the pancreas are elevated until the left side of the aorta is reached by dividing the avascular plane posterior to the pancreas and anterior to the left adrenal gland and kidney. The inferior mesenteric vein (IMV) joining the splenic vein along the inferior edge of the pancreas is preserved for subsequent venous cannulation. Division of the left gastric vessels completes the lateral to medial dissection of the pancreas.

A large Cattell maneuver is performed to elevate the small bowel mesentery and expose the retroperitoneal IVC and aorta. These are controlled with umbilical tapes or large silk ligatures for subsequent cannulation. The left renal vein, origin of the SMA, and infrahepatic cava above the right renal vein are exposed. Following mobilization of the kidneys and ureters and in coordination with the thoracic organ teams, the donor is heparinized (20,000 U) and the distal infrarenal aorta and IVC are ligated and cannulated. A portal cannula for liver perfusion is placed in the IMV, although some surgeons prefer direct cannulation of the portal vein in the hilum of the liver after it is divided to avoid overperfusion or distention of the pancreas. Following cross-clamping of the supraceliac aorta, 2 to 3 liters of cold (4°C) preservation solution are infused via aortic and portal cannulas, and crushed ice is placed in the abdominal cavity for topical cooling. University of Wisconsin (UW) solution is currently the perfusate of choice (26) (see also Chapter 16).

The liver is removed following division of the splenic artery several millimeters distal to its take-off from the celiac axis, division of the aorta above and below the origin of the celiac axis, and division of the portal vein 2 cm above the superior border of the pancreas. The duodenum is transected with a stapler proximally just distal to the pylorus and distally at the inferior border of the pancreas. The mesenteric vessels at the inferior border of the pancreas are then divided with a double row of staples and the pancreaticoduodenal graft with attached spleen is removed. Prior to packing the pancreas graft in cold storage with UW solution, the duodenal segment can be opened and flushed with amphotericin solution (50 mg/L) (Fig. 21.3).

Variations on this approach include addition of a cruciate incision and initial removal of the entire stomach to allow better exposure of the pancreas and spleen (9), en bloc removal of liver, duodenum, pancreas, and spleen with ex vivo separation of the liver and pancreas following the infusion of preservation solution (20), and a rapid en bloc technique (25).

With normal hepatic arterial anatomy, the aorta is divided between the SMA and the celiac axis, with the SMA remaining with the pancreatic graft and the celiac axis with the liver. Variations in hepatic arterial anatomy are common, with anomalies found in approximately one-quarter of liver procurements. A right hepatic artery arising from the SMA occurs in about 10% and a left hepatic artery arising from the left gastric artery in 13%, with both anomalies occurring simultaneously in about 3% of cases. None of these anomalies should preclude simultaneous liver and pancreas procurement, as several techniques are available for arterial reconstruction of either liver or pancreas allografts (27). A common arterial trunk, which is very rarely encountered, precludes simultaneous procurement.

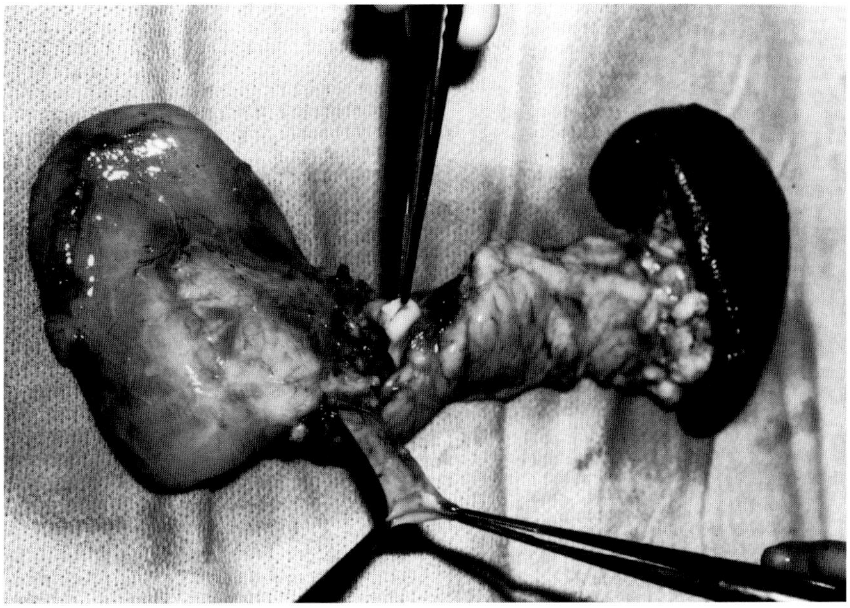

FIGURE 21.3. *A pancreaticoduodenal allograft following organ procurement. The upper forceps is holding the donor celiac and superior mesenteric artery origin. The donor portal vein is grasped by the lower forceps.*

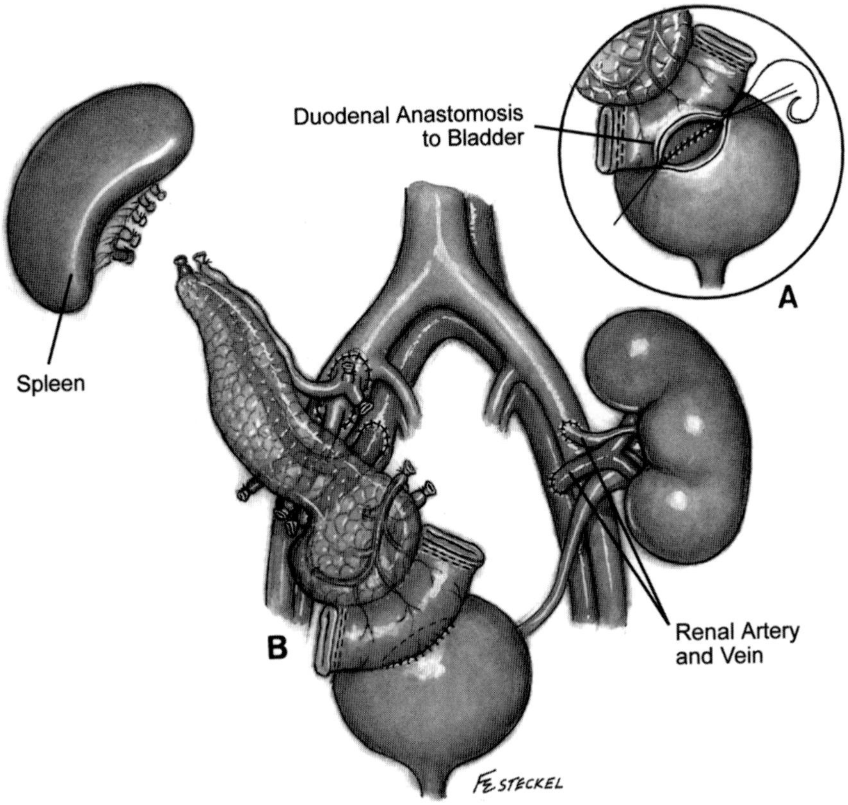

FIGURE 21.4. *Techniques of combined pancreas and kidney transplantation.* ***A.*** *The proximal and distal ends of the donor duodenal segment have been closed by staples. Bladder drainage of the pancreatic exocrine secretions is provided by the side-to-side duodenocystostomy.* ***B.*** *The renal allograft in the left iliac fossa has been revascularized via the recipient external iliac artery and vein. The ureter is drained via ureteroneocystostomy. The pancreaticoduodenal allograft in the right iliac fossa has been arterialized in this case by anastomosis of a Carrel patch of donor aorta (encompassing the origins of the celiac and superior mesenteric arteries) to recipient common iliac artery.*

Recipient Pancreas Transplantation

When performed simultaneously with a cadaver kidney transplant (88% of pancreas transplants reported to the US Registry since 1987), the pancreas is placed preferentially in the right iliac fossa (Fig. 21.4). The cecum and right colon are mobilized cephalad to expose the common iliac vessels and allow the pancreas to lie in the presacral space. For bladder-drained pancreas grafts, right-sided placement minimizes potential twisting or kinking of the graft and its vasculature. Most centers place the pancreas allograft intraperitoneally via a lower midline incision, although a transverse incision and intraperitoneal placement may also be used. Extraperitoneal placement, similar to a standard kidney transplant, is technically simpler but is associated with an increased incidence of deep wound infections

(28–30). In SPK transplants, the kidney is placed on the contralateral side, either intraperitoneally or extraperitoneally via a midline (31) or a separate flank incision. In PAK transplants, the pancreas is placed in the iliac fossa contralateral to the functioning kidney transplant.

Variations in the Techniques for Vascular Reconstruction

As noted above, following simultaneous liver–pancreas procurement, the arterial blood supply of the pancreas graft usually consists of the divided splenic artery and the SMA, including a Carrel patch of aorta. Arterial reconstruction is typically accomplished in one of two ways. A donor iliac artery Y-graft, with anastomoses between the donor external iliac artery and donor SMA and between the donor internal iliac artery and donor splenic artery, is performed on the back table and the donor common iliac artery is subsequently anastomosed to the recipient common or external iliac artery (Fig. 21.5). Alternatively, depending on the length of the donor splenic artery and SMA, the end of the donor splenic artery is anastomosed to the side of the donor SMA on the back table, with the donor SMA subsequently anastomosed to the recipient common iliac artery.

The standard technique for venous drainage of pancreas transplants is into the systemic circulation via end-to-side anastomosis of the donor portal vein with the recipient common iliac vein. As the donor portal vein is usually short (<2 cm) due to simultaneous procurement of the liver, generous mobilization of the iliac vein, in some cases including ligation and division of the hypogastric vein, may facilitate the anastomosis. The donor iliac vein should be available for a venous extension graft if there is insufficient length of portal vein, although with adequate mobilization of recipient iliac vein this is rarely necessary. In fact, using a short donor portal vein lessens the likelihood of its twisting or kinking, which can lead to graft thrombosis.

Systemic venous drainage of the pancreas allograft results in peripheral hyperinsulinemia, an independent risk factor for atherosclerosis and coronary artery disease (see below). Portal venous drainage has been used in some cases as a more physiologic approach (32). A donor iliac artery Y-graft is used for arterial reconstruction as described above. The transverse mesocolon is reflected superiorly and an end-to side anastomosis between the donor portal vein and a tributary of the recipient superior mesenteric vein inferior to the native pancreas is performed (33). In contrast to the standard bladder-drainage technique in which the head of the pancreas and duodenum are oriented inferiorly, with this technique the pancreas is oriented superiorly and enteric drainage of graft exocrine secretions is performed by anastomosis of the donor duodenum to a defunctionalized Roux-en-Y limb of the recipient (see below).

Donor splenectomy may be performed on the back table prior to transplantation, after the vascular anastomoses are completed during the transplant procedure, or just prior to closing the abdomen. Leaving the spleen permanently with the pancreas in an attempt to minimize the risk of vascular thrombosis may lead to significant hematologic complications including fatal graft-versus-host disease (34).

Variations in the Technique for Exocrine Drainage

The optimal method of draining pancreatic exocrine secretions remains controversial. Early attempts at managing exocrine secretions following pancreas transplantation included duct ligation, enterocutaneous pancreatic fistula, open drainage into the peritoneal cavity, and enteric drainage into a loop of recipient intestine. All resulted in serious surgical complications such as thrombosis, pancreatitis, anastomotic leaks, and sepsis, often culminating in graft failure and occasionally in death. Gliedman first suggested urinary drainage of pancreatic exocrine secretions by anas-

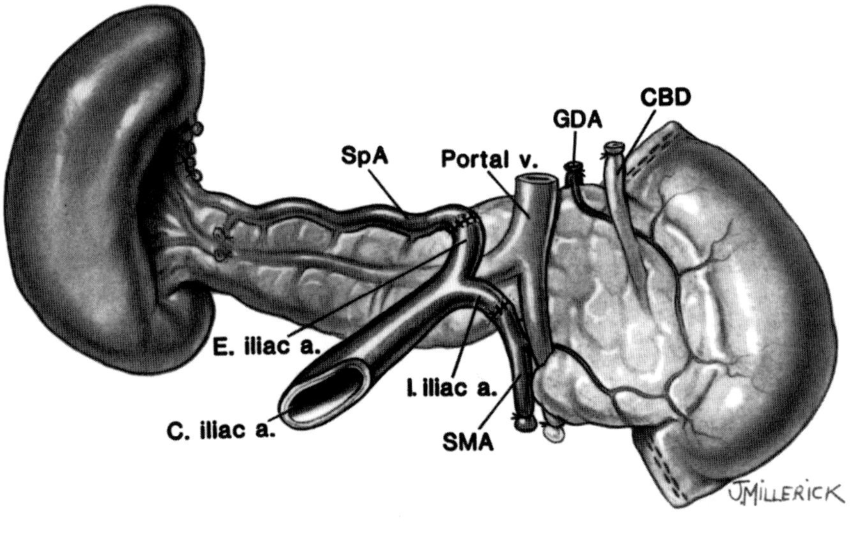

FIGURE 21.5. *Typical arterial reconstruction of the pancreas obtained from a donor from whom the liver was also removed for transplantation. A donor common iliac artery graft is utilized with the external iliac artery branch anastomosed to the splenic artery (SpA), and the internal iliac artery to the superior mesenteric artery (SMA). The donor distal common bile duct (CBD) and gastroduodenal artery (GDA) have been ligated.*

tomosing the donor pancreatic duct to the recipient ureter (35). By the early 1980s, several groups had found that direct bladder drainage of pancreatic allografts could be accomplished without leaks and without damage to the recipient bladder mucosa or fibrosis of the pancreas (6,36,37). The technique was subsequently modified to a side-to-side anastomosis between a segment of duodenum and the bladder (8,38).

Although the Stockholm group (39) and the Lyon group (87) remained proponents of enteric drainage or of duct injection, respectively, most US centers quickly adopted bladder-drainage as the standard approach because of a decrease in the incidence of postoperative complications, improved graft survival, and the ability to monitor graft function by measuring serial urinary amylase levels. Of the more than 8000 cadaver pancreas transplants in the United States reported to the International Pancreas Transplant Registry/UNOS between 1987 and 1997, over 90% were bladder-drained.

A side-to-side duodenocystostomy is performed after first stapling and turning in (with Lembert sutures) the proximal and distal ends of a short (5–10 cm) duodenal segment containing the pancreatic duct. Many surgeons perform the duodenocystostomy using a hand-sewn two-layer anastomosis, while others prefer to use an EEA stapler (40). Permanent suture material even on the outside layer of the anastomosis may serve as a nidus for bladder calculi. Minimizing the length of the duodenal segment reduces the incidence and severity of postoperative metabolic acidosis. Early experience with a duodenal button instead of a segment was associated with an increase in surgical complications and technical graft loss (7,41).

Prompted by the persistently high complications associated with bladder drainage, currently there is a resurgence of interest in enteric drainage of pancreatic exocrine secretions (42,43). While the early experience reported from both single centers and the US Registry showed significantly worse functional survival rates for enteric- versus bladder-drained pancreas grafts (44,45), excellent long-term results have been reported with enteric drainage by several centers (39). Initially, the Stockholm group used segmental grafts with the cut end of the pancreas anastomosed end-to-end to a jejunal Roux-en-Y limb with a temporary pancreatic duct catheter to divert pancreatic juice. Since 1987, pancreaticoduodenal grafts have been used, first with an anastomosis of the duodenal segment to a Roux-en-Y limb with a pancreatic duct catheter, and subsequently to a loop of small intestine without a Roux limb or duct catheter (46).

With better immunosuppression, new serologic markers to follow rejection, percutaneous pancreas biopsy techniques, and better intra-abdominal imaging and radiologic drainage techniques, several US centers have reexamined primary enteric drainage for pancreas transplantation (32,47–49). Some centers have used an end-to-end anastomosis between donor duodenum and a recipient Roux-en-Y limb (32). Others have used a side-to-side anastomosis (48).

POSTOPERATIVE MANAGEMENT AND COMPLICATIONS

General Postoperative Care

General postoperative management of pancreas recipients is similar to other organ transplant patients, with several additional organ-specific issues. Foley catheter drainage is continued for 5 to 10 days postoperatively for patients with a duodenocystostomy, and many centers obtain a cystogram before removing the catheter. Early postoperative antibiotics are also used more vigorously than for kidney transplantation alone and may include the use of systemic antifungal therapy. Most centers use some form of anticoagulation therapy, ranging from a single aspirin to the use of subcutaneous heparin and/or low-molecular-weight dextran during the first several days. Intravenous fluid replacement is initially the same as for other transplant recipients. However, the exocrine output of the pancreas gradually increases over the first 5 days, creating a requirement for sodium bicarbonate replacement, intravenously or orally, in patients with bladder drainage. Insulin therapy is not generally required postoperatively, and it is not necessary to obtain tight blood sugar control during the immediate post-transplant period. Blood sugars will be close to normal levels within 12 hours after the pancreas transplant and are almost always normal within several days as high-dose steroid therapy is reduced. Pancreas transplant recipients no longer require a diabetic diet after a successful procedure.

Immunosuppression

Since the 1980s, cyclosporine-based immunosuppression consisting of triple therapy with cyclosporine, prednisone, and azathioprine has formed the cornerstone of immunosuppressive therapy following pancreas transplantation (50). Many US centers employ quadruple immunosuppression therapy, adding a 7- to 14-day course of induction therapy with a polyclonal [anti-lymphocyte globulin (ALG), Atgam] or monoclonal (OKT-3) antilymphocyte agent (10–12). Some individual centers have reported excellent results using cyclosporine-based triple therapy without induction. Respective trials comparing Atgam and OKT-3 for induction have shown comparable patient and graft survival rates (51–53).

More recent efforts have explored the use of the newer immunosuppressive agents tacrolimus (Prograf) and mycophenolate mofetil (CellCept) in pancreas transplantation (see Chapters 9 and 10). Like cyclosporine, tacrolimus is associated with impaired glucose metabolism. Initial reports of tacrolimus as primary or rescue therapy indicated a 14% to 22% incidence of de novo diabetes mellitus following liver transplantation (54–55), and a 16% incidence of new-onset diabetes following kidney transplantation (56). Subsequent data suggested improvement in glucose intolerance with long-term use following liver transplantation (57), and several authors reported graft salvage and normal glucose metabolism with tacrolimus as rescue therapy for rejection or cyclosporine toxicity following SPK transplantation (58–59). More recently, excellent results have been reported in a multicenter analysis of the use of tacrolimus, prednisone, and azathioprine as primary therapy following pancreas transplantation (60), and many centers have begun using tacrolimus routinely as primary therapy (61).

Mycophenolate mofetil, in combination with cyclosporine and prednisone, has been shown to reduce the incidence of acute rejection following kidney transplantation compared to placebo (62) or to azathioprine (63). The main side effects appear to be leukopenia and gastrointestinal symptoms; the incidence of hyperglycemia was less than in azathioprine controls. Based on favorable data from kidney transplants alone, many centers now use cyclosporine, prednisone, and mycophenolate mofetil as standard maintenance therapy following pancreas-kidney transplantation. The results of randomized trials comparing this to other immunosuppressive regimens are only now becoming available (64,65). The combination of tacrolimus, prednisone, and mycophenolate is another approach, although the additive gastrointestinal toxicities of tacrolimus and mycophenolate mofetil may be significant. The potential role of newer immunosuppressive agents in pancreas transplantation such as sirolimus, brequinar, and 15-deoxyspergualin remains unknown (see Chapter 11).

Postoperative Monitoring

Despite advances in immunosuppression, rejection remains an important cause of pancreas graft failure (10,11,45,66). The pancreas may be more immunogenic than other solid organ allografts (64), and rejection occurs in up to 60% to 80% of cases, roughly twice as commonly as following kidney transplantation alone (12,29,45). Routine postoperative monitoring for pancreas graft rejection consists of blood sugars, serum amylase and lipase, and urinary amylase, although all of these tests lack specificity. Hyperglycemia is a relatively late sign of rejection following pancreas transplantation, and its appearance often suggests irreversible destruction of the organ. Changes in exocrine function, such as a rise in serum amylase and lipase or a fall in urinary amylase, generally precede the onset of hyperglycemia by several days. Thus, in bladder-drained grafts, initial diagnosis of rejection can sometimes be made from a 25% to 50% fall in urinary amylase and concomitant rise in serum amylase. Both events, however, can occur in the absence of rejection activity. Efforts to use urinary amylase levels to identify rejection activity require correction for urine output. Thus, this assay is best reported as amylase per unit of time rather than amylase per unit of urine volume.

Efforts have been made to identify additional markers for pancreatic rejection activity that would have better sensitivity and specificity than urinary amylase and that could be used when bladder drainage of exocrine secretions is not used. Newer serologic markers of exocrine function such as serum anodal trypsinogen (67,68) and pancreas-specific protein (69) may be more specific but are not yet available for widespread use. Urine cytology (70) and glucose disappearance rates (71) have also been reported to be helpful in diagnosing rejection in individual centers. However, at this point there is no single assay that detects early evidence of pancreatic rejection.

Biopsy is a more direct means of diagnosing rejection. Histologic criteria of pancreas rejection include an interstitial mononuclear cell infiltrate and endothelialitis of acinar tissue (72). For bladder-drained grafts it is possible to perform cystoscopic transduodenal biopsies of the pancreas (73). Experienced centers report a high yield of adequate tissue for histologic diagnosis and a low incidence of complications (74,75). Tissue yield may be increased with the use of transabdominal ultrasound guidance of cystoscopic biopsies. Complications reported include bleeding controlled with electrocautery in 8.4%, clot retention in 1%, and transient hyperamylasemia in 20% (74). Duodenal mucosal biopsies appear to correlate with pancreatic biopsies in most cases; some centers, therefore, use duodenal biopsies alone.

More recently, excellent results with percutaneous pancreas biopsy with an 18-gauge automated biopsy needle and color-flow Doppler ultrasound localization have been reported. Overlying bowel may be a problem in intra-abdominally placed pancreatic grafts, although in a large series of percutaneous pancreas biopsies (76), adequate tissue for histologic examination was obtained in 88% of cases. Two cases (2.2%) of intra-abdominal bleeding were reported, one requiring laparotomy, and there were no cases of graft pancreatitis, pancreatic fistula, or pseudocyst formation. Percutaneous pancreas biopsy allows pancreatic monitoring without the need for bladder drainage. Thus, while the ability to achieve postoperative monitoring with urinary amylase and cystoscopic pancreatic biopsies was originally thought to be a major advantage for the use of bladder-drained grafts, the development of serologic markers such as serum anodal trypsinogen and the ability to perform percutaneous biopsies have generated renewed enthusiasm for enteric drainage.

In patients with SPK transplants with both allografts from the same donor, manifestations of kidney graft rejection almost always precede significant hyperglycemia secondary to pancreas rejection. Although some authors have suggested that the kidney "protects" the pancreas from rejection following SPK, it is more likely that the kidney serves as a "sentinel" organ, allowing an earlier diagnosis and treatment for rejection. This likely accounts for the significantly improved graft survival rates following SPK versus PAK or PTA.

The use of simultaneous kidney transplants to diagnose rejection activity within the pancreas is based on the assumption that the two organs suffer immunologic rejection concordantly. On the other hand, a high incidence of discordant rejection, both in onset and severity, has been demonstrated in a pig model of simultaneous pancreas and kidney transplants from the same donor (77). Similarly, one clinical study has been performed using both cystoscopically guided pancreatic biopsies and renal biopsies in 27 SPK transplants (74). Rejection was present in both organs in 33% of cases, but discordant findings were also encountered, including renal rejection alone in 15% and pancreatic rejection alone in 15% of cases. These data suggest that pancreatic graft monitoring, both by laboratory parameters and by biopsy, may still have a role following SPK transplantation.

Postoperative Complications

The majority of surgical complications following pancreas transplantation are related to the handling of pancreatic exocrine secretions. This is particularly unfortunate because only functioning islet cells are required to treat diabetes. As with other allografts, complications are also related to the use of long-term immunosuppression. Most of the current data from US centers reporting postoperative complications include predominantly bladder-drained grafts.

Thrombosis

Pancreas graft thrombosis occurred in up to 10% to 20% of recipients in the early experience with pancreas transplants. This incidence is higher than that for other solid organ transplants, with the possible exception of pediatric livers, and may have its anatomic basis in the diminished blood flow that occurs following ligation of the distal splenic artery. Early methods to prevent thrombosis included systemic anticoagulation and attempts to increase blood flow by creating a distal arteriovenous fistula of splenic artery and vein or by leaving the spleen attached to the tail of the pancreas. Transplantation of the spleen with the pancreas resulted in hematologic complications, including fatal graft-versus-host disease, and thus that technique has been abandoned. Systemic heparinization led to a high incidence of bleeding complications, and most centers currently use only aspirin and/or subcutaneous heparin. Probably the most important determinants in avoiding vascular thrombosis are the gentle handling of the pancreas during organ procurement and achieving the proper orientation of the vascular anastomoses during transplantation. With greater experience, the incidence of vascular thrombosis has decreased considerably.

Arterial thrombosis is heralded by a sudden rise in blood sugars with a normal or stable serum amylase. The initial abdominal exam may be remarkably benign. In contrast, venous thrombosis typically presents with sudden onset of abdominal pain and tenderness and marked hyperamylasemia, with only a mild to moderate rise in blood sugars. The diagnosis can be confirmed by color flow Doppler ultrasound, radionuclide scanning, computed tomography (CT) angiogram, magnetic resonance (MR) angiogram, or selective angiography. Prompt surgical reexploration should not be delayed for radiologic confirmation, however, in the appropriate clinical setting. The graft is usually not salvageable, and transplant pancreatectomy is required. Attempts at graft salvage may result in life-threatening pancreatitis (78).

Hematuria and Cystitis

One large series found a 15.7% incidence of significant hematuria following pancreas transplantation (42). As noted above, its occurrence is in part related to the intensity of anticoagulation to prevent graft thrombosis. Hematuria may be an early sign of duodenal and pancreas rejection, but early postoperative hematuria usually subsides spontaneously and does not require blood transfusion. Initial treatment of severe hematuria is discontinuation of anticoagulation or antiplatelet therapy, followed by cystoscopy for clot evacuation and fulguration of bleeding sites, which are usually found along the duodenocystostomy or duodenal segment.

Late or chronic hematuria may also occur. It is usually due either to a stone or granulation tissue along the duodenal suture line or to the development of cystitis and urethritis from the action of pancreatic enzymes (79). Duodenal ulcerations secondary to cytomegalovirus (CMV) infection are another cause of late hematuria (80). Cystoscopy is required to determine the etiology and often to provide therapy.

The finding of a generalized cystitis and urethritis is particularly troublesome. It is not clear why a few patients develop this severe inflammation from the action of pancreas enzymes when most tolerate these potentially digestive proteins in their bladders without difficulty. The urine should be checked for infection that may have stimulated enzyme activation. Patients should then be treated with prolonged Foley catheter drainage and possibly with somatostatin analogs to reduce pancreatic enzyme secretion. Recurrent or persistent hematuria associated with cystitis can be handled by enteric conversion, as has been necessary in about 5% of patients after pancreas transplantation (42,81,82).

Bladder Leak

Bladder or duodenal segment leaks have been reported in 10% to 20% of bladder-drained pancreas transplants (30,42,83). Early leaks, usually within the first month after transplant, generally occur from the duodenocystostomy or, more commonly, from the distal duodenal staple line. Presenting symptoms include the onset of lower abdominal pain and tenderness, fever, leukocytosis, and hyperamylasemia and elevated creatinine from extravasated urine. The diagnosis can usually be confirmed by cystogram. In cases of a suspected leak with a negative contrast cystogram, a technetium-99 voiding cystourethrogram may be more sensitive (84). Initial treatment of small early leaks may be conservative, with Foley catheter drainage for several weeks. However, large early leaks require direct operative repair or enteric conversion.

Late leaks may be due to ischemia of the duodenal staple line or to ischemic or CMV ulcerations of the duodenal mucosa. Late leaks are generally best treated by enteric conversion, sometimes requiring conversion from a duodenal segment to duodenal button to remove larger ulcerations or ischemic, friable duodenal mucosa. In complicated leaks with sepsis and peritonitis, it may be advisable to defunctionalize or bypass the duodenoenterostomy.

Infection

Infections are common following pancreas transplantation, occurring in 37% to 60% of patients in most large series (11,42). Their occurrence is in part related to the type and intensity of immunosuppression. Urinary tract infections, wound infections (including intra-abdominal abscesses), and CMV infection were common in the multicenter analysis of tacrolimus after pancreas transplantation, although the incidence appears comparable to that of cyclosporine-based triple therapy.

Urinary tract infections are a common infectious complication following pancreas transplantation. There are multiple risk factors, including prolonged Foley catheter drainage to prevent bladder/duodenal leaks, retained foreign bodies such as sutures or staples from the duodenal ends or duodenocystostomy, neurogenic bladder in patients with long-standing diabetes, and proteolytic enzymes secreted from the exocrine pancreas. Urinary tract infections may be particularly serious in bladder-drained pancreatic transplants, because bacterial infection may activate the proteolytic digestive secretions of the pancreas, leading to a prolonged chemical cystitis and urethritis (85). Many centers maintain long-term antibiotic therapy for suppression of urinary tract infections.

Opportunistic infections, particularly CMV, are also common. The incidence depends on the use and type of induction therapy, preoperative serologic status of donor and recipient, number of rejection episodes, and type and intensity of antirejection treatment (11,86). CMV infection of the duodenal segment may lead to bleeding, ulceration, and perforation with urine leak.

Deep wound infections requiring drainage and parenteral antibiotics may also occur, especially in association with pancreatic allografts placed in the retroperitoneum. These infections are particularly serious when they involve fungal organisms. With intraperitoneal placement of the pancreas, the incidence of wound infection has been reduced (30); the development of intra-abdominal abscesses has been reported in 5% of bladder-drained grafts (12). The reported incidence of anastomotic leaks, pancreatic fistula, and intra-abdominal abscesses was initially quite high with enteric drainage, particularly with segmental pancreas grafts. With modification of the technique, particularly a side-to-side duodenoenterostomy using a duodenal segment, the incidence has diminished (46,48). Nonetheless, one preliminary, nonrandomized comparison of enteric and bladder drainage reported a reexploration rate for sepsis of 39% and 30%, respectively (49).

Although the use of better intra-abdominal imaging techniques and percutaneous drainage methods has simplified the management of intra-abdominal abscesses, whether from bladder-drained or enteric-drained grafts, they still represent potentially life-threatening complications that may require removal of a functioning graft for their control.

Pancreatitis

Early hyperamylasemia with or without mild pancreatitis is common in the immediate post-transplant period and is multifactorial. Ischemic injury before retrieval, excessive handling or manipulation of the pancreas, the duration of cold ischemia, and the technique for handling exocrine secretions may all contribute to early post-transplant pancreatitis. Perfusion with Collin's solution is associated with an increased risk of early graft pancreatitis compared to UW solution. Management of pancreatic exocrine secretions by ductal obliteration (87) results in higher levels of hyperamylasemia that are of longer duration than with bladder- or enteric-drained grafts. Factors that have been associated with a reduction in early graft pancreatitis include donor treatment with steroids and recipient treatment with calcium channel blockers (15).

Late allograft pancreatitis is a common complication of bladder-drained pancreases and is usually secondary to reflux of urine into the pancreatic duct (reflux pancreatitis). This may occur as a result of poor emptying of a neurogenic bladder in the formerly diabetic patient. One series of 53 intraperitoneal bladder-drained grafts reported an incidence of 36% (88). The diagnosis is made clinically by the onset of lower abdominal pain and tenderness, hyperamylasemia, the absence of a urine leak, and prompt resolution of symptoms (usually within 24 hours) after Foley catheter drainage of the bladder. A CT scan may show pancreatic edema, but this finding is nonspecific. Treatment consists of Foley catheter drainage until symptoms resolve, and pharmacologic therapy to improve bladder emptying. Enteric conversion of bladder-drained grafts for recurrent reflux pancreatitis is occasionally required (81,82). Pancreatic duct obstruction is an uncommon cause of late allograft pancreatitis, but several unusual cases have been managed with cystoscopic retrograde pancreatography and stent placement (89).

Although less often than with bladder drainage, late pancreatitis may also occur following enteric drainage, with an incidence of 15% reported in a series from Stockholm (90). In a nonrandomized comparison of bladder and enteric drainage, there was a 32% incidence of urinary retention and reflux pancreatitis with bladder drainage and a 5% incidence with enteric drainage (32). Possible explanations include transient obstruction of the pancreatic duct or reflux of enteric contents. As with native pancreatitis, symptoms generally resolve with supportive care. Additional measures may include the use of oral pancreatic extract (Pancrease) to inhibit meal-stimulated allograft exocrine secretions (91) and somatostatin to reduce exocrine secretions.

Metabolic Complications of Bladder Drainage

An important disadvantage of bladder drainage is that it generates large urinary losses of pancreatic secretions containing sodium bicarbonate. This often leads to a hyperchloremic metabolic acidosis with dehydration and orthostatic hypotension. An underlying diabetic gastropathy may impair oral fluid intake, and poor tubular concentrating mechanisms in a simultaneously transplanted kidney may exacerbate a patient's dehydration. In addition, residual diabetic neuropathy accentuates the orthostatic hypotension. As a result, patients may have recurrent episodes requiring hospitalization. Treatment is initially by intravenous fluids and by oral replacement of bicarbonate, sometimes requiring 5 to 10 grams per day. A high-salt diet and Florinef therapy may help to avoid such episodes, but chronic intractable metabolic acidosis may eventually require treatment by enteric conversion. In one series, enteric conversion was used to correct chronic metabolic acidosis in 8 of 265 (3%) bladder-drained grafts (82).

Lymphoproliferative Disorders

Development of post-transplant malignancy, particularly lymphoproliferative disorder (PTLD), is related to the intensity and duration of post-transplant immunosuppression (see Chapter 37). To the extent that the pancreas is more immunogenic than other solid organ allografts and requires additional immunosuppression, the incidence of PTLD may be increased following pancreas transplantation. To date, however, there are no data comparing the incidence of PTLD in pancreas transplant recipients to heart, liver, or kidney transplant alone recipients.

RESULTS OF PANCREAS TRANSPLANTATION

The outcome of pancreas transplantation has changed dramatically over the past 15 years, although the survival of pancreases transplanted alone continues to be substantially worse than for other organs.

Patient and Graft Survival

The 1-year patient survival rate for all pancreas recipients reported to IPTR/UNOS between 1987 and 1995 was 91%, just barely below the survival rate for recipients of cadaveric kidney transplants alone (92). The 1-year graft survival rate during this period was 78% for recipients of SPK transplants compared to about 82% for recipients of cadaveric kidney transplants. Furthermore, several large centers of pancreas transplantation have reported 1-year graft survival rates close to 90%. Thus, SPK transplantation can now be performed with a technical success rate that is essentially equivalent to that for cadaveric kidney transplantation.

In contrast to the results for combined pancreas and kidney transplantation, the results for pancreas transplantation alone have been significantly worse. The 1-year pancreas graft survival rate from 1987 to 1995 was 56% when there was not a kidney transplanted from the same donor. Furthermore, the rejection rate at 1 year was 25% for pancreases transplanted alone compared to a rejection rate of 7% at 1 year for pancreases with a simultaneous kidney (92). Although these data might suggest that the presence of a kidney protects a pancreas from immunologic injury, most investigators believe that the presence of the kidney provides a means of detecting rejection activity early enough to initiate timely immunosuppressive therapy.

Because of the less favorable survival of pancreases transplanted alone, fewer of these transplants are performed compared to combined kidney–pancreas procedures. Considering pancreas transplantation alone before a kidney transplant, the less favorable outcome and the additional need for immunosuppression usually outweigh the benefits of the procedure, except in patients with extraordinarily brittle diabetes. On the other hand, pancreas transplantation alone performed after kidney transplantation does not carry the burden of new immunosuppression except in the immediate postoperative period. Therefore, if the efficacy of new immunosuppressive agents or an improved ability to diagnose early rejection in a solitary pancreas makes it possible to achieve equivalent outcomes for pancreas-alone transplantation, then diabetic patients who have already received kidney transplants might become a large group of suitable candidates for this procedure.

Risks and Costs of the Procedure

As indicated above, combined pancreas–kidney transplantation adds substantial morbidity to that observed after kidney transplantation alone. Reoperation after the initial transplant procedure is more common, especially for drainage of peripancreatic collections. In addition, the length of the initial hospitalization is longer and the readmission rate is higher, on average, after the combined procedure. Overall, therefore, the time to achieve rehabilitation following the combined transplantation is longer than for kidney transplantation alone, and this longer postoperative recovery is associated with additional costs of medical care. Finally, most series of pancreas transplants indicate that a very small percentage of patients die from causes that can be attributed to the pancreas transplant, usually following infectious complications (93).

Exact estimates of the additional risks and costs of a combined kidney–pancreas transplant are difficult to obtain. It is probably reasonable to suggest that the hospital stay is likely to be 50% longer, the reoperation rate may be as high as 20%, the mortality risk is increased by 2% to 3%, and the overall recuperation time is twice that associated with kidney transplantation alone. These rough estimates, however, generally refer to problems during the first 3 months after the combined procedure. Even though the first several months after combined kidney–pancreas transplantation are likely to be more difficult, the eventual outcome is very nearly the same as for kidney transplantation alone.

Glucose Metabolism

Technically successful whole organ pancreas transplantation eliminates the need for insulin therapy and normalizes hemoglobin A1c levels in the recipients without the need for restrictive diabetic diets. This outcome has been documented repeatedly, as shown in Figure 21.6. Thus, patients surviving pancreas transplants can truly say that they used to have diabetes mellitus.

Because the insulin secretion of the donor pancreas is most often drained via the portal vein into the recipient's systemic circulation, glucose homeostasis is not entirely normal after pancreas transplantation. Systemic levels of insulin are higher than normal and fasting blood sugars are sometimes lower, although rarely low enough to cause symptoms. Elevated systemic levels of insulin may have their own undesirable effects on peripheral tissues (see below), and thus one technical variation for pancreas transplantation is to provide venous drainage to the portal circulation. Currently, however, this approach is not widely applied.

Quality of Life

Because pancreas transplantation is so successful in eliminating the requirement for insulin therapy, the procedure greatly improves the quality of life for diabetic recipients. Most transplant recipients regard the success of their procedure favorably, but pancreas recipients—who have generally struggled with insulin therapy for 20 or 30 years—are especially inclined to view their procedure as miraculous. The improvement in the quality of life for these patients has been documented in several studies, although often using quality-of-life instruments aimed specifically at diabetic patients (94). Such studies magnify the benefits for a group of patients who no longer take insulin, but there is little disagreement that pancreas transplantation is one of the most successful non–life-saving operations in achieving patient satisfaction.

Effects on the Secondary Complications of Diabetes

Although there is strong evidence that normalization of blood glucose levels can alter the development and progression of the secondary complications of diabetes, exactly how much benefit can be obtained when pancreas transplantation is performed relatively late in the course of diabetes remains uncertain. Addressing this issue is particularly difficult because kidney transplantation alone tends to improve or stabilize some of the neurologic and retinal abnormalities of diabetic patients. In addition, it is essentially impossible to conduct a prospective, randomized study of kidney–pancreas compared to kidney transplantation alone for diabetic patients with renal failure. Thus, all of the data that have been reported on the course of the secondary complications of diabetes after pancreas transplantation are imperfect.

Neuropathy

Several centers have reported improvement in various indexes of diabetic polyneuropathy following successful pan-

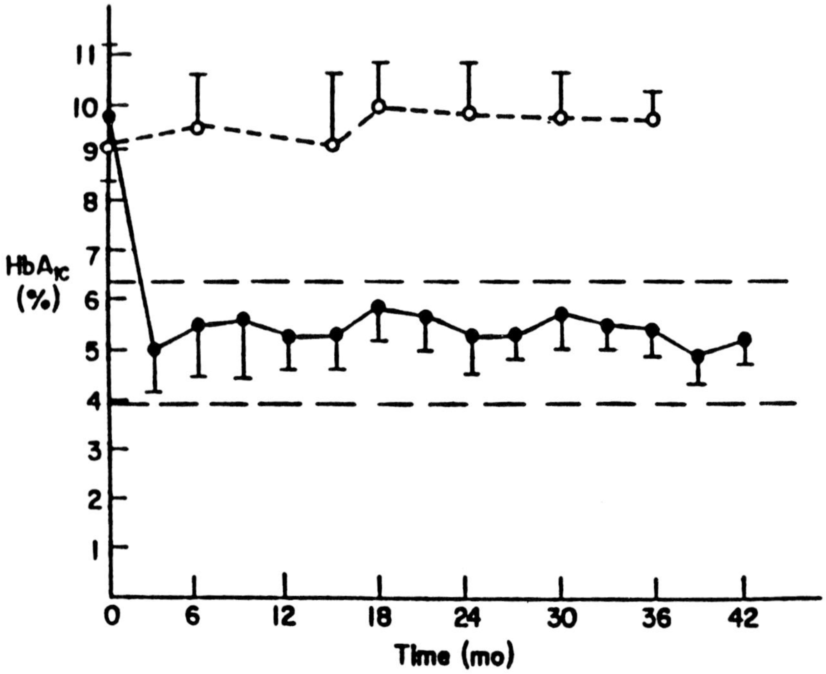

FIGURE 21.6. *Normalization of hemoglobin A1c after pancreas transplantation. The solid line depicts serial values (within normal limits of 4–6.5%) observed in recipients of SPK transplants. The dotted line (open circles) depicts values obtained in diabetic recipients of KA transplants.*

creas transplantation (95–98). For example, in one study of 61 pancreas transplant recipients, 35 of whom were nonuremic and underwent pancreas transplant alone, there was improvement in both motor and sensory indexes at 12 months and in a sensory index at 24 months compared to baseline studies pretransplant (95). In a control group of patients with type 1 diabetes studied with the same protocol, neuropathy worsened after 12 months. Other studies of combined kidney–pancreas recipients compared to kidney-alone recipients showed improved nerve conduction studies and slight improvement in autonomic nervous and gastric function 2 to 4 years after surgery in the pancreas recipients (96). Despite these apparent improvements in neurologic function following pancreas transplantation, the magnitude of the benefit has generally been relatively small, and diabetic neuropathy continues to represent a significant problem for many patients who have undergone pancreas transplantation.

Nephropathy

Diabetic nephropathy recurs in normal kidneys transplanted into diabetic recipients, although clinical manifestations of recurrent disease take many years to develop (99). There is considerable evidence that pancreas transplantation can prevent the development of these diabetic changes. Animal studies indicate that early histologic features of diabetic nephropathy are reversible by normalization of blood sugars (100). Furthermore, in a unique case report, Abouna et al (101) reported that histologic features of diabetic nephropathy resolved when kidneys from a cadaveric donor with long-standing type 1 diabetes were transplanted into nondiabetic recipients. Studies have also shown that biopsies from previously transplanted kidneys showed no progression of glomerular structural changes when subsequent pancreas transplants were performed (102), and that evidence of diabetic nephropathy did not develop in kidneys transplanted along with pancreases as they did in patients who received a kidney transplant alone (103).

Despite these findings, pancreas transplantation cannot reverse the renal failure of patients who are already approaching kidney transplantation. In addition, the clinical relevance of recurrent diabetic nephropathy in transplanted kidneys is very small. A few diabetic recipients of kidney transplants live long enough to manifest recurrent diabetic renal disease, but the majority die with functioning renal allografts, usually from their underlying cardiovascular disease (50,104).

Retinopathy

In contrast to diabetic neuropathy and nephropathy, the largest study to date failed to show improvement in retinopathy following pancreas transplantation (105). In this study, the probability of progression within 3 years in patients with successful pancreas transplants was the same as in those whose grafts failed within 3 months. Most patients in this study already had far advanced retinopathy, suggesting that the benefits of normoglycemia occur primarily in the early stages of secondary complications. A more recent series suggested that at least stabilization of retinopathy might occur following pancreas transplantation (106).

Cardiovascular Disease

Conflicting information is available regarding the impact of pancreas transplantation on the progression of cardiac and peripheral vascular disease. At least one study has demonstrated measurable improvement in cardiac function by echocardiography in pancreas–kidney recipients at 12 months after transplant, whereas stabilization of cardiac function without improvement was found in kidney-alone recipients (107). The degree of improvement in this study was small, however. No controlled data exist comparing the risk of myocardial infarction or long-term cardiac mortality in pancreas–kidney versus kidney-alone recipients.

Several preliminary studies have suggested that improvements in microangiopathy may occur following pancreas transplantation (108,109). Similarly, lipid metabolism appears to be improved following pancreas transplantation (110), but whether this will translate into fewer macrovascular complications and better clinical outcomes remains uncertain. At least one study reported a relatively low incidence of digit amputation, limb amputation, or limb revascularization in a cohort of 50 pancreas–kidney recipients with stable graft function (111). On the other hand, others have found a higher rate of peripheral vascular complications in recipients of combined kidney–pancreas transplants than in those who received kidneys alone (94,112).

Systemic venous drainage of pancreas allografts results in peripheral hyperinsulinemia, which is an independent risk factor for the development of atherosclerosis and coronary artery disease (113,114). Although fasting blood sugars and glycosylated hemoglobin are comparable with the two forms of venous drainage, portal drainage restores the physiologic first-pass degradation of insulin by the liver and results in significantly lower fasting plasma insulin and fasting C-peptide levels (32,115). Whether this approach affects long-term cardiac or peripheral vascular complications remains to be determined.

Secondary Complications of Diabetes—General Conclusions

Although the data on secondary complications are poorly controlled and often difficult to interpret, the overall conclusion at this point is that establishing normoglycemia does have an effect on the secondary complications of diabetes (consistent with the glucose hypothesis), but that the magnitude of this effect is small when these complications are as far advanced as they are in most patients who receive combined kidney and pancreas transplants. It seems likely that recipients of both organs who survive 5 to 10 years after their procedure will have a better prognosis than patients who have received only kidneys, but this benefit may be too late for many diabetic patients.

Outcomes of Pancreas Transplantation—General Conclusions

Overall, the results of pancreas transplantation performed during the past 10 years have shown that the procedure can now be performed with a likelihood of success that is very close to that for kidneys alone and for other solid organs. Furthermore, successful pancreas transplantation almost invariably normalizes blood glucose levels, eliminates the need for insulin therapy, and thereby yields a dramatic improvement in the quality of life for pancreas recipients. These benefits occur at the cost of the moderate risks associated with any form of organ transplantation, including the risks of immunosuppression, and with measurably increased morbidity compared to kidney transplantation alone. When performed in long-term diabetic patients, however, pancreas transplantation has relatively little impact on the secondary complications of diabetes, because these complications are generally too far advanced to be reversed in a clinically relevant way by normalization of blood sugar levels.

ISLET CELL TRANSPLANTATION

The central dilemma in pancreas transplantation today is that because the procedure is technically cumbersome and because it requires the use of long-term immunosuppression, its application must be delayed until late in the course of diabetes. Only when secondary complications have already developed, such as renal failure requiring kidney transplantation, is it generally accepted that pancreas transplantation is justified to stabilize these complications. However, it is unlikely that pancreas transplantation will reverse complications that have already developed at this late stage of the disease. Recognizing this dilemma, many investigators have sought ways to minimize the morbidity of the procedure and to perform it without long-term immunosuppression. For almost all of them, the transplantation of pancreatic islets has appeared to be the most promising approach. The idea of transplanting just the cellular elements needed to produce insulin and of perhaps modifying these cellular transplants so as to avoid the need for long-term immunosuppression has been especially appealing because of the relative ease with which this has been accomplished in small animal models.

Preparation of Islet Cells

Islets of Langerhans are not individual cells in suspension but rather clusters of cells of different character that are organized around a common microvasculature (Fig. 21.7). In addition to their vascular endothelium, islets are composed of β cells, which produce insulin, and alpha (α) cells, which produce other pancreatic hormones such as glucagon. Freshly isolated islets also include lymphohematopoietic cells, which can function as antigen-presenting cells (APCs). Although in theory it might be possible to treat diabetes with pure β-cell transplantation, efforts to accomplish this have generally been less successful than the use of intact islet preparations. Therefore, a key aspect in the preparation of pancreatic islets for transplantation is to separate these structures from the more abundant acinar and stromal tissues of the gland without disrupting the islets themselves.

In rodents, simple disruption of the pancreas with enzymatic digestion and Ficoll density-gradient separation allows the preparation of a relatively crude population of islets, from which it is possible manually to pick out a nearly pure preparation of islets. This approach is adequate in these small animals because only several hundred islets are needed for transplantation.

For larger animals, much larger numbers of islets are required; therefore, automated isolation procedures have been developed. A key step in this process is the infusion of collagenase into the pancreatic duct. However, differences in

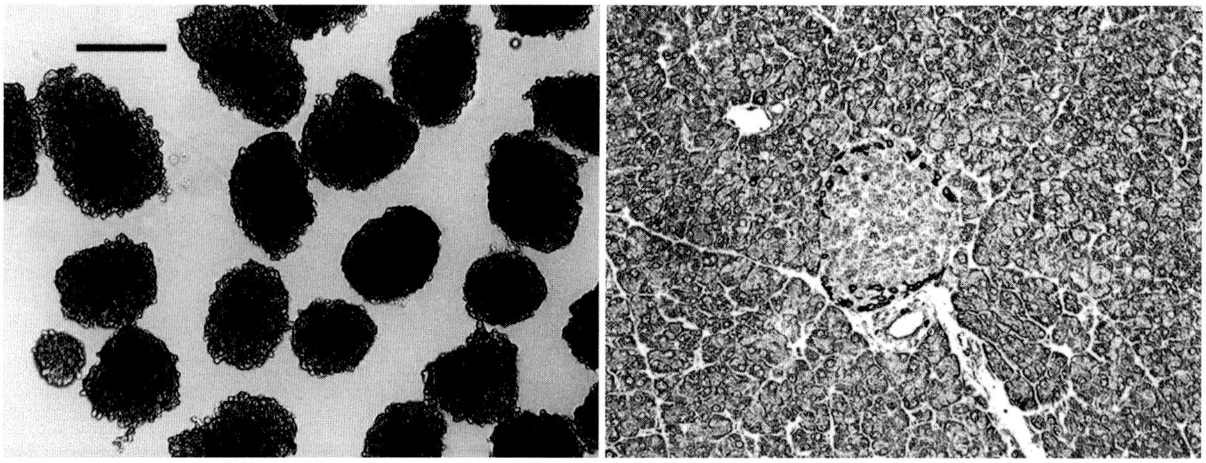

FIGURE 21.7. *Isolated pancreatic islets on the left. Microscopic section on the right emphasizes that each islet is a cluster of cells surrounding a central microvasculature.*

collagenases as well as differences in the amount of fibrosis in different pancreases continue to make islet isolation in larger animals as much an art as a science. Isolation of islets from pigs has been especially difficult, as they tend to disintegrate more easily than in other species. Despite such difficulties, several groups, following the leadership of Lacy and of Riccordi (116,117), can now generate islets from large animals that are functional when transplanted to immunoincompetent mice.

Transplantation of Islets: Experimental Studies

Transplantation of allogeneic and even xenogeneic islets into immunosuppressed mice and rats has been performed successfully for many years (116,118–120). Islets have normalized blood sugar levels when injected intraportally, when placed under the kidney capsule, or when injected intrathymically, and they have functioned appropriately even across species differences.

The mechanisms of rejection of islets have also been studied in small animal experiments. Transplanted islets are not immediately revascularized and, therefore, depend on diffusion for their initial survival. After about a week, revascularization by recipient vessels occurs. For this reason, islets do not appear to be susceptible to the processes of hyperacute rejection. Even after their revascularization, extremely high doses of antibody are required to cause their destruction, and it is currently not clear whether preformed blood group or natural antibodies represent an important immunologic barrier to islet transplantation. Cell-mediated responses, however, do cause islet rejection, involving especially the function of CD4$^+$ lymphocytes (119,121,122). In addition, islets in some species combinations appear to be susceptible to unusual mediators of tissue destruction, including nitric oxide and the function of activated macrophages (123).

Although islet transplantation in small animals is relatively easily accomplished, successful transplantation in larger species has been much harder to achieve. In part this is probably due to the technical difficulty in achieving satisfactory islet preparation in larger animals and to the difficulty in rendering large animals insulin dependent by pancreatic ablation. Successful allogeneic islet transplantation has been reported, however, in dogs, pigs, and monkeys. Xenogeneic islet transplantation has been even harder to accomplish in large animal models, and there has been essentially no long-term function of xenogeneic islets in non-human primates (120,124,125).

Transplantation of Islets: Clinical Efforts

Sporadic clinical attempts at islet transplantation have been made over the past two decades with limited success until very recently. The number of centers performing clinical transplantation for selected recipients is increasing, however, and by 1996 over 300 clinical islet transplants had been reported. Although only a handful of recipients have been rendered insulin independent for more than a year, the percentage of patients who have maintained evidence of insulin secretion based on C-peptide levels has slowly been increasing (Fig. 21.8) (126,127). Based on the analysis of patients with the best outcomes, the International Registry for Islet

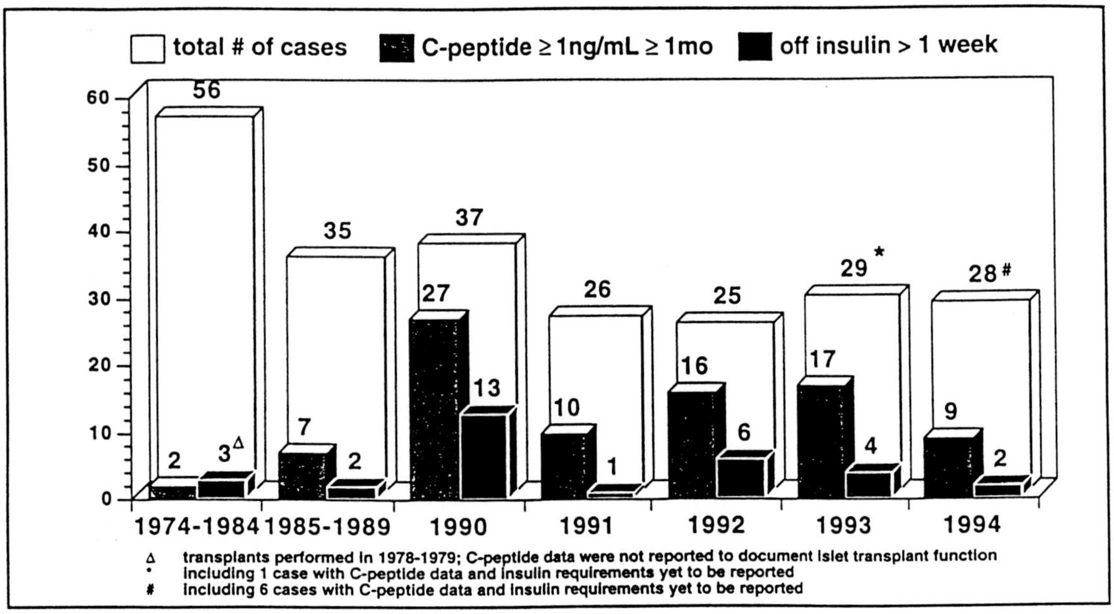

FIGURE 21.8. *Insulin independence and basal C-peptide after adult islet allotransplantation through December 31, 1994. (Reproduced from International Islet Transplant Registry Newsletter. June 1995;5(6).)*

Table 21.3. Recommended "Optimal" Conditions for Islet Transplantation

Islet mass	>8000 IEQ/kg
Islet purity	>50%
Transplant site	Liver via portal vein
Induction immunosuppression	ALG, ATG, or OKT-3
Recipient category	SIK, IAK
Postoperative management	Strict blood glucose control with IV insulin in the early postoperative period

ALG = antilymphocyte globulin; ATG = antithymocyte globulin; SIK = simultaneous islet-kidney transplant; IAK = islet after kidney transplant.

Transplantation has identified a set of features that characterize an "optimal" approach to islet transplantation (Table 21.3).

Most centers have initially maintained recipients of islet transplants on protocols for extremely tight regulation of blood sugars using exogenous insulin in the effort to minimize the stress on the newly transplanted islets. An interesting feature of clinical islet transplantation is that the best success has been achieved in nondiabetic patients undergoing combined islet-plus-liver transplantation following upper abdominal organ exenteration. These results have suggested that preexisting autoimmunity may be an important cause of the rejection of allogeneic islet transplants. On the other hand, if this is true, then it is not clear why whole organ pancreas transplantation has been so successful for diabetic patients with comparable immunosuppressive treatment.

In addition to clinical attempts at allogeneic islet transplantation, a small number of patients have received fetal pig islets at the time of allogeneic kidney transplantation. None of these patients have become insulin independent, but some have continued to show low levels of porcine C-peptide production for months after their xenogeneic transplant (128).

Immunosuppression

The list of "optimal" features for islet transplantation includes the use of anti-T cell monoclonal antibody induction therapy. As is the case for whole organ pancreas transplantation, this treatment is probably useful primarily because it is difficult to detect islet rejection episodes until it is too late to reverse the rejection process. The other standard immunosuppressive drugs have also been used for islet transplantation, although there has been particular concern that steroid therapy causes insulin resistance and that both cyclosporine and tacrolimus are diabetogenic for transplant recipients. These drugs are somewhat toxic to islets when assayed in vitro, but they have been used routinely for whole organ pancreas transplantation with excellent results (129). Therefore, it is hard to blame the poor outcome of clinical islet transplantation thus far on the toxic effects of our standard immunosuppression. Among the newer immunosuppressive drugs being investigated for clinical practice, 15-deoxyspergualin (15-DSG) has been of particular interest for those interested in islet transplantation. Perhaps because its actions include the inhibition of macrophage functions, 15-DSG has been found to lessen the incidence of early nonfunction of islet transplants in some studies.

Immunomodulation

The possibility that islet cell transplants might be more easily manipulated to avoid rejection has been a principle attraction of this variation for pancreas transplantation. One example of this approach has been the culture of islets prior to transplantation in high oxygen concentrations, a technique that causes the destruction of APCs while sparing the β cells. Pancreatic islet transplants were among the early tissues used to test the "passenger leukocyte" concept in transplantation immunology, which suggested that recipient sensitization would not occur in the absence of donor APCs. The outcomes of these experiments were variable, depending partly on the purity of the islet preparation. Ultraviolet (UV) irradiation of islet tissues, which appears to alter the function of APCs, has also been used experimentally to prolong islet survival (130). APC depletion has also contributed to prolonged survival of xenogeneic islet transplants in animal models, but by itself does not appear to be sufficient to allow successful islet transplantation without immunosuppression.

Immunomodulation of islets has also been attempted by treating the tissue with blocking antibodies directed at various co-stimulator molecules involved in T-cell activation and with antibodies designed to "mask" the class I molecules of the donor tissue (131). These strategies have been successful in small animal experiments but have not yet been adequately evaluated in more stringent large animal experiments.

Another approach to immunomodulation for islet transplantation might be to engineer genetically a regulated insulin-producing cell from autologous tissue that could then be transplanted back to a diabetic recipient. It has been possible experimentally to achieve expression of insulin by non-islet cells using gene transfection. However, regulation of insulin secretion to maintain normal glucose homeostasis is a far more challenging prospect, probably involving the transfer of multiple new genes into the target cells. It is, therefore, unlikely that genetic construction of an autologous islet cell will be clinically useful in the near future.

Immunoisolation

Because pancreatic islets can survive on the basis of diffusion, another approach to their transplantation without immunosuppression has been to isolate them from the immune system. Islets have been encapsulated in tiny chambers or in longer hollow fibers for transplantation into the peritoneal cavity, and in larger devices designed for implantation in the recipient's vascular system. In each case, the principle is to separate the islet cells from the recipient by a barrier with pore sizes that allow insulin secretion and glucose entry without allowing entry of lymphocytes or antibodies. This requires permeability that precludes diffusion of proteins greater than about 50 kd in size. The technical challenge for islet encapsulation also requires that the material be biocompatible (thus avoiding a nonspecific inflammatory response that would clog the foreign material) and that the internal environment of the device be capable of supporting islet integrity and survival over long periods of time.

These technical challenges have been met experimentally in many small animal experiments of islet encapsulation. Nonetheless, the effort to increase the scale of the transplantation of encapsulated islets to the level required for human recipients has proven to be an enormous engineering challenge. Large animal experiments have been successful for periods of many months and a small number of clinical trials have been conducted (132,133). In general, however, these efforts have not yet been successful over the long term.

While islet encapsulation can prevent a direct attack by recipient lymphocytes and antibodies, it cannot prevent the escape of small proteins and peptides from the encapsulated tissue. Such foreign molecules can stimulate a recipient's immune response by presentation in association with the MHC molecules of the recipient's APCs. T cells stimulated by this "indirect" pathway may generate the production of cytokines, which can themselves injure the encapsulated islets or be responsible for stimulating macrophages that can cause a fibrotic reaction surrounding the encapsulated transplants. Xenogeneic islet encapsulation has been especially susceptible to destruction by "indirect" effector mechanisms of graft destruction, and in this case even encapsulated islets have often required $CD4^+$ depletion of the recipient to achieve long-term survival (134).

Tolerance Induction

If not by encapsulation, the alternative approach to transplanting islets without immunosuppression is to induce tolerance to the antigens of the islet donor. Tolerance induction is one of the principle goals of all transplantation immunology, but its achievement is particularly important in pancreas transplantation to allow earlier application of the procedure before the secondary complications of diabetes become irreversible. Tolerance induction is discussed in detail in Chapter 5, and the induction of tolerance to islets is just one application of these broader principles.

In small animal studies, tolerance to islets has been accomplished more easily than for many other tissues, partly because it is easier to achieve long-term survival of islets and partly because their survival itself promotes tolerance induction. These findings have suggested that clinical achievement of tolerance induction using islets might be easily accomplished, although this has not turned out to be the case in large animal studies. Nonetheless, the success of the small animal studies demonstrates the enormous potential for pancreas transplantation in the treatment of diabetes.

Biologically, it clearly is possible to overcome the two major barriers to the more universal use of pancreas transplantation: the scope of the transplant procedure itself and the requirement that insulin therapy be replaced with immunosuppressive drugs. Although for more than 20 years the effort to translate the success of animal studies to clinical practice has been frustrating, there is no reason to think that the undertaking cannot someday be accomplished.

CONCLUSION

Technically successful pancreas transplantation took longer to accomplish in clinical practice than was the case for many other organs. However, when whole organ pancreas transplantation is performed in conjunction with kidney transplantation from the same donor, the results are now nearly equivalent to those for kidney transplantation alone. Successful pancreas transplantation eliminates the need for insulin therapy, normalizes hemoglobin A1c levels, and dramatically improves the quality of life for diabetic patients.

On the other hand, as pancreas transplantation is currently performed only after patients have suffered from diabetes for decades, and generally only when they have already manifested severe secondary complications of the disease, pancreas transplantation has had relatively little impact on the expression and progression of these secondary complications. It is generally believed that achieving the full potential benefit of pancreas transplantation will require that the procedure be performed much earlier in the course of the disease, using less technically cumbersome approaches, and without the requirement that life-long immunosuppression be substituted for insulin therapy.

Although islet transplantation would seem to offer the possibility of accomplishing these objectives, the success of small animal islet transplantation has not yet been translated into clinical practice. Even more than for other forms of organ transplantation, the full development of pancreas transplantation as a treatment for diabetes awaits the development of clinical strategies to induce donor-specific tolerance.

COMMENTARY

David E. R. Sutherland

This chapter on pancreas transplantation by Auchincloss and Shaffer reflects the remarkable advances that have occurred in the grafting of this organ since the 1970s, the current good results, the specific difficulties encountered, and the hope that, in the future, endocrine replacement therapy for diabetes can be made simpler by use of isolated islets.

The authors primarily describe the role of simultaneous pancreas and kidney transplantation (SPK) for uremic diabetic patients in whom the complications of diabetes are quite advanced. More emphasis is needed on early pancreas transplantation alone (PTA), with a more critical look at the complications and difficulties of diabetes versus the side effects of immunosuppression.

Auchincloss and Shaffer hope that eventually islet transplantation can be successfully accomplished without the need for chronic immunosuppression. However, except for the encapsulation (immunoisolation) approach, no current protocols unique to cell transplantation can eliminate the need for immunosuppression. The generic solution is tolerance, applicable to all organs including the pancreas. When a protocol will be developed that will truly eliminate the requirement for immunosuppression in humans is uncertain, but it may not be soon. Thus, it is not appropriate to delay the implementation of PTA with the thought that islet transplantation with no need for immunosuppression is just around the corner.

The authors do not really present convincing evidence that the side effects of immunosuppression are any worse than those of diabetes (1). Indeed, even with intensive insulin treatment, euglycemia is not achieved and secondary complications emerge, as documented in the Diabetes Control and Complications Trial (DCCT) to which they refer (2). If immunosuppression can be justified for kidney transplantation to get patients who are otherwise doing well off dialysis, it can be justified to eliminate the need for exogenous insulin in patients in whom the rigors of diabetes management are as onerous as those of dialysis.

What is not emphasized in the chapter is the substantial recent improvement in graft survival for solitary pancreas transplants, both in PTA and in pancreas after kidney (PAK), now at >70% at 1 year (3,4). The improved results of solitary pancreas transplantation primarily reflect a decreased rejection rate, but the technical failure rates have also decreased. The decrease in rejection probably is due to the introduction of the new immunosuppressants, tacrolimus (FK506) and mycophenolate mofetil (CellCept) (5,6). (See also Chapters 9 and 10.)

The number of pancreas transplants reported to the Pancreas Transplant Registry has increased dramatically since the late 1980s. During the mid-1990s, more than 1000 were performed per year, predominately in the United States (see Fig. 21.2). Pancreas graft survival rates (insulin independence) for US cases reported to the Registry during 1994 to 1997 are shown by category in Figure 21C.1. The rejection loss rate calculated by the Registry for technically successful cases (death with a functioning graft not included) are shown in Table 21C.1 (4). For SPK transplants, the pancreas graft loss from rejection at 1 year is now only 2% (from 1987 to 1993 it was 5% to 7% at 1 year, and 10% to 15% at 5 years) (3,4). Even for solitary pancreas transplants the 1-year graft loss from rejection is now ≤15% (from 1987 to 1993 it was 25% to 38%) (3,4). The reduction in rejection rates at 1 year will surely translate into higher long-term function rates, given the low rate of chronic rejection previously shown for pancreas grafts functioning at 5 years (7).

For these reasons, I disagree that PTA should be restricted to the labile diabetic with hypoglycemic

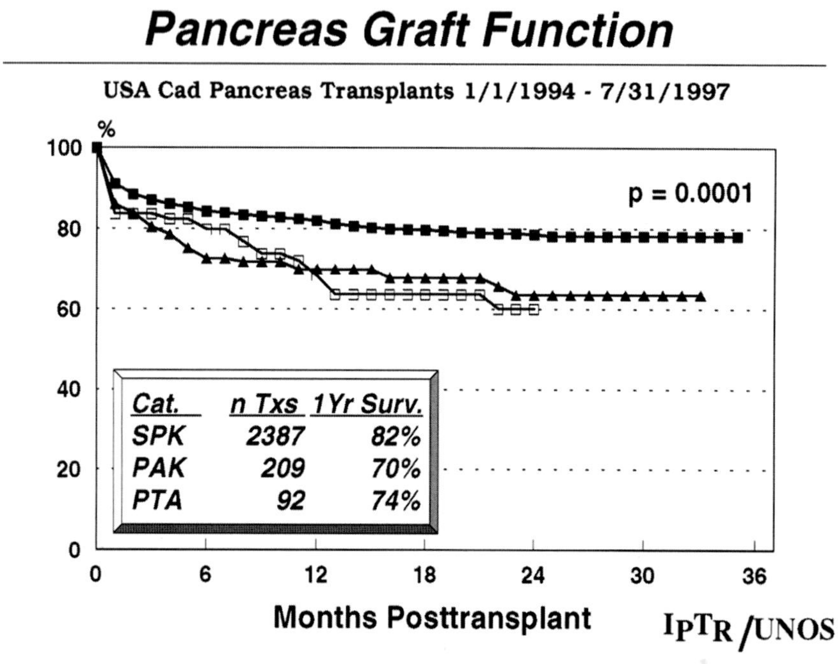

FIGURE 21C.1. *Pancreas graft functional survival rates according to recipient category for US bladder-drained cadaver pancreas transplants from 1994 to 1997. (Reproduced with permission from Gruessner A, Sutherland DER. Pancreas transplantation in the United States and Non-US as reported to the United Network for Organ Sharing (UNOS) and the International Pancreas Transplant Registry (IPTR). In: Cecka JM, Terasaki PI, eds. Clinical transplants 1996. Los Angeles, CA: UCLA Tissue Type Laboratory, 1997:47.)*

Table 21C.1. Pancreas Graft Loss Due to Rejection by Category: 1994 to 1998 Pancreas Transplant Registry Data*

Category (n)	1 Year	2 Years
SPK (2125)	2%	3%
PAK (154)	9%	14%
PTA (66)	15%	18%

* Technically successful cases. Deaths with functioning grafts were censored.

unawareness or other intractable management problems that are not well treated by exogenous insulin. The DCCT trials clearly show that the incidence and severity of secondary complications are reduced by intensive insulin treatment (2). However, it is impossible to achieve constant euglycemia with exogenous insulin; whereas, with a pancreas transplant, constant euglycemia is the norm. Presumably, secondary complications could be completely prevented by a successful pancreas transplant done early. Neuropathy, for example, clearly can improve (8). The mortality risk in advanced neuropathy is high, and it is reduced by successful transplant (9). Recent data on renal biopsies in PTA patients at the University of Minnesota show that, between 5 and 10 years, even established lesions of diabetic nephropathy are reversed (10).

For completeness, it should be noted that although pancreas transplantation is not generally used to replace exocrine function in patients with chronic pancreatitis, this has been reported (11). In patients who underwent total pancreatectomy because of chronic pancreatitis, pancreas transplantation with enteric drainage restored exocrine function, and steatorrhea as well as diabetes was abolished (11).

The authors have noted that no universally accepted solution to the technical problems of pancreas transplantation has been developed, as the bladder- or enteric-drainage and duct-injection techniques have all enjoyed success. Bladder drainage was used in more than 90% of the cases in the United States during the late 1980s and early 1990s; however, enteric drainage has seen a resurgence in popularity for SPK cases because it is physiological, and rejection can nearly always be detected by monitoring of kidney function (12,13). For solitary pancreas transplants, bladder drainage remains the technique of choice so that rejection can be monitored by urine amylase.

RATIONALE FOR PANCREAS TRANSPLANTATION

Auchincloss and Shaffer state that, except in the "rare cases" of exceptionally brittle diabetes, insulin therapy is a safer alternative in both the short and long term. Labile diabetes is not so rare (14,15). Type I diabetes affects nearly 1 million individuals in the United States today, and there are at least 30,000 new cases per year (16). If only 1% of type I diabetic patients become labile, that would be 3000 per year, approximately equivalent to the number of cadaver pancreases that should be available (currently there are 5000 cadaver donors a year). Over the long term, insulin therapy cannot be safer than immunosuppression given the 30% severe complication rate of the major organ systems (eyes, nerves, and kidney) (1). However, the justification for pancreas transplantation is not solely based on ability to prevent secondary complications. Day-to-day quality of life improves with not having to do four finger-sticks and insulin injections every day. Insulin independence per se should be sufficient reason to choose a pancreas transplant (17).

SELECTING CANDIDATES FOR PANCREAS TRANSPLANTATION

The authors state that currently no transplantation centers are willing to offer pancreas transplantation in the early stages of diabetes, but at the University of Minnesota we are willing to offer early treatment (18). We emphasize that it is a choice between long-term diabetes with the risk of secondary complications versus long-term immunosuppression with a different set of risks. In the absence of a randomized trial, it is as rational to choose one route as the other (19).

Nevertheless, currently most recipients of pancreas transplants have had long duration of diabetes. I would agree with the authors that even SPK transplants should be performed before dialysis is necessary whenever possible. We have done several SPK transplants in recipients with a serum creatinine level of 2 mg/dL or even less, particularly when renal symptoms are present in addition to their other ongoing diabetic problems.

As the authors note, SPK transplants pose the dilemma of how to allocate cadaver kidneys equitably. Most organ procurement organizations have policies that give SPK transplants a somewhat higher priority than a kidney alone, but not to the point of using one kidney with the pancreas from every donor. Since most centers currently are doing pancreas transplants in combination with a kidney, this leads to wastage of pancreases. This could be rectified by allocating the excess for solitary pancreas transplants.

On candidate selection, the authors state that for uremic diabetic patients it is reasonable to receive a living donor (LD) kidney transplant, instead of waiting for years on dialysis before receiving both organs from a cadaver donor. A cadaver pancreas can then subsequently be transplanted. The outcome of PAK transplants is now nearly as good as SPK procedures (see Fig. 21C.1). Thus, I would agree with this approach, but would also add the other option of a simultaneous kidney and segmental pancreas transplant from an LD, a procedure we have done in over 20 uremic diabetics at the University of Minnesota (20,21). The patient and renal graft survival rate is 100% in the LD SPK group, and the pancreas graft survival rate is 83% at 1 year.

SELECTING PANCREAS DONORS

In selecting pancreas donors, I would add that donor age has been found in every Registry analysis to be a factor in outcome (3,4). Thus, donors over 45 years old should be particularly scrutinized to make sure that other criteria are favorable before proceeding with a transplant.

SURGICAL PROCEDURES FOR PANCREAS TRANSPLANTATION

Regarding the technique of cadaver donor procurement, the liver dissection does not necessarily need to be performed first. Basically, the liver and pancreas transplant dissection can be done simultaneously.

The authors state that systemic venous drainage of the pancreas allograft results in peripheral hyperinsulinemia, a possible risk factor for atherosclerosis and coronary artery disease. It is not clear that peripheral hyperinsulinemia is an independent risk factor (22). The hyperinsulinemia that occurs de novo, such as in syndrome X or obesity, also includes portal hyperinsulinemia and is always associated with other risk factors such as insulin resistance. Thus, there is no conclusive evidence that simple peripheral hyperinsulinemia caused by systemic venous drainage of the pancreas allograft provides an increased risk factor for atherosclerosis and coronary artery disease. Indeed, uremic diabetic patients who receive an SPK transplant have post-transplant lipid profiles that are more favorable than those who receive a kidney alone (23,24).

It should also be mentioned that a Roux-en-Y intestinal limb for enteric drainage of pancreas grafts may not be routinely necessary. For SPK transplants, the Registry data show little difference in outcome whether or not a Roux-en-Y is constructed (4).

In regard to exocrine drainage, I agree with the authors that with SPK transplants the method of drainage does not matter too much, since isolated rejection of the pancreas is rare (25). For solitary pancreas transplantation, however, bladder drainage is nearly essential, because serum markers are not sensitive enough to detect rejection in more than 50% of the cases. Urinary amylase always declines when pancreas rejection occurs in a bladder-drained graft, even though its specificity is only 50% (26). Thus, a biopsy of the graft should ideally be obtained to confirm rejection before initiating treatment (26).

POSTOPERATIVE MANAGEMENT AND COMPLICATIONS

Today, the postoperative immunosuppressive approaches in many programs include tacrolimus or cyclosporine in combination with mycophenolate mofetil (4,6). At the University of Minnesota we use a combination of tacrolimus and mycophenolate mofetil with prednisone. Beginning at 6 months the prednisone is eliminated in patients who are stable and free of rejection episodes. It should be noted that the rejection episode rate is now more typically in the 20% range using modern immunosuppressants (4). As noted earlier in the SPK recipients, serum creatinine is the most useful marker for kidney rejection, with an increase usually preceding markers of pancreas rejection. However, isolated pancreas rejection does occur in the absence of renal allograft rejection, and thus monitoring of the pancreas is important even in this group. Also noted earlier, with PTA it is essential to monitor exocrine function, and the urine amylase still is the gold standard short of a biopsy (26). The urine amylase decrease is virtually 100% sensitive but has a specificity of only 50%. Serum enzyme monitoring is less sensitive (50%) and no more specific (50%). Using both markers gives the highest likelihood of detecting pancreas allograft rejection episodes early enough for reversal to occur (21).

Although, as the authors suggest, enteric drainage can be done with little penalty for SPK transplants, the Registry data show that there still is a slightly lower graft survival rate for enteric- versus bladder-drained SPK transplants (3,4).

As far as infections are concerned, I would disagree that long-term antibiotic therapy is justified. This can lead to super infection with opportunistic organisms. The risk of opportunistic infections is the same as for all other organs.

Pancreatitis can occur early following ischemic injury or preservation injury. Late pancreatitis, however, generally relates to urinary retention with increased pressure in the pancreatic duct, and is not necessarily the result of reflux. The authors state that pancreatic duct occlusion can result in early graft pancreatitis, but in the Minnesota series, duct injection was associated with the lowest complication rate (27).

RESULTS OF PANCREAS TRANSPLANTATION

Auchincloss and Shaffer correctly point out that the results of pancreas transplantation have improved dramatically over the past 15 years. They refer to an article from 1995 that analyzed the surgeries performed from 1987 to 1994. Two subsequent registry reports confirm this trend (3,4).

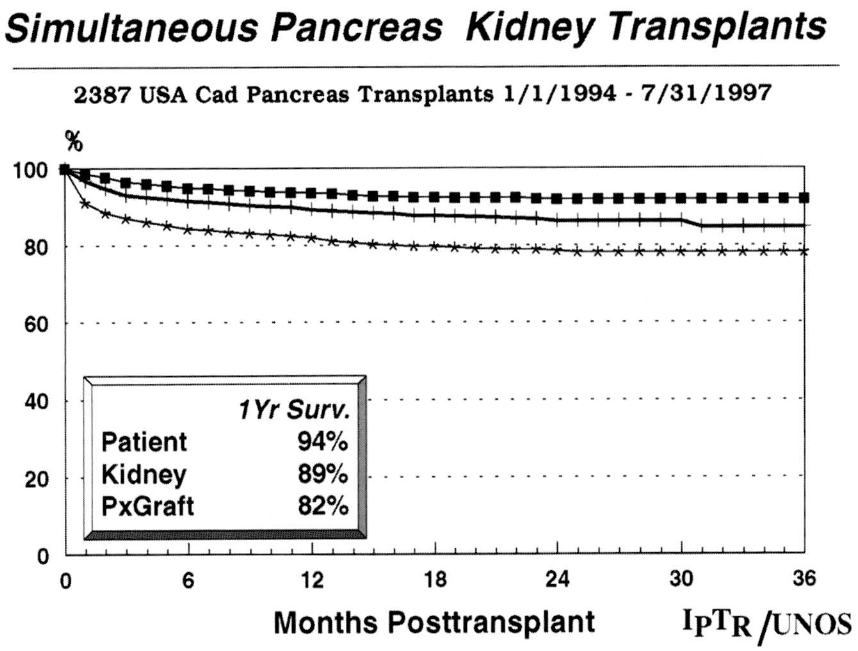

FIGURE 21C.2. *Patient survival rates and kidney and pancreas graft survival rates for US recipients of bladder-drained simultaneous pancreas–kidney (SPK) transplants from cadaver donors reported to UNOS from 1994 to 1997. (Reproduced with permission from Gruessner A, Sutherland DER. Pancreas transplantation in the United States and non-US as reported to the United Network for Organ Sharing (UNOS) and the International Pancreas Transplant Registry (IPTR). In: Cecka JM, Terasaki PI, eds. Clinical transplants 1996. Los Angeles, CA: UCLA Tissue Type Laboratory, 1997:47.)*

There could be some confusion from their reference to the 1-year graft survival rate of 78% for recipients of SPK transplants compared to about 82% for recipients of cadaver KTA. These figures compare the pancreas graft survival rate to the kidney graft survival rate in the KTA patients. Interestingly, the kidney graft survival rate has actually been higher in diabetic recipients of SPK transplants than in diabetic KTA recipients. The 1994 Registry report includes an analysis by era (4). For 1994 to 1996, in SPK (n = 2387), PAK (n = 209), and PTA (n = 92) the patient survival rates were 94%, 95%, and 93%, respectively. The pancreas graft survival rates (see Fig. 21C.1) at 1 year were 82% for SPK, 70% for PAK, and 74% for PTA. The kidney graft survival rate was 89% at 1 year for the SPK group (Fig. 21C.2), which again is slightly above that reported for KTA recipients analyzed during the same time period.

I agree with the authors that PAK transplants should be much more widely applied than they are currently. For patients receiving an LD kidney transplant, a cadaver PAK is the next logical step. As noted above, an SPK with a segmental pancreas from a LD can avoid the need for sequential transplants while retaining the advantage of eliminating the waiting time and reducing the possibility of rejection (20,21).

RISKS AND COSTS OF THE PROCEDURE

The authors state that exact figures on the additional costs and risks of the combined kidney–pancreas transplant are difficult to obtain, but they suggest that the initial hospital stay is about 50% longer. At the University of Minnesota, the mean stay for a SPK transplant is 11 days—only slightly greater than that for our patients receiving a KTA. The increased mortality risk of 2% for an SPK versus a KTA is probably an overestimate. That is not to say that there is not an increased surgical risk from adding a pancreas to the kidney transplant, but there is also a mortality risk of not adding it, particularly in patients who die of complications of hypoglycemic unawareness, a common problem in uremic diabetic patients. Finally, it can be argued that the improved quality of life is worth the extra cost of adding the pancreas, a cost that our society can well afford.

EFFECTS ON SECONDARY COMPLICATIONS OF DIABETES

The authors comment that the impact of pancreas transplantation on secondary complications has been small, because in most recipients the complications were already very advanced. Nevertheless, the effect of pancreas transplantation on diabetic neuropathy has been quite striking (8). In addition, for those with autonomic neuropathy, the patient survival rate is improved with a pancreas transplant as compared to those who do not undergo transplant or have a failed transplant (9).

Although it is clear that a pancreas transplant prevents recurrence of diabetic nephropathy in transplanted kidneys, the real question is what effect a PTA has on native kidneys with early diabetic nephropathy. In a recent study at the University of Minnesota, of 10 patients followed for more than 10 years after a PTA, a reversal of morphologic lesions was seen in serial biopsies (10). The reversal of diabetic nephropathic lesions via PTA is an outcome that has never been shown by any insulin management regimen.

In regard to retinopathy, again most pancreas recipients had preexisting advanced lesions. Patients with a long-term functioning pancreas graft tend to remain stable. It is also clear from the DCCT trial that the better the glucose control, the less likely the progression of retinopathy (2). As pointed out by the authors, there are no studies on the incidence of vascular disease in pancreas transplant recipients. However, at least two studies show that the post-transplant lipid profile is more favorable in diabetic SPK than KTA recipients (23,24).

ISLET CELL TRANSPLANTATION

Auchincloss and Shaffer seem to feel that islet transplantation will ultimately replace pancreas transplantation, perhaps even as a xenograft. Again, there is very little evidence that islet xenografts in large animal models can succeed with our current immunosuppressive regimens. The authors review both the experimental and the clinical islet transplant efforts and acknowledge that the clinical results have been very poor to date. Preexisting autoimmunity could be the cause of rejection of allogenic islet transplants, but then it is not clear why whole pancreas transplants have been so successful. That more work is needed in this area is obvious.

As far as immunosuppression for islet transplants, the authors state that the optimal regimen would include the use of anti–T cell monoclonal antibody induction. However, in the Islet Transplant Registry reports the outcome was better when a polyclonal preparation was used, perhaps because OKT-3 induces a cytokine release that is toxic to β cells. Nevertheless, I agree with the authors that it is hard to blame the poor outcome of clinical islet transplantation on the toxic effects of immunosuppression, as the same drugs have been used routinely for pancreas transplantation.

IMMUNOMODULATION

In their discussion of possible future approaches to avoid rejection, the authors include elimination of antigen-presenting cells. It should be noted that Gores et al (28) showed that complete elimination of antigen-presenting cells was still followed by rejection, and Stock et al (29) have shown that indirect presentation is effective in inducing rejection of islet allografts. It appears that only with certain mouse strain combinations can the depletion of passenger leukocytes be effective. The authors suggest that another approach might be to genetically engineer insulin-producing cells from autologous tissue. It should be cautioned that if one does induce insulin secretion from a non-β cell, the autoantigen response for autoimmunity could still be expressed.

Other approaches, such as encasing the islets in capsules or in macro devices for immunoisolation, have had only limited success in large animals (30) or humans (31).

TOLERANCE INDUCTION

The authors believe that pancreas or islet transplants alone will only be possible when immunosuppression is minimal. If this is the case, then tolerance induction will be necessary. However, tolerance is a generic problem, not one just restricted to islet or pancreas transplants. Until very recently, no regimens to induce tolerance in small animals have been successful in large animals. Hopefully, within a few years, tolerance induction in humans may be applicable to all organs or cells, including the pancreas and islets (see also Chapter 5).

CONCLUSION

I would agree with Auchincloss and Shaffer's conclusion that although pancreas transplants to date have largely been performed in patients with advanced diabetes, the future lies in performing the procedure earlier. However, I would disagree that we must wait for the development of islet transplantation without the need for immunosuppression in order to treat early diabetes. The advances made in pharmacologic immunosuppression are impressive. We should use all the pancreases available for early transplantation in diabetic patients, not only to prevent the secondary complications but also to improve the quality of life imposed on patients by intensive insulin treatment.

CHAPTER REFERENCES

1. Forte DS Jr. Diabetes complications: why is glucose potentially toxic? Science 1996;272:699–700.
2. The Diabetes Control and Complications Trial Research Group. The effect of intensive treatment of diabetes on the development and progression of long-term complications in insulin-dependent diabetes mellitus. N Engl J Med 1993;329:977–986.
3. Reichard P, Nilsson B, Rosenquist U. The effect of long-term intensified insulin treatment on the development of microvascular complications of diabetes mellitus. N Engl J Med 1993;329:304–309.
4. Gruessner RW, Sutherland DE, Najarian JS, et al. Solitary pancreas transplantation for nonuremic patients with labile insulin-dependent diabetes mellitus. Transplantation 1997;64:1572–1577.
5. Kelly WD, Lillehei RC, Merkel FK, et al. Allotransplantation of the pancreas and duodenum along with the kidney in diabetic nephropathy. Surgery 1967;61:827–837.
6. Sollinger HW, Cook K, Kamps D, et al. Clinical and experimental experience with pancreaticocystostomy for exocrine pancreatic drainage in pancreas transplantation. Transplant Proc 1984;16:749–751.
7. Sollinger HW, Stratta RJ, D'Alessandro AM, et al. Experience with simultaneous pancreas-kidney transplantation. Ann Surg 1988;208:475–483.
8. Corry RJ, Nghiem DD, Schulak JA, et al. Surgical treatment of diabetic nephropathy with simultaneous pancreatic duodenal and renal transplantation. Surg Gynecol Obstet 1986;162:547–555.
9. Sollinger HW, Knechtle SJ. The current status of combined kidney-pancreas transplantation. In: Sabiston DC. Textbook of surgery: update 6. Philadelphia: WB Saunders, 1990:83–96.

10. Sutherland DE, Dunn DL, Goetz FC, et al. A 10-year experience with 290 pancreas transplants at a single institution. Ann Surg 1989;210:274–288.
11. Stratta RJ, Taylor RJ, Bynon JS, et al. Surgical treatment of diabetes mellitus with pancreas transplantation. Arm Surg 1994;220:809–817.
12. Sollinger HW, Odorico JS, Knechtle SJ, et al. Experience with 500 simultaneous pancreas-kidney transplants. Ann Surg 1998;228:284–296.
13. Gruessner RWG, Sutherland DER. Simultaneous kidney and segmental pancreas transplants from living related donors—the first two successful cases. Transplantation 1996;61:1265–1268.
14. Sutherland DER, Goetz EC, Najarian JS. Pancreas transplants from related donors. Transplantation 1984;38:625–633.
15. Grewel HP, Garland L, Novak K, et al. Risk factors for postimplantation pancreatitis and pancreatic thrombosis in pancreas transplant recipients. Transplantation 1993;56:609–612.
16. Gores PF, Viste A, Hesse UJ, et al. The influence of donor hyperglycemia and other factors on long-term pancreatic allograft survival. Transplant Proc 1990;22:437–438.
17. Gores PF, Gillingham KJ, Dunn DL, et al. Donor hyperglycemia as a minor risk factor and immunologic variables as major risk factors for pancreas allograft loss in a multivariate analysis of a single institution's experience. Ann Surg 1992;215:217–230.
18. Shaffer D, Madras PN, Sahyoun AI, et al. Cadaver donor hyperglycemia does not impair long-term pancreas allograft survival or function. Transplant Proc 1994;26:439–440.
19. Delmonico FL, Jenkins RL, Auchincloss HJ, et al. Procurement of a whole pancreas and liver from the same cadaveric donor. Surgery 1989;105: 718–723.
20. Sollinger HW, Vernon WB, D'Alessandro AM, et al. Combined liver and pancreas procurement with Belter-UW solution. Surgery 1989;106:685–691.
21. Marsh CL, Perkins JD, Sutherland DER, et al. Combined hepatic and pancreaticoduodenal procurement for transplantation. Surg Gynecol Obstet 1989;168:254–258.
22. Simmons RL, Pinch ME, Ascher NL, Najarian JS. Manual of vascular access, organ donation, and transplantation. New York: Springer-Verlag, 1984.
23. Starzl TE, R. Shapiro R, Simmons RI. Atlas of organ transplantation. New York: Cower Medical, 1992.
24. Stanl TE, Hakala TR, Shaw BW Jr, et al. A flexible procedure for multiple cadaveric organ procurement. Surg Gynecol Obstet 1984;158:223–230.
25. Imagawa DK, Olthoff KM, Yersit H, et al. Rapid en bloc technique for pancreas-liver procurement. Transplantation 1996;61:1605–1609.
26. Wright FH, Wright C, Ames SA, et al. Pancreatic allograft thrombosis: donor and retrieval factors and early postperfusion graft function. Trans Proc 1990;22:439–441.
27. Shaffer D, Lewis WD, Jenkins ML, Monaco AP. Combined liver and whole pancreas procurement in donors with a replaced right hepatic artery. Surg Gynecol Obstet 1992;175:204–207.
28. Tesi RJ, Henry ML, Elkhammas EA, et al. Decreased wound complications of combined kidney-pancreas transplant using intraabdominal pancreas graft placement. Clin Transplant 1990;4:287–291.
29. Rosen CB, Frohnert PP, Velosa JA, et al. Morbidity of pancreas transplantation during cadaveric renal transplantation. Transplantation 1991;51:123–127.
30. Shaffer D, Madras PN, Sahyoun AI, et al. Combined kidney and pancreas transplantation: a 3-year experience. Arch Surg 1992;127:574–578.
31. Kuo PC, Shaffer D, Madras PN, et al. Retroperitoneal renal and intraperitoneal pancreatic transplantation. J Am Cell Surg 1994;179:349–350.
32. Gaber AO, Shokouh-Amiri MH, Hathaway DK, et al. Results of pancreas transplantation with portal venous and enteric drainage. Ann Surg 1995;221:613–624.
33. Gaber AO, Shokouh-Amiri H, Grewel HP, Britt LG. A technique for portal pancreatic transplantation with enteric drainage. Surg Gynecol Obstet 1993;177:417–419.
34. Deierhoi MH, Sollinger HW, Bozdech MJ, Belter FO. Lethal graft-versus-host disease in a recipient of a pancreas-spleen transplant. Transplantation 1986;41:544–545.
35. Gliedman ML, Gold M, Whittaker J, et al. Clinical segmental pancreatic transplantation with ureter-pancreatic duct anastomosis for exocrine drainage. Surgery 1973;74:171–180.
36. Cook K, Sollinger HW, Warner T, et al. Pancreaticocystostomy: an alternative method for exocrine drainage of segmental pancreatic allografts. Transplantation 1983;35:634–636.
37. Tao L, Sutherland DER, Cavallini M, et al. Duct drainage in the bladder for management of exocrine secretions or segmental pancreas grafts in dogs. Surg Forum 1983;24:376–377.
38. Nghiem DD, Corry RJ. Technique of simultaneous renal pancreaticoduodenal transplantation with urinary drainage of pancreatic secretion. Am J Surg 1987;153:405–406.
39. Groth CG, Tyden G, Ostman J. Fifteen years' experience with pancreas transplantation with pancreaticoenterostomy. Diabetes 1989;38(suppl 1):13–15.
40. Pescovitz MD, Dunn DL, Sutherland DER. Use of the circular stapler in construction of the duodenocystostomy for drainage into the bladder in transplants involving the whole pancreas. Surg Gynecol Obstet 1989;169:169–171.
41. D'Alessandro AM, Sollinger HW, Stratta RJ, et al. Comparison between duodenal button and duodenal segment in pancreas transplantation. Transplantation 1989;47:120–122.
42. Sollinger HW, Messing EM, Eckhoff DE, et al. Urological complication in 210 consecutive simultaneous pancreas-kidney transplants with bladder drainage. Ann Surg 1993;218:561–570.
43. Ploeg RJ, Eckhoff DE, D'Alessandro AM, et al. Urological complications and enteric conversion after pancreas transplantation with bladder drainage. Transplant Proc 1994;26:458–459.
44. Prieto M, Sutherland DER, Goett FC, et al. Pancreas transplant results according to the technique of duct management: bladder versus enteric drainage. Surgery 1987;102:680–691.d
45. Gruessner A, Sutherland DER. Pancreas transplants for United States (US) and non-US cases as reported to the International Pancreas Transplant Registry and to the United Network for Organ Sharing. In: Cecka JM, Terasaki PI, eds. Clinical Transplants 1997. Los Angeles: UCLA Tissue Typing Laboratory, 1998:45–59.
46. Tyden G, Tibell A, Brattstrom C, et al. Simplifying the technique for pancreaticoduodenal transplantation with enteric exocrine drainage. Trans Proc 1995;27:3027–3028.
47. Bloom RD, Olivares M, Rehman L, et al. Long-term pancreas allograft outcome in simultaneous pancreas-kidney transplantation: a comparison of enteric and bladder drainage. Transplantation 1997;64:1689–1695.
48. Nymann T, Hathaway DK, Shockouh-Amiri MH, et al. Patterns of acute rejection in portal-enteric versus systemic-bladder pancreas-kidney transplantation. Clin Transplant 1998;12:175–183.
49. Kuo PC, Johnson LB, Schweitter EJ, et al. Simultaneous pancreas-kidney transplantation—a comparison of enteric and bladder drainage of exocrine pancreatic secretion. Transplantation 1997;63:238–243.
50. Shaffer D, Simpson MA, Madras PN, et al. Kidney transplantation in diabetic patients using cyclosporine: five year follow-up. Arch Surg 1995;130: 283–288.
51. Stratta RJ, Taylor RJ, Weide LG, et al. A prospective randomized trial of OKT3 versus ATGAM induction therapy in pancreas transplant recipients. Transplant Proc 1996;28:917–918.
52. Knechtle SJ, Pirsch JD, Groshek M, et al. OKT3 vs ALG induction therapy in combined pancreas-kidney transplantation. Transplant Proc 1991;23:1581–1582.
53. Illner WD, Theodorakis J, Abendroth D, et al. Quadruple-drug induction therapy in combined renal and pancreatic transplantation—OKT3 versus ALG. Transplant Proc 1990;22:1586–1587.
54. European FK506 Multicentre Liver Study Group. 1994. Randomised trial comparing tacrolimus (FK506) and cyclosporin in prevention of liver allograft rejection. Lancet 1994;344:423–428.
55. U.S. Multicenter FK506 Liver Study Group. A comparison of tacrolimus (FK506) and cyclosporine for immunosuppression in liver transplantation. N Engl J Med 1994;331:1110–1115.
56. Shapiro R, Jordan ML, Scantlebury VP, et al. A prospective randomized trial of FK506-based immunosuppression after renal transplantation. Transplantation 1995;59:485–490.
57. Krentz AJ, Dmitrewski J, Mayer D, et al. Postoperative glucose metabolism in liver transplant recipients: a two-year prospective randomized study of cyclosporine versus FK506. Transplantation 1994;57:1666–1669.
58. Shaffer D, Simpson MA, Conway P, et al. Normal pancreas allograft function following simultaneous pancreas-kidney transplantation after rescue therapy with tacrolimus (FK506). Transplantation 1995;59:1063–1066.
59. Hariharan S, Munda R, Cavallo T, et al. Rescue therapy with tacrolimus after combined kidney-pancreas and isolated pancreas transplantation in patients with severe cyclosporine nephrotoxicity. Transplantation 1996;61:1161–1165.
60. Gruessner RWG. Tacrolimus in pancreas transplantation: a multicenter analysis. Clin Transplant 1997;11:299–312.
61. Peddi VR, Kamath S, Munda R, et al. Use of tacrolimus eliminates acute rejection as a major complication following simultaneous kidney and pancreas transplantation. Clin Transplant 1998;12;401–405.

62. European Mycophenolate Mofetil Cooperative Study Group. Placebo-controlled study of mycophenolate mofetil combined with cyclosporin and corticosteroids for prevention of acute rejection. Lancet 1995;345:1321–1325.
63. Sollinger HW for the U.S. Renal Transplant Mycophenolate Mofetil Study Group. Mycophenolate mofetil for the prevention of acute rejection in primary cadaveric renal allograft recipients. Transplantation 1995;60:225–232.
64. Stratta RJ. Immunosuppression in pancreas transplantation: progress, problems, and perspective. Transplant Immunol 1998;6:69–77.
65. Merion RM, Henry ML, Melzer JS, et al. Randomized multicenter open label comparative trial of mycophenolate mofetil versus azathioprine in simultaneous kidney-pancreas transplantation. Transplantation 1998 (in press).
66. Klassen DK, Hoehn-Saric EW, Weir MR, et al. Isolated pancreas rejection in combined kidney pancreas transplantation. Transplantation 1996;61:974–977.
67. Marks WH, Borgstrom A, Sollinger H, Marks C. Serum immunoreactive anodal trypsinogen and urinary amylase as biochemical markers for rejection of clinical whole-organ pancreas allografts having exocrine drainage into the urinary bladder. Transplantation 1990;49:122–125.
68. Perkal M, Marks C, Lorber MI, Marks WH. A three-year experience with serum anodal trypsinogen as a biochemical marker for rejection in pancreatic allografts. Transplantation 1992;53:415–419.
69. Nyberg G, Olausson M, Norden G, et al. Pancreas specific protein (PASP) monitoring in pancreas transplantation. Transplant Proc 1991;23:1604–1605.
70. Radio SJ, Stratta RJ, Taylor RJ, Linder J. The utility of urine cytology in the diagnosis of allograft rejection after combined pancreas-kidney transplantation. Transplantation 1993;55:509–516.
71. Elmer DS, Hughes TA, Hathaway DK, et al. Use of glucose disappearance rates to monitor beta-cell function of pancreas allografts. Transplant Proc 1995;27:2985–2986.
72. Sibley RK, Sutherland DER. Pancreas transplantation: an immunohistologic and histopathologic examination of 100 grafts. Am J Pathol 1987;128:151–170.
73. Lowell JA, Bynon JS, Nelson N, et al. Improved technique for transduodenal pancreas transplant biopsy. Transplantation 1994;57:752–753. Erratum. Transplantation 1994;57:1020–1028.
74. Kuhr CS, Davis CL, Parr D, et al. Use of ultrasound and cystoscopically guided pancreatic allograft biopsies and transabdominal renal allograft biopsies: safety and efficacy in kidney-pancreas transplant recipients. J Urol 1995;153:316–321.
75. Stratta RJ, Taylor RJ, Grune MT, et al. Experience with protocol biopsies after solitary pancreas transplantation. Transplantation 1995;60:1431–1437.
76. Gaber AO, Gaber LW, Shokouh-Amiri MH, Hathaway D. Percutaneous biopsy of pancreas transplantation. Transplantation 1992;54:548–550.
77. Gruessner RWG, Nakhleh R, Tzardis P, et al. Differences in rejection grading after simultaneous pancreas and kidney transplantation in pigs. Transplantation 1993;56:1357–1364. Republished with corrections. Transplantation 1994;57:1021–1028.
78. Douzdjian V, Abecassis MM, Cooper JL, et al. Pancreas transplant salvage after acute venous thrombosis. Transplantation 1993;56:222–223.
79. See WA, Smith JL. Activated proteolytic enzymes in the urine of whole organ pancreas transplant patients with duodenocystostomy. Transplant Proc 1991;23:1615–1616.
80. Stratta RJ, Taylor RJ, Bynon JS, et al. Viral prophylaxis in combined pancreas-kidney transplant recipients. Transplantation 1994;57:506–512.
81. Sollinger HW, Sasaki TM, D'Alessandro AM, et al. Indications for enteric conversion after pancreas transplantation with bladder drainage. Surgery 1992;112:842–846.
82. Stephanian E, Gruessner RW, Brayman KL, et al. Conversion of exocrine secretions from bladder to enteric drainage in recipients of whole pancreaticoduodenal transplants. Ann Surg 1992;216:663–672.
83. Ozaki CF, Stratta RJ, Taylor RJ, et al. Surgical complications in solitary pancreas and combined pancreas-kidney transplantations. Am J Surg 1992;164:546–551.
84. Eckhoff DE, Ploeg RJ, Wilson MA, et al. Efficacy of 99mTc voiding cystourethrogram for detection of duodenal leaks after pancreas transplantation. Transplant Proc 1994;26:462–463.
85. Pirsch JP, Odorico JS, D'Alessandro AM, et al. Posttransplant infection in enteric versus bladder-drained simultaneous pancreas-kidney transplant recipients. Transplantation 1998;66:1746–1750.
86. Patel R, Snydman DR, Rubin RH, et al. Cytomegalovirus prophylaxis in solid organ transplant recipients. Transplantation 1996;61:1279–1289.
87. Dubernard JM, Traeger J, Piatti PM, et al. Report of 54 human segmental pancreatic allografts prepared by duct obstruction with neoprene. Transplant Proc 1985;17:312–314.
88. Stratta RJ, Sollinger HW, Groshek M, et al. Differential diagnosis of hyperamylasemia in pancreas allograft recipients. Transplant Proc 1990;22:675–677.
89. Kuhr CS, Barr D, Healey PJ, et al. Cystoscopic management of pancreatic allograft duct obstruction. Transplant Proc 1995;27:2994–2995.
90. Groth CG. Pancreas transplantation. Philadelphia: WB Saunders, 1988.
91. Garvin PJ, Lindsey L, Aridge DL, et al. Treatment of late allograft pancreatitis with oral pancreatic extract. Transplantation 1991;52:733–735.
92. Sutherland DER, Gruessner A. Pancreas transplantation in the United States as reported to the United Network for Organ Sharing (UNOS) and analyzed by the International Pancreas Transplant Registry. In: Cecka, Terasaki, eds. Clinical Transplants 1995. Los Angeles: UCLA Tissue Typing Laboratory, 1995.
93. Stratta RJ. Mortality after vascularized pancreas transplantation. Surgery 1998;124:823–830.
94. Nathan DM, Fogel H, Norman D, et al. Long-term metabolic and quality of life results with pancreatic/renal transplantation in insulin-dependent diabetes mellitus. Transplantation 1991;52:85–91.
95. Kennedy WR, Navarro X, Goetz FC, et al. Effects of pancreatic transplantation of diabetic neuropathy. N Engl J Med 1990;322:1031–1037.
96. Solders G, Tyden G, Persson A, Groth CG. Improvement of nerve conduction in diabetic neuropathy: a follow-up study 4 years after combined pancreatic and renal transplantation. Diabetes 1992;41:946–951.
97. Hathaway DK, Abell T, Cardoso S, et al. Improvement in autonomic and gastric function following pancreas-kidney versus kidney-alone transplantation and the correlation with quality of life. Transplantation 1994;57:816–822.
98. Van der Vliet JA, Navarro X, Kennedy WR, et al. Long-term follow-up of polyneuropathy in diabetic kidney transplant recipients. Diabetes 1988;37:1247–1252.
99. Mauer SM, Steffes MW, Connett J, et al. The development of lesions in the glomerular basement membrane and mesangium after transplantation of normal kidneys to diabetic patients. Diabetes 1983;32:948–952.
100. Steffes MW, Brown DM, Basgen JM, Mauer SM. Amelioration of mesangial volume and surface alterations following islet transplantation in diabetic rats. Diabetes 1980;29:509–515.
101. Abouna GM, Al-Adnani MS, Kremer GD, et al. Reversal of diabetic nephropathy in human cadaveric kidneys after transplantation into non-diabetic recipients. Lancet 1983;2:1274–1276.
102. Bilous RW, Mauer SM, Sutherland DER, et al. The effects of pancreas transplantation on the glomerular structure of renal allografts in patients with insulin-dependent diabetes. N Engl J Med 1989;321:80–85.
103. Wiczek HE, Jaremko G, Tyden G, Groth CG. Evolution of diabetic nephropathy in kidney grafts: Evidence that a simultaneously transplanted pancreas exerts a protective effect. Transplantation 1995;59:51–57.
104. Najarian JS, Kaufman DB, Fryd DS, et al. Long-term survival following kidney transplantation in 100 type I diabetic patients. Transplantation 1989;47:106–119.
105. Ramsay RC, Goetz FC, Sutherland DER, et al. Progression of diabetic retinopathy after pancreas transplantation for insulin-dependent diabetes mellitus. N Engl J Med 1988;318:208–214.
106. Wang Q, Klein R, Moss SE, et al. The influence of combined kidney-pancreas transplantation on the progression of diabetic retinopathy: a case series. Ophthalmology 1994;101:1071–1076.
107. Gaber AO, el-Gebely S, Sugathan P, et al. Early improvement in cardiac function occurs for pancreas-kidney but not diabetic kidney-alone transplant recipients. Transplantation 1995;59:1105–1112.
108. Abendroth D, Landgraf R, Illner WD, Land W. Evidence for reversibility of diabetic microangiopathy following pancreas transplantation. Transplant Proc 1989;21:2850–2851.
109. Cheung ATW, Perez RV, Basadonna GP, et al. Microangiopathy reversal in successful simultaneous pancreas-kidney transplantation. Transplant Proc 1994;26:493–495.
110. Foger B, Konigsrainer A, Pales G, et al. Effect of pancreas transplantation on lipoprotein lipase, postprandial lipemia, and HDL cholesterol. Transplantation 1994;58:899–904.
111. Bruce DS, Newell KA, Woodie ES, et al. Long term outcome of kidney/pancreas transplant recipients with good graft function at one year. Presented at the 21st Scientific Meeting of the A.S.T.S. May 1995, Chicago, IL.
112. Morrissey PE, Shaffer D, Madras PN, Monaco AP. Progression of peripheral vascular complications after combined kidney-pancreas transplantation in diabetic patients with end-stage renal failure. Transplant Proc 1997;29: 662–663.

113. Despres JP, Lamarche B, Mauriege P, et al. Hyperinsulinemia as an independent risk factor for ischemic heart disease. N Engl J Med 1996;334:952–957.
114. Zavaroni I, Bonora E, Pagliara M, et al. Risk factors for coronary artery disease in healthy persons with hyperinsulinemia and normal glucose tolerance. N Engl J Med 1989;320:702–706.
115. Hughes TA, Gaber AO, Amiri HS, et al. Kidney-pancreas transplantation: the effect of portal versus systemic venous drainage of the pancreas on the lipoprotein composition. Transplantation 1995;60:1406–1412.
116. Ricordi C. Pancreatic islet cell transplantation. Austin, TX: RG Landes, 1992.
117. Hering BJ, Romann D, Clarius A, et al. Bovine islets of Langerhans. Potential source for transplantation? Diabetes 1989;1:206–208.
118. Inverardi L, Ricordi C. Transplantation of pancreas and islets of Langerhans: a review of progress. Immunol Today 1996;17:7–9.
119. Gill RG, Wolf L. Immunobiology of cellular transplantation. Cell Transplant 1995;4:361–370.
120. Satake M, Korsgren O, Ridderstad A, et al. Immunological characteristics of islet cell transplantation in humans and rodents. Immunol Rev 1994;141:191–211.
121. Kaufman DS, Kong CS, Shizuru J, et al. Use of anti-L3T4 and anti 1a treatments for prolongation of xenogeneic islet transplants. Transplantation 1988;46:210–215.
122. Shizuru J, Gregory AK, Chao C, Fathman CG. Islet allograft survival after a single course of treatment of recipient with antibody to L3T4. Science 1987;237:278–280.
123. Stevens RB, Ansite JD, Mills CD, et al. Nitric oxide mediates early dysfunction of rat and mouse islets after transplantation. Transplantation 1996;61:1740–1749.
124. Hamelmann W, Gray DWR, Calms DJ, et al. Immediate destruction of xenogeneic islets in a primate model. Transplantation 1994;58:1109.
125. Steele DJR, Wallstrom A, Bleier KJ, et al. Transplantation of pancreatic islets in diabetic nonhuman primates. Transplant Proc 1994;26:3317–3318.
126. Hering BJ, Browatzki CC, Schultz A, et al. Clinical islet transplantation—registry report, accomplishments in the past and future research needs. Cell Transplant 1993;2:283–305.
127. Alejandro R, Lehmann R, Ricordi C, et al. Long-term function (6 years) of islet allografts in type 1 diabetes. Diabetes 1997;46:1983–1989.
128. Groth CG, Andersson A, Korsgren O, et al. Transplantation of porcine fetal islet-like cell clusters into eight diabetic patients. Transplant Proc 1993;25:970.
129. Sandberg J, Andersson A. Toxicity in vivo of different immunosuppressive drugs in fetal porcine pancreatic islets. Transplantation 1996;61:1211–1215.
130. Hardy MA, Lau H, Weber C, Reemtsma K. Pancreatic islet transplantation: induction of graft acceptance by ultraviolet irradiation of donor tissue. Ann Surg 1984;200:441.
131. Faustman D, Coe C. Prevention of xenograft rejection by masking donor HLA class I antigens. Science 1991;252:1700–1702.
132. Aebischer P, Buchser E, Joseph JM, et al. Transplantation in humans of encapsulated xenogeneic cells without immunosuppression. Transplantation 1994;58:1275–1277.
133. Lanza RP, Beyer AM, Chick WL. Xenogeneic humoral responses to islets transplanted in biohybrid diffusion chambers. Transplantation 1994;57:1371–1375.
134. Weber CJ, Zabinski S, Koschitzky T, et al. The role of CD4+ T cells in the destruction of microencapsulated islet xenografts in mice. Transplantation 1990;49:394–404.

COMMENTARY REFERENCES

1. Krolewski AS, Warram JH, Freire MBS. Epidemiology of late diabetic complications. Endocrine 1996;25:217.
2. DCCT Research Group. Diabetes control and complications trial (DCCT): the effect of intensive diabetes treatment in long term complications in IDDM. N Engl J Med 1993;329:977.
3. Gruessner A, Sutherland DER. Pancreas transplantation in the United States as reported to the United Network for Organ Sharing (UNOS) and the International Pancreas Transplant Registry (IPTR). In: Cecka JM, Terasaki PI, eds. Clinical transplants 1997. Los Angeles, CA: UCLA Tissue Type Laboratory, 1998:45–49.
4. Gruessner A, Sutherland DER. Analysis of United States (US) and non-US pancreas transplants as reported to the International Pancreas Transplant Registry (IPTR) and to the United Network for Organ Sharing (UNOS). In: Cecka JM, Terasaki PI, eds. Clinical transplants. Los Angeles: UCLA Tissue Typing Laboratory, 1998 (in press).
5. Gruessner RWG, Burke GW, Stratta R, et al. A multicenter analysis of the first experience with FK506 for induction and rescue therapy after pancreas transplantation. Transplantation 1996;61:261.
6. Gruessner RWG, Sutherland DER, Drangstveit MD, et al. Use of FK506 in pancreas transplantation. Transplant Int 1996;9:251.
7. Sutherland DER, Gruessner A. Long-term function (>5 years) of pancreas grafts from the International Pancreas Transplant Registry database. Transplant Proc 1995;27:2977.
8. Kennedy WR, Navarro X, Goetz FC, et al. Effects of pancreatic transplantation on diabetic neuropathy. New Engl J Med 1990;322:1031.
9. Navarro X, Kennedy WR, Loewensen RB, Sutherland DER. Influence of pancreas transplantation on cardiorespiratory reflexes, nerve conduction, and mortality in diabetes mellitus. Diabetes 1990;39:802.
10. Fioretto P, Steffes M, Sutherland D, et al. Reversal of lesions of diabetic nephropathy after pancreas transplantation. N Engl J Med 1998;339:69–75.
11. Gruessner RWG, Manivel DC, Dunn DL, Sutherland DER. Pancreaticoduodenal transplantation with enteric drainage following native total pancreatectomy for chronic pancreatitis: a case report. Pancreas 1991;6:479.
12. Gaber AO, Shokouh-Amiri MH, Hathaway DK, et al. Results of pancreas transplantation with portal venous and enteric drainage. Ann Surg 1995;221:613.
13. Bartlett ST, Schweitzer EJ, Johnson LB, et al. Equivalent success of simultaneous pancreas kidney and solitary pancreas transplantation. A prospective trial of tacrolimus immunosuppression with percutaneous biopsy. Ann Surg 1996;224:449.
14. Davidson J, Paterson KR. Insulin-adverse reactions and clinical problems. Toxicol Rev 1996;15:79.
15. Patrick AW, Williams G. Adverse effects of exogenous insulin. Drug Safety 1993;8:427.
16. Harris MI. Classification, diagnostic criteria, and screening for diabetes. In: National Diabetes Data Group, eds. Diabetes in America. Washington, DC: National Institutes of Health, 1995:15.
17. Sutherland DER, Gruessner RWG. Current status of pancreas transplantation for the treatment of type I diabetes mellitus. Clin Diabetes 1997;15:152.
18. Sutherland DER, Gruessner RWG, Moudry-Munns KC, et al. Pancreas transplants alone in nonuremic patients with labile diabetes. Transplant Proc 1994;26:446.
19. Sutherland DER. Present status of pancreas transplantation alone in nonuremic diabetic patients. Transplant Proc 1994;26:379.
20. Sutherland DER, Najarian JS, Gruessner RWG. Living versus cadaver donor pancreas transplants. Transplant Proc 1998;30:2264.
21. Gruessner RWG, Kendall DM, Drangstveit MB, et al. Simultaneous pancreas-kidney transplantation from live donors. Ann Surg 1998, in press.
22. Savage PJ, Saad MF. Insulin and atherosclerosis: villain, accomplice, or innocent bystander? Brit Heart J 1993;69:473.
23. Larsen JL, Stratta RJ, Miller SA, et al. Evidence that fasting hyperproinsulinemia after combined pancreas-kidney transplantation diminishes over time. Transplantation 1993;56:1533.
24. Foger B, Konigsrainer A, Palos G, et al. Effect of pancreas transplantation on lipoprotein lipase, postprandial lipemia, and HDL cholesterol. Transplantation 1994;58:899.
25. Sutherland DER, Gruessner RWG, Moudry-Munns KC, Gruessner A. Discordant graft loss from rejection of organs from the same donor in simultaneous pancreas-kidney recipients. Transplant Proc 1995;27:907.
26. Benedetti E, Najarian JS, Gruessner A, et al. Correlation between cystoscopic biopsy results and hypoamylasuria in bladder-drained pancreas transplants. Surgery 1995;118:864.
27. Sutherland DER, Goetz FC, Elick BA, Najarian JS. Experience with 49 segmental pancreas transplants in 45 diabetic patients. Transplantation 1982;34:330.
28. Gores PF, Sutherland DER, Platt JL, Bach FH. Depletion of donor Ia+ cells before transplantation does not prolong islet allograft survival. J Immunol 1986;137:1482.
29. Stock PG, Ascher NL, Chen S, et al. Evidence for direct and indirect pathways in the generation of the alloimmune response against pancreatic islets. Transplantation 1991;52:704.
30. Soon Shiong P, Feldman E, Nelson R, et al. Long-term reversal of diabetes by the injection of immunoprotected islets. Proc Nat Acad Sci 1993;90:5843.
31. Soon-shiong P, Heintz RE, Merideth N, et al. Insulin independence in a type 1 diabetic patient after encapsulated islet transplantation. Lancet 1994;343:950.

Chapter

22

Intestinal and Multivisceral Transplantation

Farrukh A. Khan   Andreas G. Tzakis

Transplantation of the intestine was conceived and first applied as a life-saving option for patients suffering from intestinal failure by Lillehei (1,2). Starzl first described mass allotransplantation of all intra-abdominal organs in dogs (3,4). In addition to the potential application for patients in need of replacement, the multivisceral procedure was thought to offer an immunologic advantage due to the size and possible immunoprotective effect of the components of the graft, particularly the liver. Though technically successful, the early clinical trials of intestinal transplantation failed due to lack of adequate immunosuppression (5). Nevertheless, attempts continued. Of them at least two resulted in long-term life-supporting graft function and patient survival (6,7). Two recipients of multivisceral grafts also survived a stormy postoperative course only to succumb from tumor recurrence 1 year after transplantation (8) and lymphoproliferative disease 6 months after transplantation (9).

An unequivocally successful transplantation of a combined liver and intestinal graft was reported by Grant in 1989 (10). It was thought that success was due to the combination of cyclosporine-based immunosuppression and the protective effect of the simultaneously transplanted liver. A new era of intestinal transplantation started with the clinical application of tacrolimus (FK506) (see also Chapter 9). For the first time this allowed more extensive clinical trials. At the University of Pittsburgh, 104 intestinal transplants were performed in 98 patients between May 1990 and February 1997. With a mean follow-up of 32 ± 26 months, 48% of the total group survived with grafts in place. Actuarial patient survival at 1 and 5 years was 72% and 48%, respectively. The authors concluded that morbidity and mortality following intestinal transplantation remain high but selected patients (paticularly those under age 18) can be greatly benefited by the procedure (11).

RECIPIENT SELECTION

Intestinal transplantation is indicated for the treatment of chronic intestinal failure—that is, irreversible inability of the intestine to support the nutritional needs of the patient. The causes of intestinal failure include short gut syndrome resulting from resection of the intestine, and functional abnormalities leading to motility or absorption disorders. The incidence of intestinal failure is estimated to be 2 patients per million each year (12).

Total parenteral nutrition (TPN), introduced by Dudrick in 1968 (13), revolutionized the prognosis of patients suffering from intestinal failure, allowing them long-term survival and an acceptable quality of life. Nevertheless, it is expensive (the estimated cost of uncomplicated home TPN is US$100,000–US$200,000 per year) and imposes social and work restrictions that are intolerable to some patients.

In addition, TPN can result in severe, and at times life-threatening, complications such as central vein thrombosis, line sepsis, and progressive liver disease. According to OASIS (Oley ASPEN Information System) registry data, the TPN-related complication rate requiring hospitalization in the long-term clinical outcome group was 2.4 per patient per year (14). Three-year survival was 65% to 80%, with 6.7% of the deaths related to home parenteral nutrition (HPN) complications. In other studies, the overall mortality on HPN has been reported as 18% to 36% over study periods of 4 to 10 years, in part due to complications of TPN or more commonly the underlying disease (15–17).

Currently, intestinal transplantation is recommended for patients who are unable to receive TPN, usually due to depletion of access sites, or for patients who suffer severe complications from TPN and/or their disease.

Children usually suffer from congenital abnormalities such as volvulus gastroschisis, intestinal atresia, and necrotiz-

Table 22.1. Causes of Intestinal Failure

Children	Adults
Volvulus	Thrombotic disorder
Gastroschisis	Crohn's disease
Necrotizing enterocolitis	Intra-abdominal desmoid tumor
Intestinal atresia	Intestinal trauma
Pseudo-obstruction	Intestinal adhesions
Microvillus inclusion disease	Pseudo-obstruction
Intestinal polyposis	Volvulus
Hirschsprung's disease	

Source: Todo S, Reyes J, Furukawa H, et al. Outcome analysis of 71 clinical intestinal transplantations. Ann Surg 1995;222:270–282.

ing enterocolitis (18–20). Common indications in adults are short gut syndrome secondary to thrombotic disorder and trauma, Crohn's disease, and intra-abdominal desmoid tumors secondary to Gardner's syndrome (20–22). Indications for both groups are summarized in Table 22.1.

Contraindications

As with any organ transplantation, uncontrolled sepsis, AIDS, and unresectable malignancies are absolute contraindications to intestinal transplantation. Cardiovascular and respiratory compromise, cerebral edema, and multiorgan failure severely degrade the patient's prognosis.

Pretransplant Medical Evaluation

Patients who are referred for intestinal transplantation almost invariably have an extensive medical file. A detailed history, review of the medical records, and a physical examination will reveal the underlying pathology and extent of the disease. This evaluation will also provide in most cases the necessary information to determine the type of graft needed (see below). Additional pretransplant evaluation is mainly aimed at ascertaining the condition of the vital organs thought to be retainable.

Liver

Preoperatively, it is particularly important to determine whether the liver needs to be replaced due to cholestasis or involvement with other disease. The liver has also been thought by some investigators to confer immunologic tolerance if added to other allografts (see Chapter 5). The mechanism is postulated to be one of enhanced development of microchimerism, as observed with infusion of donor bone marrow cells (23–27).

Association of intestinal and liver disease is very common. TPN-related liver disease is invariably cholestatic; consequently, severe TPN-related liver disease is excluded in the absence of deep jaundice. If TPN-related liver disease is not terminal, it is believed to be reversible with successful intestinal transplantation. Experience is limited to just a few cases, but in the absence of cirrhosis or extensive fibrosis the liver most likely does not need to be replaced.

In addition to TPN-related liver disease, the native liver has to be carefully evaluated for the presence of coexisting pathology, particularly viral hepatitis. The presence of liver disease makes the diagnosis of a deficiency of the natural anticoagulants difficult or impossible to make. In these cases the diagnosis can only be established from the history. Previous records and blood samples as well as a family history of vascular thromboses and thromboembolism contribute to establishing the diagnosis.

The arterial and portal blood supply to the liver can be assessed with Doppler ultrasound or angiography. Thankfully, even in the presence of multiple previous surgeries, the extrahepatic portal vein is typically spared and can be used for the outflow of a solitary intestinal graft. To the contrary, natural anticoagulant deficiencies are frequently associated with vascular compromise. The presence of extensive collateral flow may result in falsely normal ultrasound imaging. Angiography is necessary in these cases for an accurate evaluation.

Kidneys

Evaluation of the kidneys and their function is essential. Kidneys are frequently involved in trauma, particularly if it is severe enough to injure the mesenteric vessels. They are also frequently damaged by nephrotoxic agents, most commonly nephrotoxic antibiotics. Kidney transplantation, if needed, is best performed contemporaneously in order to facilitate the perioperative course. As noted above, transplantation of the other organs, particularly the liver, also may confer an immunologic advantage to the kidney allograft.

Extra-abdominal Organs

Evaluation of the extra-abdominal organs follows the same principles as for other solid organ transplants. The cardiovascular evaluation should include delineation of the central veins with Doppler ultrasound or angiography, as some or most of them are typically clotted following prolonged periods of TPN.

Nutritional Status

The nutritional status of the patient has to be assessed, including possible vitamin and trace element deficiency.

Psychological Status

Of the psychosocial elements, drug dependency needs to be resolutely dealt with before transplantation. Patients with intestinal failure, particularly those with pseudo-obstruction, suffer from persistent abdominal pain and cramps necessitating narcotics to which they often become addicted. Compassion must be balanced with the reality that continued narcotics abuse will impair graft motility, complicate the postoperative course, and threaten the life of the recipient. Withdrawal is a formidable task, and it can only be accomplished with the full cooperation of the patient and family and with input from addiction specialists.

DONOR PROCUREMENT

Selection of the Graft

Although many centers in early trials included the liver with the graft for its possible immunoprotective effect, currently the liver is replaced only if it is irreversibly damaged (see above). Liver replacement is also indicated in the case of natural anticoagulant deficiencies. Transplantation with a phenotypically normal liver will correct the deficiency and prevent future visceral thromboses. The multivisceral graft is reserved for cases in which several intra-abdominal organs must be replaced.

Any donor suitable for liver donation can be evaluated for intestinal donation. The precondition for acceptance is a negative history of intestinal disease. The intestines are carefully inspected at the time of donation.

The donors are usually heart-beating cadavers (28), preferably of identical ABO blood group (29) and of similar or smaller size. Cytomegalovirus (CMV) seropositive donors are excluded because increased morbidity and mortality are associated with their use (see Chapter 15). In an effort to decontaminate the intestine, a mixture of polymyxin, amphotericin, and gentamicin is administered through the nasogastric tube. (The dosage of polymyxin 500,000 U, amphotericin 30 mg, and gentamicin 80 mg is mixed in 60 mL sterile water and given at 15 mL every 6 hours.) Intravenous antibiotics are also administered. Immunomanipulation of the donor is not practiced at this time in most centers.

Surgical Procedure

A midline cruciate incision is performed, extending from the suprasternal notch to the pubis and from flank to flank. Upon entering the abdomen, the surgeon ties and divides the suspensory ligament of the liver. Abnormalities of the arterial anatomy to the liver are assessed. The fundus of the gall bladder is opened, and the gall bladder is flushed with saline.

The intra-abdominal organs are mobilized en bloc (28). If kidneys are not to be included, the mobilization involves the left and right colon, duodenum, pancreas, jejunum, and spleen. The inferior mesenteric artery is divided, and the infrarenal aorta is encircled just above its bifurcation. The inferior vena cava (IVC), left renal vein, and superior mesenteric artery (SMA) are visualized. The sigmoid colon is divided. The esophagus is exposed just above the gastroesophageal junction and transected. The kidneys are carefully preserved with their blood supply and ureters intact. The aorta is cannulated just above its bifurcation and flushed with University of Wisconsin solution after systemic heparinization and proximal clamping of the thoracic or supraceliac portion. Venous decompression is through the suprahepatic cava, which at this point is transected by the cardiac surgeon retrieving the thoracic organs.

Cold slush is used for surface cooling of the graft. After the graft is cooled it is rapidly removed en bloc. The techniques used are similar to those in liver retrieval (see Chapter 19). The origin of the celiac axis and that of the SMA are removed in a common aortic patch. Particular attention is paid to the renal vessels and ureters. Iliac and subclavian vessels and a segment of the thoracic aorta are retrieved because they may be needed as interposition grafts during implantation.

The final preparation of the graft is performed on the back table (Figs. 22.1, 22.2) after a final assessment of the potential recipient's pathology is received from the transplanting team. The liver and other organs are separated as needed following Starzl's cluster principle (Fig. 22.3). According to this concept, all intra-abdominal organs are like a grape cluster. They all hang from a central stem consisting of the SMA, superior mesenteric vein (SMV), celiac axis, and portal vein. Individual clumps can be removed without jeopardizing the integrity of the remaining organs. The three main transplant possibilities based on this concept are the isolated intestinal, combined liver–intestinal, and multivisceral grafts (Figs. 22.4–22.6).

Living-related intestinal transplantation (7,30–32) has been performed on a small number of patients. The procedure is still not standardized. The majority of the trials described transplantation of the distal bowel with caval drainage of the portal vein. Stanford and Cambridge have each reported an intestinal transplantation between identical twins (30,31). The recipients recovered without any need for immunosuppression and without any evidence of rejection. There is a risk of disease in the identical twin donor in cases of congenital disease (33).

HLA Matching/Crossmatching

HLA matching is not a factor unless a perfect match is found (34). A negative lymphocytotoxic crossmatch is desirable, but a positive crossmatch does not necessarily preclude successful transplantation.

RECIPIENT SURGERY

Anesthesia

Chronic dependence on TPN usually means that perioperative placement of peripheral and central lines will be difficult, if not impossible, in the majority of patients. As already mentioned, careful preoperative mapping is helpful. Nevertheless, the anatomy may preclude placement of new central lines. The difficult task of fluid and transfusion management in such cases will depend on clinical observations at the time of surgery.

The use of intraoperative transesophageal echocardiogram (TEE) may be the single most important monitor of the intravascular fluid status. The TEE is helpful intraoperatively

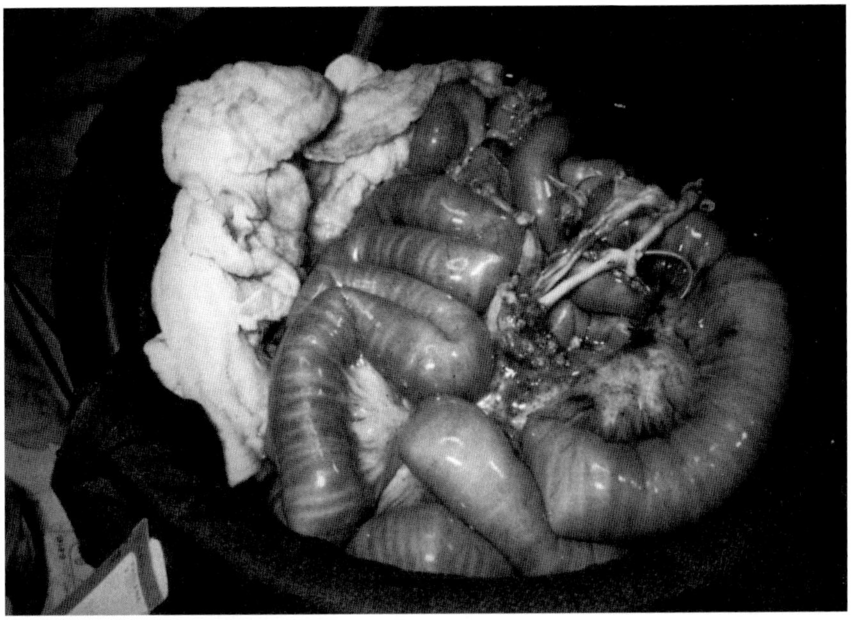

FIGURE 22.1. *Back table procedure. Donor small intestine with vessels.*

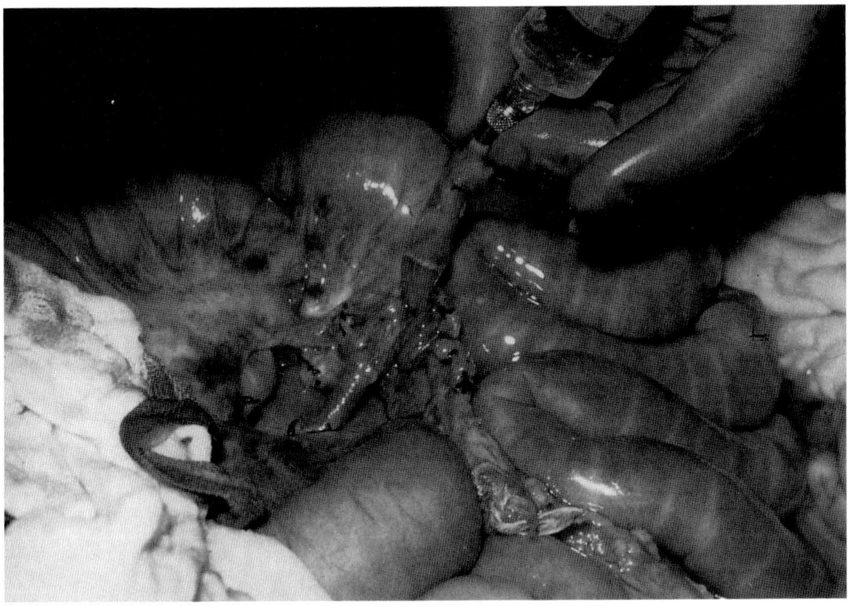

FIGURE 22.2. *Back table procedure. Donor small intestine with venous interposition graft to the superior mesenteric vein.*

to monitor left ventricular preload, ejection fraction, afterload, and contractility. Particularly in the absence of atrial septal wall reversal, TEE has a positive predictive value of 0.97 for a left atrial pressure exceeding 15 mm Hg (35,36).

If the liver is not replaced, the focus of the fluid management is on fluid shifts resulting from the extensive dissection and sequestration of fluids into the intestinal wall and lumen, as well as on replacement of the blood loss.

When transplantation includes the liver, all the additional considerations encountered in liver transplantation must be considered (see Chapter 19). The usual metabolic and physiologic parameters are monitored along with serial ionized calcium, prothrombin time, partial thromboplastin time (PTT), and thromboelastograph (TEG) (37).

The most commonly used anesthetic agent is isoflurane, with the addition of narcotics, sedatives, and atracurium. Some recipients may require large-volume transfusions due to severity of the portal hypertension, portal vein and/or SMV thrombosis, and vascularized adhesions. A rapid infusion system capable of delivering 2 to 3 liters per minute of warm blood needs to be available. The blood bank should be able to provide a large quantity of blood products at very short notice.

Implantation Technique

One of the three previously mentioned techniques—isolated intestinal, combined liver–intestinal, or multivisceral

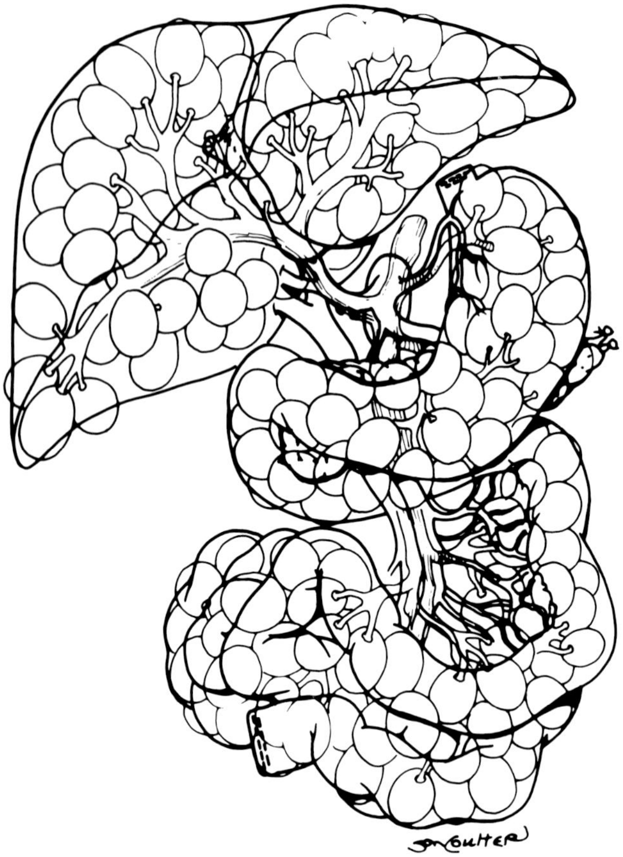

FIGURE 22.3. *Grape cluster. Starzl's principle of bunches of grapes (intra-abdominal organs) on a vine (celiac axis/SMA/SMV).*

transplantation—is usually performed, depending on the extent of pathology of the recipient's intra-abdominal viscera.

General Considerations

The abdominal incision must be carefully planned. Special consideration has to be given to the presence of multiple previous abdominal scars, as well as the location of planned feeding or decompressive stomata. In children, a generous transverse incision will suffice, but in adults a combination of midline and transverse incisions is frequently necessary.

Goals common to all variants are prevention of injury to the organs to be retained and resection of damaged ones without contamination of the peritoneal cavity. Flexibility is key, as unexpected pathology can be encountered at any time. Previous surgery is the rule and the anatomical landmarks need to be identified with care. The recipient vessels to which the new graft will be connected need to be dissected for anastomosis.

Gastrointestinal reconstruction follows general surgical principles and methods. Two-layer visceral anastomoses are preferred by most teams. Proximal and distal continuity is usually established to the remaining native jejunum and colon, respectively. Anatomical end-to-end anastomosis is preferred because it is thought to facilitate transmission of the peristaltic waves between the native and transplanted viscera. Frequently, discrepancies in size preclude the safe construction of such anastomoses, and instead the stumps are closed and continuity is established by a side-to-side anastomosis (functional end-to-end anastomosis).

The use of the graft colon is controversial (38,39). It has been suggested that inclusion of the colon in the graft degrades patient and graft survival. It has been shown that the absence of the ileocecal valve and colon precipitate water and electrolyte loss from the GI tract. Until more data are collected, inclusion of the colon should be individualized.

Access to the transplanted graft for feeding and decompression is essential. Proximally this is accomplished with a gastrostomy, a jejunostomy, or a combination, depending on the anatomy present (40,41). If safe construction of such access is not possible, then securely placed nasogastric and feeding nasojejunal tubes are necessary.

The distal end of the graft is exteriorized as an end stoma or as a Bishop-Koop–type ileostomy in order to decompress the graft and provide easy access for biopsies. These stomata are temporary except when the rectum has been already sacrificed. The transplanted intestine can be used for a pull-through procedure if indicated (42). Stomata are constructed so that later closure can be accomplished using an extraperitoneal approach. Entering the peritoneum and dissecting the viscera after intestinal transplantation can be a daunting task.

Abdominal closure is difficult because in the majority of cases there is insufficient space for the graft. Relaxing incisions and mobilization of flaps are frequently necessary. In some patients the skin may be the only layer available for closure of part of the incision. The use of prosthetic materials is not desirable because of the risk of infection, but it may be necessary.

Graft or native cholecystectomy and native and graft appendectomy are recommended to avoid future complications.

Isolated Intestinal Transplant

Arterialization of the graft is from the recipient's infrarenal aorta via side-to-end anastomosis to the donor SMA (see Fig. 22.4). The graft portal vein or SMV can be anastomosed either to the recipient's inferior vena cava or to the portal system. In the absence of IVC thrombosis, anastomosis to the IVC is technically easier. Anastomosis to the portal system provides hepatopetal flow and is more physiologic; however, it is technically more demanding if there have been previous surgical procedures involving the mesentery. It can be accomplished by an end-to-end anastomosis of the donor to the recipient SMV. End-to-side anastomosis of the donor SMV to the native extrahepatic portal vein, with or without the use of an interposition cadaveric vein graft, has been described as a practical alternative (43,44). The portal hilum is usually spared during intestinal resections, leaving the extrahepatic portal vein as a dependable outflow site even in small children.

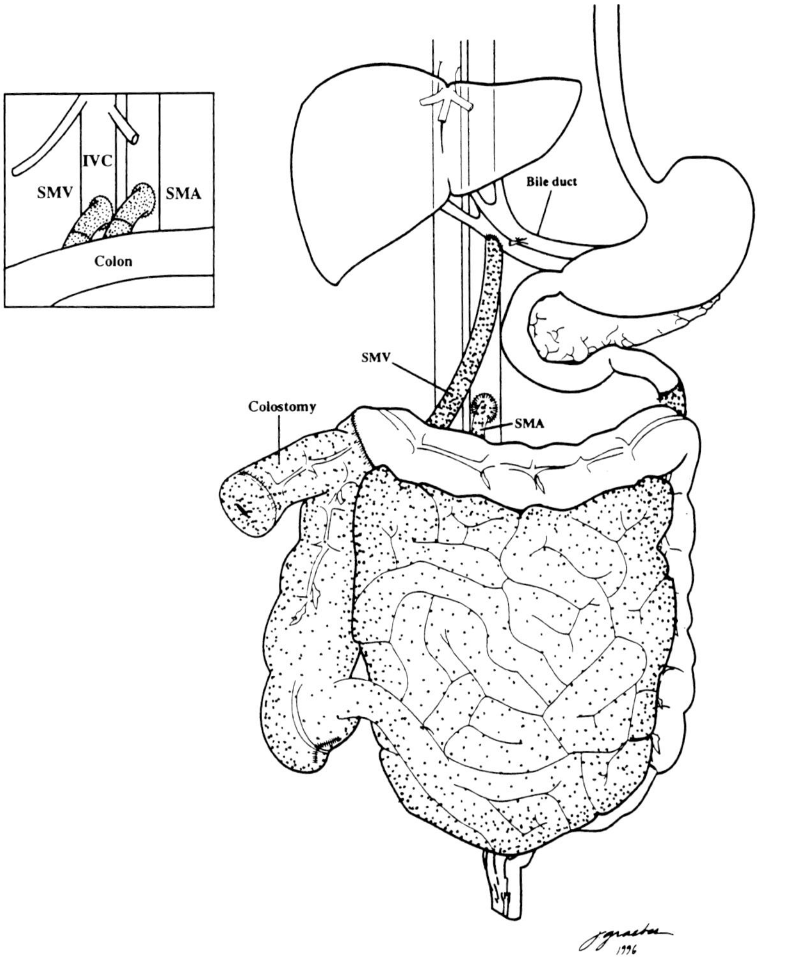

FIGURE 22.4. *Isolated intestinal transplant with SMV draining into recipient portal vein (transplanted organs are shaded). The inset shows the SMV draining into the IVC with an extension graft and the SMA anastomosed to the aorta.*

The extrahepatic portal vein is exposed by a complete Kocher maneuver of the duodenum (Fig. 22.7). An end-to-side anastomosis of the donor portal vein or SMV, with or without an interposition iliac vein graft, is performed (see Fig. 22.4). If an ectopic right hepatic artery from the SMA is encountered, the exposure takes place between the common bile duct and the ectopic artery.

Combined Liver–Intestine Transplantation

The native hepatectomy is usually performed with preservation of the native IVC. The native portal vein is anastomosed end to side to the native IVC to provide decompression of the retained viscera. This anastomosis can be taken down after the graft is implanted, and the native portal vein can then be anastomosed end to side onto the donor portal vein or end to end to the donor splenic vein (see Fig. 22.5). More commonly, this portocaval shunt is left in place permanently (see Fig. 22.5, inset) (45–47).

The duodenum is mobilized and the recipient's infrarenal aorta is exposed for arterialization of the graft. A short interposition arterial graft, usually a segment of donor thoracic aorta, is placed end to side onto the infrarenal aorta to facilitate the arterialization of the graft. Exposure is excellent at this time for the aortic anastomosis, but it becomes more difficult later because of the presence of the graft. Arterialization of the graft is achieved by anastomosis of the donor celiac artery and SMA with a common Carrel patch to the distal end of the arterial interposition graft (see Figure 22.5, inset).

The outflow of the graft is usually provided by anastomosis of the suprahepatic IVC of the graft to the joined ostia of the native suprahepatic veins, as described in liver piggyback transplantation (see Chapter 19).

Biliary reconstruction is usually performed by a Roux-en-Y choledochojejunostomy constructed with donor jejunum. Although intact, the distal native bile duct is displaced together with the mobilized duodenum. Consequently, anastomosis to the donor duct could result in obstruction from kinking. Because the biliary reconstruction in very small recipients is tedious, Langnas has suggested a near total pancreatectomy of the donor pancreas and retention of the intact bile duct for biliary drainage (48).

Multivisceral Transplantation

The first objective of the resection is to disconnect the visceral blood supply early in the dissection to avoid unnecessary bleeding. Various approaches can be used (38–47).

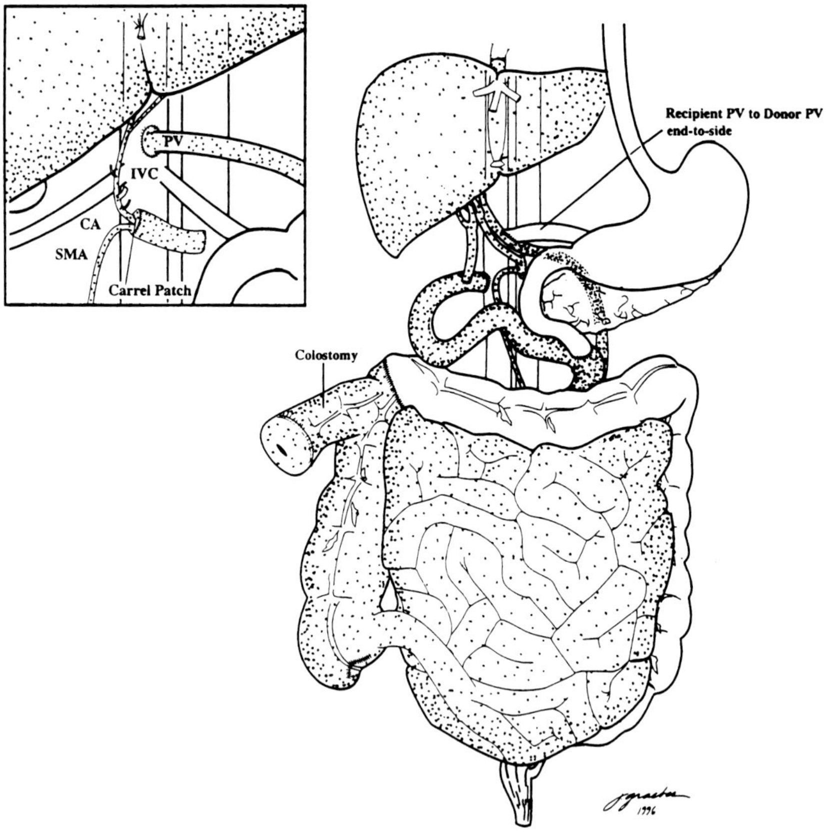

FIGURE 22.5. *Combined liver–small bowel transplant (transplanted organs are shaded). The inset shows an interposed extension graft to the recipient aorta, with native portal vein (PV) to IVC end-to-side drainage of the retained recipient viscera.*

When the lower abdomen is frozen, transection of the esophagus at the esophagogastric junction facilitates exposure of the celiac axis and SMA and early disconnection.

At times, particularly when there is complete occlusion of all portal tributaries following multiple previous surgeries, early control of the arterial inflow may be impossible. In these cases, after the patient is anesthetized he or she can be transported to the interventional radiology suite where the celiac axis and the superior and inferior mesenteric arteries are radiographically embolized and occluded. The patient is then returned to the operating theater for laparotomy and resection.

All intra-abdominal organs are removed. The retroperitoneal structures (kidneys, ureters, bladder, aorta, IVC, and iliac vessels) are carefully preserved as well as the distal esophageal and colonic stumps. Arterial inflow to the graft is with an interposition graft to the recipient suprarenal or, more commonly, infrarenal aorta. The venous outflow is to the joined ostia of the native suprahepatic veins. A Mikulicz pyloroplasty is routinely performed. The donor esophagogastric junction is oversewn. The esophago(native) gastro(graft)stomy is performed in two layers to the dome of the stomach. No biliary reconstruction is necessary (see Fig. 22.6).

Multivisceral and "domino" liver transplantation (49) has been performed once. Although the liver of the recipient was normal, it was removed, preserved, and transplanted into another patient. The first recipient received a multivisceral graft. By leaving the multivisceral graft intact, vascular anastomoses between size-discrepant vessels as well as the biliary anastomosis were avoided. It was hoped that the liver would provide an immunologic advantage to the recipient of the multivisceral graft. Unfortunately, that patient died due to severe rejection of the intestine. In the recipient of the "domino" liver graft, normal function and uneventful recovery were observed.

IMMUNOSUPPRESSION

The immunosuppressive regimens in isolated intestinal, combined liver–intestinal, and multivisceral transplantation are similar. Although cyclosporine (CsA)-based immunosuppression is still used in some centers, it appears that tacrolimus (FK506)-based immunosuppression is more potent and is the current regimen of choice (see Chapter 9).

Tacrolimus is administered intravenously until intestinal function is established. It is then gradually replaced by the enteral preparation, with the aim of achieving a 12-hour trough whole-blood level of 15–20 ng/mL. Absorption through a well-functioning intestinal graft is similar to that in the native intestine (50,51). The initial doses administered

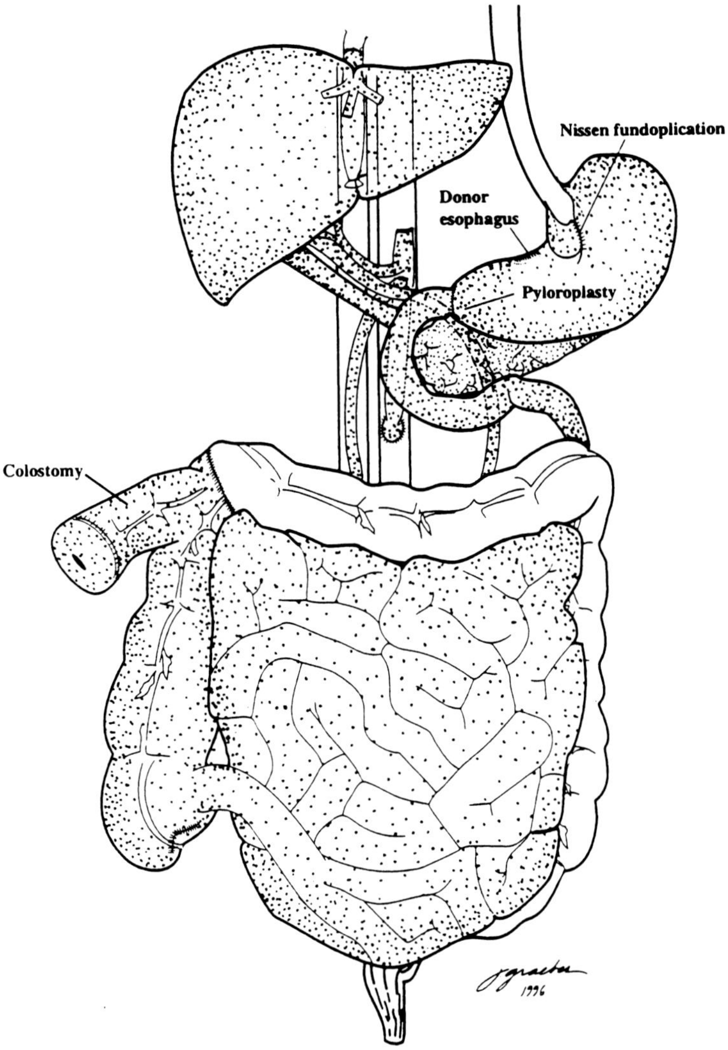

FIGURE 22.6. *Multivisceral transplant (transplanted organs are shaded).*

are 0.02–0.03 mg/kg/day for the intravenous preparation, or 0.05–0.10 mg/kg/day orally.

In addition to aiming at the desired blood levels, the tacrolimus dose is also increased in the presence of rejection or decreased in the presence of toxicity, most commonly nephrotoxicity or neurotoxicity.

Steroids

Typically, a bolus (1 gram) of intravenous methylprednisolone (Solu-Medrol) is given to adult patients after revascularization of the graft, followed by 200 mg/day in 4 divided doses tapered over 5 days to 20 mg/day as a single dose. Children smaller than 10 kg receive a bolus of hydrocortisone (1 gram) and prednisolone (100 mg) on the first postoperative day. The dose is tapered to 10 mg per day over 5 days.

Supplemental immunosuppression with azathioprine or cyclophosphamide has been used. Presently under testing is the addition of mycophenolate mofetil, at 1 gram enterally twice a day for adults, or 25 mg/kg/day in two divided doses in children.

Bone Marrow Infusion

Unmodified bone marrow infusions from the same donor are given in some centers, including those in Pittsburgh (11) and Miami (23) in an attempt to enhance chimerism and induce tolerance. Bone marrow cells are isolated from the vertebral bodies of the same cadaveric donor. At the University of Miami, 10×10^8 cells/kg equally divided in two or five infusions are given postoperatively.

POST-TRANSPLANT CARE

Immediate Postoperative Management

The patient is likely to require large volume fluid replacement during the first postoperative day because of

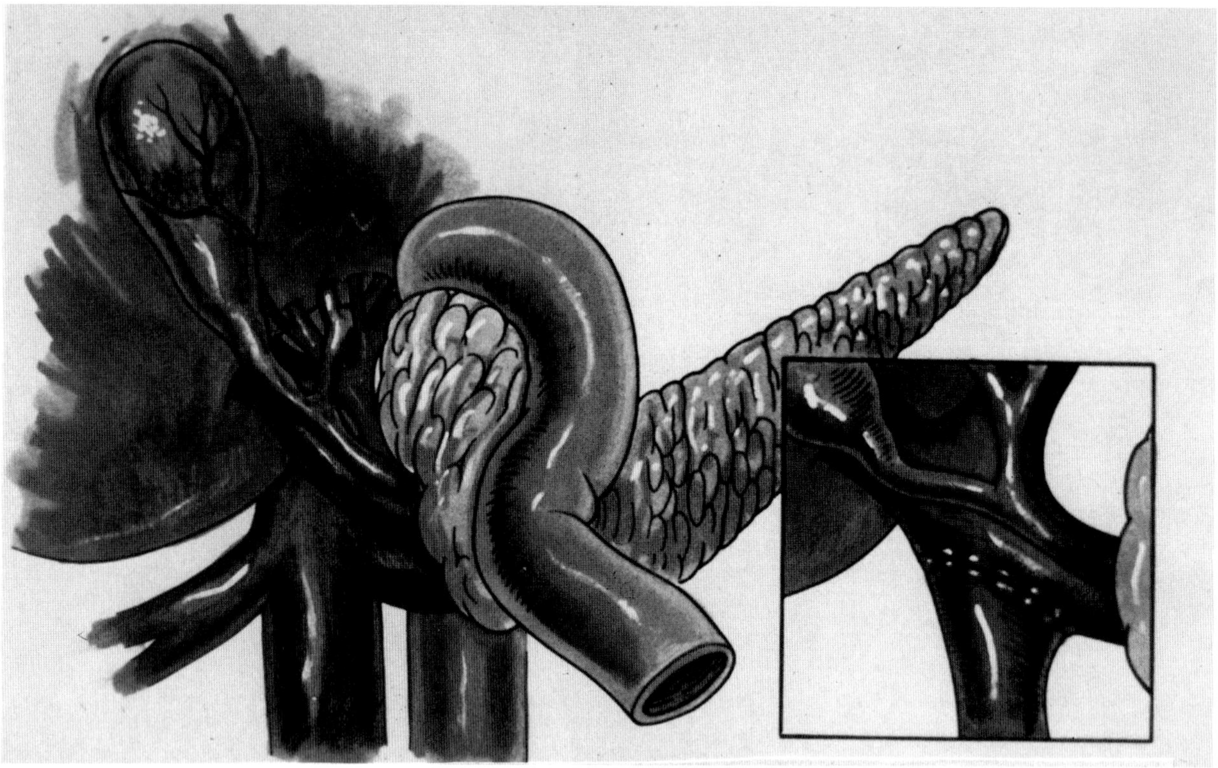

FIGURE 22.7. *Isolated intestinal transplant. The recipient duodenum has undergone an extensive Kocher maneuver. The portal vein and infrarenal aorta are exposed. The common bile duct and hepatic artery are identified. The inset shows the end-to-side anastomosis of donor portal vein or SMV to recipient portal vein. (Reproduced with permission from Tzakis AG, Todo S, Reyes J, et al. Piggyback orthotopic intestinal transplantation. Surg Gynecol Obstet 1993;176:297–298.)*

sequestration in the intestinal wall and lumen. This fluid is expected to be mobilized during the subsequent postoperative days. Gastric decompression is continued until gastric emptying is normal, at which time the patient is started on an oral diet. CMV, antifungal, and *Pneumocystis* prophylaxis as well as H_2-blockers are used routinely.

Nutrition

The TPN is continued postoperatively, and the enteral feeds are started as soon as intestinal function resumes and anastomotic integrity is established. The enteral feeds are started in the form of an elemental diet through a jejunostomy feeding tube and increased as tolerated. The TPN continues until the patient is able to satisfy nutritional needs with adequate oral or enteral feeds. The requirement is 1.5 grams protein/kg/day and 30–35 kcal/kg/day for adults, and up to 100 kcal/kg in children. Prokinetic agents or opiates and pectin–kaolin mixtures are used as needed (44).

Intestinal function is assessed clinically. Additional assessment of absorption is performed with D-xylose absorption studies (52) and serum concentrations of plasma proteins, albumin, prealbumin, vitamins, minerals, and trace elements. Acceptable tacrolimus levels are a "poor man's test" of satisfactory intestinal function.

COMPLICATIONS

Rejection

Rejection of the intestinal graft is the most common complication of intestinal and multivisceral transplantation. Virtually all recipients experience at least one episode of rejection using currently available immunosuppressive regimens. Rejection is suspected from clinical findings, and is confirmed by endoscopy and histopathology (53,54). Attempts to identify other markers of rejection, such as changes in mucosal enzyme activity, have not proved useful (55).

Clinical manifestations depend on the severity. Mild rejection presents with fever, abdominal distension, and increased or (more commonly) decreased stomal output. Severe rejection may be associated with mucosal sloughing, complete cessation of motility, and bloody discharge from the stoma. Bacterial translocation with positive blood cultures from intestinal bacteria, metabolic acidosis, respiratory distress, and septic shock can all be signs of severe rejection. Inspection of the stoma may reveal edema, redness, congestion, duskiness, and friability. In severe cases there may be ulceration, bleeding, or sloughing (33). Examination of the stoma may be misleading because rejection may involve another segment of the graft.

Endoscopy is usually performed through the stoma (colonoscopy and/or ileoscopy) (53,54). Alternatively, upper endoscopy can provide access to the stomach, duodenum, and jejunum. Common findings in rejection are mucosal edema, erythema, pseudomembrane formation, and ulceration. The mucosa may appear hyperemic, ischemic, or even necrotic, depending on the severity of rejection. There is an associated loss of fine mucosal pattern and a decrease or loss of peristalsis.

Rejection can be segmental and may be missed even by a complete endoscopy. In addition, viral infections (particularly CMV) may have exactly the same clinical and endoscopic presentation as rejection.

Pathology

In mild to moderate rejection, the biopsy reveals a mixed mononuclear infiltrate, villus blunting, cryptitis, epithelial cell necrosis, mucus, and Paneth cell depletion. Loss of mucosal pattern, hemorrhage, and sloughing can be observed in severe rejection (56,57).

Treatment

Augmentation of maintenance tacrolimus and steroid doses usually suffices for the treatment of mild rejection. Steroid boluses and OKT-3 are reserved for the treatment of moderate or severe rejection. Monitoring of the response with clinical and endoscopic observations helps to guide the treatment.

Graft-Versus-Host Disease

Graft-versus-host disease (GVHD) after isolated intestinal transplantation has been observed rarely. Transient episodes of skin rash and fevers have also been observed, which may be manifestations of GVHD. Documentation has been difficult because the histopathology of the skin has been equivocal and hard to interpret. Associated chimeric levels have varied widely. Development of technology such as in situ polymerase chain reaction (PCR) may facilitate the diagnosis in the future. Subclinical or aborted GVHD may occur more often than is diagnosed. It is clear, however, that GVHD after intestinal transplantation is not as major a problem as was once feared (53).

Other Complications

Other complications include surgical/technical complications such as hemorrhage, thrombosis, and intestinal and biliary leaks. These complications, perhaps manageable under different circumstances, usually initiate a cascade of events that inevitably lead to fatality in intestinal transplant recipients. The importance of technical perfection cannot be overemphasized. Nevertheless, infections—bacterial, fungal, or viral—commonly occur, independent of technical imperfections.

The intestine is populated with a variety of pathogens contained by the mucosal barrier. Once the barrier is damaged by ischemia, rejection, or enteritis, the bacteria translocate into the bloodstream. In the case of translocation associated with rejection, treatment with augmented immunosuppression may be necessary. This may help control the infection even though it carries the inherent risk of dissemination.

Prevention includes selective donor intestinal decontamination, as noted above. Quantitative stool cultures are performed frequently during the postoperative period. If organisms are cultured in concentrations greater than 10^6, the antibiotics are modified to control these organisms. Failure to do so typically results in translocation.

Central venous catheters are another common source of infection. These are serious infections that could be preventable. Treatment with appropriate antibiotics may suffice. Replacement of the line is not a trivial undertaking, but it may be necessary, particularly in the case of fungemia (11). Viral infections also can be the result of overimmunosuppression. Epstein-Barr virus (EBV)–related lymphoproliferative disease has affected up to 30% of recipients (58,59).

CMV infections are a major cause of morbidity in intestinal recipients (60). CMV-positive donors are particularly dangerous. The intestinal graft is considered to be a huge depository because of the lymphotropic nature of the virus. Current antiviral agents have been unable to control invasive CMV disease, particularly CMV enteritis after intestinal transplantation (11).

OUTPATIENT SURVEILLANCE

Close follow-up after discharge is essential. Patients usually need enteral feedings for several months after the transplant; they are unable to eat sufficiently due to dysmotility of native or transplanted organs, and very commonly they experience a lack of appetite. Children represent an additional problem because they often must be taught to eat after years of TPN therapy. Frequent endoscopic surveillance and intestinal function tests are needed in addition to the routine post-transplant follow-up (61). Subtle changes of the grafts need to be detected early. Chronic rejection may present as an abnormality of D-xylose absorption before it becomes clinically evident.

Rehabilitation

All clinical studies have shown excellent rehabilitation for patients with functioning intestinal grafts. Physical and mental development in children appears to be normal. Adults have been able to resume normal activities.

OUTCOME FOLLOWING INTESTINAL TRANSPLANTATION

The reported world experience was reviewed by Grant in the fall of 1995 at the Fourth International Symposium on Small Bowel Transplantation in Pittsburgh (62). At that time

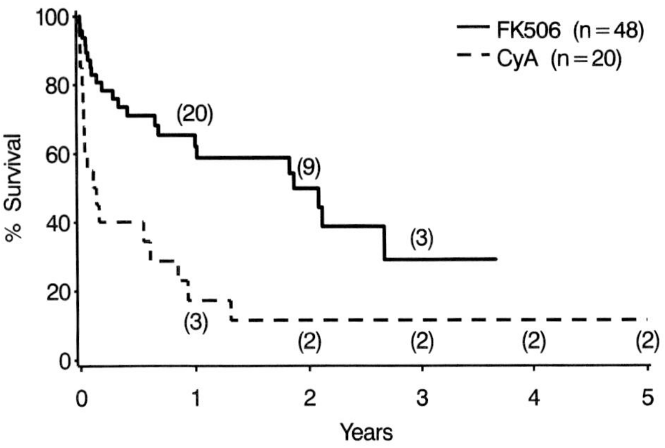

FIGURE 22.8. *International Intestinal Transplant Registry data on survival of isolated intestinal grafts according to type of maintenance immunosuppression. Numbers in parentheses indicate number of evaluable recipients at each time period. (Modified from Grant D. Current results of intestinal transplantation. Lancet 1996;347:1801–1803.)*

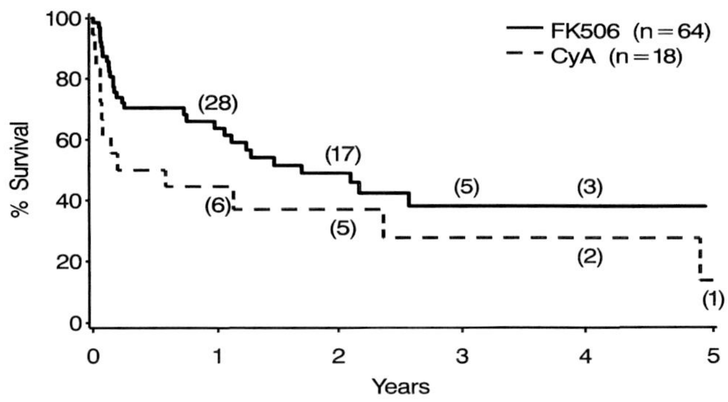

FIGURE 22.9. *International Intestinal Transplant Registry data on survival of combined intestine–liver grafts. (Modified from Grant D. Current results of intestinal transplantation. Lancet 1996;347:1801–1803.)*

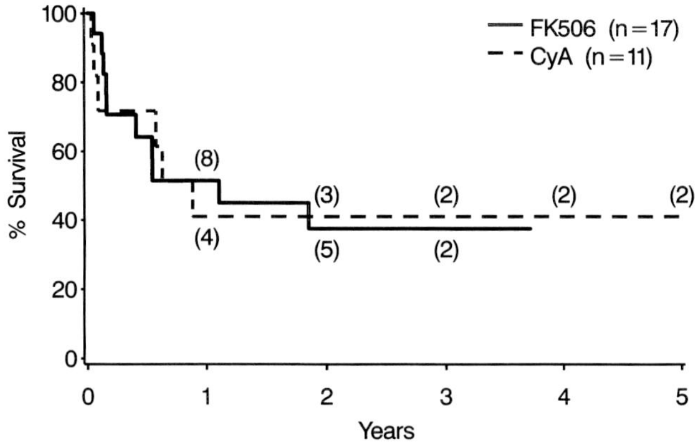

FIGURE 22.10. *International Intestinal Transplant Registry data on survival of multivisceral grafts. (Modified from Grant D. Current results of intestinal transplantation. Lancet 1996;347:1801–1803.)*

180 transplants had been performed in 170 patients in 24 centers worldwide, with more than half performed in children. The total number of transplants was composed of 38% isolated intestinal grafts, 46% combined liver–intestinal, and 16% multivisceral. The 3-year graft survival rates were 29% for small bowel (SB), 38% for small bowel–liver (SBL), and 37% for multivisceral (MV). Graft survival was better with tacrolimus-based immunosuppression, a difference that was statistically significant in isolated intestinal transplantation. Sepsis and multi-organ system failure (MOSF) accounted for more than 70% of the mortalities. A recent update (63) indicates that the Intestinal Transplant Registry now reports 273 intestinal transplants in 260 patients, of which 48% were combined liver–bowel transplants and 41% were isolated bowel transplants. The 1-year graft survival was 65%.

Contrary to what has been observed following liver or kidney transplantation, significant numbers of patient and graft losses continue in the long term after intestinal transplantation. Contemporaneous transplantation of the liver and the other intra-abdominal organs appears to diminish these late losses (Figs. 22.8–22.10).

Rehabilitation following successful surgery has been encouraging: of the survivors reported to the Registry, 78% became totally independent of any form of intravenous therapy. These observations confirmed earlier reports from the University of Pittsburgh, where tacrolimus was introduced (64–66), and emphasized that intestinal transplantation not only can be lifesaving (67), but can also reverse the impaired quality of life typically resulting from TPN (68). They also reaffirmed the conclusion that, in spite of the progress made, further development is needed for intestinal transplantation to attain the status of other solid organ transplants.

NEW IMMUNOMODULATION APPROACHES

At the University of Miami, immunomodulation is now used in all intestinal transplant recipients with unmodified bone marrow infusions. The effect of adjunctive immunosuppressive agents added to the tacrolimus-based regimen is being tested. Since the program's inception in August, 1954, 19 intestinal transplants on 11 children and 8 adults have been performed. Median length of follow-up has been 106 days (4 to 717). There were 3 isolated intestinal, 9 combined liver–intestinal, and 7 multivisceral transplants (Table 22.2). Three of the latter patients had one kidney (n = 1) or two kidneys (n = 2) included with their graft.

Table 22.2 shows the follow-up data through July 1996. All recipients of isolated grafts, 5 of the combined liver–intestinal recipients, and 3 of the recipients of multivisceral grafts are alive. All patients received tacrolimus as baseline immunosuppression, and all received or were intended to receive unmodified bone marrow infusions fol-

Table 22.2. Intestinal Transplant Patients (University of Miami)

Patient	Age (Years)	Treatment	Diagnosis	Graft	Survival (Days)
1	5	OKT-3 induction	Intestinal atresia	SBL	>717
2	2	OKT-3 induction	NEC	SBL	39
3	0.5	OKT-3 induction	Congenital abnormality of the muscularis propria	MV	44
4	32	OKT-3 induction + MMF rescue	Crohn's disease	SB[b]	>578
5	33	OKT-3 induction	Venous mesenteric occlusion	MV	20
6	7	OKT-3 induction	Mid-gut volvulus	SBL	63
7	2	Cytoxan + MMF rescue	Hirschsprung's disease	SB	>463
8	1	Cytoxan	NEC	SBL	>457
9	2	Cytoxan + MMF rescue	NEC	SBL	>422
10	28	MMF	Gardner syndrome	MV	>383
11	34	MMF	Short bowel secondary to volvulus	SBL	>368
12	25	MMF	Desmoid tumor	SB–LB	>231
13	47	MMF[a]	Crohn's disease	SBL	6
14	0.5	MMF[a]	NEC	MV	4
15	35	MMF	Mid-gut volvulus	SBL	76
16	39	MMF	Crohn's disease	SBL	>140
17	16	MMF	Intestinal pseudo-obstruction	MV	32
18	8	MMF	Megacystic microcolon	MV	>106
19	4	MMF	NEC	MV	>15

[a] Patient did not receive MMF or was only on MMF for 3 days.
[b] Graft removed at 9.5 months for recurrent Crohn's disease.
A "greater than" sign indicates the patient was still alive when follow-up data was collected.
MMF, mycophenolate mofetil; MV, multivisceral; LB, large bowel; NEC, necrotizing enterocolitis; SB, small bowel; SBL, small bowel and liver.

lowing isolation from the vertebral bodies from the same cadaveric donor. Infusions of 10×10^8 cells/kg were given in either two (postoperative days 0, 5 or 5, 11) or five (postoperative days 5, 14, 21, 28, 90) divided doses. Three adjunctive agents were tested: OKT-3, cyclophosphamide, and mycophenolate mofetil (MMF).

OKT-3

Six patients transplanted between August 1994 and January 1995 received OKT-3 induction therapy. Five patients completed the course. In 1 patient, OKT-3 was stopped after 6 doses due to fever, leukocytosis, and an infection found in the explanted liver and intestine. Four patients developed CMV (n = 3) or EBV (n = 2; one patient had both) infections that required treatment with antiviral agents. The overall incidence of rejection was 8 episodes in the 6 patients.

Patient survival was 33.3%. Mortalities were due to infectious complications: aortointestinal fistula (n = 1); intestinal perforation and MSOF (n = 1); pancreatitis, intra-abdominal sepsis, and MSOF (n = 1); and disseminated aspergillosis (n = 1). Of the surviving patients, 1 was converted to MMF therapy but later had her intestinal graft removed due to an apparent recurrence of Crohn's disease. OKT-3 induction was, therefore, discontinued for subsequent trials.

Cyclophosphamide

Three patients transplanted between April 1995 and June 1995 received cyclophosphamide. In 1 patient, cyclophosphamide was stopped after 12 days because of rejection, which required OKT-3 treatment. The patient was later treated with MMF due to persistent rejection. A second patient received cyclophosphamide for 8 days, but it was discontinued due to fever and leukocytopenia. The third patient received cyclophosphamide for about 3 months, then received OKT-3 treatment for severe rejection and was eventually converted to MMF. There were no viral infections in this group. The incidence of rejection was 6 episodes in the 3 patients. All the patients are alive.

Mycophenolate Mofetil

Ten patients transplanted between July 1995 and July 1996 were intended to receive MMF therapy at the time of transplant. Two of the patients, who had been on life support at the time of transplantation, died within 1 week after their transplant. One did not receive MMF at all, and the other received it for only 3 days. Both patients died of MSOF: one patient due to deterioration of the general condition, and the second due to diffuse abdominal sepsis that originated from an enterococcal infection in her native spleen. Of the remaining 8 patients, 6 are alive and 2 died. Two developed CMV or EBV viremia (n = 2) and CMV enteritis (n = 1) (one of these patients had both CMV viremia and CMV enteritis, diagnosed on postoperative days 106 and 177). These infections were successfully controlled with antiviral agents. The incidence of rejection was 14 episodes in the 8 patients.

Patient survival was 75%. The two mortalities resulted from a failure of the immunosuppressive regimen, which led to severe rejection in both patients. One patient was treated with multiple boluses of methylprednisolone, the other patient received OKT-3 and was converted to cyclophosphamide. This aggressive treatment caused fatal infections leading to sepsis and MSOF in both patients (POD 76 and 32).

The remaining 6 patients are currently maintained on MMF. The median length of time on MMF is 185 days (11 to 367). Side effects have been seen in 3 of these patients. Two patients developed nausea. In both cases, the nausea resolved after reduction of the dose, which was later restored successfully. One patient developed nausea, diplopia, and bacteremia with atypical mycobacteria from an apparent duodenitis. In this patient, MMF was held for a month and then restarted uneventfully.

Mycophenolate Mofetil Rescue Therapy

Three patients have been treated with MMF as a rescue agent: 1 patient had received OKT-3 induction, and 2 patients had received cyclophosphamide. All three patients are alive and have not experienced rejections or viral infections since being placed on MMF. The patient from the OKT-3 group received MMF for 286 days before her intestinal graft was removed due to a recurrence of Crohn's disease. In the patients who received cyclophosphamide, one patient is currently well on MMF (325 days). In the second case, MMF is being held at the moment due to malakoplakia (262 days on MMF).

Conclusions

All patients who are alive have well-functioning grafts, except for one patient whose graft was removed. All are maintained solely on enteral nutrition and receive no parenteral treatment whatsoever. Seven patients have resumed normal daily activities, and 3 are in the process of complete rehabilitation.

These results should not be considered as conclusive, because of the fairly short follow-up time and the relatively small number of patients. However, OKT-3 induction and the addition of cyclophosphamide did not appear to be beneficial. The incidence of rejection was lower in the OKT-3 induction patients, but it was also associated with a higher mortality rate. Although 2 of the patients in the MMF group were not salvageable because of the severity of their condition at the time of intestinal transplantation, MMF otherwise appears to be an effective adjunct immunosuppressive agent. Tacrolimus and MMF in combination appear to have a synergistic effect, and thus should be used with caution.

SUMMARY

Since the introduction of clinical intestinal transplantation by Lillehei in the 1960s, there have been remarkable advances in the immunosuppressive regimens to control rejection and in preservation techniques, anesthesia, monitoring, and critical care. Newer and more powerful immunosuppressants (cyclosporine and tacrolimus) have helped transform intestinal transplantation into a clinical reality (69).

Transplantation can be a life-saving procedure for patients with intestinal failure. Currently, it is indicated in the face of life-threatening complications of an underlying disease or from TPN. Rehabilitation in successful cases is excellent.

ACKNOWLEDGMENTS

We would like to thank the following people for their assistance in the preparation of this chapter: Ms. Pauline Bethel, Ms. Jennie Benson, Theodore Karatzas, MD, and George Fragulidis, MD. We would also like to thank David Grant, MD, of the International Intestinal Transplant Registry for providing the graphs.

COMMENTARY

David Grant

When Owen Wagenstein was asked to comment on Richard Lillehei's landmark paper published in the journal *Annals of Surgery* in 1959, he aptly described intestinal transplantation as "an adventure in search of adversity" (1). After three decades of struggle, this procedure is finally emerging as a viable clinical option.

The initial intestinal transplants failed because of technical complications, sepsis, rejection, and lymphoproliferative disease. The results have improved due to better patient selection, more reliable surgical techniques, earlier detection of rejection, and more effective immunosuppression. Nonetheless, both graft and patient survival rates are still inferior to the results of other solid organ transplants. Current controversies about small bowel grafting and potential methods to improve the outcomes are discussed below.

DONOR SUPPLY

About 25% of the patients waiting for intestinal transplants die before a donor becomes available. The use of living-related donors may improve this situation. It is known that approximately 100 to 200 cm of terminal ileum, with or without the ascending colon, can be resected with few deleterious effects. As reported by Fortner almost a decade ago (2), these segmental grafts from living donors can be revascularized using the ileocolic arcade to restore good absorptive function.

The early experience has demonstrated the technical feasibility of living donation, but more time is needed to answer the following questions:

1. What are the risk/benefit ratios for the donor and the recipient?
2. Is it better to transplant the jejunum or the ileum?
3. Can graft rejection rates be reduced by major histocompatibility complex (MHC)-matching?
4. How much bowel needs to be transplanted to achieve good long-term absorptive function?

SURGICAL TECHNIQUES

The choice of surgical procedures is also evolving. Transplantation of the small bowel alone, with or without the colon, is the preferred option because the intestinal graft can be removed if there are serious complications. Patients with severe liver dysfunction and hepatic fibrosis due to total parenteral nutrition (TPN) require combined small bowel and liver grafts. Mild to moderate liver dysfunction will reverse after transplantation of the small bowel, and it is not always clear when it is mandatory to add the liver graft. Mechanisms that may contribute to improved liver function after small bowel transplantation include stopping the noxious agent (TPN), and providing increased hepatic blood flow containing trophic nutrients from the intestinal graft.

It is particularly difficult to determine the best type of intestinal transplant for patients with motility disorders. Again, an isolated small bowel graft is preferred, but a multivisceral transplant may provide better function for those patients with severe gastric dysmotility. The choice between these two options is not easy, considering the following:

1. A multivisceral transplant is far more risky than an isolated transplant.
2. Many patients with pseudo-obstruction are taking narcotics that impair gastrointestinal motility.
3. Nuclear medicine gastric emptying scans and/or motility studies do not reliably predict functional outcomes after transplantation.

IMMUNOSUPPRESSION

Graft rejection remains the major cause of morbidity and mortality after intestinal grafting. Most centers report rejection rates of more than 80% even when tacrolimus is used as the primary immunosuppressive agent. The challenge is to identify new protocols that will reduce the frequency and severity of graft rejection without increasing the rate of infections and/or lymphoproliferative disease. Trials are currently underway to see if these goals can be achieved by combining tacrolimus with other potent immunosuppressive agents such as cyclophosphamide, rapamycin, and mycophenolate mofetil.

LONG-TERM GRAFT FUNCTION

Most patients with small bowel grafts are able to stop TPN and resume an unrestricted oral diet. However, some patients have unexplained gastric inertia, diarrhea, and/or malabsorption. Potential causes of graft dysfunction include preservation injury, disruption of the lymphatics, extrinsic denervation, the adverse effects of immunosuppressive drugs, narcotic dependency, graft rejection, and chronic cytomegalovirus (CMV) infections.

What can be done to improve the function of intestinal allografts? Studies have shown that adding a colon segment to the small bowel graft slows transit time and increases absorption without increasing the risk of rejection (3,4). However, the clinical benefits of adding a colon segment are controversial, as a recent study by Todo et al identified inclusion of the large bowel as a risk factor for poor results (5). Transplanting the ganglion tissue at the base of the small bowel mesentery is another potential method to improve graft function. Studies in rats by Kiyochi et al have shown that this technique improves gut motility due to better reinnervation of the small bowel (6,7), and clinical trials are currently underway.

FUTURE DIRECTIONS

Successful intestinal grafting enables most patients with short gut syndrome to resume a normal lifestyle. However, the results of this procedure are not reliable. To become the standard therapy for the treatment of intestinal failure, transplantation will have to provide an excellent quality of life in addition to being safe and cost-effective. Techniques are improving, and, if the current progress continues, these benchmarks may be achieved in the near future.

CHAPTER REFERENCES

1. Lillehei RC, Goott B, Miller FA. The physiological response of the small bowel of the dog to ischemia including prolonged in vitro preservation of the bowel with successful replacement and survival. Ann Surg 1959;150:543–560.
2. Lillehei RC, Idezuki Y, Feemster J, et al. Transplantation of stomach, intestine and pancreas: experimental and clinical observations. Surgery 1967;62:721–741.
3. Starzl TE, Kaupp Jr HA. Mass homotransplantation of abdominal organs in dogs. Surg Forum 1960;11:28–30.
4. Starzl TE, Kaupp Jr HA, Brock D, et al. Homotransplantation of multiple visceral organs. Am J Surg 1962;103:219–229.

5. Grant DR. Immunosuppression for small bowel transplantation. Clin Transplant 1991;5:563–567.
6. Goulet O, Revillon Y, Cerf-Bensussan N, et al. Small intestinal transplantation in a child using cyclosporin. Transplant Proc 1988;20:288–296.
7. Deltz E, Schroeder P, Gebhardt H, et al. Successful clinical bowel transplantation: report of a case. Clin Transplant 1989;3:89.
8. Margreiter R, Konigsrainer A, Schmid T, Koller J, et al. Successful multivisceral transplantation. Transplant Proc 1992;24:1226–1227.
9. Starzl TE, Rowe M, Todo S, et al. Transplantation of multiple abdominal viscera. JAMA 1989;261:1449–1457.
10. Grant D, Wall W, Mimeault R, et al. Successful small bowel/liver transplantation. Lancet 1990;335:181–184.
11. Abu-Elmagd K, Reyes J, Todo S, et al. Clinical intestinal transplantation: new perspectives and immunologic considerations. J Am Coll Surg 1998;186:512–527.
12. Pirenne J. Short bowel syndrome. Medical aspects and prospects of intestinal transplantation. Acta Chir Belg 1996;96:150–154.
13. Dudrick SJ, Wilmore DW, Vars HM, et al. Long term total parenteral nutrition with growth, development and positive nitrogen balance. Surgery 1968;169:134–142.
14. Howard L, Heaphey L, Fleming R, et al. Four years of North American home parenteral nutrition outcome data and their implications for patient management. J Parenteral Enteral Nutr 1991;15:384–393.
15. Stokes MA, Almond DJ, Pettit SH, et al. Home parenteral nutrition: a review of 100 patient years of treatment in 76 consecutive cases. Br J Surg 1988;75;481–483.
16. Chang RWS, Hatton I, Henley J, et al. Total parenteral nutrition: a four year audit. Br J Surg 1986;73:656–658.
17. Messing B, Lemann M, Landais P, et al. Prognosis of patients with nonmalignant chronic intestinal failure receiving long-term home parenteral nutrition. Gastroenterology 1995;108:1005–1010.
18. Vanderhoof JA. Short bowel syndrome in children and small intestinal transplantation. Pediatr Clin North Am 1996;43:533–550.
19. Asfar S, Atkinson C, Ghent J, et al. Small bowel transplantation. A life-saving option for selected patients with intestinal failure. Dig Dis Sci 1996;41:875–883.
20. Webb M, Tzakis A. Intestinal and multivisceral transplantation. In: Civetta J, Taylor RW, Kirby RR, eds. Critical care. 3rd ed. Philadelphia: Lippincott-Raven, 1997.
21. Frezza EE, Tzakis A, Fung JJ, Van TDH. Small bowel transplantation: current progress and clinical application. Hepato-gastroenterology 1996;43:363–376.
22. Scotti-Foglieni C, Marino IR, Cillo U, et al. Human intestinal multivisceral transplantation. In: D'Amico D, Bassi N, Tedeschi U, Cillo U, eds. Liver transplantation procedures and management. Masson, 1994:235–254.
23. Ricordi C, Karatzas T, Nery J, et al. High dose bone marrow infusions to enhance allograft survival. The effect of timing. Transplantation 1997;63:7–11.
24. Kamada N, Davies HS, Roser B. Reversal of transplantation immunity by liver grafting. Nature 1981;292:840.
25. Flye MW, Duffy BF, Phelan DL, et al. Protective effect of liver transplantation on simultaneously transplanted kidney in a highly sensitized patient. Transplantation 1990;50:1051–1053.
26. Jeyarajah DR, McBride M, Klintmalm GB, Gonwa TA. Combined liver-kidney transplantation: what are the indications? Transplantation 1997;64:1091–1096.
27. Starzl TE, Demetris AJ, Murase N, et al. Cell migration, chimerism, and graft acceptance. Lancet 1992;339:1579.
28. Starzl TE, Miller C, Broznick B, Makowka L. An improved technique for multiple organ harvesting. Surg Gynecol Obstet 1987;165:343–348.
29. Sindhi R, Landmark J, Shaw BW, et al. Combined liver/small bowel transplantation using a blood group compatible but nonidentical donor. Transplantation 1996;61:1782–1783.
30. Morris JA, Johnson DL, Rimmer JA, et al. Identical-twin small-bowel transplant for desmoid tumor. Lancet 1995;345:1577–1578.
31. Butler A, Watson C, Friend P, et al. Intestinal Isograft: functional recovery in absence of rejection, infection and immunosuppression. Presented in 5th International Symposium on Intestinal Transplantation. Cambridge, UK 1997.
32. Gruessner RWG, Sharp HL. Living related intestinal transplantation. First report of standardized surgical technique. Transplantation 1997;64:1605–1607.
33. Tzakis AG, Gruessner RWG. Future of living related small bowel transplantation in children. Pediatr Transplantation 1998;2:1–2.
34. Todo S, Tzakis A, Abu-Elmagd K, et al. Cadaveric small bowel and small bowel-liver transplantation in humans. Transplantation 1992;53:369–375.
35. Cahalan MK, Ionescu P, Melton HJ, et al. Automated real time analysis of intra operative transesophageal echocardiograms. Anesthesiology 1993;78:477–485.
36. Kusumoto FM, Muhiudeen IA, Kuecherer HF, et al. Response of the interatrial septum to transatrial pressure gradients and its potential for predicting pulmonary capillary wedge pressure: an intraoperative study using transesophageal echocardiography in patients during mechanical ventilation. J Am Coll Cardiol 1993;21:721–728.
37. Mallett SV, Cox DJA. Thromboelastography. Br J Anesth 1992;69:307–313.
38. Starzl TE, Todo S, Tzakis A, et al. The many faces of multivisceral transplantation. Surg Gynecol Obstet 1991;172:335–344.
39. Todo S, Tzakis A, Reyes J, et al. Small intestinal transplantation in humans with or without the colon. Transplantation 1994;57:840–848.
40. Todo S, Tzakis A, Abu-Elmagd K, et al. Intestinal transplantation in composite visceral grafts or alone. Ann Surg 1992;216:223–234.
41. Tzakis A, Todo S, Reyes J, et al. Intestinal transplantation in children under FK506 immunosuppression. J Pediatr Surg 1993;28:1040–1043.
42. Tzakis A, Nour B, Reyes J, et al. Endorectal pull-through of transplanted colon as part of intestinal transplantation. Surgery 1995;117:451–453.
43. Starzl TE, Todo S, Tzakis A, Fung J. The transplantation of gastrointestinal organs. Gastroenterology 1993;104:673–679.
44. Abu-Elmagd K, Todo S, Tzakis A, et al. Three years clinical experience with intestinal transplantation. J Am Coll Surg 1994;179:385–400.
45. Asfar S, Zhong R, Grant D. Small bowel transplantation. Surg Clin North Am 1994;74:1197–1210.
46. Campbell WL, Abu-Elmagd K, Furukawa H, Todo S. Intestinal and multivisceral transplantation. Radiol Clin North Am 1995;32:595–614.
47. Alessiani M, Tzakis A, Todo S, et al. Assessment of five years experience with abdominal organ cluster transplantation. J Am Coll Surg 1995;180:1–9.
48. Langnas AN, Shaw BW Jr, Antonson DL, et al. Preliminary experience with intestinal transplantation in infants and children. Pediatrics 1996;97:443–448.
49. Tzakis AG, Nery JR, Raskin JB, et al. "Domino" liver transplantation combined with multivisceral transplantation. Arch Surg 1997;132:1145–1147.
50. Jain A, Venkataramanan J, Lever V, et al. FK 506 in small bowel transplant recipients: pharmacokinetics and dosing. Transplant Proc 1994;26:1609–1610.
51. Kahan B, Ghobrial R. Immunosuppressive agents. Surg Clin North Am 1994;74:1029–1054.
52. Kadry Z, Furukawa H, Abu-Elmagd K, et al. Use of the D-xylose absorption graft in monitoring intestinal allograft. Transplant Proc 1994;26:1413.
53. Berstein CN. Small bowel transplantation (review). Scand J Gastroenterol Suppl 1995;208:118–124.
54. Gurakar A, Fagivoli S, Hassanein T, et al. Is rejection a diffuse or localized process in small bowel transplantation? Surg Endosc 1994;8:762–764.
55. Kaufman SS, Wisecarver JL, Ruby EI, et al. Correlation of mucosal disaccharidase activities with histology in evaluation of rejection following intestinal transplantation. Pediatr Transplant 1998;2:134–138.
56. Fromont G, Cerf-Bensussan N, Patey N, et al. Small bowel transplantation in children: an immunohistochemical study of intestinal grafts. Gut 1995;37:783–790.
57. White FV, Reyes J, Jaffe R, Yunis EJ. Pathology of intestinal transplantation in children. Am J Surg Pathol 1995;19:687–698.
58. Kocoshis SA. Small bowel transplantation in infants and children. Gastroenterol Clin North Am 1994;23:727–742.
59. Finn L, Reyes J, Bueno J, et al. Epstein-Barr virus infections in children after transplantation of the small intestine. Am J Surg Pathol 1998;22:299–309.
60. Manez R, Kusne S, Green M, et al. Incidence and risk factors associated with the development of cytomegalovirus disease after intestinal transplantation. Transplantation 1995;59:1010–1014.
61. Funovits M, Miller S, Kovalak, et al. Hospitalization and readmission in intestinal transplantation recipients. Transplant Proc 1994;26:1419.
62. Grant D. Current results of intestinal transplantation. Lancet 1996;347: 1801–1803.
63. Grant D. Intestinal transplantation: 1997 Report of the International Registry. Transplantation 1999 (in press).
64. Tzakis AG, Todo S, Reyes J, et al. Piggyback orthotopic intestinal transplantation. Surg Gynecol Obstet 1993;176:297–298.
65. Tzakis AG, Todo S, Starzl TE. Intestinal transplantation. Ann Rev Med 1994;45:79–91.
66. Todo S, Tzakis A, Abu-Elmagd K, et al. Current status of intestinal transplantation. Adv Surg 1994;27:295–314.
67. Di Martini A, Rovera GM, Graham TO, et al. Quality of life after small intestinal transplantation and among home parenteral nutrition patients. JPEN J Parenter Enteral Nutr 1998;22:357–362.
68. Asfar S, Atkinson P, Ghent C, et al. Small bowel transplantation. A life-saving option for selected patients with intestinal failure. Dig Dis Sci 1996;41: 875–883.

69. Kelly DA, Buckels JA. The future of small bowel transplantation. Arch Dis Child 1995;72:447–451.

COMMENTARY REFERENCES

1. Lillehei RC, Good B, Miller FA. The physiological response of the small bowel of the dog to ischemia including prolonged in vitro preservation of the bowel with successful replacement and survival. Ann Surg 1959;150:543–560.
2. Fortner JG, Sichuk G, Litwin SD, Seattle EJ. Immunological responses to an intestinal allograft with HLA identical donor-recipient. Transplantation 1972;14:531–536.
3. Hashimoto T, Zhong R, Garcia B, et al. Ileocoric allotransplantation in rats. Transplant Proc 1994;26:1533.
4. Richards WO, Golzarian J, Wasudev N, Sawyers JL. Reverse phasic contractions are present in antiperistaltic jejunal limbs up to twenty-one years postoperatively. J Am Coll Surg 1994;178:557–563.
5. Maner R, Kusne S, Green M, et al. Incidence and risk factors associated with the development of cytomegalovirus disease after intestinal transplantation. Transplantation 1995;59:1010–1014.
6. Kiyochi H, Ono A, Yamamoto N, et al. Extrinsic sympathetic reinnervation after intestinal transplantation in rats. Transplantation 1995;59:328–333.
7. Kiyochi H, Ono A, Yamamoto N, et al. Intestinal transplantation with extrinsic nerve preservation in rats. Transplantation 1995;60:387–390.

Chapter

23

Cardiac Transplantation

G. William Dec

HISTORICAL DEVELOPMENTS

Successful clinical heart transplantation began in 1967, but it was made possible by experimental studies in surgical technique, physiologic adaptation, and immunosuppression developed during the preceding 50 years. Over the last two decades, cardiac transplantation has evolved from an experimental procedure to an established therapeutic option for the management of end-stage myocardial failure. In 1905, Carrel and Guthrie demonstrated the technical feasibility of heterotopic canine transplantation (1). Mann first recognized cardiac allograft rejection as he observed that "failure of the homotransplanted heart to survive is not due to the technique of transplantation but to some biologic factor which is probably identical to that which prevents survival of other homotransplanted tissues and organs" (1). Demikhov proved that the heterotopically transplanted canine heart could independently support the circulation (1). Physiologic function of the intrathoracic cardiac allograft was clarified by Reemtsma and colleagues (1). In the early 1960s, Lower and Shumway perfected the technique for orthotopic cardiac transplantation using cardiopulmonary bypass and demonstrated long-term survival and function of the denervated heart (1).

As a prelude to human cadaveric transplantation, Hardy performed a chimpanzee xenotransplant in 1964 (2). Although technically successful, the primate heart was too small to support the circulation. The first human donor to human recipient cardiac transplant was performed in December 1967 by Barnard (3). The lack of potent, specific immunosuppressive agents and the inability to diagnose allograft rejection during its earliest stages precluded long-term survival.

During the 1970s, fewer than 50 procedures were performed each year. The development by Caves of the transvenous right ventricular endomyocardial biopsy technique for monitoring allograft rejection and the categorization of a biopsy-grading system for quantifying rejection severity by Margaret Billingham were the most significant clinical advances during this decade (4). In the early 1980s, the widespread availability of cyclosporine improved survival and prompted a virtual explosion in the number of cardiac transplant centers within the United States. During the last decade, immunosuppression has been further refined with the introduction of monoclonal antibody OKT-3, the use of steroid-free protocols, and the availability of tacrolimus. The development of satisfactory implantable circulatory assist devices, better immunosuppressive agents, and xenotropic transplantation are undergoing intense investigation and may ultimately provide new treatments for patients dying of progressive cardiac disease.

RECIPIENT SELECTION

Current Indications for Adult Transplant Listing

Selection of adult heart transplant recipients is based upon the clinical determination of which patients are most likely to exhibit substantial improvement in functional capacity and in life expectancy. Earlier patient selection guidelines have been broadened over the past two decades and are based on those preoperative characteristics associated with the best patient survival and greatest degree of rehabilitation following surgery. Intractable symptoms and a poor 1-year prognosis with conventional medical or surgical treatment are common characteristics of all patients considered for transplantation. Two consensus conferences have defined definite, probable, and inadequate indications for transplant listing (Table 23.1) (5,6).

Over 90% of adult patients are transplanted for refractory heart failure. Individuals who require continuous inotropic support or a mechanical assist device are most likely to

Table 23.1. Adult Indications for Cardiac Transplantation

Accepted Indications of Listing
- Cardiogenic shock or low output state requiring mechanical or inotropic support
- Advanced symptomatic heart failure with peak oxygen consumption (VO_2) <10 mL/kg/min with achievement of anaerobic threshold
- NYHA class IV angina pectoris or heart failure due to advanced hypertrophic or restrictive cardiomyopathy
- Refractory angina pectoris consistently limiting day-to-day activities with coronary anatomy that is not amenable to angioplasty, atherectomy, or coronary artery bypass grafting
- Recurrent symptomatic life-threatening ventricular arrhythmias uncontrolled by all appropriate medical and surgical modalities

Probable Indications for Listing
- Symptomatic heart failure with peak VO_2 between 11–16 mL/kg/min
- Recurrent or refractory heart failure symptoms unresponsive to maximal vasodilators and a flexible diuretic program
- Recurrent unstable myocardial ischemic syndromes requiring multiple hospitalizations and not amenable to coronary revascularization
- Primary cardiac tumors without evidence of metastatic disease

Inadequate Indications for Listing
- Left ventricular ejection fraction <30% with mild to moderate symptoms
- History of NYHA class IV symptoms or transient need for inotropic support on a *suboptimal* medical regimen
- Peak VO_2 >16 mL/kg/min without other clinical indications
- Prior life-threatening ventricular arrhythmias that are now controlled
- Asymptomatic nonsustained ventricular tachycardia and advanced left ventricular dysfunction

achieve an immediate benefit. In ambulatory patients with moderate heart failure symptoms (NYHA class 3), it is not yet possible to identify all patients at increased risk for death during medical therapy. Univariate predictors of reduced survival have been identified (Table 23.2) (7). Recent studies employing multivariate techniques have identified the two most consistent predictors of mortality in heart failure patients: left ventricular ejection fraction below 20%, and marked functional limitation defined by peak oxygen uptake ($\dot{V}O_2$) on cardiopulmonary exercise testing below 10 mL/kg/min (8). A peak $\dot{V}O_2$ <10 mL/kg/min predicts a 1-year mortality above 50% and is an indication for transplant listing. Conversely, when peak $\dot{V}O_2$ exceeds 18 mL/kg/min, 1-year survival is approximately 95%, suggesting that listing can be safely deferred. Although it is a powerful prognostic indicator, peak $\dot{V}O_2$ needs to be viewed in the context of other signs and symptoms as well as patient age; it should not serve as the sole indicator for listing. In all patients, medical therapy should be optimized before the final determination on the need for transplantation is made.

Refractory angina pectoris is an unusual indication for transplantation and accounts for less than 5% of patients listed. The vast majority of patients with severe angina pectoris and preserved left ventricular function will undergo coronary artery bypass surgery or angioplasty. Transplant listing should be dictated by inoperable anatomy and/or marked irreversible depression of left ventricular function (generally an ejection fraction below 20%). Inoperable anatomy may be due to poor distal vessels, lack of suitable vascular conduits, or severe coexisting valvular disease. Coronary revascularization may be associated with significant symptomatic and prognostic improvement in patients whose ejection fractions are below 30% (9,10). Patients most likely to benefit include those with symptomatic angina, reversible areas of myocardial ischemia demonstrated by positron emission tomography (PET) or thallium imaging, NYHA class 2 or 3 symptoms, and favorable distal vessels.

Life-threatening ventricular arrhythmias can usually be managed with conventional antiarrhythmic agents, radiofrequency ablation, or an automatic implantable cardioverter defibrillator (AICD). Despite electrophysiologically guided antiarrhythmic therapy and AICD placement, recurrent defibrillations rarely may require frequent hospitalizations or limit functional capacity. The majority of these patients will also exhibit advanced left ventricular dysfunction and increased short-term mortality despite AICD placement, because of progressive heart failure (see Table 23.1) (11).

Table 23.2. Predictors of Mortality in Advanced Heart Failure Populations

Clinical Features
- NYHA class IV symptoms
- Older age at presentation
- Male gender
- Ischemic etiology
- History of syncope
- Persistent S_3 gallop
- Right-sided heart failure signs

Hemodynamic and Ventriculographic Findings
- Left ventricular ejection fraction <20%
- Right ventricular dysfunction
- Pulmonary hypertension
- Right atrial pressure >8 mm Hg
- Pulmonary capillary wedge pressure >16–18 mm Hg
- Cardiac index <2.2 L/min/m^2

Neurohormonal Abnormalities
- Hyponatremia (serum sodium <137 mmol/L)
- Enhanced sympathetic tone (elevated plasma norepinephrine or resting sinus tachycardia)
- Increased plasma atrial natriuretic factor or renin

Functional Limitations
- Maximum oxygen uptake <12 mL/kg/min

Arrhythmia Pattern
- History of prior cardiac arrest
- Symptomatic or asymptomatic nonsustained runs of ventricular tachycardia
- Chronic atrial fibrillation
- Second- or third-degree AV block

Therapeutic Approach
- Inability to tolerate angiotensin-converting enzyme inhibitors
- Use of type I antiarrhythmic agents
- Use of nonglycoside-positive inotropic agents

Benign cardiac tumors such as myxomas are usually amenable to surgical resection. Heart transplantation for inoperable cardiac malignancy was first reported in 1981 and represents an extremely uncommon indication for transplantation (12). The tumors should be confined to the myocardium, and an extensive work-up to rule out metastases should be undertaken.

Contraindications to Cardiac Transplantation

Patient characteristics that increase the risk of early postoperative morbidity or mortality represent relative contraindications to transplantation (Table 23.3) (6,13).

Absolute chronologic limits are no longer desirable, but physiologic age should serve as the basis for patient selection. Although survival may be comparable, morbidity in patients above 55 years is significantly greater than it is in younger recipients (14). Diabetic candidates must be free from other end-organ damage, particularly proliferative retinopathy, severe peripheral neuropathy, proteinuria, peripheral or cerebrovascular atherosclerotic disease, chronic infections or ulcers of the extremities, or extremely brittle glucose control (14).

Table 23.3. Conditions That Increase Risk of Morbidity and Mortality Following Cardiac Transplantation

Factors Associated with a Markedly Increased Risk
Active infection
Recent malignancy (generally within the last 5 years)
Pulmonary hypertension with irreversibly high pulmonary vascular resistance (PVR >6 Wood units or 3–4 Wood units during a vasodilator trial) (orthotopic heart only)
Diabetes mellitus and evidence of significant retinopathy, neuropathy, or nephropathy
Myocardial infiltrative or inflammatory disease
Active peptic ulcer disease
Any systemic illness that would limit life expectancy or compromise functional rehabilitation
Significant pulmonary parenchymal disease
Irreversible severe renal dysfunction
Severe peripheral vascular or cerebrovascular disease
Irreversible severe hepatic dysfunction or cirrhosis
Documented medical noncompliance
Active substance abuse (including tobacco)
Noncontrolled psychiatric illness
Factors Associated with an Increased Risk
Age >60 years
Recent pulmonary embolism or infarction
Moderate pulmonary hypertension with a pulmonary vascular resistance of 4–6 Wood units or a TPG (transpulmonary gradient) >15 mm Hg (orthotopic heart only)
Insulin-dependent diabetes mellitus without end-organ dysfunction
Moderate cerebrovascular or peripheral vascular atherosclerotic disease (asymptomatic or insufficient in severity to preclude cardiopulmonary rehabilitation)
Prospective crossmatch incompatibility between donor and recipient
History of diverticulosis, ulcerative colitis, or Crohn's disease
Chronic hepatitis B or C infection
Mild-to-moderate irreversible renal, hepatic, or pulmonary disease
Severe obesity
Severe osteoporosis or arthritis
Absence of social support network

Comorbid diseases that increase transplant risk should be viewed as relative contraindications. Patients with moderate to severe hepatic dysfunction, documented cirrhosis, or renal dysfunction (creatinine clearance <30 mL/min) are generally excluded from consideration. Likewise, moderate obstructive lung disease (forced vital capacity <50% of predicted or an FEV1 <1 liter) is associated with a higher incidence of perioperative respiratory failure, impaired functional capacity, and decreased survival. Active cigarette smoking should also preclude transplantation.

High-Risk Patients

Pulmonary hypertension significantly increases the risk for early right ventricular failure. Although severe fixed pulmonary hypertension excludes orthotopic transplantation, a heterotopic approach is a possible alternative. The level of pulmonary vascular resistance (PVR) that will produce acute right heart failure in the allograft is influenced by the degree of ischemic injury that occurs during harvesting. Most centers exclude candidates whose PVR exceeds 4 to 6 Wood units (15). Elevation in PVR may demonstrate partial or complete reversibility with nitroprusside, prostaglandin E_1, or nitric oxide (16–18). If acute pharmacologic intervention fails, prolonged hemodynamic monitoring with chronic administration of dobutamine or nitroprusside may gradually reduce PVR to an acceptable range.

When PVR can be lowered below 2.5 Wood units without concomitant systemic hypotension, transplantation can be undertaken without increased risk (19). PVR indexed by body surface area is more relevant in children because of the differences in body size and absolute cardiac output. The risk of early death is quite high in congenital heart disease when the PVR index exceeds 6 (15).

Mechanical Circulatory Support

Patients selected for temporary mechanical circulatory support should be transplant candidates before device implantation and have evidence for cardiogenic shock with left atrial filling pressures >25 mm Hg, systolic blood pressure <90 mm Hg, and a cardiac index <1.8 L/min/m^2 despite pharmacologic support. Four types of mechanical support are available: intra-aortic balloon counterpulsation, left heart bypass systems, left ventricular assist devices (LVADs), and the total artificial heart.

Balloon Counterpulsation

Balloon counterpulsation has been used extensively as a bridge to transplantation for periods of days to months. Advantages include ready availability, low cost, and a non-thoracotomy approach. Prolonged use is associated with significant vascular complications, bacteremia, psychological impairment, and rapid physical deconditioning.

Left Heart Bypass Systems

Left heart bypass systems have been adapted for temporary ventricular assistance. The Bio-medicus (Bio-medicus, Eton Prairie, MN) system can provide biventricular support for adults and children. It provides nonpulsatile blood flow using a centrifugal pump. Advantages include ready availability and lower cost. Disadvantages include an increased risk of bacteremia, a need for patient immobility, and limited peak cardiac flow.

Left Ventricular Assist Devices

Left ventricular assist devices are increasingly used as a bridge to transplantation. Three pneumatically driven devices are commercially available. The Pierce-Donachy (Thoratec Laboratories, Inc., Berkeley, CA) device is composed of a flexible polyurethane blood sack and diaphragm within a rigid case; it is placed paracorporeally on the anterior abdominal wall, and is powered by pulses of compressed carbon dioxide. The Abiomed BVS 5000 system (Abiomed, Danvers, MA) can provide uni- or biventricular support. The atrial blood reservoir fills passively by gravity, and the ventricular reservoir is pneumatically driven to eject blood. Its principal advantage is that it is essentially self-regulating and does not require a dedicated technician or special care. Disadvantages include the need for thoracotomy, inability to close the chest, risk of thrombus formation, and frequent need for bed rest and ventilatory support.

The HeartMate LVAD (Thermo Cardiosystems, Inc., Woburn, MA) is a pusher-plate–designed pump driven by a portable external console using a percutaneous drive line (Fig. 23.1). A polyurethane diaphragm divides the pump into a blood chamber and an air chamber. During pulses of air, the diaphragm is displaced, propelling blood through an outflow graft to the arterial circulation. Advantages include excellent hemodynamic characteristics, ability to ambulate and exercise the patient, and low risk of thromboembolic complications despite the absence of systemic anticoagulation. Disadvantages include the need for median sternotomy, inability to provide right ventricular support or to be used in severe right heart dysfunction, and high cost.

It is imperative that LVAD support be instituted before irreversible end-organ dysfunction ensues. Factors associated with a greater likelihood of perioperative death include cardiac arrest prior to implantation, worsening hepatic dysfunction, coagulopathy, and oliguria (20). Approximately 20% of patients will not improve sufficiently to undergo transplantation. Historically, mechanically supported patients have had a 10% to 15% lower 1-year survival than less critically ill individuals. More recent data suggest that preoperative support with a HeartMate or Novacor (Baxter Healthcare Corporation, Oakland, CA) LVAD may not be associated with a decrease in post-transplant survival.

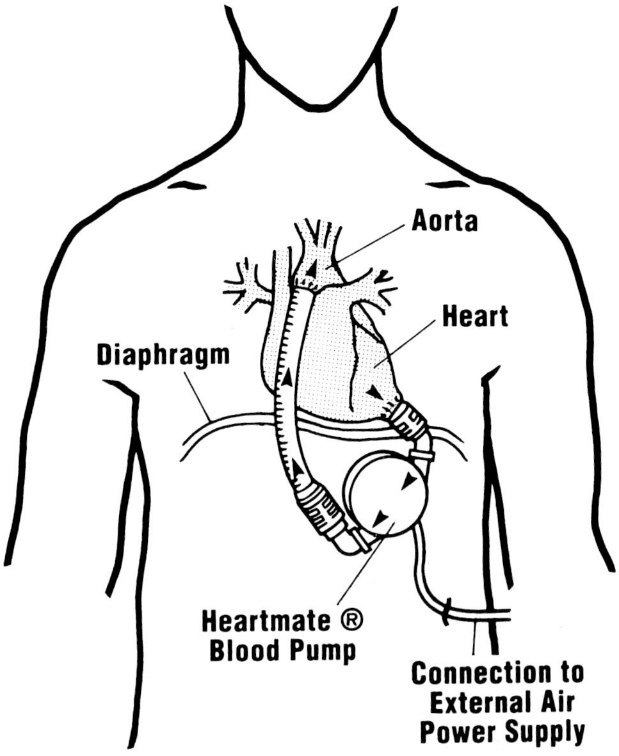

FIGURE 23.1. *Schematic drawing of a "wearable" Thermo Cardiosystems HeartMate, a pneumatically driven left ventricular assist device with an inflow cannula in the LV apex and an outflow graft in the ascending aorta. The pump is positioned in the left upper quadrant either intra-abdominally or preperitoneally. Electrical connections and the air drive line exit through a fascial tunnel. The power supply and electronics are contained on an external console or holster. (Reprinted with permission from Philips WS, et al. Surgical complications of bridging to transplantation: the Thermo Cardiosystems LVAD. Ann Thorac Surg 1992;53:482–486.)*

Total Artificial Heart

A small number of patients will require biventricular support for refractory right heart failure, and a total artificial heart may be useful in such individuals. Despite the disappointing results achieved with the Jarvik 7 artificial heart (Symbien, Inc., Salt Lake City, UT), three new devices are undergoing testing. All three artificial hearts are electrohydraulic and are designed to enable patients to lead an ambulatory lifestyle. The smaller size, more durable materials, advanced microprocessors, and less thrombogenic blood surface interfaces suggest that these second generation devices may soon undergo clinical testing.

PRETRANSPLANT EVALUATION AND MANAGEMENT

Evaluation of potential transplant recipients should be individualized (Table 23.4). Alternative medical or surgical treatment options should be considered. Right and left ventricular size and function should be assessed and correctable

Table 23.4. Recommended Transplant Evaluation

Routine Data
Comprehensive history and physical examination
Complete blood count, differential, platelet count, prothrombin time, and partial thromboplastin time
Blood chemistries including renal and hepatic function
Urinalysis
Stool guaiac × 3
24-hour urinary collection for creatinine clearance and total protein
Mammography/Papanicolaou smear*
Pulmonary function testing including diffusion capacity
Consultations (psychiatry, physical therapy, dental, social service)
Abdominal ultrasound
Carotid and peripheral Doppler vascular flow studies*
Cardiovascular Data
Electrocardiogram
Chest film
Cardiopulmonary exercise testing with oxygen consumption
Coronary angiography*
Right heart catheterization including vasodilators if needed
Echocardiography or radioventriculography
Endomyocardial biopsy*
Immunologic Data
Blood type and antibody screen
Human leukocyte antigen (HLA) typing
Panel of reactive antibodies (PRA) screen
Infectious Disease Screening
Skin testing for purified protein derivative (PPD), and control (mumps, dermatophytin)
Urine culture and sensitivity
Serologic testing for syphilis, hepatitis A, HBsAg, HBsAb, HBcAb, and hepatitis C; HIV; cytomegalovirus; toxoplasmosis; varicella titer; rubella titer; and Epstein-Barr viral capsid antibodies
Lyme titers*
Histoplasmosis and coccidioidomycosis complement-fixing antibodies*
Stool for ova and parasites × 3*

* Where clinically indicated.

valvular pathology excluded. Patients with suspected or known ischemic heart disease should undergo coronary angiography to exclude the possibility of revascularization. Exercise testing with thallium scintigraphy is often useful in this context to evaluate ischemic but potentially viable myocardium.

Many centers perform endomyocardial biopsy in patients with dilated cardiomyopathy of less than 1-year's duration in order to exclude inflammatory conditions such as sarcoidosis and myocarditis that may respond to treatment. Right heart catheterization should be undertaken in all potential recipients to evaluate and manipulate pulmonary vascular resistance as well as to evaluate the adequacy of diuretic and vasodilator treatment. The degree of functional limitation should be quantified whenever possible for outpatients to determine the prognosis and functional benefit of transplantation (8).

Comorbid conditions that increase the risks of transplantation should be excluded. Older patients or those with ischemic heart disease should undergo carotid and arterial noninvasive studies. Pulmonary function studies with diffusion capacity are mandatory in former smokers. Serum creatinine may significantly underestimate the degree of renal dysfunction in cachectic patients, so a 24-hour urine for creatinine clearance should be performed. Patients with other known diseases such as a "cured" malignancy, collagen vascular disorder, or diabetes mellitus must undergo detailed evaluation to exclude end-organ involvement. Finally, hepatic dysfunction must be evaluated to exclude the presence of chronic hepatitis or underlying cirrhosis.

Conditions that could create postoperative complications should also be diagnosed. Cholelithiasis and diverticulitis are common following transplantation in older patients (21). Preoperative identification can aid in postoperative management. Abdominal ultrasonography is performed in all patients at many centers, as is abdominal computerized tomographic (CT) imaging in individuals with any prior intra-abdominal process. Individuals who are PPD positive should be treated, either before or immediately following transplantation, to prevent disease reactivation.

Visits should occur at least monthly, and often may be increased to several times a month based on clinical stability. Hospitalizations or emergency room visits should be reviewed. The patient's symptoms, a daily record of weight, and the need for additional oral diuretics should be reviewed. A flexible diuretic program is often essential to maintain a stable volume status. For a patient who has progressive cachexia, low output symptoms, or end-organ hypoperfusion, an admission for hemodynamic monitoring, adjustment of vasodilators, or inotropic support may be indicated.

Monthly assessments should include a complete blood profile, coagulation status for anticoagulated patients, and measures of electrolytes and renal and hepatic function. Patients who have significant swings in weight or who require potent diuretics such as metolazone often will require weekly electrolytes to avoid severe hyponatremia, hypokalemia, or worsening prerenal azotemia. Chest films are typically not helpful in assessing left-sided filling pressures, but they should be performed whenever symptoms suggestive of pulmonary infection develop.

Sudden cardiac death remains the principal cause of death in outpatients awaiting transplantation. Patients with ischemic heart disease appear to be at slightly higher risk for sudden death (22). Close attention to electrolytes and avoidance of excessive diuresis are important in minimizing the risk of ventricular arrhythmias. Empiric use of antiarrhythmic therapy is ineffective in decreasing the risk of sudden death. Patients with a prior history of symptomatic ventricular arrhythmias or out-of-hospital arrest are candidates for AICD placement. Mortality in patients with an

AICD is less than 5% per year while awaiting transplantation (11). Controlled trials evaluating prophylactic AICD placement for asymptomatic ventricular tachyarrhythmias are underway.

As the pretransplant period may be quite extended, most patients report insomnia and anxiety. Many will experience frank depression with hopelessness, suicidal ideation, loss of appetite, and occasionally psychosis (23). Diazepam and lorazepam are often useful; chloral hydrate is helpful for sleep disturbances. Reactive depression often responds to tricyclic or tetracyclic agents. Psychiatric counseling and pharmacologic management are quite useful during the waiting period, establishing the basis for a therapeutic relationship following transplantation (see Chapter 34).

Reassessment of Need for Transplantation

All listed patients should be periodically reevaluated. Some patients may become too compromised by progressive end-organ dysfunction to undergo transplantation. More importantly, a significant percentage of patients will improve symptomatically (24). Patients who require inotropic support should have at least one and possibly several attempts at conversion to an oral program. Steimle et al have demonstrated that up to 30% of patients with acute onset dilated cardiomyopathy will demonstrate major improvement in left ventricular function (25). Stevenson et al have shown that peak oxygen uptake may also improve in ambulatory candidates awaiting transplantation (24). Based on initial symptoms and peak oxygen uptake <14 mL/kg/min, 30% of patients improved sufficiently to warrant inactivation from the waiting list. Two-year survival was excellent at 85% without the need for relisting. Peak oxygen uptake should therefore be reassessed every 6 months in ambulatory patients. Left ventricular ejection fraction should also be reassessed every 6 to 12 months.

IMMUNOBIOLOGY

Role of HLA Antigens

As with other solid organ allografts, Clinical heart transplantation can be successfully performed despite multiple HLA mismatches between donor and recipient (see also Chapter 4). The occurrence and severity of allograft rejection may be more dependent on how donor antigens are expressed than the actual phenotypes (26). Cell surface expression of MHC antigens is not static but is influenced by a variety of immunologic stimuli. Cellular rejection episodes are typically associated with focal or generalized expression of class I antigens on myocytes. Treatment promptly decreases MHC antigen expression in the allograft. Viral infections, particularly cytomegalovirus, also increase class I antigen expression and may initiate rejection episodes.

HLA-DR antigens are easily induced on endothelium and remain elevated throughout transplantation (26). During rejection episodes, DR expression is particularly enhanced. Because endothelial cells are the major initiation site of the host immune response, class II expression may contribute to the development of chronic rejection or graft atherosclerosis. In contrast to this differential expression of class II antigens, class I HLA-A and HLA-B antigens are routinely expressed in equal density on endothelial and interstitial cells.

HLA matching reduces the strength of the immune response and improves survival in kidney and bone marrow recipients (27). Currently, donor hearts are allocated without HLA consideration due to the severe donor shortage and the limited ability of the allograft to survive prolonged ischemia. The chance occurrence of zero or one HLA mismatch constitutes less than 2% of all cardiac transplant recipients, whereas 18% to 20% demonstrate mismatches at all six major HLA loci (28,29). Patients with two or less mismatches have a 54% incidence of freedom from rejection at 1 year, compared to 36% for patients with three or more mismatches (29). Mismatching at the HLA-DR locus also appears to increase the frequency and intensity of allograft rejection (30). While the influence of HLA mismatching on allograft survival has produced differing conclusions, the largest retrospective study by Opelz showed only a modest improvement in 3-year graft survival in partially HLA-matched recipients (28).

Hyperacute Rejection and Crossmatching

When there is a possibility of pre-formed HLA antibodies in the recipient, serum must be screened against a panel (usually 40–60) of common random antigens [panel of reactive antibodies (PRA) screen]. The percentage of antigens to which the recipient has pre-formed antibodies is reported as a "degree of sensitization." The PRA is usually less than 5% in patients without prior exposure to foreign antigens from blood transfusions, previous allografts, or pregnancies (31). A PRA consistently above 10% or isolation of an antibody against a specific HLA specificity indicates the need for a prospective cytotoxic crossmatch with donor lymphocytes and recipient serum, in order to decrease the possibility of hyperacute rejection (see Chapter 2).

The presence of circulating anti-HLA antibodies decreases the probability of long-term survival after transplantation despite a negative prospective donor-specific lymphocyte crossmatch. Although it is not predictive of the number of acute rejection episodes, a pretransplant PRA greater than 25% is associated with decreased short-term survival (32). In addition, unsensitized patients who produce anti-HLA antibodies within 6 months after transplantation exhibit increased mortality, more humoral rejection, and a greater incidence of transplant atherosclerosis than non–antibody producers (33,34).

A positive crossmatch precludes transplantation. Many highly sensitized transplant candidates, therefore, may die while awaiting a crossmatch-negative donor. Strategies to reduce the PRA are thus highly desirable. Preoperative plasmapheresis, treatment with azathioprine, or use of photochemotherapy have been advocated (35) (see also Chapter 14). Successful immunomodulation of highly sensitized heart transplant candidates has also been accomplished with intravenous immunoglobulin, alone or combined with cyclophosphamide (36,37). Post-transplant treatment with high-dose intravenous immunoglobulin (IV Ig) has also been reported to control acute humoral rejection in cardiac allograft recipients (38). Whether therapies aimed at reducing PRA before or after transplantation can improve survival remains to be proven.

ANESTHETIC MANAGEMENT: PREOPERATIVE PREPARATION

The patient should be brought to the operating room well in advance of the anticipated starting time, and an arterial catheter should be inserted in the radial artery followed by a multiport central venous line. A vitamin K preparation should be administered to anticoagulated patients. Most institutions also recommend antacids or H_2 blockers. Pulmonary artery catheters are not routinely used except in hemodynamically unstable patients or individuals with pulmonary hypertension. Benzodiazepines are used in anxious patients, and oxygen is administered by face mask.

Induction of anesthesia should be dictated by progress of the donor operation. Anesthetic techniques used for other cardiac surgical patients with impaired left ventricular function are appropriate for the transplant recipient (39). Fentanyl is the most commonly administered anesthetic, and its dosage is comparable to that used in other cardiac surgical patients. Unstable patients may require inotropic support, intra-aortic balloon counterpulsation, or rapid institution of cardiopulmonary bypass. Under ideal circumstances, the donor heart should arrive in the operating room as the recipient's ascending aorta is cannulated.

Table 23.5. Criteria for Cardiac Donors

Donor Characteristics
Age <50 years (donors between 50–60 years may be considered)
Blood type (ABO) compatibility with recipient
Normal or acceptable ventricular function after intravascular volume repletion; dopamine requirement below 10 μg/kg/min
Lack of evidence of cardiac disease or trauma
Absence of prolonged cardiac arrest (>15 min)
Absence of intracardiac injections
Lack of evidence of bacteremia
Donor body weight between 80% and 125% of recipient's body weight
Anticipated ischemic time less than 4–5 hours
Absolute Contraindications to Donor Procurement
HIV-positive serology
Death from carbon monoxide; blood carboxyhemoglobin level >20%
Intractable ventricular arrhythmias
Arterial saturation <80% on 100% oxygen and positive end-expiratory pressure (PEEP)
Documented myocardial infarction
Intracardiac tumor
Significant valvular disease
Severe global ventricular dysfunction; ejection fraction <10%–20%
Severe coronary atherosclerosis by angiography
Relative Contraindications to Donor Procurement
Hepatitis B surface antigen or hepatitis C antibody positivity
History of non–central nervous system malignancy
Significant cardiac contusion by ECG or echocardiography
Profound, prolonged hypotension requiring high-dose vasopressor support
Recurrent supraventricular arrhythmias
Prolonged cardiopulmonary resuscitation (>30 min within 24 hours of organ harvest)
Prolonged need for high-dose inotropic support (dopamine >15 μg/kg/min or comparable dosage of epinephrine, norepinephrine, or dobutamine) for more than 24 hours
Severe left ventricular hypertrophy on echocardiography
Mild to moderate global left ventricular hypokinesis by echocardiography
Noncritical coronary atherosclerotic disease
History of intravenous drug usage or high-risk behavior

SURGICAL TECHNIQUES

The Cardiac Donor

The mechanism of brain death, the occurrence of a cardiac arrest or resuscitation, and the extent of hypotension, hypoxia, or trauma should be determined for the cardiac donor. Conventional coronary risk factors (family history, obesity, hypertension, diabetes mellitus, and smoking) should be assessed in donors over the age of 30 years. Cardiac donor guidelines are summarized in Table 23.5 (see also Chapter 15). Numerous relative contraindications exist but the final decision to accept a donor organ is made on a case-by-case basis, depending on the medical urgency of the prospective recipient (40).

Acceptable age limits have gradually risen from 35 to over 60 (41). Recent reports from the International Society for Heart and Lung Transplantation (ISHLT) Registry demonstrate an incremental risk for post-transplant mortality with cardiac donors above the age of 40 (42). Early graft function may be impaired, and older donors often require significantly higher inotropic support. A threefold increase in late atherosclerosis has also been reported and argues that older donors should probably be used for older recipients whenever possible. Donor hearts with significant epicardial coronary disease have been transplanted in unusual circumstances but are associated with a high incidence of early graft nonfunction.

Donor Evaluation

A history of major medical disorders should be elicited from family members whenever possible, and a complete general physical examination should be performed. Creatine kinase (CK) and isoenzyme measurements (or troponin assessment) are important if chest trauma or cardiopulmonary resuscitation has occurred. The electrocardiogram should be relatively normal, although ST and T wave abnormalities, premature atrial contractions, or atrial fibrillation do not exclude donation. Occasionally, global "neurogenic" T wave inversions are noted in patients with head injuries. Pathologic Q waves, ST segment elevation, or severe left ventricular hypertrophy (LVH) typically preclude donation (Fig 23.2).

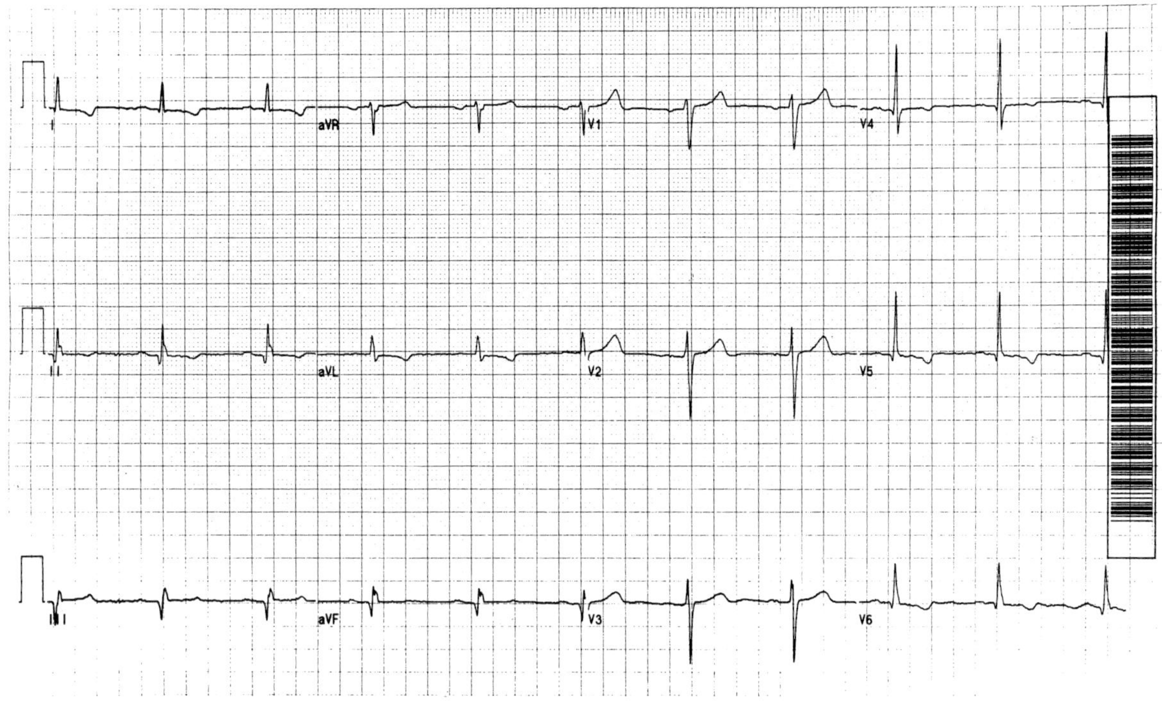

A

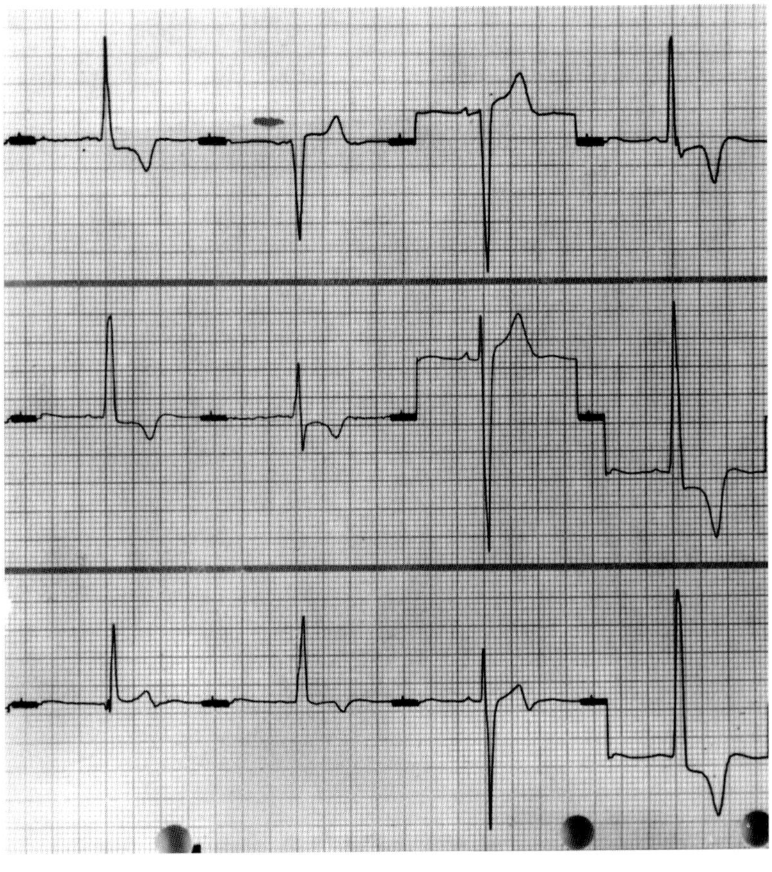

B

FIGURE 23.2. ***A.*** *Electrocardiogram from a potential donor showing evidence for a clear-cut transmural inferior myocardial infarction.* ***B.*** *Electrocardiogram from a potential donor demonstrating pronounced left vertricular hypertrophy. An echocardiogram confirmed a free wall thickness of 15 mm. The degree of hypertrophy that precludes transplantation varies among centers and is influenced by donor age, total ischemic time, and recipient stability.*

Echocardiography is an essential tool for donor evaluation, whenever it is available. Global or segmental wall motion abnormalities should be excluded. Transthoracic or transesophageal echocardiography is especially important when weaning inotropic drug support has been difficult, electrocardiographic abnormalities exist, or the donor has received CPR or chest trauma.

Mitral valve prolapse is common and need not exclude donation unless severe mitral regurgitation is present. A bicuspid aortic valve is occasionally seen. The presence of significant aortic stenosis or regurgitation generally precludes donation. Mild left ventricular hypertrophy is usually acceptable, but marked LVH (wall thickness >15 mm) usually precludes transplantation. Donors with a history of short cardiac arrest times but well-preserved cardiac function may often be used successfully, particularly pediatric donors. The circumstances that produced the arrest are of utmost importance—a hypoxic arrest due to respiratory insufficiency would not preclude donation whereas a syncopal spell or witnessed primary cardiac arrest would commonly exclude donation.

Finally, the presence of global left ventricular dysfunction or high-dose inotropic dependence increases the risk of primary graft failure. The extent of hypokinesis that will promptly reverse remains uncertain, but it is influenced by donor age and presence of other cardiac risk factors. Ischemic times up to 5 hours for adults and 8 hours for pediatric donors are not associated with increased graft loss or abnormal cardiac function (43). A young donor with mild to moderate impairment in ventricular function might be considered for local retrieval but would be less ideal for an anticipated ischemic time of 5 to 6 hours.

Coronary angiography should be performed whenever feasible in males older than 45 years, in women older than 50 years of age, or whenever significant coronary risk factors exist (40,44). Coronary angiography in older donors has expanded the potential pool and has not been associated with the development of early atherosclerosis (45).

Donor Management Prior to Cardiectomy

Monitoring of central venous pressure (CVP) is highly desirable with a goal of a CVP of 5 to 10 mm Hg and a blood pressure above 100 mm Hg. Persistent hypotension despite an adequate CVP requires inotropic support. Dobutamine (2–10 μg/kg/min) is generally effective. Inotropes can generally be weaned quite readily following volume repletion provided that profound peripheral vasomotor collapse is not present. Most centers are reluctant to use cardiac donors who require greater than 15 μg/kg/min of dopamine (or the equivalent of another α-agonist) unless echocardiography shows normal ventricular function. The use of a pulmonary artery catheter for optimization of filling pressures and assessment of peripheral vascular resistance is extremely valuable for marginal donors. Thyroxine (Synthroid, 3 μg/kg IV) is frequently administered to potential donors who are hemodynamically unstable or demonstrate impaired contractility on echocardiography, but its efficacy remains controversial (40,46).

Size-Matching Considerations

Donor and recipient have traditionally been matched to achieve a weight ratio >0.8. However, successful transplantation has been performed using donors well outside this range. Severely undersized donors may provide inadequate cardiac output and require prolonged inotropic support. Conversely, markedly oversized donors may not adequately fit into the recipient's mediastinum or may produce a high output syndrome. Oversizing is rarely a problem because the recipient usually has profound cardiomegaly and substantial size mismatches may be tolerated. Exercise hemodynamics demonstrate that recipients of undersized donors increase cardiac output at the expense of elevated filling pressures and heart rates (47,48). The use of undersized female donors for male recipients with pulmonary hypertension has been shown to increase the risk of primary graft failure.

The Donor Operation

Heart and lung procurement are generally performed as part of a multiorgan harvest and require a coordinated effort among teams to ensure donor stability and optimal organ recovery (see Chapter 15). Following standard median sternotomy, the heart is inspected for evidence of blunt trauma, occult coronary atherosclerosis, valvular disease, or congenital abnormalities. The great vessels are mobilized and encircled with umbilical tape (see Fig 23.3A) (49). The inferior vena cava is also encircled with umbilical tape and the superior vena encircled with heavy silk ligatures. The donor is heparinized, the abdominal aorta and vena cavae are cannulated, and the aorta is clamped. The inferior vena cava is then transected just below the right atrium to prevent distention of the right heart, and a pulmonary vein is incised to prevent left heart distention.

Cold crystalloid cardioplegia (10 mL/kg) is rapidly instilled via a cardioplegic needle inserted into the ascending aorta. Liberal amounts (5–6 liters) of cold saline at 4°C are applied to the heart for rapid topical cooling (49,50). The heart is then excised, beginning with division of the superior vena cava and completion of the division of the inferior vena cava. The aorta is divided at the aortic cross-clamp and the heart is retracted cephalad. The pulmonary veins are individually divided and the pulmonary artery is divided near its bifurcation. The arrested heart is immediately placed in a sterile bag of saline at 4°C. At least two sterile bags are generally used and the heart is packed in cold physiologic solution surrounded by crushed ice for transport.

Optimal preservation of the donor heart prior to restoration of coronary blood flow is a key element in successful cardiac transplantation. The right ventricle is very sensitive to the quality of myocardial protection (49). A standardized method for heart preservation that generally includes single-dose cold cardioplegia and static hypothermia has evolved (50). A variety of cardioplegic solutions, typically those used in ordinary cardiac surgery, have been successfully used. Solutions are generally slightly hyperosmolar and have an increased potassium concentration. Although University of Wisconsin solution has been adopted at many transplant centers, conflicting results exist concerning its merits compared with conventional cardioplegia (50). Intermittent warm blood cardioplegia is also under study, but concerns exist regarding the generation of free radical scavengers during reperfusion (50).

Future improvements in myocardial protection should enhance cardiac function and allow a greater possibility of HLA matching in cardiac transplantation as the period of adequate preservation is extended beyond the current 4 to 6 hours.

The Recipient Procedure/Intraoperative Considerations

Current orthotopic transplantation differs little from the original description by Lower and Shumway. The recipient heart is excised by dividing the aorta and pulmonary artery just distal to the valves. The right and left atria are excised close to the atrioventricular ring, leaving most of the intra-atrial septum in place. A generous cuff of atria (including the pulmonary veins) and intra-atrial septum are available for anastomosis to the donor heart (Fig. 23.3).

The donor heart is prepared for implantation by probing the fossa ovalis for evidence of a patent foramen ovale; if found, it is surgically closed. The left atrial anastomosis is generally performed first using a single, continuous Prolene suture (44). When the ischemic time has been long, the left-sided suture lines may be completed first, followed by removal of the aortic cross-clamp and completion of the right-sided anastomoses (49). The entire procedure is generally completed within 3 hours.

Recently, an alternate technique of bicaval anastomosis has been increasingly utilized. The bicaval technique has been shown to preserve right atrial geometry, reduce the degree of resting or exercise-induced tricuspid regurgitation, and decrease the need for permanent pacemaker implantation (51). Whether this modification improves exercise capacity or long-term cardiac function remains to be determined.

Although the first successful human transplant by Barnard used the heterotopic technique, it is rarely used today. This "piggy-back" form of transplantation is reserved for situations in which an unexpected discrepancy exists between donor and recipient size such that the donor heart could not be reasonably expected to maintain recipient circulation (44). The use of heterotopic transplantation in patients with severe pulmonary hypertension, one of its original indications, has proved disappointing; however, it is still occasionally used. Numerous disadvantages of the technique include its higher operative risk, the need for anticoagulation to prevent thromboembolism from the recipient heart, persistent angina in patients with ischemic heart disease, and greater difficulty of endomyocardial biopsy (52).

Weaning from bypass is usually straightforward. The donor heart often will begin spontaneous activity following rewarming. Isoproterenol is often required due to cardiac denervation and should be administered at 0.01–0.02 μg/kg/min and increased as necessary to maintain a heart rate above 85 beats/min. Renal dose dopamine (2 μg/kg/min) is also often administered. Temporary pacing wires are usually placed on the donor atrium and ventricle. For chronotropic unresponsiveness to isoproterenol or temporary heart block,

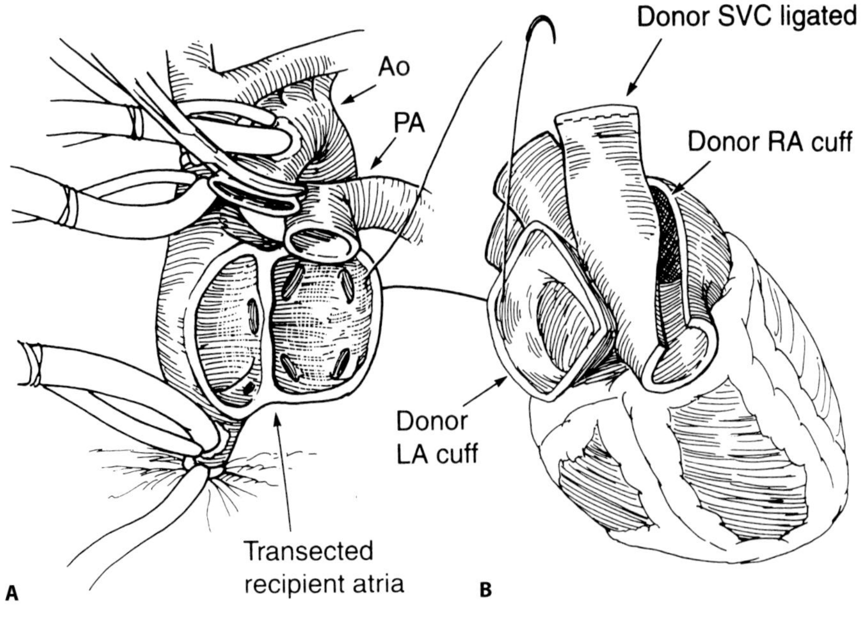

FIGURE 23.3. ***A.*** *Surgical technique for orthotopic cardiac transplantation. Following cardiectomy, the posterior portions of the right atrium, left atrium, and intra-atrial septum as well as the transected great vessels are visible. The sinoatrial node and the pulmonary veins are avoided during atrial and caval dissection.* ***B.*** *The left atrial suture line is begun first, starting near the recipient superior pulmonary vein as shown. The right atrial suture line is then completed in a similar manner. End-to-end anastomoses of the main pulmonary artery and ascending aorta complete the operation. (Reprinted with permission from Vlahakes G, Lemmer J, Behrendt D, Austen WE, eds. Handbook of patient care in cardiac surgery. Boston: Little, Brown, 1994:236.)*

atrial (AOO) or atrioventricular sequential (DDO) pacing is begun (32). Aprotinin and fresh frozen plasma are useful in patients with prior cardiac surgery, hepatic dysfunction, or coagulopathy.

Allograft function is often subnormal for the first 4 postoperative days and is particularly pronounced during the first 6 hours. This depression can usually be reversed with inotropic support. Occasionally, the donor heart is inadequate to permit weaning from bypass. Older donors, excessively cold cardioplegia, and prolonged ischemic time contribute to primary graft failure (42). Hyperacute rejection may also occasionally produce intraoperative graft dysfunction. Therapeutic options range from high-dose inotropic support to temporary mechanical support or retransplantation.

Intraoperative acute right ventricular failure is an ominous development and is most likely in patients with preexisting pulmonary hypertension. It is characterized by marked dilatation of the right ventricle, a rise in CVP >20 mm Hg, a fall in left atrial pressure <10 mm Hg, and systemic hypotension. The pulmonary artery anastomosis should be reexplored to exclude torsion or intussusception producing outflow obstruction. If no anatomic defect is identified, pharmacologic support should be instituted immediately. Isoproterenol and dobutamine may improve right ventricular contractility. Pulmonary vasodilatation is often achieved with the use of prostaglandin E_1 (0.5–5.0 μg/min) or inhaled nitric oxide (20–80 ppm). Occasionally, right ventricular assistance with an Abiomed or Biomedicus centrifugal pump may be necessary.

IMMUNOSUPPRESSIVE THERAPY

Standard Agents

Immunosuppressive agents can be used for three purposes: rejection prophylaxis, maintenance therapy, and treatment of acute rejection. No regimen can be considered ideal, as all have potential side effects and none completely inhibit lymphocyte activation against donor-specific alloantigens. During the past decade, triple-drug therapy consisting of prednisone, cyclosporine (CsA), and azathioprine has been used at most centers for chronic maintenance therapy and has been associated with improved patient survival and a decreased rate of allograft rejection (53). Use of three synergistic agents permits lower dosages, decreased side effects, and enhanced immunosuppression (Table 23.6).

Cyclosporine was first used in cardiac transplantation in 1980. Its principal benefit has been reducing the severity rather than the incidence of allograft rejection (see Chapter 6). Cyclosporine pharmacokinetics vary considerably among patients and precise dosage adjustments are required to maintain a therapeutic blood level. Since drug interactions are common, levels must be checked frequently when new drugs are added. The inhibition of CsA metabolism by agents such as ketoconazole and diltiazem can reduce cyclosporine dosage requirement and decrease cost. Azathioprine is a potent but nonspecific inhibitor of lymphocyte proliferation. The dose is generally 2 mg/kg but must be decreased if severe leukopenia, anemia, or thrombocytopenia occurs. Cyclophosphamide may replace azathioprine for intolerant patients.

Table 23.6. Massachusetts General Hospital Immunosuppressive Protocol for Maintenance Therapy During Various Phases Following Cardiac Transplantation

Phase	Agent	Protocol
Preoperative	Cyclosporine	None
	Azathioprine	None
Intraoperative	Methylprednisolone	500 mg intravenously following weaning off cardiopulmonary bypass
	Azathioprine	5 mg/kg intravenously
Postoperative	Methylprednisolone	125 mg intravenously every 8 h (× 4–6 doses)
	Prednisone	2 mg/kg daily, bid dosing; rapidly taper to 0.5 mg/kg daily prior to discharge; slowly taper to 5 mg daily as outpatient
	Azathioprine	2 mg/kg daily orally; decrease for leukocyte count <4000/mm^3
	Cyclosporine (Neoral)	4–6 mg/kg orally or per nasogastric tube given as a twice daily dose titrate to achieve a trough serum level of 200–250 ng/mL; taper to achieve a level of 150–200 ng/mL beyond 6 months; aim for long-term level <100 ng/mL in presence of chronic renal dysfunction
	OKT-3	5 mg intravenously daily (× 7–14 days) in lieu of cyclosporine in the presence of preoperative renal dysfunction (creatinine >2.5 mg/dL) or early postoperative oliguria or renal failure Premedicate for initial doses with: methylprednisolone, 500 mg intravenously acetaminophen, 650 mg orally before and 2 hours after dose diphenhydramine hydrochloride, 50 mg intravenously before and 2 hours after dose Thirty minutes after OKT-3 administration: hydrocortisone, 100 mg intravenously Monitor CD3 cell clearance

Although corticosteroid dosing protocols vary, most centers administer high-dose methylprednisolone in the immediate perioperative period and subsequently initiate oral prednisone, which is gradually tapered. Successful withdrawal of steroids can be accomplished in 30% to 50% of patients (55). Two strategies may be employed: early withdrawal, usually accomplished within 3 to 4 weeks of transplantation following administration of a course of OKT-3 or antithymocyte globulin (ATG), or late withdrawal occurring 6 to 12 months following transplantation. The latter is generally accomplished without the use of perioperative cytolytic induction therapy. Avoiding steroid-related morbidity is particularly beneficial in diabetics, in older transplant recipients at risk for progressive osteoporosis, in those with recent infections at the time of transplantation or requiring perioperative mechanical assist devices, and in pediatric recipients. Acute allograft rejection may occur following steroid withdrawal, and 8% to 30% of patients will require reinstitution of maintenance steroids (55). Steroid withdrawal does not appear to adversely affect allograft function, decrease patient survival, or lower the incidence of transplant vascular disease (56).

Corticosteroid withdrawal must be individualized. It is more likely to succeed in older individuals but has rarely been successful in female recipients (57). The desire to withdraw steroids must be balanced with the need to minimize toxicity of other immunosuppressive agents. Steroid withdrawal may be inappropriate for a patient with renal dysfunction in whom the CsA level must be kept as low as feasible. Early withdrawal is attractive because surveillance biopsies are frequently performed; however, the probability of rejection is also highest at that time. Further, some patients will display a threshold phenomenon in which rejection is absent at low doses of corticosteroids but consistently recurs following a slight dose decrement.

The role of prophylactic cytolytic therapy employing either polyclonal ATG or monoclonal OKT-3 remains controversial (see Chapter 13). Both agents decrease the rate of cellular rejection during the first 3 months following transplantation (58). OKT-3 and ATG appear equally efficacious in immunoprophylaxis. Because a 14-day course of induction therapy will often prolong hospitalization, shorter courses (5 to 7 days) have been advocated; however, this does not appear to decrease the incidence of early rejection (59).

Routine use of cytolytic therapy has some disadvantages. The agents are expensive, have a high incidence of side effects (including hemodynamic instability and pulmonary edema), and may increase the risk of cytomegalovirus (CMV) infection (60). Sensitization to OTK-3 occurs in 10% to 40% of patients and may preclude future use during acute severe rejection. The cumulative incidence of rejection, freedom from rejection, or 12-month survival do not differ between programs that do or do not employ routine cytolytic therapy. Further, the risk of post-transplant lymphoproliferative disease appears to be significantly higher when the cumulative dose of OKT-3 exceeds 75 mg (61).

Newer Immunosuppressive Agents

Several immunosuppressive agents have more recently been introduced and other novel agents are undergoing clinical trials. Tacrolimus (FK506), a potent fungal macrolide, is used either for primary immunosuppression or, more typically, for rescue therapy for refractory rejection (see Chapter 9). Armitage et al reported no difference in survival or freedom from rejection in cardiac transplant recipients receiving tacrolimus-based maintenance immunosuppression compared to historical controls who received conventional triple-drug immunosuppression (62). Fewer tacrolimus-treated patients, however, had recurrent rejection (28% vs. 48%) and only 4% required OKT-3 rescue therapy.

Tsamandas et al found no qualitative differences in the histopathologic appearance of various allograft syndromes between two groups of heart transplant recipients, one of which received tacrolimus while the other had a CsA-based regimen with ATG induction (63). The authors concluded that the histopathologic criteria used to diagnose various graft syndromes are applicable under tacrolimus immunosuppression.

In a single-center randomized trial comparing tacrolimus and CsA for the prevention of acute cardiac rejection, Meiser et al reported similar efficacy and safety profiles for the two regimens (64). They also noted a higher interpatient variance in absorption associated with oral tacrolimus during the first few days after transplantation and suggested that intravenous therapy be used during that period. In a multicenter trial performed in Europe, no significant differences in either rejection or survival rates were evident between heart transplant recipients randomly treated with either tacrolimus or CsA (65). The investigators concluded that tacrolimus provides a viable alternative to treatment with CsA, particularly when combined with antilymphocytic therapy.

Mycophenolate mofetil (MMF), mizoribine, and brequinar are more specific and potent inhibitors of DNA synthesis than is azathioprine. Uncontrolled clinical trials have shown MMF to be an effective adjunct immunosuppressive agent in cardiac transplant recipients with recurrent or persistent rejection (66). Gastrointestinal symptoms including nausea (47%), transient diarrhea (29%), and dyspepsia (12%) are common (67). A recently reported prospective randomized clinical trial comparing the efficacy of MMF to azathioprine concluded that the MMF-treated group had reduced mortality in the first year after transplantation (68). This drug is reviewed in detail in Chapter 10.

EARLY POSTOPERATIVE MANAGEMENT

ICU Management

Controlled studies of strict reverse precautions have failed to show a significant decrease in infectious complications compared to good hand washing practices and a face mask (69). Nursing coverage should not include the concomitant care of an infected patient. Standard postoperative monitoring includes an arterial line, Foley catheter, and a central venous catheter. Pulmonary artery catheterization or use of a left atrial catheter is reserved for patients with pulmonary hypertension or acute right or left ventricular dysfunction. Circulatory management should include maintenance of adequate arterial pressure, central venous pressure, and urinary output, as well as the use of blood products and aprotinin to control bleeding.

Inotropic support is routinely maintained for the first 2 to 4 postoperative days (44,49). The denervated donor heart is highly dependent upon circulating catecholamines, has a relatively fixed stroke volume and impaired diastolic relaxation, and is initially depleted of high energy metabolites (70). Isoproterenol (0.005–0.010 μg/kg/min) is administered centrally after donor reimplantation and weaned over 24 to 72 hours. Renal-dose dopamine (2–3 μg/kg/min) is also routinely employed to augment urinary output. Dobutamine or amrinone are occasionally necessary for transient right or left ventricular dysfunction. Alpha-adrenergic support is often transiently necessary in patients who have been receiving high doses of ACE inhibitors preoperatively or who require amrinone or prostaglandin E_1 to control pulmonary hypertension. Sodium nitroprusside or nitroglycerin is useful for the occasional hypertensive patient. When the CVP exceeds left atrial pressure by greater than 4 mm Hg, right ventricular dysfunction must be considered.

PVR will often increase acutely during emergence from anesthesia, and the simultaneous monitoring of left and right atrial or pulmonary artery pressures during awakening and ventilatory weaning is particularly important in patients with documented pulmonary hypertension or early right heart failure. After 24 to 48 hours of support, PVR usually falls and right ventricular function improves sufficiently to allow extubation. Occasionally, mechanical right ventricular assistance may be required.

When inotropic or vasodilator agents are no longer needed, central venous and arterial lines should be expeditiously removed to lessen the possibility of line-related bacteremia. During the initial 72 hours, daily chest x-rays, electrocardiograms, and blood specimens for complete blood count, coagulation studies, electrolytes, and renal function should be sent. Cyclosporine levels should be monitored several times per week until hospital discharge. After 2 to 5 days, stable transplant recipients are transferred to a surgical floor to begin a program of education and cardiac rehabilitation.

Bacterial and viral surveillance culturing is essential and a prophylactic strategy for minimizing infectious complications has been developed. Cephalosporin and intravenous vancomycin are administered until indwelling catheters, chest tubes, and pacing wires have been removed. Recipient and donor IgG serum titers for CMV and toxoplasmosis are compared. Those individuals who are CMV or toxoplasmosis negative and receive a positive donor are treated to prevent primary disease (71).

Cardiac Arrhythmias, Conduction Disease, and Pacing

The transplanted heart functions independently of sympathetic and vagal-mediated reflexes. Sinus node dysfunction is common and is more likely following prolonged cold ischemia or in older donors. If chronotropic response is inadequate (resting heart rate <80 to 90 beats/min), or if transient heart block is evident, atrial (AOO) or atrioventricular sequential pacing (DOO) is initiated. Preoperative amiodarone usage is associated with a higher frequency of sinus bradycardia and junctional rhythms and a greater incidence of short-term pacing (72). Although theophylline has been reported as effective in treating postoperative sinus node dysfunction, the experience of others has failed to support its beneficial effect (73). Temporary pacing is needed in approximately 27% of transplant recipients, of whom 4% to 15% will require permanent pacing (74). Since most patients return to an active lifestyle, atrioventricular (AV) synchrony and rate responsiveness are desirable pacing characteristics.

Two independent P wave foci are often seen on electrocardiogram, as a small cuff of recipient right atrium containing the sinoatrial (SA) node typically remains when noncaval anastomoses are performed. The recipient atrial activity cannot be conducted across the atrial suture line and a dissociation of recipient P wave from donor QRS may be interpreted as third-degree heart block unless the donor P waves are also evident. Conduction abnormalities occur in 70% to 75% of patients including hemiblocks (approximately 20%), right bundle branch block (RBBB) (40% to 50%), and left bundle branch block (LBBB) (<5%) (75,76). Persistent RBBB generally carries a benign prognosis, although a higher incidence of cardiac rejection and a greater in-hospital mortality have also been reported (76).

Transient supraventricular arrhythmias including isolated premature atrial contractions (PACs), atrial fibrillation, and atrial flutter occur in the majority of patients during their initial hospitalization (77,78). Likewise, premature ventricular beats and couplets are frequently evident during the perioperative period; these decrease in frequency over time, and are unrelated to allograft rejection (77). Sustained ventricular arrhythmias are quite uncommon; they respond best to treatment of the underlying cause such as hypomagnesemia or hypokalemia. Lidocaine and procainamide are safe and effective for treating ventricular arrhythmias.

The occurrence of atrial fibrillation beyond 2 weeks following transplantation may be associated with an increased risk of late mortality (78). The onset of late atrial flutter or fibrillation should prompt endomyocardial biopsy to exclude the possibility of allograft rejection.

Antiarrhythmic agents may have different effects on the denervated heart. Digoxin is occasionally useful in slowing AV node conduction, but verapamil is generally more effective in controlling a rapid ventricular response seen in atrial fibrillation. Atropine is ineffective in treating sinus bradycardia or nodal rhythms due to the absence of vagal innervation. Quinidine and procainamide exert direct effects on atrial tissue as well as on the SA and AV nodes; these agents are effective in treating supraventricular arrhythmias that fail to respond to β-adrenergic antagonists or calcium channel blockers.

ACUTE ALLOGRAFT REJECTION

Diagnosis of Cellular Rejection

Rejection remains a leading cause of mortality in transplant recipients, despite refinements in immunosuppressive therapy. Over 90% of all acute episodes occur within the first 6 months; rejection is quite rare beyond 12 months unless immunosuppression has been decreased (79). Patients who experience late rejection typically have had recurrent rejection during the first year and require more aggressive maintenance immunosuppression (80). Factors that increase the risk of acute rejection in cardiac recipients include female gender, high titers of pre- or postoperative PRA, positive donor-specific crossmatch, and preoperative myocarditis (6,79). Conversely, less rejection occurs in patients over the age of 55, presumably due to immunological downregulation.

Clinical indicators such as blood pressure, heart rate, and electrocardiographic alterations may not occur until rejection has become quite advanced. Consequently, right ventricular endomyocardial biopsy remains the most reliable method for monitoring allograft rejection. Endomyocardial biopsy is performed under fluoroscopic or echocardiographic guidance, and four to six tissue samples are obtained from the right ventricular septum. Right heart catheterization to assess filling pressures and cardiac index should also be undertaken. Endomyocardial biopsies are initially performed weekly in adults for the first month and then every 2 to 4 weeks over the next 2 months (81). Biopsy frequency is decreased to every 3 to 4 months for the remainder of the first year and less frequently during the second year in nonrejectors (82). Additional biopsies are performed for significant changes in clinical status such as unexplained tachycardia, hypotension, or echocardiographic abnormalities.

The standardized numerical grading system of the International Society for Heart/Lung Transplantation uses five numerical categories ranging from 0 to 4 (Table 23.7) (83). The two most significant histopathologic findings are the extent and type of inflammatory cellular infiltrate and the presence and degree of myocyte necrosis (Figs. 23.4–23.7 and Plates 14–17). The location of the lymphocytic infiltrate—endocardial, perivascular, or interstitial—is also important in assessing rejection severity.

Endomyocardial biopsy is subject to significant sampling error because of the small fragment size and the heterogeneous nature of acute cellular rejection. Sharples et al have reported a 14% failure to detect moderate-severe rejection

Table 23.7. Cardiac Allograft Biopsy Grading Scheme

Cellular Rejection		
ISHLT Grade	**Description**	**Nomenclature**
0	No rejection	No rejection
1A	Focal (perivascular or interstitial) cellular infiltrate without myocyte necrosis	Mild rejection
1B	Diffuse, sparse cellular infiltrate without myocyte necrosis	Mild rejection
2	Single focus with an aggressive cellular infiltrate and/or focal myocyte necrosis	"Focal" moderate rejection
3A	Multifocal aggressive infiltrates and/or myocyte necrosis	"Low" moderate rejection
3B	Diffuse cellular inflammatory process with myocyte necrosis	"Borderline" severe rejection
4	Diffuse, aggressive cellular infiltrate ± edema, ± hemorrhage, ± vasculitis with marked myocyte necrosis	Severe acute rejection

Humoral Rejection	
Grade	**Histologic Criteria**
Mild vascular rejection	LM: Endothelial cell activation, edema hemorrhage IMF: Immunoglobulin, complement deposition within vessels ± interstitial fibrin
Moderate vascular rejection	LM: Endothelial cell activation, edema, hemorrhage ± vasculitis IMF: Immunoglobulin, complement deposition within vessels ± abundant interstitial fibrin
Severe vascular rejection	LM: Extensive infiltrates of lymphocytes, plasma cells, PMNs with myocyte necrosis, edema, hemorrhage IMF: Immunoglobulin, complement deposition within vessels; interstitial leakage of immunoglobulin, complement

ISHLT, International Society for Heart and Lung Transplantation; LM, light microscopy; IMF, immunofluorescence; PMNs, polymorphonuclear neutrophils.
Source: Adapted from Olsen S, Wagoner L, Hammond E, et al. Vascular rejection in heart transplantation: clinical correlation, treatment options, and future considerations. J Heart Lung Transplant 1993;12:S135–S142.

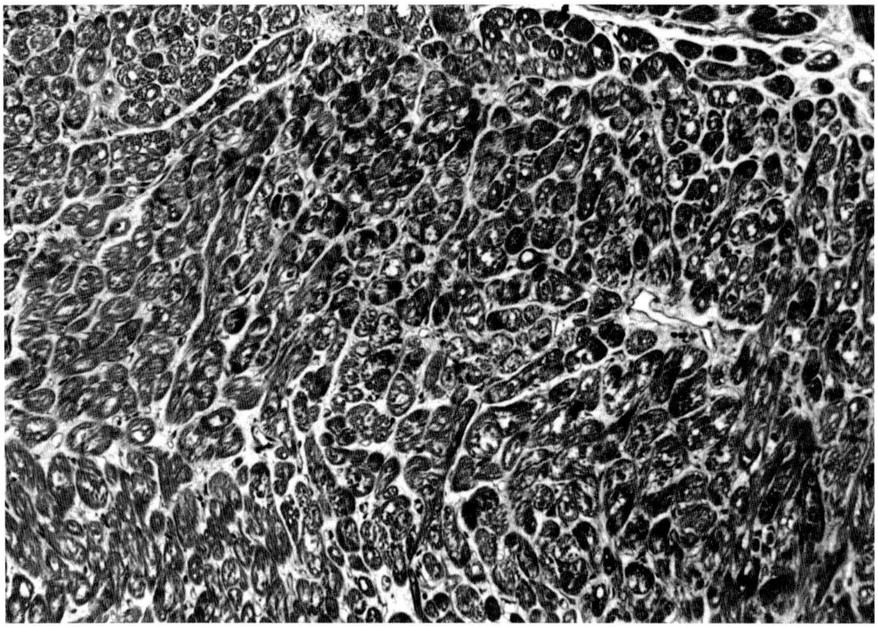

FIGURE 23.4. *ISHLT grade 0 biopsy shows no evidence for rejection (hematoxylin-eosin, ×250).*

when at least three fragments show mild rejection (84). Interobserver variability also exists in distinguishing between grade 1A and grade 3A (85). Biopsies obtained during the first 4 to 6 weeks frequently show ischemic myocardial necrosis. Although ischemic injury is usually accompanied by a less intense interstitial infiltrate and abundant macrophages and neutrophils, rejection and resolving ischemic injury may be superimposed, making histologic grading difficult. Patients who have undergone multiple prior biopsies will often have samples obtained from prior biopsy sites. An abundant inflammatory infiltrate may occasionally be present in an area of healing scar.

The use of trichrome staining is important in differentiating a healing biopsy site from an area of acute rejection (see Fig. 23.5B and Plate 15B). The "Quilty" effect has been described since the introduction of CsA and also with newer immunosuppressive drugs (86). Quilty A lesions show an abundance of subendocardial lymphocytes; Quilty B lesions show palisading of lymphocytes into the subjacent myocardium (Fig. 23.8 and Plate 18). Recent data suggest that many grade 2 biopsies may, in fact, represent en face Quilty B lesions. However, others have reported that patients with significant Quilty lesions are more likely to subsequently demonstrate allograft rejection (87). Quilty lesions do not require specific treatment.

A patient who presents with new onset heart failure or atrial flutter may require antirejection treatment despite the finding of a grade 1B biopsy. Conversely, a patient who demonstrates a grade 2 biopsy may not require additional immunosuppression if prior biopsies revealed higher rejection grades. Significant variability exists in the degree of inflammation seen on serial biopsies from the same patient. In patients receiving triple-drug immunosuppression, fewer than 25% will progress from mild (grade 1A or B) or moderate (grade 2) rejection to a higher grade of rejection on the next biopsy despite the lack of enhanced immunosuppression (88). Quantification of T-cell subtypes and immunophenotyping in serial biopsies have not been useful in predicting or managing acute rejection.

Noninvasive Diagnosis of Cellular Rejection

Monitoring the cardiac transplant recipient for allograft rejection remains challenging, as the typical recipient will experience 1.0 to 1.5 rejection episodes during the first post-transplant year (89). Fortunately, only 8% to 9% of rejection episodes present with hemodynamic compromise; over 80% respond to a single course of treatment (90). Although endomyocardial biopsy remains the current gold standard, it is invasive, costly, and subject to sampling error and misinterpretation. A variety of noninvasive methods have undergone diagnostic evaluation.

Low-grade fever, exertional dyspnea, malaise, and unexplained weight gain are common accompaniments of moderate rejection but lack specificity. Unexplained tachycardia, relative hypotension, cardiac enlargement, S_3 or S_4 gallops, and supraventricular or ventricular arrhythmias may accompany severe rejection but are uncommon in moderate rejection. Potential noninvasive screening tools include electrocardiographic findings, echocardiographic assessment, biochemical and immunologic assays, and myocardial imaging (79,91).

A fall in summated QRS voltage on surface ECG is insensitive in cyclosporine-treated patients due to the lack of significant intramyocardial edema. Intramyocardial ECG obtained from patients who have implanted pacemakers and epicardial leads may be more useful (92). A specificity of 96% has been reported for a voltage drop during daily tele-

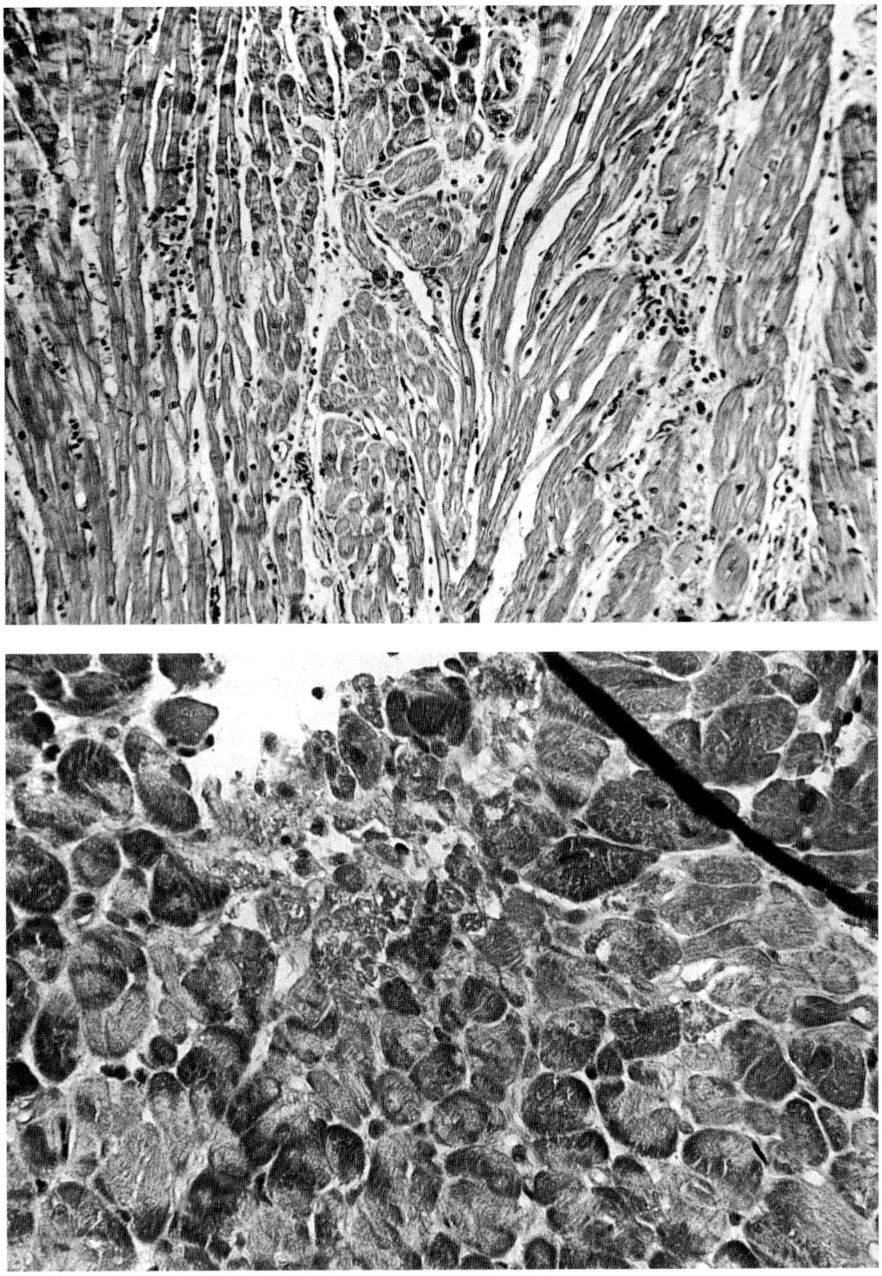

FIGURE 23.5. ***A.*** *ISHLT grade 1B biopsy shows a mild localized cellular infiltrate without evidence for myocyte necrosis (hematoxylin-eosin, ×250).* ***B.*** *Biopsy shows healing ischemic injury with myocyte loss, early granulation tissue, and an inflammatory infiltrate of mixed cellularity (hematoxylin-eosin, ×250).*

metric monitoring. The necessity of implanting a pacemaker system and the absence of confirmatory data from other groups have limited this approach. Signal-averaged ECG recording, fast-Fournier transformation of the QRS complex, and the presence of late potentials remain unproven techniques.

Systolic dysfunction on echocardiography is a late and uncommon finding in cardiac rejection. Abnormalities of diastolic function assessed using Doppler echocardiography are more sensitive and may precede histologic evidence of rejection (93). Mitral pressure half-time and isovolumetric relaxation time decrease, and early mitral flow velocity increases during acute rejection and return to baseline with enhanced immunosuppression (93,94). Although sensitivities ranging from 78% to 88% have been reported, these techniques are difficult to reproduce. In addition, because of ischemic injury, diastolic dysfunction is common early following cardiac transplantation, and may take up to 3 months to resolve. Further, late restrictive physiology after transplantation has also been recognized. Studying changes in posterior wall thickness, while quite useful in assessing rejection in infants and children, is less useful in adults.

Cytoimmunologic monitoring of T4/T8 ratios and cell surface markers is occasionally useful, but is highly influenced by viral or bacterial infections. Monitoring of transferrin receptor-positive circulating lymphocytes as well as interleukin 2 receptors (IL-2R) also correlates well with biopsy results, but is influenced by infections (91).

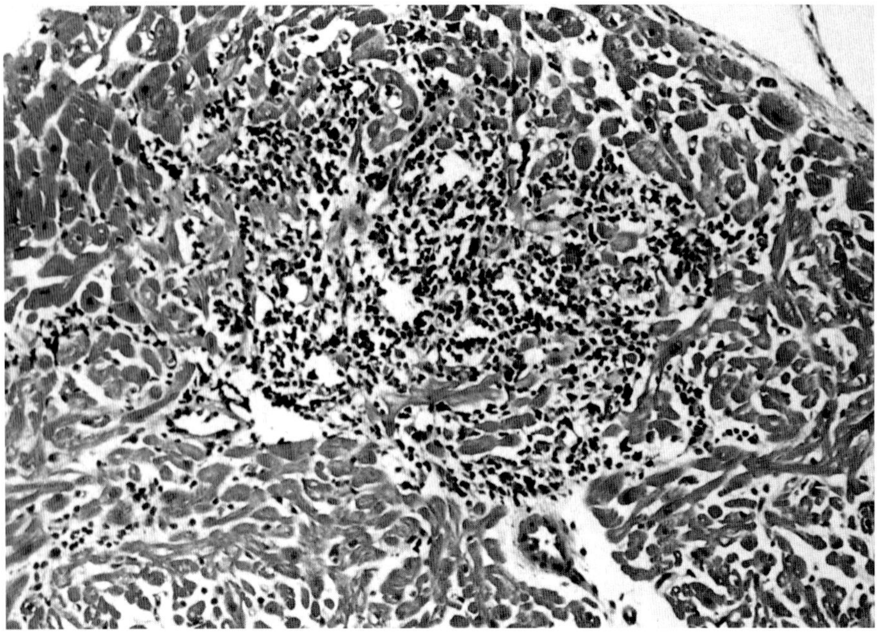

FIGURE 23.6. *ISHLT grade 2 biopsy shows focal moderate rejection with the presence of a single focus of prominent lymphocytic inflammation and/or myocyte necrosis (hematoxylin-eosin, ×250).*

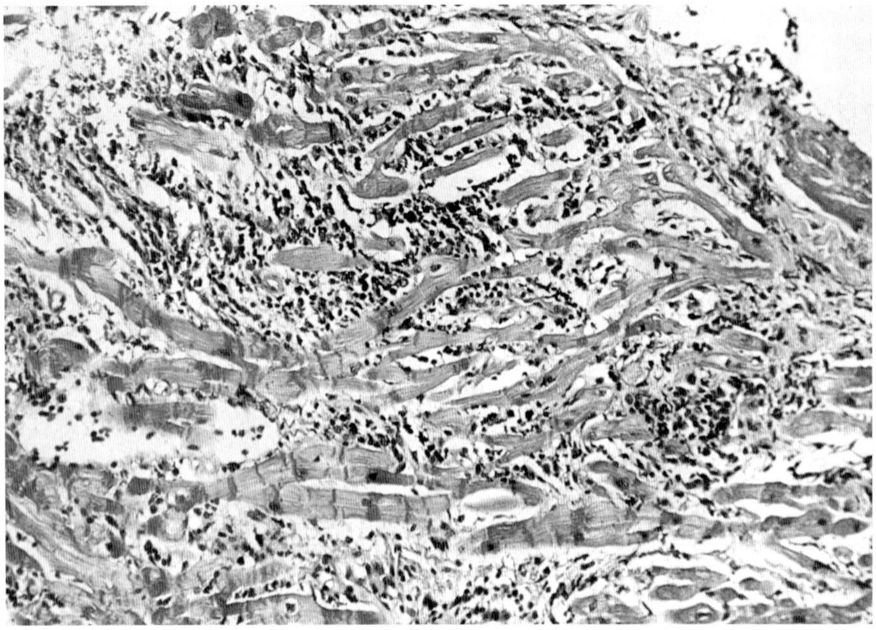

FIGURE 23.7. *ISHLT grade 3A biopsy reveals moderately severe rejection with multifocal lymphocytic infiltrates and focal myocyte necrosis. Edema and hemorrhage are absent (hematoxylin-eosin, ×250).*

Biochemical markers of immunologic activation including β_2-microglobulin, urinary polyamines (putrescine and spermidine), serum prolactin and neopterine, and breath pentane have all shown some promise, but none are routinely used (91). One potential problem with this approach is that the epiphoral markers may not reflect immunologic activity within the allograft itself.

Myocardial tissue characterization has been attempted using echocardiographic tissue density, backscatter analysis, and magnetic resonance imaging (MRI), but their clinical sensitivity and specificity remain inadequate (91). Radionuclide imaging techniques including thallium-201, technetium-99m, gallium-67, and indium-labeled leukocytes generally detect advanced rejection but have an unacceptably low sensitivity (0% to 30%) (95). Indium-111–labeled antimyosin antibody imaging has demonstrated a high sensitivity (approaching 100%), but it has a low degree of specificity. Ballester and others have shown that antimyosin uptake declines during the first year following transplantation and that a low heart–lung ratio may obviate the need for serial surveillance biopsies (96). If confirmed in larger series, a negative antimyosin scan may decrease the need for biopsies. However, its low specificity precludes it from being used to guide treatment.

Cardiac troponin T (cTnT) is an established marker of myocyte damage, and animal experiments have suggested

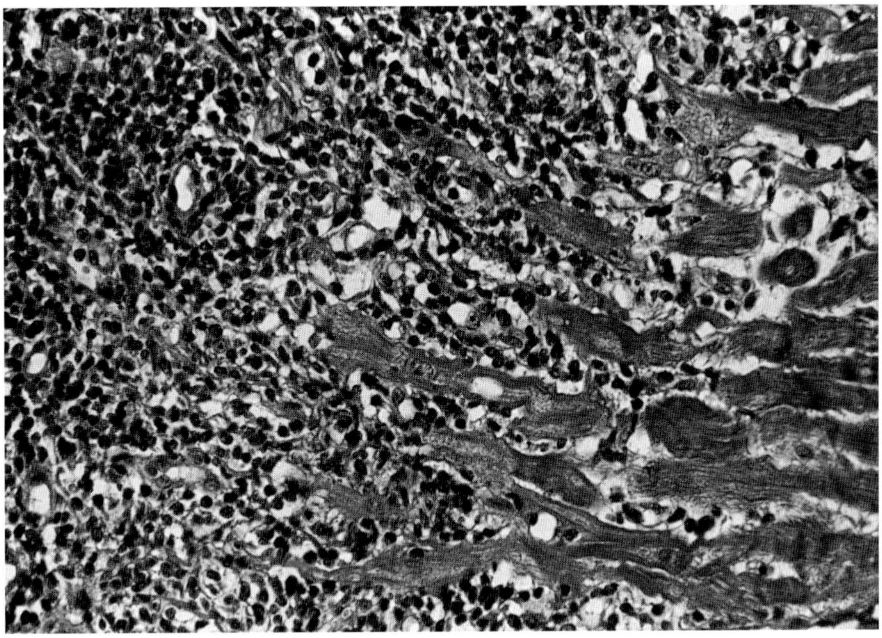

FIGURE 23.8. *Biopsy shows a "Quilty B" lesion characterized by a dense endocardial lymphocytic infiltrate extending into the subjacent myocardium (hematoxylin-eosin, ×250).*

that monitoring cTnT levels might be of value in detecting rejection. Disappointing results, however, have been reported by Alexis et al, who found cTnT to be an insensitive marker of acute rejection, both early and late after heart transplantation (97).

Diagnosis of Humoral Rejection

The main histologic features of humoral/vascular rejection are pronounced interstitial edema and endothelial cell swelling (see Table 23.7) (98). Endothelial swelling may involve capillaries, venules, and arterioles and may be subtle. More pronounced rejection may be associated with a lymphocytic or mixed cellular infiltrate. Immunoglobulin (IgG or IgM), complement, and fibrinogen deposition in linear staining patterns within the interstitium are also required for diagnosis. This form of antibody-mediated rejection typically presents within the first 3 weeks but can be seen up to 6 months following transplantation (99,100). Recently, Bonnaud concluded that immunoglobulin deposition by immunofluorescence is a nonspecific finding detected in 60% of earlier transplant recipients, thus bringing into question the utility of routine immunofluorescent studies (101). When compared to cellular rejection, humoral rejection typically occurs earlier following transplantation, is more highly associated with hemodynamic abnormalities or unexplained left ventricular dysfunction, is more resistant to augmented immunosuppression, and is associated with a higher frequency of allograft loss and mortality (102).

Cellular Rejection Treatment

Treatment is based upon associated clinical features, histologic severity, and time course during which the rejection occurs (Table 23.8) (53). Initial treatment consists of a 500- to 1000-mg pulse of methylprednisolone given intravenously for 3 days, with re-biopsy in 7 to 10 days. This approach has an 85% efficacy in reversing moderate to moderately severe rejection (79). After the initial 3 to 6 months, moderate rejection without hemodynamic compromise can be safely treated with an oral "steroid pulse" (103).

Rejection that is histologically severe (ISHLT grade 3B or 4), refractory to several courses of corticosteroids, or associated with hemodynamic compromise can usually be reversed with antilymphocyte antibody therapy. Polyclonal agents such as ATG and antilymphocyte globulin (ALG) have been largely supplanted by OKT-3, which is successful in nearly 90% of cases of rejection (104). Although randomized clinical trials comparing the efficacy of different dosage regimens are lacking, OKT-3 is usually given at 5 mg/day for 10 to 14 days, regardless of age or body size. Development by the recipient of human antimurine antibody can limit its further use. Retreatment is possible when the anti–OKT-3 titer is low and clearance of $CD3^+$ cells can be demonstrated.

Refractory and recurrent cellular rejection require alternative strategies. A change from CsA-based immunosuppression to tacrolimus is often useful (105). Methotrexate, a potent inhibitor of cellular and humoral response, may be substituted for azathioprine. The dosage should be adjusted to maintain a white blood cell count >4000 (106). Dactinomycin, 5 μg/kg every 6 weeks, may be added as a fourth immunosuppressive agent for recurrent rejection (107). Other chemotherapeutic agents including vincristine, cyclophosphamide, and mycophenolate have also been used. Total lymphoid irradiation (TLI) can be successful in highly selected patients with refractory rejection but cannot be used for urgent or rescue situations (108,109) (see Chapter

Table 23.8. Massachusetts General Hospital Protocol for Treatment of Cellular Rejection Following Cardiac Transplantation

Acute Cellular Rejection			Recurrent or Refractory Acute Cellular Rejection	
Clinical/Histologic Situation	Agent	Protocol	Clinical/Histologic Situation	Protocol
Mild rejection (ISHLT < 2)	Maintenance therapy	Rebiopsy in 7–14 days or if symptoms develop	Moderate rejection	Methylprednisolone, 1000 mg daily (×3); increase cyclosporine dosing to achieve a trough level >250 ng/dL *plus* Addition of 4th immunosuppressive agent: methotrexate or dactinomycin *or* Replace azathioprine with mycophenolate Consider replacement of cyclosporine with tacrolimus-based immunosuppression
Moderate rejection (ISHLT 2, 3A, 3B) within initial 90 days	Methylprednisolone	500–1000 mg/day × 3; rebiopsy in 7 days		
Moderate rejection (ISHLT 2, 3A, 3B) beyond 90 days	Prednisone	1.5 mg/kg day × 3; taper over 14 days to achieve 5 mg/day above prior dose; rebiopsy following taper		
Moderate or severe rejection (ISHLT 2–4) with hemodynamic compromise	Methylprednisolone + OKT-3	500–1000 mg/day × 3; 5 mg/day for 7–10 days; and rebiopsy		
			Severe rejection	Methylprednisolone, 1000 mg daily (×3); increase cyclosporine dosing to achieve a trough level >250 ng/dL *and* OKT-3, 5 mg/day (× 10–14), or ATG if OKT-3 has recently been administered or $CD3^+$ cell clearance is inadequate *and* Replacement of cyclosporine with tacrolimus-based immunosuppression *or* Consider addition of a 4th agent: methotrexate or dactinomycin *or* Consider total lymphoid radiation *or* Retransplantation for progressive left ventricular dysfunction

14). Plasmapheresis and photophoresis have also been successful in reversing recurrent rejection (21,110). When all measures fail and allograft dysfunction ensues, retransplantation is the only alternative.

Humoral Rejection Treatment

The infrequent occurrence of humoral rejection and the difficulty in diagnosis have made it difficult to evaluate the most effective form of treatment. Anecdotal reports have documented resolution with pulsed high-dose corticosteroids, cytolytic therapy with OKT-3 or ATG, cyclophosphamide, IVIg, and plasmapheresis (Table 23.9) (102). Cyclophosphamide appears to be more effective in inhibiting B-cell activity than azathioprine, and it may result in improved outcome. Intermittent therapeutic plasmapheresis is particularly important in removing circulating antibodies against HLA and endothelial antigens. Heparin administration has been proposed as useful by inhibiting vascular smooth muscle cell proliferation (102). Heparin binding to the endothelium may inhibit allogeneic recognition of receptors on the endothelial surface and improve coronary flow. Photopheresis with ultraviolet A light following treatment with 8-methoxypsoralen has been effective in treating cellular rejection in highly sensitized transplant recipients and may also be useful in reversing humoral rejection (21,110) (see Chapter 14). Selective immunoadsorption of circulating HLA class I antigens may also be beneficial (111). Despite initial resolution, humoral rejection frequently recurs and overall allograft loss exceeds 20% (102). Accelerated allograft coronary vasculopathy may also occur more frequently in these patients (112).

CARDIOVASCULAR PHYSIOLOGY

Cardiac Function at Rest

Denervation has little effect on resting allograft function. Although myocardial catecholamine stores are completely depleted within days, intrinsic myocardial contractility

Table 23.9. Massachusetts General Hospital Protocol for Treatment of Acute Humoral Rejection Following Cardiac Transplantation

Clinical/Histologic Situation	Protocol
Moderate rejection	Methylprednisolone, 1000 mg daily (×3), followed by oral prednisone pulse with taper over 14 days Increase cyclosporine dosing to achieve a trough level >250 ng/dL Replace azathioprine with cyclophosphamide, 1–2 mg/kg daily or mycophenolate mofetil 1.5–3.0 g daily Plasmapheresis (or photopheresis) 3× weekly for 2–3 weeks Consider replacement of cyclosporine with tacrolimus-based immunosuppression
Severe rejection with or without hemodynamic compromise	Methylprednisolone, 1000 mg daily (×3), followed by oral prednisone pulse with taper over 14 days Increase cyclosporine dosing to achieve a trough level >250 ng/dL Replace azathioprine with cyclophosphamide 1–2 mg/kg daily Plasmapheresis (or photopheresis) 3× weekly for 2–3 weeks OKT-3, 5 mg/day (× 10–14 days), or ATG if OKT-3 has recently been administered or $CD3^+$ cell clearance is inadequate Replace cyclosporine with tacrolimus-based immunosuppression Retransplantation for progressive left ventricular dysfunction

remains unaffected. Beta-receptor density increases and myocyte sensitivity to circulating catecholamines is enhanced. The heart rate is higher (generally 80 to 100 beats/minute) due to absence of vagal tone; the cardiac index is normal or nearly so (113). Left and right ventricular ejection fraction and stroke volume are normal and remain so over at least the first 5 years (114). Left ventricular end-diastolic volume is initially normal or slightly reduced but may increase over time (115).

Diastolic Function

Subtle abnormalities of diastolic function have been reported, including impaired rest and exercise peak filling rates, abnormal atrial transport, and restrictive physiology (113). Proposed mechanisms for abnormal diastolic filling include healed ischemic injury, myocardial fibrosis secondary to cyclosporine, and chronic fibrosis secondary to recurrent rejection. Although Valentine et al noted a 15% incidence of restrictive hemodynamics during right heart catheterization, pressure-volume loop analysis failed to confirm late restrictive hemodynamic abnormalities (114). A progressive increase in indices of isovolumetric relaxation has been shown (116). Whether abnormalities of diastolic function contribute to impaired exercise capacity remains uncertain.

Cardiac Function During Exercise

Transplant recipients exhibit elevated resting heart rates but slowed chronotropic response to exercise (113,117). Although peak heart rates may equal that of normal individuals, this may require prolonged vigorous exercise. Blood norepinephrine levels rise severalfold during exercise, with parallel increases in heart rate and cardiac index. Blood pressure rise is also damped and delayed (113). During early exercise, the stroke index increases almost entirely due to increased end-diastolic volume (113). Left ventricular end-diastolic pressure may increase >10 mm Hg during the first 2 minutes. Later during exercise, circulating catecholamines enhance contractility and further increase cardiac index (113). Cardiac output remains substantially lower in transplant recipients than it is in normal individual for any level of exercise.

Despite normal left ventricular contractility, peak oxygen uptake ($\dot{V}O_2$) and anaerobic threshold are diminished. Peak $\dot{V}O_2$ is approximately 60% of that of age-matched controls, similar to that achieved by chronic NYHA class 3 heart failure patients (118,119). Central cardiopulmonary abnormalities and peripheral skeletal muscle dysfunction partially explain the reduced exercise capacity. Cardiopulmonary abnormalities include chronotropic incompetence, reduced stroke volume consequent to diastolic dysfunction, impaired pulmonary diffusion capacity, and diminished respiratory muscle endurance (8,119–120). Peripheral factors include reduced skeletal muscle strength, diminished oxidative metabolism, and persistent peripheral vascular flow abnormalities (8,119,120). Formal exercise training can improve peak oxygen uptake by 20% or more in motivated recipients.

PEDIATRIC HEART TRANSPLANTATION

Cardiac transplantation is now an accepted therapy for infants and children with end-stage heart disease and has steadily increased as a percentage of annual transplant volume. In Chapter 24, Vricella and Bailey discuss heart transplantation in children in further detail. Currently, pediatric transplantation represents 6% to 9% of yearly US volume. Since conventional cardiac surgery provides satisfactory palliation in over 90% of patients with congenital heart disease, transplantation is generally reserved for neonates and small children with poor long-term survival, such as those with a univentricular heart or hypoplastic left heart syndrome. Although hypoplastic left heart syndrome remains the primary indication for transplantation in infants, congenital heart disease and dilated cardiomyopathy are equally represented among children aged 1 to 5 years. Familial and acquired dilated cardiomyopathies represent the principal indication for transplantation in older children and adolescents.

Traditional exclusionary criteria (see Table 23.3) also apply to children, but several special considerations deserve mention. Pulmonary vascular resistance is less likely to be reversible in individuals with congenital heart disease, and failure to respond to vasodilators should be considered a strong contraindication to orthotopic transplantation. Complex venous drainage patterns such as those that may occur in heterotaxy syndromes may preclude transplantation or necessitate extensive reconstruction during the transplant operation. Certain infiltrative diseases (i.e., Gaucher's), inborn errors of metabolism, and muscular dystrophies may either recur in the transplanted allograft or cause progressive deterioration in skeletal and respiratory muscle function and should preclude transplantation.

A wider size discrepancy may exist between pediatric donors and recipients than for adults. Significantly oversized donors (>100%) are routinely used for neonates and young children, and ischemic times up to 6 to 7 hours have become routine in many programs. Several surgical issues require additional preparation. Children who have undergone a prior Fontan operation require an additional length of superior vena cava and those with hypoplastic left heart syndrome require procurement of the entire aortic arch and a portion of the descending aorta. When complex reconstruction is considered necessary, deep hypothermia with circulatory arrest may be preferable to standard systemic hypothermia.

Postoperative immunosuppression typically consists of triple-drug therapy. Many programs are now employing steroid-free protocols. Steroids should be minimized or given on an alternate day basis to decrease growth retardation and infectious complications. Pediatric patients have a more rapid elimination of cyclosporine and often require higher (15–20 mg/kg/day) and more frequent dosing to achieve therapeutic blood levels (121).

Diagnosis of acute allograft rejection is more difficult in children who cannot relate symptoms and in whom invasive procedures are minimized. Clinical manifestations include fever, tachycardia, tachypnea, anorexia, and listlessness. Infants and small children are primarily monitored noninvasively by clinical examination, ECG, and serial echocardiography (122). The development of S_3, increased posterior wall thickness, or a fall in left ventricular fractional shortening are useful clinical indicators in children (122). Endomyocardial biopsy may be performed in infants and small children under general anesthesia, but it is usually reserved for cases unresponsive to augmented immunosuppressive therapy or when the diagnosis remains questionable. In older children, routine endomyocardial biopsies are performed according to the adult schedule. Allograft rejection is extremely common early after transplantation despite initial hopes of reduced immunologic responsiveness in neonates and children. Freedom from treated rejection episodes at 1 year averages only 22% (123).

Little improvement has occurred in pediatric heart transplant survival over the past decade (42). Early operative (30 day) mortality averages 15% to 25% for children under 5 years (42). Actuarial survival at 1, 5, and 10 years is 75%, 60%, and 50% (123). Older children (aged 6 through 18) have a 2-year survival rate approximately 10% higher than that of infants and neonates (42). Right heart failure and acute rejection are the most common causes of early death; infectious complications, rejection, and accelerated graft vasculopathy account for the majority of late deaths (123).

Although intermediate results of pediatric transplantation are encouraging, significant concerns persist regarding the consequences of lifetime immunosuppression such as growth retardation, neoplasia, hospitalizations for invasive procedures, and the need for retransplantation.

LONG-TERM COMPLICATIONS AND THEIR MANAGEMENT

Hypertension

Cyclosporine-related hypertension occurs in 60% to 100% of cardiac transplant recipients and only a prior hypertensive history predicts its development (see Chapters 6 and 30). It is more common at higher cyclosporine doses, is virtually always present in patients who develop renal insufficiency, and has several unusual features. It usually occurs within 4 to 6 weeks of transplantation and continues with little alteration over time. It may be less common in patients receiving steroid-free maintenance program protocols.

A variety of mechanisms have been postulated. Systemic vascular resistance is elevated and sympathetic nervous activity increased by twofold to sevenfold (124). Cyclosporine enhances sodium retention and increases thromboxane production, leading to a hypothesis that the hypertension is consequent to an imbalance between vasodilator and vasoconstrictor prostaglandins. Omega-3 fatty acids and fish oil, which inhibit thromboxane synthesis, appear to be beneficial (125).

Devising a drug regimen that is effective, reasonably free of major side effects, and not extraordinarily complex requires patience and ingenuity. Calcium channel antagonists, particularly amlodipine and diltiazem, are attractive because they dilate constricted afferent renal arterioles, a prominent element of CsA-related hypertension. In addition, cyclosporine's action at the cellular level is par-tially mediated through cyclophylin, which affects intracellular calcium. This might explain the superior response to calcium channel blockers over ACE inhibitors. The addition of a diuretic, ACE inhibitor, or β-blocker is often needed. Diltiazem, but not amlodipine, will significantly elevate cyclosporine levels through inhibition of hepatic metabolism of cyclosporine via the cytochrome P450 enzymatic pathway. Future strategies may lower systemic vascular resistance through the use of oral mediators of prostaglandin or endothelial function.

Obesity and Hyperlipidemia

Obesity and hyperlipidemia are common, may increase morbidity, and promote the development of accelerated coronary vasculopathy (see Chapter 31). Corticosteroids and cyclosporine elevate plasma lipids, principally low-density lipoprotein (LDL) cholesterol. Hyperlipidemia occurs in 60% to 80% of patients, frequently within 2 weeks after transplant; it peaks between 3 and 6 months (126,127). Total serum cholesterol correlates with preoperative cholesterol values, cumulative steroid dosage, glucose levels, obesity, and maintenance steroid dosage (128). Preoperative ischemic heart disease significantly increases the likelihood of postoperative hyperlipidemia (126). Triglyceride response is variable; some centers report no change, whereas others report a twofold rise in fasting triglycerides (126). The mechanism postulated for corticosteroid-mediated hyperlipidemia is via weight-related insulin resistance with a subsequent increase in hepatic synthesis of LDL cholesterol and triglycerides. Lake and others have shown that early withdrawal from corticosteroids can significantly lower plasma cholesterol and decrease postoperative weight gain (129).

Controlled trials of hyperlipidemia treatment are few (130). A low cholesterol, low saturated fat diet should be the initial treatment. Bile acid sequestrants (cholestyramine and colestipol) decrease cyclosporine absorption and should be avoided as first-line therapy. These agents may be useful in combination with other drugs when prescribed 1 hour before or 4 hours after administration of immunosuppressive agents. Nicotinic acid is useful in the mixed hyperlipidemia pattern seen after transplantation; however, it produces numerous side effects and can lead to hepatic dysfunction and elevated uric acid levels. Gemfibrozil reduces triglycerides but only modestly lowers LDL cholesterol. HMG-CoA reductase inhibitors most effectively lower serum cholesterol and should be considered first-line agents. Lovastatin reduces LDL cholesterol by 24% to 40% and also decreases triglycerides (126). Myositis and rhabdomyolysis are rarely observed in cyclosporine-treated patients. Kobashigawa et al have recently demonstrated that the prophylactic administration of pravastatin, a hydrophilic HMG co-reductase inhibitor, early following transplantation can lower serum cholesterol, decrease the frequency of hemodynamically significant rejection, decrease coronary artery intimal thickening by intravascular ultrasound, and lower the incidence of early coronary vasculopathy (127). Whether all patients including those without hyperlipidemia should receive pravastatin or other lipid-lowering compounds is undergoing further study.

Gastrointestinal Complications

Gastrointestinal complications are observed in 15% to 35% of transplant recipients, with mortality rates as high as 30% (131) (see Chapter 29). Upper gastrointestinal bleeding, usually due to peptic ulcer disease or hemorrhagic gastritis, not infrequently accompanies the stress of cardiac surgery or high-dose corticosteroids. Its incidence has decreased dramatically with the prophylactic use of H_2-blockers. Opportunistic infections including candidiasis, herpesvirus, and CMV may affect the esophagus and gastrointestinal tracts. Aggressive culture and biopsy of all lesions enhances diagnostic yield and permits prompt treatment (132). Visceral perforation suggests CMV infection, diverticular disease, or lymphoproliferative disorder of the gastrointestinal tract (131,132).

Mild transaminase elevations and hyperbilirubinemia are commonly cyclosporine-related and respond to dose reduction. Azathioprine may also produce cholestatic jaundice. Infectious causes of chronic hepatitis include hepatitis A, B, and C, herpes simplex virus, and CMV. Hepatitis C is the most prevalent form of hepatitis and is transmitted through blood transfusions or the donor allograft. Post-transplant liver disease has been observed in 20% to 48% of heart recipients receiving a hepatitis C positive donor (133). Serum transaminase typically rises within 10 to 12 weeks following transplantation in infected recipients (134). Although fulminant hepatitis is rare in both hepatitis B and C, insidious progression to frank cirrhosis may occur over 2 to 10 years following infection.

Cholelithiasis is present in 30% to 40% of transplant recipients and is twice as common as for age- and gender-matched controls (135). Gallstones develop within 2 years in 2% to 17% of patients with normal pretransplant ultrasonography (135). Although some centers advise expectant management of asymptomatic patients, biliary colic or gallstone pancreatitis are not uncommon and so many centers routinely recommend laparoscopic cholecystectomy.

Pancreatitis has been reported in 1.5% to 18% of heart transplant recipients (131). Cardiopulmonary bypass and vasopressor-mediated splanchnic vasoconstriction, and high-dose corticosteroids account for early postoperative pancreatitis; infection (CMV, viral hepatitis, mumps), ischemia, biliary tract disease, peptic ulcer perforation, and drug allergies (particularly to azathioprine) produce late pancreatitis. Nasogastric suction and total parenteral nutrition should be implemented and continued until symptoms and biochemical abnormalities resolve.

Early Infectious Complications

Infection remains the leading cause of mortality during the first post-transplant year (136). Approximately 30% of transplant recipients have one or more major infectious episodes; the cumulative incidence of infections per patient averages 0.4 at 3 months, 0.55 at 6 months, and 0.62 at 12 months (136). There are two major peaks in the incidence of infection: the early period includes the first postoperative month, which is dominated by bacterial nosocomial infections; the late post-transplant period includes all other times (Fig. 23.9). Gram-negative bacilli and staphylococcal species are the most common early pathogens. *Pseudomonas aeruginosa, Proteus*

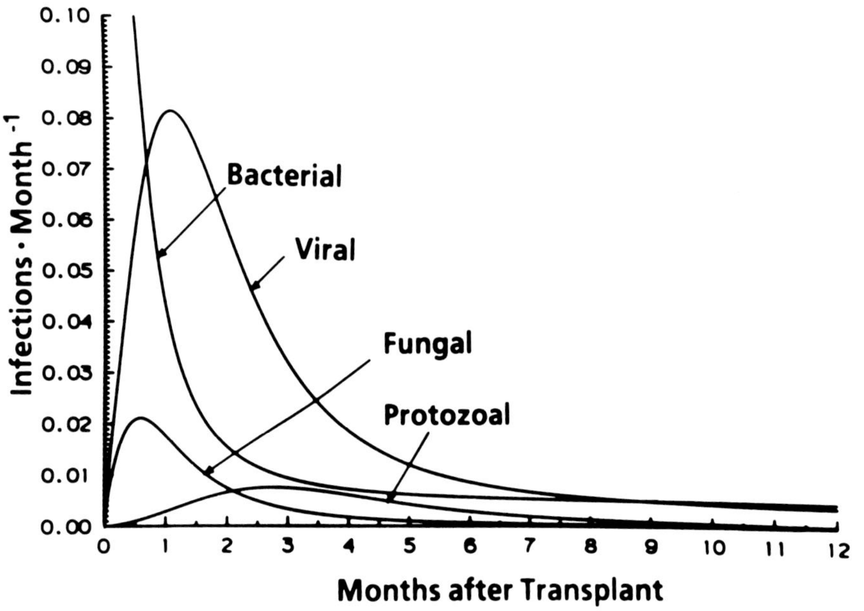

FIGURE 23.9. *Hazard function (displaying the instantaneous risk over time) for first infection by major category of infectious agent. Data are from the Transplant Cardiologist Research Database. (Reprinted with permission from Miller LW, et al. Infection after heart transplantation: a multi-institutional study. J Heart Lung Transplant 1994;13:381–393.)*

species, and *Klebsiella* are more commonly observed in transplant recipients than in routine postoperative cardiac surgical patients. In general, the more debilitated the patient or the more invasive the degree of preoperative support, the higher the likelihood of infectious morbidity (see Chapter 36).

The lung is consistently the most common site of infection; pneumonia may increase mortality by 25% (136). This increased risk may be due to chronic left-sided heart failure with pulmonary colonization, prolonged intubation, cardiac cachexia, and microaspiration. Gram-negative bacilli are the most common pathogens. When cultures and sputum gram stains fail to provide adequate culture material, tracheal aspiration or early bronchoscopy should be undertaken. Antibiotic therapy must be aggressive.

Bacteremia can be minimized through the early removal of centrally placed intravenous cannulas. Wound infections and mediastinitis are quite uncommon (<1%). When present, they occur within 2 weeks of surgery and are typically caused by *Staphylococcus* species, Enterobacteriaceae or *Pseudomonas*. Diagnosis usually requires mediastinal reexploration or aspiration, and treatment consists of a prolonged course of antibiotics, sternal débridement, and use of vascularized muscle flaps.

Late Post-transplant Infections

Infectious risk, particularly for viral and opportunistic organisms, remains high from postoperative months 1 through 6 as a result of the cumulative effects of immunosuppression. Although pulmonary infections remain common, central nervous system and gastrointestinal infections also occur. The chest x-ray appearance and the tempo of the patient's illness may provide important clues to the etiology of a pneumonia. Severe symptoms that evolve within 24 hours suggest bacterial infection or a noninfectious cause such as pulmonary edema or acute respiratory distress syndrome. A subacute presentation over several days suggests a viral infection or *Pneumocystis carinii*. An insidious onset is most characteristic of fungal infection (*Aspergillus*, *Mucor*, *Cryptococcus*), *Nocardia*, and *Mycobacterium* (136,137).

CMV infection deserves additional discussion (see Chapter 36). CMV is the most common cause of morbidity and mortality in cardiac transplant recipients; the infection rates range from 65% to 93% of patients (136,138). It typically occurs between 40 and 50 days following surgery or after antirejection therapy. OKT-3 or ATG treatment significantly increases the risk of symptomatic CMV disease. Primary infection is usually acquired from the allograft or from leukocyte-containing blood transfusions. Those with primary CMV disease often have gastrointestinal tract involvement, with fever, diarrhea, and hemorrhage. Mortality is highest when pulmonary involvement occurs. Other features may include hepatitis, CMV myocarditis, chorioretinitis, and central nervous system involvement. Many patients with reactivation disease experience only fever, malaise, and moderate leukopenia during active viremia. Symptomatic infection usually responds to treatment with ganciclovir, 5–10 mg/kg daily. Relapses are not uncommon and prolonged treatment is sometimes required. CMV interactions with host lymphocytes and macrophages increase the risk of opportunistic fungal infection and of acute allograft rejection—probably through upregulation of major histocompatibility antigens. They may also predispose the patient to angiographically severe graft vasculopathy (139).

Surveillance and Prophylaxis

Cephalosporin coverage is generally administered for 48 to 72 hours and vancomycin may also be given until central venous catheters and pacing wires have been removed.

Sputum and urine are cultured routinely during the first 2 weeks, and chest films are performed. Nystatin or clotrimazole troches are usually administered for the first 6 postoperative months. Likewise, ongoing treatment with trimethaprim/sulfa or inhaled pentamidine for *Pneumocystis* prophylaxis is recommended. Patients also receive acyclovir, 400 mg 3 times a day, for the first 4 postoperative months to decrease the incidence of herpesvirus infections.

The use of CMV-negative blood products administered through a leukopore filter may decrease the frequency of primary CMV infection. Ganciclovir (5 mg/kg intravenously 3 times weekly for the first 6 weeks) has been shown to decrease the incidence of active CMV disease in CMV-mismatched patients and to reduce the morbidity of reactivation disease (138). Hyperimmune globulin can also be used for the treatment of CMV-mismatched recipients. Patients at a high risk of primary or reactivation disease during OKT-3 or ATG treatment routinely receive prophylactic intravenous ganciclovir. The optimal dosage and duration of prophylactic therapy require additional studies.

Malignancies

The incidence of malignant tumors in transplant recipients ranges from 4% to 18% (average 6%), a 100-fold increase above the general population (140). Heart transplant recipients are at particular risk for the development of cancers of the skin and lips, as well as lymphomas. Compared to kidney transplant recipients, cardiac transplant patients have a twofold overall increase in neoplasia risk and a sixfold increase of visceral tumors (see Chapter 37). No relationship has been demonstrated between the type of maintenance immunosuppression and the risk of malignancy (141). The combination of immunosuppression and a history of prior smoking may account for the increased risk of developing lung cancer in heart transplant recipients (142).

Over 90% of post-transplant lymphomas are non-Hodgkin's type and are morphologically characterized by large B cells (see Chapter 37). The term *post-transplant lymphoproliferative disorder (PTLD)* is preferred to *lymphoma* because these tumors display a variety of morphologies, ranging from simple B-cell hyperplasia to aggressive monoclonal immunoblastic varieties. PTLD is more common in heart and heart–lung recipients than in kidney recipients, and it is more common in pediatric patients compared with adults (140). Extranodal involvement is seen in over 70% of cases; central nervous system and intra-abdominal involvement are particularly common (140,143).

Epstein-Barr virus (EBV) is believed to have a causal relationship for PTLD through induction of B-cell proliferation. Although EBV-seronegative recipients are at greater risk, PTLD may also occur during EBV reactivation (144). Augmented immunosuppression, particularly with T-cell depleting agents (ATG or OKT-3), increases the risk of PTLD. Swinnen and colleagues reported a markedly increased incidence when the cumulative OKT-3 dose exceeded 75 mg (61). Other centers have been unable to confirm such a dose-related increase in risk, but there is general consensus that cytotoxic immunosuppressive drugs may permanently eliminate T-cell clones that are necessary for controlling malignant cells or latent oncogenic viruses.

Armitage et al have described early and late PTLD clinical presentations (145). Early disease generally occurs within the first 12 months and is frequently localized or nodal disease. Focal lymphadenopathy is a common initial presentation. Early PTLD is generally polyclonal by DNA analysis and often regresses following reduction in immunosuppression. In contrast, late PTLD often presents with disseminated disease, demonstrates monoclonal B-cell proliferation, fails to respond to reduced immunosuppression, and carries a 1-year mortality rate in excess of 75% (145). Despite this general pattern, aggressive monoclonal B-cell types of PTLD may occur within the first year.

The association between PTLD and viral infections has promoted the use of antiviral prophylaxis during the early post-transplant period and during periods of augmented immunosuppression. Whether this strategy will decrease the incidence of PTLD requires longitudinal study. The mainstay of treatment is reduction in immunosuppression, as over 40% of patients will respond to this treatment. Additional treatments may include excision of the lesion if localized, localized radiation therapy for discrete masses or central nervous system lesions, or modified non-Hodgkin's chemotherapy for widespread disease. Controlled trials of acyclovir, ganciclovir, or chemotherapy in established PTLD are lacking.

Transplant Coronary Artery Disease

Accelerated transplant coronary artery disease (TCAD) is the leading cause of death in cardiac recipients who survive beyond the third year, and it remains the major limitation to multi-decade survival. It differs significantly from conventional coronary atherosclerosis in natural history and pathophysiology. Although it is uncommon during the first year, the average incidence of angiographically demonstrable TCAD is 10% to 12% per patient year and it is visible in 40% to 50% of transplant recipients by the fifth year (146,147). Children and adolescents have a similar incidence of TCAD to adult transplant recipients.

Marked fibrous intimal thickening due to smooth muscle cell proliferation, mononuclear cell infiltration, and collagen accumulation characterize the histopathology (Fig. 23.10 and Plate 19). Concentric, circumferential, and longitudinal intimal thickening affect the epicardial arteries with pruning of extramural and intramyocardial branches. Histologic similarities exist between TCAD and post-percutaneous coronary angioplasty (PTCA) restenosis.

A second distinct atheromatous lesion may also be detected in long-term allografts or from older donors (148). Such lesions are composed of dense fibrous tissue overlying lipid-rich pools of cholesterol clefts, areas of calcification,

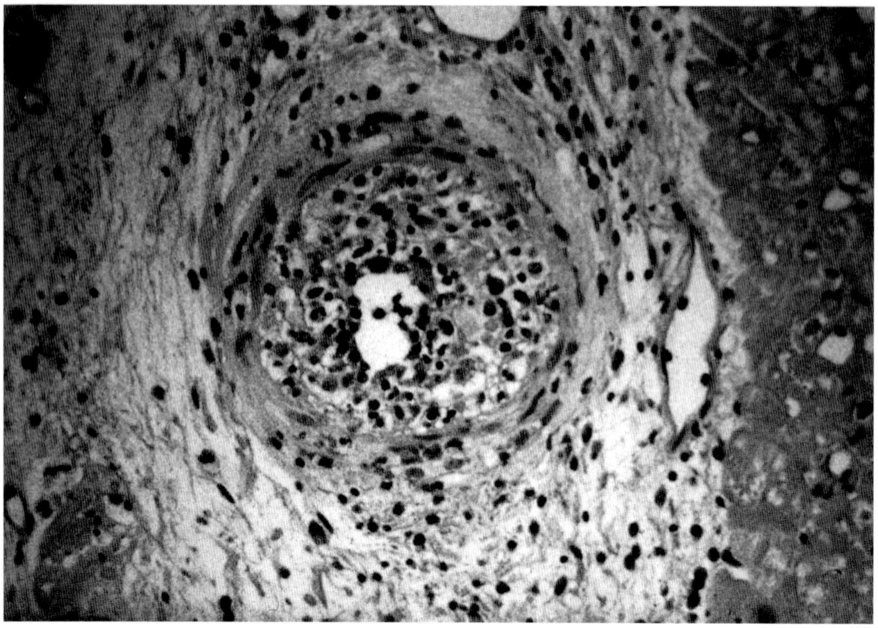

FIGURE 23.10. *Photomicrograph of an arteriole showing concentric intimal hyperplasia and an abundance of macrophages; this is the most common histopathologic lesion of transplant vasculopathy (hematoxylin-eosin, ×250).*

and disruption of the internal elastic lamina. Rarely, a diffuse necrotizing coronary vasculitis may be present during the first post-transplant year.

Identification of those recipients at higher risk for TCAD has proven problematic. Conventional coronary risk factors including hypertension, hyperlipidemia, diabetes mellitus, and tobacco usage have not been associated with the disorder. Patients transplanted for end-stage ischemic heart disease may be at increased risk for developing TCAD. A weak but consistent relation between elevated serum triglycerides and TCAD has been noted (147). Corticosteroid therapy is not an independent risk factor for TCAD.

Although the true pathogenesis of TCAD remains unknown, a vascular immunologic injury has been postulated (see Chapter 3). Endothelial injury could be either humorally or cellularly mediated. Well-controlled studies have failed to demonstrate any correlation between the number, duration, or severity of myocardial rejection episodes and subsequent development of TCAD (149,150). Libby et al have postulated that the characteristic endothelial and smooth muscle cell proliferations are due to altered local regulation of cellular proliferation. These changes may represent a chronic, localized form of delayed-type hypersensitivity to vessel-wall alloantigens. This vascular proliferative response may occur consequent to HLA class II induction on the vascular endothelium that is recognized by helper T cells (151). Deng et al have recently confirmed a correlation between HLA-DR and HLA-DQ expression and the extent of intimal hyperplasia (152). Humoral rejection may also contribute to the development of accelerated TCAD. Patients who develop anti-HLA antibodies or antiendothelial antibodies are more likely to have angiographic evidence of TCAD (34,153).

Nonimmune causes of endothelial dysfunction such as cold ischemic injury and viral infections may also contribute. CMV infection has been associated with the development of TCAD, more severe angiographic disease, and a 5-year graft loss twice that of CMV-negative patients (139,154). Recently, depletion of vascular tissue plasminogen-activator (t-PA), occurring within 3 months following transplantation, has been associated with an 8.3-fold increase in risk of the development of angiographically evident coronary disease and a greater likelihood of death or retransplantation (155).

Diagnosis of TCAD

Clinical Presentations Lacking afferent innervation, cardiac transplant recipients do not experience angina pectoris despite significant epicardial coronary disease. Initial manifestations include silent myocardial infarction and ischemic repolarization abnormalities on routine ECG. Acute myocardial infarction may have atypical presentations, including epigastric pain and a sense of impending doom. Congestive heart failure, cardiogenic shock, and death are significantly more likely in transplant recipients sustaining myocardial infarction than in nontransplant ischemic heart disease patients. Unexplained left ventricular dysfunction should also suggest the possibility of occult TCAD. Sudden cardiac death is an uncommon initial presentation but is a frequent late occurrence. An occasional patient will have anginal-like chest pain due to partial reinnervation.

Angiographic Features TCAD is angiographically characterized by diffuse concentric narrowing, particularly in middle and distal coronary vessels. The distal vessel appears disproportionately smaller than the proximal vessel; vessel tapering and "pruning" are common in secondary and ter-

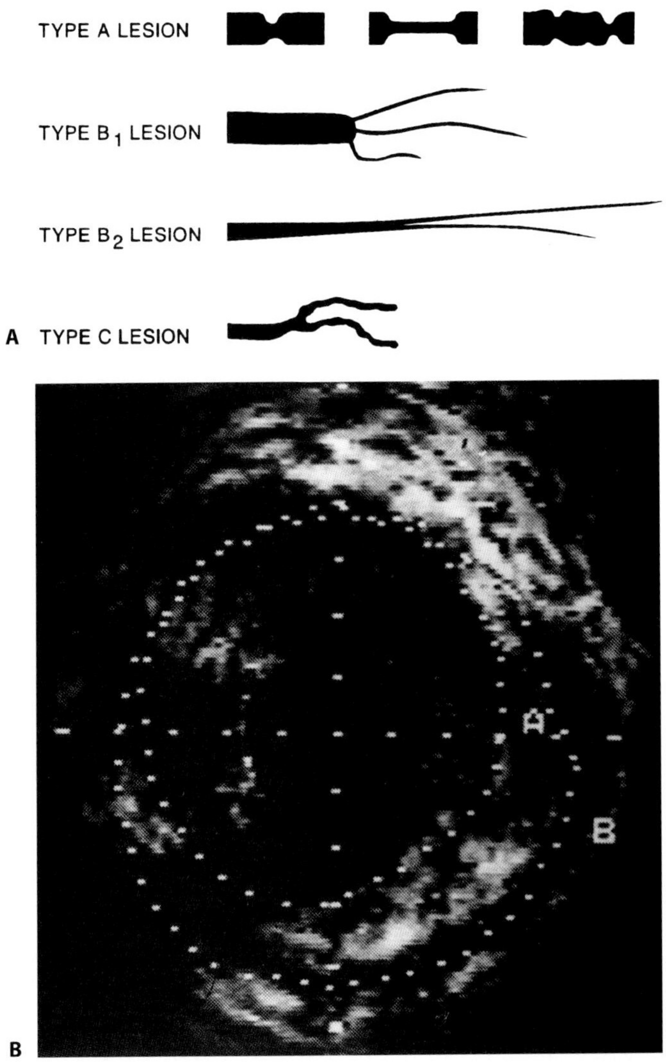

FIGURE 23.11. ***A.*** *Diagrammatic representation of angiographic patterns seen in cardiac transplant recipients with coronary artery disease. Type A lesions are focal discrete, tubular, or multiple stenoses. Type B1 lesions show abrupt transition from "normal" proximal vessels to concentrically narrowed and obliterated distal vessels. Type B2 lesions show gradual concentric tapering with preservation of some residual lumen in the distal vessel. Type C lesions are narrowed, irregular distal vessels that are squared-off rather then tapered, and terminate abruptly. (Reprinted with permission from Gao SZ, et al. Accelerated coronary vascular disease in the heart transplant patient: coronary arteriographic findings. J Am Coll Cardiol 1988;12:334–340.)* ***B.*** *Intracoronary ultrasound showing the presence of marked eccentric intimal thickening (area between* A *and* B*) of the left main coronary artery in a patient 5 years following transplantation. (Reprinted with permission from Collings CA, Pinto FJ, Valantine HA, et al. Exercise echocardiography in heart transplant recipients: a comparison with angiography and intracoronary ultrasonography. J Heart Lung Transplant 1994;13:604–613.)*

tiary epicardial branches (Fig. 23.11A). Gao et al (156) have provided the best classification scheme for disease severity (see Fig. 23.11A). Compared to nontransplant patients with coronary artery disease, transplant recipients display fewer proximal stenoses (76% vs. 100%) and more distal vessel occlusions (49% vs. 4%). The rapidity of disease progression is highlighted by the absence of collateral circulation in 92% of transplant recipients (156).

Angiographic findings provide important prognostic information. Balk et al have shown that patients with normal coronary anatomy at 12 months have a low likelihood of disease development or ischemic events during the subsequent 5 years (157). However, a qualitative normal angiogram fails to detect diffuse epicardial disease in 15% to 20% of patients (158). Serial quantitative coronary angiography is currently the most accurate way to evaluate disease presence and progression. Once mild disease has been documented progression is often rapid, with the probability of death approaching 50% over the next 3 years (159). Actuarial survival is reduced proportionate to disease severity for individuals with proximal or midvessel stenoses. Survival with single vessel disease averages 35% to 40% at 2 years, compared to less than 15% for triple-vessel disease (160).

Noninvasive Diagnostic Techniques Noninvasive assessment of TCAD is generally unreliable. Treadmill exercise testing and thallium scintigraphy are often negative, despite advanced disease (161). Exercise single-proton emission CT thallium-201 imaging (SPECT) may fail to detect multivessel disease due to the "balanced" nature of limitation in coronary blood flow (162). Studies of exercise and dobutamine stress echocardiographic techniques have yielded conflicting results in sensitivity, specificity, and negative predictive value (163,164).

Intracoronary vascular ultrasound (IVUS) is more sensitive than qualitative coronary angiography for detecting intimal thickening and is the method of choice for assessing early TCAD (165). It accurately defines cross-sectional area, delineates vessel wall thickness and morphology, and provides quantitative luminal dimensions (see Fig. 23.11B) (166). Despite "normal" angiography, IVUS often detects intimal thickening within 8 weeks of transplantation. Severe intimal thickening has been shown to predict future cardiac events despite normal coronary angiography (167). IVUS is rapidly becoming the technique of choice for serial follow-up of heart transplant recipients, and it has become particularly important in assessing strategies designed to modify TCAD progression.

Treatment of TCAD

The treatment of angiographic TCAD using antiplatelet agents, aspirin, dicumarol, heparin, or fish oil has been ineffective (168). Schroeder et al have shown that diltiazem can prevent the reduction in coronary luminal diameter seen during the first post-transplant year and decrease the incidence of symptomatic TCAD (169). Pravastatin, a lipid-lowering agent with favorable effects on natural killer cell cytotoxicity, has also been shown to lower the incidence of TCAD and improve 1-year survival (127). Angiopeptin, an inhibitor of smooth muscle cell proliferation, may decrease the onset of TCAD (170). Whether calcium channel antagonists, lipid-lowering agents, or inhibitors of smooth muscle cell proliferation can produce long-term benefits or act synergistically requires further investigation. Until confirmatory studies are available, clinicians should consider prophylactic treatment for at least the first year with one of these agents.

Coronary angioplasty, atherectomy, and bypass surgery have been performed in a limited number of cardiac transplant recipients. A multicenter registry has retrospectively assessed the effects of coronary revascularization on patient survival (171). Coronary angioplasty has a high initial rate of success in treating discrete lesions (94%) but is associated with frequent procedural complications and a restenosis rate above 50%. Coronary revascularization should be considered merely palliative.

The only definitive therapy currently available for advanced multivessel TCAD is retransplantation. Elective retransplantation should be considered when the severity of angiographic disease or its rate of progression is life threatening or when extensive left ventricular dysfunction has developed. Unfortunately, survival in retransplantation patients is decidedly inferior to initial transplantation. ISHLT Registry data report an overall 1-year survival rate of only 55% (42). Even selecting ideal candidates yields a 1-year survival rate of 74% (172). Accelerated TCAD is more likely to occur in retransplanted allografts.

OUTPATIENT SURVEILLANCE

Outpatient management should begin during the final phase of hospitalization with instruction on a "heart healthy" diet, including moderate salt and caloric restriction to maintain ideal body weight. Restriction of dietary cholesterol and saturated fats should be addressed, and cardiac rehabilitation should be emphasized. The patient and family must have an understanding of medication indications, dosing, common side effects, and particular complications related to immunosuppressive agents. Preprinted manuals and teaching aides are useful for providing a uniform approach.

The frequency and timing of early transplant outpatient visits is generally determined by the need for surveillance endomyocardial biopsies. Patients are initially seen once or twice per week; subsequently, they are seen on a less frequent basis unless complications or rejection have occurred. Each visit should begin with a review of ongoing problems and any new symptoms. For diabetics, the visit must include a careful evaluation of glucose control. Likewise, any of the common psychiatric symptoms that occur early following transplantation—particularly mood swings, depression, guilt, or euphoria—should be assessed. Each visit should include a detailed inquiry concerning all medications. Errors in immunosuppressive medications are particularly common following treatment of rejection. Other new medications, including over-the-counter drugs or those prescribed by another physician, may interact with the patient's immunosuppressive medications. The patient's compliance with, and response to, their antihypertensive program should be discussed.

Physical Examination

The patient's vital signs should be assessed, including weight, blood pressure, temperature, and pulse rate and rhythm. A moderate fall in blood pressure or new tachycardia may suggest early rejection or an inappropriate dose of an antihypertensive agent. The skin and mucous membranes should be examined for discrete lesions, such as herpetic vesicles, drug rash, or skin cancer. The lymph nodes should be examined regularly to exclude early PTLD. Examination of the thorax should check for pulmonary consolidation or effusion or the development of a new gallop rhythm, murmur, jugular venous distention, or irregularity of heart rhythm. Physical examination should also be symptom guided and focused by previous problems, such as previous hepatomegaly in a patient with liver function abnormalities.

Serum electrolytes, renal function, glucose, complete blood count, platelets, and cyclosporine levels should be determined during each visit and every 2 to 3 months during long-term follow-up. The blood cyclosporine or tacrolimus level should be checked at each visit or every 2 months. Echocardiography is performed on a surveillance basis every 6 months, and whenever hemodynamic abnormalities are detected during right heart catheterization or the patient has new symptoms suggestive of ventricular dysfunction. An electrocardiogram should be performed every 3 to 6 months and on a more frequent basis in patients with TCAD.

Endomyocardial biopsy and right heart catheterization are performed on a surveillance schedule and in patients with clinically suspected rejection or new unexplained echocardiographic abnormalities. Laboratory studies, changes in immunosuppressive medications, and biopsy results can best be tracked using a database spreadsheet.

Annual Evaluation

Most transplant recipients return annually for more extensive diagnostic studies. This provides another opportunity for review of the patient's progress. The appropriateness of current immunosuppressive and antihypertensive regimens, general health maintenance activities, and new complications should all be assessed. A complete physical examination should be performed, including rectal examination and sigmoidoscopy (where appropriate); women should undergo a gynecologic evaluation, including a Pap smear and mammogram. Complete blood studies, chest film, electrocardiogram, and echocardiogram should be performed. A complete lipid profile should also be assessed. The patient should receive dietary counseling as indicated.

Coronary angiography is the most important part of the evaluation. Most centers also perform intravascular ultrasound, right heart catheterization, and right ventricular biopsy. The necessity of these late biopsies has been called into question, as rejection is uncommon after 2 years. Exercise testing is frequently done at this time to define the patient's exercise prescription for the upcoming year.

LONG-TERM OUTCOME

The rapid growth during the 1980s in the number of cardiac transplant centers partially reflects the increasingly successful long-term outcome of heart transplantation. Statistics from the United Network for Organ Sharing (UNOS) indicate that approximately 2300 cardiac transplants are performed each year within the United States. Worldwide data from the ISHLT Registry (n > 26,000) indicate 1-, 5-, and 10-year actuarial survival rates of 80%, 65%, and 45%, respectively (39). Figure 23.12 illustrates the improvement in actuarial survival over the last two decades. Currently, many transplant programs can achieve 1-, 5-, and 10-year survival rates of 95%, 75%, and 60%. In addition, over 90% of patients are fully rehabilitated to NYHA class I or II status.

Multivariate analysis reveals several risk factors for death within the first postoperative year, including prior transplantation, preoperative ventilatory or mechanical circulatory support, recipient age less than 5 years or over 60 years, use of an older or female donor, and a prolonged ischemic time. Patients transplanted over the age of 65 experience more infectious complications, fewer episodes of rejection, and more significant residual functional impairment; their 1-year actuarial survival is significantly lower (74% vs. 84%) compared to younger transplant recipients (14,42). Regardless of age or the PRA, women have lower survival rates than men (20,57). CMV-mismatched women are at particularly high risk for poor outcome (20).

Causes of death following transplantation vary over time. Over 50% of all deaths that occur within the first 2 weeks are due to technical or primary cardiac complications, including primary graft failure, right heart failure, and hemorrhage. A higher percentage of pediatric deaths result from technical complications. Infectious complications contribute directly to 50% of deaths during the first to third postoperative months. Acute allograft rejection accounts for 25% to 35% of deaths during the first 6 months. However, rejection contributes to fewer than 20% of deaths beyond the first post-transplant year. The majority of late deaths are due to TCAD. Unexplained allograft failure and lymphoproliferative disorders account for the remainder of late deaths.

Quality of life is dramatically enhanced in most recipients (173). Over 90% of recipients achieve NYHA functional class I and 45% to 50% return to employment. As with other immunosuppressed individuals, heart transplant recipients should not be considered medically disabled but should be viewed as having specific physical limitations or restrictions that preclude certain types of work. Currently, the ability of patients to complete vocational rehabilitation and reenter the work force depends more on the employer's willingness to accept an individual with chronic heart disease than it does on any functional limitations resulting from the transplant itself.

As long-term survival has become a reality, the issue of parenting has become more common. Fetal teratogenicity is not increased by conventional immunosuppressive agents, but the effects of newer agents are unknown. Pregnancy appears to be well tolerated in most transplant recipients. Although hypertension (44%), premature labor (30%), and preeclampsia (22%) are commonly observed, no early maternal or fetal deaths or allograft dysfunctions have been reported (174). Prior recommendations for strict contraception or sterilization should be reconsidered.

Retransplantation

Retransplantation represents 2.3% of the total annual heart transplant volume (42). Significant differences in survival exist for patients retransplanted within the first 6 months compared to those retransplanted later. Early retransplantation is

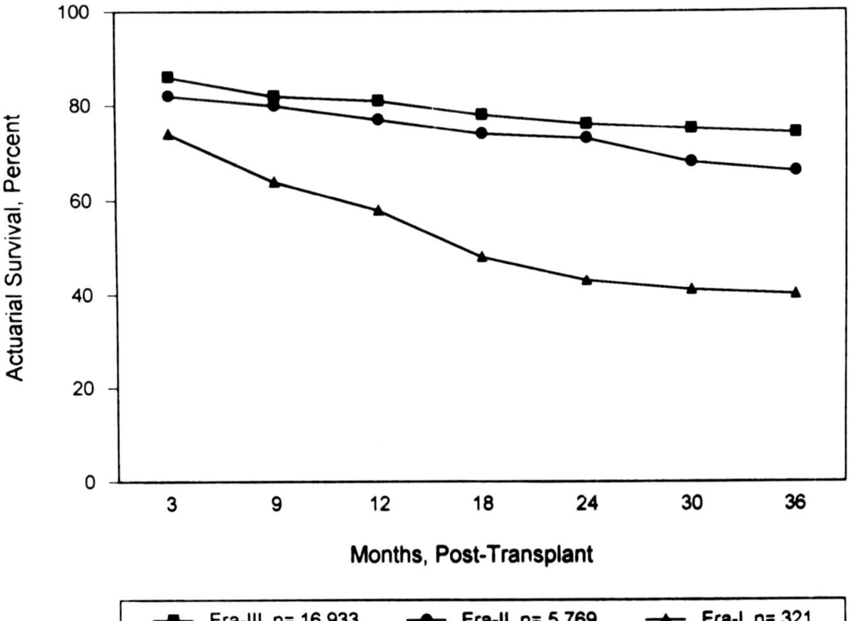

FIGURE 23.12. *Data from the International Registry of Heart Transplantation demonstrating improvement in actuarial patient survival over three eras of cardiac transplantation: Era I, 1975–1981; Era II, 1982–1987; and Era III, 1988–1994. One-year survival improved dramatically from 55% to 82% with the advent of cyclosporine-based immunosuppression. There has been modest further improvement during the most recent era, with a 1-year survival rate above 85%. (Reprinted with permission from Hosenpud JD, Novick RJ, Breen TJ, et al. The registry of the International Society for heart and lung transplantation: twelfth official report, 1995. J Heart Lung Transplant 1995;14:805–815.)*

generally due to primary graft dysfunction or refractory rejection; in these cases, the 1-year survival rate following retransplantation is only 40% (42,172). Later retransplantation is most frequently undertaken for TCAD and is associated with a 1-year survival rate of 65% (42). The poorer survival rates suggest that retransplantation be offered to only highly selected individuals, particularly those with a low degree of sensitization and normal renal function who lack complications from chronic immunosuppressive treatment.

Even with careful patient selection, 5-year survival is substantially lower for patients undergoing retransplantation (33% vs. 62%). Retransplantation also costs more than twice as much as a primary transplant (US$386,000 vs. US$162,000) (175). Given the high prevalence rate and rapid progression of TCAD, selection of patients for retransplantation represents a medical and ethical dilemma for the transplant community.

FUTURE DIRECTIONS

Cardiomyoplasty

Dynamic cardiomyoplasty involves mobilizing the latissimus dorsi with its vascular and nervous supply intact. The skeletal muscle is wrapped around the ventricle or a portion of the aorta to create a skeletalized "ventricle." If the muscle length is inadequate, a pericardial patch is sometimes used to complete the muscle wrap. Graded muscle stimulation using a cardiomyostimulator is initiated over 6 to 12 weeks. Chronic low-frequency electrical stimulation of mammalian skeletal muscle will transform fast type II muscle fibers into the slow fatigue-resistant type I fibers. Although the end result of such transformation is degeneration of adequate ATP stores for continuous working conditions, this fast to slow transformation is associated with a significant loss of muscle mass and power (176). Initial uncontrolled studies report improved functional capacity with a decline in NYHA status by one or two classes (176). A modest rise in ejection fraction is typically observed, whereas right atrial, pulmonary capillary wedge, and left ventricular end-diastolic pressures remain unchanged (176). The lack of consistent long-term hemodynamic improvement can be partially explained by the suboptimal loading of the muscle but may also reflect progressive muscle damage and fatty replacement (177).

Early operative mortality is high (15% to 23%), and 1-year survival averages only 65% to 70% (177). The procedure should not be undertaken in patients with NYH Association class IV symptoms, primarily because of the lack of sufficient time for skeletal muscle training. Currently, the procedure is only offered to patients with NYHA class III heart failure symptoms in whom conventional surgical procedures, including transplantation, are contraindicated. Benefits include each patient serving as his or her own "donor" and elimination of chronic immunosuppression. Further, maximum oxygen consumption generally increases by 4 mL/kg/min to 6 mL/kg/min (176).

Pharmacologic therapy for heart failure can be decreased in over 60% of patients following the operation (176). However, the high early surgical mortality, the unexpectedly high rate of late sudden deaths, and the uncertain durability of skeletonized muscle to support adequately the failing ventricle should restrict its use to controlled clinical studies (177,178).

Permanent Left Ventricular Assist Devices

Although interest in pneumatically driven biventricular or total artificial hearts has waned, development of totally implantable pulsatile left ventricular assist devices has progressed rapidly. Several LVADs may represent realistic alternatives to heart transplantation within the next 5 years (179). Despite the ultimate goal of permanent implantability, all current designs have been employed only as a bridge to transplantation. Both the Novacor (Baxter healthcare, Oakland, CA) and the Thermo Cardiosystems (TCI) HeartMate devices are of the pusher plate type and designed for long-term circulatory support.

The Novocor LVAD is composed of a balanced solenoid energy converter, dual pusher plate, and sack-type blood pump with a microprocessor base control and monitoring console (180). The integrated energy convertor and pump are implanted in the abdomen and connected to the patient by Dacron conduits to the LV apex and the ascending aorta. Electric energy is converted into hydraulic work, which subsequently ejects blood from the pump itself. The electric power cable is tunneled percutaneously from the right lower quadrant of the abdomen and connected to an extracorporeal console and battery power system.

The TCI HeartMate vented electric LVAD consists of a positive displacement, pusher plate pump activated by a low speed torque motor that can produce a stroke volume of 83 cc at rates varying from 50 to 120 beats/min (Figure 23.13) (180). The electromechanical actuator fits beneath the pumping diaphragm and converts the rotary motion of the torque motor into the linear motion of the pump diaphragm (181). Following initiation, the motor switches on and makes one complete revolution, pushing up the diaphragm with ejection of blood from the pump. The motor then shuts off and the pump passively refills with blood. The flexible diaphragm (blood-contacting surface) is fabricated from Biomer polyurethane and has an integrally textured fibular surface; all metal components have a sintered titanium/blood interface (179). This textured surface promotes the formation of a fiber and cellular coagulum that evolves into a blood-compatible biologic lining or pseudo-intimal layer (Figure 23.14 and Plate 20). The implanted pump is situated beneath the diaphragm in the preperitoneal cavity, and a percutaneous electric line connects the blood pump assembly to the portable system controller and battery pack. In the automatic mode, the device can increase cardiac output in response to exercise and increase venous return up to a maximum flow rate of 10 L/min.

The use of improved blood contacting surfaces and porcine valves has eliminated the need for long-term anticoagulation and reduced the incidence of thromboembolic complications to 0.2 episodes/patient/year (178). Prototypes of battery-powered LVADs are undergoing clinical evaluation. Such systems are truly "wearable," as they do not require an external drive console. Currently, energy is transmitted through a transcutaneous electrical connection, but new technology will allow transcutaneous passage through induction coils.

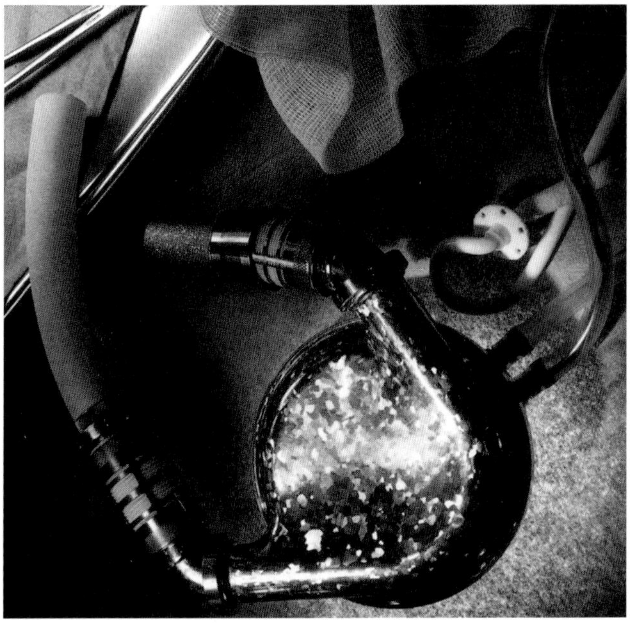

FIGURE 23.13. *Photograph of the TCI HeartMate left ventricular assist device with inflow and outflow conduits prior to preperitoneal implantation.*

Electrically powered devices have been remarkably free of infection and have supported patients for up to 1.5 years (179). Additional advances in battery technology are needed to permit long-term outpatient management. The rapid advances during the past decade in device design suggest that truly portable and permanent devices are on the horizon. The substantial cost associated with device implantation (>$120,000 per patient) and the need for intensive long-term medical follow-up suggest that strict selection criteria will be needed.

Xenotransplantation

Concordant and discordant xenografting describe transplantation between closely related (e.g., baboon to human) or distantly related species (e.g., pig to human), respectively. Concordant xenografting has the advantage of the lack of xenoreactive antibodies in the donor; it is hoped that better strategies designed to prevent cell-mediated immunity and antibody production will allow prolonged graft survival. Disadvantages include the scarcity of non-human primates, ethical concerns regarding the use of chimpanzees and monkeys, and the possibility of transmission of epizootic diseases (see Chapter 40).

Discordant xenografting, particularly using the pig, has several potential advantages, including low cost, ready donor

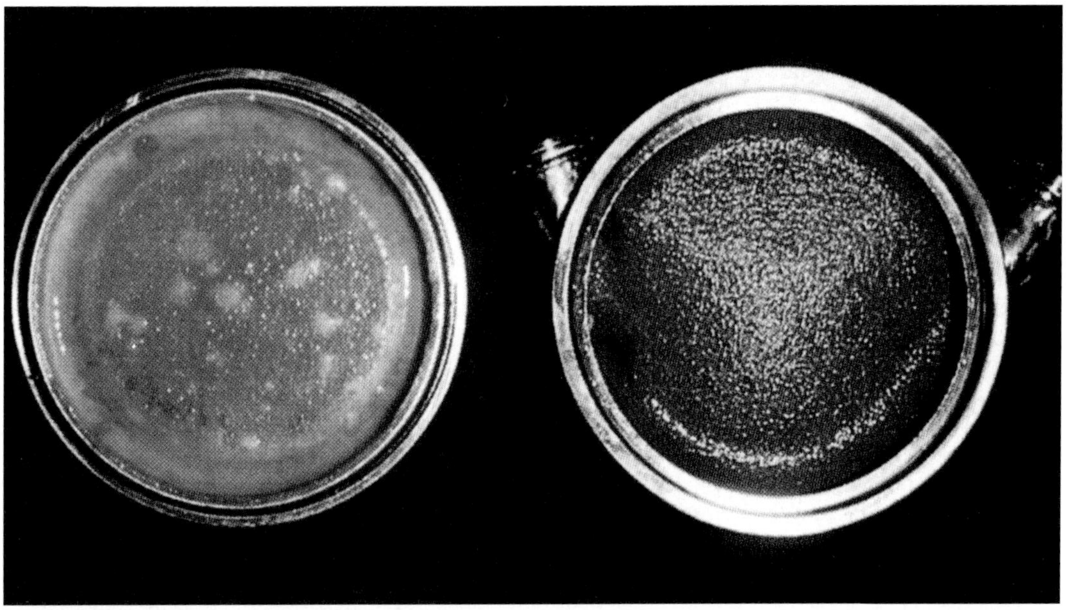

FIGURE 23.14. *Photograph of the blood contacting surface of the TCI HeartMate left ventricular assist device. The development of a pseudo-intima is evident.*

availability, the ability to select donor size for the smallest to the largest recipients, the possibility of developing pathogen-free animals, and a high degree of similarity in anatomy and physiology to humans. Rejection is uniformly vascular and generally hyperacute due to antibody-mediated complement activation. Even if hyperacute rejection can be overcome, the severity of the cellular rejection response remains to be defined.

Of the eight reported human xenotransplants, five have been concordant (non-human primates) and three have been discordant (one sheep and two pigs). The maximum survival times of concordant and discordant grafts have been 20 days and 24 hours, respectively (178).

The problem of hyperacute rejection, particularly between discordant species, remains to be solved. Despite the use of aggressive immunosuppressive strategies including monoclonal antibodies, tacrolimus, mycophenolate, total lymphoid irradiation, and plasmapheresis or photophoresis to diminish humorally mediated rejection, survival in experimental discordant xenotransplantation is still measured in days rather than months or years. Even with the use of genetically engineered donor pigs, survival has been extended to only a few months.

Cross-species transplantation may ultimately replace conventional orthotopic transplantation. However, major breakthroughs in our understanding of immunologic modulation or tolerance induction are needed to ensure the success of this approach.

CONCLUSION

The promise of human cardiac transplantation remains unfilled. Despite its remarkable success, the donor shortage limits its use to 1% to 2% of patients dying of advanced heart failure. The inability to increase the number of available donors and the high risk of patient death while awaiting transplantation argue that alternative approaches are needed. Implantable left ventricular assist devices may soon benefit selected recipients. Xenotransplantation may ultimately offer the best solution, but it appears to be at least several years away.

COMMENTARY

Dale G. Renlund

Controversy has surrounded many aspects of cardiac transplantation for years. But instead of resolving over time, the number and complexity of the controversies increase as the donor/recipient disparity worsens, heart transplant programs proliferate, and mechanical circulatory support systems develop. The use and timing of new surgical techniques such as ventricular reduction have already impacted heart transplantation, raising controversies of their own.

CONTROVERSIES IN RECIPIENT SELECTION

Advances in transplantation medicine have enabled successful transplantation in individuals who were heretofore considered inappropriate or marginal candidates. For example, selected older patients and diabetics can do well following cardiac transplantation. However, many transplant centers have established arbitrary upper age limits and routinely exclude diabetics with end-organ damage. Such exclusions present ethical and societal dilemmas because they are not based solely on medical criteria. Some have argued that these exclusions are proper, given the current donor/recipient disparity. Others justify exclusions based on ill-defined and nonquantifiable quality-of-life issues.

These and other ethical challenges face transplant physicians and surgeons daily, and they cannot be perfunctorily or nonchalantly ignored. For instance, should those with unresolved substance abuse, including tobacco use, be offered cardiac transplantation? Should those who are deemed more valuable to a community receive priority? Should patients with children to raise be given priority over patients who have no dependent children? The potential ethical dilemmas associated with recipient selection are endless and fraught with prejudice and bias.

CONTROVERSIES IN THE TIMING OF MECHANICAL CIRCULATORY SUPPORT PRIOR TO TRANSPLANTATION

With the success of mechanical circulatory support technology, consideration must be given to its earlier use in the course of end-stage heart disease. In times past, mechanical circulatory support devices were used only under dire circumstances. Now, a strong case can be made to use a left ventricular assist device instead of subjecting a patient to prolonged hospitalization with invasive monitoring. In addition, if the anticipated intensive care unit stay is longer than a month, it may be cost effective to use a ventricular assist device while awaiting a suitable donor heart. Doing so may also enable the patient to be discharged from the hospital and ultimately to become a better transplant candidate.

CONTROVERSIES IN TRANSPLANT CENTER RESTRICTION

The United States has more than 165 currently established heart transplant programs. As only 2300 heart transplants are performed in the United States each year, the average is only about one transplant per center per month. Centers performing fewer than nine heart transplant procedures each year do so with worse survival rates than do programs with higher volumes (1). Should the number of centers be limited to improve overall patient survival, to ensure continued expertise, to further develop the science and art of transplantation, and to minimize cost?

In the United States, neither the federal government nor the medical profession, believing as strongly as they do in free-market competition, will likely limit the number of transplant programs. This allows third-party insurers to create their own criteria under which transplantation will be reimbursed—criteria that may not be in the best interests of the patients or society.

ALTERNATIVES TO CARDIAC TRANSPLANTATION

The only available treatment for end-stage refractory heart disease that significantly lengthens life is cardiac transplantation. The inability to procure a sufficient supply of human donor hearts prohibits the timely application of transplantation in many excellent candidates and in many who are presently judged to be marginal candidates. Human cardiac allograft transplantation will always be inadequate in meeting the needs of those it is intended to serve, the entire population of patients with end-stage heart disease. Only through the development of viable long-term alternatives to heart allotransplantation will the needs of patients with end-stage heart disease be fully met. Indeed, the gap between the number of patients who are currently being helped and those who could and should be helped must be narrowed by looking to nonallotransplant alternatives.

Mechanical Support

Permanent mechanical circulatory support would reduce the donor/recipient disparity and limit transplantation to those who are most likely to tolerate immunosuppression. However, permanent circulatory support will be formidably expensive. Currently, the supply of donor hearts limits the total expenditure on end-stage heart failure to a significant extent. The ability to manufacture cardiac replacements will foster far greater treatment of end-stage heart failure than is currently being done with heart replacement using human donors.

Xenotransplantation

Genetically altered species with lowered antigenicity have led to speculation that xenotransplantation for humans is not far-fetched, impractical, or of theoretic interest only (see Chapter 40). Academic and commercial sponsors are actively developing xenograft products and clinical applications. As evidence of future expectations, the Department of Health and Human Services (DHHS) has recently published guidelines for infectious disease issues in xenotransplantation (2). Though the document focuses on the concerns of transmission of diseases from animals to humans, the publication foresees the emergence of routine xenotransplantation.

Government oversight of xenotransplantation may prove to be beneficial by increasing public awareness and acceptance. Successful xenotransplantation, like mechanical circulatory support, could be formidably expensive—should donors no longer be a rate-limiting factor, more patients would be eligible for treatment.

Cardiac Reduction

A new procedure, cardiac reduction, is now being discussed "amid a mixture of excitement and caution" (3). Since 1994, over 300 patients near Curitiba in southern Brazil have undergone a procedure in which the size of the left ventricle is reduced by removing an elliptical portion of the lateral left ventricular wall and sewing the ventricle back together. Dr. Randas J.V. Batista, the originator of the procedure, reports a 20% death rate in the first postoperative month and an additional 20% death rate during the remainder of the first year. Batista and others believe that the smaller left ventricular chamber size allows more effective pumping, as decreasing the ventricular radius predictably decreases wall stress.

A discussion of cardiac reduction surgery in a recent editorial noted that "if U.S. cardiac surgeons can repeat the success of Batista's best patient population (those with dilated cardiomyopathy) then this operation potentially offers new hope to some of the thousands of U.S. heart patients waiting for a suitable donor. Instead of heart transplant with its multiple attendant risks . . . some of these patients may be able to undergo ventricular remodeling and retain their own heart" (4). Cardiac reduction may obviate the need to obtain a scarce human donor heart to treat end-stage heart disease in selected patients.

Cardiac reduction procedures are being increasingly performed in the United States, Britain, and Italy with no regulation and no oversight. Despite the hype, the role of cardiac reduction in the treatment of end-stage heart failure remains undefined. Only time will tell whether the Batista operation will become a standard practice or a fad that fades. The procedure does not currently warrant acceptance without further study of the results of the ongoing trials.

CONCLUSION

As G. William Dec notes in this chapter, extraordinary progress has enabled cardiac transplantation to "evolve from an experimental procedure to an established therapeutic option for the management of myocardial failure." Other advances are on the horizon in the form of improved immunosuppressive agents and techniques. Although all who have been involved should be pleased by current progress, no one interested in the future of heart transplantation should rest comfortably or complacently until uniform survival and an excellent quality of life are achieved in all patients treated for end-stage heart disease.

CHAPTER REFERENCES

1. Rodeheffer R, McGregor C. The development of cardiac transplantation. Mayo Clin Proc 1992;67:480–484.
2. Hardy J, Chavez C, Kurrus F, et al. Heart transplantation in man: developmental studies and report of a case. J Am Med Assoc 1964;118:1132–1137.
3. Barnard C. A human cardiac transplant: an interim report of a successful operation performed at Groote Schuur Hospital, Capetown. S Afr Med J 1967;41:1271–1274.
4. Caves P, Stinson E, Billingham M, et al. Percutaneous endomyocardial biopsy in human heart recipients. Ann Thorac Surg 1973;16:325–329.
5. Mudge G, Goldstein S, Addonizio L, et al. Task Force 3: recipient guidelines/prioritization-24th Bethesda Conference on Cardiac Transplantation. J Am Coll Cardiol 1993;22:21–31.
6. O'Connell J, Bourge R, Costanzo-Nordin M, et al. Cardiac transplantation: recipient selection, donor procurement, and medical follow-up. A statement for health professionals from the Committee on Cardiac Transplantation of the Council on Clinical Cardiology, American Heart Association. Circulation 1992;86:1061–1079.
7. Vagelos R, Fowler M. Selection of patients for cardiac transplantation. Cardiol Clin 1990;8:223–238.
8. Mancini D, Kussmaul W, Mull R, et al. Value of peak oxygen consumption for optimal timing of cardiac transplantation in ambulatory patients with heart failure. Circulation 1991;83:778–786.
9. Elefteriades J, Tolis G, Levi E, et al. Coronary artery bypass grafting in severe left ventricular dysfunction: excellent survival with improved ejection fraction and functional state. J Am Coll Cardiol 1993;22:1411–1417.
10. Louie H, Laks H, Milgalter E, et al. Ischemic cardiomyopathy: criteria for coronary revascularization and cardiac transplantation. Circulation 1991;84(suppl 3):290–295.
11. Sweeney M, Ruskin J, Garan H, et al. Influence of the implantable cardioverter-defibrillator on sudden death and total mortality in patients evaluated for cardiac transplantation. Circulation 1995;92:3273–3281.
12. Goldstein D, Oz M, Rose E, Fisher P, Michler R. Experience with heart transplantation for cardiac tumors. J Heart Lung Transplant 1995;14:382–386.
13. Bourge R, Naftel D, Costanzo-Nordin M, et al. Pretransplantation risk factors for death after heart transplanation: a multiinstitutional study. J Heart Lung Transplant 1993;12:549–562.
14. Heroux A, Costanzo-Nordin M, O'Sullivan J, et al. Heart transplantation as a treatment option for end-stage heart disease in patients older than 65 years of age. J Heart Lung Transplant 1993;12:573–579.
15. Kirklin J, Naftel D, Kirklin J, et al. Pulmonary vascular resistance and the risk of heart transplantation. J Heart Transplant 1988;7:331–336.
16. Murali S, Uretsky B, Reddy S, et al. Reversibility of pulmonary hypertension in congestive heart failure patients evaluated for cardiac transplantation: comparative effects of various pharmacological agents. Am Heart J 1991;122:1375–1381.
17. Iberer F, Wasler A, Tscheliessnigg K, et al. Prostaglandin E1-induced moderation of elevated pulmonary vascular resistance. Survival on waiting list and results of orthotopic heart transplantation. J Heart Lung Transplant 1993;12:173–178.
18. Semigran M, Cockrill B, Kacmarek R, et al. Hemodynamic effects of inhaled nitric oxide in heart failure. J Am Coll Cardiol 1994;24:982–988.
19. Costard-Jackle A, Hill I, Schroeder J, Fowler M. The influence of preoperative patient characteristics on early and late survival following cardiac transplantation. Circulation 1991;84(suppl 3):329–337.
20. Rose E, Levin H, Oz M, et al. Artificial circulatory support with textured interior surfaces. A counterintuitive approach to minimizing thromboembolism. Circulation 1994;90(part 2):87–91.
21. Steck T, Costanzo-Nordin M, Keshavarian A. Prevalence and management of cholelithiasis in heart transplant patients. J Heart Lung Transplant 1991;10:1029–1032.
22. van den Broek S, van Veldhuisen D, de Graeff P, et al. Mode of death in patients with congestive heart failure: comparison between possible candidates for heart transplantation and patients with less advanced disease. J Heart Lung Transplant 1993;11:265–272.
23. Muirhead J, Meyerowitz B, Leedham B, et al. Quality of life and coping in patients awaiting heart transplantation. J Heart Lung Transplant 1992;11:265–272.
24. Stevenson L, Steimle A, Fonarow G, et al. Improvement in exercise capacity of candidates awaiting heart transplantation. J Am Coll Cardiol 1995;25:163–170.
25. Steimle A, Stevenson L, Forarow G, et al. Prediction of improvement in recent onset cardiomyopathy after referral for heart transplantation. J Am Coll Cardiol 1994;23:553–559.
26. Steihoff G, Wongeit K, Schafers H, Haverich A. Sequential analysis of monomorphic and polymorphic major histocompatibility complex antigen expression in human heart allograft biopsy specimens. J Heart Transplant 1989;8:360–370.
27. Pirsch J, D'Alessandro A, Sollinger H, et al. The effect of donor age, recipient age, and HLA match on immunologic graft survival in cadaver renal transplant recipients. Transplantation 1992;53:55–59.
28. Oplez G, Wujciak T, for the Collaborative Transplant Study. The influence of HLA compatibility on graft survival after heart transplantation. New Engl J Med 1994;330:816–819.
29. Jarcho J, Naftel D, Shroyer T, et al. Influence of HLA mismatch on rejection after heart transplantation: a multi-institutional study. J Heart Lung Transplant 1994;13:583–596.
30. Costanzo-Nordin M, Fisher S, O'Sullivan E, et al. HLA-DR incompatibility predicts heart transplant rejection independent of immunosuppressive prophylaxis. J Heart Lung Transplant 1993;12:779–789.
31. Wechsler M, Giardina E, Scuacca R, et al. Increased early mortality in women undergoing cardiac transplantation. Circulation 1995;91:1029–1335.
32. Loh E, Bergin J, Couper G, Mudge G. Role of panel-reactive antibody cross-reactivity in predicting survival after orthotopic heart transplantation. J Heart Lung Transplant 1994;13:194–201.
33. Cherry R, Nielsen H, Reed E, et al. Vascular (humoral) rejection in human cardiac allograft biopsies: relation to circulating anti-HLA antibodies. J Heart Lung Transplant 1992;11:24–30.
34. Petrossian G, Nichols A, Marboe C, et al. Relation between survival and development of coronary artery disease and anti-HLA antibodies after cardiac transplantation. Circulation 1989;80(suppl 3):122–125.
35. Rose E, Barr M, Pepino P, et al. Photochemotherapy in human heart transplant recipients at high risk for fatal rejection. J Heart Lung Transplant 1992;11:746–750.
36. Tyan DB, Li VA, Czer L, et al. Intravenous immunoglobulin suppression of HLA alloantibody in highly sensitized transplant candidates and transplantation with a histoincompatible organ. Transplantation 1994;57:553–562.
37. De Marco T, Damon LE, Colombe B, et al. Successful immunomodulation with intravenous gamma globulin and cyclophosphamide in an alloimmunized heart transplant recipient. J Heart Lung Transplant 1997;16:360–365.
38. Jordan SC, Quartel AW, Czer LSC, et al. Posttransplant therapy using high-dose human immunoglobulin (intravenous gammaglobulin) to control acute humoral rejection in renal and cardiac allograft recipients and potential mechanism of action. Transplantation 1998;66:800–805.
39. Humphrey L, Blanck T. Anesthetic management of the heart or heart-lung transplant patient. In: Baumgartner WA, Reitz BA, Achuff SA, eds. Heart and heart-lung transplantation. Philadelphia: WB Saunders, 1998:103–112.
40. Baldwin J, Anderson J, Boucek M, et al. Task Force 2: Donor guidelines. 24th Bethesda Conference on cardiac transplantation. J Am Coll Cardiol 1993;22:15–20.
41. Boucek M, Mathis C, Kanakriyeh M, et al. Donor shortage: use of the dysfunctional donor heart. J Heart Lung Transplant 1993;12:S186–S190.
42. Hosenpud J, Bennett LE, Kecle BM, et al. The registry of the international society for heart and lung transplantation: fifteenth official report-1998. J Heart Lung Transplant 1998;17:656–658.
43. Pflugfelder P, Singh N, McKenzie F, et al. Extending cardiac allograft ischemic time and donor age: effect on survival and long-term cardiac function. J Heart Lung Transplant 1991;10:394–400.
44. McGregor C. Cardiac transplantation: surgical considerations and early postoperative management. Mayo Clin Proc 1992;67:577–585.
45. Schuler S, Matschke K, Loebe M, et al. Coronary artery disease in patients with hearts from older donors: morphologic features and therapeutic implications. J Heart Lung Transplant 1993;12:100–109.
46. Jeevanandam F, Todd B, Regillo T, et al. Reversal of donor myocardial dysfunction by triiodothyronine replacement therapy. J Heart Lung Transplant 1994;13:681–687.

47. Hosenpud J, Pantely G, Morton M, et al. Relation between recipient: donor body size match and hemodynamics three months after heart transplantation. J Heart Transplant 1989;8:241–243.
48. Morely D, Boigon M, Fesniak H, et al. Posttransplant hemodynamics and exercise function are not affected by body-size matching of donor and recipient. J Heart Lung Transplant 1993;12:770–778.
49. Vlahakes G, Lemmer J, Bhrendt D, Austen WE. Transplantation. In: Handbook of patient care in cardiac surgery. Boston: Little, Brown, 1994:229–258.
50. Baldwin J. Heart graft preservation. In: Shumway SJ, Shumway NE, eds. Toracic transplantation. Cambridge, MA: Blackwell Science, 1995:67–70.
51. Deleuze P, Benvenuti C, Mazzucotelli J, et al. Orthotopic cardiac transplantation with direct caval anastomosis: is it the optimal procedure? J Thorac Cardiovasc Surg 1995;109:731–737.
52. Nankatani T, Frazier O, Lammermeier D, et al. Hetrotopic heart transplantation: a reliable option for a select group of high-risk patients. J Heart Transplant 1989;8:40–47.
53. McGoon M, Frantz R. Techniques of immunosuppression after cardiac transplantation. Mayo Clin Proc 1992;67:586–595.
54. Hunt S. Complications of heart transplantation. J Heart Transplant 1983;2:70–74.
55. Miller LE. The results of corticosteroid withdrawal in heart transplantation: a multicenter review. J Heart Lung Transplant 1992;11(part 2):S401–S434.
56. Price G, Olsen S, Taylor D, et al. Corticosteroid-free maintenance immunosuppression after heart transplantation: feasibility and beneficial effects. J Heart Lung Transplant 1992;11(suppl 2):403–414.
57. Esmore D, Keogh A, Spratt P, et al. Heart transplantation in females. J Heart Lung Transplant 1997;10:335–341.
58. Menkis A, Powell A, Novick R, et al. A prospective randomized controlled trial of initial immunosuppression with ALG versus OKT3 in recipients of cardiac allografts. J Heart Lung Transplant 1992;11:569–576.
59. Kobashigawa J, Stevenson L, Brownfield E, et al. Does short-course induction with OKT3 improve outcome after heart transplantation? A randomized trial. J Heart Lung Transplant 1993;12:250–258.
60. Macris M. Frazier O, Lammermeier D, et al. Climical experience with Moromonab-CD3 monoclonal antibody (OKT3) in heart transplantation. J Heart Transplant 1989;8:281–287.
61. Swinnen L, Costanzo-Nordin M, Fisher SG, et al. Increased incidence of lymphoproliferative disorder after immunosuppression with the monoclonal antibody OKT3 in cardiac-transplant recipients. N Engl J Med 1990;323:1723–1728.
62. Armitage J, Kormos R, Morita S, et al. Clinical trial of FK 506 immunosuppression in adult cardiac transplantation. Ann Thorac Surg 1992:54.
63. Tsamandas AC, Pham SM, Seaberg EC, et al. Adult heart transplantation under tacrolimus (FK506) immunosuppression: histopathologic observation and comparison to a cyclosporine-based regimen with lymphocytic (ATG) induction. J Heart Lung Transplant 1997;16:723–734.
64. Meiser BM, Uberfuhr P, Fuchs A, et al. Single-center randomized trial comparing tacrolimus (FK506) and cyclosporine in the prevention of acute myocardial rejection. J Heart Lung Transplant 1998;17:782–788.
65. Reichart B, Meiser B, Vigano M, et al. European multicenter tacrolimus (FK506) heart pilot study: one-year results. European Tacrolimus Multicenter Heart Study Group. J Heart Lung Transplant 1998;17:775–781.
66. Taylor D, Ensley R, Olsen S, et al. Mycophenolate mofetil (RS-61442): preclinical, clinical, and three-year experience in heart transplantation. J Heart Lung Transplant 1994;13:571–582.
67. Kirklin J, Bourge R, Naftel D, et al. Treatment of recurrent heart rejection with mycophenolate mofetil (RS-1443): initial clinical experience. J Heart Lung Transplant 1994;13:444–450.
68. Kobashigawa J, Miller L, Renlund D, et al. A randomized active-controlled trial of mycophenolate mofetil in heart transplant patients. Transplantation 1998;66:507–515.
69. Walsh T, Guttendorf J, Drummer S, et al. The value of protective isolation procedures in cardiac allograft recipients. Ann Thorac Surg 1989;47:539–545.
70. Stinson E, Caves P, Griepp R, et al. Hemodynamic observation in the early period after human heart transplantation. J Thorac Cardiovasc Surg 1975;69:264–269.
71. Keating M, Wilhelm M, Walker R. Strategies for prevention of infection after cardiac transplantation. Mayo Clin Proc 1992;67:677–683.
72. Macdonald P, Hackworthy R, Keogh A, et al. The effect of chronic amiodarone therapy before transplantation on early cardiac allograft function. J Heart Lung Transplant 1991;10:743–749.
73. Redmond J, Zehr K, Gillinov M, et al. Use of theophylline for treatment of prolonged sinus node dysfunction in human orthotopic heart transplantation. J Heart Lung Transplant 1993;12:133–139.
74. Cooper M, Smith C, Rose E, et al. Permanent pacing following cardiac transplantation. J Thorac Cardiovasc Surg 1992;104:812–816.
75. Jensen M, Olivari M, Walt M, et al. Frequency and significance of right bundle branch block after cardiac transplantation. Am J Cardiol 1994;73:1009–1011.
76. Leonelli F, Pacifico A, Young J. Frequency and significance of conduction defects early after orthotopic heart transplantation. Am J Cardiol 1994;73:175–179.
77. Scott C, Dark J, McComb J. Arrhythmias after cardiac transplantation. Am J Cardiol 1992;70:1061–1063.
78. Pavri B, O'Noonan S, Newell J, et al. Prevalence and significance of atrial arrhythmias after orthotopic cardiac transplantation. J Am Coll Cardiol 1995;25:1673–1680.
79. Miller L. Long-term complications of cardiac transplantation. Prog Cardiovasc Dis 1991;33:229–282.
80. Winters G, Costanzo-Nordin M, O'Sullivan E, et al. Predictors of late acute orthotopic heart transplant rejection. Circulation 1989;80(suppl 3):106–110.
81. Sethi G, Kosaraju S, Arabia F, et al. Is it necessary to perform surveillance endomyocardial biopsies in heart transplant recipients? J Heart Lung Transplant 1995;14:1047–1051.
82. White J, Guiraudon C, Pflugfelder P, Kostuk W. Routine surveillance myocardial biopsies are unnecessary beyond one year after heart transplantation. J Heart Lung Transplant 1995;14:1052–1056.
83. Billingham M, Cary N, Hammond M, et al. A working formulation for the standardization of nomenclature in the diagnosis of heart and lung rejection: Heart Rejection Study Group. J Heart Lung Transplant 1990;9:587–593.
84. Sharples L, Cary N, Large S, Wallwork J. Error rates with which endomyocardial biopsy specimens are graded for rejection after cardiac transplantation. Am J Cardiol 1992;70:527–530.
85. Nielsen H, Sorensen F, Nielsen B, et al. Reproducibility of the acute rejection diagnosis in human cardiac allografts. The Stanford classification and the International grading system. J Heart Lung Transplant 1993;12:239–243.
86. Forbes R, Rowan R, Billingham M. Endocardial infiltrates in human heart transplants. A serial biopsy analysis comparing four immunosuppression protocols. Hum Pathol 1990;10:850–855.
87. Costanzo-Nordin M, Winters G, Fisher S, et al. Endocardial infiltrates in the transplanted heart: clinical significance emerging from the analysis of 5026 endomyocardial biopsy specimens. J Heart Lung Transplant 1993;12:741–747.
88. Lloveras J, Escourrou G, Delisle M, et al. Evolution of untreated mild rejection in heart transplant recipients. J Heart Lung Transplant 1992;11:751–756.
89. Kirklin J, Naftel D, Bourge R, et al. Rejection after cardiac transplantation. A time-related risk factor analysis. Circulation 1992;86(suppl 2):263–241.
90. Miller L. Treatment of cardiac allograft rejection with intravenous steroids. J Heart Transplant 1990;9:283–287.
91. Kemkes B, Schutz A, Engelhardt M, et al. Noninvasive methods of rejection diagnosis after heart transplantation. J Heart Transplant 1992;11:S221–S231.
92. Wahlers T, Haverich A, Schafers H-J, et al. Changes of the intramyocardial electrogram after orthotopic heart transplantation. J Heart Transplant 1986;5:450–454.
93. Valantine H. Rejection surveillance by Doppler echocardiography. J Heart Lung Transplant 1993;12:422–426.
94. Ciliberto G, Mascarello M, Gronda E, et al. Acute rejection after heart transplantation: noninvasive echocardiographic evaluation. J Am Coll Cardiol 1994;23:1156–1161.
95. Yamamoto S, Bergsland J, Michalek S, et al. Uptake of myocardial imaging agents by rejecting and nonrejecting cardiac transplants. A comparative clinical study of thallium-201, technetium-99m, and gallium-67. J Nucl Med 1989;30:1464–1469.
96. Ballester M, Obrador D, Carrio I, et al. Early postoperative reduction of monoclonal antimyosin antibody uptake is associated with absent rejection-related complications after heart transplantation. Circulation 1992;85:61–68.
97. Alexis JD, Lao CD, Salter JC, et al. Cardiac troponin T: a noninvasive marker for heart transplant rejection? J Heart Lung Transplant 1998;17:395–398.
98. Hammond E, Yowell R, Nunoda S, et al. Vascular (humoral) rejection in heart transplantation: pathologic observations and clinical implications. J Heart Lung Transplant 1989;8:430–443.
99. Hammond E, Hansen J, Spencer L, et al. Vascular rejection in cardiac transplantation: histologic, immunopathologic, and ultrastructural features. Cardiovasc Pathol 1993;2:21–34.
100. Lones M, Czer L, Trento A, et al. Clinical-pathologic features of humoral rejection in cardiac allografts: a study in 81 consecutive patients. J Heart Lung Transplant 1995;14:151–162.

101. Bonnaud E, Lewis N, Masek M, Billingham M. Reliability and usefulness of immunofluorescence in heart transplantation. J Heart Lung Transplant 1995;14:163–171.
102. Olsen S, Wagoner L, Hammond E, et al. Vascular rejection in heart transplantation: clinical correlation, treatment options, and future considerations. J Heart Lung Transplant 1993;12:S135–S142.
103. Kobashigawa J, Stevenson L, Moriguchi J, et al. Is intravenous glucocorticoid therapy better than an oral regimen for asymptomatic cardiac rejection? A randomized trial. J Am Coll Cardiol 1993;21:1142–1144.
104. Haverty T, Sanders M, Sheahan M. OKT3 treatment of cardiac allograft rejection. J Heart Lung Transplant 1993;12:591–598.
105. Armitage J, Kormos R, Griffith B, et al. A clinical trial of FK506 as primary and rescue immunosuppression in cardiac transplantation. Transplant Proc 1991;23:1149–1152.
106. Hosenpud J, Hershberger R, Ratkovec R, et al. Methotrexate for the treatment of patients with multiple episodes of acute ardiac allograft rejection. J Heart Lung Transplant 1992;11:739–745.
107. DiSalvo T, Narula J, Cosimi AB, et al. Actinomycin D is an effective adjunctive immunosuppressive agent for recurrent allograft rejection. J Heart Lung Transplant 1995;14:955–962.
108. Hunt S, Strober S, Hoppe R, Stinson E. Total lymphoid irradiation for treatment of intractable cardiac allograft rejection. J Heart Lung Transplant 1991;10:211–216.
109. Salter M, Kirklin J, Bourge R, et al. Total lymphoid irradiation in the treatment of early or recurrent heart rejection. J Heart Lung Transplant 1992;11:902–912.
110. Costanzo-Nordin M, Hubbell E, O'Sullivan J, et al. Successful treatment of heart transplant rejection with photophoresis. Transplantation 1992;53: 808–815.
111. Olivari M, May C, Johnson N, et al. Treatment of acute vascular rejection with immunoadsorption. Circulation 1994;90(part 2):70–73.
112. Hammond E, Yowell R, Price G, et al. Vascular rejection and its relationship to allograft coronary artery disease. J Heart Lung Transplant 1992;11:S111–S119.
113. Younis L, Melin J, Schoevaerdts J, et al. Left ventricular systolic function and diastolic filling at rest and during upright exercise after orthotopic heart transplantation: comparison with young and aged normal subjects. J Heart Transplant 1990;9:683–692.
114. vonScheidt W, Ziegler U, Kemkes B, Erdmann E. Heart transplantation: hemodynamics over a five-year period. J Heart Lung Transplant 1991;10:342–350.
115. Tischler M, Lee R, Plappert T, et al. Serial assessment of left ventricular function and mass after orthotopic heart transplantation: a 4-year longitudinal study. J Am Coll Cardiol 1992;19:60–66.
116. Semigran M, Aroney C, Dec G, Fifer M. Abnormalities of diastolic function progress over time in cardiac transplant recipients. Circulation 1992;86:378.
117. Pope S, Stinson E, Daughters G, et al. Exercise response of the denervated heart in long-term cardiac transplant recipients. Am J Cardiol 1980;46: 213–218.
118. Stevenson L, Sietsema K, Tillisch J, et al. Exercise capacity for survivors of cardiac transplantation or sustained medical therapy for stable heart failure. Circulation 1990;81:78–85.
119. Kao A, VanTrigt P, Shaeffer-McCall G, et al. Allograft diastolic dysfunction and chronotropic incompetence limit cardiac output response to exercise two to six years after heart transplantation. J Heart Lung Transplant 1995;14:11–22.
120. Braith R, Limacher M, Leggett S, Pollock M. Skeletal muscle strength in heart transplant recipients. J Heart Lung Transplant 1993;12:1018–1023.
121. Canter C, Saffitz J, Moorhead S, et al. Early results after pediatric cardiac transplantation with triple immunosuppression therapy. Am J Cardiol 1993;71:971–975.
122. Chiavarelli M, Gundry S, Razzouk A, Bailey L. Cardiac transplantation for infants with hypoplastic left-heart syndrome. J Am Med Assoc 1993;270:2944–2947.
123. Sarris G, Smith J, Bernstein D, et al. Pediatric cardiac transplantation: the Stanford experience. Circulation 1994;90(part 2):51–55.
124. Scherrer U, Vissing S, Morgan B, et al. Cyclosporine-induced sympathetic activation and hypertension after heart transplantation. N Engl J Med 1990;323:693–699.
125. Ventura H, Milani R, Lavie C, et al. Cyclosporine-induced hypertension. Efficacy of w-3 fatty acids in patients after cardiac transplantation. Circulation 1993;88(part 2):281–285.
126. Ballantyne C, Radovancevic B, Framer J, et al. Hyperlipidemia after heart transplantation: report of a 6-year experience, with treatment recommendations. J Am Coll Cardiol 1992;19:1315–1321.
127. Kobashigawa J, Katznelson S, Laks H, et al. Effect of pravastatin on outcomes after cardiac transplantation. N Engl J Med 1995;333:621–627.
128. Kubo S, Peters J, Knutson K, et al. Factors influencing the development of hypercholesterolemia after cardiac transplantation. Am J Cardiol 1992;70: 520–526.
129. Lake K, Reutzel T, Pritzker M, Jorgensen C, Emery R. The impact of steroid withdrawal on the development of lipid abnormalities and obesity in heart transplant recipients. J Heart Lung Transplant 1993;12:580–590.
130. Pfugfelder P, Huff M, Oskalns R, et al. Cholesterol-lowering therapy after heart transplantation: a 12-month randomized trial. J Heart Lung Transplant 1995;14:613–622.
131. Augustine S, Yeo C, Buchman T, et al. Gastrointestinal complications in heart and in heart-lung transplant patients. J Heart Lung Transplant 1991;10: 547–556.
132. Steck T, Durkin M, Costanzo-Nordin M, Keshavarzian A. Gastrointestinal complications and endoscopic findings in heart transplant patients. J Heart Lung Transplant 1993;12:244–251.
133. Pereira B, Milford E, Kirkman R, et al. Prevalence of hepatitis C virus RNA in organ donors positive for hepatitis C antibody and in the recipients of their organs. N Engl J Med 1992;327:910–915.
134. Cadranel J, Grippon P, Lunel F, et al. Chronic liver dysfunction in heart transplant recipients, with special reference to viral B, C and non-A, non-B, non-C hepatitis. Transplantation 1991;52:645–650.
135. Peterseim D, Pappas T, Meyers C, et al. Management of biliary complications after heart transplantation. J Heart Lung Transplant 1995;14:623–631.
136. Miller L, Naftel D, Bourge R, et al. Infection after heart transplantation: a multiinstitutional study. J Heart Lung Transplant 1994;13:381–393.
137. Gentry L, Zeluff B. Infection in the cardiac transplant recipient. In: Rubin RH, Young LS, eds. Clinical approach to infection in the compromised host. 2nd ed. New York: Plenum, 1988:623–648.
138. Macdonald P, Keogh A, Marshman D, et al. A double-blind placebo-controlled trial of low-dose ganciclovir to prevent cytomegalovirus disease after heart transplantation. J Heart Lung Transplant 1995;14:32–38.
139. Gratten M, Moreno-Cabral C, Starnes V, et al. Cytomegalovirus infection is associated with cardiac allograft rejection and atherosclerosis. J Am Med Assoc 1989;261:3561–3566.
140. Penn I. Incidence and treatment of neoplasia after transplantation. J Heart Lung Transplant 1993;12:S328–S336.
141. Couetil J, McGoldrick J, Wallwork J, English T. Malignant tumors after heart transplantation. J Heart Transplant 1991;9:622–626.
142. Johnson WM, Baldrusson O, Gros TJ. Double jeopardy: lung cancer after cardiac transplantation. Chest 1998;113:1720–1723.
143. Penn I, Porat G. Central nervous system lymphomas in organ allograft recipients. Transplantation 1995;59:240–244.
144. Walker R, Paya C, Marshall W, et al. Pretransplantation seronegative Epstein-Barr virus status is the primary risk factor for posttransplantation lymphoproliferative disorder in adult heart, lung, and other solid organ transplantations. J Heart Lung Transplant 1995;14:214–221.
145. Armitage J, Kormos R, Stuart R, et al. Posttransplant lymphoproliferative disease in thoracic organ transplant patients: ten years of cyclosporine-based immunosuppression. J Heart Lung Transplant 1991;10:877–887.
146. Uretsky B, Murali S, Reedy S, et al. Development of coronary artery disease in cardiac transplant patients receiving immunosuppressive therapy with cyclosporine and prednisone. Circulation 1987;76:827–834.
147. Gao S, Schroeder J, Alderman E, et al. Clinical and laboratory correlates of accelerated coronary artery disease in the cardiac transplant patient. Circulation 1987;76(suppl 5):56–61.
148. Pucci A, Forbes C, Billingham M. Pathologic features in long-term cardiac allografts. J Heart Transplant 1990;9:339–345.
149. Gao S, Schroeder J, Hunt S, et al. Influence of graft rejection on incidence of accelerated graft coronary artery disease: a new approach to analysis. J Heart Lung Transplant 1993;12:1029–1035.
150. Stovin P, Sharples L, Schofield P, et al. Lack of association between endomyocardial evidence of rejection in the first six months and the later development of transplant-related coronary artery disease. J Heart Lung Transplant 1993;12:110–116.
151. Libby P, Salomon R, Payne D, et al. Functions of vascular cell walls related to the development of transplant-associated coronary atherosclerosis. Transplant Proc 1989;21:3677–3684.
152. Deng M, Bell S, Huie P, et al. Cardiac allograft vascular disease. Relationship to microvascular cell surface markers and inflammatory cell phenotypes on endomyocardial biopsy. Circulation 1995;91:1647–1654.
153. Crisp S, Dunn M, Rose M, Babir M, Yacoub M. Antiendothelial antibodies after heart transplantation: the accelerating factor in transplant-

associated coronary artery disease? J Heart Lung Transplant 1994;13:81–92.
154. Lowry R, Allen E, Hu C, et al. What are the implications of cardiac infection with cytomegalovirus before heart transplantation? J Heart Lung Transplant 1994;13:122–128.
155. Labarrere C, Pitts D, Nelson D, Faulk W. Vascular tissue plasminogen activator and the development of coronary artery disease in heart-transplant recipients. N Engl J Med 1995;333:1111–1116.
156. Gao S, Alderman E, Schroeder J, et al. Accelerated coronary vascular disease in the heart transplant patient: coronary angiographic findings. J Am Coll Cardiol 1988;12:334–340.
157. Balk A, Simoons M, vd Linden M, et al. Coronary artery disease after heart transplantation: timing of coronary arteriography. J Heart Lung Transplant 1993;12:89–99.
158. Evertt J, Hershberger R, Ratkovec R, et al. The specificity of normal qualitative angiography in excluding cardiac allograft vasculopathy. J Heart Lung Transplant 1994;13:142–149.
159. Sharples L, Mullins P, Cary N, et al. A method of analyzing the onset and progression of coronary occlusive disease after transplantation and its effects on patient survival. J Heart Lung Transplant 1993;12:381–387.
160. Keogh A, Valantine H, Hunt S, et al. Impact of proximal or midvessel discrete coronary artery stenoses on survival after heart transplantation. J Heart Lung Transplant 1992;11:892–901.
161. Smart F, Ballantyne C, Cocanougher B, et al. Insensitivity of noninvasive tests to detect coronary artery vasculopathy after heart transplant. Am J Cardiol 1991;67:243–247.
162. Rodney R, Johnson J, Blood D, Barr M. Myocardial perfusion scintigraphy in heart transplant recipients with and without allograft atherosclerosis: a comparison of thallium-201 and technetium 99m sestamibi. J Heart Lung Transplant 1994;13:173–180.
163. Herregods M, Anastassiou I, Cleemput J, et al. Dobutamine stress echocardiography after heart transplantation. J Heart Lung Transplant 1994;13:1039–1044.
164. Collings C, Pinto F, Valantine H, et al. Exercise echocardiography in heart transplant recipients: a comparison with angiography and intracoronary ultrasonography. J Heart Lung Transplant 1994;13:604–613.
165. Rickenbacher P, Pinto F, Chenzbraun A, et al. Incidence and severity of transplant coronary artery disease early and up to 15 years after transplantation as detected by intravascular ultrasound. J Am Coll Cardiol 1995;25:171–177.
166. St Goar F, Pinto F, Alderman E, et al. Intracoronary ultrasound imaging in cardiac transplant recipients: in vivo evidence of "angiographically silent" intimal thickening. Circulation 1992;85:979–987.
167. Mehra M, Ventura H, Stapleton D, et al. Presence of severe intimal thickening by intravascular ultrasonography predicts cardiac events in cardiac allograft vasculopathy. J Heart Lung Transplant 1995;14:632–639.
168. Gao S-Z, Hunt S, Schroeder J. Accelerated graft coronary artery disease. In: Shumway SJ, Shumway NE, eds. Thoracic transplantation. Cambridge, MA: Blackwell Scientific, 1995.
169. Schroeder J, Gao S, Alderman E, et al. A preliminary study of diltiazem in the prevention of coronary artery disease in heart-transplant recipients. N Engl J Med 1993;328:164–170.
170. Wahlers T, Mugge A, Oppelt P, et al. Preventive treatment of coronary vasculopathy in heart transplantation by inhibition of smooth muscle cell proliferation with angiopeptin. J Heart Lung Transplant 1995;14:143–150.
171. Halle A, Disciascio G, Massin E, et al. Coronary angioplasty, atherectomy, and bypass surgery in cardiac transplant recipients. J Am Coll Cardiol 1995;26:120–128.
172. Ensley R, Hunt S, Taylor D, et al. Predictors of survival after repeat heart transplantation. J Heart Lung Transplant 1992;11:S142–S158.
173. Bunzel B, Grundbock A, Laczkovics A, et al. Quality of life after orthotopic heart transplantation. J Heart Lung Transplant 1991;10:455–459.
174. Wagoner L, Taylor D, Olsen S, et al. Immunosuppressive therapy, management, and outcome of heart transplant recipients during pregnancy. J Heart Lung Transplant 1994;13:993–1000.
175. Smith J, Ribakove G, Hunt A, et al. Heart retransplantation: the 25-year experience at a single institution. J Heart Lung Transplant 1995;14:832–839.
176. Carpentier A, Chaqhues J, Acar C, et al. Dynamic cardioplasty at seven years. J Thorac Cardiovasc Surg 1993;106:42–54.
177. El Oakley R, Jarvis J. Cardiomyoplasty. A critical review of experimental and clinical results. Circulation 1994;90:2085–2090.
178. Costanzo-Nordin M, Cooper D, Jessup M, et al. Task force 6: future developments. 24th Bethesda conference on cardiac transplantation. J Am Coll Cardiol 1993;22:54–64.
179. Goldstein DJ, Oz M, Rose EA. Implantable left ventricular assist devices. N Engl J Med 1998;339:1522–1533.
180. Westaby S. The need for artificial hearts. Heart 1996;76:200–206.
181. Frazier O. First use of an untethered, vented electric left ventricular assist device for long-term support. Circulation 1994;89:2908–2914.

COMMENTARY REFERENCES

1. Hosenpud JD, Novick RJ, Bennett LE, et al. The registry of the International Society for Heart and Lung Transplantation: thirteenth official report, 1996. J Heart Lung Transplant 1996;15:655–674.
2. Department of Health and Human Services. Draft Public Heath Service (PHS) Guidelines on Infectious Disease Issues in Xenotransplantation. Federal Register 96-24448. August 1996. Filed 9-8:4.
3. Altman LK. New York Times. 14 June 1996:A16.
4. McCarthy PM. Ventricular remodeling: hype or hope? Nat Med 1996;2:859–860.

Chapter

24

Heart Transplantation in Children

Luca A. Vricella Leonard L. Bailey

During the last ten years, cardiac transplantation emerged as a reasonably durable modality for the treatment of myopathic and complex structural heart disease in neonates, infants, and children. Approximately 9% of all cardiac transplants performed annually in North America are among recipients in the pediatric age group (0 to 17 years) (1). The trend is toward transplanting more and younger patients. Currently, more than half of the pediatric recipients being treated by cardiac transplantation are those in the first 3 months of life (2).

The first pediatric heart transplantation was attempted in a new born baby with severe Ebstein's anomaly in 1968 (3). Building on experimental laboratory work with puppies, Kantrowitz performed this shortly after the first adult heart transplant was accomplished by Barnard at the Groote Shuur Hospital in Capetown, South Africa (4). Over a decade later, Behrendt reported successful heart transplantation among young children with end-stage myocardiopathy, and Frazier and Cooley became the first to achieve successful heart transplantation in an infant during the first year of life. The operation, done in 1984, was for treatment of subendocardial fibroelastosis (5). Bailey and colleagues, of Loma Linda University (LLU), performed the first successful neonatal orthotopic cardiac allotransplant in 1985. This was accomplished in a 4-day-old patient who had hypoplastic left heart syndrome (6). That recipient remains alive and well at age 12 years.

This experience with newborn recipients received broad attention in the lay press and helped create a basis for infant organ donation. Thus began the present era of heart transplantation aimed at a population of young infants with highly complex, incurable congenital heart disease, in addition to those somewhat older infants and children with end-stage myopathic illness. This chapter will focus on the aspects of cardiac transplantation that are unique to the pediatric patient, including indications for heart transplantation, management issues, and results pertaining to this evolving and challenging therapeutic intervention.

INDICATIONS

Appoximately 10% of newborns who have congenital heart disease could be potential candidates for cardiac transplantation (7). Most of these infants are palliated with more conventional methods, as donor hearts remain a scarce commodity. Nevertheless, a few, either by choice or by absolute necessity, are referred to pediatric heart transplant centers for evaluation, selection, and wait-listing with organ procurement networks. Experience at LLU suggests that 15% to 20% of potential recipients will die while awaiting a donor heart. Death is the result of severe congestive heart failure (41%) (8) and the multi-organ consequences of hypoperfusion.

Indications for pediatric heart transplantation have evolved during the experience of recent years. Complex congenital heart disease has now surpassed primary cardiomyopathy as the primary indication for transplantation in the pediatric age group (9). Figure 24.1 outlines the LLU experience with 293 pediatric patients transplanted between 1985 and 1996, and illustrates the different preoperative recipient diagnostic groups. Categorized by age, 75% of all pediatric heart transplants have been performed during the first year of life.

Hypoplastic left heart syndrome (HLHS) and its variants represent the most frequent indication for infant cardiac transplantation. HLHS is the fourth most frequent congenital heart anomaly producing symptoms in the newborn. It comprises 7.5% of all symptomatic cardiac defects, and is present in 1500 to 2000 infants born live each year in North America. It is the leading cause of death from structural heart disease in the first year of life (8,10).

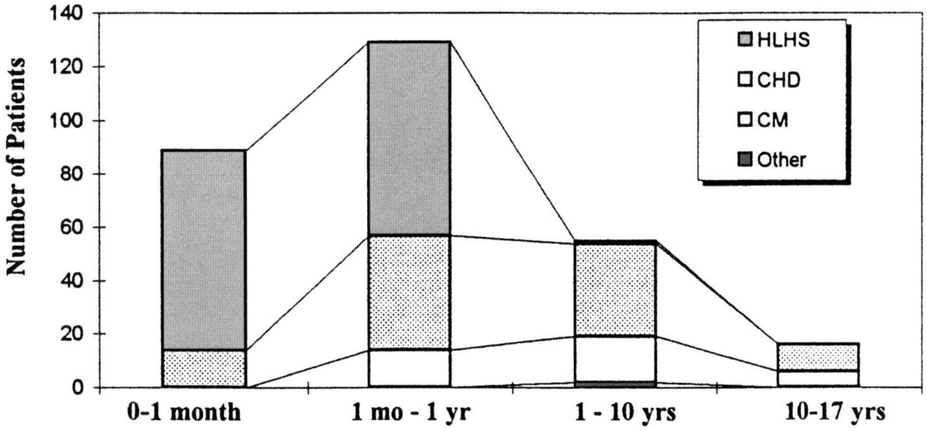

FIGURE 24.1. *Indications for cardiac transplantation by age group. Loma Linda University experience with 293 patients transplanted between 1985 and 1996.*

Debate continues regarding appropriate management of neonates with HLHS. Clearly, counseling parents to withhold therapy is quite common, although it is becoming increasingly less acceptable. In addition, the choice of surgical options remains somewhat controversial (11,12). A multistage strategy leading to lifelong "single ventricle physiology" is characterized by excessive operative mortality and interstage attrition (10,13). Those favoring cardiac transplantation as definitive therapy for these newborns point to the benefits of acceptable surgical mortality (10%), virtually normal cardiovascular physiology, and durable outcomes; however, the requirement of lifelong immunosuppression and its attendant risks accompany this form of treatment.

The information in this chapter assumes a choice in favor of cardiac transplantation. Criteria for the diagnosis of HLHS, as well as other indications for heart transplantation in children, are listed in Table 24.1.

Table 24.1. Indications for Pediatric Cardiac Transplantation Including Criteria That Define Hypoplastic Left Heart Syndrome

1. Hypoplastic Left Heart Syndrome (HLHS)
    - Primary Criteria:
        - Hypoplastic LV (LVEDV <20 mL/m^2)
        - Aortic valve stenosis, hypoplasia, or atresia (diameter <5 mm in term; infant >2.5 kg)
        - Mitral valve stenosis, hypoplasia, or atresia (diameter <8 mm in term; infant >2.5 kg)
    - Secondary Criteria:
        - Ductus-dependent systemic circulation
        - Hypoplasia of ascending aorta (diameter <5 mm)
        - Hypoplastic aortic arch
2. End-Stage Cardiomyopathy
    - Ventricular failure in spite of maximal medical therapy; refractory/unstable
    - Failure to thrive or worsening heart failure
    - Malignant arrhythmias in spite of maximal medical therapy/AICD
    - Rising pulmonary vascular resistance, precluding transplant at later date
    - Cardiomyopathy following previous intervention for congenital heart disease
3. Others (HLHS Equivalent)
    - D-TGA with hypoplastic right ventricle and aortic tract
    - Single ventricle with hypoplastic aortic tract
    - L-TGA with single ventricle and heart block
    - Shone's complex
    - Severe Ebstein's anomaly with normal pulmonary arteries
    - Multiple obstructive rhabdomyomas or fibromas
    - Pulmonary atresia with intact ventricular septum
    - A-V canal with hypoplastic left ventricle and left heart component
    - Single ventricle with subaortic obstruction (bulbo-aortic foramen)
    - Straddling A-V valve and tensor apparatus
    - Complex truncus arteriosus

LV = left ventricle; LVEDV = left ventricular end-diastolic volume; AICD = automated implantable cardioverter difibrillator; D-TGA = d-transposition of the great arteries; L-TGA = l-transposition of the great arteries; AV = atrioventricular.

DONOR ISSUES

Donor organ availability is a significant limiting factor in cardiac transplantation at any age (see Chapter 15). The pediatric age group is no exception. Although there are more than 100 deaths per day in the United States among infants less than 1 year of age, few, if any, become potential donors (7,8). Actual pediatric organ donors are usually victims of trauma, sudden infant death syndrome, or birth asphyxia (14).

The physicians caring for potential donor infants and children have ready access to their regional organ procurement network, but their sensitivity and interest in organ donation issues are critical. Brain death criteria are well established and are clinically based (15,16). The diagnosis of whole brain death does not require substantiation with sophisticated neurodiagnostic studies. Except for infants in their first week of life, the diagnosis of brain death may be established with certainty on the basis of bedside serial evaluations by two or more physicians. After death is declared, the remainder of the organ procurement process should be conducted by experienced personnel from the local or regional organ procurement agency (see also Chapter 15).

In the LLU series, 80% of donors were receiving inotropic support at the time of heart procurement. Furthermore, data suggest that transplantation of a moderately dysfunctional graft (left ventricular fiber shortening fraction of 15% to 28% or history of prolonged cardiopulmonary resuscitation) does not necessarily predict worse outcome, unless the donor heart has moderate to severe mitral insufficiency. Cardiac depression provoked by brain death appears to be fully reversible once the graft is in a more favorable milieu (7). The resilience of pediatric myocardium in particular may stem from its relative resistance to ischemia.

Donor inclusion criteria are therefore fairly liberal. Donor and recipient must be ABO compatible. HLA typing is accomplished retrospectively, but has not been a predictive factor in outcome analysis (17). Recipients with preformed reactive antibody (PRA) titers greater than 15% to 20% may require prospective crossmatch. Donor–recipient size mismatch is seldom a limiting factor in pediatric heart transplantation. Use of oversized grafts (up to a donor–recipient weight ratio of 3:1) has produced no significant increase in morbidity and mortality. Ratios of 4:1 have been accomplished, but with additional morbidity in the form of postoperative pulmonary atelectasis. Grossly undersized hearts may adversely affect pediatric host survival.

The only absolute contraindications for heart graft donation are uncontrolled sepsis, malignancy other than primary brain tumor, complex cardiac anomaly, genetic myopathic disease, hepatitis, HIV, and graft fiber shortening fraction <25% after optimization of preload and inotropic support.

DONOR OPERATION

Detailed knowledge of the recipient's cardiovascular malformations guides the extent of the donor operation. Cardiectomy is accomplished with variable en bloc removal of the great vessels. Modification of standard transplant techniques allows for successful transplantation even in the most challenging situations. Previous palliative procedures, atrial situs inversus, and complex anomalies in recipient pulmonary and systemic veins do not preclude successful transplantation (18–20).

Heart graft procurement is usually accomplished in concert with other organ procurement teams. The donor is administered methylprednisolone (25 mg/kg), heparin (5 mg/kg), dextrose (2–3 mL/kg of 50% solution), and a broad-spectrum antibiotic. The heart and great vessels are carefully isolated for en bloc procurement designed to meet recipient requirements. Cardiectomy is performed after myocardial preservation is ensured by the use of a single-dose infusion of cold crystalloid cardioplegia. The LLU graft preservation solution is 5% dextrose with 20 mEq/L of potassium, 250 mg/L of methylprednisolone, 27 mEq/L of sodium, and 3 mEq/L of magnesium, buffered with 2.25 mEq/L of sodium bicarbonate to a pH of 7.40 at 4°C (modified Roe's solution) (15). The graft is trimmed and prepared on the back table; the extent of the work is based on the recipient's malformation (1). It is packaged in cold dextrose in saline solution for transport.

The longest successful graft ischemic time in the LLU series so far is 606 minutes. Outcomes have not been adversely affected by graft ischemic times up to 10 hours using the simple procurement protocol outlined here. Specifically, recipient mortality and/or need for increased hemodynamic support have been no different among children with graft ischemic times longer than 4 hours in comparison to those children with shorter graft ischemic times. Slight loss of compliance, expressed as mild diastolic dysfunction, has been observed among those cardiac grafts subjected to 4 or more hours of cold ischemic time. Graft function normalizes within 2 weeks of the transplant procedure (21).

RECIPIENT ISSUES

Pretransplant diagnosis is established in most instances by means of transthoracic echocardiography. HLHS may be diagnosed in utero after only 17 to 20 weeks of gestation. Fetal candidates for heart transplantation may be registered with the national organ sharing network when lung maturity is adequate, usually at about 35 to 36 weeks of in utero gestation. Delivery may be induced when a donor is identified. Heart catheterization and angiography are reserved for clarification of ambiguous anomalies, and for computation of pulmonary vascular resistance.

A full neurologic evaluation, including appropriate imaging studies, is accomplished in each potential recipient. Abdominal ultrasound is used to rule out concomitant visceral malformations. Liver function assays are obtained.

Potential heart transplant recipients are excluded on the basis of the following criteria:

1. Marked prematurity (gestational age <36 weeks)
2. Low birth weight (<1.8 kg)
3. Severe neurologic deficiency
4. Irreversible pulmonary hypertension (>4 Wood units).

In addition, the heart transplant candidate should be free from life-limiting genetic abnormalities, uncontrolled infection (particularly viral pneumonia), and irreversible organ failure other than primary heart disease. Anatomic contraindications to heart transplantation include hypoplastic/atretic branch pulmonary arteries and veins.

Pretransplant mortality is 15% to 20% during a median waiting time for donor identification of 14 days (range 1.5 hours to 363 days) in the LLU series. Preoperative management focuses on maintaining hemodynamic stability and adequate nutrition, and on detecting and treating infections.

Recipient malformations characterized by pulmonary overcirculation are managed medically during the initial wait for an organ. Pulmonary artery banding is used to protect the pulmonary vascular bed from irreversible changes in infants waiting more than 4 to 6 months. Lesions with ductus-dependent circulation are palliated by continuous infusion of prostaglandin E_1 (0.01–0.05 μg/kg/min) or, as recently described, by endovascular stenting to ensure ductal patency (22).

In newborns with ductus-dependent systemic circulation awaiting transplantation, the delicate balance between systemic and pulmonary blood flow is managed by reducing inspired oxygen tension and/or increasing inhaled levels of carbon dioxide. Balloon or blade septostomy is occasionally required to ensure obligatory interatrial shunting.

Finally, those infants with complex congenital heart disease who show evidence of deterioration while waiting longer than 2 months are considered for staged surgical palliation at parental discretion (10,11). In a recent report, 21% of patients required some kind of palliative procedure in the pretransplant phase (14). Infants and children suffering from end-stage dilated cardiomyopathy may require mechanical circulatory support if deterioration is rapid and recalcitrant during their wait for a donor heart.

A continuous cyclosporine infusion (0.1 mg/kg/hour) is begun in all recipients in the immediate preoperative period. Among the ductus-dependent babies, prostaglandin E_1 is also maintained by continuous intravenous infusion. Both infusions are temporarily discontinued during the period of cardiopulmonary bypass.

RECIPIENT OPERATION

Anesthetic management of cardiac graft recipients is beyond the scope of this discussion, except to note that infants whose inspired gas mixtures have been carefully controlled in the intensive care setting prior to surgery generally should be ventilated with nothing more than room air at a rate that maintains normal partial pressure of carbon dioxide. Hyperventilation with 100% oxygen will favor net pulmonary overcirculation, coronary artery steal, and "unexplained" ventricular fibrillation among infants who have been previously stable for days and weeks.

The recipient operation in infants and children with primary cardiomyopathy is accomplished with the same steps and techniques used in adult cardiac transplantation, which are detailed in Chapter 23. A fairly demanding reoperative transplant reconstruction is required for older pediatric recipients whose heart transplantation is the final definitive intervention after multiple palliative procedures for congenital heart disease (18). Extensive reconstruction is also required during primary heart transplantation among neonates and infants with complex structural heart disease that might include anomalies of systemic and pulmonary venous connection, aortic arch hypoplasia or interruption, and/or situs inversus (12). This discussion will focus on transplantation as it is performed in infants with HLHS and its variants, and in those with other complex anomalies.

A median sternotomy is used to perform thymectomy and expose the recipient's native heart. If the donor heart is significantly larger than the native heart, the entire left pericardium anterior to the phrenic nerve is removed. Single venous and arterial cannulation is employed. In infants with ductus-dependent systemic circulation, the ductus arteriosus is isolated and cannulated for arterial perfusion through a stab incision in the distal main pulmonary artery. All aortic arch vessels are isolated with loose tourniquets during the initial cooling phase in preparation for aortic arch reconstruction.

Recently, the technique for transplantation in patients with HLHS that was previously described (1,6) has been modified. Implantation of the allograft is now accomplished with systemic hypothermia, performing the atrial anastomoses under low-flow perfusion with the pulmonary artery clamped and systemic perfusion maintained by means of the arterial cannula positioned in the ductus arteriosus. The aortic arch is then reconstructed under circulatory arrest with the arch vessel tourniquets tightened. The pulmonary artery anastomosis is completed while rewarming the patient. This modification markedly reduces the required period of hypothermic circulatory arrest.

Cardiectomy is performed while leaving behind right and left atrial cuffs and the great vessels transected just above the semilunar valve commissural posts. With the diminutive ascending aorta ligated and the pulmonary artery clamped, the donor graft is anastomosed to the recipient atrial cuff with a continuous polypropylene (6-0 or 7-0) suture technique, starting at the lowest portion of the interatrial septum and proceeding to complete the right atrial anastomosis first (Fig. 24.2). The graft is reflected toward the operating surgeon and the left atrial anastomosis is completed (Fig. 24.3).

In older children, and among those recipients at any age who have atrial situs inversus, bicaval anastomoses (as compared to atrioatrial anastomoses) are accomplished. In this setting, the left atrial anastomosis is completed first.

Both atrial chambers are filled with cold saline for air evacuation and myocardial preservation just prior to completion of the respective anastomosis. Using circulatory arrest, the ductus arteriosus is decannulated and ligated.

Over 80% of neonates and infants require extensive aortic reconstruction (14). The undersurface of the recipient's aorta is opened and the anastomosis is directed from the descending aorta toward the small, ligated ascending aorta (Fig. 24.4). The aortic cannula is then inserted into the donor innominate artery stump and cardiopulmonary bypass is reinstituted. Median hypothermic circulatory arrest time has historically been 47 minutes for this operation at LLU. Circulatory arrest has not exceeded 20 minutes when using the more recent modification outlined here. The pulmonary artery anastomosis is completed while the patient and donor graft are being reperfused and rewarmed (Fig. 24.5).

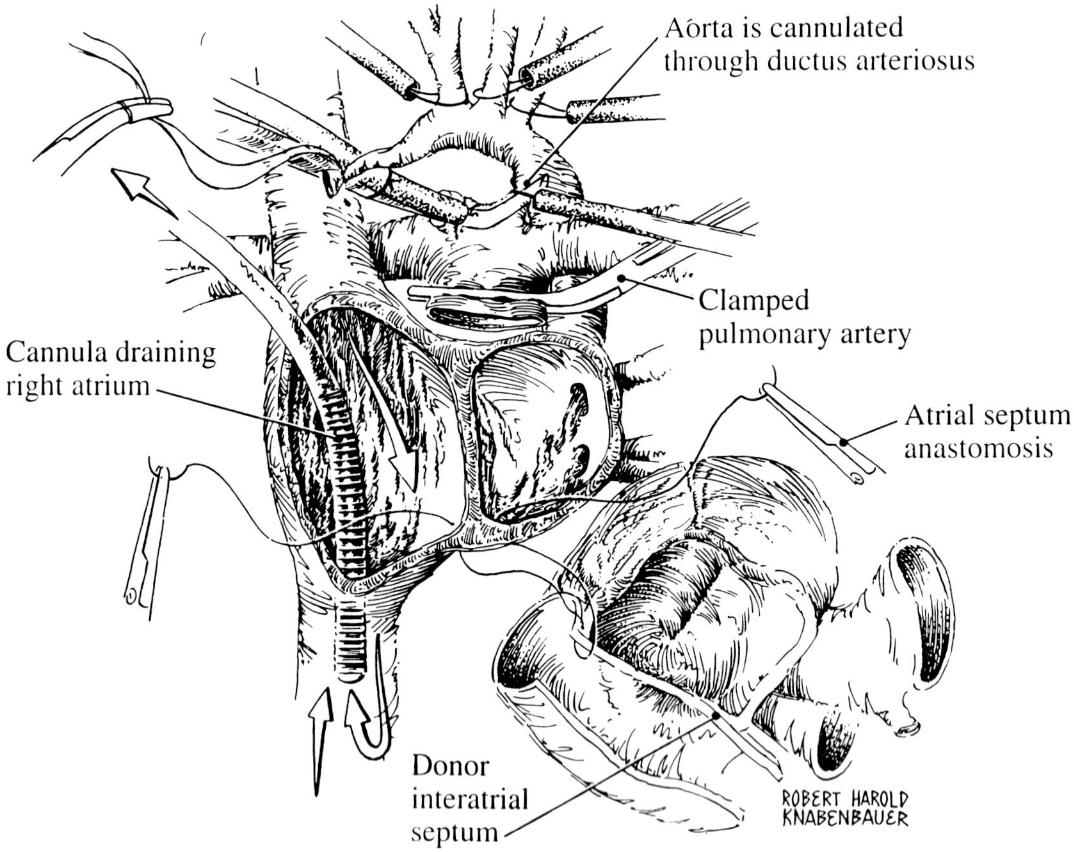

FIGURE 24.2. *The cardiac allograft anastomosis to the recipient atrial cuff is started at the inferior aspect of the interatrial septum. The pulmonary artery is clamped, and the systemic circulation is maintained by low-flow hypothermic extracorporeal perfusion through the ductus arteriosus.*

Graft reperfusion and recipient rewarming are accomplished during 60 to 90 minutes of extracorporeal circulation. Infusions of dopamine (2–3 μg/kg/min), tolazoline (0.5–1.0 mg/kg/hr), and occasionally isoproterenol (0.01–0.02 μg/kg/min) are begun after approximately 30 to 40 minutes of graft reperfusion. Prostaglandin E_1 infusion is continued initially, then weaned off over several days. Anticoagulation is reversed with protamine after discontinuation of extracorporeal circulation and decannulation of the heart graft. Primary sternotomy closure is usually feasible. Rarely, the incision is left open to avoid compression tamponade of the new graft. Delayed primary closure is accomplished after graft, mediastinal, and chest wall edema have resolved. Older patients in the LLU program who are stable prior to transplantation are typically extubated in the immediate perioperative phase of recovery. Some neonates and infants will require 24 to 48 hours of assisted ventilation before extubation may be safely accomplished.

PERIOPERATIVE MANAGEMENT

With the exception of immunosuppressive therapy, the initial postoperative course is very similar to that of infants and children undergoing conventional complex cardiac surgical procedures (1,15,23). Early extubation is usually an achievable goal. Inotropic and vasodilator support is continued for at least 24 to 48 hours. Prostaglandin E_1 infusion is weaned off over 3 to 5 days in infants with previous ductus-dependent circulation who had a prolonged waiting time. Pulmonary artery and left atrial monitoring lines are not used. Blood components are irradiated and filtered to achieve leukocyte depletion prior to administration. Broad-spectrum antibiotic coverage (cefazolin, 20 mg/kg every 12 hours) is continued until the central venous pressure line is removed. Methylprednisolone (25 mg/kg every 12 hours) is administered intraoperatively and for 48 hours following transplantation. Gastric acid antagonists are used for gastric cytoprotection, and all medications are changed to their oral equivalent once the patient is feeding well. Median length of immediate postoperative stay has been 18.9 days (range: 5 to 176 days) in the LLU experience.

EARLY COMPLICATIONS

Following transplantation, most infants and children enjoy a rather smooth postoperative course (the so-called honey-

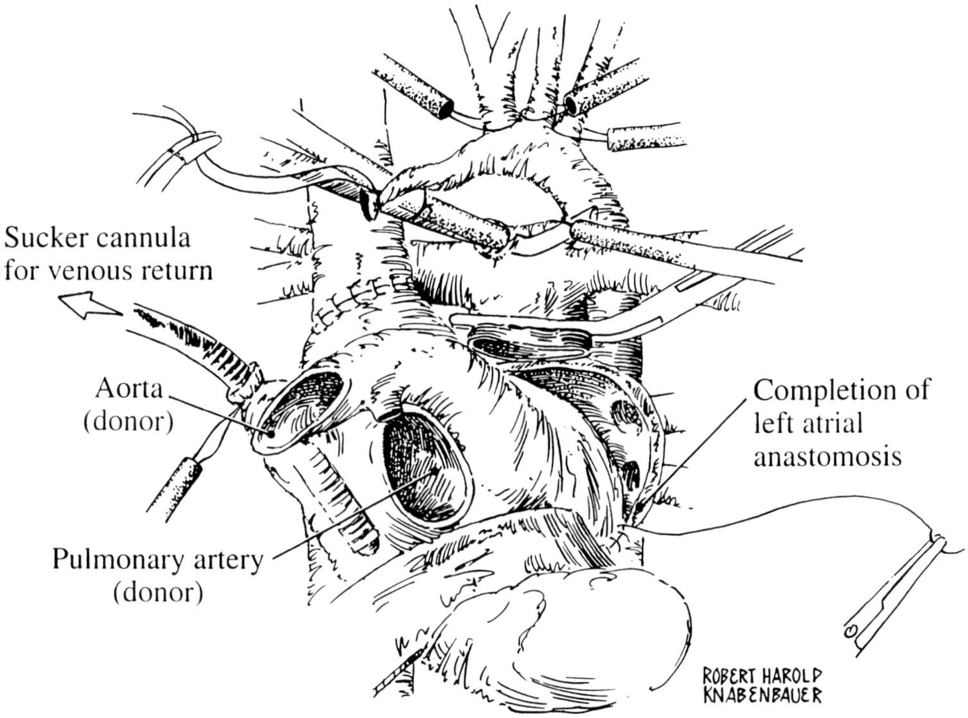

FIGURE 24.3. *Following completion of the right atrial anastomosis, the left atrial anastomosis is accomplished in a counterclockwise direction.*

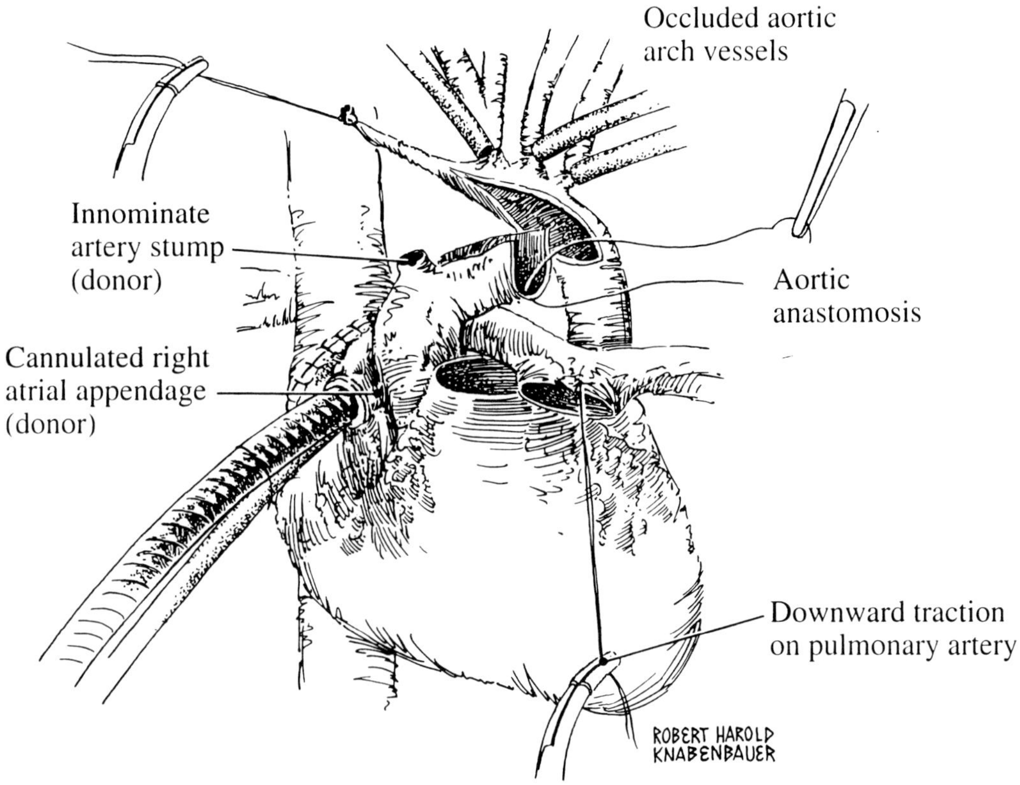

FIGURE 24.4. *The aortic arch vessels are snared and the aortic anastomosis is accomplished during a brief period of hypothermic circulatory arrest.*

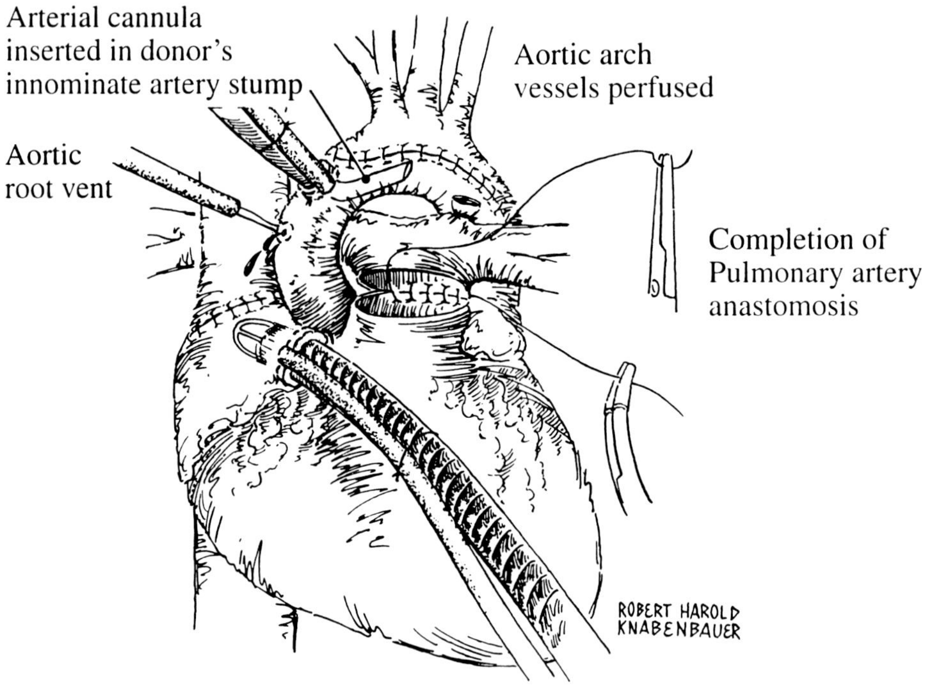

FIGURE 24.5. *The right atrial appendage and the donor innominate artery stump are cannulated and cardiopulmonary bypass is reinstituted. The pulmonary artery anastomosis is completed while the patient is being rewarmed.*

moon phase). Among the 293 pediatric transplant recipients in the LLU series, primary and secondary graft dysfunction (4% of all pediatric recipients), technical and management issues (2%), and infections (1%), were the most common causes of perioperative death. Cumulative early mortality (less than 30 days) was 9%.

Neurologic Complications

Significant early neurologic sequelae are rare, although up to 20% of patients may experience perioperative seizures, requiring short-term treatment (14). Etiology of postoperative seizure activity is multifactorial (see also Chapter 33).

1. Preoperative history of seizures
2. Use of neurotoxic drugs such as cyclosporine
3. Circulatory hyperperfusion syndrome
4. Systemic hypertension
5. Postperfusion fluid and electrolyte shifts
6. Fever
7. Hyper- or hypoglycemia, hypocalcemia, or hypomagnesemia
8. Subependymal petechial hemorrhages
9. True hypoxic/hypoperfusion or embolic cerebral injury.

Profound cerebral injury has been uncommon. None of the infants and children treated for perioperative seizures have required long-term anticonvulsant therapy in the LLU series of surviving recipients.

Hyperperfusion Syndrome

Recipients with a history of chronic low cardiac output from end-stage myocardiopathy who have received oversized donor grafts are at risk for what has been defined as "hyperperfusion syndrome." The clinical scenario is characterized by hypertension and neurologic symptoms ranging from headache and seizures to coma beginning about the third to the fifth postoperative day. Vigorous management of systemic hypertension using vasodilators and β-blockade will usually prevent permanent neurologic sequelae (24).

Renal Failure

Newborns are at risk for development of renal failure throughout the perioperative hospital course. Renal failure in this setting may be a consequence of tubular immaturity, perioperative hypoperfusion or hyperperfusion, or use of nephrotoxic drugs. In the LLU series, 22% of neonates required temporary peritoneal dialysis for treatment of acute renal failure, an incidence significantly higher than that associated with other pediatric age groups having heart transplantation. It is also a significantly higher rate than that associated with neonates having conventional repair of anomalies such as transposition of the great arteries and total anomalous pulmonary venous connection. Data indicate that early institution of peritoneal dialysis following heart transplantation results in reduced complications and improved long-term outcomes (25).

Infections

In the LLU series, 10% of all perioperative deaths (<30 days) were caused by infection, and all of these occurred during the first week after operation. Approximately half of all patients will experience at least one significant infectious complication during the first year after transplantation; the greatest risk for infections occurs during the first 3 to 4 postoperative months. There is a correlation between treatment of rejection episodes, increased immunosuppression, and occurrence of sepsis or other serious infectious illness (see Chapter 36).

Nosocomial infections, usually caused by gram-negative rods, are typically associated with prolonged preoperative hospitalization. Following discharge, the most frequently isolated microorganisms are community acquired. Scattered fungal (mainly candidiasis) and parasitic (*Pneumocystis carinii* pneumonia) infections occur, and generally respond well to conventional treatment (26).

Cytomegalovirus (CMV) prophylaxis remains somewhat debatable. Acyclovir prophylaxis (30 mg/kg/day) is used for 3 months postoperatively; ganciclovir (10 mg/kg/day for 14 to 21 days) is reserved for documented postoperative infections or those instances where the recipient is known to be CMV-negative and the donor is CMV-positive. Intravenous immunoglobulin (400 mg/kg administered 3 times in the early postoperative period) provides passive immune enhancement. Forty percent of patients will experience CMV seroconversion postoperatively, although only 16% will become symptomatic (8). Infections with respiratory syncytial virus (RSV) are common and may become lethal. Infection with RSV, which produces respiratory compromise, has responded favorably to a short course of ribavirin therapy. Increased surveillance for graft rejection (stimulated by RSV infection) is very important during recovery from this particular infection.

Children with a heart transplant do not appear to be at increased risk for common childhood illnesses including respiratory tract infections, otitis media, gastroenteritis, and bronchiolitis (26). Immunizations follow the regular schedule. Live virus vaccines (MMR) are not used in cardiac recipients, although pneumococcal vaccine is routinely administered. Asplenia is not considered a contraindication to transplantation, but it does impose the requirement for indefinite prophylaxis in the form of oral amoxicillin. Hospital readmission rates for all reasons are 1.15, 0.52, and 0.63 per patient/year at 1, 2, and 3 years postoperatively (14).

IMMUNOREGULATION

Patients experiencing cardiac allotransplantation during neonatal life appear to enjoy a so-called "window of opportunity" with regards to immune tolerance. They often experience an immunologically quiescent postoperative course. Many factors may explain the ease with which the neonatal immune system is regulated:

1. Immunosuppressive factors transferred with the colostrum.
2. Underdevelopment of newborn immune mechanisms.
3. Multiple neonatal suppressor factors.
4. Maternal anti-idiotypic antibodies and other transmissible mechanisms responsible for suppression of feto-maternal incompatibility (27).

Furthermore, the neonatal immune system is deficient in the expression of class II antigens responsible for triggering the immune response. Longer survival and less aggressive rejection patterns have been observed among newborn recipients as compared to older children (Fig. 24.6).

Though some researchers have reported beneficial effects of HLA-DR matching on freedom from rejection (28), HLA incompatibility in the LLU series has not predicted frequency and interval of rejection episodes when examined by multivariate logistic regression analysis (17,29). The only factors found to be predictive of rejection are age at time of transplantation and history of CMV infection.

The optimal immunoregulatory protocol has yet to be defined. Much debate is ongoing about the type and number of immunosuppressive agents that should be used following cardiac allotransplantation in infants and children. Most transplant protocols include the administration of cyclosporine as the basis of chronic antirejection management, although a few centers use tacrolimus as the primary agent for immunoregulation (30).

The LLU protocol uses dual therapy. Cyclosporine is started as a continuous intravenous infusion (0.1 mg/kg/hour) in the immediate preoperative setting and is withheld during cardiopulmonary bypass. The infusion is resumed postoperatively and converted to the oral form (10–20 mg/kg/day) as soon as the patient tolerates feedings. Cyclosporine trough levels are monitored closely by a

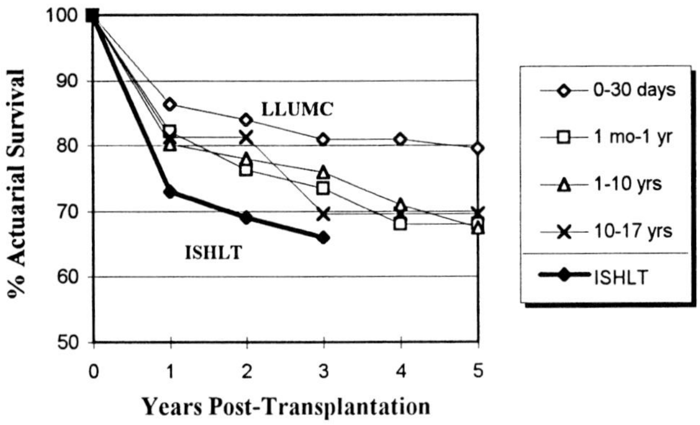

FIGURE 24.6. *Loma Linda University 5-year actuarial survival by age group, compared to cumulative pediatric outcomes collected by ISHLT (age 0 to 17, bold line). Recipients whose transplant was accomplished during the first 30 days of life appear to have a survival advantage. LLUMC, Loma Linda University Medical Center; ISHLT, International Society for Heart and Lung Transplantation.*

monoclonal antibody assay, aiming for a range between 250–300 ng/mL in the first 6 months after transplant, 150–200 ng/mL in the second 6 months, and 100–150 ng/mL thereafter. The antimetabolite azathioprine (3 mg/kg/day IV/PO) is coupled with cyclosporine. The dose is reduced to 0.5–1.0 mg/kg/day at the end of the first post-transplant year. Azathioprine is withheld in those patients who develop leukopenia (<4000 leukocytes/mm^3). A number of recipients transplanted as newborns, who have had a favorable rejection history, have been regulated with cyclosporine monotherapy, with no increase in morbidity or mortality.

Corticosteroids are used as well by many centers for the chronic prevention of rejection. Chronic oral steroid therapy is reserved, in the LLU protocol, for recalcitrant rejection based on endomyocardial biopsy. Currently, steroids are administered perioperatively (methylprednisolone, 25 mg/kg IV every 12 hours for 2 days) and during episodes of acute rejection. A protocol free of chronic steroid use has eliminated adverse side effects produced by these agents without increasing graft loss due to rejection activity.

Since 1990, rabbit-derived antithymocyte serum (Applied Medical Research, Inc., Nashville, Tennessee) has been used as induction therapy for 5 days postoperatively (0.5 mL/kg/day) in every pediatric recipient age group except newborns (8). A randomized prospective study found that the administration of ATS postoperatively decreased rejection rates from 1.38 to 0.45 per 100 patient days and increased freedom from rejection from 21% to 53% at a mean follow-up of 231 days from transplantation. Furthermore, ATS seemed to delay early rejection by an average of 20 days, allowing the recipient to be more fully recovered from transplant surgery before confronting acute rejection of the allograft (31).

Surveillance

The best modality for screening pediatric cardiac transplant recipients for rejection is the focus of ongoing debate. Adequate early and late surveillance requires an experienced and coordinated team of multidisciplinary specialists and observance of a well-defined protocol.

Detection of rejection on clinical grounds can be very challenging, for immunosuppression may mask some of the symptoms heralding rejection. At times, these children appear clinically well in the face of life-threatening rejection.

Some consider cardiac catheterization and endomyocardial biopsy to be the method of choice for diagnosing rejection (32). Though useful in older children and in clinically difficult situations, the risk/benefit ratio of endomyocardial biopsy in neonates and small infants is unfavorable (33). Because rejection rates appear to plateau at about 3 months following transplantation, routine surveillance by endomyocardial biopsy after 6 months is questioned by some clinicians because of low yield in the asymptomatic recipient (34).

Noninvasive monitoring with transthoracic echocardiography has emerged as a more versatile tool for graft surveillance (35,36). This methodology focuses on detectable changes in diastolic function. The many parameters obtained by computer-digitized M mode echocardiography are then analyzed and combined in a grading system. Potential indicators of rejection include left ventricular wall thickening and an increase in left ventricular mass secondary to lymphocytic infiltration and edema; diastolic volume reduction and diminished left ventricular shortening fraction; pericardial effusion; and atrioventricular valve dysfunction. Serial examinations are used to follow clinical improvement and monitor response to antirejection management. Echocardiographic analysis also assists in the decision for right ventricular biopsy. A sensitivity of 88% to 98%, specificity of 83%, and negative predictive value of 93% have been reported using echocardiographic surveillance (23).

Accelerated graft vasculopathy is the most frequent cause of late death in children, and periodic screening for graft vasculopathy allows for earlier detection and treatment. Preliminary data from the pediatric heart transplant program at LLU indicate that stress dobutamine echocardiography may be a more sensitive and less invasive screening test for coronary artery disease as compared to coronary arteriography. It appears that coronary artery disease screening based on yearly stress dobutamine echocardiography augmented by catheterization may become a rational surveillance protocol.

The current LLU surveillance strategy combines echocardiographic data with R-wave summation electrocardiography, chest roentgenography, cyclosporine levels, complete blood counts, and clinical assessment as a noninvasive protocol. This surveillance begins initially on a biweekly schedule, and is modified toward less frequent evaluations based on the time from transplantation and the individual rejection history (15). Endomyocardial biopsy is indicated in clinically confusing scenarios and for initial surveillance in older children (over 2 years old at transplantation). Presently, all recipients have endomyocardial biopsy 1 year after transplantation and every year thereafter as part of routine late surveillance.

Rejection Management

The vast majority of acute cardiac graft rejection episodes in children occur within the first 3 months following transplantation. Acute rejection is a relatively rare event following this interval. In the LLU series of 293 patients transplanted between 1985 and 1996, 1.3% of all patients died of acute allograft rejection during the first 30 days following transplantation. Seven percent of operative survivors have died of late acute or incessant rejection.

The majority of established rejection treatment protocols are steroid-based. High-dose methylprednisolone (25 mg/kg twice daily for 8 doses) is used. Among those recipients whose rejection episode fails to respond rapidly (within 2 to 3 days), who experience hemodynamic instability, or who experience recurrence of acute rejection within 1 week following treatment for a rejection episode, antithymocyte serum (7 to 10 day course) is added to the therapeutic regimen. Oral or intravenous methotrexate (10 mg/m^2/week) is added in the treatment algorithm if reversal of the acute episode is not forthcoming and timely (29).

Total lymphoid irradiation (TLI) is occasionally used for a pediatric recipient whose incessant rejection is unresponsive to all other measures. Results of TLI have been somewhat ambiguous (37). Both methotrexate and TLI are considered by many transplantation specialists to provide useful rescue therapy, despite bone marrow depression and risk of late cancer development.

Circulatory support using an extracorporeal membrane oxygenator (ECMO) is the last option for management of hemodynamic and respiratory failure in the setting of advanced graft rejection and failure of rescue therapy. Requirement for such support may be transient, with eventual graft recovery, or may represent a bridge to salvage retransplantation.

LATE ISSUES

Eighty-nine percent of children achieve normal neuropsychological outcome following heart transplantation (14,38,39). These results compare favorably with those obtained in patients managed by multistage surgical palliation (40). Growth curves are within the appropriate percentile for the vast majority of patients. There is a strong correlation between total number of treated rejection episodes and cumulative length of steroid-based therapy with overt growth retardation. However, when corticosteroids are discontinued, rebound growth usually occurs and the patient returns to the normal percentile range for age. Although there appears to be mild reduction in exercise tolerance among pediatric cardiac transplant recipients, oxygen consumption, maximal heart rate on treadmill testing, and pulmonary function assays are comparable to normal subjects (8).

Hypertension

The reported incidence of long-term hypertension varies in the literature between 20% and 50% (11,41). It is multifactorial in origin. Chronic cyclosporine therapy, postoperative aortic coarctation, and chronic corticosteroid therapy are some of the potential causes of this late complication. Incidence of late hypertension is low in the LLU series. This may be attributed to the steroid-free protocol used. There has been little need for prolonged antihypertensive treatment beyond the first year after transplantation (1). Aortic coarctation has occurred in 16.4% of infants following transplantation for HLHS. This late complication has responded well to balloon aortoplasty (8).

Graft Vasculopathy

Graft vasculopathy is uniformly reported as the most frequent cause of late death after cardiac transplantation in adults (see Chapter 23), and has emerged as a significant late complication in children as well (42). Graft vasculopathy is defined as luminal occlusion greater than 50% in one or more of the coronary arteries. Isolated high-grade coronary artery occlusive disease in the absence of histologic rejection has been found in 11% of autopsy specimens. Coronary stenosis may occasionally occur in the form of discrete narrowing or, most frequently, as diffuse obstructive coronary artery disease. This process has been observed angiographically as early as 18 months after transplantation.

There is evidence suggesting that graft vasculopathy may be the consequence of immune-mediated mechanisms and that it occurs more frequently in patients with aggressive rejection histories and among those requiring sustained steroid therapy. The occurrence of graft vasculopathy is unrelated to age at transplantation or to HLA matching.

Patients with graft vasculopathy may present with syncope, congestive heart failure, silent myocardial infarction, or sudden cardiac death. In a cohort study of 173 LLU pediatric recipients surviving at least 1 year following heart transplantation, accelerated graft vasculopathy was diagnosed by angiography or pathology (autopsy or retransplantation specimens) in 8% of patients (43). Freedom from graft vasculopathy was 98% and 77% at 5 and 8 years, respectively. It has been the cause of late death in 2% of 293 children transplanted at LLU.

Intravascular ultrasonography and dobutamine stress echocardiography may eventually play a significant role in the early diagnosis of this complication. Elective retransplantation provides the only known effective therapy for significant graft vasculopathy.

Retransplantation

Freedom from retransplantation is 99%, 98%, and 95% at 1, 5, and 7 years, respectively. Retransplantation has been required in 10 LLU patients whose ages ranged from 14 days to 13 years. Indications for retransplantation were coronary artery disease (n = 7) and acute graft failure (n = 3). In a multicenter study on cardiac retransplantation in the non-neonatal pediatric age group, Michler et al observed a diminished occurrence of rejection following the second engraftment. The most frequent indications for retransplantation in Michler's study were coronary artery disease (41.2%), acute rejection (23.5%), and chronic rejection with coronary artery disease (23.5%) (44). Graft vasculopathy had a tendency to recur if it was the original indication for retransplantation.

Arrhythmias

Post-transplantation arrhythmias in children have not been widely studied. Park et al from the Columbia Presbyterian Medical Center reported on a systematic study of the significance of post-transplantation dysrhythmia (45). Among 59 pediatric recipients of heart transplantation, 41% were observed to have a variety of supraventricular and/or ventricular arrhythmias discovered during either 24-hour ambulatory or 12-lead surface electrocardiography. Rejection in association with the onset of the arrhythmias occurred in 7 of 9 recipients who exhibited supraventricular tachycardia and in 6 of 7 recipients found to have ventricular tachycardia.

In addition, graft coronary artery disease was significantly associated with ventricular tachycardia. In this institutional-based patient population, graft survival was 58% among those who were arrhythmia-free. Onset of complete heart block in a recipient suffering severe acute graft rejection suggests a grave prognosis. Significant sinus bradycardia in recipients who are free of graft rejection implies injury to the sinoatrial node during the transplantation procedure. Permanent pacemakers have been used for management of sick sinus syndrome in fewer than 2% of surviving pediatric heart transplant recipients in the LLU series.

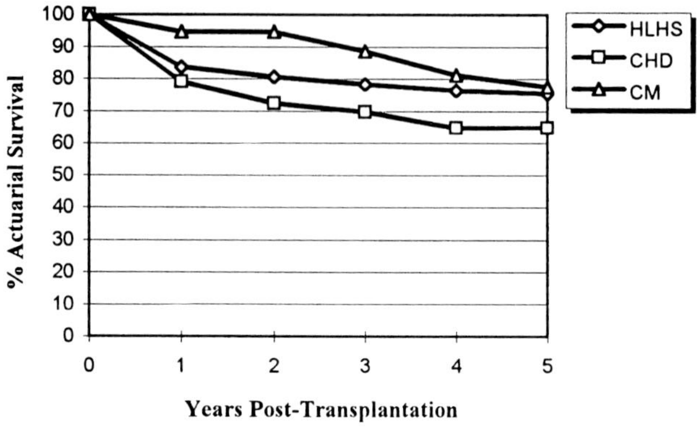

FIGURE 24.7. *The 5-year Kaplan-Meier actuarial survival curve for different diagnostic groups undergoing cardiac transplantation. HLHS, hypoplastic left heart syndrome; CHD, congenital heart disease other than HLHS; CM, cardiomyopathy.*

Renal Failure

Perioperative acute renal failure occurred in 5.4% of LLU recipients. It responded well to aggressive peritoneal dialysis. Data also indicate that 90% of transplanted children have creatinine levels below 1 mg/dL at 4.6 ± 1.7 years following transplantation, and that the average glomerular filtration rate in those children who were successfully dialyzed was within normal limits at 5 years of follow-up (25).

Neoplastic Diseases

Carcinomas occur rarely among immunosuppressed pediatric cardiac transplant recipients. In these patients, neoplastic disease is largely represented by hematopoietic malignancies and Epstein-Barr–associated lymphomas. In a series of 33 pediatric cardiac recipients with malignancy reported by Penn (46), 82% of the neoplasms were lymphomas, as compared to 41% in a comparable adult population (see also Chapter 37).

Reinterventions

Up to 43% of transplanted children will require some form of reintervention for cardiac and noncardiac-related issues at 4 years follow-up. The most frequent reintervention is balloon or operative coarctation repair (5.8%). Transplanted patients tolerate noncardiac surgical intervention for unrelated illnesses with acceptable mortality and morbidity (47). Of 293 children transplanted between 1985 and 1996 at LLU, 8 (2.7%) have undergone cardiac surgical procedures, and 39 (13.3%) required invasive cardiologic intervention. Sixty-five recipients (21%) have undergone minor and major general surgical procedures.

OUTCOMES

Experience accumulated over the last decade of pediatric heart transplantation has produced encouraging outcome data. Actuarial survival for the different diagnostic groups within the LLU series of pediatric cardiac allograft recipients aged 1.5 hours to 17 years is illustrated in Figure 24.7. Figure 24.6 compares actuarial survival from the LLU series divided by different age groups to that reported for 1996 by the International Society for Heart and Lung Transplantation (ISHLT) for all pediatric patients (9). Neonatal recipients enjoy a survival advantage over all other age groups. Furthermore, actuarial survival to 10 years for those children who have already survived 5 years is above 90%. These data are consistent with the findings of a retrospective review of the experience in pediatric heart transplantation reported by Shaffer and colleagues (48). The study found no significant difference in morbidity or mortality in patients with previous congenital heart disease compared to patients with cardiomyopathy.

Causes of mortality vary according to the time elapsed since transplantation. A 30-day operative mortality of 9.1% has not statistically correlated to preoperative age, weight, ischemic and arrest times, renal and respiratory failure, or donor/recipient weight ratio greater than 2:1. Operative mortality is usually related to technical complications or graft failure (including pulmonary hypertensive crisis), whereas rejection and infection are more remote causes of early death. Between 1 month and 1 year following transplantation, infection and graft rejection contribute to late mortality. Deaths after 1 year are related to coronary artery disease and chronic rejection.

FUTURE OF PEDIATRIC HEART TRANSPLANTATION

A decade of experience with clinical heart transplantation among infants and children has established the efficacy of this therapeutic strategy. Nevertheless, transplantation is still an imperfect technology. The future of pediatric heart transplantation rests squarely on collaborative efforts to identify and solve fundamental issues that threaten both the immediate availability and the durability of transplantation:

1. Expansion of donor graft resources
2. Improvement in the noninvasive techniques for diagnosis of early graft rejection
3. Discovery and investigation of immunoregulatory agents and protocols that reduce adverse side effects, yet help establish functional host tolerance
4. Development of a clear understanding of the molecular biology of graft vasculopathy, its identification, and, if possible, its prevention

As many as 2000 to 3000 infants and children per year would benefit from cardiac transplantation, but the current system of altruistic organ donation will never support that level of demand. Hence, alternative donor resources are currently under investigation and will require continued inquiry and careful clinical trials. It seems clear from experimental literature that infants and children suffering cardiac death might, in some instances, be a source of supply for cardiac allografts (49). A clinical protocol to implement this so-called "dead heart" type of heart donation has not been established, but perhaps should be.

Beyond human donors, the most promising additional resources lie in the area of xenotransplantation (see Chapter 40). Cardiac grafting from both closely and distantly related species is being investigated vigorously. It is possible that baboons will become a major donor organ resource for neonates and small infants who require solid organ transplantation but for whom allografts do not become available in time (50). Pig heart grafts, which have been genetically altered to humanize them, may provide the ultimate solution for an adequate and efficient donor organ supply.

A major impediment to survival of recipients following solid organ transplantation is the inability of the transplant team to reliably diagnose early graft rejection. Numerous clinical and laboratory observations are compiled in today's schema to arrive at a diagnosis of graft rejection. Regrettably, no one assay or observation, short of graft biopsy, is sufficiently reliable to allow the transplant team to establish a diagnosis of rejection before compromise of graft function becomes evident. In addition, subtle, persistent subclinical rejection is frequently overlooked and untreated. It may be this process that leads to chronic low-grade graft inflammation, ultimately reflected as graft vascular obstructive disease. Creation of new and reliable noninvasive techniques to identify early graft rejection remains a challenge.

Finally, the most threatening issue confronting transplanted patients is the evolution of graft vasculopathy. Intense research into the molecular biology of this catastrophic process should lead to a better understanding of it, and thus to its prevention. This, more than anything else, would ensure a durable outcome following heart transplantation.

It is apparent that heart transplantation provides extraordinary survival among infants and children who risk dying of either myopathic or complex structural heart disease. The LLU experience suggests that the most enduring outcomes following heart transplantation are found among neonatal recipients. This same subgroup requires the least amount of immunoregulation to achieve long-term engraftment. These features combine to provide the best functional result following heart transplantation, while minimizing the noxious side effects of immunoregulation.

Virtually all infants and children who require transplantation appear initially to benefit from this intervention. However, not all of them benefit equally. It is hoped that future laboratory and clinical research will help establish heart transplantation as a clinical reality for all children who need it, with each recipient enjoying the full benefits of the procedure.

ACKNOWLEDGMENTS

The authors would like to thank Richard Chinnock, MD, Joyce Johnston, RN, and Mrs. Dawn Huggins for their help in the preparation of this chapter.

COMMENTARY

Lori J. West

Successful extension of heart transplantation to infants and children necessitates a fundamental change in philosophy from that which has evolved for adult populations. A clinical and investigative approach solidly based in pediatric medicine is essential, not only because the diseases leading to consideration of organ replacement differ from adults, but also because the care of children before and after transplantation must encompass the complexities of immunologic development; physical growth and multisystem development; intellectual, emotional, and social maturation; and educational activities; as well as other pediatric quality-of-life parameters. Furthermore, complications of organ transplantation in children often differ in comparison to adults. Finally, donor issues can be different in the pediatric population. Thus, when compared to adults, a pediatric approach to transplantation leads to alterations in indications for transplantation, contraindications to transplantation, timing of listing for transplantation, consideration of waiting list status, complications, and resource allocation.

INDICATIONS FOR HEART TRANSPLANTATION IN INFANTS AND CHILDREN

Heart transplantation should be contemplated as life-*saving* therapy for:

- End-stage myocardial failure in the setting of cardiomyopathics, myocarditis, congenital heart disease, postcardiotomy heart failure, or malignant arrhythmias refractive to medical therapy

- Complex congenital heart malformations for which no surgical palliation is possible at acceptable risk
- Unresectable obstructive cardiac tumors
- Unresectable ventricular diverticula

Heart transplantation should also be contemplated as life-*enhancing* therapy, even when patient demise is not imminent, for treatment of excessive disability, unacceptably poor quality of life or long-term morbidity in the setting of failing myocardial function, or complex congenital heart disease. It can be a therapeutic option after failed surgical palliation of congenital heart disease, as with post-Fontan procedure complications such as protein-losing enteropathy.

CONTRAINDICATIONS TO HEART TRANSPLANTATION

As in the adult population, heart transplantation should not be performed in patients with active infection, malignancy, irreversible multi-organ failure, progressive systemic diseases with early mortality, or hypercoagulable states. In the case of concomitant profound disease of another major organ system, cardiac replacement should be contemplated as part of multi-organ transplantation. Cardiovascular contraindications to heart transplantation in children include fixed pulmonary hypertension, pulmonary vein atresia or progressive stenosis, "thread-like" hypoplastic pulmonary arteries, severe aortic hypoplasia extending to the thoracic aorta, and severe arteriovenous malformations. Total lack of venous access for performing biopsies should be considered at least a relative contraindication until noninvasive techniques allow accurate and consistent monitoring of graft rejection.

Successful pediatric heart transplantation may be achieved despite a number of complicating factors, none of which are now considered contraindications. These conditions, however, require meticulous expectant management and transplantations should be carried out only in centers with adequate experience. These include complex congenital heart disease, abnormalities of situs with associated cardiac malformations (situs inversus, situs ambiguus—the right and left "atrial isomerism" syndromes with asplenia/polysplenia), systemic venous malformations, anomalous pulmonary venous connections without stenosis, some pulmonary artery abnormalities, and previous sternotomy and/or thoracotomy (1–3). Heart transplantation is not absolutely contraindicated in the presence of nonfixed pulmonary hypertension; however, the risk of acute right ventricular failure must be anticipated. The presence of noncardiac congenital abnormalities such as tracheoesophageal fistula or duodenal atresia will complicate the clinical course but do not preclude successful heart transplantation. Likewise, kyphoscoliosis with resultant restrictive pulmonary disease as a complication of complex congenital heart disease does not preclude successful heart transplantation, but may make management difficult. Patients with nonprogressive or slowly progressive systemic diseases with life expectancies predicted into the third or fourth decade may be considered for transplantation. These systemic conditions include metabolic and/or genetic causes of cardiomyopathy such as Becker's muscular dystrophy, some myocardial mitochondrial cytopathies, and other familial cardiomyopathies. Diabetes mellitus is no longer a contraindication to cardiac replacement, though clinical management is complex because of the effects of corticosteroids and calcineurin inhibitors on glucose metabolism.

TIMING OF LISTING FOR TRANSPLANTATION AND STATUS ASSIGNMENT ON WAITING LIST

Most adult patients are of a similar size, and thus compete with each other for scarce donor organs. There are insufficient organs even for the highest status or "sickest" patients. However, in pediatric populations, size considerations subdivide the potential recipient population into smaller groups. Early listing of potential pediatric recipients is important because there may be less competition for organs from donors of a particular size range. Thus, transplantation often can be accomplished before clinical deterioration proceeds to a less optimal state. Clearly, transplantation before deterioration to a state requiring "invasion" (ventricular assistance, respiratory assistance, central lines, parenteral nutrition, dialysis, etc.) is associated with better outcomes and fewer post-transplant complications (4). With a smoother clinical course, the heavy financial burden of organ transplantation is lower. Furthermore, early listing ensures that all available organs will be used; waiting list mortality declines as more time is available to acquire an organ.

It should be noted that classification schemes for waiting list status tend to reflect the reasonably predictable course of clinical deterioration of a relatively homogeneous population of adult patients with myocardial failure secondary to ischemic heart disease or dilated cardiomyopathy. Predictors of outcome have been well studied for these patients. Clinical predictors of outcome have not been determined adequately for the pediatric population, particularly the younger patients and those with complex congenital heart disease (5). Thus, assignment of status currently is based on criteria that may not be relevant to this population.

IMMUNOLOGIC CONSIDERATIONS IN PEDIATRIC ORGAN TRANSPLANTATION

Immunologic development of the pediatric recipient, both at the time of transplantation and during subsequent stages of childhood, must be considered carefully when developing immunosuppressive drug regimens and surveillance protocols for monitoring rejection and infection. Infants undergoing transplantation during the early newborn period often exhibit less aggressive immunoreactivity toward their grafts and are more susceptible to infection (6). Attempts to minimize immunosuppressive medications are crucial. However, grafts transplanted into the relatively stimulated immune system of the toddler who frequently encounters childhood pathogens, or the adolescent undergoing the numerous physical changes of puberty, likely will encounter a more vigorous immune response. Similarly, patients who undergo transplantation after clinical deterioration to a critical state requiring invasive medical care may present an immunologic battleground to the clinician. In these children, "polypharmacy" will be the rule. The immunosuppression load required to control acute graft rejection in these patients may increase the risk of subsequent post-transplant complications such as lymphoproliferative disease and opportunistic infection; however, inadequate control may contribute to the development of chronic rejection (graft coronary artery disease).

For newborn patients, starting immunosuppression during early infancy may carry important consequences. Recent data suggest that children undergoing heart transplantation and immunosuppression prior to the age of 2 years develop a persistent defect in antibody production in response to stimulation by complex polysaccharide antigens such as pneumococcus (7). Some of these young patients may benefit from chronic antibiotic prophylaxis and/or immunoglobulin infusion, similar to patients with asplenia/polysplenia syndromes undergoing immunosuppression after heart transplantation.

COMPLICATIONS

Certain complications of transplantation are particularly problematic for children, while others present less difficulty than in adults. Post-transplant lymphoproliferative disease (PTLD) is more frequent in young patients, reported in 5% to 15% of pediatric heart transplant patients, depending on the center (8). This complication of organ transplantation, which is discussed in more detail in Chapter 37, typically occurs as a consequence of concomitant immunosuppression during primary infection with Epstein-Barr virus (EBV). It can also occur with reactivation EBV disease. As more children than adults are seronegative for EBV at the time of transplant, they will be immunosuppressed upon subsequent primary infection and are thus at greater risk. This is particularly true if the organ donor is EBV-positive, because exposure to EBV will occur during the time of maximum immunosuppression immediately following transplant. The pathology of this disorder involves uncontrolled proliferation of EBV-infected and/or transformed B lymphocytes, which can occur in any area of lymphocyte aggregation. Common sites of lymphoproliferation include tonsils, spleen, mediastinal lymph nodes, mesenteric nodes, and Peyer's patches. Restoration of T-lymphocyte function may eradicate tumors; indeed, decreasing immunosuppression alone may result in remission, although this is unlikely in the case of monoclonal, highly immunoblastic tumors, which may prove fatal. Aggressive and persistent attempts to wean immunosuppressive medications to the lowest dose necessary for control of rejection is critical in minimizing the risk of PTLD. Furthermore, as cellular and molecular targets of emerging immunomodulatory drugs are increasingly selective, some of these new agents may be helpful and need to be investigated in pediatric patients. Initiation of antiviral therapy at the time of exposure may be beneficial in reducing the viral load, which should be monitored closely with antigen detection techniques such as semiquantitative polymerase chain reaction (PCR).

The side-effects profile of specific immunosuppressive agents generally is similar in children and adult patients. However, some of these complications are perhaps more troublesome in young children and adolescents, including:

- Steroid-induced growth delay or cessation
- Steroid- and cyclosporine-induced bone loss
- Cyclosporine-induced hirsutism and gingival hyperplasia
- Exacerbation of diabetes, hypertension, obesity, and behavioral problems related to steroids

Again, timely application to the pediatric population of newer immunosuppressive drug therapies such as tacrolimus, mycophenolate mofetil, rapamycin, and interleukin 2 receptor (IL-2R) antibodies may allow amelioration of these problems. Ultimately, research toward induction of immunologic tolerance in models relevant to the immature patient may obviate the need for immunosuppressive medications altogether (9).

Surgical complications occur more commonly in small pediatric patients transplanted for complex congenital heart disease, particularly in cases of heterotaxy (1,3). These may include stenoses at sites of vascular anastomoses such as the vena cavae, as well as aberrant venous connections or reconstructed pulmonary arteries. These complications can be relieved by balloon angioplasty or by placement of endovascular stents.

Graft coronary artery disease, one of the most difficult and common complications of heart transplantation in adults, is reported with a lower but increasing incidence in pediatric recipients—typically less than 10% at most centers, but 19% in a recent multicenter analysis (10). This may reflect the consistent association of this entity with older donor age or may be an artifact of the lack of adequate diagnostic capabilities in the young pediatric patient. Recent advances allowing pediatric application of diagnostic modalities such as intravascular ultrasound and dobutamine-stress echocardiography will assist in clarifying the extent of this problem in children.

RESOURCE ALLOCATION

Organ replacement can be robust palliation for infants and children but requires meticulous long-term attention to details of clinical care, preferably in a pediatric center. In general, the quality of life is very good, particularly for children who have had life-long limitations from congenital heart disease. Constant surveillance and a high index of suspicion for transplant-related problems are necessary to improve long-term outcomes and to minimize costly complications (1–3). A multidisciplinary team approach is critical to the success of the complex pediatric care required for these patients, not only after transplantation but during the pretransplant waiting period and the perioperative phase.

Participation of pediatric subspecialty consultants with particular expertise in newly emerging transplant-related issues is invaluable. Management of issues important to adolescent patients such as self-image, compliance, contraception, athletics, and use of alcohol, tobacco, and recreational drugs requires special expertise. Specialized pediatric imaging facilities will allow safe performance of cardiac biopsies and other interventional procedures in even the smallest infants (11), and facilitate the early diagnosis of problems such as rejection, coronary artery disease (angiography, intravascular ultrasound, stress echocardiography), malignancies, and occult infection. Likewise, experienced pediatric cardiovascular anesthetists provide expertise allowing not only transplantation but also other important procedures in pretransplant patients with extremely delicate hemodynamics.

Resource allocation for pediatric heart transplantation must also include provision for psychosocial assessment and chronic support; age-appropriate educational needs for patients who require lengthy hospitalization while waiting and after transplantation; physiotherapy and occupational therapy for infants and children; and nutritionist support and pharmacy support for complex drug management. Extensive education of patient, parents, family, and community is essential. The family and patient can become a valuable source of education and awareness for the community at large about organ transplantation and donor need. Involvement and education of community practitioners and pediatricians in transplant issues further strengthens the team.

CONSIDERATIONS FOR THE FUTURE

One of the evolving challenges in pediatric heart transplantation is the emerging group of patients with complex congenital heart disease for whom earlier surgical palliation is now failing (12). This includes adolescents and young adults with complications after the total cavopulmonary connection (Fontan procedure) for malformations with single ventricle anatomy or physiology. Some of these patients have undergone numerous surgical procedures and experienced years of extreme cardiovascular disability resulting in poor growth and malnutrition, profound cyanosis, venous obstruction, and other problems. They are extremely complicated patients when transplanted in this condition. Primary transplantation during infancy could be justifiably advocated for newborns with these complex cardiac malformations, as well as those with hypoplastic left heart syndrome. These malformations can be accurately diagnosed during fetal life, whereupon listing for transplantation can proceed upon reaching a fetal age consistent with pulmonary maturity. This approach, however, is hampered by the scarcity of donor organs suitable for infants, and awaits further developments in xenotransplantation.

CHAPTER REFERENCES

1. Del Rio M, Bailey LL. Heart transplantation for congenital heart disease. In: Baue AE, Geha AS, Hammond AL, et al., eds. Glenn's thoracic and cardiovascular surgery. 6th ed. Vol 2. Stamford: Appleton & Lange, 1996:1475–1490.
2. Brown JW, Turrentine MW, Kesler KA, et al. Triple-drug immunosuppression for heart transplantation in infants and children. J Heart Lung Transplant 1993;12:S265–S274.
3. Kantrowitz A, Haller SD, Joos H, et al. Transplantation of the heart in an infant and an adult. Am J Cardiol 1968;22:782–790.
4. Barnard CN. Cardiac transplantation: an evaluation of the first two operations performed at the Groote Shuur Hospital, Cape Town. Am J Cardiol 1968;22:584.
5. Cooley DA, Frazier OH, Van Bure CT, et al. Cardiac transplantation in an 8-month-old female with subendocardial fibroelastosis. JAMA 1986;256(10):1326–1329.
6. Bailey LL, Nehlsen-Cannarella SL, Doroshow RW, et al. Cardiac allotransplantation in newborns as therapy for hypoplastic left heart syndrome. N Engl J Med 1986;315:949–951.
7. Boucek MM, Mathis CM, Kanakriyeh MS, et al. Donor shortage: use of the dysfunctional heart. J Heart Lung Transplant 1993;12:S186–S190.
8. Razzouk AJ, Chinnock RE, Gundry SR, et al. Transplantation as primary treatment for hypoplastic left heart syndrome: intermediate-term results. Ann Thorac Surg 1996;62:1–8.
9. Hosenpu JD, Novick RJ, Bennett LE, et al. The registry of the International Society for Heart and Lung Transplantation: thirteenth official report—1996. J Heart Lung Transplant 1996;15:655–674.
10. Norwood WI, Lang P, Hansen DD. Physiologic repair of aortic atresia-hypoplastic left heart syndrome. N Engl J Med 1983;308:23–26.
11. Starnes VA, Griffin ML, Pitlick PT, et al. Current approach to hypoplastic left heart syndrome. Palliation, transplantation or both? J Thorac Cardiovasc Surg 1992;104:189–195.
12. Turrentine MW, Kesler KA, Caldwell R, et al. Cardiac transplantation in infants and children. Ann Thorac Surg 1994;57:546–554.
13. Forbess JM, Cook N, Roth SJ, et al. Ten years institutional experience with palliative surgery for hypoplastic left heart syndrome. Risk factors related to stage I mortality. Circulation 1995;92(suppl 2):262–266.
14. Bailey LL, Gundry SR, Razzouk AJ, et al. Bless the babies: one hundred fifteen late survivors of heart transplantation during the first year of life. J Thorac Cardiovasc Surg 1993;105:805–815.
15. Pediatric Heart Transplantation Protocol. The Loma Linda University Medical Center, 1997.
16. Ashwal S. Brain death in early infancy. J Heart Lung Transplant 1993;12: S176–S178.
17. Alonso de Begona J, Gundry SR, Nehlsen-Cannarella SL, et al. HLA matching and its effect on infant and pediatric cardiac graft survival. Transplant Proc 1991;23(1):1139–1141.

18. Menkis AH, McKenzie FN, Novick RJ, et al. Expanding applicability of transplantation after multiple prior palliative procedures. Ann Thorac Surg 1991;52:722–726.
19. Menkis AH, McKenzie FN, Novick RJ, et al. Special considerations for heart transplantation in congenital heart disease. J Heart Lung Transplant 1990;9:602–607.
20. Bailey LL. Heart transplantation techniques in complex congenital heart disease. J Heart Lung Transplant 1993;12:S168–S175.
21. Kawauchi M, Gundry SR, Alonso de Begona J, et al. Prolonged preservation of human pediatric hearts for transplantation: correlation of ischemic time and subsequent function. J Heart Lung Transplant 1993;12:55–58.
22. Ruiz CE, Gamra H, Zhang HP, et al. Stenting of the ductus arteriosus as a bridge to cardiac transplantation in infants with hypoplastic left-heart syndrome. N Engl J Med 1993;328:1605–1608.
23. Razzouk AJ, Bailey LL. Infant heart transplantation. In: Moss AJ, Adams FH eds. Heart disease in infants, children and adolescents. 5th ed. Baltimore: Williams & Wilkins, 1995;1:510–516.
24. Reichart B. Size matching in heart transplantation. J Heart Lung Transplant 1992;11:S199–202.
25. Vricella LA, Alonso de Begona J, Gundry SR, et al. Aggressive peritoneal dialysis for treatment of acute kidney failure after neonatal heart transplantation. J Heart Lung Transplant 1992;11:320–329.
26. Bork J, Chinnock R, Ogata K, Baum MF. Infectious complications in infant heart transplantation. J Heart Lung Transplant 1993;12:S199–S202.
27. White DJ, Gilks W. The ontogeny of immune responses. J Heart Lung Transplant 1993;12:S301–S308.
28. Smith DJ, Danskine AJ, Yacoub MH. The beneficial effect of HLA-DR matching on rejection episodes following cardiac transplantation (abstract). J Heart Lung Transplant 1993;12:S76.
29. Chinnock RE, Baum MF, Larsen R, Bailey LL. Rejection management and long term surveillance of the pediatric heart transplant recipient: the Loma Linda experience. J Heart Lung Transplant 1993:S255–S264.
30. Armitage JM, Fricker FJ, del Nido P, et al. A decade (1982 to 1992) of pediatric cardiac transplantation and the impact of FK 506 immunosuppression. J Thorac Cardiovasc Surg 1993;105:464–473.
31. Boucek MM, Mathis CM, Lebeck LK, et al. Prophylactic anti-thymocyte serum reduces rejection frequency after pediatric heart transplantation (abstract). J Heart Lung Transplant 1992;11:205.
32. Billingham ME. Endomyocardial biopsy in pediatric heart recipients: the gold standard. J Heart Lung Transplant 1991;10:S841–S842.
33. Behrendt DM, Billingham ME, Boucek MM, et al. Session VI: rejection/infection: the limits of heart transplantation success. J Heart Lung Transplant 1993;12:S841–S845.
34. Baltzer DT, Moorhead S, Saffitz JE, et al. Utility of surveillance biopsies in infant heart transplant recipients. J Heart Lung Transplant 1995;14:1095–1101.
35. Boucek MM, Mathis CM, Kanakriyeh MS, Bailey LL. Noninvasive cardiac rejection surveillance in infant transplantation (abstract). Pediatr Res 1989;25(part 2):21a.
36. Tantengco MV, Dodd D, First WH, et al. Echocardiographic abnormalities with acute cardiac allograft rejection in children: correlation with endomyocardial biopsy. J Heart Lung Transplant 1993;12:S203–S210.
37. Kirklin JK, George JF, McGriffin DC, et al. Total lymphoid irradiation: is there a role in pediatric heart transplantation? J Heart Lung Transplant 1993;12: S293–S300.
38. Baum MF, Cutler DC, Fricker FJ, et al. Session VII: physiologic and psychological growth and development in pediatric heart transplant recipients. J Heart Lung Transplant 1991;10(5 Pt 2):848–855.
39. Baum MM, Chinnock RE, Ashwal S, et al. Growth and neurodevelopmental outcome in infants undergoing heart transplantation. J Heart Lung Transplant 1993;12:S211–S217.
40. Rogers BT, Msall ME, Buck GM, et al. Neurodevelopmental outcome of infants with hypoplastic left heart syndrome. J Pediatr 1995;126:496–498.
41. Starnes VA, Stinson EB, Oyer PE. Cardiac transplantation in children and adolescents. Circulation 1987;76(suppl 5):43–47.
42. Berry GJ, Rizeq MN, Weiss LM, Billingham ME. Graft coronary disease in pediatric heart and combined heart-lung transplant recipients: a study of fifteen cases. J Heart Lung Transplant 1993;12:S309–S319.
43. Bailey LL, Zuppan CW, Chinnock RE, et al. Graft vasculopathy among recipients of heart transplantation during the first 12 years of life. Transplant Proc 1995;3:1921–1925.
44. Michler RE, Edwards NM, Hsu DH, et al. Pediatric retransplantation. J Heart Lung Transplant 1993;12:S319–S327.
45. Park JK, Hsu DT, Hordof AJ, Addonizio L. Arrhythmias in pediatric heart transplant recipients. J Heart Lung Transplant 1993;12:956–964.
46. Penn I. Incidence and treatment of neoplasia after transplantation. J Heart Lung Transplant 1993;12:S328–S336.
47. Razzouk AJ. Surgical interventions in children after heart transplantation. J Heart Lung Transplant 1993;12:S195–S198.
48. Shaffer KM, Denfield SW, Showengerdt KO, et al. Cardiac transplantation for pediatric patients. With inoperable congenital heart disease. Tex Heart Inst J 1998;25:57–63.
49. Gundry SR, Alonso de Begona J, Bailey LL. Transplantation and reanimation of hearts 30 minutes after warm, asystolic "death." Arch Surg 1993;128:989–993.
50. Bailey LL, Nehlsen Cannarella SL, Concepcion W, Jolley WB. Baboon-to-human cardiac transplantation in a neonate. JAMA 1985;254:3321–3329.

COMMENTARY REFERENCES

1. Hsu DT, Quacgebeur JM, Michler RE, et al. Heart transplantation in children with congenital heart disease. J Am Coll Cardiol 1995;26:743–749.
2. Bailey LL, Gundrey SR, Razzouk AJ, et al. Bless the babies: one hundred fifteen late survivors of heart transplantation during the first year of life. J Thorac Cardiovasc Surg 1993;105:805–815.
3. Addonizio LJ. Current status of cardiac transplantation in children. Curr Opin Pediatr 1996;8:520–526.
4. Shaddy RE, Naftel DC, Kirklin JK, et al. Outcome of cardiac transplantation in children. Survival in a contemporary multi-institutional experience. Pediatric Heart Transplant Study Group. Circulation 1996;94(suppl 9):II69–73.
5. McGiffin DC, Naftel DC, Kirklin JK, et al. Predicting outcome after listing for heart transplantation in children: comparison of Kaplan-Meier and parametric competing risk analysis. Pediatric Heart Transplant Study Group. J Heart Lung Transplant 1997;16:713–722.
6. Razzouk AJ, Chinnock RE, Gundry SR, et al. Transplantation as a primary treatment for hypoplastic left heart syndrome: intermediate-term results. Ann Thorac Surg 1996;62:1–8.
7. Gennery AR, Cant AJ, Spickett GP, et al. Immunosuppression following cardiac transplantation in early childhood interrupts development of the polysaccharide antibody response. Lancet 1998;351:1778–1781.
8. Boyle GI, Michaels MG, Webber SA, et al. Post-transplantation lymphoproliferative disorders in pediatric throacic organ recipients. J Pediatr 1997;131:309–313.
9. West LJ, Morris PJ, Wood KJ. Fetal liver haematopoietic cells and tolerance to organ allografts. Lancet 1994;343:148–149.
10. Sigfusson G, Fricker FJ, Bernstein D, et al. Long-term survivors of pediatric heart transplantation: a multi-center report of 68 children who have survived longer than five years. J Pediatr 1997;130:862–871.
11. Benson LN, Burrows PE, Freedom RM. Interventional cardiac catheterization in neonates. In: Freedom RM, Benson LN, Smallhorn JF, eds. Neonatal heart disease. London: Springer-Verlag. 1992:817.
12. Somerville J. Management of adults with congenital heart disease: an increasing problem. Annu Rev Med 1997;48:283–293.

Chapter

25

Lung Transplantation

LEO C. GINNS JOHN C. WAIN

Lung transplantation has emerged over the past 15 years as a successful therapeutic intervention for a variety of end-stage pulmonary parenchymal and vascular diseases. Advances in recipient and donor selection, operative technique, and postoperative management have resulted in improved early survival. The parameters for the use of either isolated lung transplantation or heart–lung transplantation continue to be defined, with the role for heart–lung transplantation lessening over the past decade. As in all fields of transplantation, a relative shortage of donor organs has been identified as the major constraint on wider application of this therapy. In addition, chronic rejection in the pulmonary allograft, manifested as obliterative bronchiolitis, remains a major obstacle to long-term patient survival.

A decision to pursue lung transplantation stems from an understanding of the natural course of the underlying disease that not only reduces the quality of life but threatens life expectancy. Within this context, it is possible to compare the relative risks and benefits of transplantation. The suitable patient is generally understood to have a "window of opportunity" for transplantation, in which the severity of the illness justifies the risk of therapy but is not so advanced as to preclude its likely success.

A successful outcome for lung transplantation is predicated upon a knowledge of the surgical procedure and medical management of its complications, particularly the hazards associated with life-long immunosuppressive therapy. Equally important is the commitment of the patient, who must withstand the rigors of the transplant process and adhere to a complex regimen of post-transplant care and surveillance. A realistic expectation concerning functional results and survival is essential. Implicit within this outlook is the realization that the lung transplant is, in a sense, "trading in one type of a problem for another." The post-transplant patient will not be free of tests, medications, possible side effects, visits to the office, or other features of a chronic process. However, "in the bargain," there is the opportunity to function at a much higher level and for a longer life. With these principles in mind, the patient should comprehend the nature of the evaluation process. By selecting recipients with relatively more favorable prognoses, it is designed both to promote individual recovery and to optimize utilization of scarce donor organs. This chapter amplifies these concepts.

HISTORY

Pioneering efforts in experimental lung transplantation were undertaken in the 1940s and 1950s. Demikhov performed a variety of experiments involving transplantation of pulmonary lobes and heterotopic heart–lung transplantation in canine models. These experiments demonstrated the technical feasibility of such procedures. In addition, a disparate functional course was observed between the heart and the lung in heart–lung grafts, foreshadowing the differing rates of rejection of the heart and the lungs seen in combined heart–lung transplants performed clinically more than three decades later (1). Metras reported the results of left lung transplantation in a canine model and presciently emphasized technical factors that are now used clinically for isolated lung transplantation (2). Subsequent experimental studies demonstrated the potential for the transplanted lung to provide ventilation for the recipient (3).

Clinical lung transplantation was undertaken first by Hardy in 1963 (4). The procedure consisted of a left single lung transplant performed for a carcinoma involving the left hilum. The patient survived for 18 days, dying of renal failure and malnutrition. This effort demonstrated that a transplanted lung could function for the short term in a patient and stimulated further clinical and experimental efforts. However, between 1963 and 1978, at least 38 attempts were made at isolated lung transplantation and only one patient survived to hospital discharge (5). That particular patient had undergone a right single lung transplant for silicosis; he developed a bronchial anastomotic stricture and ultimately succumbed to sepsis and chronic rejection eight months after transplantation. The remaining patients in this 15-year period all died perioperatively. The major cause of mortality beyond the first postoperative week in these patients was bronchial dehiscence. In addition, the majority of patients were greatly debilitated at the time of the procedure. For many, ventilator dependence or multisystem organ failure hindered their ability to survive. It was appreciated that available immunosuppressive regimens, relying on high-dose corticosteroids, compromised postoperative healing of the bronchus and further potentiated the adverse effects of preexisting conditions in many of these patients.

The problem of bronchial healing was related to the relative ischemia of the donor bronchus following revascularization of the lung graft without re-establishing a bronchial circulation. One technical approach to this problem was the development of a procedure for combined heart–lung transplantation, allowing for maintenance of collateral bronchial circulation from the coronary circulation and mediastinal tissues. Although performed primarily for patients with end-stage cardiac failure due to pulmonary hypertension, the initial report of successful heart–lung transplantation demonstrated the feasibility of this approach in obtaining healing of the airway and confirmed the ability of the transplanted lung to provide long-term respiratory function (6). Subsequently, heart–lung transplantation has been performed for numerous pulmonary parenchymal diseases, including emphysema and bilateral septic lung diseases such as cystic fibrosis.

An alternative technique for improving bronchial healing was to optimize the bronchial-pulmonary collateral circulation by limiting the length of the donor bronchus and to revascularize the bronchial circulation extrinsically by wrapping the anastomosis with omentum. In addition to these technical measures, the avoidance of high-dose steroid immunosuppressive regimens made possible by the use of cyclosporine improved bronchial anastomotic healing (7). These advances, combined with the selection of well-conditioned recipients with pulmonary fibrosis, a disorder with a pathologic physiology favoring perfusion and ventilation of the allograft, culminated in the clinical success of isolated single lung transplantation (8). Further efforts were made to perfect a technique for isolated double lung transplantation in order to expand this approach to patients with bilateral septic lung disease. The initial clinical success of an en bloc double lung transplant procedure was tempered by the frequent occurrence of bronchial anastomotic complications (9). Further modification of the technique, however, either by direct bronchial revascularization or by performing bilateral sequential single lung transplantation has provided satisfactory results (10,11).

Despite initial concerns about the physiology of allograft ventilation, isolated single lung transplantation is also appropriate for patients with end-stage chronic obstructive pulmonary disease (COPD) (12). Isolated single and double lung transplantation has also been successfully applied to patients with primary pulmonary hypertension or Eisenmenger's syndrome (with correction of the etiologic shunt), for whom combined heart–lung transplantation was initially devised (13,14). As the utility of isolated lung transplantation for these pulmonary diseases has been demonstrated, the need for heart–lung transplantation has diminished.

The current status of lung transplantation is summarized in the 1998 report from the Registry of the International Society for Heart and Lung Transplantation. The data set includes information regarding 4777 single lung and 3278 double lung transplantations reported from 150 lung transplant centers (15). From approximately 1985 to 1993, the number of transplants performed grew strikingly (Fig. 25.1). Since 1993, however, the annual number of transplants has appeared to plateau, despite the use of increasingly older donors.

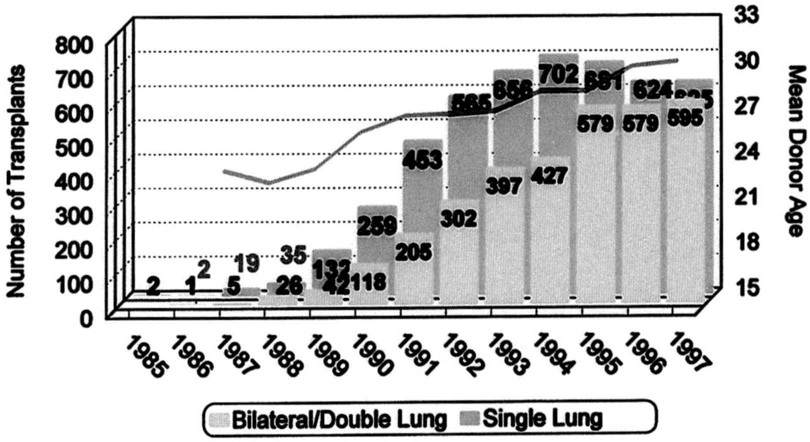

FIGURE 25.1. *Lung transplantation volumes and mean donor age from 1985 to 1997 (15).*

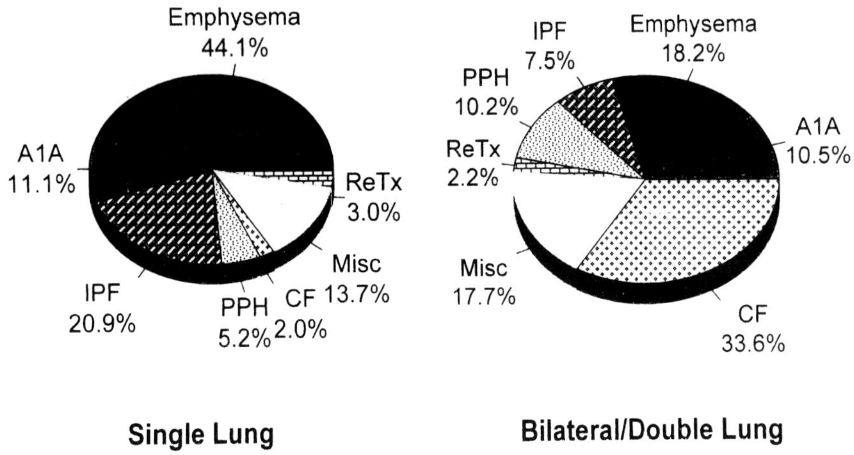

FIGURE 25.2. *Adult lung transplantation indications (15).*

The majority of lung transplants performed today are for individuals suffering from emphysema. However, cystic fibrosis is the dominant indication for bilateral/double lung transplantation (Fig. 25.2).

RECIPIENT SELECTION

General Considerations and Indications

Lung transplantation is a therapy of last resort. Potential recipients should be patients with end-stage pulmonary parenchymal and/or vascular disease who have both an unacceptable quality of life and a limited life expectancy and for whom no effective alternative therapy is available. When to list potential recipients for lung transplantation is a difficult question. There are, in fact, no universally agreed-upon standards. Instead, general guidelines have been developed that are aimed at identifying individuals whose pulmonary function and prognosis justify transplantation and whose current health will not increase the risk of the operation unnecessarily or jeopardize its long-term success.

In a joint statement, transplant physicians and surgeons representing the International Society of Heart and Lung Transplantation, the American Society of Transplant Physicians, the American Thoracic Society, the European Respiratory Society, and the Thoracic Society of Australia and New Zealand have agreed upon acceptable guidelines for lung transplant candidates (16).

Representative guidelines are shown in Table 25.1. Contraindications are listed in Table 25.2. The application of these criteria to a specific patient, however, may vary widely. A need exists to develop minimum waiting list criteria. A patient's "window of opportunity" depends upon a number of parameters, some of which are relevant to the underlying disease process, while others pertain to factors that may affect waiting time on the organ transplant waiting list. Factors that affect the candidacy of a potential recipient include: 1) the nature of the underlying disease and its severity; 2) the course of the patient's illness and the development of complications such as pulmonary hypertension,

Table 25.1. General Guidelines for Considering Lung Transplantation

Untreatable end-stage pulmonary parenchymal and/or vascular disease
Absence of other major medical illnesses
Substantial limitation of daily activities
Projected life expectancy <2 years
NYHA class III or IV functional level
Rehabilitation potential
Satisfactory psychosocial profile and emotional support system
Acceptable nutritional status
Disease specific mortality exceeding transplant specific mortality over 1 to 2 years

Table 25.2. Contraindications to Lung Transplantation

Absolute Contraindications
Current smoking, alcohol, or drug abuse
Bone marrow failure
Hepatic cirrhosis
Active malignancy precluding long-term survival
HIV infection
Other life-limiting condition
Relative Contraindications
Tobacco use within 6 months
Physiologic age
>65 for single lung transplantation
>60 for bilateral lung transplantation
>55 for heart–lung transplantation
Psychosocial instability
Weight outside of acceptable range (70% to 130% of predicted)
Prednisone use >20 mg/day or 40 mg/q.o.d.
Mechanical ventilation
Major dysfunction of other organs, especially kidney, liver, central nervous system
Coronary disease or left ventricular dysfunction
Significant peripheral vascular disease
Symptomatic osteoporosis
Severe chest wall deformity
Sputum with pan-resistant bacteria or *Aspergillus*
Active hepatitis B or C infection

right ventricular dysfunction, or cor pulmonale; 3) demographic variables such as age or gender; 4) other exposures such as smoking; and 5) comorbid conditions.

Factors that may affect waiting time, regardless of underlying conditions, include donor availability, waiting list size, and geographic area. Depending upon the population density, hospital death rate, attitudes about donation, and number and size of local transplant centers, the ability of local organ procurement agencies to obtain consent and to retrieve organs is variable and will influence the time that a patient may require before a suitable lung becomes available (see also Chapter 15). Additional considerations in the allocation of donor organs include blood group, history of prior sensitization and need for cross-matching, individual differences with respect to chest size, and even unique preference of one side versus another. All of these factors influence the acceptability of each potential lung donor, who must also pass a variety of objective standards.

The decision to list a patient for lung transplantation depends primarily on an estimate of the patient's life expectancy with continued medical management versus the projected survival following a successful transplant. The prognosis of patients at the time of transplant evaluation may be estimated from epidemiologic studies. It should be kept in mind, however, that these estimates are, at best, predictors of the average course in the population. It may not always be possible to extrapolate such data to an individual patient.

The evaluation of a potential candidate involves complete assessment of cardiopulmonary function and of the patient's general health, in addition to a thorough evaluation of psychosocial status. A battery of screening tests is required, as well as evaluation by members of the transplant team, including pulmonary physicians, cardiologists, thoracic surgeons, psychiatrists, social workers, physical therapists, and nutritionists, among select other consultants (Table 25.3). In some instances, this evaluation can be completed on an outpatient basis. For many patients, however, their respiratory disability necessitates an inpatient evaluation. A coordinated review of the results of these studies by the multidisciplinary transplant team ensures that candidates with relatively favorable long-term prognoses are accepted as potential transplant recipients.

The life expectancy of potential recipients is related to both underlying disease process and the resulting reduction in activities of daily living. The variable rates of progression of the diseases for which lung transplantation is performed and the variety of supportive therapies available dictate that many criteria relate to a specific disease state. However, with the average waiting time in the United States for donor lungs at over 550 days, a *life expectancy of approximately two years or less* is considered a critical criterion for patients who deserve further evaluation as potential transplant recipients. In addition, sufficient debility to result in a New York Heart Association class III or IV status is a general indicator of a potential transplant candidate. As physical rehabilitation is an important component of post-transplant therapy, it is important that potential recipients be able to participate in such a *rehabilitation program*. Most patients with parenchymal diseases will engage in a preoperative rehabilitation program, while patients with pulmonary vascular disease may limit their participation, due to prohibitive risk, until after the transplant procedure. In addition, an appropriate psychological and emotional context can be promoted by regular preoperative participation in a patient support group.

Table 25.3. Laboratory Evaluation for Lung Transplantation Candidate

Chemistry:	Electrolytes: Na, K, Cl, CO_2, osmolality, uric acid, amylase, LDH, CPK
Renal function:	BUN, creatinine, urinalysis, creatinine clearance
Liver function:	Total protein, albumin, bilirubin (total, direct), globulin, alkaline phosphatase, SGOT
Hematology:	Complete blood count with differential, platelet count, PT, PTT, ESR
Endocrine:	TSH, LH, FSH, PTH, vitamin D, testosterone (males), estradiol (females), glucose, triglycerides, cholesterol, HDL/LDL, Ca, Phos, Mg
Pulmonary:	Pulmonary function tests (spirometry, lung volumes, DL_{co})
	Measurement of gas exchange at rest and with exercise
	Cardiopulmonary exercise study with first-pass radionuclide angiography (if available)
	Six minute walk test
Radiology:	Chest radiograph (PA, lateral), high-resolution chest CT scan, quantitative $\dot{V}/Q$ scan, quantitative bone density, abdominal ultrasonography, sinus CT[a]
Cardiology:	ECG, echocardiogram with pulse Doppler imaging (and contrast study)[b]
	Right heart catheterization
	Left heart catheterization[c]
Infectious disease:	Sputum (Gram stain, C + S, fungal smear and culture, AFB smear and culture) serology for cytomegalovirus; hepatitis B (antigen/antibody); hepatitis C; herpes; varicella, EBV; HIV; toxoplasma; serologic test for syphilis; PPD, mumps, *Candida* skin tests
Immunology:	ABO blood type and cross-match, MHC typing, HLA sensitization (PRA screen)

[a] Septic lung disease.
[b] Patients with pulmonary hypertension.
[c] If >59 years of age, coronary artery disease or LVEF <45%, or other risk factors present.

Participation in a rehabilitation program permits the transplant candidate to undergo repeated assessment of a six-minute walk test (6MWT). The test has been identified in a retrospective analysis to have a high sensitivity and negative predictive value for death in a variety of pulmonary disorders, including emphysema, idiopathic pulmonary fibrosis, primary pulmonary hypertension, Eisenmenger's syndrome, and cystic fibrosis (17). When the test is administered in a standardized fashion, there is a reasonable correlation of distance ambulated during the 6MWT to maximum oxygen consumption ($\dot{V}o_2$ max) obtained during maximal cycle ergometry exercise testing with respiratory gas analysis (18). Such information is valuable when assessing patient response to intervention if respiratory gas analysis is unavailable or impractical. For the transplant candidate, most centers consider a distance ambulated of 100 to 1500 feet to be in an acceptable range. Patients who are unable to walk 100 feet during the 6MWT represent a high risk for a negative outcome after transplant. Patients capable of walking a distance greater than 1500 feet during the 6MWT should be scrutinized carefully for the need to undergo transplantation, in light of their underlying disease and clinical history.

Table 25.4. Recurrence Rate of Preexisting Malignancy by Tumor Type

Low (0–10%)	Intermediate (11–25%)	High (≥26%)
Incidental	Body of uterus	Bladder
Testicular	Wilm's	Sarcomas
Cervix	Colon	Melanoma
Thyroid	Prostate	Symptomatic renal
Lymphoma	Breast	Skin
		Myeloma

Contraindications

Absolute contraindications to lung transplantation are listed in Table 25.2. *Hepatic cirrhosis* is to be distinguished from reversible hepatic dysfunction due to right heart failure, which improves following lung transplantation. In exceptional circumstances, combined liver and lung transplantation may be contemplated, although the risks of such a procedure are likely to be prohibitive.

The problem of malignancy in transplantation is reviewed in depth elsewhere in this text (see Chapter 37). In considering the candidate for lung transplantation, an *active malignancy* precluding long-term survival is an absolute contraindication. The rationale is to reserve transplants for patients with a relatively favorable long-term prognosis. How to apply this rule to patients with a history of preexisting cancer is less clear. Theoretically, either a recurrence of the cancer, as part of its natural history, or its re-emergence under immunosuppression could limit life expectancy. Scientific data regarding this issue in lung transplant recipients, however, are lacking. The policy of lung transplant centers, therefore, depends upon a review of the experience in other solid organ transplants.

Penn examined the effect of immunosuppression on preexisting cancers in a large cohort of renal transplant patients (19). A decrease in the rate of recurrence accompanied an increase in the interval between treatment of the tumor and transplantation. Approximately 53% of tumor recurrences occurred in patients who had been treated within 0 to 24 months prior to transplantation, and only 13% occurred if a period of greater than 60 months had elapsed prior to transplantation. An in-depth analysis revealed certain tumor types to have a "low" recurrence rate (0% to 10%), in contrast to those with an "intermediate" rate (11% to 25%), or those with a "high" recurrence rate (26%) (Table 25.4). Another favorable prognostic factor was localized disease. Thus, it is important to consider both the natural history of the tumor and the limits to its detection clinically. A two-year waiting period between treatment of the cancer and transplantation is justified for most tumors. A waiting period beyond two years between tumor therapy and transplantation is reasonable in cases of malignant melanoma or breast or colorectal carcinoma. *Active use of tobacco products* or *illicit drugs* or *alcohol abuse* while awaiting transplantation also excludes candidates.

A host of additional factors qualify as relative contraindications to lung transplantation. The *age of the recipient* may be an important determinant of transplant outcome. Both US and international registry data show slightly lower survival rates for recipients 60 to 65 years old, compared to younger adults. Presumably, subclinical organ dysfunction associated with aging may increase the potential for postoperative complications. As the latter factor is variable among individual patients, a "physiologic age" rather than a strict chronologic criterion is appropriate. The type of planned transplant procedure also influences the impact of age as a contraindication. For example, isolated single lung transplantation is probably more suitable for older patients due to its lower operative risk. Typical guidelines for age have been less than 50 to 55 years old for heart–lung transplantation, less than 55 to 60 years old for bilateral lung transplantation, and less than 60 to 65 years for single lung transplantation.

Other contraindications include evidence of *psychosocial instability* that would preclude compliance with the necessary post-transplant regimens. *Obesity* or *cachexia* can increase the risk for perioperative morbidity, as may the chronic use of high doses of *steroid therapy* (e.g., more than 20 mg prednisone per day). Other factors such as previous cardiothoracic surgery and previous medical conditions such as diabetes mellitus, hypertension, and osteoporosis also need to be considered individually.

Respiratory failure requiring *mechanical ventilation* prior to transplantation also increases the likelihood of complications. Most centers will not consider a new patient for evaluation who is completely ventilator dependent or who has acutely deteriorated and has recently become ventilator dependent. While success has been reported, patients who are ventilator dependent have a much higher mortality rate after transplantation (20). However, patients who have chronic need for partial ventilatory assistance or patients who have been accepted as transplant candidates and require ventilation for progression of their native disease may still be considered recipients for a limited period of time. The ability to remain ambulatory is considered quite important. Prolonged mechanical ventilation results in colonization of the lower respiratory tract with significant microbiologic pathogens and a degree of deconditioning and protein wasting that enhances perioperative morbidity in these patients. Noninvasive positive pressure ventilation (NPPV), however, is an acceptable treatment that may enable a patient with end-stage lung disease to remain a viable transplant candidate. It may even be combined with a conditioning program to permit preoperative rehabilitation.

Chronic renal disease may affect eligibility for lung transplantation. All immunosuppressive regimens have some element of renal insufficiency as a complication of therapy, as do many of the antimicrobial agents required for the management of these patients. As with irreversible hepatic dysfunction, combined renal and lung transplantation may be considered, but the potential risks of the procedure, particularly in the face of a shortage of donor lungs, requires careful consideration. In most cases, severe preexisting renal insufficiency is a contraindication for lung transplantation.

Severe *peripheral vascular disease* may be a factor in selecting candidates because of the occasional need for cardiopulmonary support in the perioperative period by either partial cardiopulmonary bypass (CPB) or extra-corporeal membrane oxygenation (ECMO) via the femoral or subclavian routes. Peripheral vascular disease (PVD) is often associated with coronary or aortic disease that may greatly increase the morbidity and mortality of the lung transplant procedure. Finally, transplantation in patients with gangrenous changes in the extremities due to PVD is contraindicated because of the potential for systemic spread of the infectious process with immunosuppression.

Many candidates for lung transplantation are also at risk for *coronary artery disease (CAD).* The incidence of hemodynamically important but clinically unsuspected CAD is low in candidates without symptoms, despite the frequent occurrence of conventional coronary risk factors (21,22). Nonetheless, there is general consensus among transplant centers that the detection of CAD, as part of the pretransplant evaluation, is important in order to stratify risk as well as to develop strategies to overcome the problem. In some cases, noninvasive pharmacologic stress tests may suffice. Conventional exercise stress testing is typically not satisfactory due to the inability of transplant candidates to exercise adequately. Consequently, coronary angiography is obtained in many cases. Angiography is most likely to detect unsuspected CAD in patients with multiple coronary risk factors. Demonstration of non–life-threatening anatomy may permit listing of a subgroup of patients that might unnecessarily be excluded from transplant consideration.

Postoperatively, patients require an aggressive rehabilitation program to complete their immediate recovery and achieve their maximum functional capacity. Severe preexisting *osteoporosis* or severe *chest wall deformity* may limit these efforts due to difficulties with bone fractures, pain management, and ambulatory status. Careful consideration of such patients prior to transplantation is required. In addition, chronic steroid and cyclosporine immunosuppressive therapy will exacerbate the complications of prior osteoporosis. Close attention to bone density and calcium homeostasis (discussed in Chapter 31) is required postoperatively in all lung transplant patients.

Infectious diseases have a profound effect on the morbidity and mortality of lung transplantation (23). Colonization of the respiratory tract with potential pathogens in patients with end-stage pulmonary diseases requires careful assessment of anatomic changes in the airways and determination of antimicrobial susceptibility. Significant anatomic abnormalities that preclude mechanical drainage of secretions in either the upper or lower respiratory tract should be dealt with preoperatively (e.g., the drainage of chronic sinusitis in patients with cystic fibrosis) or at the time of the transplantation (e.g., removal of the lung containing a focal area of bronchiectasis). Most bacterial flora in transplant candidates will have a pattern of antibiotic sensitivity that can be identified preoperatively to define an effective perioperative antibiotic regimen. *Buckholderia (Pseudomonas) cepaciae*, a pathogen found in approximately 15% of patients with cystic fibrosis, or other pathogens that are highly resistant to antimicrobials are a relative contraindication to transplantation unless a suitable pattern of antibiotic sensitivity can be devised prior to transplantation (see below).

Aspergillus fumigatus and other *Aspergillus* species are also common pathogens in the sputum of patients with septic lung disease or COPD. Any history of *Aspergillus* in the sputum of a potential transplant recipient will require prophylactic perioperative therapy with amphotericin B to eliminate the potential for an invasive infection postoperatively.

Viral diseases in a potential lung transplant recipient can also have a major impact on the outcome of transplantation. Active *hepatitis B* or *C* in the lung transplant candidate increases both early and late mortality because of the effect of hepatic dysfunction on perioperative complications and the accelerated progression of these diseases in patients requiring chronic immunosuppression. Cytomegalovirus (CMV), a DNA-type virus that is incorporated into the host genome, can cause both a systemic illness and a pneumonitis in immunosuppressed patients. The serologic CMV status of the recipient is therefore an important determination to make prior to transplantation. While some centers prefer to match donor and recipient CMV status to minimize perioperative complications, the availability of ganciclovir therapy typically controls CMV disease even in seronegative recipients of seropositive organs (24). Some strains of CMV are resistant to ganciclovir, however, making it mandatory to continue surveillance for CMV based on antigenemia assays and transbronchial lung biopsy (23,25) (see Chapter 36).

Immunologic study of potential transplant candidates includes determination of ABO and major histocompatibility complex (MHC) status. Most patients are currently matched with ABO-identical donors. MHC status is assessed, primarily for use in studies of postoperative outcome such as the effect of HLA-DR mismatching or donor–recipient microchimerism on chronic rejection. Screening for sensitization to HLA antigens is also done at some centers (see Chapter 4). Pregnancy, blood transfusion, or prior transplantation can lead to HLA sensitization. Potential recipients with a PRA (panel of reactive antibodies) response of greater than 15% may warrant a direct lymphocytotoxic crossmatch with any potential donor prior to transplantation.

The importance of performing lymphocytotoxic crossmatch in lung transplant candidates with high PRA is underscored by the report by Frost et al (26) of hyperacute rejection following transplantation. The clinical diagnosis was corroborated by a positive donor-antigen–specific lymphocytotoxic crossmatch, and demonstrated histopathologic, immunofluorescent, and electron microscopic features consistent with hyperacute rejection, as described in other organs (see Chapter 2). Features of diffuse alveolar damage and neutrophilic infiltrates, as well as endothelial and epithelial damage, with IgG-fluorescent staining within alveolar spaces and septae were demonstrated. This likely represents a relatively uncommon event, as Saint-Martin et al (27) were unable to demonstrate humoral rejection in the lung in a prospective study of 55 recipients. Gammie et al (28) also concluded that humoral sensitization is uncommon in the lung transplantation population. In their study, they examined the records of 247 patients who underwent single or double lung transplantation and were unable to find an effect of modestly elevated PRA on survival or the development of acute rejection or bronchiolitis obliterans.

The influence of HLA matching on lung transplantation outcome has been the subject of several reports (29–31). Sundaresan et al (30) found that HLA-A locus mismatches and development of antibodies to HLA after lung transplantation correlate with the development of the bronchiolitis syndrome. Schulman et al (31) reported that mismatches at the HLA-DR and HLA-B loci are factors associated with early acute rejection after transplantation. These investigators concluded that the findings have implications for immunosuppressive protocols.

Table 25.5. Disease-Specific Indications for Adult Lung Transplantation

Disease	Indications
Obstructive Lung Disease	
Chronic obstructive pulmonary disease Alpha-1-antitrypsin deficiency	Postbronchodilator FEV_1 <25% predicted, and/or Pa_{CO_2} ≥55 mm Hg, and/or elevated pulmonary artery pressures with progressive deterioration (e.g., cor pulmonale)
Restrictive Lung Disease	
Idiopathic pulmonary fibrosis Other interstitial lung disease	Symptomatic progressive disease unresponsive to medical therapy Bronchodilator FVC <60% to 70% predicted Resting hypoxia (Pa_{O_2} <55 mm Hg) Hypercarbia (Pa_{CO_2} ≥45 mm Hg) Secondary pulmonary artery hypertension
Septic Lung Disease	
Cystic fibrosis Bronchiectasis	Postbronchodilator FEV_1 <30% predicted FVC ≤40% predicted resting hypoxia (Pa_{O_2} <55 mm Hg, room air) Hypercarbia (Pa_{CO_2} ≥45 mm Hg) Declining clinical course Bilateral bronchiectasis Increasing resistance of bacterial organisms
Pulmonary Vascular Disease	Symptomatic progressive disease despite optimal medical and/or surgical treatment, leaving the patient in NYHA III or IV

SPECIFIC DISEASE STATES: OBSTRUCTIVE LUNG DISEASE

The rate of progression of the specific disease state is an important factor in the assessment of potential transplant recipients. Disease-specific indications for adult lung transplantation are outlined in Table 25.5. The most common indication for lung transplantation is *obstructive lung disease.* COPD accounts for 30% of all lung transplants, with emphysema due to alpha-1-antitrypsin deficiency accounting for approximately 15% of all lung transplants. Patients with these diseases, demonstrating chronic airway obstruction on pulmonary function tests, tend to remain relatively stable for long periods of time.

COPD is most often associated with cigarette smoking and is estimated to affect at least 15 million Americans. It is the fifth leading cause of death in the United States. The death rate has risen by 22% in the past decade, and the mortality rate 10 years after diagnosis is greater than 50%. The conventional approach to patients with this disorder has emphasized the goal of minimizing the progression of COPD.

Comprehensive management programs have been based upon the need to educate patients, to retard the progression of airflow limitation, to correct secondary physiologic alterations, and to optimize functional capabilities (32). Attempts at retarding the progression of airflow limitation depend upon elimination or avoidance of risk factors. These include cigarette smoke, other environmental and behavioral factors such as air pollution, occupational exposures to particulate dusts, intravenous drug abuse, or talcosis, treatment of constitutional and genetic factors such as protease-inhibitor deficiency and bronchial hyperreactivity. A program designed to minimize airflow limitation depends upon efforts to reduce or eliminate secretions, the judicious use of bronchodilators, sympathomimetic agents, anticholinergic agents, theophylline, and corticosteroids. Correction of secondary physiologic alterations involves the use of supplemental oxygen therapy and recognition and treatment of right-sided cardiac dysfunction. Efforts to treat chronic hypercapnea focus on reducing the work of breathing by decreasing secretions and bronchoconstriction and correcting metabolic abnormalities. Ventilatory-assist devices may be beneficial.

The goals of a comprehensive pulmonary rehabilitation program are primarily to improve the patient's functional capability and quality of life, as well as to fill social, emotional, and vocational needs. The program is dependent thus on education, medical care, exercise conditioning, muscle training, and attention to nutritional and psychosocial needs.

Despite the importance of the medical therapy for COPD, the typical course pursues a gradual but relentless decline over many years. The dyspnea of patients worsens with the progression of their underlying disease; typically dyspnea limits patient's activity leading to a vicious cycle of increasing inactivity that in turn aggravates the debilitating effects of this condition. Thus, many patients remain extraordinarily limited in terms of activities of daily living.

In addition to the marked functional impairment suffered by patients with COPD, the disease results in a substantial reduction in life expectancy. Over the years, attempts have been made to assess which factors relate to survival of patients with COPD. These are listed in Table 25.6. The assessment of patients with COPD may be confounded by their treatment with oxygen therapy, which improves survival in those who have significant hypoxemia. There is thus a very wide variability in survival of individual patients whose initial findings appear to be similar (33–35).

Recognition of the severe disability and reduced life expectancy due to emphysema has prompted over the years a number of surgical interventions (36). The management surgically of emphysema has comprised a variety of procedures including costochondrectomy and transverse sternotomy; thoracoplasty and phrenic nerve paralysis; abdominal belts/pneumoperitoneum; needle aspiration of

Table 25.6. Factors Relating to Survival in COPD

Positive[a]	Negative[b]
FEV_1	Age
PaO_2	Decrease in FEV_1 on serial testing
Reversibility of airflow	Resting heart rate
Obstruction following inhaled bronchodilator	$PaCO_2$
Exercise capacity	Pulmonary artery pressure/cor pulmonale
Diffusing capacity for carbon monoxide	Total lung capacity
Vital capacity	Perceived physical disabilities dyspnea
	Continued smoking
	Malnutrition/weight loss
	Alpha-1-antitrypsin deficiency

[a] The higher the value or presence of the factor, the better the survival.
[b] The higher the value or presence of the factor, the poorer the survival.

bullae often with injection of irritant; closed thoracotomy and drainage of bullae; excision of bullae by plication, wedge, lobectomy, or pneumonectomy; parietal pleurectomy or poudrage; resection of peripheral lung tissue; reinforcement of membranous portions of the trachea and main bronchi; conventional tracheostomy, tracheal ventilation or fenestration; resection of the carotid body; or autonomic denervation procedures. Many of these procedures share the goal of reducing airflow obstruction or restoring the normal curvature of the diaphragm from its flattened position in the hyperinflated state. Other operations were devised primarily to increase the blood supply to the lung by stimulating collateral circulation. The latter operations arose from the mistaken assumption that emphysema was caused by obliterative changes within bronchial arteries.

VOLUME REDUCTION SURGERY

Brantigan proposed multiple random wedge resections of peripheral lung tissue to increase lung tension and to restore circumferential traction upon both small airways and blood vessels (37). This approach to the restoration of lung tension was considered to be a valid idea, particularly as the primary benefit derived from resection of bullae. Nonetheless the approach was criticized on the basis that it was, according to Gaensler, "difficult to believe that a disease characterized by diffuse loss of lung parenchyma could be effectively treated by resection of functioning lung."

The contrary point of view in fact was pointed out a number of years ago by Gaensler (36), who indicated that pulmonary resection performed for other reasons in patients with emphysema did not cause improvement of function, but rather led to a greater loss of function than that observed following similar resection in patients whose lungs were normal. In addition, he emphasized that while hyperinflation of a normal lung following resection did not lead to parenchymal disruption, further inflation of an already emphysematous lung caused accelerated lung disruption. Lacking objective data concerning improvement and having an unacceptably high rate of complications and mortality, the concept of volume reduction surgery (VRS) thus fell out of favor for a number of years.

The most recent and dramatic surgical treatment for COPD has been the demonstrated feasibility of isolated lung transplantation. In the last decade, a growing number of individuals with COPD have been successfully transplanted and have enjoyed excellent functional results. Consequently the number of patients being referred has continued to grow, while the number of suitable donor lungs has failed to keep pace. As a result, waiting lists for transplantation have grown longer and many patients are unable to receive this therapy.

As an alternative to lung transplantation, Cooper and colleagues revived Brantigan's work and demonstrated the feasibility of VRS or bilateral pneumonoplasty as effective treatment for selected individuals with severe COPD (38).

Based upon preliminary reports, this procedure has gained early enthusiasm but remains controversial. Typically, approximately 20% to 30% of the lung volume is removed surgically through a median sternotomy approach. The most diseased portion of the lung is resected by employing a stapler, sheathed in bovine pericardium, which serves to buttress the lung resection line and to minimize air leaks.

Early experience with VRS suggests that patients may experience a decreased sense of dyspnea, improved exercise tolerance, and generalized improvement in quality of life. Lung function studies have also shown objective improvement (39–45). The mechanism by which VRS results in these changes is unknown at this time. Possibilities include enhancement in pulmonary mechanics, improvement in gas exchange with increased effective elastic recoil of the lung (46), and/or changes in cardiopulmonary interactions. Presumably, as the diaphragm resumes its normal, dome-shaped configuration, the musculoskeletal components of the respiratory system become more efficient. It is likely that ventilation–perfusion relationships improve as well, promoting better gas exchange.

Despite these encouraging results, a number of questions remain unanswered. At the current time, selection criteria are not settled and it is not possible to gauge which patients are most likely to benefit from this therapy. Furthermore, neither the degree of benefit nor its duration can be predicted with accuracy. What effect, if any, of the procedure on the progression of the underlying emphysema is also unknown (47,48).

For many patients who suffer debilitating end-stage COPD, VRS may serve as a "bridge" to lung transplantation. For others, depending upon their course and other medical factors, this palliative treatment may become a definitive procedure. Patients need to be aware, however, that the procedure entails all the risks associated with general thoracic surgery including the risk of persistent air leak, infection, bleeding, and potentially the need for prolonged ventilatory assistance.

Although many patients may be interested in the possibility of lung reduction surgery, only a minority may turn out to be good candidates. Proposed exclusion criteria are listed in Table 25.7. A number of problems may also be considered to be relative contraindications to this procedure: high dosage steroid therapy, active wheezing or asthma, and the presence of pulmonary hypertension. Patients who may be considered to be appropriate candidates for VRS will usually have difficulty carrying out activities of daily living and will typically meet criteria listed in Table 25.8.

At the present time, evidence on chest computerized tomography (CT) of a heterogeneous pattern of emphysema is considered to be more favorable than the finding of homogeneous distribution of disease. Individuals with the most severe form of pulmonary compromise—forced expiratory volume in 1 second (FEV_1) less than 20% of that predicted or arterial P_{CO_2} greater than 55 mm Hg—represent high-risk patients whose candidacy for VRS needs to be scrutinized cautiously (45). As more experience with VRS accumulates, it is likely that selection criteria will be refined. An assessment of the impact of this therapy on patients' functional activity and on survival will also emerge (49).

In 1995, in the United States, the Health Care Financing Agency (HCFA) issued a noncoverage policy for VRS operations. In an attempt to settle the debate concerning the value of VRS, a large scale, multicenter, prospective randomized trial was set up to study the effects of VRS and pulmonary rehabilitation.

At the time of the funding withdrawal by HCFA, the St. Louis Group led by Dr. J. D. Cooper had evaluated and approved 24 patients who met their candidacy criteria for VRS. An additional 6 Medicare patients were evaluated and approved over the subsequent 11 months. Of this total of 30 patients, 8 patients chose to proceed with the operation without Medicare funding.

The remaining 22 Medicare patients selected for but denied VRS because of the Medicare support withdrawal formed the basis of a retrospective study, in which this group of patients was evaluated against 65 contemporaneous and comparable volume reduction recipients (50). Baseline physiologic characteristics were compared and longitudinal measures of pulmonary function were followed for 24 months. The authors reported that the patients denied the operation were similar to volume reduction recipients at all baseline measurements. The patients who were denied the VRS experienced a progressive worsening of function, whereas volume reduction patients experienced sustained improvements. The authors concluded that for carefully selected patients (i.e., those who had not been previously excluded from the operation because of obesity, lack of

Table 25.7. Exclusion Criteria for VRS

Currently smoking
Associated serious disorder other than the lung (such as heart disease, liver disease, kidney disease)
Active malignancy
Active infection
Inability to participate in preoperative testing and postoperative evaluation
Inability to participate in pre- and postoperative pulmonary rehabilitation program

Table 25.8. Inclusion Criteria for VRS

Long-standing history of progressive emphysema
No smoking in the past year
Age <75 years old
Prednisone <10 mg per day for 30 days prior to surgery
Otherwise in good health
Able and willing to participate in pulmonary rehabilitation
Able to undergo evaluation process prior to and following volume reduction surgery

motivation, active coronary disease, cigarette addiction, or multiple systemic diseases) the operation can be considered safe. They also contend that VRS improves survival in comparison to unselected historical controls with severe chronic lung disease.

Therapy with VRS, to date, has resulted in a substantial number of patients being removed from the transplant list and a smaller fraction bridged to transplantation (51–53). Indeed, one center has recently reported a reduced percentage of patients with a diagnosis of COPD on transplant waiting lists, demonstrating a substantial effect of reduction pneumoplasty on the timing and selection of patients for transplant (52). Some authors have used innovative combinations of volume reduction and single lung transplant to improve functional outcome (55).

Recent evidence suggests that single lung transplantation for COPD carries the same survival advantage as bilateral transplantation, despite superior improvements in function (oxygenation and exercise tolerance) after the latter procedure. There is, however, a trend toward improved late survival with bilateral transplant, possibly due to the presence of more pulmonary reserve following the onset of obliterative bronchiolitis (55). The use of larger donor allografts in transplants for COPD does not alter outcome in single lung transplantation, possibly because chronic hyperinflation accommodates larger donor organs (56), and it has been proposed that transplanting larger donor lungs should shorten waiting periods for single lung transplants. Alternatively, surgical sculpting of larger donor organs to fit a recipient thorax remains a viable option. Although the precise role for lung volume reduction surgery remains to be defined, the combined use of this new modality and the suggestion of a larger donor pool for single lung transplants may have a major impact on lung transplantation over the ensuing years. In addition, Anderson et al have proposed that unilateral VRS may be a desirable strategy in single lung transplant recipients who exhibit functional deterioration due to emphysema (57).

Despite comprehensive medical management and the option of VRS, the progressive decline experienced by some patients with COPD makes lung transplantation the most viable alternative. For these individuals, the reduction in quality of life and life expectancy justify the risk of transplantation. As with many disorders, determining the optimal timing of transplantation remains a challenge. A knowledge of the multiple factors that influence prognosis is helpful (see Table 25.6).

RESTRICTIVE LUNG DISEASES

Restrictive lung diseases (RLD) are the indication for lung transplantation in 20% of patients. The most common etiology is *idiopathic pulmonary fibrosis (IPF)*, which accounts for 15% of lung transplants, while a variety of interstitial lung diseases with mixed physiologic characteristics account for the remainder.

The interstitial lung diseases (ILDs) are a large group of heterogeneous disorders in which the major alterations occur within the alveolar supporting tissues. They are characterized by alveolitis with accumulation of various types of inflammatory and immune effector cells within the alveolar structures and air spaces, and by fibrosis with derangement and localized accumulation of interstitial collagen. In many of these disorders, airways and pulmonary arteries and veins may also be involved with similar processes (58).

In all, there are more than 150 interstitial diseases, defined by various clinical syndromes and morphologic criteria. Progressive alterations in lung parenchyma occur in all. The type of change, however, is varied. In pneumoconioses, for example, proliferative changes lead to pulmonary fibrosis; in sarcoidosis, on the other hand, granuloma are found. In still other disorders, there is a combination of fibrotic and granulomatous findings. For 25% to 30% of interstitial disorders, the causes are known; but for others the etiology is obscure. Regardless of cause, there is likely some form of initial injury to the interstitium. As a result of the injury, there is an alteration in lung cell types. This initial phase is referred to as an *acute alveolitis* and is marked by an accumulation of inflammatory and immune effector cells. Depending on a number of modulating factors, the sequence of pathogenetic events includes resolution or progression to a chronic alveolitis and alveolar injury, with subsequent derangement in interstitial collagen. As the disease progresses, many alveoli are replaced by fibrous tissue, airways become distorted and dilated, and cystic lesions develop. Thus, unchecked, these events lead to "end-stage lung." A useful classification of interstitial lung disease is presented in Table 25.9.

Pulmonary symptoms of special importance include dyspnea, nonproductive cough, and frequent constitutional symptoms (fever, arthralgia, weight loss, lassitude). Apart from the conventional past and family history, the most important aspect concerns environmental (occupational and recreational) review. This should include a summary of hobbies, recreational activities, and geographic locations, in addition to review of all materials, tools, and intermediary compounds used on the job.

Physical findings are generally nonspecific. Tachypnea is most consistent, even when dyspnea at rest is not present. Rales may be heard early. Exercise cyanosis, digital clubbing, and evidence of cor pulmonale, with or without signs of right heart failure, may occur. Patients with systemic diseases or primary cardiac problems may display the findings typical for the specific disorder.

The classic physiologic alterations in progressive, late interstitial disease are restrictive. There is a decrease in lung volumes, including vital capacity. There is reduction in the functional residual capacity (FRC), which is a better indicator of disease severity than total lung capacity (TLC). The TLC is frequently reduced more than the residual volume, such that the ratio of residual volume to total lung capacity is increased. In some instances, however, these disorders produce prominent obstructive airways defects (chronic

Table 25.9. Classification of Interstitial Lung Disease

- A. Interstitial Lung Disease of Known Etiology
  - 1. Occupational and environmental inhalants
    - a. Inorganic dusts
      Silica, silicates, aluminum, antimony, carbon, beryllium, mixed dusts, hard metal dusts
    - b. Organic dusts
      Chemical source: textile industry (orlon, polyester, acrylic)
      Living sources: moldy hay (micropolyspora faeni, thermoactinomyces vulgaris), humidifier, ducts (thermoactinomyces)
    - c. Gases, fumes, vapors, aerosols
      Gas: iatrogenic (O_2), smelting (SO_2), accidents (chlorine gas)
      Fumes: welding, foundry work, smelting, galvanizing (oxides of zinc, copper)
      Vapor: accident (mercury), rubber industry (thermosetting resins), production of polyurethane, synthetic rubber, adhesives, paints (toluene)
  - 2. Drugs
    - a. Chemotherapeutic, busulfan, bleomycin, cyclophosphamide, methotrexate
    - b. Antibiotics, nitrofurantoin, sulfonamides, penicillin
    - c. Others: gold salts, diphenylhydantion
  - 3. Poisons (paraquat)
  - 4. Radiation
  - 5. Infectious agents (schistosomiasis)
  - 6. Systemic illnesses (uremia, chronic pulmonary edema)
- B. Interstitial Lung Disease of Unknown Etiology
  - 1. Granulomatous disease
    - a. Sarcoidosis
    - b. Eosinophilic granuloma
  - 2. Idiopathic pulmonary fibrosis
  - 3. Chronic interstitial disease associated with collagen vascular disease (R.A.; PSS; SLE: polymyositis/dermatomyositis; Sjögren's; overlap)
  - 4. Lymphangioleiomyomatosis/tuberous sclerosis
  - 5. Wegener's granulomatosis
  - 6. Lymphocytic infiltrative disorders
  - 7. Pulmonary vasculitides
  - 8. Goodpasture's syndrome
  - 9. Idiopathic pulmonary hemosiderosis
  - 10. Inherited disorders

hypersensitivity pneumonitis, late sarcoidosis, eosinophilic granuloma, beryllium disease, and certain inherited diseases). Small airways dysfunction also may occasionally be a presenting feature. Nonetheless, measurements of airflow in interstitial lung disease generally are normal. Peak flow rates are preserved usually until late in the disease. Additional abnormalities secondary to the interstitial process include a loss of diffusing capacity and mild resting hypoxemia that worsens with exercise. The ratio of arterial PaO_2 to oxygen consumption during exercise may correlate with the presence of interstitial pneumonitis and/or fibrosis. A decrease in compliance also correlates with the degree of fibrosis in lung biopsy specimens. Dead space ventilation is increased and may actually increase further during exercise. Typically, there is an element of hyperventilation early in the course, although with disease progression, hypercapnea results, particularly with exercise. As a result of these alterations, patients with interstitial lung disease may display a distinctive breathing pattern characterized by rapid frequency and small tidal volumes, with increased work.

Testing of pulmonary function is not specific for the type of change within the diseased lung. Pulmonary function tests do indicate overall abnormalities within the lung, that is, those patients with the most functional impairment have the most histologic changes. Thus, for a given patient, worsening pulmonary function probably means worsening disease. Normal lung test results do not necessarily mean, however, that a patient has inactive disease. While patients with normal pulmonary function rarely have fibrosis, they may have significant alveolitis.

Knowledge of lung function abnormalities assists in the determining of pulmonary disability (59). In order to evaluate patients for disability because of pulmonary disease, criteria have been established for severe impairment. Even though mild degrees of impairment may be important, severe impairment alone precludes gainful employment. Whereas clinical and roentgenographic criteria have been inappropriate for defining impairment, physiologic measurements have been useful. Severe impairment in interstitial lung disease is generally seen in patients with a forced vital capacity 50% of predicted and a single-breath diffusing capacity of 40% of predicted. When a discrepancy between subjective symptoms, clinical findings, and physiologic testing exists, exercise testing may be useful.

Staging of disease in relation to therapy is not readily accomplished by conventional techniques. The chest x-ray is abnormal in most individuals at the time of presentation of their illness; but in one large series, about 10% of the patients had normal chest x-rays despite diagnostic lung biopsies. With the exception of hilar or mediastinal adenopathy in sarcoidosis, there is usually little to point to a specific diagnosis. Even in this disease, however, with its well-known radiographic stages, correlation between pulmonary function and roentgenographic evidence of disease is poor. The most reliable x-ray sign that alveolar fibrosis has occurred is the presence of "honeycombing," characterized by the appearance of clusters of irregular, rounded, or oval cysts, 10 mm or less in diameter.

Apart from this finding, the chest x-ray cannot stage the activity of the disease process, nor can it assess functional defects. Even when patients respond to therapy, the chest x-ray may not improve. The major usefulness of the chest x-ray in interstitial lung disease is to provide a useful anatomic guide to lung involvement.

Computerized tomography (CT) scans have been compared with pathologic determinants in pulmonary fibrosis. This is based upon the theory that intra-alveolar and interstitial cellularity would result in opacification of air spaces on CT scans. CT, especially high-resolution, thin-section CT, may aid in 1) differentiating interstitial lung disease (especially silicosis, sarcoidosis, lymphangitic carcinomatosis), 2) detecting disease (especially in patients with normal or minimally changed chest x-rays), and 3) determining localization and extent of disease (60).

In idiopathic pulmonary fibrosis, some investigators have monitored circulating levels of immune complexes. These have been reported in the blood of most patients with early stages of the process but are uncommon in individuals with more fibrotic disease. Also described in these patients are increased incidence of rheumatoid factor, autoantibodies, and antinuclear antibodies. In sarcoidosis, measurements of serum lysozyme or angiotensin converting enzyme (ACE) have been used to monitor disease activity. Of these tests, measurement of ACE levels appears to have had the widest clinical acceptance and usefulness. Nonetheless, the merit of this test comes from placing it into context with other parameters.

Because ^{67}Ga-citrate localizes in sites of inflammation, it may be useful as a scanning agent to evaluate the alveolitis of some of the interstitial disorders. This radionuclide has been used in staging idiopathic pulmonary fibrosis and sarcoidosis. In the latter condition, ^{67}Ga may also localize in nodes, lacrimal and parotid glands, as well as in lung parenchyma. The accumulation of ^{67}Ga in the lungs of patients with interstitial lung disease correlates with morphologic features of lung biopsy and analysis of lung lavage.

Quantitative analysis of inflammatory cells in lung lavage may be valuable in the diagnosis and in the study of pathogenesis of interstitial disease. In this method, small aliquots of sterile saline are instilled through a flexible fiberoptic bronchoscope that has been inserted by conventional technique into a peripheral airway; the lavage fluid, containing cells, is recovered by suction and analyzed. Diagnostically, it can be specific only in histiocytosis x or alveolar proteinosis. Otherwise, the data are nonspecific. Frequently, however, the results of cellular analysis of lung lavage allow classification of interstitial diseases into lymphocyte-predominant and polymorphonuclear cell-predominant forms of alveolitis.

The value of serial lavages in following the natural history of both treated and untreated interstitial disorders remains debatable. Quantification of lymphocytes in lung lavage is a more sensitive indicator than serum ACE level of active pulmonary sarcoidosis. In idiopathic pulmonary fibrosis, in the absence of increased lymphocytes, elevated lavage eosinophils or neutrophils appear associated with failure to respond. Increased lavage lymphocytes also correlates with a hypercellular biopsy. The response to corticosteroids may relate in part to a relative increase in glucocortocoid receptors on lavage cells in these patients. However, the promise of lavage as a clinically useful prognostic indicator remains largely unfulfilled.

In general, a more cellular lung biopsy is associated with a better prognosis than a lung biopsy in which inflammatory cells are scanty and in which there is gross destruction of architecture and extensive fibrotic scarring. This pattern of end-stage fibrosis is presumably untreatable by any medical method. In developing treatment strategies, it is thus important to distinguish between reversible and irreversible changes. Alveolitis is a potentially reversible lesion, whereas the fibrosis stage represents a permanent change, with alveolar capillary units lost forever (61).

In practice, two problems arise in staging of disease in relation to therapy. First, biopsy specimens are frequently not representative of the whole lung because the distribution and activity of the disease varies from one part of the lung to another. Second, a large number of biopsy specimens show a mixed pattern of fibrosis and inflammation and do not fall into one of the two polar categories.

Principles of therapy are aimed at reducing alveolitis and preventing fibrosis (62). In interstitial diseases of known etiology, this may be accomplished by identifying the causative agent and preventing further exposure. General supportive measures include provision of adequate oxygenation and prevention of infection. In interstitial diseases of unknown etiology, corticosteroids remain the mainstay of therapy. Cytotoxic therapy with cyclophosphamide or azathioprine is an alternative for some patients. Colchicine has been helpful in some patients. In idiopathic pulmonary fibrosis, steroids are usually more successful in patients whose biopsy shows the most cellularity and least fibrosis. High initial dose (60 mg of prednisone) may prove efficacious for some individuals. An early therapeutic response in terms of improved dyspnea, assessed four to eight weeks after the start of treatment, is said to relate to better survival. The factors relating to better survival appear to be age and less radiographic abnormality. The implication of this and other studies is that if steroids are to be effective, they have to be given early in the course of the disease and at a time when symptoms and x-ray appearance may not be severe.

Patients may have a variable course of disease progression but frequently deteriorate abruptly and severely with rapidly progressive hypoxemia and pulmonary hypertension. As a result, these patients have a mortality of over 80% while awaiting transplantation, the highest for any group of lung transplant candidates (63). Because of their high mortality rate on the waiting list, patients with IPF in the United States are awarded 90 days of waiting time at the time of listing for transplantation. The very poor overall prognosis in interstitial lung disease justifies an aggressive approach. When large groups are considered, for example, in IPF, the median survival is short—about four to five years.

Criteria for IPF patients for consideration of transplantation include severe dyspnea; forced vital capacity (FVC) less than 60% to 70% of predicted and/or diffusing capacity (corrected for alveolar volume) less than 50% to 60% of predicted; resting hypoxia or hypercarbia; and pulmonary hypertension. However, a downhill clinical course despite adequate medical therapy is the best individual indication for transplantation. Similar criteria can be used for other patients with interstitial lung disease, although the additional criterion of an FEV_1 less than 30% of predicted may be useful because a component of airway obstruction is frequently present. Three other factors in patients with interstitial lung disease patients are also important. First, many of these diseases are systemic in nature, and the cumulative effects of the disease on extrapulmonary organ systems may result in a sufficient number of relative contraindications to exclude the patient from consideration for transplantation. Secondly, many patients with end-stage interstitial disease develop cor pulmonale, making a careful assessment of right-sided hemodynamics an important feature of transplant evaluation. It may be difficult, however, to link hemodynamic parameters to prognosis (64).

A number of these diseases, including desquamative interstitial pneumonitis (DIP) (65), pulmonary alveolar proteinosis (66), sarcoidosis (67), lymphangioleiomyomatosis (LAM) (68,69), giant cell pneumonitis (70), and Langerhan's cell histocytosis (71,72), have recurred in the lung graft suggesting that lung transplantation should be undertaken only in the best potential candidates. These recipients require particularly careful postoperative monitoring by a team with expertise in pulmonary medicine.

The pretransplant assessment of patients with end-stage fibrosis associated with *sarcoidosis* is similar to that of patients with IPF. Severe progressive, restrictive lung disease possibly complicated by an obstructive physiologic defect, pronounced hypoxemia often with exercise desaturation and evidence of pulmonary hypertension are all factors leading to consideration of lung transplantation in a disabled patient. Due to the systemic nature of this disorder, evidence of involvement by noncaseating granulomata in other organ systems should be sought.

Sarcoidosis most commonly presents with respiratory tract involvement; other common sites include the thoracic lymph nodes, eyes, skin, and peripheral lymph nodes. Less frequently the disease affects the gastrointestinal tract, bones or joints, central or peripheral nervous system, heart, sinuses, kidney, reproductive tract, or bone marrow. Involvement of sites other than the lung does not necessarily exclude a candidate from transplant consideration. However, it is important to determine the functional impact, particularly on liver and heart. The potential for multiorgan involvement, varied clinical presentations, and a variable natural history, including a relatively high rate of spontaneous remission, makes it difficult to prognosticate in sarcoidosis. Up to two thirds of patients have no major, long-term sequelae. However, approximately 5% to 10% will eventually die prematurely secondary to pulmonary sarcoid. The mainstay of medical therapy is corticosteroids, although a variety of other agents have been tried. These include cytotoxic agents, cyclosporine, nonsteroidal anti-inflammatory agents, ketoconazole, radiation therapy, antimalarials, and strategies directed against cytokines. The latter have included thalidomide and other inhibitors of tumor necrosis factor (73). Unfortunately, no data exist to show convincingly that any of these therapies alter the long-term outcome of patients with sarcoidosis.

The presence of *Aspergillus* in the lung of sarcoidosis patients, particularly late in the course is not uncommon. Often, the fungus is a colonizer rather than a cause of disease, but its eradication, if possible, prior to transplant appears to be desirable. Evidence of more invasive disease and/or aspergilloma is a more serious concern, as it portends possible contamination of the pleural space with fungal organisms at the time of surgery.

The presence of a systemic disease has, in some instances, been considered a contraindication to lung transplantation. Nonetheless, for end-stage pulmonary disease associated with sarcoidosis, lung transplantation offers a potentially curative therapy. Johnson et al (67) examined a small group of individuals who received lung transplants for underlying sarcoidosis and compared them with a control group of contemporaneous transplant recipients with other respiratory diseases. The analysis led them to conclude that pulmonary transplantation appears to be an efficacious therapy for end-stage sarcoidosis. However, they noted the potential for more severe acute rejection responses, especially early after transplantation. They also detected recurrent disease in the allograft, raising concerns of long-term sequelae. In a follow-up study from the same institution in 1997, Pigula et al (74) reexamined the controversy concerning transplantation for pulmonary failure resulting from systemic disease. A relatively small group of individuals with sarcoidosis were included in this study. Overall, the data showed that survival was similar whether patients underwent transplantation for systemic or isolated pulmonary disease. The authors concluded that patients with respiratory failure resulting from systemic disorders, including sarcoidosis, could undergo transplantation with an outcome comparable to that seen in patients transplanted for isolated pulmonary disease.

Several reports have confirmed that recurrent sarcoidosis may occur in the allograft of individuals undergoing isolated lung transplantation for this disorder (67,75–78). The manifestations are not generally thought to be clinically important. However, in at least one case report, the patient's symptoms and radiographic abnormalities required increased dosage of steroid therapy (79).

Other reports have concluded that carefully selected patients with end-stage lung disease related to systemic disease, such as sarcoidosis, may benefit from single lung transplantation. A consensus has emerged that patients with end-stage pulmonary sarcoidosis who have undergone lung transplantation successfully show good short-term and intermediate-term results. Judson (80) has emphasized that candidates should have exhausted medical therapy, and that causes of pulmonary dysfunction other than pulmonary sarcoidosis, such as myocardial disease, be excluded. Commenting on the potential recurrence in the allograft, this author has emphasized that important symptoms of pulmonary dysfunction are rare as a result. There is also no evidence of an increased risk of obliterative bronchiolitis or increased mortality in patients transplanted for sarcoidosis.

Yeatman et al (81), reporting on an 11-year experience at Papworth Hospital, also have concluded that lung transplantation in patients with systemic diseases, including sarcoidosis, should be considered, with each case being judged individually. Walker et al (82), in a recent report describing medium-term results of transplantation for end-stage pulmonary sarcoidosis, also have concluded that lung transplantation is a viable option for patients with end-stage pulmonary sarcoidosis. They found that the medium-term results were comparable to those of patients undergoing transplantation for other indications.

Baughman et al (83) examined a seven-year experience at the University of Cincinnati, with respect to risk factors for death from respiratory failure due to sarcoidosis in order to predict when transplantation should be considered. Patients most at risk were those with advanced fibrotic changes on chest imaging procedures and reduced vital capacity (usually <1.5 liters).

Another ILD deserving special mention regarding lung transplantation is *lymphangioleiomyomatosis (LAM)* (84). This uncommon disease typically evolves over approximately a decade to end-stage pulmonary disease, characterized by an obstructive physiologic defect. Idiopathic in nature, LAM characteristically occurs in women, always beginning after menarche. The usual presentation occurs in women of reproductive age, with progression before occurrence of menopause. Supplemental estrogen therapy has been associated with cases of LAM occurring in postmenopausal women. Often, women diagnosed later in life have had mild or subclinical disease evident retrospectively.

The pathophysiologic hallmark of LAM is hyperplasia of smooth muscle cells leading to obstruction of small airways, venules, and lymphatics. Multiple, recurrent bilateral pneumothoraces result from spontaneous rupture of cysts that form as a consequence of progressive airway obstruction. Other presenting symptoms include hemoptysis due to venule obstruction and formation of chylous effusions due to obstruction of lymphatics. The course may be complicated by development of chylous ascites, chylopericardium, chyluria, chyloptysis, or lower extremity edema.

Diagnostically, the chest radiographic findings are variable: pneumothoraces, pleural effusions, micronodular or miliary patterns, septal lines, coarse reticular patterns, or cystic honeycombing have all been described as nonspecific features. The appearance of a coarse reticular pattern with areas of cystic dilatation in a young woman makes the diagnosis of LAM likely. Highly suggestive findings may support the diagnosis on chest high-resolution computerized tomography (HRCT).

LAM typically progresses to pulmonary insufficiency. Exposure to estrogens or pregnancy may accelerate the course. Older literature, reviewed by Manaker (34), suggests that virtually all patients die of respiratory failure within 10 years of diagnosis. More recent data, however, suggests a more variable and somewhat more favorable prognosis, with 78% of patients alive 8.5 years after diagnosis; the average time span after disease onset in survivors is 10 years (85). Examples are also noted of occasional long-term survivors. Whether this variation is due to inherent differences in the natural history of LAM among individuals or reflects intervention with therapy is not altogether clear. The pulmonary disease of LAM is strikingly similar to the clinical picture of tuberous sclerosis. This genetic disorder, however, may occur in men and chylous pleural effusions are rare. Other manifestations may include dermal angiofibroma, epilepsy, mental retardation, as well as cerebral and ventricular hamartomas that calcify, renal angiomyolipomas, cardiac rhabdomyomas, sclerotic bone, and perungual fibromas.

Medical treatment of LAM is not wholly satisfactory and has relied mainly on hormonal manipulation. Compilation of small numbers of patients for a meta-analysis has provided support for the use of progestational agents (86). Other strategies employed have included tamoxifen, long-acting analogues of luteinizing hormone-releasing hormone, immunosuppression, oophorectomy, and ovarian radiation. When the pulmonary disease advances to an end-stage, lung transplantation offers the most viable option.

Lung transplantation for LAM has been a valuable therapy (87). The procedure has included single as well as bilateral transplants in addition to heart–lung transplantation. Extensive pleural adhesions are encountered frequently and there is a tendency for the adhesions to bleed excessively. Postoperative complications have included problems related to the native disease, such as pneumothoraces and chylothorax. As noted above, recurrence of LAM in the allograft has also been reported (68,69), making it wise, perhaps, to consider continuation of progesterone following transplantation. Actuarial survival rates for LAM patients are comparable to other groups with ILD.

SEPTIC LUNG DISEASE

Septic lung disease (SLD), including cystic fibrosis and other types of bronchiectasis, accounts for 15% to 20% of patients undergoing lung transplantation. Candidates with focal or unilateral disease can frequently be managed with medical treatment or surgical resection. For a majority of patients, however, the disease is bilateral and/or systemic, and the natural history is one of recurrent infection and progressive pulmonary failure. It is important to establish an etiology for the bronchiectasis prior to transplant evaluation, if possible, because of the impact of systemic diseases on management before and after transplantation (Table 25.10).

The diagnosis of bronchiectasis rests upon a typical constellation of symptoms, physical findings, pulmonary function abnormalities, and radiographic changes. Patients typically

Table 25.10. Etiologies of Bronchiectasis

1. Congenital: cystic fibrosis, immotile cilia syndromes, Williams-Campbell syndrome, Mounier-Kuhn syndrome, Ehlers-Danlos syndrome, hypogammaglobulinemia
2. Postinflammatory tuberculosis, pertussis, rubella, respiratory syncytial virus, fungal
3. Obstruction, tumor, nodes, foreign body, allergic bronchopulmonary aspergillosis
4. Other: yellow nail syndrome.

complain of cough, purulent sputum production, and hemoptysis. The course is marked by recurrent respiratory tract infections with progressive physiologic derangement, ultimately leading to dyspnea. Physical findings are relatively nonspecific, including evidence of hyperinflation, scattered rhonchi, crackles, occasional wheezing, and digital clubbing. Pulmonary function tests characteristically demonstrate an obstructive pattern with relative preservation of the peak flow rate in contrast to other obstructive lung diseases. Most patients have relative preservation of the diffusing capacity.

Chest radiographs may show typical features of bronchiectasis, which is characterized by the presence of abnormal and permanent dilatation of the airways. There may be a loss of definition of markings with an increase in size of the airways, crowding of other areas, as well as the development of cystic spaces and honeycomb pattern in very severe disease. Presumably, this has resulted from repeated injury and inflammation of the airways (Fig. 25.3).

Histologic patterns of bronchiectasis—namely, cylindrical, varicose, and saccular (cystic)—may occur in any combination in a patient, although the cystic changes are likely to be the most severe. High-resolution computer tomography of the chest is a sensitive tool for detecting these abnormalities.

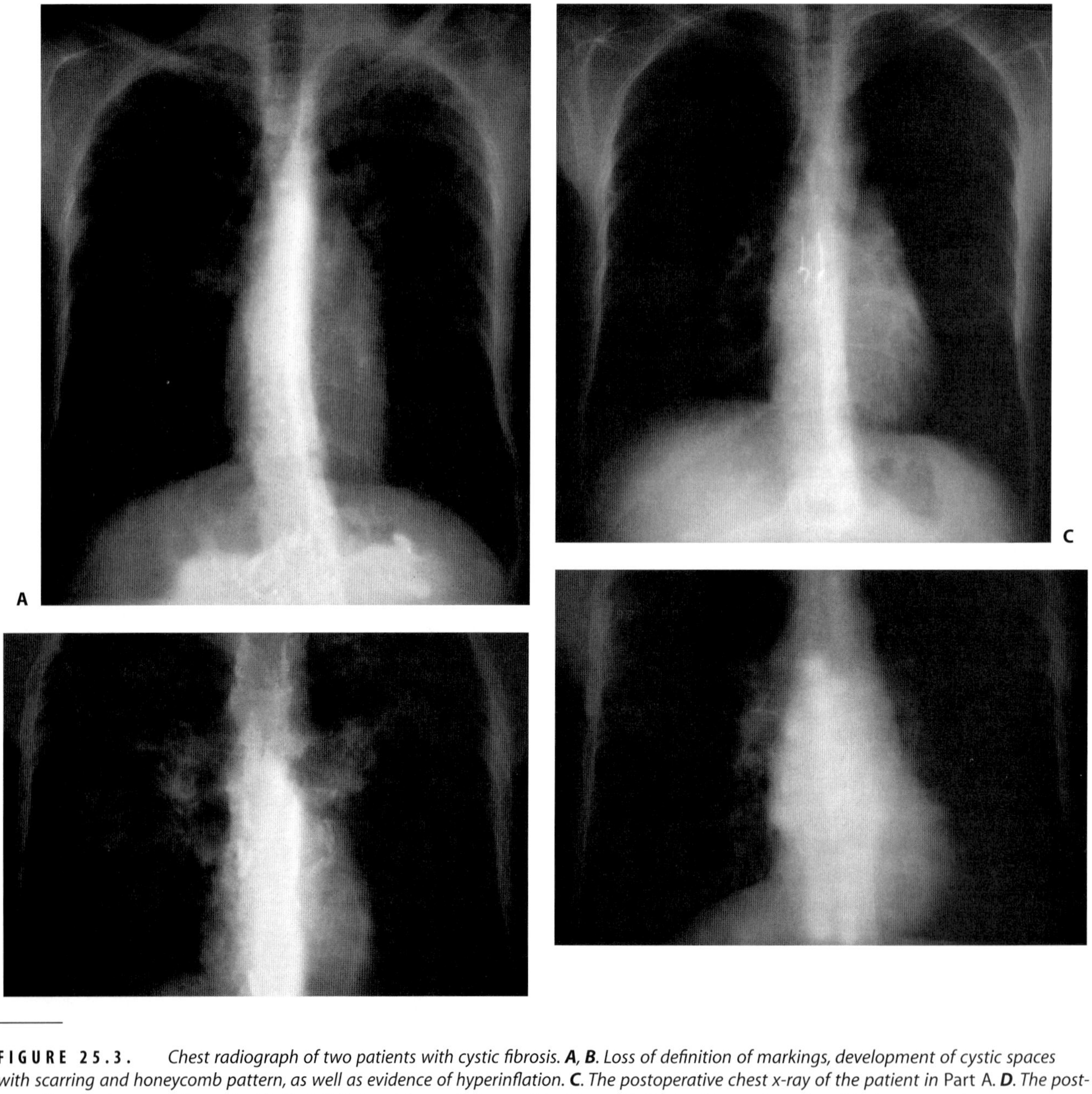

A B C D

FIGURE 25.3. *Chest radiograph of two patients with cystic fibrosis.* ***A, B.*** *Loss of definition of markings, development of cystic spaces with scarring and honeycomb pattern, as well as evidence of hyperinflation.* ***C.*** *The postoperative chest x-ray of the patient in* Part A. ***D.*** *The postoperative chest x-ray of the patient in* Part B. *Note evidence of clamshell incision with bilateral lung allografts with clear parenchyma.*

Cystic fibrosis (CF) is the most common indication for lung transplantation in individuals with bronchiectasis. It is the most common lethal inherited disorder in the white population, affecting approximately 30,000 persons in the United States. CF is an autosomal recessive disorder that has been traced to mutations in the single gene on the long arm of chromosome 7, the gene for the CF transmembrane conductance regulator (CFTR). The current understanding of CF (88,89) is that mutations in the CFTR gene result in defective chloride transport in epithelial cells of the respiratory, hepatobiliary, gastrointestinal reproductive tracts and the pancreas. The decreased chloride transport is accompanied by decreased transport of sodium and water, resulting in dehydrated, viscous secretions that are associated with luminal obstruction, destruction, and scarring of various exocrine ducts. The resulting clinical manifestations include pancreatic insufficiency, meconium ileus, diabetes mellitus, obstructive biliary disease, sinus disease, and azospermia. However, the primary cause of morbidity and mortality in patients with CF is bronchiectasis and obstructive lung disease. The latter accounts for over 90% of fatalities.

The models proposed thus far to explain the lung disease in CF have emphasized the abnormal mucus production that prevents clearance of inhaled pathogens. Recent experimental data has emerged to suggest an alternative molecular basis (90,91). This hypothesis suggests that the primary event is colonization of the airway with pathogenic bacteria that initiate cycles of infection, inflammation, airway obstruction, and destruction of lung architecture. The breach in innate immunity occurs due to the inactivation of human β-defensin-1, a naturally occurring salt-sensitive antibiotic present in epithelial lining fluid. Continued research on the β-defensin family will likely shed more light on the abnormalities of CF.

The diagnosis of CF is made when clinical features consistent with the diagnosis are combined with two sweat chloride tests with results greater than 60/mEq/L. Being homozygous for the Δ F508 deletion, the most common CF allele, is also sufficient to make the diagnosis. Although the Δ F508 mutation is responsible for approximately 70% of cases, greater than 300 mutations have been identified to date. The relationship between genotype and phenotype in CF and clinical course has been studied. Kerem et al have reported that the variable clinical course can be attributed, at least in part, to specific genotype at the locus of the CF gene (92). For example, patients homozygous with a Δ F508 allele mutation typically receive a diagnosis of cystic fibrosis at an earlier age and have a greater frequency of pancreatic insufficiency; pancreatic insufficiency is present in 99% of the homozygous patients, but only in 72% of heterozygous patients and only 36% of patients with other genotypes.

A better understanding of CF coupled with advances in medical therapy, have improved life expectancy of patients with cystic fibrosis during the past several decades. The majority, however, die in early adulthood from respiratory failure associated with pulmonary hypertension and cor pulmonale as a consequence of bronchiectasis. For these patients, lung transplantation remains not only a life-saving therapeutic option but one that has a dramatic impact upon quality of life. As with all candidates for lung transplantation, the decision as to when to list a patient and subsequently transplant a candidate depends upon understanding the natural history of the disorder and monitoring closely the individual course.

A variety of factors influence the course of patients with CF. These include general level of fitness and nutrition, frequency of infections, and the development of multiply-resistant organisms. In addition, the patient's course may be complicated by superimposed infection with nontuberculous or tuberculous mycobacteria, or fungal organisms. In some instances, allergic bronchopulmonary aspergillosis may supervene. CF patients presenting for transplant evaluation frequently suffer from osteoporosis/osteopenia, often complicated by vitamin D deficiency. There may be focal biliary fibrosis/cirrhosis, insulin-dependent diabetes mellitus, chronic sinusitis, history of hemoptysis, prior pneumothoraces, and previous thoracic surgical procedures including pleurodesis. Some patients, in addition, have been on chronic steroid therapy with its associated complications. Where such problems might once have excluded a candidate for transplantation from consideration, experience has shown that they can frequently be dealt with successfully in selected cases. Indeed, their advent may prompt the need to consider transplantation, despite the potential for higher risk.

The evaluation should document evidence of deteriorating physical condition. This is often indicated by a decreased interval of time between hospitalization for antibiotic therapy. In addition, there may also be evidence of decreasing ability to perform activities of daily living, often despite increasing oxygen supplementation. Evidence for recurring life-threatening pulmonary complications such as pneumothorax or hemoptysis should also prompt consideration of transplantation.

Of all the problems encountered in CF, it is typically chronic infection of the respiratory tract that demands the most attention. Absolute rules are difficult to define, and practice usually reflects experience that is center-specific. Colonization and infection of the lung is an important influence on survival in CF, as well as morbidity and mortality after transplantation (93). Characteristically, the prime offending organisms are gram negative and often multiply-resistant to antibiotics. These include *Pseudomonas aeruginosa*, *Stentotrophomonas* (formerly *Xanthomonas*) *maltophilia*, *Alcaligenes* (formerly *Achromobacter*) *xylosoxidans*, non-*cepacia Burkholderia* species, and *Burkholderia* (formerly *Pseudomonas*) *cepacia*. Of these microbes, the latter (*B. cepacia*) is recognized as an important determinant in the prognosis following transplantation.

Pulmonary disease secondary to *B. cepacia* reduces survival in CF (94). Infection usually occurs as a late complication after chronic infection with *P. aeruginosa*. It is often associated with a rapid, decline in airway function (95) and an increase in short-term mortality. Following transplantation, its re-emergence may cause severe and, frequently, lethal infections. In one series, 14 of 15 patients infected with *B. cepacia* had at least one serious post-transplant infection attributed to the organism, with five of the patients dying as a result (96). Similar findings have been reported in another series that underscores the high risk of lethal as well as nonfatal post-transplant infection and colonization (93,97). Genotyping studies have shown that the *B. cepacia* strains, isolated pretransplant, were responsible for the post-transplant infections and death. In addition, the data, having implications that extend beyond the individual patient to transplant programs, show that interpatient transmission of infection can occur (98).

Due to these problems associated with *B. cepacia*, many centers consider colonization by this organism to be an absolute contraindication to transplantation. Some patients harboring this microbe, however, have been transplanted successfully. This may be due to the fact that certain strains of *B. cepacia* appear to be more virulent than others and, therefore, may carry a greater risk of post-transplant infection (99). Until more is known about this organism, it is likely that transplant centers will need to assess candidates on a case-by-case basis, taking into account experience of the center, the unique clinical profile of the patients, and the antibiotic susceptibility pattern of the individual's strain.

A policy that reflects transplant center bias and experience pertains to the consideration, in general, of highly resistant organisms in lung transplant candidates. For example, some centers exclude individuals infected with pan-resistant *P. aeruginosa*. This is based upon the fact that survival is dramatically less in CF patients infected with pan-resistant organisms compared to those patients with sensitive strains (100). Other centers continue to transplant such patients, frequently relying upon testing of multiply-resistant strains for antibiotic synergy in a reference laboratory. Initial studies, based upon the demonstration of one or more synergistic combinations of intravenous or aerosolized antibiotics, have looked promising (101). In a retrospective study of 66 lung transplant recipients over a six-year period, Aris et al (102) concluded that CF patients infected with pan-resistant *P. aeruginosa* have outcomes similar to those for patients with sensitive bacteria and should not be excluded from lung transplantation based solely on this criterion.

Other organisms that should be sought with routine surveillance (sputum cultures) include methicillin-resistant *Staphylococcus aureus*, nontuberculous and tuberculous mycobacteria, and fungi. Most centers routinely treat infections with these organisms aggressively prior to transplant in an attempt to prevent dissemination of disease following transplantation with subsequent immunosuppression. These organisms do not constitute a contraindication to transplantation.

Conventional pulmonary therapy for CF relies upon alleviation of symptoms in an attempt to correct organ dysfunction. The mainstays of therapy have been pancreatic enzyme replacement (with reversal of secondary nutritional and vitamin deficiencies), clearance of lower airway secretions, and treatment of pulmonary infections. Traditionally, patients have relied upon chest physical therapy with postural drainage. It is the chief nonpharmacologic approach to enhancing clearance of pulmonary secretions. Other airway clearance techniques include forced expiratory technique (e.g., "Huff"), self-generated drainage, positive expiratory pressure, and airway oscillators (e.g., flutter). Bronchodilators including inhaled beta-adrenergic or anticholinergic agents, as well as theophylline, may be helpful in a subset of patients. Attempts to reduce viscoelasticity of sputum with a purified recombinant human deoxyribonuclease I (rhDNAse I) will benefit some patients, particularly those with purulent airway secretions. The mainstay of treatment remains judicious use of antibiotics, both for exacerbation of pulmonary infection, as well as for maintenance. In addition to systemically administered antibiotics, many CF patients receive inhaled antibiotic therapy, particularly colistin or tobramycin, with the aim of reducing the burden of *P. aeruginosa* from respiratory secretions. Furthermore, Bauldoff et al have proposed that aerosolized colistin may be a useful therapy to promote emergence of sensitive microbes from CF candidates awaiting lung transplantation with pan-resistant isolates of *Pseudomonas* (103). Other medical approaches include attempts to modulate ion transport pharmacologically. Administration of aerosolized amiloride has been attempted as a means of inhibiting sodium absorption. Drugs that stimulate chloride secretions, such as uridine triphosphate, also hold promise. Anti-inflammatory drug therapy, attempted in some patients, has met with limited success (88).

Chronic rhinosinusitis is extremely common in patients with CF. Numerous complications may develop, including nasal obstruction, congestion, sinus pain and pressure, hyposmia or anosmia, and infection. The potential "seeding" of bacteria into the lower respiratory tract is of particular concern following lung transplantation. There is no uniform opinion on the optimal management, especially preventable measures, that should be undertaken in transplant candidates. The approach tends to be center-specific, ranging from virtually no intervention to an aggressive combination of medical and surgical treatments. Advances in endoscopic sinus surgery have facilitated an aggressive approach (104).

Despite modern management, bronchiectasis in CF patients tends to progress. The challenge to the physician evaluating candidates for lung transplantation is to determine the appropriate "window of opportunity" in which to perform transplantation. Over the years, a number of clinical screening systems have been developed in order to determine prognosis. All of these clinical scoring systems are open to criticism. For example, Aitken has pointed out that the reproducibility of the Schwachman-Kulczycki (S-K) system has not been evaluated (105). A retrospective study with 142 adult patients found the S-K score, low weight percentile, and *B. cepacia* colonization to be negative prognostic indicators.

A prospective study from Toronto defined predictors of mortality in a cohort of 673 patients. In each patient, parameters of pulmonary function, blood gas values, age, and sex were analyzed for their effect on mortality. Kerem et al concluded that patients with CF should be considered candidates for lung transplantation when the FEV_1 falls below 30% of the predicted value, based upon the observation that the two-year mortality was at least 50% when spirometry fell to this level. For each 10% decline in FEV_1, there was a two-fold increase of risk of death at two years. Hypoxemia (Pa_{O_2} <55 mm Hg) and hypercapnea (P_{CO_2} = 50 mm Hg) also predicted a high mortality (92).

Ciriaco et al studied 74 patients with CF and compared those who died while on a transplant waiting list with those who survived to transplantation (106). The group with the lower FEV_1 (average 0.51 liters, 16.8% predicted) were among those who died while waiting. In contrast, those who survived had an FEV_1 on average of 0.73 liters (21.2% predicted). The results of a 6MWT were also worse among those who died waiting (290.1 m versus 391.8 m) compared to listed patients surviving to transplantation.

Hayden et al examined 25 CF patients awaiting lung transplantation and found that the percent predicted values for spirometry were significantly lower in the group of patients who died compared with those who lived (FEV_1 21 ± 5.7, FVC 37 ± 13.6 percent predicted versus FEV_1 31 ± 9.4, FVC 53 ± 11.7 percent predicted, respectively) (63). The prognostic value of exercise testing was assessed in 109 patients with CF by Nixon et al (107). Peak oxygen consumption ($\dot{V}_{O_2}$ peak) was measured in patients over an eight-year span and correlated with survival. Whether aerobic conditioning can improve life span is unproved. Short-term conditioning programs do result in better exercise tolerance, possibly by increased respiratory muscle endurance (108). A recent report has challenged the view that an absolute FEV_1 can serve as a reliable predictor of high mortality risk. Instead, the investigators concluded that the yearly rate of decline in percent predicted FEV_1 is a better parameter to identify high-risk patients (109).

Generally, impaired nutritional status is regarded as a poor prognostic sign. Although the difference was not statistically significant, Hayden et al found that the percent of ideal body weight was lower in patients who died while waiting for transplantation compared to those who survived to transplant (63). Sharples et al also found that cachexia was not a predictor of pretransplant survival, but it did correlate with poorer outcome after transplant (110). Snell et al (111) have asserted that patients with CF (particularly women) referred for lung transplantation with a body mass index (BMI) less than 18 kg/m^2 are at high risk of death over the next 12 months. With this in mind, these authors contend that such patients should not be denied transplantation unduly while attempts are made to increase weight, especially because pretransplantation BMI does not appear to influence post-transplant survival.

As noted, liver disease due to biliary cirrhosis occurs in up to 5% of CF patients. Serious liver dysfunction may increase the perioperative risk of bleeding and infection, as well as adversely affect the metabolism of drugs typically cleared by the liver. For patients with concurrent advanced disease of both organs, combined lung (or heart–lung) and liver transplantation has been accomplished (112,113). It has been reported that successful isolated lung transplants have been carried out in CF patients with liver disease and portal hypertension (114).

In sum, multiple factors play a role in determining life expectancy in CF patients. The multisystem nature of the disease and the development of multiple treatment modalities and nutritional support, as well as the variability of factors such as colonization by various infectious agents make it difficult to determine prognosis. Assessment of these factors, nonetheless, aids the decision regarding listing patients for transplantation, as well as determining their risks. Despite their potentially poor nutritional status and the presence of multiply resistant organisms, carefully selected patients with CF can undergo bilateral lung transplantation with acceptable morbidity and mortality (115).

PULMONARY VASCULAR DISEASE

Pulmonary vascular disease, either primary pulmonary hypertension (PPH) or secondary pulmonary hypertension due to Eisenmenger's syndrome, accounts for 10% to 15% of patients requiring isolated lung transplantation and for 45% to 50% of patients requiring heart–lung transplantation.

PPH is an uncommon disorder that is typically progressive and incurable. It is characterized by sustained elevations of pulmonary artery pressures without a demonstrable cause. The diagnostic criteria used in the National Institutes of Health (NIH) Registry include a mean pulmonary artery pressure of more than 25 mm Hg at rest or more than 30 mm Hg with exercise. Previous reports have described a median survival of less than four years. In the NIH Registry, PPH had a median survival of 2.8 years in a large cohort of patients followed prospectively for seven years (116,117).

In the last decade, there have been major strides in the treatment of PPH, ranging from daily oral medications to organ transplantation. The role of the various medical therapies and timing of lung transplantation are issues that continue to evolve. It is essential that physicians involved in the diagnosis and treatment of PPH have a thorough understanding of diagnostic studies and treatment options. These include anticoagulants, vasodilators, and transplantation, as well as other supportive measures including diuretics, oxygen, and cardiac drugs.

The diagnosis of pulmonary hypertension is frequently delayed due to the nonspecific nature of symptoms and the subtlety of signs of less-advanced disease. The length of time from onset of symptoms to established medical diagnosis is approximately two years. Dyspnea is the most frequent complaint occurring in approximately 60% of patients. Fatigue, angina, syncope (particularly with exertion), and Raynaud's phenomenon may also be present. In order to establish a diagnosis of PPH, secondary causes of pulmonary hypertension need to be excluded. These include parenchymal lung disease, disorders of ventilation, pulmonary vasculitides, and thromboembolic disease or obstruction of pulmonary vessels. The latter may be secondary to clot, acquired or congenital stenosis, as well as to foreign bodies, tumor, hemoglobinopathies, or schistosome eggs. Other secondary causes of pulmonary hypertension include heart disease, particularly disorders of left heart filling; congenital systemic-pulmonary shunt; HIV infection; portal hypertension; or exposure to exogenous substances including crack cocaine, L-tryptophan, toxic rape-seed oil, or anorexic agents. A familial form of PPH, inherited as an autosomal dominant trait, may also be present (118).

Essential to the rationale of medical therapy is an understanding of the key elements that combine to produce increased vascular resistance in patients with PPH. These include vasoconstriction, vascular wall remodeling, and thrombosis in situ. Vascular remodeling takes the form typically of proliferation of intimal or adventitious tissue. Pathologically, medial smooth muscle hypertrophy and plexiform lesions (representing abnormal growth of endothelial cells) are found in involved pulmonary vessels. Recent work has demonstrated that the endothelial cells in plexiform lesions in PPH are predominantly monoclonal, whereas those in secondary causes of pulmonary hypertension are polyclonal (119). Interestingly, the plexiform lesions of patients with appetite suppressant–related pulmonary hypertension also demonstrate monoclonal expansion (120). Thrombosis in situ may relate either to injury directly to endothelium, abnormal fibrinolysis, or enhanced procoagulative activity, as well as platelet abnormalities. Associated with these abnormalities, there may be altered function of the vascular endothelium. As a result, there typically is an imbalance in the thromboxane-prostacyclin ratio. There may also be a decreased synthesis of endothelium-derived relaxant factor (NO) or an increase in synthesis of endothelium-derived vasoconstrictor (endothelin) (121).

Results of the diagnostic evaluation typically are as follows: Imaging procedures show evidence of pulmonary hypertension in over 90% of cases. A chest radiograph typically reveals prominence of the main pulmonary artery or hilar vessels. In approximately half of the cases, there is pruning of distal vessels with hyperluscent lung. In the NIH Registry, approximately 6% of patients enrolled with PPH had a normal radiograph (116). The CT scan of the chest typically confirms the plain radiograph findings. In addition, there may be areas of ground-glass density interspersed amongst relatively more luscent areas of lung, owing possibly to abnormalities associated with hyperperfusion and/or edema. As a new generation of CT scanners have evolved and software has improved, these imaging techniques have also shown promise to detect central clots, potentially associated with pulmonary hypertension.

Pulmonary function studies may be normal in some patients. Others may have mild restrictive defects, small airways dysfunction, as well as impairment in gas exchange, particularly in more advanced stages of the disease. The major virtue in obtaining these studies is to detect moderate or severe physiologic abnormalities that should suggest an alternative diagnosis. Similarly, severe hypoxemia should raise the possibility of either intracardiac shunting through a patent foramen ovale or a severely depressed cardiac output.

Electrocardiographic studies ordinarily reveal right ventricular hypertrophy with secondary T wave changes on electrocardiogram, although the findings do not necessarily reflect the severity of the underlying pulmonary hypertension. Echocardiographic examination is most useful in assessing myocardial dysfunction or the presence of valvular or congenital heart disease. Doppler ultrasound is also quite useful in making a noninvasive estimation of right ventricular systolic pressure. Transesophageal echocardiography may detect abnormalities, not otherwise appreciated, of cardiac anatomy. In one study, in which 48 patients were evaluated, new diagnostic information was obtained that altered therapy in 12 of the patients (25%). The additional data included proximal pulmonary artery thrombi (3 patients), patent foramen ovale with moderate to large right to left shunt (2 patients), ASD (2 patients), double outlet right ventricle (2 patients), VSD (2 patients), and exclusion of ASD (1 patient) (122). One caveat, however, is that it is not clear that all the patients studied underwent a good quality transthoracic echocardiographic examination with contrast.

Serologic studies for connective tissue disorders are frequently abnormal in patients with PPH. Whether reflecting an underlying connective tissue disorder or simply representing an epiphenomenon, elevations in antinuclear antibodies are common. Antibodies to Ku, a DNA binding protein, found in some cases of systemic lupus erythematosus, scleroderma, myositis, and in Sjögren's syndrome, have been reported in a subset of patients with PPH. Some patients with low titer positive antinuclear antibodies (ANAs) also demonstrate hypothyroidism, raising the possibility of immunologic linkage (123). Abdominal ultrasound is useful to exclude the possibility of portal hypertension. Cardiac catheterization is considered to be an absolute requirement in confirming the diagnosis of PPH and for guiding management (121).

Therapy with vasodilators is based on the observation that vasoconstriction is a prominent feature of this disease. Since there is no way to predict clinically which patients are most likely to respond to vasodilators, the initial response to a therapeutic challenge is often employed as a means to identify those patients who are most likely to benefit from long-term oral treatment. The initial hemodynamic study is usually carried out with potent, short-acting, titratable vasodilators, such as nitric oxide, epoprostenol (prostacyclin), and adenosine. Typically, the drugs are titrated to a maximal response of the pulmonary artery pressure and pulmonary vascular resistance that is clinically tolerated. Those patients who demonstrate a reduction in pulmonary artery pressure and resistance and little change in systemic pressure or arterial oxygen saturation are felt most likely to have sustained hemodynamic and symptomatic improvement, as well as prolonged survival. With high-dose calcium channel blockers, for example, 25% of patients may show an approximate 25% reduction in both mean pulmonary artery pressure and pulmonary vascular resistance. Other patients may demonstrate a reduction in pulmonary vascular resistance as a result of increase in cardiac output without a reduction in mean pulmonary artery pressure. Many of these patients feel better and have an improved exercise tolerance, but this type of response has not been associated with improved survival (124,125). An important consideration with respect to the use of calcium antagonist therapy is that dosing needs to be adjusted carefully on the basis of symptoms or objective findings. Side effects including systemic hypotension, edema, and hypoxemia must be monitored closely.

The most widely used drugs for long-term therapy are the calcium channel blockers, nifedipine and diltiazem. In a small series of patients with PPH associated with CREST (calcinosis, Raynaud's phenomena, esophageal dysmotility, sclerodactyly, and telangiectasia) syndrome, angiotensin converting enzyme inhibitors have shown promise (126). Inhaled nitric oxide or prostacyclin (epoprostenol) has been administered to a small number of patients, but is not standard therapy (127–130). Long-term therapy with epoprostenol is an alternative strategy for patients with PPH. Given by continuous intravenous infusion via a portable infusion pump, attached to a permanent indwelling central catheter, this medication may improve hemodynamic characteristics, exercise tolerance, quality of life, as well as survival (117,131,132). Major adverse effects relate to pump and catheter problems, as well as to specific drug side effects. Of importance is the observation that long-term therapy with epoprostenol may produce sustained hemodynamic improvement, even in patients who show little or no response to acute infusion, owing possibly to the inhibitory effects of platelet aggregation as well as to the effects of vascular remodeling. Clinical experience with epoprostenol infusion in lung transplant candidates is encouraging. Conte et al (133) have suggested that this therapy is often an effective means for delaying, possibly indefinitely, the need for transplantation. When lung transplants are performed after epoprostenol therapy, excellent results can be obtained. Although their study suffers from an uncontrolled design and a retrospective nature, it is reasonable to consider this alternative prior to transplantation.

The role of anticoagulant therapy for long-term treatment of PPH is supported by clinical as well as biochemical data. Both a retrospective analysis and a small, randomized prospective study suggest that anticoagulation prolongs life (124,134). Other supportive measures include diuretics, oxygen, and digoxin, particularly to counteract the negative inotropic properties of calcium channel blockers.

Medical management of PPH is frequently not sufficient to reduce symptoms, nor to overcome the reduction of life expectancy. Surgical options for selected patients may include thromboendarterectomy (135–137), balloon septostomy (138,139), and ultimately transplantation. For PPH, heart–lung transplantation was initially preferred. Eventually, the feasibility of isolated lung transplantation, both single and bilateral (13,140–142), was demonstrated (143).

Selected criteria for pulmonary thromboendarterectomy include the following: 1) thrombus defined as accessible to surgical removal, 2) a PVR of greater than 300 dynes/sec^{-1}/cm^{-5}, 3) the absence of significant associated disease, and 4) willingness of the patient. Balloon septostomy may result in clinical and hemodynamic improvement and enhance survival in select patients with severe PPH. By creating a right-to-left shunt at the atrial level, symptoms of right heart failure may be relieved.

Lung transplantation is typically offered to patients with New York Heart Association class III or IV functional level. The exact type of isolated lung transplant remains open to discussion. The advantage of single lung transplantation is that it optimizes the use of donor organs and is less difficult technically. It is also supported by encouraging short-term results. Its potential limitation is that there may be relatively poor functional reserve and that there is likely a requirement for an excellent graft, in terms of shorter ischemic time. The choice of transplant procedure, therefore, may vary with individual transplant programs, as there are not yet sufficient scientific data upon which to base a decision. For example, it is unclear how severe or dysfunctional the right ventricle may become before it is no longer capable of improving following isolated lung transplantation (144–146). However, a right ventricle that is severely hypokinetic, with a right ventricular ejection fraction less than approximately 10% to 15%, raises concern regarding the feasibility of isolated lung transplantation. Such patients might be better considered as candidates for heart–lung transplantation (see Chapter 26). Patients with hyperbilirubinemia and/or ascites are at an advanced risk (147).

After the first report of a successful single lung transplant for Eisenmenger's syndrome, several other reports have documented encouraging hemodynamic improvement following single lung transplantation for primary and secondary pulmonary hypertension (148). However, single lung transplantation may be less optimal than bilateral lung transplantation or heart–lung transplantation. Post-transplantation pulmonary edema and hemodynamic instability are more frequent following single lung transplants for severe pulmonary hypertension than after bilateral lung or heart–lung transplantation. In addition, substantial ventilation-perfusion mismatch with resultant hypoxemia is more likely to occur in patients with single lung transplantation, owing to differences in pulmonary vascular resistance. Most of the cardiac output flows to the transplanted lung after single lung transplantation, but ventilation typically remains equally divided between the two lungs. In the series by Bando et al (148), survival after single lung transplantation was worse than after bilateral lung transplantation and heart–lung transplantation. This challenges the concept that the patient's native lung may serve as a protective "back up" and emphasizes that complications may be poorly tolerated. These findings support the concept that carefully selected patients with major intracardiac defects and pulmonary hypertension may have good early results after cardiac repair and single lung transplantation, but long-term results are considerably less favorable. However, a retrospective review of 58 lung transplants performed for pulmonary hypertension led Gammie et al (149) to conclude that single lung or bilateral lung transplants could achieve similar outcomes. These authors supported cautious preferential application of single lung transplantation for pulmonary hypertension. A limitation of these studies, however, is that the experience of each group is relatively small.

With the relative shortage of suitable heart–lung donor blocs and the high mortality of patients with severe pulmonary hypertension, an increasing number of patients with pulmonary vascular disease have undergone isolated lung transplantation. The results of isolated lung transplantation are similar to those with heart–lung transplantation for pulmonary vascular disease, provided that there is no significant left ventricular dysfunction (absence of cardiomyopathy, i.e., left ventricular ejection fraction ≥45%), right ventricular diastolic function is maintained (RVEDP ≤ 15 mm Hg), and there are no uncorrectable structural abnormalities. Interestingly, the presence of severe right ventricular systolic dysfunction (RVEF ≤ 20%) does not necessarily affect the results of isolated lung transplantation, and severe tricuspid regurgitation and pulmonary valvular regurgitation, present in virtually all patients, resolves almost immediately following lung transplantation. Thus, heart–lung transplantation is reserved for those patients with either significant biventricular dysfunction (e.g., severe valvular cardiomyopathy) or uncorrectable congenital heart defects.

Lung transplantation performed for pulmonary hypertension has an actuarial survival at years 1, 2, and 3 of approximately 66%, 60%, and 50%, respectively, for bilateral transplantation. The corresponding survival rates for isolated single lung transplants for this disorder are 58%, 52%, and 47%. In considering the risks and benefits of transplantation, it is important to recognize the natural history of PPH. The relatively rapid downhill course of PPH has been well described in the National Prospective Registry from the NIH and survival is dependent upon several parameters. These include the mean pulmonary artery and right atrial pressures, as well as cardiac index (Fig. 25.4). Other important factors, in addition to the hemodynamic parameters associated with poor survival, include New York Heart Association class III or IV status, presence of Raynaud's phe-

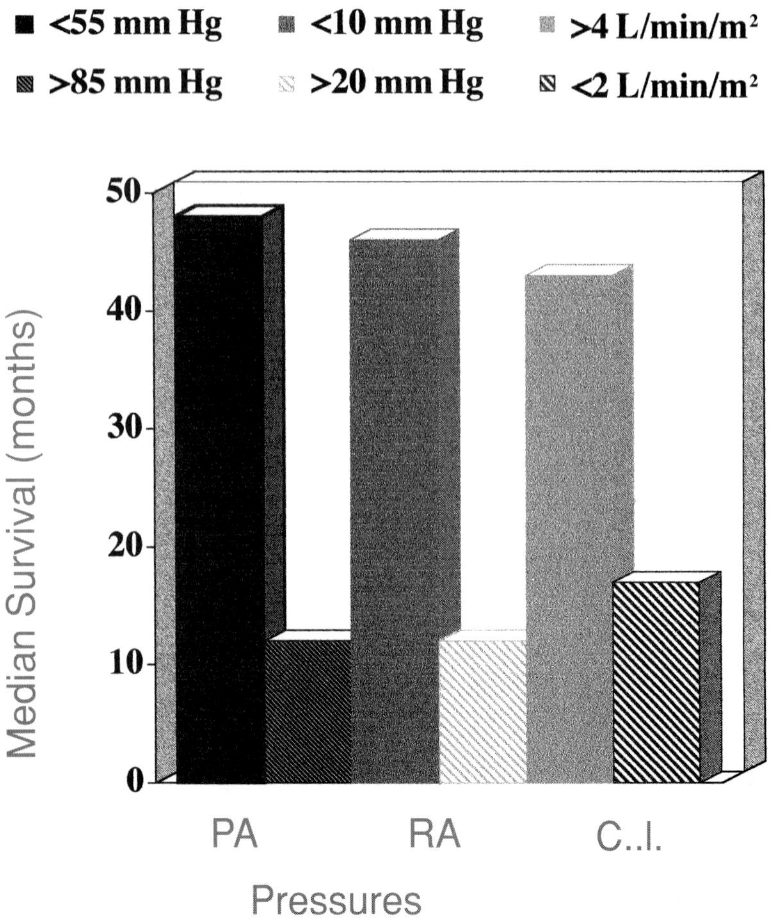

FIGURE 25.4. *Median survival in months for patients with PPH compared with three hemodynamic variables. (Modified from D'Alonzo GE, Barst RJ, Ayres SM, et al. Survival in patients with primary pulmonary hypertension: results from a national prospective registry. Ann Intern Med 1991;115:343–349.)*

nomenon, and decreased diffusing capacity of carbon monoxide (116,117).

Optimal timing of transplantation remains controversial. In order to warrant undertaking the risk of transplantation, patients should be sufficiently ill, but not so far advanced that survival following the transplant seems unlikely. The approach followed at many centers is to initiate vasodilator therapy while listing patients for transplantation, with periodic assessment of their clinical status. Patients who improve may defer, whereas those who show little or no response are more likely to proceed with transplantation. In patients whose pulmonary vascular disease is a result of Eisenmenger's physiology, determination of appropriate timing of transplantation is even more difficult. Appropriate selection criteria have not yet been defined. Traditionally, such patients have been viewed as needing to fulfill the same criteria as individuals with PPH; however, recent clinical observations of the two groups awaiting transplantation demonstrate that patients with Eisenmenger's physiology have a better survival. Six-month actuarial survival data of patients with PPH is approximately 60% in comparison to 89% for patients with Eisenmenger's syndrome (63). The relatively more-favorable prognosis is in keeping with mortality data reported by Saha et al on the basis of studying 200 patients who were followed from 1976 to 1992 (150). The study indicated that prolonged life span is possible, as the oldest patient presented at 62 years. The most common causes of death among the 20 patients who died during the course of observation were sudden cardiac deaths, congestive heart failure, and hemoptysis.

Pulmonary hypertension leads to structural and functional changes in the heart, which include interventricular septal flattening with a shift of the septum into the left ventricle as the right ventricle dilates. Lung transplantation leads to a reduction in right ventricular afterload and an improvement in systolic function. The leftward septal shift resolves and right ventricular cavitary volume decreases, while right ventricular thickness increases. Right ventricular hypertrophy eventually resolves (145).

Until these events occur, however, the patient with preoperative PPH may incur a number of postoperative problems related to hemodynamic instability, particularly as a result of right ventricular dysfunction. Patients with less severe elevation of pulmonary artery pressure, associated with other end-stage lung disease, may display similar problems to a lesser degree. Severe hypoxemia may occur, relating to ventilation-perfusion mismatch, differences in compliance, and the development of pulmonary edema. The latter may occur as a result of shifts in pulmonary blood flow and an increase in the hydrostatic forces associated with this process.

Because of the structural and functional changes in the geometry of the heart, it is important to be aware of a unique complication of transplantation in individuals with severe pulmonary hypertension. This is termed *suicidal RV*, or right ventricular outflow tract (RVOT) obstruction (151). This results from a massive right ventricular pulmonary artery gradient and may be exacerbated by inotropic agents or tachycardia. The diagnosis may be confirmed by echocardiography and/or cardiac catheterization. Management is dependent upon the use of beta blockers or diltiazem, in order to reduce contractility, improve diastolic filling, and increase diastolic function. In select cases, a surgical patch augmentation of the RVOT, with or without myectomy, may be necessary.

In the future, therapy for PPH will likely refine vasodilator treatment. Possibilities include stable prostacyclin analogues (inhaled, transdermal, or oral forms) or inhaled nitric oxide. Animal experiments have also demonstrated the feasibility of gene transfer of vasodilatory proteins that may act as pulmonary vasodilators (152). For the present, however, lung transplantation offers the most viable option for improvement in the quality of life and life expectancy for individuals suffering from severe pulmonary hypertension.

TRANSPLANT PROCEDURE SELECTION: SUMMARY

The indication for a specific lung transplant procedure depends upon the underlying disease (Table 25.11). Single lung transplantation (SLT) is optimal for the majority of end-stage pulmonary diseases requiring transplantation with the exception, as noted, of patients with bilateral septic lung disease or severe pulmonary artery hypertension (8,12,142). SLT is associated with a shorter wait for donor lungs pretransplant and a lower morbidity and mortality rate after transplant as compared to other lung transplant procedures performed for the same recipient diagnoses. The operative mortality for SLT ranges from 3% to 10% depending upon the specific transplant indication, the presence or absence of pulmonary hypertension, and the need for cardiopulmonary bypass intraoperatively.

Double lung transplantation (DLT) is the procedure of choice for patients with bilateral septic lung disease, such as cystic fibrosis, or for patients with near-systemic pulmonary

Table 25.11. Indications for Specific Lung Transplant Procedures

Single Lung Transplantation (SLT)
Obstructive lung disease
Restrictive lung disease
Unilateral septic lung disease
Primary pulmonary hypertension
Eisenmenger's syndrome with a correctable shunt defect
Double Lung Transplantation (DLT)
Obstructive lung disease (patient <50 years old)
Bilateral septic lung disease
Primary pulmonary hypertension
Eisenmenger's syndrome with a correctable shunt defect
Combined Heart–Lung Transplantation (HLT)
Refractory right ventricular diastolic dysfunction (RVEDP >15 mm Hg)
Severe intrinsic left ventricular dysfunction (LVEF <45%)
Severe coronary artery disease, not amenable to nonsurgical interventions
Eisenmenger's syndrome with an irreparable shunt defect

artery pressures from either primary or secondary causes. Some centers also favor the use of DLT for patients with emphysema who are less than 50 years of age (9). Typically, however, operative mortality rates for DLT are higher than for SLT, ranging from 10% to 15%. Operative mortality is probably higher due to the number of patients with septic lung disease treated by DLT. Such patients are at greater risk for complications. Notably, at most large centers, perioperative morbidity from other than infectious complications, including acute graft failure and bronchial dehiscence, are similar with SLT and DLT. For patients with pulmonary vascular disease, DLT is favored over SLT when there are greater elevations of pulmonary artery (PA) pressures (e.g., systolic PA ≥90 mm Hg or mean PA ≥65 mm Hg) and more advanced right ventricular dysfunction (e.g., RVEF ≤20%).

Combined heart–lung transplantation (HLT) has been used successfully for virtually all end-stage pulmonary diseases that require transplantation. However, with the perfection of the techniques of SLT and DLT and in light of the shortage of suitable donor organs, the use of HLT has focused on patients with refractory right ventricular diastolic dysfunction (e.g., right ventricular end diastolic pressure >15 mm Hg), severe intrinsic left ventricular dysfunction, Eisenmenger's syndrome, and irreparable shunt defects (9). The operative mortality for HLT at large centers is about 15%, but is typically higher than that for SLT or DLT for similar disease states (see also Chapter 26).

DONOR SELECTION

The most important factor limiting wider application of lung transplantation is the supply of donor organs. Unlike other solid organs used for transplantation, prior to brain death the lung is exposed to environmental contamination, including both microbiologic pathogens and toxic substances, which may impair its functional capabilities. The microbiologic aspects of this exposure are accentuated by the endotracheal intubation that is a necessary aspect of donor management. In addition, aspiration of oropharyngeal or gastric contents is a common occurrence during the events preceding brain death. Nearly half of all comatose patients will develop pneumonia within one week of intubation, probably due to a combination of these factors. Brain death itself may also lead to neurogenic pulmonary edema. Finally, in cases of trauma leading to brain death, either injury to the thorax and/or the fluid volume replacement, required for resuscitation, may result in a pulmonary inflammatory response, rendering the lungs unsuitable for subsequent transplantation. As a result, only about 25% of cadaveric donors of other organs are satisfactory lung donors as well.

Criteria for lung donation should identify those donors with evidence of good gas exchange in the absence of invasive infection of the airways or parenchyma (Table 25.12). A donor age of less than 60 years as well as a history of smoking for less than 20 to 30 pack years are important.

Table 25.12. Characteristics of a Suitable Lung Donor

Age less than 60 years
Cigarette smoking less than 30 pack-years
No important prior thoracic surgery on the side of the proposed donation
Normal chest radiograph of the donor lung
Adequate gas exchange of the donor lung
Pa_{O_2} >300 mm Hg on F_{IO_2} = 1.0, PEEP ≥5 cm
Bronchoscopic evaluation demonstrating absence of mucosal inflammation
No major pulmonary trauma or anatomic abnormalities

Both increasing age and prolonged tobacco abuse correlate directly with anatomic alterations in the pulmonary parenchyma that may, despite preservation of gas exchange function in the donor, result in impaired graft function in the recipient. Ideally, a chest radiograph should reveal a normal lung on the side of the proposed lung donation. Unilateral pneumonia or parenchymal trauma does not preclude use of the contralateral lung for transplantation in most circumstances. No major thoracic surgery should have been performed on the side of proposed donation, not only because of potential technical limitations, but because such a history usually suggests either a major anatomic abnormality (e.g., prior lobectomy) or pathology (e.g., malignant neoplasm) that would preclude donation. Finally, the size of the donor lungs, based on direct measurement or correlated to body surface area as estimated by donor height, is a useful parameter when selecting lungs for a particular recipient. Generally, the donor lungs should be within 25% to 30% of the *predicted* size of the recipient's lungs. Since most recipients have significant abnormalities of lung volume, the predicted size of an ideal recipient lung, estimated from the recipient's height, gender, and age, should be used for comparison. A donor lung larger than these parameters should usually be avoided.

Adequate gas exchange has been defined as a Pa_{O_2} of greater than 300 mm Hg while on mechanical ventilation, with an F_{IO_2} equal to 1.0 and positive end-expiratory pressure (PEEP) equal to 5 cm water. Minute ventilation should be adjusted to achieve normocarbia, with a tidal volume of 10 to 15 mL/kg and an appropriate respiratory rate. If a unilateral pulmonary process is present, however, a lower Pa_{O_2} may be acceptable due to mixing at the level of the left atrium. In these circumstances, intraoperative evaluation of unilateral gas exchange by sampling from the ipsilateral pulmonary vein for determination of P_{O_2} can be used to confirm the acceptability of the donor lung (153). It may be possible to improve oxygenation and increase donor lung recovery with high-dose steroid administration after brain death (154).

All lung donors will have some evidence of colonization of the lower respiratory tract by potential pathogens due to the requisite endotracheal intubation that bypasses the defense mechanisms of the upper airway. A distal tracheitis is uniformly present following 72 hours of intubation.

Therefore, a sputum gram stain revealing polymorphonuclear leukocytes or multiple bacterial forms does not necessarily imply invasive infection. For this reason, bronchoscopy is a critical step in the evaluation of any potential lung donor. Bronchoscopy allows inspection of the large airways for the presence of aspirated debris as well as assessment of the character of the secretions and the status of the bronchial mucosa. A finding of diffuse bronchial mucosal inflammation is significant, even if only a limited amount of aspirated debris or secretions are present. However, purulent secretions without significant mucosal inflammation, in the presence of a clear chest radiograph and preserved gas exchange, generally indicate a suitable lung for donation. A potassium hydroxide (KOH) smear for fungal organisms is also a part of the routine evaluation of the lung donor although, as with the Gram stain, the mere presence of fungal organisms does not preclude lung donation. In most cases, the presence of potential pathogens in the donor sputum by either Gram stain or fungal smear requires preemptive modification of the recipient antimicrobial regimen if such lungs are used for transplantation. At some centers, this treatment is begun prior to extraction of the lungs with the administration of intravenous or aerosolized antimicrobial therapy to the donor (155).

The donor evaluation is completed by an intraoperative inspection of the pleural space and lung. Occasionally, unsuspected parenchymal trauma will be evident in the form of a bloody pleural effusion or a pulmonary contusion. The donor lung should also be studied for evidence of unsuspected bullous disease or mass lesions. Excisional biopsy and intraoperative pathologic evaluation of any suspicious parenchymal lesions should be carried out. Finally, the anesthesiologist should be directed to maintain adequate tidal volumes and PEEP during intraoperative ventilation to preserve optimal function of the donor lung prior to its removal.

The appropriateness of a potential lung donor should always be interpreted in the context of the recipient's disease and clinical status. Older patients, patients with diseases such as COPD in which lung transplantation may be largely palliative, and patients with a sudden clinical deterioration, such as those who have recently been placed on mechanical ventilation, may all benefit from transplantation using a lung that does not fulfill all of the criteria of an optimal donor lung. Most frequently, the parameters regarding cigarette smoking and Pa_{O_2} are violated in these circumstances. The results have generally been satisfactory in such recipients, suggesting that the use of these marginal lung donors may partially address the problem of donor organ shortage (156). The impact of the functional status of the donor lung is greatest in the first 24 hours following transplantation; subsequent graft function depends primarily on factors related to the recipient. With respect to such issues as the incidence of rejection, the potential long-term consequences of using compromised lung is not known. However, the experience to date underscores the fact that patients with pulmonary hypertension, who are the most difficult to manage postoperatively, are best served by transplantation using noncompromised lungs from optimal donors (see Chapter 15).

LUNG PRESERVATION

The ideal method of pulmonary preservation has not yet been defined. With current techniques, however, satisfactory graft function can be obtained after ischemic intervals of as long as six to eight hours. As with other vascularized solid organ allografts, the lung consists of a heterogeneous population of cells, of which the vascular endothelial cell appears to be the most sensitive to ischemia. Ischemic injury to the pulmonary vascular endothelium increases its permeability and results in pulmonary edema, the common endpoint for assessment of injury in models of pulmonary preservation techniques. Hypothermia is the major method used clinically to limit ischemic injury to these cells. The lung also has some unique biologic and physical characteristics that distinguish it from other solid organ transplants. Although the lung has an absolute requirement for aerobic metabolism, it is capable of using ambient oxygen for the metabolism of glucose, even during the ischemic state (157). In addition, the effective size of the pulmonary vascular bed and the thermal conductivity of the lung can be manipulated by the state of lung inflation. Current clinical methods of lung preservation make use of these characteristics to optimize graft function following an ischemic interval.

Two techniques are presently being used for lung preservation: hypothermic flush perfusion and core cooling.

Hypothermic flush perfusion is the method most commonly used for pulmonary preservation in clinical practice. This technique consists of flushing the pulmonary vasculature with a cold solution after systemic heparinization of the donor, followed by extraction and transport of the lungs inflated with 100% oxygen. A cold intracellular solution with an osmolarity slightly higher than that of serum is used. Euro-Collin's solution, modified by the addition of magnesium sulfate (4 mEq/L) and 65 mL of 50% dextrose to each liter, is the most commonly used solution. University of Wisconsin (UW) solution has also been used and at some centers appears to provide superior preservation. A volume of 50 to 60 mL/kg donor body weight, delivered via a large bore pulmonary artery cannula over four to five minutes, is the preferred technique of administration (see also Chapter 16).

Extracorporeal core cooling (ECC) has been used primarily for procurement of heart–lung donor blocs, commonly in conjunction with abdominal multiorgan procurement. ECC consists of systemic heparinization of the donor and institution of full cardiopulmonary bypass (CPB) via a transpericardial approach. The donor is cooled to 15°C (rectal temperature). Ventricular fibrillation typically develops during this maneuver and the heart is decompressed via the left ventricle. CPB is then discontinued and the heart–lung bloc is harvested and transported in a cold ischemic state with the lungs inflated. No flush solutions are used, although the lungs are essentially flushed by cooled blood during the time of CPB. Safe ischemic times of six hours or more have been reported with adequate pulmonary function. Interestingly, while oxygenation in lungs preserved by ECC appears to be somewhat less optimal than in those preserved by hypothermic flush techniques, the pulmonary vascular resistance upon reperfusion of the lungs following ECC is generally lower than that seen upon reperfusion of lungs obtained by flush techniques.

The state of inflation of the lungs is an important factor in obtaining optimal perfusion of the pulmonary vasculature by the flush solution, both for the effects of rapid cooling and of direct cellular preservation by the solution itself. Intraoperatively, maintaining a tidal volume similar to that used during the initial donor assessment is important. The addition of PEEP during the procurement procedure maintains FRC and the desired state of inflation of the donor lungs. PEEP also increases the intra-alveolar release of surfactant, minimizing pulmonary compliance abnormalities after implantation of the donor lungs. Ventilation is continued throughout the period of lung perfusion to maintain the effective size of the pulmonary vascular bed. Maintenance of an FIO_2 of 1.0 during the procurement is also useful, particularly at the time of lung extraction, to provide an oxygen-rich ambient environment for metabolic activity of the lung during the ischemic interval. The lungs are extracted and transported in a state of inflation that approximates end-tidal inspiration. Some consideration should be given to the fact that the donor lungs may be transported by aircraft, where a fall in atmospheric pressure may result in further inflation of the lungs. Overinflation of the donor lungs is to be avoided, as this leads to increased capillary permeability and postimplantation pulmonary edema.

The administration of prostanoids, either prostaglandin E_1 (PGE_1) or prostacyclin, into the pulmonary circulation prior to flush perfusion improves lung preservation. The mechanism of action of prostanoids includes dilation of the pulmonary vasculature, allowing for better distribution of the flush solution, and decreased leukocyte adhesiveness, which can abrogate the initial events of reperfusion injury. In North America, PGE_1 most commonly is used as a bolus (500 μg) into the pulmonary circulation, with or without the addition of similar amounts of PGE_1 directly to the flush solution. The use of prostanoids in combination with intracellular flush solutions provides equivalent if not superior pulmonary preservation when compared to the use of extracellular type flush solutions alone.

Most flush solutions are administered at a temperature of 4°C while topical cooling is carried out by filling of the pleural cavity with iced crystalloid solution. After extraction, the lungs are immersed in crystalloid and packed in ice, resulting in a transport temperature of 1°C to 4°C. Some studies have shown that lung preservation is superior when a more moderate hypothermia with a temperature of 10°C is used. However, because of the concerns regarding the deleterious effects of flush and storage temperatures greater than 10°C and the difficulties in maintaining this temperature during the procurement procedure, clinical flush perfusion continues to be performed at the lower temperature ranges.

Experimental work has identified numerous adjuncts to the currently used technique of pulmonary preservation that have the potential for prolonging ischemic intervals. A significant part of the lung injury seen after ischemia has been shown to be due to the phenomenon of reperfusion, which is initiated by leukocyte adhesion to endothelial cells and the production of oxygen-derived free radicals and peroxides. Measures that diminish this response, in addition to the use of prostanoids, include donor leukocyte depletion, the administration of antibodies that block adhesion molecules, the use of inhaled nitric oxide, and the inclusion of oxygen radical scavengers, such as superoxide dismutase or catalase, in the flush solution. In addition, methods of increasing the resistance of cells to ischemic injury, such as the induction of heat shock proteins, have been shown to be beneficial in other organs and may be of some use in lung preservation. Evidence for an impact of these manipulations on tolerable ischemic intervals in clinical lung transplantation awaits additional study (158,159). Until more definitive results become available, clinical practice will likely continue to vary. In a recent worldwide survey of pulmonary graft preservation techniques, most centers indicated use of Euro-Collins solution (77%). Prostaglandin therapy (69%) and donor steroid treatment (32%) were included as adjuncts. Of the 125 centers polled, 15 reported use of UW solution, of which 10 (67%) also used prostaglandin and 7 (47%) employed donor steroids (160).

Whatever preservation technique is used, attempts should be made to minimize graft ischemic times with careful coordination of transport and personnel. This was the conclusion drawn by Snell et al (161) who studied the effect of prolonged pulmonary allograft ischemic time on survival after lung transplantation. They found, through multivariate analysis, that graft ischemic time was an independent predictor of survival. Subgroup analysis noted the effect to be most pronounced beyond five hours.

TECHNIQUES OF LUNG TRANSPLANTATION

Donor Procurement

Cadaver Donor Procurement

After identification of a potential donor, the final assessment of the adequacy of the lung grafts is made intraoperatively by direct inspection, as previously discussed. Most commonly, lung or heart–lung procurement is performed as part of a multiple organ procurement in coordination with a team of abdominal transplant surgeons. The approach to the intrathoracic organs is by a median sternotomy extending into the suprasternal notch, which may be extended into a midline laparotomy for the approach to the abdominal organs. The pericardium is opened vertically and the heart is inspected for evidence of unsuspected congenital anomalies, coronary disease, and wall motion abnormalities. The vena cavae are encircled intrapericardially, as is the ascending aorta. Injury to the right pulmonary artery should be avoided when the superior vena cava (SVC) is surrounded. The pleural spaces are opened sequentially for assessment of the lungs. If a significant unilateral pulmonary abnormality is identified, aspiration of blood from the contralateral superior pulmonary vein to assess gas exchange function is performed at this time.

If the lungs are appropriate for procurement, the posterior pericardium between the superior vena cava and ascending aorta is incised vertically to gain access to the mid trachea. In rare cases, it may be necessary to divide the left brachiocephalic vein to gain further exposure of the airway. A limited amount of circumferential dissection about the trachea is completed, sufficient for two applications of a mechanical stapling device to close both the proximal and distal tracheal segments. Following heparinization, a cardioplegia cannula is placed in the ascending aorta and a large-bore cannula is placed via a purse-string suture in the distal main pulmonary artery. Care should be taken to ensure that the tip of the pulmonary artery cannula does not drift into either the right or the left pulmonary artery and compromise flush perfusion of the contralateral lung (see Chapter 15).

At the time of planned extraction, discussions with the abdominal procurement team should advise them of the hypotension that will accompany prostanoid infusion and a request should be made that the hepatic perfusate be evacuated outside of the right pleural space. Following this, bolus administration of PGE or prostacyclin can be made into either the right atrial appendage or pulmonary artery followed by double ligation of the SVC above the azygous vein. As hypotension ensues, the distal ascending aorta is cross-clamped and infusion of cardioplegic solution is begun. The inferior vena cava is divided above an intrapericardial clamp in order to evacuate the cardioplegic solution. After cardioplegic arrest, the tip of the left atrial appendage is amputated and pulmonary flush is begun. Manipulation of the pulmonary cannula is sometimes necessary to ensure adequate distribution of the flush to the right and left lungs. The effluent is visually inspected and should be essentially clear of blood at the completion of the perfusion. The flush is evacuated into both pleural spaces, with additional iced crystalloid solution used to augment topical cooling of the lungs.

Following completion of flush perfusion, in most cases the heart and lungs will be used for separate recipients. Most centers prefer cardiectomy in situ. In every case, successful use of both cardiac and bilateral lung grafts is possible. The SVC is divided between ligatures, the ascending aorta is divided distal to the cardioplegia cannula and the main pulmonary artery is divided through the cannulation site. The apex of the heart is elevated and retracted to the right, allowing horizontal incision of the left atrium midway between the inferior pulmonary veins. Direct intra-atrial inspection allows completion of the division of the left atrium while preserving a 5-mm cuff of atrial tissue about the confluence of the pulmonary veins on each side. Special attention must be paid to the region of the right superior pulmonary vein, where the amount of tissue between the vein and the interatrial septum is limited, and to the region of the left superior pulmonary vein, to avoid a line of transection too close to the circumflex coronary artery (10).

Extraction of the lungs is carried out by stapling the trachea with a mechanical stapling device at two sites with the lungs in a moderate state of inflation. The stapling device may be left on the distal tracheal stump to assist in further mobilization of the donor bloc. Superior mediastinal tissues, phrenic nerves, and pericardium are divided to the level of the vertebral column on both sides of the mediastinum, as are the diaphragmatic attachments of the pericardium. If plans have been made for bronchial artery revascularization, the great vessels are transected in the anterior mediastinum and the esophagus is transected proximally and distally with a stapling device. The aorta is divided at the diaphragm, allowing removal of all mediastinal contents between the pericardium and the vertebral column, including the azygous vein. If bronchial artery revascularization is not contemplated, the planes of dissection are facilitated by reflecting the lung into the contralateral pleural space. On the right side the mediastinal pleura and other attachments are divided anterior to the esophagus and on the left side these attachments are divided anterior to the descending aorta, dividing the ligamentum arteriosum. The bloc is removed and placed in cold flush solution for subsequent packaging and transport. If both lungs are to be used at separate sites, the bloc may be divided as outlined below; if both will be used at the same recipient site, division of the bloc is performed after arrival at the recipient hospital.

If heart–lung transplantation is planned, in situ cardiectomy is not performed. The entire heart–lung bloc is excised as described above following the planes of dissection outlined for lung extraction if bronchial artery revascularization is not contemplated (see also Chapter 26). At the point of tracheal transection, care is taken to include as much pericarinal tissue as possible to preserve collateral circulation to the bronchus. Upon excision of the heart–lung bloc, inspection of the posterior mediastinal surface should be performed to identify and clip any transected vessels and to apply a topical hemostatic agent such as fibrin glue. Bleeding from the posterior mediastinal tissues following heart–lung transplantation can be a major source of postoperative morbidity.

When isolated lung transplantation is to be performed, the donor bloc is unpackaged upon return to the recipient operating room and placed in cold crystalloid solution. The attached posterior mediastinal tissues are excised and the pericardium posterior to the left atrium is divided inferiorly to superiorly. The posterior wall of left atrium is transected to provide two equal atrial cuffs. The main pulmonary artery is divided at its bifurcation and the right and left pulmonary arteries are dissected free of their pericardial attachments. The subcarinal lymph nodes are divided and the left main bronchus is transected at its origin. The left main bronchus is dissected to within 1 cm of the origin of the left upper lobe and transected. On the right side, following excision of the tracheal carina, the right main bronchus is divided 1 cm proximal to the origin of the right upper lobe bronchus. On both sides, care is taken to avoid excessive dissection of peribronchial tissues that contain important bronchopulmonary collateral circulation.

When en bloc DLT with bronchial artery revascularization is planned, following excision of the lung bloc as described above, the posterior mediastinal tissues are excised with preservation of the anterior wall of the descending thoracic aorta. The right intercostal bronchial artery (RICBA) or the bilateral bronchial artery trunks are identified and an aortic button is fashioned by excision of the remaining aortic wall about this orifice. Next, a saphenous vein graft is sutured to this aortic button for subsequent implantation onto the recipient's aorta. Injection of this vein graft prior to implantation allows identification and ligation of potential posterior mediastinal bleeding sites. For en bloc DLT, no further preparation of the excised double lung bloc is required. In the rare circumstance when SLT is planned using bronchial revascularization, in addition to division of the donor pericardium, left atrium, pulmonary artery, and main bronchus, traction on the aortic button allows mobilization and dissection of the bronchial artery vascular pedicle. In these cases, the aortic button is usually directly anastomosed to the recipient's ascending aorta following lung implantation (10). Information is limited regarding the usefulness of bronchial arterial revascularization during lung transplantation. In small series, methods of revascularization have proved successful and have been associated with good early results, but the experience is mainly with en bloc DLT (162).

Living Donor Procurement

When plans have been made for living donor lung transplantation, the operative approach is via a posterolateral thoracotomy to allow excision of either the right or left lower lobe. The division of the pulmonary fissures is performed using a mechanical stapling device. The inferior pulmonary ligament is divided and the pericardium is opened circumferentially about the inferior pulmonary vein. Dissection of the pulmonary artery is carried out proximal to the right middle lobe or lingular branches on their respective sides. Following heparinization, atraumatic vascular clamps are placed proximal to these branches of the pulmonary artery and on the left atrium distal to the inferior pulmonary venous confluence. Transection of the pulmonary artery is performed obliquely to maximize the opening available for implantation. The left atrium is divided above the vascular clamp. Bronchial transection is performed last to optimize the size of the donor bronchial orifice and to prevent compromise of the orifices of the adjacent right middle lobe or lingula on their respective sides. Following this, the donor lobe is removed, immersed in cold crystalloid solution, hand ventilated using a sterile endotracheal tube and flushed with an intracellular flush solution. The lobe remains in cold crystalloid solution until implantation and no further surgical preparation is required prior to its implantation. The proximal pulmonary artery and left atrium in the donor are closed with running sutures. In some circumstances, the inferior subsegmental branch of the pulmonary artery to the lingula may require ligation (163). The bronchial closure is best performed using a technique of interrupted absorbable sutures followed by coverage with a flap of vascularized tissue (see also Chapter 15).

Anesthetic Management of the Recipient

Proper perioperative management of the recipient is crucial to obtaining the best outcome following lung transplantation. Close cooperation and understanding between the anesthesiology and surgical teams is essential. An appreciation of the unique aspects of the physiology of the various types of lung transplant recipient is also important. Following endotracheal intubation, for example, extreme care should be taken in patients with *COPD* to allow adequate expiratory time for emptying of the lungs, thus avoiding the cardiovascular instability caused by "pulmonary tamponade" due to progressive air trapping in the lungs and reduction of ventricular filling. Tension pneumothorax due to rupture of bullae can also occur but is relatively uncommon. Recipients with pulmonary hypertension or cor pulmonale may not tolerate occlusion of the pulmonary artery during implantation of the donor lung without the support of CPB. Careful and repeated assessment of filling pressures and cardiac output is required to allow prompt interventions in such patients. Oxygen therapy should be continued throughout the time of preoperative preparation and line placement to avoid abrupt right heart dysfunction. Because these patients have normal pulmonary mechanics, they will generally tolerate mechanical ventilation well. It is important to remember that patients with Eisenmenger's syndrome are well adapted to chronic hypoxemia. In these patients, supplemental oxygen will not reverse their hypoxemia and may even worsen their oxygen vasodilation and increased right to left shunting. Those recipients with *septic lung disease* demonstrate primarily an obstructive pulmonary physiology with a less severe tendency to air trapping than COPD patients. However, these recipients have copious, purulent secretions that can exacerbate air trapping and also contribute to marked $\dot{V}/Q$ abnormalities, particularly during single lung ventilation. Careful management of double lumen endotracheal tubes to avoid contamination of the contralateral lung graft and attention to bronchopulmonary hygiene to avoid obstruction of the lumen of these tubes is needed in these patients. Finally, recipients with *pulmonary vascular disease* presenting for transplantation will have marginally compensated cor pulmonale and will be extremely dyspneic and anxious.

Monitoring of multiple physiologic parameters is essential for the management of patients during lung transplantation. A radial arterial line, central venous line, thermodilution pulmonary artery catheter (with oximetry and right ventricular ejection fraction capabilities if possible), and Foley catheter are required. An epidural catheter for postoperative pain management may also be placed if the patient appears to be unlikely to require CPB during the procedure. Placement of the pulmonary artery catheter is preferably done with the patient in a semi-Fowler position, awake and breathing spontaneously so that monitoring of right heart function is possible during the induction of anesthesia. A femoral arterial line may also be needed, particularly in patients who will require CPB. Many centers routinely use transesophageal echocardiography (TEE) to monitor cardiac performance during the procedure. TEE is particularly useful in patients with evidence of cor pulmonale preoperatively. Finally, a variety of vasopressor and vasodilator substances should be mixed and ready prior to the induction of anesthesia. The anesthesiologist must react swiftly to any evidence of cardiovascular instability to avoid a rapid decompensation and cardiovascular collapse.

Endotracheal intubation is carried out after induction of anesthesia using a large single lumen endotracheal tube that allows for flexible bronchoscopy of the recipient. Inspection of the airways, aspiration of as many secretions as possible, particularly in bronchiectasis patients, and lavage to obtain a specimen for microbiologic study are carried out. Following this, in most patients, a left-sided double lumen tube is placed. This provides optimal isolation of the lungs and management of these patients during the procedure. However, when the recipient is of relatively short stature or in pediatric recipients, it may be necessary to use a single lumen endotracheal tube and a Fogarty venous embolectomy catheter as a bronchial blocker to obtain lung isolation (164). The Fogarty catheter is passed into the trachea outside of the cuff of the endotracheal tube and positioned into the appropriate bronchial lumen by flexible bronchoscopy. In all patients, availability of a flexible bronchoscope that can be passed through the endotracheal tube used during the implantation procedure is required to allow for frequent aspiration of secretions and confirmation of tube position.

Induction of anesthesia should be cautious and gradual, as the abrupt withdrawal of the endogenous catecholamine support in these chronically stressed patients may precipitate cardiovascular collapse. After preoxygenation, a routine intravenous induction agent is administered, followed by a synthetic narcotic and a nondepolarizing muscle relaxant. Administration of small amounts of anxiolytic agents is useful during the initial placement of monitoring equipment and continued administration of these agents throughout the procedure will assist in the maintenance of both anesthesia and amnesia. Administration of 100% oxygen throughout the procedure is advisable as is the avoidance of nitrous oxide. Careful use of mechanical ventilation is possible, using the guidelines previously described based on the recipient's underlying disease. A capnograph, which allows assessment of flow volume loops, may be useful in assessing pulmonary compliance and emptying of the lungs during ventilation. There is frequently no substitute, however, for ventilation by the hand of an experienced anesthesiologist to assess changes in pulmonary compliance and to ascertain the optimal pattern of ventilation with respect to oxygenation and hemodynamic parameters. For patients with COPD, it is most useful to use a moderate tidal volume (8 to 10 mL/kg) and higher respiratory rate (15 to 25 bpm), increasing the peak inspiratory flow as needed to optimize expiratory times and lower I:E ratios. Alternatively, for patients with RLD, high peak inspiratory pressures and high respiratory rates are required to maintain effective oxygenation. In most cases, hemodynamics will be optimized by minimizing intrathoracic pressures and augmenting cardiac output by the cautious administration of volume and the use of balanced alpha and beta sympathomimetic agents (e.g., ephedrine or levophed). Excessive β-adrenergic stimulation should be avoided due to concomitant increases in pulmonary vascular resistance. Vasodilator agents should be used cautiously, particularly in patients with Eisenmenger's syndrome. Inhaled nitric oxide (NO) offers the unique advantage, unlike an alternative agent PGE_1, of being a highly selective pulmonary vasodilator with a very limited systemic effect.

Following implantation of the lung graft, hand ventilation to obtain complete reinflation of the lung graft and maintenance of PEEP will maximally reduce pulmonary vascular resistance and can be useful in minimizing postimplantation pulmonary edema. At the conclusion of the transplant procedure, patients are most commonly reintubated with a single lumen endotracheal tube, rebronchoscoped, and transported to the intensive care unit in a sedated, ventilated condition.

All lung transplant procedures should be performed with CPB on standby availability. However, CPB is best avoided in cases of SLD or when there are known extensive intrapleural adhesions to avoid excessive bleeding complications. If CPB is required, the routine use of aprotonin infusions will reduce the likelihood of postoperative hemorrhage due to excessive fibrinolysis and the requirement for transfusion (56). No specific preoperative factors can be used to predict the need for CPB with the exception of either PPH or Eisenmenger's syndrome. For other lung transplant recipients, assessment of the need for CPB is best made intraoperatively by trial clamping of the pulmonary artery followed by assessment of hemodynamic parameters, oximetry, and, if available, ventricular function by TEE. A progressive deterioration in these parameters without stabilization requires unclamping of the pulmonary artery and an attempt to optimize factors such as preload, inotropic support, PaO_2, and pulmonary vascular resistance. If repeat trial clamping of the pulmonary artery is still not tolerated, plans for CPB are made. Cannulation after systemic heparinization is typically via the femoral vessels for SLT and via a transpericardial approach for patients undergoing DLT or HLT.

Single Lung Transplantation

The approach to SLT requires an initial decision regarding the side of implantation. Most commonly, the native lung with the least pulmonary function based on preoperative $\dot{V}/Q$ scans is excised. However, specific technical factors, such as prior pleurodesis, may supersede this factor in some cases. When pulmonary function of the two lungs is equal or when the need for CPB is anticipated, the right side is preferred for the relative ease of surgical exposure of the ascending aorta and right atrium. A right-sided approach also facilitates exposure for closure of intracardiac defects in patients with Eisenmenger's syndrome. Despite the potential differences in size of the right and left hemithorax, there does not appear to be any long-term difference in outcome following right or left SLT.

The exposure for SLT is commonly via a generous posterolateral thoracotomy through the fifth intercostal space or the bed of the excised fifth rib. When elective CPB via the right hemithorax is planned, the use of a fourth interspace may facilitate placement of the cannulae. The ipsilateral groin is included in the operative field in the event that cannulation of the femoral vessels is required for partial CPB. While the use of femoral sites for cannulation requires repair of the vessels after removal of the cannulae, it does provide a site for additional venous drainage when using intrathoracic cannulation sites. Femoral cannulation sites also provide access for conversion to extracorporeal membrane oxygenation (ECMO) support if acute graft failure occurs immediately after implantation. Occasionally, a median sternotomy may be used for right SLT in patients with Eisenmenger's syndrome, when the repair of an associated intracardiac defect requires an anterior approach.

Upon entry into the pleural space, intrapleural adhesions are carefully divided with attention to obtaining hemostasis, particularly when CPB requiring systemic heparinization is contemplated. Following division of the inferior pulmonary ligament, circumferential hilar dissection is completed, carefully avoiding injury to the phrenic and recurrent laryngeal nerves. The pulmonary veins may be either individually isolated or their left atrial confluence may be surrounded intrapericardially at this time. Isolation of the pulmonary artery is completed extrapericardially and assessment is made of the potential need for CPB by trial clamping of the pulmonary artery as outlined previously. Following this, easily accessible upper lobe branches of the pulmonary artery are ligated. This maneuver allows eventual anastomosis of the donor pulmonary artery to a more distal segment of the recipient pulmonary artery, which is frequently a better size match, and also provides a landmark for orientation of the pulmonary artery anastomosis.

After the donor lung is brought to the recipient operating room and inspected, recipient pneumonectomy can be completed. The pulmonary veins are controlled by either individual ligatures or by a clamp on the left atrium prior to their division. A vascular clamp is placed on the proximal pulmonary artery and it is transected. There may be vigorous bleeding from the distal pulmonary artery from collateral bronchial circulation, which is controlled by clamping or ligation of the distal pulmonary artery orifice. Transection of the bronchus is performed at the upper lobe bronchial origin after dissection and ligation of bronchial artery branches and other peribronchial tissue. The recipient bronchus is dissected within the peribronchial tissues to a point within 1 cm of the tracheal carina and then divided.

The donor lung is prepared for implantation, wrapped in sponges soaked with cold crystalloid solution, and placed into the hemithorax. The bronchial anastomosis is performed first. A variety of techniques have been described, but the essential points are to minimize the length of both the donor and recipient bronchus to preserve collateral blood supply and to achieve some degree of anastomotic overlap. The smaller bronchus, most commonly the donor bronchus, is telescoped into the larger bronchus using either a technique of interrupted sutures or a combination of running suture on the membranous wall and interrupted sutures on the anterior wall in a figure-of-eight or horizontal mattress fashion. Polyfilament absorbable suture (e.g., 4-0 polypropylene) may be used. The anastomosis is covered by either local peribronchial tissue or local pedicled flaps of thymic tissue or pericardial fat. See Figure 25.5.

The order of the vascular anastomoses can be varied, although the pulmonary artery anastomosis is frequently the more technically difficult to perform. A continuous 5-0 polypropylene suture is used for each anastomosis, leaving the ends untied for de-airing upon reperfusion of the lung. For the pulmonary artery anastomosis, the length of the donor and recipient vessels requires careful assessment to avoid kinking. For the left atrial anastomosis, the confluence of the recipient pulmonary veins is incised to create a left atrial cuff. Occasionally, dissection in the interatrial groove is required to allow more proximal placement of the vascular clamp on the recipient left atrium. See Figure 25.6. After completion of these anastomoses, the lung is gently reinflated. Perfusion of the lung graft is re-established, initially in an antegrade fashion, evacuating air via the left atrial suture line. The atrial clamp is removed with the atrial suture line under a fluid level to prevent entrainment of air into the left heart. Ventilation of the donor lung is resumed and, after allowing the vascular suture lines to adapt for a few minutes to the distention caused by increased flow, these suture lines are secured. Hemostasis is obtained, two chest tubes are placed and the chest is closed in a standard fashion. Following reintubation with a single lumen tube, flexible bronchoscopy is completed to inspect the bronchial anastomosis and to clear the airway of blood or residual secretions.

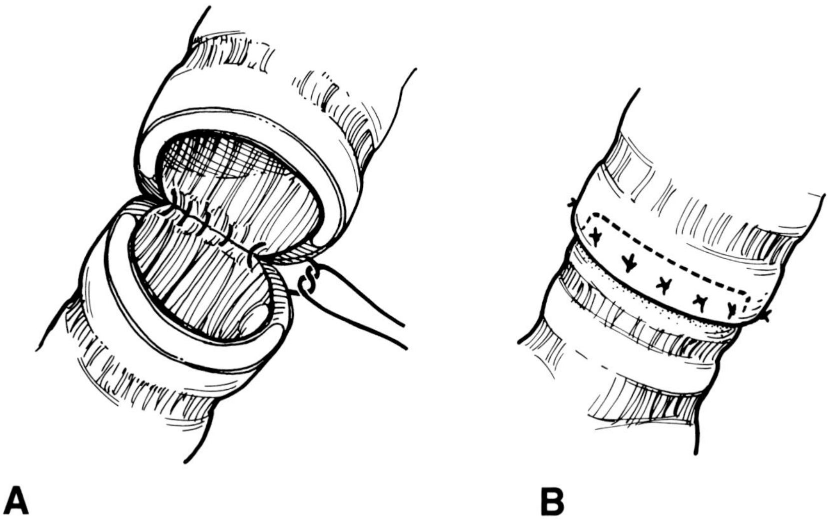

FIGURE 25.5. *Bronchial anastomosis.* ***A****. The blood supply of the donor bronchus is derived from peribronchial collateral vessels communicating with the donor pulmonary vasculature. The recipient bronchus is supplied by the bronchial arterial circulation. For anastomosis, the donor bronchus is shortened to preserve its collateral blood supply and then approximated to the recipient bronchus by initial suturing of the coapted membranous walls.* ***B****. The remainder of the anastomosis is completed by an interrupted suture technique to achieve intussusception of the donor bronchus into the lumen of the recipient bronchus. The recipient bronchus essentially functions as a wrap of vascularized tissue about the anastomotic site (dashed line).*

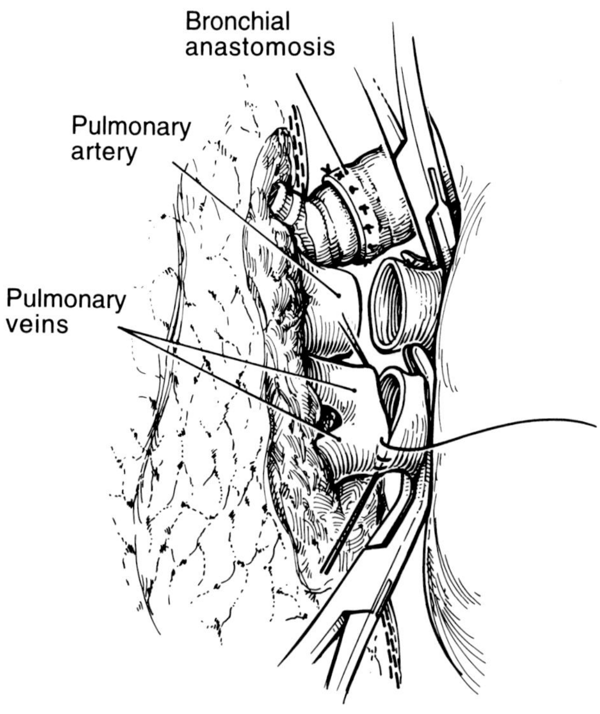

FIGURE 25.6. *Implantation of the lung graft. The recipient bronchus, pulmonary artery, and left atrium containing the pulmonary venous confluence are mobilized within the mediastinum. Bronchial anastomosis is performed first, followed by left atrial and pulmonary arterial anastomosis. The lung graft is reinflated prior to reperfusion, which is carried out in an antegrade fashion initially to minimize reperfusion injury to the graft.*

Double Lung Transplantation

The most frequently performed DLT procedure is a bilateral sequential single lung transplantation. This procedure has a significantly lower incidence of bronchial complications than the en bloc DLT procedure and is technically less difficult to perform than en bloc DLT with simultaneous bronchial artery revascularization. The exposure for bilateral sequential lung transplantation is via bilateral anterior lateral thoracotomies through the fourth or fifth intercostal space, connected by a transverse sternotomy [the so-called clam shell incision (Fig. 25.7)]. The incision provides adequate exposure for mobilization of intrapleural adhesions, even after previous pulmonary resections or pleurodesis, and also provides excellent access for institution of CPB and for correction of intracardiac defects. In most cases, the entire incision is made at the beginning of the procedure and both lungs are completely mobilized. For patients with emphysema undergoing DLT, however, the contralateral hemithorax may be left closed until after implantation of the first lung graft to minimize the tendency to overinflation of the native lung that may occur during the initial implantation procedure. The mobilization and pneumonectomy of the native lung and the implantation of the lung graft are conducted in the same manner as described for SLT. Thymic and anterior mediastinal tissue on a superiorly based vascular pedicle may be mobilized for coverage of the bronchial anastomoses (11,165).

CPB can be instituted via a transpericardial approach using the right atrial appendage for venous drainage and the distal ascending aorta for arterial inflow. It is usually performed at normothermic temperatures. CPB is required in all patients with pulmonary hypertension who undergo DLT and is usually instituted after mobilization of both lungs, prior to pneumonectomy. Maintaining a mean arterial pressure of 60 mm Hg or greater while on CPB may be useful for these patients to preserve perfusion of their thickened ventricular myocardium. When repair of an associated intracardiac defect is required, this is typically done at the start of CPB while the remainder of the implantation procedure is being completed. CPB may be required in some

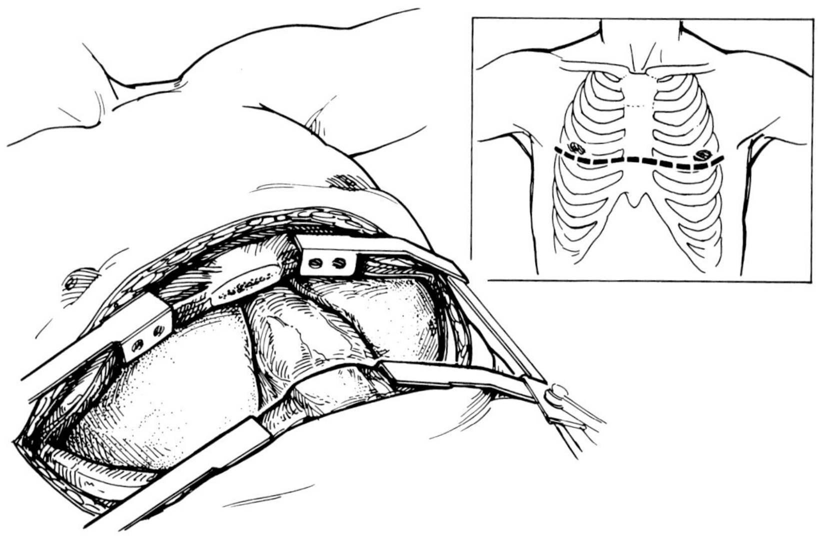

FIGURE 25.7. *Operative approach for double lung transplant. A bilateral anterior transsternal thoracotomy ("clamshell incision") is used, entering the chest through the fourth intercostal space. Following sternal transection, bilateral retractors allow exposure of both hila and pleural spaces. Central access for cardiopulmonary bypass is also available with this exposure.*

patients with septic lung disease or emphysema, usually following implantation of the first lung graft. In these cases, the allograft appears to be unable to tolerate perfusion with the entire cardiac output, with increasing pulmonary artery pressures and interstitial pulmonary edema. Achieving maximal air inflation of the lung graft and aggressive use of vasodilators, such as inhaled nitric oxide, may be useful in these circumstances. Early institution of CPB is recommended in most cases, however, rather than waiting until an emergent situation develops.

Living Donor Transplantation

Living donor lung transplantation is most commonly performed as a bilateral sequential transplant procedure using the "clam shell" incision. CPB is instituted electively after mobilization of the recipient native lungs. Each of the donor lobes is implanted at the recipient hilum. There is typically little size discrepancy between the lobar bronchus and pulmonary vein of the donor, usually an adult, and the main bronchus and left atrium of the typically smaller recipient. The order of the anastomoses (bronchus first) and technique is the same as for cadaveric SLT and DLT. Overinflation of the lobar graft is more likely than with a cadaveric allograft and may contribute to postoperative pulmonary edema. A marked size discrepancy between the lobar allograft and the recipient hemithorax is uncommon, but if present should be treated conservatively—for example, by avoiding chest tube suction—rather than by aggressive surgical measures such as thoracoplasty. In all cases, sufficient remodeling of the thorax and/or hyperinflation of the lobar grafts will occur to obliterate any residual pleural space (163).

The procedure of en bloc DLT as initially described had a 40% incidence of bronchial complications, presumably due to ischemia in the watershed region of the collateral circulation located at the origin of the left main bronchus. However, when en bloc DLT is performed with concomitant bronchial artery revascularization, the incidence of bronchial complications is similar to that of the bilateral sequential type of DLT. A "clam shell" incision or a median sternotomy may be used and only a single lumen endotracheal tube is required. After mobilization of the recipient lungs, incisions are made bilaterally posterior to the phrenic nerves to connect the posterior pericardium and the pleural spaces. After institution of CPB via the right atrium and ascending aorta, bilateral pneumonectomy is carried out by transection of the distal trachea and intrapericardial stapling of the pulmonary veins and left and right pulmonary arteries. The donor lungs are passed into the pleural spaces via the retrophrenic pericardial incisions and a distal tracheal anastomosis is completed. Cardioplegic arrest is achieved and the recipient left atrium is opened, allowing completion of a left atrial anastomosis and, after trimming of the recipient main pulmonary artery, an end-to-end pulmonary artery anastomosis. The donor bronchial arterial circulation is revascularized by either saphenous vein or internal mammary artery grafting to the aortic button containing the origin of the bronchial arteries or by direct implantation of this orifice onto the recipient ascending aorta. The technical requirements of donor procurement for this procedure, as previously described, are formidable and the requisite need for CPB during the implantation procedure increases the perioperative morbidity of this approach. Because of these limitations, wider application of en bloc DLT with bronchial artery revascularization will require demonstration of a significant long-term advantage relative to the technically easier and less morbid bilateral sequential technique of DLT (10).

Heart–Lung Transplantation

The topic of heart–lung transplantation is reviewed in detail in Chapter 26. Either a standard median sternotomy or a "clam shell" incision may be used for HLT. The latter provides better access for mobilization of intrapleural adhesions and is particularly useful for recipients with septic lung disease or prior pulmonary procedures. A single lumen endotracheal tube is used. Normothermic CPB is instituted using bicaval cannulation via the right atrium and cannulation of the distal ascending aorta after mobilization of intrapleural adhesions. Aprotinin infusions are helpful to minimize perioperative bleeding complications. As with CPB for DLT, maintenance of a perfusion pressure of greater than 65 mm Hg is recommended, as is maintaining a cardiac index greater than 2.6 L/min/m^2 and a perfusion hematocrit of greater than 35% by priming the pump circuit with blood. The aorta is transected at the level of the aortic valve commissures and the main pulmonary artery at its midpoint. The right atrial wall and the atrial septum are incised at the atrioventricular junction. After division of the left atrial wall, the heart is removed. The opening of bronchial veins in the posterior wall of the left atrium are oversewn by sutures. The lungs are removed by an extrapericardial approach using successive stapling of the bronchovascular structures at the pulmonary hila. The pulmonary artery stumps are usually left in situ to avoid injury to surrounding nerves, particularly the recurrent laryngeal nerve on the left. The central portions of the main bronchi are mobilized by careful dissection posterior to the phrenic nerve. The airway is not divided until the time of implantation to minimize bacterial contamination. Retrophrenic transpericardial incisions are created, posterior to the stumps of the right pulmonary veins and anterior to the stumps of the left pulmonary veins. The use of stapling devices to perform these maneuvers appears to decrease the incidence of postoperative bleeding.

The donor heart–lung bloc is procured as previously described and inspected upon arrival in the operating room. The donor right atrium is incised from the inferior vena cava to the right atrial appendage. Inspection is made for the presence of an atrial septal defect and for adequate closure of the SVC. If ischemic time has been prolonged, a dose of cardioplegic solution may be administered at this juncture. The donor bloc is positioned by passing the lungs into the pleural spaces via the retrophrenic pedicles. If a supracarinal anastomosis is planned, the posterior pericardium is incised between the ascending aorta and superior vena cava to expose the distal trachea. After trimming the donor and recipient tracheas, a distal tracheal anastomosis is performed. Some centers prefer bilateral bronchial anastomoses at the mediastinal pleural reflection, using a telescoping technique as described for SLT. This approach avoids the need for dissection in the posterior mediastinum and may be associated with fewer anastomotic complications. A line is placed in the left atrial appendage to fill the cardiac chambers and the right atrial anastomosis is completed, followed by aortic anastomosis. The aortic cross clamp is removed and, after reinflation of the lungs, the heart is de-aired via the pulmonary artery and left ventricle. After defibrillation, the patient is weaned from CPB. Inspection for adequate hemostasis is made, with particular attention to bleeding sites from the posterior mediastinum. A pulmonary artery catheter may be inserted for use in monitoring of postoperative hemodynamics (6).

POSTOPERATIVE MANAGEMENT

Monitoring

Patients are transferred to the intensive care unit (ICU) following reintubation with a single lumen endotracheal tube. Universal precautions, including hand washing, masks, and gloves are indicated. Although not a requisite, an isolation room with HEPA-filtration of the ambient air is desirable. The use of these facilities may limit the incidence of fungal infections from extrinsic sources in transplant patients (see Chapter 36). Monitoring should include electrocardiogram, intra-arterial line, pulmonary artery catheter, Foley catheter, and continuous pulse oximetry.

Ventilation

Ventilatory management in most cases follows standard criteria. The FIO_2 is adjusted to maintain a PaO_2 greater than 65 mm Hg. Standard volume ventilation is used with a tidal volume of 12 to 15 mL/kg and PEEP of 5 to 7.5 cm water. Significant barotrauma due to increased airway pressures is extremely uncommon after lung transplantation and higher airway pressures may have a beneficial effect in minimizing postoperative pulmonary edema. Transitioning from volume ventilation to pressure support ventilation prior to extubation may be useful to decrease the work of breathing and serves to minimize compliance differences between the native lung and allograft following SLT. Appropriate management of postoperative pain is also helpful in weaning these patients from the ventilator. A functional thoracic epidural catheter is useful, although intravenous narcotics administered via a patient-controlled analgesia approach may be used after the patient achieves a conscious state. Anti-inflammatory adjuncts to control pain are best avoided because of potential additive nephrotoxicity with the perioperative antimicrobial and immunosuppressive regimen. Extubation is performed when the patient has a normal mental status and has achieved a reasonable rate of ventilation and spontaneous tidal volume, typically 48 to 72 hours after the procedure. Maintaining good bronchopulmonary hygiene with frequent endotracheal aspiration of secretions and physiotherapy is important in achieving and maintaining extubation in these patients.

Patients with emphysema who undergo SLT are an exception to the above guidelines. These patients require particular attention to airway pressures and the compliance differential between the allograft and the native lung. Hyperinflation of the native lung will not only result in compromise of cardiac filling, but will progressively interfere with ventilation of the allograft. Efforts to control hyperinflation of the native lung include using slightly lower tidal volumes (9 to 12 mL/kg) accompanied by higher respiratory rates to preserve minute ventilation and lower levels of PEEP (1 to 3 cm water). Positioning of the patient with the native lung down may further increase the impedance of that hemithorax and limit hyperinflation, although increased blood flow to the native lung induced by this maneuver may require adjustment of ventilatory parameters to maintain satisfactory gas exchange. In rare circumstances, when marked edema has occurred in the allograft, independent lung ventilation using a double lumen endotracheal tube may be needed (Fig. 25.8). In such cases, more rapid ventilation of the allograft with smaller tidal volumes, using PEEP and higher inspiratory flow rates, will provide carbon dioxide clearance while ventilation of the native lung at very low rates (e.g., four breaths per minute), with standard volumes and no PEEP, will maintain oxygenation but minimize hyperinflation.

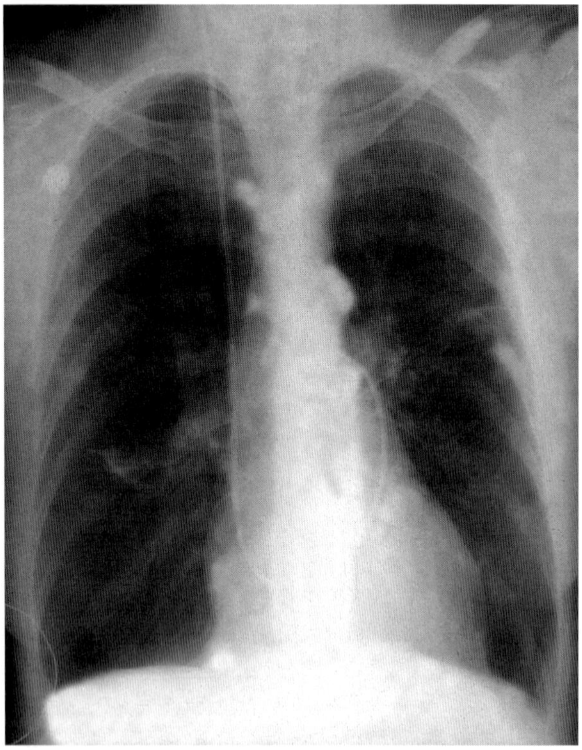

A

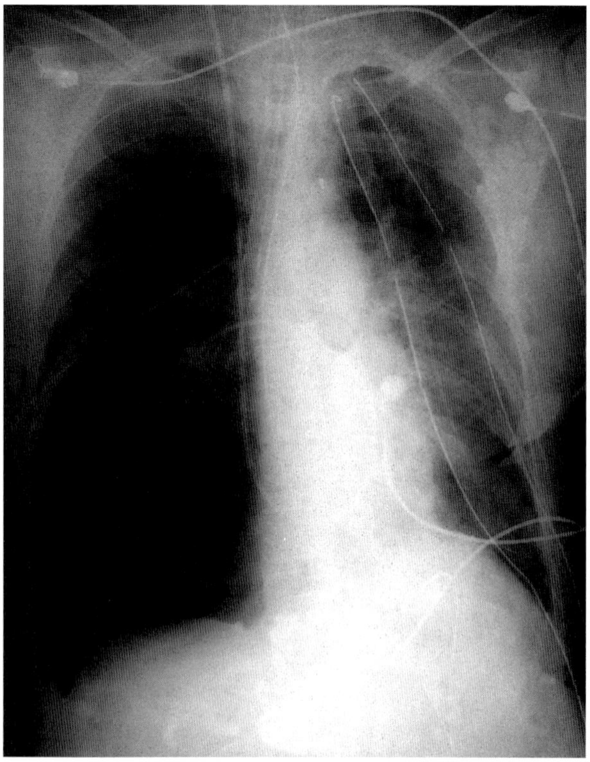

B

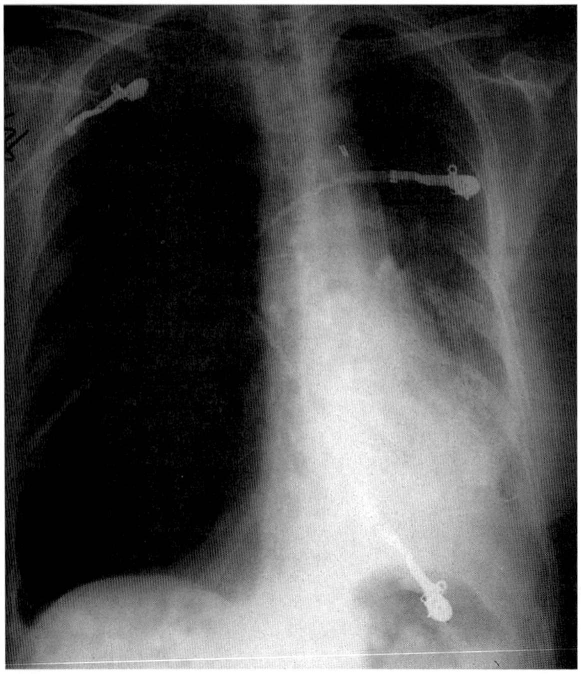

C

FIGURE 25.8. *Chest radiographs of a patient with emphysema. Treated with dual asynchronous mechanical ventilators following acute graft dysfunction.* ***A****. Preoperative radiograph of patient with end-stage emphysema secondary to alpha-1-antitrypsin deficiency. Note hyperinflation and bullous disease mainly at bases.* ***B****. Postoperative radiograph of patient shown in* ***A****, with acute allograft dysfunction in the left lung. Independent ventilation using a double lumen endotracheal tube allowed for high level PEEP therapy, low tidal volumes, and relatively higher respiratory rate in the poorly compliant allograft. The native lung was ventilated at lower level of PEEP, with larger tidal volumes and at a slower rate. Complications due to auto-PEEP were minimized.* ***C****. Radiograph of patient in* ***A*** *and* ***B*** *three days later. The patient was converted to a single ventilator as she improved. Eventually, she recovered completely.*

Patients with significant pulmonary hypertension who undergo lung transplantation have a unique postoperative physiology, as noted above. The right ventricles in these patients have been conditioned to generate peak systolic pressures against a markedly elevated pulmonary vascular resistance (PVR). Following lung transplantation, an abrupt near-normalization of the PVR occurs accompanied by improved ventricular hemodynamics. With minimal catecholamine stimulation, as seen upon awakening from anesthesia or weaning from a ventilator, the right ventricle in these patients responds by generating a peak systolic pressure similar to that required preoperatively. The resultant abrupt rise in pulmonary artery pressure, in combination with increased capillary permeability (due to ischemia and reperfusion injury) and the absence of lymphatic continuity, causes rapid fluid accumulation in the donor lung. This pulmonary edema is typically of very rapid onset and results in hypoxia and additional rises in pulmonary artery pressure. Preemptive treatment for this condition is necessary and involves maintaining a high degree of sedation, or even of muscular paralysis, in the first three to five days postoperatively. This approach serves to minimize catecholamine stimulation during the time in which the ischemic and reperfusion injury in the allograft is resolving. Minimizing other stimuli to right ventricular output, such as hypercarbia or hypoxia, within the first few days following transplantation is also beneficial. Following this period, patients can be cautiously awakened and ventilatory weaning can proceed using standard methods while closely monitoring cardiac output, blood gases, and pulmonary artery pressures. In some cases, additional measures such as low dose beta blockade to diminish myocardial contractility or intravenous anxiolytic therapy may be required if significant hemodynamic abnormalities persist.

Fluid Management

The goal of fluid management following lung transplantation is to minimize the accumulation of edema fluid in the implanted lung while maintaining optimal cardiac function. As previously noted, the effects of ischemia, reperfusion injury, and lymphatic discontinuity all contribute to a tendency toward pulmonary edema in the lung graft. Pulmonary artery pressures and pulmonary artery occlusion ("wedge") pressures need to be kept as low as possible postoperatively without compromising ventricular preload. Continuous hemodynamic monitoring and accurate intake-output measurements are needed during this early postoperative period to make the necessary adjustments in rates of fluid administration, pressor, and diuretic therapy to achieve this goal. Most patients have an increase in total body water immediately postoperatively, but may be relatively depleted intravascularly. Transfusion with red blood cells and colloid is recommended to maintain a hematocrit greater than 30% and a serum albumin level greater than 3.0 g/dL as initial measures in these circumstances. For most patients, the effects of a reduction in PVR almost immediately following lung transplantation results in improved right ventricular, and secondarily left ventricular, performance. Some inotropic support may be required, however, in patients who have preexisting right ventricular hypertrophy, particularly when pressure overload of the right ventricle occurs during the implantation procedure or following CPB. In these cases, inotropic stimulation is required, using pure beta agents such as dobutamine or balanced alpha and beta agents such as dopamine or levophed, to optimize cardiac output in the face of a reduced preload relative to the preoperative state.

Concomitant renal dysfunction as a result of the preoperative status of the recipient may further complicate fluid management postoperatively. A low cardiac output state, prolonged central venous hypertension, or the chronic use of nephrotoxic antibiotics or diuretics prior to transplantation may have adverse effects on glomerular filtration rate. The liberal use of diuretic therapy and the use of agents to improve renal perfusion (e.g., low-dose dopamine or venodilators) are helpful in the management of these patients. After stabilization and extubation of the lung transplant patient, ongoing loss of lean body mass occurs as expected for patients in a postoperative stress state. At this point, daily recording of body weight is useful in assessing fluid balance. Weight loss of up to 10% of preoperative lean body mass is typical in the first four weeks following lung transplantation. Continued diuretic therapy is usually required during this interval to maintain a nonedematous state.

Antimicrobial Therapy

Bacterial prophylaxis involves prophylaxis against gram-positive organisms in combination with a broad spectrum antibiotic to provide appropriate coverage for organisms identified preoperatively from the sputum of the recipient. Recipients who have been recently hospitalized and, therefore, exposed to respiratory therapy equipment, or those with cystic fibrosis, will require coverage for *Pseudomonas*, usually with ceftazidime. For CF patients, ongoing surveillance of sputum flora and determination of antibiotic sensitivities is important in the waiting period prior to transplantation to develop an appropriate multidrug antimicrobial regimen for use perioperatively. The addition of inhaled antimicrobial therapy, either tobramycin or colistin, can have additive effects in the management of *Pseudomonas* in these patients. Postoperative antibacterial coverage should be modified if pathogens are identified in the sputum of the donor that are not already covered by the recipient-specific regimen.

Routine prophylaxis for fungal organisms is useful when preoperative recipient sputum cultures have demonstrated the presence of *Aspergillus* at any time preceding the transplant procedure, when there has been evidence of heavy overgrowth of yeast (e.g., *Candida*) in the donor sputum culture, or when cytolytic induction immunosuppression is used. In the case of *Aspergillus*, prophylactic therapy requires the use of amphotericin B, while in the latter instances fluconazole or low-dose ketoconazole therapy is effective.

The incidence of herpes simplex infection, including mucosal ulceration and pneumonitis, has been eliminated by the routine use of acyclovir prophylaxis after lung transplantation. Cytomegalovirus (CMV) infection, however, remains a significant problem following lung transplantation. Infection with CMV results in incorporation of the viral DNA into the host genome. Immunosuppression induces the replication of CMV in tissues that have been previously infected with the virus, and this virus may then spread to other uninfected tissues. The incidence of CMV infection following lung transplantation is related to the preoperative CMV status of both the donor (D) and recipient (R). A discordant CMV status between the donor and the recipient may result in either primary infection of the donor lungs by the recipient (in the case of D−/R+) or in the more serious circumstance of primary systemic CMV infection (in the case of D+/R−). In either case, the incidence of acute and chronic rejection and of mortality is higher in mismatched patients than among patients in whom CMV status is concordant. For this reason, many centers prefer to match D and R status. However, the use of ganciclovir prophylaxis decreases the incidence of primary disease and improves the outcome of CMV-disparate lung transplants. Prophylactic ganciclovir therapy should be resumed whenever immunosuppression is augmented to treat episodes of acute rejection in CMV-disparate patients. At some centers, CMV-negative recipients who receive lungs from CMV-positive donors also are treated with CMV hyperimmune globulin, given their high risk of developing severe disease.

Pneumocystis carinii pneumonia (PCP) in lung transplant patients has been markedly reduced by the routine use of sulfamethoxazole-trimethoprim (Bactrim, one single-strength tablet every day) beginning one week postoperatively. Alternative treatments recommended for patients with sulfa allergy, such as aerosolized pentamidine, appear to be less effective. Figure 25.9 is an example of failure of aerosolized pentamidine to prevent PCP in a patient following SLT for emphysema. In this case, the infection involved the native emphysematous lung, but not the allograft. Presumably, the differential distribution of ventilation, and hence drug delivery, favors the well functioning graft, leaving the native lung vulnerable to infection. Sulfa desensitization is frequently possible in these patients and is recommended given the efficacy of sulfa prophylaxis (see also Chapter 26).

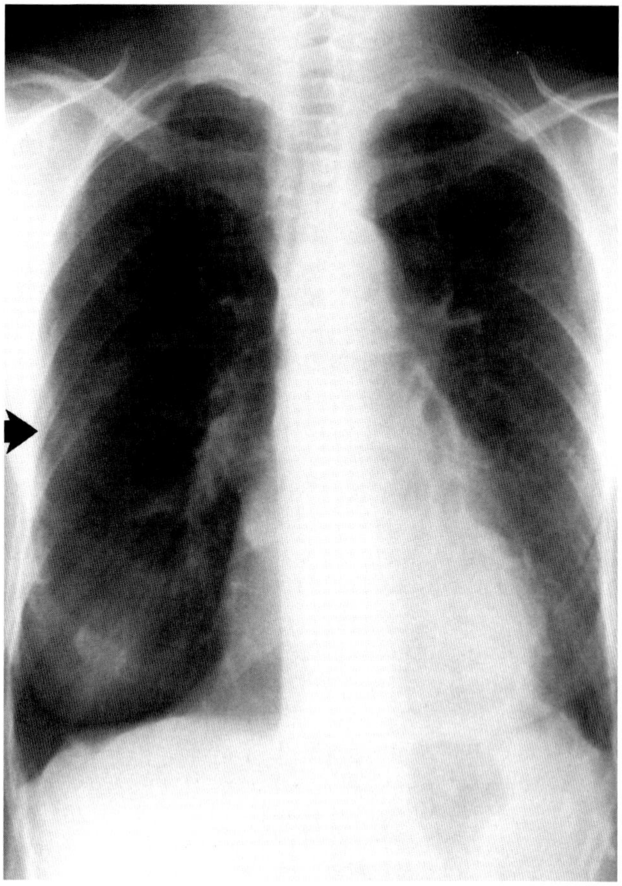

FIGURE 25.9. *Chest radiograph of a patient with* Pneumocystis carinii *pneumonia (PCP) in native lung. The patient underwent isolated single left lung transplant for emphysema. She was allergic to sulfa and unable to be desensitized. Aerosolized pentamidine was therefore used as prophylaxis against PCP. This figure illustrates an irregular infiltrate in the native right lung* (arrow) *at a time when the patient developed fever and dyspnea, and had a decline in lung function. Bronchoalveolar lavage and transbronchial lung biopsy led to the diagnosis of PCP for which she was treated with systemic therapy with success.*

Nutrition

Maintaining optimal nutrition in the postoperative period is a useful adjunct for improving operative outcomes. Most patients can resume oral intake following extubation, although dietary consultation should be obtained by the second postoperative week to assess the adequacy of caloric intake. Frequently, the addition of liquid nutritional supplements (e.g., Ensure) will be required to meet caloric requirements for the postoperative state. When prolonged ventilatory support is required, the use of intravenous hyperalimentation or, preferably, enteral alimentation via a nasogastric feeding tube is mandatory. Patients with cystic fibrosis will often have a malabsorptive syndrome that will require resumption of preoperative pancreatic enzyme supplementation. These patients have difficulty absorbing medications such as cyclosporine, a circumstance that may be improved by the intake of bile salts (e.g., ursodeoxycholic acid 300 mg prior to each cyclosporine dose). Finally, CF patients are prone to both gastroparesis and meconium ileus equivalent, both of which may be avoided by the use of promotility agents (e.g., metaclopramide 10 mg IV four times a day) and a cathartic bowel regimen (e.g., Go-Lytely 300–500 mL twice a day).

Immunosuppression

The induction of a state of relatively nonspecific immune suppression by pharmacologic means has been the key to successful clinical lung transplantation. While the ideal method would be to achieve specific, permanent tolerance of the allograft without the need for chronic medication, this is presently not possible (see Chapter 5). As a result, while the current regimens lead to satisfactory control of most acute rejection processes, the combined side effects of these medications and their incomplete ability to control chronic rejection in the lung account for the major long-term morbidity and mortality associated with lung transplantation.

The immunosuppressive regimens used for lung transplantation are based on the successful protocols that have evolved for renal and heart transplantation. Virtually all centers use a three-drug regimen for immunosuppression, with the hope of obtaining additive effects in terms of immune suppression while limiting drug toxicities. While most centers use a combination of cyclosporine (CYA), azathioprine (AZA), and steroids for this purpose, a recent report substituting tacrolimus (FK-506) for cyclosporine has suggested a greater efficacy with this combination in the control of rejection (166). Most lung transplant programs use steroids as part of the regimen for the induction of immunosuppression, although some centers have used cytolytic therapies for this purpose and have subsequently found a reduced incidence of episodes of acute rejection in these patients.

Intraoperatively, methylprednisolone (10–15 mg/kg) is typically administered prior to reperfusion of the lung graft. Postoperatively, in the absence of cytolytic induction therapy, moderate dose corticosteroid therapy (methylprednisolone 0.5–1.0 mg/kg/day IV) is used in combination with CYA and AZA for induction immunosuppression. A dose of prednisone (0.5 mg/kg/day IV) is used in combination with CYA and AZA for induction immunosuppression. An oral dose of prednisone (0.5 mg/kg/day) is usually begun on postoperative day 5 to 7. Although corticosteroids have profound inhibitory effects on wound healing, their use in the immediate postoperative period in this fashion has not adversely affected the outcomes of lung transplantation. The prednisone dosage is gradually reduced over the first 9 to 12 months postoperatively to achieve a dose of 0.2–0.25 mg/kg every other day.

Various antilymphocytic antibody preparations, so-called cytolytic therapies, have been used in clinical lung transplantation. Both polyclonal preparations, such as antilymphocyte globulin (ALG) and antithymocyte globulin (ATG), and a murine monoclonal antibody to the CD3 complex of human lymphocytes (OKT-3) have been used (see Chapter 13). Initially, it was felt that strict avoidance of steroids in the early postoperative period was needed to ensure satisfactory healing of the bronchial anastomosis. As a result, cytolytic therapy was felt to be necessary to induce immunosuppression prior to the initiation of steroid therapy in the second postoperative week. The subsequent demonstration that moderate dose corticosteroid therapy was well tolerated immediately after lung transplantation, as described above, as well as concerns regarding the risks of cytolytic therapy resulted in the majority of centers reserving the use of these agents for the treatment of refractory acute rejection. All of these cytolytic preparations are associated initially with fever, chills, and an increased capillary permeability that may predispose to pulmonary edema (see Chapter 30). With the polyclonal preparations, leukopenia and thrombocytopenia may be also be seen, as well as a serum sickness-like reaction consisting of skin rash and arthralgias (see Chapter 13). With OKT-3, the proportional lymphocyte count will usually fall to less than 3% of the total white blood cell count, although assays of T-cell subsets are needed to document specifically a therapeutic effect. Occasionally, the initial dose of OKT-3 (5 mg/day IV) may need to be increased depending on the results of these studies. An antimouse antibody response will occur with OKT-3 administration, which limits its effectiveness after 10 to 14 days of therapy and effectively prevents its use for a second course of therapy in most instances.

The two major concerns regarding the use of cytolytic therapy have been the increased incidence of CMV disease and the incidence of post-transplant lymphoproliferative disorder (PTLD). CMV disease can be effectively eliminated by several strategies, including matching of donor and recipient CMV status and the use of prophylactic ganciclovir, as discussed previously. The incidence of PTLD may also be minimized by the use of ganciclovir, which has additional effects against the Epstein-Barr virus, the likely etiology of PTLD in most cases (23,167) (see also Chapter 37).

Tacrolimus (FK506) is a macrolide compound with a mechanism of action similar to that of CYA, through an immunophilin protein called the FK binding protein (FKBP). It is discussed in detail in Chapter 9. As noted, tacrolimus is 100 times as potent as CYA in inhibiting the mixed lymphocyte reaction and concentrates in tissues, leading to levels in the lung that are eight-fold those of the plasma. Tacrolimus has been used for induction immunosuppression in lung transplant recipients as part of a three-drug regimen with AZA and steroids, and as a rescue therapy for patients with refractory rejection on a standard three-drug regimen (CYA, AZA, steroids). Tacrolimus is usually begun immediately postoperatively at a dosage of 0.025 mg/kg/d IV by continuous infusion and adjusted to achieve a blood level of 10 to 20 ng/mL by commercial assay (Abbott Inc.). Oral dosage is 0.15 mg/kg twice a day, adjusting for similar blood levels. Toxicity is similar to CYA and includes reversible renal dysfunction, hypertension, and neurotoxicity. New-onset diabetes mellitus has also been reported. Hypertrichosis and gingival hyperplasia have not been seen with tacrolimus. In a randomized trial in lung transplant patients of three-drug regimens containing either CYA or tacrolimus, the incidence of postoperative fungal infections was higher in patients receiving tacrolimus.

Despite immunotherapy, some patients may suffer from refractory acute allograft rejection or develop the syndrome of chronic rejection, including bronchiolitis obliterans. These complications, discussed in detail below, call for adjustment in immune suppression. High doses of "pulsed" methylprednisolone are frequently employed and acute cellular rejection may be ameliorated but, in some cases, not completely reversed (168). In selected instances, cytolytic therapy may reverse or at least stabilize the decrement in lung function that occurs in this setting (169). An alternative strategy is to use tacrolimus in those patients who have not previously received this treatment. In a multicenter US trial that included 15 lung transplant recipients, tacrolimus was used as a "rescue" immunosuppressant with some success (170). Rose et al (171) also found stabilization of spirometric indices in some patients who were converted to a tacrolimus-based regimen as rescue therapy for obliterative bronchiolitis after lung transplantation. Horning et al (172) also have concluded, on the basis of a retrospective analysis of a small number of patients, that tacrolimus is a viable alternative to cyclosporine when rejection problems persist. Other options reported for treating steroid-resistant acute rejection of the lung include total lymphoid irradiation (173) and photopheresis (174), which are discussed in Chapter 14, as well as methotrexate (175) and aerosolized cyclosporine (176,177).

Other immunosuppressive drugs currently undergoing clinical trials include rapamycin and mycophenolate mofetil (MMF). Experience with lung transplant patients is limited, however. Extensive review of these drugs is found in Chapters 10 and 11.

MMF is an ester prodrug of the active immunosuppressant mycophenolic acid. The latter is a noncompetitive reversible inhibitor of the enzyme inosine monophosphate dehydrogenase, which is necessary for de novo synthesis of guanosine nucleotides. T and B lymphocytes are dependent on this pathway for purine biosynthesis, whereas most other proliferating cells can also utilize the "salvage" pathway. In this way, MMF can selectively inhibit T- and B-cell proliferation, providing a theortical advantage over AZA. Preliminary experience with MMF suggests that it may be useful both as primary therapy after transplantation and rescue treatment for patients with recurrent episodes of acute rejection.

Ross et al (178) conducted a pilot two-center concurrent cohort study to assess MMF versus AZA in a triple drug immunosuppressive regimen after lung transplantation. The MMF group received 2.0 g/day in two divided doses beginning immediately after transplantation, whereas the AZA group received 1–2 mg/kg/day to maintain an absolute white blood cell count of 4000 or greater. The principal findings of this study were a decreased incidence of acute cellular rejection for the MMF versus AZA cohort and better spirometric function in the MMF group during the first 12 months. A trend was noted for decreased bronchiolitis obliterans syndrome in the MMF-treated group. Limitations to this study include the rather small number of patients and lack of randomization.

A potential role for MMF in reducing the rate of acute rejection episodes after lung transplantation was supported by O'Hair et al (179) in their preliminary experience. Thirteen patients received MMF as primary therapy immediately after transplantation and had a lower rate of acute rejection in the first 3 postoperative months than did historical controls treated with AZA-based immunosuppression. Nonetheless, limitations of this study must be recognized, including the small number of patients, lack of randomization, and lack of blinding of the investigators.

Lack of rigorously designed scientific studies hinder knowledge regarding the use of MMF for patients with bronchiolitis obliterans syndrome. Nonetheless, Whyte et al (180) have suggested that the use of MMF in this setting is generally well tolerated and associated with stabilization of pulmonary function.

COMPLICATIONS OF LUNG TRANSPLANTATION

Complications of lung transplantation can be classified into three broad categories: 1) complications of the operation itself, 2) immunologic complications, and 3) complications of the immunosuppressive agents used to prevent rejection, including infection, malignancy, and direct side effects of the medications. The accumulation of experience with lung transplant patients has allowed for delineation of the usual clinical presentations of the major complications in each of these categories, as well as of their usual times of presentation, which are presented in Table 25.13. The remainder of this chapter describes the clinical presentations of the major lung transplant-related complications, as well as strategies for their prevention, early diagnosis, and treatment.

Complications of the Operation Itself

In the first two weeks following lung transplantation, the greatest cause of morbidity and mortality are complications due to the transplant operation itself (181). These early complications include those related to the lung transplant operations specifically, such as the reimplantation response and airway anastomotic complications, and those complications related to thoracic surgical operations generally. The latter include pain, phrenic nerve dysfunction, retained bronchial secretions and mucous plugging, atelectasis, pneumonia, persistent air leaks, tension and nontension pneumothoraces, hemorrhage, respiratory failure, and cardiac and hemodynamic complications (182,183). Therapies of certain of these general thoracic surgical complications must be modified for the lung transplant recipient. For example, concern about healing of the airway anastomosis limits endotracheal suc-

Table 25.13. Timing of Major Complications Following Lung Transplantation

Time Postoperatively	Complications of Operation General to Thoracic Surgery	Complications of Operation Specific to Lung Transplantation	Rejection	Infection	Malignancy
0 to 4 weeks	Retained bronchial secretions and mucous plugging Atelectasis Persistent air leaks Pneumothorax Hemorrhage Atrial arrhythmias Myocardial infarction Cardiac arrest	Reimplantation response Airway dehiscence Systemic hypotension Adynamic ileus Diaphragmatic hernia	Hyperacute rejection Acute rejection	Bacterial pneumonia Fungal infections Wound and line infections	
2 to 3 months		Airway stenosis	Acute rejection	Bacterial pneumonia Fungal infections	Post-transplant lymphoproliferative disorder
4 to 6 months				Viral infections, including CMV and RSV *Pneumocystis carinii* pneumonia	
>6 months			Acute rejection Chronic rejection	Mycobacterial infections	

tioning to the airways proximal to the anastomosis. Retained bronchial secretions and mucous plugging distal to the anastomosis are treated instead with frequent therapeutic flexible bronchoscopies, usually performed daily, or even more frequently, in the early postoperative period.

Surgical Procedure Complications

Major technical complications following lung transplantation have become increasingly rare with improvements in operative technique and perioperative management. *Pulmonary artery obstruction* can occur as a result of anastomotic stenosis, kinking, or extrinsic compression. Persistent pulmonary hypertension and unexplained hypoxemia may be evident in these cases. Attention to anatomic factors, such as the length of the donor and recipient pulmonary artery and division of the pericardial attachments surrounding the donor pulmonary artery, as well as awareness of the potential for a flap wrapping the bronchial anastomosis to compress the adjacent anastomosis helps to avoid these problems. *Left atrial anastomotic obstruction* can also occur due to faulty anastomotic technique or to extrinsic compression by clot, pericardium, or an omental flap. This problem results in more severe abnormalities than pulmonary artery obstruction, including marked pulmonary hypertension and ipsilateral pulmonary edema. Diagnostic methods for these vascular anastomotic complications include routine intraoperative measurement of anastomotic gradients and TEE, which is particularly helpful in assessing the left atrial anastomosis. Postoperatively, diagnostic measures include contrast angiography and ventilation/perfusion scanning. Reoperation and correction of the anastomosis is indicated if clinical compromise is apparent, which is particularly likely if there is significant left atrial anastomotic obstruction.

Hemorrhage

The underlying pulmonary disease of lung transplant recipients frequently leads to the formation of dense pleural adhesions and the hypertrophy of the bronchial circulation. These changes may promote hemorrhage following the removal of the recipient's native lung(s). Any degree of hemorrhage that occurs can be exacerbated by the anticoagulation necessary for cardiopulmonary bypass, which is required during some transplant operations. The incidence of major hemorrhage has been reduced by the use of aprotinin as a hemostatic and the use of a transverse, or "clamshell," incision rather than a median sternotomy in double lung transplant recipients, which allows better visualization of the pleural surface and posterior mediastinum (184).

Reimplantation Response

The reimplantation response has been defined broadly as "the morphologic, roentgenographic, and functional changes that occur in a lung transplant in the early postoperative period as a result of surgical trauma, ischemia, denervation, lymphatic interruption, and other injurious processes (exclusive of rejection) that are unavoidable aspects of the transplant operation." The reimplantation response presents with the triad of worsened gas exchange, decreased lung compliance, and alveolar and interstitial infiltrates, typically most extensive in perihilar regions. It is extremely common, occurring in the majority of patients (185,186), and present within hours to days of operation. A perihilar infiltrate in

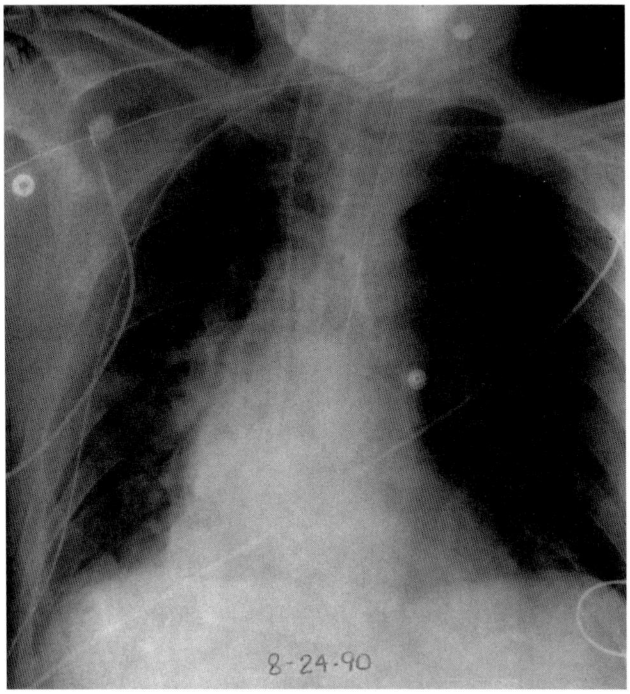

FIGURE 25.10. *Chest x-ray of a patient with perihilar infiltrate in transplanted right lung on postoperative day 3. The infiltrates and the timing of its occurrence are typical of the "reimplantation response."*

the transplanted right lung typical of the reimplantation response is demonstrated in Figure 25.10, which shows the chest x-ray of a patient on postoperative day 3. The same patient's chest x-ray on postoperative day 1, prior to the development of the reimplantation response, is shown in Figure 25.11 for comparison.

Treatment is supportive, with mechanical ventilation, and diuretics and fluid-restriction as tolerated. Although the reimplantation response can cause severe hypoxemia and prolong the need for mechanical ventilation, the typical course is marked by progressive clearing to complete resolution within several days to several weeks. Figure 25.12 shows the chest x-ray of the patient described above on postoperative day 4, demonstrating early resolution of the previously seen reimplantation response with supportive care, including the judicious use of diuretics. However, a minority of patients who develop the reimplantation response go on to develop adult respiratory distress syndrome (ARDS) attributed to the initial reperfusion injury (187). Development of ARDS unilaterally in single lung transplant recipients can make the ventilatory requirements of the transplanted lung differ dramatically from those of the remaining native lung. Some of these patients have benefited from the use of two separate ventilators to ventilate independently each lung.

Some transplanted lungs will demonstrate *acute graft dysfunction*, even without evidence of vascular anastomotic complications. As many as 20% of patients will have severe

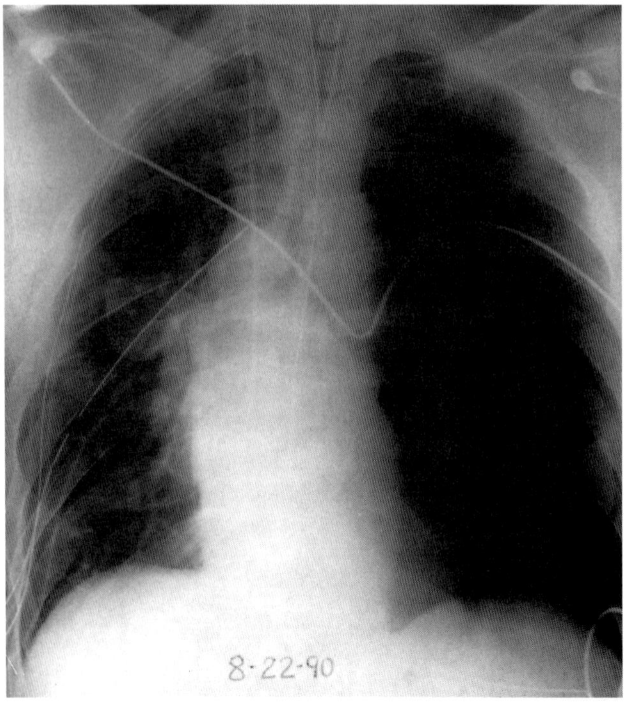

FIGURE 25.11. *Chest x-ray of the same patient as in Figure 25.10 on postoperative day 1 following single lung transplantation of the right lung. The patient's severe underlying emphysema is demonstrated in the hyperexpanded left lung. The transplanted right lung appears clear.*

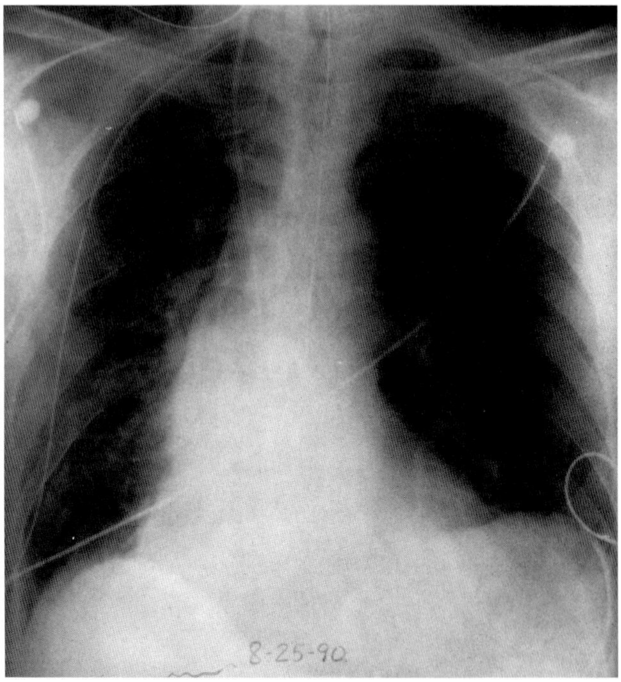

FIGURE 25.12. *Chest x-ray of the same patient as in Figures 25.10 and 25.11 on postoperative day 4, demonstrating resolution of the reimplantation response seen previously in the transplanted right lung, with supportive care, including the judicious use of diuretics.*

early abnormalities of lung function, with rapidly progressive pulmonary edema, persistent pulmonary hypertension, and a markedly diminished pulmonary compliance occurring rapidly after graft implantation. This process is to be differentiated from the reimplantation response, described above, which is seen in almost all patients at 36 to 96 hours post-transplant and consists of perihilar and peribronchiolar edema. Acute graft dysfunction is due in some cases to unsuspected donor lung abnormalities, such as aspiration or contusion, while in other cases it may be due to inadequate pulmonary preservation. Most commonly, however, no etiology is found. Management includes evaluation of the vascular anastomoses, to rule out a potentially correctable, technical complication, and maintenance of oxygenation using volume ventilation and PEEP. As previously noted, excluding patients with emphysema who have undergone SLT, increases in airway pressures are unlikely to induce barotrauma following lung transplantation and may serve to limit the accumulation of edema fluid in the lung graft. Minimizing elevations in pulmonary artery pressures by correction of blood gas and acid-base abnormalities and by pharmacologic interventions such as the use of inhaled nitric oxide (which also improves intrapulmonary $\dot{V}/Q$ matching) are beneficial. The use of sedation with or without muscular paralysis can also aid in optimizing lung function and ventilatory support. Despite these maneuvers, acute graft dysfunction (or *primary graft failure*) can be an extremely serious complication. Christie et al (188) have noted that it is associated with a high mortality rate, lengthy hospitalization, and protracted and often compromised recovery among survivors.

When there is a marked compliance difference between the native lung and the lung graft, independent lung ventilation using a double lumen endotracheal tube, as mentioned above, should be considered. ECMO will be needed for the management of less than 5% of these patients. ECMO, instituted using arteriovenous routes, provides optimal gas exchange and allows decompression of the pulmonary circulation. Complete diversion of pulmonary arterial flow via the ECMO circuit should be avoided, however, as the lung graft will not have a native bronchial arterial circulation and some antegrade pulmonary flow is required to maintain graft viability. In most cases, regardless of the supportive measure required, the process will resolve over several days with satisfactory long-term graft function (189).

Pleural Complications

Pleural space complications are not uncommon after lung transplantation, although they are usually of minor importance. *Pneumothorax* may occur on either the side of a lung graft or on the side of a native lung. Pneumothoraces that arise from the lung graft are of greatest concern because of the possibility of airway dehiscence communicating with the pleural space. Fortunately, this is a rare occurrence, but flexible bronchoscopy is always indicated for diagnostic purposes in patients presenting with this problem. In most cases, placement of a chest tube with re-expansion of the lung will limit the process acutely. More commonly, pneumothorax is the result of rupture of a bullous lesion in an emphysematous native lung after SLT. Conservative management with intercostal tube drainage is indicated. Occasionally, pneumothoraces will be noted after DLT when a significant size discrepancy exists between the donor lungs and the recipient thorax. In these cases, the space will resolve spontaneously over a short period of time and specific interventions are not required.

Pleural effusions are common after lung transplantation, particularly when a large size disparity exists between the donor lungs and the thorax. Continued chest tube drainage following the primary procedure is not indicated as a preventative measure for these effusions and may actually lead to secondary infection and empyema. Management of these effusions is best done conservatively, with diuretic therapy and dietary salt restriction. Invasive measures, such as thoracentesis or tube drainage, are indicated only for effusions complicated by a delayed pneumothorax, for enlarging effusions, or for large effusions that persist for more than four weeks postoperatively.

Empyema is uncommon after lung transplantation. It is most frequently seen when a persistent pleural space due to a prolonged airleak, a chronic effusion, or an incompletely expanded lung is secondarily infected, usually with sputum flora. Management is initially conservative, with tube drainage and antibiotic therapy. In some cases, local drainage by rib resection or Eloesser flap will allow for adequate resolution. However, when the etiologic agent has a limited antimicrobial sensitivity (e.g., *B. cepacia* or *Aspergillus*) more aggressive measures such as transposition of muscle flaps or limited thoracoplasty to obliterate the space may be indicated (23).

Airway Complications

The door to successful lung transplantation was opened by the demonstration that wrapping the airway anastomosis with a protective flap of well-vascularized tissue, such as intestinal omentum, can provide an adequate blood supply for healing. The omental wrap was used in the first successful series of single lung transplants (190). Subsequently, some transplant centers have reported a low incidence of airway complications using the alternative technique of a telescoping anastomosis, without an omental wrap (191). Instead of an end-to-end anastomosis, the telescoping anastomosis employs the intussusception of the donor bronchus into that of recipient.

Airways anastomotic complications are diagnosed by direct visualization with bronchoscopy (192). Their presence also can be signaled by changes in follow-up spirometry indicative of unilateral mainstem bronchial obstruction (193,194). Anastomotic narrowing due to granulation tissue can be treated with rigid bronchoscopy and surgical debridement, or with bronchoscopic ND:YAG laser ablation (195,196). Narrowing due to stricture formation can be managed with bronchoscopic dilatation or stent placement (196,197).

Airway complications are significantly less common in the recent experience with lung transplantation. Bronchial ischemia is the most common cause of postoperative airway complications. The most common methods of lung transplantation do not provide direct revascularization of the bronchial arterial circulation and the donor bronchus must rely entirely on collateral perfusion from the pulmonary circulation in the initial postimplantation period. Airway ischemia at this time leads to mucosal ulceration, followed by progressive mural necrosis. Localized bronchomalacia is frequently present adjacent to this region. A spectrum of abnormalities ranging from anastomotic dehiscence to submucosal fibrosis may occur as a result. Most commonly, partial anastomotic dehiscence occurs followed by formation of granulation tissue and eventually some degree of anastomotic stenosis.

The reduced incidence of these complications has been attributed to methods of anastomosis that limit the length of the donor bronchus, minimizing the amount of airway for which collateral perfusion is required. Most anastomotic techniques emphasize trimming the donor bronchus to within 2 rings of the upper lobe orifice and the preservation of peribronchial tissues containing the collateral circulation. Telescoping the bronchi and covering the anastomosis with vascularized tissue are also useful adjunctive measures. The use of omentum does not appear to be a critical factor in most cases, although in patients who require prolonged mechanical ventilation because of graft dysfunction or in whom anastomotic dehiscence develops, the presence of an omental wrap will help minimize the morbidity of these complications. The effect of improved methods of lung preservation and of more specific immunosuppression on the decrease in airway complications is difficult to quantitate, but these factors are likely of some importance in the reduced incidence of this problem.

Diagnosis of airway complications is most commonly obtained by flexible bronchoscopy. Tomographic scanning (Fig. 25.13) may be useful in initial identification or assessment of the effects of the dehiscence by delineating the scope of inflammatory change or emphysema in the surrounding mediastinal tissues. At later times in the postoperative course, anastomotic stenoses may be identified on the basis of an unexplained drop in FEV_1 or an early plateau in the expiratory limb of the flow-volume loop. In patients with emphysema, however, there is routinely a "plateau" of the maximal expiratory flow volume curve (MEFV) and a "biphasic" MEFV, following single lung transplantation. In this instance, neither of these findings necessarily reflects anastomosis pathology (198).

The overall incidence of airway complications in all lung transplant patients is 15% to 20%. In approximately half of these cases, the diagnosis is made by endoscopic surveillance. Healing frequently occurs without further treatment or secondary complication. In the remainder, the airway complication requires more specific management and may lead to secondary complications. Of these patients, 70% will require anastomotic dilatation or stent placement and 20% will develop a bronchopleural fistula that will require a chest tube and perhaps reoperation. Death due to extensive airway necrosis or secondary infectious complications occurs in 10% of patients who develop symptomatic airway complications.

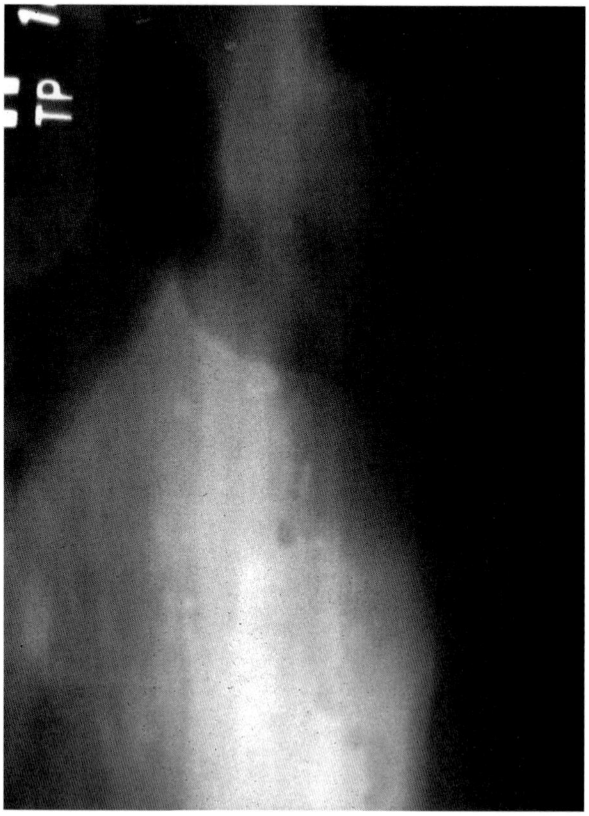

FIGURE 25.13. *Radiograph of airway showing narrowing of left main bronchus due to stenosis. The patient underwent airway dilatation via bronchoscopy.*

Treatment of airway complications in most cases is conservative and expectant. Patients in whom an asymptomatic complication develops can be managed by endoscopic surveillance alone at two-to-four-week intervals until healing is complete. Even when regions of contained dehiscence are identified, most of these will heal without major interventions. Membranous wall defects usually heal without stenosis, while cartilaginous wall defects typically heal with the development of some granulation tissue. Anastomotic granulation tissue can interfere with the clearance of secretions from the distal lung and can serve as a nidus for colonization by pathogens. Figure 25.14 (see also Plate 21), for example, shows an example of the fungus *Aspergillus fumigatus* invading an airway anastomosis. For these reasons, significant granulations should be excised by rigid bronchoscopy or laser excision, sometimes repeatedly, until healing is complete. Ultimately, areas of granulation tissue heal by fibrosis, which may cause anastomotic stenosis if it involves more than 50% of the anastomotic circumference.

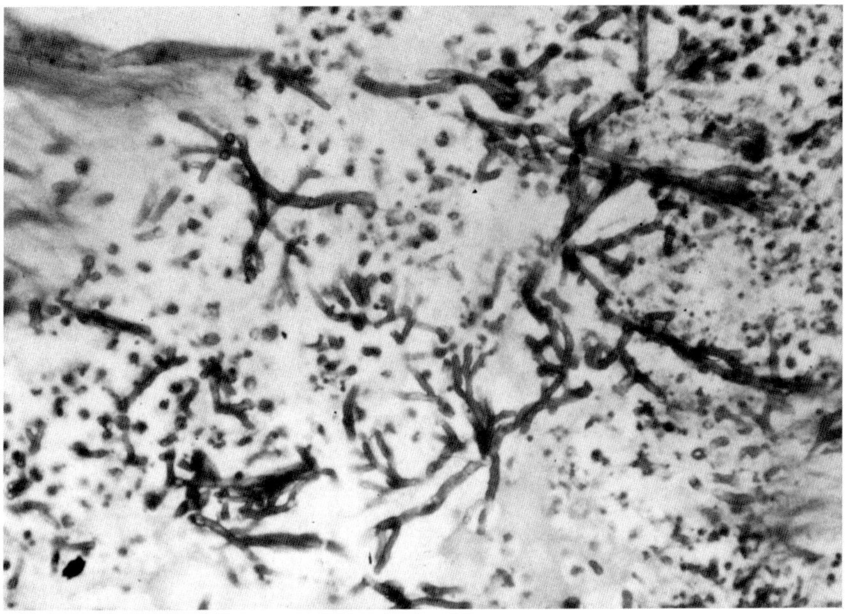

FIGURE 25.14. *Biopsy of granulation tissue at airway anastomosis demonstrating fungal invasion. Microbiologic culture confirmed identity of the organism as* Aspergillus fumigatus. *The disease resolved completely with antifungal therapy.*

These stenoses are amenable to dilatation by the rigid bronchoscope or by endobronchial balloon dilatation. Most will require the temporary placement of endobronchial stents for several months until sufficient remodeling of the fibrous tissue has occurred to create a stable anastomosis. Silastic self-retaining stents are used in most cases. Single lumen stents are used for most isolated lung transplant procedures, while Y-type stents are useful for stenoses occurring after HLT or en bloc DLT. These stents are tolerated well, although patients require daily N-acetyl cysteine nebulizer treatments to minimize secretion accumulation within the lumen of the stent. Wire stents are generally to be avoided unless complete epithelization is present at the anastomotic site, as granulation tissue can continue to grow within the interstices of these stents.

In circumstances where free communication occurs between the anastomotic site and the pleural space or the mediastinum, reinflation of the lung by chest tube insertion and/or mediastinal drainage via a mediastinoscopy incision will usually result in healing. When there is complete dehiscence and massive airleak or mediastinal contamination, surgical revision is rarely possible because of the short length of donor bronchus. Urgent retransplantation has been successfully performed for these patients in some cases.

Cardiac and Hemodynamic Complications

Both perioperative myocardial infarctions and cardiac arrests have occurred in lung transplant recipients, though relatively infrequently (199). More common cardiac and hemodynamic complications are atrial arrhythmias and episodes of systemic hypotension. Postoperative atrial arrhythmias, including atrial fibrillation and flutter, are not unexpected given that atrial clamps are applied intraoperatively and that some handling of the heart is inevitable. Most convert spontaneously or with medical therapy (199), making the need for DC cardioversion infrequent.

Systemic hypotension requiring vasopressor and inotropic support also is common in the first week following transplant (184,200). The hemodynamic profile seen typically includes a severely depressed systemic vascular resistance with a normal or diminished cardiac index. This complication has been associated with the reimplantation response. Postoperative hemodynamic instability also has been common in patients with underlying pulmonary hypertension. In the first week post-transplant, minimal activity, suctioning, or pain can cause wide swings in the pulmonary artery pressures in these patients, which can result in episodes of systemic hypotension or hypertension, as well as oxygen desaturations.

Gastrointestinal Complications

As previously reported with heart and heart–lung transplant recipients, the incidence of gastrointestinal (GI) complications in lung transplant recipients substantially exceeds that observed in patients undergoing nontransplantation thoracic operations (201). Common GI complications occurring early after transplant include the development of a diaphragmatic hernia through the defect created to allow passage of the omental pedicle used to wrap the bronchial anastomosis, and the development of a prolonged adynamic ileus requiring nasogastric suction and parenteral nutritional support. A postoperative ileus developing in a transplant recipient may be potentiated by drug toxicities described.

GI complications occurring later after transplant may present atypically (201). Transplant patients may fail to manifest the usual symptoms and signs of intra-abdominal pathologic processes due to their immunosuppressive medications, which reduce their ability to mount inflammatory responses.

This can result in delays in diagnosis and lead to poorer outcomes. For this reason, a high index of suspicion and liberal use of diagnostic studies has been recommended in evaluating abdominal complaints post-transplant. Additionally, pretransplant GI imaging to identify preexisting abdominal conditions can be extremely helpful in post-transplant management (see also Chapter 29).

A GI complication unique to patients with underlying CF is the development of a meconium ileus equivalent. In this syndrome, inspissated intestinal contents in the distal ileum and proximal colon cause small bowel obstruction, presenting with pain, distention, constipation, and bilious vomiting (202). The syndrome is likely related to malabsorption due to the exocrine pancreatic insufficiency commonly occurring in CF patients. Preventive strategies center around the resumption of supplemental pancreatic enzymes as soon as bowel function permits. Some centers also add N-acetylcysteine to the enteral feedings of these patients (203).

Rejection

As previously noted, placing a donor organ from one individual into a genetically different recipient is referred to as *allogeneic transplantation*, that is, transplantation between members of the same species who nonetheless possess different copies (alleles) of multiple genes (204). These genetic differences between donor and recipient result in rejection of the graft by the recipient's immune system, owing mainly to differences in histocompatibility antigens. There are multiple immunologic processes that can produce a spectrum of rejection responses to transplanted organs. This spectrum can be subdivided into hyperacture, acute, and chronic rejection. Each of these categories can be characterized in terms of its causative immunologic mechanism(s), as well its typical mode and timing of clinical presentation (see Chapter 2).

Hyperacute Rejection

Hyperacute rejection, when it occurs, is noted within minutes to hours after transplantation (205). This form of rejection was described in kidney transplant recipients and has been documented following lung transplantation as well (26). It is caused by preexisting antibodies in a recipient to antigens on donor vascular endothelium, including HLA antigens and ABO blood group antigens. Such antibodies may be present in a recipient due to prior exposure to these antigens through blood transfusion, pregnancy, or previous transplantation. These antibodies bind to the vascular endothelium of graft, and activate inflammatory and coagulation cascades. This results in rapid and extensive thrombosis of graft vessels, which causes graft failure.

Acute Rejection

Acute rejection typically occurs in the first three months following transplantation, although the risk of this form of rejection persists thereafter and late episodes are not unusual (206,207). Acute rejection is caused by the recipient's cellular immune responses against the graft's HLA antigens. Although this response is complex and involves multiple cell types and soluble mediators, the key cell is the T lymphocyte as outlined above. The T lymphocyte consequently is the target of both preventive and therapeutic measures for this form of rejection. In keeping with the central role of the lymphocyte in its etiology, the key pathologic feature of acute rejection is a perivascular lymphocytic infiltrate, which may also be accompanied by a lymphocytic bronchitis or bronchiolitis (208). Acute rejection is graded pathologically in terms of severity, from grade one, minimal acute rejection, to grade four, severe acute rejection (160). The full classification is depicted in Table 25.14. Examples are shown in Figure 25.15 (see also Plate 22).

The current pathologic classification of lung allograft rejection recognizes that the vasculature and airways can be affected in both acute and chronic rejection. In 1990, an international grading scheme was developed to provide guidelines for the histologic diagnosis of rejection. In 1995, Yousem led a group of international pathologists to revise the original proposal (209). Based primarily upon analysis of transbronchial biopsies, the group emphasized that acute rejection is "characterized by perivascular and subendothelial mononuclear infiltrates and by lymphocytic bronchitis and bronchiolitis. Chronic rejection, by definition, manifests as bronchiolitis obliterans—dense eosinophilic fibrous scarring of the bronchioles—and accelerated vascular sclerosis affecting pulmonary arteries and veins."

Table 25.14. Classification of Lung Transplant Rejection

A. Acute rejection: perivascular inflammation	*with/without*	B. Airway inflammation: lymphocytic bronchitis/bronchiolitis—documented with acute rejection
Grade 0—None		Grade 0—None
Grade 1—Minimal: Infrequent perivascular infiltrate		Grade 1—Minimal
Grade 2—Mild: Frequent perivascular infiltrates		Grade 2—Mild
Grade 3—Moderate: Dense perivascular infiltrates extending into alveolar septae		Grade 3—Moderate
Grade 4—Severe: Diffuse perivascular, interstitial, and alveolar infiltrates; pneumocyte damage; and parenchymal necrosis, infarction, or necrotizing vasculitis		Grade 4—Severe
C. Chronic airway rejection: bronchiolitis obliterans, active or inactive		
D. Chronic vascular rejection: accelerated graft vascular sclerosis		

Despite the emphasis on the anatomic hallmarks of rejection, it is essential to the interpretation of all biopsy specimens that the clinical context be taken into account. In particular, infection must be excluded since infection and rejection often occur together and can be confused histologically (201). Another limitation to the pathologic assessment is that perivascular and interstitial mononuclear infiltrates are not specific for acute rejection. Other conditions that simulate or mimic alloreactive injury include the following: CMV pneumonitis, pneumocystis carinii pneumonia, post-transplant lymphoproliferative disease, bronchial-associated lymphoid tissue, previous biopsy sites, recurrent primary disease, ischemia (preservation injury) (209).

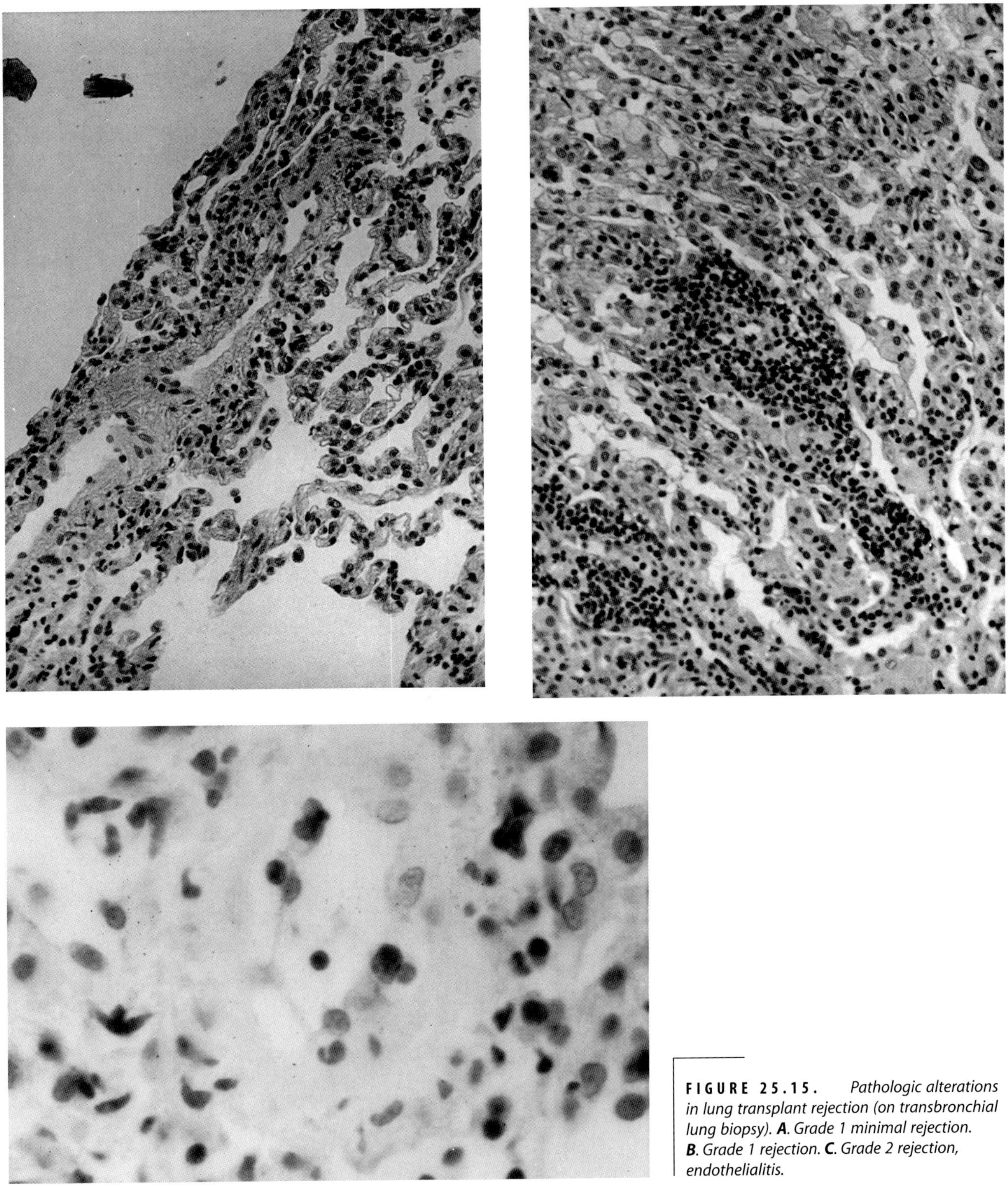

A B C

FIGURE 25.15. *Pathologic alterations in lung transplant rejection (on transbronchial lung biopsy).* ***A.*** *Grade 1 minimal rejection.* ***B.*** *Grade 1 rejection.* ***C.*** *Grade 2 rejection, endothelialitis.*

D
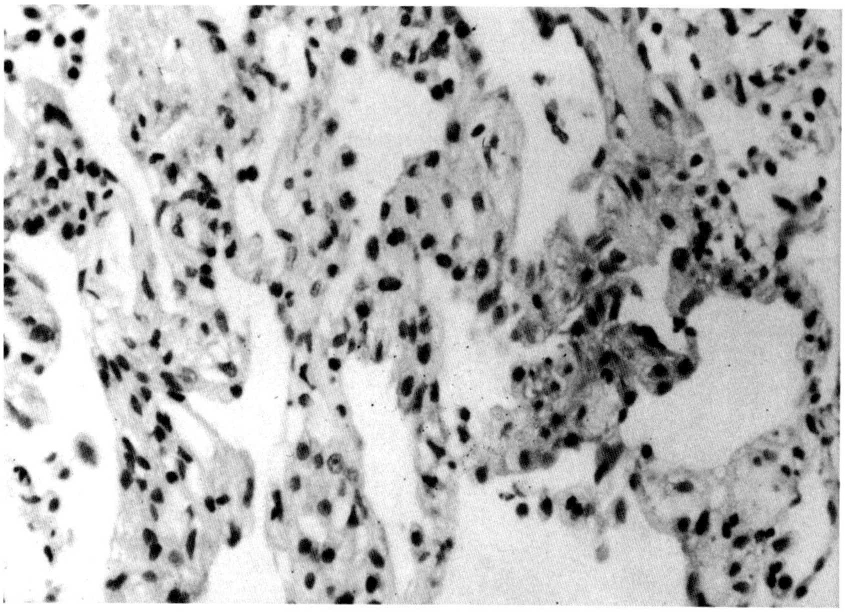

E
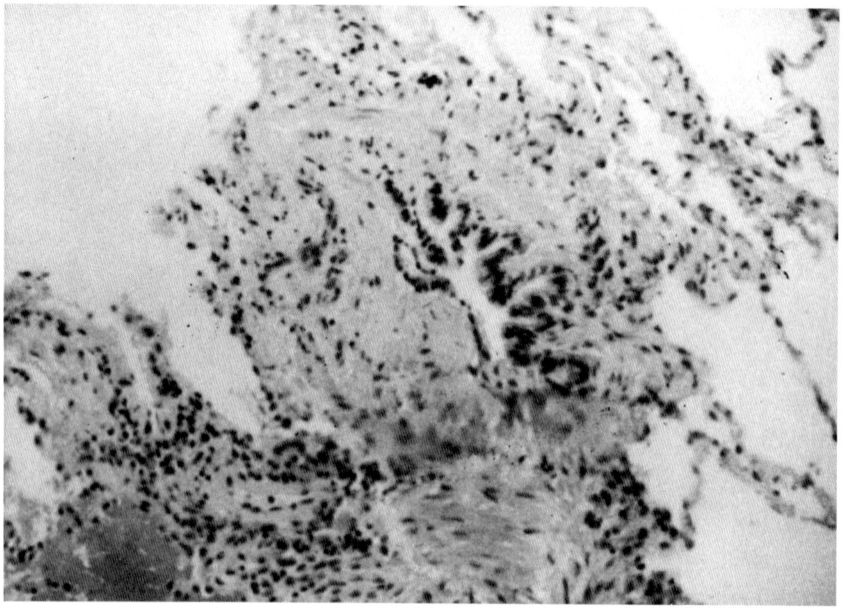

FIGURE 25.15. ***D.*** *Grades 3–4 rejection.* ***E.*** *Chronic rejection, obliterative bronchiolitis.*

A variety of nonspecific pathologic changes, unrelated to rejection, may occur in the lung allograft (Table 25.15). Although they are unlikely to be confused with rejection, it is important to recognize their potential contribution to allograft dysfunction.

The lymphocytic infiltrate characteristic of grade one acute rejection is demonstrated in Figure 25.15B (see also Plate 22B), which shows lung tissue taken from a transbronchial biopsy of a patient during an episode of acute rejection. Although the severity of the perivascular infiltrate determines the "grade" of acute rejection, the bronchial inflammation may be an important factor in predicting the later development of chronic rejection involving the airways (209,211).

Symptoms of acute rejection include cough, dyspnea, and fatigue, although a substantial number of patients may be asymptomatic (212). Physical signs include rales and wheezes. The presence of acute rejection may also be indicated by a rise in temperature of greater than 0.5°C above a stable baseline, a fall in oxygenation of greater than 10 mm Hg below a stable baseline, or a fall in FEV_1 of greater than 10% below a stable baseline. Radiographic findings associated with acute rejection include increased septal lines, new or increased pleural effusions, and new or increased air-space disease (213). The increased septal lines seen are felt to be the radiographic correlates of the lymphocytic infiltrates that are characteristic of acute rejection histologically. Figure 25.16 shows the chest x-ray of the same patient previously shown developing the reimplantation response, who developed an episode of acute rejection on postoperative day 12. At this time, the patient's chest x-ray demonstrates a diffuse interstitial and alveolar infiltrate, including increased septal

Table 25.15. Pathologic Alterations in the Lung Allograft Not Related to Rejection

Diffuse alveolar damage/patchy acute alveolar injury—usually a manifestation of ischemic/reperfusion injury or other perioperative insults
Acute alveolar hemorrhage
Alveolar hemosiderosis
- Related to previous biopsy site
- Resolved high-grade endotheliolitis
- Prior infection
- Coagulation defect

Infection
Post-transplant lymphoproliferative disorder
Emboli
Recurrence of native disease
Unrecognized donor disease
Smoker's macrophages

Source: Adapted from Yousem SA, Berry GJ, Cagle PT, et al. Revision of the 1990 Working Formulation of the Classification of Pulmonary Allograft Rejection: Lung Rejection Study Groups. J Heart Lung Transplant 1996;15:1–15.

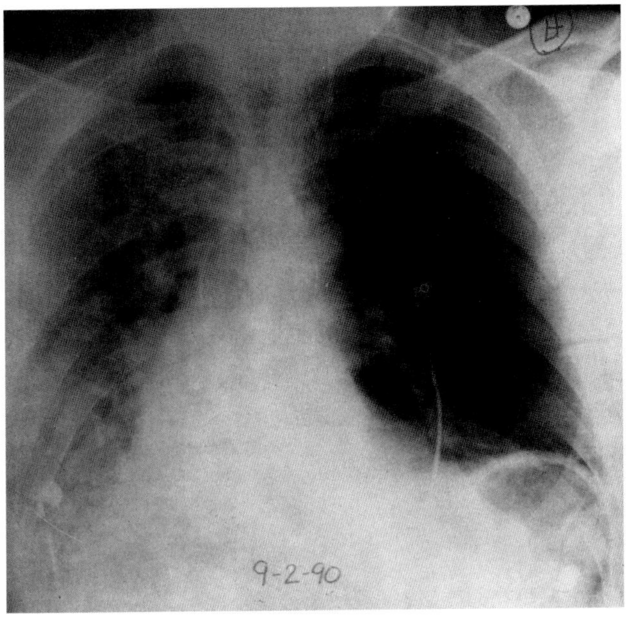

FIGURE 25.16. *Chest x-ray of the same patient as in Figures 25.10–25.12 on postoperative day 12, showing diffuse interstitial and alveolar infiltrate, and increased septal lines. At this time the patient's WBC was elevated, oxygenation declined, and bronchoscopy revealed no evidence of infection. The clinical diagnosis was acute allograft rejection.*

lines. Despite this potentially characteristic radiographic appearance, a substantial number of patients with acute rejection may have no chest x-ray abnormalities (214). In some of these patients, an increase in septal lines can still be appreciated on chest CT scan, as demonstrated in Figure 25.17A, which shows the scan of another patient during an episode of acute rejection in the transplanted right lung. For comparison, Figure 25.17B shows the chest CT scan of a single lung transplant patient doing well at the time of routine follow-up. However, these chest CT findings also can be nonspecific, and establishing the diagnosis of acute rejection generally requires ruling out possible infectious complications with bronchoalveolar lavage and transbronchial biopsy. Unfortunately, despite preventive measures, acute rejection is an almost universal occurrence in the first several months following lung transplantation (215,216).

Lung grafts contain a large population of immunocompetent cells including lymphocytes and macrophages within the parenchyma, hilar and pulmonary lymph nodes, and the bronchus-associated lymphoid tissue (BALT). The majority of these cells are memory T cells. Studies have suggested that a prominent interaction occurs between donor and recipient immune cells in the early time period after implantation. Analysis of cells obtained by bronchoalveolar lavage (BAL) during the first months post-transplant demonstrates donor-specific lymphocyte proliferation, suggesting in vivo mixed lymphocyte reactivity at a time when both donor and recipient immune competent cells are present (217). Subsequently, a rapid replacement of donor lymphocytes and macrophages occurs. By 90 days post-transplant, the majority of the intraparenchymal cells are of recipient origin and the BALT has been markedly depleted (218). In view of these rapid and profound changes in immune cell populations, it is not surprising that rejection is common in lung allografts and that, in the case of heart–lung grafts, lung rejection may occur more frequently than, and independent of, rejections of the heart. A protocol of routine transbronchial biopsy of the lung for identification of histologic evidence of lung rejection is usually recommended for both heart–lung and isolated lung transplants because of the likelihood of rejection that may occur with minimal clinical symptoms. Typically, surveillance bronchoscopy is performed at 3 weeks, 6 weeks, 3 months, 6 months, 9 months, and 12 months postoperatively. Not all centers, however, adhere to such a protocol, reserving biopsy only for events that are clinically suspicious. Bronchoscopy and biopsy is, of course, also performed for clinical symptoms or changes in lung spirometry such as a decrease in FEV_1. Bronchoalveolar lavage is most useful in excluding infection and is not generally helpful in confirming rejection.

Attempts to diagnose rejection noninvasively have, to date, been disappointing. Measurements of pulmonary function, together with radiologic and clinical examination are typically relied upon, but have their shortcomings. An alternative approach has been to focus on monitoring of the immune system. Tissue culture techniques, using BAL cells for example, are unsatisfactory for clinical purposes because the results are not available until several days after the episode. Investigators have turned to measuring levels of various cytokines: tumor necrosis factor (TNF), gamma interferon (IFNγ), and soluble interleukin 2 receptor (IL-2R).

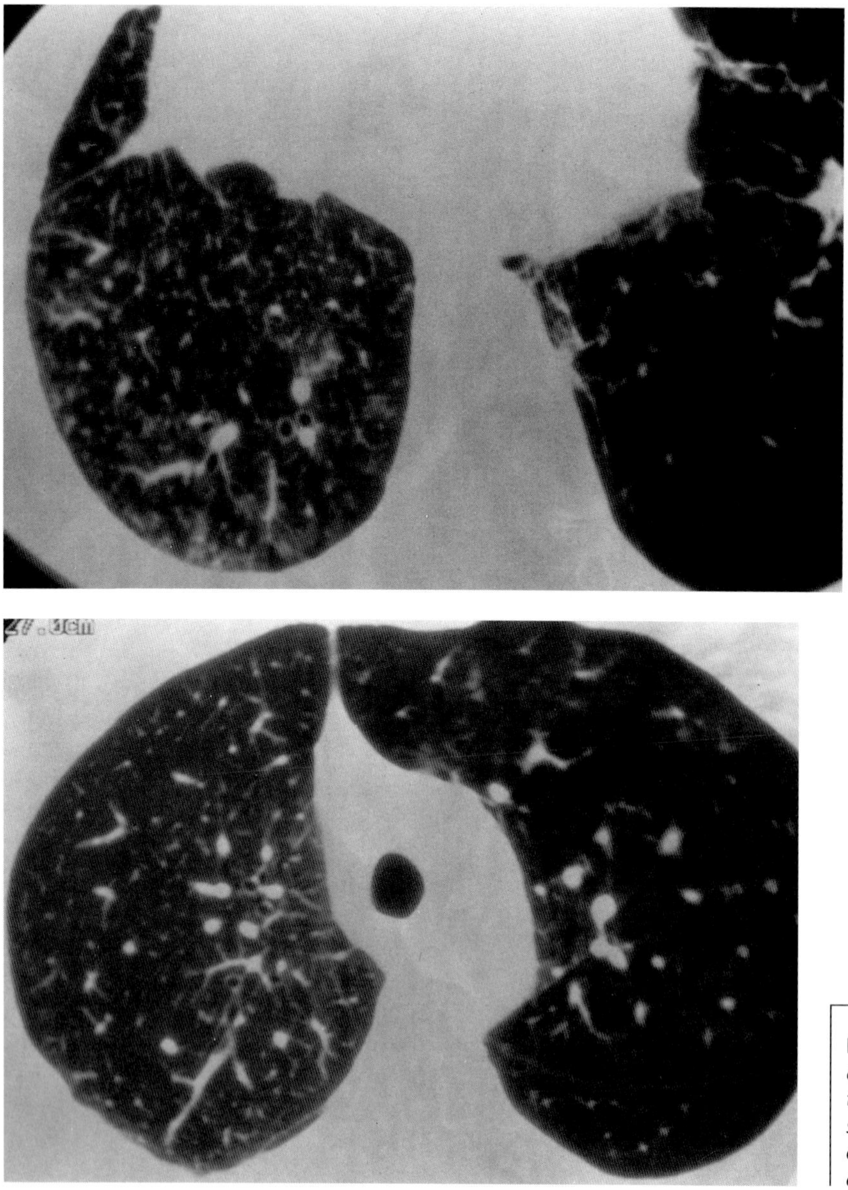

A

B

FIGURE 25.17. ***A.*** *Chest CT scan of another patient during an episode of acute rejection in the transplanted right lung.* ***B.*** *Chest CT scan of a different patient doing well at the time of routine follow-up. The patient's severe underlying emphysema is demonstrated in the native left lung.*

These are all elevated during episodes of acute rejection, but the findings suffer from lack of sensitivity and specificity (219).

Because the incidence of acute rejection in the first three weeks after lung transplantation is high, antirejection therapy is usually administered empirically for recently transplanted patients with the appropriate clinical syndrome, even in the absence of confirmatory biopsy findings, if no infectious etiology is found by BAL. The initial treatment, typically, is the administration of a brief course of high-dose corticosteroids (e.g., methylprednisolone 500 mg IV every day for 3 days). Ganciclovir prophylaxis (5 mg/kg twice a day tapered over six weeks) is indicated for all patients with CMV disparate donor/recipient status when antirejection therapy is initiated in order to prevent reactivation. Symptomatic and radiographic improvement occurs usually within 48 hours in most cases, as shown in Figure 25.18, the chest x-ray of the patient described above with acute rejection. Following this, the maintenance dose of steroids is ordinarily increased for several weeks before reducing it gradually to the prerejection levels. Typically, it is not necessary to repeat transbronchial biopsy to confirm resolution of the acute rejection unless symptoms or radiographic abnormalities persist. Occasionally, some patients with persistent findings will require a second course of steroids. Centers differ in their approach to this problem. One option is to administer high doses of corticosteroids as previously described; an alternative is to provide a slightly longer course of oral therapy (i.e., "recycling" beginning with prednisone 200 mg/day and reducing the dosage by 40 mg/day to return to a maintenance dosage 10 mg/day higher than the dosage on which rejection occurred). For the rare patient in whom these

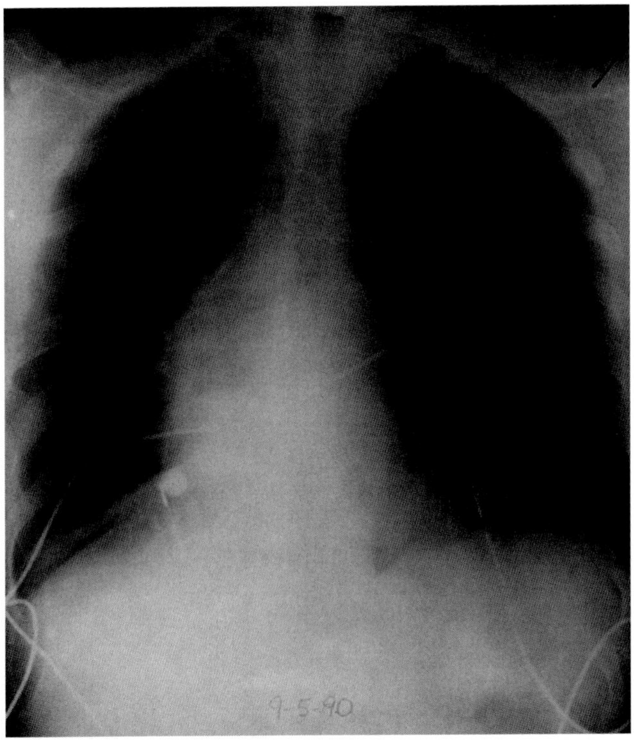

FIGURE 25.18. *Chest x-ray of the same patient as in Figures 25.10–25.12 and 25.16, previously diagnosed as having acute allograft rejection in the right lung. This radiograph, taken on postoperative day 15, shows complete clearance of rejection following high-dose intravenous steroid therapy (methylprednisolone 500 mg/day).*

methods do not result in resolution of the process, repeat bronchoscopy for BAL and transbronchial biopsy is recommended to confirm the diagnosis. If persistent acute rejection is identified, cytolytic therapy with OKT-3 or ATG should be considered.

Chronic Rejection

Chronic rejection is a poorly understood process that affects all solid transplants, leading to chronic graft dysfunction and late graft failure (see Chapter 3). This form of rejection typically occurs more than one year after lung transplantation but has been described as early as two months following operation (220). The etiology of chronic rejection is unclear. Hypothesized causes include the cumulative effect of recurrent episodes of acute rejection, chronic arterial insufficiency and progressive graft ischemia, and an ongoing subclinical host immune response against graft (212,221). Some studies have suggested that the use of OKT-3 for induction immunosuppression or the use of tacrolimus as part of a three-drug immunosuppressive regimen has been associated with a lower incidence of chronic rejection of the lung involving the airways (166,222).

Pathologically, for all solid organ transplants, "the common denominator of (chronic rejection) entails development of obliterative fibrosis of hollow structures within the graft, regardless of whether they are vessels, bronchioles, or bile ducts" (221). Histologically, chronic rejection of the lung is identified as bronchiolitis obliterans and consists of dense eosinophilic scarring of the membranous and respiratory bronchioles (see Fig. 25.15E and Plate 22E). Further progression of this process leads to worsening dyspnea and bronchiectasis with secondary infection. In the transplanted lung, chronic rejection thus causes: 1) bronchiolitis oblilterans, characterized by submucosal scarring of membranous and respiratory bronchioles, which causes subtotal or total obliteration of the bronchiolar lumens, and 2) chronic vascular rejection, characterized by fibrointimal thickening of arteries and veins (208). These changes are analogous to the chronic rejection identified in many isolated cardiac allograft recipients. In fact, when this type of chronic rejection is identified in the lungs of heart–lung transplant recipients, it appears to correlate with similar changes in the coronary arteries of these patients (209). In one study, patients with a pretransplant diagnosis of PPH were found to have an increased risk for development of obliterative bronchiolitis (OB) (223).

The central clinical feature of chronic rejection is the development of physiologic airway obstruction. Although the diagnosis of chronic rejection may be confirmed by a transbronchial biopsy demonstrating the changes described above, the key diagnostic criterion is a 20% decline in the FEV_1 from a previously established post-transplant baseline for which no other cause (e.g., infection or acute rejection) can be found (224). Clinically, chronic rejection often presents insidiously, with the first manifestation typically being a nonproductive or minimally productive cough. Dyspnea is a relatively late manifestation of this form of rejection, occurring up to several months later and reflecting extensive airway disease (225). Bronchomalacia has been described in association with OB.

The term *bronchiolitis obliterans syndrome (BOS)* identifies patients with chronic rejection of the lung involving the airways. The presence of an unexplained fall in expiratory flow rates and progressive symptoms are the hallmarks of this process. Because of sampling errors with transbronchial biopsy, some patients with chronic rejection may not have histologic proof of bronchiolitis obliterans despite a course of progressive deterioration. The diagnosis of BOS, therefore, is based on symptoms and objective changes in pulmonary function and does not require histologic evidence of bronchiolitis obliterans (Table 25.16). Detection of air trapping by expiratory high-resolution computed tomography (HRCT) of the chest may be supportive. The clinical condition of patients with BOS is graded on a scale from 0 to 3. Some patients with BOS will remain stable within a given grade, but most will demonstrate evidence of disease progression (226). Rarely, a patient may improve clinically, despite persistence of bronchioliltis obliterans pathologically.

Some evidence exists to suggest that augmented immunosuppression may stabilize the BOS process, particularly if initiated early in its evolution. Treatment is usually

Table 25.16. Staging Classification of Bronchiolitis Obliterans Syndrome

Stage	Severity	FEV_1 (% of baseline)
0	No symptoms	>80%
1	Mild	66–80%
2	Moderate	51–65%
3	Severe	≤50%

All stages may be subcategorized according to the presence (subcategory a) or absence (subcategory b) of histologic evidence of bronchiolitis obliterans.

directed to patients with symptomatic BOS (grades 1 to 3). Augmented corticosteroid therapy, including the use of inhaled steroids or cyclosporine, cytolytic agents, tacrolimus and MMF have all been used for this purpose, as discussed above. Whether there is a specific benefit to any type of therapy as compared to another in the treatment of this syndrome is not yet clear. Unfortunately, despite preventive strategies, chronic rejection affects approximately one half of lung transplant recipients and is a major cause of late mortality. The mortality rate at three years after diagnosis is 40% or higher.

Management of progressive BOS in its later stages is mostly palliative. At its most advanced stage, BOS is essentially an acquired form of septic lung disease and management is similar to that required for other patients with septic lung disease awaiting lung transplantation. Retransplantation has been performed for some patients with BOS. The results demonstrate a significantly increased perioperative mortality for such patients. One-year survival is approximately 45%, less than half that of primary lung transplantation. Approximately 40% of patients surviving retransplantation develop recurrent BOS within three years, an incidence of BOS similar to that following primary lung transplantation (227).

Infections

The immunosuppressive agents used to prevent and to treat rejection also suppress transplant patients' immunologic defenses against infection. Consequently, infections are a principal source of morbidity and mortality in recipients of all solid organ transplants (see Chapter 36). However, the rate of infectious complications is even higher in lung-transplant patients than in recipients of other solid organs (184). There are multiple factors contributing to this higher infection rate. First, the possibility of organ donation is established by virtue of donors' brain death, and hence donors are intubated and mechanically ventilated. This exposes all donor lungs to aspiration, airway colonization, and parenchymal infection (228). Second, lung transplant recipients are commonly intubated for longer periods of time after their operation than other solid organ transplant recipients, further increasing their risk of pneumonia. Third, the lung allografts, like the bowel (see Chapter 22), are unique among organ transplants in that they are exposed continuously to the external environment, and consequently, to potential pathogens. Finally, two important pulmonary defense mechanisms, the cough reflex (229) and mucociliary clearance (229,230) are impaired in transplanted lungs. All of these factors increase lung transplant patients' susceptibility to pulmonary infections and, in fact, the lung is the site of the majority of their post-transplant infections (231).

An aggressive approach to the evaluation of all new pulmonary infiltrates, in either the lung graft or the native lung, is required in these patients. Flexible bronchoscopy with BAL and/or protected brushing is needed to diagnose properly pulmonary infections after lung transplantation. BAL specimens from both lungs should be routinely sent for Gram stain, fungal smear, and acid-fast bacilli smear as well as for culture of these organisms. In addition, analysis of the BAL for *Pneumocystis carinii, Legionella* spp., and viruses is required.

Bacterial Pneumonia

The majority of infections in lung transplant recipients are caused by bacteria, and the most common bacterial infection in these patients is pneumonia. Bacterial pneumonias occur most frequently in the early postoperative period, within two months of transplant. Gram-negative bacilli are the most common causative organisms (231). Clinically, these infections present with fever, new or increased radiographic infiltrates, and the presence of a new or newly predominant organism by sputum Gram stain and culture (232). The diagnosis frequently is confirmed by bronchoscopy. Patients are treated with culture-directed antibiotics for two to four weeks, often accompanied by a modest reduction in immunosuppression. When a limited spectrum of antimicrobial sensitivity is available, the use of aerosolized antimicrobial therapy in addition to intravenous therapy may be helpful. Unfortunately, despite therapy, these infections remain a leading cause of mortality.

Potential host sources of contamination of the respiratory tract should be evaluated, particularly in patients with CF or recurrent pneumonias. Since chronic sinusitis is common in CF patients and may act as a source for contamination of the lower respiratory tract, careful otolaryngologic evaluation and sinus drainage is indicated in selected patients. Gastroesophageal reflux is common in both CF patients and patients with COPD and can lead to recurrent aspiration pneumonias in dependent regions of the lungs. Conservative treatment with elevation of the head of the bed and the administration of promotility agents, in addition to the H_2 blocking agents taken by most transplant recipients, will control the reflux in most cases. In SLT patients, the native lung may occasionally be a site of graft contamination or, more commonly, may become the site of a pneumonia or a lung abscess. Standard therapy is recommended for such cases, although a localized area of anatomic abnormality in the native lung (e.g., focal bronchiectasis) may require surgical excision if it proves to be the source of recurrent infection.

Cytomegalovirus Infections

Although CMV usually does not cause clinically important disease in immunocompetent persons, it is a chief opportunistic infection in lung transplant recipients and the second most frequent infection in these patients overall. Following a primary infection, CMV is not cleared from the body but remains present in a latent state. Consequently, CMV disease in lung transplant recipients can result from either: 1) reactivation of a latent CMV infection acquired by the recipient prior to transplant, or 2) transmission of CMV to the recipient following transplant, from either the donor lung or transfused blood products, resulting in a new primary infection. The frequency of CMV disease, therefore, depends on whether the recipient and donor carry latent CMV, which is determined by the presence or absence of antibodies to CMV. Post-transplant infections are most frequent in recipients positive for CMV antibodies, indicative of prior CMV exposure, regardless of CMV status of donor (232). CMV infections in these patients are felt to be due to reactivation of their own latent infections, due to their immunosuppressive therapy (233). However, CMV infections are most severe in recipients negative for CMV antibodies who receive lungs from CMV-positive donors. CMV infections in these patients are felt to be due to primary infections with virus transmitted from the allograft, which has been documented to occur in renal transplant recipients (234). Primary infections have been associated with more severe manifestations of disease, and higher mortality rates, than reactivation of latent infections (235,236).

In most cases of CMV disease, the infection is generalized, involving multiple organ systems, although clinically apparent disease may not be present in all organ systems affected (237). The most damaging site of disease is the lung, where CMV pneumonitis can present with fever, dyspnea, hypoxemia, and diffuse radiographic infiltrates (232). In a significant minority of lung transplant patients, the primary site of clinically apparent disease is the GI tract. These cases present with anorexia, weight loss, epigastric pain, and/or diarrhea. CMV also can present with a nonspecific complex of symptoms and signs, including fevers, chills, malaise, and myalgias, which can be accompanied by leukopenia, with greater than 3% atypical lymphocytes in the peripheral blood smear (232,238). Prior to the use of ganciclovir preventively, CMV disease typically presented in the second month post-transplant. In addition to reducing the frequency of CMV disease, the use of ganciclovir preventively has delayed the usual time of presentation of CMV disease until four to six months post-transplant.

The ability to diagnose rapidly the presence of CMV infection has improved dramatically (237,239). CMV early antigen can be assayed for in bronchoalveolar lavage fluid and urine, and its presence indicates active CMV replication. A test for the rapid detection of CMV antigenemia in peripheral blood also is now available and appears to be a sensitive early marker for CMV infection (see Chapter 36). Additionally, positive culture results can be obtained decidedly earlier with the use of a shell-vial system in place of traditional viral culture methods. However, even in immunosuppressed patients, CMV *infection* can be asymptomatic, and the documentation of clinically significant *disease* due to CMV requires biopsy of the organ(s) suspected to be involved, with demonstration of intracellular inclusions typical of the virus in the biopsied tissue (Fig. 25.19 and Plate 23) (232).

Without treatment, the mortality of CMV pneumonitis approaches 100% (239). Fortunately, the introduction of ganciclovir has led to successful treatment outcomes in most

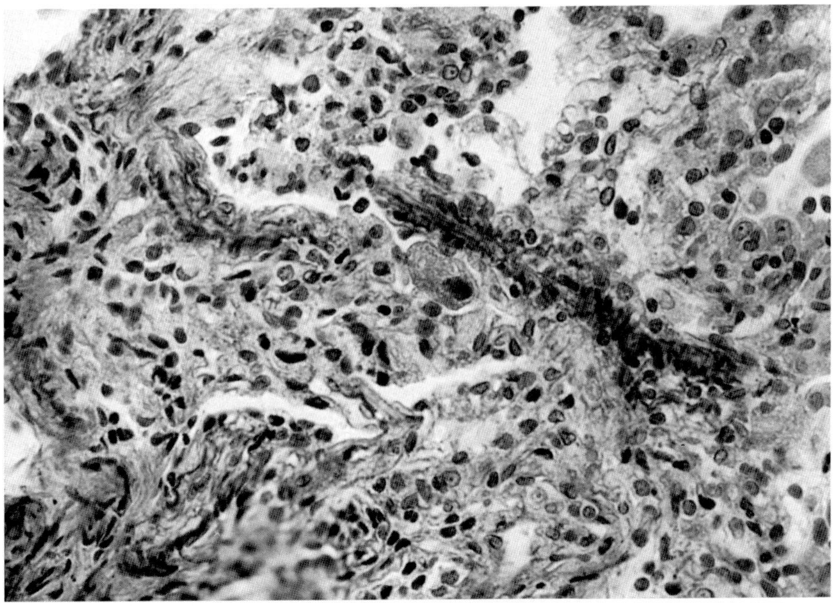

FIGURE 25.19. *Photomicrograph of transbronchial lung biopsy demonstrating CMV pneumonia with characteristic cytopathic changes including intranuclear inclusions.*

cases (240). In a few cases, ganciclovir resistance calls for alternative agents. However, lung transplant patients surviving CMV pneumonitis still appear to be subject to multiple long-term sequelae, including reduced lung function, increased rates of subsequent bacterial or fungal pneumonias, increased rates of chronic rejection, and lower two-year survival (25).

Other Viral Infections

Herpes simplex virus (HSV) can cause necrotizing tracheobronchitis and esophagitis, and less frequently, pneumonitis in the early weeks post-transplant, but these infections have become uncommon with the widespread use of prophylactic acyclovir or ganciclovir (235). Epstein-Barr virus (EBV), which can cause pharyngitis and mononucleosis in immunocompetent persons, rarely has been reported to cause fever, malaise, pharyngitis, and adenopathy in lung transplant patients (248). However, EBV also has been implicated in the pathogenesis of posttransplant lymphoproliferative disorders, a severe complication of transplantation described in detail in Chapter 37. Respiratory syncytial virus (RSV), which causes tracheobronchitis, bronchiolitis, and pneumonia in immunocompetent children, recently has been implicated as causing a broad spectrum of respiratory illness in lung and other solid organ transplant recipients, ranging from isolated rhinitis to fatal ARDS (241). Aerosolized ribavirin and RSV hyperimmune globulin have been used to treat these infections, with successful outcomes reported (235,242,243). Adenovirus has also been reported as a cause of late fatal pneumonitis following lung transplantation (244).

Fungal Infections

Fungal infection of the lung transplant recipient is relatively rare. *Aspergillus* spp. are the most common cause of fungal infection following lung transplantation. *Aspergillus* may present as part of the resident flora of the recipient or it may cause an invasive infection, either an ulcerative tracheobronchitis involving the anastomosis and airways or a disseminated illness with pneumonitis and fungemia. *Aspergillus* airway colonization is not uncommon after lung transplantation, and in most cases is transient. Invasive *Aspergillus* disease, in contrast, is less common but frequently fatal (245). An ulcerative trancheobronchitis due to *Aspergillus* and involving the anastomotic site and large airways also has been described and appears to be highly specific to lung and heart–lung transplantation (246). Unfortunately, symptoms are often minimal or absent in these infections initially, which can lead to a delay in diagnosis. Consequently, fungal infections are frequently disseminated at the time of recognition and are associated with high mortality rates (132,246).

Although sputum colonization may be treated with itraconazole or inhaled amphotericin B, such therapy rarely is able to clear the airway of fungus. In the absence of symptoms, a specific anatomic abnormality (e.g., airway granulation tissue or bronchiectasis), or radiographic changes suggesting pneumonitis, most patients with sputum colonization can be managed without specific antifungal therapy. When invasive *Aspergillus* infection is identified, therapy with amphotericin B (25–35 mg/day IV to a total dose of 1000 mg) is required, followed by itraconazole therapy or possibly liposomal amphotericin for 6 to 12 weeks. In severe cases, invasive *Aspergillus* infection is frequently fatal.

Candida albicans may also cause invasive pneumonia following lung transplantation. The fungal source is usually the donor trachea. The use of prophylactic fluconazole (100 mg IV each day) initially, regardless of donor sputum flora, and clotrimazole (10 mg PO four times a day) subsequently has virtually eliminated this problem.

Pneumocystis carinii *Pneumonia*

Infection with *P. carinii* initially was extremely common in lung transplant recipients, but the frequency of this infection has been markedly reduced by the adoption of prophylactic therapy with oral trimethoprim-sulfamethoxazole (239). Interestingly, many transplant patients from whom *P. carinii* has been recovered have been asymptomatic, and clinically important pneumonias, with fever, cough, dyspnea, hypoxia, and radiographic infiltrates, have represented the minority of cases (239,247). Treatment of pneumonias with standard high-dose regimens of intravenous trimethoprim-sulfamethoxazole has been largely successful. The incidence of this infection peaks three to six months posttransplant, but cases have occurred greater than one year following transplant in the setting of recently increased immunosuppressive therapy with high-dose corticosteroids for the treatment of rejection (248).

Mycobacterial Infections

Immunosuppression also makes lung transplant recipients prone to infection with *Mycobacterium tuberculosis* (249). Although reported cases have been infrequent to date, the recent resurgence of tuberculosis in the general population may make this a more common problem in transplant patients in the future. Tuberculosis can occur in transplant patients due to: 1) reactivation of latent infections acquired pretransplant, 2) transmission from donor lungs, or 3) posttransplant exposures to persons with active tuberculosis. The time of presentation of reported cases has ranged from 3 to 20 months post-transplant. Most cases have been pulmonary infections, presenting with fevers, constitutional symptoms, and chest radiographic abnormalities, including parenchymal infiltrates, pulmonary nodules, hilar adenopathy, and/or pleural effusions. These cases have responded well to antituberculous antibiotics. One case of disseminated tuberculosis has been reported, which was fatal. A fatal case of infection with the nontuberculous mycobacterium *M. chelonae* also has been reported in a heart–lung transplant recipient (250).

Malignancies

In addition to the increased risk of infections described above, immunosuppression also causes an increased risk of certain malignancies in recipients of solid organ transplants, as reviewed elsewhere in this text (see Chapter 37). This increased risk is confined to specific cancers, including non-Hodgkin's lymphomas and other post-transplant lymphoproliferative disorders, squamous cell cancers of the lip and skin, Kaposi's sarcomas, soft tissue sarcomas, carcinomas of the vulva and perineum, carcinomas of the kidney, and hepatobiliary tumors (19). Lung transplant recipients, however, have no increased risk of most cancers common in the general population, including carcinomas of the lung, breast, colon, and prostate, and invasive carcinomas of the uterine cervix.

A clinically and morphologically diverse group of B-cell lymphoid proliferations may occur in immunosuppressed patients after transplant. These proliferations were initially felt to all be malignant non-Hodgkin's lymphomas. They do not always meet the criterion of monoclonality necessary to be classified as such, however, and hence have become referred to by the broad term of *post-transplant lymphoproliferative disorders (PTLD)* (251). These disorders represent a significant source of morbidity and mortality in lung transplant recipients, and in some series represent the third leading cause of mortality outside of the perioperative period, after infections and rejection (167). Their hypothesized mechanism of pathogenesis relates to EBV infection of B lymphocytes whose subsequent proliferation is increased due to patients' immunosuppression. A causative role of EBV is supported by serologic evidence of EBV infection in almost all patients with PTLDs (252), and DNA evidence of EBV infection in lymphoid cells in almost all pathologic specimens of PTLDs (253).

Clinically, a distinction can be made between PTLDs presenting early, defined as less than one year post-transplant, and those presenting later than one year post-transplant (167). PTLDs occurring early tend to present with localized disease, tend to respond favorably to reductions in immunosuppression as their sole treatment, and are associated with lower mortality. PTLDs occurring late frequently present with disseminated disease, do not respond to reductions in immunosuppression, require cytotoxic chemotherapy for treatment, and are associated with higher mortality. In a large series of thoracic organ transplant patients, all PTLDs occurring in lung transplant patients occurred early, between two and four months after transplant.

Pickhardt et al (254) used chest radiography as a predictor of outcome in PTLD in lung transplant recipients. They observed that a solitary pulmonary nodule (seen in 50% of patients in their series) was the most common finding. Other findings included multiple nodules, multifocal alveolar infiltrates, and hilar and mediastinal adenopathy. CT scans of the chest detected additional nodules and lymph nodes, but did not show occult disease in any case where the chest x-ray appeared normal. Patients with solitary nodules, the authors found, have a better prognosis in the first year after diagnosis than do patients with other presentations.

Direct Toxicities of Immunosuppressive Medications

In addition to increasing patients' risks of infection and malignancy, immunosuppressive medications also have direct toxicities potentially affecting almost all organ systems. These toxicities can be a source of major morbidity, and even mortality, for lung transplant recipients.

Nephrotoxicity

Impaired renal function is the most troublesome toxicity of cyclosporine (255). This topic is reviewed in detail in Chapters 6 and 35. In a study of patients with nonrenal disease, cyclosporine treatment has been shown to cause significant decreases in renal blood flow, glomerular filtration rate, and creatinine clearance, associated with significant elevations in serum creatinine (256). There is evidence that these effects are reversible up to 12 months after the initiation of cyclosporine treatment, but eventually irreversible anatomic damage occurs (257). Renal function with these chronic changes can remain compromised but stable for prolonged periods of time. But renal deterioration can progress to end-stage renal disease requiring dialysis, and death from renal failure has been reported in one lung transplant patient over six years post-transplant (258). Multiple drugs can exacerbate cyclosporine nephrotoxicity, including furosemide, amphotericin B, ganciclovir, acyclovir, trimethoprim-sulfamethoxazole, and the aminoglycosides (255,259). Prevention and treatment of cyclosporine nephrotoxicity requires careful monitoring of both renal function and cyclosporine levels. If a decline in renal function is noted, it generally can be ameliorated by a reduction in cyclosporine dose. Additionally, treatment with misoprostrol, a prostaglandin E_1 analogue, has been shown to improve renal function in a small number of cyclosporine-treated kidney transplant patients (260).

Cyclosporine nephrotoxicity also can cause hypertension, at least in part by causing sodium retention and subsequent extracellular volume expansion (257). Corticosteroids also cause sodium retention, and these may contribute to hypertension in transplant patients. Dietary sodium restriction has been shown to significantly reduce the blood pressure of cycloporine-treated patients with hypertension (261). However, a minority of lung transplant patients will require medications to control their blood pressure (255).

Cyclosporine also induces renal magnesium wasting, which results in moderate to severe hypomagnesemia requiring chronic replacement therapy in almost one half of lung transplant patients (255). Finally, cyclosporine causes potassium retention (257). This results in hyperkalemia in only a minority of patients, however, and has been managed successfully with dietary modification and avoidance of potassium-sparing diuretics (255).

Gastrointestinal Toxicity

Immunosuppressive medications have multiple potential GI toxicities. Corticosteroids disrupt the cytoprotective gastric mucosal barrier and can thereby contribute to the development of gastroduodenal ulceration and bleeding (262). Cyclosporine has been associated with gastric atony, causing anorexia, nausea and vomiting, and erratic drug absorption in at least one third of lung transplant patients (215,255). Both cyclosporine and azathioprine can cause elevations in serum bilirubins and transaminases (263). The prevalence of cholelithiasis in heart transplant patients has been noted to be more than twice that expected for age- and gender-matched controls, and the cholestatic properties of cyclosporine and azathioprine may be contributory (262). Azathioprine, high-dose corticosteroids, and possibly cyclosporine also can cause pancreatitis (264) (see Chapter 29).

Musculoskeletal Toxicity

Corticosteroids can cause a myopathy that can involve both respiratory and proximal limb muscles (265). This weakness is fully reversible when steroids are discontinued or dosages are reduced. Rehabilitative conditioning programs appear to be the most effective treatment (266).

Corticosteroids also cause reduced bone formation and increased bone resumption, which can lead to osteoporosis (267). Steroid-induced osteoporosis affects trabecular bone more than cortical bone, typically resulting in fractures of the vertebrae, ribs, distal radius, and proximal femur. The incidence of fractures in steroid-treated individuals ranges from 11% to 20%. Bone mineral density is determined in lung transplant candidates prior to transplant to identify those with low bone mass who will be particularly at risk for steroid-induced osteoporosis. Multiple therapies are being investigated to determine their ability to prevent and/or treat osteoporosis, but the optimal management of this problem has not yet been established. For further discussion of this topic, the reader is referred to Chapter 31.

Central Nervous System Toxicity

Fifteen to forty percent of patients treated with cyclosporine experience neurologic side effects (268). The most common of these is tremor. A variety of other motor syndromes—including hemiparesis, paraparesis, and quadraparesis—have been reported. Cyclosporine is also epileptogenic, causing seizures in 2% to 6% percent of patients. A variety of encephalopathies can be caused by cyclosporine, with two syndromes being described most frequently. The first of these is characterized by a depressed level of consciousness, confusion, cortical blindness, and visual hallucinations. The second syndrome is characterized by ataxia, cerebellar tremor, focal weakness, and an altered mental status. Finally, cyclosporine can cause peripheral neuralgias and neuropathies, particularly paresthesias, dysesthesias, and hyperesthesias of the distal extremities, especially the hands. Fortunately, nearly all of these neurologic side effects are reversible with discontinuation or reduction in dosage of cyclosporine. Tacrolimus, like cyclosporine, is capable of inducing fulminant leukoencephalopathy after single lung transplantation. Improvement in neurologic symptoms, including seizures, is typically noted after discontinuation of the drug, with resolution of changes seen in neuroimaging (269) (see Chapter 33).

Psychiatric Toxicity

In addition to the neurologic toxicities described above, cyclosporine also has been associated with an organic anxiety disorder (270,271). Corticosteroids have been associated with delirium; organic mood disturbances, particularly euphoria, mania, and depression; and psychotic reactions, characterized by delusions, hallucinations, stupor, and catatonia (270,272). Lithium and clonazepam have been reported to be helpful in managing mania secondary to steroid use in transplant recipients; phenothiazines have been reported to be effective in treating psychiatric side effects of steroid use in general patient populations. These side effects typically resolve without specific psychiatric therapy if steroids are able to be discontinued.

Hematologic Toxicity

Azathioprine causes bone marrow suppression, which can result in leukopenia and, less frequently, anemia and thrombocytopenia (273). These effects on patients' peripheral blood counts are delayed, typically being noted 7 to 14 days after the initiation of treatment. Leukopenia, when it occurs, further increases patients' risk for opportunistic infections. It is reversible with discontinuation or reduction in dosage of azathioprine. Occasionally, colony stimulating factor is required to address neutropenia. Ganciclovir, as well as CMV infection, also can cause bone marrow suppression. Unexplained neutropenia should prompt a search for these causes. Finally, a chronic anemia associated with depressed levels of erythropoietin has been reported in solid organ transplant recipients, possibly due to cyclosporine (274). This form of anemia has been ameliorated in lung transplant patients by treatment with recombinant erythropoietin (275) (see Chapter 32).

Endocrine Toxicity

Corticosteroids can cause both hypercholesterolemia and hyperglycemia. Hypercholesterolemia has been noted in the majority of patients following lung transplantation (255). Hyperglycemia has been noted most commonly when high doses of steroids are employed, both in the early postoperative period and with treatment of episodes of acute rejection (276). Animal studies indicate that cyclosporine is also diabetogenic. Hyperglycemia is usually adequately controlled by diet or oral hypoglycemic agents, but occasionally requires treatment with insulin. Weight gain is very common with corticosteroid therapy and is due to both increased calorie intake and abnormal metabolism (see Chapter 31).

Dermal Toxicity

Corticosteroids can cause acne, dermal atrophy, and a redistribution of subcutaneous fat. Steroid-induced dermal atrophy can result in skin so thin and fragile that even slight trauma may cause significant bruising (277). Steroid-induced redistribution of subcutaneous fat causes the typical cushingoid appearance of central obesity and moon faces. Cyclosporine frequently causes gingival hyperplasia (278) and hypertrichosis (279). Cyclosporine-induced hypertrichosis is characterized by thick, pigmented hair developing on the trunk, back, shoulders, arms, neck, ears, forehead, and malar areas of the face.

OUTCOME

Despite the limitations of lung transplantation, many patients benefit greatly from this therapy. Individuals who were previously totally disabled, unable to carry out activities of daily living without enormous difficulty, are usually able to resume an active life-style and enjoy an enhanced life expectancy. They typically are more active and mobile and are able to travel, to resume work, or to return to school. For the individual patient, faced with the almost overwhelming complexity of transplantation and its potential attendant complications, the image of restoration to a markedly improved health status is important to emphasize. For society, the importance of defining additional measures of utility cannot be overlooked. As the population of recipients surviving for an extended period increases, more research data on this topic is likely to accrue.

Assessment of lung transplant recipients' status after transplantation may take several forms. Factors to consider include subjective well-being, alterations in pulmonary physiology and functional capacity, actuarial survival, and cost.

Survival

Operative mortality following lung transplantation has decreased markedly over the past decade. The reason for this reduction is probably multifactorial and is likely the result of technical improvements in the procedure, of improved recipient selection and preoperative management, and of increasing experience in perioperative management of these patients. In most recent series, operative mortality following lung transplantation is between 10% to 15%. DLT has an operative mortality rate ranging from 10% to 15% as compared to SLT, which is usually associated with an operative mortality rate of 10% or less. This difference is attributable in large part to the increased likelihood of postoperative infectious complications in patients with septic lung disease who require DLT. Operative mortality following HLT is usually slightly higher than for patients undergoing DLT, probably due to the more advanced disease state in those patients who require HLT as compared to isolated lung transplantation. Most centers have not noted a marked difference in operative mortality for patients undergoing SLT for different diseases, although preoperative pulmonary hypertension in these patients will usually increase the risk of postoperative morbidity (23,142,164).

Infection is the leading cause of early mortality in lung transplant recipients, accounting for 30% to 45% of deaths. The likelihood of pulmonary infection is greatest in the first 100 days after transplantation, before restoration of recipient defense mechanisms (e.g., cough) has occurred. Risk factors for infection in this time period include a positive sputum culture from the donor, a lower Pa_{O_2} in the donor lung (less than 350 mm Hg on F_{IO_2} of 1.0), a prolonged ischemic time (more than 6 hours), a recipient age of more than 40 years, and CMV disease as the result of donor/recipient mismatching without ganciclovir prophylaxis. Postoperative graft failure with diffuse alveolar damage may also contribute to early mortality in as many as 15% of patients. Unfortunately, there do not appear to be any specific risk factors for acute graft failure. However, with newer methods of management (e.g., inhaled nitric oxide) and increased skill in treating these patients, the mortality rate of this complication has been greatly reduced. Cardiovascular decompensation, termed *heart failure,* is the third leading cause of early death. In most cases, this process occurs in the clinical setting of ARDS and persistent pulmonary hypertension with secondary cardiac dysfunction. Coronary artery disease or myocardial infarction is uncommon in these patients (142).

Long-term survival data indicates a cumulative survival rate of 70% to 80% at one year. Later survival curves can vary significantly beyond one year depending upon the disease for which transplantation was performed. Patients with emphysema and patients with pulmonary vascular disease appear to have a survival advantage over patients with restrictive lung disease or septic lung disease, in whom infectious complications or recurrence of native disease in the lung graft may be seen. By three years, survival ranges from 75% in the former group to 55% in the latter group. At this interval, BOS begins to have a significant impact on survival as well, leading to an overall survival rate of only 50% at five years. Causes of death in this time period include infection, which has another peak of increased incidence throughout the second postoperative year, and BOS, which can be identified in half of patients surviving to three years. Malignancy, usually PTLD, is the third most common cause of late mortality following lung transplantation (23,142,227).

Functional Results

The majority of patients surviving lung transplantation have a dramatic improvement in their functional capability as compared to their preoperative state. Typically, patients can resume an exercise program without oxygen supplementation by six weeks after transplantation. In some patients, however, who have required muscular paralysis for management of postoperative graft failure, a demyelinating process may occur that will delay full recovery for two to three months. Eventually complete resolution is seen in the majority of these cases.

Improvements are seen regardless of the native disease that led to transplantation. Functional capacity remains stable for at least three years by the standards of reproducible exercise testing, unless symptomatic BOS occurs. Controversy exists over the potential benefit of SLT as compared to DLT for younger patients with emphysema. Although spirometry is obviously better in DLT recipients, exercise tolerance is similar in both groups initially. Whether a significant later advantage exists for DLT recipients that would offset the increased perioperative risk of the procedure remains to be seen. Similarly, functional results following SLT or DLT for pulmonary vascular disease demonstrate little objective difference between the two approaches. However, DLT may provide a slight advantage when preoperative pulmonary artery pressures approach systemic levels because such an approach provides the maximum reduction of PVR. In addition, because the allograft receives up to 95% of the blood flow after SLT for this indication, the development of BOS, even at grade 1, will have profound functional implications. The development of BOS in patients who have undergone DLT for pulmonary vascular disease is associated with less immediate hemodynamic compromise because of the similarity of blood flow among the two lungs (13,23,142).

As previously noted, exercise tolerance in patients with COPD is compromised by high ventilatory demand relative to capacity. Lung transplantation improves gas exchange, pulmonary mechanics, and exercise capacity. Despite the removal of the ventilatory limit to exercise, however, peak oxygen consumption ($\dot{V}O_2$ peak) does not reach predicted normal values after transplant. The $\dot{V}O_2$ at which ventilatory and lactate thresholds occur is also decreased in most lung transplant recipients (280–283). Some of the decrease in exercise capacity may be accounted for by abnormal systemic oxygen delivery. Specifically, anemia and submaximal heart rate may be limiting factors after transplantation. An alternative explanation is suggested by investigation of skeletal muscle oxidative capacity after lung transplantation by magnetic resonance spectroscopy (^{31}P-MRS). The data support the concept of a peripheral abnormality during exercise in lung transplant recipients by demonstrating abnormal skeletal muscle acid-base regulation and relating it to a reduced $\dot{V}O_2$ max. Speculatively, an acquired impaired mitochondrical oxidative capacity, related to cyclosporine, may best explain the abnormal skeletal muscle acid-base regulation and impaired aerobic capacity following lung transplantation (284).

A number of other interesting physiologic changes have been observed following lung transplantation. Some of these may reflect the effects of pulmonary denervation.

Both the cough reflex and mucociliary clearance are impaired after lung transplantation (285–288), which leads to the need for frequent bronchoscopies in order to promote better pulmonary hygiene in the immediate post-transplant period. Airway reactivity, as reflected by results of methacholine challenge tests, histamine, and distilled water has been hyperactive in some, but not all, studies (20). Some patients deserve a trial of inhaled bronchodilators and/or steroids for that reason. Minor variations in the control of breathing have been reported, such as the ventilatory response to hypercapnea, but the importance of these observations is unclear (20).

Quality of Life and Cost-Effectiveness

Several studies have documented improvement in measures of quality of life after heart–lung and lung transplantation. The data thus far, however, remain preliminary. Reports have generally been limited by relatively small numbers of patients, retrospective data accumulation, and by cross-sectional rather than longitudinal design. Ramsey et al (289) compared 21 recipients on a waiting list with 23 transplant recipients. Health-related quality of life was rated as superior after transplantation compared with before transplantation; however, the average time of assessment was only 9.3 months. Gross et al (290) reported similar findings after comparing a group of 44 candidates for lung transplantation with 54 allograft recipients. The development of BOS, not surprisingly, was associated with diminished quality of life. Nonetheless, Chaparro et al (291) found that most recipients who have survived beyond five years have acceptable lung function, are active, and are generally working, despite the frequent occurrence of BOS.

In a prospective longitudinal study of 24 Dutch lung transplant recipients, Ten Vergert et al concluded that lung transplantation not only improves survival but contributes positively to quality of life (292). Compared to their pre-transplant status, the recipients reported an improvement in mobility, energy, sleep, dyspnea, and capacity to perform activities of daily living. The improvements were rated approximately four months after transplantation and were maintained for the following 15 months. Despite the methodologic limitations of this and other studies, general agreement exists that lung transplantation improves survival and quality of life. Further research will likely substantiate this finding and focus on issues of cost-effectiveness.

The cost and cost-effectiveness of lung transplantation is an important issue, particularly in the context of managed care, the advent of global fees, and capitated systems. Many limitations presently prevent firm policy implications from being drawn from the pilot studies available, however. Gartner et al (293) have attempted to address the direction of research in this area, emphasizing the need to define carefully the utility measures used.

Retransplantation

Pulmonary retransplantation has been undertaken with increasing frequency in recent years. Retransplantation is used either as a method to correct an acute complication, such as graft failure or diffuse airway necrosis, or as a treatment for a chronic process in the graft, such a BOS or airway stenosis. At the present time, BOS appears to be the most common indication. A variety of approaches have been used, including redo ipsilateral SLT, contralateral SLT, or DLT following either a prior SLT or DLT. These are technically challenging procedures, with an operative mortality, in 1993, of nearly 50%. Factors contributing to a more favorable outcome include an ambulatory status prior to retransplantation, the use of ABO identical grafts, and prior institutional experience with retransplantation. Retransplantation with a seronegative CMV donor is also associated with a favorable outcome. Until recently, the long-term results of this approach were considered much worse than with initial lung transplantation. In 1993, one-year survival was about 45%, and two-year survival was 35%. BOS occurred with a frequency similar to that seen with primary lung transplantation and could be identified in one third of patients at two years following retransplantation (228).

Recently, Novick (294) reported that the results of retransplantation have improved considerably. Compared to the approximately 25% gap in survival between first and repeat lung transplants in 1993, he noted that in 1995 the one-year survival rate of approximately 60% for retransplantation was only 10% less than that for first transplants.

Therefore, offering retransplantation to carefully selected patients seems justified. However, controversy persists, much of it based on issues of individual and collective ethics. In the face of a scarce resource of donor organs, debate continues on how best to allocate them and to serve patient and societal needs (295).

REFERENCES

1. Demikhov VP. In: Experimental transplantation of vital organs. New York: Consultants Bureau Enterprises, 1962.
2. Metras H. Note preliminaire sur la greffe totale du poumon chez le chien. C R Acad Sci Paris 1950;231:1176–1178.
3. Hardin CA, Kittle CF. Experience with transplantation of the lung. Science 1954;119:87–89.
4. Hardy JD. Lung homotransplantation in man. JAMA 1963;186:1065–1066.
5. Derome F, Barbier F, Ringoir S, et al. Ten month survival after lung homotransplantation in man. J Thorac Cardiovasc Surg 1971;61:835–846.
6. Reitz BA, Wallwork JL, Hunt SA, et al. Heart–lung transplantation: successful therapy for patients with pulmonary vascular disease. N Engl J Med 1982;306:557–564.
7. Goldberg M, Lima O, Morgan E, et al. A comparison between cyclosporine A and methylprednisolone plus azathioprine on bronchial healing following canine lung autotransplantation. J Thorac Cardiovasc Surg 1983;85:821–826.
8. Toronto Lung Transplant Group. Unilateral lung transplantation for pulmonary fibrosis. N Engl J Med 1986;314:1140–1145.
9. Patterson GA, Cooper JD, Goldman B, et al. Technique of successful clinical double-lung transplantation. Ann Thorac Surg 1988;45:626–633.
10. Couraud L, Baudet E, Martigne C, et al. Bronchial revascularization in double lung transplantation. A series of 8 patients. Ann Thorac Surg 1992;53:88–94.
11. Pasque MK, Cooper JD, Kaiser LR, Haydock DA, et al. Improved technique for bilateral lung transplantation: rationale and initial clinical experience. Ann Thorac Surg 1990;49:785–791.
12. Mal H, Andreassian B, Pamela F, et al. Unilateral lung transplantation in end-stage pulmonary emphysema. Am Rev Respir Dis 1989;140:797–802.
13. Pasque MK, Trulock EP, Kaiser LR, Cooper JD. Single lung transplantation for pulmonary hypertension: three month hemodynamic follow-up. Circulation 1991;84:2275–2279.
14. Fremes SE, Patterson GA, Williams WG, et al. Single lung transplantation and closure of patent ductus arteriosus for Eisenmenger's syndrome. J Thorac Cardiovasc Surg 1990;100:1–5.
15. Hosenpud JD, Bennett LE, Keck BM, et al. The registry of the international society for heart and lung transplantation: fifteenth official report 1998. J Heart Lung Transplant 1998;17:651–668.
16. Joint Statement of ASTP, ATS, ERS, ISHLT. International guidelines for the selection of lung transplant candidates. Am J Respir Crit Care Med 1998;158:335–339.
17. Kadikar A, Maurer J, Kesten S. The six-minute walk test: a guide to assessment for lung transplantation. J Heart Lung Transplant 1997;16:313.
18. Cahalin L, Pappagianopoulos P, Prevost S, et al. The relationship of the 6-minute walk test to maximal oxygen consumption in transplant candidates with end-stage lung disease. Chest 1995;108:452–459.
19. Penn I. Neoplastic complications of transplantation. Semin Respir Infect 1993;8:233–239.
20. Trulock EP. State of the art lung transplantation. Am J Respir Crit Care Med 1997;155:789–818.
21. Liebowitz DW, Caputo AL, Shapiro GC, et al. Coronary angiography in smokers undergoing evaluation for lung transplantation: is routine use justified? J Heart Lung Transplant 1994;13:701–703.
22. Thaik CM, Semigran MJ, Ginns LC, et al. Evaluation of ischemic heart disease in potential lung transplant recipients. J Heart Lung Transplant 1995;14:257–266.
23. Bando K, Paradis IL, Komatsu K, et al. Analysis of time-dependent risks for infection, rejection and death after pulmonary transplantation. J Thorac Cardiovasc Surg 1995;109:49–57.
24. Arbustini E, Morbini P, Grasso M, et al. Human cytomegalovirus early infection, acute rejection and major histocompatibility class II expression in transplanted lung. Transplantation 1996;61:418–427.
25. Duncan SR, Paradis IL, Yousem SA, et al. Sequelae of cytomegalovirus pulmonary infections in lung allograft recipients. Am Rev Respir Dis 1992;146:1419–1425.
26. Frost AE, Jammal CT, Cagle PT. Hyperacute rejection following lung transplantation. Chest 1996;110:559–562.
27. Saint-Martin GA, Reddy VB, Garrity ER, et al. Humoral (antibody-mediated) rejection in lung transplantation. J Heart Lung Transplant 1996;15:1217–1222.
28. Gammie JS, Pham SM, Colson YL, et al. Influence of panel-reactive antibody on survival and rejection after lung transplantation. J Heart Lung Transplant 1997;16:408–415.
29. Wisser W, Wekerle T, Zlabinger G, et al. Influence of human leukocyte antigen matching on long-term outcome after lung transplantation. J Heart Lung Transplant 1996;15:1209–1216.
30. Sundaresan S, Mohanakumar T, Smith MA, et al. HLA-A locus mismatches and development of antibodies to HLA after lung transplantation correlate with the development of bronchiolits obliterans syndrome. Transplantation 1998;65:648–653.
31. Schulman IL, Weinberg AD, McGregor C, et al. Mismatches at the HLA-DR and HLA-B loci are risk factors for acute rejection after lung transplantation. Am J Respir Crit Care Med 1998;157:1833–1837.
32. Ferguson GT, Cherniack RM. Management of chronic obstructive pulmonary disease. N Engl J Med 1993;328:1017–1022.
33. Kesten S. End-stage lung disease and prediction of mortality. Semin Respir Crit Care Med 1996;17:423–435.
34. Manaker S, Tino G. Natural history and prognosis of advanced lung disease. Clin Chest Med 1997;18:433–455.
35. Edelman JD, Kotloff RM. Lung transplantation. A disease-specific approach. In: Kotloff R, Hansen-Flascher J, eds. Clin Chest Med 1997;18:627–644.
36. Gaensler EA, Cugell DW, Knudson RJ, et al. Surgical management of emphysema. In: Snider GL, ed. Clinics in Chest Medicine. Vol. 4. Philadelphia: WB Saunders, 1983.

37. Brantigan OC, Mueller E. Surgical treatment of pulmonary emphysema. Am Surg 1957;23:789–804.
38. Cooper JD, Trulock EP, Triantafillou AN, et al. Bilateral pneumonectomy (volume reduction) for chronic obstructive pulmonary disease. J Thorac Cardiovasc Surg 1995;109:106–119.
39. McKenna RJ, Brenner M, Fischel RJ, et al. Should lung volume reduction for emphysema be unilateral or bilateral. J Thorac Cardiovasc Surg 1996;112:1331–1339.
40. Keenan RJ, Landreneau RJ, Sciurba FC, et al. Unilateral thoacoscopic surgical approach for diffuse emphysema. J Thorac Cardiovasc Surg 1996;111:308–316.
41. Miller JI, Lee RB, Mansour KA. Lung volume reduction surgery: lessons learned. Ann Thorac Surg 1996;61:1464–1469.
42. Argenziano M, Moazami N, Thomashow B, et al. Extended indications for lung volume reduction surgery in advanced emphysema. Ann Thorac Surg 1996;62:1588–1597.
43. Wisser W, Tschernko E, Senbaklavaci O, et al. Functional improvement after volume reduction: sternotomy versus videoendoscopic approach. Ann Thorac Surg 1997;63:822–828.
44. Bingisser R, Zollinger A, Hauser M, et al. Bilateral volume reduction surgery for diffuse pulmonary emphysema by video-assisted thoracoscopy. J Thorac Cardiovasc Surg 1996;112:875–882.
45. Szekely LA, Oelberg DA, Wright CD, et al. Preoperative predicators of operative morbidity and mortality in COPD patients undergoing bilateral volume reduction surgery. Chest 1997;111:550–558.
46. Sciurba FC, Rogers RM, Keenan RJ, et al. Improvement in pulmonary function and elastic recoil after lung-reduction surgery for diffuse emphysema. N Engl J Med 1996;334:1095–1099.
47. Cooper JD, LeFrak SS. Editorial: Is volume reduction surgery appropriate in the treatment of emphysema? Yes. Am J Respir Crit Care Med 1996;153:1201–1204.
48. Make BJ, Fein AM. Editorial: Is volume reduction surgery appropriate in the treatment of emphysema? No. Am J Respir Crit Care Med 1996;153:1205–1207.
49. Snider GL. Pulmonary perspective: health-care technology assessment of surgical procedures: the case of reduction pneumoplasty for emphysema. Am J Respir Crit Care Med 1996;153:1208–1213.
50. Meyers BF, Yusen LD, Lefrak SS, et al. Outcome of Medicare patients with emphysema selected for, but denied, a lung volume reduction operation. Ann Thorac Surg 1998;66:331–336.
51. Zenati M, Keenan RJ, Sciurba FC, et al. Role of lung reduction in lung transplant candidates with pulmonary emphysema. Ann Thorac Surg 1996;62:994.
52. Bavaria JE, Pochettino A, Kotloff RM, et al. Effect of volume reduction on lung transplant timing and selection for chronic obstructive pulmonary disease. J Thorac Cardiovasc Surg 1998;115:9.
53. Gaissert HA, Trulock EP, Cooper JD, et al. Comparison of early functional results after volume reduction or lung transplantation for chronic obstructive pulmonary disease. J Thorac Cardiovasc Surg 1996;111:296.
54. Todd TR, Perron J, Winton TL, et al. Simultaneous single-lung transplantation and lung volume reduction. Ann Thorac Surg 1997;63:1468.
55. Sundaresan RS, Shiraishi Y, Trulock EP, et al. Single or bilateral lung transplantation for emphysema. J Thorac Cardiovasc Surg 1996;112:1485.
56. Hayden AM, Scarlett MV, Fox K. Relationship between donor/recipient lung size mismatch and functional outcome in single lung transplantation for COPD. J Transpl Coord 1996;6:155.
57. Anderson MB, Kriett JM, Kapelanski DP, et al. Volume reduction surgery in the native lung after single lung transplantation for emphysema. J Heart Lung Transplant 1993;16:752–757.
58. Reynolds HY. Diagnostic and management strategies for diffuse interstitial lung disease. Chest 1998;113(1):192–202.
59. Epler GR, Saber FA, Gaensler EA. Determination of severe impairment (disability) in interstitial lung disease. Rev Respir Dis 1980;121:647–660.
60. Raghu G. Interstitial lung disease: a diagnostic approach. Am J Respir Crit Care Med 1995;151:909–914.
61. Carrington CB, Gaensler EA, Coutu RE, et al. Natural history and treated course of usual and desquamative interstitial pneumonia. N Engl J Med 1978;298:801–809.
62. Hunninghake GW, Kalica AR. Approaches to the treatment of pulmonary fibrosis. Am J Respir Crit Care Med 1995;151:915–918.
63. Hayden AM, Robert RC, Kreitt JM, et al. Primary diagnosis predicts prognosis of lung transplant candidates. Transplantation 1993;55:1048.
64. Harari S, Simonneau G, DeJuli E, et al. Prognostic value of pulmonary hypertension in patients with chronic interstitial lung disease referred for lung or heart-lung transplantation. J Heart Lung Transplant 1997;16:460–463.
65. King MB, Jessurun J, Hertz MI. Recurrence of desquamative interstitial pneumonia after lung transplantation. Am J Respir Crit Care Med 1997;156:2003.
66. Parker LA, Novotny DB. Recurrent alveolar proteinosis following double lung transplantation. Chest 1997;111:1457–1458.
67. Johnson BA, Duncan SR, Ohori NP, et al. Recurrence of sarcoidosis in pulmonary allograft recipients. Am Rev Respir Dis 1993;148:1373.
68. Nine JS, Yousem SA, Paradis IL, et al. Lymphangioleiomyomatosis: recurrence after lung transplantation. J Heart Lung Transplant 1994;13:714–719.
69. O'Brien JD, Lium JH, Parosa JF, et al. Lymphangioleiomyomatosis recurrence in allograft after single-lung transplantation. Am J Respir Crit Care Med 1995;151:2033–2036.
70. Frost AE, Keller CA, Brown RW, et al. Giant cell interstitial pneumonitis disease recurrence in the transplanted lung. Am Rev Respir Dis 1993;148:1401–1404.
71. Habib SB, Congleton J, Carr D, et al. Recurrence of recipient Langerhans' cell histiocytosis following bilateral lung transplantation. Thorax 1998;53:323–325.
72. Etienne B, Bertocchi M, Gamondes JP, et al. Relapsing pulmonary Langerhans cell histiocytosis after lung transplantation. Am J Respir Crit Care Med 1998;157:288–291.
73. Lynch III JP, Kazerooni EA, Gay SE. In: Sharma OP, ed. Clinics in Chest Medicine. Pulmonary sarcoidosis. Vol. 4. Philadelphia: Saunders, 1997.
74. Pigula FA, Griffith BP, Zenati MA, et al. Lung transplantation for respiratory failure resulting from systemic disease. Ann Thorac Surg 1997;64:1630–1634.
75. Scott J, Higenbottam T. Transplantation of the lungs and heart and lung for patients with severe pulmonary complications from sarcoidosis. Sarcoidosis 1990;7:9–11.
76. Bjortuft O, Foerster A, Boe J, et al. Single lung transplantation as treatment for end-stage pulmonary sarcoidosis: Recurrence of sarcoidosis in two different lung allografts in one patient. J Heart Lung Transplant 1994;13:24.
77. Muller C, Briegel J, Haller M, et al. Sarcoidosis recurrence following lung transplantation. Transplantation 1996;61:1117–1119.
78. Kazerooni EA, Jackson C, Cascade PN. Sarcoidosis: Recurrence of primary disease in transplanted lungs. Radiology 1994;192:461.
79. Martinez F, Orens JB, Deeb M, et al. Recurrence of sarcoidosis following allogeneic lung transplantation. Chest 1994;106:1597–1599.
80. Judson MA. Lung transplantation for pulmonary sarcoidosis. Eur Respir J 1998;11:738–744.
81. Yeatman M, McNeil K, Smith JA, et al. Lung transplantation in patients with systemic diseases: an eleven year experience at Papworth Hospital. J Heart Lung Transplant 1996;15:144–149.
82. Walker S, Mikhail G, Banner N, et al. Medium term results of lung transplantation for end stage pulmonary sarcoidosis. Thorax 1998;53:281–284.
83. Baughman RP, Winget DB, Bowen EH, Lower EE. Predicting respiratory failure in sarcoidosis patients. Sarcoidosis Vasc Diffuse Lung Dis 1997;14:154–158.
84. Kalassian KG, Doyle R, Kao P, et al. Lymphangioleiomyomatosis: new insights. Am J Resp Crit Care Med 1997;155:1183–1186.
85. Taylor DR, Ryu J, Colby TV, et al. Lymphangioleiomyomatosis. N Engl J Med 1990;323:1254–1260.
86. Eliasson AH, Phillips YY, Tenholder MF. Treatment of lymphangioleiomyomatosis: a meta-analysis. Chest 1989;196:1352–1355.
87. Boehler A, Speich R, Russi EW, et al. Lung transplantation for lymphangioleiomyomatosis. N Engl J Med 1996;335:1275.
88. Ramsey BW. Management of pulmonary disease in patients with cystic fibrosis. N Engl J Med 1996;335(3):179–188.
89. Davis PB, Drumm M, Konstan MW. State of the art. Cystic fibrosis. Am J Respir Crit Care Med 1996;154:1229–1256.
90. Goldman MJ, Anderson GM, Stolzenberg ED, et al. Human B-defensin-1 is a salt-sensitive antibiotic in lung that is inactivated in cystic fibrosis. Cell 1997;88:553–560.
91. Smith JJ, Travis SM, Greenberg EP, et al. Cystic fibrosis airway epithelia fail to kill bacteria because of abnormal airway surface fluid. Cell 1996;85: 229–238.
92. Kerem E, Corey M, Kerem B, et al. The relation between genotype and phenotype in cystic fibrosis—analysis of the most common mutation (ΛF508). N Engl J Med 1990;323:1517–1522.
93. Flume PA, Egan TM, Paradowski LJ, et al. Infectious complications of lung transplantation: impact of cystic fibrosis. Am J Respir Crit Care Med 1994;149:1601–1607.
94. Tablan OC, Martone WJ, Doershuk CF, et al. Colonization of the respiratory tract with *Pseudomonas cepacia* in cystic fibrosis. Chest 1987;91:527–532.

95. Lewin LO, Byard PJ, Davis PB. Effect of *Pseudomonas cepacia* colonization on survival and pulmonary function of cystic fibrosis patients. J Clin Epidemiol 1990;43:125–131.1
96. Snell G, de Hoyos A, Krajden M, et al. *Pseudomonas cepacia* in lung transplantation recipients with cystic fibrosis. Chest 1993;103:466.
97. Egan T, Detterbeck F, Mill M, et al. Improved results of lung transplantation for patients with cystic fibrosis. J Thorac Cardiovasc Surg 1995;109:224.
98. Steinbach S, Sun L, Jiang R, et al. Transmissibility of *Pseudomonas cepacia* infection in clinic patients and lung-transplant recipients with cystic fibrosis. N Engl J Med 1994;331:981.
99. Sun L, Jiang R, Steinbach S, et al. The emergence of a highly transmissible lineage of cbl$^+$ *Pseudomonas (Burkholderia) cepacia* causing CF centre epidemics in North America and Britain. Nat Med 1995;1:661.
100. Griffith B, Hardesty R, Armitage J, et al. A decade of lung transplantation. Ann Surg 1993;218:310.
101. Saiman L, Mehar F, Niu W, et al. Antibiotic susceptibility of multiply resistant *Pseudomonas aeruginosa* isolated from patients with CF including candidates for transplant. Clin Infect Dis 1996;23:532–537.
102. Aris RM, Gilligan PH, Neuringer IP, et al. The effects of panresistant bacteria in cystic fibrosis patients on lung transplant outcome. Am J Respir Crit Care Med 1997;155:1699–1704.
103. Bauldoff GS, Nunley DR, Manzetti JD, et al. Use of aerosolized colistin sodium in cystic fibrosis patients awaiting lung transplantation. Transplantation 1997;64:748–752.
104. Davidson TM, Murphy C, Mitchell M, et al. Management of chronic sinusitis in cystic fibrosis. Laryngoscope 1995;105:354–358.
105. Aitken ML, Burke W, McDonald G, et al. Nontuberculous mycobacterial disease in adult cystic fibrosis patients. Chest 1993;103:1096–1099.
106. Ciriaco P, Egan T, Cairns E, et al. Analysis of cystic fibrosis referrals for lung transplantation. Chest 1995;107:1323–1326.
107. Nixon PA, Orenstein DM, Kelsey SF, et al. The prognostic value of exercise testing in patients with CF. N Engl J Med 1992;327:1785–1788.
108. Orenstein DM, Kaplan RM. Measuring quality of well-being in cystic fibrosis and lung transplantation. Chest 1991;100:1016–1018.
109. Milla CE, Warwick WJ. Risk of death in cystic fibrosis patients with severely compromised lung function. Chest 1998;113:1230–1234.
110. Sharples L, Hathaway T, Dennis C, et al. Prognosis of patients with cystic fibrosis awaiting heart and lung transplantation. J Heart Lung Transplant 1993;12:669–674.
111. Snell GI, Bennetts K, Bartolo J, et al. Body Mass Index as a predictor of survival in adults with cystic fibrosis referred for lung transplantation. J Heart Lung Transplantation 1998;17:1097–1103.
112. Couetil JP, Houssin DP, Soubrane O, et al. Combined lung and liver transplantation in patients with cystic fibrosis: a $4^1/_2$ year experience. J Thorac Cardiovasc Surg 1995;110:1415.
113. Dennis CM, McNeil KD, Dunning J, et al. Heart–lung-liver transplantation. J Heart Lung Transplant 1996;15:536.
114. Klima LD, Kowdley KV, Lewis SL, et al. Successful lung transplantation in spite of cystic fibrosis-associated liver disease: a case series. J Heart Lung Transplant 1997;16:934–938.
115. Egan TM, Detterbeck FC, Mill MR, et al. Lung transplantation for cystic fibrosis: effective and durable therapy in a high-risk group. Ann Thorac Surg 1998;66:337–346.
116. Rich S, Dantzker DR, Ayres SM, et al. Primary pulmonary hypertension. A national prospective study. Ann Intern Med 1987;107:216–223.
117. D'Alonzo GE, Barst RJ, Ayres SM, et al. Survival in patients with primary pulmonary hypertension: results from a national prospective registry. Ann Intern Med 1991;115:343–349.
118. Rubin LJ, Barst RJ, Kaiser LR, et al. ACCP consensus statement. Primary pulmonary hypertension. Chest 1993;104:236–250.
119. Lee SD, Shroyer KR, Markham CD, et al. Monoclonal endothelial cell proliferation is present in primary but not secondary pulmonary hypertension. J Clin Invest 1998;101:927–934.
120. Tuder RM, Radisavljevic Z, Shroyer K, et al. Monoclonal endothelial cells in appetite suppressant-associated pulmonary hypertension. Am J Resp Crit Care Med 1998;158:1999–2001.
121. Rubin LJ. Primary pulmonary hypertension. N Engl J Med 1997;336: 111–117.
122. Gorcsan III J, Edwards TD, Ziady GM, et al. Transesophageal echocardiography to evaluate patients with severe pulmonary hypertension for lung transplantation. Ann Thorac Surg 1995;59:717–722.
123. Badesch DB, Wynne KM, Bonvallet S, et al. Hypothyroidism and primary pulmonary hypertension: an autoimmune pathogenetic link? Ann Intern Med 1993;119:44–46.
124. Rich S, Kaufmann E, Levy PS. The effect of high doses of calcium-channel blockers on survival in primary pulmonary hypertension. N Engl J Med 1992;327:76–81.
125. Rich S. Medical treatment of primary pulmonary hypertension: a bridge to transplantation? Am J Cardiol 1995;75:63A–66A.
126. Alpert MA, Pressly TA, Mukerji V, et al. Short- and long-term hemodynamic effects of captopril in patients with pulmonary hypertension and selected connective tissue disease. Chest 1992;102:1407–1412.
127. Adatia I, Perry S, Landzberg M, et al. Inhaled nitric oxide and hemodynamic evaluation of patients with pulmonary hypertension before transplantation. J Am Coll Cardiol 1995;25:656–664.
128. Snell GI, Salamonsen RF, Bergin DS, et al. Inhaled nitric oxide used as a bridge to heart–lung transplantation in a patient with end-stage pulmonary hypertension. Am J Respir Crit Care Med 1995;151:1263–1266.
129. Olschewski H, Walmrath D, Schermuly R, et al. Aerosolized prostacyclin and iloprost in severe pulmonary hypertension. Ann Intern Med 1996;124:820–824.
130. Channick RN, Newhart JW, Johnson FW, et al. Pulsed delivery of inhaled nitric oxide to patients with primary pulmonary hypertension. Chest 1996;109:1545–1549.
131. Rubin LJ, Mendoza J, Hood M, et al. Treatment of primary pulmonary hypertension with continuous intravenous prostacyclin (epoprostenol). Ann Intern Med 1990;112:485–491.
132. Barst RJ, Rubin LJ, Long WA, et al. A comparison of continuous intravenous epoprostenol (prostacyclin) with conventional therapy for primary pulmonary hypertension. N Engl J Med 1996;334:296–301.
133. Conte JV, Gaine SP, Orens JB, et al. The influence of continuous intravenous prostacyclin therapy for primary pulmonary hypertension on the timing and outcome of transplantation. J Heart Lung Transplant 1998;17: 679–685.
134. Fuster V, Steele PM, Edwards WD, et al. Primary pulmonary hypertension: natural history and the importance of thrombosis. Circulation 1984;70:580–587.
135. Bengtsson L, Henze A, Holmgren A, Bjork VO. Thromboendarterectomy in chronic pulmonary embolism. Scand J Thorac Cardiovasc Surg 1986;20:67–70.
136. Daily PO, Dembitsky WP, Iversen S, et al. Risk factors for pulmonary thromboendarterectomy. J Thorac Cardiovasc Surg 1990;99:670–678.
137. Simonneau G, Azarian R, Brenot F, et al. Surgical management of unresolved pulmonary embolism: a personal series of 72 patients. Chest 1995;107:52S–55S.
138. Rothman A, Beltran D, Kriett JM, et al. Graded balloon dilation atrial septostomy as a bridge to lung transplantation in pulmonary hypertension. Am Heart J 1993;125:1763–1766.
139. Kerstein D, Levy PS, Hsu DT, et al. Blade balloon atrial septostomy in patients with severe primary pulmonary hypertension. Circulation 1995;91:2028–2035.
140. Levine SM, Gibbons WJ, Bryan CL, et al. Single lung transplantation for primary pulmonary hypertension. Chest 1990;98:1107–1115.
141. Maurer JR, Winton TL, Patterson GA, Williams TR. Single-lung transplantation for pulmonary vascular disease. Transplant Proc 1991;23:1211–1212.
142. Cooper JD, Patterson GA, Trulock EP, et al. Results of single and bilateral lung transplantation in 131 consecutive recipients. J Thorac Cardiovasc Surg 1994;107:460–471.
143. Chapelier A, Vouhe P, Macchiarini P, et al. Comparative outcome of heart–lung and lung transplantation for pulmonary hypertension. J Thorac Cardiovasc Surg 1993;106:299–307.
144. Carere R, Patterson GA, Liu P, et al. Right and left ventricular performance after single and double lung transplantation. J Thorac Cardiovasc Surg 1991;102:115–123.
145. Ritchie M, Waggoner AD, Davila-Roman VG, et al. Echocardiographic characterization of the improvement in right ventricular function in patients with severe pulmonary hypertension after single-lung transplantation. J Am Coll Cardiol 1993;22:1170–1174.
146. Kramer MR, Valantine HA, Marshall SE, et al. Recovery of the right ventricle after single-lung transplantation in pulmonary hypertension. Am J Cardiol 1994;73:494–500.
147. Kramer MR, Marshall SE, Tiroke A, et al. Clinical significance of hyperbilirubinemia in patients with pulmonary hypertension undergoing heart–lung transplantation. J Heart Lung Transplant 1991;10:317–321.
148. Bando K, Armitage JM, Paradis IL, et al. Indications for and results of single, bilateral, and heart–lung transplantation for pulmonary hypertension. J Thorac Cardiovasc Surg 1994;108:1056–1065.

149. Gammie JS, Keenan RJ, Pham SM, et al. Single versus double lung transplantation for pulmonary hypertension. J Thorac Candiovasc Surg 1998;115:397–402.
150. Saha A, Balakrishnan KG, Jaiswal PK, et al. Prognosis for patients with Eisenmenger's syndrome of various aetiology. Int J Cardiol 1994;45:199–207.
151. Kirshbom PM, Tapson VF, Harrison JK, et al. Delayed right heart failure following lung transplantation. Chest 1996;109:575–577.
152. Janssens SP, Bloch KD, Nong Z, et al. Adenoviral-mediated transfer of the human endothelial nitric oxide synthase gene reduces acute hypoxic pulmonary vasoconstriction in rats. J Clin Invest 1996;98:317–324.
153. Puskas JD, Winton TL, Miller JD, et al. Unilateral donor lung dysfunction does not preclude successful contralateral single-lung transplantation. J Thorac Cardiovasc Surg 1992;103:1015–1018.
154. Follette DM, Rudich SM, Babcock WD. Improved oxygenation and increased lung donor recovery with high-dose steroid administration after brain death. J Heart Lung Transplant 1998;17:423–429.
155. Low DE, Kaiser LR, Haydock D, et al. The donor lung: infectious and pathologic factors affecting outcome in lung transplantation. J Thorac Cardiovasc Surg 1993;106:614–620.
156. Sundaresan S, Semenkovich J, Ochoa J, et al. Successful outcome of lung transplantation is not compromised by the use of marginal donor lungs. J Thorac Cardiovasc Surg 1995;109:1075–1079.
157. Date H, Matsamura A, Manchester JK, et al. Evaluation of lung metabolism during successful twenty-four hour canine lung preservation. J Thorac Cardiovasc Surg 1993;105:480–491.
158. Christie NA, Waddell TK. Lung preservation. Chest Surg Clin North Am 1993;3:29–43.
159. Novick RJ. New trends in lung preservation: a collective review. J Heart Lung Transplant 1992;11:377–385.
160. Hopkinson DN, Bhabra MS, Hooper TL. Pulmonary graft preservation: a worldwide survey of current clinical practice. J Heart Lung Transplant 1998;17:525–531.
161. Snell GI, Rabinov M, Griffiths A, et al. Pulmonary allograft ischemic time: an important predictor of survival after lung transplantation. J Heart Lung Transplant 1996;15:160–168.
162. Norgaard MA, Olsen PS, Svendsen, et al. Revascularization of the bronchial arteries in lung transplantation: an overview. Ann Thorac Surg 1996;62:1215–1221.
163. Starnes VA, Barr ML, Cohen RG. Lobar transplantation. Indications, technique and outcome. J Thorac Cardiovasc Surg 1994;108:403–410.
164. Spray TL, Mallory GB, Canter CB, Huddleston CB. Pediatric lung transplantation. Indications, techniques and early results. J Thorac Cardiovasc Surg 1994;107:990–1000.
165. Ramirez JC, Patterson GA, Winton TL, et al. Bilateral lung transplantation for cystic fibrosis. J Thorac Cardiovasc Surg 1992;103:287–294.
166. Keenan RJ, Konishi H, Kawai A, et al. Clinical trial of tacrolimus versus cyclosporine in lung transplantation. Ann Thorac Surg 1995;60:580–585.
167. Armitage JM, Kormos RL, Stuart SR, et al. Posttransplant lymphoproliferative disease in thoracic organ transplant patients: ten years of cyclosporine-based immunosuppression. J Heart Lung Transplant 1991;10:877–887.
168. Ross DJ, Marchevsky A, Kramer M, et al. Refractoriness of airflow obstruction associated with isolated lymphocytic bronchiolitis/bronchitis in pulmonary allografts. J Heart Lung Transplant 1997;16:832–838.
169. Snell GI, Esmore DS, Willams TJ. Cytolytic therapy for the bronchiolitis obliterans syndrome complicating lung transplantation. Chest 1996;109:874–878.
170. Mentzer Jr RM, Jahania MS, Lesley RD. Tacrolimus as a rescue immunosuppressant after heart and lung transplantation. The U.S. multicenter FK506 study group. Transplantation 1998;65:109–113.
171. Ross DJ, Lewis MI, Kramer M, et al. FK506 rescue immunosuppression for obliterative bronchiolitis after lung transplantation. Chest 1997;112:1175–1179.
172. Horning NR, Lynch SP, Sundaresan SR, et al. Tacrolimus therapy for persistent or recurrent acute rejection after lung transplantation. J Heart and Lung Transplant 1998;17:761–767.
173. Valentine VC, Robbins RC, Wehner JH, et al. Total lymphoid irradiation for refractory acute rejection in heart-lung and lung allografts. Chest 1996;109:1184–1189.
174. Andrew G, Achkar A, Coutil JP, et al. Extracorporeal photochemotherapy treatment for acute lung rejection episode. J Heart Lung Transplant 1995;14:793–796.
175. Cahill BC, O'Rourke MK, Strasburg KA, et al. Methotrexate for lung transplant recipients with steroid-resistant acute rejection. J Heart Lung Transplant 1996;15:1130–1137.
176. Iacano AT, Keenan RJ, Duncan SR, et al. Aerosolized cyclosporine in lung recipients with refractory rejection. Am J Respir Crit Care Med 1996;153:1451–1455.
177. Iacano AT, Smaldone GC, Keenan RJ, et al. Dose-related reversal of acute lung rejection by aerosolized cyclosporine. Am J Respir Crit Care Med 1997;155:1690–1698.
178. Ross DJ, Waters PF, Levine M, et al. Mycophenolate mofetil versus azathioprine immunosuppressive regimens after lung transplantation: preliminary experience. J Heart Lung Transplant 1998;17:768–774.
179. O'Hair DP, Cantu E, McGregor C, et al. Preliminary experience with mycophenolate mofetil used after lung transplantation. J Heart Lung Transplantation 1998;17:864–868.
180. Whyte RI, Rossi SJ, Mulligan MS, et al. Mycophenolate mofetil for obliterative bronchiolitis syndrome after lung transplantation. Ann Thorac Surg 1997;64:945–948.
181. Kriett JM, Kaye MP. The registry of the International Society for Heart and Lung Transplantation: eighth official report—1991. J Heart Lung Transplant 1991;10:491–498.
182. Pairolero PC, Payne WS. Postoperative care and complications in the thoracic surgery patient. In: Baue AD, Geha AS, Hammond GL, et al., eds. Glenn's thoracic and cardiovascular surgery. Norwalk: Appleton and Lange, 1991:31–44.
183. Wolfe WG, ed. Complications in thoracic surgery: Recognition and management. St. Louis: Mosby-Year Book, 1992.
184. de Hoyos A, Maurer JR. Complications following lung transplantation. Semin Thorac Cardiovasc Surg 1992;4:132–146.
185. Anderson DC, Glazer HS, Semenkovich JW, et al. Lung transplant edema: chest radiography after lung transplantation—the first 10 days. Radiology 1995;195:275–281.
186. Sleiman C, Mal H, Dubois F, et al. Pulmonary reimplantation response in single lung transplantation. Am Rev Respir Dis 1992;145:A305.
187. Chaparro C, Chamberlain D, Maurer J, et al. Acute lung injury in lung allografts. J Heart Lung Transplant 1995;14:267–273.
188. Christie JD, Bavaria JE, Palevsky HI, et al. Primary graft failure following lung transplantation. Chest 1998;114:51–60.
189. Haydock DA, Trulock EP, Kaiser LR, et al. Management of dysfunction in the transplanted lung: experience with 7 clinical cases. Ann Thorac Surg 1992;53:635–641.
190. Morgan E, Lima O, Goldberg M, et al. Improved bronchial healing in canine left lung reimplantation using omental pedicle wrap. J Thorac Cardiovasc Surg 1983;85:134–139.
191. Calhoon JH, Grover FL, Gibbons WJ, et al. Single lung transplant: alternative indications and technique. J Thorac Cardiovasc Surg 1991;101:816–825.
192. Shennib H, Massard G. Airway complications in lung transplantation. Ann Thorac Surg 1994;57:506–511.
193. Anzeuto A, Levine SM, Tillis WP, et al. Use of the flow-volume loop in the diagnosis of bronchial stenosis after single lung transplantation. Chest 1994;105:934–936.
194. Neagos GR, Martinez FJ, Deeb GM, et al. Diagnosis of unilateral mainstem bronchial obstruction following single-lung transplantation with routine spirometry. Chest 1993;103:1255–1258.
195. Cavaliere S, Foccoli P, Farina RL. Nd:YAG laser bronchoscopy: a five year experience with 1,396 applications in 1,000 patients. Chest 1988;94:15–21.
196. Colt HG, Janssen JP, Dumon JF, et al. Endoscopic management of bronchial stenosis after double lung transplantation. Chest 1992;102:10–16.
197. Dumon JF. A dedicated tracheobronchial stent. Chest 1990;97:328–332.
198. Herlihy JP, Venegas JG, Systrom DM, et al. Expiratory flow pattern following single-lung transplantation in emphysema. Am J Respir Crit Care Med 1994;150:1684–1689.
199. Haydock DA, Trulock EP, Kaiser LR, et al. Lung transplantation: analysis of thirty-six consecutive procedures performed over a twelve-month period: the Washington University Lung Transplant Group. J Thorac Cardiovasc Surg 1992;103:329–340.
200. Mal H, Sleiman C, Jebrak G, et al. Early hemodynamic complications after lung transplantation. Am Rev Respir Dis 1992;145:A702.
201. Smith PC, Slaughter MS, Petty MG, et al. Abdominal complications after lung transplantation. J Heart Lung Transplant 1995;14:44–51.
202. Littlewood JM. Gastrointestinal complications. Brit Med Bull 1992;48:847–859.
203. Jenkinson SG, Levine SM. Lung transplantation. Disease-A-Month 1994;40:1–38.
204. Hutchinson I. Transplantation and rejection. In: Roitt IM, Brostoff J, Male DK, eds. Immunology. Vol. 23. London: Mosby-Year Book Europe, 1993:1–14.

205. Auchincloss Jr H, Sachs DH. Transplantation and graft rejection. In: Paul WE, ed. Fundamental immunology. New York: Raven, 1993:1099–1142.
206. de Hoyos A, Chamberlain D, Schvartzman R, et al. Prospective assessment of a standardized pathologic grading system for acute rejection in lung transplantation. Chest 1993;103:1813–1818.
207. Paradis IL, Duncan SR, Dauber JH, et al. Distinguishing between infection, rejection, and the adult respiratory distress syndrome after human lung transplantation. J Heart Lung Transplant 1992;11:S232–S236.
208. Yousem SA, Berry GJ, Brunt EM, et al. A working formulation for the standardization of nomenclature in the diagnosis of heart and lung rejection: lung rejection study group. J Heart Transplant 1990;9:593–601.
209. Yousem SA, Berry GJ, Cagle PT, et al. Revision of the 1990 working formulation for the classification of pulmonary allograft rejection: lung rejection study group. J Heart Lung Transplant 1996;15:1–15.
210. Tazelaar HD. Perivascular inflammation in pulmonary infections: implications for the diagnosis of lung rejection. J Heart Lung Transplant 1991;10:437–441.
211. Yousem SA. Lymphocytic bronchitis/bronchiolitis in lung allograft recipients. Am J Surg Pathol 1993;17:491–495.
212. Trulock EP. Management of lung transplant rejection. Chest 1993;103:1566–1576.
213. Bergin CJ, Castellino RA, Blank N, et al. Acute lung rejection after heart–lung transplantation: correlation of findings on chest radiographs with lung biopsy results. AJR 1990;155:23–27.
214. Millet B, Higenbottam TW, Flower CD, et al. The radiographic appearances of infection and acute rejection of the lung after heart-lung transplantation. Am Rev Respir Dis 1989;140:62–67.
215. Griffith BP, Bando K, Hardesty RL, et al. A prospective randomized trial of FK506 versus cyclosporine after human pulmonary transplantation. Transplantation 1994;57:848–851.
216. Griffith BP, Hardesty RL, Armitage JM, et al. Acute rejection of lung allografts with various immunosuppressive protocols. Ann Thorac Surg 1992;54:846–851.
217. Westaby S. Aprotonin in perspective. Ann Thorac Surg 1993;55:1033–1041.
218. Hruban RH, Beschorner WE, Baumgartner WA, et al. Depletion of bronchus-associated lymphoid tissue with lung allograft rejection. Am J Pathol 1988;132:6–10.
219. Dark JH. Clinical diagnosis of rejection and the development of obliterative bronchiolitis after lung transplantation. In: Rose ML, Yacomb MH, eds. Immunology of heart and lung transplant. London: Edward Arnold, 1993.
220. Keller CA, Cagle PT, Brown RW, et al. Bronchiolitis obliterans in recipients of single, double, and heart–lung transplantation. Chest 1995;107:973–980.
221. Tilney NL, Whitley WD, Diamond JR, et al. Chronic rejection—an undefined conundrum. Transplantation 1991;52:389–398.
222. Bando K, Paradis IL, Similo S, et al. Obliterative bronchiolitis after lung and heart–lung transplantation. An analysis of risk factors and management. J Thorac Cardiovasc Surg 1995;110:4–14.
223. Kshettry VR, Kroshus TJ, Savik K, et al. Primary pulmonary hypertension as a risk factor for the development of obliterative bronchiolitis in lung allograft recipients. Chest 1996;110:704.
224. Cooper JD, Billingham M, Egan T, et al. A working formulation for the standardization of nomenclature and for clinical staging of chronic dysfunction in lung allografts. J Heart Lung Transplant 1993;12:713–716.
225. Theodore J, Starnes VA, Lewiston NJ. Obliterative bronchiolitis. Clin Chest Med 1990;11:309–321.
226. Sundaresan S, Trulock EP, Mohanakumar T, et al. Prevalence and outcome of bronchiolitis obliterans syndrome after lung transplantation. Ann Thorac Surg 1995;60:1341–1346.
227. Novick RJ, Kaye M, Patterson GA, et al. Redo lung transplantation: a North American-European experience. J Heart Lung Transplant 1993;12:5–16.
228. Judson MA. Clinical aspects of lung transplantation. Clin Chest Med 1993;14:335–357.
229. Hathaway T, Higenbottam T, Lowry R, et al. Pulmonary reflexes after human heart–lung transplantation. Respir Med 1991;85:17–21.
230. Shankar S, Fulsham L, Read RC, et al. Mucociliary function after lung transplantation. Tranplant Proc 1991;23:1222–1223.
231. Maurer JR, Tullis DE, Grossman RF, et al. Infectious complications following isolated lung transplantation. Chest 1992;101:1056–1059.
232. Paradis IL, Williams P. Infection after lung transplantation. Semin Respir Infect 1993;8:207–215.
233. Smyth RL, Scott JP, Borysiewicz LK, et al. Cytomegalovirus infection in heart–lung transplant recipients: risk factors, clinical associations, and response to treatment. J Infect Dis 1991;164:1045–1050.
234. Chou S. Acquisition of donor strains of cytomegalovirus by renal-transplant recipients. N Engl J Med 1986;314:1418–1423.
235. Avery RK, Longworth DL. Viral pulmonary infections in thoracic and cardiovascular surgery. Semin Thorac Cardiovasc Surg 1995;7:88–94.
236. Duncan AJ, Dummer JS, Paradis IL, et al. Cytomegalovirus infection and survival in lung transplant recipients. J Heart Lung Transplant 1991;10:638–646.
237. Hayden FG, Gwaltney Jr JM. Viral infections. In: Murray JF, Nadel JA, eds. Textbook of respiratory medicine. Philadelphia: WB Saunders, 1994:977–1035.
238. Dauber JH, Paradis IL, Dummer JS. Infectious complications in pulmonary allograft recipients. Clin Chest Med 1990;11:291–308.
239. Morris DJ. Opportunities for diagnosing cytomegalovirus in pulmonary infections. Thorax 1995;50:9–13.
240. Ettinger NA, Bailey TC, Trulock EP, et al. Cytomegalovirus infection and pneumonitis: impact after isolated lung transplantation. Am Rev Respir Dis 1993;147:1017–1023.
241. Krinzman S, Basgoz N, Kradin R, et al. Respiratory syncytial virus-associated infections in adult recipients of solid organ transplants. J Heart Lung Transplant 1998;17:202–210.
242. Krinzman S, Basgoz N, Bhalla M, et al. RSV associated pneumonitis in recipients of solid organ transplantation. Am J Respir Crit Care Med 1995;151:A81.
243. Murris-Espin M, Didier A, Carre P, et al. Continuous aerosolised ribavirin for respiratory syncytial virus infection in lung transplant recipients. Lancet 1993;341:897.
244. Simsir A, Greenbaum E, Nuovo G, et al. Late fatal adenovirus pneumonitis in a lung transplant recipient. Transplantation 1998;65:592–594.
245. Cahill BC, Hibbs JR, Savik K, et al. Aspergillus airway colonization and invasive disease after lung transplantation. Chest 1997;112:1160–1164.
246. Kramer MR, Denning DW, Marshall SE, et al. Ulcerative tracheobronchitis after lung transplantation. Am Rev Respir Dis 1991;144:552–556.
247. Gryzan S, Paradis IL, Zeevi A, et al. Unexpectedly high incidence of Pneumocystis carinii infection after lung–heart transplantation. Am Rev Respir Dis 1988;137:1268–1274.
248. Kramer MR, Stoehr C, Lewiston NJ, et al. Trimethoprim-sulfamethoxazole prophylaxis for pneumocystis carinii infections in heart–lung and lung transplantation—how effective and for how long. Transplantation 1992;53:586–589.
249. Miller RA, Lanza LA, Kline JN, et al. Mycobacterium tuberculosis in lung transplant recipients. Am J Respir Crit Care Med 1995;152:374–376.
250. Trulock EP, Bolman RM, Genton R. Pulmonary disease caused by mycobacterium chelonae in a heart–lung transplant recipient with obliterative bronchiolitis. Am Rev Respir Dis 1989;140:802–805.
251. Knowles DM, Cesarman E, Chadburn A, et al. Correlative morphologic and molecular genetic analysis demonstrates three distinct categories of posttransplantation lymphoproliferative disorders. Blood 1995;85:552–565.
252. Nalesnik MA, Jaffe R, Starzl TE, et al. The pathology of posttransplant lymphoproliferative disorders occurring in the setting of cyclosporine A-prednisone immunosuppression. Am J Pathol 1988;133:173–192.
253. Berg LC, Copenhaver CM, Morrison VA, et al. B-cell lymphoproliferative disorders in solid-organ transplant patients: detection of Epstein-Barr virus by in situ hybridization. Hum Pathol 1992;23:159–163.
254. Pickhardt PJ, Siegel MJ, Anderson DC, et al. Chest radiography as a predictor of outcome in post-transplantation lymphoproliferative disorder in lung allograft recipients. Am J Roentgenol 1998;171:375–382.
255. Maurer JR. Therapeutic challenges following lung transplantation. Clin Chest Med 1990;11:279–290.
256. Tegzess AM, Doorenbos BM, Minderhoud JM, et al. Prospective serial renal function studies in patients with nonrenal disease treated with cyclosporine A. Transplant Proc 1988;20:530–533.
257. Sturrock ND, Lang CC, Struthers AD. Cyclosporine-induced nephrotoxicity and hypertension. Brit J Hosp Med 1992;48:483–489.
258. de Hoyos AL, Patterson GA, Maurer JR, et al. Pulmonary transplantation: early and late results. J Thorac Cardiovasc Surg 1992;103:295–306.
259. Lake KD. Management of drug interactions with cyclosporine. Pharmacotherapy 1991;11:110S–118S.
260. Moran M, Mozes MF, Maddux MS, et al. Prevention of acute graft rejection by the prostaglandin E1 analogue misoprostol in renal-transplant recipients treated with cyclosporine and prednisone. N Engl J Med 1990;322:1183–1188.
261. Curtis JJ, Luke RG, Jones P, et al. Hypertension in cyclosporine-treated renal transplant recipients is sodium dependent. Am J Med 1988;85:134–138.
262. Frist WH. Management of complications. In: Shumway SJ, Shumway NE, eds. Thoracic transplantation. Cambridge: Blackwell Science, 1995:226–251.
263. Klintmalm GB, Iwatsuki S, Starzl TE. Cyclosporine A hepatotoxicity in 66 renal allograft recipients. Transplantation 1981;32:488–489.

264. Kawanishi H, Rudolph E, Bull FE. Azathioprine-induced acute pancreatitis. N Engl J Med 1973;289:357.
265. Decramer M, Lacquet LM, Fagard R, et al. Corticosteroids contribute to muscle weakness in chronic airflow obstruction. Am J Respir Crit Care Med 1994;150:11–16.
266. Hollister JR. The untoward effects of steroid treatment on the musculoskeletal system and what to do about them. J Asthma 1992;29:363–368.
267. Jenkinson T, Bhalla AK. A reappraisal of steroid-induced osteoporosis. Brit J Hosp Med 1993;50:472–476.
268. Patchell RA. Neurological complications of organ transplantation. Ann Neurol 1994;6:688–703.
269. Thyagarajan GK, Cobanoglu A, Johnston W. FK506 induced fulminant leukoencephalopathy after single lung transplantation. Thoracic Surg 1997;64:1461–1464.
270. Trzepacz PT, DiMartini A, Tringali R. Psychopharmacologic issues in organ transplantation. Part 1: pharmacokinetics in organ failure and psychiatric aspects of immunosuppressants and anti-infectious agents. Psychosomatics 1993;34:199–207.
271. Trzepacz PT, Levenson JL, Tringali RA. Psychopharmacology and neuropsychiatric syndromes in organ transplantation. Gen Hosp Psychiatry 1991;13:233–245.
272. Milgrom H, Bender BG. Psychologic side effects of therapy with corticosteroids. Am Rev Respir Dis 1993;147:471–473.
273. Min DI, Monaco AP. Complications associated with immunosuppressive therapy and their management. Pharmacotherapy 1991;11:119S–125S.
274. Frost AE, Keller C, for the Multi-organ Transplant Group. Anemia and erythropoietin levels in recipients of solid organ transplants. Transplantation 1993;56:1008–1011.
275. End A, Ringl H, Grimm M, et al. Chronic anemia after lung transplantation: treatment with human recombinant erythropoietin. Transplantation 1994;57:1142.
276. Shumway SJ, Frist WH. Immunosuppressants. In: Shumway SJ, Shumway NE, eds. Thoracic transplantation. Cambridge: Blackwell Science, 1995:55–66.
277. Oikarinen A, Autio P. New aspects of the mechanism of corticosteroid-induced dermal atrophy. Clin Exper Derm 1991;16:416–419.
278. Wysocki GP, Gretzinger HA, Laupacis A, et al. Fibrous hyperplasia of the gingiva: a side effect of cyclosporine A therapy. Oral Surg 1983;55:274–278.
279. Bencini PL, Montagnino G, Sala F, et al. Cutaneous lesions in 67 cyclosporine-treated renal transplant recipients. Dermatologica 1986;172:24–30.
280. Gibbons WJ, Levine SM, Bryan CL, et al. Cardiopulmonary exercise responses after single lung transplantation for severe obstructive lung disease. Chest 1991;100:106–111.
281. Miyoshi S, Trulock EP, Schaefers HJ, et al. Cardiopulmonary exercise testing after single and double lung transplantation. Chest 1990;97:1130–1136.
282. Williams TJ, Patterson GA, McClean PA, et al. Maximal exercise testing in single and double lung transplant recipients. Am Rev Respir Dis 1992;145:101–105.
283. Ross DJ, Waters PF, Mohsenifar Z, et al. Hemodynamic responses to exercise after lung transplantation. Chest 1993;103:46–53.
284. Evans AB, Al-Himyary AJ, Hrovat MI, et al. Abnormal skeletal muscle oxidative capacity after lung transplantation by ^{31}P-MRS. Am J Respir Crit Care Med 1997;155:615–621.
285. Higenbottam T, Jackson P, Woolman R, et al. The cough response to ultrasonically nebulized distilled water in heart–lung transplantation patients. Am Rev Respir Dis 1989;140:58–61.
286. Herve P, Silbert J, Cerrina G, et al. Impairment of bronchial mucociliary clearance in long-term survivors of heart/lung and double-lung transplantation. Chest 1993;103:59–63.
287. Read RC, Shanker A, Rutman C, et al. Ciliary beat frequency and structure of recipient and donor epithelia following transplantation. Eur Respir J 1991;4:796–801.
288. Veale D, Glasper PN, Gascoigne A, et al. Ciliary beat frequency in transplanted lungs. Thorax 1993;48:629–631.
289. Ramsey S, Patrick D, Lewis S, et al. Improvement in quality of life after lung transplantation: a preliminary study. J Heart Lung Transplant 1995;14:870–877.
290. Gross C, Savik K, Bolman M, Hertz M. Long-term health status and quality of life outcomes of lung transplant recipients. Chest 1995;108:1587–1593.
291. Chaparro C, Scavuzzo M, Winton T, et al. Status of lung transplant recipients surviving beyond five years. J Heart Lung Transplant 1997;16:511–516.
292. TenVergert EM, Essink-Bot ML, Geertsma A, et al. The effect of lung transplantation on health-related quality of life. Chest 1998;113:358–364.
293. Gartner SH, Sevick MA, Keenan RJ, Chen GJ. Cost-utility of lung transplantation: a pilot study. J Heart Lung Transplant 1997;16:1129–1134.
294. Novick RJ. Heart and lung retransplantation: should it be done? J Heart Lung Transplant 1998;17:635–642.
295. Mentzer SJ, Reilly JJ, Caplan AL, et al. Ethical considerations in lung transplantation. J Heart Lung Transplant 1994;13:56–58.

Chapter

26

Heart–Lung Transplantation

George V. Letsou John C. Baldwin

Nearly 100 years ago, Alexis Carrel and Charles Guthrie began the first experimental work in combined heart–lung transplantation. In the presentation of their work before the John Hopkins Medical Society, it was noted that the operation had been successful technically but that the lungs became edematous and the right ventricle distended (1,2). Since this initial experimental report, a century of experimental and clinical work has been directed toward making heart–lung transplantation a clinical reality.

Until the advent of combined heart and lung transplantation, the treatment of advanced end-stage pulmonary vascular disease in combination with cardiac failure was difficult and frustrating. Such patients had few medical treatment options. The introduction of combined heart and lung transplantation as well as cyclosporine, however, improved the prospects for survival and effective rehabilitation for properly selected patients with a variety of cardiopulmonary syndromes such as primary pulmonary hypertension, congenital heart disease with Eisenmenger's physiology, fibrotic and emphysematous lung disease with associated cor pulmonale, and cystic fibrosis.

HISTORY

The history of heart–lung transplantation is intimately related to that of cardiac transplantation. Pioneering efforts in both fields were made by Alexis Carrel at the turn of the twentieth century. His work involving vascular anastomoses as well as heart–lung transplantation eventually led to his receipt of the Nobel Prize. Carrel's work demonstrated that cardiac transplantation was technically feasible, that all four chambers of the heart would function properly, and that the heart and lungs could be moved from one mammal to another. Other important findings continued through the early part of the twentieth century. Mann et al demonstrated eight-day survival in a mammalian model of cardiac transplantation in 1933 (3). Demikhov, working in the Soviet Union in the 1950s, performed several successful heart–lung transplants. However, it was not until Lower and Shumway's landmark report of experimental canine orthotopic cardiac transplantation, in which five of eight animals survived for 21 days, that thoracic transplantation became feasible (4). Experimental work culminated in the first human orthotopic cardiac transplantation, which was performed by Barnard in 1967 based on the experimental work of Lower and Shumway and on observations in Lower's laboratory (5). Subsequently, continued clinical work with orthotopic cardiac transplantation in conjunction with the development of techniques for safe cardiopulmonary bypass, effective myocardial preservation using hypothermia, the rapid and early diagnosis of myocardial rejection, and the introduction of the immunosuppressant cyclosporine made isolated cardiac transplantation a clinical success and widely accepted in the 1980s.

With the success of clinical isolated orthotopic cardiac transplantation, the large population of end-stage cardiac patients with associated pulmonary vascular disease or primary pulmonary problems presented a difficult treatment dilemma. It became obvious that patients with elevated pulmonary vascular resistances above eight Wood units were poor candidates for isolated cardiac transplantation. Attempts to circumvent this problem by transplanting the heart and lungs as a unit culminated in the first successful clinical orthotopic heart–lung transplant reported by Reitz and colleagues at Stanford (6).

Since this landmark report, heart–lung transplantation has become an accepted technique for the treatment of combined heart and lung pathology. Suitable organ donors, however, have become increasingly hard to identify. The rise of isolated lung transplantation as a technique for treating isolated lung pathology has made suitable heart–lung donors even more scarce (see Chapter 25). Heart–lung transplantation, isolated heart transplantation, and isolated lung transplantation have overlapping therapeutic roles, but offer a broad variety of patients extremely effective treatment.

RECIPIENT SELECTION

Heart–lung transplantation offers good prospects for survival in patients with a variety of cardiopulmonary syndromes. These include primary pulmonary hypertension, congenital heart disease with Eisenmenger's physiology, fibrotic and emphysematous lung disease with cor pulmonale, and cystic fibrosis. Potential recipients should have severe life-threatening symptoms and limited life expectancy of less than six months to one year (although the natural history of these various diseases is unpredictable). All other modes of conventional medical and surgical therapy should be exhausted prior to listing a patient for transplantation. Because of the shortage of donor organs and the relatively favorable experience with younger recipients, heart–lung transplantation is usually limited to recipients who are less than 60 years of age. Contraindications include the presence of other systemic diseases. The renal dysfunction (prerenal azotemia) seen with heart failure is not considered a contraindication, however, and the passive hepatic congestion present in patients with right-sided heart failure is also not a strict contraindication. Established systemic infection resulting in elevated white blood cell counts or fever is a contraindication. Major previous thoracic surgery, such as formal posterolateral thoracotomy, is a contraindication, although more limited incisions such as those necessary for lung biopsy are not. Patients with insulin-dependent diabetes mellitus should be considered carefully because of the expected exacerbation with postoperative steroid immunosuppressants.

All patients must be stable psychologically and able to comply with the rigid postoperative protocol of immunosuppressants as well as the difficult, prolonged preoperative waiting times necessary for heart–lung transplantation.

Evaluation of recipients preoperatively should be directed at detecting the potential recipient's severity of illness and the presence of relative or absolute contraindications. Basic assessments of cardiac and pulmonary function are mandatory. All patients should have a detailed assessment of pulmonary function including forced expiratory volume at one second, forced vital capacity, total lung capacity, and diffusing capacity of oxygen. Pulmonary malignancies or abnormalities should be ruled out by routine chest radiograph and computerized tomography (CT) or magnetic resonance imaging (mRI) as indicated. Patients with cystic fibrosis must have a careful analysis of pulmonary pathogens; those patients with untreatable or highly resistant bacterial strains (most commonly *Pseudomonas*) should be excluded from transplantation. Patients with resistant fungal species in the sputum are not good candidates. Bronchoscopy may be necessary for adequate pulmonary evaluation, but it is not mandatory. This assessment is similar to that described in detail, for isolated lung transplant candidates, in Chapter 25.

Preoperative cardiac evaluation usually is directed at ascertaining whether pulmonary transplantation in conjunction with cardiac transplantation is necessary. Right heart catheterization is necessary for the determination of pulmonary vascular resistance. Nuclear cardiac scanning is very useful for determining right ventricular function. Cineangiography of the coronary arteries is not mandatory.

Preoperative evaluation of the remaining organ systems is directed at determining whether other irreversible systemic illnesses are present. The evaluation is directed first at those systems commonly affected by cardiac failure. Azotemia and hepatic dysfunction as evidenced by mild elevation in renal or liver function tests are not uncommon and, while not absolute contraindications for surgery, they do mandate a more careful approach and thorough evaluation.

MANAGEMENT OF THE RECIPIENT AND DONOR PERIOPERATIVELY

As in all thoracic transplantation, organs are matched through size, weight, and ABO blood group compatibility. Donors should be within 20% of the receipient's size and weight. It is particularly important to ascertain an appropriate thoracic size match between donor and recipient in heart–lung transplantation. Significant technical difficulties during implantation of grafts have been encountered when large donors have been matched with relatively small recipients and the chest cavity cannot contain the organs. Other problems—persistent air space and pleural fluid collections—have been encountered when inappropriately small grafts are placed into larger recipients. An ideal size match is one in which the donor thoracic dimensions are slightly smaller than those of the proposed recipient; this facilitates graft implantation and allows for full lung expansion.

Although HLA typing is typically performed prior to thoracic organ transplantation, retrospective reviews of HLA matching in cardiac transplantation reveal only slightly improved survival rates with closer compatibility. This slight improvement in survival rates has not been felt to warrant HLA matching as a part of the preoperative workup (7). HLA data are collected for retrospective analysis.

Appropriate donors are difficult to identify (see Chapter 15). The rate-limiting factor in clinical heart–lung transplantation is the continuing and acute shortage of suitable donor organs. The problem is particularly acute in the case of heart–lung donors because of the propensity for neurogenic pulmonary edema, atelectasis, pneumonia, and other pulmonary complications in brain-dead, ventilated patients. Also, the current thoracic organ regulations of the United Network for Organ Sharing (UNOS) somewhat discriminate against the use of combined heart–lung donors in favor of single-lung donors. Nevertheless, current criteria for the appropriate heart–lung donor are those donors who have been declared brain-dead under appropriate local criteria and who are less than 35 years of age. Older donors may be used, but a thorough examination of the heart including echocardiography and, if necessary, cineangiography and cardiac catheterization should be performed. There should be no history of preexisting cardiopulmonary disease and any smoking history should be remote. If the donor died because of a high–kinetic energy accident, there should be no evidence of pulmonary or cardiac contusion by electrocardiogram (EKG), enzymes, or radiograph. Donors should not require maintenance with high-dose pressors (greater than 5 μg/kg/min of dopamine). There should be no requirement for high concentrations of inspired oxygen. All donors should have a Po_2 greater than 100 mm Hg when being appropriately ventilated on an Fio_2 of 0.40. An "oxygen challenge" with an Fio_2 of 1.0 should result in a Po_2 of greater than 400 mm Hg. Cultures of any sputum obtained through endotracheal suctioning should not reveal gross contamination, markedly abnormal numbers of white cells, or gross bacterial infection.

The medical management of combined heart–lung donors is one of the most challenging aspects of organ procurement. Such donors require careful attention to pulmonary toilet, inspired oxygen concentrations, and fluid administration. They should be kept on an Fio_2 of less than 0.40. Administered fluid should be kept to an absolute minimum to avoid pulmonary edema. Peak inspiratory airway pressure should be kept below 30 cm H_2O.

Once a suitable donor is identified, the recipient must be notified and prepared for the operation. Appropriate immunosuppressants (discussed below) are administered and the patient is brought to the operating room. Induction of anesthesia in the heart–lung recipient is straightforward and uses the techniques common to all cardiovascular procedures. Cardiopulmonary bypass and the attendant invasive monitoring are necessary. Double lumen endotracheal intubation is not necessary for heart–lung transplantation and a single lumen endotracheal tube is used. Most recipients will require only a central venous catheter and a central venous pressure measurement for appropriate management intraoperatively.

OPERATIVE TECHNIQUE

Donor Operation

The donor operation is performed via a median sternotomy, usually in conjunction with abdominal organ procurement. The thoracic organs are examined first and both pericardium and pleura are opened. The heart is inspected carefully for signs of trauma (Fig. 26.1); the coronary arteries are palpated to ensure the absence of lesions. Manipulation of the lungs is kept to a minimum, but both are inspected to verify the absence of traumatic injuries or other abnormalities. The lungs should be free of the chest wall as the presence of adhesions will make lung procurement difficult.

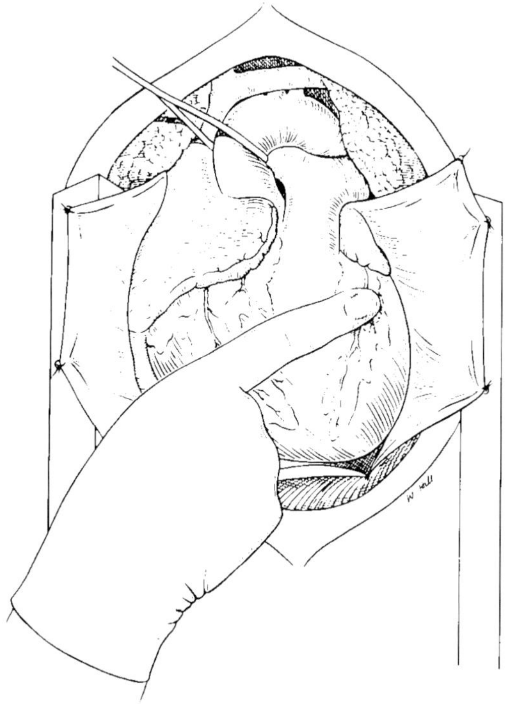

FIGURE 26.1. *The heart is carefully inspected for evidence of coronary artery disease, valvular disease, unrecognized trauma, and unrecognized congenital disease. (Reproduced by permission from Baldwin JC. Heart–lung and lung graft preservation. In: Shumway SJ, Shumway NE, eds. Thoracic transplantation. Cambridge, MA: Blackwell Science, 1995.)*

As in isolated cardiac harvests, the superior vena cava and the inferior vena cava are encircled and controlled (see also Chapter 23). The anterior pleura are opened for their entire course. The ascending aorta and the pulmonary artery are inspected and cleared of surrounding tissues to allow aortic cross-clamping as high as possible. The main trachea is exposed and controlled, approaching it anteriorly between the superior vena cava and the ascending aorta. Blunt and sharp dissection is used to encircle the trachea, taking care not to injure the underlying esophagus or the posterior membranous portion of the trachea.

At this point, other organ procurement teams complete their dissection of the abdominal organs. Once they have completed their work, the patient is systemically heparinized with 20,000 to 30,000 units of heparin given intravenously through a central venous catheter that is then removed. For pulmonary preservation, prostaglandin E_1, a relatively selective pulmonary vasodilator, is administered intravenously. Infusion begins at 20 ng/kg/min. The dose is increased gradually over 15 minutes to the range of 70–100 ng/kg/min, as blood pressure tolerates. The actual procurement begins at this point. The superior vena cava is ligated and divided. The inferior vena cava is widely incised, allowing blood to egress from the right side of the heart. The left atrial

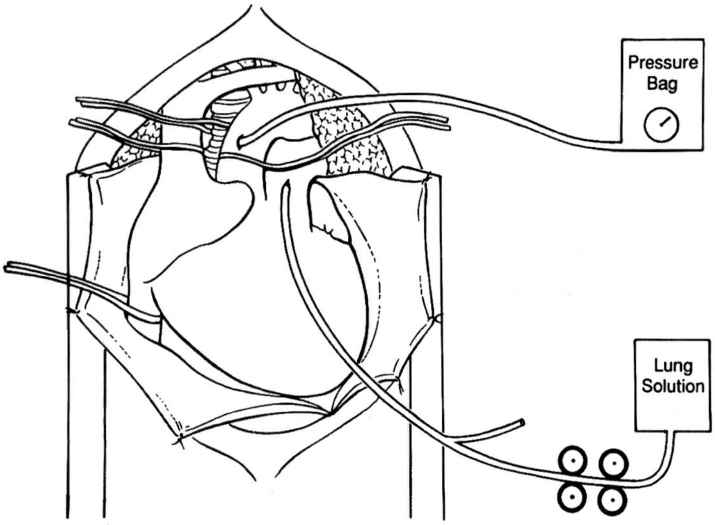

FIGURE 26.2. *The 14-gauge sump catheter for infusion of the pulmonary preservation solution is inserted via a stab wound in the main pulmonary artery and connected to the rollerhead pump apparatus for delivery of the solution. Cardioplegic solution is delivered via a simple pressure bag arrangement. (Reproduced by permission from Baldwin JC. Heart–lung and lung graft preservation. In: Shumway SJ, Shumway NE, eds. Thoracic transplantation. Cambridge, MA: Blackwell Science, 1995.)*

appendage is incised to allow egress of the blood from the left side of the heart. The heart is allowed to beat five or six times, allowing it to empty completely before the aorta is cross-clamped. After aortic occlusion, 1000 cc of standard cold crystalloid cardioplegia is infused via the ascending aortic root.

Pulmonary preservation is continued using an infusion of Euro-Collins solution at 4°C via a cannula in the main pulmonary artery (Fig. 26.2). The solution is administered via gravity drainage taking care to keep the infusion pressure less than 20 cm H_2O. During this infusion, it is particularly important to continue slow ventilation of the lungs to ensure adequate distribution of the pulmonary perfusate and adequate preservation. With continued slow ventilation of the lungs, the lungs eventually blanch to white, indicating adequate preservation.

The heart and lungs are then excised as a block. The inferior vena cava is completely divided. The lungs are deflated and rotated to expose the tissue posterior to the pulmonary veins. Dissection is carried up along the anterior esophagus and is continued out to the level of the division of the main trachea, taking care not to injure the membranous portion of either of the main bronchi. The ascending aorta is divided, taking care not to injure the pulmonary artery. The lungs are inflated to two-thirds of total lung capacity and the main trachea is stapled closed. The heart and lungs are excised as a block (Fig. 26.3). The graft is placed in Euro-Collins solution at 4°C, wrapped in several sterile cellophane bags, and placed in a hard container packed in ice for transport.

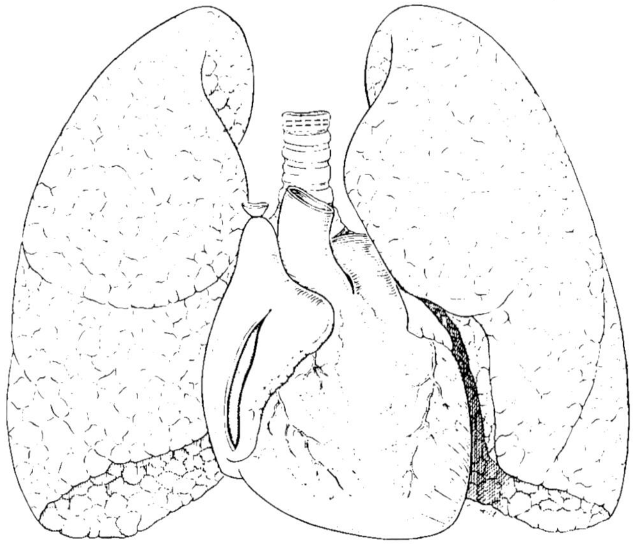

FIGURE 26.3. *The intact heart–lung graft is withdrawn from the chest. The high application of the TA 55 stapler on the trachea results in continued expansion of the lungs at the level of normal tidal volume. (Reproduced by permission from Baldwin JC. Heart–lung and lung graft preservation. In: Shumway SJ, Shumway NE, eds. Thoracic transplantation. Cambridge, MA: Blackwell Science, 1995.)*

Recipient Operation

The central features of the recipient operation include avoidance of injury to the phrenic nerves, avoidance of injury to the vagus nerves, avoidance of injury to the recurrent laryngeal nerve, and avoidance of bleeding in the posterior mediastinum, which is extremely difficult to control after the graft is placed. The operation is performed through a median sternotomy. After the establishment of cardiopulmonary bypass, both vena cavae are snared and the aorta is cross-clamped. The patient is systemically cooled to 32°C. The native heart is removed by dividing the aorta and pulmonary artery at the supravalvular level and the atria at the mid atrial level. On the left, a phrenic nerve pedicle includ-

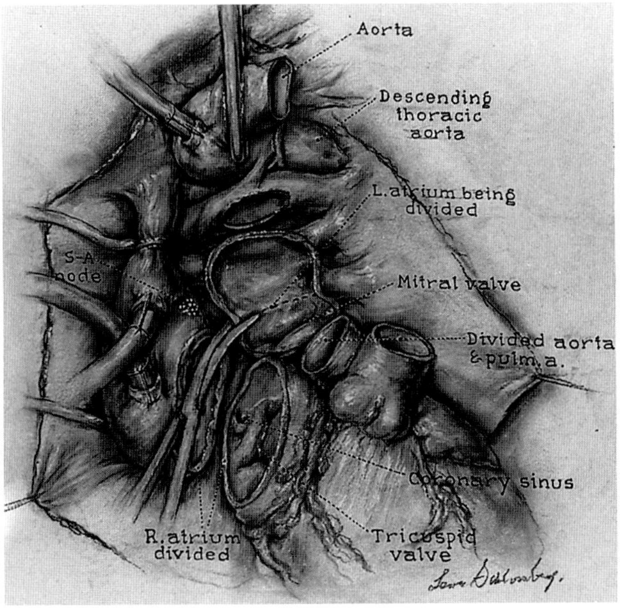

FIGURE 26.4. *The recipient heart is being excised; the final division is along the left atrium. (Reproduced by permission from Shumway SJ. Operative techniques in heart–lung transplants. In: Shumway SJ, Shumway NE, eds. Thoracic transplantation. Cambridge, MA: Blackwell Science, 1995.)*

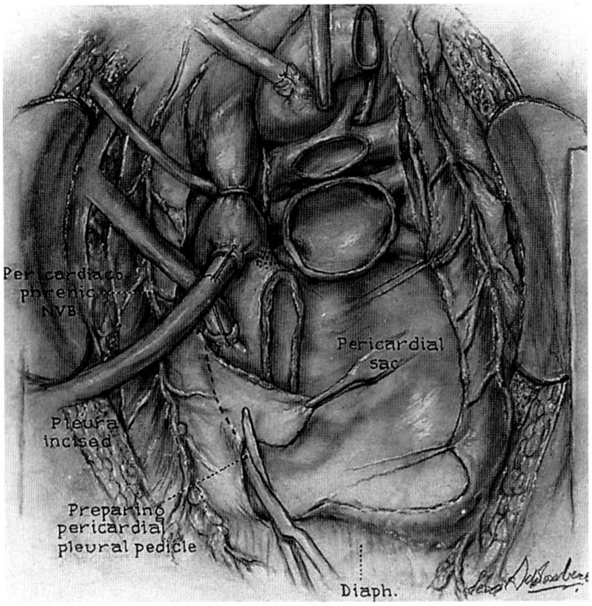

FIGURE 26.5. *Bilateral phrenic nerve pedicles, or pericardiacophrenic neurovascular bundles, are developed. (Reproduced by permission from Shumway SJ. Operative techniques in heart–lung transplants. In: Shumway SJ, Shumway NE, eds. Thoracic transplantation. Cambridge, MA: Blackwell Science, 1995.)*

ing 3 cm of pericardium anteriorly and as much as possible posteriorly is created sharply. Use of cautery should be avoided as this is potentially dangerous to the nerve.

The pericardium is incised posteriorly from the level of the pulmonary artery to the diaphragm to establish this pedicle. A vertical incision is made in the oblique sinus of the left atrium and the left-sided pulmonary veins are dissected, reflecting them into the left pleural space (Fig. 26.4). The left pulmonary ligament is divided as is the left pulmonary artery. The left main bronchus is stapled and divided. On the right, a pericardial pedicle for the phrenic nerve is established in a similar fashion (Fig. 26.5). An incision in the left atrium is made from the lateral approach as for mitral valve replacement. This allows a reflection of the right pulmonary veins into the right pleural space. After division of the pulmonary ligament, the pulmonary artery is divided, and the bronchus is stapled and divided as on the left (Fig. 26.6).

The pulmonary arterial remnant is removed leaving a button approximately 2 cm in diameter in the area of the ductus diverticulum, thus avoiding injury to the recurrent laryngeal nerve. Clamps are placed on the two stapled bronchi, and downward traction facilitates dissection of the bronchial tree proximally. During this phase of the operation, very careful attention must be given to hemostasis in the bronchial circulation. Application of metal clips to each vessel is usually sufficient; it is important to maintain a perfusion pressure of at least 60 mm Hg during this phase in order to mimic postoperative aterial pressure and thus to unmask any potential bleeding sites. The dissection is carried up to the carina and the trachea is divided at that level (Fig. 26.7). Proximal dissection of the trachea is to be avoided as it compromises tracheal blood supply and tracheal anastomotic healing.

The graft is brought onto the field and the donor trachea is opened. It is divided one or two rings above the carina and the tracheobronchial tree is carefully irrigated with normal saline and any residual secretions are removed. The graft is lowered into place and the right lung is placed under the phrenic pericardial pedicle and the right atrial remnant. The left lung is placed under the left phrenic pericardial pedicle. It is important to avoid twisting of the pulmonary hilum at this junction. Next, the anastomoses are begun. The tracheal anastomosis (Fig. 26.8) is performed using an end-to-end running 3-0 polypropylene suture. No reinforcement or buttressing of this anastomosis is necessary. After completion of the tracheal anastomosis, topical cooling of both lungs is instituted, and a third cooling line is placed in the tip of the left atrial appendage to enhance endomyocardial cooling and to exclude air from the left side of the graft.

The donor right atrium is opened from the inferior vena cava up toward the base of the right atrial appendage, avoiding the area of the sinal atrial node. The right atrial anastomosis is performed, beginning posteriorly in the area of the recipient atrial septum (which is now the posterior edge of the recipient right atrium). This anastomosis is carried out using a continuous running 3-0 polypropylene suture. Rewarming is ordinarily begun during performance of the

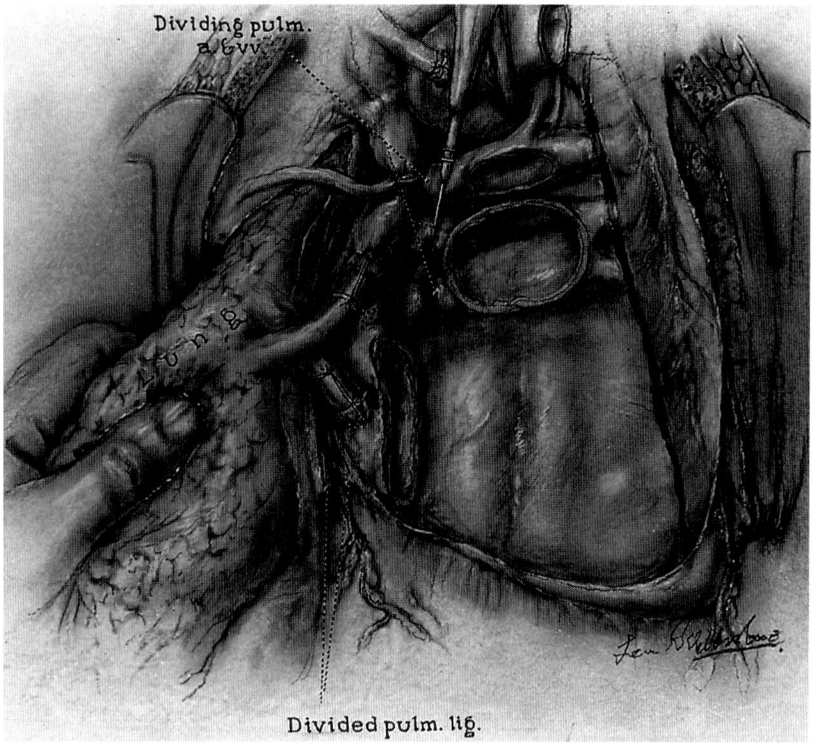

FIGURE 26.6. *The intrapericardial pulmonary arteries and veins are divided, as are the inferior pulmonary ligaments bilaterally. (Reproduced by permission from Shumway SJ. Operative techniques in heart–lung transplants. In: Shumway SJ, Shumway NE, eds. Thoracic transplantation. Cambridge, MA: Blackwell Science, 1995.)*

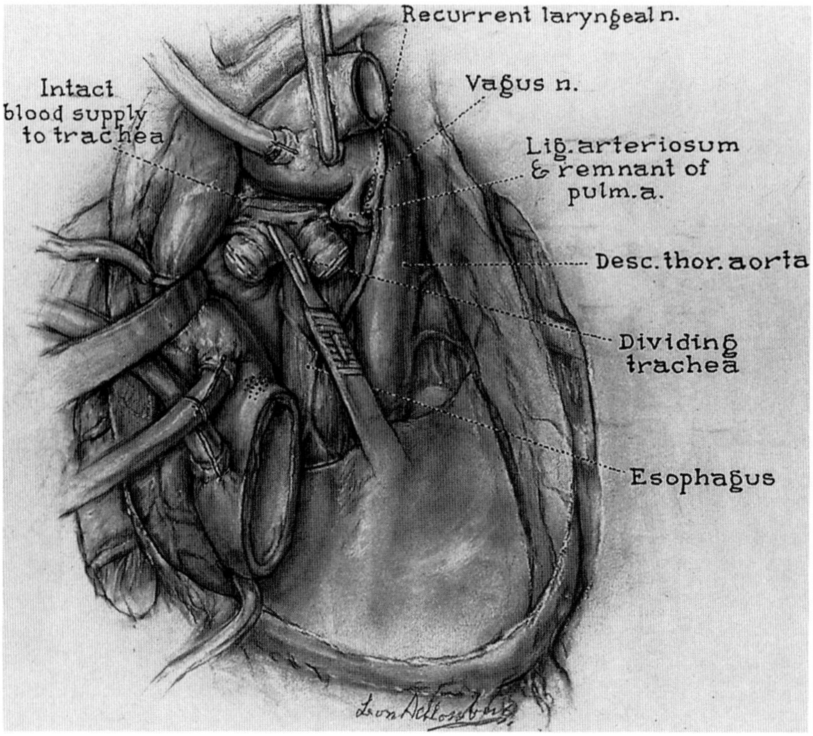

FIGURE 26.7. *The trachea is divided just about the carina. Care is taken not to injure the vagus nerve or the recurrent laryngeal nerve. (Reproduced by permission from Shumway SJ. Operative techniques in heart–lung transplants. In: Shumway SJ, Shumway NE, eds. Thoracic transplantation. Cambridge, MA: Blackwell Science, 1995.)*

right atrial anastomosis. The aortic anastomosis is performed last, using a running 4-0 polypropylene suture. The use of the left atrial catheter eliminates the need for elaborate maneuvers to evacuate air.

All anastomoses are now completed, and the heart is gradually resuscitated as the lungs are ventilated with 40% inspired oxygen and 5 cm H_2O of positive and expiratory pressure. Approximately 30 minutes after removal of the aortic cross-clamp, the patient is weaned from cardiopulmonary bypass on low-dose isoproterenol for chronotropic support of the heart. Temporary epicardial pacing wires are left in place on the donor right atrium and right ventricle.

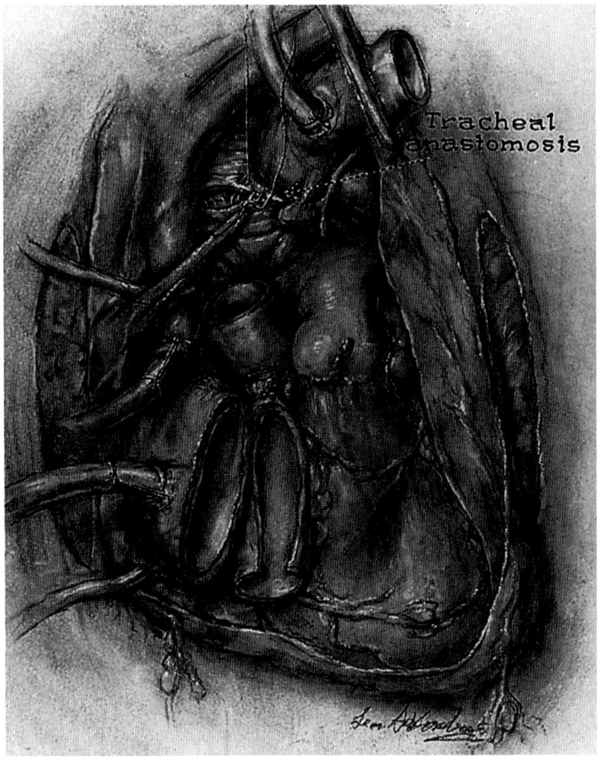

FIGURE 26.8. *The tracheal anastomosis is performed first. (Reproduced by permission from Shumway SJ. Operative techniques in heart–lung transplants. In: Shumway SJ, Shumway NE, eds. Thoracic transplantation. Cambridge, MA: Blackwell Science, 1995.)*

IMMUNOSUPPRESSION

The introduction of cyclosporine in the 1980s revolutionized heart and heart–lung transplantation (see Chapter 6). The immunosuppressive regimen for heart–lung transplantation differs from that used in orthotopic cardiac transplantation in that steroids are minimized to enhance tracheal healing. A typical regimen includes a single preoperative dose of cyclosporine orally. Azathioprine is also given at this time. After graft implantation, 500 mg of methylprednisolone is given as a bolus on discontinuation of cardiopulmonary bypass. Intravenous methylprednisolone is continued for the first 24 hours after operation (125 mg every 8 hours). Thereafter, steroids are withheld for three weeks to enhance early tracheal healing. Oral cyclosporine therapy is continued postoperatively to maintain a level of approximately 300 ng/mL. After the first month, the cyclosporine level may be lowered. Azathioprine is given at a dose of 1–2 mg/kg/day depending on the white blood cell count. Azathioprine is usually continued indefinitely. Corticosteriods are begun three weeks postoperatively; usually at a dose of 0.1 mg/kg/day.

Recently, the introduction of a new gel formulation of cyclosporine, Neoral, has allowed for better bioavailability. Nephrotoxicity secondary to cyclosporine is a common problem with long-term cyclosporine use and renal function must be closely monitored in all recipients (see Chapter 6). The main side effect of azathioprine is leukopenia; if the white blood cell (WBC) count drops, azathioprine must be decreased, and at WBC levels of less than 5000 cells per microliter, the drug should be withheld.

In cases of rejection resistant to pharmaceutical-based interventions, plasmapheresis and photopheresis may be considered. Both are potentially useful in dealing with humoral rejection episodes (see Chapter 14).

POSTOPERATIVE MANAGEMENT

The management of postoperative heart–lung recipients is very similar to that of any open-heart surgery patient. Extubation can often be accomplished within 6 to 12 hours. Early mobilization and ambulation is especially important for pulmonary toilet. For severely debilitated patients who have had prolonged waits for suitable organs, a period of reconditioning may be necessary, but should not hinder early mobilization. Usually, isoproterenol is administered intravenously for four to five days for its chronotropic effects. After five to seven days, if the heart rate does not return spontaneously to 80 or greater, a permanent pacemaker is inserted. The typical stay in intensive care ranges from two to five days. Oral nutrition usually can begin within 48 hours of surgery in most cases. Good hand washing and common-sense prevention of contact with family members with viral infections, especially children, is important.

An uncomplicated heart–lung transplant patient can be discharged from the hospital as early as seven to ten days postoperatively. Usually, the results of the first endomyocardial biopsy are obtained prior to discharge.

REJECTION

Cardiac and pulmonary rejection can occur asynchronously. Special vigilance for both types of rejection is very important. Cardiac rejection is detected and treated in a fashion similar to orthotopic cardiac transplant (see Chapter 23). Endomyocardial biopsies are performed routinely for each of the first three weeks. The frequency is decreased to every other week for three weeks if no rejection episodes occur, and then every month for three months. Cardiac rejection is graded on the same international grading scale as for isolated cardiac rejection. Rejection with evidence of myocardial necrosis is treated with a pulse of steroids (500 mg to 1 g of methylprednisolone for each of one, two, or three days). Milder rejection is treated with augmented cyclosporine or oral steroids.

The diagnosis of pulmonary rejection is more difficult and subtle to ascertain than cardiac rejection. Pulmonary rejection is usually manifested by radiographic changes, fever, and/or dyspnea (see Chapter 25). Transbronchial biopsy is helpful in making the diagnosis, but the reliability of transbronchial biopsy does not approach that of endomyocardial biopsy in detecting cardiac rejection. Significant pulmonary rejection resulting in subjective dyspnea or a decrease in pulmonary function is treated in a fashion similar to that of cardiac rejection, with a pulse of steroids being given over one to three days. Augmented oral immunosuppression is warranted for lesser degrees of rejection. After the treatment of cardiac or pulmonary rejection, repeat biopsy is necessary within five to seven days to follow the results of treatment.

LONG-TERM RESULTS

Combined heart–lung transplantation is a proven technique. International accumulated data from the Registry of the International Society for Heart and Lung Transplantation documents a 1-year survival of approximately 60% in all recipients and a 5-year survival of 40 to 50% (8) (Fig. 26.9). The survival rate at 11 years is approximately 21%. A multicenter logistic regression analysis shows that pretransplant ventilator dependence and low center volume are significant risk factors for death after heart–lung transplantation. Risk also increases with advanced age.

In the first month following transplantation, acute rejection and infection are the most common complications. Acute rejection accounts for approximately 30% of all deaths and infection for another 20%. In the first three months after transplantation, 70% to 80% of recipients will have an episode of acute rejection. After one year, the incidence of acute rejection decreases. Less than 10% of recipients will have an episode of acute rejection each year after the first year. Early after transplantation, other factors including technical problems, hemorrhage, and nonspecific graft failure account for the remainder of deaths. From 1 month to 1 year after transplant, infection is the leading cause of death. After 1 year, both infection and bronchiolitis obliterans are the primary causes.

The number of heart–lung transplants performed annually peaked in 1990 and has declined thereafter (Fig. 26.10), though donor age continued to rise. The three most common indications for these procedures currently include pulmonary hypertension, congenital heart disease, and cystic fibrosis. Most of the recipients have been in the range of 18 to 49 years of age.

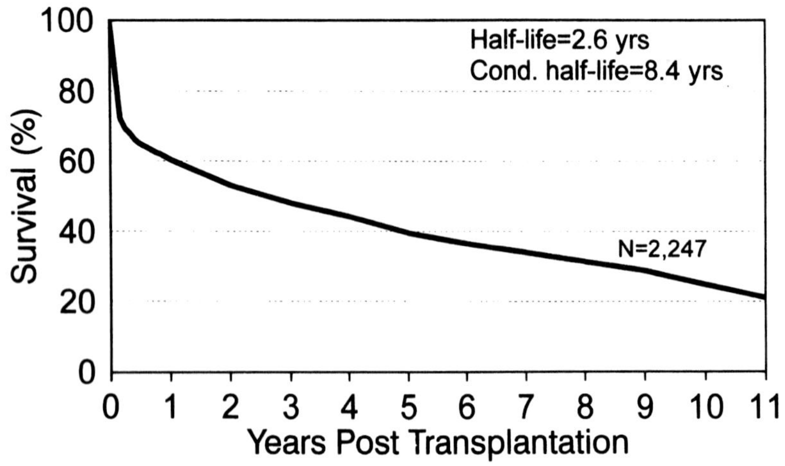

FIGURE 26.9. *Heart–lung transplantation actuarial survival. (Reproduced by permission from Hosenpud JD, Bennett LE, Berkeley MK, et al. The Registry of the International Society for Heart and Lung Transplantation: fifteenth official report 1998. J Heart Lung Transplant 1998;17:656–668.)*

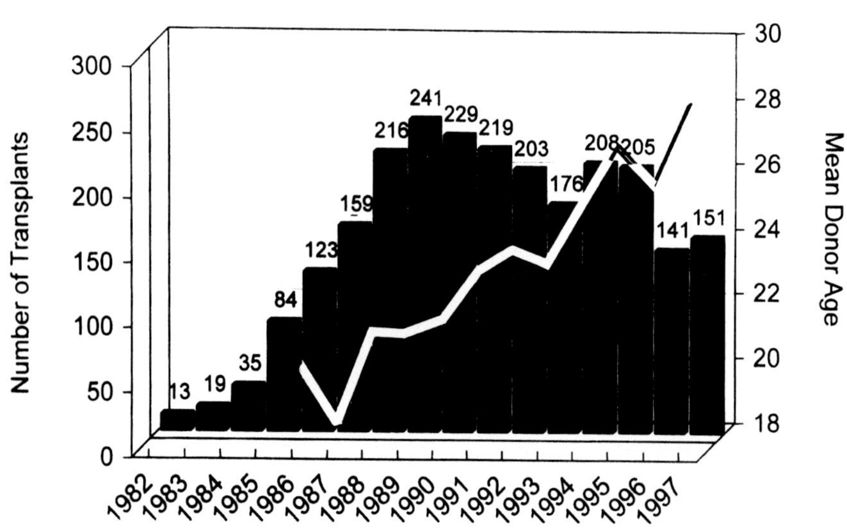

FIGURE 26.10. *Heart–lung transplantation volume and donor age from 1982 through 1997.*

The introduction of endomyocardial biopsy revolutionized the early detection of cardiac rejection and allows early treatment. Usually the right internal jugular vein is used for percutaneous access to the heart. Biopsies are taken in several locations from the right ventricle under fluoroscopic guidance. Since rejection can be patchy, several biopsies are required on each occasion. Right ventricular pressures are also measured at the time of biopsy. Histologic analysis of the specimens is performed and usually rejection can be diagnosed within 8 to 12 hours of biopsy.

Several scales have been developed for the grading of rejection. The most widely used is the international system in which rejection is graded on a scale of 0 to 4. The hallmark of rejection that requires treatment is myocyte necrosis. Lymphocytic infiltration is indicative of lesser rejection and can be treated with orally augmented immunosuppression. Myocyte necrosis with extramyocardial hemorrhage is indicative of severe rejection and myocardial damage; it requires early aggressive intervention.

Because the diagnosis of pulmonary rejection is often unclear, treatment with pulse steroids may be initiated on the basis of radiographic and clinical symptoms alone. Improvement is empiric evidence of rejection. As noted above transbronchial biopsy can be helpful. Lymphocytic infiltration from the pulmonary vasculature is indicative of rejection. Bronchoscopy can also be helpful in ruling out infection.

Although rejection is the most common problem, infection is a potentially lethal complication in the first months after operation in these immunocompromised patients (see Chapter 36). Perhaps the most useful aspect of cardiac and pulmonary biopsies is the ability to exclude rejection and thus avoid treatment with aggressive immunosuppression that may exacerbate infection. Any heart–lung patient with signs of a fever or other abnormal clinical findings should be thoroughly cultured, especially the sputum. Pathogenic organisms should be treated empirically until the diagnosis of rejection or infection is certain.

As with other organs, chronic rejection is the primary unsolved problem in cardiac and pulmonary transplantation (see Chapter 3). The heart–lung transplant recipient is susceptible to the graft atherosclerosis that affects the heart or the bronchiolitis obliterans that affects the lungs. Both are felt to be related to immunologic incompatibility and long-term exposure to foreign antigens. An association with cytomegalovirus infection has been documented, but, as yet, antiviral treatment directed against this agent has not been shown to lessen the incidence of chronic rejection in either the heart or the lung. Coronary arteries are the primary sites of cardiac graft atherosclerosis. They develop a diffuse narrowing not amenable to standard interventions for coronary atherosclerotic disease. This coronary artery disease often develops extraordinarily rapidly and is often not detected on routine yearly cardiac catheterization (see Chapter 23). Bronchiolitis obliterans is a slowly progressive, relentless disease resulting in severe dyspnea, x-ray findings of pulmonary fibrosis, and eventual clinical deterioration (see Chapter 25).

CONCLUSION

Heart–lung transplantation is an extremely effective treatment for combined end-stage cardiac and pulmonary disease. Survival rates in excess of 70% after one year can be anticipated in younger, healthier patients. The donor shortage is the most critical problem in cardiopulmonary transplantation and it is especially acute in this population requiring combined organ transplantation. The number of heart–lung transplants has plateaued to less than 100 per year in the United States and is unlikely to rise in the absence of any improvement of donor supply. Nevertheless, cardiac and pulmonary transplantation offers an extremely effective treatment for the management of combined cardiopulmonary disease and should be offered to appropriate recipients.

REFERENCES

1. Lansman S, Ergin MA, Griepp RB. The history of heart and heart-lung transplantation. In: Shumway SJ, Shumway NE, eds. Thoracic transplantation. Cambridge, MA: Blackwell Science, 1995.
2. Carrel A. The surgery of blood vessels, etc. Bull Johns Hopkins Hosp 1907;18:18–28.
3. Mann FC, Priedny JT, Markowitz J, Yater YM. Transplantation of the intact mammalian heart. Arch Surg 1933;26:219–224.
4. Lower RR, Shumway NE. Studies in orthotopic homotransplantation of the canine heart. Surg Forum 1960;11:18–19.
5. Lower RR. Foreword. In: Shumway SJ, Shumway NE, eds. Thoracic transplantation. Cambridge, MA: Blackwell Science, 1995.
6. Reitz BA, Wallwork JL, Hunt SA, et al. Heart–lung transplantation: successful therapy for patients with pulmonary vascular disease. N Engl J Med 1982;306:557–564.
7. Pfeffer PF, Fuerster A, Froysaker T, et al. HLA-Dr mismatch and histologically evaluated rejection episodes in cardiac transplants can be correlated. Transplant Proc 1988;20:367–368.
8. Hosenpud JD, Bennett LE, Berkeley MK, et al. The Registry of the International Society for Heart and Lung Transplantation: Fifteenth Official Report 1998. J Heart Lung Transplant 1998;17:656–768.

Chapter 27

Bone Marrow Transplantation

THOMAS R. SPITZER STEVEN L. MCAFEE

HISTORY

While the medicinal potential of animal bone marrow has been discussed since ancient times, the function of the bone marrow as the primary site of blood cell production was not demonstrated until 1868 by Neumann and Bizzozero (1,2). Early hypotheses regarding an ancestral stem cell include the description by Ehrlich in 1879 of a large mononuclear cell (a "myelocyte"), and the description of a primitive mononuclear cell ("lymphoidocyte") in 1900 by Pappenheim, who believed this cell to be a totipotential stem cell and to be derived from the bone marrow (1,2).

The first published case of an attempted bone marrow transplantation (BMT) as corrective therapy for a primary bone marrow stem cell disorder was by Osgood and colleagues in 1939 (3). A 19-year-old female with severe aplastic anemia received 43 whole blood transfusions in 52 days along with 18 mL of sternal bone marrow infused five days prior to her death. While anemia was corrected by this aggressive transfusional support (and in fact a peak hematocrit of 52% was achieved), no significant white blood cell or platelet recovery occurred. At autopsy, however, scattered islets of regenerating marrow were seen, raising at least the possibility that early engraftment had occurred.

The next 30 years were an exercise in transplantation futility. In 1970 Bortin summarized the outcomes of the first 203 published human bone marrow transplants (4). In only 11 of the 203 cases was any degree of chimerism established. At the time of publication only five patients were alive, and two of those patients subsequently died. Given that the major histocompatibility locus in humans—human leukocyte antigen (HLA)—was not defined as a two-locus complex until 1967 (the great majority of those 203 transplants were from donors in whom no histocompatibility typing was attempted) and, further, that there was a scarcity of experimental bone marrow transplant experience (resulting in lack of knowledge of adequate preparative therapy or cell doses), it is hardly surprising that these early transplants were almost uniformly unsuccessful.

Of note, however, in Bortin's series was the inclusion of two patients whose successful transplants had been previously reported by Good and his colleagues and Bach et al, respectively, in 1968 (5,6). Good and colleagues reported the successful transplant of a 5-month-old child with thymic alymphoplasia and agammaglobulinemia with peripheral blood buffy coat and bone marrow from an HLA-A-identical (as determined by mixed lymphocyte culture and lymphocytotoxic assay) sibling donor (5). Bach and colleagues described a 2-year-old patient with Wiskott-Aldrich syndrome who underwent an allogeneic transplant from her HLA-identical sister (6). In both cases, mixed allogeneic chimerism was demonstrated.

The decade of 1960 to 1970 was also notable for a series of elegant animal experiments documenting the capacity of allogeneic stem cells to reconstitute lethally irradiated recipients (7,8). Vital to the future success of clinical transplantation was information regarding successful conditioning regimens, correlation of the number of infused stem cells with subsequent regeneration of marrow, and pharmacologic graft-versus-host disease (GVHD) prophylaxis. With the availability of HLA typing and these important experimental data, Thomas and colleagues at the Fred Hutchinson Cancer Center in Seattle began their pioneering investigations in clinical BMT. In 1977 Thomas reported the results of the first 100 patients with advanced leukemia who received an allogeneic BMT from an HLA-identical related donor (9). Six patients died before engraftment, while one patient had transient engraftment followed by graft failure. Of the remaining 93 patients, 50 developed moderate to severe acute GVHD and 54 developed interstitial pneumonitis predominantly due to cytomegalovirus (CMV). Thirty-one patients experienced a relapse of their leukemia. Despite the initial high mortality risk in this group of patients with largely advanced refractory leukemia, 13 patients became long-term disease-free survivors. Many early lessons were learned from this initial experience including the fact that nearly uniform engraftment resulted in patients with advanced leukemia, provided sufficiently intense chemoradiotherapeutic conditioning was administered, and the possibility, although remote, of long-term disease-free survival among patients whose leukemia was resistant to conventional chemotherapy. Other problems that were observed in this early experience have subsequently been addressed or remain a focus of intensive investigation. Prevention of severe acute GVHD and interstitial pneumonitis has significantly improved through a variety of therapeutic inventions including pharmacologic GVHD prophylaxis with cyclosporine and early detection and treatment of CMV infections (10–13). Improved patient selection and overall supportive care have at least modestly improved the long-term survival of patients currently receiving bone marrow transplants (14,15). Relapse, however, remains a formidable problem and a large obstacle to dramatic improvement in the long-term outcomes of BMT. For his pioneering clinical investigations in bone marrow transplantation, Dr. E. Donnell Thomas was awarded the Nobel Prize in Medicine in 1992.

RECIPIENT SELECTION

Indications

Bone marrow or peripheral blood stem cell transplantation (PBSCT) is indicated for a heterogeneous group of congenital and acquired disorders (Table 27.1). The donor source for transplantation (see below) is dependent on the underlying disease, availability of a suitably HLA-matched donor, and the quality of the stem cell product. Bone marrow transplantation fulfills a dual function: 1) as replacement for lymphohematopoietic disorders arising from the pluripotential stem cell, and 2) as a hemopoietic rescue following myeloablative doses of chemoradiotherapy.

The latter function of BMT is based on the experimentally well-demonstrated dose–response relationship of chemotherapy and radiation therapy (16,17). Ablative conditioning regimens are necessary to eradicate residual malignancy in the case of neoplastic disease, to provide sufficient immunosuppression to prevent rejection following allogeneic BMT, and most likely to "create space" for lymphohematopoietic stem cell engraftment.

Common features of this very heterogeneous group of indications for BMT include: 1) the life-threatening and often imminently fatal outcome of the underlying disease, and 2) the potential cure of an otherwise incurable disease by the delivery of tumor-eradicating doses of chemoradiotherapy and/or reconstitution of a diseased (or che-

Table 27.1. Indications for BMT/PBSCT

	Allogeneic	Autologous
Hematologic Malignancies		
AML		
CR1	S	S
1st relapse/CR2	S	S
Advanced (>CR2, primary refractory)	S	S
ALL		
CR1	P	U
CR2	S	S
Advanced (>CR2)	S	S
Non-Hodgkin's lymphoma		
Primary refractory	P	P
Chemosensitive relapse	S	S
Chemoresistant relapse	U	U
Hodgkin's lymphoma		
Chemosensitive relapse	S	S
Chemoresistant relapse	U	U
Multiple myeloma		
Primary refractory	U	U
≥CR1/PR1	P	P
CLL	P	P
CML		
CP	S	P
AP	S	P
BP	S	P
Solid Tumors		
Breast cancer		
Stage II (>10 lymph nodes)		U
Stage III (inflammatory)		P
Stage IV (metastatic)		P
Neuroblastoma		P
Bone/soft tissue sarcoma		P
Germ cell tumor		P
Small-cell lung cancer (LD)		P
Acquired, Nonmalignant Stem Cell Disorders		
Severe aplastic anemia	S	
Paroxysmal nocturnal hemoglobinuria	P	
Congenital Stem Cell Disorders		
Thalassemia major	S	
Sickle cell disease	S	
Severe combined immunodeficiency disease	S	
Metabolic storage disorders	S	
Osteopetrosis	S	

S = Standard: proof of benefit from phase III trial, established curative potential for an otherwise incurable disease, and/or ≥50% long-term disease-free survival probability; P = Promising: improved disease-free or overall survival compared with historical controls, preliminary analysis from phase III trials suggests benefit, and/or possibly curative therapy with lower (≤50%) long-term disease-free survival; U = Unproven: benefit compared with standard therapy not established or curative potential not established. CR = complete remission; AML = acute myelogenous leukemia; ALL = acute lymphoblastic leukemia; CLL = chronic lymphocytic leukemia; CML = chronic myelogenous leukemia; CP = chronic phase; AP = accelerated phase; BP = blast phase; LD = limited disease.

moradiotherapeutically ablated) bone marrow by normal lymphohematopoietic pluripotential stem cells. Thus, some disorders such as the acute leukemias benefit from both the high-dose chemoradiotherapy given in an attempt to overcome resistance to conventional dose chemotherapy and the replacement of the diseased marrow with healthy (hopefully tumor free) autologous or allogeneic stem cells. Other neoplastic diseases such as breast cancer may benefit from high-dose chemotherapy, with autologous stem cell support serving merely a "rescue" function. A variety of congenital lymphohematopoietic stem cell disorders may also benefit by replacement of their dysfunctional stem cell population. An illness like osteopetrosis, for example, demonstrates how a defective osteoclast compartment (which in turn is derived from the monocyte/macrophage cell lineage) can be at least partially corrected by transplantation of normal pluripotential lymphohematopoietic stem cells (18).

Contraindications

Factors influencing eligibility for BMT include age, disease status (remission status in the case of neoplastic disease), performance status, visceral organ function, and psychosocial status.

Age

An upper age limit for transplant eligibility is usually recommended. For allogeneic BMT, an upper age limit of 40 years was usually recommended in the pre-cyclosporine era (19). With improved GVHD prophylaxis and supportive care, an upper age limit of 55 to 60 years has been adopted by most transplant centers. For autologous transplantation, upper age limits of 65 to 70 years have been adopted by most centers. While transplant-related morbidity (and acute GVHD risk in the case of allogeneic transplantation) is likely to be increased in patients over 55 to 60 years of age, survival probabilities in the 40- to 50-year-old age group no longer differ significantly from those of younger patients (20,21).

Disease Status

For most malignant diseases, long-term disease-free and overall survival probabilities correlate well with remission status at the time of the transplant. For the acute leukemias and lymphomas, for example, patients in first or second remission have long-term disease-free survival probabilities following allogeneic transplantation in the 30% to 50% range (22). Patients transplanted in refractory relapse, however, have only a 10% to 15% long-term disease-free survival probability (22). For inherently chemoresistant solid tumors (e.g., colorectal cancer or non-small-cell lung cancer), high response rates are seen following high-dose chemotherapy and autologous BMT (23,24). Durable responses are, however, rarely seen. For more chemotherapy-sensitive solid tumors (e.g., breast cancer), long-term disease-free survival probabilities following high-dose chemotherapy and autologous bone marrow or PBSCT are dependent on tumor chemosensitivity at the time of the transplant. Whereas an approximately 20% long-term disease-free survival probability is achieved following high-dose chemotherapy and bone marrow or PBSCT for chemosensitive metastatic breast cancer, there is no realistic possibility of durable disease control for chemoresistant disease (23,25,26).

Performance Status

Performance status, or overall "clinical condition," much like its importance in predicting survival following conventional chemotherapy, is an important prognostic determinant of survival following BMT (9). Most transplant protocols require patients to have a Karnofsky performance status of greater than or equal to 70% or an Eastern Cooperative Oncology Group (ECOG) performance status of 0 or 1. Poorer performance status is associated with increased transplant-related morbidity and mortality.

Organ Function

Visceral organ function as measured by a series of evaluations including pulmonary function tests and radionuclide ventriculogram is also an important determinant of outcome following BMT (see Chapters 28, 30). Some controversy exists regarding minimum necessary parameters for these evaluations. Investigators at the Fred Hutchinson Cancer Research Center, for example, showed that early survival following allogeneic BMT for patients with left ventricular ejection fractions of less than 40%, as determined by left radionuclide ventriculogram, were similar to those of patients with ejection fractions of greater than 40% (27). The feasibility of autologous stem cell transplants for patients with myeloma and renal failure using a busulfan/cyclophosphamide conditioning regimen has also been demonstrated (28). Nonetheless, the realization of at least a transient decline in cardiac function in many patients following BMT makes it prudent to consider minimum necessary organ function for transplant eligibility. These values may vary according to the type of transplant (autologous versus allogeneic) and the preparative regimen employed (e.g., consideration of a higher level of pulmonary function for patients receiving total body irradiation). Organ function may also influence metabolism or excretion of frequently used drugs. Delivery of crucial drugs such as cyclosporine and amphotericin B depend on adequate renal function.

Infectious Disease Status

The presence of uncontrolled infection is a contraindication to bone marrow transplantation. A progressive invasive fungal infection, for example, would be associated with a prohibitively high transplant-related mortality risk. A series of viral serologies are also obtained prior to transplantation. A positive hepatitis B surface antigen assay is often considered to be a contraindication to BMT, given the concern about fulminant liver injury following high-dose chemoradiotherapy. Similarly, a positive HIV assay is usually a contraindication to BMT. The importance of a positive hepatitis C antibody assay in predicting transplant-related complications is controversial, with some series demonstrating a very high transplant-related mortality risk but others showing no significant impact on survival (29,30).

Psychosocial Status

Given the well-demonstrated impact of BMT on a number of activities of daily living, sexual function, and self esteem, it is recommended that patients be evaluated by a social worker prior to transplant. Psychiatric intervention is often important to assist in evaluation of baseline psychiatric disorders and in designing a behavioral and potentially a pharmacologic plan of management during the transplant.

Pretransplant Medical Evaluation

A representative evaluation that is performed within two weeks prior to conditioning therapy is as follows:

1. Complete medical history with details of the patient's previous diagnostic studies and treatment response
    a. Patient exposure to chemotherapy (including total dosage and duration of therapy) and radiation therapy (including radiation ports with dose fractions and total dose)
    b. Prior transfusion history including history of transfusion reactions, alloantibody formation, and whether the patient received irradiated blood products
    c. Drug allergies, including a description of any reaction (? allergy versus intolerance); this will be particularly important in designing future antibiotic strategies
    d. Detailed history of prior medical illnesses and surgeries, anesthesia exposure, and complications
2. Complete physical examination; baseline weight should be obtained and a Karnofsky or ECOG performance status assigned
3. Evaluation of disease status
    a. Flow cytometric and cytogenetic studies of malignant cells if appropriate
    b. Lumbar puncture to rule out leptomeningeal leukemia/lymphoma (and administration of intrathecal therapy as clinically indicated)
    c. Extent of disease evaluation to include computerized tomography (CT) scans of chest, abdomen, and pelvis, as well as bone scan, gallium scan, or other imaging techniques as clinically indicated
    d. Marrow aspiration and biopsy with flow cytometry and cytogenetics as indicated both for staging purposes and for evaluation of baseline bone marrow architecture and cellularity
4. Evaluation of medical eligibility
    a. Infectious disease screening
        1. Hepatitis B surface antigen and antibody, hepatitis B core antibody, HSV, CMV, HIV1 and 2, HTLV-1, toxoplasmosis antibody titers, VDRL
        2. Cultures of blood, stool, urine, nose, and throat for pathogenic bacterial viruses and fungi
    b. Organ function
        1. Pulmonary function tests with baseline room air arterial blood gas
        2. Radionuclide ventriculogram
        3. Liver function tests
        4. 24-hour urine for creatinine clearance
    c. General
        1. Dental evaluation including Panorex films
        2. Chest x-ray
        3. Electrocardiogram
5. Immunologic studies
    a. Allogeneic transplants
        1. ABO and/or Rh typing and red blood cell cross-match with donor
        2. HLA-A, B, DR typing of patient and donor
        3. Mixed leukocyte culture and lymphocytotoxic cross-match between patient and prospective donor (related donors)
        4. DNA oligotyping of recipient and potential donor(s), (unrelated and mismatched related marrow donor(s), matched donors when DR typing of the patient is not feasible)
        5. Storage of recipient and donor cells for future chimerism studies

DONOR SOURCE

Graft Composition

Regardless of donor source, the central feature of all bone marrow and peripheral blood transplants is the infusion of a sufficient number of pluripotential stem cells for reconstitution of the hematopoietic and immune systems of an intensively conditioned recipient. In contrast to solid organ transplantation, the stem cell "graft" cannot be easily quantified. Murine experimental data have demonstrated an early progenitor cell (colony forming unit-spleen or CFU-S) that has self-renewal and differentiation capacities (31,32). These transplantable lymphohematopoietic progenitor cells have been shown to copurify with lymphocytes (33). Selection of human lymphohematopoietic progenitor cells by exposure to 4-hydroperoxycyclophosphamide or 5-fluorouracil (which eliminates proliferating cells but spares noncycling stem cells) has similarly shown these early cells to have morphologic characteristics of a lymphocyte (34).

Recent evidence, however, suggests that the murine CFU-S cells do not represent the true pluripotential stem cell. A more primitive progenitor cell with competitive repopulative capacity may in fact constitute the true stem cell compartment (35). Immunophenotypic and biologic analyses of very early human progenitor cells have been performed (Table 27.2). Characteristic features of these cells include expression of the glycoprotein CD34 antigen, the absence of expression of lineage-committed antigens (CD33, CD38, CD71, etc.), and growth in a variety of long-term bone marrow culture systems (long-term culture-initiating cell (LTC-IC) or cobblestone area-forming cell assay) (34,36–38).

The practical definition of a successful collection of an adequate number of bone marrow or peripheral blood progenitor cells relies on quantification of CD34 antigen–positive cells and/or assays of in vitro stem cell growth (e.g., colony forming unit-granulocyte monocyte or CFU-GM assays). CD34+ cells constitute approximately 1% to 3% of normal marrow cells but a negligible percentage of steady-state peripheral blood white blood cells (39). Following myelosuppressive chemotherapy, a transient but significant increase in the number of circulating CD34+ cells occurs. Similarly, recombinant human myeloid growth factors can induce a significant rise in circulating CD34+ cells. The concomitant use of chemotherapy and recombinant growth factors results in an even greater increment in the number of these cells (40,41). Consequently, strategies have been developed to "mobilize" bone marrow CD34+ cells into the peripheral circulation. These cells can then be collected by one or more leukophereses, thus avoiding an intraoperative bone marrow harvest procedure.

Despite advancement in the characterization of the phenotypic and biologic properties of the stem cell, clinical experience continues to dictate the criteria for establishment of a successful bone marrow harvest. For example, a target number of allogeneic nucleated blood cells of more than 3 $\times 10^8$/kg of recipient body weight is generally accepted and is based on a long-standing record of successful engraftment following HLA-matched allogeneic BMT with this number of cells. The data from one study showed an increased risk of graft rejection following transplantation for severe aplastic anemia with fewer than 3×10^8/kg nucleated cells (42). While other analyses have not confirmed this threshold dose of allogeneic bone marrow stem cells (43) and engraftment can be reliably achieved with a considerably smaller number of cells, particularly if selection of mononuclear cells or more specifically CD34+ cells (resulting in a one or two log reduction in cell numbers, respectively) is undertaken, similar target cell numbers guide the practice of most bone marrow transplant centers. In the case of HLA-mismatched related or matched or partially mismatched unrelated donor transplants, particularly if T-cell depletion is undertaken, considerably more than 3×10^8/kg nucleated cells are frequently harvested.

Extrapolation of data from animal transplant experiments suggests that a minimum of 1×10^8/kg nucleated cells are necessary for successful engraftment following autologous bone marrow transplantation (44). While this number generally constitutes the minimum number of cells that are acceptable for autologous transplantation, engraftment has also been reliably achieved when one (following mononuclear cell separation) or two (following CD34+ cell selection) log marrow nucleated cell depletions are performed (45,46). Correlation of engraftment with surrogate markers of stem cell content and function, namely CD34+ cell content or growth in progenitor colony assays, has not been well substantiated in the autologous bone marrow transplant setting.

Table 27.2. Functional and Phenotypic Characterization of Human "Stem Cells"

Pluripotential Stem Cells			Lineage Committed Progenitor Cells	
Phenotype	**Functional Assays**		**Phenotype**	**Functional Assays**
CD34+	LTC-IC		CD34+	GFU-GEMM/CFU-MIX
CD38–	CFU-blast		CD33+ (myeloid)	CFU-GM
CD45RA–	Cobblestone forming assay		CD71+ (erythroid)	CFU-E/BFU-E
DR–	In vivo assays (SCID hu mice, etc)	→	CD41+ (megakaryocyte)	CFU-Mega
Thy1+			CD19+, CD20+ (B lymphoid)	Mitogenic stimulation (pokeweed mitogen)
Rhodamine dull			CD5+, CD7+ (T lymphoid)	Mitogenic stimulation (PHA)
Lineage		→		
CD33–				
CD71–				
CD19–, CD20–				
CD5–, CD7–				

Peripheral Blood Stem Cells

An alternative source of lymphohemopoietic progenitor cells for transplantation is the peripheral blood. Chemotherapy and/or recombinant growth factor mobilized peripheral blood stem cells are notable for a several-fold increase in CD34+ cell content compared with harvested marrow and clinically by the significantly more rapid hematologic reconstitution following peripheral blood stem cell transplantation compared with BMT (47,48). Concerns about the true stem cell content of these products, given the possibility that most of these cells are committed to a specific lymphohemopoietic lineage, have been raised (49,50). In vitro assays of early multipotential cell content such as the percent of CD34+ lineage negative cells and growth in the LTC-IC, however, have shown comparable percentages of these cells to normal bone marrow (51). Concerns about late engraftment failure following peripheral blood stem cell transplantation have also not been substantiated (52). A rapidly emerging experience with allogeneic peripheral blood stem cell transplantation is also underway. Normal donors have in most instances received granulocyte colony stimulating factor for mobilization. Despite the collection of a log more in CD3+ T-cells, the incidence of acute GVHD does not appear to be increased above that of HLA-matched donor allogeneic bone marrow transplants. Engraftment, moreover, is rapid and appears to be sustained (53–56).

Syngeneic Donors

Of the three types of donors potentially available to donate stem cells—syngeneic donors (identical twin donors), autologous donors (self donors), and allogeneic donors (nonself donors)—transplants from syngeneic donors are the least common (less than 2% of all marrow transplants) owing to the infrequent availability of an identical twin. Nonetheless, analyses of these transplants are important when comparisons of outcomes are made with either HLA-matched donor allogeneic or autologous transplants. An analysis of syngeneic transplants for "standard" risk leukemia [acute myelogenous leukemia (AML) or acute lymphoblastic leukemia (ALL) in first complete remission or chronic myelogenous leukemia (CML) in chronic phase] was recently undertaken by Gale and colleagues of the International Bone Marrow Transplant Registry (57). An increased relapse probability for syngeneic recipients with AML or CML compared with a cohort of HLA-identical sibling allogeneic bone marrow transplant recipients was observed. Although loss of a graft-versus-leukemia effect was considered as a possible explanation for this result, the increased relapse rate was found to persist even after adjustment for GVHD. A comparison of relapse probability can also be made with autologous transplant recipients. Given the tumor-free stem cell product of a syngeneic donor, any difference in relapse rates can presumably be attributed to tumor contamination of autologous grafts.

Autologous Donors

Autologous marrow or PBSC transplants are performed for a variety of hematologic malignancies and solid tumors. Historically, bone marrow demonstrated morphologically to be tumor-free was a potential source for an autologous transplant. Based on a concern of tumor cell contamination in diseases such as acute leukemia and non-Hodgkin's lymphoma, however, attempts have been made to "purge" the marrow of malignant cells (58–62). A variety of techniques have been employed toward this end (Table 27.3). These techniques can effectively eliminate up to several logs of malignant cells in vitro, and normal stem cells, at least in sufficient numbers to permit engraftment, are generally preserved.

The role of ex vivo purging of autologous marrow, however, remains controversial. Evidence in support of purging include: 1) the correlation of disease-free survival probability with reduction in CFU-GM content and increased time to engraftment following 4-hydroperoxycyclophosphamide purged autologous marrow in acute myeloid leukemia (59), 2) an increased probability of disease-free survival for certain subsets of patients with acute myeloid or lymphoblastic leukemia who had autologous marrow treated with mafosfamide (as determined by a retrospective analysis by the European Bone Marrow Transplant Group) (58,62), and 3) improved disease-free survival probabilities following autologous bone marrow transplantation for patients with no detectable bcl-2 genomic abnormality by polymerase chain reaction (PCR) analysis following purging of low-grade non-Hodgkin's lymphoma with multiple anti-B-cell monoclonal antibodies compared with patients who had residual bcl-2 abnormality detected (61). Arguments against the routine use of purging include favorable disease-free survival probabilities shown in some autologous transplant series of patients with acute leukemia and lymphoma with unpurged bone marrow (63) and the potential injury that may occur from the purging process, thereby resulting in prolonged time to engraftment and increased risk of infections and bleeding. Unfortunately, no prospective randomized trials have been conducted to definitively evaluate the value of ex vivo purging in the outcome of autologous bone marrow or PBSC transplantation.

An alternative source of stem cells for autologous transplantation is the peripheral blood. Chemotherapy and/or recombinant myeloid growth factors are used to mobilize PBSC and presently constitute the source of stem cell rescue following autologous transplantation in the majority of autologous transplant centers. Autologous PBSC transplants are associated with significantly shorter durations of neutropenia and thrombocytopenia and, in some studies, fewer days of febrile neutropenia, fewer infections, less mucositis, earlier hospital discharge, and reduced cost. Controversy exists as to whether peripheral blood stem cell transplants are associated with faster immunologic reconstitution (64–66). Preliminary data suggesting a decreased probability

Table 27.3. Methods of Ex Vivo Purging of BM/PBSC

Agent	Method	Target Cell(s)	Principal Disease
Negative Selection			
Monoclonal antibody (Mab)	Mab + complement	B cell (CD19, CD20, etc)	B-cell non-Hodgkin's lymphoma
	Mab + immunomagnetic beads	T cell (CD3, CD5, etc)	T-cell non-Hodgkin's lymphoma
	Mab-immunotoxin	Myeloid (CD14, CD15, etc)	AML
		Epithelial (UJ 13A, 223.8, etc) (HMFG-1, 2, etc)	Neuroblastoma
		K19	Breast cancer
Cytotoxic chemotherapy	Incubation with drug(s)/wash	Lymphohemopoietic malignant cells	AML, ALL, non-Hodgkin's lymphoma
4 hydroperoxy-cyclophosphamide (4- HC)			
Etoposide (VP-16)			
Vincristine			
Combinations			
Corticosteroids	Incubation with drug(s)/wash	Lymphohemopoietic malignant cells	AML, ALL, non-Hodgkin's lymphoma
Positive Selection			
Monoclonal antibody (anti-CD34)	Mab/column immunoadsorption	CD34+ normal hemopoietic progenitor cells	Breast cancer
Mab/immunomagnetic depletion	Mab/flask "panning"		Non-Hodgkin's lymphoma
	Mab/immunomagnetic depletion		Multiple myeloma

of relapse following PBSC for non-Hodgkin's lymphoma compared with autologous bone marrow transplants are encouraging but require confirmation (67).

Allogeneic Donors

Allogeneic donors may be either related or unrelated and HLA-matched or partially mismatched. Crucial to the selection of an allogeneic donor is HLA typing of the patient, the patient's siblings, and parents, if possible, to fully define family haplotypes.

Human Leukocyte Antigen Complex

The HLA system comprises a series of genes on the p21 portion of chromosome 6 that encode for a series of cell surface glycoprotein antigens that are critical in antigen presentation and immune responsiveness (68,69). The classic transplantation antigens can be divided into two classes (70). Class I antigens are transmembrane glycoproteins that form heterodimers with β_2-microglobulin. HLA-A, B, C, E, F, and G antigens have been identified. Only HLA-A and B genes have clearly defined roles in bone marrow transplantation. Class II molecules are also heterodimers comprised of alpha and beta genes, with HLA-DR, DQ, and DP being the major loci. The function of both class I and class II molecules is antigen presentation to T cells (see also Chapter 4).

The time-honored and most widely utilized method of HLA typing involves a serologic determination of the HLA-A, B, and DR alleles. This methodology involves highly HLA-specific antisera obtained from multiparous women and a complement-dependent microcytotoxicity assay (71). Whereas class I molecules are expressed on virtually all cells, class II antigens are limited to B cells, cells of monocyte/macrophage lineage, and activated T cells. A B-cell enriched population of mononuclear cells must therefore be prepared for serologic testing of class II antigens. The ability to serologically test for class II antigens, therefore, requires a suitable peripheral blood mononuclear cell count; in addition, class II typing may be affected by contaminating malignant cells (usually leukemic blasts).

Based on the results of HLA typing, family haplotypes can be determined. Inheritance of these haplotypes occurs in a mendelian fashion. Hence, there is a 25% chance that a patient and sibling will be HLA genotypically identical. Based on current average US family size, only 35% of patients will have an HLA-identical sibling donor (69). Therefore, alternative donor sources are required to meet the needs of the majority of patients who require an allogeneic bone marrow transplant. Among these alternate donor sources are extended family members and voluntary unrelated bone marrow donors.

In approximately 5% of cases, an appropriate allogeneic extended family donor can be identified (70). This includes HLA phenotypically matched donors as well as one-antigen mismatched donors (based on similar survival outcomes from these donors compared with the survivals of transplants from HLA genotypically identical sibling donors for hematologic malignancies) (72). Searching for a suitably matched donor within the extended family is a reasonable strategy, particularly if a rare familial haplotype is present.

The strategy of utilizing voluntary unrelated donors arose from a knowledge of the HLA system in which significant polymorphism was recognized but the number of antigens identified as finite. The mechanism of linkage disequilibrium, moreover, results in an increased probability of certain class I and II alleles being inherited on the same haplotype compared to chance alone. Hence, provided there is an ample pool of potential unrelated donors and the haplotype frequency within the population in question is sufficiently high, there is a reasonable chance of finding a suitably matched donor.

Based on these considerations, several unrelated donor registries have been organized. The largest of these registries, the National Marrow Donor Program (NMDP), was initiated in 1987 with the tasks of donor recruitment, coordination of donor searches, and facilitation of donor collection for unrelated bone marrow donor transplants (73). Starting with a small number of predominantly regular platelet donors in 1987, there has been an immense expansion of the potential unrelated donor pool recruited by the NMDP. As of February 1996, there had been recruitment of more than 2 million potential donors in the United States. Approximately 100 transplants per month from voluntary unrelated donors were being performed in the United States in 1996.

The realization that there is extensive polymorphism within broad serologic HLA specificities has led to the use of alternative methods of typing of unrelated donors. Molecular typing of class II alleles utilizing sequence-specific oligonucleotide probes (SSOPs) and PCR technology has become routine in the identification and selection of unrelated donors. With this technology, for example, 11 molecular variants have been identified for the serologically determined DR4 antigen (74). Molecular matching has had significant clinical application as well. The incidence of moderate to severe acute GVHD is less for recipients of marrow from donors who are class II antigen–matched by molecular methods, compared with transplants from donors who are serologically class II antigen–identical but molecularly disparate (75). Molecular typing for class I alleles is not yet routinely performed in most laboratories. Isoelectric focusing gel electrophoresis may identify structural variants of class I molecules. While the potential value of identifying microvariants of class I alleles with isoelectric gel focusing was demonstrated by a case of graft rejection occurring after an unrelated marrow transplant in which host cytotoxic T cells were identified against a microvariant disparity of the HLA-B44 allele of the recipient (76), the technique remains logistically difficult and it is not routinely utilized for donor screening. Similarly, PCR technology is capable of identifying molecular variants of class I alleles, but its use in selection of unrelated donors is not presently routine (77).

Allogeneic Peripheral Blood Stem Cell Transplantation

Initial concerns about using peripheral blood as a source of allogeneic stem cells included concerns about an inadequate number of pluripotential stem cells available for sustained engraftment and treatment of normal donors with recombinant DNA growth factors. Experience with granulocyte colony stimulating factor (G-CSF) administration to normal syngeneic donors showed the tolerability of this approach and the high yield of CD34+ progenitors that could be collected (78). Early engraftment occurred in all five syngeneic transplants in which PBSC were the sole source of lymphohemopoietic support. Subsequently, multiple series have confirmed that G-CSF administration to normal donors is well tolerated and capable of mobilizing sufficient numbers of lymphohematopoietic progenitors for successful allogeneic bone marrow transplantation (53–56). Of note, there has been an approximate one log increase in CD3+ T cells collected by this method compared with bone marrow harvest. However, there has been no appreciable increase in the incidence of acute GVHD compared with historical bone marrow transplant recipients. Potential advantages of peripheral blood stem cell use are the avoidance of anesthesia and an operative procedure and potentially faster engraftment after transplant. Disadvantages of this approach include the uncertain long-term effects of administration of a recombinant DNA molecule to normal donors, immediate G-CSF–related side effects such as bone pain, and the potential need for central venous access if peripheral access is inadequate.

Umbilical Cord Stem Cells

A potentially attractive source of stem cells for allogeneic transplantation is umbilical cord blood. These cells have been shown to be enriched for CD34+ progenitors and, theoretically, in view of containing relatively naive immune effector cells, are less capable of causing GVHD. The feasibility of this approach has been documented (79,80). Transplants involving umbilical cord blood stem cells have been remarkable for sustained engraftment in most cases, including in recipients of HLA-mismatched donor cells. Grade III to IV GVHD incidence is acceptably low (<10%). Based on an overall low (average 10^7/kg) number of nucleated blood cells procured from umbilical cord, transplants have been largely limited to recipients weighing less than 20 to 30 kg. Purported advantages of an umbilical cord source of stem cells include the potentially ready availability of a large inventory of HLA-matched or partially mismatched unrelated donors (with an improved representation by minority donors) and the lack of risk to the donor. In addition, immunologically naive T cells may be less capable of causing GVHD. Given the relatively low overall number of CD34+ progenitors in an umbilical cord harvest, reliable methods of ex vivo stem cell expansion will likely be required before umbilical cord stem cells are widely applicable to an adult recipient population. The demonstration of small numbers of contaminating maternal cells, theoretically capable of causing a third-party graft-versus-host reaction, is of concern and needs to be further evaluated (81).

BONE MARROW/PBSC HARVESTING

Bone Marrow Harvest

The procurement of bone marrow for transplantation is undertaken in the operating room under sterile conditions. General or regional anesthesia is performed, depending on donor preference and any underlying medical condition.

After suitable anesthesia is obtained, the donor is placed in the prone position. Using 11- to 12-gauge aspiration needles and heparinized syringes, multiple bone marrow aspirations are performed along the posterior iliac crest. Generally, the posterior superior iliac spine is the initial site of puncture. Subsequent punctures are performed in a superolateral direction along the iliac crest. Practice varies as to whether each puncture into the iliac crest is through a separate skin puncture site or whether it is sufficient to use several (usually three to five) skin puncture sites overlying each iliac crest, with punctures of underlying bone over an area several centimeters in diameter from each puncture site. Individual aspirations of 5 cc or less are generally recommended. Increased volumes of aspirate are associated with decreased nucleated cell and CD34+ cell counts and increased T-cell contamination (82). The desired cell count and marrow volume are based on recipient body weight. Generally accepted guidelines for harvested marrow include a volume of 10 to 15 cc/kg of recipient body weight and 3×10^8/kg or more of nucleated cells.

In order to avoid the need for homologous red blood transfusion, normal bone marrow donors generally have autologous red blood cells collected prior to the procedure. This strategy is effective in avoiding heterologous red blood cell transfusions in 99% of harvests. Autologous bone marrow donors may receive salvaged autologous red blood cells prepared during a mononuclear cell preparation procedure. On occasion, the anterior iliac crests or the sternum may be used for additional bone marrow aspirations. In the great majority of harvests, however, the posterior iliac crest areas are sufficient for collecting the desired number of nucleated marrow cells.

Following completion of the aspirations, the operative site is cleansed and a pressure dressing is applied. Postoperative management consists of pain medications (usually parenteral meperidine or morphine sulfate or oral codeine or Oxycodone) as needed or, for patients who had an epidural anesthesia, maintenance of the epidural catheter for 12 to 24 hours and use of an epidural analgesic. Pain control is generally easily achieved, and bone marrow harvests on strictly an outpatient basis are becoming more routine (83).

Complications

Soreness, bruising, and mild oozing from the puncture sites are nearly universal for the first 24 to 48 hours following a bone marrow harvest. Occasionally (probably less than 5% of procedures), a transient nerve root related symptom (numbness or pain) develops likely due to either local bleeding (and hematoma formation and compression of a nerve root or irritation of the nerve root from extravasated blood) or possibly direct needle injury to a nerve root. Rare cases of long-lasting (longer than one year) and possibly permanent sciatic nerve root injury have been reported (84). Other reported complications of bone marrow harvesting include pelvic fracture, phlegmon formation, and fat embolus syndrome. On rare occasions (less than 1% of harvests), life-threatening complications occur. These may include anaphylactic reactions to anesthetic agents, cardiac arrhythmias, and septic shock (84,85).

Complications of bone marrow harvesting, particularly duration and severity of pain, have been shown to correlate with length of anesthesia in an analysis of volunteer unrelated donors (86). Other factors likely to contribute to operative risk include those medical conditions (e.g., cardiac or pulmonary disease) that may increase anesthetic risk.

Leukopheresis

Peripheral blood stem cells are collected using a continuous flow cell separator apparatus programmed to enrich for mononuclear cells. Adequate venous access is required for this procedure. For normal donors, peripheral venous access has sufficed in most cases. Patients undergoing autologous PBSC collections usually require a central venous catheter for access. In order to achieve optimal draw and infusion rates, a large-bore, stiff-walled pheresis or dialysis catheter should be utilized.

Initial attempts to harvest autologous PBSC under "steady state" (nonmobilized) conditions often required 8 to 10 phereses. With combined chemotherapy and recombinant myeloid growth factor stem cell mobilization, knowledge of the optimal timing for stem cell collection (peripheral white blood count $\geq 5–10 \times 10^9$/L), and the routine use of large volume leukophereses (20 to 25 liters in four to six hours), adequate collections of hemopoietic progenitors for transplantation have often been procured from one or two procedures. Normal allogeneic donors receive growth factor(s) (usually G-CSF) alone for PBSC mobilization. One to two leukophereses starting on days 4 or 5 of G-CSF administration are generally sufficient to collect the targeted number of hemopoietic progenitor cells. Based on engraftment profiles following high-dose chemotherapy and peripheral blood stem cell transplantation, target cell numbers that have been adopted by most transplant centers are $\geq 5 \times 10^8$/kg mononuclear cells and $\geq 5 \times 10^6$/kg CD34 antigen–positive cells. While successful engraftment has been achieved with lower numbers of cells, delayed or incomplete (particularly failure to achieve normal platelet production) engraftment has been correlated with lower numbers of CD34-positive cells (87).

Risks of Leukopheresis

Leukopheresis is generally well tolerated. Aside from possible complications of hemorrhage or pneumothorax from central venous catheter insertion, most of the risks are due to citrate toxicity. Donors commonly experience peripheral and perioral paresthesias. On occasion, hypocalcemia may lead to neuromuscular irritability, tetany, seizures, or arrhythmias. To prevent these complications, pheresis programs use at a minimum oral calcium tablets for treatment of hypocalcemic related complications. Prophylactic oral or IV calcium may be used with monitoring of free ionic calcium levels.

Other complications of the pheresis procedure may include infection and hemodynamic instability, including rare fatal complications owing to arrhythmias or hemodynamic collapse.

CARE OF THE TRANSPLANT PATIENT

Physical Environment

Transplant patients are usually admitted to private rooms in which some form of reverse isolation is utilized. High-efficiency particulate air (HEPA) filtration has been shown to reduce airborne fungal spore content and, in retrospective analyses, incidence of *Aspergillus* infection (880). It has been recommended as a standard of care by the American Society of Hematology and the American Society of Clinical Oncology (89). Strict laminar air flow (LAF) with gut decontamination and sterile food and water has been shown to reduce the risk of bacterial infections and, in one randomized trial of patients undergoing transplantation for severe aplastic anemia, to improve survival (90). However, no benefit has been demonstrated following transplantation for malignant disease. Given the expense and possible psychological deprivation associated with LAF environments, this form of isolation has not been widely adopted. Given the significantly reduced duration of neutropenia following mobilized PBSC transplantation (and the resultant reduction in infection risk), efforts have been made to perform at least a portion of these transplants on an outpatient basis. New guidelines will be required to address the issues of protective isolation in terms of degree of immunosuppression and length of cytopenias.

Table 27.4. Conditioning Regimens for BMT

	Principal Use(s)	Dose-Limiting Toxicities
TBI-Based Regimens		
TBI + CY	HM	Pulmonary
TBI + VP-16	HM	Hepatic
TBI + CY + VP-16	HM	Mucosal
TBI + BU + VP-16	HM	Hepatic
TBI + MEL	HM	Mucosal
TBI + ara-C	HM	Skin, gastrointestinal
TBI + ara-C + CY	HM	Gastrointestinal, pulmonary
Non-TBI-Based Regimens		
MEL	MM	Gastrointestinal
BU + CY_1	HM	Hepatic
BU + CY_2	HM	Hepatic
BU + VP-16 + CY	HM	Hepatic
BU + VP-16	HM	Hepatic
BU + TT + MEL	BC	Gastrointestinal
BCNU + cDDP + CY	BC, ST	Hepatic
CARBO + TT + CY	BC, ST	Mucosal
TT + CY	BC, ST	Hepatic
CARBO + CY	BC, ST	Hepatic
BCNU + VP-16 + CY	NHL, HD	Pulmonary
BCNU + ara-C + VP-16 + CY	NHL, HD	Hepatic
BCNU + ara-C + VP-16 + MEL	NHL, HD	Hepatic
IFOS + CARBO + VP-16	HM, BC, ST	Mucosal, hepatic
CARBO + VP-16	GCT	Mucosal, hepatic

TBI = total body irradiation; VP-16 = etoposide; ara-C = cytosine arabinoside; BU = busulfan; MEL = melphalan; CY = cyclophosphamide (CY_1 = 120 mg/kg; CY_2 = 200 mg/kg); HM = hematologic malignancies; MM = multiple myeloma; BC = breast cancer; ST = solid tumor; NHL = non-Hodgkin's lymphoma; HD = Hodgkin's disease; GCT = germ cell tumors.

Conditioning Therapy

Intensive, usually multi-agent conditioning therapy is used prior to bone marrow or peripheral blood stem cell transplantation. This therapy serves the purposes of: 1) immunosuppression to prevent graft rejection (allogeneic transplantation), 2) treatment of an underlying malignancy, and 3) "creation of space" for lymphohemopoietic cell engraftment. The most commonly utilized conditioning regimens and associated dose-limiting toxicities are listed in Table 27.4. Total body irradiation (TBI), by virtue of its myeloablative and potent immunosuppressive properties, has been widely utilized in transplant conditioning regimens. Early conditioning regimens used single-fraction TBI in a dose of 950–1000 cGy. Fractionated TBI regimens (1200–1320 cGy in 6 to 11 fractions) are associated with decreased toxicity (particularly interstitial pneumonitis) and no apparent increased risk of relapse (91). Cyclophosphamide has been shown to be well tolerated when used with TBI and also has potent myelosuppressive and immunosuppressive properties (92). For patients unable to receive TBI (e.g., previous radiation therapy where additional TBI would exceed tolerance of an involved organ), the radiomimetic alkylating agent busulfan has been shown to be an acceptable substitute. While busulfan is not as immunosuppressive as TBI in experimental animal transplant models, when combined with cyclophosphamide it is associated with similarly low (≤1%) graft rejection risk following HLA-matched allogeneic bone marrow transplantation (93). Preliminary experience with busulfan for non-HLA genotypically identical donor transplants suggests a slightly increased risk of engraftment failure (94). Busulfan is available orally only. With the most commonly administered dosage (1 mg/kg every six hours for 16 doses), absorption and pharmacokinetic parameters are highly variable (95). Increased busulfan levels may correlate with toxicities, particularly hepatic veno-occlusive disease (95,96). The addition of chemotherapy agents such as etopside to TBI/cyclophosphamide or busulfan/cyclophosphamide regimens has resulted in increased toxicity but no proven benefit in terms of diminished relapse. Prospective randomized trials comparing busulfan/cyclophosphamide with TBI/cyclophosphamide regimens have shown conflicting disease-free survival probabilities (97–100). On balance, however, the evidence seems to show no significant difference in probability of graft rejection, relapse, or survival.

A wide variety of alternative chemotherapeutic agents have been evaluated in the BMT setting. Most of these drug regimens consist of one or more alkylating agents, based on the logarithmic dose–response cytotoxicity profile that has been demonstrated experimentally for these agents and the ability to escalate many of these agents to very high doses before nonmarrow toxicity becomes dose limiting. Commonly used combinations of these drugs are listed in Table 27.4. Preparative regimens for autologous transplantation frequently employ drugs that have significant activity against the tumor in standard doses [e.g., ifosfamide, carboplatin, and etoposide (ICE) for germ cell tumors]. The immunosuppressive potential of the preparative regimen for autologous transplantation is not a relevant issue. Hence, drugs with limited (or untested) immunosuppressive potential are included in these regimens.

Recently, efforts have been made to use nonmyeloablative conditioning regimens for allogeneic BMT (101,102). Potential advantages of this approach include less transplant-related toxicities, thereby allowing transplantation of older patients or patients with coexistent medical illnesses. Preliminary clinical trials with these nonmyeloablative chemotherapy regimens (e.g., using fludarabine-based regimens or cyclophosphamide alone) have demonstrated the feasibility of this approach. Based on murine transplant experiments in which an initial state of mixed lymphohematopoietic chimerism can be converted to a fully donor chimeric state without clinical GVHD by delayed donor leukocyte infusions (103), clinical trials are underway to evaluate the toxicities and efficacy of this strategy. Preliminary results are remarkable for the development of an at least transient mixed chimeric state in all cases and striking antitumor responses that have been observed in a group of patients with chemoradiotherapy refractory hematologic malignancies (102).

Bone Marrow/PBSC Infusion

Following postchemotherapy intervals sufficient to allow for clearance of the drug(s), bone marrow and/or PBSC are infused intravenously. This interval varies according to the drug(s) used but is generally in the range of 36 to 72 hours. Allogeneic bone marrow (or PBSC) infusions are performed as soon as possible following their collection. In the case of major red blood cell ABO incompatibility, a red blood cell depletion step via a density gradient sedimentation method or cell separator apparatus is used. For patients with high titer antidonor isoagglutinins (e.g., >1:16 IgM antibodies) plasmapheresis may also be utilized. In the case of a minor ABO blood group incompatibility, plasma removal is performed prior to infusion of the bone marrow or PBSC. When ex vivo T-cell depletion is performed, the marrow or PBSC are usually infused immediately following the depletion step. Marrow or PBSC are infused intravenously as quickly as tolerated. Volume considerations and heparin content may influence the speed of the infusion. Complications of allogeneic bone marrow infusion include volume overload, hypertension, and transfusion reactions (fevers, chills, noncardiogenic pulmonary edema). With proper processing of the marrow or PBSC prior to infusion, life-threatening transfusion reactions due to ABO incompatibility are exceedingly rare.

Cryopreservation of allogeneic bone marrow has historically been discouraged out of concern for stem cell loss. Recent experience, however, has demonstrated insignificant loss of stem cell viability and comparable rates of sustained engraftment (104). This strategy may prove useful. Cryopreservation of unrelated bone marrow (or potentially PBSC) harvests may, for example, obviate the frequent logistical problems of scheduling and transport of marrow or PBSC in these situations (105).

Autologous bone marrow or PBSC are usually cryopreserved in liquid nitrogen. Marrow or PBSC are thawed in a 37°F water bath, then infused as rapidly as possible. In this situation, a balance exists between the desire to minimize exposure of stem cells to dimethyl sulfoxide (DMSO) and the need to avoid the toxicities of DMSO by too rapid an infusion. Toxicities of DMSO-cryopreserved bone marrow or PBSC include nausea, vomiting, and flushing. Hemodynamic changes include bradycardia, hypertension, and (rarely) respiratory decompensation (85).

Post-transplant Supportive Care

Prophylactic oral broad spectrum antibiotics have been shown to reduce the risk of documented gram-negative bacterial infections but not to improve overall survival (106). The quinolone antibiotic ciprofloxacin has been shown in a randomized trial of patients receiving intensive chemotherapy for acute leukemia to be superior to co-trimoxazole and colistin in terms of prevention of gram-negative infections (107). Antifungal prophylaxis with fluconazole has been shown in a prospective randomized placebo-controlled trial to reduce superficial and hematogenous candidiasis (108). Acyclovir is routinely used for prevention of herpes simplex virus reactivation. High-dose acyclovir (500 mg/m^2 IV every eight hours) has been shown to reduce the risk of cytomegalovirus disease in one prospective randomized placebo-controlled trial (109). For *Pneumocystis carinii* prophylaxis, co-trimoxazole is usually used. Therapy is frequently discontinued at the time of transplant, however, then resumed following engraftment (given its potential myelosuppressive potential). CMV infection prophylaxis strategies consist of: 1) administration of CMV-seronegative blood products (or blood products infused through third-generation white blood cell depletion filters) to CMV-seronegative bone marrow transplant recipients, 2) high-dose intravenous immunoglobulin (500 mg/kg) weekly to prevent CMV disease in CMV-seropositive allogeneic bone marrow transplant recipients, 3) monitoring for early

CMV reactivation using CMV antigenemia assays or shell viral cultures and preemptive therapy with ganciclovir with evidence of infection (12,13,110,111). It has been suggested that patients at higher risk for CMV disease (e.g., seropositive recipients of unrelated donor allogeneic marrow transplants) may benefit from prophylactic ganciclovir administration (i.e., the routine administration of ganciclovir at the time of engraftment) (112).

Transfusion Support

Recipients of ABO-incompatible allogeneic marrow transplants will undergo a change in their ABO blood group to that of the donor. Persistent antidonor ABO blood group isoagglutinins may persist, however, for weeks to months after transplant. In order to minimize risks of hemolysis following ABO-mismatched marrow transplantation, recipients should receive group O blood following their transplant.

All cellular blood products (i.e., excluding fresh frozen plasma and cryoprecipitate) should be irradiated to a dose of approximately 2500 cGy to prevent transfusion-induced GVHD. Third-generation white blood cell depletion filters capable of a 3 to 4 log white cell depletion have been shown in some studies to: 1) reduce or delay onset of alloimmunization, 2) reduce incidence of febrile nonhemolytic transfusion reactions, and 3) reduce risk of CMV transmission. They are common practice in the bone marrow transplant setting. Based on a similarly low risk of CMV infection and disease in CMV-seronegative transplant recipients receiving either screened CMV-negative blood products or filtered blood products (110), the latter are believed to be an acceptable alternative to CMV-screened blood products.

The most commonly recommended platelet count for prophylactic platelet transfusions has been 10×10^9/L. However, bone marrow recipients are at increased risk of bleeding because of complications such as severe mucositis, hemorrhagic cystitis, stress (or corticosteroid-induced) gastritis and gastrointestinal GVHD. Higher prophylactic threshold counts (e.g., 20×10^9/L) are therefore often employed in the bone marrow transplant setting. Individual threshold platelet counts, however, may need to be established based on bleeding complications and the platelet count at the time of the bleeding.

Intensive Care Unit

Transfer to the intensive care unit (ICU) is required in 10% to 20% of BMT admissions. Reasons for transfer to the ICU include: 1) pressor-dependent hypotension, frequently as a result of septic shock; 2) respiratory insufficiency requiring mechanical ventilation; and 3) hemodynamic monitoring for regimen-related cardiac toxicity. ICU care is often discouraged because of less favorable quality of air than is found in transplant rooms and the psychological stresses imposed on patients and their families by the unfamiliar environment and restricted visiting privileges. The mortality associated with admission to the ICU for BMT patients is very high. For patients requiring mechanical ventilation, mortality risk is in excess of 95% (113).

Nutrition

Maintenance of positive nitrogen balance is an appropriate nutritional goal for marrow transplant recipients. Factors that lead to a diminished oral intake during transplant hospitalizations include nausea, vomiting, and alimentary tract mucositis. Supplemental nutrition is often required for marrow transplant recipients. Total parenteral nutrition (TPN) was shown to increase survival following allogeneic BMT in one randomized trial (114). Oral feeding via a feeding tube was shown in one study to be equivalent to TPN and can be considered in selected patients with intact alimentary tract mucosa (115). Caution should be observed, however, with the use of TPN. Patients appear to be at increased risk of TPN hepatotoxicity, probably because of multiple potentially hepatotoxic insults (e.g., hepatic veno-occlusive disease, hepatic GVHD, and cyclosporine toxicity).

Physical Therapy

An evaluation by a physical therapist prior to BMT is an important part of the treatment plan. Development of an individual exercise program, which is supervised on an ongoing basis by the therapist is useful to maintain muscle tone and strength. A stationary bicycle or light weights are useful in this regard. Attention must be paid to factors that might limit exercise in this setting, such as severe thrombocytopenia or persistent nausea. Patients receiving intensive corticosteroid therapy for GVHD are particularly prone to develop muscle weakness and atrophy and osteoporosis. Ongoing consultation with the physical therapist is mandatory. A posthospital exercise plan should also be coordinated with the physical therapist prior to discharge.

Nursing

Crucial to a successful BMT is the coordination of a treatment plan with the nursing staff. Ideally, transplant candidates should be evaluated by a BMT nurse specialist prior to admission in order to assess medical and psychological suitability for the transplant and to provide additional education regarding the transplant as well as post-transplant recovery. An assessment of the medical status and likely future needs of the patient is also undertaken by a primary nurse following hospital admission. Formulation of a nursing plan, interaction with the patient's family, delivery of intensive inpatient nursing care, and recording of all relevant clinical data are among the vital responsibilities of the nursing staff in establishing a successful transplant. Long-term relationships with the patient and their family are important in facilitating the complete recovery of patients following their transplant. The nursing staff are also often involved in collaborative clinical investigative efforts. These duties often include the development of protocols and the collection and analysis of clinical data.

Social Service

All transplant candidates should meet with the BMT social workers as early in the course of evaluation as possible. Inquiries regarding insurance coverage of transplant-related costs including outpatient medications and home nursing services are made during this initial evaluation in an effort to ease the financial burdens imposed by a bone marrow transplant. An evaluation of the patient's and his or her family's psychosocial status is very important as well. This triage function serves to identify potential emotional problems for which intensive support from the social worker or psychiatric intervention is warranted. Participation in multidisciplinary BMT team meetings is crucial to full understanding of the emotional needs of the patient. The social worker assumes a leadership role in coordinating family meetings and facilitating transplant-related home care.

COMPLICATIONS AND THEIR MANAGEMENT

Early Versus Late Transplant-Related Complications

Complications following BMT can be considered as either early (within the first 100 days following transplantation) or late (more than 100 days following transplantation) events. Early complications are generally either conditioning regimen–related toxicities or immunologic complications of the transplant (rejection and GVHD). Late complications include chronic GVHD, prolonged immunoincompetence (often related to underlying chronic GVHD), and secondary malignancies.

Rejection

Engraftment failure may be either a primary event (failure to restore a level of functional hematopoiesis) or a secondary phenomenon (initial engraftment followed by loss of the graft). Following HLA genotypically identical donor non-T-cell–depleted allogeneic BMT for hematologic malignancies, the incidence of engraftment failure is approximately 1% to 2% (116). Following non-HLA genotypically identical transplants, the incidence of engraftment failure is considerably higher, ranging from 5% to 10% following HLA genotypically identical unrelated donor transplantation to 21% following HLA two- to three-antigen mismatched related donor transplantation (116). An increased risk of engraftment failure (approximately 10% to 15%) has been observed after HLA-identical donor BMT for aplastic anemia (43). Transplants in which the marrow has been depleted ex vivo of T cells are accompanied by a higher risk of engraftment failure, particularly after HLA nongenotypically identical donor transplants (117–121).

Engraftment failure is associated with a very high mortality rate. Second transplants are often required following primary engraftment failure; however, given the compromised state of the recipient (because of prior conditioning therapy and prolonged pancytopenia), second transplants are often poorly tolerated. Recently, transplantation of G-CSF mobilized allogeneic peripheral blood stem cells have been associated with prompt restoration of hematopoiesis in selected cases (120). Treatment of secondary engraftment failure varies according to the underlying cause. Cytomegalovirus disease, for example, can be treated with ganciclovir with or without high-dose intravenous immunoglobulin. Severe pancytopenia, a result of GVHD, in which residual host hematopoiesis can be documented, can sometimes be managed with "booster" bone marrow infusions without intensive conditioning therapy. Administration of recombinant hematopoietic growth factors (particularly granulocyte/monocyte colony-stimulating factor or granulocyte colony-stimulating factor) has been associated with at least partial restoration of hematopoiesis in some cases.

Graft-Versus-Host Disease

Acute GVHD occurs within the first 100 days following transplantation (although clinical manifestations are usually apparent within the first 30 days after the transplant) (121,122). The pathogenesis of GVHD involves the recognition by immunocompetent donor T cells of disparate host histocompatibility antigens. While T cells are crucial to the development of GVHD, and ex vivo T-cell depletion (provided that the number of T cells is reduced to less than a threshold level of approximately 1×10^5/kg) can essentially eliminate the risk of acute GVHD, the eventual manifestations of GVHD are probably mediated by a complex interaction of multiple effector cells and cytokines. Not surprisingly, once GVHD is well established anti-T-cell therapies are often ineffective.

Clinically, acute GVHD is characterized primarily by skin, gastrointestinal (GI), and hepatic manifestations (Table 27.5). Concomitant with or shortly after engraftment, a skin rash is often the first sign of GVHD. An erythematous, macular, though sometimes morbilliform, eruption develops typically over the scalp, ears, neck and upper chest, palms, and/or soles. The rash, however, may involve any skin site and a high index of suspicion for the diagnosis of GVHD should be kept, particularly following alloengraftment. Gastrointestinal manifestations of GVHD usually include diarrhea, although an upper gastrointestinal form of GVHD (characterized predominantly by nausea and vomiting) has also been described. Hepatic abnormalities are usually cholestatic in nature. High bilirubin levels, predominantly conjugated bilirubin, out of proportion to elevation of transaminase and alkaline phosphatase levels, is characteristic of hepatic GVHD. Other potential sites of acute GVHD

Table 27.5. Clinical Manifestations of GVHD

Site	Clinical Manifestation
Acute GVHD	
Skin	Rash
Gastrointestinal	Nausea, vomiting, diarrhea
Liver	Cholestatic hepatitis
Lymphohematopoietic system	Immunodeficiency, cytopenia(s)
Other	
Oral/vaginal mucosa	Mucositis
Conjunctiva	Conjunctivitis
Lung	Diffuse pneumonitis
Chronic GVHD	
Skin	Rash, xeroderma, sclerodermatous change
Mouth/conjunctiva	Sicca complex
Esophagus	Dysmotility/dysphagia
Liver	Mixed cholestatic, hepatocellular abnormalities
Gastrointestinal tract	Malabsorption
Muscle/joint	Polymyositis/polyarthritis
Nerve	Peripheral neuropathy
Kidney	Minimal change nephrotic syndrome
Bladder	Cystitis
Lymphohematopoietic system	Immunodeficiency/cytopenias
Lung	Lymphocytic bronchitis/pulmonary fibrosis/ bronchiolitis obliterans

include lung, conjunctiva, oral and vaginal mucosa, and the lymphohematopoietic system. The latter injury is more difficult to measure and may be overlooked. The resulting cytopenias and dysfunctional immune system may ultimately be the cause of the patient's demise. A grading system for GVHD, in which the primary sites of involvement (skin, GI tract, liver) are scored on a 1+ to 4+ basis depending on severity, has been developed and has prognostic significance (123).

Histologically, GVHD is characterized by extensive epithelial injury (Figs. 27.1, 27.2 and Plates 24, 25). Scattered apoptotic keratinocytes accompanied by satellitosis, vacuolization of the basal layer, and lymphocytic infiltration is commonly seen in cutaneous GVHD. Focal necrotic epithelial cells, crypt abscesses, and eventually total denudation of the intestinal mucosa may be manifestations of gastrointestinal GVHD. Hepatic GVHD involves injury to bile duct epithelium. Late in the course of the disease, however, the histologic picture in hepatic GVHD can be quite nonspecific. Diffuse cholestasis with bile duct dropout may be the only significant findings.

A GVHD-like syndrome has been described following approximately 5% to 10% of syngeneic and autologous transplants. Clinical and histologic features may be indistinguishable from GVHD following allogeneic transplants, although they are typically less severe. A transient imbalance between autoreactive and suppressor T-cell populations, likely induced by thymic injury from the chemoradiotherapeutic conditioning regimen, is thought to be the

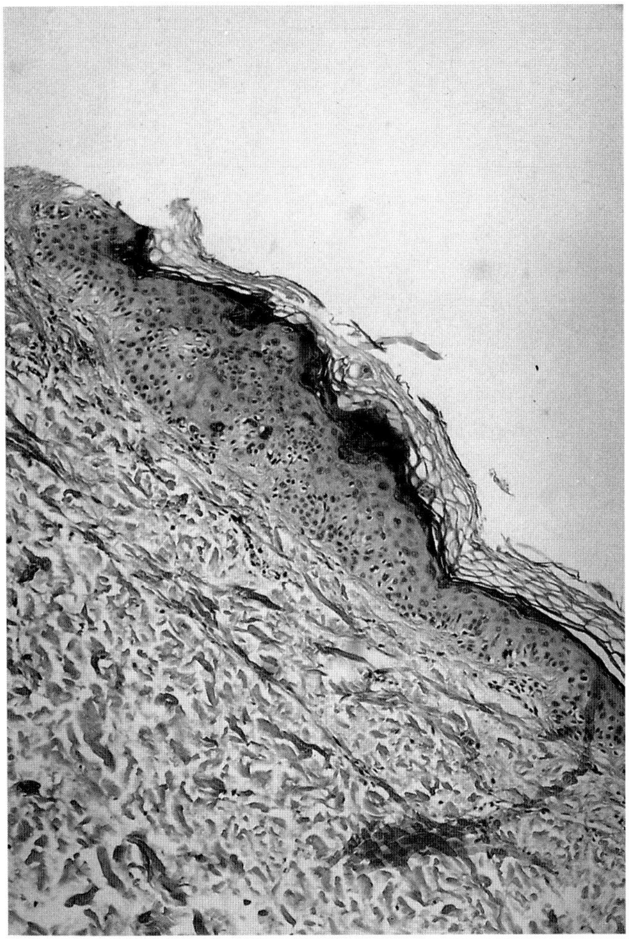

FIGURE 27.1. *Cutaneous GVHD (day 14 after BMT). Vacuolar interface dermatitis with sparse superficial perivascular lymphocytic infiltrate and scattered necrotic keratinocytes.*

mechanism of this syndrome. Induction of autologous GVHD by cyclosporine, in an attempt to produce a graft-versus-leukemia (GVL) effect, has been described (122).

Prevention of GVHD can be accomplished by either pharmacologic means or by ex vivo T-cell depletion. A combination of cyclosporine with methotrexate or corticosteroids is associated with an approximately 30% to 40% incidence of grade II–IV GVHD following HLA genotypically identical donor BMT. With progressive HLA antigen disparity, the risk of GVHD increases. Following HLA two-to three-antigen–mismatched donor allogeneic transplantation, the incidence of GVHD may be greater 80%. The incidence of grade II or higher GVHD following transplantation with ex vivo T-cell–depleted marrow is typically less than 10%. Ex vivo T-cell depletion, however, is associated with increased risks of engraftment failure and relapse of the underlying malignancy, particularly in chronic myelogenous leukemia (118,119,124).

Treatment of acute GVHD has been largely unsatisfactory. Intensive corticosteroid therapy is the mainstay of

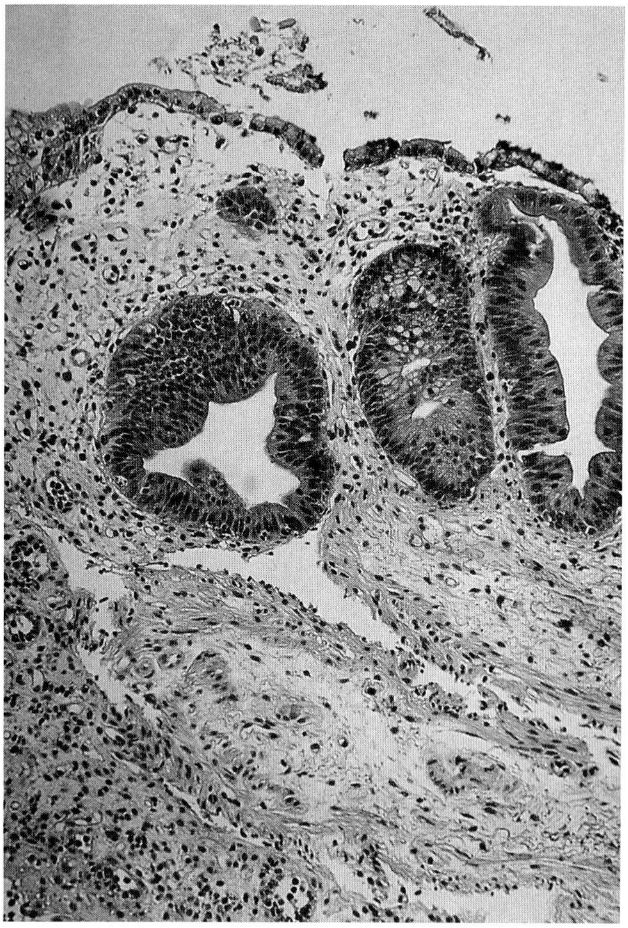

FIGURE 27.2. Colonic GVHD (day 8 after HLA-mismatched donor BMT). Mucosal atrophy with focally reactive colonic epithelium and cellular apoptosis.

treatment. Nonrelapse mortality of patients with grade II or higher GVHD who do not achieve a complete remission with GVHD therapy is greater than 50% (125). Patients with grades III or IV GVHD have mortality risks in excess of 60% and 90%, respectively. New therapies that have shown some promise in the management of moderate to severe acute GVHD have included monoclonal antibodies directed against putative effector cells (e.g., anti-natural killer cell antibodies) or cytokines (e.g., anti-IL-1 or antitumor necrosis factor antibodies).

Regimen-Related Toxicities

Virtually every organ system can be affected by high-dose chemoradiotherapeutic preparative regimens. Some of these toxicities may lead to significant short-term morbidity but are completely reversible (e.g., oral pharyngeal mucositis, gastroenteritis). Other toxicities, however, may be irreversible and life threatening (e.g., progressive hepatic failure from veno-occlusive disease or interstitial pneumonitis). Certain toxicities may be more common after allogeneic transplantation (e.g., interstitial pneumonitis) owing to the immunologic influences that contribute to the pathogenesis of the injury. The more profound immunocompromise that accompanies allogeneic bone marrow transplantation may also lead to an increased incidence of infection, particularly with organisms that are ordinarily controlled by an intact cell-mediated immunity. The most common, potentially life-threatening complications that occur following BMT include infection or hemorrhage secondary to severe pancytopenia, hepatic veno-occlusive disease, diffuse interstitial pneumonitis, and cardiac toxicity.

Infection

Early infectious complications following either autologous or allogeneic transplantation are due primarily to severe neutropenia. There has been a shift in the spectrum of bacterial infections that occur following transplantation, from predominantly gram-negative bacteria to gram-positive bacteria and fungal organisms. This change has been attributed to the routine use of indwelling silastic central intravenous catheters, the common use of prophylactic broad spectrum oral antibiotics, and increasingly intensive conditioning regimens leading to more severe mucosal injury. The use of quinolone antibacterial prophylaxis, for example, is associated with a very low incidence of gram-negative infections. However, infections with coagulase-negative staphylococci and other gram-positive organisms are common. Candidal infections are considerably less common when prophylactic fluconazole is used. *Aspergillus* infections appear to be less common since peripheral blood stem cells have been used routinely. The incidence of *Aspergillus* infections is related to the duration of neutropenia; hence, with durations of severe neutropenia of only approximately one week after peripheral blood stem cell transplantation, opportunistic fungal infections have become less common.

With resolution of neutropenia, infectious complications are uncommon after autologous peripheral blood stem cell transplantation. Following allogeneic transplantation, however, cell-mediated immunity may be significantly impaired. *Pneumocystis carinii* pneumonia, CMV disease, and other herpes virus related illnesses are potentially problematic. Routine antipneumocystis prophylaxis is employed, as are intravenous immunoglobulin and early preemptive ganciclovir use for patients with evidence of CMV reactivation.

Hemorrhage

Severe thrombocytopenia occurs following intensive chemoradiotherapeutic preparative therapy. While guidelines for using prophylactic platelet transfusions for platelet counts of less than 10,000/µL have been proposed, patients undergoing bone marrow transplantation often may require more aggressive platelet support to prevent or treat bleeding. Bleeding from injured mucosal surfaces, hemorrhagic cystitis, cyclosporine-induced hypertension, and stress gastritis are all common after BMT and warrant aggressive platelet transfusional therapy. Maintenance of platelet counts greater than 20,000/μL is often necessary, and in patients who do have hemorrhagic manifestations, maintenance of considerably higher platelet counts may be necessary. Single-donor apheresis platelets may delay alloimmunization and are a preferred source of transfusional support in most transplant centers. Related platelet donors, particularly HLA-matched donors, may be an ideal source of platelet support.

Hepatic Veno-Occlusive Disease

Hepatic veno-occlusive disease (VOD) occurs in approximately 20% to 50% of patients following BMT (126,127). This syndrome is believed to result from chemoradiotherapy-induced injury to hepatocytes and vascular endothelium in zone three of the liver acinus, local hypercoagulability, and microvenular/sinusoid hepatic vascular obstruction secondary to thrombosis and fibrosis (Fig. 27.3 and Plate 26). Clinically, the syndrome is characterized by hyperbilirubinemia, right upper quadrant pain/tenderness and hepatomegaly, and weight gain (with or without ascites). The differential diagnosis of hepatic VOD disease is shown in Table 27.6. Risk factors for VOD include antecedent liver disease (with elevated transaminase levels at the time of transplant), multialkylator conditioning regimens [particularly those that contain high-dose carmustine (BCNU)], and second transplants. Strategies that have been shown at least in some studies to be effective for the prevention of VOD include ursodeoxycholic acid (128), and low-dose heparin

A

B

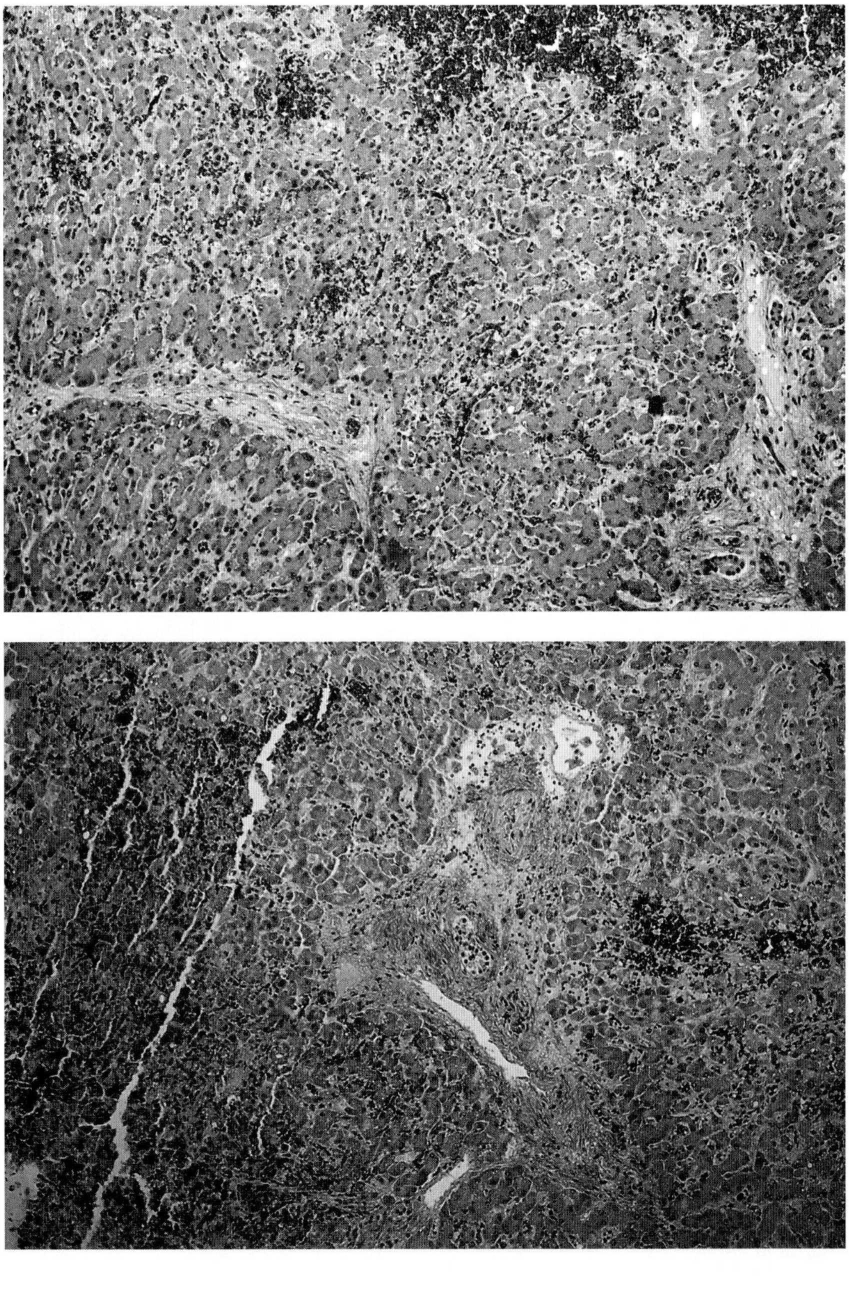

FIGURE 27.3. *Hepatic veno-occlusive disease (autopsy specimen day 39 after HLA-mismatched donor BMT).* ***A.*** *Hematoxylin and eosin stain showing global occlusion of centrilobular veins with amorphous eosinophilic material, surrounding centrilobular hemorrhage, and focal necrosis.* ***B.*** *Trichrome stain showing collagen deposition in the centrilobular veins.*

(129) or low-molecular-weight heparin (130). Since most cases of VOD resolve spontaneously, supportive care alone may be sufficient. For patients with severe VOD, characterized by very high bilirubin levels (>25 dL), massive weight gain, and other signs of multiorgan dysfunction, low-dose tissue plasminogen activator (t-PA) has been effective in approximately half of the cases. Because patients with hepatic failure and severe thrombocytopenia are at very high risk of bleeding complications, t-PA is reserved for patients who are believed to have a very high mortality risk from their underlying VOD. Ultimate mortality is often, however, a manifestation of multiorgan system failure (126).

Interstitial Pneumonitis and Acute Lung Injury Syndromes

Interstitial pneumonitis occurs more frequently after allogeneic than autologous transplantation (131). The peak risk period for interstitial pneumonitis occurs 50 to 80 days following transplantation. The majority of cases of interstitial pneumonitis were originally understood to be caused by CMV. With more effective CMV prophylaxis strategies, the majority of cases are now idiopathic. Among the latter group of cases are likely a mixture of conditioning-therapy–related lung injuries (particularly with BCNU-containing regimens) and pulmonary GVHD. Earlier lung injuries may occur in relation to engraftment and include noncardiogenic pulmonary edema secondary to capillary leak syndrome (132) and diffuse alveolar hemorrhage (Fig. 27.4 and Plate 27) (133). Management of acute lung injury and interstitial pneumonitis is dictated by the underlying cause. Early administration of high-dose corticosteroids and aggressive platelet transfusional support may be effective in the management of engraftment-related acute lung injury syndrome. Corticosteroid therapy may also be important in the manifestation of later (after one month following transplantation) interstitial pneumonitis. Exclusion of an infectious cause for the pneumonitis, however, is imperative prior to aggressive corticosteroid therapy (see Chapter 28).

Table 27.6. Differential Diagnosis of Cholestatic Hepatitis Following Allogeneic BMT

Disease	Onset Post-transplant	Distinguishing Features(s)
Veno-occlusive disease	1–3 weeks	Tender hepatomegaly, weight gain ± ascites
Acute GVHD	2–12 weeks	Skin ± GI GVHD common
Cyclosporine toxicity	2–6 weeks	More prominent with elevated cyclosporine levels
Parenteral nutrition	2–6 weeks	More prominent elevation of alkaline phosphatase, transaminase levels
Cholangitis lenta	Time independent	Associated sepsis

Cardiac Toxicity

High-dose cyclophosphamide is associated with significant cardiac toxicity in a small percentage of patients (134,135). In approximately 1% to 5% of patients receiving more than 120 mg/kg of cyclophosphamide, an acute cardiac injury occurs. The acute myopericarditis that may result may be heralded by loss of voltage on electrocardiogram (EKG), the development of a pericardial friction rub, and/or signs of tamponade. The mortality of patients with severe acute myopericarditis with cardiac decompensation and refractory hypotension is very high. Patients with more subtle forms of disease, particularly those with a pure pericarditis variant

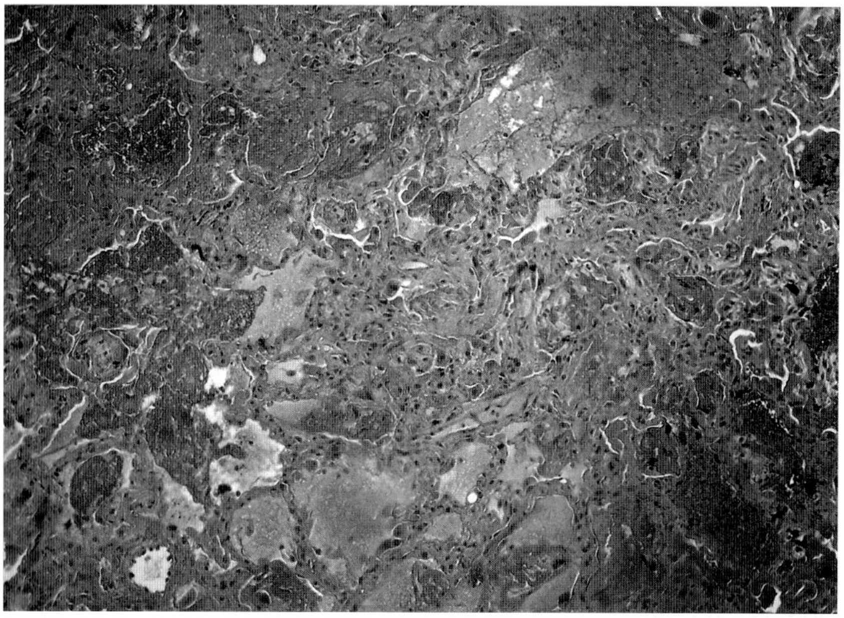

FIGURE 27.4. *Diffuse alveolar injury and hemorrhage day 23 after busulfan, cyclophosphamide, and autologous PBSCT for Hodgkin's disease.*

of cyclophosphamide-induced cardiac injury have a more favorable prognosis. Prospective series using more sensitive methods of cardiac evaluation have documented a considerably higher incidence of cardiac abnormalities after BMT (134). More than half of transplant recipients have at least transient EKG abnormalities or evidence of myocardial dysfunction.

Late Complications

Late complications include infections, chronic GVHD, infertility, and secondary malignancy. Pediatric BMT recipients may also have growth retardation and impairment in the development of secondary sexual characteristics. Other complications that may result from intensive chemoradiotherapeutive preparative regimens include cataract formation (in 20% to 30% patients receiving fractionated total body irradiation) and radiation-induced pulmonary or pericardial fibrosis. Complications of intensive corticosteroid therapy for earlier GVHD include osteoporosis, hypertension, and diabetes mellitus.

Infection

Late infectious complications of autologous bone marrow or peripheral blood stem cell transplantation are unusual. An approximately 20% to 40% incidence of herpes zoster occurs after autologous transplantation. *Pneumocystis* prophylaxis is usually not necessary beyond the first three to six months following autologous transplantation. Late infectious complications following allogeneic BMT are associated with the lack of establishment of immunocompetence. Patients with GVHD, particularly those requiring immunosuppressive therapy, are at high risk for infections caused by encapsulated bacteria (hence the frequent indication for penicillin prophylaxis). *Pneumocystis carinii*, fungal organisms, and viral infections (particularly CMV and adenovirus) are also not uncommon in this setting (see also Chapter 36).

Chronic Graft-Versus-Host Disease

Chronic GVHD occurs in approximately one third to one half of patients undergoing allogeneic BMT (136). The most important risk factor for chronic GVHD is the presence of acute GVHD. Older recipient age, non-T-cell–depleted marrow, and the use of supplemental donor buffy coat cells (and possibly the use of peripheral blood stem cells rather than bone marrow) also contribute to the development of chronic GVHD. Chronic GVHD appears to be mediated by autoreactive T cells directed against an HLA class II common determinant (122). Clinical manifestations of chronic GVHD are related to the multiorgan system involvement that the disease may cause. Many of these manifestations are similar to the clinical sequelae of collagen vascular diseases including sclerodermatous skin changes, a sicca complex similar to Sjögren's syndrome, and clinical and histologic hepatic abnormalities similar to primary biliary cirrhosis. The treatment of chronic GVHD consists of immunosuppressive therapy, usually corticosteroids in conjunction with cyclosporine or azathioprine. Thalidomide has shown promise for the treatment of refractory chronic GVHD (137). The prognosis of chronic GVHD is dependent on severity (limited versus extensive) of disease and bone marrow function (patients with severe thrombocytopenia have a particularly poor prognosis).

Infertility

Restoration of fertility usually occurs following cyclophosphamide preparative therapy for severe aplastic anemia. However, following TBI or multialkylator-containing preparative regimens, sterility is almost universal in males and occurs in the majority of females (138). In female transplant recipients, age at the time of the transplant is the most important determinant for risk of sterility. Attempts to protect the ovaries by using oral contraceptives or luteinizing hormone-releasing hormone (LHRH) antagonists have not proved to be successful. Cryopreservation of sperm or ova for in vitro fertilization following the transplant, if feasible, has been successful in some cases.

Secondary Malignancies

A small but significant risk of secondary malignancy occurs following BMT. Two large series of more than 2000 patients each have shown 6.6- and 11.6-fold increases in the incidence of malignant neoplasms compared with the general population (139,140). Included among these malignancies is post-transplant lymphoproliferative disease. The risk factors for this malignancy are ex vivo T-cell depletion, HLA-mismatched donor transplantation, the use of antithymocyte globulin, and primary immunodeficiency. The risk factors for the development of other second cancers may include use of TBI in the conditioning regimen, allogeneic versus autologous marrow transplantation, and the presence of chronic GVHD (particularly for the development of skin cancer). Recently, an actuarial 6% to 18% incidence of myelodysplastic syndrome has been seen following TBI-containing conditioning therapy and autologous transplantation for malignant lymphoma (141). In B-cell lymphoproliferative disease and occasional cases of recurrent leukemia, a donor cell origin of the malignancy has been demonstrated.

RESULTS

General Principles

Survival after bone marrow or stem cell transplantation is a function of early transplant-related mortality, the probability of relapse of the underlying disease, and late complications such as secondary malignancy. Representative Kaplan-Meier survival probability curves from the International Bone Marrow Transplant Registry/Autologous Bone Marrow Transplant Registry (IBMTR/ABMTR) for AML following allogeneic and autologous bone marrow transplantation are shown in Figures 27.5 and 27.6. Early transplant-related

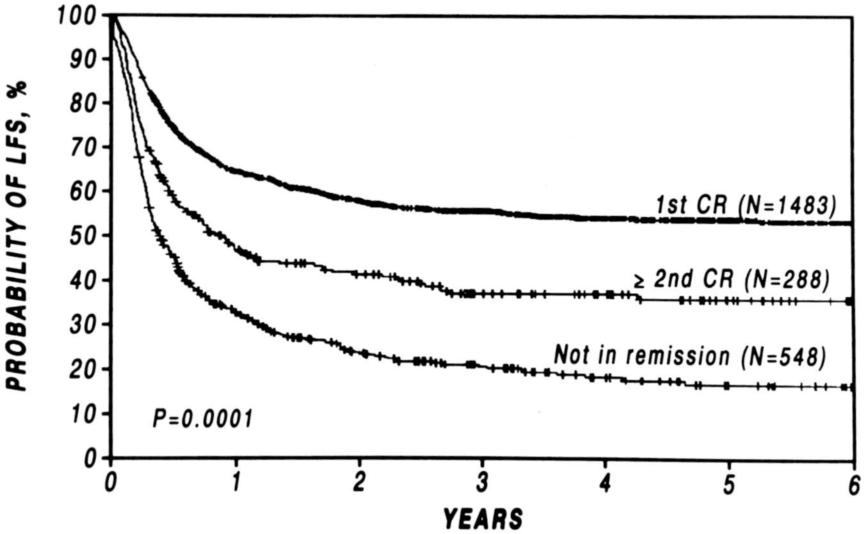

FIGURE 27.5. *Probability of leukemia-free survival after HLA-identical sibling transplants for acute myelogenous leukemia, 1987 to 1994. (Data from the IBMTR/ABMTR.)*

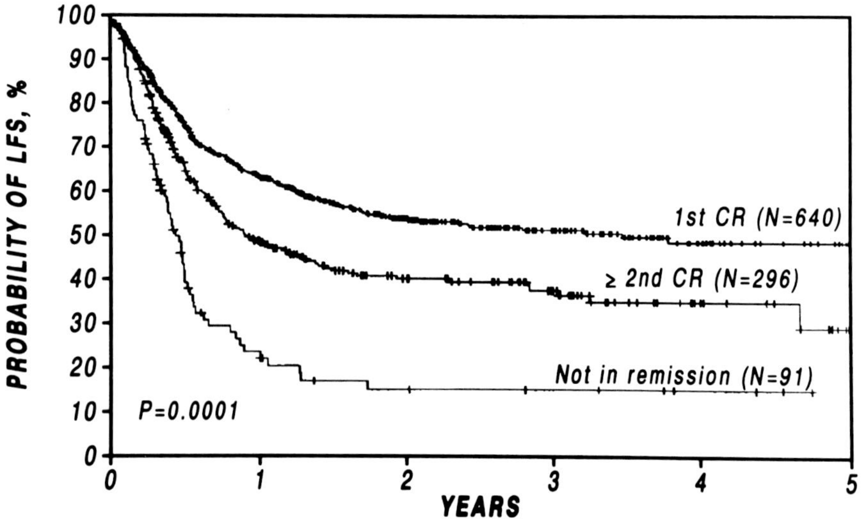

FIGURE 27.6. *Probability of leukemia-free survival after autotransplants for acute myelogenous leukemia, 1989 to 1994. (Data from the IBMTR/ABMTR.)*

mortality, generally defined as death from causes other than relapse within 100 days of transplantation, accounts for the steep fall in survival probability within the first several months following transplantation. The more moderate decline in survival from three months to approximately two years after transplant reflects the probability of relapse, while the plateau in survival after two years is indicative of the probability of long-term disease-free survival (or in some malignancies, cure). In AML, long-term disease-free survival probabilities following allogeneic or autologous transplantation in first complete remission are approximately 50% (142,143). In first relapse/second remission or refractory relapse, disease-free survival probabilities following allogeneic transplantation are approximately 25% and 10% to 15%, respectively (142,144). The latter survival probability is similar to that reported by Thomas and colleagues in 1977 (9). While early transplant-related mortality has lessened with improved supportive care and GVHD prophylaxis, relapse probability for those patients who now live long enough to be evaluated for remission status remains very high. Similar disease-free survival probabilities are seen in other hematologic malignancies. In CML, for example, disease-free survival probabilities for patients in chronic phase, accelerated phase, and blast phase of their disease are approximately 45% to 60%, 15% to 25%, and 10%, respectively (142,145).

Transplant-Related Mortality

Owing to improvements in supportive care and GVHD prophylaxis, early transplant-related mortality has diminished significantly over the past two decades. Following allogeneic BMT from HLA genotypically identical sibling donors, transplant-related mortality is now approximately 15% to 20%. With the introduction of cyclosporine for GVHD prophylaxis, the incidence of clinically significant (grade II to IV) GVHD has been reduced from approximately 70% to a range of 30% to 40%. With this improved management of

GVHD, the upper age limit for allogeneic BMT from HLA-identical donors has increased from 40 years in most centers in 1980 to 55 to 60 years at the present time. With the use of alternative donors (HLA phenotypically matched unrelated donors or partially mismatched related donors), transplant-related mortality is considerably higher. With incidences of grade III to IV GVHD as high as 30% to 40% in some series, transplant-related mortality may be as high as 40% to 60% (146). Factors that influence the risk of transplant-related mortality following allogeneic BMT include age, disease status (remission/chemosensitive versus advanced/chemorefractory), histocompatibility of donor and recipient, and the presence or absence of comorbid disease.

The reduction in transplant-related mortality following autologous bone marrow or stem cell transplantation has been even more dramatic over the past two decades. Contributing to this reduction in mortality has been the use of peripheral blood stem cells rather than bone marrow as the source of hematopoietic rescue. A correlation between the markedly shortened duration of neutropenia with peripheral blood stem cells and a reduction in infectious complications, mucositis, and hepatic VOD have been observed. Transplant-related mortality following autologous bone marrow transplantation for advanced solid malignancies was previously reported to be as high as 15% to 25%. Transplant-related mortality in modern series utilizing PBSC support has ranged from approximately 1% to 5% (146,148). Concomitant with the recent introduction of peripheral blood stem cells, however, has been a change in patient selection for transplant trials. Recent series involving autologous bone marrow or stem cell transplantation for metastatic breast cancer, for example, include patients mostly without heavy pretreatment and almost entirely with chemotherapy-sensitive disease (as compared with previous series in which heavily pretreated patients with chemoresistant disease were often included).

Survival Probabilities According to Disease

Hematologic Malignancies

Similar long-term disease-free and overall survival probabilities have been seen following allogeneic BMT for AML and ALL (Table 27.7) (142,149). Patient selection for transplantation in these two diseases is quite different, however. Outside of the setting of randomized trials, patients with AML are often chosen for transplantation in first-year remission if they have unfavorable prognostic features such as an antecedent hematologic disorder or an adverse cytogenic abnormality. Patients with ALL who receive a transplant while in first-year remission are almost exclusively adult patients (given the excellent prognosis of children with ALL), also with adverse albeit different prognostic factors such as a high white blood count at diagnosis and the presence of the Philadelphia chromosome.

For the chronic leukemias, the decision to proceed with transplantation often creates a therapeutic dilemma. In CML, for example, median survival probabilities of three to four years are achieved with minimal therapy. This dilemma is compounded by data showing improved long-term disease-free survival probabilities when transplantation from HLA-matched related donors is carried out within one to two years after diagnosis (145). An emerging experience with allogeneic transplantation for chronic lymphocytic leukemia (CLL) has created an additional question regarding timing of transplantation (150,151). Patients with CLL often have a long duration (sometimes in excess of 10 years) of indolent disease. With more advanced disease, patients may not be eligible for transplantation due to either advanced age or the presence of disease complications such as opportunistic infection. Nonetheless, an approximately 40% long-term disease-free survival has been achieved following allogeneic BMT for CLL, suggesting a possibly curative role for transplantation (151).

The curative potential of allogeneic BMT for other hematologic malignancies, including malignant lymphoma (both non-Hodgkin's and Hodgkin's type), multiple myeloma, and myelodysplastic syndrome has also been established (152–166). Given the differences in patient selection compared with patients who undergo autologous bone marrow or stem cell transplantation for these diseases (e.g., patients who are younger or have more bone marrow involvement by their underlying disease possibly being favored for this approach), the roles of allogeneic BMT for these diseases remain unclear.

Table 27.7. Estimated Disease-Free or Event-Free Survival (DFS/EFS) Following Allogeneic BMT

Disease	Remission Status	% DFS/EFS (References)
AML	1st CR	45–60% (22,98,142)
	1st relapse/2nd CR	23–30% (22,142,144)
	>2nd CR	10–18% (9,22,142)
ALL	1st CR	28–43% (22,142,152)
	2nd/subsequent CR	25–30% (22,142)
	Relapse/refractory	10–15% (9,22,142)
CML	Chronic phase	45–60% (22,99,142,145)
	Accelerated phase	15–25% (22,142,145)
	Blast phase	10–15% (22,142,145)
MDS	RA/RARS	50–63% (159,162)
	RAEB/RAEB-T	30–40% (159,162)
Non-Hodgkin's/Hodgkin's lymphoma	Relapsed/refractory	15–25% (152,165)
Multiple myeloma		20–35% (153,164)
CLL		30–40% (151)
SAA		52–69% (184,185,186)

AML = acute myelogenous leukemia; ALL = acute lymphoblastic leukemia; CML = chronic myelogenous leukemia; MDS = myelodysplastic syndrome; CLL = chronic lymphocytic leukemia; SAA = severe aplastic anemia; RA/RARS = refractory anemia/refractory anemia with ringed sideroblasts; RAEB/RAEB-T = refractory anemia with excess blasts/refractory anemia with excess blasts in transformation.

Autologous Bone Marrow/PBSC Transplantation

For diseases in which a bone marrow remission can be achieved with conventional therapy, autologous BMT or PBSCT provides an alternative treatment option for some transplant candidates (Table 27.8). Comparable long-term disease-free survival probabilities have been demonstrated in multiple phase II trials evaluating autologous bone marrow or stem cell transplantation for AML in first complete remission compared with allogeneic BMT. In a multicenter prospective randomized trial comparing allogeneic or autologous BMT with conventional therapy for AML, no statistically significant difference was seen between allogeneic and autologous BMT in terms of disease-free survival probability (161). While both forms of transplantation resulted in superior disease-free survival probability compared with conventional chemotherapy, overall survival was not affected. This latter outcome reflects primarily the potential for "salvage" BMT therapy for patients who relapse following conventional chemotherapy.

Autologous bone marrow or stem cell transplantation for non-Hodgkin's lymphoma constitutes the treatment of choice for patients with relapsed chemotherapy-sensitive intermediate- to high-grade histology. The Parma trial, a randomized prospective study evaluating the efficacy of autologous bone marrow transplantation compared with conventional chemotherapy, demonstrated disease-free and overall survival advantages for the transplanted group (160). Overall, approximately 30% to 40% of patients who receive an autologous bone marrow transplant for intermediate-grade non-Hodgkin's lymphoma in second remission achieve long-term disease-free survival (152,157,160). Similar long-term disease-free survival probabilities can be achieved following autologous bone marrow or stem cell transplantation for Hodgkin's disease (152,158). Questions regarding optimal timing of autologous transplantation for Hodgkin's lymphoma have been raised. Long-term follow-up of patients treated with salvage conventional chemotherapy for relapsed disease has suggested a lower cure rate than previously had been believed. An important role of autologous transplantation for relapsed Hodgkin's lymphoma, particularly for relapse within two years after initial diagnosis, has been realized. In multiple myeloma, increased probabilities of complete remission (22% versus 5%), event-free survival (28% versus 10%), and overall survival (52% versus 12%) have been demonstrated for patients undergoing autologous BMT for newly diagnosed multiple myeloma compared with patients receiving conventional chemotherapy alone (163)

Solid Tumors

The role of high-dose chemotherapy and autologous bone marrow or stem cell transplantation for solid tumors remains less well defined than for hematologic malignancies. Nonetheless, the possibility of durable disease control has been demonstrated for a number of inherently chemosensitive malignancies (see Table 27.8) (23,25,26,167–176). A

Table 27.8. Estimated Disease-Free or Event-Free Survival (DFS/EFS) Following Autologous BMT/PBSCT

Disease	Remission Status	% DFS/EFS (References)
Hematologic Malignancy		
AML	1st CR	40–54% (58,62,143)
	2nd/subsequent CR	25–30% (62,63)
ALL	1st CR	40–45% (62)
	2nd/subsequent CR	20–30% (62)
NHL	Low grade	50–55% (1,154)
	Intermediate–high grade	30–50% (152,157,160)
HD		40–50% (152,158)
Multiple myeloma	1st PR/CR	30–60% (163,164,166)
	>1st PR/CR	15–30% (153)
Solid Tumors		
Breast cancer	Stage II–III (adjuvant)	70–80% (26,169)
	Stage IV (chemosensitive)	15–34% (23,25,26,170,171)
Ovarian cancer	Stage III–IV (relapsed/chemosensitive)	20–30% (174)
Germ-cell tumor	Relapsed	15–51% (172,173)
Neuroblastoma	Stage IV (1st PR/CR)	40–53% (175,176)
Small-cell lung cancer	Limited disease (1st PR/CR)	20–40% (167,168)

AML = acute myelogenous leukemia; ALL = acute lymphoblastic leukemia; NHL = non-Hodgkin's lymphoma; HD = Hodgkin's disease.

striking increase in the number of autologous transplants performed for breast cancer has been seen in the last decade. As adjuvant therapy for high-risk breast cancer (such as inflammatory breast cancer or in patients with more than 10 involved axillary lymph nodes), high-dose chemotherapy and autologous bone marrow or stem cell transplantation has been associated with long-term disease-free survival probabilities of 70% to 80% (26,169). Multicenter prospective, randomized trials are now underway to determine whether autologous transplantation offers a survival advantage over conventional chemotherapy in some of these patient subgroups. Approximately 20% of patients undergoing high-dose chemotherapy and autologous bone marrow or stem cell transplantation for metastatic breast cancer achieve durable disease control (greater than two-year disease-free survival probability) (23,25,26,166,167). Improvements in complete remission probability and disease-free and overall survival probabilities have been suggested in a prospective randomized trial comparing autologous BMT with conventional chemotherapy (170). Other prospective randomized trials are in progress in order to better define the impact of high-dose chemotherapy/autologous transplantation strategies for metastatic breast cancer. Improved patient selection may also lead to improve long-term survival probabilities. Patients who are in complete remission at the time of their transplant, have limited sites of nonvisceral disease, and are of younger age may, for example, have improved outcomes following autologous transplantation.

High-dose chemotherapy/autologous transplantation strategies for other solid tumors, such as relapsed germ cell tumors or ovarian cancer, are also being developed. Long-term disease-free survival probabilities of 15% to 50% have been realized in a number of series evaluating autologous transplantation in relapsed disease (172,173). Once again, prior therapy and chemosensitivity at the time of the transplant affect survival probabilities. In some centers, the role of high-dose chemotherapy and autologous bone marrow or stem cell transplantation for patients with poor-prognosis metastatic disease (e.g., stage IIIC ovarian cancer) in first remission is being evaluated (174).

For pediatric solid tumors, such as metastatic neuroblastoma and rhabdomyosarcoma, high-dose chemotherapy/autologous transplantation also may have a role. A suggestion of improved long-term disease-free survival following autologous transplantation for metastatic neuroblastoma in the first remission has been raised by several retrospective analyses (175,176).

Despite impressive response rates (including complete response rates in some series) following high-dose chemotherapy and autologous BMT for more chemoresistant solid tumors (such as colorectal cancer or melanoma), the lack of durable responses has led to abandonment of this strategy. In malignant melanoma, for example, overall and complete response rates of 60% and 30%, respectively, have been reported (177). However, median response durations were less than one year.

Graft-Versus-Leukemia (Graft-Versus-Malignancy) Effect

Several lines of evidence exist for the presence of a graft-versus-malignancy effect; that is, a lesser probability of relapse following allogeneic transplantation compared with autologous or syngeneic marrow/stem cell transplantation (178,179). Allogeneic bone marrow transplantation is associated with a lower relapse probability in AML and malignant lymphoma than is autologous marrow transplantation. The most striking evidence for a graft-versus-malignancy effect occurs in CML. Patients receiving a syngeneic or T-cell–depleted allogeneic marrow transplant for CML have relapse probabilities as high as 60% to 80% compared with a 20% relapse probability following non-T-cell–depleted allogeneic bone marrow transplantation. Patients relapsing after an allogeneic BMT for CML have a high probability (75% to 80%) of achieving a sustained cytogenic and molecular remission following adoptive immunotherapy with donor leukocytes (180,181). An intermediate probability of relapse following allogeneic BMT for hematologic malignancy in recipients of non-T-cell–depleted transplants who do not develop clinically evident GVHD compared with patients with clinical GVHD and those who receive a syngeneic or T-cell–depleted transplant provides clinical evidence for a separation of GVHD and GVL effects (182).

Source of Allogeneic Donor

Allogeneic bone marrow transplants from non-HLA genotypically identical donors are associated with an increased risk of GVHD and, in some series, transplant-related mortality (145). Patients receiving HLA single-antigen mismatched related donor or phenotypically matched unrelated donor transplants for hematologic malignancy have had comparable survival to patients receiving HLA genotypically identical related donor transplants (183). These similar long-term outcomes, despite increased risks of severe GVHD and transplant-related mortality, reflect potent graft-versus-malignancy effects, since relapse probabilities are significantly lower following these non-HLA genotypically identical donor transplants. Allogeneic bone marrow transplants from two- or three-HLA-antigen–disparate donors have been associated with distinctly inferior survival probabilities owing to prohibitively high risks of life-threatening GVHD and high risks of engraftment failure (183).

Nonmalignant Disease

Acquired Lymphohematopoietic Stem Cell Disorders

The prototype acquired stem cell disorder for which BMT has had an important impact is severe aplastic anemia. Long-term survival rates of 52% to 69% have been demonstrated following HLA genotypically identical donor bone marrow transplantation for severe aplastic anemia (184–186). These results compare favorably to alternative therapy, usually with immunosuppressants such as antithymocyte globulin (ATG) with or without cyclosporine. A recent retrospective analysis from Seattle has supported the importance of BMT as a potentially curative therapy for severe aplastic anemia. An actuarial survival of 69% at 15 years was observed in 168 recipients of an HLA-identical donor transplant (186). Patients who received immunosuppressive therapy had an actuarial survival of 39% at 15 years. Moreover, a 10% incidence of clonal hematopoietic neoplasms was observed in recipients of immunosuppressive therapy. While other series have shown comparable survivals between BMT and immunosuppressive therapy, the lack of curative potential of immunosuppressive therapy and the late risk of clonal disorders favor allogeneic BMT as the treatment of choice for severe aplastic anemia in patients less than 40 years of age. Transplants from HLA phenotypically matched donors have resulted in similar survivals to recipients of HLA genotypically identical donor transplants (187). However, HLA-mismatched related and HLA genotypically matched or minor-mismatched unrelated donor transplants have been associated with inferior survival. Transplants from alternative donors are largely reserved for patients who do not respond to immunosuppressive therapy. Successful allogeneic BMT has also been performed for paroxysmal nocturnal hemoglobinuria (188).

Congenital Lymphohematopoietic Stem Cell Disorders

Allogeneic BMT has been a successful and potential curative therapy for a number of congenital lymphohematopoietic stem cell disorders starting with the successful transplants by Good and his team and Bach et al of infants with combined immunodeficiency syndromes in 1968 (5,6,189–193). A common feature of these disorders is the potential to replace a defective stem cell population or immune system by the infusion of normal lymphohematopoietic pluripotential stem cells. Disorders of hemoglobin production, as a result of abnormal hemoglobin production (e.g., sickle cell anemia) or inadequate alpha or beta globin chain synthesis (the thalassemic disorders), can also be corrected by replacement of a normal erythrocytic stem cell compartment. A wide variation in preparative therapy required for transplantation, types of donors that have been effectively used for transplantation, and results of transplantation exist for the various congenital stem cell disorders. Low-dose cyclophosphamide (20 mg/kg), for example, is effectively used as conditioning therapy for Fanconi's anemia, given the impaired DNA repair mechanisms that exist following alkylating agent exposure in that disease (192). High-dose busulfan and cyclophosphamide have most commonly been used as conditioning therapy for thalassemia major and sickle cell anemia (190,193). In sickle cell anemia, approximately 75% of children are cured following HLA genotypically identical donor allogeneic BMT. Complications following transplantation for sickle cell anemia include early transplant-related mortality (5% to 10%), graft rejection or recurrence (20%), and GVHD (10%) (193). While event-free survivals of 70% to 90% following bone marrow transplantation for selected congenital stem cell disorders are encouraging, further progress in alleviating transplant-related acute and chronic toxicities is required.

COMMENTARY

John M. Goldman

The remarkable evolution of allogeneic bone marrow transplantation from a dream treated with incredulity by many to a near-routine clinical procedure is well documented in the chapter by Spitzer and McAfee. At a time when clinicians throughout the world are aware that bone marrow transplantation is a sophisticated technique that can cure selected patients with leukemia, aplastic anemia, and certain other hematologic disorders, it is difficult to realize that a mere 30 years ago the notion that hematopoietic stem cells could be collected from one person and transfused to another in a manner that would permit durable engraftment was for most people the material of which medical "science fiction" was constructed. As the authors note, clinicians had little preclinical data on which to base their clinical studies, they knew virtually nothing of the biology of the now still-elusive stem cell, the existence of the HLA system had barely been recognized, and the optimal approach to immune suppression to permit engraftment was entirely unexplored. Even the technology of how to collect stem cells, how many marrow cells one would need, and how best to administer these to the patient were matters for speculation and then cautious experimentation.

It is in some ways regrettable, though perhaps understandable, that the Nobel Prize for medicine is in fact seldom awarded for the contribution that an individual or team of individuals makes in the realm of clinical medicine. This reflects no doubt the fact that it is usually difficult to delineate with any accuracy the precise contribution of just one or two individuals in a given clinical field that may have developed very significantly in 10 or 20 years. It is much easier to recognize and acclaim the contribution of the man or woman who unravels a fundamental pathway in signal transduction, who conceives the strategy for designing monoclonal antibodies, or who discovers the microbial or molecular cause of a previously mysterious disease. E. Donnall Thomas has been a happy exception to this general rule. It was his team uniquely that built on the early studies of Robert Good and colleagues in Minneapolis and perfected the combination of radiotherapy and cytotoxic drugs, rather euphemistically called "conditioning," that is now used to induce immune suppression in the patient and simultaneously to destroy residual leukemia cells. His team went on to demonstrate that patients with aplastic anemia or leukemia could in some cases be cured by chemotherapy and transplantation of allogeneic stem cells. None doubted that Thomas was a worthy recipient of the

Nobel Prize in 1992; many wondered why it had taken so long to recognize his seminal contributions.

Progress in this field in the last few years has slowed. We still face some formidable problems, of which the greatest is perhaps the intractability of graft-versus-host disease (GVHD). For an adult patient with leukemia who receives a conventional allogeneic transplant with unmanipulated marrow cells from an HLA-identical sibling donor, the risk of sustaining severe GVHD is still 10% to 20% and it carries an appreciable mortality. The demonstration that depletion of T cells in donor marrow would reduce significantly the incidence of GVHD appeared at first to be a major contribution to the field, but it then became clear that there was a high price to be paid in terms of graft failure, impaired immune recovery, and increased risk of relapse. A landmark event was the demonstration that transfusions of lymphoid cells collected from the original transplant donor could be effective in treating leukemia in relapse after bone marrow transplantation, albeit most effective in chronic myeloid leukemia (CML), which was important confirmation of the existence and power of the previously somewhat ill-defined graft-versus-leukemia (GVL) effect. But in terms of patient survival, probably the most important single development in the last 10 years was the introduction of drugs, ganciclovir and foscarnet, that are active against cytomegalovirus (CMV) infection (see Chapter 36). The judicious use of these agents has virtually eliminated one major cause of morbidity and mortality after sibling transplants.

The success with sibling transplants in the 1980s led logically to the question: Can the pool of donors be expanded such that patients who lack HLA-identical siblings can also be transplanted successfully? The report from Seattle that a patient with leukemia had been transplanted successfully using a "matched" unrelated donor (1) had constituted a major conceptual advance, but the donor in this case had been identified fortuitously and no formal system existed for identifying volunteer donors. In fact, a volunteer donor panel had been established in London in 1974, but it was relatively small and little used. In the late 1980s, the London panel was reconstituted and expanded, still retaining the title of the patient, Anthony Nolan, in whose name it was founded. At the same time, the National Marrow Donor Program was established in the United States to collate tissue type data from a number of volunteer donor panels (2). Other countries rapidly followed the leads established in Britain and the United States. Today there are donor panels in more than 30 countries, and the computer files of the agency Bone Marrow Donors Worldwide show that more than 5 million persons have been tissue typed and all would in theory give marrow stem cells for a patient in need. In practice, an appreciable proportion of the persons classified as volunteers are not actually available to donate when targeted as prospective donors, and donor panels must continue to add volunteers in order to maintain numbers. Moreover, identifying a suitably matched donor is still a relatively slow procedure; but in extreme circumstances the interval between search initiation and marrow donation can be as short as one week (3).

What then of the future for bone marrow transplantation? Many lines of evidence suggest that the alloreactive lymphoid cells that engender GVHD can in principle be separated from those that mediate the GVL effect. The most urgent need is for a technology that would permit eradication of the former while maintaining the latter intact. One might even imagine that GVL cells could in certain circumstances be isolated and exploited outside the context of a formal allograft. Another pressing need is for more effective methods of combating infection, which remains a major complication of transplant procedures, especially those involving the use of alternative donors. Thus, an effective drug for prophylaxis of *Aspergillus* infection would be most valuable; agents that suppress the proliferation of viruses other than CMV such as polyoma, parainfluenza, adenovirus, and respiratory syncytial virus would also help to improve the results of transplants using unrelated donors.

Another development that would contribute greatly to the technology of bone marrow transplantation would be the ability to "expand" hematopoietic stem cells reliably in vitro. One of the interesting aspects of clinical transplantation has been the observation that although occasionally a graft fails within the first few months after transplant, this is almost always attributable to immunologic mechanisms. Late graft failure, attributable presumably to stem cell exhaustion, is exceedingly rare. This must mean that in most cases the stem cells in the original transfusion have expanded in vivo in a manner that permits the maintenance of hematopoiesis in the patient for years or more probably for decades. Can this expansion be simulated in vitro? Such an achievement might permit collection of relatively small numbers of donor stem cells, and equally important, it might provide a mechanism for depleting or eliminating the cells that mediate GVHD. At present there is ample evidence that progenitor cells can be expanded in vitro, often many hundred-fold, but little convincing evidence exists for stem cell expansion, which must theoretically be possible.

Finally, comment should be made about autografting. Although Spitzer and McAfee provide data showing clearly that autografting can be valuable in some circumstances, for the great majority of tumors for which high-dose chemotherapy followed by autografting has been tested, there is still little evidence of clinical benefit. This must relate in part to the fact that harvested marrow cells are frequently contaminated with tumor cells and in part to the fact that the techniques for eradicating tumor in the patient even with high-dose therapy remain imperfect. Real progress in both areas could pave the way for effective therapy for a variety of the more common solid tumors, including cancers of breast, ovary, and lung, which of course pose the greatest challenge for the oncologist today.

CHAPTER REFERENCES

1. Lajtha LG. The common ancestral cell. In: Wintrobe MW, ed. Blood, pure and eloquent. New York: McGraw-Hill, 1980:81–95.
2. Cirenza E. Peripheral blood stem cells: a historical perspective. J Infus Chemother 1996;6:4–8.
3. Osgood EE, Riddle MC, Mathews TJ. Aplastic anemia treated with daily transfusions and intravenous marrow; case report. Ann Intern Med 1939;13:357–367.
4. Bortin MM. A compendium of reported human bone marrow transplants. Blood 1970;9:571–587.
5. Gatti RA, Allen HD, Meuwissen JH, et al. Immunological reconstitution of sex-linked lymphopenic immunological deficiency. Lancet 1968;2:1366–1369.
6. Bach FH, Albertini RJ, Joo P, et al. Bone marrow transplantation in a patient with Wiskott-Aldrich syndrome. Lancet 1968;2:1364–1366.
7. Goodman JR, Hodgson GS. Evidence for stem cells in the peripheral blood of mice. Blood 1962;19:702–714.
8. Cavins JA, Scheer SC, Thomas ED, Ferrebee JW. The recovery of lethally irradiated dogs given infusions of autologous leukocytes preserved at –80°C. Blood 1964;23:38–43.
9. Thomas ED, Buckner CD, Banaji M, et al. One hundred patients with acute leukemia treated by chemotherapy, total body irradiation, and allogeneic marrow transplantation. Blood 1977;49:511–533.
10. Storb R, Deeg HJ, Farewell V, et al. Marrow transplantation for severe aplastic anemia: methotrexate alone compared with a combination of methotrexate and cyclosporine for prevention of acute graft-versus-host disease. Blood 1986;68:119–125.
11. Storb R, Deeg HJ, Whitehead J, et al. Methotrexate and cyclosporine compared with cyclosporine alone for prophylaxis of acute graft-versus-host disease after marrow transplantation for leukemia. N Engl J Med 1986;314:729–735.
12. Schmidt GM, Horak DA, Niland JC, et al. A randomized controlled trial of prophylactic ganciclovir for cytomegalovirus pulmonary infection in recipients of allogeneic bone marrow transplants. N Engl J Med 1991;324:1005–1011.
13. Goodrich JM, Mori M, Gleaves CA, et al. Early treatment with ganciclovir to prevent cytomegalovirus disease after allogeneic bone marrow transplantation. N Engl J Med 1991;325:1601–1607.
14. Bortin MM, Horowitz MM, Gale RP, et al. Changing trends in allogeneic bone marrow transplantation for leukemia in the 1980's. JAMA 1992;268:607–612.
15. Frassoni F, Labopin M, Gluckman E, et al. Results of allogeneic bone marrow transplantation for acute leukemia have improved in Europe with time—a report of the Acute Leukemia Working Party of the European Group for Blood and Marrow Transplantation. Bone Marrow Transplant 1996;17:13–18.
16. Frei III E, Canellos GP. Dose: a critical factor in cancer chemotherapy. Am J Med 1980;69:585–594.
17. Weischelbaum RR, Greenberger JS, Schmidt A, et al. In vitro radiosensitivity of human leukemia cell lines. Radiology 1981;139:485–487.
18. Coccia PF, Krivit W, Cervenka J, et al. Successful bone marrow transplantation for infantile malignant osteopetrosis. N Engl J Med 1980;302:701–708.
19. Thomas ED. Marrow transplantation for malignant diseases. J Clin Oncol 1993;1:517–531.
20. Ringden O, Horowitz MM, Gale RP, et al. Outcome after allogeneic bone marrow transplant for leukemia in older adults. JAMA 1993;270:57–60.
21. Clift RA, Buckner CD, Storb R, et al. The influence of patient age on the outcome of transplantation during chronic phase of chronic myeloid leukemia. Blood 1995;86(suppl 1):617a.
22. Advisory Committee of the International Bone Marrow Transplant Registry. Report from the International Bone Marrow Transplant Registry. Bone Marrow Transplant 1989;4:221–228.
23. Antman K, Gale RP. Advanced breast cancer. High-dose chemotherapy and bone marrow autotransplants. Ann Intern Med 1988;108:570–574.
24. Cheson BD, Lacerna L, Leyland-Jones B, et al. Autologous bone marrow transplantation. Ann Intern Med 1989;110:51–65.
25. Antman K, Ayash L, Elias A, et al. A phase II study of high-dose cyclophosphamide, thiotepa and carboplatin with autologous marrow support in women with measurable advanced breast cancer responding to standard-dose therapy. J Clin Oncol 1992;10:102–110.
26. Spitzer TR, Cirenza E, McAfee S, et al. Phase I-II trial of high-dose cyclophosphamide, carboplatin and autologous bone marrow or peripheral blood stem cell rescue. Bone Marrow Transplant 1995;15:537–542.
27. Bearman SI, Petersen FB, Schor RA, et al. Radionuclide ejection fraction in the evaluation of patients being considered for bone marrow transplantation: risk for cardiac toxicity. Bone Marrow Transplant 1990;5:173–177.
28. Ballester O, Zorsky P, Janssen W, et al. High dose therapy with autologous peripheral blood stem cell transplantation in patients with multiple myeloma and end-stage renal failure. Blood 1995;86(suppl 1):208a.
29. Frickhofer N, Wiesneth M, Jainta C, et al. Hepatitis C virus infection is a risk factor for liver faiulure from veno-occlusive disease after bone marrow transplantation. Blood 1994;13:417–422.
30. Locasciulli A, Bacigalupo A, Van Lint MT, et al. Hepatitis C virus infection and liver failure in patients undergoing allogeneic bone marrow transplantation. Bone Marrow Transplant 1995;16:407–410.
31. Becker AJ, McCullouch EA, Till JE. Cytological demonstration of the clonal nature of spleen colonies derived from transplanted mouse marrow cells. Nature 1963;197:452–455.
32. Magli MC, Iscove NN, Odartchenko N. Transient nature of early hemopoietic spleen colonies. Nature 1982;295:527–529.
33. Morrison JH. Separation of lymphocytes of rat bone marrow by combined glass-wool filtration and dextran-gradient centrifugation. Br J Haematol 1967;13:229–235.
34. Scott MA, Gordon MY. In search of the haemopoietic stem cell. Br J Haematol 1995;90:738–743.
35. Szilvassy SJ, Hoffman R. Enriched hematopoietic stem cells: basic biology and clinical utility. Biol Blood Marrow Transplant 1995;1:3–17.
36. Sutherland HJ, Eaves CJ, Eaves AC, et al. Characterization and partial purification of human marrow cells capable of initiating long-term hematopoiesis in vitro. Blood 1989;74:1563–1570.
37. Landsdorp PM, Sutherland HJ, Eaves CJ. Selective expression of CD45 isoforms on functional subpopulations of CD34+ hemopoietic cells from human bone marrow. J Exp Med 1990;172:363–366.
38. Skour EF, Brandt JE, Briddell RA, et al. Human CD34+ HLA-DR bone marrow cells contain progenitor cells capable of self renewal, multilineage differentiation and long term in vitro hematopoiesis. Blood Cells 1991;17:287–295.
39. Sutherland DR, Stewart AK, Keating A. CD34 antigen: molecular features and potential clinical applications. Stem Cells 1993;11:50–57.
40. Lasky LC. Hemotopoietic reconstitution using progenitors recovered from blood. Transfusion 1989;29:552–557.
41. Socinski MA, Cannistra SA, Elias A, et al. Granulocyte-macrophage hemopoietic progenitor cell compartment in man. Lancet 1989;1:1194–1198.
42. Storb R, Pretice RL, Thomas ED. An analysis of factors associated with graft rejection. N Engl J Med 1977;296:61–66.
43. Champlin RE, Horowitz MM, van Bekkum DW, et al. Graft failure following bone marrow transplantation for severe aplastic anemia: Risk factors and treatment results. Blood 1989;73:606–613.
44. Vriesendorp HM, van Bekkum DW. Role of total body irradiation in conditioning for bone marrow transplantation. Haematol Bluttransfus 1980;25:349–364.
45. Areman EM, Cullis H, Spitzer T, Sacher R. Automated processing of human bone marrow results in a purified population of mononuclear cells capable of achieving engraftment following transplantation. Transfusion 1991;31:724–730.
46. Shpall EJ, Jones RB, Bearman SI, et al. Transplantation of enriched CD34-positive autologous marrow into breast cancer patients following high-dose chemotherapy: Influence of CD34-positive peripheral blood progenitors and growth factors on engraftment. J Clin Oncol 1994;12:28–36.
47. Bensinger W, Singer J, Appelbaum F, et al. Autologous transplantation with peripheral blood mononuclear cells collected after administration of recombinant granulocyte colony-stimulating factor. Blood 1993;81:3158–3163.
48. Byer J, Schwella N, Zingsem J, et al. Hematopoietic rescue after high-dose chemotherapy using autologous peripheral-blood progenitor cells or bone marrow: a randomized comparison. J Clin Oncol 1995;113:1328–1335.
49. Williams DA. Ex vivo expansion of hematopoietic stem and progenitor cells—robbing Peter to pay Paul? Blood 1993;81:3169–3172.
50. Goldman J. Peripheral blood stem cells for allografting. Blood 1995;85:1413–1415. Editorial.
51. Pettengell R, Testa NG, Swindell R, et al. Transplantation potential of hematopoietic cells released into the circulation during routine chemotherapy for non-Hodgkin's lymphoma. Blood 1993;82:2239–2248.
52. Haas R, Witt B, Möhle R, et al. Sustained long-term hematopoiesis after myeloablative therapy with peripheral blood progenitor cell support. Blood 1995;85:3754–3761.

53. Bensinger WI, Weaver CH, Appelbaum FR, et al. Transplantation of allogeneic peripheral blood stem cells mobilized by recombinant human granulocyte colony-stimulating factor. Blood 1995;85:1655–1658.
54. Schmitz N, Dreger P, Suttorp M, et al. Primary transplantation of allogeneic peripheral blood progenitor cells mobilized by filgrastim (granulocyte colony-stimulating factor). Blood 1995;85:1666–1672.
55. Korbling M, Przepiorka D, Huh YO, et al. Allogeneic blood stem transplantation for refractory leukemia and lymphoma: potential advantage of blood over marrow allografts. Blood 1995;85:1659–1665.
56. Russell JA, Luider J, Weaver M, et al. Collection of progenitor cells for allogeneic transplantation from peripheral blood of normal donors. Bone Marrow Transplant 1995;15:111–115.
57. Gale RP, Horowitz MM, Ash RC, et al. Identical twin bone marrow transplants for leukemia. Ann Intern Med 1994;120:646–652.
58. Gorin NC, Aegerter P, Auvert B, et al. Autologous bone marrow transplantation for acute myelocytic leukemia in first remission: a European survey of the role of marrow purging. Blood 1990;75:1606–1614.
59. Rowley SD, Zuehlsdorf M, Braine HG, et al. CFU-GM content of bone marrow graft correlates with time to hematologic reconstitution following autologous bone marrow transplantation with 4-hydroperoxycyclophosphamide-purged bone marrow. Blood 1987;70:271–275.
60. Rowley SD, Jones RJ, Piantodose S, et al. Variability in 4-hydroperoxycyclophosphamide activity during clinical purging for autologous bone marrow transplantation. Blood 1987;70:1490–1494.
61. Gribben JG, Freedman A, Neuberg D, et al. Immunologic purging of marrow assessed by PCR before autologous bone marrow transplantation for B-cell lymphoma. N Engl J Med 1991;325:1525–1533.
62. Gorin NC, Labopin M. European survey on 1688 autografts for consolidation of acute leukemia: further evidence that marrow purging with mafosfamide is effective in acute myelocytic leukemia. Blood 1990;76(suppl 1):542a. Abstract.
63. Chopra R, Goldstone AH, McMillan AK, et al. Successful treatment of acute myeloid leukemia beyond first remission with autologous bone marrow transplantation using busulfan/cyclophosphamide and unpurged marrow: the British Autograft Group Experience. J Clin Oncol 1991;9:1840–1847.
64. Roberts MM, To LB, Gillis D, et al. Immune reconstitution following peripheral blood stem cell transplantation, autologous bone marrow transplantation and allogeneic bone marrow transplantation. Bone Marrow Transplant 1993;15:469–475.
65. Fegan C, Thomas H, Bailey-Wood R, et al. In vitro LAK (lymphokine activated killer) activity following autologous peripheral blood stem cell is significantly greater than that following autologous bone marrow and allogeneic bone marrow transplantation. Bone Marrow Transplant 1995;16:277–281.
66. Takaue Y, Okamoto Y, Kawano Y, et al. Regeneration of immunity and varicella-zoster virus infection after high-dose chemotherapy and peripheral blood stem cell autografts in children. Bone Marrow Transplant 1994;14:219–223.
67. Vose J, Anderson J, Kessinger A, et al. High-dose chemotherapy and autologous hematopoietic stem-cell transplantation for aggressive non-Hodgkin's lymphoma. J Clin Oncol 1993;11:1846–1851.
68. Hansen JA, Choo SY, Geraghty DE, Mickelson E. The HLA system in clinical marrow transplantation. Hematol Oncol Clin N Am 1990;4:507–515.
69. Beatty PG. The use of unrelated donors for bone marrow transplantation. In: Sullivan K, Koppa SD, eds. Marrow transplantation reviews. Charlottesville: Kluge Corden Jennings, 1995:53–57.
70. Mickelson EM, Hansen JA. HLA matching in marrow transplantation. In: Sullivan K, Koppa SD, eds. Marrow transplantation reviews. Charlottesville: Kluge Carden Jennings, 1995:45–50.
71. Zmijewski CM. HLA antigens and their detection. In: Hackel E, Mallory, eds. Theoretical Aspects of HLA. Arlington, VA: American Association of Blood Banks, 1982:33–50.
72. Beatty PG, Clift RA, Mickelson EM, et al. Marrow transplantation from related donors other than HLA-identical siblings. N Engl J Med 1985;313:765–771.
73. Stroncek D, Bartsch G, Perkins HA, et al. The National Marrow Donor Program. Transfusion 1993;33:567–577.
74. Petersdorf EW, Smith AG, Mickelson EM, et al. Ten HLA-DR4 alleles defined by sequence polymorphisms within the DRB1 first domain. Immunogenetics 1991;33:267–275.
75. Petersdorf EW, Longton GM, Anasetti C, et al. The significance of HLA-DRB1 matching on clinical outcome after HLA-A, B, DR identical unrelated donor marrow transplantation. Blood 1995;86:1606–1613.
76. Fleischauer K, Kernan NA, O'Reilley RJ, et al. Bone marrow allograft rejection by host-derived allocytotoxic T lymphocytes recognizing a single amino acid at position 15b of the HLA-B44 class I antigen. N Engl J Med 1990;323:1818–1822.
77. Baxter-Lowe LA. Molecular techniques for typing unrelated marrow donors—potential impact of molecular typing disparity on donor selection. Bone Marrow Transplant 1994;14(suppl 4):42–50.
78. Weaver CH, Buckner CD, Longin K, et al. Syngenic transplantation with peripheral blood mononuclear cells collected after the administration of recombinant human granulocyte colony-stimulating factor. Blood 1993;82:1981–1984.
79. Wagner JE, Kernan NA, Steinbuch M, et al. Allogeneic sibling umbilical-cord blood transplantation in children with malignant and non-malignant diseases. Lancet 1995;346:214–219.
80. Kurtzberg J, Laughlin M, Graham M, et al. Placental blood as a source of hematopoietic stem cells for transplantation into unrelated recipients. N Engl J Med 1996;335:157–166.
81. Lingenfetter P, Adams SL, Lasser D, et al. Detection of maternal cells in human umbilical cord blood using fluorescence in situ hybridization. Blood 1995;86:2829–2832.
82. Spitzer TR, Areman E, Cirenza E, et al. The impact of harvest center on quality of marrow collected from unrelated donors. J Hematother 1994;3:65–70.
83. Bolwell BJ, Maurer W, Anderson J, et al. Outpatient bone marrow harvest: the Cleveland Clinic experience. Bone Marrow Transplant 1995;16:703–705.
84. Buckner CD, Clift RA, Sanders JE, et al. Marrow harvesting from normal donors. Blood 1984;64:630–634.
85. Davis JM, Rowley SD, Braine HG, et al. Clinical toxicity of cryopreserved bone marrow graft infusion. Blood 1990;75:781–786.
86. Stroncek DF, Holland PV, Bartch G, et al. Experience of the first 493 unrelated marrow donors in the National Marrow Donor Program. Blood 1993;81:1940–1946.
87. Bensinger W, Appelbaum F, Rowley S, et al. Factors that influence collection and engraftment of autologous peripheral blood stem cells. J Clin Oncol 1995;13:2547–2555.
88. Sherertz RJ, Belani A, Kramer BS, et al. Impact of air filtration on nosocomial *Aspergillus* infections. Unique risk of bone marrow transplant recipients. Am J Med 1987;83:709–718.
89. The American Society of Clinical Oncology and American Society of Hematology recommended criteria for the performance of bone marrow transplantation. J Clin Oncol 1990;8:563–564.
90. Storb R, Prentice RL, Buckner CD, et al. Graft-versus-host disease and survival in patients with aplastic anemia treated by marrow grafts from HLA-identical siblings. Beneficial effect of a protective environment. N Engl J Med 1983;308:302–307.
91. Thomas CD, Clift RA, Hersman J, et al. Marrow transplantation for acute nonlymphoblastic leukemia in first remission using fractionated or single-dose irradiation. Int J Rad Oncol Biol Phys 1982;8:817–821.
92. Buckner CD, Rudolph RH, Fefer A, et al. High dose cyclophosphamide therapy for malignant disease. Cancer 1972;29:357–365.
93. Santos GW, Tutschka PJ, Brookmeyer R, et al. Marrow transplantation for acute nonlymphocytic leukemia after treatment with busulfan and cyclophosphamide. N Engl J Med 1983;309:1347–1353.
94. Mehta J, Powles RL, Mitchell P, et al. Graft failure after bone marrow transplantation from unrelated donors using busulphan and cyclophosphamide for conditioning. Bone Marrow Transplant 1994;13:583–587.
95. Slattery JT, Sanders JE, Buckner CD, et al. Graft-rejection and toxicity following bone marrow transplantation in relation to busulfan pharmacokinetics. Bone Marrow Transplant 1995;16:31–42.
96. Grochow LB, Jones RJ, Brundreh RB, et al. Pharmacokinetics of busulfan: correlation with veno-occlusive disease in patients undergoing bone marrow transplantation. Cancer Chemother Pharmacol 1989;25:55–61.
97. Blume KG, Kopecky KJ, Henslee-Downey JP, et al. A prospective randomized comparison of total body irradiation—etoposide versus busulfan-cyclophosphamide as preparatory regimens for bone marrow transplantation in patients with leukemia who were not in first remission: a Southwest Oncology Group Study. Blood 1993;81:2187–2193.
98. Blaise D, Maraninchi D, Archimbaud E, et al. Allogeneic bone marrow transplantation for acute myeloid leukemia in first remission: a randomized trial of busulfan–Cytoxan versus Cytoxan–total body irradiation as preparative regimen: a report from the groupe d' Etudes de la Greffe de Moelle Osseuse. Blood 1992;79:2578–2582.
99. Clift RA, Buckner CD, Thomas ED, et al. Marrow transplantation for chronic myeloid leukemia: a randomized study comparing cyclophosphamide and total body irradiation with busulfan and cyclophosphamide. Blood 1994;84:2036–2043.

100. Ringden O, Ruutu T, Remberger M, et al. A randomized trial comparing busulfan vs total body irradiation in allogeneic marrow transplants with hematological malignancies. Transplant Proc 1994;26:1831–1832.
101. Giralt S, Estey E, Albitar M, et al. Engraftment of allogeneic hematopoietic progenitor cells with purine analog containing chemotherapy: harnessing graft-versus-leukemia without myeloablative therapy. Blood 1997;89:4531–4536.
102. Spitzer TR, McAfee SL, Saidman S, et al. Clinical remission of refractory non-Hodgkin's lymphoma induced by allogeneic bone marrow transplantation with mixed chimerism in non-myeloablated recipients. Blood 1997;90(suppl I):418a.
103. Pelot MR, Pearson DA, Swenson K, et al. Lymphohematopoietic graft-versus-host reactions can be induced without graft-versus-host disease. Biol Blood Marrow Transplant 1999 (in press).
104. Stockschläder M, Krüger W, Kroschke G. Use of cryopreserved bone marrow in allogeneic bone marrow transplantation. Bone Marrow Transplant 1995;15:569–572.
105. Korbling M, Przepiorka D, Gajewski J, et al. With first successful allogeneic transplantation of apheresis-derived hematopoietic progenitor cells reported, can the recruitment of volunteer matched unrelated stem cell donors be expanded substantially? Blood 1995;86:1235–1239.
106. Momin F, Chandrasekar PH. Antimicrobial prophylaxis in bone marrow transplantation. Ann Intern Med 1995;123:205–215.
107. Dekker AW, Rozenberg-Arska M, Verhoef J. Infection prophylaxis in acute leukemia: a comparison of ciprofloxacin with trimethoprim-sulfamethoxazole and colistin. Ann Intern Med 1987;106:7–12.
108. Goodman JL, Winston DJ, Greenfield RA, et al. A controlled trial of fluconazole to prevent fungal infections in patients undergoing bone marrow transplantation. N Engl J Med 1992;326:845–851.
109. Myers JD, Reed EC, Shepp DH, et al. Acyclovir for prevention of cytomegalovirus infection and disease after allogeneic marrow transplantation. N Engl J Med 1988;318:70–75.
110. Sullivan KM, Kopecky KJ, Jocom J, et al. Immunomodulatory and antimicrobial efficacy of intravenous immunoglobulin in bone marrow transplantation. N Engl J Med 1990;323:705–712.
111. Bowden RA, Slichter SJ, Sayers M. A comparison of filtered leukocyte-reduced and cytomegalovirus seronegative blood products for the prevention of transfusion-associated CMV infection after marrow transplant. Blood 1995;86:3598–3603.
112. Ward KN, Roberts IAG, vanRhee F. Ganciclovir and the prevention of CMV disease after allogeneic BMT: policy at the Hammersmith Hospital. Bone Marrow Transplant 1994;13:230–231. Letter.
113. Faber-Langendoen K, Caplan AL, McGlave PB. Survival of adult bone marrow transplant recipients receiving mechanical ventilation: a case for restricted use. Bone Marrow Transplant 1993;12:501–507.
114. Weisdorf SA, Lysne J, Wind D, et al. Positive effect of prophylactic total parenteral nutrition on long-term outcome of bone marrow transplantation. Transplantation 1987;43:833–838.
115. Szeluga DJ, Stuart RK, Brookmeyer R, et al. Nutritional support of bone marrow transplant recipients: a prospective, randomized clinical trial comparing total parenteral nutrition to an enteral feeding program. Cancer Res 1987;47:3309–3316.
116. Anasetti C, Amos D, Beatty P, et al. Effect of HLA compatibility on engraftment of bone marrow transplants in patients with leukemia or lymphoma. N Engl J Med 1989;320:197–204.
117. Bozdech MJ, Sondel PM, Trigg ME, et al. Transplantation of HLA-haploidentical T-cell depleted marrow for leukemia. Addition of cytosine arabinoside to the pretransplant conditioning prevents rejection. Exp Hematol 1985;13:1201–1210.
118. Mitsuyasu RT, Champlin RE, Gale RP, et al. Treatment of donor bone marrow with monoclonal anti-T-cell antibody and complement for the prevention of graft-versus-host-disease. Ann Intern Med 1986;105:20–26.
119. Kernan NA, Bordignon C, Heller G, et al. Graft failure after T-cell-depleted human leukocyte antigen identical marrow transplants for leukemia: I. Analysis of risk factors and results of secondary transplants. Blood 1989;74: 2227–2236.
120. Dreger P, Suttorp M, Haferlach T, et al. Allogeneic granulocyte colony-stimulating factor-mobilized peripheral blood progenitor cells for transplant of engraftment failure after bone marrow transplantation. Blood 1993;81:1404–1407.
121. Ferrara JLM, Deeg HJ. Graft-versus-host disease. N Engl J Med 1991;324:667–674.
122. Vogelsang GB, Hess AD. Graft-versus-host disease: new directions for a persistent problem. Blood 1994;84:2061–2067.
123. Thomas ED, Storb R, Clift RA, et al. Bone marrow transplantation. N Engl J Med 1975;292:823–843, 895–902.
124. Goldman JM, Gale RP, Horowitz MM, et al. Bone marrow transplantation for chronic myelogenous leukemia in chronic phase: increased risk of relapse associated with T-cell depletion. Ann Intern Med 1988;108:806–814.
125. Martin PJ, Schoch G, Fisher L, et al. A retrospective analysis of therapy for acute graft-versus-host-disease: initial treatment. Blood 1990;76:1464–1472.
126. McDonald GB, Hinds MS, Fisher LD, et al. Veno-occlusive disease of the liver and multiorgan failure after bone marrow transplantation: a cohort study of 355 patients. Ann Intern Med 1993;118:255–267.
127. Bearman SI. The syndrome of hepatic veno-occlusive disease after marrow transplantation. Blood 1995;85:3005–3020.
128. Essell J, Schroeder M, Thompson J, et al. A randomized double-blind trial of prophylactic ursodeoxycholic acid vs. placebo to prevent veno-occlusive disease of the liver in patients undergoing allogeneic bone marrow transplantation. Blood 1994;84(suppl I):250a.
129. Attal M, Huquet F, Rubie H, et al. Prevention of hepatic veno-occlusive disease after bone marrow transplantation by continuous infusion of low-dose heparin: a prospective, randomized trial. Blood 1992;79:2834–2840.
130. Or R, Nagler A, Shpilgerg O, et al. Low molecular weight heparin for the prevention of veno-occlusive disease of the liver in bone marrow transplantation patients. Transplantation 1996;61:1067–1071.
131. Weiner RS, Bortin MM, Gale RP, et al. Interstitial pneumonitis after BMT. Assessment of risk factors. Ann Intern Med 1986;104:168–175.
132. Cahill RA, Spitzer TR, Mazumder A. Marrow engraftment and clinical manifestations of capillary leak syndrome. Bone Marrow Transplant 1996;18:177–184.
133. Robbins RA, Linder J, Stahl MG, et al. Diffuse alveolar hemorrhage in autologous bone marrow transplant recipients. Am J Med 1989;87:511–518.
134. Gottdiener JS, Appelbaum FR, Ferrans VJ, et al. Cardiotoxicity associated with high-dose cyclophosphamide therapy. Arch Intern Med 1981;141:758–763.
135. Cazin B, Gorin NC, Laporte JP, et al. Cardiac complications after bone marrow transplantation. A report on a series of 63 consecutive transplantations. Cancer 1986;57:2061–2069.
136. Atkinson K. Chronic graft-versus-host disease. Bone Marrow Transplant 1990;5:69–82.
137. Vogelsang GB, Farmer ER, Hess AD, et al. Thalidomide for the treatment of chronic graft-versus-host disease. N Engl J Med 1991;326:1055–1058.
138. Sanders JE, the Seattle Marrow Transplant Team. The impact of marrow transplant preparative regimens on subsequent growth and development. Semin Hematol 1991;28:244–249.
139. Witherspoon RP, Fisher LD, Schoch G, et al. Secondary cancers after bone marrow transplantation for leukemia or aplastic anemia. N Engl J Med 1989;321:784–789.
140. Bhatia S, Ramsay NKC, Steinbuch M, et al. Malignant neoplasms following bone marrow transplantation. Blood 1996;87:3633–3639.
141. Stone RM. Myelodysplastic syndrome after autologous transplantation for lymphoma: the price of progress? Blood 1994;83:3437–3440.
142. Sullivan KM, Witherspoon RP, Storb R, et al. Long term results of allogeneic bone marrow transplantation. Transplant Proc 1989;21:2926–2928.
143. Cassileth PA, Anderson J, Lazarus HM, et al. Autologous bone marrow transplant in acute myeloid leukemia in first remission. J Clin Oncol 1992;10:1723–1729.
144. Clift RA, Buckner CD, Appelbaum FR, et al. Allogeneic marrow transplantation during untreated first relapse of acute myeloid leukemia. J Clin Oncol 1992;10:1723–1729.
145. Clift R, Appelbaum F, Thomas E. Bone marrow transplantation for chronic myelogenous leukemia. Blood 1993;82:1954–1956.
146. Beatty PG, Hansen JA, Longton GM, et al. Marrow transplantation from HLA-matched unrelated donors for treatment of hematologic malignancies. Transplantation 1991;51:443–447.
147. Stemmer SM, Cagnoni PJ, Shpall EJ, et al. High-dose paclitaxel, cyclophosphamide, and cisplatin with autologous hematopoietic progenitor-cell support: a Phase I trial. J Clin Oncol 1996;14:1463–1472.
148. Meisenberg BR, Miller WE, McMillan R, et al. Outpatient high-dose chemotherapy with autologous stem-cell rescue for hematologic and non hematologic malignancies. J Clin Oncol 1997;15:11–17.
149. Zhang MJ, Hoelzer D, Orowitz M, et al. Long-term follow-up of adults with acute lymphoblastic leukemia in first remission treated with chemotherapy or bone marrow transplantation. Ann Intern Med 1995;123:428–431.
150. Rabinowe SN, Soiffer RJ, Gribben JG, et al. Autologous and allogeneic bone marrow transplantation for poor prognosis patients with B-cell chronic lymphocytic leukemia. Blood 1993;82:1366–1376.

151. Michallet M, Archimbaud E, Bandini G, et al. HLA-identical sibling bone marrow transplantation in younger patients with chronic lymphocytic leukemia. Ann Intern Med 1996;124:311–315.
152. Armitage JD. Bone marrow transplantation in the treatment of patients with lymphoma. Blood 1989;73:1749–1758.
153. Barlogie B, Gahrton G. Bone marrow transplantation in multiple myeloma. Bone Marrow Transplant 1991;7:71–79.
154. Freedman AS, Ritz J, Neuberg D, et al. Autologous bone marrow transplantation in 69 patients with a history of low-grade B-cell non-Hodgkin's lymphoma. Blood 1991;77:2524–2529.
155. Bensinger WI, Buckner CD, Clift RA, et al. Phase I study of busulfan and cyclophosphamide in preparation for allogeneic marrow transplant for patients with multiple myeloma. J Clin Oncol 1992;10:1492–1497.
156. Bastion Y, Brice P, Haioun C, et al. Intensive therapy with peripheral blood progenitor cell transplantation in 60 patients with poor-prognosis follicular lymphoma. Blood 1995;86:3257–3262.
157. Mills W, Chopra R, McMillan A, et al. BEAM chemotherapy and autologous bone marrow transplantation for patients with relapsed or refractory non-Hodgkin's lymphoma. J Clin Oncol 1995;13:588–595.
158. Nademanee A, O'Donnell MR, Snyder DS, et al. High dose chemotherapy with or without total body irradiation followed by autologous bone marrow and/or peripheral blood stem cell transplantation for patients with relapsed and refractory Hodgkin's disease: results in 85 patients with analysis of prognostic factors. Blood 1995;85:1381–1390.
159. O'Donnell MR, Long GD, Parker PM, et al. Busulfan/cyclophosphamide as conditioning regimen for allogeneic bone marrow transplantation for myelodysplasia. J Clin Oncol 1995;13:2973–2979.
160. Phillip T, Guglielmi C, Hagenbeek A, et al. Autologous bone marrow transplantation as compared with salvage chemotherapy in relapses of chemotherapy sensitive non-Hodgkin's lymphoma. N Engl J Med 1995;333:1540–1545.
161. Zittoun RA, Mandelli F, Willemze R, et al. Autologous or allogeneic bone marrow transplantation compared with intensive chemotherapy in acute myelogenous leukemia. N Engl J Med 1995;332:217–223.
162. Anderson JE, Applebaum FR, Schoch G, et al. Allogeneic marrow transplantation for refractory anemia: a comparison of two preparative regimens and analyses of prognostic factors. Blood 1996;87:51–58.
163. Attal M, Arousseau JL, Stoppa AM, et al. A prospective, randomized trial of autologous bone marrow transplantation and chemotherapy in multiple myeloma. N Engl J Med 1996;335:91–97.
164. Bjorkstrand B, Ljungman P, Svensson H, et al. Allogeneic bone marrow transplantation versus autologous stem cell transplantation in multiple myeloma: a retrospective case-matched study from the European Group for Blood and Marrow Transplantation. Blood 1996;88:4711–4718.
165. Gajewski JL, Phillips GL, Sobocinski KA, et al. Bone marrow transplants from HLA-identical siblings in advanced Hodgkin's disease. J Clin Oncol 1996;14:572–578.
166. Barlogie B, Jagannath S, Vesole DH, et al. Superiority of tandem autologous transplantation over standard therapy for previously untreated multiple myeloma. Blood 1997;89:789–793.
167. Hamblet Y, Syman M, Bosley A, et al. Late intensification chemotherapy with autologous bone marrow transplantation in selected small cell carcinoma of the lung: a randomized study. J Clin Oncol 1987;5:1864–1873.
168. Elias AD, Ayash L, Frei III E, et al. Intensive combined modality therapy for limited stage small cell lung cancer. J Natl Cancer Inst 1993;85:559–566.
169. Peters WP, Ross M, Vredenburg JJ, et al. High-dose chemotherapy and autologous bone marrow support as consolidation after standard-dose adjuvant therapy for high-risk primary breast cancer. J Clin Oncol 1993;11:1132–1143.
170. Bezwoda WR, Seymour L, Dansey RD. High-dose chemotherapy with hematopoietic rescue as primary treatment for metastatic breast cancer: a randomized trial. J Clin Oncol 1995;13:2483–2489.
171. Brown ER, Sridhara R, Sledge GW, et al. Tandem autotransplantation for the treatment of metastatic breast cancer. J Clin Oncol 1995;13:2050–2055.
172. Siegert W, Beyer J, Strobscheer I, et al. High-dose treatment with carboplatin, etoposide, and ifosfamide followed by autologous stem cell transplantation in relapsed or refractory germ cell cancer—a phase I/II study. J Clin Oncol 1994;12:1223–1231.
173. Beyer J, Kramer A, Mandanas R, et al. High-dose chemotherapy as salvage treatment in germ cell tumors—a multivariate analysis of prognostic variables. J Clin Oncol 1996;14:2638–2645.
174. Shpall EJ, Jones RB, Bearman SI, et al. Future strategies for the treatment of advanced epithelial ovarian cancer using high-dose chemotherapy and autologous bone marrow support. Gyn Onc 1994;54:357–361.
175. Phillip T, Zucker JM, Bernard JL, et al. Improved survival at 2 and 5 years in the LMCE1 unselected group of 72 children with stage IV neuroblastoma older than 1 year of age at diagnosis: is cure possible in a small subgroup? J Clin Oncol 1991;9:1037–1044.
176. Saarinen UM, Wilkström S, Mäkipernaa A, et al. In vivo purging of bone marrow in children with poor-risk neuroblastoma for marrow collection and autologous bone marrow transplantation. J Clin Oncol 1996;14:2791–2802.
177. Lazarus HM, Herzig RH, Wolff SN, et al. Treatment of metastatic malignant melanoma with intensive melphalan and autologous bone marrow transplantation. Cancer Treat Rep 1985;69:473–477.
178. Butturini A, Bortin MM, Gale RP. Graft-versus leukemia following bone marrow transplantation. Bone Marrow Transplant 1987;2:233–242.
179. Champlin R. Graft-versus-leukemia without graft-versus-host disease: an elusive goal of bone marrow transplantation. Semin Hematol 1972;29(suppl 2):46–52.
180. Mackinnon S, Papadopoulos EP, Carabasi MH, et al. Adoptive immunotherapy evaluating escalating doses of donor leukocytes for relapse of chronic myeloid leukemia following bone marrow transplantation: Separation of graft-versus-leukemia responses from graft-versus-host disease. Blood 1995;86:1261–1268.
181. Porter DL, Roth MS, McGarigle C, et al. Induction of graft-versus-host disease as immunotherapy for relapsed chronic myeloid leukemia. N Engl J Med 1994;330:100–106.
182. Horowitz MM, Gale RP, Sondel PM, et al. Graft-versus-leukemia reactions after bone marrow transplantation. Blood 1990;75:555–562.
183. Beatty PG, Clift RA, Mickelson FM, et al. Marrow transplantation from related donors other than HLA-identical siblings. N Engl J Med 1985;313:765–791.
184. Bacigalupo A, Hows J, Gluckman E, et al. Bone marrow transplantation (BMT) versus immunosuppression for the treatment of severe aplastic anemia (SAA): a report of the EBMT SAA Working Party. Br J Haematol 1988;70:177–182.
185. Paquette RL, Tebyani N, Frane M, et al. Long-term outcome of aplastic anemia in adults treated with antithymocyte globulin: comparison with bone marrow transplantation. Blood 1995;85:283–290.
186. Doney K, Leisenring W, Storb R, et al. Primary treatment of acquired aplastic anemia: outcomes with bone marrow transplantation and immunosuppressive therapy. Ann Intern Med 1997;126:107–115.
187. Beatty PG, DiBartolomeo P, Storb R, et al. Treatment of aplastic anemia with marrow grafts from related donors other than HLA genotypically-matched siblings. Clin Transplant 1987;1:117–124.
188. Kawahara K, Witherspoon RP, Storb R. Marrow transplantation of paroxysmal nocturnal hemoglobinuria. Am J Hematol 1992;39:283–288.
189. O'Reilly RJ, Brochstein J, Dinsmore R, Kirkpatrick D. Marrow transplantation for congenital disorders. Semin Hematol 1984;21:188–221.
190. Lucarelli G, Galimberti M, Polchi P, et al. Bone marrow transplantation in patients with thalassemia. N Engl J Med 1990;322:417–421.
191. Filipovich AH, Shapiro RS, Ramsey NKC, et al. Unrelated donor bone marrow transplantation for correction of lethal congenital immunodeficiencies. Blood 1992;80:270–276.
192. Gluckman E, Auerbach AD, Horowitz MM, et al. Bone marrow transplantation in Fanconi anemia from the International Bone Marrow Transplant Registry. Blood 1995;86:2586–2862.
193. Walters ML, Patience M, Leisenring W, et al. Bone marrow transplantation for sickle cell disease. N Engl J Med 1996;335:369–376.

COMMENTARY REFERENCES

1. Hansen JA, Clift RA, Thomas ED, et al. Transplantation of marrow from an unrelated donor to a patient with acute leukemia. N Engl J Med 1980;305:565–567.
2. Confer DL. Unrelated marrow donor registries. Curr Opin Hematol 1997;4:408–412.
3. Oudshoorn M, Falkenburg JHF, Ebeling LJ, et al. Unrelated bone marrow transplantation as a rescue procedure following inadvertent loss of an autologous bone marrow graft. Bone Marrow Transplant 1996;18:461–463.

Part V

Systemic Considerations of Organ Transplantation

Chapter

28

Pulmonary Considerations of Organ Transplantation

Sanjiv Tewari Janet Maurer

This chapter focuses on the pulmonary considerations of solid organ transplantation and bone marrow transplantation. In an exhaustive review of this topic in 1991, Ettinger and Trulock divided the pulmonary considerations of organ transplantation into pretransplant, intraoperative, and post-transplant categories (1–3). A similar format is followed in this chapter, with particular emphasis on developments that have emerged since their article.

Solid organ transplantation affects the lungs in several ways. The underlying disease necessitating the transplant can have pulmonary manifestations that need to be assessed and managed preoperatively. Early postsurgical pulmonary complications reflect the effects of anesthesia, surgical site, intraoperative difficulties, postoperative respiratory care, and prophylaxis for thromboembolism. Late pulmonary sequelae include progression or recurrence of the underlying disease with respiratory involvement and novel infectious or noninfectious pulmonary diseases in the context of immunosuppression.

Although bone marrow transplantation or peripheral stem cell infusion does not involve a surgical procedure that can directly compromise lung function, the underlying hematologic disease or malignancy responsible for the transplant can have pulmonary manifestations. More commonly, pulmonary complications, both infectious and noninfectious, will arise after transplantation due to consolidation chemotherapy, radiation, and immunosuppressive medications.

This chapter is divided into three sections. In the first section, the diagnostic modalities used to investigate pulmonary disease in organ transplant recipients are reviewed. The second section details the noninfectious pulmonary considerations in liver, renal, cardiac, and bone marrow transplantation. The third section discusses the etiology and manifestations of pulmonary infections in transplant recipients.

DIAGNOSTIC MODALITIES USED IN PULMONARY DISEASE

In the transplant recipient on immunosuppressive medications, it is often very difficult to differentiate clinically infectious from noninfectious pulmonary disease. Pulmonary infections in this setting can progress rapidly and, therefore, rapid exclusion of infection is paramount (4). This discussion focuses on imaging modalities including chest radiography and computed tomography, sputum culture, and invasive techniques including bronchoscopy, thoracoscopy, open-lung biopsy, percutaneous fine-needle biopsy, mediastinoscopy, and transbronchial needle aspiration. A diagnostic algorithm is presented in Figure 28.1.

Chest radiography is essential to define both the location and the nature of a pulmonary abnormality and to choose an appropriate diagnostic procedure. The process should be localized if possible to the lung parenchyma, the mediastinum, the airways, the pleura, or the chest wall. A particular pulmonary disease may affect many different locations in the chest; these patterns of involvement help to narrow down the potential etiologies (5). Parenchymal lesions should be further characterized as being either focal or diffuse, unilateral or bilateral, and peripheral or central in distribution.

The nature of the infiltrate refers to whether it is alveolar, reticular, nodular, reticulonodular, mass-like, or a combination. The radiographic pattern reflects the site of the pathologic process in the lung and is useful in formulating a differential diagnosis and in choosing a diagnostic strategy. Although atypical radiographic presentations of pulmonary diseases are frequently encountered in the context of organ transplantation, certain radiographic features can suggest certain disorders. Alveolar infiltrates are generally seen with pneumonia caused by bacteria or *Pneumocystis carinii*,

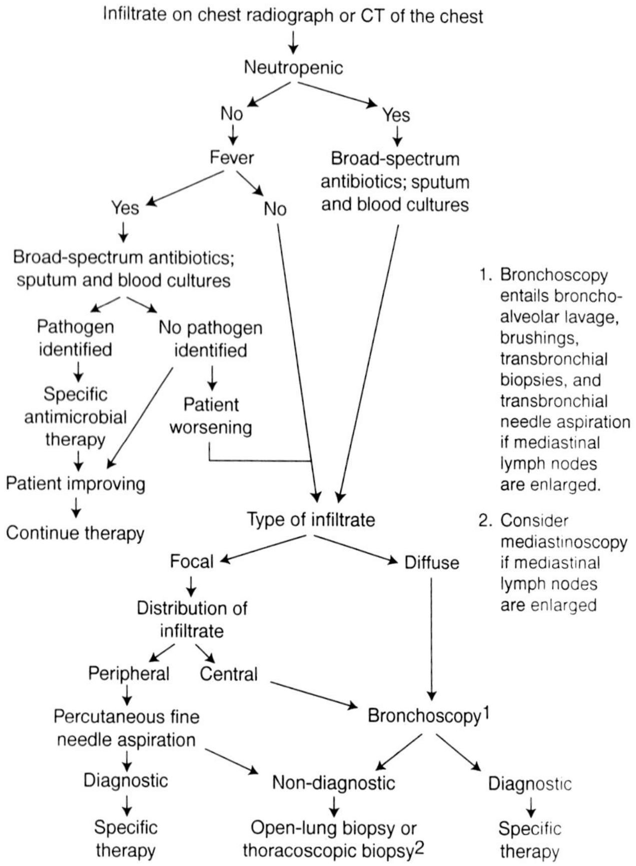

FIGURE 28.1. *Diagnostic algorithm for pulmonary infiltrates in an immunocompromised host. The diagnostic strategy for each patient must be individualized depending on the problem. Neutropenic patients with a pneumonia can deteriorate rapidly and, therefore, a more aggressive diagnostic work-up is suggested.*

cardiogenic and noncardiogenic pulmonary edema, and alveolar hemorrhage. Reticular infiltrates suggest viral pneumonia, radiation pneumonitis, or drug-induced lung injury. Nodules in the chest most often indicate disseminated fungal or mycobacterial disease or metastatic malignancy. Masses occurring after transplantation should raise the possibility of a primary lung neoplasm, a metastatic malignancy, or a lymphoma.

High-resolution computed tomography (HRCT) of the chest may be a useful adjunct to chest radiography in transplant recipients. In the immunocompromised host with symptomatic pulmonary disease, the chest radiograph is normal in 10% of cases (6). In a patient with a normal or nonspecific chest radiograph, HRCT will better delineate parenchymal abnormalities and will help to guide the site of potential diagnostic procedures (7,8). Even when abnormalities are present on the chest radiograph, HRCT is useful to precisely localize them and to look for additional disease in the chest that may not be evident on the chest radiograph.

Table 28.1. Organisms Identified in Sputum With a High Positive Predictive Value of Causing Pulmonary Infection

Organisms
Legionella
Mycobacterium tuberculosis
Aspergillus
Mucormycosis
Dimorphic fungi
Strongyloides

Source: Adapted with permission from the ATS Board of Directors. Clinical role of bronchoalveolar lavage in adults with pulmonary disease. Am Rev Respir Dis 1990;142:481–496.

Sputum examination for microbiologic diagnosis is the first step in evaluating pulmonary infiltrates. The isolation of certain pathogens portends a high likelihood of actual pulmonary disease as these organisms are not ordinarily part of the normal flora (Table 28.1) (9–11). Sputum culture is, unfortunately, often unrewarding in transplant recipients for three reasons (12). First, these patients often produce only scant amounts of sputum and, therefore, the sensitivity of the test is low. Second, the sputum produced has a paucity of neutrophils, particularly if the patient is neutropenic. A satisfactory sputum sample should have greater than 25 polymorphonuclear leukocytes per high power field on Gram's stain. The specificity of the examination is lowered if the patient does not expectorate neutrophils, as respiratory secretions can be mistaken for saliva and vice versa. Third, the upper airway of these patients is often colonized with many organisms that may contaminate a sputum sample. Differentiating colonization from true infection using such a specimen may be extremely difficult or impossible. Finding greater than 10 epithelial cells per high power field suggests that the sample is saliva rather than sputum. Sputum induction in patients unable to adequately expectorate can increase the diagnostic yield (13).

A variety of invasive procedures are useful in determining the etiology of pulmonary infiltrates, both focal and diffuse (Table 28.2). There are four established invasive methods to obtain lung specimens: bronchoscopy, thoracoscopic biopsy, open-lung biopsy, and percutaneous biopsy. Transtracheal aspiration of pulmonary secretions is not used by most centers due to its attendant morbidity in this population and will not be discussed. Many factors must be considered when choosing a procedure to investigate a pulmonary abnormality: the distribution and type of lung disease; the severity and progression of the illness; the extent to which the patient is immunocompromised; the sensitivity and specificity of the procedure; the therapeutic impact of confirming a suspected diagnosis; and the risks of the procedure to a particular patient. Provided that the benefits outweigh the risks, the diagnostic procedure should be employed rapidly, as a delay in diagnosis can be fatal in an immunocompromised patient.

Table 28.2. Invasive Procedures to Evaluate Lung Infiltrates in Immunocompromised Patients

Procedure	Indication	Diagnostic Yield	Risks	References
BAL	Focal or diffuse infiltrates	31–55%	Hypoxemia during procedure; fever after procedure	15, 19, 22, 26
TBB	Focal/central or diffuse infiltrates	45–67%	Hemorrhage; pneumothorax	15, 19
PFNA	Focal/peripheral infiltrates	53–82%	Hemorrhage; pneumothorax	31
OLB	Focal or diffuse infiltrates	55–95	Hemorrhage; prolonged airleak	26, 27
TLB	Focal or diffuse infiltrates	Unknown	Unknown	—

BAL = bronchoalveolar lavage; TBB = transbronchial biopsy; PFNA = percutaneous fine-needle aspiration; OLB = open-lung biopsy; TLB = thoracoscopic lung biopsy; TBNA = transbronchial needle aspiration.

Bronchoscopy is frequently used in the evaluation of pulmonary infiltrates in these patients. Either the transoral or the transnasal approach can be used safely, even in patients with significant thrombocytopenia (14). In addition to evaluating the upper airway and tracheobronchial mucosa, there are a number of procedures that can be employed to confirm infectious and noninfectious diagnoses.

Pulmonary infections can be confirmed through the use of bronchoalveolar lavage, protected specimen brushing, and tissue cultures (15–17). Bronchoalveolar lavage involves wedging the bronchoscope into the affected lung segment and instilling and then aspirating normal saline or sterile water. Bacterial infection is likely if there are greater than 10^4 colony-forming units (CFU)/mL on culture of the fluid. A protected specimen brush can increase the likelihood of recovering organisms; a positive test is defined by growth of organisms on culture exceeding 10^3 CFU/mL. Transient arterial desaturation can be anticipated during the procedure and is most pronounced in patients with abnormal spirometries or severe roentgenographic abnormalities (18). Postprocedure fever occurs in 10% to 50% of patients depending on the lobe lavaged and the volume of saline instilled. Transbronchial biopsies can increase the diagnostic yield by up to 33% and are useful to demonstrate tissue invasion by organisms (19). The major risk of biopsy is bleeding that occurs in 2.5% of cases. Patients who have a coagulopathy, thrombocytopenia, or uremia are at higher risk for significant bleeding. The mortality associated with the procedure is 0.2% (9).

Noninfectious pulmonary diseases are evaluated bronchoscopically by examining the cells recovered in respiratory secretions and by performing biopsies on the lung parenchyma or the mediastinum. A cell count and a cytologic analysis can be performed on bronchoalveolar lavage fluid. The normal cell population in the lavage fluid consists primarily of alveolar macrophages. A neutrophilic, lymphocytic, or eosinophilic predominance can be associated with various pulmonary diseases. The finding of hemosiderin-laden macrophages can be a useful marker for alveolar hemorrhage (20,21). The fluid from a lavage or from simple bronchial washings can from cytologic analysis suggest or confirm a pulmonary malignancy (22).

Table 28.3. Thoracoscopic Procedures in Immunocompromised Patients

Indication	Thoracoscopic Procedure
Pulmonary infiltrates	Wedge biopsy
Pleural effusions	Pleural biopsy
Loculated effusions	Breaking up loculations and drainage
Malignant effusions	Drainage, biopsy, talc insufflation
Pneumothorax	Bleb stapling, pleurectomy, pleurodesis
Pericardial effusions	Pericardial drainage

Source: Adapted with permission from Feiins RH. The role of thoracoscopy in the AIDS/immunocompromised patient. Ann Thorac Surg 1993;56:650.

Bronchoscopic biopsies can be taken endobronchially or transbronchially. Endobronchial biopsies are used when there is an endobronchial abnormality, usually either infection or malignancy in the setting of organ transplantation. Transbronchial biopsies are used more frequently both in focal parenchymal disease that is accessible to the forceps and in diffuse parenchymal disease. A central distribution of infiltrates on chest CT is associated with a greater diagnostic yield (23). Bronchocentric or alveolar disease is evaluated better by this modality than interstitial disease. The latter group of diseases generally requires more tissue on the biopsy specimen to make a definitive diagnosis. Furthermore, interpretation of specimens obtained by transbronchial biopsy is difficult because they are frequently crushed. Nevertheless, transbronchial biopsy is far less invasive than either thoracoscopic or open-lung biopsy and, therefore, it serves often as the initial biopsy procedure of choice.

Thoracoscopic lung biopsy and open-lung biopsy represent the gold standards for obtaining lung tissue. The former is comparable to the latter in terms of diagnostic yield, but carries less morbidity (24,25). Thoracoscopic evaluation permits direct visualization of the pleural surfaces and allows the operator to perform a number of different procedures (Table 28.3) while sparing the patient an open thoracotomy. A direct comparison of these two procedures has not been done in immunocompromised patients. In either procedure, biopsies are performed in areas that appear grossly abnormal. The transbronchial biopsy, in contrast, is a blind procedure. In the deteriorating patient, either open-lung biopsy or thoracoscopic lung biopsy should be employed early in the course of the illness to rapidly confirm a diagnosis. Aggressive diagnostic interventions at this early stage may be associated with a better outcome (26–30).

Percutaneous biopsy is an alternative to these procedures, particularly in situations where the lung disease is focal, peripheral, or cavitary (31). A fine needle is used to obtain a cytologic specimen and a sample for Gram's stain and culture. Histologic specimens cannot be obtained with this needle and, therefore the procedure is less suited for diffuse lung disease. Although larger needles have been used to obtain more tissue, they are associated with an unacceptable rate of complications, in particular pneumothorax. This complication occurs in 8% to 44% of cases depending upon the size of the needle used, the location of the lesion, and whether the patient has bullous emphysema (9).

Mediastinal abnormalities can be evaluated if present with bronchoscopy or mediastinoscopy. The use of transbronchial needle aspiration with either a 22-gauge needle for cytologic aspiration of tracheobronchial lymph nodes or an 18-gauge needle for a histology specimen can obviate the need for mediastinoscopy, which involves the administration of a general anesthetic.

NONINFECTIOUS PULMONARY CONSIDERATIONS OF ORGAN TRANSPLANTATION

Liver Transplantation

Pretransplant Considerations

Chronic liver disease from a wide variety of causes can be associated with pulmonary abnormalities (32). The preoperative screening of liver transplantation (LT) candidates should therefore include a comprehensive assessment of respiratory function. Although not well validated, performing certain baseline tests are helpful to document abnormalities and to optimize pulmonary function prior to transplantation (33). These studies should include chest radiography, arterial blood gas analysis, and pulmonary function testing including spirometry, measurement of lung volumes, and diffusing capacity. Some institutions now perform physiologic shunt studies and bubble echocardiography using agitated saline to confirm and quantify the presence of intrapulmonary shunts.

The rationale for performing these examinations becomes evident as one appreciates the frequency of respiratory signs and symptoms in this population. In a prospective analysis of 116 patients with end-stage liver disease of differing etiologies, dyspnea was present in 39% of patients on exertion and in 14% of patients at rest (34). Platypnea, or dyspnea in the upright position, was seen in 7% of patients and reflects orthodeoxia, arterial desaturation in the upright position. Intravascular pulmonary dilations (IVPDs) at the lung bases act as intrapulmonary shunts and are perfused to a greater extent in the upright position.

Physical examination may reveal diminished lung volumes and evidence of atelectasis or effusions. The presence of cyanosis and clubbing suggests hypoxemia often in the context of the hepatopulmonary syndrome. Spider nevi were found in 71% of patients (34). The presence of cutaneous spider nevi correlates with the presence of IVPDs and with impaired hypoxic pulmonary vasoconstriction (35,36).

The pretransplant pulmonary evaluation requires knowledge of the following pulmonary problems that occur in liver failure patients:

- Abnormal pulmonary function tests
- Atelectasis
- Pleural effusions
- Acute respiratory distress syndrome
- Specific lung–liver disorders:
    - Primary biliary cirrhosis
    - Chronic active hepatitis
    - Sclerosing cholangitis
    - α1-Antitrypsin deficiency
    - Cystic fibrosis
    - Hepatopulmonary syndrome
    - Pulmonary hypertension
- Malignancy

Abnormal Pulmonary Function Tests Abnormal pulmonary function tests are observed in the majority of patients with advanced liver disease. Whether those patients with abnormal preoperative tests are at increased risk for postoperative pulmonary complications is unknown.

The most frequent abnormality is a reduced diffusing capacity, which is often, but not necessarily, accompanied by an elevated alveolar-to-arterial (A-a) gradient (32). Patients with more severe liver dysfunction as assessed by the Child's classification have lower values for diffusing capacity (37), perhaps because of atelectasis, aspiration, pleural effusions, and lower lung volumes because of ascites. Hypoxemia is observed in 13% to 22% of patients while an elevated A-a oxygen gradient occurs in 45% to 69% of patients (34,38). Pulse oximetry may underestimate the true oxygen saturation due to hyperbilirubinemia because some biosynthetic pigments have similar spectrophotometric wavelengths as oxygenated blood (39). Arterial blood gas analysis is, therefore, the preferred tool for detecting hypoxemia. The potential causes of hypoxemia in this setting are summarized in Table 28.4, and a diagnostic algorithm is presented in Figure 28.2.

Restriction is observed in one quarter of patients with cirrhosis presenting for transplantation (34). An inverse correlation between total lung capacity and bilirubin concentration has been noted, perhaps because higher concentrations of the latter are associated with ascites and respiratory muscle weakness (34).

Atelectasis Chest radiographs are frequently abnormal in patients with significant liver disease. The most frequent findings include diminished lung volumes in over 50% of patients and pleural effusions in approximately 20% of patients (34).

Atelectasis was present in nearly one quarter of patients awaiting liver transplantation in a recent series (40) and is usually subsegmental. Ascites, immobility, encephalopathy, and pleural effusions in patients with decompensated cirrhosis are contributing factors. Respiratory muscle weakness, perhaps from deconditioning and malnutrition, was additionally documented in 71% of these patients (34). Patients with atelectasis preoperatively should be watched carefully in the perioperative period for worsening of this abnormality. These patients should be targeted for aggressive respiratory care in the perioperative period consisting of a combination of incentive spirometry, percussion and postural drainage, and aerosolized beta-2 agonists.

Table 28.4. Causes of Hypoxemia in Liver Disease

Mechanism	Clinical Problem
Diffusion defect	Intravascular pulmonary dilatations
Ventilation–perfusion mismatch	Early airway closure, pleural effusions, pulmonary hypertension, aspiration
Shunt	Atelectasis, pneumonia, ARDS
Hypoventilation	Respiratory muscle weakness, encephalopathy

Pleural Effusions The development of pleural effusions due to cirrhosis of the liver is referred to as hepatic hydrothorax. Effusions are present in 18% of patients and are usually transudative and nonhemorrhagic (40). They occur more often on the right side than the left side. Microscopic wrents in the diaphragm allow the passage of ascitic fluid into the relatively low-pressure pleural space. Even subclinical ascites may produce effusions by this mechanism. The diagnosis is often not clinically apparent, however, but can be confirmed by radionuclide scanning. The pleural fluid should be sampled at least once prior to transplantation to exclude other causes of effusion such as malignancy or infection. Large effusions that are symptomatic or that cause hypoxemia require drainage and often pleurodesis either through a tube thoracostomy or under direct visualization during thoracoscopy (41). Diaphragmatic defects can effectively be sealed using thoracoscopy by applying biologic glue or by closure with sutures.

Acute Respiratory Distress Syndrome (ARDS) ARDS frequently complicates the course of liver failure (42) and carries a mortality approaching 100% in this population.

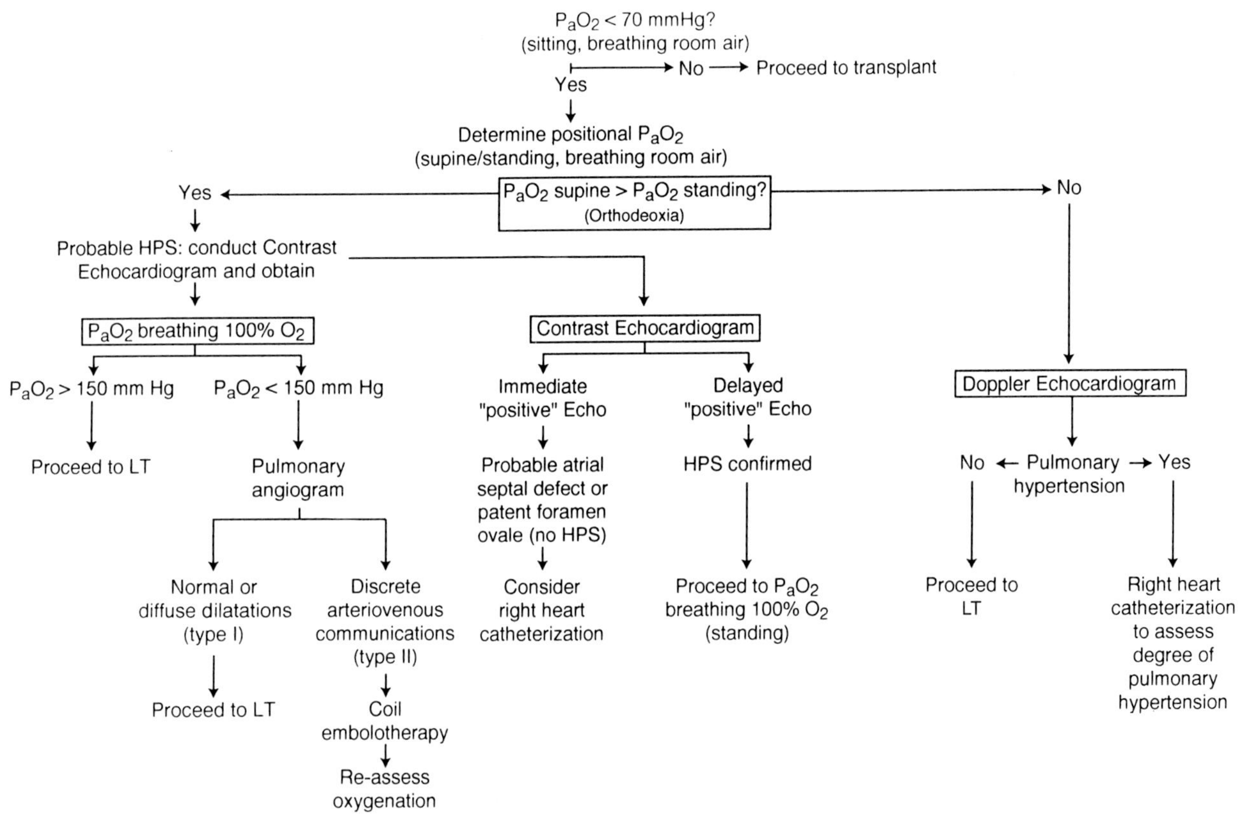

FIGURE 28.2. *Pulmonary evaluation of liver transplant candidates with significant hypoxemia and suspected pulmonary vascular abnormalities. (Adapted with permission from Poterucha JJ, Krowka MJ, Dickson ER, et al. Failure of hepatopulmonary syndrome to resolve after liver transplantation and successful treatment with embolotherapy. Hepatology 1995;21:96–99.)*

Hepatic encephalopathy, upper gastrointestinal (GI) bleeding, and increased intra-abdominal pressure from ascites favor aspiration that can lead to a chemical pneumonitis, ARDS, or an anaerobic pneumonia.

The mechanism of lung injury is not clear but may involve the failure of the diseased liver to metabolize gut-derived endotoxins, which may in turn lead to lung injury. A high endotoxin level before LT has been associated with a longer requirement for mechanical ventilation following surgery (43). LT interestingly has resulted in resolution of ARDS in a small retrospective series (44). If transplantation is being considered in such a case, a bronchoscopy should be performed to exclude a pulmonary infection.

Malignancy Because cirrhotics are at higher risk to develop hepatoma, the discovery of nodules in the chest suggests the possibility of occult metastases (45). Liver transplantation is an accepted treatment modality for locally confined hepatic malignancies but is contraindicated in patients with pulmonary metastases (46). This tumor metastasizes to the lung with a frequency approaching 70% in some autopsy series (33). Symptomatic lung metastases occur much less commonly and are often not apparent on routine chest radiography. High-resolution computed tomography of the chest may be useful to exclude subclinical metastases in a patient with a suspected hepatoma or in a patient with a confirmed hepatoma awaiting LT. The finding of nodular densities should also prompt consideration of fungal or mycobacterial infection, lymphoma, or, rarely, pulmonary varices (47,48). The diagnosis can be confirmed by percutaneous fine-needle aspiration in peripheral lesions or by bronchoscopy in central lesions.

Specific Lung–Liver Disorders The following diseases have diverse respiratory manifestations that may or may not preclude successful LT. The decision whether to list such patients for transplantation must be individualized. Combined liver–lung transplantation has been successfully performed for patients with severe disease affecting both organs (49).

Primary biliary cirrhosis. Primary biliary cirrhosis is a granulomatous liver disease associated with the presence of antimitochondrial antibodies in over 95% of patients (50). Interstitial lung disease, obstructive airways disease, chest wall deformities, pulmonary hemorrhage, the hepatopulmonary syndrome, and pulmonary hypertension are seen. Although frank interstitial lung disease is rare, subclinical alveolitis occurs in many patients (50). This alveolitis is characterized by a high concentration of T-helper lymphocytes and activated macrophages, virtually identical to the findings observed in sarcoidosis. Sjögren's syndrome frequently accompanies primary biliary cirrhosis and accounts for many of the pulmonary abnormalities observed (51). Some patients have associated progressive systemic sclerosis or the CREST syndrome and can develop pulmonary fibrosis or pulmonary hypertension. Transplantation of the liver, heart, and lungs has been performed on a patient with primary biliary cirrhosis and pulmonary hypertension (52).

Chronic active hepatitis. Chronic active hepatitis occasionally precedes the development of interstitial pneumonitis and pleuritis (39). Whether a causal link actually exists is debated in the literature. In addition, novel therapies for the treatment of viral hepatitis C such as interferon alfa may also produce a pneumonitis.

Sclerosing cholangitis. Sclerosing cholangitis is seen most commonly in association with inflammatory bowel disease, particularly ulcerative colitis. Chronic bronchitis and bronchiectasis rarely complicate the course of sclerosing cholangitis (39). LT in patients with bronchiectasis could, theoretically, lead to suppurative pulmonary infections postoperatively. HRCT is a sensitive method to detect bronchiectasis and should be employed in patients with copious sputum production.

α1-Antitrypsin deficiency. α1-Antitrypsin deficiency is an autosomal codominant disorder characterized by diminished hepatic production of this neutrophil elastase inhibitor. Clinically evident panacinar emphysema results, particularly in smokers, by the fourth or fifth decade in the majority of patients. Children with cirrhosis from this disease generally do not have airflow obstruction. LT in children tends to normalize α1-antitrypsin levels and, theoretically, over time could protect against the development of emphysema (39).

In contrast, adults should be carefully screened for obstructive pulmonary disease with spirometry. In a retrospective review by Rakela et al, seven of eight patients with cirrhosis from α1-antitrypsin deficiency had emphysema (53). Patients older than 18 with the PiZZ phenotype with α1-antitrypsin levels less than 80 mg/dL and obstructive lung disease are candidates for therapy with intravenous α1-antitrypsin from pooled serum preparations. The therapeutic efficacy of this preparation is currently being validated. The hepatitis B vaccine should be administered prior to such supplementation. A preoperative FEV_1 less than 50% of the predicted normal is associated with a higher incidence of postoperative pulmonary complications in patients undergoing abdominal surgery. For those patients with severe emphysema and cirrhosis, combined liver and lung transplantation has been successfully performed (49).

Cystic fibrosis. Cirrhosis is seen in approximately 7% of patients with cystic fibrosis and tends to occur in adolescence (54). In cirrhotics with impaired lung function, combined heart-lung-liver transplantation has been successfully reported (54). Isolated liver transplantation has been performed in patients with cirrhosis from cystic fibrosis who have relatively well-preserved lung function (55,56). Interestingly, some of these patients have post-transplant improvement in their respiratory symptoms. Colonization of the airways with *Aspergillus* and *Pseudomonas* is not infrequent and must be aggressively treated in the peritransplant period (19). Problems with the absorption of cyclosporine may also be noted.

Hepatopulmonary syndrome. The term hepatopulmonary syndrome refers to the presence of hypoxemia due to intravascular pulmonary dilatations in the setting of cir-

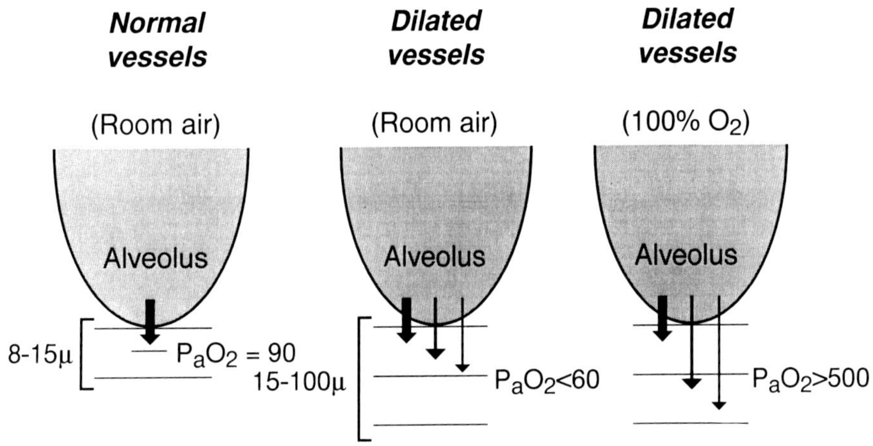

FIGURE 28.3. *The diffusion–perfusion impairment. Schematic of the pulmonary vascular abnormality suspected in the hepatopulmonary syndrome. Blood in the center of the lumen of a normal blood vessel is readily oxygenated by oxygen-rich air in the alveolus. With dilatation of the vessel, however, this blood is oxygenated to a lesser extent, a situation that is exacerbated by the hyperdynamic circulation seen with liver failure. This diffusion–perfusion impairment is corrected by the administration of 100% oxygen because of the increased driving pressure of the alveolar oxygen. (Adapted with permission from Krowka MJ, Cortese DA. Severe hypoxemia associated with liver disease: Mayo Clinic experience and the experimental use of almitrine bismesylate. Mayo Clin Proc 1987;62:164–173.)*

rhosis. The features of the syndrome have been reviewed in detail recently (57–59). Precapillary dilation of pulmonary vessels and the hyperdynamic circulation associated with liver disease produces a situation in which erythrocytes in the middle of the engorged pulmonary vessel cannot become adequately oxygenated (Fig. 28.3). This problem, termed the diffusion–perfusion defect, responds as would be expected to the administration of 100% oxygen. The dilatation itself is thought to occur because of an imbalance between endogenous pulmonary vasodilators and vasoconstrictors.

As described by Krowka et al (60), two radiographic presentations of the hepatopulmonary syndrome may be seen. In the type 1 minimal pattern, dilated pulmonary blood vessels appear as fine reticular infiltrates. Resolution of hypoxemia with oxygen administration is expected with this abnormality. The type 1 minimal form may progress to a type 1 advanced pattern that has a blotchy angiographic appearance and is correlated with a worse response to oxygen administration. The type 2 pattern refers to discrete arteriovenous malformations, which functionally act as pure anatomic shunts.

The diagnosis is confirmed by the presence of platypnea, orthodeoxia, clubbing, and the demonstration of intrapulmonary vascular dilations. They are confirmed by the presence of an elevated shunt fraction on physiologic shunt study, a positive bubble contrast echocardiogram demonstrating microbubbles on the left side of the heart after 3 to 6 beats postinfusion, or a technetium-99 macroaggregated albumin body scan showing uptake over the brain, kidneys, or liver. Transesophageal echocardiography, although used rarely for this purpose, may be more sensitive than surface echocardiography. Angiography can occasionally be useful to delineate discrete arteriovenous malformations that could be amenable to coil embolization (61).

Treatment of the hepatopulmonary syndrome has thus far been disappointing. A wide variety of agents including almitrine bimesylate, cyclooxygenase inhibitors, tamoxifen, somatostatin analogues, garlic, methylene blue, and others have been used with variable success. The role of hepatic transplantation in the treatment of hepatopulmonary syndrome is evolving (62). The pretransplantation predictors of successful resolution of the hepatopulmonary syndrome are still not well defined. Some patients have dramatic resolution of hypoxemia whereas others remain with persistent gas exchange abnormalities (63).

Pulmonary hypertension. Pulmonary hypertension occurs in 2% to 12% of patients and usually follows the development of portal hypertension and portosystemic collaterals (64,65) (see Chapter 30). Endogenous vasodilators and vasoconstrictors bypass the diseased liver in this fashion leading to an imbalance. This theory is supported by the development or worsening of pulmonary hypertension that has been recently observed in a patient following transjugular intrahepatic portosystemic shunting, which increases the amount of blood bypassing the liver in an effort to reduce portal pressures (66). The endothelial cell is key in the pathogenesis of this disorder (67). Damage to the endothelium leads to vascular remodeling that effectively reduces the cross-sectional area of the pulmonary vascular bed and exacerbates pulmonary hypertension.

The degree of elevation of the pulmonary artery pressure is important. Patients with severe pulmonary hypertension are at higher risk for intraoperative and perioperative death. In contrast, patients with mild or moderate hypertension who underwent LT were found to have a mortality comparable to those without pulmonary hypertension (68). For this reason, quantification of pulmonary artery pressures with cardiac catheterization preoperatively is essential in patients with suspected pulmonary hypertension. A vasodilator trial can be performed at this time, although most of these patients do not improve significantly. Thereafter, serial determinations of the pulmonary artery pressure and right ventricular function can be accurately assessed noninvasively while the patient is on the waiting list using echocardiography. Because of the hemodynamic shifts occurring intraoperatively, normal right ventricular function is essential to undergo the procedure.

Some patients have resolution of their pulmonary hypertension whereas others, likely due to vascular remodeling, have persistence. As with the hepatopulmonary syndrome, the clinical factors predicting the resolution of pulmonary hypertension following LT are currently unknown.

Intraoperative Considerations

The two major intraoperative concerns from a pulmonary perspective during LT include pulmonary edema and pulmonary embolism (69). During stage 1, the period before explantation of the recipient's liver, bleeding may be significant and, consequently, large volumes of fluids are infused. Nevertheless, the pulmonary capillary wedge pressure usually declines at this time. In stage 2, the recipient's liver is removed, the donor liver is inserted, and the vascular anastamoses are completed. The use of veno-venous bypass at this stage has attenuated the otherwise dramatic decrease in preload caused by cross-clamping the inferior vena cava (see Chapter 19). Stage 3 is characterized by reperfusion of the donor liver and a marked decrease in afterload that improves cardiac output. Pulmonary capillary wedge pressures may not accurately reflect left ventricular end diastolic volume as left ventricular compliance decreases (70). Transesophageal echocardiography has indicated that hypotensive patients at this stage have under-filled ventricles, suggesting that intravascular volume depletion is present. Pulmonary edema can occur at any stage of this process but is more likely postoperatively as patients mobilize extravascular fluid gains during surgery. Massive blood transfusion may also produce the adult respiratory distress syndrome by causing pulmonary microemboli.

Air, thrombi, or platelet aggregates may embolize to the pulmonary circulation and present as intraoperative catastrophes. Although tumor and fat emboli have also been reported in patients with LT for hepatic malignancy and fatty liver, respectively, these are less frequent. Air embolism can occur with the use of veno-venous bypass if the connections allow air to be entrained (71). The use of nitrous oxide for anesthesia is avoided as this gas may actually increase the size of the air embolus (69). The pump used for bypass can also serve as a nidus for thrombi, which may then dislodge into the venous circulation (72). Massive fatal thromboembolism from a pulmonary artery catheter has also been reported following aprotinin administration intraoperatively (73). Lastly, platelet aggregates have been observed postmortem in the pulmonary arteries of 10 children who died suddenly intraoperatively (74). In another study involving 100 adults, three patients that died immediately after transplantation had similar abnormalities (75). The cause of these platelet aggregates is unclear.

Post-transplant Considerations

The noninfectious pulmonary problems associated with liver transplantation can be divided anatomically into the following areas:

- Pulmonary parenchymal complications
- Pleural complications
- Diaphragmatic complications

Pulmonary Parenchymal Complications The lung parenchyma can be affected in several different ways after transplantation. Atelectasis and the adult respiratory distress syndrome may be seen in the early post-transplant period whereas pulmonary calcification and malignancies occur in the late post-transplant period.

Atelectasis. Atelectasis is one of the most common post-transplant complications and occurs in up to 75% of patients (40). Bilateral subsegmental atelectasis is the most common presentation. Because of the diaphragmatic trauma that occurs during right upper quadrant dissection, the right lung is more involved than the left lung. Factors favoring atelectasis include postoperative pain causing shallow breathing, overzealous narcotic administration causing hypoventilation, postoperative diaphragm dysfunction, restriction caused by ascites, and the presence of pleural effusions.

A variety of methods have been used to deal with this problem. Periodic rotation of a bed to prevent secretions from pooling in dependent areas has been attempted, a strategy known as chronic lateral rotational therapy. One prospective study showed a trend toward resolution of atelectasis using this modality; however, the difference did not reach statistical significance (76). Postoperative incentive spirometry, bronchodilators, and early ambulation are the most effective interventions. Rarely, bronchoscopy may be required for lobar atelectasis unresponsive to conservative measures.

ARDS. The incidence of the adult respiratory distress syndrome is 5% to 15% following LT with a mortality approaching 80% (33). Sepsis, aspiration, transfusions, allograft rejection, intravenous cyclosporine use, and OKT3 use have all been associated with acute lung injury (77,78). Trimethoprim-sulfamethoxazole, used for *Pneumocystis carinii* prophylaxis, may also produce an acute hypersensitivity reaction with peripheral eosinophilia that radiographically can mimic ARDS (79). Treatment is primarily supportive and death most commonly occurs as a result of infection. Successful resolution has been reported with the use of extracorporeal membrane oxygenation and retransplantation when ARDS occurs in association with graft rejection (77,80).

Pulmonary calcification. Pulmonary calcification is a rare complication of LT and presents weeks following as asymptomatic nodular infiltrates on the chest radiograph (33). Blood transfusions and excessive calcium infusion have been associated with the development of this problem. The diagnosis is confirmed by technetium scanning, CT scan, or by transbronchial biopsy or open-lung biopsy. No treatment is necessary for the majority of patients. The rare patient with significant symptoms and restrictive lung disease should have blood transfusions and calcium infusions minimized (81).

Malignancy. Lymphoma and metastatic hepatoma need to be considered in the evaluation of post-transplant pulmonary nodules or masses. The latter is discussed above in the section on preoperative complications of LT. The incidence of lymphoma in liver transplant recipients is 2.2% to 4% (33); the Epstein-Barr virus has been implicated in the pathogenesis of these neoplasms. Reduction of immunosuppression effectively aborts many such tumors (82) (see Chapter 37).

Pleural Complications Pleural complications following LT include the development of pleural effusions that occur in 77% to 100% of patients (40,83). Right-sided effusions are more common, reflecting trauma to the diaphragmatic pleura during right upper quadrant dissection. Volume overload, hypoalbuminemia, ascites, and atelectasis are contributing factors. The majority of these effusions are transudates. The recovery of hemorrhagic or bilious pleural fluid should raise the possibility of a diaphragm rupture and a biliopleural fistula, respectively. The majority of effusions will resolve spontaneously over a few weeks. Symptomatic effusions should be drained by a thoracentesis or a thoracostomy tube. Persistent effusions should also be sampled to exclude an empyema (84).

Diaphragmatic Complications Trauma to the diaphragm during surgery can impair its mobility postoperatively; a more serious concern is that of intraoperative phrenic nerve injury. In a prospective study of 48 patients, right phrenic nerve injury documented by nerve conduction study was found in 79% of patients following LT (85). The left phrenic nerve was normal in all patients. The right diaphragm was completely paralyzed in 38% of patients. Injury to the phrenic nerve likely occurs from application of the suprahepatic caval clamp during surgery. Most patients, including those with complete absence of phrenic nerve conduction, recovered motor function after several months. The diagnosis of right hemidiaphragm paralysis should be suspected in any liver transplant patient who is difficult to wean from the mechanical ventilator. The diagnosis can be confirmed by using fluoroscopy to look for paradoxical diaphragmatic motion while breathing spontaneously. In weaning these patients off the ventilator, they should be sitting and not supine. Occasionally, plication of the hemidiaphragm is needed.

Renal Transplantation

Pretransplant Considerations

Because of the distance of the kidneys from the lungs, renal transplantation (RT) is not associated with pulmonary complications arising specifically from the site of the surgery as in the case of LT. Nevertheless, these patients experience pulmonary problems for two reasons. First, many of the diseases necessitating RT can affect extrarenal sites including the lungs either before or after RT. Second, many of the patients presenting for RT have significant comorbidities including chronic obstructive pulmonary disease (COPD) from prior smoking and impaired left ventricular function from coronary artery disease. For these reasons, noninfectious or infectious pulmonary complications occur after transplant in 37% of recipients (86) and are the most common cause of death in the first three years following RT.

In light of the frequency of pulmonary complications, certain baseline tests may be useful. A chest radiograph and an arterial blood gas determination are adequate for most patients. Formal pulmonary function testing should be reserved for patients with specific pulmonary–renal syndromes or underlying pulmonary disease for which these indices may be useful to follow disease activity or progression.

In the pulmonary evaluation of a potential renal transplant recipient, the following problems may be encountered:

- Abnormal pulmonary function tests
- Atelectasis
- Pleural effusions
- Metastatic calcification
- Pulmonary fibrosis
- Pulmonary hypertension
- Pulmonary edema
- Malignancy

Abnormal Pulmonary Function Tests Although pulmonary function tests are not routinely indicated in these patients, there is a high likelihood of abnormal results if these tests are done. Diminished lung volumes and a decreased diffusing capacity are found in the majority of these patients whether they are on hemodialysis or on chronic ambulatory peritoneal dialysis (87). Interestingly, these abnormalities persist even after RT, reflecting the irreversible changes in lung architecture that result from repeated bouts of fluid overload, pulmonary hemosiderosis, calcium deposition, and infection prior to transplantation.

Although resting hypoxemia is uncommon in adequately dialyzed chronic renal failure patients, desaturation commonly occurs during hemodialysis (88,89) and over time may contribute to the development of pulmonary hypertension. Hypoxemia is present because of hypoventilation and because of ventilation–perfusion mismatching. Carbon dioxide loss through the dialysis membrane and decreased carbon dioxide production when using acetate-based dialysates decreases the minute ventilation required to maintain a physiologic pH. Ventilation–perfusion mismatching arises because leukocytes are activated by the dialysis membrane and are then sequestered in the lung where they release a variety of vasoactive mediators (90).

Atelectasis Rounded atelectasis has been reported infrequently in patients with end-stage renal disease. The clinician must be careful not to confuse this entity with a mass in the chest as radiographically they share a similar appearance (91). Rounded atelectasis occurs in areas of passive atelectasis that have formed a fibrinous adhesion to the surrounding pleura, in effect trapping the atelectatic segment. Radiographic differentiation from a mass relies on demonstrating stability of the lesion over time and by specific radiologic features of atelectasis such as a curvilinear distribution of blood vessels around the lesion. Computed tomography may be required in ambiguous cases to obviate other invasive biopsy procedures that are otherwise required to investigate a mass lesion.

Pleural Effusions The etiology of pleural effusions in these patients is multifactorial. Pleural effusions arise from volume overload or uremic pleuritis and are typically small to moderate in size and can involve either hemithorax. The pleural fluid in the former is transudative whereas in the latter it is exudative and, possibly, hemorrhagic. Massive hydrothorax from instillation of fluid for peritoneal dialysis has been reported, presumably because of passage of fluid through microscopic wrents in the diaphragm. A diagnostic thoracentesis should be performed at least once to exclude entities, such as malignancy and empyema, that would represent a contraindication to RT.

The therapy depends upon the underlying cause. Dialysis will decrease the size of effusions from volume overload, but has little effect on uremic effusions, which tend to resolve spontaneously in a few weeks. Chronic pleural inflammation from uremia can lead to an empyema or a fibrinous peel that requires decortication (87).

Pulmonary Edema The pulmonary edema associated with renal failure usually occurs due to volume administration with impaired urinary output or left ventricular dysfunction. As such, pulmonary vascular permeability assessed by radiolabeled transferrin is normal (92). The contribution of uremia itself to the development of pulmonary edema is unclear. Perihilar alveolar infiltrates with or without accompanying pleural effusions are characteristic. Intravascular volume as assessed by pulmonary artery catheterization is elevated. Oxygen, diuretics, and hemodialysis are the mainstays of therapy. The institution of positive pressure ventilation noninvasively with mask continuous positive airway pressure (CPAP) can avert endotracheal intubation while these measures are being instituted.

Metastatic Calcification The term *pulmonary calcification* refers to the deposition of calcium in normal lung and can occur before or after RT, usually in association with an elevated calcium-phosphate product. Deposition is greatest in the lung apices because of the relatively alkaline pH in this area. Pulmonary calcifications may form on the alveolar septa, known as metastatic pulmonary calcification, or in the alveolar spaces, known as alveolar microlithiasis (93). Although symptomatic disease is uncommon, autopsy studies reveal that the majority of patients with chronic renal failure have intraparenchymal pulmonary calcifications. Rarely, patients will develop significant restrictive lung disease with cor pulmonale. Similarly, postmortem examinations of RT recipients have clearly demonstrated the presence of pulmonary calcifications in some patients, particularly those who have a rapid demise after transplantation (94). This finding may reflect the often severe imbalances in calcium homeostasis that result from renal failure and other severe metabolic abnormalities.

Nodular or alveolar infiltrates result in either case (95). As a rule, however, the chest radiograph is insensitive for the diagnosis (96). Computed tomography of the chest showing intraparenchymal calcifications or radiolabeled technetium scans with uptake in the lungs support the diagnosis, which can be confirmed with a transbronchial biopsy. Because of the characteristic radiographic appearance on CT, however, a biopsy is unnecessary in the majority of patients.

The treatment is currently supportive. Efforts should be made to reduce the calcium-phosphate product with phosphate binders and vitamin D supplements should be provided. The presence of metastatic pulmonary calcification should not exclude patients for RT as this abnormality may actually reverse following successful transplantation (97).

Pulmonary Fibrosis Pulmonary fibrosis associated with repeated bouts of infection, pulmonary edema, pulmonary hemorrhage, and uremia appears on the chest radiograph as interstitial infiltrates or cystic lucencies similar to honeycombs. Although highly prevalent in autopsy studies (98), the pulmonary fibrosis seen in the context of renal disease has been poorly characterized and is only rarely symptomatic. Significant pulmonary fibrosis should raise the possibility of a pulmonary–renal syndrome, in particular a collagen vascular disease. RT in the setting of pulmonary fibrosis is not advisable given the overall poor prognosis of these patients.

Malignancy Because RT is being offered to patients with renal malignancies, the pretransplant pulmonary evaluation of these patients should focus on excluding metastatic disease to the chest. The treatment required for Wilm's tumor including surgical excision of the kidneys, chemotherapy, and radiation treatment, can lead to renal failure, for which RT is a therapeutic option in some centers (99). Wilm's tumor can metastasize to the lungs even years after the initial diagnosis. The presence of such metastases does not preclude transplantation provided that the lung metastases have been successfully treated, usually with resection or chemotherapy. Confining transplantation to the group of patients who are disease free for at least one year following treatment for the malignancy has been suggested (100).

Pulmonary Hypertension Pathologic vascular changes suggesting pulmonary hypertension are seen postmortem in many patients with chronic renal failure. Left ventricular dysfunction, pulmonary fibrosis and calcification, and excessive levels of parathyroid hormone likely contribute to this problem (101). Parathyroid hormone, in particular, may play a significant role in the pathogenesis of pulmonary hypertension. This hypothesis has been studied in an animal model. In mongrel dogs with chronic renal failure, those animals with an intact parathyroid glands had higher levels of parathyroid hormone, a greater content of calcium in the lungs, higher pulmonary artery pressures, and a greater degree of right ventricular hypertrophy than animals having had parathyroidectomies. Whether the same pathophysiology is present in humans is unknown.

Specific Pulmonary–Renal Syndromes RT is performed for renal failure secondary to diseases that may have prominent pulmonary manifestations. Patients with antiglomerular basement membrane disease (anti-GBM disease), Wegener's granulomatosis, and sarcoidosis must be carefully evaluated for pulmonary abnormalities. Although systemic lupus erythematosis can also affect both organs, this disease will not be discussed as those patients are generally not RT candidates if active multisystem disease is present.

Antiglomerular basement membrane (anti-GBM) disease. Pulmonary hemorrhage is a feature of anti-GBM disease in 60% to 90% of patients (102). Pulmonary involvement occurs most frequently in young males. The mere presence of the anti-GBM antibody does not correlate with the development of pulmonary disease. Additional lung injury, for example from smoking or a viral upper respiratory infection, is needed to cause pulmonary hemorrhage in a susceptible individual. Patients present with hemoptysis and perihilar alveolar infiltrates or subtle interstitial infiltrates with a tendency to spare the apices. A normal chest radiograph does not exclude the diagnosis (103). The diffusing capacity may be a noninvasive way of determining the presence of alveolar hemorrhage and is often elevated in this situation. Treatment consists of corticosteroids and plasmapheresis. RT should be delayed until the disease is quiescent in the lungs and until titers of anti-GBM antibody are at low levels (1).

Wegener's granulomatosis. This necrotizing granulomatous vasculitis most commonly affects the lungs, upper airway, and the kidneys. Pulmonary manifestations include cavitary nodular infiltrates, diffuse alveolar hemorrhage, and stenotic lesions involving the airways (104). Mild restrictive lung disease with a diffusing capacity that is decreased varies with the presentation. The presence of a cytoplasmic neutrophilic antibody (c-ANCA) strongly supports the diagnosis, although it is neither sensitive nor specific for Wegener's granulomatosis. Cyclophosphamide and corticosteroids constitute the mainstays of therapy for this disorder. Even the presence of active pulmonary disease should not preclude RT because the risk of relapse postoperatively has been low in the experience, albeit limited, with these patients (105). Patients on immunosuppressive regimens without cyclophosphamide may be at higher risk to develop recurrent lung disease. A rising antineutrophil antibody titer will often be a harbinger of disease recurrence (106).

Sarcoidosis. Renal failure complicating sarcoidosis is extremely rare whereas pulmonary involvement is almost universal. RT for the small subset of patients with renal involvement may be life saving (107). In the lungs, bilateral hilar adenopathy, interstitial infiltrates, or pulmonary fibrosis may be seen. Even with a normal chest radiograph, transbronchial biopsy reveals noncaseating granulomas in 70% to 80% of cases. Treatment consists of corticosteroids and rarely cytotoxic therapy for symptomatic, progressive, or multisystem disease. As with other organs, late recurrence of sarcoidosis in the renal allograft has been reported (108).

Intraoperative Considerations

Aside from the usual risks of general anesthesia, there are no particular pulmonary risks associated with RT in the operating room. For this reason, most of these surgeries are done without intraoperative pulmonary artery catheterization.

Post-transplant Considerations

The noninfectious pulmonary problems of RT recipients can be divided anatomically into the following areas:

- Pulmonary parenchymal complications
- Pulmonary vascular complications
- Malignancies

Pulmonary Parenchymal Complications

Pulmonary edema. Acute pulmonary edema postoperatively occurs in 17% of patients (86). Acute and chronic allograft rejection or nonfunction of the graft are possible risk factors. Cardiac dysfunction, either systolic or diastolic, is implicated in 10% of patients with pulmonary edema. Postoperative fluid administration should be judicious in these conditions. The presentation and management are described in the treatment of this disorder prior to RT.

Drug-induced lung injury. Drug-induced pneumonitis, although not unique to RT recipients, must be recognized and treated rapidly. A capillary leak syndrome has been described with OKT3 (109) and can mimic pulmonary edema caused by fluid overload (see Chapters 13 and 30). Although somewhat controversial (110), alveolar hemorrhage has been described with the use of nitrofurantoin in RT recipients (111). Cyclophosphamide and azathioprine have been associated with interstitial pneumonitis in a few case reports (112,113). The toxicity of the latter may be potentiated by allopurinol, which raises azathioprine levels (114).

Malignancy Malignancies including Kaposi's sarcoma and non-Hodgkin's lymphoma complicate the late postoperative course of some RT recipients. They both present as solitary or multiple masses in the chest and may be associated with the Epstein-Barr virus (115). Kaposi's sarcoma occurs 500 times more commonly in RT recipients than in the general population (116) and tends to have a greater predilection for visceral and lymph node involvement. Patients on cyclosporine are particularly at risk (117). In the chest, interstitial and alveolar infiltrates, mediastinal adenopathy, or pleural effusions are seen (118). Withdrawal of immunosuppression may lead to spontaneous resolution in some patients (116).

Like Kaposi's sarcoma, non-Hodgkin's lymphoma represents a significant problem for these patients accounting for 10% to 14% of all malignancies post-RT (119). As in other organ transplant recipients, some of these tumors respond to a reduction in immunosuppression.

Pulmonary Vascular Complications

Clinically significant venous thromboembolism is exceedingly rare in patients with renal failure because of qualitative and quantitative platelet abnormalities induced by uremia (120). In a retrospective study of 2255 autopsies, no macroscopic thrombi were discovered in the 95 patients with chronic renal failure (97).

The risk of venous thromboembolism increases substantially following RT. In Edelstein's series, 4.5% of RT recipients were diagnosed with a pulmonary embolism (86). The prevalence may in fact be much higher, as this group represents only those patients who had symptomatic emboli. In fact, in an autopsy study detailing pulmonary pathology following RT, the prevalence of pulmonary thromboembolism was 20% (86). The source of the thrombi is usually from the lower extremities or less commonly the renal veins ipsilateral to the allograft.

The clinician must maintain a high index of suspicion for venous thromboembolism. The diagnosis should be entertained in patients with unexplained pleurisy or hypoxemia, especially if the chest radiograph is normal. Duplex ultrasonography and ventilation–perfusion scanning are often the initial diagnostic modalities. A normal ventilation–perfusion scan excludes a pulmonary embolism whereas a high-probability scan in this setting confirms this diagnosis (121). All other results must be followed by duplex ultrasonography of the lower extremities or the renal veins or angiography depending upon the degree of clinical suspicion for a pulmonary embolism. Because these patients are postsurgical, anticoagulation or thrombolysis is frequently not a therapeutic option. A vena caval filter should therefore be considered in all such cases. This device must be placed proximal to the site of thrombus and generally does not interfere with allograft function, even if placed in a suprarenal location for renal vein thrombi (122).

Cardiac Transplantation

Pretransplant Considerations

Often pulmonary and cardiac symptomatology overlap and distinguishing cardiac from pulmonary disease can be exceedingly difficult. This distinction is important because many changes in the lungs secondary to cardiac dysfunction improve following cardiac transplantation (CT), whereas primary pulmonary disease would not be expected to improve and, in fact, can complicate the postoperative course. The clinician, in approaching these patients before transplantation, must therefore have a complete understanding of the changes in lung physiology and architecture that result from advanced cardiac disease to avoid misdiagnosis.

Complicating the preoperative assessment even further is the fact that many patients have both cardiac and pulmonary diseases. The risk factors for ischemic cardiomyopathy including increased age and smoking are also risk factors for pulmonary diseases such as COPD and lung cancer.

The preoperative pulmonary evaluation of these patients should focus on their operability from a pulmonary standpoint, on distinguishing cardiac from pulmonary disease, and on appreciating any cardiac-induced pulmonary derangements that may preclude transplantation. These goals can be achieved in most cases by performing an arterial blood gas, a chest radiograph, a pulmonary function test, and a cardiopulmonary exercise test. The most common abnormalities disclosed by these tests and other preoperative pulmonary issues that pertain to cardiac transplantation are discussed below. This section is divided into the following topics:

- Abnormal pulmonary function tests and cardiopulmonary exercise testing
- Pulmonary hypertension
- Pulmonary thromboembolism
- Sleep apnea
- Pulmonary edema and pleural effusions
- Pulmonary effects of cardiac medications

Abnormal Pulmonary Function Tests and Cardiopulmonary Exercise Testing Pulmonary function tests performed on patients awaiting cardiac transplantation show abnormalities in 67% to 88% of cases (123,124). In patients with compensated cardiac failure, usually of a chronic nature, a reduced diffusing capacity is the most frequent abnormality followed by a restrictive abnormality (124). The reduction in diffusing capacity is thought to occur because of fibrosis and thickening of alveolar septae as a consequence of repeated bouts of pulmonary edema and, in some patients, because of chronic pulmonary emboli. Restriction is present because of cardiomegaly, interstitial edema, and pleural effusions and may resolve after transplantation (125). In the absence of chronic obstructive pulmonary disease, an obstructive ventilatory impairment is uncommon in patients with chronic heart failure. In contrast, 48% of patients with acute heart failure demonstrate obstructive physiology (124). Peribronchiolar fluid accumulation and prior smoking likely account for this finding.

Obstructive lung disease also occurs in these patients because of bronchial hyperreactivity (126). In one study evaluating patients with chronic left ventricular failure, bronchial hyperresponsiveness to methacholine was found in 21 of 23 patients (127). This bronchospasm is reversible with the administration of bronchodilators (127).

Despite the high frequency of pulmonary abnormalities in patients with chronic heart failure, their significance is uncertain. Various criteria have been proposed but have not been validated. In the only study specifically addressing this question, no correlation between preoperative pulmonary function tests or arterial blood gases and subsequent pulmonary complications or mortality could be found (128). The mean FEV_1 was 86% of the mean predicted FEV_1 for the population studied. The two factors that portended an increased mortality were an increased age at transplantation and an elevated pulmonary vascular resistance (PVR).

Because this study evaluated patients with relatively good lung function, a value for the FEV_1 that precludes successful transplantation is not available. Extrapolating from the literature in patients undergoing a thoracotomy for other indication, an FEV_1 of greater than 50% of the predicted normal value is desirable.

Exercise testing has been used to indicate the optimal timing of cardiac transplantation and to stratify these patients in terms of intraoperative risk (129). A peak oxygen consumption ($\dot{V}O_2$ max) of less than 10 to 14 mL/kg/min is associated with a high short-term mortality and indicates the need for transplantation as soon as possible. In interpreting this test, it is important to ensure that the limitation to achieving the predicted $\dot{V}O_2$ max is cardiac rather than pulmonary in origin.

Pulmonary Hypertension The mean pulmonary artery pressures (PAPs) of patients with chronic heart failure awaiting transplantation is approximately 30 to 35 mm Hg (123,124,128). Left ventricular failure is responsible for most cases of this mild-to-moderate pulmonary hypertension. In patients with a low cardiac output, the mean pulmonary artery pressure may underestimate the degree of pulmonary hypertension. The pulmonary vascular resistance (PVR) [(mean PAP − left atrial pressure)/cardiac output] in this situation may be a more accurate reflection of the degree of pulmonary vasoconstriction.

An elevated PVR before transplantation correlates with a higher postoperative mortality (128). A PVR exceeding 4 mm Hg/L/min portends a higher risk of death whereas a value above 5 to 6 mm Hg/L/min should preclude transplantation (128). This view is strengthened by the observation that patients with high preoperative PVRs have right ventricular failure by echocardiographic criteria in the early postoperative period (128). Patients with an elevated PVR who demonstrate a reduction in the PVR with vasodilators may, however, have a more favorable outcome (130,131). A lack of response to vasodilators implies that the pulmonary hypertension is fixed; orthotopic CT is contraindicated in this setting.

One strategy that has been suggested is the use of heterotopic CT in patients with a markedly elevated PVR. This approach is controversial given the generally poor outcome of these patients (132–135). Implantation of an oversized cardiac replacement, domino heart transplantation, or heart–lung transplantation may be an alternative in this subset of patients.

Despite the common occurrence of pulmonary hypertension in these patients, the clinician must be wary of other potential causes of secondary pulmonary hypertension. Pulmonary thromboembolism and sleep apnea, in particular, occur in this population.

Pulmonary Thromboembolism Pulmonary emboli from lower extremity or intracardiac thrombi occur frequently in patients with chronic heart failure. In a study of pediatric patients with dilated cardiomyopathy not on systemic anticoagulation, the prevalence of pulmonary infarction was 10% (136). Because the majority of adult patients are anticoagulated, the incidence is likely lower.

Pulmonary emboli are especially dangerous to these patients for two reasons. First, they are more prone to pulmonary infarction because many patients have atherosclerotic disease involving their bronchial artery circulation, which serves as collateral circulation to the lung. Embolism of a pulmonary artery branch in this setting causes infarction of the lung parenchyma subtended by the vessel. These infarcts frequently become infected after transplantation and can produce lung abscesses, bronchopleural fistulas, and empyemas (137). For this reason, a recent pulmonary infarction is considered by some to represent a contraindication to transplantation. Surgical resection of the infarcted areas both before and after transplantation has been described to treat and to avoid these complications (137–139).

The second major risk posed by pulmonary emboli in these patients is that of sudden death. Because they have preexisting pulmonary hypertension from left ventricular dysfunction, even a small pulmonary embolism can produce marked pulmonary hypertension acutely and can lead to right ventricular collapse and death.

A high index of suspicion must be maintained for this diagnosis. Although not systematically studied, angiography and portable ventilation scans may have a decreased sensitivity in this population, but nevertheless are the diagnostic tests of choice. These studies should be supplemented by duplex ultrasonography and echocardiography as required.

The treatment of acute pulmonary emboli in these patients consists of anticoagulation or thrombolysis. The latter should be considered in the face of hypotension or new-onset right ventricular dysfunction.

Sleep Apnea Sleep disordered breathing and nocturnal hypoxemia has been observed in 45% and 20% of patients awaiting CT, respectively (140). These individuals can have either central or obstructive sleep apnea. Nocturnal desaturations and hypoventilation over time can produce pulmonary hypertension and right ventricular dysfunction as well as left ventricular dysfunction and hypoxemia-induced arrhythmias. Patients or their spouses describe excessive snoring and daytime somnolence. The diagnosis is readily confirmed by polysomnography. Treatment consists of oxygen, noninvasive positive pressure ventilation, surgery, or respiratory stimulants depending upon the type of apnea present (141,142). Early recognition and treatment of this problem is essential before transplantation to optimize cardiac function during the waiting period and to minimize potentially fatal arrhythmias at night. The normal weight gain experienced after transplantation can worsen or unmask sleep apnea (141).

Pulmonary Edema and Pleural Effusions The etiology of pulmonary edema arising in the context of chronic, compensated left ventricular failure includes excessive salt intake, noncompliance with medications, infections, and worsening cardiac function. These inciting factors are often readily identifiable clinically. Cardiac medications including preload and afterload reducing agents and inotropes should be optimized prior to transplantation.

Pleural effusions were reported in 34% of patients awaiting CT and occur because of elevated pulmonary venous and lymphatic hydrostatic pressures (124). These effusions are transudative and most often bilateral. If unilateral, they are more common on the right side. Diuretic therapy can occasionally alter the characteristics of the fluid and transform it into an exudate. The albumin gradient can be useful in this situation (2,143). An albumin gradient of greater than 1.2 g/dL between the serum and the pleural fluid albumin generally signifies the presence of a transudate. A large unilateral effusion should raise suspicion for a complicating factor such as a malignancy, a pulmonary embolism, or an infection and mandates a thoracentesis.

Pulmonary Effects of Cardiac Medications A number of cardiac medications can cause pulmonary toxicity. A complete discussion of this topic can be found in several recent reviews (144,145). Pulmonary toxicity has been clearly described with amiodarone, procainamide, and tocainide. Amiodarone used in doses below 400 mg/day is not associated with an increased likelihood of pulmonary complications after cardiac transplantation (146).

Intraoperative Considerations

Pulmonary complications arising intraoperatively vary with the type of transplantation performed. In orthotopic CT, the left lung is manipulated and the left pleura traumatized to allow removal of the native heart and implantation of the donor heart. As anticipated, three postoperative problems that need to be watched for are bronchopleural fistulas, intrapleural bleeding, and atelectasis. Heterotopic CT entails placement of the donor heart in the right side of the chest. Both pleural spaces are traumatized in an effort first to place the donor heart in the right chest and subsequently to anastamose it to the left side of the heart. Pneumothoraces and hemothoraces in this operation can be bilateral. The theoretical advantage of this procedure is to avoid right ventricular collapse of the transplanted heart when faced with a high pulmonary vascular resistance. The utility of this operation has been questioned even in this population with pulmonary hypertension because of a higher mortality when compared with orthotopic CT (134).

Both orthotopic and heterotopic CT employ cardiopulmonary bypass. The latter generally necessitates a greater length of time on bypass. Cardiopulmonary bypass has been associated with enhanced pulmonary capillary permeability and intraoperative air or thromboembolism (71,72).

Post-transplant Considerations

In a retrospective study, the frequency of both infectious and noninfectious respiratory complications approached 20% (155). The noninfectious pulmonary problems of CT can be divided anatomically into the following areas:

- Parenchymal complications
- Pleural complications
- Diaphragmatic complications
- Pulmonary vascular complications

Parenchymal Complications The significant parenchymal problems following CT include pulmonary edema, atelectasis, and neoplasms.

Pulmonary edema. Cardiogenic pulmonary edema in the immediate postoperative period suggests primary graft failure. This problem is increasingly uncommon because of stringent donor criteria (147). Biventricular failure is present on echocardiography. The treatment consists of mechanical assists to increase cardiac output and retransplantation in refractory cases.

Atelectasis. Atelectasis is a common occurrence in the postoperative period although the precise frequency in this population is unknown. The left lung is involved more commonly in orthotopic transplants. Retraction of the left lung and damage to the left phrenic nerve intraoperatively from direct trauma or cold cardioplegia are responsible. Right lower lung atelectasis is common in heterotopic transplants reflecting the site of surgery. The size of the implanted heart in orthotopic transplants in children does correlate with the subsequent development of atelectasis. Oversized hearts produce more atelectasis; however, they do not seem to increase the length of time of mechanical ventilation (148). Postoperative incentive spirometry should be used routinely in the postoperative period. Failing conservative methods of treatment, bronchoscopy is sometimes required for extensive atelectasis.

Neoplasms. Lung neoplasms are common in CT recipients. Lung nodules were present in 9.7% of patients in one series (149). Approximately 75% were of infectious etiology whereas 25% were of noninfectious etiology. Among the noninfectious causes of lung nodules, bronchogenic carcinoma and lymphomas must be considered.

Because older patients and former smokers are being offered CT, the risk of bronchogenic carcinoma likely will increase in this population (150). In one report, 70% of patients smoked within 10 years of the time of transplant. Limited experience with these patients suggests that these tumors can progress rapidly perhaps because of the disinhibiting influence of immunosuppression. Surgical resection of these tumors has been used to achieve long-term cure (150). Whether screening chest radiography is useful in high-risk patients has yet to be established.

Post-transplant lymphoproliferative disorder (PTLD) occurs in 1.8% to 11.4% of cardiac transplant recipients (Fig. 28.4) (151). Risk factors for the development of PTLD include transplantation for cardiomyopathy, cyclosporine use,

A

B

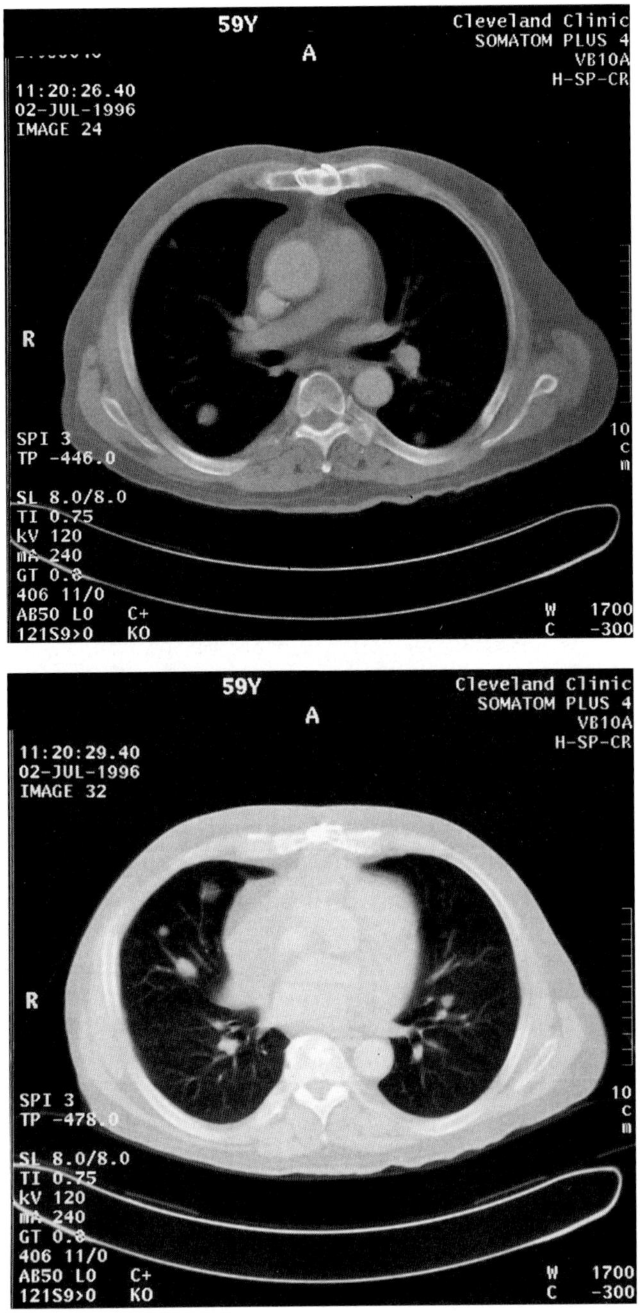

FIGURE 28.4. *Multifocal nodules of non-Hodgkin's lymphoma in a cardiac transplant recipient involving the right and left lower lobes **(A)** and the right middle lobe **(B)**. The Epstein-Barr virus has been implicated in the pathogenesis of many of these neoplasms. (Photographs courtesy of M. Meziane, MD, Cleveland Clinic Foundation.)*

and the administration of OKT3 (151,152). The early PTLD occur within a year of transplantation and are felt to be strongly linked to Epstein-Barr virus induced monoclonal or oligoclonal B-cell proliferation (153). Diminishing immunosuppression often effectively treats these neoplasms. The late-occurring lymphomas, in contrast, tend to be less responsive to such therapy and are more often disseminated at presentation (see Chapter 37). Extranodal involvement is relatively common in PTLD, particularly in the GI tract and the lung. Interestingly, extranodal presentation in these locations is associated with a more favorable prognosis (151). Chest radiographs reveal solitary or multiple pulmonary nodules with indistinct borders or an interstitial pattern in the event of lymphangitic spread of tumor. Although the diagnosis can occasionally be obtained using bronchoscopy, a surgical biopsy is usually required. As in PTLD in other transplant groups, the mainstay of therapy is a reduction in immunosuppression. Acyclovir, monoclonal B-cell antibodies, and chemotherapy have all been used with variable success (153).

Pleural Complications

Pleural effusions. Significant pleural effusions were present in 8 of 94 patients in one series (153). Small effusions occur almost uniformly after CT because of pleural trauma, pleural bleeding, and seepage of cold cardioplegia or iced saline through pleural tears created by surgery. Atelectasis, pulmonary emboli, and malignancy are other possible etiologies in this population. Most simple postoperative effusions resolve spontaneously weeks to months following transplantation.

Diaphragmatic Complications

Diaphragmatic paralysis. Although diaphragmatic paresis and paralysis are common after CT, most data regarding this complication are derived from patients having other types of cardiac surgery. The frequency of this complication is reported to be 2% to 20% in patients having open heart surgery (154). The phrenic nerve is damaged by direct surgical trauma or from the effects of cold cardioplegia. Most often the paralysis is unilateral and confined to the left hemidiaphragm although occasionally it can be bilateral. Unilateral diaphragmatic paralysis is evident under fluoroscopy as the patient "sniffs." Patients with bilateral diaphragmatic paralysis have abdominal paradox while supine. Diaphragmatic function usually takes months to fully recover.

Pulmonary Vascular Complications

Venous thromboembolism. The precise incidence of thromboemboli after CT is unknown. In one series in which patients were not systematically screened for, 5 of 94 patients had clinically evident pulmonary emboli (155). Unfortunately, the diagnosis was made postmortem in four of the patients. A high frequency of pulmonary emboli is not surprising given the fact that these patients are at high risk for such events preoperatively. The diagnosis is even more difficult to make after transplant because of the wide spectrum of pulmonary abnormalities that develop. Treatment options are more limited after transplant because these patients have a relative contraindication to anticoagulation and, therefore, the placement of a vena caval filter should be considered.

Bone Marrow Transplantation

Pretransplant Considerations

Hematologic disease for which bone marrow transplantation (BMT) is required can have a wide spectrum of pulmonary abnormalities. Because of the high prevalence of pulmonary abnormalities induced by BMT, certain baseline studies such as pulmonary function testing, arterial blood gas analysis, and a chest radiograph should be routinely performed (156). In evaluating the potential risk for the development of pulmonary complications, the following considerations are important:

- Results of pulmonary function tests
- Presence of focal or cavitary infiltrates on the chest radiograph
- Chemotherapeutic regimen employed
- Total radiation dose and the method by which it is delivered
- Type of transplant being performed, allogeneic or autologous, to assess the likelihood of graft-versus-host disease (GVHD)

The first three of these considerations are discussed in this section, whereas the latter two are discussed under post-transplant considerations.

Role of Pulmonary Function Tests Abnormal pulmonary function tests occur in approximately one third of prospective BMT candidates (157). Patients with a prior thoracotomy, chest irradiation, or pulmonary metastases have a relatively high incidence of such abnormalities (158). Mild restriction and a mild reduction in diffusing capacity are seen. In addition, at least 40% of these patients have evidence of bronchial hyperreactivity (159). Those patients with abnormal pulmonary function tests have a higher incidence of both infectious and noninfectious pulmonary complications (160,161). Some authors have advocated serial pulmonary function tests to screen for the onset of interstitial pneumonitis prior to the onset of clinical symptoms and radiographic abnormalities to permit early diagnosis and treatment (160). The efficacy of this approach in improving the outcome of this syndrome has yet to be demonstrated.

Focal or Cavitary Pulmonary Infiltrates Patients presenting for BMT are often immunosuppressed because of hematological malignancies, aplasia or infiltration of the bone marrow, or conditioning regimens consisting of chemotherapeutic agents and total body irradiation. These patients occasionally develop a focal infiltrate, which may cavitate. Exclusion of infection, particularly fungal or mycobacterial infection, is essential. The most common pathogen in this setting is *Aspergillus*. Recovery of organisms in sputum, bronchoalveolar lavage fluid, or lung biopsies mandates therapy with amphotericin B intravenously. Resection of the involved area should be considered before BMT (162). If resection is to be performed, perioperative amphotericin B and postoperative itraconazole therapy should be considered in these patients.

Other noninfectious causes of a focal infiltrate in this scenario need to be considered. Pulmonary infarcts exceeding 4 cm in size can cavitate (163). Malignancy, bacterial pneumonia, and necrotizing vasculitis are other possibilities.

Pretransplant Chemotherapeutic Regimen A variety of chemotherapeutic agents may be administered during the conditioning preceding BMT (see Chapter 27). These agents may be used to eradicate the hematopoietic cells populating the host's marrow and to eradicate any neoplastic cells if present. Cyclophosphamide is most commonly used for this purpose. A number of other agents may be used, particularly in light of the expanding indications for BMT. Many of these agents can have acute as well as chronic pulmonary toxicities (Table 28.5). A full discussion of these problems can be found in several recent reviews (164,165).

Additionally, certain subgroups of patients with hematological disease may be particularly at risk for these problems. For example, patients with aplastic anemia due to dyskeratosis congenita, an inherited syndrome of ectodermal dysplasia, have a high likelihood of developing pulmonary fibrosis (167). In one series, 50% of patients surviving more than two weeks after BMT developed pulmonary fibrosis.

Table 28.5. Cytotoxic Agents Associated With Lung Injury

Agents
Alkylating Agents
Cyclophosphamide
Busulfan
Melphalan
Chlorambucil
Antimetabolites
Methotrexate
Cytosine arabinoside
Azathioprine
6-Mercaptopurine
Cytotoxic Antibiotics
Bleomycin
Mitomycin-C
Neocarzinostatin
Nitosoureas
Carmustine (BCNU)
Lomustine (CCNU)
Semustine (Methyl-CCNU)
Cholorozotocin
Vinca Alkaloids
Vinblastine
Vindesine
Other Agents
Procarbazine
Teniposide (VM-26)
Etoposide (VP-16)
Ifosphamide
Interleukin-2

Source: Adapted with permission from Twohig KJ, Matthay RA. Pulmonary effects of cytotoxic agents other than bleomycin. Clin Chest Med 1990;11:32.

Intratransplant Considerations

Following conditioning with radiation and chemotherapy, the host marrow is eradicated and the donor marrow is infused. In autologous transplants, the marrow is obtained from the patient prior to conditioning and treated with chemotherapeutic agents or T-cell–depleting antibodies and then reinfused into the host. Allogeneic BMT involves the infusion of another patient's marrow elements without purging as in autologous transplants. In peripheral stem cell infusion, selected hematopoietic precursors are infused. Patients with allogeneic BMT have the highest incidence of GVHD and, consequently, the highest incidence of pulmonary complications, both infectious and noninfectious.

Approximately 150 to 200 cc of marrow is infused. Transient hypoxemia and a fall in the vital capacity can occur with infusion of the cryopreserved marrow. Dimethylsulfoxide, a cryopreservative, has been implicated as the offending agent in most cases (168). This compound causes histamine release and may cause direct pulmonary endothelial injury or may activate neutrophils. Diffuse alveolar hemorrhage has been reported following the administration of dimethylsulfoxide. Patients with a prior episode of diffuse alveolar hemorrhage immediately following BMT may be at higher risk for this problem and, therefore, they should receive washed marrow that is free of dimethylsulfoxide (168).

Post-transplant Considerations

After BMT, the types of pulmonary complications change as the length of time from transplantation increases (see Chapter 27). The initial period prior to engraftment of the donor bone marrow is characterized by severe neutropenia and thrombocytopenia. Patients are susceptible to opportunistic infections, pulmonary edema, and diffuse alveolar hemorrhage. After engraftment and hematological recovery, interstitial pneumonitis from chemotherapy, radiation, GVHD, and infection poses a significant risk to these patients. The importance of infection and GVHD in producing pulmonary complications cannot be overstated. These entities are central to the pathogenesis of and can complicate the course of many pulmonary diseases encountered by the BMT recipient (Fig. 28.5).

The noninfectious complications of BMT may be divided anatomically into the following areas:

- Parenchymal complications
- Malignancy
- Pulmonary alveolar proteinosis
- Airway disease
- Pulmonary vascular disease

Parenchymal Pulmonary Disease The most significant pulmonary complication arising after BMT is interstitial pneumonia, which may be primary (idiopathic) or secondary to a number of different causes. These patients may also develop bronchiolitis obliterans with organizing pneumonia (BOOP), diffuse alveolar hemorrhage (DAH), and interstitial edema or frank pulmonary edema. The pulmonary effects of the various chemotherapeutic agents have been discussed in the section on pretransplant pulmonary complications.

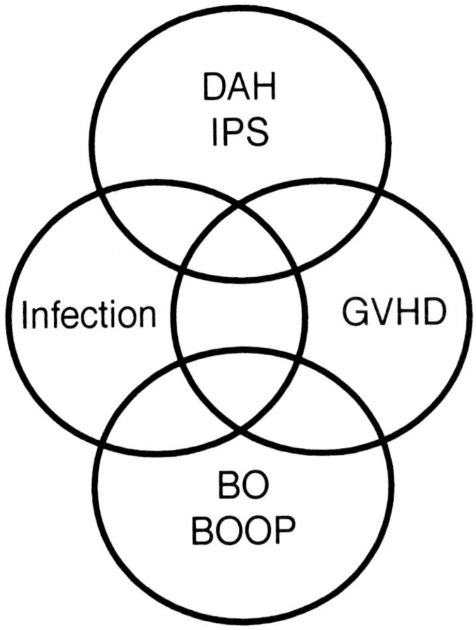

FIGURE 28.5. *Central role of GVHD and infection in the development of pulmonary complications after BMT. Many pulmonary complications of BMT arise in the context of GVHD and can be complicated or precipitated by infection.*

Table 28.6. Proposed Definition of the Idiopathic Pneumonia Syndrome

Evidence of widespread alveolar injury manifested by multilobar infiltrates with clinical evidence of a pneumonia or a restrictive pulmonary abnormality.
Absence of lower respiratory tract infection by bronchoalveolar lavage, preferably with a transbronchial biopsy, and lack of response to broad spectrum antibiotics.
Absence of respiratory pathogens identified on repeat bronchoalveolar lavage or open-lung biopsy at 2 to 14 days following initial procedure.

Source: Adapted with permission from Clark JG, Hansen JA, Hertz MI, et al. Idiopathic pneumonia syndrome after bone marrow transplantation. Am Rev Respir Dis 1993;147:1603.

Idiopathic pneumonia syndrome (IPS). The incidence of IPS following autologous and allogeneic BMT is 5% and 12%, respectively (169,170). The disease typically occurs 42 to 49 days after transplantation. The pathologic correlates of IPS include interstitial pneumonitis and diffuse alveolar damage. These pathologic entities may have a number of potential causes, however, including infection and drug toxicities. To make the diagnosis of IPS, these other entities must be excluded; a proposed definition of this syndrome is presented in Table 28.6 (169).

Clinically, the presentation of IPS is nonspecific. It resembles pulmonary edema or diffuse infectious pneumonia. Patients typically are dyspneic, may have a nonproductive cough, and develop fever and tachypnea. The laboratory evaluation is characterized by evidence of hypoxemia, hyperventilation, and chest radiographic findings consisting of diffuse alveolar or interstitial infiltrate. Prior to 1992, this constellation was termed *idiopathic pneumonia.* Since that time, the entity has been known as IPS and includes the condition *diffuse alveolar hemorrhage* within the syndrome.

In order to determine if IPS has the same incidence and risk factors as described previously for idiopathic pneumonia, Kantrow et al (171) undertook a case series review of 1165 consecutive marrow recipients at a single center from 1988 to 1991. These authors documented IPS in 85 recipients (7.3%) by bronchoalveolar lavage (n = 68), open-lung biopsy (n = 3), or autopsy (n = 14). The incidence calculated for IPS within 120 days after BMT was 7.7%. Median time to onset was approximately 21 days. Hospital mortality was 74% and 53 BMT recipients died with progressive respiratory failure. IPS resolved in 22 patients (26%); 18 patients (21%) survived to discharge. Mechanical ventilation was required by 59 BMT recipients (69%) within a median of 2 days for onset of infiltrates.

Although the study found no difference in incidence between autologous and allogeneic marrow recipients, risks were identified only for the latter: malignancy other than leukemia and grade 4 graft-versus-host disease. No factors were associated with recovery.

The authors concluded that the incidence of IPS seems lower, the onset earlier, and the risk factors different from those previously reported. The major risks seem to be regimen-related toxicity and multiorgan dysfunction associated with alloreactive processes.

The pathogenesis of IPS is complex. Abnormalities in alveolar lymphocytes and macrophages and the local alveolar production of immunoglobulins have been identified (172–174). Clinical risk factors for the development of IPS include an increased age or weight, the presence of GVHD, the use of bleomycin during conditioning or methotrexate as GVHD prophylaxis, the use of total body irradiation (TBI), conditioning chemotherapy, and a low Karnofsky score before transplantation (175–181). The contribution of radiation to the development of IPS can be reduced by minimizing total radiation dosages or by using fractionated regimens (182,183).

With improvements in the detection of micro-organisms, a large number of cases of interstitial pneumonitis, previously though to represent IPS, may now be understood to be due to viruses such as cytomegalovirus (CMV) or human herpes virus 6 (HHV6) (184–187). As methods of viral detection improve, the numbers of cases of interstitial pneumonitis presently classified as idiopathic may diminish.

The prognosis of IPS is poor. These patients have a 71% mortality rate in the hospital (170). Long-term survivors occasionally develop pulmonary fibrosis (188). High levels of transforming growth factor beta (TGFβ) prior to transplant can identify a subset of patients at high risk to develop pulmonary fibrosis (189). The treatment of IPS is currently supportive and, therefore, all efforts should be directed at identifying a potentially treatable etiology. Single lung transplantation should be considered in patients with progressive disease (190).

Delayed pulmonary toxicity syndrome. The term *delayed pulmonary toxicity syndrome (DPTS)* has been proposed to describe a condition of interstitial pneumonitis seen in women undergoing high-dose chemotherapy and autologous BMT for primary breast cancer. The condition results in a restrictive lung defect accompanied by cough and dyspnea, but does not conform to the definition of IPS. Steroid therapy may be helpful (191).

BOOP. Bronchiolitis obliterans with organizing pneumonia occurs in BMT recipients most often in association with GVHD. Nevertheless, there are a few case reports of so-called idiopathic BOOP occurring in the absence of GVHD (192). The pathologic features of BOOP include a lymphocytic pneumonitis with polypoid plugs of fibroconnective tissue in the small airways. Chest radiography reveals diffuse alveolar or interstitial infiltrates with hyperinflation. Pulmonary function tests show a mixed pattern of obstruction and restriction. Although IPS can present with similar radiologic patterns, hyperinflation and obstruction are generally absent.

The diagnosis is confirmed on a lung biopsy specimen. Many infections can produce a BOOP-like picture and they need to be excluded with appropriate cultures. This differentiation is important because idiopathic BOOP is treated with high doses of corticosteroids, which could be disastrous in the infected patient not on antimicrobial therapy.

DAH. Diffuse alveolar hemorrhage is seen in 5% to 21% of cases following BMT and carries a mortality of 80% (193–196). Patients tend to develop this problem in the first few weeks following transplant coincident with the recovery of their neutrophil counts (196).

Risk factors for the development of DAH include the presence of GVHD, TBI, increased age, solid tumors, high fevers, severe mucositis, and renal insufficiency (195,196). Neutrophil- and lymphocyte-mediated endothelial injury is felt to play a central role in the pathogenesis of this disorder. Elevated numbers of neutrophils and eosinophils before BMT on bronchial washings portend the development of DAH (194). Bronchial inflammation may, therefore, antedate frank alveolar hemorrhage.

Patients can present with or without hemoptysis and have diffuse airspace disease on the chest radiograph. The diffusing capacity for carbon monoxide is elevated. The diagnosis is made using bronchoscopy. The recovery of progressively bloodier aliquots on bronchoalveolar lavage from the affected subsegment suggests the presence of alveolar hemorrhage. Finding hemosiderin-laden macrophages implies more chronic alveolar hemorrhage from any one of a number of causes including DAH. Infection can complicate or masquerade as DAH and, therefore, appropriate cultures must be sent from the lavage fluid.

Supporting the hypothesis that this is an inflammatory disorder is the efficacy of corticosteroids (193). The dosage used is important. In one study, the mortality was lower in those patients who received high dosages of corticosteroids (197). The authors recommended a dosage of methylprednisolone of 120–250 mg every six hours for five days with a slow taper over two to four weeks. This treatment recommendation has not been prospectively validated.

Pulmonary edema. Pulmonary edema from cardiogenic and noncardiogenic factors frequently complicates BMT. During and after conditioning chemotherapy, these patients receive large amounts of fluids to avoid renal toxicity. The tremendous volume of some intravenous antibiotics exacerbates fluid overload. Some agents such as adriamycin and cyclophosphamide can be cardiotoxic (198). Other chemotherapeutic drugs have been associated with a pulmonary capillary leak syndrome. In short, these patients become volume overloaded with leaky capillaries and may have an inability to excrete this excess fluid by virtue of renal or cardiac impairment.

Careful monitoring of volume status is essential. Diuretics should be used aggressively in patients who are steadily gaining weight to avert pulmonary edema (198). Close attention should be paid to the patients' renal function with such therapy.

Malignancy With the increasing numbers of bone marrow transplants being performed for malignancies, recurrence in the chest is a concern. Primary lung neoplasms, such as bronchogenic carcinoma, and neoplasms with lung metastases, such as osteogenic sarcoma and Hodgkin's disease, can present as nodules or masses in BMT recipients (199–202). Secondary malignancies, including non-Hodgkin's lymphoma, leukemias, and solid tumors, must also be considered as BMT recipients are clearly at higher risk (203). Total body irradiation, acute GVHD, and antithymocyte globulin use are associated with a higher likelihood of developing a secondary malignancy.

Pulmonary Alveolar Proteinosis Pulmonary alveolar proteinosis can rarely cause respiratory failure in BMT recipients (204). Diffuse pulmonary infiltrates develop, typically prior to engraftment. Bronchoalveolar lavage is diagnostic showing a proteinaceous material, paradoxically composed primarily of phospholipids, which stains with periodic acid-Schiff. Although bronchoalveolar lavage is effective for primary or idiopathic alveolar proteinosis, the utility of this therapy for alveolar proteinosis in association with BMT is unclear.

Airway Disease

Bronchiolitis obliterans (BO). Bronchiolitis obliterans occurs in 3.9% to 5% of adults and 26% of children after BMT, primarily in those patients with allogeneic transplants and chronic GVHD (205–207). Patients with BO after BMT have a much higher mortality than patients without BO.

Unmasking of major histocompatibility class II antigens after BMT may lead to bronchial inflammation (208). Alternatively, such inflammation could potentially arise because of chronic aspiration or occult viral infection involving the airways (206). Risk factors for the development of BO include the presence of chronic GVHD, the use of methotrexate for GVHD prophylaxis, and increased age (208). Protective factors include the use of cyclosporin A (209). Notably, TBI does not predispose to this problem.

Patients with BO present three months or more after BMT (210). The clinical manifestations include dyspnea and wheeze and patchy areas of hypoattenuation and bronchial dilatation best seen on HRCT (211). Spirometry typically reveals an obstructive pattern. As mentioned, the majority of cases occur in allogeneic transplants although cases have been reported with autologous transplants. This finding supports the hypothesis that BO is multifactorial in etiology rather than just being a manifestation of GVHD.

The diagnosis is confirmed by transbronchial biopsy or an open or thoracoscopic lung biopsy. Sampling the lung tissue is also necessary to exclude infection, which frequently complicates the course of BO. The airways involved are the bronchioles, whose walls are infiltrated by lymphocytes. This entity has been distinguished from lymphocytic bronchitis, which affects the larger airways in a similar fashion and is felt by some to be a manifestation of chronic GVHD (212).

The treatment of BO following BMT is not uniform between institutions. One treatment protocol is given in Table 28.7 (208). For patients with progressive disease, lung transplantation should be considered early in the course of the disease (213,214). Interestingly, BO in the transplanted lung can recur, underscoring the similarities that exist

Table 28.7. Recommended Treatment Approach for Airflow Obstruction After Marrow Transplantation

1. Control any associated chronic GVHD with pharmacologic immunosuppression.
2. Prophylaxis for *Pneumocystic carinii* pneumonia during immunosuppression.
3. Treat intercurrent respiratory infection with broad spectrum antibiotics.
4. Augment low immunoglobulin levels by administration of intravenous immunoglobulin G.
5. Administer aerosolized adrenergic agents for symptomatic patients.
6. Prednisone (or its equivalent) in daily doses of 1–1.5 mg/kg (up to 100 mg/day) for four to six weeks.
7. Repeat chest roentgenograms and pulmonary function tests monthly.
8. If improvement is not noted within one month of corticosteroid therapy or deterioration continues during treatment, begin adjunctive immunosuppression with azathioprine (up to 3 mg/kg/day, 200 mg/day maximum).
9. Repeat diagnostic evaluation, including fiberoptic bronchoscopy with bronchoalveolar lavage, if clinical deterioration develops at any point in the treatment course.

Source: Reproduced by permission from Crawford SW, Clark JG. Bronchiolitis associated with bone marrow transplantation. Clin Chest Med 1993;14:747.

between BO in BMT recipients and lung transplant recipients (215).

Pulmonary Vascular Disease In addition to the endothelialitis observed in DAH, pulmonary embolism and pulmonary veno-occlusive disease constitute the other pulmonary vascular complications of BMT.

Venous thromboembolism. Pulmonary emboli in these patients can be marrow elements or thrombus. The former typically occurs with the infusion of donor marrow and consists of fat and bone spicules (216,217). These emboli are usually insignificant clinically.

Pulmonary thromboembolism, in contrast, is an infrequent yet potentially fatal problem (218). The source of venous thrombi are classically the lower extremities; however, in patients with vascular catheters the thrombi can occur in the upper extremities. Dyspnea, pleuritic chest pain, or hypoxemia with an unimpressive chest radiograph suggest the diagnosis, which is confirmed by ventilation–perfusion scanning or angiography. The treatment consists of anticoagulation, thrombolysis, or a filter proximal to the source of the embolus. Thrombolysis in the setting of thrombocytopenia can occasionally cause fatal hemorrhage (219).

Pulmonary veno-occlusive disease. Pulmonary veno-occlusive disease is an extremely rare complication of BMT (220). Chemotherapy and radiation may be etiologic factors (221). The clinical exam suggests the presence of pulmonary hypertension. The diagnosis is confirmed by an open or thoracoscopic lung biopsy showing fibrous plugging of the small venules. In one small series, corticosteroid treatment was effective (222).

INFECTIOUS PULMONARY CONSIDERATIONS OF ORGAN TRANSPLANTATION

Epidemiology of Pulmonary Infections in Organ Transplantation

The pulmonary infections affecting organ transplant recipients are often protean in their manifestations and can be exceedingly difficult to diagnose and to treat. Because these patients are immunosuppressed, the classic signs of a respiratory infection such as sputum production and fever may be absent. The chest radiograph can even be normal in the early stages of a pneumonia in this population, particularly in neutropenic patients.

The frequency of pulmonary infections after organ transplantation is difficult to determine. Studies assessing the epidemiology of pulmonary infections even within specific organ transplant recipients differ in the case definitions of pneumonia used, the methods by which a pneumonia is confirmed, the immunosuppressive regimens, the use of prophylactic antimicrobials, and the length of follow-up. Of course, differences between different organ transplant recipients are expected given the differences in operative technique and in the subsequent management in terms of immunosuppression and prophylaxis of infections. The epidemiologic differences in the frequency and outcome of pneumonia in these groups is summarized in Table 28.8.

There are several important host factors that determine a patient's likelihood of developing a pulmonary infection (Table 28.9). Considerable overlap exists among these different risk factors. For example, the extent of immunosuppression depends in large part on the time from transplantation. In the initial period following solid organ transplantation, the doses of immunosuppressives are high to avoid acute cellular rejection. Similarly, the doses of immunosuppressives are increased during periods of acute rejection or acute GVHD.

Studies examining risk factors for pneumonias in organ transplant recipients are plagued by this inability to clearly distinguish these different issues. Rather than discussing each risk factor in detail, therefore, this section is devoted to identifying clinically useful temporal trends that emerge in the development of pulmonary infections in this heterogeneous population. Thereafter, specific pathogens are discussed under the headings of bacterial, viral, fungal, and parasitic infections. Salient differences in the epidemiology, presentation, treatment, and prophylaxis of these infections between organ transplant recipients will be emphasized. Cytomegalovirus (CMV) is considered to be the most common pathogen responsible for pneumonia in organ transplant recipients and is discussed in detail (see also Chapter 36).

Table 28.8. Frequency and Mortality of Pneumonia in Transplant Patients*

Transplant Group	Frequency	Mortality	References
LT	15–44%	28–53%	235, 241, 242, 352
RT	7–24%	7–21%	86, 353
CT	14–24%	11–42%	155, 237, 238
BMT	4–25%	50–75%	239, 243, 275

* Length of follow-up, method of diagnosis, immunosuppression, and prophylaxis for infections were different among studies.

Table 28.9. Epidemiologic Factors Important in the Development of Pneumonia in Transplant Patients

Time from transplantation
Extent of immunosuppression
Type of immunosuppression
Presence or absence of rejection or GVHD
Presence or absence of underlying pulmonary disease or previous pulmonary infections
Mental status of the patient as it relates to the risk of aspiration
Use of specific antimicrobial prophylaxis
Immunization history of the patient
Patient's environment (the home or the hospital) and the geographic location
Serologic status of the donor and recipient for CMV

Evolution of Pulmonary Infections After Solid Organ and Bone Marrow Transplantation

Infections following solid organ transplantation occur with a predictable temporal sequence because of alterations in host defense, initially because of the surgery and later because of immunosuppression. In order to understand the evolution of pulmonary infections after organ transplantation, one must appreciate the changes in the immune system that occur both locally in the lungs and systemically.

The various lineages of immune cells have different fates following organ transplantation. Neutrophil function is not significantly impaired except in BMT recipients. These patients become profoundly neutropenic prior to engraftment, which normally takes three to four weeks. Lymphocyte and humoral abnormalities, in contrast, occur uniformly in all organ transplant recipients, although the duration of such abnormalities varies. There is a lowering of the CD4:CD8 ratio and a decrease in immunoglobulin synthesis both in the lungs and elsewhere (223). Bronchoalveolar lavage shows a lymphocytosis with a preponderance of CD8 and CD16 lymphocytes (224).

After solid organ transplantation, cellular and humoral immunity eventually recovers to near normal levels in the majority of patients. A subset of patients can, however, acquire a combined variable hypogammaglobulinemia perhaps secondary to the administration of azathioprine (225). This problem has, thus far, been reported in renal transplant recipients. Recurrent bacterial infections in this setting should prompt the clinician to measure antibody titers, which, if low, warrant a trial of intravenous immunoglobulin.

Bone marrow transplant recipients follow the same time frame for reconstruction of the immune system in general. The presence of chronic GVHD can profoundly impede this recovery in several different ways. First, cellular and humoral immunity can remain persistently abnormal in patients with this complication. As in the case of solid organ transplantation, hypogammaglobulinemic patients benefit from immunoglobulin supplementation. Second, chronic GVHD causes splenic dysfunction in the presence of an intact spleen, a condition known as *functional asplenia* (226). Because of these abnormalities, patients with chronic GVHD are particularly susceptible to infections with encapsulated organisms such as *Streptococcus pneumoniae* (227,228).

In the immediate postoperative period, patients acquire nosocomial infections, primarily with gram-positive and gram-negative bacteria aerobic. Patients aspirating before or after the procedure are at risk for anaerobic pulmonary infections as well.

In solid organ transplantation, specific prophylactic strategies are frequently employed that decrease the risk of bacterial infections. Prophylactic antibiotics are given preoperatively and postoperatively and probably diminish the risk of bacterial pneumonia while administered. In LT recipients, the use of selective bowel decontamination effectively eliminates colonization with *Candida* and with aerobic gram-negative pathogens. As most centers now employ selective bowel decontamination with enteral antibiotics and antifungals prior to liver transplantation, infection with aerobic gram-positive bacteria predominates in the early post-transplant period (229). Despite the reduction in gram-negative and fungal infections, selective bowel decontamination has not been convincingly shown to decrease systemic endotoxemia nor mortality in this population (230,231). Selective bowel decontamination is not used in cardiac or renal transplant recipients.

Bone marrow transplant recipients are susceptible to the same nosocomial pathogens, especially prior to engraftment. During the neutropenic period, they are highly susceptible to both bacterial and fungal pathogens. Two strategies have been used to decrease the incidence of such infections: 1) nonselective decontamination of the skin and mucous membranes with topical or nonabsorbable enteral antibiotics, or 2) selective inhibition of the aerobic gut flora with absorbable enteral antibiotics. The efficacy of the latter approach was affirmed in a recent study in which the use of ciprofloxacin prophylactically significantly reduced the incidence of bacterial infections (232). Unlike trimethoprim-sulfamethoxazole, which has also been used for this purpose, ciprofloxacin does not increase the duration of neutropenia. In spite of prophylaxis, bacterial pneumonia still poses a danger for these patients, although the aggressive use of broad spectrum antibiotics at the first febrile episode has likely diminished the morbidity and mortality from bacterial pneumonia. Interestingly, recent evidence suggests that the use of granulocyte macrophage colony-stimulating factor (GM-CSF) does not result in an improved outcome (233).

The period from 30 days to 6 months after transplantation is characterized by pulmonary infections with opportunistic pathogens because immunosuppression is still maintained at a relatively high level (248). Patients are at risk for viral infections, particularly with the herpes virus group and opportunistic fungi and bacteria. Many of these infections such as *Pneumocystis carinii* and *Nocardia* are effectively prevented by the use of trimethoprim-sulfamethoxazole. CMV is the most frequently isolated organism and is believed to be immunomodulating in itself, predisposing to other infections. Many strategies have been proposed to diminish the likelihood of developing CMV pneumonia and these are discussed below in the section on CMV.

After six months, community acquired organisms become more significant pathogens as the immune system begins to reconstitute. Influenza, the endemic fungi, and bacterial pathogens prevalent in the community cause pulmonary disease (234). The clinician must remember that intensification of immunosuppression, particularly with cytolytic therapy, makes the patient once again susceptible to opportunistic pathogens. Reinstitution of prophylaxis for CMV and for *Pnemocystis carinii* pneumonia (PCP) should be considered in susceptible patients.

Bacterial Infections

In this section, the nosocomial pulmonary infections developing immediately after transplantation are discussed first. Then the opportunistic bacteria that typically develop one to six months following transplantation are considered. Finally, the community acquired bacteria that are responsible for many bacterial infections six months or more after transplantation are discussed.

Immediately following organ transplantation, patients are at risk for developing nosocomial pneumonias. The most frequently identified pathogens are *Staphylococcus aureus* and aerobic gram-negative rods (235–239). *Legionella* has, likewise, been documented in hospital outbreaks and should be considered in the differential diagnosis. Anaerobic infections should be suspected in a patient with a history suggestive of aspiration. Risk factors for the development of nosocomial pneumonia vary across transplant groups. The following factors are associated with the development of nosocomial pneumonia: the use of high-dose corticosteroids, azathioprine rather than cyclosporine-based immunosuppression, a neutrophilic alveolitis perhaps from subclinical aspiration before transplant, reintubation following transplant, and preoperative pulmonary infarction (137,238,240–242). BMT recipients with prolonged neutropenia and mucositis are at higher risk as are LT recipients with severe liver disease as assessed by the Child-Pugh score before transplant or recurrent hepatitis C infections after transplant (242).

Fever and sputum production, if present, support the diagnosis; however, the absence of these symptoms does not exclude a bacterial pulmonary infection. This caveat is particularly important in BMT recipients who are neutropenic in the first few weeks after transplantation. Focal or diffuse infiltrates are present, most often assuming an alveolar pattern; however, cavitation is not infrequent. Multiple cavitary lesions in a patient with an indwelling catheter should raise the possibility of septic emboli to the lungs. Pleural effusions occurring in the presence of an infiltrate mandate sampling of the fluid to exclude an empyema. The diagnosis of nosocomial pneumonia is often apparent and empiric antibiotics and sputum cultures are reasonable initial steps. Failure to improve rapidly mandates bronchoscopy to exclude other nonbacterial infections (243). The treatment consists of antibiotics directed against the pathogen for at least two weeks. Profoundly immunosuppressed or neutropenic patients may need to have antibiotics continued until these abnormalities resolve.

From one to six months after transplantation and during periods of heightened immunosuppression, opportunistic bacteria can cause fulminant pulmonary disease. Impaired T-cell function during these periods predisposes to these infections. The clinician must be particularly aware of the possibility of the following organisms that have a propensity to infect immunocompromised patients: *Legionella*, *Bartonella*, *Nocardia*, *Rhodococcus*, and *Mycobacteria*.

Patients having organ transplantation are particularly susceptible to *Legionella* pneumonia, most often caused by *Legionella pneumophila* (244). The organism is water borne and can be aerosolized by air conditioners and water heaters. Once inhaled into the lungs, the bacteria replicates in alveolar macrophages. Clues to the diagnosis include the presence of encephalopathy, relative bradycardia with fever, diarrhea, hepatic dysfunction, and hyponatremia (245). Rapidly progressive alveolar infiltrates and lobar consolidation, at times cavitary, can develop and culminate in respiratory failure. The organism is detected by direct fluorescent antibody staining or culture of respiratory secretions. The legionella urinary antigen is a very sensitive test for the detection of *Legionella pneumophila* serogroup 1 and remains positive despite treatment for weeks (245). Serologic evaluation using acute and convalescent titers can confirm the diagnosis in retrospect, but is of little value in managing the patient. Coinfection with other organisms is not uncommon and should be considered in all cases (246). The mainstay of therapy is erythromycin with or without rifampin for synergy for three weeks. Both drugs affect the metabolism of cyclosporine and, therefore, levels need to be monitored carefully. Routine culture of the water supply in hospitals performing organ transplantation is prudent to detect *Legionella* because various disinfection strategies do exist (245).

Bartonella hensalae can cause nodular infiltrates, pleural effusions, mediastinal adenopathy and endobronchial lesions (247) in immunocompromised hosts. A recent exposure to cats, which can transmit the bacteria, suggests the diagnosis. Culturing the organism can be difficult and, therefore, the laboratory needs to be alerted to the possibility of this infection. Treatment consists of doxycycline, often for a period of several weeks.

Nocardia is a filamentous gram-positive, weakly acid fast organism that is typically found in the soil. *Nocardia asteroides* is responsible for most nocardial disease observed in the transplant patient. Metastatic infection to the skin and nervous system is common. Findings in the chest include peripheral nodules that can cavitate, extend to the pleura, or invade the chest wall (248). The organism is difficult to culture and the laboratory should be notified if the diagnosis is suspected. Trimethoprim-sulfamethoxazole is effective prophylaxis against nocardial infection and accounts for the rarity with which nocardial disease is now observed in the transplant population. In higher doses, trimethoprim-sulfamethoxazole is also the recommended treatment. Relapses are frequent and, therefore, high-dose therapy should be continued for at least one year and prophylaxis should be given indefinitely to these individuals (249–251).

Rhodococcus equi is a common pathogen in the acquired immunodeficiency syndrome and has recently been reported in a CT recipient (Fig. 28.6) (252). The organism is a gram-positive rod that, like *Nocardia*, is weakly acid fast. An exposure to farm animals is present in the majority of cases. Nodular infiltrates, with or without cavitation, are typical. The organism is readily cultured from respiratory secretions.

A

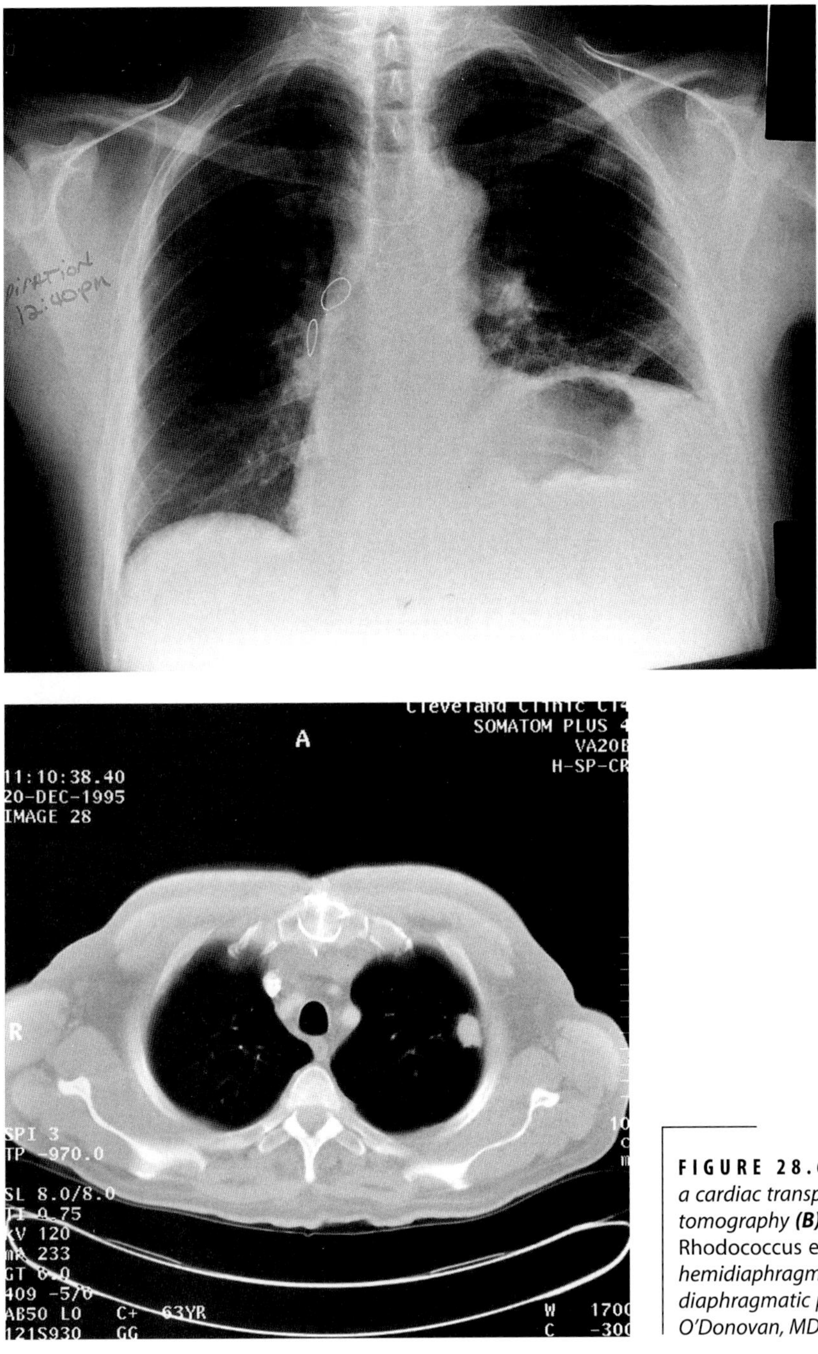

B

FIGURE 28.6. *A nodular lesion, seen in the left upper lobe of a cardiac transplant recipient on radiography* ***(A)*** *and computed tomography* ***(B)*** *of the chest, was confirmed by biopsy to represent* Rhodococcus equi. *In addition, the patient has an elevated left hemidiaphragm and linear atelectasis of the left lower lobe from diaphragmatic paresis postoperatively. (Photographs courtesy of P.B. O'Donovan, MD, Cleveland Clinic Foundation.)*

An extended duration of therapy, up to six months, is required with at least two lipophilic antibiotics such as vancomycin and ciprofloxacin.

Disease with *Mycobacterium tuberculosis* occurs with greater frequency in this population although the incidence will depend upon the type of transplant and the prevalence of tuberculosis in the community. Liver and renal transplant recipients are especially prone to these infections. The prevalence in RT recipients can vary from 0.5% in North America to 21.0% in India (253,254). Atypical mycobacteria only rarely cause lung disease in transplant patients and will not specifically be discussed (255,256).

Many patients prior to organ transplantation will have a positive Mantoux test (257). Generally, isoniazid should be administered to these patients to avoid reactivation of the organism after transplantation. This recommendation is most controversial in LT recipients because they may be at greater risk for isoniazid-induced hepatotoxicity and because they have a generally favorable response to multidrug therapy for tuberculosis if required (258). Nevertheless, prophylaxis of patients with a positive Mantoux test with close monitoring of liver function seems prudent (259).

The radiographic features of pulmonary tuberculosis are variable. Upper lung zone consolidation is the most frequent radiographic presentation although a miliary pattern, nodules, pleural effusions, and mediastinal adenopathy may be seen (260). Disseminated disease occurs in 40% of cases (261,262). The diagnosis is confirmed by examination of expectorated sputum, bronchoscopy, or rarely percutaneous fine-needle aspiration. Given the increasing prevalence of multidrug-resistant tuberculosis, therapy for active tuberculosis should be initiated with a four-drug regimen consisting of isoniazid, rifampin, ethambutol, and pyrazinamide until the drug susceptibilities of the organism are known (263). Treatment may be complicated by the interaction of rifampin and isoniazid with cyclosporine (264,265). Notably, although cyclosporine levels diminish, the concentrations of these antituberculous drugs do not change significantly. Agents such as streptomycin and ethambutol may be useful agents as they do not interfere with the cytochrome P450 system (266). Despite the generally favorable response to treatment observed in LT recipients, the mortality associated with tuberculosis RT recipients despite antibiotics remains high (267).

With the gradual re-establishment of host immunity, community-acquired organisms tend to cause the majority of sinopulmonary disease. Hypogammaglobulinemia and functional asplenia, in BMT recipients, place these patients at risk for bacterial infections. The use of trimethoprim-sulfamethoxazole likely reduces the incidence of otherwise common pathogens in the community such as *Streptococcus pneumoniae* and *Haemophilus influenzae*. Vaccinations against both *Streptococcus pneumoniae* and *Haemophilus influenzae* type B should be offered to these patients although subsequent antibody titers may be variable (268–270). Other organisms that are prevalent in the community, however, such as *Legionella*, *Mycoplasma*, and *Chlamydia TWAR* are not prevented by the use of this agent. The clinical and radiographic presentation of these infections is highly variable and respiratory cultures are often unrevealing. Empiric therapy with antimicrobial agents effective against typical and atypical pathogens is essential and effective in the majority of patients.

Viral Infections

Cytomegalovirus is the single most important pathogen causing pneumonia in transplant recipients. Infection most commonly occurs because of transmission of the virus in the allograft or because of reactivation of latent virus in a previously infected recipient. Disease produced by transmission of the virus is most severe in patients who are seronegative for CMV. Less severe disease results from viral transmission to a seropositive host or from viral reactivation. Blood transfusions represent another source for the transmission of CMV.

Clinical disease produced by CMV reflects both infection and immunologic injury elicited by the virus (271). Interleukin-2–mediated cytotoxic T-cell activity in the bone marrow is increased (272). These natural killer cells, once activated, migrate to the lung tissue where they cause damage to both infected and noninfected lung parenchyma. Local stimulation of cytotoxic T-cells in the lungs themselves is unlikely given the absence of interferon-alpha or interleukin-2 in bronchoalveolar lavage fluid (273).

The incidence of CMV pneumonia differs between transplant groups and, within these groups, varies depending upon the serologic status of the donor and the recipient and the use of prophylaxis (Table 28.10) (274–278). CMV pneumonia is most common in CT and BMT recipients and is associated with a high mortality in these groups. The median time to the development of CMV pneumonia is 60 days after transplantation, but cases even prior to engraftment have been reported in BMT recipients (279). The risk factors for CMV pneumonia are summarized in Table 28.11 (280,281).

The radiographic picture of CMV pneumonia is consistent throughout the different transplant groups (Fig. 28.7). Reticular or nodular infiltrates are most commonly seen, however, a normal chest radiograph does not exclude the diagnosis (282). Gallium scanning or indium scanning may be useful in the latter setting to confirm lung involvement.

The diagnosis of CMV pneumonia is made by detecting or culturing CMV from respiratory secretions or blood and by demonstrating tissue invasion by CMV. Bronchoscopy

Table 28.10. Frequency of CMV Pneumonia in Transplant Recipients in the Absence of Prophylaxis

Transplant	Frequency	References
LT	2–5%	235, 236, 278
RT	5–8%	297, 353
CT	10–16%	238, 277
BMT—Allogeneic	3.3%	274
BMT—Autologous	12–13%	274

Table 28.11. Risk Factors for the Development of CMV Pneumonia in Transplant Recipients

Seropositivity of recipient
Seropositivity of donor
CMV excretors
Increased age
OKT-3
Anti-lymphocyte globulin (ALG)
Transfusions
Allogeneic BMT
Graft-versus-host disease
T-cell–depleted marrow infusion
Total body irradiation

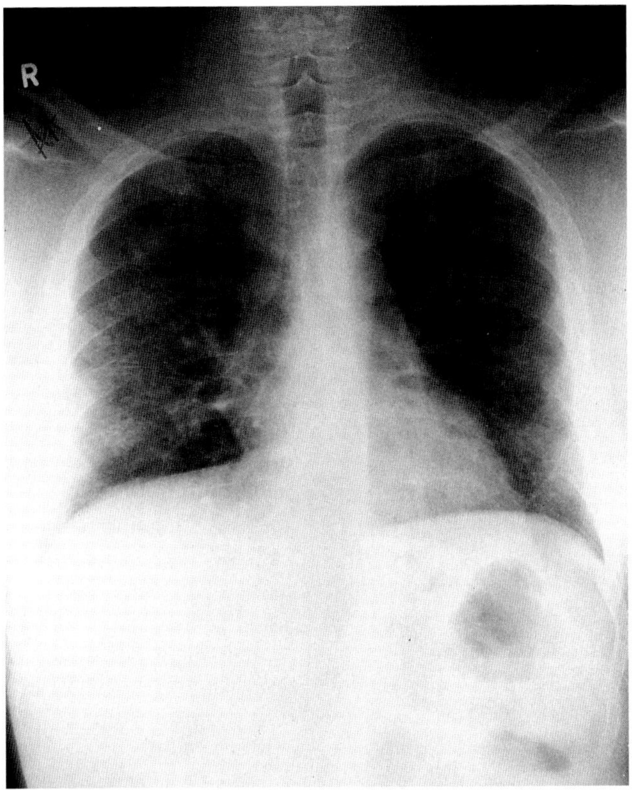

FIGURE 28.7. *Diffuse reticulonodular infiltrates in a renal transplant recipient with CMV infection. (Photograph courtesy of P.B. O'Donovan, MD, Cleveland Clinic Foundation.)*

with bronchoalveolar lavage and transbronchial biopsies suffices most of the time; however, occasionally open or thoracoscopic lung biopsy is required.

The virus is detected in bronchoalveolar lavage specimens or from blood by a variety of techniques. The fluid can be used to culture cells that, when infected, show characteristic cytopathic changes after two to three weeks of growth. The shell vial technique uses a monoclonal antibody to an early antigen to confirm the presence of CMV after only 16 hours of incubation (283). Antigen detection of the p65 antigen expressed in infected peripheral leukocytes using specific antibodies has been used and appears more sensitive than the shell vial assay to detect asymptomatic CMV excretion (284). The polymerase chain reaction (PCR) is the most sensitive modality but only indicates the presence of the organism and not whether it is causing disease. The specificity is enhanced when combined with CMV immunostaining of alveolar cells obtained on bronchoalveolar lavage. The use of both techniques together has a sensitivity and specificity approaching 100% for the diagnosis of CMV pneumonia (285). PCR has been employed, similarly, to detect otherwise occult CMV viremia, which is often a harbinger of pneumonia (286,287). The use of CMV-specific mouse monoclonal antibodies and immunomagnetic beads conjugated with sheep antimouse IgG offers another rapid technique for the detection of CMV with a reported sensitivity of 100% and a specificity of 92% (288). Bronchoalveolar lavage samples with CMV demonstrate rosettes around the organisms under light microscopy using this technique.

Tissue invasion is suggested by the presence of infected alveolar cells on lavage or by finding characteristic histopathology on lung biopsy. Bronchoalveolar lavage is used to look for the characteristic intranuclear or intracytoplasmic inclusions in alveolar cells on cytologic examination. As mentioned, alveolar cell immunostaining can be a useful adjunct although it is not widely available. Lung biopsy specimens show interstitial pneumonitis or, less commonly, diffuse alveolar damage with inclusion bodies. The clinician should remember that CMV pneumonia is heterogeneous in its distribution and, therefore, sampling errors can occur leading to falsely negative biopsies.

Much interest has focused on the use of these tests to predict which patients are at high likelihood of developing CMV pneumonia. Effective prophylaxis is needed in these patients because of the high mortality associated with CMV pneumonia despite treatment. The two most powerful predictors of subsequent CMV pneumonia are the presence of viremia and the excretion of CMV in respiratory secretions (289,290).

Although prophylaxis is used with a number of different strategies and agents, who should receive prophylaxis and the duration of therapy necessary are still unclear. Seronegative transplant recipients should receive CMV-negative blood transfusions or should have transfusions using a leukocyte filter. Studies in BMT recipients have suggested that prophylactic ganciclovir given to asymptomatic excretors of CMV from any site after transplantation or in bronchoalveolar lavage fluid at day 35 after transplant is associated with a reduced incidence of CMV pneumonia and a reduced mortality (290,291). Data in other transplant groups, with the exception of lung transplant, is not as convincing. Intravenous acyclovir administered to allogeneic BMT patients seems to decrease the incidence of CMV infection, but interestingly this salutary effect is not observed in autologous BMT recipients (292,293). Acyclovir seems to decrease the likelihood of CMV infection in RT as well (294). Intravenous immunoglobulin has, similarly, decreased the incidence and severity of CMV associated interstitial pneumonitis in BMT (295,296). Human interferon seems to delay the onset of CMV excretion, but does little to decrease the overall incidence of CMV infection (297).

The treatment of CMV pneumonia consists of intravenous ganciclovir with or without standard immunoglobulin (298–300). BMT recipients should receive both agents as survival is clearly improved (301). The data supporting the use of both agents are less convincing in other transplant patients and, therefore, those patients should be initially treated with ganciclovir alone (302). Despite treatment, the survival rate in BMT recipients is 31% to 35% and underscores the need for effective prophylactic strategies. Foscarnet is an option for patients unable to tolerate ganciclovir or for ganciclovir-resistant strains of CMV (303). In treating these patients, the clinician must bear in mind that other organisms such as *Pneumocystis* and *Aspergillus* can coinfect with CMV.

In addition to CMV, the other herpes viruses including the Epstein-Barr virus, varicella zoster, herpes simplex types 1 and 2, and the human herpes viruses type 6 cause pulmonary disease in transplant patients. The role of the Epstein-Barr virus in the pathogenesis of post-transplant lymphoproliferative disease has been discussed in the section on cardiac transplantation. Herpes simplex 1 or 2 and varicella causes hemorrhagic tracheobronchitis or pneumonia. Mucocutaneous vesicles in the mouth, genitals, or on the skin suggest the diagnosis. Acyclovir is used for the treatment and prophylaxis of these infections (304). Human herpes virus 6 may represent a previously unrecognized cause of interstitial pneumonia. This virus causes fevers and rashes in over 90% of children, who thereafter acquire antibodies directed against it (187). Viral DNA was discovered by PCR in high concentrations in patients with interstitial pneumonitis thought initially to be idiopathic.

Respiratory syncytial virus (RSV) has been associated with upper and lower respiratory tract disease in transplant recipients and can cause outbreaks of infection (305,306). Pneumonia caused by RSV carries a 78% mortality and presents most commonly as bilateral interstitial infiltrates (306). The presence of otitis and sinusitis can help in differentiating this entity from CMV (307). The virus can be isolated from nasopharyngeal swabs or respiratory secretions. Early treatment with ribavirin can be beneficial (306,308). Cross-transmission of the organism between patients can be avoided through the use of stringent hand-washing, gloves, and masks and gowns (307).

Parainfluenza, usually type 3, occurs in 2% to 3% of BMT recipients (309,310). Pneumonia caused by this agent is associated with a 50% mortality. Like RSV, upper respiratory tract involvement is prominent. Although ribavirin has been used for this infection, its efficacy has not been established (310).

Adenoviral infections have been reported to occur in 4.9% and 10% of BMT recipients and LT recipients, respectively (311,312). Infection may occur by reactivation of latent virus or by de novo infection. Elevated liver enzymes are seen in the majority of infected patients; however, most of them also have chronic GVHD (311). Pneumonia is the most serious consequence of infection. On lung biopsy, characteristic histopathology in the form of "smudge cells" or intranuclear inclusions may be present. PCR and in situ hybridization offer more sensitive means of diagnosis, however; treatment is currently supportive (313).

Influenza pneumonia can be life threatening in immunocompromised patients (314). Patients present with upper respiratory tract symptoms and constitutional symptoms including myalgias and arthralgias. Amantadine given within 48 to 72 hours can shorten the course of pneumonia caused by influenza A. Immunization should be provided yearly to all transplant patients. Antibody titers achieve protective levels for influenza A and B in the majority of patients (315).

Fungal Infections

PCP occurs in 5% to 20% of transplant recipients who do not receive prophylaxis with trimethoprim-sulfamethoxazole, dapsone, or pentamidine (316–318). Infection is very unlikely in patients receiving adequate prophylaxis, although the length of such prophylaxis that is required is unclear (319–323). The organism can reactivate or be transmitted by droplet spread (324,325). The clinical presentation is characterized by rapidly progressive diffuse infiltrates and hypoxemia (Fig. 28.8) (326). A normal chest radiograph does not exclude the diagnosis (327); radionuclide scanning can assist in this setting followed by bronchoscopy if there is increased tracer uptake in the lungs.

The organism can be recovered in induced sputum or bronchoalveolar lavage fluid using the silver-methenamine stain. Because these patients may not have a large load of organisms, transbronchial biopsies may need to be performed to increase the diagnostic yield of bronchoscopy. The use of bronchoalveolar lavage solely will miss 15% of cases of PCP (328). Coinfection with other viral pathogens is not uncommon (329).

Treatment consists of intravenous trimethoprim-sulfamethoxazole or pentamidine and corticosteroids if the alveolar-arterial oxygen gradient exceeds 35 mm Hg or if the PaO_2 is less than 70 mm Hg (330). The recommendation for steroid treatment is derived from studies performed in patients infected with the human immunodeficiency virus rather than transplant patients, most of whom are on corticosteroids anyway (331).

Pulmonary infection with *Aspergillus*, a ubiquitous dimorphic fungus, occurs uncommonly but carries an extremely high mortality (332). Invasive aspergillosis occurs in 5.6% of BMT recipients and is associated with a mortality of 82% (333). Hemoptysis and high fevers are characteristic but not always present. Both the larger cartilaginous airway and the pulmonary parenchyma can be involved (334,335). Radiographically, the *halo sign* is seen in the neutropenic period after BMT and refers to an area or halo of intermediate density surrounding a focal infiltrate. With resolution of the neutropenia, the infiltrate retracts and an area of hyperlucency forms, which is referred to as the *air crescent sign* (336). Cavitation may be seen at this time. Single or multiple nodules are present typically, although areas of pulmonary infarction can occur because the organism is angioinvasive (Fig. 28.9).

Other opportunistic fungi such as *Mucor* and *Dactylaria* need to be considered in the differential diagnosis (Fig. 28.10). Infection with the latter has only recently been described in a CT recipient (337). *Mucormycosis*, like

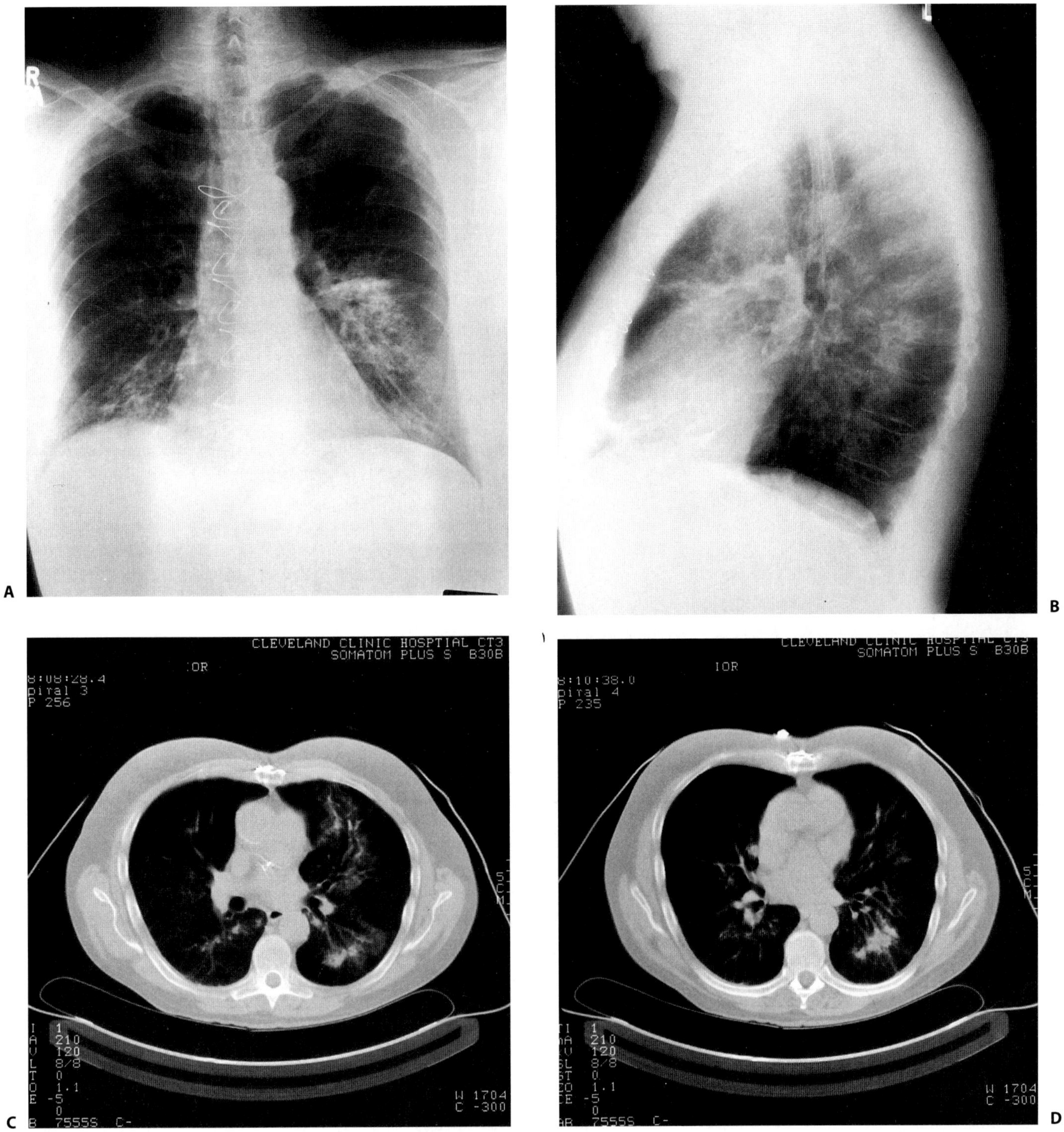

FIGURE 28.8. *Bilateral perihilar and lower lobe alveolar infiltrates in a cardiac transplant recipient from* Pneumocystis carinii *on chest radiograph PA and lateral projections* ***(A,B)****. The CT scan images* ***(C,D)*** *show clear air bronchograms and nodularity or coalescence of the infiltrate. (Photographs courtesy of L.S. Goldstein, MD, Cleveland Clinic Foundation.)*

Aspergillus, is angioinvasive and is associated with a high mortality.

Establishing a diagnosis of invasive aspergillosis can be difficult. Bronchoscopy with a bronchoalveolar lavage and biopsies are often used initially. Percutaneous fine-needle aspiration has been used successfully to diagnose *Aspergillus* infection (338). Occasionally, an open or thoracoscopic biopsy is needed to demonstrate tissue invasion. Present methods of detection of the organism are sensitive; however, demonstrating that the organism is causing invasive disease

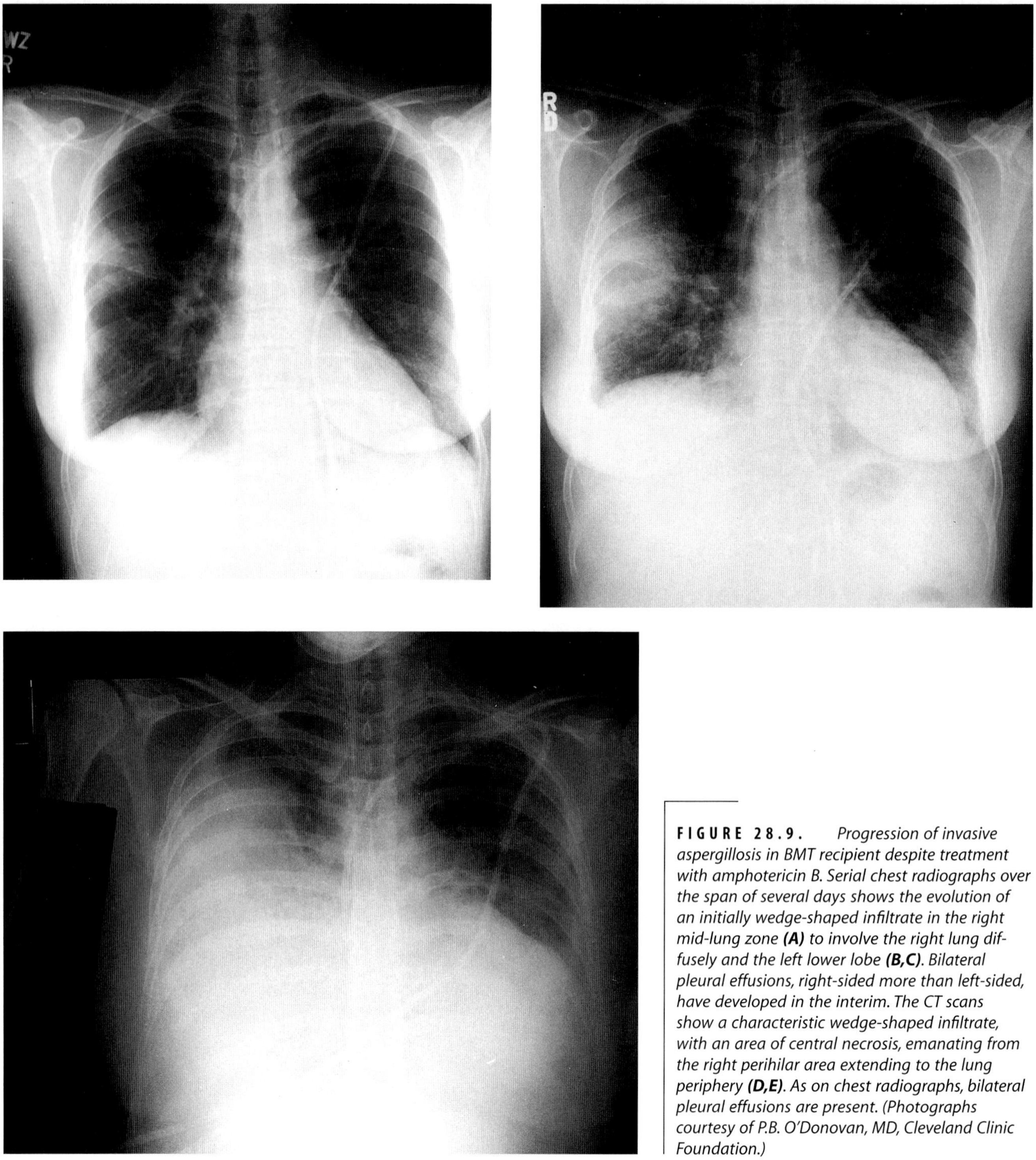

A B C

FIGURE 28.9. *Progression of invasive aspergillosis in BMT recipient despite treatment with amphotericin B. Serial chest radiographs over the span of several days shows the evolution of an initially wedge-shaped infiltrate in the right mid-lung zone* ***(A)*** *to involve the right lung diffusely and the left lower lobe* ***(B,C)****. Bilateral pleural effusions, right-sided more than left-sided, have developed in the interim. The CT scans show a characteristic wedge-shaped infiltrate, with an area of central necrosis, emanating from the right perihilar area extending to the lung periphery* ***(D,E)****. As on chest radiographs, bilateral pleural effusions are present. (Photographs courtesy of P.B. O'Donovan, MD, Cleveland Clinic Foundation.)*

is problematic. Unfortunately, many patients still have the diagnosis confirmed definitively only at autopsy (333).

The finding of *Aspergillus* species in respiratory secretions on sputum analysis or bronchoalveolar lavage in an organ transplant recipient with an unexplained infiltrate mandates treatment with amphotericin B (339). Itraconazole has been used for the treatment of invasive aspergillosis; however, amphotericin B intravenously remains the mainstay of therapy (340). Resection should be considered for focal infiltrates that fails to clear with systemic antifungals (341–343).

Because of the high mortality associated with this infection, many prophylactic measures have been attempted. Inhaled amphotericin B, low-dose intravenous amphotericin

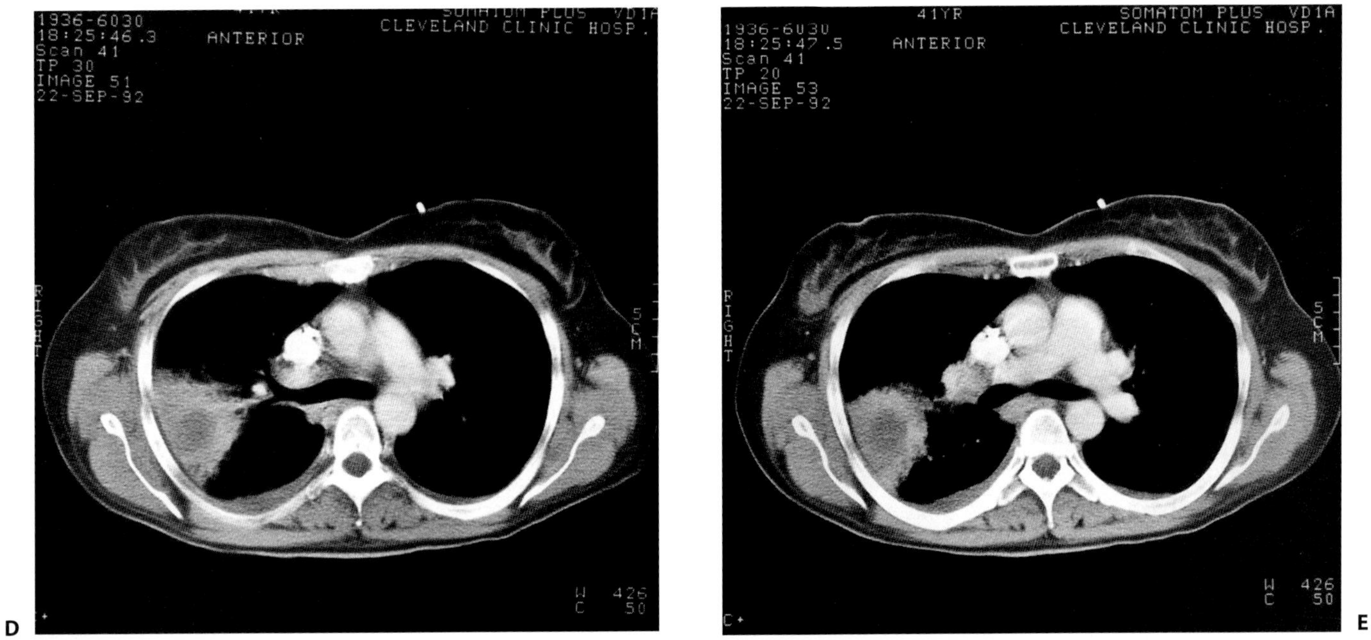

FIGURE 28.9. *Continued*

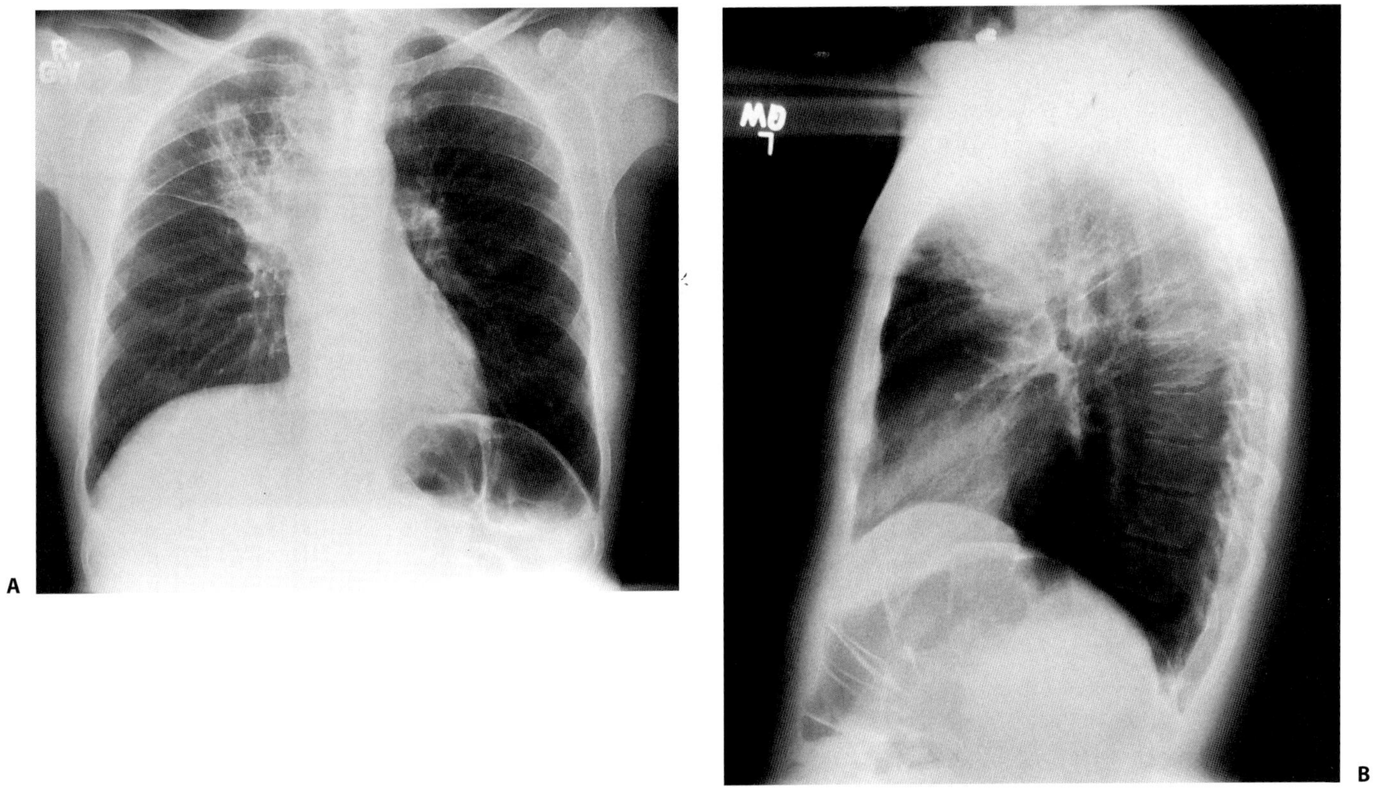

FIGURE 28.10. *A right upper lobe infiltrate is present with volume loss of the right upper lobe in a renal transplant recipient* ***(A,B)****. CT images show an infiltrate in the right upper lobe with rapid tapering of the bronchus to the anterior segment, suggesting the presence of an endobronchial lesion* ***(C,D)****. Bronchoscopy showed a markedly inflamed and narrowed right upper lobe orifice with endobronchial biopsies and washings positive for* Mucor *species. In addition to amphotericin B treatment, surgical resection of the right upper lobe was undertaken; however, a pneumonectomy had to be performed because the infection was encasing the right pulmonary artery. The patient died postoperatively. (Photographs courtesy of L.S. Goldstein, MD, Cleveland Clinic Foundation.)*

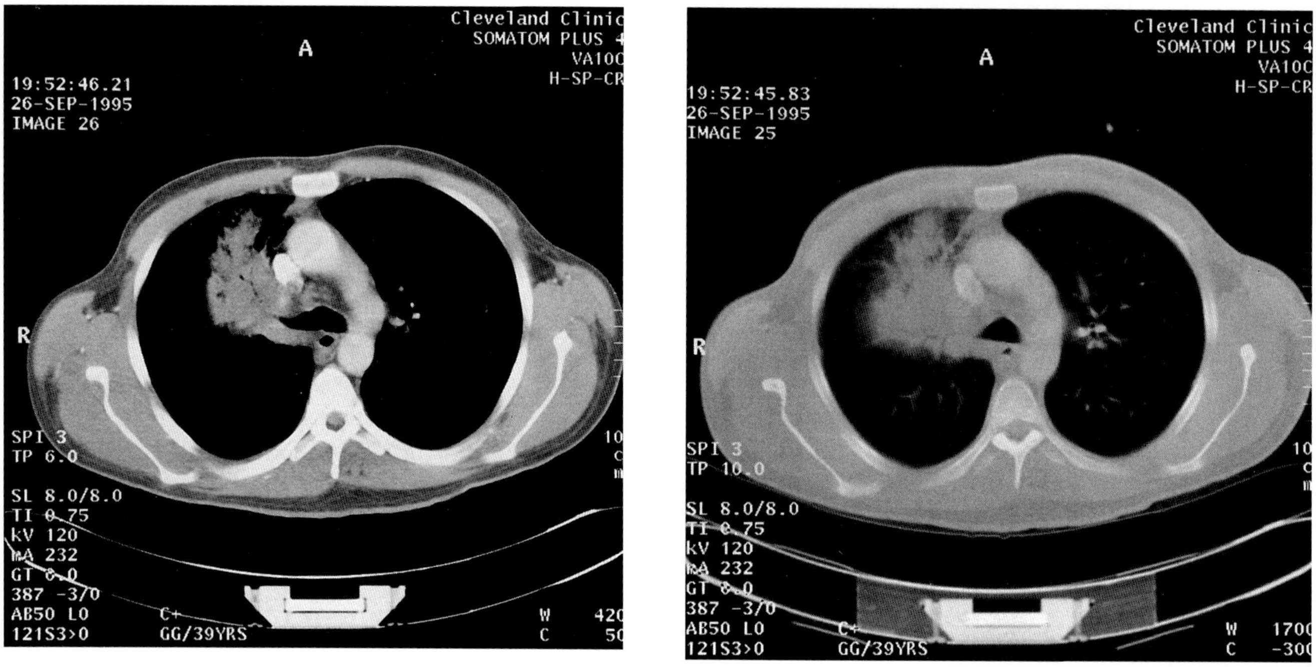

C D

FIGURE 28.10. *Continued*

B, or itraconazole can be used for prophylaxis. Precise recommendations regarding the optimal agent and the indications, however, are still evolving (345,346).

Fungi such as *Histoplasma*, *Coccidioides*, or *Blastomyces* may reactivate or cause primary disease in transplant recipients and should be considered in areas where they are endemic (346). The use of corticosteroids and other immunosuppressants is the major predisposing factor. Nodular or interstitial infiltrates are observed. Therapy consists of amphotericin B or one of the azole antifungals depending upon the severity of the disease.

Parasitic Infections

Parasitic disease need to be entertained in patients having LT for Echinococcal infestation of the liver (347). Parasitic recurrence likely occurs from microscopic subdiaphragmatic foci that can subsequently invade the right lower lobe and the liver. IgG to *Echinococcus granulosus* antigen extract is a useful marker of disease.

Pneumonia caused by *Toxoplasma gondii* is seen most commonly in CT recipients by transmission of the organism in the donor heart in infected myocytes. Infected blood products can also transmit the organism or reactivation disease can occur in patients with prior infections. Disseminated disease is common in seronegative patients who become infected (348). The chest radiograph shows diffuse interstitial infiltrates most commonly. Bronchoalveolar lavage demonstrating trophozoites, cysts, or pseudocysts is diagnostic, although a lung biopsy may be required in some cases. Despite antiparasitic treatment, usually with pyrimethamine and sulfadiazine, the mortality is high (349). Prophylactic therapy with pyrimethamine and folic acid should be considered for seronegative recipients of cardiac transplants from a seropositive donors (350).

Stongyloides stercoralis is a nematode that resides in soil contaminated with human feces and has a propensity to invade the skin and the venules. The organism can affect the lungs in two different ways: 1) an acute infection can occur with transmigration of the larvae from the intestines to the lungs, or 2) an allergic reaction to the organisms can occur consisting of an eosinophilic pneumonia (351). The former presentation is more severe because large numbers of parasites can migrate to the lungs, often accompanied by bacteria originating from the intestines, and is known as the *hyperinfection syndrome*. Meningitis is seen commonly in these patients with this large parasite burden. The diagnosis of *Strongyloides* pneumonia is confirmed by visualizing filariform larvae in respiratory secretions. The treatment consists of thiabendazole (351).

CONCLUSION

Pulmonary considerations arise frequently in transplant medicine. The purpose of this chapter has been to present a systematic approach to those problems encountered specifically in nonthoracic solid organ and bone marrow transplantation. Hopefully, timely and appropriate diagnostic studies and therapeutic intervention can be derived from such orderly appraisal.

REFERENCES

1. Ettinger NA, Trulock EP. Pulmonary considerations of organ transplantation. Part 1. Am Rev Respir Dis 1991;143:213–223.
2. Ettinger NA, Trulock EP. Pulmonary considerations of organ transplantation. Part 2. Am Rev Respir Dis 1991;143:433–451.
3. Ettinger NA, Trulock EP. Pulmonary considerations of organ transplantation. Part 3. Am Rev Respir Dis 1991;143:1386–1405.
4. White DA. Pulmonary infection in the immunocompromised host. Semin Thorac Cardiovasc Surg 1995;7:78–87.
5. McLoud TC, Naidich DP. Thoracic disease in the immunocompromised host. Radiol Clin North Am 1992;30:525–554.
6. Primack SL, Muller N. High-resolution computed tomography in acute disease in the immunocompromised patient. Radiol Clin North Am 1994;32:731–744.
7. Barloon TJ, Galvin JR, Mori M, et al. High-resolution ultrafast chest CT in the clinical management of febrile bone marrow transplant patients with normal or nonspecific chest roentgenograms. Chest 1991;99:928–933.
8. Graham NJ, Muller NL, Miller RR, Shepherd JD. Intrathoracic complications following allogeneic bone marrow transplantation: CT findings. Radiology 1991;181:153–156.
9. Levine SJ. An approach to the diagnosis of pulmonary infections in immunosuppressed patients. Semin Respir Infect 1992;7:81–95.
10. Wilson JP, Turner HR, Kirchner KA, et al. Nocardial infections in renal transplant patients. Medicine 1989;68:38–57.
11. Horvath JA, Dummer S. The use of respiratory tract cultures in the diagnosis of invasive aspergillosis. Am J Med 1996;100:171–178.
12. Wilson WR, Cockerill FR, Rosenow EC. Pulmonary disease in the immunocompromised host (Part 2). Mayo Clin Proc 1985;60:610–631.
13. Foot ABM, Caul EO, Rome AP, et al. An assessment of sputum induction as an aid to diagnosis of respiratory infections in the immunocompromised child. J Infect 1992;24:49–54.
14. Weiss SM, Hert RC, Gianola FJ, et al. Complications of fiberoptic bronchoscopy in thrombocytopenic patients. Chest 1993;104:1025–1028.
15. Ekdahl K, Eriksson L, Rollof J, et al. Bronchoscopic diagnosis of pulmonary infections in a heterogenous nonselected group of patients. Chest 1993;103:1743–1748.
16. Baughman RP. Use of bronchoscopy in the diagnosis of infection in the immunocompromised host. Throrax 1994;49:3–7.
17. McCubbin MM, Trigg ME, Hendricker CM, Wagener JS. Bronchoscopy with bronchoalveolar lavage in the evaluation of pulmonary complications of bone marrow transplantation in children. Pediatr Pulmonol 1992;12:43–47.
18. Verra F, Hmouda H, Rauss A, et al. Bronchoalveolar lavage in immunocompromised patients. Chest 1992;101:1215–1220.
19. Cazzadori A, Di Perri G, Todeschini G. Transbronchial biopsy in the diagnosis of pulmonary infiltrates in immunocompromised patients. Chest 1995;107:101–106.
20. Grebski E, Hess T, Hold G, et al. Diagnostic value of hemosiderin-containing macrophages in bronchoalveolar lavage fluid. Chest 1992;102:1794–1799.
21. Lassence AD, Fleury-Feith F, Escudier E, et al. Alveolar hemorrhage: diagnostic criteria and results in 194 immunocompromised hosts. Am J Respir Crit Care Med 1995;151:157–163.
22. Pisani RJ, Wright AJ. Clinical utility of bronchoalveolar lavage in immunocompromised hosts. Mayo Clin Proc 1992;67:221–227.
23. Janzen DL, Adler BD, Padley SPG, Muller NL. Diagnostic success of bronchoscopic biopsy in immunocompromised patients with acute pulmonary disease: predictive value of disease distribution as shown on CT. AJR 1993;160:21–24.
24. Feins RH. The role of thoracoscopy in the AIDS/immunocompromised patient. Ann Thorac Surg 1993;56:649–650.
25. Mack MJ, Aronoff RJ, Acuff TE, et al. Present role of thoracoscopy in the diagnosis and treatment of diseases of the chest. Ann Thorac Surg 1992;54:403–409.
26. Ellis ME, Spence D, Bouchama A. Open lung biopsy provides a higher and more specific diagnostic yield compared to broncho–alveolar lavage in immunocompromised patients. Scand J Infect Dis 1995;27:157–162.
27. Bove P, Ranger W, Pursel S, et al. Evaluation of outcome following open lung biopsy. Am Surg 1994;60:564–570.
28. Wagner JD, Stahler C, Knox S, et al. Clinical utility of open lung biopsy for undiagnosed pulmonary infiltrates. Am J Surg 1992;164:104–108.
29. Shah SS, Tsang V, Goldstraw P. Open lung biopsy: a safe, reliable and accurate method for diagnosis in diffuse lung disease. Respiration 1992;59:243–246.
30. Gururangan S, Lawson RA, Jones PH, et al. Evaluation of the usefulness of open lung biopsies. Pediatr Hematol Oncol 1992;9:107–113.
31. Utz JP, Perrella MA, Rosenow EC. Lung biopsy. Adv Intern Med 1992;37:337–361.
32. Krowka MJ, Cortese DA. Pulmonary aspects of chronic liver disease and liver transplantation. Mayo Clin Proc 1985;60:407–418.
33. O'Brien JD, Ettinger NA. Pulmonary complications of liver transplantation. Clin Chest Med 1996;17:99–114.
34. Hourani JM, Bellamy PE, Tashkin DP, et al. Pulmonary dysfunction in advanced liver disease: frequent occurrence of an abnormal diffusing capacity. Am J Med 1991;90:693–700.
35. Rodriguez-Roisin R, Agusti AGN, Roca J, et al. Gas exchange and pulmonary vascular reactivity in patients with liver cirrhosis. Am Rev Respir Dis 1987;135:1085–1092.
36. Agusti AGN, Roca J, Rodriquez-Roisin R. Mechanisms of gas exchange impairment in patients with liver cirrhosis. Clin Chest Med 1996;17:49–66.
37. Krowka MJ, Dickson ER, Weisner RH, et al. A prospective study of pulmonary function and gas exchange following liver transplantation. Chest 1992;102:1161–1166.
38. Fahy JV, Kerr KM, Lake JR, Gold WM. Pulmonary function before and after liver transplantation. Am Rev Respir Dis 1992;143:A303. Abstract.
39. Krowka MJ. Recent pulmonary observations in alpha-one antitrypsin deficiency, primary biliary cirrhosis, chronic hepatitis C and other hepatic problems. Clin Chest Med 1996;17:67–82.
40. Afessa B, Gay PC, Plevak DJ, et al. Pulmonary complications of orthotopic liver transplantation. Mayo Clin Proc 1993;68:427–434.
41. Mouroux J, Perrin C, Venissac N, et al. Management of pleural effusion of cirrhotic origin. Chest 1996;109:1093–1096.
42. Matuschak GM, Rinaldo JE, Pinsky MR, et al. Effects of end-stage liver failure on the incidence and resolution of the adult respiratory distress syndrome. J Crit Care 1987;2:162.
43. Miyata T, Todo S, Selby R, et al. Endotoxaemia, pulmonary complications, and thrombocytopenia in liver transplantation. Lancet 1989;2:189.
44. Doyle HR, Marino IR, Miro A, et al. Adult respiratory distress syndrome secondary to end-stage liver disease—successful outcome following liver transplantation. Transplantation 1993;55:292–296.
45. Tsai G, Liu J, Siauw C, et al. Throracic roentgenologic manifestations in primary carcinoma of the liver. Chest 1984;86:430–434.
46. Maddrey WC, Van Thiel DH. Liver transplantation: an overview. Hepatology 1988;8:948–959.
47. Man KM, Keefe EB, Brown CR, et al. Pulmonary varices presenting as a solitary lung mass in a patient with end-stage liver disease. Chest 1994;106:294–296.
48. Youssef AI, Escalante-Glersky S, Bonnet RB, Chen YK. Hemoptysis secondary to bronchial varices associated with alcoholic liver disease and portal hypertension. AJG 1994;9:1562–1563.
49. Bund M, Seitz W, Schaefers HJ, et al. Anesthesiologic management of combined lung and liver transplantation. Anesthetist 1994;43:322.
50. Wallaert B, Bonniere P, Prin L, et al. Primary biliary cirrhosis: subclinical inflammatory alveolitis in patients with normal chest roentgenograms. Chest 1986;90:842–848.
51. Rodriguez-Roisin R, Pares A, Bruguera M, et al. Pulmonary involvement in primary biliary cirrhosis. Thorax 1982;36:208–212.
52. Wallwork J, Williams R, Calne RY. Transplantation of liver, heart, and lungs for primary biliary cirrhosis and primary pulmonary hypertension. Lancet 1987;2:182.
53. Rakela J, Goldschmeidt M, Ludwig J. Late manifestations of chronic liver disease in adults with alpha-one antitrypsin deficiency. Dig Dis Sci 1987;32:1358.
54. Feigelson J, Anagnostopoulos C, Poquet M, et al. Liver cirrhosis in cystic fibrosis—therapeutic implications and long-term follow-up. Arch Dis Child 1993;68:653–657.
55. Noble–Jamieson G, Valente J, Barnes ND. Liver transplantation for hepatic cirrhosis in cystic fibrosis. Arch Dis Child 1004;71:349–352.
56. Williams SGJ, Westaby D, Tanner MS, Mowat AP. Liver and biliary problems in cystic fibrosis. Br Med Bull 1992;48:877–892.
57. Lange PA, Stoller JK. The hepatopulmonary syndrome. Ann Intern Med 1995;122:521–529.
58. Krowka MJ. Hepatopulmonary syndrome: an evolving perspective in the era of liver transplantation. Hepatology 1990;11:138–141.
59. Castro M, Krowka MJ. Hepatopulmonary syndrome: a pulmonary vascular complication of liver disease. Clin Chest Med 1996;17:35–48.
60. Krowka MJ, Dickson ER, Cortese DA. Hepatopulmonary syndrome. Clinical observations and lack of therapeutic response to somatostatin analogue. Chest 1993;1104:515–521.

61. Poterucha JJ, Krowka MJ, Dickson ER, et al. Failure of hepatopulmonary syndrome to resolve after liver transplantation and successful treatment with embolotherapy. Hepatology 1995;21:96–99.
62. Lange PA, Stoller JK. The hepatopulmonary syndrome: effect of liver transplantation. Clin Chest Med 1996;17:115–123.
63. Stoller JK, Lange PA, Westveer MK, et al. Prevalence and reversibility of the hepatopulmonary syndrome after liver transplantation: the Cleveland Clinic experience. West J Med 1995;163:133–138.
64. Donovan CL, Marcowitz PA, Punch JD, et al. Two-dimensional and dobutamine stress echocardiography in the pre-operative assessment of patients with end-stage liver disease prior to orthotopic liver transplantation. Transplantation 1996;61:1180–1188.
65. Lebrec D, Capron JP, Dhumeaux D, Benhamou JP. Pulmonary hypertension complicating portal hypertension. Am Rev Respir Dis 1979;120:849–856.
66. Van Der Heijde RMJL, Lameris JS, Van Den Berg B, et al. Pulmonary hypertension after transjugular intrahepatic portosystemic shunt (TIPS). Eur Respir J 1996;9:1562–1564.
67. Mandell MS, Groves BM. Pulmonary hypertension in chronic liver disease. Clin Chest Med 1996;17:17–33.
68. Castro M, Krowka MJ, Schroeder R, et al. Frequency and clinical implications of increased pulmonary artery pressures in liver transplant patients. Mayo Clin Proc 1996;71:543–551.
69. Rettke SR, Chantigian RC, Janossy TA. Anesthesia approach to hepatic transplantation. Mayo Clin Proc 1989;64:224–231.
70. Rettke SR, Janossy TA, Chantigian RC. Hemodynamic and metabolic changes in hepatic transplantation. Mayo Clin Proc 1989;64:232–240.
71. Khoury GF, Mann ME, Porot MJ, et al. Air embolism associated with veno-venous bypass during orthotopic liver transplantation. Anesthesiology 1987;67:848–851.
72. Navalgund AA, Kang Y, Sarner JB, et al. Massive pulmonary thromboembolism during liver transplantation. Anesth Analg 1988;67:400–402.
73. Baubillier E, Cherqui D, Dominique C, et al. A fatal thrombotic complication during liver transplantation after aprotinin administration. Transplantation 1994;57:1664–1666.
74. Gosseye S, Obbergh LV, Weynand B, et al. Platelet aggregates in small vessels and death during liver transplantation. Lancet 1991;338:532–534.
75. Sankey EA, Crow J, Mallett SV, et al. Pulmonary platelet aggregates: possible cause of sudden perioperative death in adults undergoing liver transplantation. J Clin Pathol 1993;46:222–227.
76. Whiteman K, Nachtmann L, Kramer D, et al. Effects of continuous lateral rotation therapy on pulmonary complications in liver transplant recipients. Am J Crit Care 1995;4:133–139.
77. Matuschak GM, Shaw BW. Adult respiratory distress syndrome associated with acute liver allograft rejection: resolution following hepatic retransplantation. Crit Care Med 1987;15:878–881.
78. Powell-Jackson PR, Carmichael JL, Calne RY, Williams R. Adult respiratory distress syndrome and convulsions associated with administration of cyclosporine in liver transplant recipients. Transplantation 1984;38:341–343.
79. Pirsch JD, Kalayoglu M, D'Allessandro, et al. Pulmonary infiltrates and eosinophilia in an FK506 liver transplant recipient. Transplant Proc 1991;23:3195–3196.
80. Jeng LB, Cheng MH, Lee WC, et al. Extracorporeal membrane oxygenation therapy for adult respiratory distress syndrome developing post liver transplantation. Transplant Proc 1994;26:2237–2238.
81. Munoz SJ, Nagelberg SB, Green PJ, et al. Ectopic soft-tissue calcium deposition following liver transplantation. Hepatology 1988;8:476–483.
82. Cherqui D, Duvoux C, Plassa F, et al. Lymphoproliferative disorder of donor origin in a liver transplant recipient: complete remission after drastic reduction of immunosuppression without graft loss. Transplantation 1993;56:1023–1026.
83. Plevak DJ, Southorn PA, Narr BJ. Intensive-care unit experience in the Mayo liver transplantation program: the first 100 cases. Mayo Clin Proc 1989;64:433–445.
84. Krom RA, Wiesner RH, Rettke SR, et al. The first 100 liver transplantations at the Mayo Clinic. Mayo Clin Proc 1989;64:84–94.
85. McAlister VC, Grant DR, Roy A, et al. Right phrenic nerve injury in orthotopic liver transplantation. Transplantation 1993;55:826–830.
86. Edelstein CL, Jacobs JC, Moosa MR. Pulmonary complications in 110 consecutive renal transplant recipients. S Afr Med J 1995;85:160–163.
87. Bush A, Gabriel R. Pulmonary function in chronic renal failure: effects of dialysis and transplantation. Thorax 1991;46:424–428.
88. Lee HY, Stretton TB, Barnes AM. The lungs in renal failure. Thorax 1975;30:46–53.
89. Pitcher WD, Diamond SM, Henrich WL. Pulmonary gas exchange during dialysis in patients with obstructive lung disease. Chest 1989;96:1136–1141.
90. Bush A, Gabriel R. The lungs in uremia: a review. J R Soc Med 1985;78:849–855.
91. Yao L, Killam DA. Rounded atelectasis associated with end-stage renal disease. Chest 1989;96:441–443.
92. Rocker GM, Morgan AG, Pearson D, et al. Pulmonary vascular permeability to transferrin in the pulmonary oedema of renal failure. Thorax 1987;42:620–623.
93. Richardson J, Slovis B, Miller G, Dummer S. Development of pulmonary alveolar microlithiasis in a renal transplant recipient. Transplantation 1995;59:1056–1057.
94. Fairshter RD, Vaziri ND, Farooqui S, Martin D. Pulmonary pathology in renal transplant recipients. Int J Artif Organs 1984;7:327–330.
95. Brodeur FJ, Kazerooni EA. Metastatic pulmonary calcification mimicking air-space disease. Chest 1994;106:620–622.
96. Hartman TE, Muller NL, Primack SL. Metastatic pulmonary calcification in patients with hypercalcemia: findings on chest radiographs and CT scans. AJR 1994;162:799–802.
97. Fulladosa X, Gonzalez MT, Cruzado JM. Metastatic pulmonary calcification in severe secondary hyperparathyroidism: evolution after renal transplantation. Transplant Proc 1995;27:2272–2276.
98. Fairshter R, Vaziri N, Mirahmadi M. Lung pathology in chronic hemodialysis patients. Int J Artif Organs 1982;5:97–100.
99. Hamida BM, Bedrossian J, Pruna A, et al. Wilms tumor and renal transplantation: a case report and literature review. Transplant Proc 1993;25:2346–2347.
100. Pais E, Pirson Y, Squifflet JP, et al. Kidney transplantation in patients with Wilms' tumor. Transplantation 1992;53:782–785.
101. Akmal M, Barndt RR, Ansari AN, et al. Excess PTH in CRF induces pulmonary calcification, pulmonary hypertension, and right ventricular hypertrophy. Kidney Int 1995;47:158–163.
102. Herody M, Bobrie G, Gouarin C, et al. Anti-GBM disease: predictive value of clinical, histological, and serological data. Clin Nephrol 1993;40:249–255.
103. Primack SL, Miller RR, Muller NL. Diffuse pulmonary hemorrhage: clinical, pathologic, and imaging features. AJR 1995;164:295–300.
104. Boubenider SA, Akhtar M, Alfurayh O, et al. Late recurrence of Wegener's granulomatosis presenting as tracheal stenosis in a renal transplant patient. Clin Transpl 1994;8:5–9.
105. Schmitt WH, Haubitz M, Mistry N, et al. Renal transplantation in Wegener's granulomatosis. Lancet 1993;342:860.
106. Rosenstein ED, Ribot S, Ventresca E, Kramer N. Recurrence of Wegener's granulomatosis following renal transplantaion. Br J Rheumatol 1994;33:869–871.
107. Hakaim AG, Stilmant MM, Kauffman J, et al. Successful renal transplantation in a patient with systemic sarcoidosis and renal failure due to focal glomerulosclerosis. Am J Kidney Dis 1992;19:493–495.
108. Shen SY, Hall-Craggs M, Posner JN, Shabazz B. Recurrent sarcoid granulomatous nephritis and reactive tuberculin skin test in a renal transplant recipient. Am J Med 1986;80:699–702.
109. Rowe PA, Rocker GM, Morgan AG, Shale DJ. OKT3 and pulmonary capillary permeability. BMJ 1987;295:1099–1100.
110. Vincent F, Bensousan TA. Letter to the editor. J Urol 1995;154:214–215.
111. Meyer MM, Meyer RJ. Nitrofurantoin-induced pulmonary hemorrhage in a renal transplant recipient receiving immunosuppressive therapy: case report and review of the literature. J Urol 1994;152:938–940.
112. Brown AL, Corris PA, Ashcroft T, Wilkinson R. Azathioprine-related interstitial pneumonitis in a renal transplant recipient. Nephrol Dial Transplant 1992;7:362–364.
113. Queffeulou G, Ducloux D, Faucher C, et al. Fatal cyclophosphamide-induced interstitial pneumonitis in a renal transplant patient. Nephrol Dial Transplant 1994;9:1655–1657.
114. Murnaghan DJ. Letter to the editor. Nephrol Dial Transplant 1992;7:1166.
115. Drut R, Drut RM. EBV-associated Kaposi's sarcoma in a pediatric renal transplant recipient. Pediatr Pathol 1994;14:863–872.
116. Margolius L, Stein M, Spencer D, Bezwoda WR. Kaposi's sarcoma in renal transplant recipients. S Afr Med J 1994;84:16–17.
117. Khan GA, Klapper P. Pulmonary haemorrhage following renal transplantation. Thorax 1995;50:98–99.
118. Mandel C, Silberstein M, Hennessy O. Case report: fatal pulmonary Kaposi's sarcoma and Castleman's disease in a renal transplant recipient. Br J Radiol 1993;66:264,265.
119. Hayashi K, Hoshida Y, Ohnoshi T. Primary pulmonary non-Hodgkin's lymphoma in a Japanese renal transplant recipient. Int J Hematol 1993; 57:245–250.

120. Mossey RT, Kasabian AA, Wilkes BM. Pulmonary embolism: low incidence in chronic renal failure. Arch Intern Med 1982;142:1646–1648.
121. PIOPED Investigators. Value of the ventilation/perfusion scan in acute pulmonary embolism: results of the prospective investigation of pulmonary embolism diagnosis (PIOPED). JAMA 1990;263:2753–2759.
122. Milano S, Niccoli L, Cristinelli L, Mombelloni G. Vena cava filter and renal transplant. Ann Thorac Surg 1988;45:350.
123. Naum CC, Sciurba FC, Rogers RM. Pulmonary function abnormalities in chronic severe cardiomyopathy preceding cardiac transplantation. Am Rev Respir Dis 1992;145:1334–1338.
124. Wright TS, Levine MS, Bellamy PE, et al. Ventilatory and diffusion abnormalities in potentital heart transplant patients. Chest 1990;98:816–820.
125. Hosenpud JD, Stibolt TA, Atwal K, Shelley D. Abnormal pulmonary function specifically related to congestive heart failure: Comparison of patients before and after cardiac transplantation. Am J Med 1990;88:493–496.
126. Sasaki F, Ishizaki T, Mifune J, et al. Bronchial hyperresponsiveness in patients with chronic congestive heart failure. Chest 1990;97:534–538.
127. Cabanes LR, Weber SN, Matran R, et al. Bronchial hyperresponsiveness to methacholine in patients with impaired left ventricular function. N Engl J Med 1989;320:1317–1322.
128. Bussieres LM, Cardella CJ, Daly PA, et al. Relationship between preoperative pulmonary status and outcome after heart transplantation. J Heart Transplant 1990;9:124–128.
129. Weisman IM, Connery SM, Belbel RJ, Zeballow RJ. The role of cardiopulmonary exercise testing in the selection of patients for cardiac transplantation. Chest 1992;102:1871–1874.
130. Torre-Amione G, Kapadia S, Short III D, Young JB. Evolving concepts regarding selection of patients for cardiac transplantation: assessing risks and benefits. Chest 1996;109:223–232.
131. Taylor AJ, Bergin JD. Cardiac transplantation for the cardiologist not trained in transplantation. Am Heart J 1996;129:578–592.
132. Kirklin JK, Naftel DC, McGriffin DC, et al. Analysis of morbid events and risk factors for death after cardiac transplantation. J Am Coll Cardiol 1988;11:917–924.
133. Kawaguchi A, Gandjbakhch I, Pavie A, et al. Cardiac transplant recipients with preoperative pulmonary hypertension. Circulation 1989;80(suppl):90–96.
134. Kawaguchi A, Gandjbakhch I, Pavie A, et al. Factors affecting survival after heterotopic heart transplantation. J Thorac Cardiovasc Surg 1989;98:928–934.
135. Baumgartner WA. Heterotopic transplantation: is it a viable alternative? Ann Thorac Surg 1992;54:401–402.
136. Hsu DT, Addonizio LJ, Hordof AJ, Gersony WM. Acute pulmonary embolism in pediatric patients awaiting heart transplantation. J Am Coll Cardiol 1991;17:1621–1625.
137. Cavarocchi NC, Carp NZ, Mitra A, et al. Successful heart transplantation in recipients with recent preoperative pulmonary emboli. J Heart Transplant 1989;8:494–498.
138. Loria KM, Salinger MH, Frohlich TG, et al. Right lower lobectomy for pulmonary infarction before orthotopic heart transplantation. J Heart Lung Transplant 1991;10:325–328.
139. Young JN, Yazbeck J, Esposito G. The influence of acute preoperative pulmonary infarction on the results of heart transplantation. J Heart Transplant 1986;5:20–22.
140. Lofaso F, Verschueren P, Rande JLD, et al. Prevalence of sleep-disordered breathing in patients on a heart transplant waiting list. Chest 1994;106:1689–1694.
141. Klink ME, Sethi GK, Copeland JG, Quan SF. Obstructive sleep apnea in heart transplant patients: a report of five cases. Chest 1993;104:1090–1092.
142. Collop NA. Cheyne–Stokes ventilation converting to obstructive sleep apnea following heart transplantation. Chest 1993;104:1288–1289.
143. Roth BJ, O'Meara TF, Cragun WH. The serum-effusion albumin gradient in the evaluation of pleural effusions. Chest 1990;98:546–549.
144. Martin WJ. Mechanisms of amiodarone pulmonary toxicity. Clin Chest Med 1990;11(1):131–138.
145. Kennedy JI. Clinical aspects of amiodarone pulmonary toxicity. Clin Chest Med 1990;11(1):119–130.
146. Chelimsky-Fallick C, Middlekauff HR, Stevenson WG, et al. Amiodarone therapy does not compromise subsequent heart transplantation. J Am Coll Cardiol 1992;20:1556–1561.
147. Miller LW, Schlant RC, Iobashigawa J, et al. Task force 5: complications. J Am Col Cardiol 1993;22:41–54.
148. Fullerton DA, Gundry SR, Alonso de Begona J, et al. The effects of donor–recipient size disparity in infant and pediatric heart transplantation. J Thorac Cardiovasc Surg 1992;104:1314–1319.
149. Haramati LB, Schulman LL, Austin JH. Lung nodules and masses after cardiac transplantation. Radiology 1993;188:491–497.
150. Fleming RH, Jennison SH, Naunheim KS. Primary bronchogenic carcinoma in the heart transplant recipient. Ann Thorac Surg 1994;57:1300–1301.
151. Chen JM, Chadburn A, Frizzera G, et al. Management of lymphoproliferative disorders after cardiac transplantation. Ann Thorac Surg 1993;56:527–538.
152. Reyes CV, Jensen JA, Chinoy M. Pulmonary lymphoma in cardiac transplant patients treated with OKT3 for rejection: diagnosis by fine-needle aspiration. Diagn Cytopathol 1995;2:32–36.
153. Schwend M, Tiemann M, Kreipe HH, et al. Rapidly growing Epstein-Barr virus-associated pulmonary lymphoma after heart transplantation. Eur Respir J 1994;7:612–616.
154. Alldrich TK, Rochester DF. The lungs and neuromuscular diseases. In: Murray JF, Nadel JA, eds. Textbook of respiratory medicine. 2nd ed. Philadelphia: WB Saunders, 1994:2495.
155. Schulman LL, Smith CR, Drusin R, et al. Respiratory complications of cardiac transplantation. Am J Med Sci 1988;296:1–10.
156. Quabeck K. The lung as a critical organ in marrow transplantation. Bone Marrow Transplant 1994;14:19S–28S.
157. Ghalie R, Szidon JP, Thompson L, et al. Evaluation of pulmonary complications after bone marrow transplantation: the role of pretransplant pulmonary function tests. Bone Marrow Transplant 1992;10:359–365.
158. Carlson K, Backlund L, Smedmyr B, et al. Pulmonary function and complications subsequent to autologous bone marrow transplantation. Bone Marrow Transplant 1994;14:805–811.
159. Krowka MJ, Staats BA, Hoagland HC. A prospective study of airway reactivity before bone marrow transplantation. Mayo Clin Proc 1990;65:5–12.
160. Milburn HJ, Prentice HG, Du Bois RM. Can lung function measurements be used to predict which patients will be at risk of developing interstitial pneumonitis after bone marrow transplantation? Thorax 1992;47:421–425.
161. Horak DA, Schmidt GM, Zaia JA, et al. Pretransplant pulmonary function predicts cytomegalovirus-associated interstitial pneumonia following bone marrow transplantation. Chest 1992;102:1484–1496.
162. Richard C, Romon I, Baro J, et al. Invasive pulmonary aspergillosis prior to BMT in acute leukemia patients does not predict a poor outcome. Bone Marrow Transplant 1993;12:237–241.
163. Morgenthaler TI, Ryu JH, Utz JP. Cavitary pulmonary infarct in immunocompromised host. Mayo Clinic Proc 1995;70:66–68.
164. Rosenow III EC. Drug-induced pulmonary disease. Dis Month 1994;40:253–310.
165. Twohig KJ, Matthay RA. Pulmonary effects of cytotoxic agents other than bleomycin. Clin Chest Med 1990;11:31–54.
166. Zitnik RJ. Drug-induced lung disease: cancer chemotherapy agents. J Respir Dis 1995;16:855–865.
167. Langston AA, Sanders JE, Deeg J, et al. Allogeneic marrow transplantation for aplastic anemia associated with dyskeratosis congenita. Br J Haematol 1996;92:758–765.
168. Corso S, Vukelja SJ, Wiener D, Baker WJ. Diffuse alveolar hemorrhage following autologous bone marrow infusion. Bone Marrow Transplant 1993;12:301–303.
169. Clark JG, Hansen JA, Hertz MI, et al. Idiopathic pneumonia syndrome after bone marrow transplantation. Am Rev Respir Dis 1993;147:1601–1601.
170. Crawford SW, Hackman RC. Clinical course of idiopathic pneumonia after bone marrow transplantation. Am Rev Respir Dis 1993;147:1393–1400.
171. Kantrow SP, Hackman RC, Bueckh M, et al. Idiopathic pneumonia syndrome. Changing spectrum of lung injury after marrow transplantation. Transplantation 1997;63:1079–1086.
172. Milburn HJ, Prentice HG, Grundy JE. IgG subclasses in the lungs of patients with interstitial pneumonitis following bone marrow transplantation. Eur Respir J 1993;6:944–950.
173. Milburn HJ, Prentice HG, Poulter LW. Abnormal alveolar macrophage populations in bone marrow transplant populations in bone marrow transplant recipients with pneumonitis. Eur Respir J 1993;6:1295–1300.
174. Leblond V, Zouabi H, Sutton L, et al. Late CD8+ lymphocytic alveolitis after allogeneic bone marrow transplantation and chronic graft-versus-host disease. Am J Respir Crit Care Med 1994;150:1056–1061.
175. Ozsahin M, Schwartz LH, Pene F, et al. Is body weight a risk factor of interstitial pneumonitis after bone marrow transplantation? Bone Marrow Transplant 1992;10:97. Letter.
176. Crawford SW, Longton G, Storb R. Acute graft-versus-host disease and the risks for idiopathic pneumonia after marrow transplantation for severe aplastic anemia. Bone Marrow Transplant 1993;12:225–231.

177. Kurisu K, Taniguchi M, Kamikonya N, et al. Interstitial pneumonitis after allogeneic bone marrow transplantation following total body irradiation. Radiat Med 1991;9:118–121.
178. Latini P, Aristei C, Aversa F. Interstitial pneumonitis after hyperfractionated total body irradiation in HLA-matched T-depleted bone marrow transplantation. Int J Radiat Oncol Biol Phys 1992;23:401–404.
179. Socie G, Devergie MD, Girinsky T. Influence of the fractionation of total body irradiation on complications and relapse rate for chronic myelogenous leukemia. Int J Radiat Oncol Biol Phys 1991;20:397–403.
180. Hartsell WF, Czyzewski EA, Ghalie R, Kaizer H. Pulmonary complications of bone marrow transplantation: a comparison of total body irradiation and cyclophosphamide to busulfan and cyclophosphamide. Int J Radiat Ocol Biol Phys 1995;33:69–73.
181. Gogna NK, Morgan G, Downs K, et al. Lung dose rate and interstitial pneumonitis in total body irradiation for bone marrow transplantation. Australas Radiol 1992;36:317–320.
182. Latini P, Aristei C, Aversa F. Lung damage following bone marrow transplantation after hyperfractionated total body irradiation. Radiother Oncol 1991;22:127–132.
183. Kader HA, Khanna S, Hutchinson RM, et al. Pulmonary complications of bone marrow transplantation: the impact of variations in total body irradiation parameters. Clin Oncol 1994;6:96–101.
184. Schmidt U, Metz KA, Soukou C, Quabeck K. The association of pulmonary CMV infection with interstitial pneumonia after bone marrow transplantation. Zentralbl Pathol 1993;139:225–230.
185. Burgart LJ, Heller MJ, Reznicek MJ, et al. Cytomegalovirus detection in bone marrow transplant patients with idiopathic pneumonitis. Am J Clin Pathol 1991;96:572–576.
186. Carrigan DR, Drobyski WR, Russler SK, et al. Interstitial pneumonitis associated with human herpes virus-6 infection after marrow transplantation. Lancet 1991;38:147–149.
187. Cone RW, Hackman RC, Huang MW, et al. Human herpes virus 6 in lung tissue from patients with pneumonitis after bone marrow transplantation. N Engl J Med 1993;329:156–161.
188. Kaplan EB, Pietra GG, August CS. Interstitial pneumonitis, pulmonary fibrosis, and chronic graft-versus-host disease. Bone Marrow Transplant 1992;9:71–75.
189. Anscher MS, Peters WP, Reisenbichler H, et al. Transforming growth factor *B* as a predictor of liver and lung fibrosis after autologous bone marrow transplantation for advanced breast cancer. N Engl J Med 1993;328:1592–1598.
190. Boas SR, Noyes BE, Kurland G, et al. Pediatric lung transplantation for graft-versus-host disease following bone marrow transplantation. Chest 1994;105:1584–1586.
191. Wilczynski SW, Erasmus JJ, Petro WP, et al. Delayed pulmonary toxicity syndrome following high-dose chemotherapy and bone marrow transplantation for breast cancer. Am J Respir Crit Care Med 1998;157:565–573.
192. Przepiorka D, Abu-Elmagd K, Huaringa A, et al. Bronchiolitis obliterans organizing pneumonia in a BMT patient receiving FK506. Bone Marrow Transplant 1993;11:502.
193. Chao NJ, Duncan SR, Long GD, et al. Corticosteroid therapy for diffuse alveolar hemorrhage in autologous bone marrow transplant recipients. Ann Intern Med 1991;114:145–146.
194. Sisson JH, Thompson AB, Anderson JR, et al. Airway inflammation predicts diffuse alveolar hemorrhage during bone marrow transplantation in patients with Hodgkin disease. Am Rev Respir Dis 1992;146:439–443.
195. Wojno KJ, Vogelsang GB, Beschorner WE, Santon GW. Pulmonary hemorrhage as a cause of death in allogeneic bone marrow recipients with severe acute graft-versus-host disease. Transplantation 1994;57:88–92.
196. Robbins RA, Linder J, Stahl MG, et al. Diffuse alveolar hemorrhage in autologous bone marrow transplant recipients. Am J Med 1989;87:511–518.
197. Metcalf JP, Rennard SI, Reed E, et al. Corticosteroids as adjunctive therapy for diffuse alveolar hemorrhage associated with bone marrow transplantation. Am J Med 1994;96:327–334.
198. Dickout WJ, Chan CK, Hyland RH, et al. Prevention of acute pulmonary edema after bone marrow transplantation. Chest 1987;92:303–309.
199. Lazarus HM. Autologous bone marrow transplantation for the treatment of lung cancer. Semin Oncol 1993;20:72–79.
200. Elias AD, Ayash L, Frei III E, et al. Intensive combined modality therapy for limited-stage small-cell lung cancer. J Natl Cancer Inst 1993;85:559–566.
201. Grimwade DJ, Chopra R, King A, et al. Detection and significance of pulmonary Hodgkin's disease at autologous bone marrow transplantation. Bone Marrow Transplant 1994;13:173–179.
202. Esartia PT, Deichman GI, Kluchareva TE, et al. Allogeneic bone-marrow transfusion suppresses development of lung metastases in osteogenic sarcoma patients after radical surgery. Int J Cancer 1993;54:907–910.
203. Witherspoon RP, Fisher LD, Schoch G. Secondary cancers after bone marrow transplantation for leukemia or aplastic anemia. N Engl J Med 1989;321:784–789.
204. Cordonnier C, Fleury-Feith J, Escudier E, et al. Secondary alveolar proteinosis is a reversible cause of respiratory failure in leukemic patients. Am J Respir Crit Care Med 1994;149:788–794.
205. Paz HL, Crilley P, Topolsky DL, et al. Bronchiolitis obliterans after bone marrow transplantation: the effect of preconditioning. Respiration 1993;60:109–114.
206. Schultz KR, Fernandez CV, Israel DM, et al. Association of gastroesophageal reflux with obstructive lung disease in children after allogeneic bone marrow transplantation. Blood 1995;85:3763–3765.
207. Schultz KR, Green GJ, Wensley D, et al. Obstructive lung disease in children after allogeneic bone marrow transplantation. Blood 1994;9:3212–3220.
208. Crawford SW, Clark JG. Bronchiolitis associated with bone marrow transplantation. Clin Chest Med 1993;14:741–749.
209. Payne L, Chan CK, Fyles G, et al. Cyclosporine as possible prophylaxis for obstructive airways disease after allogeneic bone marrow transplantation. Chest 1993;104:114–118.
210. Soubani AO, Miller KB, Hassoun PM. Pulmonary complications of bone marrow transplantation. Chest 1996;109:1066–1077.
211. Sargen MA, Cairns RA, Murdoch MJ, et al. Obstructive lung disease in children after allogeneic bone marrow transplantation: evaluation of high-resolution CT. AJR 1995;164:693–696.
212. Beschorner WE, Saral R, Hutchins GM, et al. Lymphocytic bronchitis associated with graft-versus-host disease in recipients of bone marrow transplants. N Engl J Med 1978;299:1030–1036.
213. Dark J. Lung transplants in patients with prior bone marrow transplants. Chest 1994;105:327. Letter.
214. Svendson UG, Aggestrup S, Heilmann C. Transplantation of a lobe of lung from mother to child following previous transplantation with maternal bone marrow. Eur Respir J 1995;8:334–337.
215. Philit F, Wiesendanger T, Archimbaud E, et al. Post-transplant obstructive lung disease ("bronchiolitis obliterans"): a clinical comparative study of bone marrow and lung transplant patients. Eur Respir J 1995;8:551–558.
216. Lipton JH, Russell JA, Burgess KR, Hwang WS. Fat embolization and pulmonary infiltrates after bone marrow transplantation. Med Pediatr Oncol 1987;15:24–27.
217. Abrahams C, Catchatourian R. Bone fragment emboli in the lungs of patients undergoing bone marrow transplantation. Am J Clin Pathol 1983;79:360–363.
218. Uderzo C, Marraro G, Riva A, et al. Pulmonary thromboembolism in leukaemic children undergoing bone marrow transplantation. Bone Marrow Transplant 1993;11:201–203.
219. Otheo de Tejada E, Maldonado MS, Camarero C, Munoz A. Fatal hemorrhage after recombinant tissue plasminogen activator therapy for hepatic veno-occlusive disease complicating autologous BMT. Bone Marrow Transplant 1994;14:176–177. Letter.
220. Williams LM, Fussell S, Veith RW, et al. Pulmonary veno-occlusive disease in an adult following bone marrow transplantation. Chest 1996;109:1388–1391.
221. Doll DC, Yarbo JW. Vascular toxicity associated with antineoplastic agents. Semin Oncol 1992;19:580–596.
222. Hackman RC, Madtes DK, Peterson FB, Clark JG. Pulmonary venoocclusive disease following bone marrow transplantation. Transplant 1989;47:989–992.
223. Cunningham I. Pulmonary infections after bone marrow transplantation. Semin Respir Infect 1992;7:132–138.
224. Bowden RA, Mori M, Dobbs S, et al. Mononuclear cell reconstitution in the lung after marrow transplantation. Transplantation 1993;55:557–561.
225. Miller BW, Brennan DC, Korenblat PE, et al. Common variable immunodeficiency in a renal transplant patient with severe recurrent bacterial infection: a case report and review of the literature. Am J Kidney Dis 1995;25:947–951.
226. Kalhs P, Panzer S, Kletter K, et al. Functional asplenia after bone marrow transplantation. Ann Intern Med 1988;109:461–464.
227. Rege K, Mehta J, Treleaven J, et al. Fatal pneumococcal infections following allogeneic bone marrow transplant. Bone Marrow Transplant 1994;14:903–906.
228. Martino R, Altes A, Nomdedeu J, et al. Atypical presentation of pneumococcal pneumonia in a patient undergoing bone marrow transplantation for Hodgkin's disease. Bone Marrow Transplant 1994;14:174–175. Letter.

229. Paya CV, Hermans PE, Washington JA, et al. Incidence, distribution, and outcome of episodes of infection in 100 orthotopic liver transplantations. Mayo Clin Proc 1989;64:555–564.
230. Wiesner RH, Hermans PE, Rakela J. Selective bowel decontamination to decrease gram-negative aerobic bacterial and candida colonization and prevent infection after orthotopic liver transplantation. Transplantation 1988;45:570–574.
231. Bion JF, Badger I, Crosby HA, et al. Selective decontamination of the digestive tract reduces gram-negative pulmonary colonization but not systemic endotoxemia in patients undergoing elective liver transplantation. Crit Care Med 1994;22:40–49.
232. Lew MA, Kehoe K, Ritz J. Prophylaxis of bacterial infections with ciprofloxacin in patients undergoing bone marrow transplantation. Transplantation 1991;51:630–636.
233. Anaissie EJ, Vartivarian S, Bodey GP, et al. Randomized comparison between antibiotics alone and antibiotics plus granulocyte-macrophage colony-stimulating factor (*Escherichia coli* derived) in cancer patients with fever and neutropenia. Am J Med 1996;100:17–23.
234. Dominquez EA. Long-term infectious complications of liver transplantation. Semin Liver Dis 1995;15:133–137.
235. Kusne S, Dummer JS, Singh N, et al. Infections after liver transplantation. Medicine 1988;67:132–143.
236. Colonnna JO, Winston DJ, Brill JE, et al. Infectious complications in liver transplantation. Arch Surg 1988;23:360–364.
237. Miller LW, Naftel DC, Bourge RC, et al. Infection after heart transplantation: a multiinstitutional study. J Heart Lung Transplant 1994;13:381–393.
238. Gorensek MJ, Stewart RW, Keys TF, et al. A multivariate analysis of risk factors for pneumonia following cardiac transplantation. Transplantation 1988;46:860–865.
239. Pannuti CS, Gingrich RD, Pfaller MA, Wenzel RP. Nosocomial pneumonia in adult patients undergoing bone marrow transplantation: a 9 year study. J Clin Oncol 1991;9:77–84.
240. Dummer JS, Hardy A, Poorsattar A, Ho M. Early infections in kidney, heart, and liver transplant recipients on cyclosporine. Transplantation 1983;36:259–267.
241. Thompson AB, Rickard BW, Shaw RP. Pulmonary complications and disease severity in adult liver transplant recipients. Transplant Proc 1988;20:646–649.
242. Singh N, Gayowski T, Wagener M, et al. Pulmonary infections in liver transplant recipients receiving tacrolismus. Transplantation 1996;61:396–401.
243. Campbell JH, Blessing N, Burnett AK, Stevenson RD. Investigation and management of pulmonary infiltrates following bone marrow transplantation: an eight year review. Thorax 1993;48:1248–1251.
244. Ampel NM, Wing EJ. *Legionella* infection in transplant patients. Semin Respir Infect 1990;5:30–37.
245. Nguyen MLT, Yu VL. *Legionella* infection. Clin Chest Med 1991;12:257–268.
246. Humphreys H, Marshall RJ, Mackay I, Caul EO. Pneumonia due to *Legionella bozemanii* and *Chlamydia spittaci*/TWAR following renal transplantation. J Infect 1992;25:67–71.
247. Caniza MA, Granger DL, Wilson KH. *Bartonella hensalae*: etiology of pulmonary nodules in a patient with depressed cell-mediated immunity. Clin Infect Dis 1995;20:1505–1511.
248. Rubin RH. Infectious disease complications of renal transplantation. Kidney Int 1993;44:221–236.
249. Perschak H, Gubler J, Speich R, Russi E. Pulmonary nocardiosis with *Pneumocystis carinii* pneumonia in two patients undergoing immunosuppressive therapy. J Infect 1991;23:183–185.
250. King C, Chapman SW, Butkus DE. Recurrent nocardiosis in a renal transplant recipient. South Med J 1993;86:225–227.
251. Shearer C, Chandrasekar PH. Pulmonary nocardiosis in a patient with a bone marrow transplant. Bone Marrow Transplant 1995;15:479–481.
252. Segovia J, Pulpon LA, Crespo MG, et al. *Rhodococcus equi*: first case in a heart transplant recipient. J Heart Lung Transplant 1994;13:332–335.
253. Ip MS, Yuen KY, Chiu EK, et al. Pulmonary infections in bone marrow transplantation: the Hong Kong experience. Respiration 1995;62:80–83.
254. Ho KJ. Galloping caseous pneumonia with miliary dissemination in a renal transplant recipient: emphasis on pretransplant detection and prophylaxis. Nephron 1992;62:363–364.
255. Peters EJ, Morice R. Miliary pulmonary infection caused by *Mycobacterium terrae* in an autologous bone marrow transplant patient. Chest 1991;100:1449–1450.
256. LeMense GP, VanBakel AB, Crumbley III AJ, Judson MA. *Mycobacterium scrofulaceum* infection presenting as lung nodules in a heart transplant recipient. Chest 1994;106:1918–1920.
257. Mitwalli A. Tuberculosis in patients on maintenance dialysis. Am J Kidney Dis 1991;18:579–582.
258. Stoblen F, Neuhaus R, Neumann K, et al. Tuberculosis in liver transplant recipients: recurrence after transplantation. Transplant Proc 1994;26:3604–3605.
259. Dummer S, Kusne S. Liver transplantation and related infections. Semin Respir Infect 1993;8:191–198.
260. Hall CM, Willcox PA, Swanepoel CR, et al. Mycobacterial infection in renal transplant recipients. Chest 1994;106:435–439.
261. Quinibi WY, Al-Sibai MB, Taher S, et al. Mycobacterial infection after renal transplantation—report of 14 cases and review of the literature. Q J Med 1990;282:1039–1060.
262. Mat O, Abramowicz D, Peny MO. Tuberculosis presenting as acute hepatitis in a renal transplant recipient. Transplant Int 1994;7:67–69.
263. Tomford JW, Rice TW. The diagnosis and medical management of pulmonary parenchymal mycobacterial diseases. Semin Thorac Cardiovasc Surg 1995;7:104–107.
264. Tantawichien T, Suwangool P, Suvanapha R. Tuberculosis in renal transplant recipients. Transplant Proc 1994;26:2187–2188.
265. Peschke B, Ernst W, Gossmann J, et al. Antituberculous drugs in kidney transplant recipients treated with cyclosporine. Transplantation 1993;56:236–238.
266. Chen CH, Hsieh H, Lai MK. Pulmonary tuberculosis or MOTT infection in kidney transplant recipients. Transplant Proc 1994;26:2136–2137.
267. Sundberg R, Shapiro R, Darras. A tuberculosis outbreak in a renal transplant program. Transplant Proc 1991;23:3091–3092.
268. Ljungman P, Cordonnier C, de Bock R, et al. Immunisations after bone marrow transplantation: results of a European survey and recommendations from the infectious diseases working party of the European group for blood and bone marrow transplantation. Bone Marrow Transplant 1995;15:455–460.
269. Avery RK. Infections and immunizations in organ transplant recipients: a preventive approach. Cleve Clin J Med 1994;61:386–392.
270. Somani J, Larson RA. Reimmunization after allogeneic bone marrow transplantation. Am J Med 1995;98:389–398.
271. Chien SM, Chan CK, Kasupski G, et al. Long-term sequelae after recovery from cytomegalovirus pneumonia in allogeneic bone marrow transplant recipients. Chest 1992;101:1000–1004.
272. Duncombe AS, Grundy JE, Prentice HG, Brenner MK. IL2 activated killer cells may contribute to cytomegalovirus induced marrow hypoplasia after bone marrow transplantation. Bone Marrow Transplant 1991;7:81–87.
273. Slavin M, Dobbs S, Crawford S, Bowden R. Interleukin-2, interferon-gamma and natural killer cell activity in bronchoalveolar lavage fluid from marrow transplant recipients with cytomegalovirus pneumonia. Bone Marrow Transplant 1993;11:113–118.
274. Enright H, Haake R, Weisdorf D, et al. Cytomegalovirus pneumonia after bone marrow transplantation: risk factors and response to therapy. Transplantation 1993;55:1339–1346.
275. Gentile G, Micozzi A, Girmenia C, et al. Pneumonia in allogeneic and autologous bone marrow recipients: a retrospective study. Chest 1993;104:371–375.
276. Ljungman P, Biron P, Bosi A. Cytomegalovirus interstitial pneumonia in autologous bone marrow transplant recipients. Infectious disease working party of the European group for bone marrow transplantation. Bone Marrow Transplant 1994;209–212.
277. Schulman LL, Reison DS, Sustin JHM, Rose EA. Cytomegalovirus pneumonitis after cardiac transplantation. Arch Intern Med 1991;151:1118–1124.
278. Singh N, Dummer S, Kusne S, et al. Infections with CMV and other herpes viruses in 121 liver transplant recipients: transmission by donated organ and the effect of OKT3 antibodies. J Infect Dis 1988;158:124–131.
279. Nagler A, Elishoov H, Kapelushnik Y, et al. Cytomegalovirus pneumonia prior to engraftment following T-cell depleted bone marrow transplantation. Med Oncol 1994;11:127–132.
280. Webster A, Blizzard B, Pillay D, et al. Value of routine surveillance cultures for detection of CMV pneumonitis following bone marrow transplantation. Bone Marrow Transplant 1993;12:477–481.
281. Foot ABM, Caul EO, Roome AP, et al. Cytomegalovirus pneumonitis and bone marrow transplantation: identification of a specific high risk group. J Clin Pathol 1993;46:415–419.
282. Chinsky K, Goodenberger DM. Use of indium 111-labeled white blood cell scan in the diagnosis of CMV pneumonia in a renal transplant recipient with a normal chest roentgenogram. Chest 1991;99:761–763.
283. Paya CV, Smith TF, Ludwig J, Hermans PE. Rapid shell vial culture and tissue histology compared with serology for the rapid diagnosis of CMV infection in liver transplantation. Mayo Clin Proc 1989;64:670–675.

284. Boeckh M, Bowden RA, Goodrich JM, et al. Cytomegalovirus antigen detection in peripheral blood leukocytes after allogeneic marrow transplantation. Blood 1992;80:1358–1364.
285. Cathomas G, Morris P, Pekle K, et al. Rapid diagnosis of cytomegalovirus pneumonia in marrow transplant recipients by bronchoalveolar lavage using the polymerase chain reaction, virus culture and the direct immunostaining of alveolar cells. Blood 1993;81:1909–1914.
286. Aspin MM, Gallez-Hawkins GM, Giugni TD, et al. Comparison of plasma PCR and bronchoalveolar lavage fluid culture for detection of cytomegalovirus infection in adult bone marrow transplant recipients. J Clin Microbiol 1994;32:2266–2269.
287. Erice A. Diagnosis of cytomegalovirus pneumonia after bone marrow transplantation: is PCR the answer? Am J Clin Pathol 1991;96:564–567.
288. Heurlin N, Markling L, Barkholt L, et al. Rapid detection of cytomegalovirus antigen on alveolar cells in bronchoalveolar fluid from transplant patients with cytomegalovirus pneumonia. Clin Transplant 1994;8:466–473.
289. Slavin MA, Gooley TA, Bowden RA. Prediction of cytomegalovirus pneumonia after marrow transplantation from cellular characteristics and cytomegalovirus culture of bronchoalveolar lavage fluid. Transplantation 1994;58:915–919.
290. Schmidt GM, Horak DA, Niland JC, et al. A randomized, controlled trial of prophylactic ganciclovir for cytomegalovirus pulmonary infection in recipients of allogeneic bone marrow transplants. N Engl J Med 1991;324:1005–1011.
291. Goodrich JM, Mori M, Gleaves CA, et al. Early treatment with ganciclovir to prevent cytomegalovirus disease after allogeneic bone marrow transplantation. N Engl J Med 1991;325:1601–1607.
292. Boeckh M, Gooley TA, Reusser P, et al. Failure of high-dose acylovir to prevent cytomegalovirus disease after autologous marrow transplantation. J Infect Dis 1995;172:939–943.
293. Meyers JD, Reed EC, Shepp DH, et al. Acyclovir for prevention of cytomegalovirus infection and disease after allogeneic marrow transplantation. N Engl J Med 1988;318:70–75.
294. Balfour Jr HH, Chace BA, Stapleton JT, et al. A randomized, placebo-controlled trial of oral acyclovir for the prevention of cytomegalovirus disease in recipients of renal allografts. N Engl J Med 1989;320:1381–1387.
295. Krischer J, Elfbein G, Babington R, et al. Risk factors for cytomegalovirus pneumonia following allogeneic bone marrow transplantation after prophylaxis with intravenous immunoglobulin. Semin Hematol 1992;29:89–95.
296. Sullivan MP, Kopecky KJ, Jocom J, et al. Immunomodulatory and antimicrobial efficacy of intravenous immunoglobulin in bone marrow transplantation. N Engl J Med 1990;323:705–712.
297. Luis F, Ali AA, Grundy JE, et al. Double-blind placebo controlled trial of human lymphoblastoid interferon prophylaxis of cytomegalovirus infection in renal transplant recipients. Nephrol Dial Transplant 1992;7:1230–1237.
298. Ljungman P, Engelhard D, Link H, et al. Treatment of interstitial pneumonitis due to cytomegalovirus with ganciclovir and intravenous immune globulin: experience of European Bone Marrow Transplant Group. Clin Infect Dis 1992;14:831–835.
299. Emanuel D, Cunningham I, Jules-Elysee K, et al. Cytomegalovirus pneumonia after bone marrow transplantation successfully treated with the combination of ganciclovir and high-dose intravenous immune globulin. Ann Intern Med 1988;109:777–782.
300. Paya CV, Hermans PE, Smith TF, et al. Efficacy of ganciclovir in liver and kidney transplant recipients with severe CMV infection. Transplantation 1988;46:229–234.
301. Foramn SJ, Zaia JA. Treatment and prevention of cytomegalovirus pneumonia after bone marrow transplantation: where do we stand? Blood 1994;83:2392–2398.
302. Zaia JA. Prevention and treatment of cytomegalovirus pneumonia in transplant recipients. Clin Infect Dis 1993;17(suppl):392–399.
303. Drobyski WR, Knox KK, Carrigan DR, Ash RC. Foscarnet therapy of gancyclovir resistant cytomegalovirus in marrow transplantation. Transplantation 1991;52:155–157.
304. Avery RK, Longworth DL. Viral pulmonary infections in thoracic and cardiovascular surgery. Semin Thorac Cardiovasc Surg 1995;7:88–94.
305. Berberi N, Johnson DH, Cunha BA. Respiratory syncytial virus pneumonia in a heart transplant recipient presenting as fever of unknown origin diagnosed by gallium scan. Heart Lung 1995;24:257–259.
306. Harrington RD, Hooton TM, Hackman RC, et al. An outbreak of respiratory syncytial virus in a bone marrow transplant center. J Infect Dis 1992;165:987–993.
307. Fouillard L, Mouthon L, Laporte JJP, et al. Severe respiratory syncytial virus pneumonia after autologous bone marrow transplantation: a report of three cases and review. Bone Marrow Transplant 1995;9:97–100.
308. Win N, Mitchell D, Pugh S, Russell NH. Successful therapy with ribavirin of late onset respiratory syncytial virus pneumonitis complicating allogeneic bone transplantation. Clin Lab Haematol 1992;14:29–32.
309. Whimbey E, Vartivarian SE, Champlin RE, et al. Parainfluenza virus infection in adult bone marrow transplant recipients. Eur J Clin Microbiol Infect Dis 1993;12:699–701.
310. Wendt CH, Weisdorf DJ, Jordan C, et al. Parainfluenza virus respiratory infection after bone marrow transplantation. N Engl J Med 1992;326:921–926.
311. Shields AF, Hackman RC, Fife KH, et al. Adenovirus infections in patients undergoing bone-marrow transplantation. N Engl J Med 1985;312:529–533.
312. Michaels MG, Green M, Wald ER, Starzl TE. Adenovirus infection in pediatric liver transplant recipients. J Infect Dis 1992;165:170–174.
313. Matsuse T, Matsui H, Shu C-Y, et al. Adenovirus pulmonay infections identified by PCR and in situ hybridisation in bone marrow transplant recipients. J Clin Pathol 1994;47:973–977.
314. Apalsch AM, Green M, Ledesma-Medina J, et al. Parainfluenza and influenza virus infections in pediatric organ transplant recipients. Clin Infect Dis 1995;20:394–399.
315. Mauch TJ, Crouch NA, Freese DK, et al. Antibody response of pediatric solid organ transplant recipients to immunization against influenza virus. J Pediatr 1995;127:957–960.
316. Olsen SL, Renlund DG, O'Connell JB, et al. Prevention of *Pneumocystis carinii* pneumonia in cardiac transplant recipients by trimethoprim-sulfamethoxazole. Transplantation 1993;56:359–362.
317. Link H, Vohringer HF, Wingen F, et al. Pentamidine aerosol for prophylaxis of *Pneumocystis carinii* pneumonia after BMT. Bone Marrow Transplant 1993;11:403–406.
318. Colombo JL, Sammut PH, Langnas AN, Shaw BW. The spectrum of *Pneumocystis carinii* infection after liver transplantation in children. Transplantation 1992;54:621–624.
319. Elinder CG, Andersson J, Bolinder G, Tyden G. Effectiveness of low-dose cotrimoxazole prophylaxis against *Pneumocystis carinii* pneumonia after renal and/or pancreas transplantation. Transplant Int 1992;5:81–84.
320. Przepiorka D, Selvaggi K, Rosenzweig PQ, et al. Aerosolized pentamidine for prevention of *Pneumocystis* pneumonia after allogeneic marrow transplantation. Bone Marrow Transplant 1991;7:324–325. Letter.
321. Mahon FX, Sadoun A, Benz-Lemoine E, et al. Possible prevention of *Pneumocystis carinii* pneumonia by pentamidine aerosol after bone marrow transplantation. Bone Marrow Transplant 1991;8:64–65.
322. Hibberd PL, Tolkoff-Rubin NE, Doran M, et al. Trimethoprim-sulfamethoxazole compared with ciprofloxacin for the prevention of urinary tract infection in renal transplant recipients. A double-blind, randomized controlled trial. Online J Clin Trials Doc. No. 15, 1992.
323. Saukkonen K, Garland R, Koziel H. Aerosolized pentamidine as alternative primary prophylaxis against *Pneumocystis carinii* pneumonia in adult hepatic and renal transplant recipients. Chest 1996;109:1250–1255.
324. Hennequin C, Page B, Roux P, et al. Outbreak of *Pneumocystis carinii* pneumonia in a renal transplant unit. Eur J Clin Microbiol Infect Dis 1995;14:122–126.
325. Chave JP, David S, Wauters JP, et al. Transmission of *Pneumocystis carinii* from AIDS patients to other immunosuppressed patients: a cluster of *Pneumocystis carinii* pneumonia in renal transplant recipients. AIDS 1991;5:927–932.
326. Harmon WE. Opportunistic infections in children following renal transplantation. Pediatr Nephrol 1991;5:118–125.
327. Kinsmore SF, Schwab SJ. Pneumonia due to *Pneumocystis carinii* in a transplant recipient with normal arterial oxygen tension and normal radiographic findings. South Med J 1993;86:1052–1053.
328. Tuan IZ, Dennison D, Weisdorf DJ. *Pneumocystis carinii* pneumonia following bone marrow transplantation. Bone Marrow Transplant 1992;10:267–272.
329. Grossi P, Ippoliti GB, Goggi C, et al. *Pneumocystis carinii* pneumonia in heart transplant recipients. Infection 1993;21:75–79.
330. Saigenji H, Kaneko M, Rhenmen B, et al. *Pneumocystis carinii* pneumonia after heart transplantation. Ann Thorac Surg 1991;52:107–111.
331. The National Institute of Health: University of California expert panel for corticosteroids as adjunctive therapy for *Pneumocystis* pneumonia in the acquired immunodeficiency syndrome. N Engl J Med 1990;322:161–165.
332. Brown RS, Lake JR, Katzman BA, et al. Incidence and significance of *Aspergillus* cultures following liver and kidney transplantation. Transplantation 1996;61:666–669.
333. Saugier-Veber P, Devergie A, Sulahian A, et al. Epidemiology and diagnosis of invasive pulmonary aspergillosis in bone marrow transplant patients: results of a 5 year retrospective study. Bone Marrow Transplant 1993;12:121–124.

334. Hummel M, Schuler S, Hempel S, et al. Obstructive bronchial aspergillosis after heart transplantation. Mycoses 1993;36:425–428.
335. Putnam JB, Dignani MC, Mehra RC, et al. Acute airway obstruction and necrotizing tracheobronchitis from invasive mycosis. Chest 1994;106:1265–1267.
336. Mori M, Galvin JR, Barloon TJ, et al. Fungal pulmonary infections after bone marrow transplantation: evaluation with radiography and CT. Radiology 1991;178:721–726.
337. Mancini MC, McGinnis MR. Dactylaria infection of a human being: pulmonary disease in a heart transplant recipient. J Heart Lung Transplant 1992;11:827–830.
338. McCalmont TH, Silverman JF, Geisinger KR. Cytologic diagnosis of aspergillosis in cardiac transplantation. Arch Surg 1991;126:394–396.
339. Kusne S, Torre-Cisneros J, Manez R, et al. Factors associated with invasive lung aspergillosis and the significance of positive aspergillus culture after liver transplantation. J Infect Dis 1992;166:1379–1383.
340. Denning DW, Stepan DE, Blume KG, Stevens DA. Control of invasive pulmonary aspergillosis with oral itraconazole in a bone marrow transplant patient. J Infect 1992;24:73–79.
341. Wang SS, Chu SH, Lee YC, et al. Successful treatment of invasive pulmonary aspergillosis in heart transplantation. Transplant Proc 1994;26:2329–2332.
342. Mayer JM, Nimer L, Carroll K. Isolated pulmonary aspergillar infection in cardiac transplant recipients: case report and review. Clin Infect Dis 1992;15:698–700.
343. Robinson LA, Reed EC, Galgraith TA, et al. Pulmonary resection for invasive *Aspergillus* infections in immunocompromised patients. J Thorac Cardiovasc Surg 1995;109:1182–1197.
344. Lupinetti FM, Behrendt DM, Giller RH, et al. Pulmonary resection for fungal infection in children undergoing bone marrow transplantation. J Thorac Cardiovasc Surg 1992;104:684–687.
345. Rousey SR, Russler S, Gottlieb M, Ash RC. Low-dose amphotericin B prophylaxis against invasive *Aspergillus* infections in allogeneic marrow transplantation. Am J Med 1991;91:484–492.
346. Warnock DW. Fungal complications of transplantation: diagnosis, treatment, and prevention. J Antimicrob Chemother 1995;36(suppl):73–90.
347. Bresson-Hadni S, Miguet JP, Lenys D, et al. Recurrence of alveolar echinococcosis in the liver graft after liver transplantation. Hepatology 1992;16:279–280.
348. Gordon SM, Gal AA, Gertzler GL, et al. Diagnosis of pulmonary toxoplasmosis by bronchoalveolar lavage in cardiac transplant recipients. Diagn Cytopathol 1993;9:650–654.
349. Pomeroy C, Filice GA. Pulmonary toxoplasmosis: a review. Clin Infect Dis 1992;14:863–870.
350. Petri WA. Infections in heart transplant recipients. Clin Infect Dis 1994;18:141–148.
351. Armstrong D, Paredes J. Strongyloidiasis. In: Shelhamer J, Pizzo PA, Parrillo JE, Masur H, eds. Respiratory disease in the immunosuppressed host. Philadelphia: Lippincott, 1991:428–432.
352. Jensen WA, Rose RM, Hammer SM, et al. Pulmonary complications of orthotopic liver transplantation. Transplantation 1986;42:484–490.
353. Carmellini M, Romagnoli J, Pietrabissa A, et al. Evaluation of infections in renal transplant recipients treated with cyclosporine. Transplant Proc 1994;26:2658–2659.

Chapter

29

Gastroenterologic Considerations of Organ Transplantation

Philip L. Shields James M. Neuberger

This chapter reviews the gastroenterologic aspects and complications of organ transplantation. Most complications, especially those related to immunosuppression, are common to all organs. Other complications may depend on the organ that is grafted. Particular problems that will be reviewed include the following:

- Opportunistic infections of the gastrointestinal tract and liver
- Complications of immunosuppressive therapy
- Gastrointestinal manifestations of graft-versus-host disease (GVHD)
- Biliary complications of liver transplantation
- Gastrointestinal bleeding, pancreatitis, and colonic complications
- Gastrointestinal malignancy after transplantation
- Preexisting gastrointestinal disease and organ transplantation
- Chronic viral hepatitis and primary disease recurrence following liver transplantation

Gastrointestinal (GI) symptoms (Table 29.1) are common after organ transplantation and are important to recognize as there may often be a serious underlying cause, especially in the immunosuppressed patient, resulting in a significant increase in mortality.

GASTROINTESTINAL AND HEPATIC COMPLICATIONS OF THERAPY ASSOCIATED WITH ORGAN TRANSPLANTATION

Immunosuppressive Therapy

The main complications of immunosuppressive therapies used to treat allograft rejection are infections, and these are discussed elsewhere in this chapter and in Chapter 36. Drug-specific GI and hepatic complications are considered in this section.

Corticosteroids

A mainstay of immunosuppressive therapy, corticosteroids have a number of potentially adverse effects (see also Chapter 8). The role of steroids in the etiology of peptic ulceration remains controversial. In an analysis of 3064 patients in 71 clinical trials (1), the incidence of peptic ulceration was higher in patients taking steroids than in controls (1.8% versus 0.8%). The incidence appeared to correlate with the dose of steroid. Gastrointestinal hemorrhage was more common in patients taking steroids (2.25% versus 1.6%). It is important that the clinician be aware that steroids may mask the symptoms associated with peptic ulcer disease.

High-dose corticosteroids have been associated with the development of bacterial overgrowth resulting in diarrhea (2). Pancreatitis is also associated with long-term steroid therapy.

Fatty infiltration of the liver, mainly in the centrilobular region, is reported with steroid treatment. The pathogenesis is not completely understood but possibly relates to increased lipid synthesis and reduced formation of very-low-density lipoproteins (VLDL) with reduced clearance from hepatocytes (3). It is rarely of clinical importance but may give a bright echogenic liver.

Azathioprine

Azathioprine commonly causes nausea that may often be relieved by food, suggesting that azathioprine may have a direct irritant effect on gastric mucosa (Glaxo, personal communication). It may also be associated with pancreatitis.

Azathioprine is associated with liver damage that may be characterized by cholestatic/hepatocellular injury. Abnormalities of liver tests, especially of the serum transaminases, may occur in up to 10% of patients. Rarely, cirrhosis has been reported. Several reports implicate azathioprine and the chemically related compound mercaptopurine as a cause of veno-occlusive disease (4). Most of these cases involve renal

Table 29.1. Common Gastrointestinal Symptoms Complicating Organ Transplantation and Their Causes

Mouth Ulceration/Sore Throat
- Herpes simplex virus (HSV)
- Cytomegalovirus (CMV)
- GVHD
- Candidiasis

Odynophagia/Dysphagia
- Candidiasis
- CMV
- HSV
- GVHD
- Ulceration or abscess formation with stricturing following variceal sclerotherapy

Abdominal Pain
- Constipation
- Peptic ulceration
- Pancreatitis
- Bowel perforation
- CMV colitis
- GVHD
- Small bowel lymphoma

Gastrointestinal Bleeding
- Fungal infection
- CMV ulceration
- Peptic ulceration/stress ulceration
- Roux loop anastamotic bleed
- Lymphoma
- Hemobilia—post liver biopsy
- Infectious diarrhea

Diarrhea
- Drugs
  - Antibiotic therapy
  - H2 blockers
  - Proton pump inhibitors
- High osmolality enteral feed

Infectious Diarrhea
- Viral
  - CMV colitis
  - HSV
  - Adenovirus
  - Coxsackievirus
- Bacterial
  - *Salmonella*
  - *Clostridium difficile* (Pseudomembranous colitis)
- Fungal
  - *Candida albicans*
- Parasites
  - *Cryptosporidium*
  - *Microsporidium*
  - *Isospora belli*
  - *Strongyloides*
- Lymphoma
- GVHD

Jaundice
- Infection
  - Viral
    - Hepatitis A, B, C, D, E
    - CMV
    - Epstein-Barr virus (EBV)
    - HSV
    - Adenovirus
- Bacterial
  - Cholangitis
- Pancreatitis
- Total parenteral nutrition
- GVHD of the liver
- Sepsis-related cholestasis
- Hemolysis
- Drug-related
  - Antibiotics
  - H2 blockers
- Lymphoma

Associated with Liver Transplantation
- Biliary complications
- Primary nonfunction/preservation injury
- Acute and chronic rejection
- Hepatic artery thrombosis

transplant recipients concurrently receiving steroids, and there is also preponderance of males in this group. The onset is often delayed for at least six months after beginning therapy but may occur within three months of therapy or years later. Presentation varies from that associated with veno-occlusive disease due to other causes, with more prominent jaundice and histologic features of both cholestasis and centrilobular necrosis. Sinusoidal and perivenular fibrosis, peliosis hepatis, and nodular regenerative hyperplasia may be seen as associated pathologic lesions. One study has implicated veno-occlusive disease in 12 (2%) of 500 renal allograft recipients.

Mycophenolate Mofetil

Mycophenolate mofetil (MMF) selectively inhibits proliferation of T and B lymphocytes by inhibition of inosine monophosphate dehydrogenase (see Chapter 10). Its side effect profile is similar to that of azathioprine, although studies reported a higher incidence of GI symptoms in those taking MMF compared to azathioprine, particularly on higher doses (5). The principal manifestations were diarrhea, abdominal pain, vomiting, and GI infection. MMF-induced diarrhea usually starts quite rapidly after treatment is initiated and also disappears relatively soon after cessation of therapy. Late-onset diarrhea has been reported in association with villous atrophy (6).

More severe problems in 164 renal transplant patients receiving 3 g MMF daily included enteric infection (n = 9), colitis (n = 3), and hepatitis (n = 5). These were the predominant events leading to discontinuation or interruption of the drug. The more severe GI adverse events occurred beyond one month after renal transplantation in the MMF group, unlike the experience with azathioprine in which most complications developed within one month (7).

Cyclosporine

Cyclosporine has been associated with a severe nonspecific colitis in a renal transplant patient, manifesting as vomiting and bloody diarrhea that proved unresponsive to intravenous steroids. There were extensive vascular thromboses in the colonic submucosa (8). Hepatotoxicity and cholestatic jaundice may also occur (9). The side effects are dose dependent and are characterized by elevation of serum alkaline phosphatase and transaminases. Rarely, cyclosporine may precipitate in the biliary tree. As with other forms of immunosuppression, cyclosporine has been associated with an increased incidence of malignancy, notably lymphoma (10) (see Chapter 6).

Murine Monoclonal CD3 Antibody (OKT-3)

OKT-3 is efficacious when used in the treatment of early post-transplant rejection episodes (see Chapter 13). Its side effects include a combination of symptoms including fever, chills, shortness of breath, and bronchospasm. Gastrointestinal symptoms also occur and include nausea, vomiting, and diarrhea. These usually occur within one hour of the dose and may last several hours or even days. Acute pancreatitis has also been reported in association with OKT-3 administration in a heart transplant patient. It has been proposed that these side effects may be due to the release of vasoactive cytokines after lysis of opsonized T cells (11).

Tacrolimus

Tacrolimus (Prograf or FK506) is a macrolide compound isolated from *Streptomyces tsukabaensis* that has potent immunosuppressive properties (see Chapter 9). It inhibits the mixed lymphocyte reaction. Gastrointestinal symptoms associated with tacrolimus include severe prolonged vomiting, diarrhea, and also constipation. Less frequent associations include abnormal liver function tests, hepatomegaly, jaundice, cholangitis, pancreatitis, and liver failure.

In the European multicenter study in liver transplant patients, diarrhea was reported in 37% of tacrolimus-treated patients versus 26% of those treated with cyclosporine. It was reported as serious in 3 patients in the tacrolimus group (1.1%) and led to withdrawal of therapy in 1 case. Nausea occurred in 32% of the tacrolimus group, versus 27% of those taking cyclosporine, but did not lead to withdrawal of treatment in any patient (12). In the US study, diarrhea, dyspepsia, nausea, and vomiting were reported more frequently in the tacrolimus group (13).

Obviously these symptoms are often multifactorial and difficult to interpret due to the number of concurrent medications and in the setting of hepatic surgery.

Diarrhea Associated with Antibiotic Therapy

Almost all antibiotics can cause diarrhea. In the majority of cases, the cause of diarrhea is not clear. In some, infection due to *Clostridium difficile* is the cause; in others there is a drug-specific cause, for example the inactivation of lipase by tetracycline, the acceleration of GI transit by erythromycin, or the binding of bile salts by neomycin.

GASTROINTESTINAL AND HEPATIC COMPLICATIONS OF NUTRITIONAL SUPPORT IN THE TRANSPLANT PATIENT

Enteral Nutrition

Enteral nutrition is the most common and preferred method of providing nutritional support to the malnourished, often severely ill post-transplant patient. It is complicated, however, by diarrhea in up to 68% of cases (14). Other adverse GI effects include gastric distention, abdominal cramping, nausea, and vomiting.

Potential causes of diarrhea in enterally fed patients include malnutrition and malabsorption, hyperosmotic formulas, lactose intolerance, bacterial contamination of formulas, and the use of antibiotics including penicillins, cephalosporins, and clindamycin. Hypoalbuminemia as a result of malnutrition may cause bowel mucosal edema and impair absorption leading to diarrhea. Several studies have demonstrated an association between hypoalbuminemia and intolerance of enteral feed. Although osmolality may be a significant factor in patients with hypoalbuminemia, administration of hypertonic formulas does not correlate with diarrhea in healthy controls.

There is little consistent data regarding the use of supplementary fiber in enteral feeds to reduce the incidence of diarrhea, although such a practice is associated with a decreased stool frequency and improved stool consistency (15).

The association between contaminated formulas and diarrhea remains controversial, although some intervention studies have suggested that manual manipulation of feeding formula and the administration bag promotes bacterial contamination and possibly development of diarrhea (14).

Total Parenteral Nutrition

In addition to mechanical complications and sepsis arising from insertion of feeding lines, and metabolic derangements, total parenteral nutrition (TPN) may be associated with alterations in GI structure and function (16). Small intestinal mucosal atrophy with a fall in brush border enzyme activity and reduced absorption may occur. Absence of luminal nutrients also results in impaired barrier function and increased intestinal permeability, and allows translocation of bacteria and endotoxin from the gut lumen into the portal circulation, increasing the incidence of septicemia (17). When supplemented to TPN solutions, glutamine, an amino acid essential for the production of nucleotides, which are a prime energy source for the enterocyte, may partially reverse mucosal atrophy and brush border enzyme activity. In a double-blind, randomized study, bone marrow transplant recipients received TPN with or without glutamine supplementation. There were reduced sepsis and microbial colonization, a better nitrogen balance, and a shorter inpatient stay in the glutamine-supplemented group (18).

The exact incidence of liver dysfunction in those given TPN is not known, although 90% of those receiving a lipid-free formula for one week developed elevated alanine transferase and aspartate aminotransferase levels. Transaminase rises are more likely to occur if parenteral nutrition is given for longer than three weeks. Reversible steatosis and later cholestasis, chronic active hepatitis, fibrosis, and cirrhosis can occur. Biliary sludge accumulation and gallstones may occur and may be associated with an enlarged atonic gallbladder. This may result from atrophy of intestinal mucosa and reduction in GI secretion of hormones such as gastrin and cholecystekinin. Bacterial translocation and endotoxemia of the portal system may account for hepatic dysfunction (19) and this dysfunction may be more common in those with preexisting sepsis, liver disease, or concurrent bowel disease. Management of hepatic dysfunction includes cycling of TPN with administration for 12 hours per day to avoid prolonged hyperglycemia and hyperinsulinemia (20). It may take two to three weeks before improvement occurs. Reduction of lipid to only 30% of total daily calorie intake and to less than 3 g/kg/day may also be beneficial. The role of ursodeoxycholic acid in the prevention and treatment of TPN-related liver disease is currently under evaluation.

INFECTIONS

Allograft recipients are susceptible to several systemic, GI, and hepatic infections that are rare in the immunocompetent subject. Detailed discussions of those infectious complications are presented elsewhere in this book (see Chapter 36), and only clinically important bacterial, fungal, viral, and parasitic infections manifesting with GI symptoms in the post-transplant period are discussed here. Although other enteric infections such as campylobacter, shigella, giardia, and amebiasis may occur in transplant patients, they are not reported to occur with increased frequency in the transplant setting and are beyond the scope of this chapter.

Bacterial Infection

Clostridium difficile *(Pseudomembranous Colitis)*

Pseudomembranous colitis due to *Clostridium difficile* infection is an important problem in hospitalized transplant patients and most commonly results as a consequence of antibiotic therapy (Fig. 29.1 and Plate 28). Almost any antibiotic may allow emergence of *C. difficile* infection but those with activity against enteric bacteria are the most common culprits.

C. difficile is carried by 1% of healthy adults but after recent therapy with antibiotics this figure rises to 25% (21). The majority of patients are asymptomatic, although they act as an important reservoir for spread throughout the environment. Symptomatic *C. difficile* infection commonly causes lower abdominal cramps and mild to moderate diarrhea that may occur shortly after antibiotic therapy but is occasionally delayed several weeks. Stopping the antibiotic may improve the diarrhea; however, many clinicians institute specific therapy as summarized below.

More severe colitis may occur, often with pseudomembrane formation, and produce debilitating diarrhea,

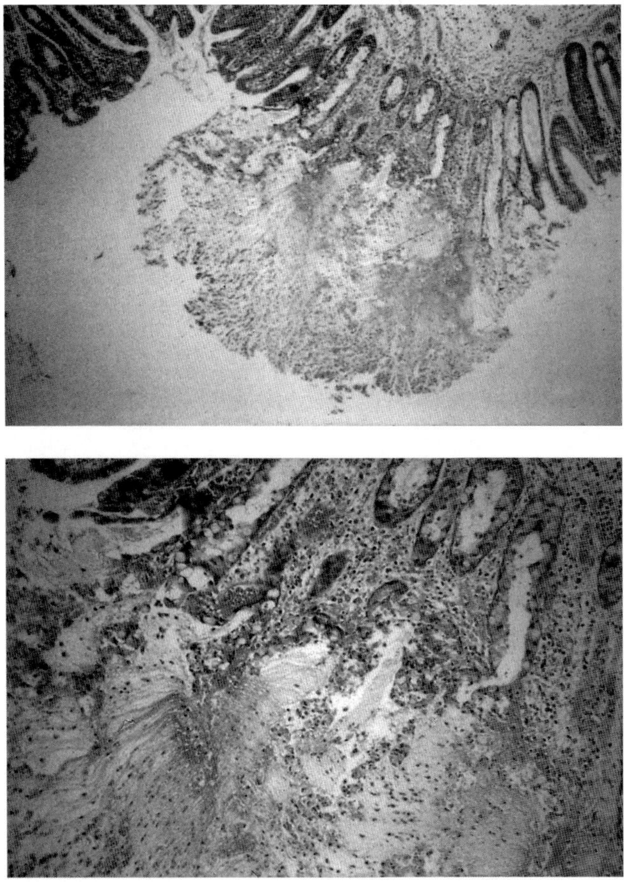

A

B

FIGURE 29.1. *Photomicrographs of colonic biopsy taken from a patient with lower abdominal cramps, fever, and diarrhea, showing histologic changes of pseudomembranous colitis.*

abdominal pain, and distention. Sigmoidoscopy usually provides the diagnosis; however, in approximately 10% of cases colitis is confined to the more proximal colon and may be missed by the sigmoidoscope. Detection of *C. difficile* toxin in stool specimens by the highly sensitive and specific stool cytotoxin test is useful but requires overnight incubation. Treatment is with oral metronidazole or vancomycin for seven days. Relapse may occur, which can be effectively treated by a repeat course. Patients who are unable to tolerate oral medication can be effectively treated with intravenous metronidazole, although intravenous vancomycin is not appropriate as there is minimal excretion of this agent into the intestinal lumen.

Nontyphoid Salmonella

Nontyphoid salmonella infection has been reported to occur in up to 5% of patients after renal transplantation (22), with an annual incidence 20 times that in the normal adult population (23). In most studies of patients after transplantation, *Salmonella typhimurium* (group B salmonella) is the most common serotype to cause infection.

In the largest reported series in post-transplant patients, the most common presentation was with fever (77%) and diarrhea (58%). Focal manifestations such as abscesses, arthritis, cholecystitis, and peritonitis were also more common than in the immunocompetent. There was an associated mortality of 5% (23). Treatment with amoxycillin, 1 g four times a day, or with ciprofloxacin is usually successful. Recurrence of nontyphoid salmonellosis is common in the immunosuppressed, with relapse in approximately 35% in one series (23). The source of persistent infection may be the biliary tract, urinary tract, colonic diverticuli, a chronically inflamed jejunum, lymph nodes, or spleen. Chronic carriers should be treated with oral ciprofloxacin for six weeks. Cholecystectomy for enteric carriers, or bilateral nephrectomy for renal transplant patients who are urinary carriers, particularly in those with structural abnormalities, should be considered.

Parasitic Infection

Cryptosporidiosis

Cryptosporidia are coccidial parasites spread by feco-oral transmission that may colonize the small and large bowel, occupying an intracellular but extracytoplasmic location in intestinal epithelial cells (24). It is well recognized as a cause of traveler's diarrhea (3% to 15%) and is common in the immunosuppressed, particularly those with HIV infection (25). There are several reports of cryptosporidiosis after organ transplantation, particularly after bone marrow (26,27) and renal transplantation (28,29).

Patients present with chronic, profuse watery diarrhea. Microscopy of stained stool specimens and histologic examination of small or large intestinal mucosal biopsies should give the diagnosis. Fecal antigen enzyme-linked immunosorbent assay (ELISA) for *C. parvum* is also now available (25). Patients should be isolated to prevent spread of infection and treatment consists of reduction in immunosuppression. No antimicrobial agents have consistently been effective although some report resolution with spiramycin (27).

Strongyloidiasis

Strongyloides stercoralis is an intestinal nematode occurring predominantly in the tropics and subtropics. The parasite can complete its life cycle in its host and thus can survive within subjects unnoticed for many years. Immunosuppression may result in dissemination of the disease in carriers and may be fatal. All transplant patients potentially exposed to the organism should be examined for parasites and preemptive therapy given to any carriers or those with a history of travel to endemic areas. There are several reports of *Strongyloides* infection after organ transplantation mainly in renal allograft recipients. This presented with a tropical enteropathy in one case (29), and disseminated and fatal disease in another (30).

Gastrointestinal symptoms include upper abdominal discomfort and diarrhea. It has also been associated with protein-losing enteropathy and edema. In the immunosuppressed, unchecked autoinfection and migration of worms from the bowel may cause a hyperinfection syndrome. Intestinal penetration results in bowel wall edema and ulceration, and is accompanied by severe abdominal pain with ileus, small bowel obstruction, and occasionally peritonitis. Bacterial or fungal infection carried from the bowel lumen may result in septic shock. Passage of larvae to the lungs results in bronchospasm and pulmonary bacterial superinfection. Eosinophilic meningitis may also occur.

Diagnosis may be made by microscopy of stool, duodenal fluid, or sputum. Several stool specimens should be examined in order to confidently exclude disease as even five or more examinations will only detect 80% of infection. Serology for *S. stercoralis* by ELISA is also available. Small bowel biopsies may reveal an inflammatory infiltrate of mononuclear cells and eosinophils and partial villous atrophy. Treatment is with thiabendazole 25 mg/kg daily for up to one week. Repeated courses of therapy may be necessary in the immunosuppressed. Other agents include mebendazole and albendazole.

Microsporidiosis

Microsporidia are obligate intracellular protazoan parasites that may cause enteritis, hepatitis, cholangitis, and peritonitis when associated with the human immunodeficiency virus. Infection is unusual in the post-transplant setting but has been reported after liver transplantation, resulting in nausea, malaise, watery diarrhea, and weight loss. Diagnosis may be made by stool and duodenal aspirate microscopy, and small bowel biopsies may show partial villous atrophy. There is good response to metronidazole (32).

Fungal Infection

Candida may produce significant inflammatory lesions in any part of the GI tract. Infections usually result from *Candida albicans* and *Candida tropicalis*. The esophagus is a common site of infection in immunosuppressed patients and usual presentation is with odynophagia or dysphagia, with or without oral thrush. Less commonly patients have fever, heartburn, epigastric pain, or GI bleeding. The stomach, duodenum, and small bowel and colon may also be involved (33). Visible lesions include superficial erosions, white nodules or plaques, ulceration, and even tumor-like masses. Perforation with tracheoesophageal fistula formation has also been described (34).

Fungal colonization of the small intestine and colon most commonly occurs in immunosuppressed, debilitated patients. Other risk factors include antibiotic use, GVHD, and cytomegalovirus (CMV) infection (35). Clinical manifestations of fungal enteritis include abdominal pain, diarrhea, perforation, peritonitis, and mass lesions (33).

Diagnosis is best made by endoscopic brushings and biopsy (36). Culture of brush or biopsy specimens may identify unusual fungal infection such as blastomycosis (37). In patients with diarrhea, large numbers of yeast may be seen in fecal smears (38). Treatment is with oral nystatin for oral thrush. Fluconazole (200–400 mg/day) is indicated for esophageal, gastric, and bowel involvement. It is highly effective and less hepatotoxic than agents such as ketoconazole. In more severe infections, intravenous amphotericin is used, with liposomal amphotericin being reserved for those patients with moderate or severe renal impairment.

Viral Infection

Herpes Simplex Virus

Herpes simplex virus (HSV) may cause a spectrum of disease varying from GI tract ulceration to hepatitis (Fig. 29.2 and Plate 29). HSV esophagitis may result in discrete vesicles, ulceration with raised edges, and coalescent necrosis in the distal esophagus (39). Duodenojejunal ulcers are less common. Herpes virus colitis has also been described resulting in diarrhea (40).

Herpes hepatitis is uncommon after organ transplantation with one study suggesting an incidence of approximately 0.01% (3 of 348 liver transplant patients), with infection developing on average 14 days after transplantation (41). In 2 of 3 patients, hepatitis was associated with previous OKT-3 therapy for rejection and with disseminated herpes virus infection. Fatal fulminant herpes simplex hepatitis has also been reported after renal transplantation (42).

The diagnosis of HSV may be made by inspection of lesions; however, it is more accurately diagnosed by culture or by finding typical inclusion-bearing or multinucleate epithelial cells on biopsy (Fig. 29.3 and Plate 30). In addition, HSV antigens may be demonstrated in epithelial cells

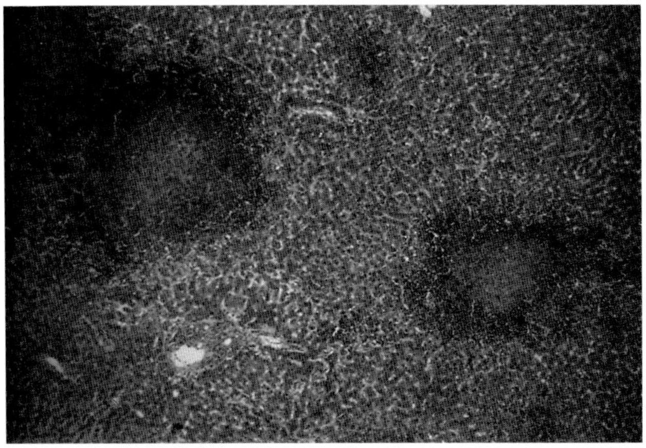

FIGURE 29.2. *Photomicrograph of herpes simplex hepatitis.*

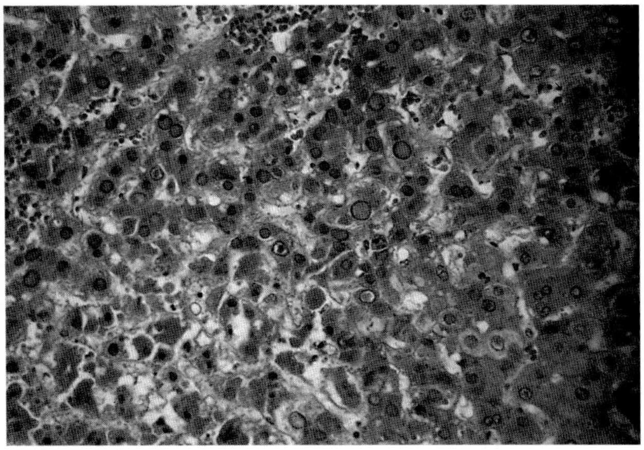

FIGURE 29.3. *Photomicrograph of herpes simplex hepatitis demonstrating characteristic nuclear inclusion on biopsy.*

by immunofluorescence (Fig. 29.4 and Plate 31) (43). Treatment is with acyclovir, normally taken orally, 400 mg five times daily for five days. More severe infection, particularly hepatitis, warrants intravenous therapy.

Epstein-Barr Virus

Epstein-Barr virus (EBV) infection is common in the general population with primary infection occurring in childhood, when it is often subclinical, or from mid-teens onward, when it can present with infectious mononucleosis. It follows that in the transplant population children are more likely to develop primary infection than adults. Reactivation under immunosuppression may also occur.

After transplantation EBV infection may arise as a result of transfused blood or from the donor organ. In one large study (44), 1117 (92%) of 1214 adults and 126 (50%) of 253

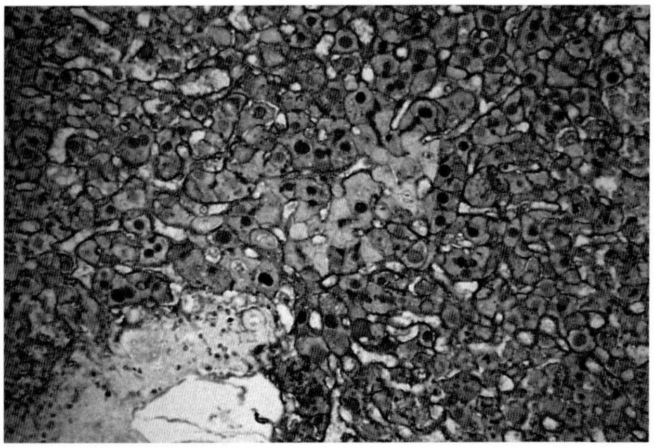

FIGURE 29.4. *Photomicrograph of liver biopsy with immunoperoxidase staining demonstrating HSV antigens in epithelial cells.*

children had serologic evidence of past EBV infection at transplant. Primary infection occurred in 82% and 77% of seronegative adults and children, respectively, whereas reactivation occurred in 33% and 48% of seropositive adults and children, respectively. The mean incubation time was 66 days for primary infection and 61 days for reactivation after liver transplantation.

EBV can cause a range of illnesses including pharyngitis, tonsillitis, hepatitis, and lymphoproliferative disease. Risk factors for post-transplant EBV-related disorders include the use of immunosuppressants, polyclonal antilymphocyte globulin, and the monoclonal antibody OKT-3.

EBV Hepatitis EBV hepatitis is a relatively uncommon problem with a reported incidence of 2% to 3% after liver transplantation (45). It most commonly occurs within six months of liver transplantation (46) and presents with liver graft dysfunction and nonspecific elevation of liver enzymes. This may often occur promptly following an episode of acute rejection where immunosuppression was increased. This supports the rationale to repeat the liver biopsy promptly when an improvement in graft function is not seen after antirejection therapy. Serial biopsies often show a characteristic transition from acute rejection to EBV hepatitis or lymphoproliferative disorder (47). Histologically, the most obvious features are loss of eosinophils from the inflammatory infiltrate and increased plasmacytic lymphocytes and immunoblasts in the portal areas. There may be mild bile duct changes but no bile duct destruction. The inflammatory infiltrate varies from portal area to portal area and may or may not expand beyond the limiting plate into the surrounding parenchyma.

The histologic diagnosis may be confirmed by detection of EBV DNA in liver by the polymerase chain reaction (PCR) (46). Diagnosis of EBV infection can be made serologically by detection of EBV viral capsid antigen (VCA) IgM or a four-fold increase in EBV VCA IgG. Treatment of EBV disease in transplant patients involves reduction or withdrawal of immunosuppression in addition to the use of antiviral agents such as acyclovir and ganciclovir, either alone or in combination. Acyclovir is administered at a dosage of 10 mg/kg every eight hours, ganciclovir at a dosage of 5 mg/kg every 12 hours. Controlled clinical trials supporting the use of either of these agents are limited.

Cytomegalovirus

Cytomegalovirus (CMV), a herpesvirus that commonly infects humans, is typically harmless in healthy individuals. However, it is one of the most important opportunistic pathogens in the immunosuppressed, particularly in the organ transplant setting, occurring in 60% to 70% of kidney, liver, bone marrow, heart, and lung transplant recipients (48) (see Chapter 36). This may be as a result of primary infection, which usually occurs when a seronegative recipient receives an organ from a seropositive donor, or secondary infection, which may result from reactivation in latently infected seropositive recipients during immunosuppression. In addition to the direct infectious processes caused by CMV, it also has an immunomodulatory effect causing an increased incidence of rejection and superinfection.

Risk factors for CMV infection and disease include the serologic status of the donor organ and the transplant recipient and the use of anti-T-cell therapy such as OKT-3 for allograft rejection (49). Reports detailing the incidence of CMV GI tract infection are scarce, but in one study examining renal transplant patients with CMV infection, 9 out of 12 patients had evidence of large bowel ulceration. CMV infection may affect any part of the GI tract from the mouth to the anus, with variable appearances, but most commonly ulceration. Description of some of the features associated with CMV infection follow.

1. **Ulcers.** These may be superficial, punched-out lesions or deeper, penetrating ulcers. Appearances resembling Crohn's disease with skip lesions have been reported affecting bowel (50). CMV infection has been shown to result in deep, linear ulceration in the esophagus (51) and giant ulceration in the esophagus and stomach. A solitary ulcer due to CMV has been described in the ascending colon (52).
2. **Hemorrhagic proctocolitis.** A colitis resembling infectious or ulcerative colitis may occur and cases of toxic megacolon, one case associated with a severe CMV vasculitis, have been described (52). Pseudomembrane formation due to CMV has been demonstrated, affecting the cecum and ascending colon.
3. **Lesions mimicking neoplasia.** Case reports have described inflammatory masses resembling tumors in the gastric antrum (53) and ileocecal area. One described a stenosing ulcerative lesion in the colon that clinically, radiologically, and macroscopically resembled a neoplasm (54).

4. **Appendicitis.** CMV infection of the appendix causing perforation has been described (55).

5. **Perforation.** Perforations may occur in any part of the GI tract but most commonly between the distal ileum and the splenic flexure (56).

6. **Pneumatosis intestinalis.** Pneumatosis was associated with CMV colitis in one renal transplant recipient (57).

7. **Biliary tract lesions.** CMV has been implicated as the cause of lesions in the biliary tree. Cholangitis (58), acalculous cholecystitis (59), and papillary stenosis (60) have been associated with CMV, and CMV diseases of the pancreas and the spleen have also been described.

8. **Hepatitis.** CMV is the most frequent viral pathogen to affect the liver with one study suggesting an incidence of 12% following liver transplantation. The mean time for developing primary CMV infection was found to be 37 days, and 46 days for developing reactivation or reinfection (41). CMV hepatitis has been associated with a significantly higher incidence of chronic rejection after liver transplantation (61).

Symptoms of CMV Clinical symptoms vary in severity depending on the nature and extent of the CMV lesions and their site in the GI tract. In organ transplant recipients with GI involvement, bleeding due to ulceration and occasionally perforation are the most common modes of presentation. Other symptoms are as follows:

- Fever
- Abdominal pain
- Abdominal distention
- Diarrhea—loose, bloody
- Hematochezia
- Hematemesis
- Dysphagia
- Weight loss

Diagnosis of CMV The onset of fever, leukopenia, and any of the above symptoms may suggest the diagnosis. It can be confirmed by the development of a high titer of IgM antibodies or a four-fold rise in IgG antibodies, although measurement and interpretation of rising antibody titers is often difficult in the context of immunosuppression. Detection of immediate early antigens by monoclonal antibodies is a more sensitive and specific test, allowing early diagnosis of active CMV infection from peripheral blood neutrophils and monocytes (62). This provides a useful marker of disease activity and for the monitoring of response to treatment. CMV can be cultured in human embryo fibroblast cell cultures. Successful isolation of CMV does not necessarily mean active disease as the virus may be excreted for years after primary infection (63). Endoscopic biopsies either of the upper GI tract in those with upper GI symptoms or of the rectum or large bowel in those with diarrhea may provide the diagnosis (Fig. 29.5 and Plate 32). Histology demonstrates "owl's eye" intranuclear inclusions in vascular endothelium, mucosal epithelium, and connective tissue stromal cells (Fig. 29.6 and Plate 33). Immunohistochemistry can demonstrate virus antigens, and PCR to detect CMV nucleic acid is also available as a research tool (Fig. 29.7 and Plate 34).

Treatment of CMV Ganciclovir is a virustatic agent and treatment with 5 mg/kg intravenously every 12 hours is effective in treating GI CMV disease (64). Clinical relapse of CMV infection may occur in up to a quarter of patients after completion of the treatment course, however (65). Foscarnet has also been used and shown to be effective in CMV disease of the GI tract (66).

CMV hyperimmune globulin obtained from plasma donors who have high titers of CMV antibody may be used in conjunction with drug therapy in those with life-

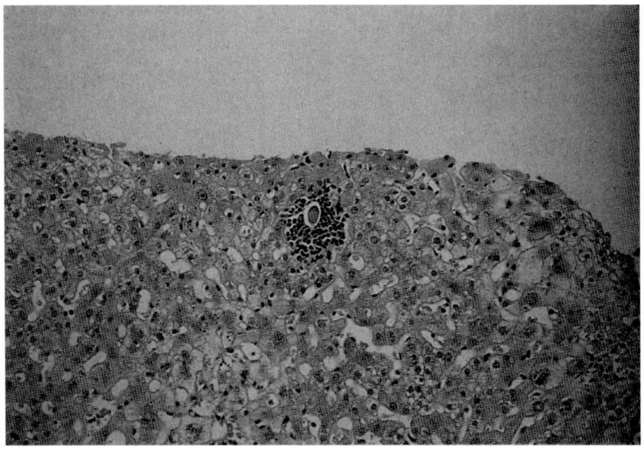

FIGURE 29.5. *Photomicrograph of liver biopsy demonstrating a microabscess in CMV hepatitis.*

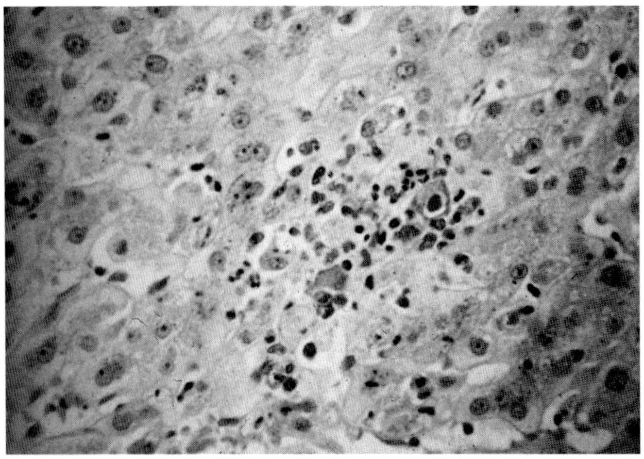

FIGURE 29.6. *Photomicrograph of liver biopsy in a case of CMV hepatitis with characteristic nuclear inclusion.*

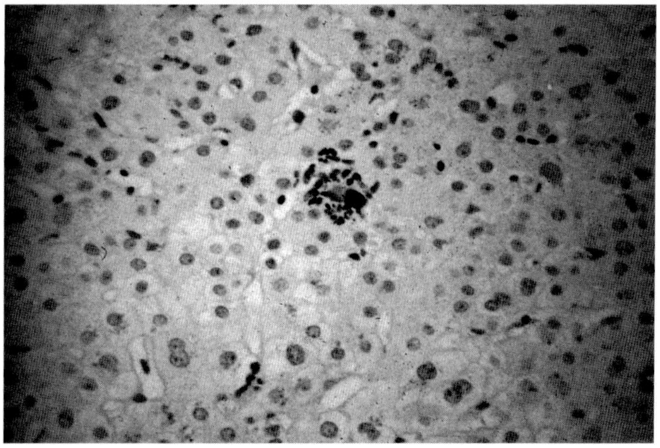

FIGURE 29.7. *Photomicrograph of liver biopsy in a case of CMV hepatitis diagnosed by positive stain of immunoperoxidase.*

threatening disease or in those slow to respond to ganciclovir therapy.

Adenovirus

Adenovirus infections may cause serious disease in immunocompromised post-transplant patients and are a recognized cause of GI and hepatic complications in bone marrow, renal, and liver transplant recipients. Gastrointestinal manifestations include gastroenteritis, colitis, and hepatitis (67), which may be severe enough to cause fulminant hepatic necrosis (68) (Figs. 29.8, 29.9, and Plates 35 and 36). In immunosuppressed patients, adenovirus disease has been attributed to both primary infection and reactivation of endogenous latent infection (69). There is also evidence to suggest adenovirus transmission from donor organ to recipient (70).

The incidence of adenovirus infection is between 3.8% and 20.9%, with clinical disease in 0.04% to 6.5% of bone marrow transplant recipients depending on the study (67). The incidence is higher in pediatric patients than in adults. Moderate to severe acute GVHD and isolation of adenovirus from two or more sites were significant risk factors for adenovirus disease, which carried a significant mortality (67). Gastrointestinal symptoms include prolonged diarrhea lasting up to 12 days, vomiting, and fever (71).

Diagnosis can be made by stool culture and electron microscopy. Intranuclear inclusion bodies may be seen in histologic samples and the diagnosis may be confirmed by immunohistochemical staining (68). There is currently no known effective therapy for adenovirus infection.

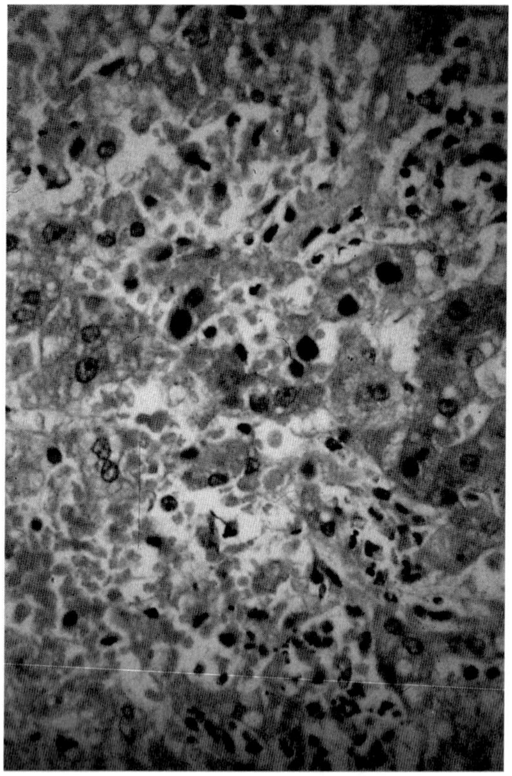

FIGURE 29.8. *Photomicrograph of liver biopsy showing hepatitis due to adenovirus infection. Note presence of "smudge" cells.*

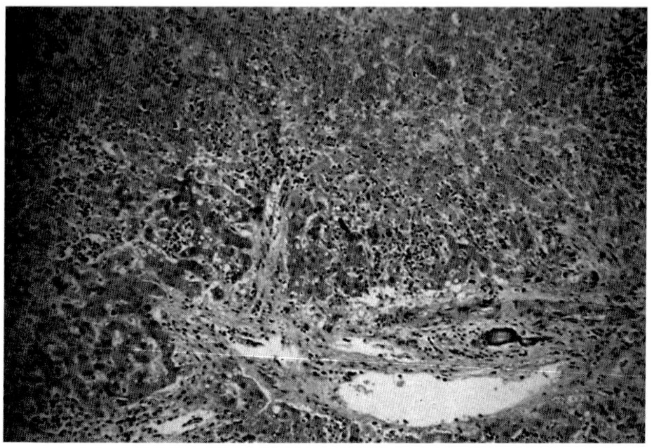

FIGURE 29.9. *Photomicrograph of liver biopsy revealing hemorrhagic necrosis of the allograft due to adenovirus infection.*

Varicella Zoster Virus

Primary infection with the varicella zoster virus (VZV) causes chickenpox, whereas reactivation in those previously infected results in shingles. Approximately 95% of healthy adults have been exposed to VZV in childhood. VZV infections can be life threatening in immunosuppressed patients (72). Typically, infection occurs three to six months after transplantation.

Gastrointestinal manifestations have been reported and include necrotizing esophagitis (43), gastritis (73), and hepatitis (74), usually appearing in association with a characteristic rash and disseminated disease. Hepatitis and even fulminant hepatic failure have been reported without the classic skin lesions, however, leading to delays in diagnosis and treatment (75). Approximately 10% to 15% of cases result in visceral dissemination, which has a reported mortality of 9% (76).

The diagnosis can be made from routine histologic stains of brushings and biopsy specimens, showing epithelial cell changes similar to those in HSV infection. Immunohistochemistry and PCR can be used to confirm the diagnosis (75). Where close contact between an immunocompromised VZV seronegative patient to chickenpox or shingles occurs, it has been advocated that varicella zoster immune globulin therapy 125 mg/kg body weight (max 625 mg) and oral acyclovir 800 mg five times a day be given for the duration of the incubation period (74). Treatment of VZV infection is with intravenous acyclovir 10 mg/kg body weight every eight hours.

Hepatitis B Virus

Hepatitis B virus (HBV) is a significant cause of liver disease after organ transplantation. The natural course of HBV infection in transplant recipients may be distinct from that in the normal population, with immunosuppressive therapy having a negative effect on the rate of natural clearance, disease progression, and survival in these patients. In the case of liver transplantation, recurrent HBV infection may run an accelerated course. The outcome after other organ transplants is slightly more controversial.

Hepatitis B and Renal Transplantation Preexisting HBV infection has been shown in several studies to have a negative impact on long-term morbidity and mortality due to liver disease in renal transplant recipients (77–79). This has not been the universal experience, however, as other researchers have found similar rates of survival in HBsAg-positive and -negative patients (80).

Fibrosing cholestatic hepatitis due to HBV infection has been described after renal transplantation in a patient demonstrated to have developed a precore HBV mutation (81) and may also occur with the wild-type virus.

Hepatitus B and Bone Marrow Transplantation Hepatitis B virus may account for liver dysfunction in patients undergoing bone marrow transplantation with exacerbation of existing disease occurring under immunosuppression. In particular, reactivation of hepatitis B has been described where patients with evidence of past infection (anti-HBs, anti-HBe, and anti-HBc) developed reduced titers of these antibodies in association with reappearance of HBsAg. Fulminant HBV hepatitis (82) and fibrosing cholestatic hepatitis (83) have also been described in association with bone marrow transplantation. Transplantation of bone marrow from healthy HBV-immune donors to nonexposed immunosuppressed recipients has recently been demonstrated to result in acquired immunity to HBV in recipients (84). This raises the possibility of an innovative approach to the prevention of HBV infection and the treatment of chronic viral hepatitis.

Hepatitis B and Liver Transplantation

Natural history of hepatitis B infection. The natural history of HBV infection in liver transplant patients without preventive therapy was studied by Todo et al (85), who demonstrated HBV recurrence in 82% of patients and worse survival in HBV-infected than in HBV-immune patients after 60 days (45% and 63%, respectively). HBV infection led to 73% of all deaths among these patients after 60 days (Table 29.2) (see also Chapter 19).

Pretransplantation HBV replicative state was an important factor in predicting viral recurrence. In patients with HBV cirrhosis, the presence of HBV DNA at the time of transplantation was associated with a recurrence rate of 83% compared to 58% in those without HBV DNA and HBeAg (86). The high recurrence rate of hepatitis B after transplant can be explained if one considers that viral replication occurs in several extrahepatic sites and in an extensive range of cell types (87). HBV has been demonstrated in lymph nodes, spleen, the GI tract, kidneys, skin, central nervous system, and gonads (88). The recurrence rate is lower after fulminant hepatitis B, as these patients present during a period of active elimination of the virus, often with no detectable serum HBV DNA at the time of transplantation (86). Reactivation of hepatitis B infection may occur after liver transplantation where the liver donor had serologic evidence of past infection and immunity to HBV. It has been recommended to avoid using organs from donors who are positive for anti-HBs and anti-HBc (89).

Pathology. A number of histologic findings have been reported in post-transplantation infection. Commonly there is progression from acute to chronic active hepatitis and cirrhosis. A minority of patients develop a histologic pattern resembling a chronic carrier state with little inflammation and ground-glass hepatocytes. Early histologic changes include HBcAg staining in the cytoplasm, often without inflammation or necrosis. By five months there is hepatitis with hepatocyte swelling, necrosis, and lobular disarray, often with less inflammatory changes than in nonimmunosuppressed patients. By nine months there has often been a transition to chronic active hepatitis and even cirrhosis. Cirrhosis has been reported to occur within 200 days of liver transplantation (85). As many as 25% of patients with recurrent disease may develop fibrosing cholestatic hepatitis. Although there is only a modest elevation of aminotransferase levels, the liver's synthetic function becomes grossly abnormal and there is a picture of fulminant liver failure as

Table 29.2. Predictors of Posttransplant Outcome in HBV Infection

Reduced Recurrence	Increased Survival
Pretransplantation HBeAg negative, HBV DNA negative	Pretransplantation HBeAg, HBV DNA negative
Fulminant hepatitis	Delta agent coinfection
Delta agent coinfection	Immunoprophylaxis
Long-term immunoprophylaxis	

Source: Samuel D, Bismuth A, Mathieu D, et al. Passive immunoprophylaxis after liver transplantation in HBsAg-positive patients. Lancet 1991;337:813–815.

the graft fails. Histologically this is characterized by ballooning degeneration of hepatocytes, cholestasis, a paucity of inflammatory response, and periportal fibrosis (90).

Strategies to Prevent HBV Recurrence Associated with Liver Transplantation Several therapeutic strategies have been used to inhibit viral replication prior to liver transplantation in order to reduce the incidence of graft reinfection with HBV and improve survival.

Interferon (IFN) alpha. There have been a few reports that considered the efficacy of IFN in patients with decompensated HBV cirrhosis (91). IFN is poorly tolerated in those patients whose liver disease is advanced enough to warrant transplantation, provoking exacerbations of their disease and serious bacterial infections. In one study, however, low doses of IFN produced a sustained loss of HBV DNA in 33% of patients treated and resulted in improvement in synthetic function (92).

New antiviral agents. Newer antiviral agents such as lamivudine (3TC), a nucleoside analogue that suppresses HBV DNA, are currently being evaluated in trials aimed at prevention of recurrence of hepatitis B after transplantation. This has so far been demonstrated to be a safe and well-tolerated oral therapy at a dose of 100 mg/day (93). When administered to those with high-replicative HBV infection (HBeAg positive, HBV DNA positive) undergoing liver transplantation, HBV DNA rapidly becomes undetectable by the liquid hybridization assay, although not always by PCR. Early results in this setting have been promising, although there are already reports of hepatitis B mutations occurring in the usually conserved YMDD motif in the RNA-dependent DNA polymerase (94). These have resulted in resistance to lamivudine and may possibly limit its long-term success. Early reports suggest that resistant strains developing during lamivudine prophylaxis may rapidly progress with histologic features consistent with fibrosing cholestatic hepatitis (FCH) (Shields et al, unpublished). The exact management of these patients remains a challenge at the present time, although in the short term withdrawal of immunosuppression and ganciclovir therapy has been shown to reverse the histologic changes of FCH in two cases.

Ganciclovir, another nucleoside analogue, when given for 3 to 10 months has been shown to reduce HBV replication and result in biochemical and histologic improvement in HBV infection in post-transplant immunosuppressed patients. Withdrawal of the drug resulted in return to pretreatment HBV replication (95). Both these drugs and famciclovir are currently in trial and it remains to be seen if they hold any promise for the long-term prevention of recurrent HBV infection, either alone or in combination with HBs-immunoglobulin.

Immunoprophylaxis. Use of anti-hepatitis B surface immunoglobulin to neutralize circulating HBV has been widely practiced to avoid graft reinfection. Low-dose therapy used in the immediate postoperative period proved ineffective; however, higher doses given perioperatively and for six months postoperatively delayed HBV recurrence, particularly in the absence of pretransplantation viral replication (96). Further studies have shown risk of HBV recurrence to be significantly reduced by long-term (>6 months) immunoprophylaxis compared to no immunoprophylaxis and short-term therapy (recurrence rates of 36%, 75%, and 74%, respectively) (86). The use of long-term anti-HBs immunoglobulin in those seropositive for HBV DNA was not beneficial. One protocol for prophylaxis is 5000 IU given intravenously during the anhepatic phase and then daily for the first week after surgery. Repeated doses in order to maintain the anti-HBs levels above 100 IU/L are given, usually monthly in the first year and approximately eight times yearly thereafter.

Strategies to Treat HBV Recurrence in the Transplant Patient Recurrence of HBV in the liver graft is a serious problem carrying a significant mortality. Unfortunately there are limited therapeutic possibilities at the present time. Long-term immunotherapy with anti-HBsAg is one option but there is little data in the literature to suggest its appropriate duration. Initial experience so far suggests that most patients who do develop recurrent HBV infection in their graft, while treated with anti-HBs, will do so in the first year after transplantation. A few cases have been reported after two years (86). The issue of whether therapy can be discontinued after one year or two years must be further researched.

Very little data exists regarding the use of interferon for HBV recurrence after transplantation. Irreversible acute rejection of renal grafts has been reported with interferon, and enhanced HLA expression on hepatocytes caused by interferon may in theory precipitate liver allograft rejection. In a small study considering this question, interferon had little effect on HBV replication, although reassuringly there were no reported cases of rejection (97).

Data regarding the role of lamivudine to treat recurrent hepatitis B after liver transplantation is sparse. One case report, however, describes persistent inhibition of HBV DNA and a reduction in alanine transaminase (ALT) by lamivudine in one patient who developed recurrent hepatitis B four months after liver transplantation (see also Chapter 19).

Hepatitis D Virus

Hepatitis D (delta) virus (HDV) is a defective virus or virusoid that requires the helper functions of hepatitis B for its transmission. The delta particle uses HBsAg to make its own coat. After liver transplantation, HBV recurrence is reduced by coinfection with HDV and hepatitis is less severe than in patients with HBV alone (86). Survival is increased after liver transplantation in those with HDV coinfection. These effects are likely to be a result of the inhibitory effects of HDV on HBV replication. Low HBV DNA levels pretransplant result in decreased recurrence rates, and low levels after transplant result in attenuated disease (98).

Long-term prophylaxis with anti-HBs is the best therapy for chronic HDV infection; it has a three-year recurrence rate of 17% compared to 56% in those having short-term prophylaxis and 70% in those with no therapy (86).

Early data suggests that interferon alpha may reduce HDV replication in reinfected liver grafts (99).

Hepatitis C Virus

In 1989, the hepatitis C virus (HCV) was identified as the major cause of parenterally transmitted non-A, non-B hepatitis and since then has also been recognized as the main cause of liver disease after organ transplantation. Transplant recipients are at risk of developing post-transplantation hepatitis C from progression of their already existing disease under immunosuppression, or from infection acquired at the time of transplantation from blood products or from infected cadaveric organ donors.

In a study considering the risk of hepatitis C transmission by organ transplantation (100), post-transplantation prevalence of anti-HCV and HCV RNA was 67% and 96% among recipients of HCV-infected donor organs compared to 20% and 18% in the recipients of noninfected donor organs. The incidence of post-transplant hepatitis was 55% in those who had received an infected graft versus 16% in those who had not been infected. The screening of blood products for hepatitis C has almost eliminated the risk of post-transfusion HCV infection and most transplant centers now ban the use of organs from donors with anti-HCV.

Renal transplant patients have been shown to have a high incidence of hepatitis C with reports suggesting that up to 46% of patients are infected. This is independently associated with the amount of transfused blood products and duration of hemodialysis (101). HCV infection has been associated with an increased risk of adverse outcomes after renal transplantation (102). Recipients with pretransplantation HCV infection had a 3.3-fold increased risk of death and a 9.9-fold increased risk of death due to sepsis after a mean follow-up of 45 months. Not all studies have shown such an adverse effect and this may reflect variation in the severity of liver disease at the time of renal transplantation.

HCV and Liver Transplantation HCV-associated liver cirrhosis is an increasingly common indication for liver transplantation. However, HCV infection recurs after liver transplantation in almost all patients with pretransplantation infection (103,104). Immunosuppression after transplantation is associated with a fall in anti-HCV relative to other antibody titers (105), whereas HCV RNA levels have been shown to increase to 16 times their pretransplant levels (104).

The long-term consequences of recurrent hepatitis C after liver transplantation remain to be defined (106), but interestingly only half of patients with detectable viremia one year after transplantation have histologic hepatitis (107). In a series of 149 patients transplanted for hepatitis C cirrhosis with a median follow-up of 36 months (108), the cumulative five-year survival rates were almost identical to those transplanted for non-HCV related causes. Of 130 patients with HCV surviving more than six months, 12% had no evidence of chronic hepatitis, 54% had mild and 27% had moderate chronic hepatitis, and 8% had cirrhosis. Graft loss occurred in 27 of the 149 patients (median graft survival 303 days). Five patients had HCV-related cirrhosis and three developed fibrosing cholestatic hepatitis. Genotype 1b was associated with more severe liver injury. Others have described aggressive post-transplantation HCV infection (109).

Treatment of HCV Infection After Transplantation There is to date little definitive information regarding the use of interferon or other antiviral agents in the treatment of hepatitis C infection after liver or organ transplantation. In one small study of interferon after liver transplantation (110), 5 patients (28%) had a complete response whereas 13 (72%) were nonresponders. After stopping treatment, the ALT remained normal in 4 of 5 responders but serum HCV levels returned to pretreatment levels. There was no significant change in histologic score with therapy.

Another study (111) demonstrated an increased incidence of rejection in IFN-treated patients (15), leading to retransplantation in three individuals. There was one episode of rejection in 32 patients in the untreated group. Only one treated patient had a long-term response to IFN. The role of interferon therapy in the post-transplant period is thus questionable and it should certainly only be used with extreme caution.

Combination therapy with ribavirin and interferon may be more effective in preventing progression of HCV-related graft disease after liver transplantation (112). Of 14 patients with recurrent hepatitis C, there was normalization of ALT in all patients after six months of treatment, with nine patients becoming HCV RNA negative. Eighteen months later all but one patient had a normal ALT and 12 of 13 achieved a histologic benefit. There were no episodes of graft rejection in this study. It remains to be seen whether larger studies with longer periods of follow-up can confirm these initially promising results with combination therapy.

GRAFT-VERSUS-HOST DISEASE

Graft-versus-host disease (GVHD) is induced by immunologically competent T cells of donor origin damaging host tissues. The clinical importance of GVHD is therefore determined by the amount of lymphoid tissue in the transplanted organ. It is particularly prevalent after bone marrow transplantation (see Chapter 27) and is becoming increasingly recognized after small bowel transplantation, where there is a considerable amount of lymphoid tissue contained in mesenteric lymph nodes, Peyer's patches, and the lamina propria (see Chapter 22). It is uncommon after liver transplantation, with few cases but a high mortality reported. The incidence of GVHD in decreasing order is: bone marrow transplantation, small bowel, liver, heart–lung, pancreas, kidney, heart. The risk and severity of this immune-mediated condition are directly related to the degree of genetic mismatch between host and donor organ (113).

The syndrome of acute GVHD usually starts 20 to 70 days after transplantation and consists of dermatitis, enteritis, and liver disease (114). Chronic GVHD usually develops after 100 days and may affect up to 30% of long-term survivors after allogeneic bone marrow transplantation (115). Sites of involvement, histologic changes, and response to treatment differ from acute GVHD patients. The majority of patients with chronic GVHD have already had preceding acute GVHD that has either resolved or evolved into chronic GVHD. Twenty to thirty percent of those with chronic GVHD have de novo late-onset disease. Esophageal and hepatic involvement are common (116).

Acute GVHD

Gastrointestinal symptoms are common with diarrhea, colicky lower abdominal pain, nausea, anorexia, vomiting, and intestinal bleeding. Diarrhea is usually profuse and watery, with a green mucoid appearance. Exfoliated epithelial and inflammatory cells are passed as strands of flesh-like material. Abdominal pain is often worse with food. Signs of peritonitis may occur if transmural bowel wall edema and perforation of the intestine develop (116). On the other hand, some patients with intestinal GVHD may have little in the way of symptoms.

Upper GI acute GVHD has been increasingly recognized with incidences of 22% being reported after bone marrow transplantation (117). Small bowel involvement may present with a rapidly falling albumin and protein-losing enteropathy (118). The diagnosis of GVHD is dependent on the exclusion of infectious causes of enteritis. The severity of intestinal GVHD parallels that affecting skin and liver; however, GI symptoms may occur in the absence of other organ involvement (119)

Endoscopic appearances of GVHD range from normal to patchy erythema to extensive mucosal sloughing. As GVHD is most prominent in the ileum, cecum, and ascending colon, gastric and rectal mucosa are often grossly normal. However, microscopic changes of GVHD are usually evident in these sites if there is extensive midgut disease, and upper GI endoscopy and sigmoidoscopy with biopsy are important tools in the diagnosis of acute GVHD (120).

Diagnostic histologic findings of acute GVHD are present only in relatively intact mucosa and are less specific once the disease has reached the stage of total mucosal denudation (116). Apoptosis of individual cells in intestinal crypts is the first change on light microscopy. Necrosis of individual epithelial cells may also be seen in the esophagus and stomach. Debris from cell necrosis is enveloped in spaces at the bottom of crypts giving rise to accumulations known as *apoptotic bodies*. There is no lymphocytic infiltrate in the lamina propria and microorganisms should be absent. This is in contrast to conditions such as infectious colitis and inflammatory bowel disease and after chemoradiation therapy, where there is significant inflammatory cell infiltrate. There may be a progression to involvement of whole crypts with crypt cell flattening, drop out of entire crypts, and eventually total denudation of the epithelium. The small bowel demonstrates ulceration of the lamina propria, loss of villous architecture, submucosal edema and fibrosis, and deep ulceration extending into the submucosa. There may be lymphocyte and plasma cell infiltration into the lamina propria and smooth muscle layers.

Chronic GVHD

Gastrointestinal manifestations of chronic GVHD include oral mucositis, oral sicca, esophagitis, and intestinal involvement with fibrosis. Liver involvement may occur either as part of an extensive chronic GVHD or as a more favorable limited disease involving just the skin and the liver. Oral involvement in chronic GVHD occurs frequently and occasionally is the manifestation of greatest concern to the patient (121). Erythema, striations resembling those seen in lichen planus, and severe generalized ulceration involving the buccal mucosa and tongue may occur.

Esophageal chronic GVHD disease may present with dysphagia, odynophagia, retrosternal pain, aspiration, anorexia, and weight loss. One third of patients with severe chronic GVHD may develop such symptoms (115). Lesions include desquamation of the mucosa ranging in severity from superficial epithelial peeling to mucosal sloughing, where mucosa hangs in shreds in the lumen of the esophagus. This particularly involves the upper and mid esophagus. Fibrous webs of the upper esophagus that may be eccentric and occlude the lumen may occur. Short symmetrical ring-like narrowings associated with desquamation and long tapering strictures have been clearly demonstrated radiologically. Interestingly, the distal esophagus is relatively spared by chronic GVHD (43).

In contrast to the histologic findings in the intestine, endoscopic biopsy reveals desquamation of the surface epithelium; infiltration of the esophageal mucosa with neutrophils, eosinophils, and lymphocytes; necrosis of individual squamous cells in the basal layer; and submucosal fibrosis. These findings are analogous to the histologic findings of chronic GVHD in the oral mucosa and skin (122).

Intestinal fibrosis has been reported in untreated chronic GVHD leading to malabsorption, diarrhea, and abdominal pain. Histopathology revealed patchy fibrosis of the lamina propria and marked fibrosis of the submucosa and serosa with involvement of most of the GI tract. The overlying mucosa appeared normal (123).

GVHD of the Liver

GVHD of the liver usually presents with cholestatic jaundice and pruritus. There is often mild hepatomegaly, and skin and intestinal manifestations of GVHD may also be present. Hepatocellular failure with accompanying ascites and portal hypertension is rare, although it is recognized particularly in those with prolonged severe multisystem GVHD and may be an indication for liver transplantation.

There is a rise in serum alkaline phosphatase of up to 20 times normal paralleled by a hyperbilirubinemia. A transaminitis also occurs but is less marked with values rarely exceeding 10 times normal. Histologic changes in the early stages of the disease include a nonspecific lobular hepatitis. Beyond two weeks, cholestasis, mild panlobular hepatocellular injury, and degenerative changes in small septa are seen with lymphocytic infiltration in portal zones. Limiting plates are intact. Abnormal interlobular bile ducts are the most characteristic feature of liver GVHD, but with disease progression bile duct loss with development of a vanishing bile duct syndrome can occur. Cholestasis becomes more profound with hepatocyte ballooning degeneration, hepatocyte dropout, sinusoidal fibrosis, and Kupffer cell hyperplasia. There may be bridging necrosis with portal-to-central or portal-to-portal bands, piecemeal necrosis with erosion of the limiting plates, and fibrosis eventually leading to portal hypertension.

Prevention and Treatment of Acute and Chronic GVHD

Therapy to prevent and to treat acute and chronic GVHD includes systemic immunosuppressive drugs, including steroids (2 mg/kg/day) in combination with prophylactic therapy such as cyclosporine, tacrolimus (FK506), and methotrexate. These agents are generally more effective as preventive than therapeutic agents possibly because, in the early stages of GVHD, fewer cells that are reactive to alloantigens need to be suppressed as they have not yet fully expanded and differentiated.

Prednisolone induces a complete and sustained remission of GI symptoms in 50% to 70% of patients with GVHD. Lack of response warrants therapy with higher-dose prednisolone, antithymocyte globulin, and investigational anti-T-cell (CD3, CD5) or IL-2 receptor monoclonal antibodies (see Chapter 13).

Studies have suggested the use of topical therapies including dexamethasone and more recently cyclosporin A administered as an oral rinse in patients with oral GVHD with good response (121). Oral bethamethasone dipropionate, a potent topically active corticosteroid, has been used in mild to moderate intestinal GVHD with significant improvements in appetite, oral intake, nausea, and diarrhea (72% overall response rate) (124).

ORAL COMPLICATIONS IN THE TRANSPLANT PATIENT

The main oral and dental problems in organ transplant recipients include side effects of immunosuppressive therapy, periodontal disease, infections, and oral GVHD. Dental assessment of potential transplant patients is important to assess oral hygiene and to treat caries. Dental extraction and even total clearance may be indicated if it is anticipated that immunosuppression may result in dental infections and abscess formation. Often a febrile patient is assessed for a source of sepsis and no source other than dental infection can be identified. Occult sinusitis is another potential source of sepsis in such patients (125).

The unwanted effects of immunosuppression include gingival overgrowth due to cyclosporine therapy. It has been estimated that 30% of dentate organ transplant patients develop gingival hyperplasia. Children appear to be more susceptible to this problem than adults (126). Gingival overgrowth may occur within three months of initiating drug therapy and predominantly affects the labial aspects of the upper and lower anterior teeth (127). The pathogenesis is unknown but possible factors include dose and duration of therapy, oral hygiene, existing periodontal status, the patient's age, and genetic predisposition. Some studies have suggested that blood and salivary concentrations are important determinants of expression of gingival overgrowth; others, however, have failed to substantiate these findings (128). Histopathology shows a chronic fibrous hyperplasia. Squamous cell carcinoma has been reported in association with cyclosporine-induced gingival overgrowth (129). Nifedipine and other calcium channel blockers are also associated with gingival overgrowth. Their effects appear to be additive with cyclosporine as the two drugs in combination result in a 40% prevalence of overgrowth (130).

In the past, gingival overgrowth may have been of sufficient magnitude to warrant surgical excision (gingivectomy) or laser therapy (131). Recurrence, however, was common and the procedure needed to be repeated. Currently, most clinicians first replace cyclosporine with tacrolimus, which often resolves the problem.

Periodontal disease is influenced by immunosuppressive agents and there is some evidence that they inhibit the response of the periodontal tissues to bacterial plaque, although this does not appear to be influenced by drug dosage or duration of therapy (132). Therefore, gingival inflammation is not commonly seen when oral hygiene is poor. Longitudinal studies of transplant patients suggest that this reduced gingival inflammation has no effect on the rate of periodontal breakdown or bone loss (132).

Oral ulceration may occur with infections such as HSV and CMV, and also with fungal infections. GVHD may also cause ulceration, stomatitis, and a lichenoid eruption.

GASTROINTESTINAL ULCERATION AND BLEEDING

Minor upper GI hemorrhage due to stress ulceration is common in critically ill or postoperative transplant patients; however, the incidence of serious hemorrhage that is accompanied by a high degree of morbidity and mortality is significantly lower. The use of high-dose steroids for moderate to severe acute cellular allograft rejection may contribute to the development of peptic ulceration in post-transplant patients (1). Other contributing factors include coagulopathy immediately after liver transplantation often associated with large blood transfusions, immunosuppression-induced thrombocytopenia, and the use of heparin for dialysis in patients with renal impairment.

Duodenal ulcers rarely present classically in these patients and abdominal pain may be absent. More often hemorrhage or perforation may be the presenting feature. Less commonly upper GI hemorrhage may result from severe fungal or viral esophageal infection and ulceration or due to lymphoproliferative disease.

Gastrointestinal hemorrhage has been reported in 20% of patients following renal transplantation and carries a high mortality (133). One study in renal transplant patients demonstrated a 9.6% incidence of gastroduodenal ulcer despite the use of prophylactic H2 receptor antagonists (134). Stuart et al (135) showed a 5% incidence of gastroduodenal perforation with a 50% mortality rate after renal transplantation. This was reduced to 0.8% with H2 receptor antagonist prophylaxis. Similarly, one earlier study showed that prophylactic use of antacids reduced mortality from 22% to 0% (136).

Gastrointestinal bleeding after bone marrow transplantation was reported in 6% of recipients, all of whom were taking H2 receptor antagonist prophylaxis (137). Most of these cases occurred within three weeks of transplantation and all bleeds were self limiting and did not contribute to overall mortality.

Past history of ulcer disease is an important factor governing recurrence after organ transplantation, with prior ulcer history giving a 70% to 80% chance of relapse in one study.

Gastric and duodenal ulceration is described after cardiopulmonary bypass surgery with GI hemorrhage accounting for between 35% and 61% of abdominal complications in two series (138,139). In a further series of 429 patients undergoing heart or heart–lung transplantation, 8 developed peptic ulceration (6 duodenal, 2 gastric) manifesting as hemorrhage or epigastric pain with a mean time of presentation after transplantation of 14 days (140).

Prophylaxis with H2 receptor antagonists significantly decreased stress ulceration and significant bleeding in critically ill patients (141). Cimetidine prophylaxis in patients with fulminant hepatic failure reduced the incidence of GI hemorrhage to 3%, compared with 54% in controls, with a reduction in transfusion requirements in the treated group (142). The data support the use of prophylactic H2 receptor antagonists for liver transplant recipients.

The role of *Helicobacter pylori* in the etiology of peptic ulceration is currently unclear. In one study, the incidence of *H. pylori* in dyspeptic patients with chronic renal failure undergoing renal transplantation was higher than the general population (143). Increased colonization was seen, but there were less gastritis and ulceration particularly in those receiving triple immunosuppression, suggesting that immunosuppression may alter the natural history of this infection.

Low-grade lymphomas associated with *H. pylori* infection (maltoma) have occasionally been reported after transplantation and under immunosuppression. These did not behave like the lymphomas often associated with immunosuppression (144). The role of *H. pylori* in the etiology of such tumors in this setting will need further study before a direct causal link is established, however.

Sclerotherapy of esophageal varices prior to liver transplantation may result in sclerotherapy ulceration and bleeding after transplantation. Recurrent variceal hemorrhage is uncommon, as portal hypertension is immediately reversed following liver transplantation; it may, however, occur in association with acute portal vein thrombosis. This is often related to purse stringing and stricture of the anastomosis (145). Excessive length of the portal vein may lead to kinking, which can also lead to thrombosis. Pancreatitis following liver transplantation may cause splenic vein thrombosis, leading to left-sided portal hypertension, gastric varices, and hemorrhage.

PANCREATITIS

Pancreatitis following renal transplantation is well described and the incidence has been reported to be between 0.4% and 7.0%, with an associated mortality of between 20% to 70% (146). Possible causes include immunosuppressive drugs (steroids, azathioprine, cyclosporine), viral infections, postoperative hyperparathyroidism, vasculitis, and intraoperative pancreatic trauma. Pancreatitis has complicated heart and heart–lung transplantation, particularly when cardiopulmonary bypass was used (147).

Pancreatitis has been described after liver transplantation with retrospective analyses suggesting an incidence as high as 5.9% with a mortality in this group of 33% (148). The etiology in these cases may be multifactorial, although an association with hepatitis B infection has been suggested (145). Other factors thought to be important include extensive surgical dissection around the pancreas, type of biliary reconstruction, number of liver grafts, duration of venovenous bypass, and the quantity of intravenous calcium chloride administered intraoperatively (149).

Pancreatitis should be treated aggressively in the transplant setting as in any other, with intravenous fluids, pancreatic rest, and cautious refeeding. The use of immunosuppressive agents, in particularly azathioprine, should be re-evaluated.

GASTROINTESTINAL MALIGNANCY AFTER ORGAN TRANSPLANTATION

There is an increased incidence of malignancy associated with immunodeficiency, whether this is due to HIV infection, a congenital disorder, or immunosuppressive therapy (see Chapter 37). Uncontrolled growth of neoplastic cells following somatic mutations or an oncogenic viral infection may arise through impaired immune surveillance. The largest and most complete record of malignancies occurring after transplantation comes from Australia and New Zealand, relating to renal transplant patients (6067 renal allograft recipients with a mean follow-up of 7 years) (150). There is a higher incidence of all tumors after transplantation, including GI malignancies that account for 20% of the total. A summary of this experience is shown in Table 29.3.

Table 29.3. Malignancies of the Digestive Organs

Tumor Type	Observed	Expected	Risk Ratio
Buccal cavity	10	4.8	2.1
Pharynx	2	1.0	2.0
Esophagus	8	1.0	8.0
Stomach	5	3.7	1.4
Small intestine	1	0.3	3.2
Colon	25	9.2	2.7
Rectum and anus	13	6.1	2.1
Liver	6	0.7	9.2
Biliary	2	1.1	1.9
Pancreas	5	2.1	2.3

Source: Shiel AGR. Development of malignancy following renal transplantation in Australia and New Zealand. Transplant Proc 1992;24:1275–1279.

POST-TRANSPLANT LYMPHOPROLIFERATIVE DISORDER

Post-transplant lymphoproliferative disorder (PTLD) is usually B cell in origin and is almost always associated with Epstein-Barr virus (EBV) infection. Numerous in situ hybridization studies have demonstrated that essentially all PTLD lesions contain detectable EBV genomes within transformed B cells. PTLD occurs more commonly after primary infection in a seronegative subject than after secondary infection in one who is seropositive. The higher incidence of primary infections in children and the higher number of seronegative recipients account for the higher frequency of PTLD in childhood (4% of pediatric children transplant recipients compared to 1% of adults) (49). The type of organ transplanted has an impact on the frequency of PTLD: 1% to 3% of bone marrow, kidney, and liver recipients, and 5% to 13% of heart and heart–lung recipients.

PTLD may produce a broad range of symptoms and signs including GI symptoms in 30% of patients. Common sites of involvement include lymph nodes, liver, bowel, spleen, bone marrow, kidney, tonsils, adrenals, and the central nervous system. Histopathology usually shows a polymorphic lymphoblastic proliferation. Cytologic features thought to predict an aggressive course include atypical nuclei, the presence of necrosis, and invasion beyond the capsule of the involved organ (Figs. 29.10, 29.11, and Plates 37, 38). Other adverse prognostic factors include a longer interval after transplantation, monoclonality, karyotype abnormalities, multiple extranodal sites of disease, and occurrence of PTLD after heart or bone marrow transplantation (151). In one collective review overall survival was 31% (152).

Reduction of immunosuppressive therapy may cause complete regression in approximately 42% of patients (151). Additional therapies such as interferon alpha, gamma globulin, and acyclovir have been tried with limited success. Chemotherapy and radiotherapy have been described as curative, but overall survival from meta-analyses is still only about 20% (153). Serotherapy using anti-B-cell monoclonal antibody (anti-CD21 and anti-CD24) produced an 89% complete response rate in patients who were unresponsive to reduction in immunosuppression and whose disease was oligoclonal. Those patients with monoclonal disease failed to respond (154). Surgical therapy and local excision of nodes has cured some patients with localized lymphoproliferation, although many of these patients had concomitant reduction in immunosuppressive therapy (155).

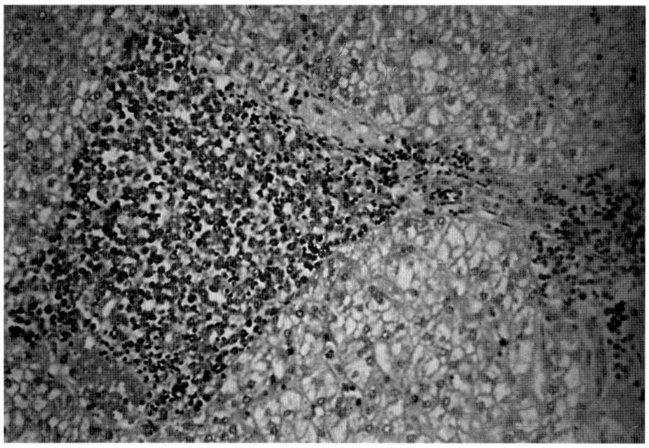

FIGURE 29.10. *Photomicrograph demonstrating post-transplant lymphoma.*

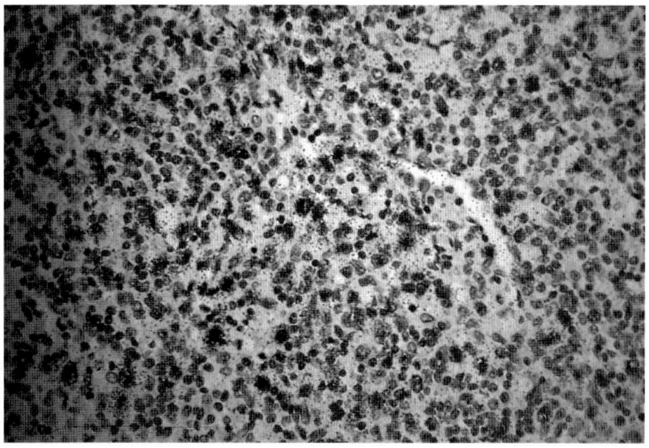

FIGURE 29.11. *Photomicrograph of lymph node biopsy demonstrating PTLD disease, in this case related to EBV.*

MECHANICAL INTESTINAL OBSTRUCTION AND PSEUDO-OBSTRUCTION (NONOBSTRUCTING COLONIC DILATATION)

Bowel obstruction as a result of adhesions may occur, especially after liver transplantation. Conservative management by nasogastric decompression may be successful, although the threshold for surgical exploration should be low, especially with evidence of vascular compromise to the bowel. Other causes of mechanical obstruction include incarceration in an umbilical hernia and more rarely herniation of small bowel through the mesenteric defect formed during construction of a Roux-en-Y choledochojejunostomy (156).

Nonobstructing colonic dilatation (pseudo-obstruction) has been reported rarely after renal transplantation, usually within a short time after transplantation, and is associated with poor graft function. Colonic decompression using a colonoscope was successful in treating 5 of 6 patients in one series (157). Unrelieved nonobstructing colonic dilatation may lead to colonic perforation with a high reported mortality (158). It has been suggested that distention and transmural tension results in compromise to the venous drainage and ischemia, which in turn may result in perforation (159).

Pmeumatosis intestinalis is described after renal and liver transplantation. It has been associated with CMV infection, although in most cases the etiology is unclear.

INTESTINAL AND COLONIC PERFORATION FOLLOWING TRANSPLANTATION

Early in the postoperative period, intestinal perforations may arise as a result of anastomotic leakage in the case of liver transplantation, or due to inadvertent iatrogenic perforation of the bowel wall. In a series of 246 pediatric patients undergoing orthotopic liver transplantation (160), 24 patients developed bowel perforation most commonly presenting at around 10 days following surgery. Most affected patients had biliary atresia and had undergone previous upper abdominal surgery, most often a Kasai portoenterostomy, which was thought to be the main risk factor for development of perforation. Other groups have found the incidence of bowel perforations to be more common in the pediatric than adult population (161). Perforations were often multiple and in most cases no specific etiology could be determined. Other potential causes of bowel perforation in transplant recipients include nonobstructing colonic dilatation (157), CMV colitis, mesenteric ischemia, fecal impaction, and erosion into the bowel wall of an intra-abdominal abscess. Uremic enterocolitis may rarely lead to perforation in renal transplant patients. The use of nonselective immunosuppression such as azathioprine and steroids has been associated with perforation, primarily in the sigmoid colon in patients with diverticular disease. Steroids lead to impairment of wound healing by inhibition of ground substance, reducing turnover of mucosal cells and the reparative activity of fibroblasts. They can also induce atrophy of lymphoid aggregates with subsequent thinning of the bowel wall, possibly increasing the risk of perforation (161).

TRANSPLANTATION AND EXISTING GASTROINTESTINAL DISEASE

Inflammatory Bowel Disease

Primary sclerosing cholangitis (PSC) is now a common indication for liver transplantation and, as 70% to 80% of these patients have concomitant ulcerative colitis (UC), experience of UC in the post-transplant setting is increasing. Pouchitis after a restorative colectomy and ileal pouch anal anastomosis is more prevalent in colitis with PSC than without PSC, and so this may also pose a clinical problem following liver transplantation.

The incidence of recurrent inflammatory bowel disease (IBD) in the post-transplant setting is low due to the use of immunosuppressive therapy. There are a few studies reporting the course of IBD after transplantation. In one study of 24 patients with IBD, symptoms improved after transplantation in 62.5%, were unchanged in 16.6%, and were worse in 20.8%. In another study of 46 patients transplanted for PSC, the majority of patients with IBD had improvement in their symptoms (62.5% for UC, 100% for Crohn's disease). Of five patients with UC whose symptoms were worse after liver transplantation, four received colectomy for moderate UC symptoms of which one had an early incidental carcinoma. No transplanted patients with PSC without a history of IBD prior to transplantation developed IBD afterwards (162). Rowley et al (163) described four patients undergoing restorative proctocolectomy and pouch anal anastomosis for ulcerative colitis after liver transplantation (performed for primary sclerosing cholangitis). Significant early complications occurred in these patients including hemorrhage in three and hepatic artery thrombosis in one. One patient later developed chronic pouchitis.

In patients with primary sclerosing cholangitis who have had a colectomy and ileal pouch anal anastomosis prior to their liver transplant, liver transplantation and immunosuppression do not seem to alter the disease course of pouchitis (164).

There has been concern over the long-term risk of malignancy in patients with IBD after transplantation, as a complication of long-term immunosuppressive therapy. Two studies have demonstrated a raised incidence of rapidly occurring colorectal tumors in IBD patients after liver transplantation for PSC. In one study, 2 of 31 patients developed colorectal cancer despite no detectable severe dysplasia on biopsies performed at pretransplant colonoscopy (165). In another, 3 of 27 patients whose duration of ulcerative colitis was 9, 22, and 27 years, respectively, developed colorectal neoplasms at 9, 12, and 13 months after transplant (166). This apparent increased incidence of colorectal neoplasms may reflect either sampling error in the pretransplant biopsies or that small lesions were missed at screening colonoscopy. It may also be explained by a report that patients with PSC and UC represent a subset of patients with UC who are at a significantly increased risk of colonic dysplasia (167). It would therefore seem sensible to recommend careful colonoscopic follow-up in these patients after transplantation.

Celiac Disease

In patients with celiac disease undergoing organ transplantation, it is sensible to ensure that the disease is controlled by gluten-free diet prior to grafting so that the patient is as nutritionally replete as possible and that malabsorption and diarrhea will not impair drug and enteral nutrient absorption after transplantation. This is particularly important for immunosuppressive therapy such as cyclosporine where consistent absorption is important to predict drug levels.

Although lymphomatous change in the small bowel is a complication of celiac disease particularly under immunosuppression, this is not a problem experienced in clinical practice.

It is standard practice in some centers to actively look for concurrent celiac disease in those undergoing liver transplantation. This is particularly relevant in the case of primary biliary cirrhosis where there is a recognized association (168). At least four biopsies taken endoscopically from the second part of the duodenum are usually enough to exclude the condition.

Infections

Strongyloides stercoralis infection, although rare, is an important pathogen to recognize and eradicate in carriers prior to transplantation. It may persist within subjects for many years and reactivate under immunosuppression with fatal consequences. All patients with potential exposure to the organism should have a careful examination for GI parasites prior to transplantation and be given preemptive therapy.

Diverticular Disease

Although there is a high incidence of diverticular disease in the general population (5% to 50%) (169) and debatably an increased incidence in patients with chronic renal failure, particularly among those undergoing renal transplantation for adult polycystic kidney disease (170), diverticulitis is a recognized but uncommon complication of organ transplantation. McCune et al (170) screened 100 renal transplant recipients over 50 years of age (10% of total transplanted) for colonic disease by either colonoscopy or barium enema. Twenty of the patients had diverticular disease (7 of 14 with polycystic kidney disease) prior to transplantation. The incidence of diverticulitis in the total population transplanted was low with only four cases, all of whom were over the age of 50 and on low-dose immunosuppression, and in most cases it occurred remotely after transplantation. Each was managed with either left hemicolectomy or sigmoid colectomy.

Others have reported perforation of diverticuli with intra-abdominal abscess formation following organ transplantation (171).

SPECIFIC COMPLICATIONS OF LIVER TRANSPLANTATION

Biliary Complications

Biliary tract complications are a major source of morbidity after orthotopic liver transplantation, occurring in 7% to 34% of patients (172,173). Biliary obstruction and bile leakage account for the majority of complications (Table 29.4).

Table 29.4. Biliary Tract Complications Following Orthotopic Liver Transplantation

Biliary Tract Complications
Biliary obstruction
Anastomotic stricture
Intrahepatic stricture
Stent-related obstruction
Anastomotic leakage
Necrosis or dehiscence of biliary anastomosis
Bile leak from surface of split liver
Biliary fistula
Hepatic artery
Portal vein
Cholangitis
Cholangiocarcinoma
Hemobilia following liver biopsy
Mucocele of the cystic duct
Sphincter of Oddi dysfunction/papillary stenosis

Bile Leak

The most common site of bile leak is at the biliary anastomosis and is usually associated with technical factors. It is seen most often in the early postoperative period and is thought to be related to ischemia. The common bile duct receives a dual blood supply from the right hepatic artery and the gastroduodenal artery. In the liver transplant patient, the donor liver common bile duct and the retained recipient common bile duct have tenuous end artery blood supplies that may be disrupted by excessive dissection or cauterization, causing ischemic complications. Bile duct ischemia and subsequent leakage above the anastomosis may occur with hepatic artery thrombosis as the donor common bile duct receives its blood supply from the hepatic artery. In addition, tension on the anastomosis or poorly placed sutures may result in local ischemia and an anastomotic leak.

Leakage from the T-tube entry site can be seen following liver transplantation, but these leaks usually cause no symptoms and, if small, will settle conservatively.

Symptoms of bile leak include abdominal pain, distention, fever, and constipation. There may be leukocytosis, rising bilirubin, alkaline phosphatase, and gamma-glutamyltranspeptidase levels, and bile drainage from abdominal drains.

T-tube cholangiogram, percutaneous cholangiogram, or endoscopic retrograde cholangiopancreatography (ERCP) is required to visualize the site of leak, and surgical repair should be considered if it is found to be significant. Repair may be made with placement of one or two sutures or the leaking segment can be excised and the biliary anastomosis converted to a roux-en-Y choledochojejunostomy.

Bile leakage from a choledochojejunostomy anastomosis should be revised by closing the previous jejunal enterostomy and performing a new anastomosis at least 1 cm distal on the jejunal limb.

Biliary Stricture

Biliary strictures often occur later in the postoperative period than bile leaks. The etiology of early biliary obstruction includes stricture, retained biliary stent, biliary sludge or stones, common duct redundancy, and mucocele of the cystic duct. Discrepancy between the recipient and donor ducts at transplantation can cause biliary obstruction. Anastomotic strictures probably account for less than half of cases of biliary strictures. The main etiologic factors include technical failure, ischemia and scarring with traction of the anastomosis, and narrowing. The development or recurrence of cholangiocarcinoma is encountered rarely.

Nonanastomotic biliary strictures are more common in the later postoperative period and are often the result of ischemia. Hepatic artery thrombosis may be associated with a diffuse biliary tract injury and the development of multiple strictures throughout the biliary system. It is also associated with a discrete stricturing. Similar lesions have been seen after successful revascularization of the hepatic artery. The process of liver preservation after donor removal may also result in biliary stricturing. A cold ischemic time of greater than 15 hours with storage in University of Wisconsin preservation solution has been associated with a "chain of lakes" appearance of the biliary system. This is complicated by infection and often requires retransplantation. ABO-incompatible grafts may undergo a process of arteriopathic rejection that has been associated with nonanastomotic biliary strictures.

Patients with a Roux anastomosis to the liver, which is routinely performed in patients transplanted for primary sclerosing cholangitis, have a raised incidence of biliary complications including cholangitis, sludge formation, and obstruction (174).

Disease Recurrence Following Liver Transplantation

With our growing experience and with greater numbers of patients surviving longer after liver transplantation, it has become evident that certain diseases may recur. Recurrence of viral hepatitis is obviously of major importance and may, in the case of hepatitis B, have a profound effect on early graft function and patient survival. In other conditions such as primary biliary cirrhosis, primary sclerosing cholangitis, and autoimmune chronic active hepatitis, the question of recurrence has been less easy to answer. Criteria used to define the disease in the native liver may be inappropriate when applied to the allograft, as both the natural history and the histologic features may be modified after transplantation. Hence the effects of possible recurrence may be subtle, with the patient remaining well and with little noticeable compromise of quality of life.

Primary Biliary Cirrhosis

There is considerable debate in the literature as to whether primary biliary cirrhosis recurs after liver transplantation. Most researchers do agree, however, that if it does occur it is unlikely to have an adverse effect on patient outcome, at least for the first decade. In one study (175) of 83 patients transplanted for primary biliary cirrhosis, 13 had histologic features suggestive of recurrent disease that were not seen in any biopsy taken from 105 patients grafted for other reasons. One of these developed progressive damage resulting in early cirrhosis. In another series (176), 5 of 60 patients two to six years following liver transplant developed typical histology suggestive of recurrent primary biliary cirrhosis. All these were asymptomatic, had normal liver function tests, and only 2 of 5 had persistent antimitochondrial antibodies after transplantation.

Histologic findings in these patients should be viewed with some caution. Interpretation of the allograft is often difficult owing to such factors as rejection, infections such as CMV (which can cause bile duct damage), and biliary tract complications such as an anastomotic stricture.

Primary Sclerosing Cholangitis

Although recurrence of primary sclerosing cholangitis (PSC) has been suspected after liver transplantation (177), proving recurrence has been impossible. Histologic features of PSC are rarely specific and may be missed on liver biopsy. Also, differentiation between primary and secondary sclerosing cholangitis may be impossible and bile duct changes characteristic of PSC may be seen as a consequence of other conditions such as recurrent cholangitis, bile duct ischemia, and CMV infection. Formation of a Roux loop, which is common practice in patients transplanted for PSC, is in itself associated with an increased incidence of cholangitis, biliary sludge formation, and obstruction, further confusing the issue (174).

Autoimmune Chronic Active Hepatitis

Recurrence of autoimmune chronic hepatitis after liver transplantation has been described in isolated reports. In one case (178), the patient developed clinical, biochemical, immunologic, and histologic features of recurrence on stopping prednisolone. Reintroduction of corticosteroid resulted in resolution of the abnormal features.

A retrospective study has also demonstrated that 11 of 43 patients developed histologic features of recurrence after liver transplantation (107). It therefore seems possible that autoimmune chronic hepatitis can recur in the graft and that there is good clinical response to increased immunosuppression.

Cholangiocarcinoma

Several studies demonstrate high recurrence rates of cholangiocarcinoma after liver transplantation, and in general transplantation is not recommended for the treatment of cholangiocarcinoma or indeed of metastatic disease to the liver (179). Ismail et al (180) did not observe any survivors beyond one year in 42 patients with cholangiocarcinoma. Small incidental cholangiocarcinomas found in approximately 10% of patients with PSC at transplant have been associated with a slightly better prognosis, with a 54% two-year survival. This study showed a 28.6% two-year mortality in those patients in whom the diagnosis of cholangiocarcinoma had been made preoperatively (181).

Hepatocellular Carcinoma

Recurrence of hepatocellular carcinoma has a significant impact on survival after liver transplantation and therefore it is important to thoroughly assess patients known to have a hepatoma before transplantation. The size and number of intrahepatic lesions and the presence of extrahepatic disease govern suitability for transplantation. In one series, unifocal tumors smaller than 5 cm recurred in 7% of patients compared to 62% with larger lesions (182); the five-year disease-free survival was 71% compared with 29%. Patients with single tumors had a mean survival of 68 months compared with 37 months in those with two or more.

The presence of lymph node involvement is an important prognostic indicator, with a mean survival of 10 months in lymph node–positive patients compared with 49 months in those with clear lymph nodes (183). Pichlmayr (184) showed a two-year survival of 75% (with clear nodes) compared with 11% (with nodes involved).

Vascular invasion is associated with a poor prognosis after transplantation. Those with invasion only on microscopic examination had a 50% tumor-free survival at five years, compared to 12% in patients with macroscopic vascular invasion. Complete absence of invasion is associated with a tumor-free survival of 95% at five years (185).

REFERENCES

1. Messer J, Reitman D, Sacks HS, et al. Association of adrenocorticosteroid therapy and peptic ulcer disease. N Engl J Med 1983;309:21–24.
2. Dennison H, Wallerstedt S. Bacterial overgrowth after high-dose corticosteroid treatment. Scand J Gastroenterol 1989;24:561.
3. Thaler H. Fatty change. Baillieres Clin Gastroenterol 1988;2:453.
4. Haboubi NY, Ali HH, Whitwell HL, Ackrill P. Role of endothelial cell injury in the spectrum of azathioprine-induced liver disease after renal transplant:light microscopy and ultrastructural observations. Am J Gastroenterol 1988;83:256.
5. Sollinger HW for the U.S. Renal Transplant Mycophenylate Mofetil Study Group. Mycophenylate mofetil for the prevention of acute rejection in primary cadaveric renal allograft recipients. Transplantation 1995;60:225–232.
6. Ducloux D, Ottignon Y, Semboun-Ducloux S, et al. Mycophenolate mofetil-induced villous atrophy. Transplantation 1998;66:1115–1116.
7. Innes A, Rowe PA, Foster MC, et al. Cyclosporin toxicity and colitis. Lancet 1988;2:957.
8. Innes. Complete information not available.
9. Klintmalm GBH, Iwatsuki S, Starlz TE. Cyclosporin A hepatotoxicity in 66 renal allograft recipients. Transplantation 1981;32:488.
10. Penn I. Cancers following cyclosporine therapy. Transplantation 1987;43:32–35.
11. Scheinin S, Radovancevic B, Frazier OH. Acute pancreatitis complicating OKT3 administration for resistant cardiac rejection. Transplant Proc 1993;25:2368–2369.
12. Europeon FK506 Multicentre Liver Study Group. Randomized trial comparing tacrolimus and cyclosporin in the prevention of liver allograft rejection. Lancet 1994;344:423–428.
13. U.S. Multicenter FK506 Liver Study Group. A comparison of tacrolimus and cyclosporine for immunosuppression in liver transplantation. N Engl J Med 1994;331:1110–1115.
14. Mickschl DB, Davidson LJ, Flournoy GJ, Parker DE. Contamination of enteral feeding and diarrhea in patients in intensive care units. Infect Dis Crit Care 1990;15:362–370.
15. Burns PE, Jairath N. Diarrhea and the patient receiving enteral feeding: a multifactorial problem. J Wound Ostomy Continence Nurses Soc 1994;21:257–263.
16. Jenkins AP, Thompson RPH. Enteral nutrition and the small intestine. Gut 1994;35:1765–1769.
17. Moore F, Feliciano D, Andrassy R, et al. Enteral feeding reduces postoperative septic complications. J Parent Ent Nutr 1991;15(suppl):22S.
18. Zeigler TR, Young LS, Benfell K, et al. Clinical and metabolic efficacy of glutamine-supplemented parenteral nutrition after bone marrow transplantation: a randomized, double-blind controlled study. Ann Intern Med 1992;116:821–828.
19. Mok KT. Etiology and outcome of total parenteral nutrition induced liver dysfunction. Am Surg 1993;53:650–655.
20. Fein BI, Holt PR. Hepatobiliary complications of total parenteral nutrition. J Clin Gastroenterol 1994;18:62–66.
21. Kelly CP, Pothoulakis C, Lamont JT. *Clostridium difficile* colitis. N Engl J Med 1994;330:257–262.
22. Huang JY, Huang MK, Lai MK, et al. Salmonella infection in renal transplant recipients. Transplant Proc 1994;26:2147.
23. Dhar JM, Al Khader AA, Al Sulaiman, Al Hasam MK. Nontyphoid salmonella in renal transplant recipients: a report of twenty cases and a review of the literature. Q J Med 1991;287:235–250.
24. Zu S-X, Fang G-D, Fayer R, Guerrant RL. Cryptosporidiosis:pathogenesis and immunology. Parasitology Today 1992;8:24–27.
25. Manivel C, Filipovich A, Snover DC. Cryptosporidiosis as a cause of diarrhea following bone marrow transplantation. Dis Colon Rectum 1985;28:741–742.
26. Manivel. Complete information not available.
27. Collier AC, Miller RA, Joel D, Meyers MD. Cryptosporidiosis after marrow transplantation: person to person transmission and treatment with spiramycin. Ann Intern Med 1984;101:205–206.
28. Roncoroni AJ, Gomez MA, Mera J, et al. *Cryptosporidium* infection in the renal transplant patient. J Infect Dis 1989;160:559.
29. Weisburger WR, Hutcheon DF, Yardley JH, et al. Cryptosporidiosis in an immunocompromised renal transplant recipient with IgA deficiency. Am J Clin Pathol 1979;72:473–479.
30. Acharya UN, Kishnan R, Kondpalle VK, Almeida AF. *Strongyloides stercoralis* infestation producing tropical enteropathy in a renal transplant patient. Dial Transplant 1995;24:468–469.
31. Scoden E, Scaffner W, Stone W. Overwhelming strongyloidiasis. An unappreciated opportunistic infection. Medicine 1978;57:527–544.
32. Sax PE, Rich JD, Pieciak WS, Trnka YM. Intestinal microsporidiosis occurring in a liver transplant recipient. Transplantation 1995;60:617–618.
33. Eras P, Goldstein M, Sherlock P. *Candida* infection of the gastrointestinal tract. Medicine 1972;51:367–379.
34. Obrecht WF, Richter JE, Olympio GA, Gelfand DW. Tracheoesophageal fistula; a serious complication of infectious esophagitis. Gastroenterology 1984;87:1174–1179.
35. Meyers JD, Thomas ED. Infection complicating bone marrow transplantation. In: Rubin RH, Young LS, eds. Clinical approach to infection in the compromised host. New York: Plenum, 1981:507–551.
36. Young JA, Elias E. Gastro-oesophageal candidiasis: diagnosis by brush cytology. J Clin Pathol 1985;38:293–296.
37. McKensie R, Khakoo R. Blastomycosis of the esophagus presenting with gastrointestinal bleeding. Gastroenterology 1985;88:1271–1273.
38. Kane JG, Chretien J, Garagusi V. Diarrhea caused by *Candida*. Lancet 1976;i:335–336.
39. Buss DH, Scharyj M. Herpes virus infection of the esophagus and other visceral organs in adults. Incidence and clinical significance. Am J Med 1979;66:457–461.
40. Boulton AJM, Slater DN, Hamock BW. Herpes virus colitis; a new cause of diarrhea in a patient with Hodgkin's disease. Gut 1982;23:247–249.
41. Markin RS, Langnas AN, Donovan JP, et al. Opportunistic viral hepatitis in liver transplant recipients. Transplant Proc 1991;23:1520–1521.
42. Anuras S, Summers R. Fulminant herpes simplex hepatitis in an adult: report of a case in renal transplant recipient. Gastroenterology 1976;70:425–428.

43. McDonald GB, Sharma P, Hackman RC, et al. Esophageal infections in immunosuppressed patients after marrow transplantation. Gastroenterology 1985;88:1111–1120.
44. Ho M, Jaffe R, Muller G, et al. The frequency of Epstein-Barr virus infection and associated lymphoproliferative syndrome after transplantation and its manifestations in children. Transplantation 1989;45:719–727.
45. Cox KL, Lawrence-Miyasaki LS, Garcia-Kennedy R, et al. An increased incidence of Epstein-Barr virus infection and lymphoproliferative disorder in young children on FK506 after liver transplantation. Transplantation 1995;59:524–529.
46. Langnas AN, Markin RS, Inagaki M, et al. Epstein-Barr virus hepatitis after liver transplantation. Am J Gastroenterol 1994;89:1066–1070.
47. Howard TK, Klintmalm GB, Stone MJ, et al. Lymphoproliferative disorder masquerading as rejection in liver transplant recipients—an early aggressive tumor with atypical presentation. Transplantation 1992;53:1145–1147.
48. Ponteil-Noble C, EcoChard R, Landrivon G, et al. Cytomegalovirus infection—an etiological factor for rejection? Transplantation 1993;55:851.
49. Ho M. Risk factors and pathogenesis of posttransplant lymphoproliferative disorders. Transplant Proc 1995;27:S1:S38–S40.
50. Knapp AB, Horst DA, Eliopoulos G, et al. Widespread cytomegalovirus gastroenterocolitis in a patient with AIDS. Gastroenterology 1983;85:1399–1402.
51. Connelly GM, Hawkins D, Harcourt Webster JN, et al. Oesophageal symptoms, their causes, treatment and prognosis in patients with AIDS. Gut 1989;230:1033–1039.
52. Orloff JJ, Saito R, Laskey S, Dave H. Toxic megacolon in cytomegalovirus colitis. Am J Gastroenterol 1989;84:794–797.
53. Elta G, Turnage R, Eckhauser FE, et al. A submucosal antral mass caused by cytomegalovirus infection in a patient with AIDS. Am J Gastroenterol 1986;81:714–717.
54. Lewis-Jones HG, Ward RG, Garvey C. Cytomegalovirus infection masquerading as colonic neoplasia. Br J Radiol 1990;63:573–574.
55. Dieterich DT, Kim MH, McMeeding A, Rotterdam H. Cytomegalovirus appendicitis in a patient with AIDS. Am J Gastroenterol 1991;86:904–906.
56. Kram HB, Shoemaker WC. Intestinal perforation due to cytomegalovirus in patients with AIDS. Dis Colon Rectum 1990;33:1037–1040.
57. Van Son WJ, van der Jagt EJ, van der Woude FJ, et al. Pneumatosis intestinalis in patients after cadaveric kidney transplantation: possible relationship with an active cytomegalovirus infection. Transplantation 1984;38:506–510.
58. Agha FP, Nostrant PP, Abrams GD, et al. Cytomegalovirus cholangitis in a homosexual man with the acquired immune deficiency syndrome. Am J Gastroenterol 1986;81:1068–1072.
59. Aaron JS, Wynter CD, Kirton OC, Simko V. Cytomegalovirus-associated acalculous cholecystitis in a patient with acquired immune deficiency syndrome. Am J Gastroenterol 1988;83:879–881.
60. Schneiderman DJ, Cello JP, Laing FC. Papillary stenosis and sclerosing cholangitis in the acquired immunodeficiency syndrome. Ann Intern Med 1987;106:546–549.
61. Bronsther O, Manez R, Kusne S, et al. Posttransplant B, non A, non B and cytomegalovirus hepatitis increase the risk of developing chronic rejection after liver transplantation. Transplant Proc 1995;27:1206–1207.
62. Van der Bij W, Torensma R, van Son WJ, et al. Rapid immunodiagnosis of active CMV infection by monoclonal antibody staining of blood leucocytes. J Med Virol 1988;25:179–188.
63. Gregory WW, Menegus MA. Practical protocol for cytomegalovirus isolation: use of MRC-5 cell monolayers incubated for two weeks. J Clin Microbiol 1983;17:605–609.
64. Erice A, Jordan MC, Chace BA, et al. Ganciclovir treatment of cytomegalovirus disease in transplant recipients and other immunocompromised hosts. JAMA 1987;257:3082–3087.
65. Stratta RJ, Shaefer MS, Markin RS, et al. Clinical patterns of CMV disease after liver transplantation. Arch Surg 1989;124:1443–1450.
66. Drobyski WR, Knox KK, Carrigan DR, Ash RC. Foscarnet therapy of ganciclovir resistant CMV in bone marrow transplantation. Transplantation 1991;52:155.
67. Flomenberg P, Babbitt J, Drobyski W, et al. Increasing incidence of adenovirus disease in bone marrow transplant recipients. J Infect Dis 1994;169:775–781.
68. Berteau P, Parquet N, Ferchal F, et al. Fulminant adenovirus hepatitis after allogeneic bone marrow transplantation. Bone Marrow Transplant 1996;17:295–298.
69. Myerowitz RL, Stalder H, Oxman MN, et al. Fatal disseminated adenovirus infection in a renal transplant recipient. Am J Med 1975;59:591–598.
70. Koneru B, Atchison R, Jaffe R, et al. Serological studies of adenovirus hepatitis following pediatric liver transplantation. Transplant Proc 1990;22:1547–1548.
71. Uhnoo I, Wadell G, Svensson L, et al. Importance of enteric adenoviruses 40 and 41 in acute gastroenteritis in infants and young children. J Clin Microbiol 1984;20:365–372.
72. Bradley JR, Wreghitt TG, Evans DB, et al. Chickenpox in adult renal transplant patients. Nephrol Dial Transplant 1987;1:242.
73. McCluggage W, Fox JD, Baillie K, et al. Varicella zoster gastritis in a bone marrow transplant recipient. J Clin Pathol 1994;47:1054–1056.
74. Kusne S, Pappo O, Pazin G, et al. Varicella zoster virus hepatitis and a suggested management plan for prevention of varicella zoster virus infection in adult liver transplant recipients. Transplantation 1995;60:619–621.
75. Roger SY, Irving W, Harris A, Russell NH. Visceral varicella zoster infection after bone marrow transplantation without skin involvement and the use of PCR for diagnosis. Bone Marrow Transplant 1995;15:805–807.
76. Lockesley R, Flournoy N, Sullivan K, et al. Infection with varicella zoster virus after bone marrow transplantation. J Infect Dis 1989;152:1172–1181.
77. Grekas D, Dioudis C, Mandravelli K, et al. Renal transplantation in asymptomatic carriers of hepatitis B surface antigen. Nephron 1995;69: 267–272.
78. Parfrey PS, Farge D, Forbes RD, et al. Chronic hepatitis in end stage renal disease: comparison of HBsAg negative and HBsAg positive patients. Kidney Int 1985;28:959–967.
79. Pirson Y, Alexander G, Strihou C. Long-term effect of HBsAg antigenaemia on patient survival after renal transplantation. N Engl J Med 1977;269:194–196.
80. Berne TV, Fitzgibbons TJ, Silbernian H. The effect of hepatitis B antigenemia on long-term success and hepatic disease in renal transplant recipients. Transplantation 1977;24:412–415.
81. Booth JC, Goldin R, Brown J, et al. Fibrosing cholestatic hepatitis in a renal transplant recipient associated with the hepatitis B virus precore mutant. J Hepatol 1995;22:500–503.
82. Devergie A, Brechot C, Schenmetzler C, Bernuau J. Fulminant hepatitis due to reactivation of chronic hepatitis B virus infection after allogeneic bone marrow transplantation. Dig Dis Sci 1988;33:1185–1189.
83. Ilan Y, Nagler A, Naparstek E, et al. Adoptive transfer of immunity to hepatitis B virus after T cell-depleted allogeneic bone marrow transplantation. Hepatology 1993;18:246–252.
84. Ilan. Complete information not available.
85. Todo S, Demetris AJ, Van Thiel D, et al. Orthotopic liver transplantation for patients with hepatitis B related liver disease. Hepatology 1991;13:619–626.
86. Samuel D, Muller R, Alexander G, et al. Liver transplantation in European patients with the hepatitis B surface antigen. N Engl J Med 1993;329:1842–1847.
87. Mason A, Wick M, White H, Perillo R. Hepatitis B virus replication in diverse cell types during chronic hepatitis B infection. Hepatology 1993;18:781–789.
88. Yoffe B, Burns DK, Bhatt HS, Combes B. Extrahepatic hepatitis B virus DNA sequences in patients with acute hepatitis B infection. Hepatology 1990;12:187–192.
89. Lowell JA, Howard TK, White HM, et al. Serological evidence of past hepatitis B infection in liver donor and hepatitis B infection in liver allograft. Lancet 1995;345:1084–1085.
90. Davies SE, Portmann BC, O'Grady JG, et al. Hepatic histological findings after transplantation for chronic hepatitis B virus infection, including a unique pattern of fibrosing cholestatic hepatitis. Hepatology 1991;13:150–157.
91. Lavine JE, Lake JR, Ascher NL, et al. Persistent hepatitis B virus following interferon alpfa therapy and liver transplantation. Gastroenterology 1991;100:263–267.
92. Hoofnagle JH, Di Bisceglie AM, Waggoner JG, Park Y. Interferon alpha for patients with clinically apparent cirrhosis due to hepatitis B. Gastroenterology 1993;104:1116–1121.
93. Grellier L, Mutimer D, Ahmed M, et al. Lamivudine prophylaxis against reinfection in liver transplantation for hepatitis B cirrhosis. Lancet 1997;348:1212–1215.
94. Ling R, Mutimer D, Ahmed M, et al. Selection of mutations in the hepatitis B virus polymerase during therapy of transplant recipients with lamivudine. Hepatology 1996;24:711–713.
95. Gish RG, Lau JYN, Brooks L, et al. Ganciclovir treatment of hepatitis B virus infection in liver transplant recipients. Hepatology 1996;23:1–7.
96. Lauchart W, Muller R, Pichlmayr R. Immunoprophylaxis of hepatitis B virus reinfection in recipients of human liver allografts. Transplant Proc 1987;19:2387–2389.
97. Wright HL, Gavaler JS, Van Thiel DH. Preliminary experience with a-2b-interferon therapy of viral hepatitis in liver graft recipients. Transplantation 1992;53:121–124.

98. Lucey MR, Graham DM, Martin P, et al. Recurrence of hepatitis B and delta hepatitis after orthotopic liver transplantation. Gut 1992;33:1390–1396.
99. Hopf U, Neuhaus P, Lobeck H, et al. Follow-up of recurrent hepatitis B and delta infection in liver allograft recipients after treatment with recombinant interferon alpha. J Hepatol 1991;13:339–346.
100. Genesca J, Vila J, Cordoba J, et al. Hepatitis C virus infection in renal transplant recipients: epidemiology, clinical impact, serological confirmation and viral replication. J Hepatol 1995;22:272–277.
101. Genesca. Complete information not available.
102. Pereira BJG, Wright TL, Schmit CH, Levey AS. The impact of pretransplantation hepatitis C infection on the outcome of renal transplantation. Transplantation 1995;60:799–805.
103. Wright HL, Bou-Abboud C, Hassanein T, et al. Disease recurrence following liver transplantation for autoimmune chronic active liver disease. Transplantation 1992;53:136–139.
104. Chazouillieres O, Kim M, Combs C, et al. Quantitation of hepatitis C virus RNA in liver transplant recipients. Gastroenterology 1994;106:994–999.
105. Hsu HH, Wright TL, Tsao SC, et al. Attenuated antibody response to hepatitis C virus after liver transplantation. Am J Gastroenterol 1994;89:1109–1114.
106. Araya V, Rakela J, Wright T. Hepatitis C after orthotopic liver transplantation. Gastroenterology 1997;1132:575–582.
107. Wright TL, Donegan E, Hsu HH, et al. Recurrent and acquired hepatitis C viral infection in liver transplant recipients. Gastroenterology 1992;103:317–322.
108. Gane EJ, Portmann BC, Naoumov N, et al. Long-term outcome of hepatitis C infection after liver transplantation. New Engl J Med 1996;334:815–820.
109. Martin P, Munoz SJ, Di Biscegli AM, et al. Recurrence of hepatitis C virus infection after orthotopic liver transplantation. Hepatology 1991;13:719–721.
110. Wright HL, Combs C, Kim M, et al. Interferon therapy for hepatitis C virus infection following liver transplantation. Hepatology 1994;20:773–779.
111. Gayowski T, Singh N, Wanstedt CF, et al. Interferon alpha therapy for hepatitis C virus recurrence after liver transplantation. Long-term response with maintenance therapy. Hepatology 1995;22:103.
112. Bizollon T, Ducert C, Trepo C. New approaches to the treatment of hepatitis C virus infection after liver transplantation using ribavirin. J Hepatol 1995;23:22–25.
113. Sullivan KM. Graft versus host disease. In: Forman SJ, Blume KG, Thomas ED, eds. Bone marrow transplantation. Cambridge, MA: Blackwell Scientific, 1994:339.
114. Glucksberg H, Storb R, Fefer A, et al. Clinical manifestations of graft versus host disease in human recipients of marrow from HLA matched sibling donors. Transplantation 1974;18:295–304.
115. Sullivan KM, Shulman HM, Storb R, et al. Chronic graft versus host disease in 52 patients: adverse natural course and successful treatment with combination immunosuppression. Blood 1981;57:267–276.
116. McDonald GB, Shulman HM, Sullivan K, Spencer G. Intestinal and hepatic complications of bone marrow transplantation. Part II. Gastroenterology 1986;90:770–784.
117. Weisdorf D, Snover D, Haake R, et al. Acute upper gastrointestinal graft versus host disease: clinical significance and response to immunosuppressive therapy. Blood 1990;76:624–629.
118. Serota FT, Rosenberg HK, Rosen J, et al. Delayed onset of gastrointestinal disease in the recipients of bone marrow transplants. A variant graft-versus-host reaction. Transplantation 1982;34:60–64.
119. Serota. Complete information not available.
120. Roy J, Snover D, Weisdorf S, et al. Simultaneous upper and lower endoscopic biopsy in the diagnosis of intestinal graft versus host disease. Transplantation 1991;51:642–646.
121. Epstein JB, Reece DE. Topical cyclosporine A treatment of oral chronic graft versus host disease. Bone Marrow Transplant 1994;13:81–86.
122. Schubert MM, Sullivan KM, Morton TH, et al. Oral manifestations of chronic graft versus host disease. Arch Intern Med 1984;144:1591–1595.
123. Shulman HM, Sullivan KM, Weiden PL, et al. Chronic graft versus host syndrome in man. A long-term clinicopathological study of 20 Seattle patients. Am J Med 1980;69:204–217.
124. Baehr P, Levine D, Bouvier M, et al. Oral beclomethasone dipropionate for the treatment of human intestinal graft versus host disease. Transplantation 1995;60:1231–1238.
125. Baddour H, Gurakar A, Hassanein T, et al. Sinus disease: a source of unsuspected pathology in patients with end-stage liver disease. Meeting of the American Gastroenterological Association, New Orleans, Louisiana, May 15–18, 1994.
126. Daley TD, Wysocki GP, May C. Clinical and pharmacological correlations in cyclosporine-induced gingival hyperplasia. Oral Surg 1986;62:417–421.
127. Hassell TM, Hefti A. Drug-induced gingival overgrowth: old problem, new problem. Crit Rev Oral Biol Med 1991;2:103–137.
128. Seymour RA, Jacobs DJ. Cyclosporine and the gingival tissues. J Clin Periodontol 1992:19:1–11.
129. Varga E, Tyldesley WR. Carcinoma arising in cyclosporin-induced gingival hyperplasia. Br Dent J 1991;171:20–27.
130. Thomason JM, Seymour RA, Rice N. The prevalence and severity of cyclosporine and nifedipine induced gingival overgrowth. J Clin Periodontol 1993;20:37–40.
131. Seymour RA, Smith DG, Rogers SR. The comparative effect of azathioprine and cyclosporine on some gingival health parameters of renal transplant patients. J Clin Periodontol 1987;14:610–613.
132. Thomason JM, Seymour RA, Ellis JS. The periodontal problems and management of the renal transplant patient. Ren Fail 1994;16:731–745.
133. Komorowski RA, Cohen EB, Kamiffman HM. Gastrointestinal complications in renal transplant recipients. Am J Clin Pathol 1986;86:161–167.
134. Benoit G, Moukarzel M, Verdelli G, et al. Gastrointestinal complications in renal transplantation. Transplant Int 1993;6:45–49.
135. Stuart FP, Reckard CR, Schulak JA, Ketel BL. Gastroduodenal complications in kidney transplant recipients. Ann Surg 1981;194:339–344.
136. Kaur S, Cooper G, Fakult S, Lazarus HM. Incidence and outcome of overt gastrointestinal bleeding in patients undergoing bone marrow transplantation. Dig Dis Sci 1996;41:598–603.
137. Kaur. Complete information not available.
138. Heikkinen LO, Ala-Kulju K. Abdominal complications following cardiopulmonary bypass in open heart surgery. Scand J Thorac Cardiovasc Surg 1987;21:1–7.
139. Hanks JB, Curtis SE, Hanks BB. Gastrointestinal complications after cardiopulmonary bypass surgery. Surgery 1982;92:394–400.
140. Watson CJE, Jamieson NV, Johnston PS, et al. Early abdominal complications following heart and heart–lung transplantation. Br J Surg 1991;78:699–704.
141. Cook DJ, Witt LG, Cook RJ, Guyatt GH. Stress ulcer prophylaxis in the critically ill: a meta-analysis. Am J Med 1991;91:519–527.
142. Macdougall BRD, Bailey RJ, Williams R. H2 receptor antagonists and antacids in the prevention of acute gastrointestinal haemorrhage in fulminant hepatic failure. Lancet 1977;1:617–619.
143. Hruby Z, MyszkaBijak K, Gosciniak G, et al. *Helicobacter pylori* in kidney allograft recipients: high prevalence of colonization and low incidence of active inflammatory lesions. Nephron 1997;75:25–29.
144. Wotherspoon AC, Diss TC, Pan L, et al. Low-grade gastric lymphoma of mucosa-associated lymphoid tissue in immunocompromised patients. Histopathology 1996;28:129–134.
145. Calleja IJ, Polo JR, Garcia-Sabrido JL, et al. Two-clamp method to avoid portal anastamotic stenosis in liver transplantation. Am J Surg 1993;165:367.
146. Alexander J, Demetrius AJ, Gavaler JS, et al. Pancreatitis following liver transplantation. Transplantation 1988;45:1062–1065.
147. Huddy S, Joyce W, Pepper J. Gastrointestinal complications in 4473 patients who underwent cardiopulmonary bypass surgery. Br J Surg 1991;78:293–296.
148. Camargo CA, Greig PD, Levy GA, Clavien PA. Acute pancreatitis following liver transplantation. J Am Coll Surg 1995;181:249–255.
149. Krokos N, Karavias D, Tzakis A, et al. Acute pancreatitis after liver transplantation: incidence and contributing factors. Transpl Int 1995;8:1–7.
150. Shiel AGR. Development of malignancy following renal transplantation in Australia and New Zealand. Transplant Proc 1992;24:1275–1279.
151. Cohen JI. EBV lymphoproliferative disease associated with acquired immunodeficiency. Medicine 1990;70:137–160.
152. D'Amore ESG, Manivel JC, Gajl-Peczalska KJ, et al. B cell lymphoproliferative disorders after bone marrow transplant. Cancer 1991;68:1285–1295.
153. Benkerrou M, Durandy A, Fischer A. Therapy for transplant-related lymphoproliferative diseases. Hematol Oncol Clin N Am 1993;7:467–475.
154. Fischer A, Blanche S, Lebidois J, et al. Anti-B-cell monoclonal antibodies in the treatment of severe B cell lymphoproliferative syndrome following bone marrow and organ transplantation. N Engl J Med 1991;324:1451–1456.
155. Ozaki CF, Katz SM, Monsour HP Jr, et al. Surgical complications of liver transplantation. Surg Clin North Am 1994;74:1155–1167.
156. Ozaki. Complete information not available.
157. Koneru B, Selby R, O'Hair D, et al. Nonobstructing colonic dilatation following renal transplantation. Arch Surg 1990;125:610–613.
158. Wojtalik RS, Lindenauer SM, Kahn SS. Perforation of the colon associated with adynamic ileus. Am J Surg 1973;125:601–606.
159. Wangensteen OH. Intestinal obstructions. 3rd ed. Springfield, Ill: Charles C Thomas, 1955.
160. Shaked A, Vargas J, Csete M, et al. Diagnosis and treatment of bowel perforation following pediatric orthotopic liver transplantation. Arch Surg 1993;128:994–999.

161. Marujo W, Stratta RJ, Langnas AN, Wood P. Syndrome of multiple bowel perforations in liver transplant recipients. Am J Surg 1991;162:594–597.
162. Stephens J, Goldstein R, Crippin J, et al. Effects of orthotopic liver transplantation and immunosuppression on inflammatory bowel disease in primary sclerosing cholangitis patients. Transplant Proc 1993;25:1122–1123.
163. Rowley S, Candinas D, Mayer AD, et al. Restorative proctocolectomy and pouch anal anastamosis for ulcerative colitis following orthotopic liver transplantation. Gut 1995:37:845–847.
164. Zins BJ, Sandborn WJ, Penna C, et al. Pouchitis disease course after orthotopic liver transplantation in patients with primary sclerosing cholangitis and an ileal pouch anal anastamosis. Am J Gastroenterol 1995;90:2177–2181.
165. Higashi H, Yanaga K, Marsh JW, et al. Development of colon cancer after liver transplantation for primary sclerosing cholangitis associated with ulcerative colitis. Hepatology 1990;11:477–480.
166. Bleday R, Lee E, Jessurun J, et al. Increased risk of early colorectal neoplasms after hepatic transplant in patients with inflammatory bowel disease. Dis Colon Rectum 1993;36:908–912.
167. Brentnall TA, Haggitt R, Rabinovitch P, et al. Risk and natural history of colonic neoplasia in patients with primary sclerosing cholangitis and ulcerative colitis. Gastroenterology 1996;110:331–338.
168. Lohr M, Lotterer E, Hahn EG, Fleig WE. Primary biliary cirrhosis associated with coeliac disease. Eur J Gastroenterol Hepatol 1994;6:263–267.
169. Almy TP, Howell DA. Diverticular disease in the colon. N Engl J Med 1980;302:324.
170. McCune TR, Nylander WA, Vanburen DH, et al. Colonic screening prior to renal transplantation and its impact on posttransplant colonic complications. Clin Transplant 1992;6:91–96.
171. Abramson SJ, Berdon WE, Laffey K, et al. Colonic diverticulitis in young patients with chronic renal failure and transplantation. Pediatr Radiol 1991;21:352–354.
172. Colonna JO, Shaked A, Gomes AS, et al. Biliary strictures complicating liver transplantation: incidence, pathogenesis, management and outcome. Ann Surg 1992;216:344.
173. Van Thiel DH, Fagiuoli S, Wright HI, et al. Biliary complications of liver transplantation. Gastrointest Endosc 1993;39:455.
174. Leturneau JG, Day JL, Hunter DW, et al. Biliary complications after liver transplantation in patients with preexisting sclerosing cholangitis. Radiology 1988;167:349–351.
175. Hubscher S, Elias E, Buckels JAC, et al. Primary biliary cirrhosis. Histological evidence of disease recurrence after liver transplantation. J Hepatol 1993;18:173–184.
176. Harrison RF, Davies MH, Neuberger JM, Hubscher SG. Fibrous and obliterative cholangitis in liver allografts: evidence of recurrent primary sclerosing cholangitis? Hepatology 1994;20:356–361.
177. Harrison. Complete information not available.
178. Neuberger J, Portmann B, Calne R, Williams R. Recurrence of autoimmune chronic active hepatitis following orthotopic liver transplantation. Transplantation 1984;37:363–365.
179. Olthoff KM, Millis JM, Rosose MH, Goldstein L. Is liver transplantation justified for the treatment of hepatic malignancies? Arch Surg 1990;125: 1261–1268.
180. Ismail T, Angrisani L, Gunson BK, et al. Primary hepatic malignancy: the role of liver transplantation. Br J Surg 1990;77:983–987.
181. Abu Elmagd KM, Selby R, Iwatsuki S, et al. Cholangiocarcinoma and sclerosing cholangitis: clinical characteristics and the effect on survival after liver transplantation. Transplant Proc 1993;25:1124–1125.
182. Koneru B, Cassavilla A, Bowman J, et al. Liver transplantation for malignant tumours. Gastroenterol Clin N Am 1988;17:177–193.
183. Yokoyama I, Todo S, Iwatsuki S, Starzl TE. Liver transplantation in the treatment of primary liver cancer. Hepatogastroenterology 1990;37:188–193.
184. Pichlmayr R. Is there a place for liver grafting for malignancy? Transplant Proc 1988;20(suppl):478–482.
185. Yokoyama I, Carr B, Saitsu H, et al. Accelerated growth rates of recurrent hepatocellular cancer after liver transplantation. Cancer 1991;68:2095–2100.

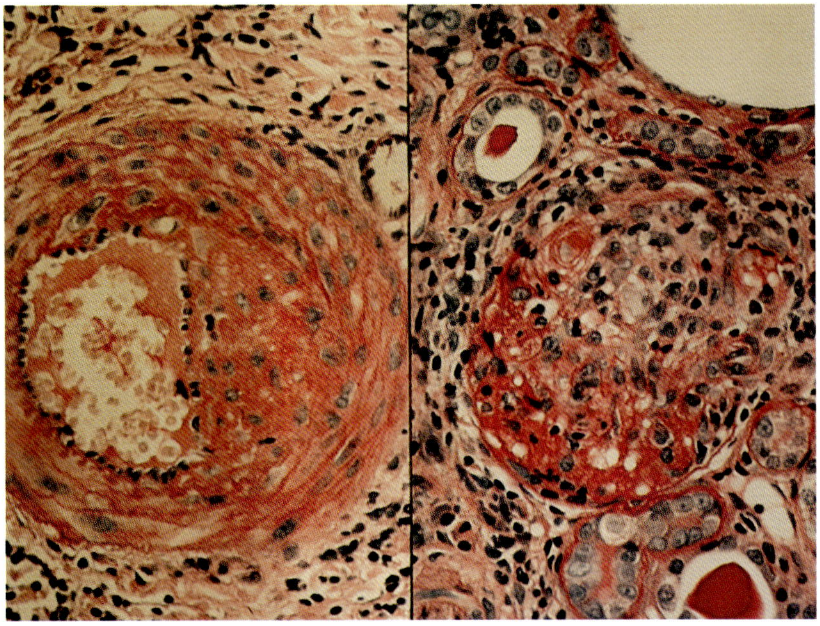

PLATE 1. *The typical lesions of chronic rejection are here demonstrated in a kidney, showing both arterial and glomerular involvement. The arterial lesion is virtually identical to that seen in the coronary vessels of heart allografts. In the glomerulus, there is mesangial proliferation and occlusion of capillary spaces, leading to gradual glomerulosclerosis.*

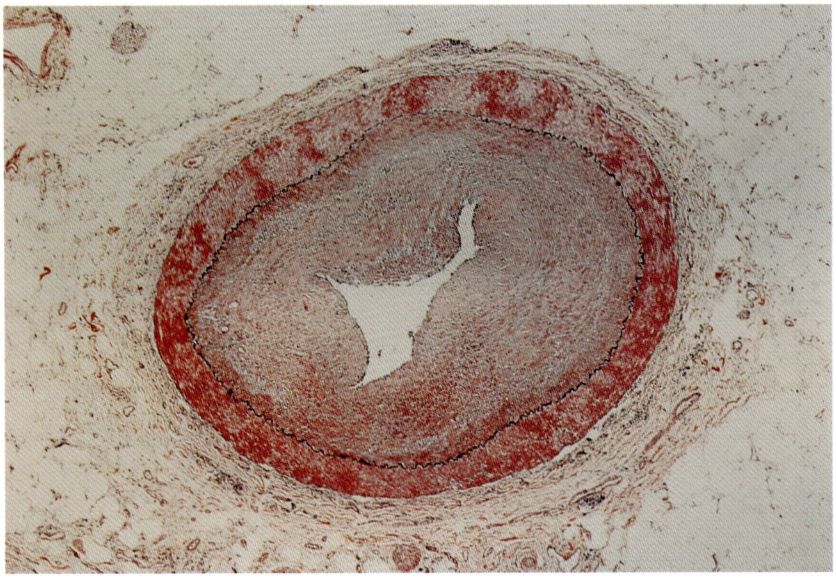

PLATE 2. *Graft arteriosclerosis of cardiac allografts, the primary manifestation of chronic rejection in this organ, involves concentric myointimal proliferation involving the entire coronary arterial tree.*

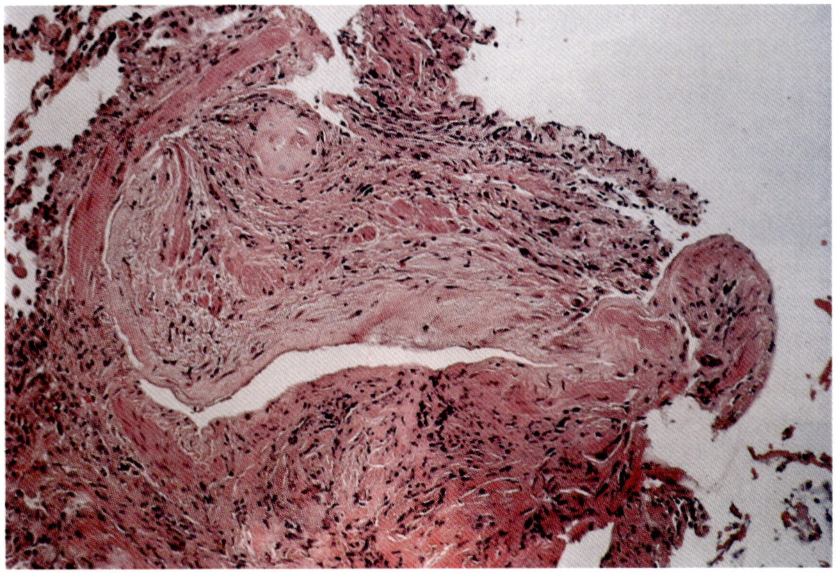

PLATE 3. *Bronchiolitis obliterans is the most common manifestation of chronic rejection of lung allografts. Like graft arteriosclerosis, it involves gradual luminal obliteration of bronchi and bronchioles, with inflammatory cells, granulations, and hypertrophy of smooth muscle.*

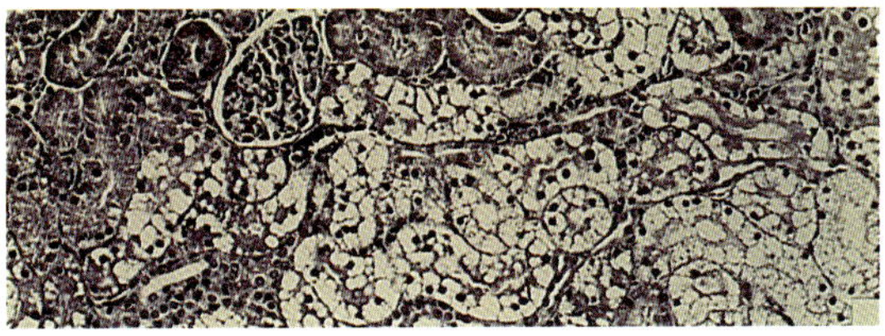

PLATE 4. *Acute CsA nephrotoxicity in a patient with allograft dysfunction 3 weeks after initiation of CsA therapy. The extensive proximal tubular vacuolization and sparse cellular infiltrate are characteristic of CsA nephrotoxicity rather than acute rejection.*

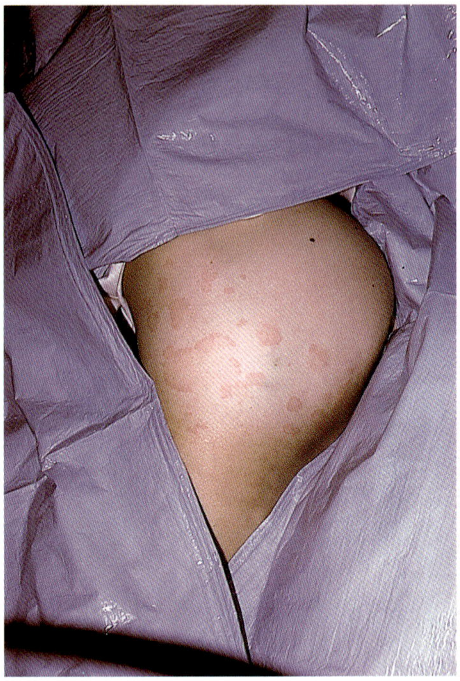

PLATE 6. *Skin rash in an ATG-treated patient. The maculopapular, blotchy eruption developed primarily over the recipient's thighs and buttocks six days after initiating ATG therapy. The 12-day course of treatment, required to reverse the patient's acute rejection episode, was completed without complications following administration of antihistamines for symptomatic relief.*

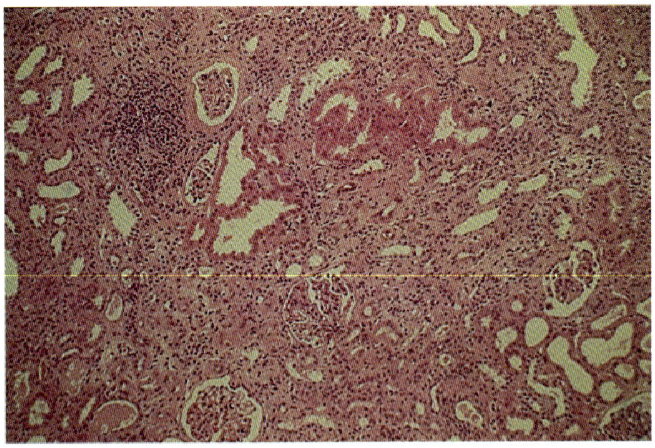

PLATE 5. *Chronic CsA nephrotoxicity. Note the severe ("striped") interstitial fibrosis and diffuse cellular infiltrate. Although intimal proliferation in this biopsy is not dramatic, the histopathologic changes of chronic rejection are often quite similar.*

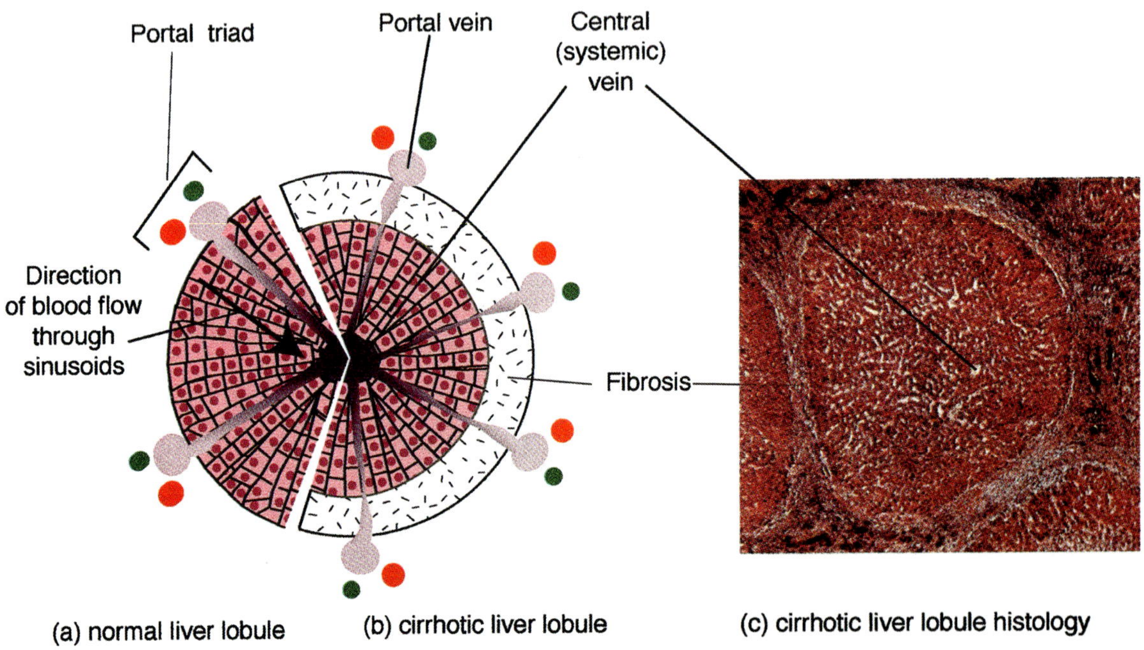

PLATE 7. *Cirrhosis is a histopathologic diagnosis describing the end-stage liver scarring due to a wide variety of liver diseases. Its hallmarks are diffuse hepatic fibrosis and nodule formation. The hepatic fibrosis, by impeding portal venous inflow, results in portal hypertension.*

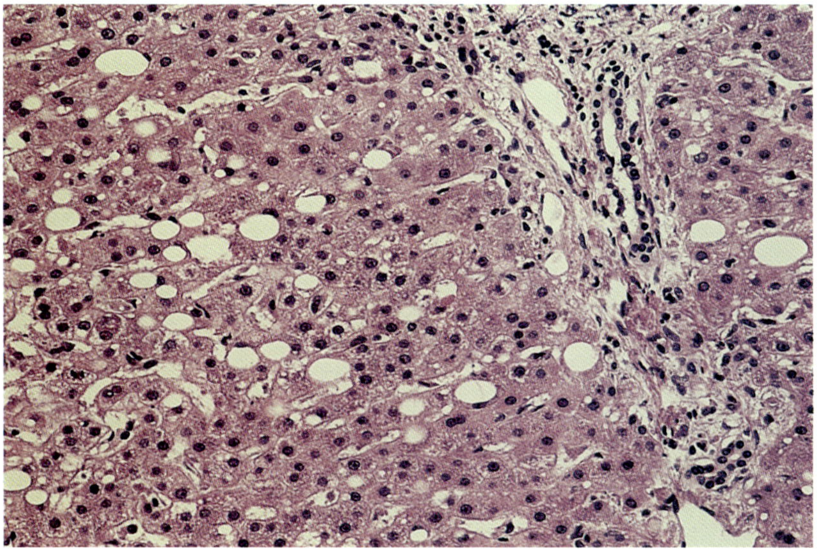

PLATE 8. *Macrovesicular steatosis in the donor liver. Many of the hepatocytes contain one or more vesicles that displace the nucleus and occupy the majority of the cytoplasm.*

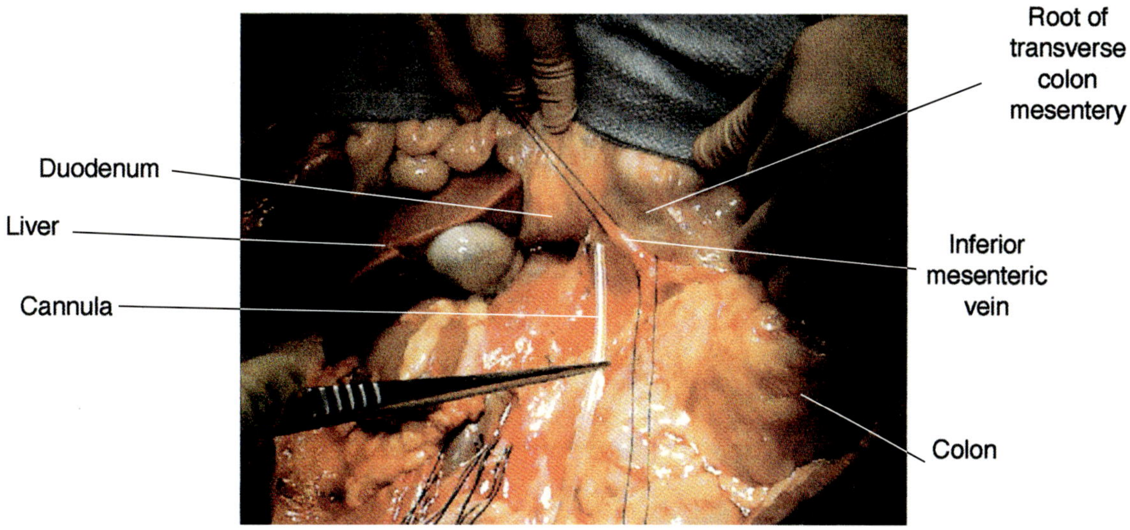

PLATE 9. *The inferior mesenteric vein is found at the base of the distal transverse colon mesentery and can be cannulated to perfuse the portal vein.*

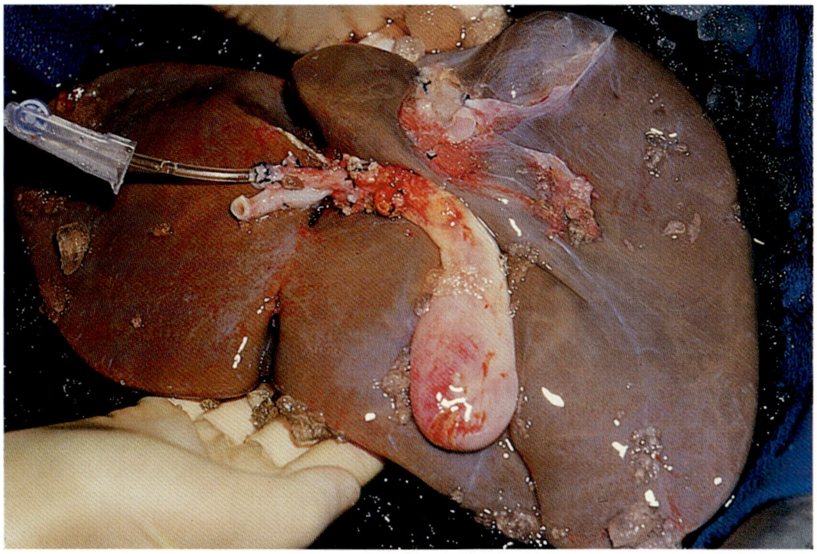

PLATE 10. *A procured liver's inferior surface. The cannula for portal perfusion is still in place. After back-table flushing of the portal vein, hepatic artery, and common bile duct, the liver is packed in preservation fluid and stored in a bag surrounded by ice-cold solution.*

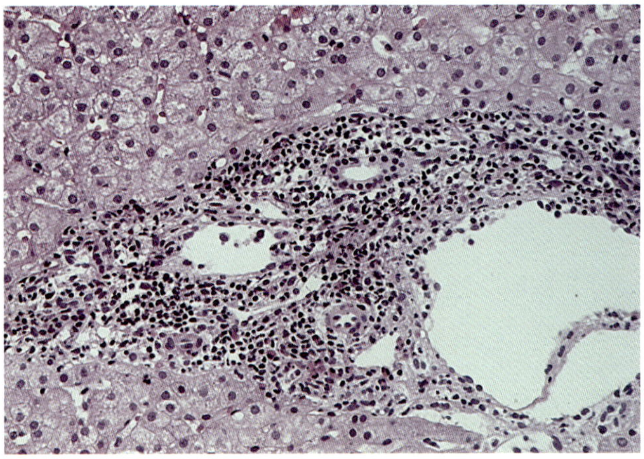

PLATE 11. *Acute cellular rejection in liver allograft. A mixed cellular infiltrate is typically seen in the portal tract (portal vein at right of specimen). Such nondestructive lesions are typically reversible.*

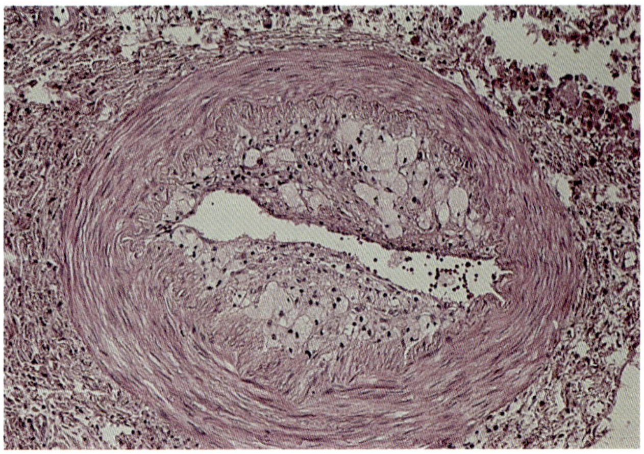

PLATE 12. *Chronic liver allograft rejection. Note artery with severe fibrous intimal thickening and lipid-containing foam cells in the thickened intima. (Courtesy of Dr. A. Bhan.)*

A

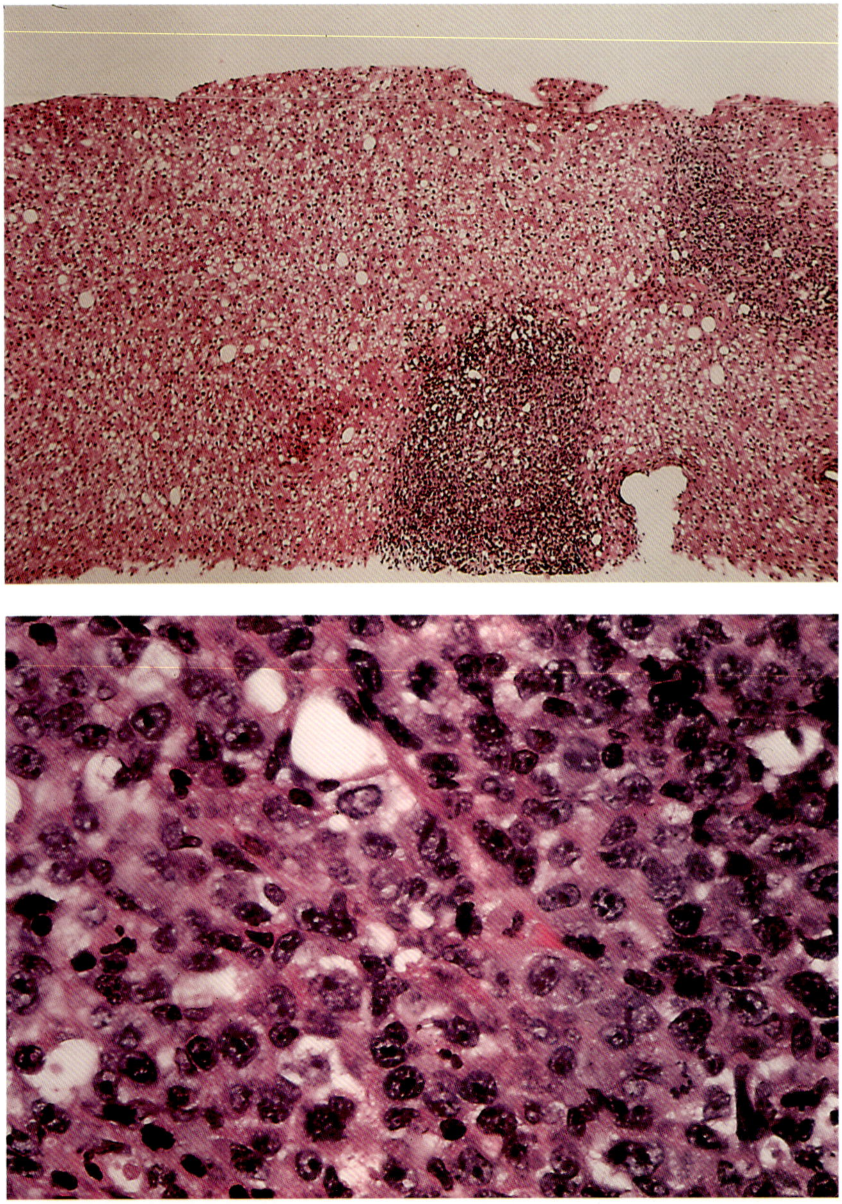

B

PLATE 13. *The histologic appearance of post-transplant lymphoproliferative disease (PTLD) in a liver allograft is shown.* ***A.*** *Note the infiltrating lymphocytes in the triad, which may be confused with rejection (low-power view).* ***B.*** *A feature of note for distinguishing PTLD from rejection is the monomorphous infiltrate of large immature lymphocytes (high-power view).*

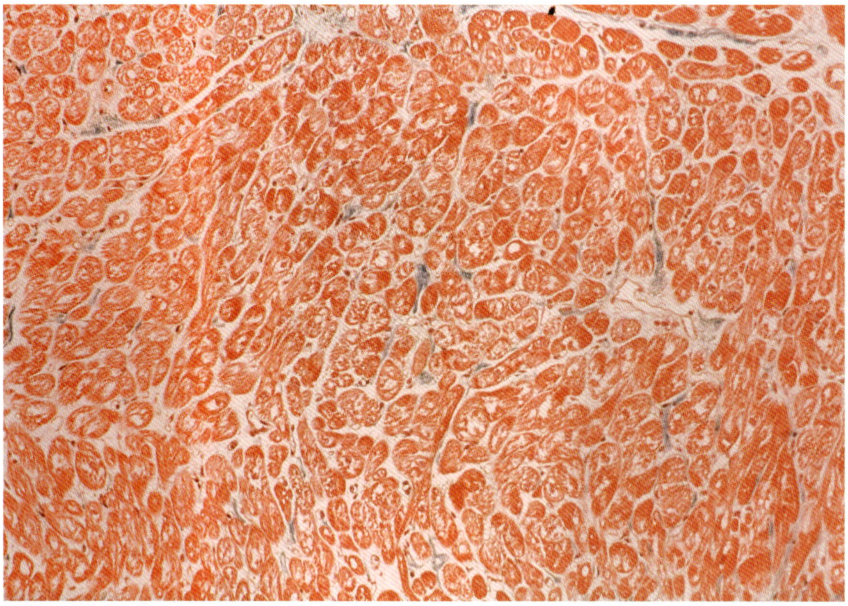

PLATE 14. *ISHLT grade 0 hearttallograft biopsy shows no evidence for rejection (hematoxylin-eosin, ×250).*

A

B

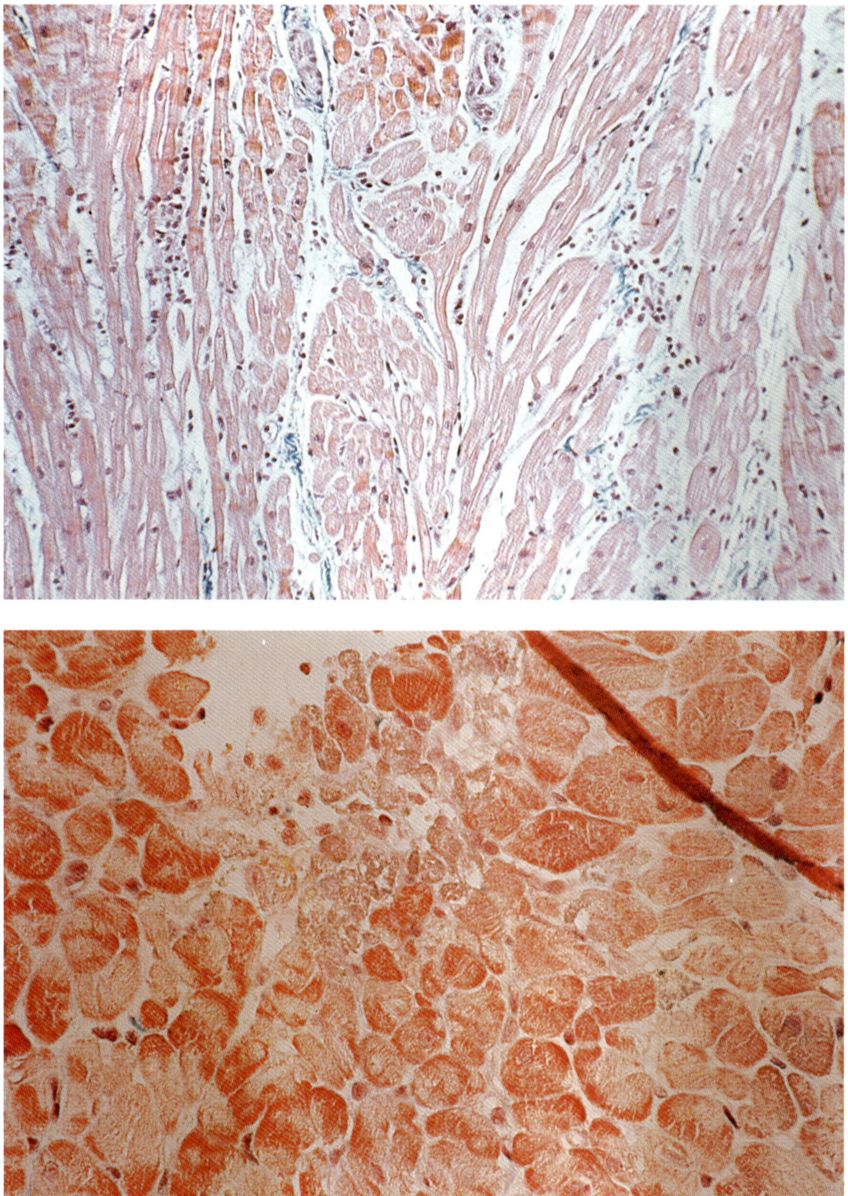

PLATE 15. ***A.*** *ISHLT grade 1B biopsy shows a mild localized cellular infiltrate without evidence for myocyte necrosis (hematoxylin-eosin, ×250).* ***B.*** *Biopsy shows healing ischemic injury with myocyte loss, early granulation tissue, and an inflammatory infiltrate of mixed cellularity (hematoxylin-eosin, ×250).*

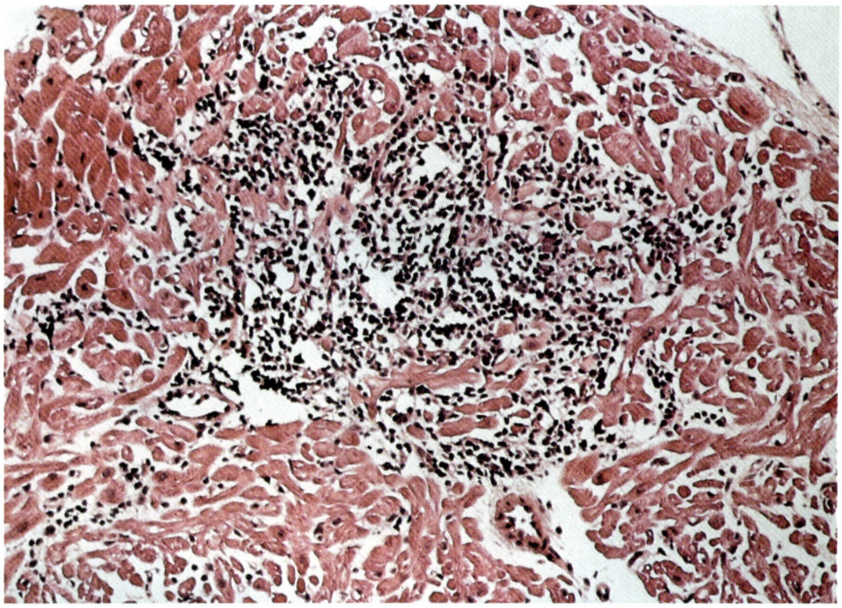

PLATE 16. *ISHLT grade 2 biopsy shows focal moderate rejection with the presence of a single focus of prominent lymphocytic inflammation and/or myocyte necrosis (hematoxylin-eosin, ×250).*

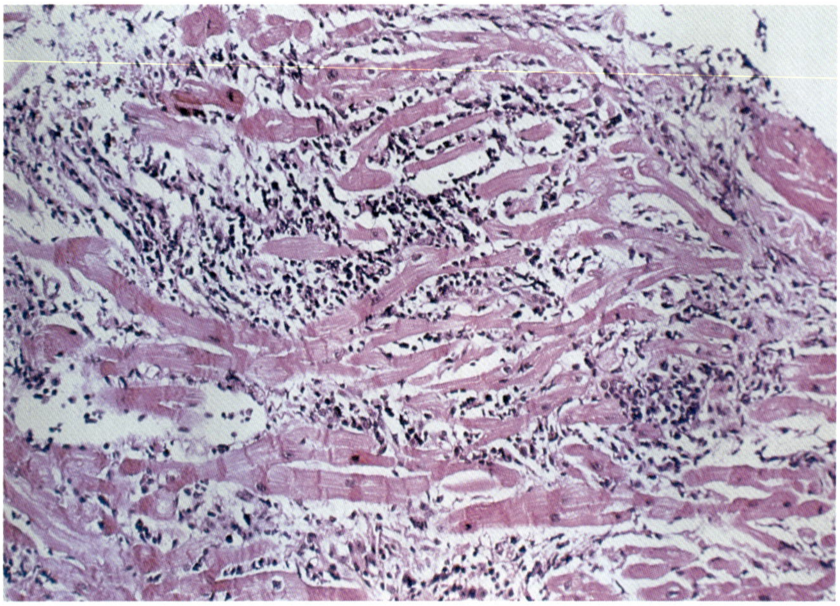

PLATE 17. *ISHLT grade 3A biopsy reveals moderately severe rejection with multifocal lymphocytic infiltrates and focal myocyte necrosis. Edema and hemorrhage are absent (hematoxylin-eosin, ×250).*

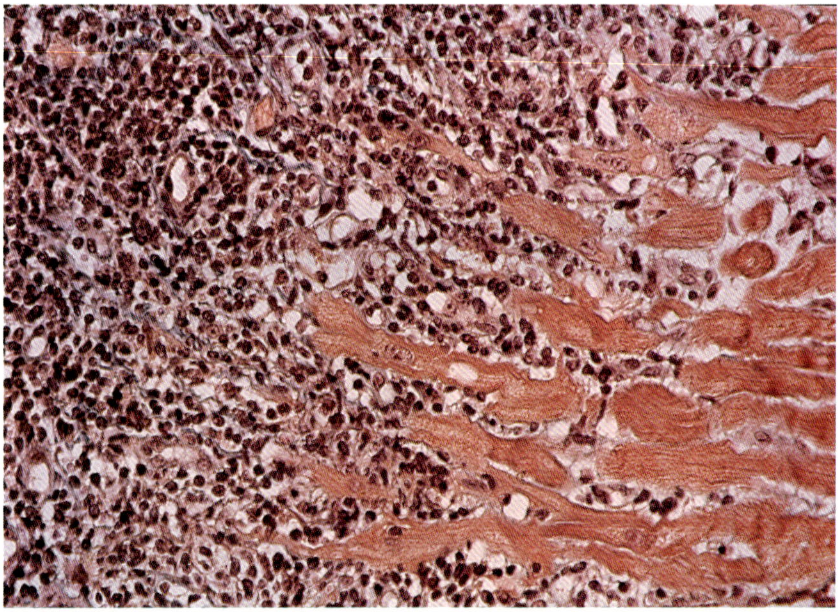

PLATE 18. *Biopsy shows a "Quilty B" lesion characterized by a dense endocardial lymphocytic infiltrate extending into the subjacent myocardium (hematoxylin-eosin, ×250).*

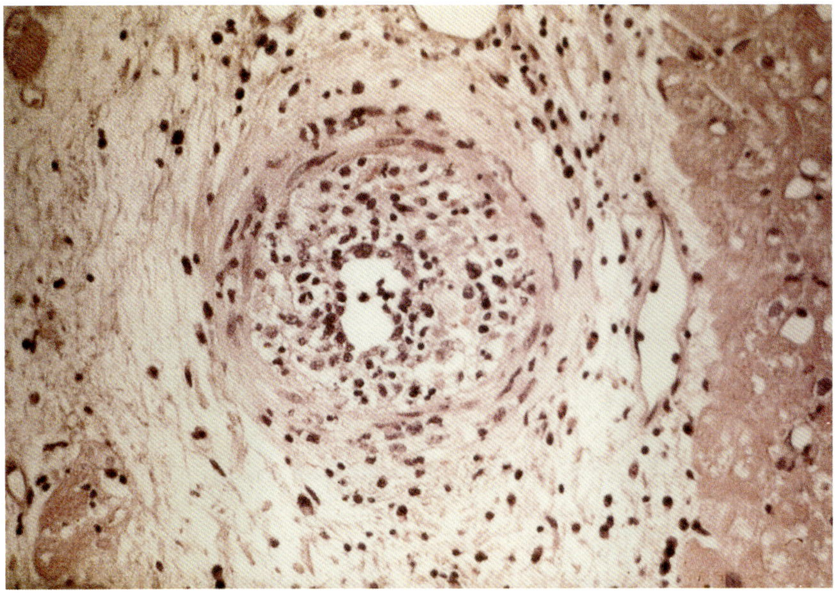

PLATE 19. *Photomicrograph of an arteriole showing concentric intimal hyperplasia and an abundance of macrophages; this is the most common histopathologic lesion of transplant vasculopathy (hematoxylin-eosin, ×250).*

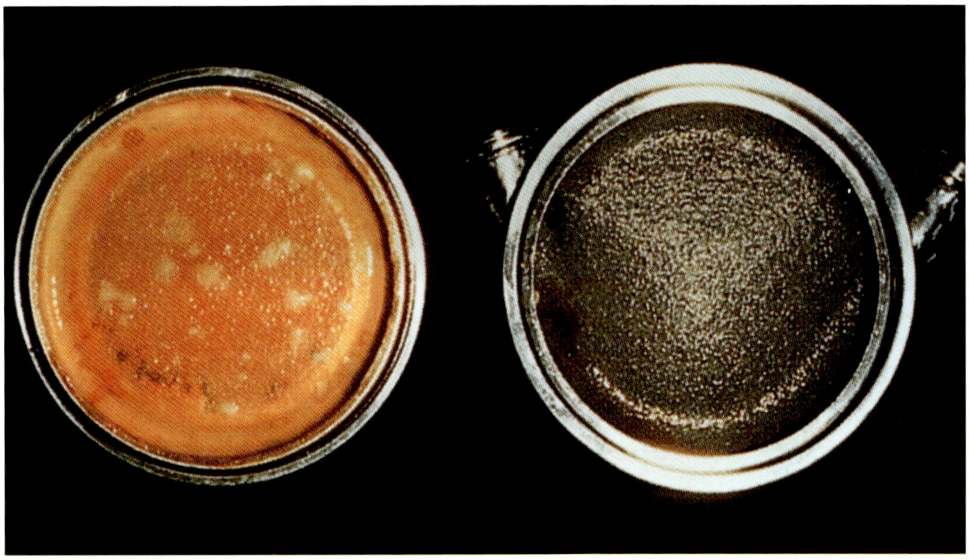

PLATE 20. *Blood contacting surface of the TCI HeartMate left ventricular assist device. A pseudo-intima is evident.*

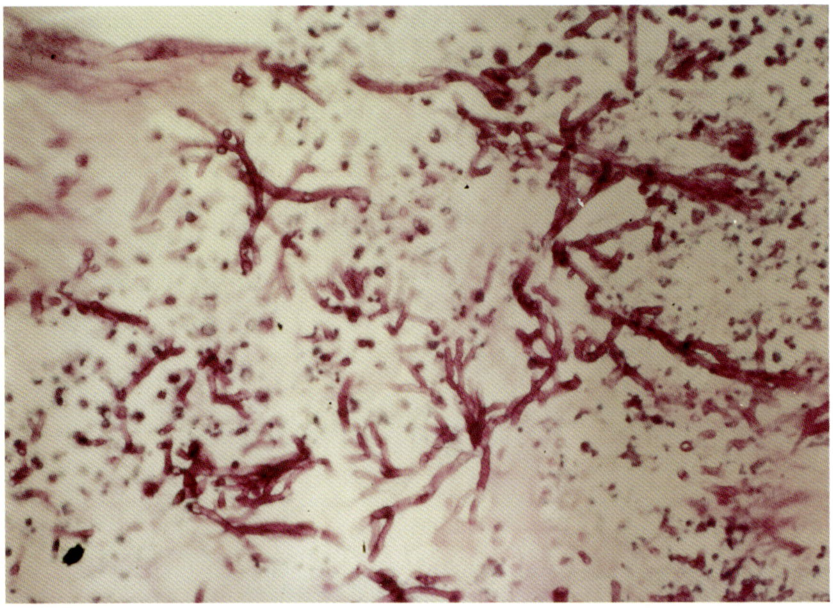

PLATE 21. *Biopsy of granulation tissue at airway anastomosis demonstrating fungal invasion. Microbiologic culture confirmed the organism was* Aspergillus fumigatus. *The disease resolved completely with antifungal therapy.*

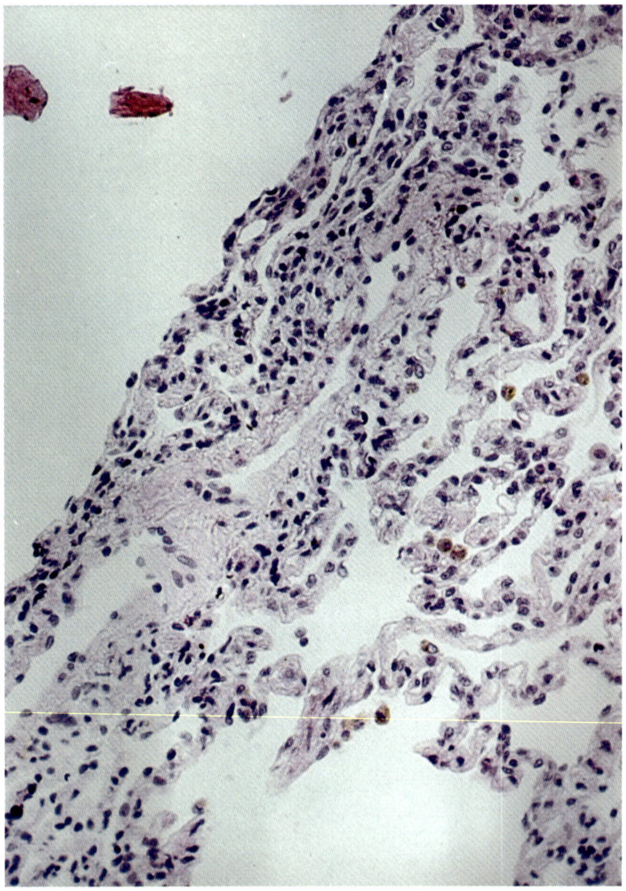

A

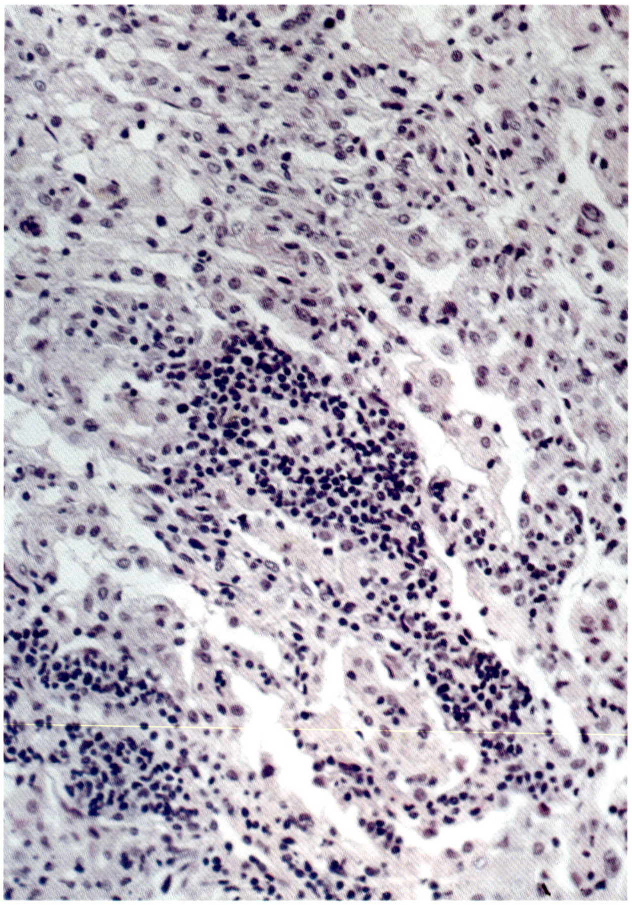

B

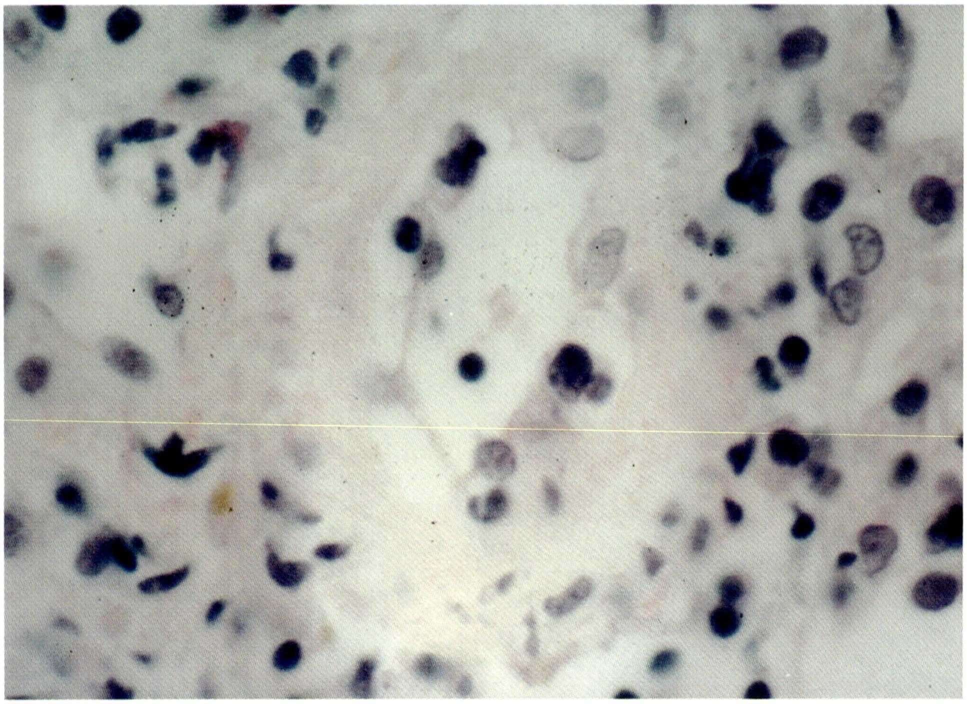

C

PLATE 22. *Pathologic alterations in lung transplant rejection (on transbronchial lung biopsy).* ***A****. Grade 1 minimal rejection.* ***B****. Grade 1 rejection.* ***C****. Grade 2 rejection, endothelialitis.* ***D****. Grades 3–4 rejection.* ***E****. Chronic rejection, obliterative bronchiolitis. (Courtesy of Dr. R. Kradin.)*

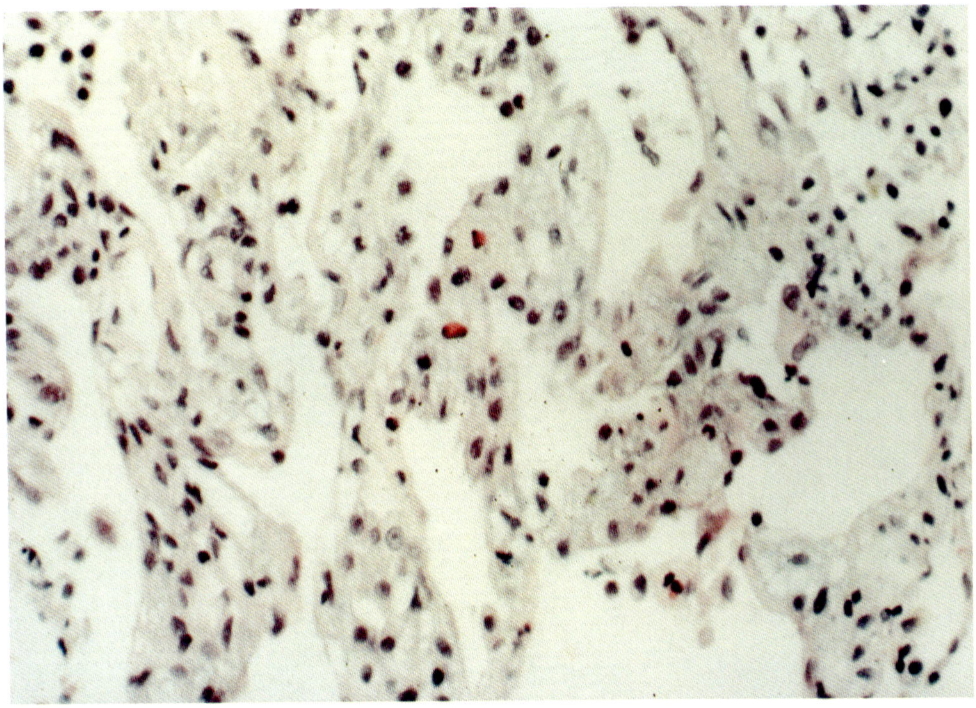

D

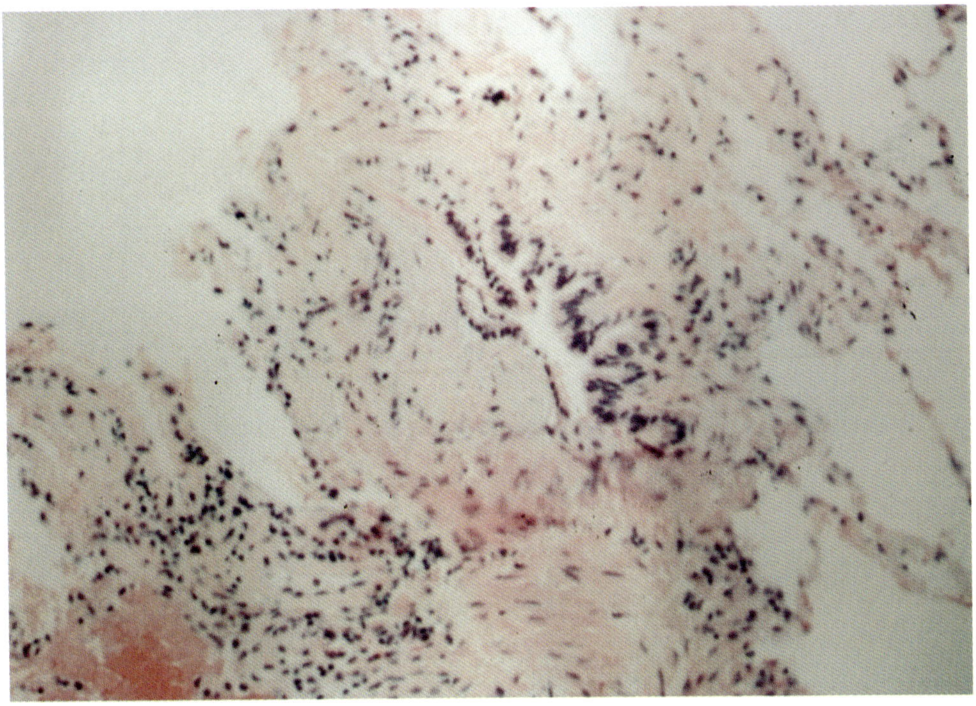

E

PLATE 22. *Continued.*

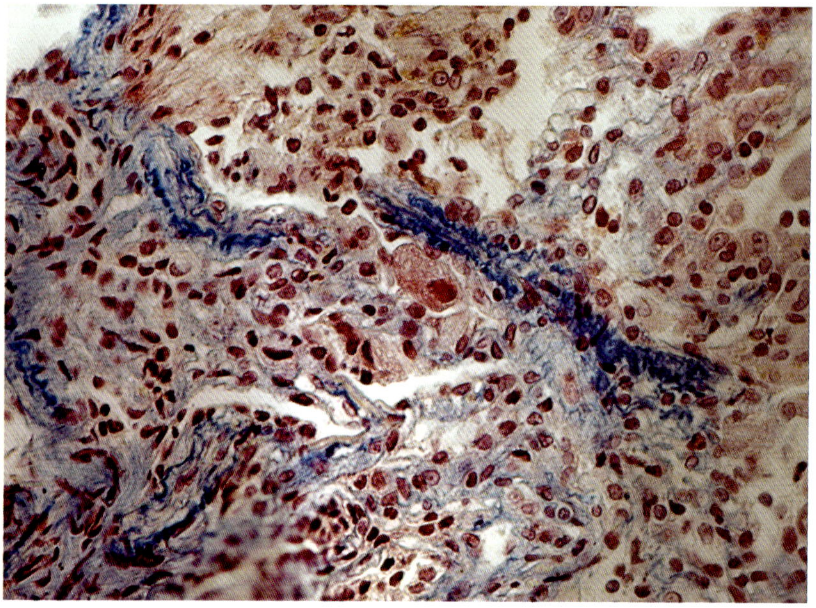

PLATE 23. *Photomicrograph of transbronchial lung biopsy demonstrating CMV pneumonia with characteristic cytopathic changes including intranuclear inclusions.*

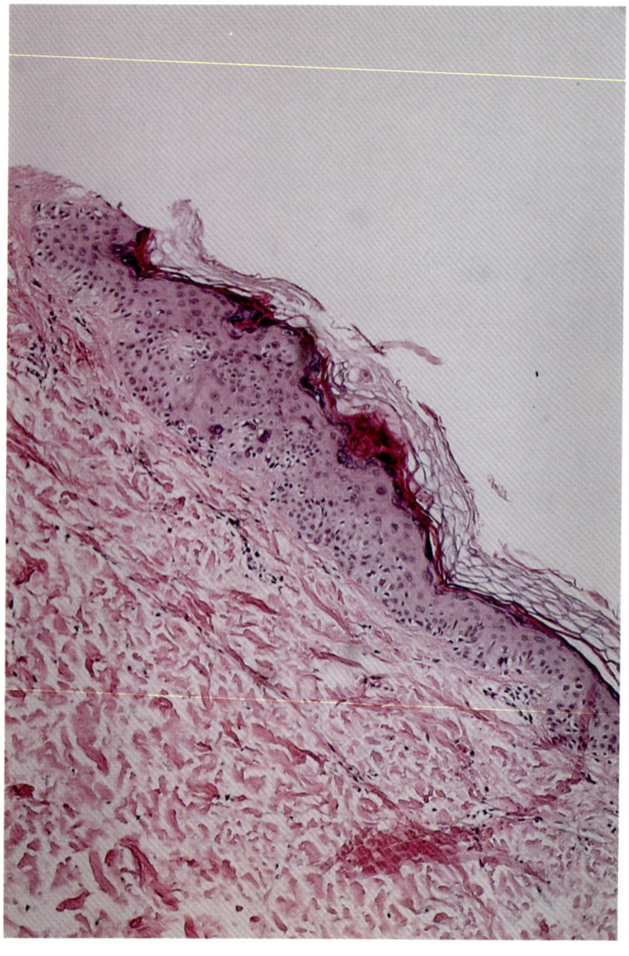

PLATE 24. *Cutaneous GVHD (day 14 after BMT). Vacuolar interface dermatitis with sparse superficial perivascular lymphocytic infiltrate and scattered necrotic keratinocytes.*

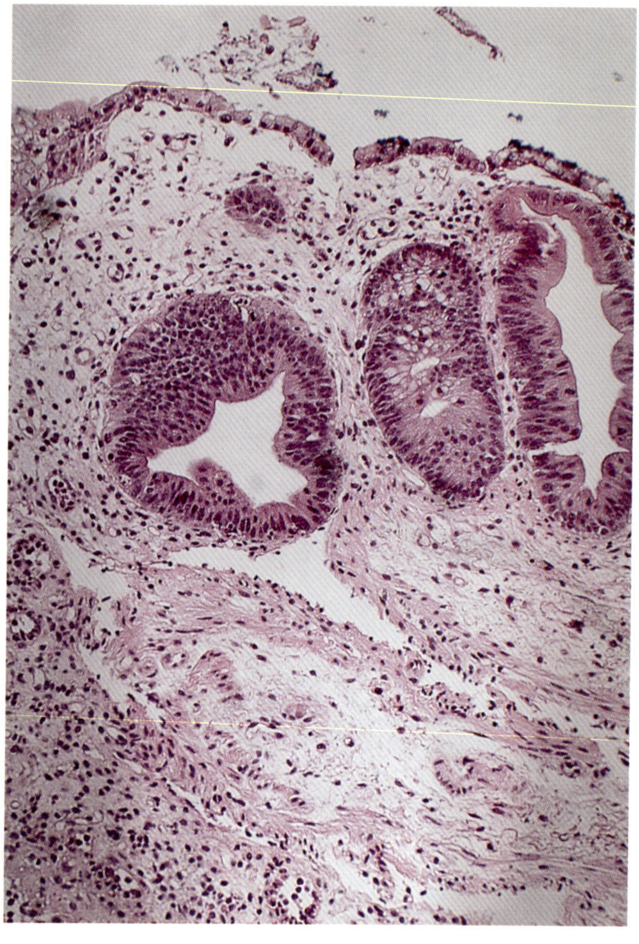

PLATE 25. *Colonic GVHD (day 8 after HLA-mismatched donor BMT). Mucosal atrophy with focally reactive epithelium and cellular apoptosis.*

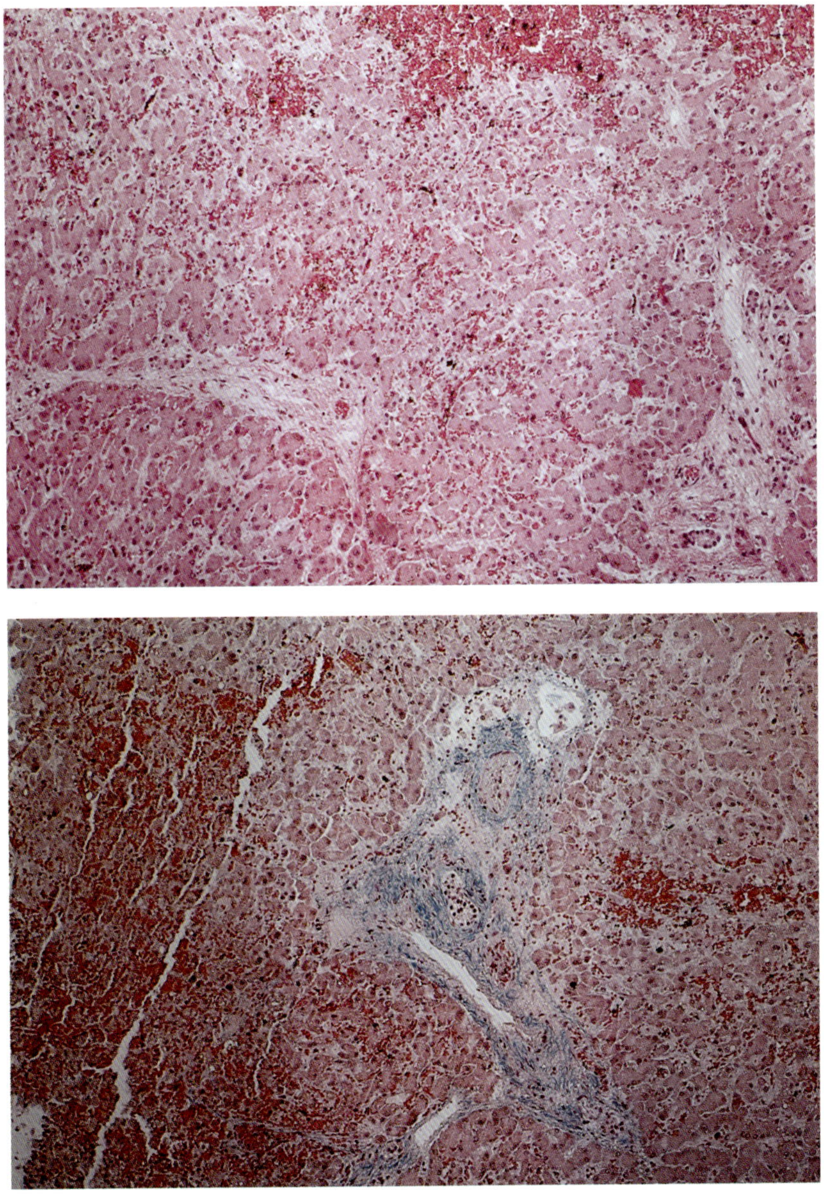

A

B

PLATE 26. *Hepatic veno-occlusive disease (autopsy specimen day 39 after HLA-mismatched donor BMT).* ***A.*** *Hematoxylin and eosin stain showing global occlusion of centrilobular veins with amorphous eosinophilic material, surrounding centrilobular hemorrhage, and focal necrosis.* ***B.*** *Trichrome stain showing collagen deposition in the centrilobular veins.*

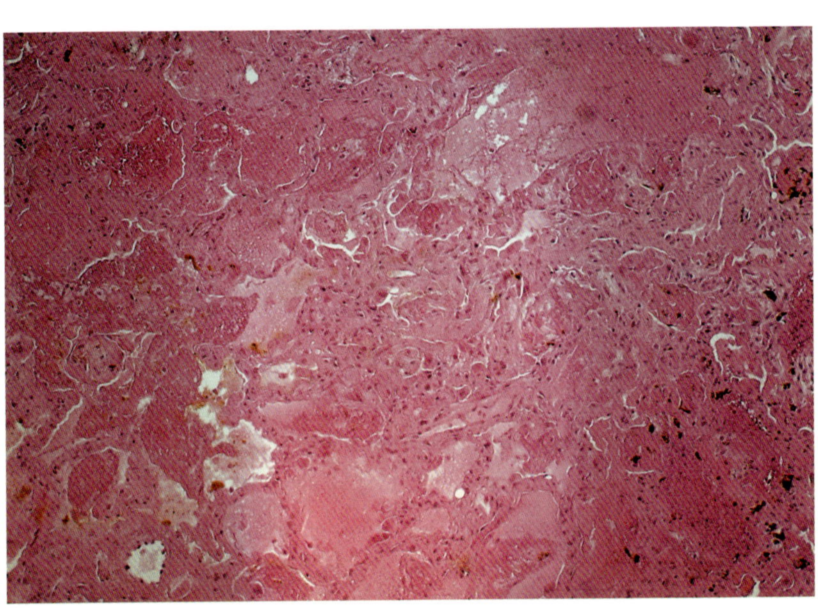

PLATE 27. *Diffuse alveolar injury and hemorrhage day 23 after busulfan, cyclophosphamide, and autologous PBSCT for Hodgkin's disease.*

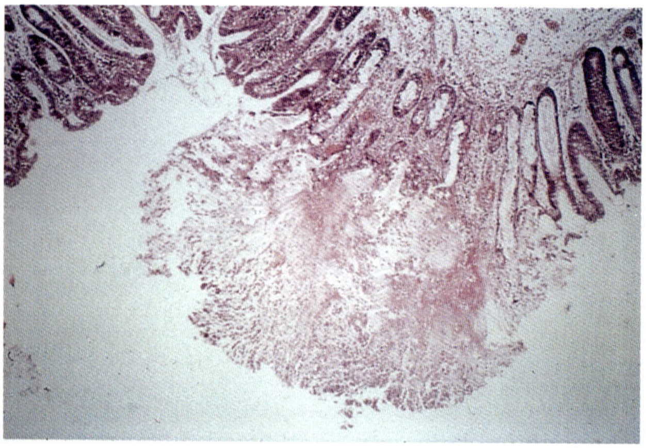

A

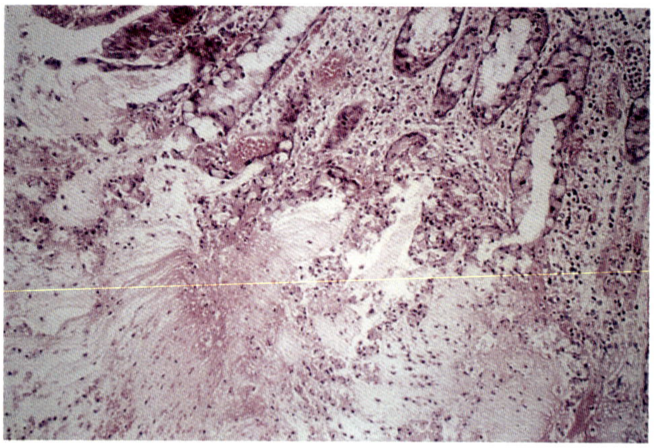

B

PLATE 28. *Photomicrographs of colonic biopsy taken from a patient with lower abdominal cramps, fever, and diarrhea, showing histologic changes of pseudomembranous colitis.* ***A****. Low power view.* ***B****. High power.*

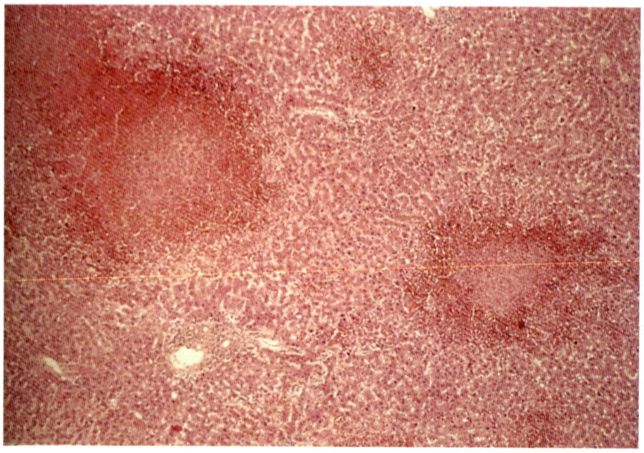

PLATE 29. *Photomicrograph of herpes simplex hepatitis.*

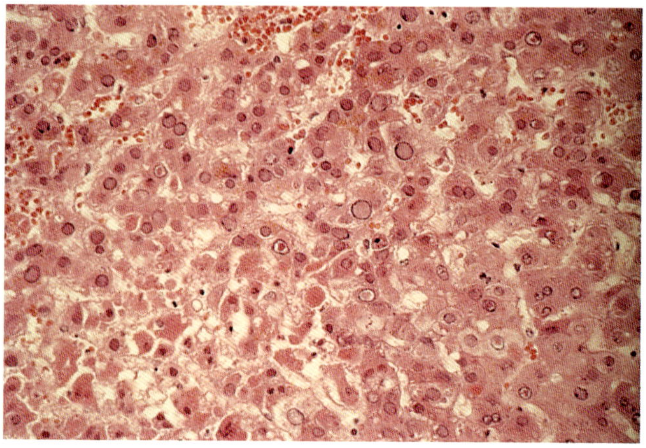

PLATE 30. *Photomicrograph of herpes simplex hepatitis demonstrating characteristic nuclear inclusion on biopsy.*

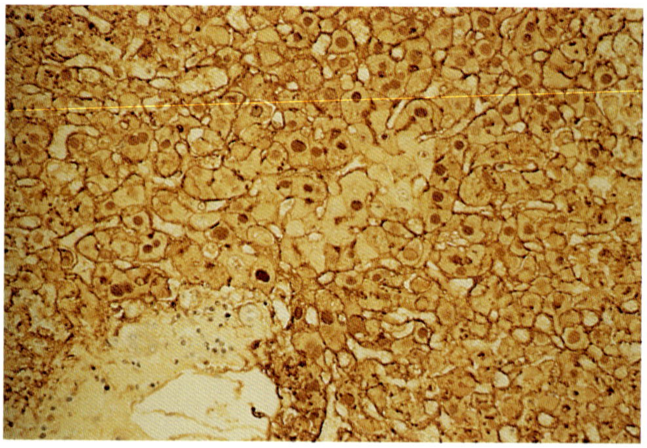

PLATE 31. *Photomicrograph of liver biopsy with immunoperoxidase staining demonstrating HSV antigens in epithelial cells.*

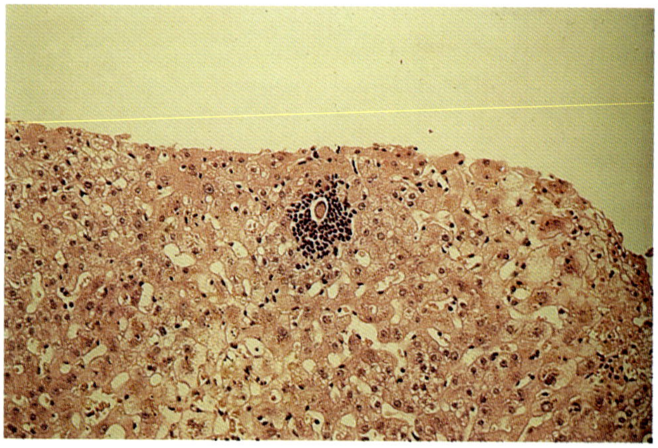

PLATE 32. *Photomicrograph of liver biopsy demonstrating a microabscess in CMV hepatitis.*

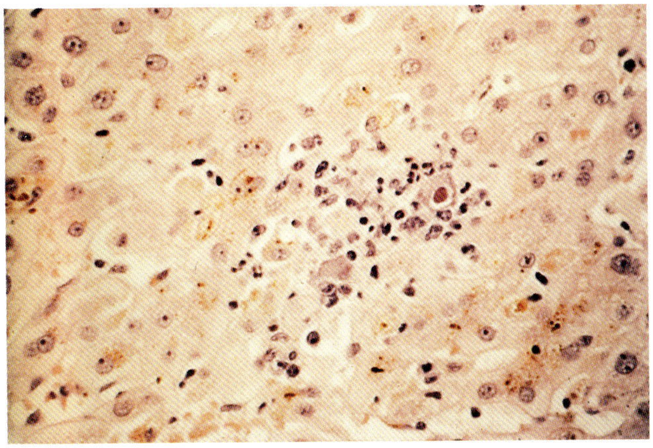

PLATE 33. *Photomicrograph of liver biopsy in a case of CMV hepatitis with characteristic nuclear inclusion.*

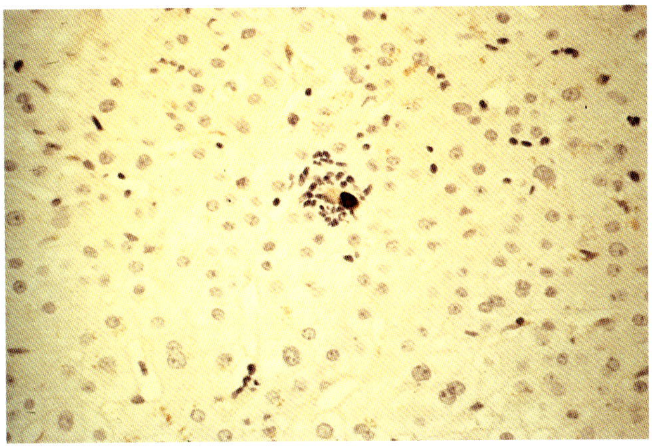

PLATE 34. *Photomicrograph of liver biopsy in a case of CMV hepatitis diagnosed by positive stain of immunoperoxidase.*

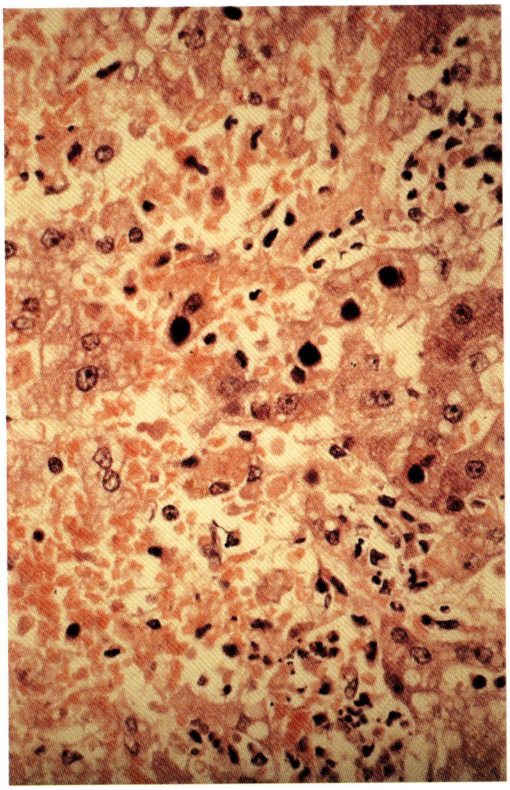

PLATE 35. *Photomicrograph of liver biopsy showing hepatitis due to adenovirus infection. Note presence of "smudge" cells.*

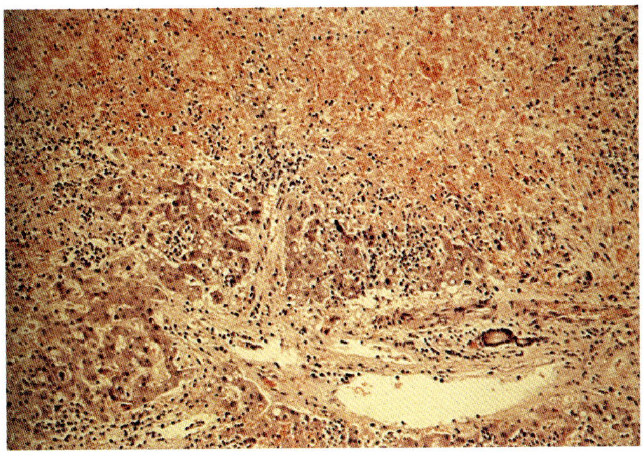

PLATE 36. *Photomicrograph of liver biopsy revealing hemorrhagic necrosis of the allograft due to adenovirus infection.*

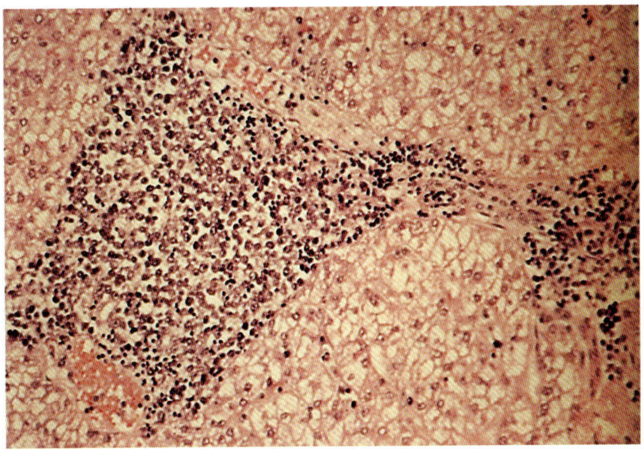

PLATE 37. *Photomicrograph demonstrating post-transplant lymphoma.*

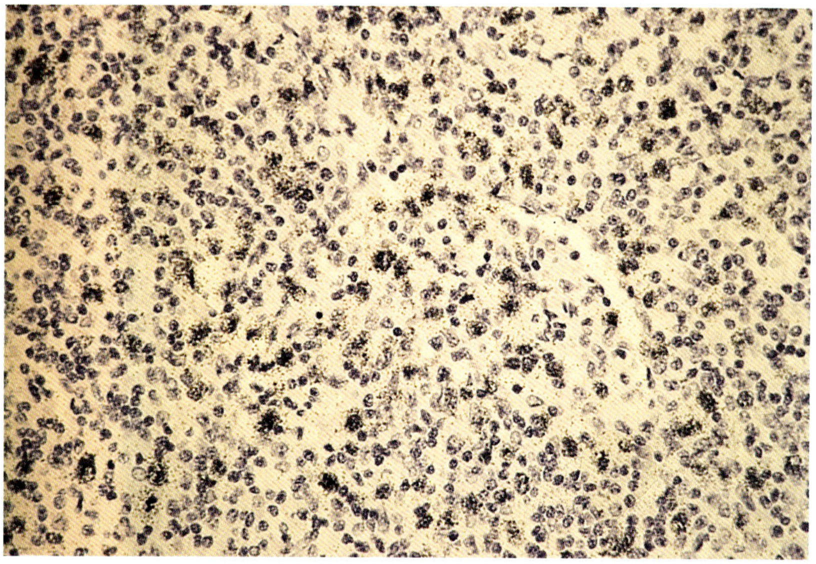

PLATE 38. *Photomicrograph of lymph node biopsy demonstrating PTLD disease, in this case related to EBV.*

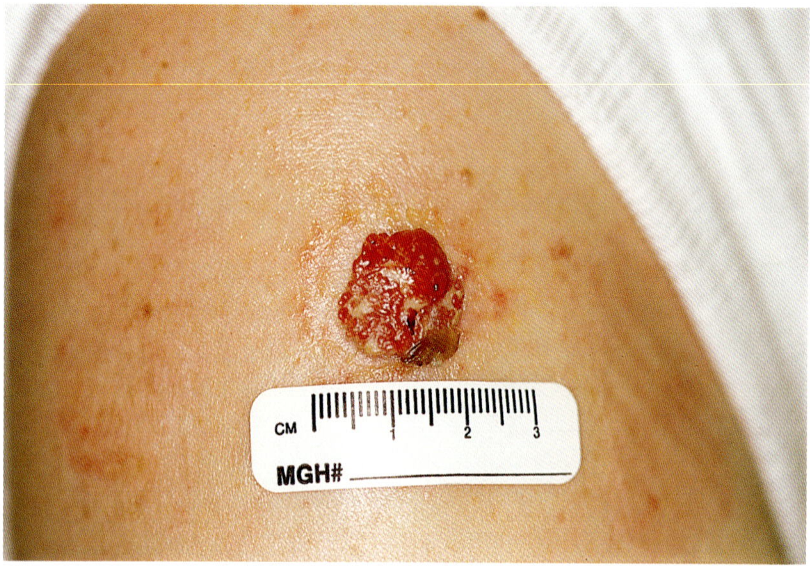

PLATE 39. *Squamous cell carcinoma on the lateral upper arm in sun-damaged skin. This 52-year-old woman had undergone lung transplantation 7 years earlier and was being maintained on cyclosporine, azathioprine, and prednisone immunosuppression.*

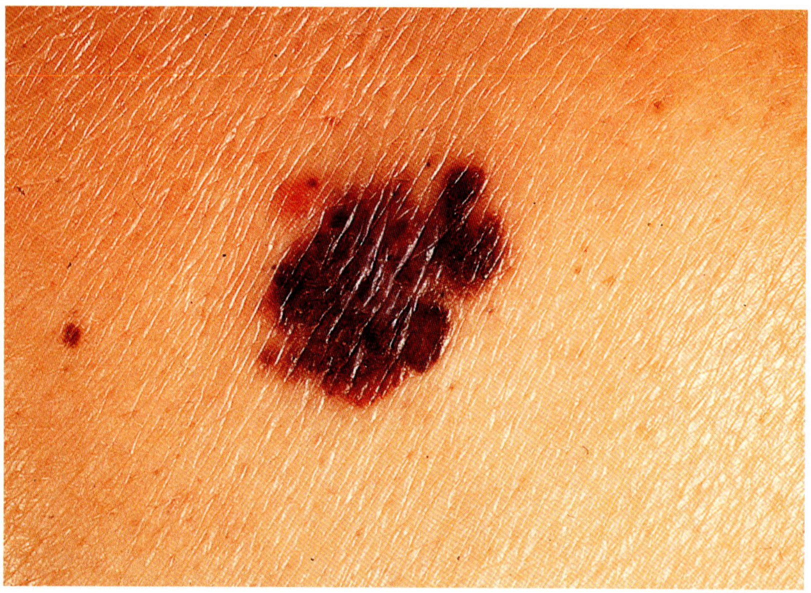

PLATE 40. *Early superficial spreading melanoma on the back of a kidney transplant recipient receiving azathioprine and prednisone. Note the irregularly scalloped borders and central hypopigmentation that distinguish this lesion from a benign nevus.*

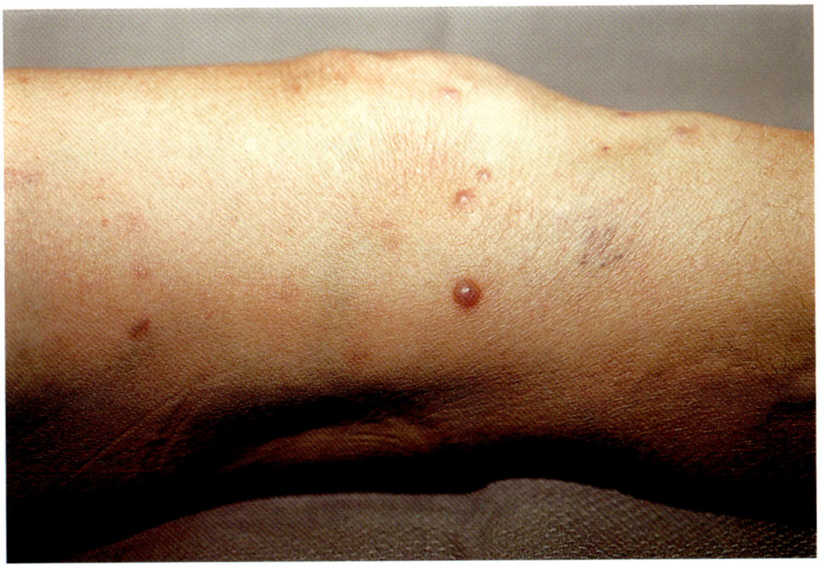

PLATE 41. *Typical clinical appearance of reddish, elevated, nodular Kaposi's sarcoma lesion of the skin. This 57-year-old liver allograft recipient had received tacrolimus, azathioprine, and steroid induction therapy and was then maintained on tacrolimus–prednisone suppression.*

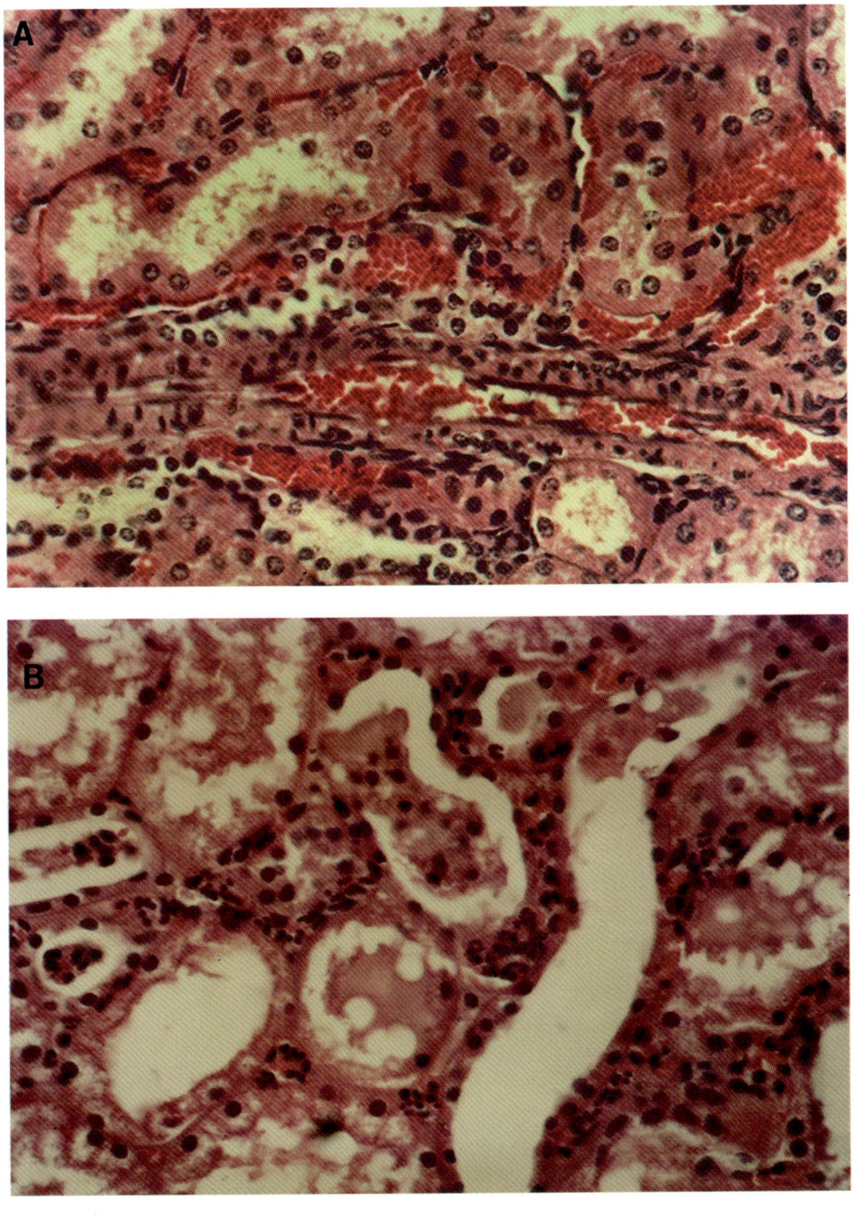

PLATE 42. *Hyperacute xenograft rejection.* ***A.*** *Intravascular thrombosis and hemorrhage in a renal xenograft (sheep-to-dog). This has been likened to a Shwartzman-type reaction.* ***B.*** *Polymorphonuclear granulocyte accumulation in capillaries in the renal xenograft.*

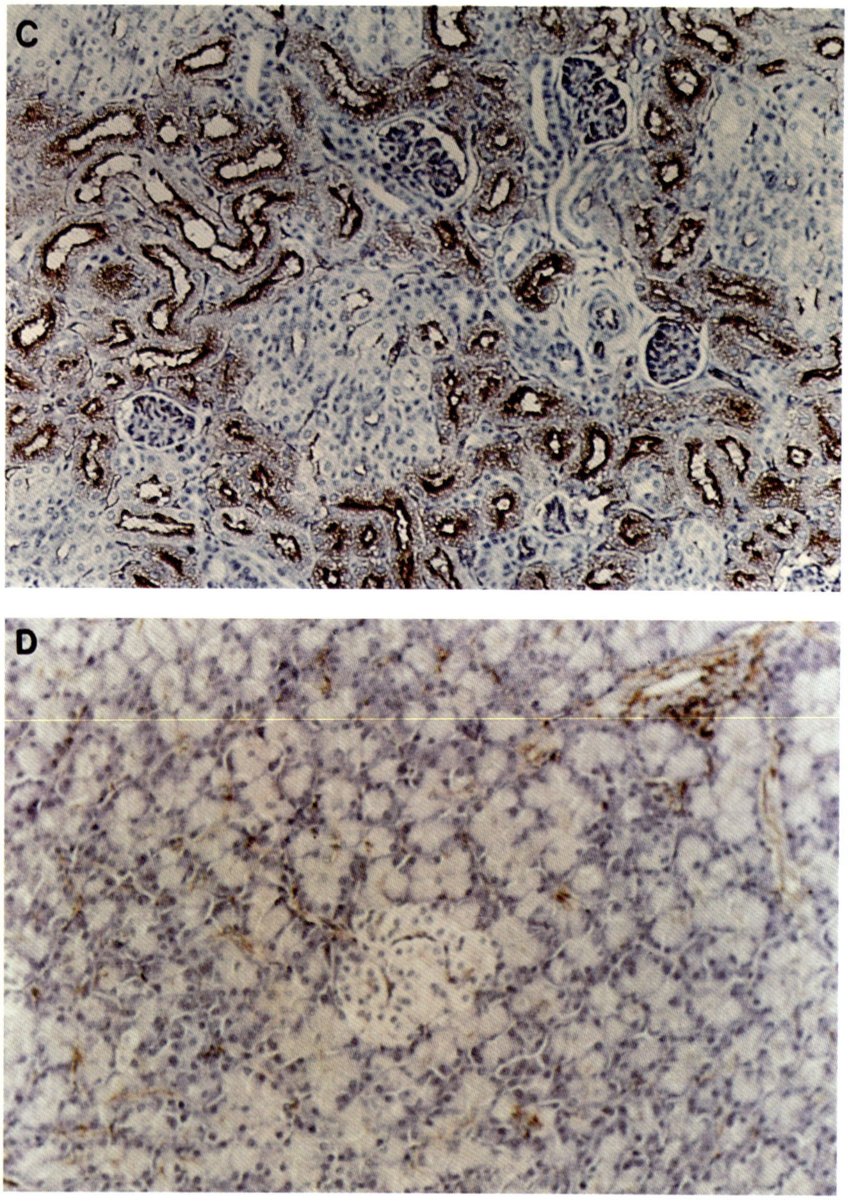

PLATE 42. ***C.*** *The expression of Galα(1,3)Gal in a pig kidney. Staining with the lectin IB4 and the immunoperoxidase method: brown staining [Galα(1,3)Gal] is lining tubules (proximal convoluted), collecting ducts, and capillary endothelium.* ***D.*** *Lack of expression of Galα(1,3)Gal in an adult pig islet cell (see* ***C*** *for details); the minimal staining is in capillary endothelium and in pancreatic ducts, but not in acini or islet cells.*

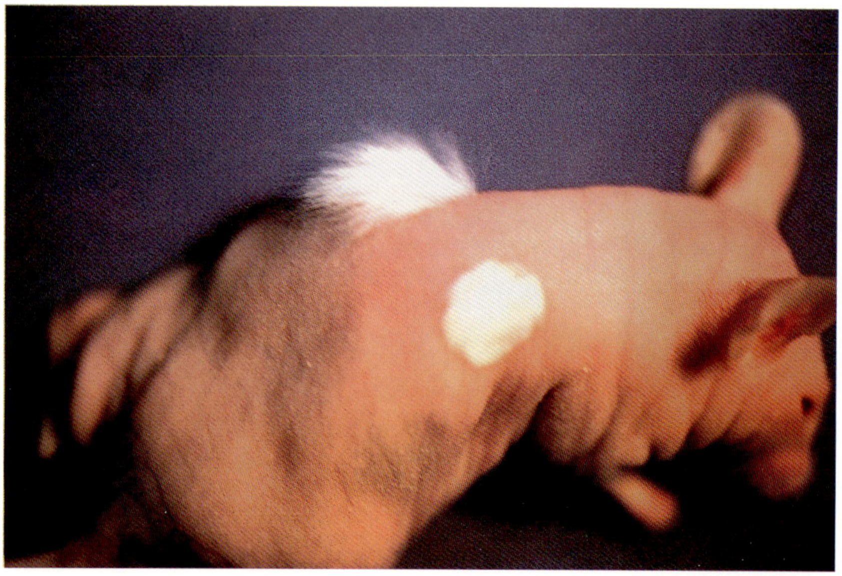

PLATE 43. *Nude mouse with long-surviving allogeneic mouse and xenogeneic monkey skin grafts.*

Chapter 30

Cardiovascular Considerations of Organ Transplantation

Marc J. Semigran

Transplantation cardiology has emerged as a specialized role among cardiac practitioners wherein a fundamental knowledge of cardiology is linked to the unique cardiovascular considerations of organ transplantation. These include immunosuppressive drug effects on the heart and blood pressure, cardiac malignancies, and organ-specific issues related to extrathoracic transplants. This chapter provides a framework for dealing with these considerations, both as part of the pretransplant evaluation and as part of managing post-transplant complications.

EFFECT OF IMMUNOSUPPRESSIVE DRUGS ON THE HEART

Corticosteroids

Corticosteroids have long been used as immunosuppressive agents in transplantation and for the treatment of collagen vascular disease (see Chapter 8). As a result, much is known regarding their deleterious effects on the cardiovascular system. Unfortunately, the side effects of steroid therapy of hypertension, diabetes, and hyperlipidemia can significantly worsen the risk factor profile for the development of coronary heart disease. Despite this, corticosteroid therapy remains central to the maintenance of immunosuppression in transplant recipients. Its effects on the heart are difficult to differentiate from those of other medications; however, studies of patients with rheumatologic diseases have compared the natural history of cardiovascular manifestations to those occurring in patients on steroid therapy, thus shedding light on the specific effects of prednisone.

Bulkley and Roberts reported that systemic hypertension, accompanied by left ventricular hypertrophy, was fivefold more common in steroid-treated patients with systemic lupus erythematosus than in patients treated during the pre-steroid era (1). The development of heart failure was eightfold more common in steroid-treated patients, and increased epicardial fat was observed only in the steroid-treated group. It is not surprising to find that most series report an 8% to 9% prevalence of coronary artery disease in steroid-treated lupus patients despite their young age and female sex (2).

The development of hypertension in patients on corticosteroid therapy appears to be multifactorial. The administration of corticosteroids causes an increase in plasma volume and an increase in cardiac output and systemic arterial pressure, despite a decrease in peripheral vascular resistance. There is also an increase in the sensitivity of the peripheral vasculature to the vasoconstrictive effects of norepinephrine (3). Corticosteroids also stimulate the synthesis of renin substrate, causing an increase in angiotensin production that leads to further sodium retention and vasoconstriction. More support for a unique hypertensive effect of steroid therapy comes from the observation that withdrawal of steroid therapy can lead to a reduction in mean arterial pressure despite the need to continue therapy with cyclosporine. This reduction in blood pressure has been shown to be confined largely to those patients who are hypertensive; little change in mean arterial pressure occurs in previously normotensive patients (4). Merely the use of alternate-day steroid therapy has been shown to be related to a lower incidence of arterial hypertension (5). Despite efforts to lower the dosage of steroid therapy, transplant recipients will usually be obligated to observe sodium restriction in their diets and to use diuretics and/or vasodilator therapy to control their blood pressure.

Corticosteroids also have potent effects on lipid metabolism, which can hasten the development of coronary and peripheral vascular atherosclerosis (see Chapter 31). It has been observed that the withdrawal of prednisone in patients on cyclosporine-based immunosuppressive therapy lowers serum cholesterol levels independent of the effects of cyclosporine (6). Prednisone and cyclosporine have differing effects on lipoprotein metabolism. The increase in cholesterol associated with prednisone is associated with an increase in both high-density lipoprotein (HDL) and low-density lipoprotein (LDL) cholesterol (7), while cyclosporine therapy leads to an increase in both total and LDL-cholesterol with little effect on HDL-cholesterol (8).

Thus, although total cholesterol would be expected to decrease as the prednisone dose is decreased in transplant recipients on cyclosporine-based immunosuppression, it is not certain that this would have a beneficial effect on the risk of cardiovascular disease. A study of prednisone withdrawal in renal transplant recipients who continued to be treated with cyclosporine alone found that serum HDL cholesterol decreased by 27% and triglycerides increased by 49% (9). As the ratio of total/HDL cholesterol increased in these transplant recipients as they withdrew from steroids, it would be predicted that their risk of cardiovascular disease actually increased as a result of prednisone withdrawal. Thus, lipid profiles need to be regularly assessed in transplant recipients as their steroid dose is decreased, because the protective effect of a high HDL-cholesterol (defined as an HDL-cholesterol >65 mg/dL) may "disappear" at lower steroid doses.

As discussed in Chapter 31, transplant recipients with hyperlipidemia may benefit from the salutary effects of cholesterol-lowering agents. Pravastatin has been demonstrated to have a beneficial effect on the incidence of allograft coronary vascular disease in cardiac transplant recipients (10). Further study is necessary to determine if the beneficial preventative effects that lipid lowering agents have on cardiovascular disease in hyperlipidemic patients in the general population can be extended to transplant recipients.

Corticosteroids can also adversely affect tissue healing after injury by modulating the transmembrane signals induced by growth factors. The ramifications for patients recovering from general surgery are well known. The high prevalence of coronary disease in transplant recipients necessitates an increased frequency of invasive cardiovascular procedures, which can also be complicated by corticosteroid therapy. A study of stent placement during coronary angioplasty revealed a 32% incidence of arterial aneurysm formation in patients who were simultaneously on steroid therapy. This was associated with a 50% restenosis rate (11). The altered vascular healing in these patients suggests that caution must be used during interventional procedures such as atherectomy and high-pressure balloon angioplasty.

Cyclosporine

Cyclosporine is a potent immunosuppressive agent, but its cardiovascular side effects of hypertension and hyperlipidemia, which are commonly encountered in transplant recipients receiving therapeutic doses, may cause long-term morbidity (see Chapter 6).

The development of hypertension has been described in 70% to 90% of solid-organ transplant recipients receiving cyclosporine. This has also been described in patients with other immunologic disorders, such as psoriasis and primary biliary cirrhosis, where it is used for therapeutic effect (12–14). Some transplant recipients, particularly those with end-stage renal disease (ESRD), may have hypertension prior to transplantation; however, the incidence clearly increases after the initiation of cyclosporine therapy (Table 30.1). Despite the eventual reduction of cyclosporine and prednisone doses, blood pressure remains elevated in over 90% of transplant recipients (15).

The exact mechanism by which cyclosporine produces hypertension is not known. Two different syndromes of hypertension have been described and may be related to different physiologic effects of the drug. An acute elevation in arterial pressure frequently occurs during initiation of cyclosporine therapy and is accompanied by an increase in heart rate and a slight increase in vascular resistance. These effects resolve after several doses. Animal and human studies have shown that they are related to increased sympathetic neural outflow, which can be blocked by central or ganglionic sympatholytic agents (16,17). Chronic administration of cyclosporine is usually associated with the occurrence of hypertension after at least 4

Table 30.1. Incidence of Hypertension Associated with Various Transplant Procedures Before and After the Availability of Cyclosporine

Organ Transplanted	Hypertension (%) Before CsA	After CsA	Clinical Features
Bone marrow	5–10	33–60	Intracerebral hemorrhage Hemolysis Encephalopathy
Heart	10	71–100	Stroke
Kidney	45–55	67–86	Renovascular thrombosis
Liver	N/A	65–85	Hemolytic-uremic syndrome
Lung	N/A	66	Possible later development of coronary disease

to 8 weeks of therapy; this is often, though not always, associated with renal dysfunction (18). Disturbances in circadian patterns of blood pressure lead to loss of the normal nocturnal decline, a feature that magnifies hypertensive end-organ effects. Elevation of arterial pressure occurs with variable effects on heart rate; in most animal models a slight increase is seen. In addition, cardiac output decreases during the development of hypertension consistent with an increase in peripheral vascular resistance (19).

There appear to be several mechanisms for the increase in vascular resistance observed. Cyclosporine itself has a direct contractile effect on vascular smooth muscle when studied in isolated vascular segments in vitro (20). This appears to be related to a direct augmentation of cellular uptake of calcium, as an increase of calcium influx in smooth muscle cells cultured in the presence of cyclosporine has been observed in response to exogenously administered vasoconstrictor substances (such as angiotensin II) (21). This effect may be particularly important when it occurs in the afferent renal arteriole (18), as renal reabsorption of sodium is enhanced in transplant recipients on cyclosporine and blood pressure is certainly sensitive to dietary sodium intake. Activation of the renin-angiotensin-aldosterone axis appears to be less important. Investigations in both non-renal solid organ recipients (22,23) and renal (24) transplant recipients have shown either a decrease or no change of plasma renin activity despite the increase in afferent renal arteriolar tone. In fact, impairment of the release of renin in response to sympathetic stimulation has been described (23).

The endothelial cell may also be a target for the vasoconstrictive effects of cyclosporine. Cyclosporine is strongly lipophilic and readily passes through cell membranes, including those of the vascular endothelium. Thus, it can directly affect endothelial cell function, including the release of vasoconstrictor and vasodilator substances. Endothelin is produced by endothelial cells and is a potent vasoconstrictor. Cyclosporine administration acutely stimulates the release of endothelin by endothelial cells. Its vasoconstrictor effects can be reversed in vitro by the pretreatment with antiendothelin antibodies, although blocking endothelin in this manner does not completely reverse the hypertensive effects of cyclosporine (25). The binding affinity of vascular smooth muscle for endothelin is increased in animals when they are chronically administered cyclosporine (26). The role of endothelin in mediating cyclosporine-induced hypertension in humans remains under investigation.

The vasoconstrictive effects of cyclosporine are reversed by the administration of L-arginine, suggesting that the response of smooth muscle cells to nitric oxide is intact and that the endothelial nitric oxide release is inhibited. The vasoconstrictive effects of cyclosporine are more pervasive than can be explained only by the inhibition of endothelial nitric oxide synthase, as direct inhibitors of the enzyme such as nitro-L-arginine methyl ester will vasoconstrict only a portion of the renal microvasculature affected by cyclosporine (27).

In summary, the effects of cyclosporine on the vascular endothelium and smooth muscle cell are likely interdependent. The effects of small increases in endothelin concentration and binding to smooth muscle cells may be augmented by inhibition of nitric oxide synthesis or release, particularly if the ability of the contractile apparatus of the cell to take up calcium is directly augmented.

It has been thought that cyclosporine might have a direct effect on cardiac tissue, related to the observation of myocardial hypertrophy and fibrosis in endomyocardial biopsies taken from cardiac transplant recipients who were treated with cyclosporine in the absence of the diagnosis of allograft rejection. Studies of isolated fibroblasts have not been able to demonstrate any direct effect on collagen metabolism by cyclosporine (28). It appears that the morphologic changes observed are likely related either to the effects of chronic hypertension or to a graft rejection process that is not appreciated by standard diagnostic techniques.

Hyperlipidemia is common in transplant recipients, and the finding that withdrawal of steroid therapy may actually worsen the lipoprotein profile by increasing the ratio of total cholesterol to HDL-cholesterol has emphasized the contribution of cyclosporine to this problem (7). Studies of animal models of accelerated atherosclerosis and of transplant recipients have elucidated the role of cyclosporine in hyperlipidemia.

Cyclosporine was shown by Emeson and colleagues to be atherogenic in animal models of vascular disease, much to the surprise of these investigators who thought that T-cell activation was important in the pathogenesis of atherosclerotic lesions (29,30). The atherogenic effect of cyclosporine appears to be related to its ability to elevate plasma LDL and total cholesterol and depress HDL cholesterol in these animals. Animals fed an extremely low-fat diet were protected from developing an increase in LDL cholesterol while on cyclosporine, and no atherosclerotic lesions were seen.

In an effort to avoid the confounding effects of concomitant corticosteroid therapy, Ballantyne and colleagues studied the lipoprotein profiles of patients with amyotrophic lateral sclerosis who were treated in a randomized fashion with cyclosporine as a sole immunosuppressive agent. During cyclosporine treatment a 21% increase in total cholesterol as well as a 31% increase in LDL cholesterol was demonstrated in those patients with therapeutic levels of cyclosporine (31). No effect of cyclosporine on serum HDL cholesterol was observed in these patients, and the adverse effects on plasma lipoproteins persisted with continued cyclosporine use for 2 months.

The mechanism for the effect of cyclosporine on LDL cholesterol may be related to its inhibitory effects on bile acid synthesis in the liver. Cyclosporine blocks bile acid synthesis in cultured rat and human hepatocytes by inhibiting the hydroxylation of cholesterol to β-muricholic acid, the first step in the pathway of chenodeoxycholic acid synthesis (32). This did not appear to have any effect on the overall quantity of bile acid synthesis, but a shift to alternative pathways of cholesterol degradation may be less efficient or effective in limiting de novo cholesterol synthesis by the liver.

The West of Scotland Coronary Prevention Study recently demonstrated that a 20% reduction of cholesterol in men with hypercholesterolemia led to a 31% reduction in cardiovascular mortality (33). As atherosclerotic cardiovascular disease is the primary cause of mortality among renal transplant recipients and is a significant problem in other solid-organ recipients as well, it would be expected that treatment of hyperlipidemia is an important part of decreasing cardiovascular mortality.

Tacrolimus

Tacrolimus is a potent immunosuppressive agent that is structurally different from cyclosporine, although the two agents share many features in modulation of T-cell function (see Chapter 9). Hypertension and hyperlipidemia are observed with tacrolimus, though they are less severe than with therapeutic levels of cyclosporine. The development of hypertrophic cardiomyopathy, a side effect not seen with cyclosporine, has been described in a few pediatric transplant recipients treated with tacrolimus.

Despite its different structure, tacrolimus does have renal vasoconstrictive effects that are similar to, but may be less potent than, those of cyclosporine (see Chapter 35). In a study of liver transplant recipients, Textor et al found that urinary excretion of 6-keto-$PGF_{1\alpha}$, a metabolite of the intrinsic vasodilator prostacyclin, was lower in tacrolimus-treated patients than in a similar group of cyclosporine patients, suggesting that the vasoconstrictive effect of tacrolimus is *more* potent (34). Despite this, arterial pressure was lower in the tacrolimus-treated patients and a noninvasive measurement of stroke volume was higher, leading to the conclusion that systemic vascular resistance was lower in tacrolimus patients. It has been hypothesized that tacrolimus may affect resistance vessels outside of the kidney differently than cyclosporine; however, further study of the mechanism of its effects on the vasculature is necessary. Similar findings of a lower incidence of hypertension in transplant recipients on tacrolimus-based immunosuppression have been described by other groups (35–37).

The conclusion that tacrolimus is less likely to produce hypertension in transplant recipients is confounded by the fact that in all clinical studies thus far corticosteroid doses are lower in the tacrolimus patients than in those on cyclosporine immunosuppression. Furthermore, the decreased prevalence of hypertension appears only to be a finding within the first year after transplantation; a long-term study comparing tacrolimus and cyclosporine found that the incidence of hypertension is equal in tacrolimus- and cyclosporine-treated patients by 2 years after transplantation (34).

Studies of liver (38) and cardiac (39) transplant recipients have demonstrated lower serum total and LDL-cholesterol levels with tacrolimus-based immunosuppression than with the use of cyclosporine. As with the finding of less hypertension in tacrolimus-treated patients, this is probably related to both a true effect of tacrolimus and a secondary effect of the lower prednisone doses required for tacrolimus patients.

Several pediatric transplant recipients have been observed to develop hypertrophic cardiomyopathy while on tacrolimus-based immunosuppression after liver and/or bowel transplant. In two of these patients, left ventricular outflow tract obstruction developed and subsequently regressed after cyclosporine was substituted for tacrolimus (40). The mechanism of the development of this cardiomyopathy is not known, although tacrolimus has been reported to bind to a protein associated with the ryanodine-receptor/calcium-release channel isolated from canine heart sarcoplasmic reticulum (41). The functional significance of that interaction is not known, but it is possible that an alteration in cytoplasmic calcium related to tacrolimus could lead to the initiation of cellular genetic programs for hypertrophy.

A case report of QT prolongation and torsades de pointes has also been described in a pediatric liver transplant recipient on tacrolimus. Echocardiographic study did not reveal any structural abnormalities in this patient (42).

Cyclophosphamide

The cardiotoxicity of cyclophosphamide is reviewed later in this chapter. In brief, cyclophosphamide is an alkylating agent shown to have potent immunosuppressive effects. It is most commonly used in preparation for bone marrow transplantation. In lower doses, it has also been used as an adjuvant agent for solid-organ transplants. Animals given doses of 240 mg/kg of cyclophosphamide have a greater than 75% incidence of cardiomyopathy, marked by biventricular dilation and dysfunction (43). In humans, cyclophosphamide doses greater than 120–270 mg/kg appear to be cardiotoxic. Mortality from heart failure caused by cyclophosphamide has been reported as high as 43% to 60% (44). Thus, the dose of cyclophosphamide given in preparation for bone-marrow transplantation should be minimized, and cardiac function in patients given doses approaching the toxic range must be monitored (see also Chapter 27).

Antilymphocytic Antibodies

Antilymphocytic antibodies, including the monoclonal antibody OKT-3, are highly effective agents for reversing rejection and inducing immunosuppression in appropriate circumstances (see also Chapter 13). After a brief acute adrenergic release, the predominant cardiovascular effects of these agents are attributable to the subsequent release of cytokines and other inflammatory mediators following T-cell activation and lysis, effects particularly noticeable after the first and second doses.

Many cytokines have been observed to be released during cytolytic antibody administration, but the best documented are tumor necrosis factor α (TNF-α), interferon gamma (INF-γ), and interleukin 2 (IL-2). The interactions among immune cells, cytokines, and tissues that cause the cardiovascular and pulmonary effects associated with OKT-3 are summarized in Figure 30.1. After OKT-3 administration, serum TNF-α levels peak at 1 hour, interferon and interleukin levels peak at 4 hours (45), and the time course of cytokine release closely parallels that of the observed cardiovascular abnormalities. The early hyperdynamic cardiovascular response seen after OKT-3 administration is related to the vasodilatory effects of TNF-α. Pulmonary and systemic arterial pressures fall and cardiac output increases at the same time that TNF-α plasma levels increase (see also Chapter 12).

Complement activation also appears to play a role in the development of pulmonary symptoms during OKT-3 administration. Plasma levels of the products of complement activation increase within 15 minutes of OKT-3 administration, coincident with the appearance of activated granulocytes in the lungs and prior to the development of elevated cytokine levels (46). In a recent study of kidney and lung transplant recipients, OKT-3 administration rapidly produced all complement activation fragments (C4d, Bb, ¡C3b, and Sc5b-9), indicating activation of both the classic and the alternative pathways. The activation of complement was associated with increased expression of adhesion molecules and with pulmonary hemodynamic changes. These results support the theory that OKT-3–induced complement activation leads to rapid sequestration of neutrophils in the lungs, a phenomenon that in turn can cause lung injury, hypoxemia, and pulmonary hemodynamic changes (47).

An intraoperative study by Robinson et al of the hemodynamic effects of OKT-3 administration in patients with simultaneous pulmonary artery monitoring demonstrated an initial rise in systemic vascular resistance of 16% at 10 minutes after OKT-3 administration, coincident with an acute sympathetic effect. This was followed by a 21% fall at 105 minutes after administration. Pulmonary vascular resistance fell slightly, although there was no change in systemic blood pressure (48). In general, patients may develop hypotension and tachycardia; as myocardial oxygen consumption increases, angina may occur, particularly in patients with coronary artery disease. TNF-α release stimulates IL-1 release from monocytes and endothelial cells. TNF-α and IL-1 synergistically have a negative inotropic effect on the myocardium; an exacerbation of the hypotension can occur, as the already present vasodilation is now accompanied by a low cardiac output. Supportive evidence for this direct negative inotropic effect comes from observations made

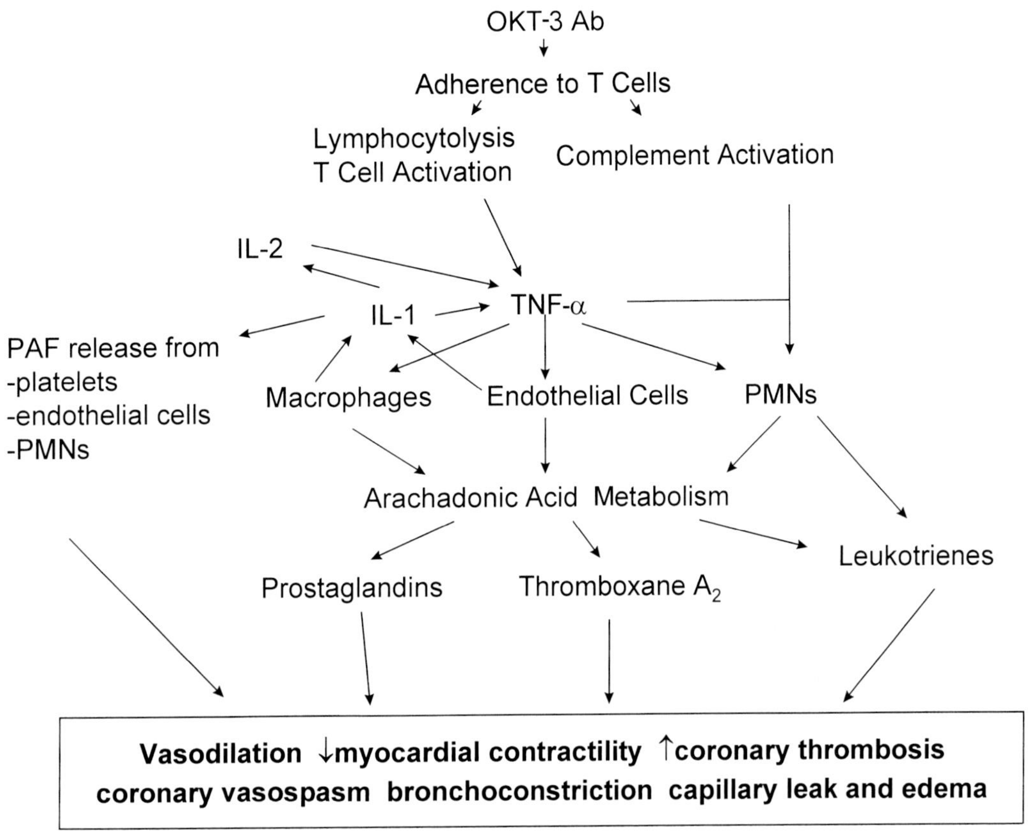

FIGURE 30.1. *Cytokine pathways of the cardiovascular and pulmonary effects of OKT-3 monoclonal antibody. Ab, antibody; IL, interleukin; TNF, tumor necrosis factor; PAF, platelet activating factor; PMNs, polymorphonuclear leukocytes.*

during the use of OKT-3 in cardiac transplant recipients. During OKT-3–induced hypotension, the administration of fluid to expand intravascular volume resulted in left ventricular dilation, despite a decreased systemic vascular resistance (49). TNF-α, IL-1, and IL-2 also adversely affect endothelial cell function, causing extravascular fluid accumulation. Patients with graft dysfunction who are volume overloaded can develop edema, including acute interstitial pulmonary edema leading to bronchospasm and respiratory distress (50). These symptoms are usually accompanied by fever, although there is a temporal dissociation between the peak of fever (which occurs at 3 hours) and the lowest arterial pressure (which occurs at 5 hours) (49,51). This may be explained by the additive effects of the release of IFN-γ to the vasodilatory and negative inotropic effects of TNF-α and IL-2.

The abnormalities in myocardial function can lead to an increase in pulmonary venous pressures. The increased pressure combines with the increase in vascular permeability to lead to pulmonary edema, the major acute clinical complication of OKT-3 administration. This complication usually occurs after the administration of the first OKT-3 dose, coinciding with the greatest cytokine release, particularly TNF-α (52). The role of increased endothelial permeability in this complication has been directly demonstrated by studies showing the extravasation into lung tissue of isotopically labeled transferrin co-administered with OKT-3 (53). The occurrence of cardiac depression and altered vascular permeability is sufficient to lead to OKT-3–induced pulmonary edema, as both hypoxemia and interstitial pulmonary edema have been observed in the absence of volume overload. Nonetheless, intravascular volume overload in the immediate pretreatment period certainly increases the risk of pulmonary edema. Pulmonary edema was described during OKT-3 administration in 5 of 39 renal transplant recipients who had a more than 3% weight gain prior to its initiation and in none of the 197 patients who had no such weight gain (54).

Strategies to prevent and treat the OKT-3–associated cardiovascular and pulmonary effects should therefore include efforts to limit volume overload prior to its administration. Pharmacologic efforts to inhibit the release of cytokines are also of benefit in ameliorating these side effects. High doses of intravenous corticosteroids given before OKT-3 administration can significantly reduce the production of TNF-α, IL-2, and INF-γ by OKT-3–activated T cells (see Chapters 12 and 13). As some of the OKT-3–associated hemodynamic effects such as vasodilation and myocardial depression are mediated by cytokine-induced release of prostaglandins, the addition of agents that inhibit prostaglandin effects (such as acetaminophen) may be helpful. Cyclooxygenase inhibitors such as indomethacin may also be effective, because they inhibit the conversion of arachidonic acid to prostaglandins such as PGE_1 and PGE_2, both of which are vasodilators. Unfortunately, cyclooxygenase inhibitors can have deleterious effects on renal perfusion, which may be particularly disadvantageous in the setting of a decreased cardiac output (55). In rare cases of severe OKT-3–associated cardiovascular and pulmonary effects, inotropic support, as well as mechanical ventilatory and circulatory support, may be needed.

The cardiovascular complications of antithymocyte globulin (ATG) appear to be less severe than those of OKT-3. In one study of 38 renal transplant recipients randomly given either OKT-3 or ATG, changes in blood pressure and heart rate were observed only in the OKT-3–treated patients. One of the 20 patients given OKT-3 developed pulmonary edema during a hypertensive crisis, but no pulmonary edema occurred in ATG-treated patients (56). Thus, ATG may not cause a release of vasoactive cytokines comparable to that observed with OKT-3.

HYPERTENSION IN THE TRANSPLANT RECIPIENT

The near universal development of hypertension among transplant recipients (see Table 30.1) leads to the need for long-term antihypertensive therapy in approximately 80% of patients (15) (see Chapter 35). The development of end-organ manifestations of hypertension such as renal dysfunction, cardiac hypertrophy, and strokes, as well as other coronary risk factors such as hyperlipidemia, mandates that clinicians make efforts to adequately treat elevated blood pressure when it occurs. Furthermore, at least in renal recipients, uncontrolled hypertension can be deleterious to the graft itself. A study of 135 renal transplant recipients treated with cyclosporine-based immunosuppression revealed that lack of control of hypertension was the only predictor of long-term graft survival other than age and postoperative glomerular filtration rate (GFR) (57).

Prior to initiation of drug therapy for hypertension in the transplant recipient, all causes must be considered (Table 30.2). Excessive levels of cyclosporine or tacrolimus have been associated with severe vasodilator-resistant hypertension, complicated by encephalopathy and intracranial bleeding. In the pre-cyclosporine era, chronic rejection was the most common cause of hypertension in renal recipients, and it was usually accompanied by proteinuria and a progressive decline in graft function. Nephrotoxicity from drugs commonly given to transplant recipients (other than cyclosporine) can also lead to hypertension. Offending agents can include antibiotics such as aminoglycosides, antifungal agents such as amphotericin, and nonsteroidal anti-inflammatory agents.

Transplant renal artery stenosis can magnify the vasoconstriction associated with cyclosporine therapy, and its relief can have a significant beneficial effect on both blood pressure and allograft function. Its development is marked by an acute decline in renal function and the appearance of a new bruit over the transplant. The possibility of this diagnosis can be noninvasively assessed using magnetic resonance angiography. Treatment by revascularization usually leads to improvement in both graft function and hypertension.

The prevalence of atherosclerotic coronary vascular disease as the etiology of heart failure in patients undergoing cardiac transplantation also identifies them as prime candidates for the development of renovascular disease. A recent study of 118 patients with hypertension and/or renal insufficiency undergoing coronary angiography identified significant renal arterial stenosis in 23% (58). Renin release from the native kidneys causes hypertension in a small group of hypertensive patients and may also induce severe hypertension after transplantation. When antihypertensive therapy does not lead to adequate control of blood pressure, surgical nephrectomy may be necessary (59). Endocrine causes of hypertension should also be considered, if appropriate.

Table 30.2. Causes of Persistent Hypertension in the Transplant Recipient

Cause	Type of Transplant
Cyclosporine or tacrolimus toxicity	All
Renal dysfunction	
Chronic allograft rejection	Renal
Drug-induced (immunosuppressive, antibiotic)	All
Transplant renal artery stenosis	Renal
Native renal artery stenosis	Extrarenal (particularly if a history of vascular disease is present)
Recurrent essential hypertension	All
High renin output from native kidneys	Renal
Endocrinopathies	
Aldosteronism	All
Pheochromocytoma	
Hypercalcemia	

A review of the patient's diet prior to the initiation of medical antihypertensive therapy is important, as restriction of sodium intake is the mainstay of any program to control blood pressure. This may be particularly true in cardiac transplant recipients, in whom a unique blunted diuretic and natriuretic response to volume expansion has been observed that is not present in other organ recipients receiving similar immunosuppression (60). Even when sodium restriction is not effective by itself, it does decrease intravascular volume, making any pharmacologic therapy more effective. Obesity, which is particularly common in transplant recipients on steroid therapy, can also lead to hypertension. Weight loss is an important adjunct to therapy; however, the efficacy of weight loss in controlling blood pressure is less in transplant recipients than in the general population.

Several general principles can be used to guide the selection of antihypertensive therapy from the choices in Table 30.3.

The occurrence of vasoconstriction (particularly of the renal circulation) in the pathophysiology of cyclosporine-induced hypertension suggests that vasodilator therapy should be effective in its treatment. Calcium channel antagonists are frequently the first drug of choice because of their effectiveness at smooth muscle relaxation. The dihydropyridine class of calcium channel blockers, which appears to be particularly potent, includes the drugs nifedipine, isradipine, amlodipine, felodipine, nitrendipine, and nicardipine. They have been found to be effective in reducing systemic arterial vasoconstriction and appear to reduce the renal

Table 30.3. Antihypertensive Drug Therapy in the Transplant Recipient

Class of Drug (Specific Agents)	Hemodynamic Effect	Adverse Effects	Effect on CsA Level
Calcium channel blockers			
Dihydropyridines (e.g., nifedipine, amlodipine)	Vasodilator, may reverse CsA renal vasoconstriction	Edema	Slight ↑
Benzothiazepine (e.g., diltiazem)	Vasodilator	Edema	↑↑
Papaverine-like (e.g., verapamil)	Vasodilator Inotrope Dromotrope	AV block, CHF	↑
Adrenergic blockers			
β-blockers (e.g., atenolol, metoprolol)	↓ Cardiac output, ↓ heart rate	CHF, fatigue, bronchospasm, ↓ HDL cholesterol	None
α- and β-blockers (e.g., labetalol, carvedilol)	↓ Cardiac output, ↓ heart rate, vasodilator	CHF, fatigue, bronchospasm, ↓ HDL cholesterol	None
α-blockers (e.g., doxazosin, prazosin)	Vasodilator	Orthostasis	None
Inhibitors of renin-angiotensin axis			
Converting enzyme inhibitors (e.g., captopril, enalapril)	Vasodilator	Azotemia (esp. if renal artery stenosis), ↑ K^+, cough	None
Angiotensin II antagonists (e.g., losartan)	Vasodilator	Azotemia (esp. if renal artery stenosis), ↑ K^+	None
Diuretics			
Thiazides (e.g., HCTZ, indapamide)	↓ Intravascular volume	Azotemia, gout	None
Loop (e.g., furosemide)	↓↓ Intravascular volume	Azotemia, gout	None

vasoconstriction in transplant recipients, with a predominant vasodilator effect on the preglomerular arteriole.

One study of the use of amlodipine found that a 10% decrease in arterial pressure was accompanied by a 10% increase in GFR and a 23% decrease in renal vascular resistance (61). Two long-term studies have shown a particular beneficial effect of nifedipine on long-term renal allograft function when compared with other agents, particularly angiotensin-converting enzyme (ACE) inhibitors in hypertensive recipients (62,63). This is due, presumably, to the effect of these agents on reversing the renal vasoconstriction produced by cyclosporine. The beneficial effects of calcium channel antagonists may also extend beyond their vasodilator properties to alterations in the immune response. Verapamil, a calcium channel blocker derived from papaverine, not only has a hypotensive effect in transplant recipients but has been demonstrated to have an inhibitory effect in vitro on the activation and function of human peripheral blood monocytes (64). The implications of this effect on graft rejection have not been well defined.

The effects of an antihypertensive agent on cyclosporine or tacrolimus levels must be considered when selecting therapy. Calcium channel blockers vary in their effects on cyclosporine metabolism. The dihydropyridine calcium antagonists, with the exception of nicardipine, do not substantially alter cyclosporine metabolism. Diltiazem appears to decrease cyclosporine metabolism by altering cytochrome P450 activity, and the dose of cyclosporine required to maintain therapeutic levels is decreased by 30% to 40% (65,66). Diltiazem may also improve cyclosporine absorption, an effect that may be beneficial in patients in whom it is poorly absorbed, such as lung transplant recipients with cystic fibrosis (67). The effects of diltiazem on tacrolimus metabolism are less well characterized; however, preliminary animal studies and case reports suggest that diltiazem's effects are more potent, necessitating a 60% to 70% decrease in tacrolimus dose (68,69). The effects of verapamil on cyclosporine metabolism are intermediate, between those of diltiazem and nifedipine; one report describes a 15% increase in whole blood cyclosporine levels with initiation of verapamil therapy (70).

ACE inhibitors can be effective vasodilator agents in transplant recipients, but they must be used with caution. The unique arterial blood supply to the renal allograft makes it certain that ACE inhibition will provoke graft dysfunction in the presence of transplant renal artery stenosis, an effect noted soon after the availability of this class of drugs (71–73). A fall in GFR has been reported in renal transplant recipients even in the absence of renal artery stenosis (74). This is not surprising in light of the vasoconstrictive effect that cyclosporine has on the afferent arteriole of the renal vasculature. It would be expected that glomerular perfusion pressure, and hence GFR, would tend to be maintained by angiotensin II–dependent constriction of the efferent arteriole. The effect of an ACE inhibitor would be to interfere with this autoregulatory response, leading to a fall in filtration rate. This effect may not be clinically significant; a randomized, 2.5-year trial of the ACE inhibitor lisinopril versus nifedipine for the treatment of hypertension in renal transplant patients revealed that a lower filtration fraction in the lisinopril-treated patients was not accompanied by a difference in GFR (75).

ACE inhibitors can be effective agents for the control of hypertension in renal transplant patients without renal arterial stenosis and in other organ recipients. However, renal function and serum potassium must be monitored during therapy. ACE inhibitors may be less effective vasodilators than calcium channel antagonists, given the already low renin physiology of cyclosporine-induced hypertension.

The severity of the hypertension seen in transplant recipients is such that a second agent frequently has to be administered to achieve the goal of an arterial pressure less than 140/90. β-Adrenergic blockers can be useful in this regard (75), because they can add to the negative inotropic effect of calcium channel antagonists; they can have beneficial effects on myocardial oxygen demand in patients with concomitant coronary artery disease. They are usually not effective as single agents due to the low renin state of the hypertension that occurs. The use of combination α- and β-adrenergic blockers such as carvedilol and labetalol can be effective as monotherapy in transplant recipients. The α-blocking activity of carvedilol has a beneficial renal vasodilating effect similar to that seen with the dihydropyridine calcium channel antagonists (76). α-Adrenergic blockers have been used, but their use is accompanied by orthostatic symptoms (77), and they are of limited efficacy.

INFECTIONS OF THE HEART, INCLUDING ENDOCARDITIS

Transplant recipients are at increased risk of infection, and this risk extends to the cardiovascular system. Many of the mechanisms that are used to protect against infective endocarditis are diminished by immunosuppressive therapy. Furthermore, transplant recipients usually have indwelling catheters for intravenous medication administration, and most liver, lung, and cardiac recipients will undergo invasive hemodynamic monitoring at some point. These catheters will provide a portal for entry of microorganisms, and their injurious effect on endothelium may provide a nidus for the initiation of an infection.

Normal endothelium is a poor site for attachment of most bacteria and fungi, and the development of native valve endocarditis usually requires the presence of organisms with a tenacious ability to adhere to endothelium. Thus, denuded endothelial surfaces in the heart are an important factor in the development of most cases of infectious endocarditis. Such surfaces usually occur at sites beyond which a high velocity jet stream passes (i.e., on the left ventricular surfaces of an incompetent aortic valve or the atrial surface of an incompetent mitral or tricuspid valve), but they can also occur where foreign bodies are in contact with the vessel wall. Thus, intravascular catheters passing through the right side of the heart (such as Swan-Ganz catheters) can injure the endocardium, as can cannulae used in cardiopulmonary bypass (78). Patients undergoing liver and lung transplantation are at particular risk for the development of a denuded endothelial surface due to the frequent use of invasive hemodynamic monitoring and extracorporeal circulation during their surgery. Indeed, several cases have been reported of tricuspid valve fungal endocarditis in liver transplant recipients within 1 month of their surgery (79,80). In each case, the patient had undergone right heart catheterization for hemodynamic monitoring during the perioperative period.

Work in rabbits has revealed the rapid deposition of clumps of fibrin and platelets at the site of denuded endothelium, forming sterile vegetations called "nonbacterial thrombotic endocarditis" (81,82). These sterile vegetations appear to be essential for the colonization of the heart with microorganisms; they form a protected site into which phagocytic cells penetrate poorly, thus microorganisms survive, proliferate, and lead to the development of bacterial endocarditis (83). Immunosuppressive therapy can impair the ability of neutrophil and macrophage defense systems to eliminate organisms located in vegetations. This may account for the high frequency of patients on corticosteroid therapy who have native valve endocarditis caused by organisms that usually have low virulence, such as *Corynebacterium* (84) and fungi (85).

Transplant recipients may also be more likely to experience episodes of transient bacteremia or fungemia, conditions essential for the infection of a sterile vegetation. Certainly, the need for invasive monitoring and the slower wound healing seen in patients on immunosuppressive therapy heightens the acute risk associated with surgery. Chronic corticosteroid therapy can lead to thinning of the skin and loss of its integrity as a barrier to microorganisms. Gingivitis is a complication of cyclosporine therapy that doubles the risk of bacteremia during dental procedures (86). A 3% to 13% bacteremia rate with pneumococci and gram-negative rods after liver biopsy has also been reported (87).

Fungal endocarditis poses a significant risk in transplant recipients, as an increased burden of mycotic organisms is associated with higher incidences of colonization and primary infection (see Chapter 36). Fungal endocarditis from *Candida albicans* and *Candida tropicalis* has been reported to occur in increased frequency in transplant recipients (85). Not only is there a higher quantitative burden of these organisms due to the patient's defects in cell-mediated immunity, but also *Candida* species have surface receptors for fibronectin (87), which can enhance their adherence to a site of vascular injury. *Aspergillus* species have also been reported as infective endocarditis pathogens in a higher than expected frequency in patients who have undergone organ transplantation; these infections are always associated with another (usually pulmonary) site of primary infection (88). Invasive aspergillosis occurs almost exclusively in immunocompromised patients. Once an infection is established, this organism's ability to invade the vessel wall and subsequently to adhere to normal endothelium makes the risk of endocarditis significant. This risk is evident even in patients who do not have hemodynamic lesions that would predispose them to the denudation of endothelium and the formation of sterile thrombotic vegetations.

Most transplant recipients are relatively free from the intracardiac hemodynamic lesions or prosthetic valves that would predispose them to endocarditis, a factor that tends to decrease the potential incidence of this disease. Nonetheless, this diagnosis should be considered in a patient with the insidious onset of constitutional symptoms including a low-grade fever, a new heart murmur, or episodes of embolic phenomena. In those instances, the diagnostic evaluation should include culturing a larger-than-usual volume of blood, as fungemia may be transient and the concentrations of organisms low.

CARDIAC MALIGNANCIES

Tumors occur at an increased frequency in transplant patients receiving immunosuppressive therapy (see Chapter 37). Skin and lip tumors, lymphomas, and Kaposi's sarcoma occur most commonly (89). In the general population, primary tumors of the heart—which are almost always sarcomas—are extremely rare, with a frequency at postmortem examination 0.05%; this frequency does not appear to be any greater in transplant recipients. A rhabdomyosarcoma of the left ventricle has been described in a patient at postmortem examination 17 years after renal transplantation (90); given the rarity of such reports, immunosuppression does not appear to play a causative role.

Metastatic tumors of the heart are 16 times more common than primary tumors. Most commonly these involve carcinoma of the breast and lung, malignant melanoma, leukemia, and lymphoma. A case of B-cell lymphoma occurring in the heart has been described 3 years after renal transplantation in a patient presenting with sepsis and a right ventricular mass; this tumor also involved the allograft kidney as well as other abdominal organs (91). A B-cell lymphoma isolated to the heart has also been identified during a postmortem examination (92). Malignant renal cell carcinomas of both the host kidney and the allograft itself have been described in transplant recipients. Because renal cell carcinomas have a proclivity for invading large veins and, by direct extension, the right atrium, the occurrence of metastatic disease in the heart might be expected. In fact, the sudden death of a renal transplant recipient 10 years after transplantation has been ascribed to intracardiac metastases of a renal cell carcinoma causing obstruction of the right ventricular outflow tract (93).

In summary, while reports of metastatic disease to the heart in transplant recipients are few, this diagnosis should be considered in a patient presenting with the onset of new heart failure or a new cardiac murmur and a mass visualized by echocardiography. Percutaneous endomyocardial biopsy may be useful in providing tissue for pathologic analysis when this diagnosis is suspected (94).

The remainder of this chapter is devoted to a discussion of organ-specific considerations of extrathoracic transplantation and the cardiovascular system. Chapter 25 presents additional discussion of the cardiovascular considerations of pulmonary transplantation, including pulmonary hypertension.

ORGAN-SPECIFIC CONSIDERATIONS OF TRANSPLANTATION AND THE HEART

Renal Transplantation

Cardiovascular disease is commonly associated with many of the conditions that can lead to end-stage renal disease (ESRD) such as diabetes mellitus, hypertension, and atherosclerotic vascular disease. The evaluation of a patient for renal transplantation must therefore include a consideration of the possible presence and severity of cardiac disease. As several of the conditions that could lead to cardiac comorbidity are actually exacerbated by the immunosuppression used after transplantation, the treatment of cardiac disease in the renal transplant recipient is a subject with which the transplant physician needs to be familiar.

Evaluation of the Cardiac Status of the Patient with End-Stage Renal Disease.

Refinement of the care of renal transplant recipients over the past 20 years has resulted in a decrease in allograft loss from rejection and in patient loss from infection, while cardiovascular deaths have increased (95). Because cardiac disease comprises approximately 50% of patient mortality after renal transplantation, assessing the presence and severity of cardiac disease *before* transplantation is important in predicting how much real benefit the patient will receive *after* transplantation.

The relative increase in mortality in transplant recipients has occurred during a time period in which overall cardiovascular mortality in the general population has actually fallen. The decrease in cardiovascular mortality has been ascribed to a number of factors, including risk factor control, sophisticated techniques to diagnose cardiac disease, and an increasingly aggressive approach to therapy that includes pharmacologic agents, interventional techniques, and cardiac surgical procedures. A similarly aggressive approach to the identification and treatment of cardiac disease before and after transplantation is the only means of achieving a significant reduction in allograft loss and patient mortality.

Mortality from coronary disease in transplant recipients is 25-fold that of an age- and sex-matched population (96); therefore, it must be identified and treated aggressively. Furthermore, pretransplant ischemic heart disease has been shown to be the most important predictor of the development of cerebral and peripheral vascular disease (97). The relative risk of developing a major transplant cerebrovascular event is increased fivefold in recipients who had coronary disease preoperatively (97). Thus, the identification of coronary artery disease in patients with ESRD being considered for transplantation is of considerable importance, as it predicts both future cardiac complications as well as vascular complications in other organ systems. In patients with ESRD, coronary artery disease and cardiomyopathy are the most frequently encountered cardiac disorders. The presence and severity of coronary disease must be assessed in these patients, as it is the most common cause of death in long-term renal transplant survivors. Cardiomyopathy secondary to uremia also occurs in patients with ESRD, but it appears to improve after transplantation (98); its presence may affect perioperative management, but it should not be considered a major contraindication to proceeding with transplantation.

The initial cardiovascular evaluation of a patient being considered for transplantation should, of course, consist of a careful history and clinical examination. It is likely that most patients with a documented history of ischemic heart disease will need to proceed to a full evaluation by a cardiologist, which will likely include cardiac catheterization. Cardiac catheterization permits an assessment of the number and severity of coronary stenoses, as well as allows the measurement of overall cardiac function. This information, at times combined with a functional assessment, may prompt coronary revascularization by either the surgical or percutaneous route. Injury to the allograft by radiocontrast agents or inadequate perfusion during or after cardiopulmonary bypass can be avoided if revascularization is performed prior to transplantation.

In patients without a known history of coronary disease, identification of risk factors for coronary disease is an important first step in stratifying recipients who will need further testing. The risk factors include increased age, male sex, atherosclerotic disease in other vascular beds, a family history of premature coronary disease before age 55, smoking, excess weight, a sedentary life style, hypercholesterolemia (particularly elevation of the LDL cholesterol to >160 mg/dL or depression of the HDL cholesterol below 35 mg/dL), hypertension, and diabetes. Among these risk factors, diabetes is particularly important for two reasons: diabetics have a significant prevalence of asymptomatic coronary disease, and the sensitivity of the commonly available noninvasive tests for coronary disease is low in these patients (see below).

It has long been acknowledged that diabetic patients are at increased risk of "silent" myocardial infarctions, during which they do not experience the typical antecedent symptoms of chest pain (99). The asymptomatic nature of their ischemic heart disease does not signify a lesser extent or a better prognosis. An angiographic study of 21 azotemic patients with juvenile-onset diabetes found that the anatomic distribution of lesions was similar to that seen in symptomatic nondiabetic patients (100). The 2-year survival of the asymptomatic patients (none of whom underwent a revascularization procedure) was only 22%. A larger, nonangiographic study of 58 diabetic men used ambulatory electrocardiogram (ECG) monitoring corroborated by thallium scintigraphy to identify myocardial ischemia in 17% of the patients studied (101).

Upon completion of the initial risk factor assessment, a decision must be made whether to proceed with further screening studies for an asymptomatic patient or to proceed directly to coronary arteriography. A disease prediction chart such as the one in Table 30.4, developed in the Framingham Heart Study, can be useful for identifying patients at high risk of having coronary disease based on their risk factors (102). In patients calculated as having a high probability of coronary disease, it may be best to proceed directly to coronary angiography. Otherwise, the use of a noninvasive test may be helpful in stratifying patients.

Despite the addition of "points" to increase the estimated risk of coronary disease when diabetes is present, general risk calculations such as those in Table 30.4 still tend to underestimate the risk of coronary disease in diabetic men with ESRD. A recent study by Manske and colleagues using coronary angiography identified significant coronary stenoses in 88% of type I diabetic renal transplant candidates age 45 or older. This is an example of a population in which the high prevalence of the coronary disease should lead to coronary angiography regardless of the results of noninvasive testing. Manske found that in patients younger than the age of 45, a low risk group of patients could be identified. These were patients who had had diabetes for less than 25 years, had a smoking history of less than 5 pack years, and did not have resting ST-T wave abnormalities on ECG. Coronary disease was absent in 22 of 23 patients with this profile (96%). As opposed to those patients aged ≥45 years, younger patients meeting these criteria can likely avoid coronary angiography if a noninvasive study is negative (103).

Table 30.4. Coronary Heart Disease Risk Prediction Chart

Age (If Female)		Age (If Male)				HDL Cholesterol (mg/dL)			
Age	Points	Age	Points	Age	Points	HDL	Points	HDL	Points
30	1	30	−2	48–49	9	25–26	7	67–73	−4
31	2	31	−1	50–51	10	27–29	6	74–80	−5
32	3	32–33	0	52–54	11	30–32	5	81–87	−6
33	4	34	1	55–56	12	33–35	4	88–96	−7
34	5	35–36	2	57–59	13	36–38	3		
35	6	37–38	3	60–61	14	39–42	2		
36	7	39	4	62–64	15	43–46	1		
37	8	40–41	5	65–67	16	47–50	0		
38	9	42–43	6	68–70	17	51–55	−1		
39	10	44–45	7	71–73	18	56–60	−2		
40	11	46–47	8	74	19	61–66	−3		

Total Cholesterol (mg/dL)				Systolic Blood Pressure (mm Hg)					
Chol	Points	Chol	Points	SBP	Points	SBP	Points	Other Factors	Points
139–151	−3	220–239	2	98–104	−2	140–149	3	Smoking	4
152–166	−2	240–262	3	105–112	−1	150–160	4	Diabetes	
167–182	−1	263–288	4	113–120	0	161–172	5	Male	3
183–199	0	289–315	5	121–129	1	173–185	6	Female	6
200–219	1	316–330	6	130–139	2			ECG-LVH	9

	Total Points	5-Year Probability of CAD	Total Points	5-Year Probability of CAD
Age	1–10	1.5%	27–29	18%
+SBP	11–16	4%	30–32	24%
+HDL chol.	17–20	7%		
+Total chol.	21–23	10%		
+Other Factors = **Total Points**	24–26	15%		

Modified from Anderson KM, Wilson PWF, Odel PM, Kannel WB. An updated coronary risk profile: a statement for health professionals. Circulation 1991;83:356–362.

Noninvasive Exercise Testing

Exercise-based screening tests have been traditionally used to assess both the diagnosis and extent of coronary disease (Table 30.5). The sensitivity and specificity of the tests rely on the ability of the patient to exercise to a workload that is no less than 75% of that predicted for the patient's age and gender. A patient's ability to achieve this workload can be estimated by assessing his or her maximal heart rate response in a given exercise protocol. An adequate workload can be assumed to have been achieved if a patient's maximum heart rate is 85% of that predicted for age by the following equation ($HR_{maximum} = 210 - \text{age in years}$). When patients are unable to exercise to that extent, as is not infrequent in patients with ESRD, the predictive power of the test is unacceptably low, and pharmacologic stress testing should be considered.

Even when patients are able to perform an exercise test to an acceptable workload, the sensitivity and specificity of the test or the detection of coronary disease can vary with the presence of comorbid conditions such as diabetes (see Table 30.5). For example, the exercise thallium test has a sensitivity of 84% in patients without diabetes, but in uremic patients with diabetes the sensitivity is only 67%. This may be related to the diffuse nature of the coronary disease that develops in these patients, which alters thallium uptake in most myocardial segments studied on planar imaging. Because the analysis of thallium imaging relies on a comparison of uptake in different segments, a disease that involves multiple vessels or left main coronary disease might give a false-negative thallium result. Thus, it is precisely those patients one would most like to identify on the basis of noninvasive testing who will not be recognized as having coronary disease. The use of single photon emission computed tomography (SPECT) imaging may improve the sensitivity of thallium testing in diabetics with ESRD, but the sensitivity of this technique remains to be completely evaluated in uremic patients.

Table 30.5. Sensitivity and Specificity of Noninvasive Tests for Coronary Artery Disease

	Sensitivity %	Specificity %
Exercise Tests		
Electrocardiography (138)	65	85
Thallium 201:		
Planar, without diabetes (138)	84	87
Planar, with uremia and diabetes (139)	67	62
SPECT	96	83
Pharmacologic Tests		
Dipyridamole thallium 201:		
Patients without diabetes (140)	79	76
Patients with uremia and diabetes (141)	37	73
Adenosine thallium 201 (142)	83	75
Dipyridamole positron emission tomography:		
Patients without diabetes (140)	95	82
Patients with left ventricular hypertrophy (143)	55	60
Dipyridamole echocardiography (144)	60	93
Dobutamine echocardiography (106)	82	88

Noninvasive Pharmacologic Diagnostic Testing

For transplant candidates who are unable to achieve an appropriate workload in an exercise test, a variety of pharmacologic stress tests are available. Two categories of agents are used to alter coronary blood flow to allow the imaging of the myocardium supplied by diseased arteries. Drugs such as dipyridamole create a "steal" phenomenon by preferentially improving blood flow in normal coronary arteries. Drugs such as dobutamine increase myocardial oxygen demand without exercise and allow for the identification of ischemic myocardial segments.

The intravenous infusion of dipyridamole blocks cellular resorption of adenosine, increasing the intravascular concentration of this endogenous vasodilator. As areas supplied by diseased arteries are already maximally vasodilated, the additional intravenous infusion of dipyridamole, or adenosine itself, does not affect coronary blood flow in these areas. On the other hand, areas of myocardium supplied by normal coronary arteries increase their coronary blood flow 3 to 5 times above baseline levels. A heterogeneity of myocardial blood flow is thus created and can be imaged by a radionuclide such as thallium 201 or technetium 99m sestamibi.

Unfortunately, dipyridamole thallium imaging is subject to some of the same limitations in sensitivity in patients with diabetes and uremia as is exercise thallium imaging (see Table 30.5); patients with diffuse coronary disease may not have a normally perfused segment to serve as a basis for identifying a defect in an abnormally perfused segment. Furthermore, the high resting levels of adenosine seen in patients with ESRD may reduce the vascular responsiveness to dipyridamole or intravenously administered adenosine, resulting in a high false-negative rate for resting exercise testing in these patients (104). Adding to the low utility of pharmacologic stress thallium testing can be the presence of left ventricular hypertrophy, a not uncommon finding in hypertensive ESRD patients. The rate of false-positive thallium tests in the presence of left ventricular hypertrophy is high, and the specificity of a positive dipyridamole scan is only 60% (105). This may be due to real inhomogeneities in coronary perfusion from abnormalities of microcirculatory regulation in these patients.

During dobutamine infusion at as high a dose as 40 μg/kg/min, heart rate and myocardial contractility increase. An increase in myocardial oxygen demand results, and myocardial dysfunction occurs in regions receiving an inadequate blood supply. Echocardiography performed simultaneously can reveal segments of myocardium that do not augment their contractility normally, thus providing for both the diagnosis and assessment of the extent of coronary disease present. This technique offers the potential for the accurate diagnosis of coronary disease in patients with ESRD without the need for radionuclides or sophisticated imaging equipment. A preliminary study by Nally and colleagues reported that dobutamine echocardiography has an 86% sensitivity for the detection of coronary disease. This sensitivity was similar to that found in a control population matched for age, gender, and coronary disease but lacking ESRD (106).

Coronary Arteriography

Coronary arteriography remains the gold standard for both the diagnosis and assessment of the extent of coronary disease. It may be appropriate to use it directly in a patient with known ischemic heart disease or a high probability of having it. Of course, coronary angiography is essential for definitive studies prior to coronary artery bypass surgery and for interventions to revascularize the heart. Unfortunately, in patients with severe renal disease, coronary angiography is accompanied by a risk of clinically significant nephrotoxicity. The risk may be decreased with the use of nonionic, low osmolar radiocontrast agents such as iopamidol, but no decrease in nephrotoxic effect has been demonstrated in patients who also have diabetes (107). For this reason, it may be prudent to wait until a patient requires dialysis before proceeding with an angiographic study, particularly if coronary angioplasty is anticipated, as it requires a greater dye load than does diagnostic angiography.

An Algorithm for the Detection of Coronary Disease in Patients with End-Stage Renal Disease

Patients in whom the diagnosis of coronary disease is clear should undergo coronary angiography at some point prior to transplantation. This will allow for the definitive identification both of the amount of myocardial damage already present and of the myocardium at risk in a future coronary occlusion. In those ESRD patients who do not have symptoms of myocardial ischemia, several algorithms for the identification of occult coronary disease have been proposed (103,108,141). These algorithms use clinical criteria to categorize patients as either low risk or high risk.

Le et al have proposed an effective algorithm for the identification of patients who are at a low risk of cardiac events after renal transplantation (109). In their study of ESRD patients in an urban, university-based transplant program, patients were considered high risk if they had a history compatible with angina or previous myocardial infarction, diabetes, and age of greater than 50 years, or an abnormal ECG. The remaining patients, considered low risk, constituted half of the study population; they underwent no further cardiac investigations. Only 1 of the 94 patients classified as low risk suffered a cardiac death during a 5-year follow-up; the patient died 45 months after evaluation and had not undergone transplantation. High-risk patients underwent noninvasive stress testing with radionuclide scintigraphy; those with positive studies proceeded to coronary angiography.

An alternative algorithm to that of Le and associates makes more aggressive use of coronary angiography in high-risk patients, and is based on the findings of other centers of an unacceptably low sensitivity with noninvasive stress thallium imaging (Fig. 30.2) (138,139). In asymptomatic patients who are nondiabetic or are diabetic and younger than 45 years, a noninvasive screening test is performed. In patients who can exercise to at least 75% of their maximum predicted heart rate for age, a negative thallium scan may predict a low cardiac mortality of less than 10% over 5 years (108); these patients may be transplanted without coronary angiography. Impaired exercise tolerance in this population makes it likely that the majority of asymptomatic high-risk patients will also require coronary angiography. Dobutamine echocardiography may eventually have a role in avoiding coronary angiography in these patients, but its sensitivity remains to be fully defined in this population, particularly with diabetics. High-risk patients who are unable to exercise to at least 75% of their maximum predicted heart rate for age should be considered for coronary angiography prior to transplantation.

When coronary angiography demonstrates occlusive disease in a major epicardial artery of greater than 70% in severity, the patient's status must be evaluated: Is coronary angioplasty or bypass grafting appropriate prior to transplantation, or is transplantation too great a risk because of the diffuseness and severity of the disease and the degree of left ventricular dysfunction? There may be a few patients in whom the occlusive lesion does not supply a significant amount of myocardium, and in whom transplantation can proceed without revascularization, but the risk of progression due to an exacerbation of coronary risk factors by current immunosuppressive therapy usually indicates the need for revascularization of even single-vessel disease.

Liver Transplantation

Considerations of coexisting cardiac disease in the patient with end-stage liver disease are based on the changes in the pulmonary and systemic circulation that can accompany the disease, the existence of inherited disorders of metabolism involving both the liver and the heart, and the risk factor profile for coronary disease. The possible coexistence of cardiac disease with liver failure is an important factor in the evaluation of potential liver transplant recipients.

Circulatory Changes Occurring in Liver Failure

Changes occur in both the pulmonary and systemic circulations in patients with liver failure accompanied by portal hypertension (see Chapter 28). Pulmonary hypertension can occur in a small number of patients with liver failure, and its consequences can be fatal when it is not identified preoperatively. On the other hand, systemic vasodilation occurs in the majority of patients with liver failure; although the increase in vascular tone that occurs after surgery often requires monitoring of the cardiovascular system, it rarely has adverse consequences.

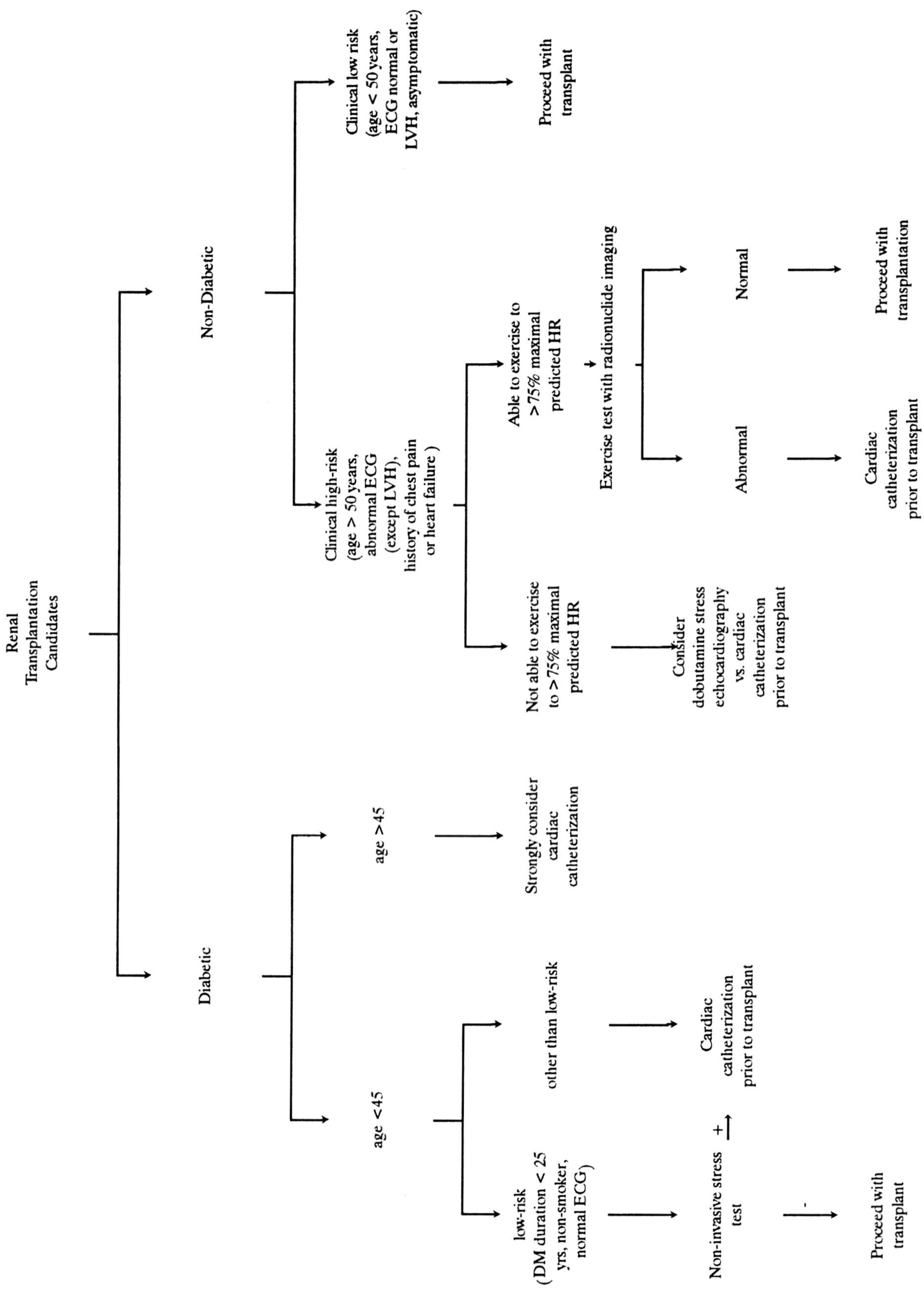

FIGURE 30.2. *Algorithm for the detection of coronary disease in patients with end-stage renal disease. DM, diabetes mellitus; ECG, electrocardiogram; HR, heart rate; LVH, left ventricular hypertrophy.*

Pulmonary hypertension, defined as a resting mean pulmonary artery pressure greater than 25 mm Hg, occurs with an increased prevalence in patients with portal hypertension or cirrhosis. The exact incidence of pulmonary hypertension in this population has been difficult to ascertain. A review of 1205 patients with end-stage liver disease being evaluated for transplantation revealed a prevalence of pulmonary hypertension of 8.5% (110). The degree of pulmonary hypertension was mild in the majority of these patients. In 2.2% of the patients it was moderate or severe (systolic pulmonary artery pressure >45 mm Hg). In those patients who underwent transplantation, survival was unaffected by mild or moderate pulmonary hypertension; however, in patients with severe hypertension (systolic pulmonary artery pressure >60 mm Hg), the 9-month post-transplant survival was decreased at 58%, and 36-month survival was only 29%.

Primary pulmonary hypertension is more common among women than men, but there does not seem to be a sex-linked bias in pulmonary hypertension related to liver disease (111), suggesting that the mechanism for the development of pulmonary hypertension may differ between the two diseases. On the other hand, the pathologic appearance of the pulmonary arteriopathy seen in both diseases is similar: medial hypertrophy of the "muscular" sized arteries extending into the arterioles with narrowing of the vessel lumen.

The diagnosis of pulmonary hypertension in potential liver recipients needs to be based on careful use of physical and laboratory examinations, as 60% of patients will be asymptomatic (112). Cardiac examination will reveal a widening and increase in intensity of the pulmonary component of the S_2. The presence of a right ventricular S_3 (which can be differentiated from a left ventricular S_3 by position and changing intensity with respiration) indicates that right ventricular dysfunction has developed. Chest radiography in patients with pulmonary hypertension and end-stage liver disease may reveal prominence of the central pulmonary arteries with pruning of the distal pulmonary vasculature. Right ventricular enlargement may also be seen on the lateral chest radiograph. The ECG of a patient with pulmonary hypertension can show right axis deviation and right ventricular hypertrophy with secondary T wave changes.

Echocardiography is the most important screening test to identify pulmonary hypertension in potential liver transplant candidates. Multiple findings of pulmonary hypertension can be identified echocardiographically, and the systolic pulmonary artery pressure itself can be estimated from the Doppler velocity of the tricuspid regurgitation jet. The echocardiogram can also be used to measure right ventricular dimensions and systolic function, albeit with less precision than is possible with the left ventricle. If evidence of pulmonary hypertension is present, the echocardiogram can also exclude some other etiologies such as the presence of intracardiac left-to-right shunting.

Right heart catheterization should be considered an absolute requirement in all cases of suspected pulmonary hypertension. Catheterization will allow confirmation of the diagnosis and estimation of the severity of the pulmonary hypertension, as well as allow for a trial of vasodilators to temporarily reverse the process. This is particularly important for identifying potential recipients who have the hyperdynamic circulation that develops in patients with end-stage liver disease: an elevation of the pulmonary artery pressure but also an elevated cardiac output and thus a normal pulmonary vascular resistance. This group of patients with normal pulmonary resistance does not have an adverse outcome after transplantation (113). For patients with an elevated pulmonary resistance, vasodilators such as nitroprusside, prostacyclin, and nifedipine have been administered, but they often are ineffective—systemic hypotension develops prior to any pulmonary vasodilator effect (114). Nevertheless, favorable results have been reported in a small series of patients. Kuo et al (115) administered epoprostenol (formerly known as prostacyclin or prostaglandin I_2) to 4 patients with portopulmonary hypertension over 6 to 14 months. They found a 29% to 46% decrease in pulmonary artery pressure, a 22% to 71% decline in pulmonary vascular resistance, and a 25% to 75% increase in cardiac output.

Preliminary work suggests that inhaled nitric oxide is also ineffective as a pulmonary vasodilator in patients with cirrhosis, despite its potent vasodilator effects in patients with primary pulmonary hypertension or collagen vascular disease (116). However, acute intraoperative therapy with inhaled nitric oxide has been used successfully to reduce pulmonary artery pressure (117). It may be that patient selection accounts for some of these differences.

Hemodynamic evaluation of the patient with cirrhotic liver disease will reveal systemic vasodilation and a decrease in the response of the periphery to vasoconstrictors far more commonly than it will reveal pulmonary hypertension (118). After transplant, a vasoconstrictor state develops, which can place an unusual stress on the cardiovascular system, particularly if its reserve is diminished by disease. In a study of 113 consecutive liver transplant recipients, Nasraway et al identified an increased cardiac index and a decreased systemic vascular resistance in patients prior to transplantation (119). Both cardiac index and systemic vascular resistance fell during the first two postoperative days. A fall during the first 12 hours in left ventricular stroke work index, a marker of myocardial contractile function, occurred only in those patients who would not survive their postoperative course. This suggests that patients with marginal cardiac reserve may not be able to tolerate the increase in afterload that presumably occurs with the restoration of hepatic function.

The problems associated with liver transplantation in the patient with cardiovascular disease suggest that every potential recipient's initial evaluation should include a physical and laboratory examination with an emphasis on the cardiovascular system, and that echocardiographic screening should be liberally used to identify abnormalities in ventricular function or pulmonary hypertension (see Chapter 19).

Cardiac Involvement in Systemic Disorders

Several causes of end-stage liver disease, such as hemochromatosis, glycogen storage disorders, familial hypercholesterolemia, Gaucher's disease, and familial amyloidosis, can also affect the heart and its function. The salient features of the most common indications for liver transplantation that can cause cardiac involvement are listed in Table 30.6.

Cirrhosis

Alcohol abuse as a cause of cardiomyopathy as well as hepatic cirrhosis has been well described. Even in alcoholic cirrhosis patients without symptoms or signs of cardiac disease at rest, abnormalities of cardiac function can be present. The response of cardiac stroke volume to pressure or volume overload is impaired in approximately one-half of patients who have alcoholic cirrhosis without known cardiac disease (120). A decrease in the usual augmentation of contractility with exercise also occurs in patients with alcoholic cirrhosis (121). This subclinical abnormality in cardiac function may become manifest during the stress of liver transplantation, and may account for the relatively high frequency with which pulmonary edema and hypotension have been observed in these patients (122).

Hemochromatosis

Post-transplant survival in patients with hemochromatosis has been identified as diminished in liver recipients because of the development of cardiomyopathy, despite preoperative evaluation including two-dimensional echocardiography (123). Even though liver transplantation may correct the abnormality of iron metabolism present in patients with hemochromatosis, a case in which cardiac dysfunction progressed despite regression of previously identified myocyte hemosiderin deposits has been reported (124). As noninvasive assessment by echocardiography may underestimate the severity of cardiac involvement by hemochromatosis, endomyocardial biopsy may be appropriate for all patients with this disease being considered for liver transplantation, with combined heart–liver transplantation undertaken in patients with involvement of both organs (125) (see also Chapter 23).

Table 30.6. Cardiovascular Complications of Diseases Causing Severe Hepatic Dysfunction

Disorder Causing Hepatic Dysfunction	Cardiovascular Complication
Alcoholic cirrhosis	Dilated cardiomyopathy Hypertension
Hemochromatosis	Mixed dilated and restrictive cardiomyopathy
Sarcoidosis	Dilated cardiomyopathy Atrioventricular block Ventricular arrhythmia
Glycogen storage disorders (Pompe's disease, branching enzyme deficiency)	"Pseudohypertrophic" restrictive cardiomyopathy Left ventricular outflow obstruction Short PR interval (Pompe's)
Familial hypercholesterolemia	Coronary artery disease Atherosclerosis of the aorta, mesenteric, and peripheral vasculature
Familial amyloidosis	Restrictive cardiomyopathy Atrioventricular and intraventricular conduction defects Orthostatic hypotension

Glycogen Storage Diseases

Other infiltrative diseases that can cause hepatic failure can also cause heart failure, and they should be considered when evaluating a potential liver transplant recipient. Patients with glycogen storage disorders, particularly types I (Pompe's disease) and IV (branching enzyme deficiency), can develop a "pseudohypertrophic" cardiomyopathy. The walls of both ventricles are thickened not from myocardial cell hypertrophy, but from cellular or interstitial infiltration. Heart failure develops due to abnormalities of systolic and diastolic function, and outflow obstruction may occur. The conduction system can also be affected, as shortening of the PR interval is seen in ECGs taken in patients with Pompe's disease.

Glucocerebrosidase deficiency (Gaucher's disease) can also lead to an infiltrative cardiomyopathy from interstitial infiltration of myocytes by macrophages. A constrictive pericarditis can develop, as can right ventricular failure due to pulmonary hypertension. Again, echocardiography can be helpful in both the identification and staging of the severity of cardiac involvement in patients with Gaucher's.

Concern is appropriate regarding potential cardiac involvement in these diseases, but there is potential for the reversal of their systemic complications due to the development of "microchimerism." Both immunohistochemistry and the polymerase chain reaction (PCR) have been used to identify infiltration of the heart by donor cells in patients undergoing liver transplantation (126). Furthermore, regression of cardiac amylopectin deposition has been noted in a liver transplant recipient with type IV glycogen storage disease (126).

Amyloidosis

Familial amyloidosis can lead to dysfunction of multiple organ systems as a result of transthyretin protein overload, a condition that improves after liver transplantation (127). Familial amyloidosis usually presents with a neuropathy and renal dysfunction, and it is only occasionally associated with cardiac involvement. This differs from light-chain amyloidosis associated with immunocyte dyscrasia, which often causes a fatal cardiomyopathy.

Nonetheless, patients with significant cardiac transthyretin amyloid infiltration can develop a restrictive cardiomyopathy in which symptoms of right heart failure such as edema will predominate. These cardiac amyloid patients may also have orthostatic hypotension and even angina owing to amyloid involvement of the coronary arteries (128). Their ECGs will show depression of QRS voltage and the prolongation of the PR and QRS intervals, as conduction system involvement is relatively common in these patients.

The echocardiographic appearance of a "speckled" myocardium, as well as abnormalities in Doppler indices of left ventricular filling (129), probably provides the best means of identifying cardiac involvement in patients with familial amyloidosis being considered for liver transplant (128,129). A definitive diagnosis can be made by right ventricular endomyocardial biopsy, which can be positive even when samples of other tissues such as fat pad and gingiva are negative (130).

Identification of cardiac involvement prior to transplantation is important, as the treatment of heart failure due to infiltrative restrictive cardiomyopathy is generally unsatisfactory. The diastolic pressure-volume relationship in these patients is generally quite steep, and small increases or decreases in intravascular volume can rapidly lead to congestion or a low cardiac output, respectively. Agents that provide inotropic support, such as dobutamine or phosphodiesterase inhibitors, are usually ineffective, as is digoxin. Calcium antagonists may lead to an exacerbation of the patient's heart failure, and vasodilators may lead to hypotension. The difficulty of managing a patient with a restrictive myopathy through the intravascular volume shifts and autonomic lability that occur during liver transplantation should lead to a consideration of combined heart-liver transplantation if evidence of cardiomyopathy is present.

Hypercholesterolemia

Liver transplantation or combined cardiac and liver transplantation can be lifesaving in patients with familial hypercholesterolemia, because there is a near 100% risk of their developing premature coronary atherosclerosis and myocardial infarction, even with pharmacologic therapy (131). The surgeon should expect that there may be atherosclerotic disease of the aorta and hepatic artery as well as in the coronary vasculature, but post-transplant progression of this disease is slowed by the marked reduction in LDL and total cholesterol levels seen in these patients (131).

Screening for Coronary Disease in the Potential Liver Transplant Recipient

As the age restrictions for the use of orthotopic liver transplantation to treat end-stage liver disease have been liberalized, the possible coexistence of age-related cardiac diseases such as coronary heart disease must be considered prior to liver transplantation. Furthermore, patients with cholestatic liver disease might be expected to have an even greater prevalence of coronary disease from hyperlipidemia, which accompanies their hepatic dysfunction. One series of end-stage liver disease patients over age 50 who did *not* have symptoms of cardiac disease and underwent coronary angiography as part of their transplant evaluation identified moderate or severe coronary disease in 13.3% (132). Diabetes has been an important predictor of occult coronary disease, as it has been with ESRD patients.

The postoperative implications of coronary disease during liver transplantation are found in a series of liver recipients studied by Dec et al. The study found a 52% incidence of major intraoperative and postoperative complications in liver recipients with known preoperative cardiac disease (122). Myocardial ischemia and infarction were most common, with pulmonary edema and ventricular arrhythmia also occurring. Although 6-month postoperative survival was not diminished in patients having these complications, long-term (4-year) survival was lower in the patients who had a major cardiac complication.

The studies have reinforced the importance of careful evaluation. If necessary, cardiac disease in transplant recipients should be treated when they are initially evaluated. This will allow perioperative cardiac complications to be anticipated and appropriately dealt with so that they do not alter overall survival. The fact that there is a relatively high prevalence of coronary disease in the liver transplant population with no real impact on survival suggests that appropriate management of these patients can lead to a successful post-transplant result.

Management begins with a preoperative coronary risk assessment. The usual risk factors of age, sex, smoking, history of diabetes or hyperlipidemia, or family history of premature coronary disease should guide further assessment. Exercise testing is the preferred study to exclude coronary disease. If general debility or encephalopathy preclude maximal exercise, pharmacologic stress testing using either dipyridamole or adenosine radionuclide imaging or dobutamine stress echocardiography should be performed. Coronary angiography may be useful for patients with a positive exercise study or patients who have had prior cardiac events or undergone previous coronary revascularization to define their coronary anatomy. Diabetic patients, particularly over the age of 50 years, should undergo coronary angiography as a part of their transplant evaluation because of the high prevalence of occult coronary disease (132) and the uncertain sensitivity of noninvasive stress testing in this population.

Bone Marrow Transplantation

Cardiac complications of bone marrow transplantation were initially quite frequent and limited the early success of the procedure (see Chapter 27). The cardiac complications of bone marrow transplantation fall into two categories: myopathic effects of the immunosuppressive regimen used to achieve successful bone marrow engraftment, and transient arrhythmias and hemodynamic instability that occur during infusion of donor stem cells or marrow.

The immunosuppressive regimen given to bone marrow recipients prior to transplantation frequently includes cyclophosphamide (an alkylating agent) and ionizing radiation. Both of these can be injurious to the myocardium (133), but most programs have found that cyclophosphamide is the more significant cardiotoxic agent. Gottdiener et al found that heart failure developed in 28% of bone marrow recipients who received a preconditioning dose of 180 mg/kg of cyclophosphamide over 4 days prior to bone marrow transplant (44). Echocardiographic study revealed that the majority of patients who received this regimen had a decline in left ventricular systolic function, even if they did not develop heart failure. Strikingly, two-thirds of those who did develop heart failure died during the early post-transplant period. Postmortem examination of the heart revealed endothelial injury and a severe hemorrhagic myopericarditis (44).

If the cyclophosphamide dose is calculated according to the recipient's body surface area, cardiotoxicity may be more easily avoided. Only 3% of patients receiving a dose of less than 1.55 g/m^2/day for 4 days developed heart failure, as opposed to 25% of those receiving a higher dose (134).

As a result of this initial experience, total body irradiation has been combined with cyclophosphamide in an effort to reduce the cardiotoxicity of the alkylating agent. Successful engraftment has been reported in patients receiving cyclophosphamide doses as low as 120 mg/kg in addition to 10 to 12 Gy of total body irradiation (133). Heart failure still occurred in 9% of patients, and was fatal in all. Echocardiography identified adverse changes in both systolic and diastolic myocardial function in the majority of patients given this regimen, including an 11% fall in fractional shortening and a 12% increase in left ventricular mass. These changes resolved by 1-year in survivors.

Cardiac arrhythmias, including sinus bradycardia, second-degree atrioventricular block, and complete heart block, have been reported at the time of donor marrow or stem cell infusion (135,136). Ventricular arrhythmias are rare, and reports describe them as limited to premature ventricular contractions. Bradycardia, secondary either to sinus bradycardia or to atrioventricular block, has been generally asymptomatic and is accompanied by hypertension rather than hypotension (135,136). Dimethylsulfoxide, which is commonly used in the marrow or stem cell infusate as a cryopreservative, has been shown to have negative chronotropic effects on the sinus and atrioventricular nodes, and to induce the release of histamine, which can cause conduction system block (137). The use of the antihistamine diphenhydramine appears to decrease the incidence of heart block (135).

SUMMARY

It is important for health care professionals caring for transplant candidates and recipients to be aware of the cardiovascular implications of many aspects of transplant surgery and immunosuppressive therapy. Caution is necessary when using agents that appear effective in the general population but have not been tested in immunosuppressed patients. The increased incidence of rhabdomyolysis observed with "statin" therapy in recipients taking cyclosporine demonstrates the problem.

On the other hand, transplant candidates and recipients should not be denied the recent advances in preventative and interventional cardiology that have decreased cardiac morbidity and mortality over the past 10 years. Judicious use of the latest advances in cardiology will require the joint efforts of members of the transplant community and cardiologists who are aware of the particular needs of the transplant patient taking immunosuppressive therapy.

REFERENCES

1. Bulkley BH, Roberts WC. The heart in systemic lupus erythematosus and the changes induced in it by corticosteroid therapy. A study of 36 necropsy patients. Am J Med 1975;58:243–264.
2. Petri M, Spence D, Bone LR, Hochberg MC. Coronary artery disease risk factors in the Johns Hopkins lupus cohort. Medicine 1992;71:291–302.
3. Sudhir K, Jennings GL, Esler MD, et al. Hydrocortisone induced hypertension in humans: pressor responsiveness and sympathetic function. Hypertension 1989;13:416–421.
4. Hricik DE, Lautman J, Bartucci MR, et al. Variable effects of steroid withdrawal on blood pressure reduction in cyclosporine treated renal transplant recipients. Transplantation 1992;53:1232–1235.
5. Curtis JJ, Galla JH, Catch TA, Luke RG. Prevalence of hypertension in a renal transplant population on alternate-day steroid therapy. Clin Nephrol 1976;5:123–127.
6. Hricik DE, Mayes JT, Schulak JA. Independent effects of cyclosporine and prednisone on post-transplant hypercholesterolemia. J Am Kidney Dis 1991;18:353–358.
7. Hricik DE, Bartucci MR, Mayes JT, Schulak JA. The effects of steroid withdrawal on the lipoprotein profiles of cyclosporine treated kidney and kidney-pancreas transplant recipients. Transplantation 1992;54:868–871.
8. Raine AEG, Carter R, Mann JL. Increased plasma LDL cholesterol after renal transplantation associated with cyclosporine immunosuppression. Transplant Proc 1987;19:1820–1821.
9. Hildbrands LD, Demacker PN, Hoitsma AJ, et al. The effects of cyclosporine and prednisone on serum lipid and (apo)lipoprotein levels in renal transplant recipients. J Am Soc Nephrol 1995;5:2073–2081.
10. Kobashigawa JA, Katznelson S, Laks H, et al. Effect of pravastatin on outcomes after cardiac transplantation. N Engl J Med 1995;333:621–627.
11. Rab ST, King SB, Carlin S, et al. Coronary aneurysms after stent placement: a suggestion of altered vessel wall healing in the presence of anti-inflammatory agents. J Am Coll Cardiol 1991;18:1524–1528.
12. Canadian Multicenter Transplant Study Group. A randomized clinical trial of cyclosporine in cadaveric renal transplantation. N Engl J Med 1983;309:809–815.
13. European Multicenter Trial Group. Cyclosporine in cadaveric renal transplantation: one-year follow-up of a multicenter trial. Lancet 1983;2:986–989.
14. O'Grady JG, Forbes A, Rolles K, et al. An analysis of cyclosporine efficacy and toxicity after liver transplantation. Transplantation 1988;45:575–579.
15. Textor SC, Cazanello VJ, Taler SJ, et al. Cyclosporine induced hypertension after transplantation. Mayo Clin Proc 1994;69:1182–1193.
16. Scherrer U, Vissing SF, Morgan BJ, et al. Cyclosporine-induced sympathetic activation and hypertension after heart transplantation. N Engl J Med 1990;323:693–699.
17. Morgan BJ, Lyson T, Scherrer U, Victor RG. Cyclosporine causes sympathetically mediated elevations in arterial pressure in rats. Hypertension 1991;18:458–466.
18. Curtis JJ, Luke RG, Dubovsky E, et al. Cyclosporine in therapeutic doses increases renal allograft vascular resistance. Lancet 1985;2:477–479.
19. Gerkens JF. Cyclosporine treatment of normal rats produces a rise in blood pressure and decreased renal vascular responses to nerve stimulation, vasoconstrictors and endothelium-dependent dilators. J Pharmacol Exp Ther 1989;250:1105–1112.

20. Xue H, Bukowski RD, McCarron DA, Bennett WM. Induction of contraction in isolated rat aorta by cyclosporine. Transplantation 1987;43:715–718.
21. Meyer-Lehnart H, Schreier RW. Potential mechanism for cyclosporine induced vascular smooth muscle contraction. Hypertension 1989;13:352–360.
22. Bellet M, Cabrol C, Sassano P, et al. Systemic hypertension after cardiac transplantation: effect of cyclosporine on the renin-angiotensin-aldosterone system. Am J Cardiol 1985;56:927–931.
23. Held P, Yusuf S, Mathias C, et al. Renin response to sympathetic stimulation in cyclosporine-treated heart-transplant patients. Am J Cardiol 1989;63:1142–1144.
24. Bantle JP, Nath KA, Sutherland DE, et al. Effects of cyclosporine on the renin-angiotensin-aldosterone system and potassium excretion in renal transplant recipients. Arch Intern Med 1985;145:505–508.
25. Perico N, Dadan J, Remuzzi G. Endothelin mediates the renal vasoconstriction induced by cyclosporine in the rat. J Am Soc Nephrol 1990;1:76–83.
26. Fozard JR, Menninger K, Schoeffter P. Cardiovascular effects of cyclosporine A and OG37–325 after chronic administration to conscious rats: role of endothelin. Transplant Proc 1994;26:3006–3009.
27. Bloom IT, Bentley FR, Spain DA, Garrison RN. An experimental study of altered nitric oxide metabolism as a mechanism of cyclosporine-induced renal vasoconstriction. Br J Surg 1995;82:195–198.
28. Eleftheriades EG, Ferguson AG, Samarel AM. Cyclosporine A has no direct effect on collagen metabolism by cardiac fibroblasts in vitro. Circulation 1993;86:1368–1377.
29. Emeson EE, Shen ML. Accelerated atherosclerosis in hyperlipidemia mice treated with cyclosporine A. Am J Pathol 1993;142:1906–1915.
30. Frens M, Reidy M, Ross R. Vascular effects of cyclosporine in vivo and in vitro. Am J Pathol 1990;137:403–413.
31. Ballantyne CM, Podet EJ, Harati Y, et al. Effects of cyclosporine therapy on plasma lipoprotein levels. JAMA 1989;262:53–56.
32. Princen HN, Neijar P, Wolthers BG, et al. Cyclosporine A blocks bile acid synthesis in cultured hepatocytes by specific inhibition of chenodeoxycholic acid synthesis. Biochem J 1991;275:501–505.
33. Shepherd J, Cobbe SM, Ford I, et al. Prevention of coronary heart disease with pravastatin in men with hypercholesterolemia. N Engl J Med 1995;333:1301–1307.
34. Textor C, Weisner R, Wilson DJ, et al. Systemic and renal hemodynamic differences between FK-506 and cyclosporine in liver transplant recipients. Transplantation 1993;55:1332–1339.
35. The US Multicenter FK-506 Liver Study Group. A comparison of tacrolimus and cyclosporine for immunosuppression in liver transplantation. N Engl J Med 1994;331:1110–1115.
36. Swenson JM, Fricker FJ, Armitage JM. Immunosuppression switch in pediatric heart transplant recipients: cyclosporine to FK 506. J Am Coll Cardiol 1995;25:1183–1188.
37. Ellis D, Shapiro R, Jordan ML, et al. Comparison of FK-506 and cyclosporine regimens in pediatric renal transplantation. Pediatric Nephrol 1994;8:193–200.
38. Abouljoud MS, Levy MF, Klintmalm GB. Hyperlipidemia after liver transplantation: long-term results of the FK506/cyclosporine A US Multicenter trial. US Multicenter Study Group. Transplant Proc 1995;27:1121–1123.
39. Swenson JM, Fricker FJ, Armitage JM. Immunosuppression switch in pediatric heart transplant recipients: cyclosporine to FK 506. J Am Coll Cardiol 1995;25:1183–1188.
40. Atkison P, Joubert G, Barron A, et al. Hypertrophic cardiomyopathy associated with tacrolimus in pediatric transplant patients. Lancet 1995;345:894–896.
41. Timerman AP, Jayaraman T, Weiderrecht G, et al. The ryanodine receptor from canine heart sarcoplasmic reticulum is associated with a novel FK-506 binding protein. Biochem Biophys Res Comm 1994;198:701–706.
42. Johnson MC, So S, Marsh JW, Murphy AM. QT Prolongation and torsades de pointes after administration of FK-506. Transplantation 1992;53:929–930.
43. Storb R, Buckner CD, Dillingham LA, Thomas ED. Cyclophosphamide regimens in rhesus monkeys with and without marrow infusion. Cancer Research 1970;30:2195–2200.
44. Gottdiener JS, Appelbaum FR, Ferrans VJ, et al. Cardiotoxicity associated with high-dose cyclophosphamide therapy. Arch Intern Med 1981;141:758–763.
45. Chatenoud L, Ferran C, Legendre C, et al. In vivo cell activation following OKT3 administration. Systemic cytokine release and modulation by corticosteroids. Transplantation 1990;49:697–702.
46. Raasveld MH, Bemelman FJ, Schellekens PT, et al. Complement activation during OKT3 treatment: a possible explanation for respiratory side effects. Kidney Int 1993;43:1140–1149.
47. Vallhonrat H, Williams W, Cosimi AB, et al. In vivo generation of C4d, Bb, iC3b, and 5c5b-9 after OKT3 administration in kidney and lung transplant recipients. Transplantation 1999;67:253–258.
48. Robinson ST, Barry JM, Norman DJ. The hemodynamic effects of intraoperative injection of muromonab CD3. Transplantation 1993;56:356–358.
49. Hosenpud JD, Norman DJ, Pantely GA. OKT3-induced hypotension in heart allograft recipients treated for steroid-resistant rejection. J Heart Transplant 1989;8:159–165.
50. Ortho Multicenter Transplant Study Group. A randomized clinical trial of OKT3 monoclonal antibody for acute rejection of cadaveric renal transplants. N Engl J Med 1985;313:337–342.
51. Costanzo-Nordin MR. Cardiopulmonary effects of OKT-3: determinants of hypotension, pulmonary edema and cardiac dysfunction. Transplant Proc 1993;25:21–24.
52. Gaston RS, Deierhoi MH, Patterson T, et al. OKT3 first-dose reaction: association with T cell subsets and cytokine release. Kidney Int 1991;39:141–148.
53. Rowe PA, Rocker GM, Morgan AG, Shale DJ. OKT-3 and pulmonary capillary permeability. BMJ 1987;295:1099–1100.
54. Cosimi AB. OKT3: first-dose safety and success. Nephron 1987;46(suppl 1):12–18.
55. Deierhoi MH, Barber WH, Curtis JJ. A comparison of OKT-3 monoclonal antibody and corticosteroids in the treatment of acute renal allograft rejection. Am J Kidney Dis 1988;11:86–93.
56. Spieker C, Barenbrock M, Buchholz B, et al. Cardiovascular effects of ATG and OKT-3 in renal allograft recipients. Transplant Proc 1992;24:2594–2595.
57. Vianello A, Mastrosimone S, Calconi G, et al. The role of hypertension as a damaging factor for kidney grafts under cyclosporine therapy. Am J Kidney Dis 1993;21:79–83.
58. Vetrovec GW, Landwehr DM, Edwards VL. Incidence of renal artery stenosis in hypertensive patients undergoing coronary angiography. J Interven Cardiol 1989;2:2–8.
59. Curtis JJ, Diethelm AG, Jones P, et al. Benefits of removal of native kidney in hypertension after renal transplantation. Lancet 1985;2:739–742.
60. Braith RW, Mills RM, Wilcox CS, et al. Breakdown of blood pressure and body fluid homeostasis in heart transplant recipients. J Am Coll Cardiol 1996;27:375–383.
61. van der Schaaf MR, Hene RJ, Floor M, et al. Hypertension after renal transplantation. Calcium channel or converting enzyme blockade? Hypertension 1995;25:77–81.
62. Morales JM, Rodriguez-Paternina E, Araque A, et al. Long-term protective effect of a calcium antagonist on renal function in hypertensive renal transplant patients on cyclosporine therapy: a 5-year prospective randomized study. Transplant Proc 1994;26:2598–2599.
63. Hauser AC, Derfler K, Stockenhuber F, et al. Effect of calcium-channel blockers on renal function in renal graft recipients treated with cyclosporine. N Engl J Med 1991;324:1517.
64. Weir MR. Therapeutic benefits of calcium channel blockers in cyclosporine-treated organ transplant recipients: blood pressure control and immuno-suppression. Am J Med 1991;90(5A):32S–36S.
65. Smith CL, Hampton EM, Pederson JA, et al. Clinical and medicoeconomic impact of the cyclosporine-diltiazem interaction in renal transplant recipients. Pharmacotherapy 1994;14:471–481.
66. Patton PR, Brunson ME, Pfaff WW, et al. A preliminary report of diltiazem and ketoconazole. Their cyclosporine-sparing effect and impact on transplant outcome. Transplantation 1994;57:889–892.
67. Shennib H, Auger JL. Diltiazem improves cyclosporine dosage in cystic fibrosis lung transplant recipients. J Heart Lung Transplant 1994;13:292–296.
68. Xioshan R, Flowers J, Warty SW, Venkataramahan R. Drug interactions with FK506. Pharm Res 1992;9(suppl 10):S314.
69. Jaracz E. Fujisawa Inc. Personal communication.
70. Henricsson S, Lindholm A. Inhibition of cyclosporine metabolism by other drugs in vitro. Transplant Proc 1988;20(suppl 2):569–571.
71. Curtis JJ, Luke RG, Whelchel JD, et al. Inhibition of angiotensin-converting enzyme in renal-transplant recipients with hypertension. N Engl J Med 1983;308:377–381.
72. Hays R, Aquino A, Lee BB, et al. Captopril-induced acute renal failure in a kidney transplant recipient. Clin Nephrol 1983;19:320–321.
73. van der Woude FJ, van Son WJ, Tegzess AM, et al. Effect of captopril on blood pressure and renal function in patients with transplant renal artery stenosis. Nephron 1985;39:184–188.

74. Curtis JJ, Laskow DA, Jones PA, et al. Captopril induced fall in glomerular filtration rate in cyclosporine treated hypertensive patients. J Am Soc Nephrol 1993;3:1570–1574.
75. Mourad G, Ribstein J, Mimran A. Converting enzyme inhibitor versus calcium antagonist in cyclosporine treated renal transplants. Kidney Int 1993;43:419–425.
76. Leeman M, Vereerstraeten P, Uytdenhoef M, Degaute JP. Systemic and renal hemodynamic responses to carvedilol and metoprolol in hypertensive renal transplant patients. J Cardiovasc Pharmacol 1993;22:706–710.
77. Curtis JR, Bateman FJ. Use of prazosin in management of hypertension in patients with chronic renal failure and in renal transplant recipients. BMJ 1975;4:432–434.
78. Becker AE, Becker MG, Martin FH, Edwards JC. Bland thrombosis and infection in relation to intracardiac catheters. Circulation 1972;4–6:200–203.
79. Egawa H, Woodley S, Keeffe EB, et al. Aortic valve endocarditis after orthotopic liver transplantation. Transplantation 1994;58:732–733.
80. Welty FK, McLeod GX, Ezratty C, et al. Pseudallescheria Boydii endocarditis of the pulmonic valve in a liver transplant recipient. Clin Infect Dis 1992;15:858–860.
81. Baddour LM. Production and progress of endocarditis in rabbits. Br J Exp Pathol 1973;54:142–156.
82. Lopez JA, Ross RS, Fishbein MC, Siegal RJ. Nonbacterial thrombotic endocarditis, a review. Am Heart J 1987;113:773–776.
83. Ferguson DJP, McColm AA, Savage TJ. A morphologic study of experimental rabbit staphylococcal endocarditis and aortitis. Br J Exp Pathol 1986;67:667–678.
84. David CA, Horowitz MD, Burke GW. Aortic valve endocarditis in a liver transplant recipient-successful management by aortic valve replacement. Transplantation 1992;53:1366–1367.
85. Walsh TJ, Hutchins GM, Bulkley BH, Mendelsohn G. Fungal infections of the heart: analysis of 51 autopsy cases. Am J Cardiol 1980;45:357–366.
86. Everett ED, Hirschmann JV. Transient bacteremia and endocarditis prophylaxis, a review. Medicine 1987;56:61–82.
87. Skerl KG, Calderone R, Segal E. In vitro binding of *Candida albicans* T-cells to human fibronectin. Can J Microbiol 1984;30:221–226.
88. Woods GL, Wood RP, Shaw BW. *Aspergillus* endocarditis in patients without prior cardiovascular surgery: report of a case in a liver transplant recipient and review. Rev Infect Dis 1989;11:263–272.
89. Penn I. Tumors of the immunocompromised patient. Ann Rev Med 1988;39:63–77.
90. Rheeder P, Simpson IW, Mentis H, Karusseit VO. Cardiac rhabdomyosarcoma in a renal transplant patient. Transplantation 1995;60:204–205.
91. Case records of the Massachusetts General Hospital. Weekly clinicopathological exercises. Case 4-1985. A 36-year-old man with a cardiac mass three years after renal transplantation. N Engl J Med 1985;312:226–237.
92. Rodenburg CJ, Kluin P, Maes A, Paul LC. Malignant lymphoma confined to the heart, 13 years after a cadaver kidney transplant. N Engl J Med 1985;313:122.
93. Reynen K, Bachmann K, Weber M, et al. Right ventricular metastasis of renal cell carcinoma 10 years after kidney transplantation. Z Kardiol 1995;84(2):163–168. German.
94. Flipse TR, Tazelaar HD, Holmes DR Jr. Diagnosis of malignant cardiac disease by endomyocardial biopsy. Mayo Clin Proc 1990;65:1415–1422.
95. Schweitzer EJ, Matas AJ, Gillingham KJ. Causes of renal allograft loss: progress in the 1980s, challenges for the 1990s. Ann Surg 1991;214:679–688.
96. Mahony JF. Long-term results and complications of transplantation: the kidney. Transplant Proc 1989;21:1433–1434.
97. Kasiske BL, Guijarro C, Massy ZA, et al. Cardiovascular disease after renal transplantation. J Am Soc Nephrol 1996;7:158–165.
98. Parfrey PS, Harnett JD, Foley RN, et al. Impact of renal transplantation on uremic cardiomyopathy. Transplantation 1995;60:908–914.
99. Bradley RF, Schonfeld A. Diminished pain in diabetic patients with acute myocardial infarction. Geriatrics 1962;17:322–326.
100. Weinrauch LA, D'Elia JA, Healy RW, et al. Asymptomatic coronary artery disease: angiography in diabetic patients before renal transplantation. Ann Int Med 1978;88:346–348.
101. Langer A, Freeman MR, Josse RG, et al. Coronary artery disease: detection of silent myocardial ischemia in diabetes mellitus. Am J Cardiol 1991;16:1073–1077.
102. Anderson KM, Wilson PWF, Odel PM, Kannel WB. An updated coronary risk profile: a statement for health professionals. Circulation 1991;83:356–362.
103. Manske CL, Thomas W, Wang Y, Wilson RF. Screening diabetic transplant candidates for coronary artery disease: identification of a low risk subgroup. Kidney Int 1993;44:617–621.
104. Melissinos K, Delidou A, Grammeno US, Markopoulos P. Study of the activity of lymphocyte adenosine deaminase in chronic renal failure. Clin Chim Acta. 1983;135:9–12.
105. Marwe TH, Cook SA, Lafont A, et al. Influence of left ventricular mass on the diagnostic accuracy of myocardial perfusion imaging using positron emission tomography with dipyridamole stress. J Nucl Med 1991;32:2221–2228.
106. Nally J, Mairesse G, Grimm R. Dobutamine echocardiography is an effective screening tool for coronary artery disease in ESRD. J Am Soc Nephrol 1993;4:255.
107. Cotaliercio CP, Vlietstra RE, Ilstrup DM, et al. A randomized comparison of the nephrotoxicity of iopamidol and diatrizoate in high risk patients undergoing cardiac angiography. J Am Coll Cardiol 1991;17:384–390.
108. Brown KA, Rimmer J, Haisch C. Noninvasive cardiac risk stratification of diabetic and nondiabetic uremic renal allograft candidates using dipyridamole-thallium-201 imaging and radionuclide ventriculography. Am J Cardiol 1989;64:1017–1021.
109. Le A, Wilson R, Douek K, et al. Prospective risk stratification in renal transplant candidates for cardiac death. Am J Kidney Dis 1994;24:65–71.
110. Ramsay MAE, Simpson BR, Nguyen AT, et al. Severe pulmonary hypertension in liver transplant candidates. Liver Transplant Surg 1997;3:494–500.
111. Robatino BD, Moodie DS. Association between primary pulmonary hypertension and portal hypertension: analysis of its clinical, laboratory and hemodynamic manifestations. J Am Coll Cardiol 1991;17:492–498.
112. Hadengue A, Behnayoun MK, Lebrec D. Pulmonary hypertension complicating portal hypertension, prevalence and relation to splanchnic hemodynamics. Gastroenterology 1991;100:520–526.
113. Castro M, Krowka MJ, Schroder DR, et al. Frequency and clinical implications of increased pulmonary artery pressures in liver transplant patients. Mayo Clin Proc 1996;71:543–551.
114. Praeger MC, Cauldwell CA, Ascher NL. Pulmonary hypertension associated with liver disease is not reversible after liver transplantation. Anesthesiology 1992;77:375–378.
115. Kuo PC, Johnan LB, Plotkin JS, et al. Continuous intravenous infusion of epoprostenol for the treatment of portopulmonary hypertension. Transplantation 1997;63:604–606.
116. Cockrill BA, Kacmarek R, Thompson BT, et al. Nitric oxide is a selective pulmonary vasodilator in patients with pulmonary vascular disease. J Am Coll Cardiol 1993;21:368A.
117. Mendell MS, Duke J. Nitric oxide reduces pulmonary hypertension during hepatic transplantation. Anesthesiology 1994;81:1538.
118. Blendis LM. Circulation in liver disease. Transplant Proc 1993;25:1741–1743.
119. Nasraway SA, Klein RD, Spanier TB, et al. Hemodynamic correlates of outcome in patients undergoing orthotopic liver transplantation. Chest 1995;107:218–224.
120. Ahmed SS, Howard M, ten Hove W, et al. Cardiac function in alcoholics with cirrhosis: absence of overt cardiomyopathy—myth or fact? J Am Coll Cardiol 1984;3:696–702.
121. Kelbaek H, Eriksen J, Brynjolf I, et al. Cardiac performance in patients with asymptomatic alcoholic cirrhosis of the liver. Am J Cardiol 1984;54:852–855.
122. Dec GW, Kondo N, Farrell ML, et al. Cardiovascular complications following liver transplantation. Clin Transplant 1995;9:463–467.
123. Farrell FJ, Nguyen M, Woodley S, et al. Outcome of liver transplantation in patients with hemochromatosis. Hepatology 1994;20:404–410.
124. Westra WH, Hruban RH, Baughman KL, et al. Progressive hemochromatic cardiomyopathy despite reversal of iron deposition after liver transplantation. Am J Clin Pathol 1993;99:39–44.
125. Gore JM, Fallon JT. Case records of the Massachusetts General Hospital: weekly clinicopathological exercises: case 31-1994: a 25-year-old man with the recent onset of diabetes mellitus and congestive heart failure. N Engl J Med 1994;331:460–466.
126. Starzl TE, Demetris AJ, Trucco M, et al. Chimerism after liver transplantation for type IV glycogen storage disease and type 1 Gaucher's disease. N Engl J Med 1993;328:745–749.
127. Holmgren G, Ericzon BG, Groth CG, et al. Clinical improvement and amyloid regression after liver transplantation in hereditary transthyretin amyloidosis. Lancet 1993;341:1113–1116.
128. Hongo M, Ikeda SI. Echocardiographic assessment of the evolution of amyloid heart disease: a study with familial amyloid polyneuropathy. Circulation 1986;73:249–256.
129. Kinoshita O, Hongo M, Yamada H. Impaired left ventricular diastolic filling in patients with familial amyloid polyneuropathy: a pulsed Doppler echocardiographic study. Br Heart J 1989;61:198–203.

130. Pellikka PA, Holmes DR Jr, Edwards WD, et al. Endomyocardial biopsy in 30 patients with primary amyloidosis and suspected cardiac involvement. Arch Int Med 1988;148:662–666.
131. Valdivielso P, Escolar JL, Cuervas-Mons V, et al. Lipids and lipoprotein changes after heart and liver transplantation in a patient with homozygous familial hypercholesterolemia. Ann Intern Med 1988;108:204–206.
132. Carey WD, Dumot JA, Pimental RR, et al. The prevalence of coronary artery disease in liver transplant candidates over age 50. Transplantation 1995:59;859–864.
133. Kupari M, Volin L, Suokas A, et al. Cardiac involvement in bone marrow transplantation: serial changes in left ventricular size, mass and performance. J Int Med 1990;227:259–266.
134. Goldberg MA, Antin JH, Guinan EC, Rappeport JA. Cyclophosphamide cardiotoxicity: an analysis of dosing as a risk factor. Blood 1986;68:1114–1118.
135. Styler MJ, Topolsky DL, Crilley PA, et al. Transient high grade heart block following autologous bone marrow infusion. Bone Marrow Transplant 1992;10:435–438.
136. Keung YK, Lau S, Elkayam U, et al. Cardiac arrhythmia after infusion of cryopreserved stem cells. Bone Marrow Transplant 1994;14:363–367.
137. Shlafer M. Cardiac pharmacology of dimethylsulfoxide and its postulated relevance to organ preservation in ischemic or hypoxic states. Ann NY Acad Sci 1983;411:170–179.
138. Kotler TS, Diamond GA. Exercise thallium 201 scintigraphy in the diagnosis and prognosis of coronary artery disease. Ann Intern Med 1990;113:684–702.
139. Holley JL, Fenton RA, Arthur RS. Thallium stress testing does not predict cardiovascular risk in diabetic patients with end-stage renal disease undergoing cadaveric renal transplantation. Am J Med 1991;90:563–570.
140. Go RT, Marwick TH, Macintyre WJ, et al. A prospective comparison of rubidium 82 PET and thallium 201 SPECT myocardial perfusion imaging in detecting coronary artery disease. J Nucl Med 1990;31:1899–1905.
141. Marwick TH, Steinmuller DR, Uderwood DA, et al. Ineffectiveness of dipyridamole Spect thallium imaging as a screening technique for coronary artery disease in patients with end-stage renal disease. Transplantation 1989;49:100–103.
142. Coyne EP, Belvedere DA, Vandestreek PR, et al. Thallium 201 scintography after intravenous infusion of adenosine compared with exercise thallium testing in the diagnosis of coronary artery disease. J Am Coll Cardiol 1991;17:1289–1294.
143. Marwick TH, Cook SA, Lafont A, et al. Influence of left ventricular mass on the diagnostic accuracy of myocardial perfusion imaging using positron emission tomography with dipyridamole stress. J Nucl Med 1991;32:2224–2228.
144. Mazeika P, Nihoyannopoulos P, Joshi J, Oakley CM. Uses and limitations of high dose dipyridamole stress echocardiography for evaluation of coronary artery disease. Br Heart J 1992;67:144–149.

Chapter

31

Endocrine and Metabolic Considerations of Organ Transplantation

Maria A. Rodino Neil Shachter Elizabeth Shane

Organ transplant recipients manifest a variety of endocrinologic and metabolic abnormalities. While some of these antedate transplantation as they are associated with chronic illness in general or factors unique to the patient's underlying disease, most are direct effects of immunosuppressive therapy. This chapter focuses on several disturbances that commonly develop in the post-transplant period (Table 31.1).

HYPERLIPIDEMIA

Background

An increase in occlusive vascular disease is commonly observed in the post-transplant setting. After rejection and infection, coronary artery disease (CAD) is one of the common conditions limiting survival after solid organ transplantation.

Etiology and Pathogenesis

The etiology and pathogenesis of arteriosclerosis after cardiac transplantation are incompletely understood and most likely multifactorial (see Chapter 23). The pathology of the arterial lesions is distinct from typical coronary artery atherosclerosis and involves a uniform intimal thickening without lipid accumulation (1). However, despite the absence of lipid accumulation, the conventional lipid risk factors (Table 31.2) of elevated cholesterol and triglycerides and obesity have been shown to be highly predictive of the development of these lesions (2,3), regardless of whether patients were transplanted for ischemic or nonischemic cardiomyopathy (4). Furthermore, hypercholesterolemia is observed in 60% to 80% of cardiac transplant recipients (5). Increased levels of lipoprotein(a), a form of low-density lipoprotein (LDL) in which the structural protein apoB is covalently linked to another protein apo(a), have also been associated with CAD in cardiac transplant recipients (4).

Hyperlipidemia is also commonly observed after renal transplantation. Pretransplant hypercholesterolemia is associated with a greater risk of graft loss, and post-transplant hypercholesterolemia has been strongly associated with lower glomerular filtration rate (GFR) and more pronounced albuminuria (6). Although hypertriglyceridemia is proposed by some to be a strong independent predictor of graft failure (7), others do not find a correlation between cardiovascular risk factors and chronic rejection (8). The importance of dyslipidemia in renal transplant recipients is underscored by the observations that cardiovascular disease is now the major cause of death in this population (9), and hyperlipidemic renal transplant recipients have markedly increased carotid atherosclerosis (10).

The etiology of hyperlipidemia in the post-transplant setting is related to the use of cyclosporine (11,12). Triglycerides and Lp(a) levels were significantly higher, and high-density lipoprotein (HDL) cholesterol levels lower, in cyclosporine-treated renal transplant patients compared to those treated with azathioprine (11). In contrast, prednisone withdrawal led to increased triglycerides and decreased HDL, though these changes may have been exacerbated by the development of central obesity related to corticosteroid therapy (11). Brattström et al (13) recently reported that long-term treatment with sirolimus in combination with cyclosporine and corticosteroids may increase the risk of hypertriglyceridemia. Cyclosporine blood levels have been shown to correlate directly with total plasma cholesterol, LDL cholesterol, and apoB; they correlate inversely with HDL cholesterol and apoA-I (the anti-atherogenic protein component of HDL). Moreover, highly significant correlations with the total cholesterol/HDL ratio and cyclosporine

Table 31.1. Endocrine and Metabolic Complications of Organ Transplantation

Hyperlipidemia
Diabetes mellitus
Osteoporosis
Avascular necrosis
Hypogonadism

Table 31.2. Risk Factors for Coronary Artery Disease After Organ Transplantation

Elevated total cholesterol
Elevated triglycerides
Low HDL
Elevated lipoprotein(a)
Obesity

levels have been reported (12). Triglyceride levels did not correlate with cyclosporine levels in this study (12). These correlations were independent of other determinants of plasma lipid levels in stepwise regression analysis. Direct pro-atherogenic effects of cyclosporine, independent of dyslipidemia, have also been observed in experimental systems (14).

Prevention and Management

The benefits of cholesterol reduction in patients with coronary artery disease and in high-risk patients without established coronary artery disease are well established. All-cause mortality is markedly and significantly reduced owing to a dramatic reduction in coronary end points (15,16). No randomized trial has examined the issue of treatment of hyperlipidemia in renal transplant recipients with regard to clinical end points. However, the benefit of treatment of hyperlipidemia in heart transplant recipients has been defined recently by Kobashigawa et al in a randomized trial of 97 patients using the 3-hydroxy-3-methylglutaryl coenzyme A (HMG-CoA) reductase inhibitor pravastatin (17). Pravastatin, at doses of 20–40 mg daily, was well tolerated and produced a 22% lowering of total plasma cholesterol. There was no change in the number of episodes of rejection, but there was a dramatic reduction in episodes of rejection associated with hemodynamic compromise, as well as a marked improvement in survival. There was also a lower incidence of coronary vasculopathy, as determined by angiography or intravascular ultrasound. The mechanism of this effect is most likely related to cholesterol reduction. However, a significant decrease was noted in the cytotoxicity of natural killer cells, suggesting that an immunologic mechanism may contribute to the effectiveness of this intervention. Despite the potential for rhabdomyolysis in patients receiving HMG-CoA reductase inhibitors together with cyclosporine, no elevations of creatine kinase, transaminases, myositis, or rhabdomyolysis were documented over the 12-month study.

Table 31.3. Management of Hyperlipidemia After Organ Transplantation

Diet
HMG-CoA reductase inhibitors
Bile acid sequestrants

The therapeutic approach to hyperlipidemic post-transplant patients differs only slightly from standard recommendations (Table 31.3) (18). HMG-CoA reductase inhibitors are currently the first line of therapy for hypercholesterolemia, and all currently available HMG-CoA reductase inhibitors have been shown to be safe in transplant recipients taking cyclosporine (19,20). Blood levels of these drugs are higher, so it is generally recommended that doses be restricted to the lower end of the recommended dosing range (21).

Bile acid sequestrants (cholestyramine, colestipol), which may have side effects of constipation and bloating, are now often limited to combination regimens with HMG-CoA reductase inhibitors, with which they have fully additive effects. They have not been extensively used in transplant patients because of concern that they may interfere with the absorption of other drugs, particularly cyclosporine. In this regard, the pharmacokinetics of cyclosporine have been investigated in a small number of patients administered cholestyramine. Although no differences were observed (22), standard recommendations to administer other drugs at the beginning and end of the day and the bile acid sequestrant in the middle of the day still apply.

It has been suggested that the triglyceride-lowering drug gemfibrozil may have the potential for harmful interaction with cyclosporine (10). Niacin has been used to treat hypertriglyceridemia in patients on cyclosporine, though patients should be followed for evidence of rhabdomyolysis or myositis.

DIABETES MELLITUS

Background

In the past three decades, diabetes mellitus (DM) has emerged as a significant problem after organ transplantation. The first report of "steroid diabetes" in previously nondiabetic renal transplant patients appeared in 1964 (23). Since then, there have been several other reports of new onset diabetes mellitus in transplant recipients treated with other immunosuppressive regimens.

Incidence

The reported incidence of post-transplant diabetes mellitus (PTDM) has varied widely (from 2% to 46%), largely due

Table 31.4. Diagnosis of Diabetes Mellitus in Adults: World Health Organization Criteria

Fasting blood glucose >140 mg/dL on two or more occasions
Random plasma glucose >200 mg/dL with symptoms (polydipsia, polyuria, weight loss, etc)
Plasma glucose >200 mg/dL both at 2 hours and at some other time between 0 and 2 hours after an oral tolerance test with a 75-g glucose load

to variations in the criteria used to define DM after transplantation (24). Some investigators have followed the World Health Organization criteria (Table 31.4) (25) used to identify diabetes in the general adult population; others have defined their own standards (26). WHO criteria are probably the most sensitive means of diagnosing PTDM in transplant recipients.

Etiology and Pathogenesis

The onset of diabetes mellitus after organ transplantation is related to immunosuppressive therapy. Endogenous glucocorticoid excess is a well-known cause of impaired glucose tolerance. Soon after the introduction of corticosteroids as therapeutic agents, it became evident that exogenous glucocorticoids also cause DM in predisposed individuals (27). Most authorities agree that insulin resistance is the major cause of steroid-induced DM (26). Glucocorticoids impair both hepatic and extrahepatic actions of insulin, probably at the postreceptor level as neither binding of insulin to its receptor nor the number of insulin receptors is affected by glucocorticoid administration (28). Furthermore, in addition to insulin resistance, Ekstrand et al demonstrated impaired first-phase, second-phase, and glucagon-mediated insulin secretion in their PTDM patients (29). However, some of these patients were also receiving cyclosporine, which itself has been shown to impair insulin secretion.

In 1985, Yamamoto and co-workers noted a striking increase in the incidence of PTDM when azathioprine was replaced by cyclosporine, despite reduced methylprednisolone dosage (30). Sakhuja et al also demonstrated a higher incidence of PTDM in patients receiving triple-drug immunosuppression (cyclosporine 3 mg/kg/d, azathioprine 2 mg/kg/d, and prednisolone 15 mg/d) than in those receiving conventional immunosuppression (prednisolone 10–15 mg/d and azathioprine 2.0–2.5 mg/kg/d) (31). Since then, several animal studies have demonstrated that cyclosporine interferes with glucose metabolism (see also Chapter 6). In the rat, cyclosporine accumulates in pancreatic islet cells causing decreased B-cell volume, diminished insulin secretion, and hyperglycemia (32). These effects are reversible with discontinuation of the drug (33). In addition, cyclosporine may potentiate the diabetogenic effects of glucocorticoids by decreasing their clearance, as both drugs are metabolized by the cytochrome P450 system (34).

Because of its steroid-sparing effects, tacrolimus was expected to reduce the incidence of PTDM. However, Krentz et al observed that glucose intolerance was more pronounced in liver transplant recipients treated with tacrolimus than in those treated with cyclosporine (35). Studies in several animal models have shown that tacrolimus has a direct toxic effect on pancreatic islet cells similar to that of cyclosporine (26). Nevertheless, further experience has shown that the tacrolimus dosages used in the early clinical trials were unnecessarily high. With more conservative therapy, this agent can be effectively used without an excessive risk of diabetes (see Chapter 9).

Clinical Features

PTDM has been best characterized in renal transplant recipients. Risk factors for PTDM in these patients include obesity, older age, first-degree relative with non-insulin-dependent diabetes, and cadaveric transplant (24). The development of PTDM appears to be dose related, with low-dose steroid regimens (20 mg prednisone per day, immediately postoperatively) associated with a lower incidence of PTDM (36). The incidence of PTDM is not related to original renal disease, number of rejection episodes, or graft function (24).

The peak onset of PTDM in renal transplant recipients is during the first year after transplantation, particularly the first 2 to 3 months. The majority of patients are asymptomatic at presentation and are found to be hyperglycemic on routine blood testing. Approximately 40% to 50% of patients ultimately require insulin therapy (31).

Prevention and Management

Although there have been no long-term studies on the effects of PTDM on the cardiovascular system, nervous system, kidney, and retina, it is reasonable to assume that these would be similar to those encountered in the general diabetic population. The widely reported results of the Diabetes Control and Complications Trial (37) have demonstrated that tight glucose control can significantly reduce the risk of microvascular complications. Therefore, patients with PTDM should be closely monitored with measurements of blood glucose and glycosylated hemoglobin and tightly controlled with multiple daily injections of insulin if necessary.

In some patients, adequate glycemic control may be accomplished with oral hypoglycemic agents. However, because most of these compounds or their metabolites are partially excreted by the kidney, they may be undesirable in transplant recipients who often have fluctuating renal function. The exception is glipizide; although its metabolites are eliminated by the kidney, they are essentially inactive. However, glipizide does interfere with the metabolism of cyclosporine, so its use requires close monitoring of cyclosporine blood levels and possible reduction in dose (38).

Table 31.5. Management of Post-transplant Diabetes Mellitus

Patient education
Dietary management
Exercise
Insulin
Oral hypoglycemic agents (glipizide)
Screen for and treat microalbuminuria and hyperlipidemia
Regular ophthalmologic and podiatry examinations

In addition to glucose management, other measures are important to prevent diabetic complications in patients with PTDM. Urine should be screened for microalbuminuria (30–300 mg albumin/day), a predictor of diabetic nephropathy. Patients with microalbuminuria may be candidates for treatment with angiotensin-converting enzyme (ACE) inhibitors. A lipid profile should be obtained, and hyperlipidemia should be treated appropriately. Regular ophthalmology and podiatry examinations should be encouraged. Finally, patient education, particularly with regard to proper diet and exercise, should be the standard of care (Table 31.5).

OSTEOPOROSIS

Background

Osteoporosis is a disease characterized by low bone mass, resulting in an increased risk of fracture. In recent years, this disease has been recognized as an important public health problem in the United States. The majority of cases of osteoporosis result from postmenopausal estrogen deficiency and/or age-related bone loss and are classified as primary osteoporosis. Secondary causes of osteoporosis include a variety of endocrine disorders, genetic diseases, and medications, as well as conditions such as multiple myeloma, vitamin D deficiency, alcohol abuse, and chronic hepatic, renal, and pulmonary disease. Among secondary causes of osteoporosis, the most common is therapeutic use of corticosteroids (39).

Organ transplant recipients are at particular risk for developing osteoporosis. In part, this may be related to osteopenia that antedates transplantation. It could also be associated with disease of the transplanted organ, as well as with immobilization, poor nutrition, and exposure to medications that may cause bone loss. In addition, several of the drugs used to prevent rejection after transplantation have adverse effects on the skeleton.

Etiology and Pathogenesis

Glucocorticoids

Glucocorticoids are well known to cause osteoporosis. These agents suppress osteoblast function and inhibit bone formation; inhibit intestinal calcium absorption and stimulate renal calcium excretion, which may lead to secondary hyperparathyroidism and increased osteoclastic bone resorption; decrease the production of certain skeletal growth factors; and alter the hypothalamic-pituitary-gonadal axis, causing hypogonadism (40).

Bone loss occurs in most patients exposed to long-term, high-dose glucocorticoid therapy. Postmenopausal women, children, and patients over 50 years old are at greatest risk. The most rapid demineralization occurs during the first 12 to 18 months of therapy, with less rapid bone loss thereafter. The amount of bone loss is directly related to dose and duration of exposure: as little as 7.5–10.0 mg of prednisone daily or its equivalent may result in demineralization. Fracture prevalence varies from 30% to 50% (41).

Cyclosporines

Cyclosporines recently have been shown to affect bone and mineral metabolism in ways that could contribute to bone loss after transplantation. In the rat, Epstein and colleagues have consistently shown that the administration of doses comparable to, or somewhat higher than, those used in patients after organ transplantation is associated with profound bone loss (42,43). The bone loss is characterized histologically by increases in both bone resorption and bone formation, is partially reversible after the drug is discontinued, and can be prevented by agents that inhibit bone resorption (calcitonin, estrogen, bisphosphonates) (44,45). Because the most frequent clinical use of cyclosporine has been in association with glucocorticoids, its effects in human subjects have not been clearly defined. However, there are data suggesting that bone turnover is increased in patients managed with cyclosporine (46).

Tacrolimus (FK506)

Tacrolimus also causes bone loss in the rat model, accompanied by biochemical and histomorphometric alterations similar to those observed with cyclosporine (47). As is the case with cyclosporine, tacrolimus is generally used in conjunction with glucocorticoids, so its effects in humans have not been well defined. Although regimens that include tacrolimus generally permit less exposure to glucocorticoids, which in turn results in less bone loss, recent cross-sectional data suggest that the bone loss in cardiac transplant recipients treated with tacrolimus is similar to the loss in patients treated with cyclosporine (48).

Azathioprine

Short-term administration of azathioprine does not appear to influence bone volume (49).

Sirolimus (Rapamycin)

Although sirolimus is structurally similar to tacrolimus, it has had no direct adverse effects on bone in rat studies (50). However, in large doses, sirolimus caused hypogonadism that resulted in severe osteopenia with fractures (47).

Clinical Features

Kidney Transplantation

The majority of patients who undergo kidney transplantation have significant pretransplant bone disease. The type of renal osteodystrophy varies among individuals and may include hyperparathyroidism, with or without osteitis fibrosa; osteomalacia; low turnover or adynamic bone disease due to aluminum accumulation (or other as yet poorly understood factors); osteosclerosis, particularly of the vertebral bodies; and β-macroglobulin amyloidosis. Other factors that may affect skeletal integrity in patients with end-stage renal disease include hypogonadism, diseases such as systemic lupus erythematosus and diabetes mellitus, and drugs such as loop diuretics, aluminum-containing phosphate binders, glucocorticoids, or cyclosporine (47). Thus, many candidates for renal transplantation have already sustained significant bone loss.

Several studies have documented a decline in bone mineral density (BMD) following renal transplantation (51,52). The amount of bone loss varies from 6% to 18% and is greatest during the first 6 months after transplantation. Bone loss is most apparent at skeletal sites enriched with cancellous bone. The amount of bone loss and the incidence of fractures after renal transplantation may be somewhat less than observed in liver and cardiac transplantation. The reasons for this difference are unclear, but may be related to the lower doses of glucocorticoids and cyclosporine used for immunosuppression after kidney transplantation (53).

Cardiac Transplantation

Although end-stage cardiac disease has not been associated with a well-defined skeletal disorder, candidates for cardiac transplantation frequently have low BMD. Risk factors for osteopenia in patients with severe cardiac disease include tobacco and alcohol use, treatment with loop diuretics, physical inactivity, hypogonadism, dietary calcium and vitamin D deficiency, hepatic congestion, and prerenal azotemia due to diminished perfusion (47).

After cardiac transplantation, the majority of studies have documented that lumbar spine BMD declines by 8% to 10%, mainly during the first 6 months following transplantation (54,56). In addition, Shane et al have reported that femoral neck BMD continues to decline during the second half of the first post-transplant year (56). Bone loss essentially ceases after the initial year, and some authors have reported recovery of BMD during the second and third post-transplant years (56,57).

Fractures are a major cause of morbidity after cardiac transplantation (55,58). The incidence of fracture ranges from 5% to 36% (55,59). The fractures most commonly involve the spine and occur during the first 6 months after transplantation (Fig. 31.1). Women are at increased risk to sustain a fracture, perhaps because their pretransplant BMD is lower than men. However, even patients with normal pretransplant BMD fracture frequently (55). No pretransplant biochemical or densitometric measurement reliably predicts fracture in the individual patient.

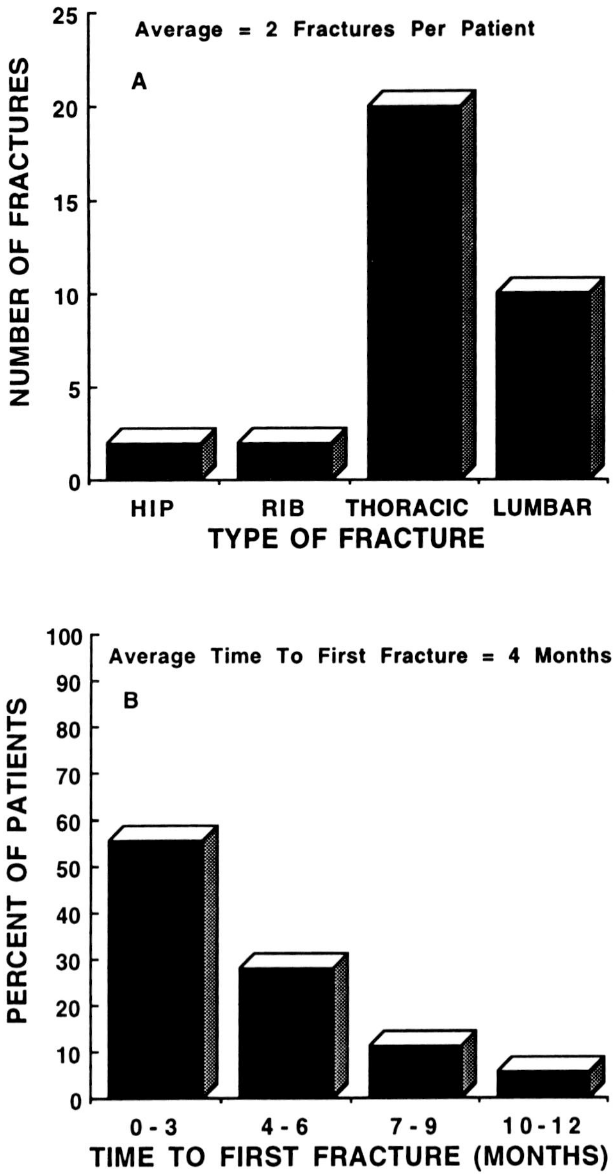

FIGURE 31.1. ***A.*** *Sites of fracture in men and postmenopausal women during the first year after cardiac transplantation. The most common site of fracture was the thoracolumbar spine.* ***B.*** *Time to first fracture in men and postmenopausal women during the initial year after cardiac transplantation. Among the patients who had fractures, 85% sustained the initial fracture within the first 6 months.*

Liver Transplantation

Patients with end-stage liver disease often have very severe osteoporosis that antedates transplantation (see Chapter 19). Chronic cholestatic liver diseases such as biliary cirrhosis are associated with severe osteoporosis, possibly related to selective impairment of osteoblast activity (60).

Patients with alcoholic cirrhosis may also have low bone mass prior to transplantation, likely related to hypogonadism and excess iron deposits in bone (61). Osteoporosis has also been described in patients with hemochromatosis (62) and steroid-treated autoimmune chronic active hepatitis (63).

Liver transplant recipients probably experience more bone loss and a higher incidence of fracture after transplantation than do renal or cardiac transplant patients (53). This may be because their dosages of immunosuppressive drugs are larger than those commonly employed for renal transplantation. In addition, pretransplant osteopenia may be more severe. Similar to cardiac and renal transplant recipients, in liver recipients the bone loss and fractures are concentrated during the initial 6 months of the first post-transplant year. Fracture incidence varies from 24% to 65% (47).

Lung Transplantation

Candidates for lung transplantation may also have severe osteoporosis (64,65). Glucocorticoid therapy in patients with chronic obstructive pulmonary disease and sarcoidosis is an important predisposing factor. Adults with cystic fibrosis also have low BMD (66). The etiology is multifactorial and includes hypogonadism, malnutrition, vitamin D deficiency, and possibly glucocorticoid therapy.

A cross-sectional study of lung transplant recipients indicates that vertebral fractures are also very common in this population (65). Moreover, sacral insufficiency fractures have also been reported after lung transplantation (67).

Bone Marrow and Pancreas Transplantation

Recipients of other common transplants such as bone marrow and pancreas may also be at risk for osteoporosis. However, little data has been published on these populations (68).

Prevention and Management

Pretransplant Evaluation

Because bone disease is common in patients awaiting renal, cardiac, liver, and lung transplantation, a skeletal evaluation should be performed prior to transplantation so that potentially reversible abnormalities may be addressed (Table 31.6). The history should emphasize risk factors for osteoporosis such as family history, thyroid and parathyroid disease, prolonged immobilization, dietary calcium deficiency, and drugs associated with bone loss. In women, premature menopause, postmenopausal status, and a history of anorexia nervosa or prolonged amenorrhea are important risk factors. In men, hypogonadism is a major cause of osteoporosis.

Despite observations that patients with normal pretransplant BMD fracture after transplant (55), studies in postmenopausal women have shown that risk of future fracture is greater in individuals with a prevalent vertebral fracture and in those with BMD measurements more than 2.5 standard deviations below peak normal bone mass. Therefore, the most important tests to obtain prior to transplantation are BMD of the spine and hip and plain radiographs of the thoracic and lumbar spine. Biochemical evaluation should include serum calcium, thyroid function tests, an intact parathyroid hormone level, a 25-hydroxyvitamin D level to assess body stores of vitamin D, and testosterone (in men). Markers of bone formation (bone-specific alkaline phosphatase, serum osteocalcin) and resorption (urinary pyridinium crosslinks, or N-telopeptides from collagen degradation) can also be measured, although they are primarily useful in the research setting.

Table 31.6. Pretransplant Osteoporosis Evaluation

1. History and physical examination with attention to risk factors for osteoporosis
2. Bone densitometry by dual energy x-ray absorptiometry
3. Thoracic and lumbar spine radiographs
4. Serum for calcium, parathyroid hormone, thyroid function tests, vitamin D metabolites, and testosterone
5. Urine for calcium and markers of bone resorption

During the pretransplant waiting period, physical therapy should be prescribed as tolerated. Patients should receive supplementation with the recommended daily allowance of vitamin D (400 IU) and elemental calcium (1000–1500 mg, depending on dietary intake and menopausal status). Hormone replacement should be considered in postmenopausal women and hypogonadal men without contraindications to such therapy. Patients in whom osteoporosis is diagnosed by pretransplant BMD measurements should be treated with antiresorptive therapy (hormone replacement, bisphosphonates, or calcitonin) prior to transplantation, according to standard medical practice.

Even very aggressive pharmacologic efforts to prevent bone loss and fractures may be ineffective in patients with extremely severe osteoporosis. Therefore, serious consideration should be given to the advisability of transplanting individuals with BMD measurements more than 3 to 4 standard deviations below the mean of a young normal population or those with multiple osteoporotic fractures.

Management After Transplantation

Recommendations for the treatment of transplantation osteoporosis are similar to those for other types of osteoporosis (Table 31.7). In general, preventing the bone loss that accompanies transplantation is more likely to be effective than treating established osteoporosis.

Pharmacologic strategies to prevent bone loss and fractures should be instituted as soon as is practical after transplantation, as these complications occur most commonly during the first year. Because there have been few controlled prospective studies that support any particular therapy for transplantation osteoporosis, the recommendations described here are based on experience with glucocorticoid-induced osteoporosis or on supportive experimental and clinical

Table 31.7. Approaches to Management of Osteoporosis After Organ Transplantation

General
Multivitamin
Calcium supplements
Exercise
Pharmacologic
Hormone replacement
Estrogen and progesterone
Testosterone
Inhibition of bone resorption
Calcitonin (nasal spray or injectable)
Bisphosphonates (etidronate, pamidronate, alendronate)
Bone-forming agents
Fluoride
Mechanism uncertain
Pharmacologic doses of vitamin D metabolites

evidence. Whether or not these therapies have important effects in immunity or other unique aspects of allograft function is not known.

Vitamin D Pharmacologic doses of vitamin D or its analogs are commonly recommended after transplantation. Vitamin D may be prescribed as the parent compound in doses of 50,000 IU once a week, as 25-hydroxycholecalciferol (calcidiol, 20–50 μg daily) (69), or as 1,25-dihydroxycholecalciferol (calcitriol, 0.25–0.75 μg daily). Calcitriol has been shown to prevent bone loss in patients treated with glucocorticoids (70), perhaps by overcoming the glucocorticoid-induced inhibition of gastrointestinal calcium absorption. Hypercalcemia and hypercalciuria are common side effects of therapy with these agents; thus, frequent monitoring of urinary and serum calcium is required. Vitamin D toxicity from calcitriol resolves more rapidly, because it is more polar than either parent vitamin D or calcidiol and there is less accumulation in body fat stores. Thus, calcitriol may be the preferred metabolite.

Hormone Replacement In postmenopausal women or premenopausal women with amenorrhea or irregular menses, estrogen replacement should be recommended provided that there are no contraindications. This recommendation is based on the observation that estrogen prevents cyclosporine-induced osteopenia in the oophorectomized rat (44). Moreover, a protective effect of estrogen and progesterone in women with glucocorticoid-induced osteoporosis (40) has also been described. Estrogen therapy may be administered orally or transdermally. Progesterone must also be prescribed to prevent endometrial cancer in patients with an intact uterus. Continuous, rather than cyclical, therapy is preferred after transplantation as estrogen enhances hepatic metabolism of cyclosporine (and presumably tacrolimus).

Hypogonadism is common in men with hepatic, renal, or cardiac failure (see below). In addition, high doses of both glucocorticoids and cyclosporine suppress the hypothalamic-pituitary-gonadal axis and produce hypogonadism. After successful transplantation, serum testosterone levels frequently normalize, but testosterone deficiency both before and after transplantation may contribute to bone loss and fractures (40). For this reason, some experts prescribe testosterone in men after transplantation.

Testosterone may be administered transdermally or as a long-acting depot injection. The potential risks of testosterone therapy include acceleration of hyperlipidemia in patients already prone to atherosclerosis from hypertension, diabetes, and/or glucocorticoid and cyclosporine therapy (47). In addition, prostatic hypertrophy and liver abnormalities are side effects of androgen therapy. These risks may be minimized by maintaining serum testosterone concentrations below 500 ng/dL. Monitoring should include measurement of serum lipids and hepatic enzymes monthly as well as regular prostate examinations. It is important to recognize that hypogonadism may be transient, lasting only a few weeks or months, and that there is a great deal of controversy surrounding the issue of hormone replacement therapy in this clinical situation.

Calcitonin Calcitonin has been used successfully in patients with glucocorticoid-induced osteopenia (71). Experimental work in the rat model has demonstrated that calcitonin can prevent cyclosporine-induced bone loss (45). Moreover, this drug may have an analgesic effect in patients with painful fractures. The usual dose is synthetic salmon calcitonin, 100 units daily by subcutaneous injection. Recently available is a new intranasally administered preparation; the dose is 200 units daily.

In a recent report, Grotz et al (72) concluded that cyclical treatment of osteopenia and osteoporosis with calcitonin after renal transplantation holds promise. These investigators found that calcitonin induced a gain in bone mineral density at the lumbar spine in patients with low bone mass after transplantation. However, the effect was small and not significantly different from the control group, which recovered bone density spontaneously. The authors noted that the major limitation of the study was the relatively small number of patients. Nonetheless, they identified no adverse effect on graft function and side effects were minimal.

Bisphosphonates Bisphosphonates have been shown to prevent glucocorticoid-induced bone loss (73). These compounds, including etidronate, pamidronate, tiludronate, and alendronate, act by inhibiting bone resorption and constitute a promising approach to the prevention and treatment of this form of osteoporosis. One study (74) has shown that bone loss after cardiac transplantation was largely prevented by administration of a single infusion of intravenous pamidronate (60 mg) within 2 weeks of transplantation followed by 1 year of cyclic etidronate (400 mg for the first 14 days of every third month). However, a recent study by Riemens et al suggested that bone loss and fractures occurred at rates similar to those in the literature despite therapy with cyclic etidronate, calcium, and calcitriol D (75).

Clinical trials are currently underway with other, more potent bisphosphonates. Preliminary data show, for example, an effect of clodronate similar to that described above for calcitonin (72).

Fluoride Fluoride therapy has been used extensively outside the United States to treat osteoporosis. Meunier et al have demonstrated that disodium monofluorophosphate, when administered to patients with glucocorticoid-induced osteoporosis, resulted in a 63% increase in trabecular bone mass (76). In an uncontrolled study of cardiac transplant recipients, Meys et al (69) showed that disodium monofluorophosphate, elemental calcium, and calcidiol resulted in an increase in bone mass compared with those patients receiving calcium and calcidiol alone. However, increases in BMD in response to fluoride therapy are not consistently associated with improvement in bone quality and strength or reduction in fracture rates.

AVASCULAR NECROSIS

Background

Avascular necrosis, which may also be referred to as aseptic, ischemic, or idiopathic necrosis, is a form of ischemic bone disease caused by regional interruption of blood flow to the skeleton (77). When ischemia is sufficiently severe and prolonged, death of bone and cartilage cells results. Avascular necrosis may be idiopathic or familial or may be associated with a variety of medical illnesses. Among the associated conditions are Cushing's syndrome and glucocorticoid therapy, alcohol abuse, gout, osteomalacia, and collagen vascular disorders. In addition, local trauma such as dislocation or fracture may ultimately result in avascular necrosis of the involved area. This is most commonly encountered in the femoral head after a fracture of the femoral neck or in dislocation of the femoral capital epiphysis.

Avascular necrosis of the femoral head was initially reported in renal transplant recipients in 1964 (78). Since that original description, avascular necrosis has become a well-recognized complication of renal transplantation (77). Early studies of renal transplant recipients with a minimum graft survival of 12 months put the prevalence of this complication at 11% to 18% (79–81). It is not clear whether the incidence lowered after 1980, when the introduction of cyclosporine permitted reduced exposure to glucocorticoids. In recent years reported rates have ranged from 4.5% to 20.2% (82–85). The prevalence rate of avascular necrosis after cardiac transplantation is 3% to 6% (86–88), and it has also been reported after liver (89) and bone marrow transplantation (90,91).

Etiology and Pathogenesis

Disruption of the microvasculature of the skeleton predisposes bone, particularly subchondral bone, to infarction. However, the pathogenesis of disrupted blood flow in nontraumatic avascular necrosis is not well understood. Some types of nontraumatic avascular necrosis (alcohol abuse, glucocorticoid therapy, Cushing's syndrome) appear to be associated with replacement of red marrow with fat, resulting in a corresponding decrease in marrow blood flow. Increased fat within the nondistensible marrow spaces may compress sinusoids and lead to infarction of bone. Fat embolization and hemorrhage at the sites of involvement predispose the patient to both nontraumatic and traumatic avascular necrosis. Similarly, avascular necrosis may develop at sites where there are underlying abnormalities in bone microarchitecture, such as the microfractures encountered in patients with osteoporosis or osteomalacia. Bone infarction is followed by revascularization and, in some cases, by resorption of necrotic bone with reparative new bone formation upon the surfaces of infarcted trabeculae. These processes of skeletal death and repair may be occurring simultaneously in different areas within an affected site.

Clinical Features

Avascular necrosis may develop at any time after transplantation. Pain is the predominant symptom of early avascular necrosis, although the condition may also be asymptomatic (77). The pain is of a nagging quality, is often not related to weight bearing, and may be particularly troublesome at night. It may persist indefinitely or resolve spontaneously. Over time, the changes of skeletal disintegration and repair may result in increased risk of fracture and ultimately in arthritis secondary to joint deformation.

The specific symptoms depend on the age of the patient, the site of involvement, and the size of the compromised region. Several studies have addressed the risk factors for avascular necrosis in transplant recipients. Direct associations have been reported with glucocorticoid exposure, cyclosporine, the number of transplants, the presence of hyperparathyroidism, low bone mass, and fractures (81).

The radiologic features of avascular necrosis vary, depending on when the films are taken relative to the onset of symptoms and the relative prominence of necrosis, revascularization, deposition of new and resorption of infarcted bone, joint deformation, and collapse. Plain radiographs are of limited usefulness in the diagnosis of early avascular necrosis. Changes in the density of necrotic bone do not appear before 10 to 14 days, and radiolucent bands from revascularization and resorption of infarcted bone are often not visible for 6 to 8 weeks (77). Bone scintigraphy with technetium 99m diphosphonate can detect avascular necrosis before changes become apparent on plain radiographs; tracer accumulation in the infarcted region is decreased before and increased after revascularization occurs. Magnetic resonance imaging (MRI) is the most sensitive test for detecting early avascular necrosis; computed tomography (CT) is particularly useful for the femoral head.

Management

Therapy of avascular necrosis varies according to site of involvement, the size of the lesion, and the degree of disability. At present there is no effective medical therapy. Osteonecrosis of the femoral head has received the most attention, perhaps because it is the most common site of involvement and the sequelae can be associated with significant disability.

When there is collapse of the femoral head or disabling pain requiring use of crutches or a wheelchair, total hip arthroplasty may be the only effective therapy. Unfortunately, many transplant recipients are young relative to the typical candidate for joint replacement, and prosthetic hips have a finite life span with an actuarial 10-year revision-free interval of only 78%.

Precollapse osteonecrosis may be treated by either observation or surgical intervention. As results of surgery are considered by some to be favorable in earlier stages of disease, some recommend intervention as soon as the disease is diagnosed. However, recent reports of an early reversible stage of avascular necrosis raise the question of whether all patients with MRI changes require surgical intervention (83,92–94). Moreover, the optimal surgical procedure remains controversial.

The most widely studied procedure is core decompression, in which a cylindrical core of bone is removed from the femoral head and neck, thereby reducing the elevated bone marrow pressure with improvement of blood flow. However, this procedure is variably successful and may weaken the structure of the femoral head, resulting in collapse (95,96). Other available procedures, such as bone grafting, electrical stimulation, and femoral osteotomy, have been less well studied.

GONADAL DYSFUNCTION

Background

Sexual function is controlled by the hypothalamic-pituitary-gonadal (HPG) axis. The hypothalamus produces gonadotropin-releasing hormone (GnRH), which is released into the hypophyseal-portal circulation and stimulates production of the gonadotropins, follicle-stimulating hormone (FSH), and luteinizing hormone (LH) by the anterior pituitary. In men, LH is responsible for testosterone production by the Leydig cells of the testes; in conjunction with testosterone, FSH stimulates spermatogenesis. In women, FSH stimulates growth of ovarian follicles and estrogen formation, while the surge in LH at midcycle triggers ovulation. Primary gonadal failure results in deficiencies in estrogen and testosterone, which in turn cause elevations in FSH and LH due to loss of negative feedback inhibition on the hypothalamus and pituitary. Hypothalamic and/or pituitary dysfunction, on the other hand, results in reduced levels of all hormones within this system.

It is difficult to generalize about the effects of organ transplantation on the hypothalamic-pituitary-gonadal axis. A variety of factors may be operative, including the extent of pretransplant gonadal dysfunction, the types and doses of immunosuppressive agents, and the degree of organ recovery after transplantation. It is also important to consider the effects of long-standing renal, hepatic, respiratory, and cardiac disease on the HPG axis.

Sexual dysfunction, particularly in men, is nearly universal in chronic renal failure. Uremia is associated with subnormal levels of testosterone and elevated levels of LH (97), impaired spermatogenesis (98), gynecomastia (97), and impotence (99). Women with severe renal failure frequently develop menstrual irregularities and loss of libido or orgasm. The rarity of pregnancy in both undialyzed and dialyzed uremic women suggests that anovulation is common, and this is confirmed by the absence of ovulatory surges of serum LH and luteal elevations of serum progesterone. Hypothalamic dysfunction is thought to be central to these problems (97,100).

In men, hepatic cirrhosis, including non-alcoholic forms, is classically associated with signs of hypogonadism and feminization such as testicular atrophy with loss of germ cells, impotence, reduced axillary and pubic hair, and gynecomastia. Specific hormonal abnormalities include decreased total and free testosterone levels, increased estrone and estradiol levels, and, except in severely ill patients, normal or elevated LH and FSH. These defects are believed to result from both primary testicular dysfunction and hypothalamic/pituitary dysfunction (101). In women, amenorrhea and infertility are frequent sequelae of chronic liver disease (102).

Men with chronic obstructive lung disease have been shown to suffer from a relative testosterone deficiency that correlates strongly with the degree of hypoxia (103). Whether hypoxia acts directly on the testis or suppresses the hypothalamic-pituitary axis is presently unknown. The effects of restrictive lung disease and cyanotic heart disease also await further study.

While formal studies of the effects of congestive heart failure (CHF) on sexual function are not available, it is well known that both chronic illness and acute myocardial infarction are associated with depression of the hypothalamic-pituitary axis (104). Moreover, a number of drugs used to treat cardiac disease adversely affect sexual function. Beta-blockers, methyldopa, and clofibrate have been associated with decreased libido and erectile dysfunction in men. Spironolactone has been shown to cause impotence in men and irregular menses or amenorrhea in women. Finally, long-term administration of digitalis may lead to gynecomastia in men and breast enlargement in women, probably due to its chemical similarity to gonadal hormones (105).

Etiology and Pathogenesis

Both glucocorticoids and cyclosporine have been shown to disturb gonadal function. In men, chronic administration of glucocorticoids has been associated with loss of libido and erectile dysfunction, lower plasma testosterone levels (106), and significant reduction in sperm count and motility (107). Even a single dose of intravenous hydrocortisone (100 mg) has been shown to reduce plasma testosterone (108), while as little as 30 mg of cortisol (7.5 mg prednisone) given orally suppresses the normal nocturnal rise in plasma testosterone. In men, glucocorticoids both alter hypothalamic GnRH secretion (106) and directly inhibit testicular LH receptor activity (109). Although fewer studies are available in women, chronic steroid use has been shown to cause menstrual abnormalities by altering anterior pituitary function, as demonstrated by a blunted LH response following administration of GnRH (110).

In animal studies, cyclosporine has been shown to suppress the HPG axis. Rajfer et al demonstrated that rats given 15 mg/kg/day of cyclosporine for 28 days had significant reductions in serum testosterone compared to controls with similar renal function, and that this effect was attributable to pituitary dysfunction (111). Seethalakshmi et al demonstrated similar hormonal suppression as well as a 50% reduction in sperm count and motility and a 60% reduction in fertility in rats treated with a much smaller dose of cyclosporine (1–2 mg/kg/d) (112). Although little is known about the effects of cyclosporine on human gonadal function, Rivas et al demonstrated a negative correlation between cyclosporine levels and serum testosterone concentrations in male heart transplant recipients (113). Such an effect may help explain why gynecomastia occurs with increased frequency in cyclosporine-treated patients (114), although the mechanism is still unknown. In women, hirsutism is a commonly observed side effect of cyclosporine, but this is thought to result from a direct effect of cyclosporine on hair follicles rather than on hormone levels (115).

Although azathioprine has been found to be teratogenic in mice, it does not appear to affect fertility in animals or humans (116). Lange et al noted no depression in spermatogenesis in men with chronic active hepatitis treated for over 4 years with up to 150 mg/day of this agent (117).

Clinical Features

Despite the effects of drug treatments, there is increasing evidence that sexual function actually improves after successful organ transplantation. Lim and Fang studied young adult men before and after renal transplantation (98). Prior to transplantation, these patients uniformly suffered from impotence, decreased libido, testosterone deficiency, and abnormally low sperm count and motility. Six months after transplantation, while these patients received on average 25 mg of prednisone and 150 mg of azathioprine daily, all of these abnormalities were reversed.

Samojlik et al studied renal transplant recipients receiving a triple-drug immunosuppression regimen that included cyclosporine. One month after transplantation, all hormone levels were suppressed. By 3 months the levels began to rise, and by 12 months they had normalized. The investigators concluded that cyclosporine (in doses sufficient to maintain serum concentrations of 150–250 ng/mL) with daily prednisone (at doses of 10 mg/day) does not suppress the HPG axis (118). However, Handelsman showed that gonadal function in men steadily improves but does not quite reach normal levels by 12 months after successful liver

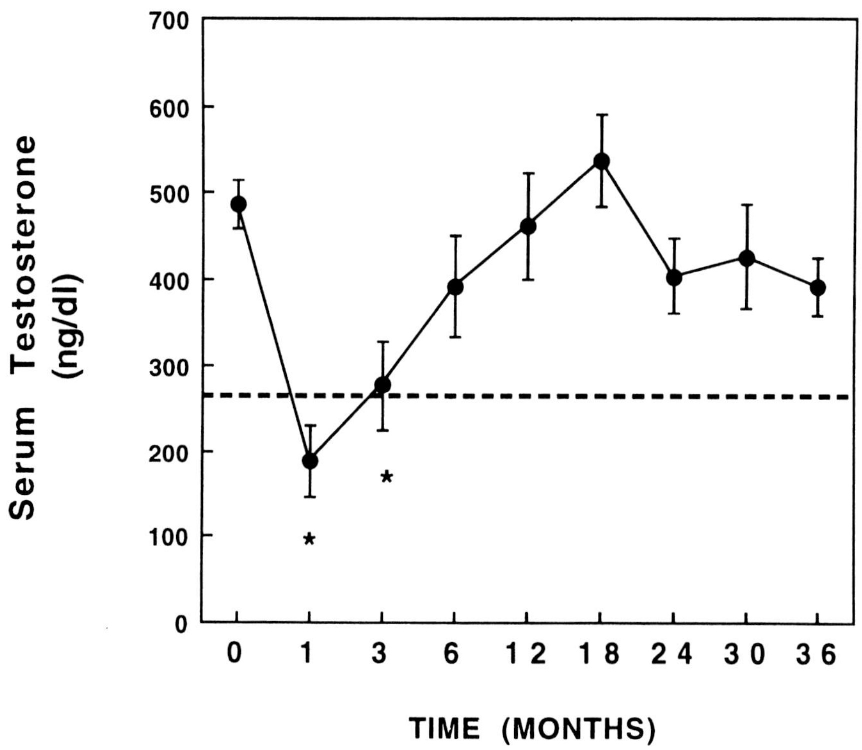

FIGURE 31.2. *Total serum testosterone concentrations in 52 men during the first three years after cardiac transplantation.*

transplantation when the patients were maintained on doses of 7.5 mg/day of prednisone, 50 mg/day of azathioprine, and 300 mg/day cyclosporine (119).

In two studies of heart transplant recipients receiving prednisone, azathioprine, and cyclosporine, testosterone levels diminished significantly in the first month following transplantation but returned to baseline by 3 months and remained at that level over the next 12 months (Fig. 31.2) (56,120). However, Rivas et al observed that by 2 years after cardiac transplantation approximately 25% of men had low serum testosterone levels (113).

Management

Perhaps because gonadal status frequently improves following successful organ transplantation, there are currently no well-established guidelines for hormonal replacement therapy in transplant recipients. Moreover, many experts disagree on the advisability of hormone replacement therapy early in the post-transplant period. Most authorities believe that postmenopausal women should receive hormone replacement therapy both before and after transplantation according to currently accepted guidelines. However, for premenopausal women and men, in whom hypogonadism is likely to be transient, the situation is less clear cut.

Hormonal replacement therapy, in addition to providing patients with a sense of sexual well-being, may be beneficial in a number of ways. Androgens increase lean body mass and hemoglobin levels, and both androgens and estrogens increase bone density—all of which may be reduced in chronically ill patients receiving immunosuppressive therapy (121). There is also evidence that testosterone enhances the immunosuppressive activity of cyclosporine, thus increasing graft survival time (122), and that estrogens raise HDL and lower LDL cholesterol. In contrast, high doses of androgens adversely affect serum lipid levels, which may have serious implications in a transplant population already prone to hyperlipidemia. In addition, estrogen/progesterone therapy has been shown to alter both glucocorticoid and cyclosporine metabolism (123).

Until the appropriate studies are performed, a reasonable approach might be to treat hypogonadal men and premenopausal women only if gonadal status does not improve following transplantation when their regimen has been tapered to minimal doses of steroids and cyclosporine. In contrast, all postmenopausal women, except those in whom obvious contraindications exist, should be considered for hormone replacement therapy. They will obviously remain hypogonadal, and the benefits of such therapy in the normal population have been clearly demonstrated. In women, constant daily dosing of estrogen and progesterone (rather than cyclic regimens) may result in fewer fluctuations in cyclosporine levels. In men treated with testosterone, maintaining serum testosterone at levels less than 500 ng/dL may help to avoid hyperlipidemia.

REFERENCES

1. Lin H, Wilson JE, Kendall TJ, et al. Comparable proximal and distal severity of intimal thickening and size of epicardial coronary arteries in transplant arteriopathy of human cardiac allografts. J Heart Lung Transplant 1994;13:824–833.
2. Eich D, Thompson JA, Ko D, et al. Hypercholesterolemia in long-term survivors of heart transplantation: an early marker of accelerated coronary artery disease. J Heart Lung Transplant 1991;10:45–49.
3. Winters GL, Kendall TJ, Radio SJ, et al. Posttransplant obesity and hyperlipidemia: major predictors of severity of coronary arteriopathy in failed human heart allografts. J Heart Lung Transplant 1990;9:364–371.
4. Barbir M, Kushwaha S, Hunt B, et al. Lipoprotein(a) and accelerated coronary artery disease in cardiac transplant recipients. Lancet 1992;340:1500–1502.
5. Miller LW, Schlant RC, Kobashigawa JA, et al. 24th Bethesda Conference: Cardiac Transplantation Task Force 5: complications. J Am Coll Cardiol 1993;22:41–54.
6. Dimeny E, Wahlberg J, Lithell H, Fellstrom B. Hyperlipidaemia in renal transplantation—risk factor for long-term graft outcome. Euro J Clin Invest 1995;25:574–583.
7. Guijarro C, Massy ZA, Kasiske BL. Clinical correlation between renal allograft failure and hyperlipidemia. Kidney Int 1995;52:S56–S59.
8. Hegemann RL, Hunzicker LG. Chronic rejection in renal allografts: importance of cardiovascular risk factors. Clin Transplant 1995;9:135–139.
9. Wanner C, Bartens W, Galle J. Clinical utility of antilipidemic therapies in chronic renal allograft failure. Kidney Int 1995;52:S60–S62.
10. Jogestrand T, Fehrman-Ekholm I, Angelin B, et al. Increased prevalence of atherosclerotic wall changes in patients with hyperlipidemia after renal transplantation. J Int Med 1996;239:177–180.
11. Hilbrands LB, Demacker PN, Hoitsma AJ, et al. The effects of cyclosporine and prednisone on serum lipid and (apo) lipoprotein levels in renal transplant recipients. J Am Soc Nephrol 1995;5:2073–2081.
12. Kuster GM, Drexel H, Bleisch JA, et al. Relation of cyclosporine blood levels to adverse effects on lipoproteins. Transplantation 1994;57:1479–1483.
13. Brattström C, Wilczek H, Tydén G, et al. Hyperlipidemia in renal transplant recipients treated with sirolimus (Rapamycin). Transplantation 1998;65:1272–1274.
14. Bellon JM, Bujan MJ, Jurado F, et al. Atherogenic effects of cyclosporine in an experimental model of arterial autograft. Transplantation 1995;60:407–414.
15. Scandinavian Simvastatin Survival Study Group. Randomised trial of cholesterol lowering in 4444 patients with coronary heart disease: the Scandinavian Simvastatin Survival Study (4S). Lancet 1994;344:1383–1389.
16. Shepherd J, Cobbe SM, Ford I, et al. Prevention of coronary heart disease with pravastatin in men with hypercholesterolemia. N Engl J Med 1995;333:1301–1307.
17. Kobashigawa JA, Katznelson S, Laks H, et al. Effect of pravastatin on outcomes after cardiac transplantation. N Engl J Med 1995;333:621–627.
18. Summary of the second report of the National Cholesterol Education Program (NCEP) expert panel on detection, evaluation, and treatment of high blood cholesterol in adults (Adult Treatment Panel II). JAMA 1993;269:3015–3023.
19. Traindl O, Reading S, Franz M, et al. Treatment of hyperlipidemic kidney graft recipients with lovastatin: effect on LDL-cholesterol and lipoprotein(a). Nephron 1992;62:394–398.
20. Martinez Hernandez BE, Persaud JW, Varghese Z, Moorhead JF. Low dose simvastatin is safe in hyperlipidemic renal transplant. Nephrol Dial Transplant 1993;8:637–641.
21. Cheung AK, DeVault GA Jr, Gregory MC. A prospective study on treatment of hypercholesterolemia with lovastatin in renal transplant patients receiving cyclosporine. J Am Soc Nephrol 1993;3:1884–1891.
22. Jensen RA, Lal SM, Diaz-Arias A, et al. Does cholestyramine interfere with cyclosporine absorption? A prospective study in renal transplant patients. ASAIO J 1995;41:M704–M706.
23. Starzl TE, Marchioro TL, Rifkin D, et al. Renal homotransplantation: late function and complications. Ann Int Med 1964;61:470–477.
24. Koselj M, Koselj KM, Kveder R. Posttransplant diabetes mellitus in renal allograft recipients. Transplant Proc 1992;24:2756–2757.
25. National Diabetes Data Group. Classification and diagnosis of diabetes mellitus and other categories of glucose intolerance. Diabetes 1979;28:1039–1057.
26. Jindal RM. Posttransplant diabetes mellitus—a review. Transplantation 1994;58:1289–1298.

27. Bookman JJ, Drachman SR, Schafer LE, Adlersberg D. Steroid diabetes in man: the development of diabetes during treatment with cortisone and corticotropin. Diabetes 1953;2:100.
28. Rizza RA, Mandarino LJ, Gerich JA. Cortisol-induced insulin resistance in man: impaired suppression of glucose production and stimulation of glucose utilization due to a postreceptor defect of insulin action. J Clin Endocrinol Metab 1982;54:131–138.
29. Ekstrand AV, Eriksson JG, Gronhagen-Riska C, et al. Insulin resistance and insulin deficiency in the pathogenesis of posttransplantation diabetes mellitus in man. Transplantation 1992;53:563–569.
30. Yamamoto H, Akazawa S, Yamaguchi Y, et al. Effects of cyclosporin A and low dosages of steroid on posttransplantation diabetes in kidney transplant recipients. Diabetes Care 1991;14:867–870.
31. Sakhuja V, Sharma UK, Jha V, et al. High incidence of posttransplant diabetes mellitus in renal transplant recipients on triple-drug immunosuppression. Transplant Proc 1995;27:2728–2730.
32. Hahn HJ, Dunger A, Laube F, et al. Toxic effects of cyclosporine on the endocrine pancreas of Wistar rats. Transplantation 1986;41:44–47.
33. Hahn HJ, Dunger A, Laube F, et al. Reversibility of the acute toxic effect of cyclosporin A on pancreatic B cells of Wistar rats. Diabetologia 1986;29:489–494.
34. Ost L. Effects of cyclosporin on prednisone metabolism. Lancet 1984;451.
35. Krentz AJ, Dousset B, Mayer D, et. al. Metabolic effects of cyclosporine A and FK-506 in liver transplant recipients. Diabetes 1993;42:1753–1759.
36. McGeown MG, Douglas JF, Brown WA, et al. Advantages of low dose steroid from the day after renal transplantation. Transplantation 1980;29:287–289.
37. DCCT Research Group. The effect of intensive treatment of diabetes on the development and progression of long-term complications in IDDM. N Engl J Med 1993;329:977–986.
38. Chidester PD, Connito DJ. Interaction between glipizide and cyclosporine: report of two cases. Transplant Proc 1993;25:2136–2137.
39. Tohme J, Cosman F, Lindsay R. Osteoporosis. In: Becker K. Principles and practice of endocrinology and metabolism. 2nd ed. Philadelphia: JB Lippincott, 1995:567–585.
40. Lukert BP. Glucocorticoid-induced osteoporosis. In Marcus R, Feldman D, Kelsey J, eds. Osteoporosis. New York: Academic Press, 1996:801–820.
41. Shane E, Epstein S. Immunosuppressive therapy and the skeleton. Trends Endocrinol Metabol 1994;5:169–175.
42. Movsowitz C, Epstein S, Fallon M, et al. Cyclosporin A in vivo produces severe osteopenia in the rat: effect of dose and duration of administration. Endocrinology 1988;123:2571–2572.
43. Schlosberg M, Movsowitz C, Epstein S, et al. The effects of cyclosporin A administration and its withdrawal on bone mineral metabolism in the rat. Endocrinology 1989;124:2179–2184.
44. Joffe I, Katz I, Jacobs T, et al. B-estradiol prevents osteopenia in the oophorectomized rat treated with cyclosporin A. Endocrinology 1992;130:578–586.
45. Stein B, Takizawa M, Katz I, et al. Salmon calcitonin prevents cyclosporin A induced high turnover bone loss. Endocrinology 1991;129:92–98.
46. Bourbigot B, Moal MC, Cleder J. Bone histology in renal transplant patients receiving cyclosporin. Lancet 1988;1:1048–1049.
47. Epstein S, Shane E. Transplantation osteoporosis. In: Marcus R, ed. Osteoporosis. San Diego, CA: Academic Press, 1996:947–957.
48. Stemple HU, Wehr U, Meiser B, et al. Effect of FK506 (tacrolimus) on trabecular bone loss shortly after cardiac transplantation. J Bone Miner Res 1996;11:5127A.
49. Bryer HP, Isserow JA, Armstrong EC, et al. Azathioprine alone is bone sparing and does not alter cyclosporine A induced osteopenia in the rat. J Bone Miner Res 1995;10:1–6.
50. Joffe I, Katz I, Sehgal S, et al. Lack of change of cancellous bone volume with short term use of the new immunosuppressant rapamycin in rats. Calcif Tissue Int 1993;53:45–52.
51. Julian BA, Laskow DA, Dubovsky J, et al. Rapid loss of vertebral bone density after renal transplantation. N Engl J Med 1991;325:544–550.
52. Horber FF, Casez JP, Steiger LL, et al. Changes in bone mass early after kidney transplantation. J Bone Miner Res 1994;9:1–9.
53. McDonald JA, Dunstan CR, Dilworth P, et al. Bone loss after liver transplantation. Hepatology 1991;14:613–619.
54. Rivas M, Kim TS, Staron RS, et al. Bone loss and fractures occur within 6 months of heart transplantation. J Bone Miner Res 1992;8:601A.
55. Shane E, Rivas M, Staron R, et al. Fracture after cardiac transplantation: a prospective longitudinal study. J Clin Endocrinol Metab 1996;81:1740–1746.
56. Shane E, Rivas M, McMahon DJ, et al. Bone loss and turnover after cardiac transplantation. J Clin Endocrinol Metab 1997; 82:1497–1506.
57. Henderson NK, Sambrook PN, Kelly PJ, et al. Bone mineral loss and recovery after cardiac transplantation. Lancet 1995;2:905.
58. Shane E, Rivas M, Silverberg S, et al. Osteoporosis after cardiac transplantation. Am J Med 1993;94:257–264.
59. Muchmore JS, Cooper DKC, Ye Y, et al. Loss of vertebral bone density in heart transplant patients. Transplant Proc 1991;23:1184–1185.
60. Hodgson SR, Dickson ER, Wahner HW, et al. Bone loss and reduced osteoblast function in primary biliary cirrhosis. Ann Int Med 1980;103:855–860.
61. Bikle DD, Genant MD, Conn C, et al. Bone disease in alcohol abuse. Ann Intern Med 1985;103:42–48.
62. Diamond T, Stiel D. Osteoporosis in hemochromatosis: iron excess, gonadal deficiency, or other factors? Ann Intern Med 1989;110:430–436.
63. Stellon AJ, Davies A, Compston J. Bone loss in autoimmune chronic active hepatitis on maintenance corticosteroid therapy. Gastroenterology 1985;89:1078–1083.
64. Shane E, Silverberg SJ, Donovan D, et al. Osteoporosis in lung transplantation patients with end-stage pulmonary disease. Am J Med 1996;101:262–269.
65. Aris R, Neuringer I, Weiner M, et al. Severe osteoporosis before and after lung transplantation. Chest 1996;109:1176–1183.
66. Bachrach LK, Loutit CW, Moss RB, Marcus R. Osteoporosis in adults with cystic fibrosis. Am J Med 1994;96:27–34.
67. Schulman LL, Addesso V, Staron RB, et al. Insufficiency fractures of the sacrum: a cause of low back pain after lung transplantation. J Heart Lung Transplant 1997;16:1081–1085.
68. Kelly PJ, Atkinson K, Ward RL, et al. Reduced bone mineral density in men and women with allogeneic bone marrow. Transplantation 1990;50:881–883.
69. Meys E, Terreaux-Duvert F, Beaume-Six T, et al. Effects of calcium, calcidiol, and monofluorophosphate on lumbar bone mass and parathyroid function in patients after cardiac transplantation. Osteoporosis Int 1993;3:329–332.
70. Sambrook PN, Birmingham J, Kelly P. Prevention of corticosteroid osteoporosis: a comparison of calcium, calcitriol, and calcitonin. N Engl J Med 1993;328:1747–1752.
71. Montemurro L, Schiraldi G, Fraioli P, Rizzato G. Prevention of corticosteroid-induced osteoporosis with salmon calcitonin. Calcif Tissue Int 1991;49:71–76.
72. Grotz WH, Rump LC, Niessen A, et al. Treatment of osteopenia and osteoporosis after kidney transplantation. Transplantation 1998;66:1004–1008.
73. Reid IR, King AR, Alexander CJ, Ibberston HK. Prevention of steroid-induced osteoporosis with (3-amino-1-hydroxypropylidene)-1,1 bisphosphonate. Lancet 1988;1:143–146.
74. Shane E, Jacobs S, Papadopoulos A, et al. Antiresorptive therapy prevents bone loss after cardiac transplantation. J Bone Miner Res 1996;11:5340A.
75. Riemens SC, Oostdijk A, van Doormaal J. Bone loss after liver transplantation is not prevented by cyclical etidronate, calcium, and alphacalcidiol. Osteoporosis Int 1996;6:213–218.
76. Meunier PJ, Brancon D, Chavassieux P, et al. Treatment with fluoride. In: Christiansen C, Johansen JS, Riis BJ, eds. Osteoporosis. Copenhagen: Osteopress, 1987:824–828.
77. Whyte MP. Ischemic bone disease. In: Favus MF, ed. Primer on the metabolic bone diseases and disorders of mineral metabolism. 3rd ed. Philadelphia, Lippincott-Raven, 1996:399–403.
78. Starzl TE, Marchioro TL, Porter KA, et al. Renal homotransplantation: late function and complications. Ann Int Med 1964;61:470–477.
79. Arfi S, Moreau F, Heuclin C, et al. L'osteonecrose aseptique de la transplantation renale. A propos be 29 cas. Rev Rheum Mal Osetoartic 1975;42:167.
80. Springfield DS, Enneking WJ. Surgery for aseptic necrosis of the femoral head. Clin Orthop 1978;130:175.
81. Elmstedt E, Szahn T. Skeletal complications following renal transplantation. Acta Orthop Scand 1981;52:279–286.
82. Fryer JP, Granger DK, Leventhal JR, et al. Steroid-related complications in the cyclosporine era. Clin Transplant 1994;8:224–229.
83. Ternoven O, Mueller DM, Matteson EL, et al. Clinically occult avascular necrosis of the hip: prevalence in an asymptomatic population at risk. Radiology 1992;182:845–847.
84. Le Parc JM, Andre T, Helenon O, et al. Osteonecrosis of the hip in renal transplant recipients. Changes in functional status and magnetic resonance imaging findings over three years in three hundred five patients. Rev Rheum Engl Ed 1996;63:413–420.
85. Naiker IP, Govender S, Naicker S, et al. Avascular necrosis of bone following renal transplantation. S Afr Med J 1993;83:646–649.

86. Lee AH, Mull RL, Keenan GF, et al. Osteoporosis and bone morbidity in cardiac transplant recipients. Am J Med 1994;96:35–41.
87. Bradbury G, Benjamin J, Thompson J, et al. Avascular necrosis of bone after cardiac transplantation. Prevalence and relationship to administration and dosage of steroids. J Bone Joint Surg Am 1994;76:1385–1388.
88. Foley-Nolan D, Daly C, Barry C, et al. Avascular necrosis of the femoral head post heart-transplantation and steroid dosage. Ir Med J 1992; 85:138–139.
89. Strasser S, Sheil AG, Gallagher ND, et al. Liver transplantation for primary sclerosing cholangitis versus primary biliary cirrhosis. J Gastroenterol Hepatol 1993;8:238–243.
90. Russell JA, Blahey WB, Stuart TA, et al. Avascular necrosis of bone in bone marrow transplant patients. Med Pediatr Oncol 1989;17:140–143.
91. Bizot P, Witvoet J, Sedel L. Avascular necrosis of the femoral head after allogeneic bone-marrow transplantation. A retrospective study of 27 THAs with a minimal two-year follow-up. J Bone Joint Surg Br 1996; 78:878–883.
92. Kopecky KK, Braunstein EM, Brandt KD, et al. Apparent avascular necrosis of the hip: appearance and spontaneous resolution of MR findings in renal allograft recipients. Radiology 1991;179:523–527.
93. Mulliken BD, Renfrew DL, Brand RA, Whitten CG. The prevalence and natural history of early osteonecrosis (ON) of the femoral head. Iowa Orthop J 1994;14:115–119.
94. Siddiqui AR, Kopecky KK, Wellman HN, et al. Prospective study of magnetic resonance imaging and SPECT bone scans in renal allograft recipients: evidence for a self-limited subclinical abnormality of the hip. J Nucl Med 1993;34:381–386.
95. Mont MA, Hungerford DS. Non-traumatic avascular necrosis of the femoral head. J Bone Joint Surg 1995;77:459–473.
96. Mankin HJ. Nontraumatic necrosis of bone (osteonecrosis). N Engl J Med 1992;326:1473–1479.
97. Handelsman DJ. Hypothalamic-pituitary gonadal dysfunction in renal failure, dialysis, and renal transplantation. Endocr Rev 1985;6:151–182.
98. Lim VS. Fang VS. Gonadal dysfunction in uremic men. Am J Med 1975;58:655–662.
99. Procci WR, Goldstein DA, Adelstein J, Massry SG. Sexual dysfunction in the male patient with uremia: a reappraisal. Kidney Int 1981;19:317.
100. Zingraff J, Jungers P, Pelissier C, et al. Pituitary and ovarian dysfunction in women on haemodialysis. Nephron 1982;30:149–153.
101. Griffin J, Wilson J. Disorders of the testes and the male reproductive tract In: Wilson JD, Foster DW, eds. Williams textbook of endocrinology. 8th ed. Philadelphia: WB Saunders, 1992:799–852.
102. Cello JP, Sleisenger MH. The liver in systemic conditions. In Zakim D, Boyer T, eds. Hepatology. Philadelphia: WB Saunders, 1982:1221–1249.
103. Semple PD, Beastall GH, Watson WS, Hume R. Serum testosterone depression associated with hypoxia in respiratory failure. Clin Sci 1980;58:105–106.
104. Woolf PD, Hamill RW, McDonald JV, et al. Transient hypogonadotropic hypogonadism caused by critical illness. J Clin Endocrinol Metab 1985;60:444–450.
105. Papadopoulos C. Cardiovascular drugs and sexuality: a cardiologist's review. Arch Intern Med 1980;140:1341–1345.
106. MacAdams MR, White RH, Chipps BE. Reduction of serum testosterone levels during chronic glucocorticoid therapy. Ann Intern Med 1986;104:648–651.
107. Mancini RE, Lavieri JC, Muller F, et al. Effect of prednisone upon normal and pathologic human spermatogenesis. Fertil Steril 1966;17:500–508.
108. Cumming DC, Quigley ME, Yen SSC. Acute suppression of circulating testosterone levels by cortisol in men. J Clin Endocrinol Metab 1983;57:671–673.
109. Bambino TH, Hsueh AJW. Direct inhibitory effect of glucocorticoids upon testicular luteinizing hormone receptor and steroidogenesis in vivo and in vitro. Endocrinology 1981;108:2142–2148.
110. Sakakura M, Takebe K, Nakagawa S. Inhibition of luteinizing hormone secretion induced by synthetic LRH by long-term treatment with glucocorticoids in human subjects. J Clin Endocrinol Metab 1975;40:774–779.
111. Rajter J, Sikka S, Lemmi C, Koyle M. Cyclosporine inhibits testosterone biosynthesis in the rat testes. Endocrinology 1987;121:586–589.
112. Seethalakshmi L, Flores C, Carboni A, et al. Cyclosporine: its effects on testicular function and fertility in the prepubertal rat. J Androl 1990;11:17–24.
113. Rivas M, Hembree WC, Kim TS, et al. Hypogonadism, bone mass, and fractures in men after cardiac transplantation. J Bone Miner Res 1994;8:S267(A).
114. Jacobs U, Klein B, Klehr H. Cumulative side effects of cyclosporine and calcium antagonists: hyperprolactinemia, mastadenoma, and gynecomastia. Transplant Proc 1994;26:3122.
115. Schmidt J, Gebbart W, Kopsa H, Spona J. Does cyclosporin A enhance sex hormone level? Exp Clin Endocrinol 1986;88:207–211.
116. Rosenkrantz JG, Githens JH, Cox SM, Kellum DL. Azathioprine (Imuran) and pregnancy. Am J Obst Gynec 1967;97:387–394.
117. Handelsman DJ, McDowell IFW, Caterson ID, et al. Testicular function after renal transplantation: comparison of cyclosporin A with azathioprine and prednisone combination regimens. Clin Nephrol 1981;22:144–148.
118. Samojlik E, Kirschner MA, Ribot S, Szmal E. Changes in the hypothalamic-pituitary-gonadal axis in men after cadaver kidney transplantation and cyclosporin therapy. J Androl 1992;13:332–336.
119. Handelsman DJ, Strasser S, McDonald JA, et al. Hypothalamic-pituitary-testicular function in end-stage non-alcoholic liver disease before and after liver transplantation. Clin Endocrinol 1995;43:331–337.
120. Sambrook PN, Kelly PJ, Fontana D, et al. Mechanics of rapid bone loss following cardiac transplantation. Osteoporos Int 1994;4:273–276.
121. Bagatell CJ, Bremner WJ. Androgens in men—uses and abuses. N Engl J Med 1996;334:707–714.
122. Hirasawa K, Enosawa S. Effects of sex steroid hormones on sex-associated differences in the survival time of allogeneic skin grafts in rats. Transplantation 1990;50:637–641.
123. Deray G, LeHoang P, Cacoub P, et al. Oral contraceptive interaction with cyclosporine. Lancet 1987;1:158–159.

Chapter

32

Hematologic Considerations of Organ Transplantation

JOHAN F. VANWALLEGHEM   YVES F. CH. VANRENTERGHEM

Hematologic complications reported in organ transplant recipients may affect all three bone-marrow–derived blood cell components—erythrocytes, leukocytes, and platelets—as well as the coagulation system. Although they frequently reflect drug toxicity, either of specific immunosuppressive drugs or of other agents, they also may be more organ specific and be related to the underlying original disease responsible for the organ failure. Red blood cell abnormalities in renal transplant recipients in particular may be related to the underlying renal failure. A thorough history, meticulous physical examination, and a few laboratory tests are the basic steps to a correct diagnosis.

The complex interactions between the various hematologic abnormalities and possible etiologies in organ transplantation are shown in Figure 32.1. Several aspects of blood transfusions are discussed at the end of this chapter. Organ transplant recipients also show an increased incidence of lymphoproliferative and other hematologic malignancies; but these complications are discussed in detail in Chapter 37.

ANEMIA

Erythropoietin and Iron in Kidney Transplantation

Inadequate production of erythropoietin by failing native kidneys and inhibition of erythropoiesis by uremic toxins are essential factors in the anemia of chronic renal failure, whereas shortened red blood cell survival seems to play a lesser role (1,2). Kidney transplantation reverses these abnormalities. Erythropoietin production and subsequent reticulocytosis increase within the week after early onset of renal function, and anemia is corrected during the first months (3,4). Serum erythropoietin—measured by radioimmunoassay—returns to normal as the hematocrit level rises above 32%. Thereafter, erythropoiesis is sustained by normal erythropoietin levels. This could be explained by the disappearance of uremic inhibitors or stimulation by other factors besides erythropoietin (4). The normal process of erythropoiesis will be interrupted by acute rejection (5).

The hematopoietic response results in a rapid decrease in iron stores, reflected in a fall in the serum ferritin levels. Frequent blood sampling in the early post-transplant period contributes to this, and iron deficiency anemia may eventually develop (6–8). Such patients need iron replacement therapy, comparable to the situation of hemodialysis patients receiving recombinant human erythropoietin (rHuEPO). Considering the few reports in the literature, this topic is a neglected one. In cases of unexplained iron deficiency, chronic gastrointestinal blood loss has to be excluded. Another factor to keep in mind is the presence of severe pretransplantation hyperparathyroidism, which can delay the correction of anemia either by bone marrow fibrosis or by the direct inhibitory effect of parathormone (PTH) on erythropoietin (9). Deficiencies of vitamin B_{12} or folate are not particular problems after renal transplantation (10).

Treatment with rHuEPO After Kidney Transplantation

Continuing anemia is common early after renal transplantation, as the transplanted kidney may have delayed function. Later after renal transplantation, when impaired graft function persists or when graft function progressively decreases due to so-called chronic rejection, renal anemia is frequently seen. In these cases, several single-center studies have shown that treatment with rHuEPO is effective in correcting the anemia despite immunosuppressive therapy (11–13). This results in a significant improvement in quality of life, similar to what has been seen in the hemodialyzed

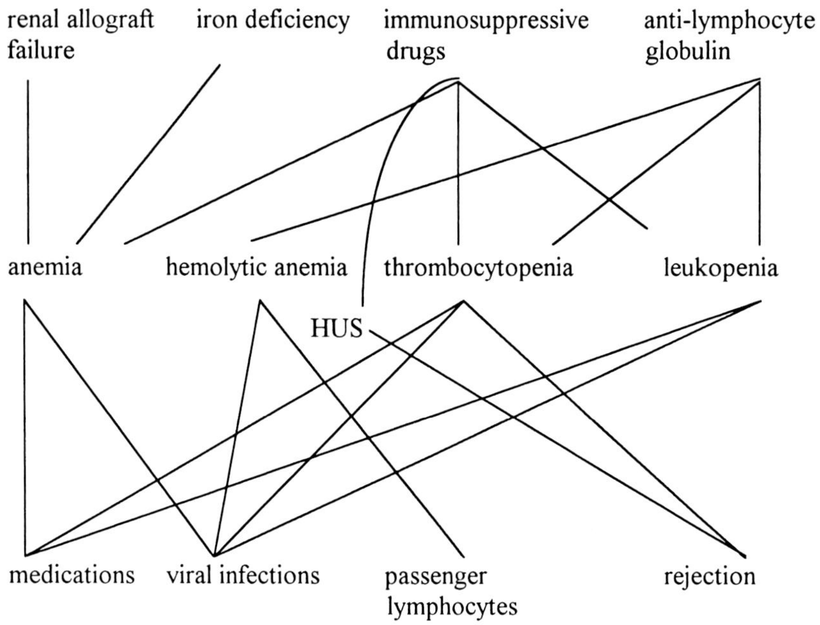

FIGURE 32.1. *Hematologic abnormalities and etiologies in organ transplantation.*

patients. It also enables abstention from blood transfusions, therefore reducing the risks of developing viral hepatitis, acquired immunodeficiency syndrome (AIDS), transfusion reactions, iron overload, and anti-HLA sensitization (14).

A negative effect of rHuEPO treatment may be an exacerbation of hypertension, which is often already a major problem in advanced graft failure. In the study by Muirhead et al, 18 patients out of 40 had a significantly increased need for antihypertensive drugs (12). Another concern with rHuEPO therapy is the possibility of accelerated graft failure. There is no clear evidence that this occurs, but experience is still limited. In predialysis patients, accelerated deterioration of renal function with rHuEPO administration has not been substantiated (15). Maintenance of adequate iron stores in patients undergoing rHuEPO therapy is provided by oral supplements, because it is impractical to give parenteral iron to patients who are not yet on dialysis.

Further studies are necessary to determine the long-term clinical benefits, safety, target hemoglobin levels, and economic implications of rHuEPO therapy. In evaluating the cost-effectiveness one also has to consider the possibility that improved well-being of patients with deteriorating graft function will postpone the initiation of dialysis.

Myelotoxicity

Macrocytosis is present in a majority of renal allograft recipients treated with azathioprine, and the leukocyte count in peripheral blood is used to monitor dosage. Selective erythroid toxicity of azathioprine is rare but potentially hazardous (16–18). The underlying mechanism of azathioprine-induced erythroid hypoplasia is poorly understood. Similar cases of transient pure red-cell aplasia have occurred after antilymphocyte globulin treatment, caused by antibodies against erythroid progenitors (19).

In contrast, cyclosporine does not depress the bone marrow. Of the newer immunosuppressive agents, tacrolimus (FK506) also appears to have no effect on bone marrow. In the large experience with tacrolimus in the multicenter liver study, no hematopoietic side effects were reported (20). Recently, however, two cases have been described of severe anemia in patients receiving tacrolimus (21,22). Mycophenolate mofetil (MMF) selectively blocks the de novo or ribose-derived purine synthesis pathway, so it should not have a major effect on the cell proliferation, except of lymphocytes. In spite of this prediction, there was a similar incidence of anemia reported in the U.S. and European MMF trials as was seen with azathioprine (23,24). Recombinant human erythropoietin also has been used to correct the anemia caused by immunosuppressive drugs in nonrenal organ transplantation (25,26).

Other possible erythrotoxic medications after transplantation include the angiotensin-converting enzyme (ACE) inhibitors (see Chapter 30). They are now frequently used for the treatment of post-transplant hypertension, in which it is recognized that the renin-angiotensin system plays an important part. Anemia with ACE inhibitors initially was not even a reported side effect (27), although small decreases in hematocrit had been observed in patients treated for hypertension (28). Recent reports have noted that enalapril can account for otherwise unexplained anemia in renal transplant recipients (29,30). The combination of ACE inhibitors with azathioprine might even result in quite severe anemia (31). A possible explanation lies in the interrelationship between the renin-angiotensin-aldosterone system and erythropoietin. In rats the administration of renin has been shown to increase erythropoietin levels, while the continuous infusion of angiotensin II prevented the suppression of erythropoietin seen after ACE inhibition (32). These experiments suggest that angiotensin II stimulates the production of erythropoietin, either directly or indirectly, by decreasing renal perfusion. Also, in humans it has been shown that the administration of rHuEPO in normotensive dialysis patients suppresses renin (33).

In the differential diagnosis of unexplained anemia in a transplant recipient, persistent viral infections such as the hepatitis B and C viruses, herpes viruses, or parvovirus B19 should be considered (34). The chronic anemia caused by parvovirus B19 can be explained by its cytotoxic effect on late erythroid progenitor cells (35); treatment with intravenous immunoglobulin has been used successfully (34,36). Young patients after liver transplantation for acute non-A, non-B hepatitis appear to be a particularly high-risk group for developing aplastic anemia (37,38). The causative agent in this situation is yet to be identified.

Hemolysis

Autoimmune hemolytic anemia caused by autoantibodies against the ABO blood group A or B antigen is a very rare condition. In the early post-transplant period, its occurrence may be due to autoantibodies produced by "passenger" donor lymphocytes in some kind of graft-versus-host disease (39–41). In most reported cases, blood group A, B, or AB recipients received an organ from blood group O donors (39,42–44). This has been reported after kidney, lung, liver, and pancreas transplantation (45,46). Also, the presence of anti-Rh antibodies in Rh-positive patients who received a renal transplant from a Rh-sensitized cadaver donor has been documented (47).

The development of autoantibodies after ABO isogroup kidney transplantation is very unusual (48–50). These disorders seem to be more frequent in cyclosporine-treated patients, perhaps because cyclosporine does not prevent B cells from mounting secondary immune responses (43).

Management includes transfusion with red blood cells negative for the antibody in question. The antibody formation and hemolysis is usually self-limiting, but in severe cases switching of immunosuppressive therapy from cyclosporine to azathioprine is recommended (42).

Thrombotic Microangiopathy

The hemolytic uremic syndrome (HUS) is characterized by a triad of acute hemolytic anemia of the microangiopathic type, thrombocytopenia, and acute renal failure (51). Oligoanuria is frequently accompanied by hypertension. It is most common in children, in whom renal failure generally recovers spontaneously and prodromal symptoms of respiratory or diarrheal illness are present. In adults the outcome is less favorable, often leading to end-stage renal failure. It may be precipitated by pregnancy, oral contraceptives, malignant hypertension, systemic sclerosis, and certain chemotherapeutic agents (52–54).

Thrombotic thrombocytopenic purpura (TTP) is a related syndrome with systemic and neurologic signs that are often difficult to distinguish from HUS (55). Since the pathogenetic mechanism is the same, Remuzzi and Ruggenenti suggested that the term "thrombotic microangiopathy" should be preferred (56).

Examination of the peripheral smear reveals fragmented erythrocytes with the aspect of burr cells or schistocytes. Markers of hemolysis include high levels of lactate dehydrogenase and low haptoglobin. Renal biopsy is helpful if the diagnosis is not clear on clinical grounds, as it allows a prediction of prognosis (57). The pathogenesis is complex and probably multifactorial. Endothelial damage seems to be a central feature. Other hypothetical causal factors, including increased levels of plasminogen activator inhibitor type I (58), defective prostacyclin activity (59), or large factor VIII:von Willebrand factor multimers (60), may indeed only reflect endothelial cell dysfunction. Glomerular deposits of C3 and IgM can be seen, probably without pathogenetic significance (51).

Some cases of recurrence of HUS after renal transplantation have been described (61–63), but the overall risk is difficult to determine. The transplant biopsy of a female patient with thrombotic microangiopathy after delivery of her first child is shown in Figure 32.2. Recurrences have been seen under immunosuppression with azathioprine (64), cyclosporine (65,66), ATG (62), OKT-3 (67), and FK506 (68) without convincing evidence that these agents contributed to the recurrence. As for the newer immunosuppressive agents such as deoxyspergualin, rapamycin, and mycophenolate mofetil, recurrent hemolytic uremic syndrome has not been reported yet, but experience is still very limited (69).

In the post-transplant setting, a differential diagnosis, including malignant hypertension, acute vascular rejection, or cyclosporine nephrotoxicity, can be very difficult to establish on clinical and pathological grounds (61,70). Severe vascular rejection can simulate the HUS clinical picture by sequestration of platelets in the kidney leading to thrombus formation in intralobular vessels and cortical ischemia (71). Distinguishing between rejection and HUS is important to prevent needless aggressive immunosuppressive therapy. The absence of graft tenderness or fever and the presence of central nervous system symptoms are important clues for a correct diagnosis.

Treatments with aspirin, antiplatelet agents, steroids, or heparin have been advocated, but the value of these therapies is doubtful (56,72,73). The overall graft outcome is poor. Plasma exchange or infusions are universally accepted as the most appropriate treatment, although there are no controlled trials evaluating their efficacy after transplantation. Plasma exchange may be effective because it removes a platelet-activating substance, or because it restores a deficient plasma factor that prevents platelet activation.

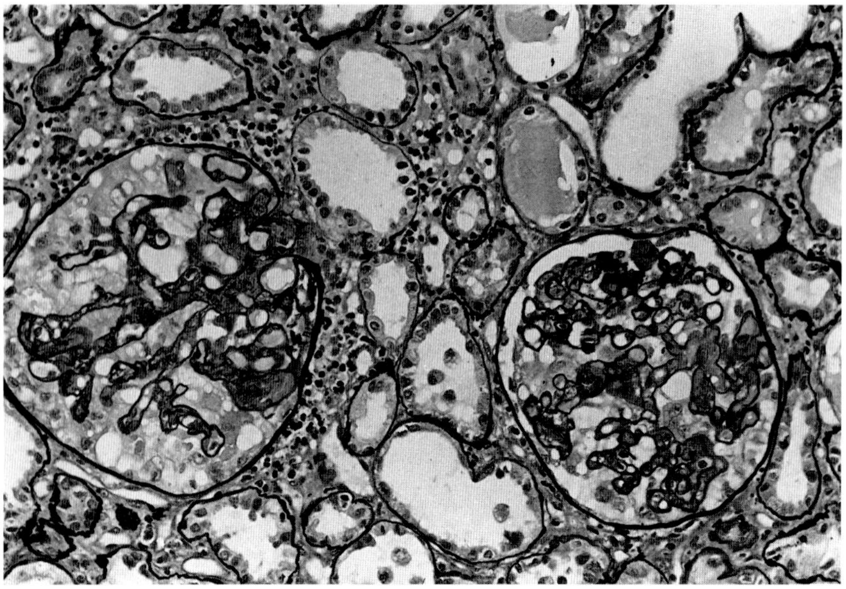

FIGURE 32.2. *Transplant biopsy of a female patient with thrombotic microangiopathy after delivery of her first child. She had a relapse in two consecutive grafts. Two glomeruli with thrombosis of some capillary loops and partial collapse of the other loops, surrounded by hypertrophic visceral epithelial cells, are also evident. The mesangia show increase of matrix. The tubules contain desquamated cells (methenamine silver, ×250). (Courtesy of Dr. B. Van Damme.)*

Other important supportive measures include blood pressure control, cautious use of blood transfusions, and dialysis if necessary. Allograft nephrectomy is the ultimate therapy for refractory cases. The occurrence in siblings suggests a genetic predisposition, so caution is indicated when considering a family member as a living-related donor (73,74).

HUS not only may recur after renal transplantation, but may even arise as a de novo presentation independent of the prior history (75). Also, in these cases an etiologic role for cyclosporine has been proposed, as similar conditions are seen in liver (76) and bone marrow (77) transplant recipients. However, the pathogenesis remains unknown. Some authors describe resolution after dose reduction or withdrawal of the drug (78,79). Recently we have seen a complete resolution after switching from cyclosporine to FK506 in a combined kidney-pancreas recipient who developed a de novo hemolytic uremic syndrome 6 months after transplantation.

The different causes of thrombotic microangiopathy after renal transplantation are summarized in Table 32.1.

Table 32.1. Causes of Thrombotic Microangiopathy After Transplantation

Recurrence
Pregnancy
Oral contraceptives
Malignant hypertension
Immunosuppressive drugs
Azathioprine
Cyclosporine
Polyclonal antithymocyte globulin (ATG)
OKT-3
Tacrolimus (FK506)
De Novo
Immunosuppressive drugs
Cyclosporine?
Rejection

ERYTHROCYTOSIS

After successful renal transplantation, the hemoglobin concentration rapidly returns to normal. In some patients, however, the hematocrit continues to rise until erythrocytosis develops (see Chapter 17). True erythrocytosis represents a state of increased red blood cell mass with normal plasma volume. Because red blood cell mass studies are not routinely available in the clinical setting, it is usually defined as a hematocrit greater than 51% on two or more consecutive determinations (80,81). It is a frequent pathology occurring in 5% to 20% of renal transplant recipients (80,82,83).

The initial scarce reports suggested transplant renal artery stenosis (84,85), hydronephrosis, rejection (86), or overzealous use of diuretics (87) as possible causes, but recent studies have indicated that, surprisingly, erythrocytosis often occurs in patients with good renal function and without these conditions (82). Also, it has been considered to be a consequence of increased erythropoietin release by the native kidneys, while the allograft worked within the normal range of feedback regulation (88). The pathophysiology, however, remains poorly understood, and thus the etiologic role of elevated levels of erythropoietin is speculative (82,89,90). About half of the patients with post-transplant erythrocytosis have undetectable erythropoietin levels (91).

In a recent report, Brox et al (92) have suggested that the secondary erythrocytosis results from increased levels of insulin-like growth factor-1 (IGF-1) and its major binding proteins, IGF-1-binding proteins (IGFBP) 1 and 3. These investigators found that renal transplant recipients have elevated serum levels of IGF-1 and IGFBP3 compared to normal individuals. When they compared transplant recipients with and without post-transplant erythrocytosis, the former group had significantly greater IGFBP1 and IGFBP3. There were no differences for other parameters, including EPO levels. The authors contend that this data is consistent with the theory that IGF-1 and its major binding proteins are important regulators of erythropoiesis.

Whatever the pathogenetic mechanism, erythrocytosis is not a harmless laboratory finding, but rather is associated with increased blood viscosity and an increased incidence of thromboembolic events. Wickre reported stroke, transient ischemic attack, pulmonary embolus, or phlebitis in 11 out of 53 patients (22%) with post-transplant erythrocytosis (81). Treatment options include repeated phlebotomies, native nephrectomy in selected cases (93), and more recently the administration of theophylline (94) or ACE inhibitors (91,95–97). Theophylline has too many side effects to be of practical use, whereas ACE inhibitors offer the additional benefit of lowering the often associated post-transplant hypertension.

When used with caution in renal transplant recipients (i.e., with creatinine and potassium control soon after drug administration begins), both captopril and enalapril are safe, without major side effects (98,99). Their mechanism of action remains obscure, and is not necessarily dependent on circulating erythropoietin levels (99,100). In the study by Perazella et al there was no correlation between mean circulating erythropoietin levels and hematocrit or between changes in these parameters during enalapril therapy (100). The ACE inhibitors possibly have a direct inhibitory effect at the level of the bone marrow.

LEUKOPENIA, THROMBOCYTOPENIA, AND PANCYTOPENIA

Direct Myelotoxicity

Leukopenia in the post-transplant setting has many possible causes, including immunosuppressive drugs or associated medications and bacterial or viral infections. Azathioprine has a well-documented myelosuppressive toxicity. After oral administration, azathioprine is rapidly converted to 6-mercaptopurine, which in turn undergoes extensive metabolism. One important catabolic route is thiol methylation catalyzed by the enzyme thiopurine methyltransferase. The activity of this enzyme is controlled by genetic polymorphism, and inherited differences in drug metabolism may explain interindividual variations in azathioprine toxicity (101). Very low activity of thiopurine methyltransferase results in severe leukopenia or pancytopenia, appearing shortly after administration of azathioprine (101).

5-Nucleotidase deficiency is another possible cause of azathioprine-induced bone marrow toxicity (102). In most cases, however, the leukopenia is easily reversed by adjusting the dose. Another catabolic pathway of azathioprine is oxidation catalyzed by the enzyme xanthine oxidase. Also, xanthine oxidase inhibitors such as allopurinol substantially enhance the risk of azathioprine-related bone marrow toxicity, sometimes leading to severe pancytopenia (103).

Some clinicians recommend that only 25% of the dose of azathioprine be given to patients also receiving allopurinol (104,105), while others recommend that azathioprine not be used in combination with allopurinol. Although transplant physicians are well aware of the potential toxicity of this combination, physicians who only occasionally care for these patients may be unaware of the consequences. Because patients with liver disease are more susceptible to the myelosuppressive effects of azathioprine, they should also receive lower doses (103). Severe myelodysplastic syndromes after kidney grafting have been described. After withdrawal of azathioprine, some of the syndromes are reversible (106), but others are not (107).

Although mycophenolate mofetil is said to be lymphocyte specific because it does not block the salvage purine synthesis pathway present in most nucleated cells except lymphocytes, some hematologic side effects have been seen (see Chapter 10). In the European MMF cooperative study, leukopenia and anemia were more frequently reported in the group treated with mycophenolate mofetil than in the control group, with a few cases of pancytopenia and agranulocytosis, all of which resolved within a week (23).

The effect of the commonly used immunosuppressive agents on various hematologic components is listed in Table 32.2.

Other common medications, some of them used for prophylactic purposes, such as trimethoprim-sulfamethoxazole, ganciclovir, and acyclovir, have to be kept in mind as possible causes of leukopenia (108,109). In kidney transplant recipients, trimethoprim-sulfamethoxazole in a prophylactic dose is usually tolerated very well without major myelosuppression (110,111). Randomized trials have shown that the same is true for acyclovir (112) and ganciclovir (113).

As neutropenia in transplant recipients may increase the susceptibility to opportunistic infections, treatments with granulocyte-stimulating factor and granulocyte-macrophage colony-stimulating factor have been used in this setting. A major concern is that such a treatment might contribute to

Table 32.2. The Effects of Commonly Used Immunosuppressive Drugs on Hematologic Components

Drug	Anemia	Leukopenia	Thrombocytopenia
Azathioprine	+	++	+
Cyclosporine	*	–	–
Tacrolimus (FK506)	*	–	–
Rapamycin	*	–	–
Mycophenolate mofetil	+/–	+	+/–
ATG	+/–	+	+

* Hemolytic-uremic syndrome reported.

allograft rejection. The available reports in kidney (114,115), kidney–pancreas (116), liver (117), and cardiac (118) transplantation suggest that colony-stimulating factors can be used safely. However, these are basically uncontrolled observations, so the real risk remains unknown.

Viral infections in transplant recipients may result in a profound bone marrow suppression. Cytomegalovirus (CMV) infection, especially, has been implicated as a cause of leukopenia, with associated morbidity and mortality (119). Human herpesvirus 6 is a newly recognized opportunistic pathogen that has attracted a great deal of interest. Infection occurs in 31% to 55% of solid organ transplant recipients (120–122). It is an important cause of pneumonitis and marrow dysfunction in bone marrow transplant recipients, but the clinical importance in solid organ transplants remains to be elucidated. Thrombocytopenia with rash and encephalopathy in a liver transplant recipient (123) has been reported. The as-yet poorly understood mechanisms of marrow suppression involve direct viral-mediated cell destruction (124,125) (see also Chapter 36).

Immune-Mediated Cytopenia

Polyclonal antithymocyte globulin (ATG) is used for prophylaxis or treatment of allograft rejection (see Chapter 13). The name is misleading because ATG is not specific for thymocytes but also reacts with circulating lymphocytes, granulocytes, and platelets (126). Decreases in platelet and granulocyte number may thus occur in patients treated with ATG, in addition to the almost complete disappearance of lymphocytes. This effect might depend more on induction of platelet aggregation and release, rather than on complement-involved mechanisms (127,128). Pretreatment with high-dose steroids prevents most granulocyte and platelet destruction (129). Thrombocytopenia seems to be less frequent with OKT-3 than with ATG (130,131). It is important to keep in mind, however, that thrombocytopenia may be indicative of ongoing vascular rejection.

Viral infections cause hematologic problems by suppressing the bone marrow, as already discussed. Recent data suggest that autoimmune mechanisms may also be operative. For example, CMV derives a CD13 protein from infected cells, resulting in the formation of CD13-specific antibodies in bone marrow transplant patients (132). Autoantigens associated with virus particles is an appealing theory to explain the association between virus infections and autoimmune manifestations.

HEMOSTATIC CHANGES

An increased incidence of both venous and arterial thromboembolic complications has been described in renal transplant patients. In the literature, the prevalence ranges between 1% to 24%, but this frequency is probably even underestimated as most of the reports were retrospective and the diagnoses were mainly based on clinical parameters (133–136). Factors that have been implicated in producing an increased risk of thromboembolism in the early postoperative period include the use of high doses of corticosteroids with its associated hyperlipidemia (137), the overcorrection of the coagulation abnormalities of uremia after successful transplantation (138), and the decreased fibrinolytic activity with prolonged high blood levels of fibrinolytic inhibitors (139,140). Juvenile diabetes mellitus is also considered as a major risk factor for the development of deep vein thrombosis after transplantation (135).

In 1985, the results of a retrospective analysis indicated a significantly higher incidence of thromboembolic complications in cyclosporine-treated renal transplant recipients as compared to azathioprine-treated controls (141). Although the findings were confirmed later by other authors (142,143), several subsequent studies could not demonstrate a higher incidence of thromboembolic phenomena in cyclosporine-treated patients. In fact, some studies even demonstrated a lower incidence than in azathioprine-treated patients (144–146). It has become clear that cyclosporine has complex effects on coagulation—some effects enhancing coagulation, others more antithrombotic. Cyclosporine has been reported to increase factor VIII coagulant activity (141), factor VIII antigen (147,149), von Willebrand factor (148), and plasma fibrinogen (141), all of which enhance coagulation. Furthermore, cyclosporine increases ADP-induced platelet aggregation (141,149), enhances the synthesis of procoagulant activity on monocytes and blood mononuclear cells (150), increases the release of thromboxane A_2 from platelets (148), and suppresses the prostacyclin release from endothelial cells. On the other hand, cyclosporine has some antithrombotic effects, such as the increase of protein C and of antithrombin III levels (141). The clinical situation is complicated further by the association of other immunosuppressive drugs, as well as other agents that may also affect coagulation. For example, corticosteroids increase plasminogen activator inhibitor activity, resulting in a reduced fibrinolytic activity, as shown recently in stable renal transplant recipients (140).

Hemostatic changes caused by chronic liver failure are frequently seen in the perioperative liver transplant period, but they are beyond the scope of this review.

BLOOD TRANSFUSIONS AND ORGAN TRANSPLANTATION

Blood transfusion in allograft recipients, which can result in infectious and serological problems, has been linked to allograft outcome. Infection may occur as a reactivation of a previous infection, or may occur as a result of transmission of the virus from the transplanted organ or blood products (119,152,153).

CMV infection is a major cause of increased morbidity and mortality for immunocompromised transplant recipients. Due to the shortage of donors and the short time between donor identification and transplantation, donor-receptor matching with respect to CMV is usually not feasible. The use of CMV-seronegative screened blood reduces the incidence of infection in seronegative bone marrow (154,155) and cardiac transplant recipients (153); therefore, using CMV-seronegative blood has become the standard practice for CMV-seronegative bone marrow transplant recipients with seronegative donors. In these patients, leukocyte reduction by filtration has been an equally effective alternative to CMV-seronegative blood products in preventing transfusion-associated CMV disease (156). In solid-organ transplant recipients, filtered blood products probably also offer some benefit, but so far no studies have been performed.

Pre-transfusion testing problems in allograft recipients are rare. A positive direct antiglobulin test is possible in ABO-mismatched organ transplantation (40–46). Hemagglutinating antibodies may also be detected in patients receiving antilymphocyte globulin. These agents may be insufficiently absorbed during their preparation and may therefore contain red cell agglutinins, resulting in incompatible crossmatches (157,158).

Transfusion Effect

Blood transfusions have profound immunomodulatory properties. In 1973 a retrospective analysis by Opelz et al suggested that cadaveric kidney grafts survived better in patients who had been transfused before transplantation (159). Subsequently, over a hundred papers have confirmed this so-called blood transfusion effect. The transfusion effect was also seen with donor-specific transfusion in living-related renal transplantation (160) and cardiac transplantation (161).

The number, type, HLA-matching, and timing of blood transfusion all seemed to have an impact on the observed effect. The timing of blood transfusion remains a controversial issue. Large retrospective data suggest that transfusions during operation do not prolong allograft survival (162,163), although smaller studies mentioned opposite results (164,165). Iwaki et al reported that transfusions appear to play the greatest role in HLA-DR–mismatched transplants, with no effect in zero HLA-DR–mismatched transplants (166).

Since the improvement of graft survival with the advent of cyclosporine in the 1980s, the transfusion effect seemed to diminish or even disappear (167–170). Very recently, however, the results of a large prospective randomized trial organized by Opelz with his Collaborative Transplant Study became available. They clearly show that in the cyclosporine era there is still a 10% kidney graft survival benefit in the transfused group (171). The fundamental mechanism of this beneficial effect remains elusive despite intensive research. Various hypotheses have been advanced, including induction of a suppressor cell response (172,173), clonal deletion (174), Fc receptor blocking (175), or anti-idiotypic antibodies (176–178). Blood transfusions in which the donor and the recipient have HLA antigens in common may induce mixed chimerism (179,180). From the perspective of the complexity of the immune response, several of these mechanisms are probably operative, but all are unproven to date. There remains the risk of sensitization and infection. At present, the potential benefits of transfusion appear to outweigh the risks. Thus, administration of one to three units of packed red blood cells to renal transplant candidates is appropriate, in the opinion of many centers.

Surgical Hemostasis

An increased risk of perioperative bleeding accompanies thoracic organ transplantation. A number of factors likely contribute to this problem, including the nature of the underlying disease, presence of adhesions, and increased collateral vessels from the bronchial circulation. Activation of the clotting and fibrinolytic systems, particularly following cardiopulmonary bypass (CPB), also seems to play a role. Gu et al (181) found that the concentration of the clotting marker thrombin/antithrombin III complex is increased significantly during the early phase of CPB surgery. The levels remained elevated until the completion of surgery. Tissue-type plasminogen activator released by injured endothelium also increased in the early phase of the procedure, followed by a rise in fibrin degradation products. Aprotinin, a serine protease inhibitor, reduced activation of clotting and fibrinolysis during the early phase, but not the late phase, of the transplant procedure. In a later study conducted by Spray (182), the efficacy and safety of pediatric thoracic transplant operations were investigated further. Aprotinin appeared to be particularly valuable in patients who had previous sternotomy or transplantation. It appeared to be safe, and it reduced blood loss.

SUMMARY

The hematologic considerations in solid organ transplantation depend on a unique interplay of the underlying disease, the specific organ transplanted, and the bone marrow effects of immunosuppressive agents and other drugs. This chapter has emphasized management principles that rest on these considerations. Issues pertaining to bone marrow transplantation are reviewed in Chapter 27.

ACKNOWLEDGMENT

We thank Prof. Dr. B. Van Damme for the reproduction of the renal biopsy and Mrs. J. Gorter for secretarial assistance.

REFERENCES

1. Fisher JW. Mechanism of the anemia of chronic renal failure. Nephron 1980;25:106–111.
2. McGonigle RJS, Wallin JD, Shadduck RK, Fisher JW. Erythropoietin deficiency and inhibition of erythropoiesis in renal insufficiency. Kidney Int 1984;25:437–444.

3. Besarab A, Caro J, Jarrell B, et al. Effect of cyclosporine and delayed graft function on posttransplantation erythropoiesis. Transplantation 1985;40:624–631.
4. Sun CH, Ward HJ, Paul WL, et al. Serum erythropoietin levels after renal transplantation. N Engl J Med 1989;321:151–157.
5. Besarab A, Caro J, Jarrell BE, et al. Dynamics of erythropoiesis following renal transplantation. Kidney Int 1987;32:526–536.
6. Lataste A, Renoult P, Lederlin P, Kessler M. Analysis of serum ferritin changes after kidney transplantation: a prospective study of 123 cases. Transplant Proc 1994;26:2001–2005.
7. Teruel JL, Lamas S, Vila T, et al. Serum ferritin levels after renal transplantation: a prospective study. Nephron 1989;51:462–465.
8. Tornero F, Prats D, Alvarez-Salsa JL, et al. Iron deficiency anemia after successful renal transplantation. J Urol 1993;149:1398–1400.
9. Cotorruelo JG, De Francisco ALM, Canga E, et al. The role of secondary hyperparathyroidism in the recovery of anemia after kidney transplantation. Transplant Proc 1990;22:1412–1413.
10. Milman N. Serum vitamin B12 and erythrocyte folate in chronic uraemia and after renal transplantation. Scand J Haematol 1980;25:151–157
11. Jindal KK, Hirsch DJ, Belitsky P, Whalen MA. Low-dose subcutaneous erythropoietin corrects the anaemia of renal transplant failure. Nephrol Dial Transplant 1992;7:143–146.
12. Muirhead N, Cattran DC, Zaltzman J, et al. Safety and efficacy of recombinant human erythropoietin in correcting the anemia of patients with chronic renal allograft dysfunction. J Am Soc Nephrol 1994;5:1216–1222.
13. Traindl O, Barnas U, Franz M, et al. Recombinant human erythropoietin in renal transplant recipients with renal anemia. Clin Transplant 1994;8:45–48.
14. Ettenger RB, Marik J, Grimm P. The impact of recombinant human erythropoietin therapy on renal transplantation. Am J Kidney Dis 1991;27:57–61.
15. The US Recombinant Human Erythropoietin Predialysis Study Group. Double-blind, placebo-controlled study of the therapeutic use of recombinant human erythropoietin for anemia associated with chronic renal failure in predialysis patients. Am J Kidney Dis 1991;18:50–59.
16. McGrath BP, Ibels LS, Raik E, et al. Erythroid toxicity of azathioprine. Q J Med 1975;44:57–63.
17. Old CW, Flannery EP, Grogan TM, et al. Azathioprine-induced pure red blood cell aplasia. JAMA 1978;240:552–554.
18. Pruijt JFM, Haanen JBAG, Hollander AAMJ, den Ottolander GJ. Azathioprine-induced pure red-cell aplasia. Nephrol Dial Transplant 1996;11:1371–1373.
19. Schaffner A, Thomann B, Zala GF, et al. Transient pure red cell aplasia caused by antilymphoblast globulin after cadaveric renal transplantation. Transplantation 1991;51:1018–1023.
20. H. Bismuth for the European FK-506 multicenter liver study group. Comparison of FK-506- and cyclosporine-based immunosuppression: FK-506 therapy significantly reduces the incidence of acute, steroid-resistant, refractory, and chronic rejection whilst possessing a comparable safety profile. Transplant Proc 1995;27:45–49.
21. Suzuki S, Osaka Y, Nakai I, et al. Pure red cell aplasia induced by FK-506. Transplantation 1996;61:831–832.
22. Winkler M, Schulze F, Jost U, et al. Anaemia associated with FK 506 immunosuppression. Lancet 1993;I:1035–1036.
23. European Mycophenolate Mofetil Cooperative Study Group. Placebo-controlled study of mycophenolate mofetil combined with cyclosporin and corticosteroids for prevention of acute rejection. Lancet 1995;I:1321–1325.
24. H. W. Sollinger for the U.S. renal transplant mycophenolate mofetil study group. Mycophenolate mofetil for the prevention of acute rejection in primary cadaveric renal allograft recipients. Transplantation 1995;60:225–232.
25. End A, Ringl H, Grimm M, et al. Chronic anemia after lung transplantation: treatment with human recombinant erythropoietin. Transplantation 1994;57:1142.
26. End A, Stift A, Ringl H, et al. The use of recombinant human erythropoietin in lung transplantation. Wien Klin Wochenschr 1995;107/6:181–183.
27. Williams GH. Converting-enzyme inhibitors in the treatment of hypertension. N Engl J Med 1988;319:1517–1525.
28. Griffing GT, Melby JC. Enalapril (MK-421) and the white cell count and haematocrit. Lancet 1982;I:1361.
29. Loftus WK, Ierino F, Mathew TH. Enalapril and anaemia. Med J Aust 1988;148:209–210.
30. Vlahakos DV, Canzanello VJ, Madaio MP, Madias NE. Enalapril-associated anemia in renal transplant recipients treated for hypertension. Am J Kidney Dis 1991;17:199–205.
31. Gossmann J, Kachel HG, Schoeppe W, Scheuermann EH. Anemia in renal transplant recipients caused by concomitant therapy with azathioprine and angiotensin-converting enzyme inhibitors. Transplantation 1993;56:585–589.
32. Gould AB, Goodman S, DeWolf R, et al. Interrelation of the renin system and erythropoietin in rats. J Lab Clin Med 1980;96:523–534.
33. Yaqoob M, Morris K, Bell GM, Ahmad R. Suppression of the renin-angiotensin-aldosterone axis with erythropoietin therapy by a negative feedback loop. Nephrol Dial Transplant 1992;7:125–128.
34. Sturm I, Watschinger B, Geissler K, et al. Chronic parvovirus B19 infection-associated pure red cell anaemia in a kidney transplant recipient. Nephrol Dial Transplant 1996;11:1367–1370.
35. Young NS, Mortimer PP, Moore JG, Humphries RK. Characterization of a virus that causes transient aplastic crisis. J Clin Invest 1984;73:224–230.
36. Nour B, Green M, Michaels M, Reyes J, et al. Parvovirus B 19 infection in pediatric transplant patients. Transplantation 1993;56:835–838.
37. Cattral MS, Langnas AN, Markin RS, et al. Aplastic anemia after liver transplantation for fulminant liver failure. Hepatology 1994;20:813–818.
38. Tzakis AG, Arditi M, Whitington PF, et al. Aplastic anemia complicating orthotopic liver transplantation for non-A, non-B hepatitis. N Engl J Med 1988;319:393–396.
39. Ahmed KY, Nunn G, Brazier DM, et al. Hemolytic anemia resulting from autoantibodies produced by the donor's lymphocytes after renal transplantation. Transplantation 1987;43:163–164.
40. Mangal AK, Growe GH, Sinclair M, et al. Acquired hemolytic anemia due to "auto"-anti-A or "auto"-anti-B induced by group O homograft in renal transplant recipients. Transfusion 1984;24:201–205.
41. Lundgren G, Asaba H, Bergstrom J, et al. Fulminating anti-A autoimmune hemolysis with anuria in a renal transplant recipient: a therapeutic role of plasma exchange. Clin Nephrol 1981;16:211–214.
42. Nyberg G, Sandberg L, Rydberg L, et al. ABO-autoimmune hemolytic anemia in a renal transplant patient treated with cyclosporine. A case report. Transplantation 1984;37:529–530.
43. Povlsen JV, Rasmussen A, Hansen HE, et al. Acquired haemolytic anaemia due to isohaemagglutinins of donor origin following ABO-minor-incompatible kidney transplantation. Nephrol Dial Transplant 1990;5:148–151.
44. Stevens J, Callender CO, Jilly PN. Emergence of red blood cell agglutinins following renal transplantation in a patient with systemic lupus erythematosus. Transplantation 1981;32:398–400.
45. Bird GWG, Wingham J. Formation of blood group "autoantibodies" after transplantation. Transfusion 1982;22:400.
46. Swanson J, Sastamoinen R, Steeper T, Sebring E. Production of anti-A and B by donor lymphocytes following transplantation of group O organs to ABO incompatible patients receiving cyclosporin A. Transfusion 1984;24:231.
47. Ramsey G, Israel L, Lindsay GD, et al. Anti Rh(D) in two Rh-positive patients receiving kidney grafts from an Rh-immunized donor. Transplantation 1985;41:67–69.
48. De Vecchi A, Zanella A, Egidi F, Ponticelli C. Autoimmune hemolytic anemia in a cadaveric renal transplant recipient treated with cyclosporine. Acta Haemat 1985;73:216–218.
49. McMillan MA, Muirhead CSM, Lucie NP, et al. Autoimmune haemolytic anaemia related to cyclosporin with ABO-compatible kidney donor and recipient. Nephrol Dial Transplant 1991;6:57–59.
50. Rougier JP, Viron B, Ronco P, et al. Autoimmune haemolytic anaemia after ABO-match, ABDR full match kidney transplantation. Nephrol Dial Transplant 1994;9:693–697.
51. Kaplan BS, Drummond KN. The hemolytic-uremic syndrome is a syndrome. N Engl J Med 1978;298:964–966.
52. Brown CB, Robson JS, Thomson D, et al. Haemolytic uraemic syndrome in women taking oral contraceptives. Lancet 1973;I:1479.
53. Hauglustaine D, Van Damme B, Vanrenterghem Y, Michielsen P. Recurrent hemolytic uremic syndrome during oral contraception. Clin Nephrol 1981;15:148–153.
54. Ramos EL, Tisher CC. Recurrent diseases in the kidney transplant. Am J Kidney Dis 1994;24:142–154.
55. Neild GH. Haemolytic-uraemic syndrome in practice. Lancet 1994;II: 398–401.
56. Remuzzi G, Ruggenenti P. The hemolytic uremic syndrome. Kidney Int 1995;47:2–19.
57. Morel-Maroger L, Kanfer A, Solez K, et al. Prognostic importance of vascular lesions in acute renal failure with microangiopathic hemolytic anemia (hemolytic-uremic syndrome): clinicopathological study in 20 adults. Kidney Int 1979;15:548–558.

58. Bergstein JM, Riley M, Bang NU. Role of plasminogen-activator inhibitor type 1 in the pathogenesis and outcome of the hemolytic uremic syndrome. N Engl J Med 1992;327:755–759.
59. Remuzzi G, Marchesi D, Mecca G, et al. Haemolytic-uraemic syndrome: deficiency of plasma factor(s) regulating prostacyclin activity? Lancet 1978;II:671–872.
60. Moake JL, Rudy CK, Troll JH, et al. Unusually large plasma factor VIII: Von Willebrand factor multimers in chronic relapsing thrombotic thrombocytopenic purpura. N Engl J Med 1982;307:1432–1435.
61. Eijgenraam FJ, Donckerwolcke RA, Monnens LAH, et al. Renal transplantation in 20 children with hemolytic-uremic syndrome. Clin Nephrol 1990;33:87–93.
62. Hebert D, Sibley RK, Mauer SM. Recurrence of hemolytic uremic syndrome in renal transplant recipients. Kidney Int 1986;30:S51–S58.
63. van den Berg-Wolf MG, Kootte AMM, Weening JJ, Paul LC. Recurrent hemolytic uremic syndrome in a renal transplant recipient and review of the Leiden experience. Transplantation 1988;45:248–251.
64. Grino JM, Caralps A, Carreras L, et al. Apparent recurrence of hemolytic uremic syndrome in azathioprine-treated allograft recipients. Nephron 1988;49:301–304.
65. Leithner C, Sinzinger H, Pohanka E, et al. Recurrence of haemolytic uraemic syndrome triggered by cyclosporin A after renal transplantation. Lancet 1982;I:1470.
66. Leithner C, Sinzinger H, Pohanka E, et al. Occurrence of hemolytic uremic syndrome under cyclosporine treatment: accident or possible side effect mediated by a lack of prostacyclin-stimulating plasma factor? Transplant Proc 1983;15:2787–2789.
67. Doutrelepont JM, Abramowicz D, Florquin S, et al. Early recurrence of hemolytic uremic syndrome in a renal transplant recipient during prophylactic OKT3 therapy. Transplantation 1992;53:1378–1379.
68. Holman MJ, Gonwa TA, Cooper B, et el. FK-506-associated thrombotic thrombocytopenic purpura. Transplantation 1993;55:205–206.
69. Agarwal A, Mauer SM, Matas AJ, Nath KA. Recurrent hemolytic uremic syndrome in an adult renal allograft recipient: current concepts and management. J Am Soc Nephrol 1995;6:1160–1169.
70. Remuzzi G, Bertani T. Renal vascular and thrombotic effects of cyclosporine. Am J Kidney Dis 1989;23:261–272.
71. Kohler TR, Tilney NL. Microangiopathic hemolytic anemia associated with hyperacute rejection of a kidney allograft. Transplant Proc 1982;14:444–446.
72. Keusch G, Baumgartner D, Gmur J, et al. Successful plasmapheresis for cyclosporin (Cs)-induced hemolytic uremic syndrome (HUS) in two renal allograft recipients. Kidney Int 1985;28:377. Abstract.
73. Mathew TH. Recurrence of disease following renal transplantation. Am J Kidney Dis 1988;12:85–96.
74. Kaplan BS. Hemolytic uremic syndrome with recurrent episodes: an important subset. Clin Nephrol 1977;8:495–498.
75. Wolfe JA, McCann RL, Sanfilippo F. Cyclosporine-associated microangiopathy in renal transplantation: a severe but potentially reversible form of early graft injury. Transplantation 1986;41:541–544.
76. Bonser RS, Adu D, Franklin I, McMaster P. Cyclosporin-induced haemolytic uraemic syndrome in liver allograft recipient. Lancet 1984;II:1337–1338.
77. Shulman H, Striker G, Deeg HJ, et al. Nephrotoxicity of cyclosporin A after allogeneic marrow transplantation. N Engl J Med 1981;305:1392–1395.
78. Van Buren D, Van Buren CT, Flechner SM, et al. De novo hemolytic uremic syndrome in renal transplant recipients immunosuppressed with cyclosporine. Surgery 1984;98:54–62.
79. Verpooten GA, Paulus GJ, Roels F, De Broe ME. De novo occurrence of hemolytic-uremic syndrome in a cyclosporine-treated renal allograft patient. Transplant Proc 1987;19:2943–2945.
80. Gaston RS, Julian BA, Curtis JJ. Posttransplant erythrocytosis: an enigma revisited. Am J Kidney Dis 1994;24:1–11.
81. Wickre CG, Norman DJ, Bennison A, et al. Postrenal transplant erythrocytosis: a review of 53 patients. Kidney Int 1983;23:731–737.
82. Qunibi WY, Barri Y, Devol E, et al. Factors predictive of post-transplant erythrocytosis. Kidney Int 1991;40:1153–1159.
83. Tatman AJ, Tucker B, Amess JAL, et al. Erythaemia in renal transplant recipients treated with cyclosporin. Lancet 1988;I:1279.
84. Schramek A, Adler O, Hashmonai, et al. Hypertensive crisis, erythrocytosis, and uraemia due to renal-artery stenosis of kidney transplants. Lancet 1975;I:70–71.
85. Bacon BR, Rothman SA, Ricanati ES, Rashad FA. Renal artery stenosis with erythrocytosis after renal transplantation. Arch Intern Med 1980;140:1206–1211.
86. Westerman MP, Jenkins JL, Dekker A, et al. Significance of erythrocytosis and increased erythropoietin secretion after renal transplantation. Lancet 1967;II:755–757.
87. Pollak R, Maddux MS, Cohan J, et al. Erythrocythemia following renal transplantation: influence of diuretic therapy. Clin Nephrol 1988;29:119–123.
88. Thevenod F, Radtke W, Grutzmacher P, et al. Deficient feedback regulation of erythropoiesis in kidney transplant patients with polycythemia. Kidney Int 1983;24:227–232.
89. Lamperi S, Carozzi S, Manca F, Valente U. Erythropoietin-independent erythropoiesis in polycythemic transplanted patients. Transplant Proc 1986;23:86–88.
90. Rostaing L, Demur C, Huyn A, et al. Erythrocytosis after renal transplant: study of erythroid progenitors and response to enalapril. Transplant Proc 1994;26:280–281.
91. Gaston RS, Julian BA, Barker CV, et al. Enalapril: safe and effective therapy for posttransplant erythrocytosis. Transplant Proc 1993;25:1029–1031.
92. Brox AG, Margel J, Hanley JA, et al. Erythrocytosis after renal transplantation represents an abnormality of insulin-like growth factor-1 and its binding proteins. Transplantation 1998;66:1053–1058.
93. Friman S, Nyberg G, Blohmé I. Erythrocytosis after renal transplantation; treatment by removal of the native kidneys. Nephrol Dial Transplant 1990;5:969–973.
94. Bakris GL, Sauter ER, Hussey JL, et al. Effects of theophylline on erythropoietin production in normal subjects and in patients with erythrocytosis after renal transplantation. N Engl J Med 1990;323:86–90.
95. Pisani F, Tisone G, Alciati E, et al. Role of ACE inhibitors in the treatment of erythrocytosis in patients with renal allograft. Transplant Proc 1994;26:2602–2603.
96. Rell K, Koziak K, Jarzyo I, et al. Correction of posttransplant erythrocytosis with enalapril. Transplantation 1994;57:1059–1063.
97. Torregrosa JV, Campistol JM, Montesinos M, et al. Efficacy of captopril on posttransplant erythrocytosis. Transplantation 1994;58:311–314.
98. Curtis JJ, Luke RG, Whelchel JD, et al. Inhibition of angiotensin-converting enzyme in renal transplant recipients with hypertension. N Engl J Med 1983;308:377–381.
99. Gaston RS, Julian BA, Diethelm AG, Curtis JJ. Effects of enalapril on erythrocytosis after renal transplantation. Ann Intern Med 1991;115:954–955.
100. Perazella M, McPhedran P, Kliger A, et al. Enalapril treatment of posttransplant erythrocytosis: efficacy independent of circulating erythropoietin levels. Am J Kidney Dis 1995;3:495–500.
101. Lennard L, Van Loon JA, Weinshilboum RM. Pharmacogenetics of acute azathioprine toxicity: relationship to thiopurine methyltransferase genetic polymorphism. Clin Pharmacol Ther 1989;46:149–154.
102. Kerstens PJSM, Stolk JN, Hilbrands LB, et al. 5-nucleotidase and azathioprine-related bone-marrow toxicity. Lancet 1993;II:1245–1246.
103. Kaplan SR, Calabresi P. Drug therapy—immunosuppressive agents—purine antimetabolites. N Engl J Med 1973;289:1234–1236.
104. Murrell GAC, Rapeport WG. Clinical pharmacokinetics of allopurinol. Clin Pharmacokin 1986;11:343–353.
105. Chocair P, Duley J, Simmonds HA, et al. Low-dose allopurinol plus azathioprine/cyclosporin/prednisolone, a novel immunosuppressive regimen. Lancet 1993;II:83–84.
106. Bammatter F, Binswanger U, Fehr J. Reversibles azathioprin assoziiertes dysmyeloproliferatives Syndrom nach Nierenallotransplantation. Klin Wochenschr 1987;65:620–624.
107. Ihle BU, Constable J, Gordon S, Mahony JF. Myelodysplasia in cadaver renal allografts: a report of four cases. Am J Kidney Dis 1985;5:251–257.
108. Hulme B, Reeves DS. Leucopenia associated with trimethoprim-sulfamethoxazole after renal transplantation. Br Med J 1971;3:610–611.
109. Winston DJ, Wirin D, Shaked A, Busuttil RW. Randomised comparison of ganciclovir and high-dose acyclovir for long-term cytomegalovirus prophylaxis in liver-transplant recipients. Lancet 1995;346:69–74.
110. Higgins RM, Bloom SL, Hopkin JM, Morris PJ. The risks and benefits of low-dose cotrimoxazole prophylaxis for pneumocystis pneumonia in renal transplantation. Transplantation 1989;47:558–560.
111. Maki DG, Fox BC, Kuntz J, et al. A prospective, randomized, double blind study of trimethoprim-sulfamethoxazole for prophylaxis of infection in renal transplantation. J Lab Clin Med 1992;119:11–24.
112. Balfour HH, Chace BA, Stapleton JT, et al. A randomized placebo-controlled trial of oral acyclovir for the prevention of cytomegalovirus disease in recipients of renal allografts. N Engl J Med 1989;320:1381–1387.

113. Hibberd PL, Tolkoff-Rubin NE, Conti D, et al. Preemptive ganciclovir therapy to prevent cytomegalovirus disease in cytomegalovirus antibody-positive renal transplant recipients. A randomized controlled trial. Ann Intern Med 1995;123:18–26.
114. Peddi VR, Hariharan S, Schroeder TJ, First MR. Role of granulocyte colony stimulating factor (G-CSF) in reversing neutropenia in renal allografts recipients. Clin Transplant 1996;10:20–23.
115. Page B, Morin MP, Mamzer MF, et al. Use of granulocyte-macrophage colony-stimulating factor in leukopenic renal transplant recipients. Transplant Proc 1994;26:283.
116. Squiers EC, Elkhammas EA, Henry ML. Use of granulocyte-macrophage colony-stimulating factor for reversal of neutropenia following combined kidney-pancreas transplantation. Transplant Proc 1995;27:3092–3093.
117. Colquhoun SD, Shaked A, Jurim O, et al. Reversal of neutropenia with granulocyte colony-stimulating factor without precipitating liver allograft rejection. Transplantation 1993;56:1593–1595.
118. Patel HDL, Anderson JR, Duncombe AS, et al. Granulocyte colony-stimulating factor: a new application for cytomegalovirus-induced neutropenia in cardiac allograft recipients. Transplantation 1994;58:863–867.
119. Marker SC, Howard RJ, Simmons RL, et al. Cytomegalovirus infection: a quantitative prospective study of three hundred twenty consecutive renal transplants. Surgery 1981;89:660–671.
120. Herbein G, Strasswimmer J, Altieri M, et al. Longitudinal study of human herpesvirus 6 infection in organ transplant recipients. Clin Infect Dis 1996;22:171–173.
121. Singh N, Carrigan DR. Human herpesvirus-6 in transplantation: an emerging pathogen. Ann Intern Med 1996;124:1065–1071.
122. Yoshikawa T, Suga S, Asano Y, et al. A prospective study of human herpesvirus-6 infection in renal transplantation. Transplantation 1992;54:879–883.
123. Singh N, Carrigan DR, Gayowski T, et al. Variant B human herpesvirus-6 associated febrile dermatosis with thrombocytopenia and encephalopathy in a liver transplant recipient. Transplantation 1995;60:1355–1357.
124. Burd EM, Knox KK, Carrigan DR. Human herpesvirus-6-associated suppression of growth factor-induced macrophage maturation in human bone marrow cultures. Blood 1993;81:1645–1650.
125. Knox KK, Carrigan DR. In vitro suppression of bone marrow progenitor cell differentiation by human herpesvius 6 infection. J Infect Dis 1992;165:925–929.
126. Greco B, Bielory L, Stephany D, et al. Antithymocyte globulin reacts with many normal human cell types. Blood 1983;62:1047–1054.
127. Lekas N, Rosenberg JC. Release, aggregation and lysis of human platelets by antilymphocyte globulin and antiplatelet serum. Thromb Haemost 1976;36:411–423.
128. Rosenberg JC, Lekas N, Lysz K, Morrell R. Effect of antithymocyte globulin and other immune reactants on human platelets. Surgery 1975;77:520–529.
129. Gratama JW, Brand A, Jansen J, et al. Factors influencing platelet survival during antilymphocyte globulin treatment. Br J Haemat 1984;57:5–15.
130. Bock HA, Gallati H, Zürcher RM, et al. A randomized prospective trial of prophylactic immunosuppression with ATG-Fresenius versus OKT3 after renal transplantation. Transplantation 1995;59:830–840.
131. Ortho Multicenter Transplant Study Group. A randomized clinical trial of OKT3 monoclonal antibody for acute rejection of cadaveric renal transplants. N Engl J Med 1985;313:337–342.
132. Söderberg C, Karuppan SS, Ljungman P, Möller E. CD13-specific autoimmunity in cytomegalovirus-infected immunocompromised patients. Transplantation 1996;61:594–600.
133. Rao KV, Smith EJ, Alexander JW, et al. Thromboembolic disease in renal allograft recipients. Arch Surg 1976;111:1086–1092.
134. Arnadottir M, Bergentz SE, Bergqvist D, et al. Thromboembolic complications after renal transplantation. World J Surg 1983;7:757–761.
135. Bergqvist D, Bergentz SE, Bornmyr S, et al. Deep vein thrombosis after renal transplantation: a prospective analysis of frequency and risk factors. Eur Surg Res 1985;17:69–74.
136. Brunkwall J, Bergqvist D, Bergentz SE, et al. Postoperative deep vein thrombosis after renal transplantation. Effects of cyclosporine. Transplantation 1987;43:647–659.
137. Patrassi GM, Dal Bo Zanon R, Boscaro M, et al. Further studies on the hypercoagulate state of patients with Cushing's syndrome. Thromb Haemost 1985;54:518–520.
138. von Kaulla KN, von Kaulla E, Wasantapruck S, et al. Blood coagulation in uremic patients before and after hemodialysis and transplantation of a kidney. Arch Surg 1966;92:184–191.
139. Seitz R, Michalik R, Karges HE, et al. Impaired fibrinolysis and protein C increase after cadaveric transplantation. Thromb Res 1986;42:277–288.
140. Patrassi GM, Sartori M, Rigotto P, et al. Reduced fibrinolytic potential one year after kidney transplantation. Transplantation 1995;59:1416–1420.
141. Vanrenterghem Y, Roels L, Lerut T, et al. Thromboembolic complications and haemostatic changes in cyclosporin-treated cadaveric kidney transplant allograft recipients. Lancet 1985;I:999–1002.
142. Rigotti P, Flechner SM, Van Buren CT, et al. Increased incidence of renal allograft thrombosis under cyclosporine immunosuppression. Int Surg 1986;71:38–41.
143. Jones RM, Murie JA, Ting A, et al. Renal vascular thrombosis of cadaveric renal allografts in patients receiving cyclosporin, azathioprine and prednisolone triple therapy. Clin Transplant 1988;44:775–778.
144. Gruber SA, Pescovitz MD, Simmons RL, et al. Thromboembolic complications in renal allograft recipients. Transplantation 1987;44:775–778.
145. Leitha T, Graninger W, Zazgornik J. Cyclosporine A does not increase the frequency of thromboembolic events. Transplant Proc 1988;20:436–438.
146. Glicklich D, Tellis VA, Matas AJ, et al. No association between post-transplant erythrocytosis, thromboembolic events and cyclosporine therapy. Transplant Proc 1989;21:2141–2142.
147. Huser B, Lämmle B, Landmann J, et al. Von Willebrand factor and factor VIII in renal transplant recipients under immunosuppression with cyclosporine and steroids. Clin Nephrol 1990;34:214–222.
148. Brown Z, Neild G, Willoughby JJ, et al. Increased factor VIII as an index of vascular injury in cyclosporine nephrotoxicity. Transplantation 1986;42:150–153.
149. Grace AA, Barradas A, Mikhailidis DP, et al. Cyclosporine A enhances platelet aggregation. Kidney Int 1987;32:889–895.
150. Thomson AW, Webster LM, Alridge RD, Morrice LN. Cyclosporin and leucocyte procoagulant activity. Lancet 1985;I:1396.
151. Neild GH, Rocchi G, Imberti L, et al. Effect of cyclosporin A on prostacyclin synthesis by vascular tissue. Thromb Res 1983;32:1178–1180.
152. Ho M, Suwansirikul S, Dowling JN, et al. The transplanted kidney as a source of cytomegalovirus infection. N Engl J Med 1975;293:1109–1112.
153. Preiksaitis JK, Rosno S, Grumet C, Merigan TC. Infections due to herpesviruses in cardiac transplant recipients: role of the donor heart and immunosuppressive therapy. J Infect Dis 1983;147:874–981.
154. Bowden RA, Sayers M, Flournoy N, et al. Cytomegalovirus immune globulin and seronegative blood products to prevent primary cytomegalovirus infection after marrow transplantation. N Engl J Med 1986;314:1006–1010.
155. Verdonck LF, de Graan-Hentzen YCE, Dekker AW, et al. Cytomegalovirus seronegative platelets and leukocyte-poor red blood cells from random donors can prevent primary cytomegalovirus infection after bone marrow transplantation. Bone Marrow Transplant 1987;2:73–78.
156. Bowden RA, Slichter SJ, Sayers M, et al. A comparison of filtered leukocyte-reduced and cytomegalovirus (CMV) seronegative blood products for the prevention of transfusion-associated CMV infection after marrow transplant. Blood 1995;86:3598–3603.
157. Ballas SK, Draper EK, Dignam CM. Pre-transfusion testing problems caused by anti-lymphocyte globulin and their solution. Transfusion 1984;25:254–256.
158. Swanson JL, Issitt CH, Mann EW, et al. Resolution of red cell compatibility testing problems in patients receiving anti-lymphoblast or anti-thymocyte globulin. Transfusion 1984;24:141–143.
159. Opelz G, Sengar DPS, Mickey MR, Terasaki PI. Effect of blood transfusion on subsequent kidney transplants. Transplant Proc 1973;5:253–259.
160. Salvatierra O, Vincenti F, Amend W, et al. Deliberate donor-specific blood transfusions prior to living related renal transplantation. A new approach. Ann Surg 1980;192:543–552.
161. Katz MR, Barnhart GR, Goldman MH, et al. Pretransplant transfusions in cardiac allograft recipients. Transplantation 1987;43:499–501.
162. Opelz G, Terasaki PI. Importance of preoperative (not peroperative) transfusions for cadaver kidney transplants. Transplantation 1981;31:106–108.
163. Opelz G for the Collaborative Transplant Study. Current relevance of the transfusion effect in renal transplantation. Transplant Proc 1985;27:1015–1022.
164. Stiller CR, Lockwood BL, Sinclair NR, et al. Beneficial effect of operation-day blood-transfusions on human renal-allograft survival. Lancet 1978;I:169–170.
165. Williams KA, Ting A, French ME, et al. Peroperative blood-transfusions improve cadaveric renal-allograft survival in non-transfused recipients. Lancet 1980;I:1104–1106.
166. Iwaki Y, Cecka M, Terasaki P. The transfusion effect in cadaver kidney transplants—yes or no. Transplantation 1990;49:56–59.

167. Editorial. Time to abandon pre-transplant blood transfusion? Lancet 1988;I:567–568.
168. Lundgren G, Albrechtsen D, Flatmark A, et al. HLA-matching and pretransplant blood transfusions in cadaveric renal transplantation—a changing picture with cyclosporin. Lancet 1986;II:66–69.
169. Melzer JS, Husing RM, Feduska NJ, et al. The beneficial effect of pretransplant blood transfusions in cyclosporine-treated cadaver renal allograft recipients. Transplantation 1987;43:61–64.
170. Opelz G for the Collaborative Transplant Study. Improved kidney graft survival in nontransfused recipients. Transplant Proc 1987;19:149–152.
171. Opelz G, Vanrenterghem Y, Kirste G, et al. Prospective evaluation of pretransplant blood transfusions in cadaver kidney recipients. Transplantation 1997;63:964–967.
172. Quigley RL, Wood KJ, Morris PJ. Investigation of the mechanism of active enhancement of renal allograft survival by blood transfusion. Immunology 1988;63:373–381.
173. Quigley RL, Wood KJ, Morris PJ. Transfusion induces blood donor-specific suppressor cells. J Immunol 1989;142:463–470.
174. Terasaki PI. The beneficial transfusion effect on kidney graft survival attributed to clonal deletion. Transplantation 1984;37:119–125.
175. MacLeod AM, Mason RJ, Shewan WG, et al. Possible mechanisms of action of transfusion effect in renal transplantation. Lancet 1982;II:468–470.
176. Barkley SC, Sakai RS, Ettenger RB, et al. Determination of antiidiotypic antibodies to anti-HLA IgG following blood transfusions. Transplantation 1987;44:30–34.
177. Burlingham WJ, Sollinger HW. Action of donor-specific transfusions: analysis of three possible mechanisms. Transplant Proc 1986;18:685–689.
178. Reed E, Hardy M, Benvenisty A, et al. Effect of antiidiotypic antibodies to HLA on graft survival in renal-allograft recipients. N Engl J Med 1987;316:1450–1455.
179. van Twuyver E, Mooijaart RJD, ten Berge IJM, et al. Pretransplantation blood transfusion revisited. N Engl J Med 1991;325:1203–1205.
180. de Waal LP, van Twuyver E. Blood transfusion and allograft survival: is mixed chimerism the solution for tolerance induction in clinical transplantation? Crit Rev Immunol 1991;10:417–425.
181. Gu YJ, de Haan J, Brenken UP, et al. Clotting and fibrinolytic disturbance during lung transplantation: effect of low-dose aprotinin. Groningen Lung Transplant Group. J Thorac Cardiovasc Surg 1996;112:599–606.
182. Spray TL. Use of aprotinin in pediatric organ transplantation. Ann Thorac Surg 1988;65:S71–S73, S74–S76.

Chapter

33

Neurologic Considerations of Organ Transplantation

MICHAEL DONAGHY

NEUROLOGIC SYNDROMES IN TRANSPLANT RECIPIENTS

Neurologic disorders are a major contributor to the morbidity and mortality of transplantation. Often these disorders develop months or years after transplantation and may never be seen by the surgical team who performed the engraftment. The range of neurologic disease encountered in transplant recipients is enormous. A few particular conditions occur regularly: cerebral lymphoma, stroke, infections, polyneuropathy, and drug complications. The diagnosis and management of these disorders often requires combined attention from neurologists, neuroradiologists, neurosurgeons, neuropathologists, oncologists, and microbiologists. Accurate diagnoses are crucial for definitive therapy, particularly for neurologic infections. Diagnostic confusion may be generated by the remnants of previous neurologic disease, by the coexistence of multiple illnesses, and by attenuation of normal inflammatory responses by immunosuppression. Neurologic disorders can result from recurrence or continuation of the underlying disease process that initially caused organ failure, such as systemic lupus erythematosus, systemic vasculitis, atherosclerosis, diabetes mellitus, alcoholism, leukemia, or lymphoma.

The initial diagnostic step requires the patient's disorder to be categorized into one of these broad syndromes: diffuse encephalopathy, focal cerebral abnormality, seizure disorder, or peripheral nerve damage. Then one should investigate the diseases most commonly encountered in transplant recipients who have that particular syndrome (Table 33.1). Certain problems are particularly common in the immediate postoperative period, particularly perioperative damage to peripheral nerves, electrolyte disturbances, hypertension, and cyclosporine toxicity.

Diffuse Encephalopathy

Encephalopathy may range from mild personality change, confusion, drowsiness, or ataxia to deep coma. Headache, seizures, or meningeal irritation may be present also, depending on the underlying cause.

Drugs are a potent cause of encephalopathy. Cyclosporine toxicity usually becomes evident within the first 3 months after transplantation, and the resultant encephalopathy often includes tremors, seizures, or visual disturbances (1). Tacrolimus treatment can produce a similar encephalopathy. OKT-3 monoclonal antibody treatment for rejection can produce aseptic meningitis lasting a few days, with photophobia and headache. Occasionally these symptoms are accompanied by mild encephalopathy.

Infective meningoencephalitis should always be suspected in patients with diffuse encephalopathy. One should be aware that signs of meningeal irritation, such as neck stiffness or photophobia, are often absent in the immunosuppressed transplant recipient (2). *Listeria monocytogenes* causes a meningoencephalitis that develops over a few days, and often includes signs of brainstem dysfunction such as eye movement disorders or dysarthria. *Cryptococcus neoformans* meningitis usually develops 6 months or more after transplantation, and the symptoms may be nonspecific and insidiously progressive. Encephalopathy may be a remote effect of systemic sepsis, sometimes accompanied by seizures or focal signs (3).

An entity termed "rejection encephalopathy" has been proposed based upon observations of 13 renal transplant recipients with a reversible acute encephalopathy coinciding with severe acute rejection (4). Young transplant recipients seemed especially susceptible. Varying combinations of seizures, headache, confusion, irritability, and papilledema

Table 33.1. Neurological Syndromes in Transplant Recipients

Diffuse encephalopathy
Meningitis
Encephalitis
Electrolyte disturbances
Rejection encephalopathy
Hypertensive encephalopathy
Hypoxic, hypotensive encephalopathy
Remote effects of systemic sepsis
Multifocal cerebral lymphoma
Pulmonary, liver, or renal failure
Cyclosporine toxicity
Tacrolimus toxicity
OKT-3 antibody meningoencephalopathy
Focal neurologic abnormalities
Cerebral lymphoma
Ischemic stroke
Intracerebral hematoma
Focal cerebral infection
Central pontine myelinolysis
Seizures
Cyclosporine toxicity
Hypomagnesemia
Hyponatremia
Rejection encephalopathy
Cerebral lymphoma
Meningitis/encephalitis
Neuromuscular disease
Perioperative nerve damage
Guillain-Barré syndrome
Chronic inflammatory demyelinating polyneuropathy
Tacrolimus neuropathy
Critical illness polyneuropathy
Polymyositis
Myasthenia gravis
Rhabdomyolysis

were noted. Only one of these patients was receiving cyclosporine. Nonencephalopathic patients with acute graft rejection exhibited similar degrees of hypertension. It should be noted that a similar syndrome occurs after transplantation of other organs, and that hypertension is considered to play a major part. In these patients, the encephalopathy apparently resolves satisfactorily with antihypertensive therapy and little or no reduction in cyclosporine dosage (5).

It is unclear whether so-called rejection encephalopathy should be regarded as a direct consequence of graft rejection, or whether it merely reflects the cumulative physiologic and metabolic insults at the time. Patients developing encephalopathy during acute graft rejection should be assessed for cyclosporine toxicity, electrolyte disorders, fluid overload, severe uremia, systemic sepsis, and malignant hypertension. If the rejection has been delayed more than a few weeks after transplantation, neurologic infection and cerebral lymphoma should be considered as well.

A diffuse encephalopathy due to operative or postoperative hypoxia or hypotension is particularly likely in pulmonary or cardiac transplant recipients. In the first 6 weeks after bone narrow transplantation accompanied by high-dose chemotherapy for Hodgkin's disease, 30% of patients develop encephalopathy, often as a result of associated pulmonary or renal failure (6). Deterioration in cognitive abilities or personality change is common in the first weeks after liver transplantation (7).

Prompt and thorough investigation for potentially treatable causes is necessary in encephalopathic transplant recipients. Brain imaging with computed tomography (CT) or magnetic resonance imaging (MRI) will detect multiple cerebral mass lesions masquerading as diffuse encephalopathy, a particular problem with multifocal cerebral lymphoma. The spinal fluid should be examined for tuberculosis, fungi, and conventional bacteria if the brain scan is normal. Blood-CSF glucose ratios of more than 2:1 point to meningeal infection or malignant meningitis; this test can be valuable if spinal fluid microscopy is inconclusive.

Hyponatremia can be a nonspecific feature of chronic meningitis or other intracranial diseases and should not be accepted as a definitive explanation for encephalopathy in its own right. Only rarely does the clinical and laboratory assessment point so convincingly to cyclosporine toxicity, hypertension, dilutional hyponatremia, or hypoxic-hypotensive encephalopathy that other diagnostic tests can be avoided.

Focal Cerebral Abnormalities

Hemiparesis, dysphasia, or homonymous hemianopia are frequently encountered in transplant recipients. When focal disorders cause disturbed memory, disrupted spatial orientation, or a speech disorder, they are often misinterpreted as diffuse encephalopathies.

Transplant recipients with focal neurologic disturbances should be investigated initially with CT or MRI brain scans. Focal mass lesions usually require neurosurgical biopsy with both histologic and microbiologic examination of the specimen.

Ischemic stroke is common during the long-term follow-up of renal and heart-lung transplant recipients. It usually presents with an abrupt onset of neurologic deficit and little or no headache (8). CT scans may show no abnormality during the first 24 to 48 hours following small ischemic strokes. Intracerebral hematoma is particularly common in bone marrow and liver transplant recipients. It causes a rapidly worsening, rather than instantaneous, neurologic deficit such as a hemiparesis, often with headache (9,10).

The risk of primary cerebral lymphoma is greatly increased in transplant recipients. By the time of diagnosis, symptoms of focal cerebral damage have usually been progressively worsening for weeks and months. Surprisingly, headache seems to be a relatively late feature (11). Cerebral lymphoma may be multifocal and masquerade as a diffuse encephalopathy.

Focal cerebral infections are usually due to aspergillosis or, less often, to toxoplasmosis. Symptomatic *Aspergillus* or *Toxoplasma* brain infection may occur within 2 weeks of transplantation; most *Aspergillus* infections are seen within the first 6 months following transplantation (12). In contrast, *Nocardia* brain abscesses tend to present more than 3 months following transplantation. Many patients with these focal cerebral infections do not exhibit the expected headache or fever.

Benign intracranial hypertension or pseudotumor cerebri, with papilledema and headache, has been reported in children after renal transplantation (12) or bone marrow transplantation (13), possibly related to cyclosporine usage. On clinical grounds such patients may be suspected of harboring a focal cerebral mass lesion, but the brain scan will be normal.

Central pontine myelinolysis usually presents with paralysis of all four limbs progressing over hours or days. It is particularly likely in hepatic transplant recipients (14). The cranial musculature can be affected, causing loss of speech; and the resultant "locked-in state" may be mistaken for coma. Central pontine myelinolysis usually occurs in the postoperative period a few days after unduly rapid correction of chronic hyponatremia (15).

Convulsions

Convulsions are frequent in transplant recipients. Cyclosporine appears to reduce seizure thresholds (1), and hypomagnesemia appears to predispose patients toward cyclosporine-induced seizures (16). Multiple factors often act in combination to cause convulsions in transplant recipients (17). Focal cerebral lesions such as lymphoma, infection, or infarction should be sought with CT or MRI brain scans. The possibilities of meningitis, systemic sepsis, and graft rejection should be considered. Hypoglycemic convulsions can occur in transplanted diabetics. Blood levels of cyclosporine, sodium, and magnesium should be estimated in transplant recipients with seizures.

Seizures seem particularly likely following liver transplantation—they occurred in 25 to 42% of patients in series from the mid-1980s, usually during the first postoperative week (18–20). Various explanations for seizures should be sought in this setting. Many patients will have evidence of hyponatremia, cerebrovascular disease, or infection (21). Intolerance of cyclosporine is probably a factor in the incidence of seizures and other encephalopathic neurologic complications after transplantation, but the risk is lessened by a readiness to withdraw cyclosporine at the onset of mental changes or dysarthria (19).

Neuromuscular Disease

Focal Peripheral Nerve Damage

Femoral nerve lesions can be caused by self-retaining retractor blades during renal transplantation if the surgeon has not checked that the femoral artery remains pulsatile after positioning the retractor (22–24). Symptoms of femoral neuropathy often fail to become apparent until the patient tries to walk postoperatively. The examination will show unilateral weakness of knee extension and loss of the knee jerk, as well as sensory disturbance on the anterior thigh or medial calf. These perioperative femoral nerve lesions usually resolve over months, although sometimes incompletely.

Diabetics undergoing renal transplantation seem to be vulnerable to a presumed ischemic lesion of the lumbosacral plexus when the internal iliac arteries are used for revascularization of the graft (25). These patients present postoperatively with weakness of the leg below the knee and buttock pain. Recovery may be incomplete.

Lung transplantation can lead to unilateral or bilateral phrenic nerve lesions. The resultant diaphragm paralysis and respiratory difficulties could lead to prolonged postoperative ventilator dependence (26).

Various perioperative mononeuropathies can complicate liver transplantation; most often seen is a brachial plexus injury attributable to arm malpositioning (27). Perioperative palsies of the peroneal, radial, and cutaneous branch of the femoral nerves, and a Horner's syndrome related to cervical sympathetic chain damage have also been recorded in liver transplant recipients (7,28). In general these perioperative compressive neuropathies recover either partially or completely.

Polyneuropathy

Generalized muscle weakness in transplant recipients has various causes, and is usually seen in bone marrow or hepatic transplantation (28,29). An acute polyneuropathy presenting as an areflexic tetraparesis evolving over 4 to 6 weeks is typical of Guillain-Barré syndrome. Critical illness polyneuropathy usually presents in patients with sepsis and multiple organ failure as difficulty in weaning from the ventilator; patients usually recover with treatment of the underlying general medical problems (30). Chronic inflammatory demyelinating polyneuropathy can develop in the months following liver transplantation. It responds well to plasma exchange or intravenous immunoglobulin (31). A neuropathy indistinguishable from chronic inflammatory demyelinating polyneuropathy can follow a few weeks after starting tacrolimus immunosuppression in liver transplant recipients (32,33). If neuropathy occurs in bone marrow graft recipients with underlying hematologic malignancies, a contribution from cytotoxic drug treatments such as *Vinka* alkaloids (34) or etoposide (35) should be suspected. Tinglings in fingers and toes are common during cyclosporine administration, but nerve conduction studies are normal and no clinical evidence of polyneuropathy develops. A true polyneuropathy is rarely if ever attributable to cyclosporine; neurotoxic effects of other drugs or metabolic contributions have been difficult to exclude in the few postulated cases (36,37).

Myopathy

Myopathies can occur in bone marrow or liver transplant recipients. Polymyositis causing proximal muscle weakness has been recorded in chronic graft-versus-host disease 18 months after bone marrow transplantation (38,39). Fatigable weakness and ptosis typical of myasthenia gravis, associated with antiacetylcholine receptor antibodies, has occurred in chronic graft-versus-host disease (39,40). Although these myopathies should be treated in their own right, their ultimate prognosis depends on effective suppression of the graft-versus-host disease.

Severe quadriplegia, sometimes due to proven rhabdomyolysis, may occur in liver transplant recipients but tends to recover well; its cause is unknown (28).

SPECIFIC DISEASES REGULARLY ENCOUNTERED IN TRANSPLANT RECIPIENTS

Cerebral Lymphoma

From the early days of renal transplantation, a marked incidence of lymphoproliferative disorders has been noted (41,42). From the outset, it was recognized that primary lymphomas of the central nervous system were the predominant component of this increase (43), an impression repeatedly confirmed by more recent studies (11). The incidence of primary cerebral lymphoma is increasing rapidly both in the immunocompetent normal population (44) and in the immunocompromised patient (45). The risk of cerebral lymphoma in transplant recipients is estimated at 2%, between 30 and 350 times higher than in the general population (45,46). This risk may be highest in cardiac and hepatic transplant recipients, and lowest after bone marrow transplantation (see also Chapter 37).

Primary cerebral lymphoma is much more common than cerebral or meningeal spread from systemic lymphoma in transplant recipients. Most primary cerebral lymphomas are non-Hodgkin's monoclonal B lymphocyte proliferations. Primary cerebral lymphoma seems to be caused by Epstein-Barr virus (EBV), given the serum antibody responses, the immunostaining and DNA hybridization studies of biopsy specimens, and the evidence of clonal proliferation from a single EBV-infected progenitor cell in a case of HIV-related cerebral lymphoma (47–51).

The median interval from transplantation to clinical detection of primary cerebral lymphoma in transplant recipients is 9 months, with a range of 5.5 to 46 months (11). It remains to be seen whether the widespread introduction of cyclosporine and other new immunosuppressant agents since the mid-1980s will influence the incidence or timing of cerebral lymphoma in transplant recipients.

Primary cerebral lymphoma is multifocal in a third of patients, and it affects the cerebral hemispheres about 3.5 times as frequently as it affects the brainstem or cerebellum (11,52). It can invade the meninges, but lymphomatous meningitis more often represents spread from a systemic primary. Primary cerebral lymphoma usually presents with a focal neurologic deficit, which worsens over a few weeks or months. Typical symptoms and signs include hemiparesis, aphasia, hemianopia, or cerebellar ataxia. Patients with multifocal cerebral lymphoma may develop features more suggestive of diffuse encephalopathy, such as convulsions, personality change, or dementia. Headache is usually a late symptom, reflecting raised intracranial pressure or meningeal infiltration (11). Rarer neurologic presentations of lymphomas include spinal cord lesions due to localized intradural masses, visual disturbance due to ocular deposits, and malignant meningitis (11).

MRI or CT brain scan detects the vast majority of primary central nervous system lymphomas (Figs. 33.1, 33.2). Sensitivity is increased by contrast enhancement, that also helps reveal the smaller lesions in multifocal disease. Cerebral lymphoma is often situated periventricularly and usually appears as a homogeneously contrast-enhancing mass with relatively little surrounding edema, quite unlike the ring-enhancing lesions surrounded by marked edema that are so typical of malignant glioma or secondary carcinoma deposits. If it is suspected after brain scanning, the diagnosis of primary intracerebral lymphoma should be confirmed by prompt neurosurgical biopsy, preferably stereotactically guided. High-dose steroid therapy should be avoided before obtaining the biopsy specimen, as dexamethasone can shrink cerebral lymphomas dramatically within a few days and interfere with the reliability of histologic diagnosis (see Fig. 33.1) (53,54).

The approach to treatment and prognosis of primary cerebral lymphoma is based mainly on studies of the immunocompetent normal population or of HIV-infected individuals. Neurosurgical resection of primary intracerebral lymphoma should not be attempted, because this does not enhance long-term survival and marked neurologic deficits will follow attempts to resect deep-sealed tumor masses (54). In immunocompetent cases, dramatic initial responses can be achieved with steroids and cranial radiotherapy, but the median survival is only 10 to 18 months. Improved survival has been reported when high-dose cytosine arabinoside and intrathecal methotrexate are combined with radiotherapy (54).

The prognosis is generally poorer in HIV-infected individuals or immunosuppressed transplant recipients with primary cerebral lymphoma (45). Radiotherapy is the mainstay of treatment, with or without chemotherapy (see Fig. 33.2). The effect upon prognosis of continuing the

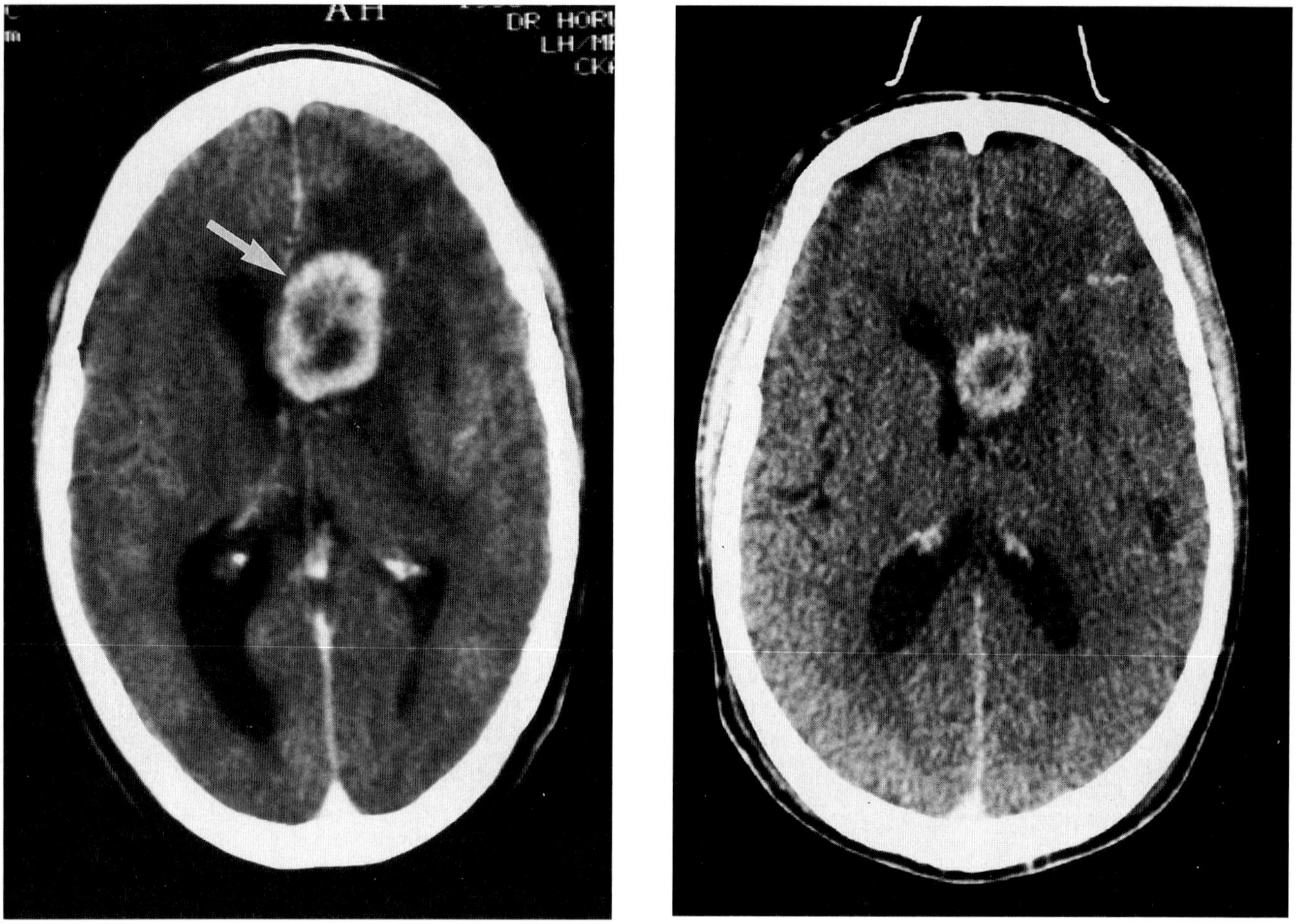

A B

FIGURE 33.1. *Primary cerebral lymphoma* (arrow) *shown on enhanced CT scans.* ***A.*** *Before steroids.* ***B.*** *After 5 days of dexamethasone therapy.*

immunosuppressant drug therapy is unknown in transplant recipients. Logic dictates that immunosuppressant drug dosages should be minimized, but the benefits of such a change remain unknown.

Cerebrovascular Disease

Stroke is a prominent cause of morbidity and mortality following transplantation, both in the early months and in the years that follow successful transplantation.

Ischemic Stroke

A 6-year follow-up study of the early renal transplants found that 3% of deaths were caused by ischemic stroke, a risk estimated to be more than 100 times higher than for the normal population (55). Later studies showed stroke to account for 12% of deaths during 10 years of follow-up. Stroke or transient cerebral ischemic attacks had occurred in 8.5% of the 10-year survivors of renal transplantation (56). Thromboembolic disease is second only to infection as the cause of death in the early years following transplantation (57,58). Thromboembolic disease is the major cause of death or illness in those surviving into their second decade of engraftment (59).

A variety of factors contribute to the huge incidence of ischemic stroke after renal transplantation, which particularly affects transplant recipients aged 40 years and older (8,55). Diabetes mellitus, systemic lupus erythematosus, hypertensive renal failure, and polycystic renal disease have all been associated with an increased risk of subsequent stroke in transplant recipients (8,55). Accelerated atherosclerosis may be due to the hyperlipidemia that occurs in renal failure and following transplantation (60). Long-term prednisolone therapy may accelerate the development of atherosclerosis. It will be interesting to see whether the incidence of ischemic stroke now has fallen following the introduction of cyclosporine, which is steroid sparing.

Patients with ischemic stroke usually develop a sudden focal neurologic deficit such as aphasia, hemiparesis, clumsiness, or homonymous hemianopia. Headache, if present, is rarely severe. If the neurologic deficit recovers within 24 hours it is termed a transient cerebral ischemic attack rather

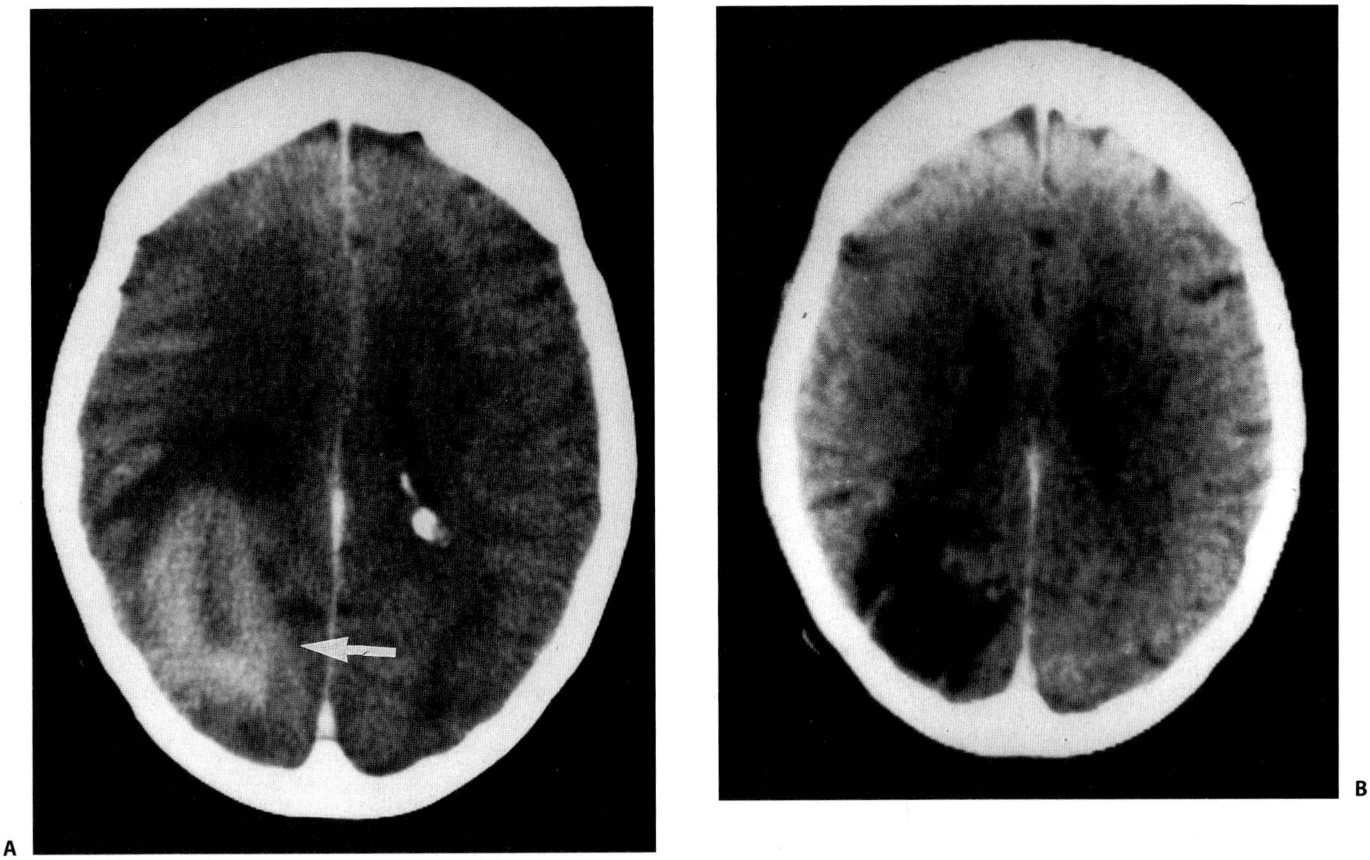

FIGURE 33.2. *Primary cerebral lymphoma* (arrow). ***A.*** *Before radiotherapy (contrast-enhanced CT scan).* ***B.*** *After radiotherapy (unenhanced CT scan).*

than a completed stroke. Patients with transient ischemic attacks should be investigated for potentially reversible risk factors and treated with low-dose aspirin (75–150 mg daily) to reduce the risk of future stroke.

Potentially reversible risk factors include hypertension, diabetes mellitus, smoking, syphilis, polycythemia, and thrombocythemia. Patients with a history of systemic lupus erythematosus may have anticardiolipin antibodies. Cerebral vasculitis, meningeal fungal infection with *Aspergillus*, or mucormycosis should be considered in patients with multiple strokes, fever, prominent headache, seizures, or a lymphocytic spinal fluid examination. Cerebral vasculitis has occurred in an immunosuppressed transplant recipient (61).

Atheromatous stenosis of the internal carotid artery should be sought by carotid duplex scanning when stroke occurs in transplant recipients. If the stenosis exceeds 70%, carotid endarterectomy is known to produce a small but significant improvement in long-term stroke-free survival in the nonimmunosuppressed population (62,63). However, one cannot presume that the recommendations from these trials can be translated automatically to transplant recipients affected by stroke. Transplant recipients would be expected to have a higher risk of stroke in other arterial territories, a higher risk of ischemic cardiac disease, and a higher risk of other factors affecting overall prognosis. These factors might offset the small benefits otherwise expected from carotid endarterectomy.

Perioperative ischemic stroke during heart transplantation is thought to result from air embolism from the chambers of the grafted heart, or from dislodgment of solid emboli during operation, or from perioperative cerebral hypoperfusion (64). Many patients will have been chronically hypotensive due to cardiac failure, and it is possible that successful transplantation elevates blood pressure to an extent exceeding the threshold of cerebral autoregulation, thus resulting in stroke (65). Cerebral infarction can occur both early and late after bone marrow or liver transplantation, and may reflect underlying endocarditis (7,66,67). However, after bone marrow or liver transplantation, cerebral infarction is generally overshadowed by the noteworthy incidence of hemorrhagic strokes.

Intracranial Hemorrhage

Hemorrhagic stroke, with immediate development of an intracerebral hematoma or subdural hematoma visible on unenhanced CT scan, seems to be particularly common in bone marrow and liver transplant recipients and also occurs following renal transplantation (Fig. 33.3). Intracerebral hemorrhage after liver transplantation usually occurs in the frontal or parietal lobes, and is often associated with bacteremia or fungemia, or with thrombocytopenia (10). Intracranial hemorrhage may occur either early or late after bone marrow transplantation for Hodgkin's disease (6). Subdural hematoma, or less often intracerebral hematoma, has occurred particularly in the leukemic subgroup of a heterogeneous population of bone marrow transplant recipients (9). If patients with sickle cell anemia have suffered cerebral infarction prior to transplantation, the risk of post-transplant intracranial bleeding was found to be as high as 38% (68). An autopsy series showed no evidence of graft-versus-host disease affecting the central nervous system in bone marrow transplant recipients with hemorrhagic or ischemic stroke (67). Subarachnoid hemorrhage occurs relatively infrequently in transplant recipients, even in those with underlying polycystic renal disease who have a high risk of cerebral aneurysm (8).

Patients with intracranial hemorrhage should be investigated for a potentially correctable coagulation deficit. Subdural hematomas should be evacuated surgically if sufficiently large to cause impaired consciousness or focal signs such as hemiparesis. Often, smaller subdural hematomas can be managed conservatively. Endocarditis and other bacteremias or fungemias should be sought in patients with intracerebral hematoma, particularly if mycotic aneurysms are discovered on cerebral angiography. Surgical evacuation is unlikely to improve the outcome from intracerebral hematoma except in the rare situation of potentially life-threatening brainstem compression due to a cerebellar hemorrhage. Overall, many transplant recipients die from intracranial hemorrhage.

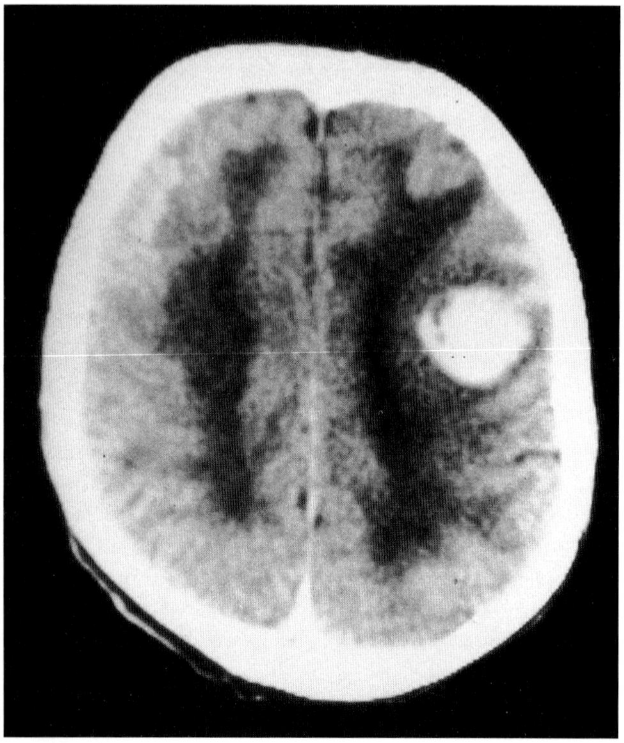

FIGURE 33.3. *Primary intracerebral hematoma in a renal transplant recipient (unenhanced CT scan).*

Neurologic Infections

Varied neurologic infections occur in transplant recipients (2,69,70) (see Chapter 36). Diagnoses are often elusive, and require close cooperation between transplant clinicians, neurologists, microbiologists, and neuropathologists. During the 1970s, 7% of renal transplant recipients developed central nervous system infection during a 10-year period with a resultant mortality of nearly 50% (2). *Cryptococcus*, *Aspergillus*, and *Listeria* infections accounted for 90% of these infections. Since the introduction of cyclosporine immunosuppression, a wider range of nervous system infections seems to be occurring, with increasingly frequent diagnoses of *Nocardia* and *Toxoplasma* infection in particular. Central nervous system infection should be considered in transplant recipients who experience headache, undiagnosed fever, confusion, altered consciousness, focal symptoms, or convulsions. Brain imaging will detect focal lesions, which can be biopsied. The spinal fluid should be examined if there is no cerebral mass lesion to contraindicate lumbar puncture.

Three main syndromes of central nervous system infection will be encountered. First, meningitis can be caused by *Listeria*, *Cryptococcus*, or conventional bacteria. Less commonly, meningitis can be caused by tuberculosis, lymphoma, or coccidioidomycosis (in endemic areas such as Arizona) (71). Aseptic meningitis may follow OKT-3 antibody therapy for rejection or administration of high-dose intravenous human immunoglobulin. Focal brain abscesses are generally caused by *Aspergillus* or *Nocardia*, and less commonly by *Toxoplasma* or *Candida*. A diffuse encephalitic picture can be caused by aspergillosis or toxoplasmosis, which will usually show focal lesions on MRI scan.

Less frequently, infective encephalopathy is due to progressive multifocal leukoencephalopathy or cytomegalovirus (CMV) encephalitis, which both show as diffuse, patchy destruction of the cerebral hemisphere white matter on MRI scan. Herpes simplex encephalitis is surprisingly uncommon in the immunosuppressed, but does occur in bone marrow transplant recipients. It should be considered if there are signal changes in the medial temporal lobes on MRI scan, and the polymerase chain reaction for herpesvirus should be performed on the cerebral spinal fluid (67).

Acanthamoeba meningoencephalitis has caused rapidly progressive mental deterioration, coma, and seizures, with eventual death in two bone marrow transplant recipients (72). The source of infection is thought to be the upper respiratory tract; there may be a history of sinusitis, or pulmonary infiltrates may be evident on chest x-ray. Mucormycosis is particularly common in diabetics receiving transplants. Fungal infection in the paranasal sinuses causes periorbital edema; subsequent fungal invasion of the intracavernous carotid artery can cause fatal cerebral emboli and stroke (73).

Diagnosis of the infection usually requires brain biopsy of focal lesions or repeated spinal fluid examinations. Generally these infections cause a lymphocytic spinal fluid pleocytosis, often with a low glucose level. The spinal fluid should be examined microscopically and cultured for conventional bacteria, microbacteria, and fungi. Fungal serology is most reliable if performed on both serum and spinal fluid. Cryptococcal antigen may be detected immunologically in the spinal fluid.

Often, patients are too acutely ill with meningitis to await definitive bacteriological diagnosis. If so, empiric ampicillin treatment should be started immediately after lumbar puncture; this will cover listeriosis pending a definitive diagnosis.

Listeria monocytogenes

Listeria causes meningitis, and less commonly, focal cerebral infection or meningoencephalitis (74). The fever and headache develop subacutely. Impaired consciousness and typical signs of meningism or focal neurologic deficits are encountered in less than half of cases (75). It is rare for *Listeria* infection to present within the first month after transplantation; thereafter, it must be a prominent consideration (2).

It is easiest to diagnose *Listeria* meningitis in those with purely meningitic syndromes in whom there is a high chance of positive blood or spinal fluid cultures. The spinal fluid white cell count may vary from less than 10 to many thousands per mm^3, and may be predominantly polymorphonuclear or lymphocytic. The spinal fluid glucose level is reduced in approximately half of cases (74). Proving the diagnosis may be difficult in those with focal neurologic signs, but the combination of brainstem dysfunction and a cellular spinal fluid should raise a particular suspicion of listeriosis.

Combined ampicillin and gentamicin therapy is recommended. Trimethoprim and sulfamethoxazole provide an alternative (70). Listeriosis proves fatal in nearly a quarter of renal transplant recipients (74).

Cryptococcus neoformans

Cryptococcus produces an indolent chronic lymphocytic meningitis that rarely presents earlier than 6 months following transplantation (2). Mild headache and fever are the usual early symptoms. Severely depressed consciousness or focal signs are rare.

In suspected cases, it is recommended that antibody detection of cryptococcal antigen in the spinal fluid be undertaken, as this allows prompt and reliable diagnosis. Spinal fluid contains up to 500 lymphocytes per mm^3 with a low glucose level, and the pressure is often increased.

The infection can be eradicated in most patients using a combination of intravenous amphotericin B and/or fluconazole without reducing the immunosuppression (2,76).

Cytomegalovirus

Proven cytomegalovirus encephalitis is rare in transplant recipients, although it is often suspected (77). Clinical experience of this condition has been derived mainly from AIDS patients (78). Patients usually present with a meningoencephalitis in which confusion and memory loss are prominent. Other features such as headache or retinitis may be present. MRI brain scan can be normal, or it may show atrophy, white matter abnormalities, or meningeal enhancement. Spinal fluid can be normal or lymphocytic. A positive polymerase chain reaction seems to be a reliable indicator of central nervous system infection (79).

After a positive diagnosis, treatment is initiated with ganciclovir or foscarnet; also, the immunosuppressant drug regimen is reduced (77,79). The prognosis of cytomegalovirus encephalitis is poor, at least in AIDS patients.

Aspergillus fumigatus

Focal *Aspergillus* infection of the brain usually develops within the first few months following transplantation (2). Generally patients develop sudden focal neurologic deficits or seizures, fever, and evidence of lung infiltration (80). Brain scans show focal lesion with a paucity of contrast enhancement and relatively little mass effect. Spinal fluid is often normal, but may contain an excess of lymphocytes with a normal glucose concentration.

Fungal invasion of cerebral blood vessels with distal embolization accounts for the stroke-like onset of some symptoms. Multiple cerebral lesions may be present. A purely meningitic syndrome may result from rupture of cerebral abscesses into the subarachnoid space. The diagnosis can be proved by lung or cerebral biopsy.

Most patients progressively deteriorate. Many die, despite antifungal therapy with amphotericin B (2,80,81).

Nocardia asteroides

Nocardia brain abscesses in transplant recipients are usually derived from a pulmonary focus of infection. Nocardial infections may occur in clusters in transplant units (82). The abscesses usually occupy much of a cerebral hemisphere, causing hemianopia, hemiparesis, aphasia, or confusion, accompanied by fever and headache. Subcutaneous lesions may be palpable and their biopsy may prove the diagnosis.

Brain scans reveal the abscesses. Aspiration is necessary to prove the diagnosis, and also is generally recommended as treatment. High-dose sulphonamide therapy should be given.

Central Pontine Myelinolysis

Pontine myelinolysis consists of acute or subacute demyelination of the mid-brainstem, particularly affecting the corticospinal tracts as they pass through the pons (83). Over hours or a few days patients develop symmetrical limb weakness with extensor plantar responses. Sometimes the bulbar and facial musculature is also paralyzed. A locked-in state develops in severe cases—such patients remain fully conscious and yet no voluntary movements are possible apart from vertical eye movements. The latter condition is often misinterpreted as coma. Central pontine myelinolysis usually causes death; full recovery is rare, and usually survivors are chronically disabled. MRI clearly demonstrates the demyelination within the brainstem (Fig. 33.4).

Hyponatremia has been present in many patients developing central pontine myelinolysis, particularly in those with alcoholic liver disease, with inappropriate antidiuretic hormone secretion, and under thiazide diuretic therapy. In transplant recipients it is most common following liver transplantation (15,85), but also occurs after renal engraftment (86,87). Central pontine myelinolysis is usually noted a few days after intravenous fluid correction of chronic hyponatremia at rates that raise the serum sodium by more than 12 mmol/L/day. Many cases of this disastrous neurologic disorder seem to be iatrogenic, and it is recommended that the serum sodium concentration be increased by no more than 8 mmol/L/day (15,87,88).

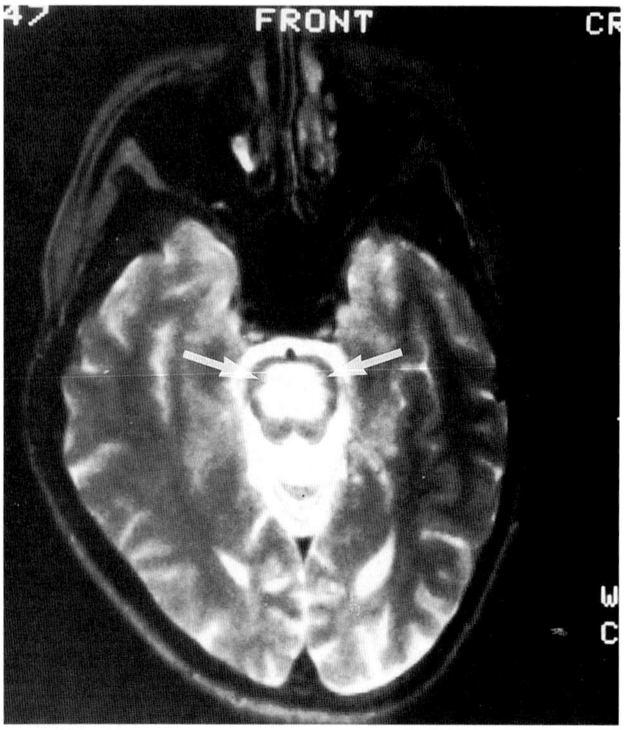

FIGURE 33.4. *Central pontine myelinolysis* (arrows) *shown on MRI scan.*

Guillain-Barré Syndrome

A Guillain-Barré polyneuropathy is encountered most usually in bone marrow transplant recipients, but it has been recorded following renal transplantation. It produces rapidly progressive limb muscle paralysis, with areflexia and variable sensory loss, reaching its worst by 4 to 6 weeks. In many patients severe respiratory or bulbar muscle paralysis requires temporary endotracheal intubation and ventilation. The clinical picture is usually diagnostic, but supporting evidence for the diagnosis comes from demonstrating a raised protein in an otherwise acellular cerebrospinal fluid, and from demonstrating a demyelinating neuropathy on nerve conduction studies.

Guillain-Barré syndrome following renal transplantation is usually thought to result from transmitted CMV infection or reactivation of latent CMV (89,90). In bone marrow transplant recipients Guillain-Barré syndrome or chronic inflammatory demyelinating polyneuropathy may be associated with graft-versus-host disease (29,91), or with reactivation of CMV infection (92,93) or *Campylobacter jejuni* bacteremia (94). The patient usually recovers from the neuropathy or improves substantially following treatment of the graft-versus-host disease. The usual treatment for Guillain-Barré syndrome should be given—either plasma exchange or intravenous immunoglobulin.

NEUROLOGIC SIDE EFFECTS OF IMMUNOSUPPRESSANT DRUGS

Cyclosporine

Drug-induced neurologic side effects are most common with cyclosporine and range from tremors, fits, or paresthesia to a severe leukoencephalopathy (see Chapter 6). Neurologic complications attributable to cyclosporine occurred in roughly 20% of renal transplant recipients in the early days of its use (1,95), but they have become much less common with more experienced use of the drug. Nowadays, cyclosporine side effects are most common in liver transplant recipients, occurring in one-tenth (96), possibly as a result of associated hypocholesterolemia and hyponatremia (18,97).

Limb tremor, often minor, is the most common neurologic side effect, being noted at some time by as many as 20% of patients. This tremor is usually most prominent in the first 3 months, and is generally asymptomatic a few years after transplantation (1). Burning paresthesia of the limbs is a common complaint in patients taking cyclosporine, but these patients have no objective evidence of peripheral neuropathy on clinical and electrophysiologic testing. Visual hallucinations or cortical blindness have been associated with high blood cyclosporine levels (19,98,99). Some cyclosporine recipients develop psychological disorders such as depression or sleepiness (1). Tremor, paresthesia, visual hallucinations, and cortical blindness are usually dose-related side effects of cyclosporine and recover or improve with dosage reduction, or after switching to an alternative immunosuppressant. Generally the MRI brain scan is normal in these dose-related side effects (96). Most occurrences of paresthesia or tremor are not sufficiently disabling to warrant stoppage or reduction of effective immunosuppressive therapy.

Mutism (expressive aphasia) is a rare but distressing complication occurring within the first postoperative fortnight after liver transplantation. The MRI brain scan is usually normal, and speech returns after stopping cyclosporine (100,101).

Recurrent throbbing headaches, sometimes unilateral with nausea and photophobia and a visual aura, and typical of migraine, have been noted in liver transplant recipients treated with cyclosporine. They may improve with reduction in dosage (102).

Leukoencephalopathy, visible on MRI scanning, is a rare but serious side effect of cyclosporine most commonly seen in bone marrow and liver transplant recipients (19,97,103). Coma, confusion, cerebellar syndromes, hemiplegia, and flaccid quadriparesis have all been described. Combinations of these features have been termed a "cerebrocerebellar syndrome" (19).

Leukoencephalopathy is most likely to develop within the first 3 months of cyclosporine therapy. Although cyclosporine levels are usually elevated, they can be normal. Diffuse white matter abnormalities are visible in the cerebral hemispheres on MRI scan (Fig. 33.5). The spinal fluid protein can be elevated. The leukoencephalopathy usually improves after stopping cyclosporine or reducing the dosage if blood levels were high (Fig 33.6).

Seizures can be precipitated by cyclosporine, particularly in hypomagnesemic patients (16,18). Other coincidental factors need to be considered when seizures occur, including hyponatremia, graft rejection, hypotension, high-dose steroid therapy, cerebral infections, or lymphomas. Seizures probably occur in 1.5% of cyclosporine-treated renal transplant recipients (95). After chronic renal dialysis, chronic aluminum overload prior to transplantation may predispose to seizures (104). If seizures occur, the dosage should be reduced if blood cyclosporine levels are high. Other precipitating factors should be corrected. When seizures persist despite these measures, choosing an anticonvulsant drug is difficult. Phenytoin, carbamazepine, and phenobarbitone all induce enzymes, which poses problems in achieving adequate blood levels of cyclosporine (17,36). Thus, sodium valproate is the recommended anticonvulsant in patients also receiving cyclosporine (105).

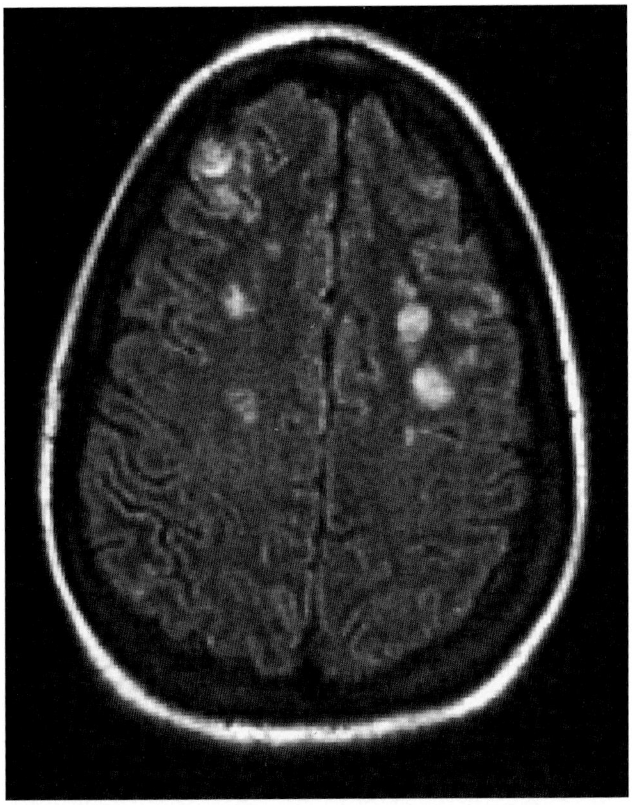

FIGURE 33.5. *Bilateral while matter lesions in cyclosporine-treated liver allograft recipient with confusion and seizures.*

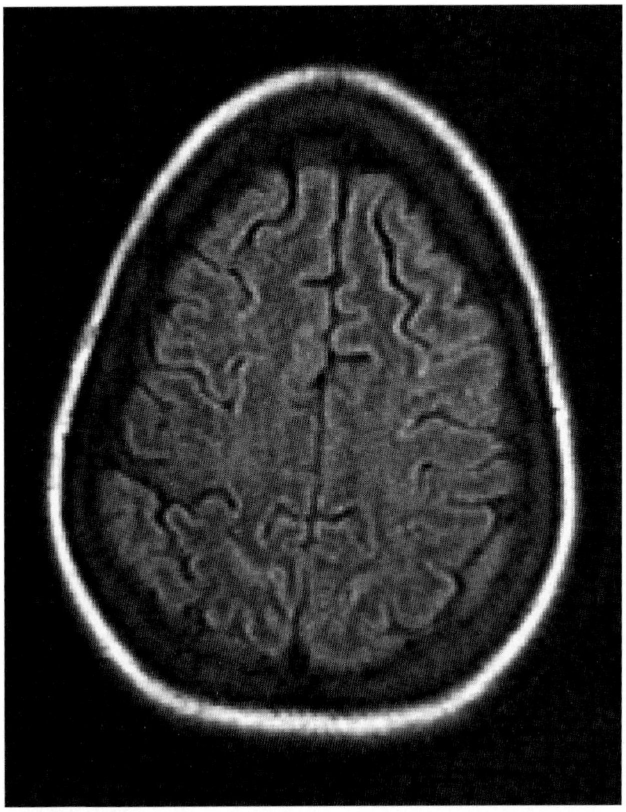

FIGURE 33.6. *Resolution of MRI-detected lesions and clinical symptoms 3 weeks after discontinuing cyclosporine.*

Tacrolimus

Tacrolimus is used as an alternative immunosuppressant to cyclosporine, and is usually a satisfactory replacement in cases of severe cyclosporine-associated neurologic side effects (see Chapter 9). However, tacrolimus itself does have neurotoxic side effects in 20% to 30% of patients (106,107). These usually occur within the first months of therapy, and are more common at higher doses (106). Speech disturbances, generalized seizures, tremor and ataxia, encephalopathy, and nightmares and agitation have occurred. Most complications resolve with dosage reduction, but mild tremor or speech disturbance may persist.

A leukoencephalopathy with white matter abnormalities on MRI scan affecting the parietooccipital regions and centrum semiovale can occur. It closely resembles the cyclosporine-associated leukoencephalopathy (108). This syndrome usually presents with occipital headache, nausea and vomiting, followed by a seizure, and there may be visual disturbances. Tacrolimus blood levels may be high, although not invariably. The disorder resolves with dosage reduction.

A severe demyelinating sensory motor peripheral neuropathy resembling chronic inflammatory demyelinating polyneuropathy has been associated with tacrolimus (32,33).

OKT-3 Antibody

The use of OKT-3 monoclonal antibody therapy to suppress acute graft rejection is occasionally followed by aseptic meningitis a few days later. Fever, photophobia, and headache are associated with an aseptic spinal fluid lymphocytosis. Fourteen percent of patients treated with OKT-3 experience such symptoms, but the meningitis resolves spontaneously even with continued OKT-3 therapy (109). Reversible encephalopathy with prominent myoclonic jerking has occurred following OKT-3 (110). Milder encephalopathic changes with altered mentation are seen in many patients with OKT-3-induced aseptic meningitis (111). This aseptic meningitis is similar to that seen in a proportion of patients treated with high-dose intravenous immunoglobulin in settings other than transplantation (112).

Steroids

High-dose steroid therapy may alter mood, and occasionally causes a psychosis requiring major tranquilizers. Steroid-induced proximal myopathy is seen less frequently now that cyclosporine has reduced the long-term dosage of prednisolone (see Chapter 8).

CONCLUSION

A systematic approach, as emphasized in this chapter, is required to evaluate neurologic problems in organ transplant recipients. Knowledge of the most common difficulties encountered in specific types of transplantation may also be helpful. For example, a recent autopsy series of 16 patients who died following orthotopic liver transplantation revealed that the most common neuropathology was related to ischemia and infarction. Other central nervous system findings included infection, which was most commonly a cause of death (113). In a 4-year prospective review of 1730 consecutive liver transplant recipients, 60 patients (3.5%) developed CNS lesions. Vascular events (52%), infections (18%), and immunosuppression-associated leukoencephalopathy (12%) were the predominant etiologies (114). As mentioned above, focal peripheral nerve damage may complicate liver transplantation. In a prospective series, 10% of liver transplant recipients were noted to have focal peripheral nerve lesions in the postoperative period. The ulnar nerve was most frequently involved, possibly due to intraoperative compression or postoperative trauma (115).

In a retrospective chart review of lung transplant recipients, central nervous system complications were common, but functional outcome was generally favorable (116). Of the 100 transplant recipients studied over 5 years, 26 patients had a central nervous system event; 5 patients had more than one event. Severe headaches were most common (n = 14 patients), followed by seizures (n = 10), stroke (n = 5), and confusion (n = 3). Most of the events were thought to be related to cyclosporine toxicity or infection. A separate report by Stang et al (117) has noted the unique possibility of atrial anastomotic thrombus causing neurologic deficits in a lung transplant recipient.

The importance of drug toxicity causing neurologic problems in transplant recipients cannot be overemphasized. While some of the effects on the nervous system may be readily apparent, others may be more subtle, such as the effect of cyclosporine on cognitive function (118). The mechanism of the changes is not fully elucidated, but includes potential disruption of the blood-brain barrier, as well as hypoxic or vascular cortical injury. Interestingly, investigators have also proposed that immune factors may play a role in cyclosporine toxicity. Following allogeneic bone marrow transplantation, Zimmer et al (119) reported that cyclosporine-induced neurotoxicity was seen more frequently in HLA-mismatched and unrelated donor transplants.

Early recognition of and timely intervention in neurologic problems in transplant recipients is essential in order to reduce morbidity and mortality. The proper perspective requires attention to the underlying disease, the unique aspects of the organ transplanted, and a thorough familiarity with the toxicities and drug interactions of the immunosuppressive regimen.

REFERENCES

1. Kahan ED, Flechner SM, Lorber MI, et al. Complications of cyclosporine-prednisone immunosuppression in 402 renal allograft recipients exclusively followed at a single center for from one to five years. Transplantation 1987;43:197–204.

2. Hooper DC, Pruitt AA, Rubin RH. Central nervous system infections in the chronically immunosuppressed. Medicine 1982;61:166–188.
3. Jackson AC, Gilbert JJ, Young GB, Bolton CF. The encephalopathy of sepsis. Can J Neurol Sci 1986;12:303–307.
4. Gross MLP, Sweny P, Pearson RM, et al. Rejection encephalopathy. J Neurol Sci 1982;56:23–34.
5. Schwartz RE, Brave SM, Klufas RA, et al. Cyclosporine neurotoxicity and its relationship to hypertensive encephalopathy: CT and MRI findings in 16 cases. Am J Radiol 1995;165:627–631.
6. Snider S, Bashir R, Bierman P. Neurological complications after high-dose chemotherapy and autologous bone marrow transplantation for Hodgkin's Disease. Neurology 1994;44:681–684.
7. Menegaux F, Keeffe EB, Andrews BT, et al. Neurological complications of liver transplantation in adult versus pediatric patients. Transplantation 1994;58:447–450.
8. Adams HP, Dawson G, Coffman TJ, Corry RJ. Stroke in renal transplant recipients. Arch Neurol 1986;43:113–115.
9. Pomeranz S, Naparstek E, Ashkenazi E, et al. Intracranial hematomas following bone marrow transplantation. J Neurol 1994;241:252–256.
10. Wijdicks EF, de Groen PC, Wiesner RH, Krom RA. Intracerebral hemorrhage in liver transplant recipients. Mayo Clinic Proc 1995;70:443–446.
11. Hochberg FH, Miller DC. Primary central system lymphoma. J Neurosurg 1988;68:835–853.
12. Sheth KJ, Kivlin JD, Leichter HE, et al. Pseudotumour cerebri with vision impairment in two children with renal transplantation. Pediatr Nephrol 1994;8:91–93.
13. Avery R, Jabs DA, Saral R, et al. Optic disc edema after bone marrow transplantation. Possible role of cyclosporine toxicity. Ophthalmology 1991;98:1294–1301.
14. Winnock S, Janvier G, Parmentier F, et al. Pontine myelinolysis following liver transplantation: a report of two cases. Transplant Int 1993;6:26–28.
15. Wszolek ZK, McComb RD, Pfeiffer RF, et al. Pontine and extrapontine myelinolysis following liver transplantation. Relationship to serum sodium. Transplantation 1989;48:1006–1012.
16. Thompson CB, June CH, Sullivan KM, Thomas ED. Association between cyclosporine neurotoxicity and hypomagnesaemia. Lancet 1984;2:1116–1120.
17. Gilmore RL. Seizures and antiepileptic drug use in transplant patients. Neurol Clin 1988;6:279.
18. Adams DH, Ponsford S, Gunson B, et al. Neurological complications following liver transplantation. Lancet 1987;1:949–951.
19. Stein DF, Lederman RJ, Vogt DP, et al. Neurological complications following liver transplantation. Ann Neurol 1992;31:644–649.
20. Vogt DP, Lederman RJ, Carey ND, Broughan TA. Neurologic complications of liver transplantation. Transplantation 1988;45:1057–1061.
21. Estol CJ, Lopez O, Brenner RP, Martinet AJ. Seizures after liver transplantation: a clinicopathologic study. Neurology 1989;39:1297–1301.
22. Meech PR. Femoral neuropathy following renal transplantation. Aust N Z J Surg 1990;60:117–119.
23. Pontin AR, Donaldson RA, Jacobson JE. Femoral neuropathy after renal transplantation. S Afr Med J 1978;53:376.
24. Vasiri ND, Barton CH, Ravikumar GR, et al. Femoral neuropathy: a complication of renal transplantation. Nephron 1981;28:30–31.
25. Hefty TR, Nelson KA, Hatch TR, Barry JM. Acute lumbosacral plexopathy in diabetic women after renal transplantation. J Urol 1990;143:107–109.
26. Maziak DE, Maurer JR, Kesten S. Diaphragmatic paralysis: a complication of lung transplantation. Ann Thoracic Surg 1996;61:170–173.
27. Katirji MB. Brachial plexus injury following liver transplantation. Neurology 1989;39:736–738.
28. Wijdicks EFM, Litchy WJ, Wiesner RH, Krom RAF. Neuromuscular complications associated with liver transplantation. Muscle Nerve 1996;19:696–700.
29. Amato AA, Barohn RJ, Sahenk Z, et al. Polyneuropathy complicating bone marrow and solid organ transplantation. Neurology 1993;43:1513–1518.
30. Zochodne DW, Bolton CF, Wells GA, et al. Critical illness polyneuropathy: a complication of sepsis and multiple organ failure. Brain 1987;110:819–842.
31. Taylor BV, Wijdicks EF, Poterucha JJ, Weisner RH. Chronic inflammatory demyelinating polyneuropathy complicating liver transplantation. Ann Neurol 1995;38:828–831.
32. Wilson JR, Conwit RA, Eidelman PH, et al. Sensorimotor neuropathy resembling CIDP in patients receiving FK506. Muscle Nerve 1994;17:528–532.
33. Bronster DJ, Yonover P, Stein J, et al. Demyelinating sensorimotor polyneuropathy after administration of FK506. Transplantation 1995;59:1066–1068.
34. Donaghy MJ. Vincristine and neuropathies. Prescribers J 1996;36:116–119.
35. Imrie KR, Couture F, Turner CC, et al. Peripheral neuropathy following high dose Etoposide and autologous bone marrow transplantation. Bone Marrow Transplant 1994;13:77–79.
36. Walker RW, Brochstein JA. Neurologic complications of immunosuppressive agents. Neurol Clin 1988;6:261–278.
37. Blin O, Desnuelle C, Pelliessier J-F, et al. Neuropathie peripherique et ciclosporine. Therapie 1989;44:55–57.
38. Urbano-Marquez A, Estruch R, Grau JM, et al. Inflammatory myopathy associated with chronic graft-versus-host disease. Neurology 1986;36:1091–1093.
39. Nelson KR, McOuillen MP. Neurologic complications of graft-versus-host disease. Neurol Clin 1988;6:389–404.
40. Shimoda K, Gondo H, Harada M, et al. Myasthenia gravis after allogeneic bone marrow transplantation. Bone Marrow Transplant 1994;14:155–156.
41. Hoover R, Fraumeni JF. Risk of cancer in renal transplant recipients. Lancet 1973;2:55–57.
42. Penn I. Cancer in immunosuppressed patients. Transplant Proc 1984;2:492–494.
43. Schneck SA, Penn I. De-novo brain tumours in renal transplant recipients. Lancet 1971;1:983–986.
44. Eby NL, Grufferman S, Flannelly CM, et al. Increasing incidence of primary brain lymphoma in the US. Cancer 1988;62:2461–2465.
45. Jellinger RA, Paulus W. Primary central nervous system lymphomas—an update (editorial). J Cancer Res Clin Oncol 1992;119:7–27.
46. Patchell RA. Primary central nervous system lymphoma in the transplant patient. Neurol Clin 1988;6:297–303.
47. Hochberg FH, Miller G, Schooley RT, et al. Central nervous system lymphoma related to Epstein-Barr virus. N Engl J Med 1983;309:745–748.
48. Hanto DW, Gajl-Peczalska JG, Frizzera G, et al. Epstein-Barr virus (EBV) induced polyclonal and monoclonal B-cell lymphoproliferative diseases occurring after renal transplantation. Ann Surg 1983;198:356–369.
49. Ho M, Miller G, Atchison RW, et al. Epstein-Barr virus infections and DNA hybridisation studies in pro-transplantation lymphoma and lymphoproliferative lesions: the role of primary infection. J Infect Dis 1985;152:879–886.
50. Bashir RM, Harris NL, Hochberg FH, Singer RM. Detection of Epstein-Barr virus in CNS lymphomas by in-situ hybridisation. Neurology 1989;39: 813–817.
51. Vital C, Merlio JP, Rivel J, et al. Three cases of primary cerebral lymphoma in AIDS patients: detection of Epstein-Barr virus by in-situ hybridisation and Southern blot technique. Acta Neuropathol 1992;84:331–334.
52. Murray K, Kun L, Cox J. Primary malignant lymphoma of the central nervous system. Results of treatment of 11 cases and review of the literature. J Neurosurg 1986;65:600–607.
53. Singh A, Strobes RJ, Singh BM, et al. Steroid-induced remissions in CNS lymphoma. Neurology 1982;32:1267–1271.
54. DeAngelis LM, Yahalom J, Heinemann M-H, et al. Primary CNS lymphoma: combined treatment with chemotherapy and radiotherapy. Neurology 1990;40:80–86.
55. Ibels LS, Stewart JH, Mahoney JF, Shell AGR. Deaths from occlusive arterial disease in renal allograft recipients. BMJ 1974;3:552–554.
56. Mahoney JF, Shell AGR, Etheridge SB, et al. Delayed complications of renal transplantation and their prevention. Med J Aust 1982;2:426–429.
57. Rao KV, Smith EJ, Alexander JW, et al. Thromboembolic disease in renal allograft recipients. Arch Surg 1976;111:1086–1092.
58. Blohme I, Ahlmen J. Late complications after successful renal transplantation. Scand J Urol Nephrol Suppl 1977;42:173–175.
59. Rao KV. Renal transplantation: complications and results in the second decade. Transplant Proc 1987;19:3758–3759.
60. Ibels LS, Simons LA, King JO, et al. Studies on the nature and causes of hyperlipidaemia in uraemia, maintenance haemodialysis and renal transplantation. Q J Med 1975;44:601–614.
61. Rothenberg RJ. Isolated angiitis of the brain. Am J Med 1985;79:629–632.
62. European carotid surgery trialists' collaborative group. MRC European carotid surgery trial: interim results for symptomatic patients with severe (70–99%) or with mild (0–29%) carotid stenosis. Lancet 1991;337:1235–1243.
63. North American Symptomatic Carotid Endarterectomy Trial Collaborators. Beneficial effect of carotid endarterectomy in symptomatic patients with high-grade carotid stenosis. N Engl J Med 1991;325:445–453.
64. Hotson JR, Pedley TA. The neurological complications of cardiac transplantation. Brain 1976;99:673–694.
65. Montero CG, Martinet AJ. Neuropathology of heart transplantation: 23 cases. Neurology 1986;36:1149–1154.

66. Wiznitzer M, Packer RJ, August CS, Burkey FD. Neurological complications of bone marrow transplantation in childhood. Ann Neurol 1984;16:569–576.
67. Patchell RA, White CL, Clark AW, et al. Neurologic complications of bone marrow transplantation. Neurology 1985;35:300–306.
68. Welters MC, Sullivan KM, Bernaudin F, et al. Neurologic complications after allogenic marrow transplantation of sickle cell anaemia. Blood 1995;85:879–884.
69. Gallis HA, Berman RA, Gate TR, et al. Fungal infection following renal transplantation. Arch Intern Med 1975;135:1163–1172.
70. Petersen PK, Anderson RC. Infection in renal transplant recipients. Current approaches to diagnosis, therapy and prevention. Am J Med 1986;81(suppl 1A):2–10.
71. Cohen IM, Galgiani JN, Potter D, Ogden DA. Coccidioidomycosis in renal replacement therapy. Arch Int Med 1982;142:489–494.
72. Anderlini P, Przepiorka D, Luna M, et al. Acanthamoeba meningoencephalitis after bone marrow transplantation. Bone Marrow Transplant 1994;14:459–461.
73. Carbone KM, Pennington LR, Gimenez LF, et al. Mucormycosis in renal transplant patients—a report of two cases and review of the literature. Q J Med 1985;57:825–831.
74. Stamm AM, Dismukes WE, Simmons BP, et al. Listeriosis in renal transplant recipients: report of an outbreak and review of 102 cases. Rev Infect Dis 1982;4:665–682.
75. Pollock SS, Pollock TM, Harrison MJG. Infection of the central nervous system by Listeria monocytogenase: a review of 54 adult and juvenile cases. Q J Med 1984;211:331–340.
76. Watson AJ, Russell RP, Cabreja RF, et al. Cure of cryptococcal infection during continued immunosuppressive therapy. Q J Med 1985;55:169–172.
77. Bamborschke S, Wullen T, Huber M, et al. Early diagnosis and successful treatment of acute cytomegalovirus encephalitis in a renal transplant recipient. J Neurol 1992;239:205–208.
78. Holland NR, Power C, Mathews VP, et al. Cytomegalovirus encephalitis in acquired immunodeficiency syndrome (AIDS). Neurology 1994;44:507–514.
79. Cohen BA. Prognosis and response to therapy of cytomegalovirus encephalitis and meningomyelitis in AIDS. Neurology 1996;46:444–450.
80. Beal MF, O'Carroll CP, Kleinman GM, Grossman RI. Aspergillosis of the nervous system. Neurology 1982;32:473–479.
81. Weiland D, Ferguson RM, Peterson PK, et al. Aspergillosis in 25 renal transplant patients. Ann Surg 1983;198:622–629.
82. Baddour LM, Baselski VS, Herr MJ, et al. Nocardiosis in recipients of renal transplants: evidence for nosocomial transmission. Am J Infect Control 1986;18:214–219.
83. Wright DG, Laureno R, Victor M. Pontine and extrapontine myelinolysis. Brain 1979;102:361–385.
84. Miller GM, Baker HL, Okazaki H, Whisnant JP. Central pontine myelinolysis and its imitators. Radiology 1988;168:795–802.
85. Estol CJ, Paris AA, Martinet AJ, Ahdab-Barmada M. Central pontine myelinolysis after liver transplantation. Neurology 1989;39:493–498.
86. Schneck SA. Neuropathological features of human organ transplantation: II central pontine myelinolysis and neuroaxonal dystrophy. J Neuropath Exp Neurol 1966;25:18–39.
87. Norenberg MD, Leslie KO, Robertson AS. Association between rise in serum sodium and central pontine myelinolysis. Ann Neurol 1982;11:128–135.
88. Sterns RH, Riggs JE, Schochet SS. Osmotic demyelination syndrome following correction of hyponatremia. N Engl J Med 1986;314:1535–1542.
89. Bale JF, Rote NS, Bloomer LC, Bray PF. Guillain-Barré-like polyneuropathy after renal transplant. Possible association with cytomegalovirus infection. Arch Neurol 1980;37:788.
90. Donaghy M, Gray JA, Squier W, et al. Recurrent Guillain-Barré syndrome after multiple exposures to cytomegalovirus. Am J Med 1989;87:339–341.
91. Liedtke W, Quabeck K, Beelen DW, et al. Recurrent acute inflammatory demyelinating polyradiculitis after allogeneic bone marrow transplantation. J Neurol Sci 1994;125:110–111.
92. Ferry A, Mehta J, Iveson T, et al. Guillain-Barré syndrome after bone marrow transplantation. Bone Marrow Transplant 1994;14:165–167.
93. Myers SE, Williams SF. Guillain-Barré syndrome after autologous bone marrow transplantation for breast cancer: report of two cases. Bone Marrow Transplant 1994;13:341–344.
94. Hagensee ME, Benyunes M, Miller JA, Spach DH. *Campylobacter jejuni* bacteraemia and Guillain-Barré syndrome in a patient with GVHD after allogenic BMT. Bone Marrow Transplant 1994;13:349–351.
95. O'Sullivan DP. Convulsions associated with cyclosporin A. BMJ 1985;290:858.
96. Wijdicks EF, Wiesner RH, Krom RA. Neurotoxicity in liver transplant recipients with cyclosporine immunosuppression. Neurology 1995;45:1962–1964.
97. De Green PC, Aksamit AJ, Rakela J, et al. Central nervous system toxicity after liver transplantation: the role of cyclosporine and cholesterol. N Engl J Med 1987;317:861–866.
98. Katirji MB. Visual hallucinations and cyclosporine. Transplantation 1987;43:768–769.
99. Edwards LL, Wszolek ZK, Narnrand MM. Neurophysiologic evaluation of cyclosporine toxicity associated with bone marrow transplantation. Acta Neurol Scand 1995;92:423–429.
100. Bronster DJ, Boccagni P, O'Rourke M, et al. Loss of speech after orthotopic liver transplantation. Transplant Int 1995;8:134–237.
101. Valldeoriola F, Graus F, Rimola A, et al. Cyclosporine-associated mutism in liver transplant patients. Neurology 1996;46:252–254.
102. Steiger MJ, Farram T, Rolles K, et al. Cyclosporin associated headache. J Neurol Neurosurg Psychiatr 1994;57:1258–1259.
103. Hinchey J, Chaves C, Appiguani B, et al. A reversible posterior leukoencephalopathy syndrome. N Engl J Med 1996;334:494–500.
104. Nordal KP, Talseth T, Dahl F, at al. Aluminum overload, a predisposing condition for epileptic seizures in renal transplant patients treated with cyclosporine? Lancet 1985;2:153–154.
105. Hillebrand G, Castro LA, Van Scheidt W, et al. Valproate for epilepsy in renal transplant recipients receiving cyclosporine. Transplantation 1987;43:915–916.
106. Wijdicks EFM, Wiesner RM, Dahlke LJ, Krom RAF. FK506-induced neurotoxicity in liver transplantation. Ann Neurol 1994;35:498–501.
107. Mueller AR, Platz KP, Bechstein WO, et al. Neurotoxicity after orthotopic liver transplantation. A comparison between cyclosporine and FK506. Transplantation 1994;58:155–170.
108. Small SL, Fukui MB, Bramblett GT, Eidelman BM. Immunosuppression-induced leukoencephalopathy from tacrolimus (FK506). Ann Neurol 1996;40:575–580.
109. Martin MA, Massanari RM, Nghiem DD, et al. Nosocomial aseptic meningitis associated with administration of OKT3. J Am Med Assn 1988;259:2002–2005.
110. Coleman AE, Norman DJ. OKT3 encephalopathy. Ann Neurol 1990;28:837–838.
111. Adair JC, Woodley SL, O'Connell JB, et al. Aseptic meningitis following cardiac transplantation. Neurology 1991;41:249–252.
112. Watson JDG, Gibson J, Joshua DE, Kronenberg H. Aseptic meningitis associated with high-dose intravenous immunoglobulin therapy. J Neurol Neurosurg Psychiatr 1991;54:275–274.
113. McCarron KF, Prayson RA. The neuropathology of orthotopic liver transplantation: an autopsy series of 16 patients. Arch Pathol Lab Med 1998;122:726–731.
114. Bonham CA, Dominguez EA, Fukui MB, et al. Central nervous system lesions in liver transplant recipients: prospective assessment of indications for biopsy and implications for management. Transplantation 1998;66:1596–1604.
115. Campellone JV, Lacomis D, Giuliani MJ, et al. Mononeuropathies associated with liver transplantation. Muscle Nerve 1998;21:896–901.
116. Goldstein LS, Haug MT III, Perl J II, et al. Central nervous system complications after lung transplantation. J Heart Lung Transplant 1998;17:185–191.
117. Stang MR, Hinderliter AL, Gott KK, et al. Atrial anastomotic thrombus causes neurologic deficits in a lung transplant recipient. Transplantation 1996;62:693–695.
118. Grimm M, Yeganehfar W, Laufer G, et al. Cyclosporine may affect improvement of cognitive brain function after successful cardiac transplantation. Circulation 1996;94:1339–1345.
119. Zimmer WE, Hourihane JM, Wang HZ, et al. The effect of human leukocyte antigen disparity on cyclosporine neurotoxicity after allogeneic bone marrow transplantation. AJNR Am J Neuroradiol 1998;19:601–610.

Chapter

34

Psychiatric Considerations of Organ Transplantation

Owen S. Surman

Organ transplantation has flourished in the past three decades. Rejection and the complications of antirejection therapy are the principal biologic limitations to transplantation. Societal limits are posed by the shortage of cadaveric organs and, in some parts of the world, by the absence of brain-death criteria essential to cadaveric transplantation. Transplantation candidacy is provided to patients with end organ failure who appear healthy enough to survive meaningfully and to comply with the demands of postoperative care. The cost and the relative scarcity of organ transplantation impose a special demand for thoughtful selection and support of recipients.

Patient selection and organ donor selection are two areas that require psychiatric support. In some centers, there is a specific transplantation psychiatrist assigned to this task. Many transplant centers, however, use a general hospital psychiatric consultation service, and in other centers, psychologists and social workers perform the principal evaluation of recipients and donors.

Perioperative psychiatric support of transplant candidates requires an appreciation of the special needs of patients with end organ failure and an understanding of the psychiatric aspects of surgical care (1). Mental health professionals endeavor to predict and shape patient compliance and to treat preoperative and postoperative psychiatric syndromes. Postoperative sequelae unique to transplantation are posed by allograft rejection and by requirements for immunosuppressive medication. Many clinicians refer to the experience of transplantation as a roller-coaster, with its mixture of hope and uncertainty (2).

RECIPIENT SELECTION

Ethical models applied to patient selection are inevitably in conflict if each is taken to its logical end point (3). Assignment may be made on a basis that is egalitarian or utilitarian in nature. If the decision to transplant is primarily driven by patient demand, candidates with a poor risk will be included and the pool of recipients will be larger than if the decision is made on the basis of potential outcome and societal benefit (4). When time waiting is the predominant consideration, patients in most acute need will not survive long enough to receive an organ, and those who are most healthy will be at greater risk when they reach the top of the list. "Tragic Choices," the title of a thought-provoking text in medical ethics by Calabrese and Bobbit (5), is thus an apt phrase for the challenge posed by the limitation of resources for solid organ transplantation.

A rational approach to solid organ transplantation must be multicameral in nature (6). Current selection procedures are based on both urgency and time waiting. Priority among renal transplant recipients is given to availability of a six antigen match in histocompatibility (HLA) typing. Some candidates for solid organ transplantation are chosen despite their high-risk status. For example, the one-year survival rate for retransplantation of heart and liver recipients is approximately 38%, yet many centers perform second transplants. Multiple organ recipients and patients with challenging psychosocial profiles are other subgroups who are often included in the pool of recipients despite their high-risk status.

Another difference in patient candidacy among various types of solid organ transplantation is the priority given to mechanical support. Ventilator support is a contraindication to transplantation for potential lung transplant recipients, whereas heart and liver candidates have priority listing in such circumstances unless there are additional complications such as active infection.

Prioritization in solid organ transplantation has evolved from the more selective or parajuridical "lifeboat ethics" philosophy of the 1960s to our current, more egalitarian approach. It is principally, however, a societal consideration. Individual transplant centers do vary in their assessment of a given candidate, but the ultimate decision is driven by a medical model (7). The transplant center must determine which patients will benefit within the context of currently accepted norms for selection. When prospective patients are at greater risk, the team must determine whether a favorable outcome can be achieved by additional perioperative intervention.

Psychiatric Screening

The psychiatrist and allied mental health professionals are asked to determine whether the patient is sufficiently able, motivated, and socially supported to follow through with the demands of transplantation. Unfortunately, there is a lack of valid and reliable predictive data. Freeman et al used the designation "reservation about suitability for transplantation" for 19 of 70 patients who were psychiatrically screened for heart transplantation. Of 19 patients who met DSM-III criteria for a psychiatric disorder, 14 had postoperative surgical or psychiatric complications (8). Olbrisch and Levenson showed that transplant centers differ in their acceptance of patients with specific psychiatric disorders. Some centers do not accept patients with active schizophrenia. Most transplant units deny access to patients who manifest active substance abuse, dementia, current suicidality or past multiple suicide attempts, and severe mental retardation. Mild mental retardation, affective disorder, and commission of a felony are other possible causes for exclusion, especially in cardiac and lung transplant programs, which tend to be more selective (9). Olbrisch developed the Psychosocial Assessment of Candidates for Transplantation (PACT) in an effort to standardize patient evaluation and selection. The PACT rates each of four categories—social support, psychological health, lifestyle factors, and understanding of transplantation and follow-up—along a five-point semantic differential (10).

Factors that influence the variability in selection among transplant centers include case volume, outcome statistics, and availability of psychiatric expertise. Larger centers with good results tend to tolerate higher risk patients. Anecdotal success has been experienced in select patients with major depression, personality disorder, substance abuse, bipolar affective disorder, and moderate mental retardation. One patient with chronic schizophrenia, who had been turned down at another major center because of her psychiatric diagnosis, has continued to do well several months following liver transplantation. Her treating physicians have been impressed by her perseverance and by her family support.

Flexibility in transplant decisions derives from a diagnostic and behavioral inventory that identifies areas of risk for noncompliance. The ultimate selection of transplant candidates depends on a perception by the team that a given patient can be medically managed after transplant. Operationally, the problem areas in a given case are elucidated and interventions are established that might diminish risk. The development of a workable therapeutic relationship and the availability of stabilizing psychosocial supports suggest that successful transplantation is feasible.

Continuity in psychiatric consultation is especially advantageous. Through active participation with the transplant unit, the mental health professional gains knowledge about the specific concerns that team members bring to the selection process. Patient compliance is an obvious concern. The social worth of the candidate is another (11). Some who come to transplant evaluation are unattractive candidates because they are contentious or antisocial or have personality disorders that are taxing to available medical resources. Team members may also perceive greater tragedy when they have participated in the long-term care of a patient who has experienced multiple setbacks or rejection of a previous allograft.

A psychiatrist can perform an important role in the continuing medical education of the transplant team by sharing current practice standards in psychiatric care and prognostication and by participating in ethical review of complex clinical events.

Noncompliance

Noncompliance causes graft loss in up to 5% of renal transplant recipients (12). It may present with missed appointments, failure to make a timely report of important clinical changes, or dietary abuse and missed medications. Noncompliance may be inferred from unexpectedly low blood levels of cyclosporine or of other required medications; however, there may also be a metabolic basis for such variations. Another clue to noncompliance is evident in patients with recurrent rejection who repeatedly stabilize with surprising rapidity following hospital admission and routine monitoring of medications.

Depression, substance abuse, cognitive impairment, and personality disorder are the leading psychiatric factors in noncompliance. Patients are also at increased risk when they live at a distance from the transplant center and when there is insufficient social and financial support. Youth is another well-established risk factor. Young people are often prone to denial and tend to be more distressed by the cosmetic complications of immunosuppressant medication (13).

It is difficult to prognosticate with certainty in individual cases, but the patient's past and current history of compliance is the most valuable clue to future behavior (14,15). Patients who are at risk by virtue of psychiatric history or social turmoil should have an extended period of follow-up, when feasible, with the understanding that documentation of compliance must precede active consideration for transplantation. Reasonable efforts should be undertaken at the transplant center or through the patient's primary care provider to treat psychiatric disorders and to improve social support.

End-Stage Alcoholic Liver Disease

As Levenson and Olbrisch have documented in their surveys, there is considerable variation among transplant centers in psychosocial criteria for recipient selection (16). Transplant groups worldwide vary in how they deal with this scarce resource. The stakes are especially high in the setting of thoracic transplantation. Approximately 20% of those awaiting heart transplantation die before an organ becomes available. Lung transplantation is even less accessible. Evans reported the annual need for liver transplantation to be 14,400 in the United States. Alcoholism accounts for approximately half of the cases of hepatic failure.

Inevitably, comparisons are made, whether they are articulated or not, between patients whose disease is the result of an intemperate lifestyle and those who are passive victims. Siegler and Moss argued that past inattention to substance abuse is ethically an individual's responsibility (17). Those who hold to a medical model of alcoholism are less inclined to see its sequelae as related to behavioral choice.

If fault is assigned to the patient with end-stage alcoholic liver disease, second-class status is inevitable for this subgroup. A risk of using such logic in a health care system that is government regulated or subject to managed care is that all who seek medical care may become hostage to their past and subject to exclusion (18). In the American health system, unequal access within a specific category independent of prognosis is considered to be a form of discrimination incompatible with federally mandated protection for the disabled (19).

Confounding the rational selection of alcoholic end-stage liver disease is a presumed but unproved association between substance abuse and graft loss from noncompliance. Active drinking ultimately will take its toll on a new liver, but hepatitis C or a recurrence of cancer may cause comparable morbidity. Other chronic conditions such as diabetes mellitus, connective tissue disorders, arteriosclerotic cardiovascular disease, and cystic fibrosis also limit both duration and quality of survival.

The diagnosis and care of alcoholic patients is confounded by the absence of reliable biologic markers and pathognomonic biopsy findings for alcoholic end-stage liver disease, the lack of consistently applied criteria for substance abuse, and the difficulty in obtaining reliable historical data from patients and families intent on obtaining advanced medical care (Gastfriend DR, personal communication, 1996). Close family may be in denial about the problem or they may feel obliged to withhold information that would apparently prejudice care.

If, as is generally done, clinicians accede to the logic that continued alcohol abuse threatens compliance and is hepatotoxic, there remains the challenge of prognostication. Faced with the complexities of alcoholic liver disease, some groups consult with a psychiatrist who is also certified in addictionology.

An example of generally accepted inclusion criteria are those developed at the Massachusetts General Hospital in conjunction with the Massachusetts Ethics Committee for Organ Transplantation. They require a confirmed history of medical compliance, the presence of adequate social support for continued sobriety, the absence of dementia or comorbid alcoholic cardiomyopathy, and active participation in substance abuse counseling and treatment for those perceived to be at risk for relapse or who presented with less than a year of established sobriety. Patients who are actively drinking, who are involved in illicit drug abuse, and who cannot be helped to achieve sufficient psychosocial stability are excluded. Criteria are not based on length of sobriety, since there is almost always an opportunity to follow patients closely during the pretransplant waiting period. Most patients have had at least six months of sobriety prior to receiving a liver. Those with a prior history of polysubstance abuse are included if they appear otherwise stable. Patients in methadone maintenance programs are not excluded unless there are additional contraindications.

Transplantation psychiatrist Thomas Beresford of the University of Colorado Medical Center has advocated a system of inclusion based on Valliant's prognostic criteria. Beresford et al (20) assessed the extent to which patients and their families recognize alcohol dependence, the current degree of social stability, and the likelihood of lifestyle change conducive to long-term sobriety. Yates et al (21) prognosticated with attention to the amount of alcohol consumed and to the frequency and success of prior rehabilitation efforts. Knechtle et al (22), at the University of Wisconsin Medical Center, used more liberal criteria, performing liver transplantation in a group of patients whose families advocated transplantation despite failure of the patient to meet criteria for abstinence. Knechtle reported that these patients had outcomes similar to those with established abstinence (Knechtle SJ, personal communication, 1995).

Reported rates of recidivism among individuals with a history of alcoholism vary following transplantation for end-stage alcoholic liver disease. Accumulating evidence suggests that patient survival and graft survival for this patient population are comparable to other etiologic groups of liver failure (23–26). As is the case in other psychiatric disorders, the patient's capacity to develop an effective therapeutic bond to the transplant center is very important. Patients with past alcohol or drug abuse may begin to heed medical advice for the first time when faced with the rigors of transplantation and formal preoperative evaluation. A higher risk is to be expected if the patient presents in hepatic coma following a period of active drinking, or if he or she is only recently sober but too ill to benefit from treatment of substance abuse.

Selection of transplantation candidates among those with alcoholic liver disease is, in some ways, comparable to selection of patients with primary hepatic cancer. By analogy, one attempts to exclude those with unmanageable alcohol-related psychosocial morbidity. While transplant centers will continue to have differing selection criteria, there should be a clear pretransplant agreement about postoperative alcohol use. Some centers subscribe to a formal signed statement of intent regarding future alcohol use. The therapeutic advantage of such an approach is not known. Subspecialized psychiatric care for patients and their families must take into account that alcoholism tends to be chronic and that "slips" may occur that are amenable to supportive care. Because of the risk of recidivism, it is advisable to request that patients with a history of alcoholism consent to monitoring of blood, urine, or saliva at appropriate intervals. When patients are excluded from transplantation because of substance abuse or other psychiatric consideration, they should be given opportunity to obtain a second opinion from another transplant center.

Tobacco Abuse

As in the case of end-stage alcoholic liver disease, smoking is a primary etiologic agent among some patients with heart failure or pulmonary failure. Smoking as an exclusion criterion varies among centers internationally. Tobacco abuse has historically been tolerated more in Europe than in the United States. If abstinence from tobacco products is a prerequisite for transplantation, serial determination of urinary cotinine levels may assist evaluation of compliance. Referral to a hospital-based smoking cessation program is advisable where such services are available. Antidepressant agents, behavior therapy, and use of nicotine replacement systems when medically acceptable have each been beneficial for some who are striving for smoking cessation.

It is especially important to be aware of negative reactions that some staff members may experience in regard to past nicotine use. While members of the transplant community have customarily had opportunity to discuss such considerations, others in the general hospital may be less familiar with the ethics of transplant candidate selection. Timely teaching may help to diminish unfavorable reactions when former smokers undergoing pretransplantation evaluation are admitted to the general medical or surgical service.

ORGAN ALLOCATION

Organ donation comes from living or cadaveric sources. Living donors are usually closely related to the intended recipient, although transplantation from distant relatives or from unrelated donors has increased in recent years. Cadaveric donation proceeds under the supervision of organ procurement organizations (OPOs) (see Chapter 41). Patterns of organ distribution vary with geographic region and with the type of allograft. For example, hearts have a shorter ischemic survival time than kidneys and are available for distribution within a 500-mile radius. Organs are obtained with family consent following brain death. By societal definition and agreement, death occurs when brain function ceases. Non–heart-beating (asystolic) cadaveric donors are an alternative, if limited, source of availability, principally for renal allografts. Other organ systems are less able to withstand ischemic injury. Non–heart-beating donors do not experience a different kind of death, but their availability for organ retrieval is restricted to cessation of cardiovascular activity (29) (see Chapter 15).

Many transplant centers fund an organ donation coordinator, typically a registered nurse, who forms a liaison between the transplant team and the OPO, conducts in-service teaching, and assists with bereavement support and the request for organs.

Ethical limits to organ donorship in the United States are governed by the National Organ Transplant Act, which proscribes sale of organs. Interest is developing in the ethics of xenografting, as that new therapeutic option appears on the horizon (28,29) (see Chapter 40).

Mechanisms for Increasing Organ Donation

Efforts have been made worldwide to increase the availability of organs for transplantation (see Chapter 42). In America, required consent laws, championed by ethicist Arthur Caplan, exist in most states.

Presumed consent has been legalized in some countries. Those who choose not to participate must opt to be excluded from organ donation should they experience future brain death. Mandatory consent requires all adults to give consent for postmortem donation or to provide their written objection (30). Neither presumed nor mandatory consent has found favor in the United States.

A variety of incentives have been proposed to stimulate organ donation. A market approach to cadaveric organ donation in the United States is specifically outlawed by the National Organ Transplant Act. Preferred status for organ donors who may have future need of a transplant procedure is another option that has been reviewed by a special subcommittee of the United Network for Organ Sharing (UNOS) Ethics Committee. The major concerns about such inducements to donation relate to the potential for coercion or breach of individual autonomy and to the fear of societal backlash (31).

Innovative procedures including split-liver transplantation and reduced-size grafts for pediatric recipients have found some limited application (32).

Ethical Aspects of Living-Related Organ Donation

Death of a living donor is fortunately a rare event and serious, treatable complications are uncommon (33). American law provides support for organ donation based on the potential for emotional benefit to the donor (34). An improved sense of self esteem among donors has been documented in several psychiatric studies (35,36). Yet the experience of organ donation is painful and costly, despite free coverage of medical expenses, and there may be stress on previously troubled marriages (37). Difficulty may arise when conflict exists for a potential donor who faces objections from an anxious spouse, or for an ambivalent donor who feels unduly pressured by the recipient. Gouge et al (38), using standard measures, did not find enhanced quality of life in a retrospective study of kidney donors, but almost all of those studied were glad to have given a kidney.

For transplantation to proceed, the donor, recipient, and surgeon must all consent. Not all transplant surgeons support living donor participation, in which event the donor and recipient should be offered consultation at another center.

Donor Assessment

There is an inherent conflict of interest for the medical specialist who wishes to see a patient avoid the potentially life-endangering wait for cadaveric transplantation. If an available donor is healthy, enthusiastic, and sufficiently informed about the potential risks of surgery, there is little reason for delay. When the donor is ambivalent or there are concerns about the donor's welfare, however, it is important to enlist the advocacy of a specialist uninvolved in the direct care of the recipient.

Routine psychiatric interviews should be performed for all living pulmonary and hepatic donors and for all unrelated renal transplant donors. Ad hoc psychiatric intervention is routine when the donor has a history of important past or current psychiatric illness and when there is a psychosocial conflict regarding donation. Sometimes it is necessary for the transplant team to excuse a potential donor while helping to maintain family standing and self worth. It may be tempting in such instances to fabricate biologic incompatibility, but in addition to ethical considerations, there is always the possibility that circumstances may change at some future time and allow for appropriate donation. It is better to inform the recipient that current medical factors make donation unfavorable and to stress that organ donation is an exceptional event reserved for ideal circumstances.

When the donor has a known psychiatric condition, the treating psychiatrist, psychologist, or social worker should be included in the process of evaluation. Potential donors who experience active substance abuse or psychiatric symptomatology may benefit from a treatment program, which can be followed by reevaluation. Mild adjustment disorders caused by preoperative anxiety may respond to short-term behavioral intervention and anxiolytics. Occasionally, donor evaluation may provide a fortuitous opportunity for secondary prevention.

Living Donation in Kidney Transplantation

In the United States, approximately one in four renal transplants are from living donors, and donor nephrectomy is the only occasion for living-unrelated donation of a solid organ. Criteria for unrelated organ donation may include documentation of a close bond between donor and recipient, evidence of altruistic intent on the part of the donor, and lack of apparent coercion. Among those who have been unrelated kidney donors there have been distant relatives, friends, spouses, and, in one documented instance, a home health worker.

Potential kidney donors benefit from participation in a pretransplant "family meeting" attended by the primary nephrologist, the surgical chief of the renal transplant program, the nurse coordinator, a social worker, the consulting psychiatrist, and a representative from the tissue typing laboratory. Such meetings are best preceded by an education and information gathering session with the social worker and nurse coordinator. Additional formal psychiatric evaluation should be done for unrelated donors and for related donors with current emotional difficulties or a significant past psychiatric history. The donor's medical evaluation should include a standard self-report questionnaire to screen for substance abuse. All cases can be reviewed at weekly transplant work rounds as new information becomes available.

One-year cadaveric allograft survival statistics in many centers are comparable to the results of live donor transplantation. For example, at the Massachusetts General Hospital, these were 82.3% and 94.5%, for cadaveric and live donor grafts respectively, for calendar years 1995–1998. At three years after transplant, 75.8% of cadaveric grafts were functioning compared to 90.2% of living-related kidneys (Delmonico F, personal communication, 1996). In general, patients currently wait for a cadaveric donor kidney for an average of two years. Availability of a living donor considerably shortens the wait for transplantation and provides a marked reduction in the risk of ischemic injury followed by acute tubular necrosis in the early postoperative period (see Chapter 17).

Living Donation in Lung Transplantation

Living organ donation is an option for some individuals with pulmonary failure who are unlikely to survive until a cadaveric source becomes available (see Chapter 25). Two individuals may volunteer, each undergoing lobectomy to provide sufficient pulmonary function for the recipient. Full recovery and return to customary activities is anticipated. Psychiatric consultation as well as ethical consultation is essential for this relatively novel technology. As with other organ donor situations, ethical principles of autonomy, beneficence, and nonmalfeasance apply.

Living Donation in Liver Transplantation

Parent-to-child liver transplantation is performed in some centers with partial donor hepatectomy (see Chapter 19).

Postoperative complication rates are higher than in the setting of nephrectomy for living renal transplantation (39,40). The ethics of this procedure were explored by Singer et al (41), and it has subsequently become an accepted approach. Habib et al (42) reported the first case of living-related liver transplantation in Africa, thereby demonstrating the suitability of this technology in countries where cadaveric organ transplantation is unavailable by law and social custom.

THE TRANSPLANT EVENT

The transplant team's first encounter with a new patient occurs most often at the time of evaluation for transplantation candidacy. Functional decline, role loss, and impairment of mental acuity are evident in varying degree among patients experiencing end organ failure. For many who come to evaluation, transplantation represents a prospect for improved autonomy and prolongation of life. On the other hand, a documented need for transplantation eliminates the possibility of a spontaneous remission from organ failure. At the same time that the patient seeks acceptance for transplantation, there is also an element of grief that varies in intensity with the acuteness of the organ failure and with the patient's style of adaptive function and available supports.

The patient's social network is an important factor in both the level of suffering that occurs during the wait for transplantation and the patient's capacity for medical compliance following the operation. Those who are close to the patient share the burden of progressive illness. One man who presented with fulminant hepatitis in stage IV hepatic coma did remarkably well after receiving a cadaveric liver, even though he was so ill at the time he was placed on the list that his family members were preparing funeral arrangements (43).

The wait for transplantation is often extremely stressful. For cardiac transplant candidates in intensive care, the wait for a heart is like watching a pot that never boils. Lung transplant candidates, who typically wait in excess of two years for an allograft, may express a feeling of having been forgotten. For some, a lengthy wait for transplantation may be followed by a call to the hospital for an organ that never materializes. Such false starts are typically occasioned by unsuitability of the potential allograft.

At the time of transplant evaluation, patients often express feelings of guilt about the stress that their illness imposes on family members. Transplant candidates may also experience guilt about their need for an organ that can only be a product of another's death. Patients with heredofamilial disorders may be saddened by the inability of a loved one to obtain a successful allograft. Many patients who have formed a bond with other transplant candidates empathize with those who continue to wait for a graft or who encounter serious post-transplantation complications.

Except in kidney transplantation, solid organ transplant recipients do not have a reliable backup system of medical support. Some are open in stating their fear of dying. Others with a strong spiritual base speak of being "in God's hands." For example, a priest who underwent liver transplantation referred to this adaptive perspective as "surrender" (43).

Patient expectation regarding surgical outcome plays an important role in successful adaptation to transplantation candidacy. For example, patients with polycystic kidney disease are likely to be influenced by the medical experiences of other afflicted family members. Patients may also have specific therapeutic expectations, as in the case of one middle-aged man with end-stage alcoholic liver disease and tense ascites, who became depressed and angry while awaiting a donor during an extended hospital stay. He was upset about the team's reluctance to proceed with therapeutic paracentesis and interpreted this as evidence of disinterest in his welfare. When paracentesis was reinitiated for its psychological benefit, the patient's mood improved dramatically.

Preoperative Psychiatric Syndromes

Adjustment disorders, depression, anxiety disorders, and encephalopathy are common psychiatric events in the preoperative period.

Depression has been traditionally thought to predispose to postoperative morbidity (44), but post-transplant reversal of organ failure significantly improves mood for most patients. The distinction between treatable and intractable depression is best clarified through assessment of premorbid psychiatric history. When there is past history of affective disorder, it is important to ascertain to what extent exacerbations have affected compliance with prescribed medications and procedures.

Among cadaveric transplant recipients, the hopeful anticipation of donor organ availability is typically followed by anxiety when the team calls with news about an allograft. Rarely, an anxious patient may decline transplantation. Urgent psychiatric consultation may be helpful if there is an established relationship between patient and psychiatrist.

There has been little formal research on preoperative anxiety among transplant patients. Johnston found that preoperative anxiety levels were high among orthopedic and gynecologic patients and tended to persist for several days following the operation (45). Some people approach surgery with minimal apprehension; however, frank denial is problematic for the individual who mistakenly expects that transplant will be immediately beneficial and uneventful. Psychiatric intervention is recommended for those with unrealistic expectations, as well as for patients with debilitating anxiety and for those with premorbid anxiety disorders or phobias specific to the planned procedure (1).

Because trust and rapport between the patient and the transplant team is essential for successful organ transplantation, personality-disordered patients present a higher risk for transplantation. These individuals have a pattern of strained relationships that is usually evident from psychological evaluation and from the patient's interaction with the primary care physician and other medical personnel. Most transplant procedures occur in a time course that allows the team to get to know the patient and to establish a successful therapeutic alliance. The best predictor of postoperative compliance is preoperative compliance (14,15). When relations with the patient are shaky in advance of surgery, one must anticipate similar difficulties in the postoperative period and take whatever steps might realistically ameliorate the situation.

Substance abuse may be a cause or exacerbant of end organ dysfunction. Careful screening is essential in the preoperative period. One bedside technique is the standard "CAGE" test. Patients are asked if they have perceived a need to *c*ut down ("C") on the amount they drink, if they have been *a*ngry or annoyed ("A") at others who complain about their drinking, if they have felt *g*uilty ("G") about substance abuse, and if they have ever had a morning drink or "*e*ye opener" ("E"). Those with two or more positive responses have a greater than 90% likelihood of problem drinking. It is best in such cases to involve an addictive disorders expert and to obtain further historical data from the family and the primary care physician. While there is no specific test for alcoholism, there is no excuse for failing to inquire.

Encephalopathy is another common preoperative psychiatric disorder. Its pathophysiology and treatment differs depending on the specific organ system that is involved. Some additional psychiatric aspects of kidney, heart, liver, and lung failure are also of pretransplantation interest and are discussed below.

Psychiatric Aspects of Kidney Failure

Among renal failure patients, systemic diseases such as diabetes mellitus are associated with relatively greater morbidity than disorders isolated to the kidneys, and this is reflected in preoperative incidence of psychiatric difficulties.

Those with inherited diseases such as polycystic kidney disease are less likely to have an available family donor, and their fears and expectations are influenced by impact of the disease on other relatives.

Lithium-induced nephropathy is rare. When it does occur, anticonvulsants, especially valproate, can often stabilize bipolar mood disorder. Infrequently, it is necessary to continue treatment with lithium despite the progression of renal pathology.

Availability of dialytic treatment, the feature that most distinguishes renal failure from other types of end organ disease, has been associated with increased incidence of depression. Depression is more frequent in those who present with higher levels of morbidity, which can be quantified on the Endstage Renal Disease Severity Index (46). Depression has also been found to increase mortality in the dialysis population (47). Factors contributing to mood change include abnormality in endocrine function, especially hyperparathyroidism, and alteration of neurotransmission (48).

Encephalopathy is a concomitant condition of uremia but may also occur in response to activation of cytokines secondary to immunologic reaction by synthetic dialysis membranes (Rubin NT, personal communication, 1998). A change in mental status may be an indication for initiation of dialysis and is sometimes mistaken for depression. Knowledge of the patient and the results of a brief mental status examination are usually sufficient in the differential. Neuropsychiatric syndromes specific to renal failure include dialysis dysequilibrium and, rarely, dialysis dementia, which is most commonly ascribed to aluminum encephalopathy and theoretically might benefit from transplantation (49). Seizures are common in uremia and complex partial seizures can be responsible for behavioral change including agitation and, in one extreme instance, for catatonia that proved responsive to anticonvulsant therapy (49,50).

The benefits of one or another form of end-stage renal disease therapy vary with medical circumstance. Overall, it is evident that transplant patients do best. For example, in the pre-erythropoietin era, Evans et al (51) reported that 115 (80%) of 144 kidney transplant recipients and 343 to 429 (48% to 60%) of 715 dialysis patients were functioning at a near-normal level, depending on the type of dialysis. However, a successful vascular anastomosis may not be possible in a patient who has advanced atherosclerosis. Nor will transplant offer improved life quality if the patient is unable to secure funding for immunosuppressant medications. Access to an established transplant center is another consideration. Also, some nephrologic centers may be biased toward dialytic treatment (52). Some highly sensitized patients may be unable to obtain a suitable match. Diabetic patients are less tolerant of hemodialysis and are threatened by acceleration of retinopathy. For some diabetics, combined pancreas and kidney transplantation offers a significant advantage in eliminating the need for insulin therapy despite increased risk of postoperative morbidity.

Psychiatric Aspects of Heart Failure

Coronary artery disease and cardiomyopathy are the principal disorders encountered by patients in need of heart transplantation. The vast majority of patients are male. Alcoholic cardiomyopathy is an infrequent finding among those undergoing transplant evaluation and may improve substantially with effective addictive disorders treatment and sustained abstinence.

Prolonged intensive care unit stays have been the rule prior to heart transplantation because medical selection criteria are prioritized by urgency. Unfortunately, many relatively high-functioning younger patients, with a risk of death from sudden arrhythmia, have lengthier waiting times as outpatients because they are not critically ill at the time of evaluation.

Remarkably, the type of stress encountered by cardiac patients prior to transplantation is similar to the stressors known to exacerbate heart disease in the general population. There is a significant adverse impact from role loss and from family separation (53–56). The potential unavailability of transplantation among the heart transplant population is also a source of anticipatory bereavement.

Patients who are initially interviewed for heart transplantation express a combination of willingness to proceed coupled with the sense that they have "no other choice." For many, anger and anxiety, each of which has a known association to cardiovascular morbidity, occurs to an increased degree as patients sense that time is running out (57).

Encephalopathy is often evident in this patient population and has been studied in detail by Riether et al (58). Contributing to central nervous system impairment are decreased cerebral blood flow, metabolic disorder, and toxic medication effects. For example, xylocaine and other beta-blocking agents may produce cognitive impairment (59).

Delirium is common among cardiac patients who require intra-aortic balloon pump therapy. Hypotensive and microembolic events may be responsible and possibly there may be a role played by cytokine activation, although to our knowledge this aspect has not yet been studied.

Psychiatric Aspects of Liver Failure

Alcoholic cirrhosis is the greatest single cause of liver failure. Although alcoholics are among the most frequent transplant recipients, the vast majority of alcoholics in need of liver transplantation are never referred for transplant evaluation.

Hepatic Encephalopathy The principal cause of hepatic encephalopathy is absorption of toxic metabolites from the intestine. One possibility is that false neurotransmitters may be a factor in the attendant central nervous system depression. Grading of hepatic encephalopathy has traditionally been done with Parsons–Smith criteria (60). Some patients present in frank stupor and one occasionally encounters a transplant recipient who has no recall of preoperative medical preparation. More subtle evidence of cognitive dysfunction may be evident on standard mental status examination or in behavioral oddities and memory impairment apparent to the attending medical and nursing staff. It is especially important for the psychiatrist to be aware of premorbid functioning, since the presence of even subclinical hepatic encephalopathy may make patients look less functional than they are likely to be following transplantation (61). Neurologic improvement following transplantation may be slower for some patients but is associated in general with significant improvement in quality of life (61,62).

Medical management is the primary approach to these patients. Control of bleeding and infection, reduction of protein intake, and administration of lactulose constitute the standard approach. Anxiolytic and sedative agents must be used with great care since they are hepatically metabolized and may precipitate obtundation when used in relatively modest dosage (63).

Psychiatric Aspects of Pulmonary Failure

Etiologic Considerations Genetic disorders such as cystic fibrosis and α1-antitrypsin deficiency are frequent among lung transplantation candidates. Cystic patients sometimes learn of their condition with the onset of pulmonary symptoms during young adulthood. More often, they are seasoned warriors with childhood onset of disease and a life-long history of recurrent hospitalization. Many of these patients maintain a surprising level of activity. One limiting variable is the acquisition of resistant microbial infection, especially *Pseudomonas* (see Chapter 25).

Idiopathic pulmonary disorders such as primary pulmonary hypertension, lymphangioleiomyomatosis (LAM), and idiopathic pulmonary fibrosis are acquired causes of end-stage lung disease that often occur in previously healthy individuals unaccustomed to medical restriction. Among these patients, one may see denial and resistance to the need for transplant. Alternatively, those who have recognized the threatening progression of their pathology may be actively grieving the attendant loss of independent function at the time of transplant evaluation. Feelings of guilt are commonly encountered among those with chronic obstructive pulmonary disease (COPD) exacerbated by past tobacco dependence.

The Waiting Period End-stage lung disease patients often arrive at clinic with a portable oxygen supply that makes them look like interplanetary travelers. The wait for lung transplantation is especially demanding because of the relative infrequency with which lungs become available. Unlike heart transplant patients, the wait is principally an outpatient event. Patients on advanced life support are considered poor candidates for pulmonary transplant surgery.

Encephalopathy in this population may be a product of hypercapnia or hypoxia. Increased anxiety and agitation in a formerly stable patient may represent an acute change in pulmonary function.

Anxiety disorders are especially common among pulmonary patients. Pollack et al (64) reported a 17% (20/115) incidence of panic disorder among patients referred for pulmonary function testing. Anxiety symptoms were not associated with objective findings of airway obstruction and might represent a catastrophic response to perceived change in pulmonary function.

PREOPERATIVE PSYCHIATRIC INTERVENTION

Informed Consent

Teaching and informed consent are the cornerstone of preoperative care. In addition to a declaration of clinical goals and methods for their accomplishment, preoperative discussions between the patient and the transplant team form the basis of a bond that will be important during the difficult times that occur in the course of solid organ transplantation. The opportunity to shape expectation is especially important. Transplant patients need to understand that hospital care may be prolonged and that recurrent admissions may be necessitated by rejection and infection and other post-transplant complications. The need for indwelling catheters and drains, the nature of the incision, special diets, and the experience and approach to postoperative pain must all be addressed. Transplant recipients should be acquainted with the need for strict compliance with medications, with the frequency of postoperative clinic visits, and with the financial demands of transplantation. The process of selection, the likely amount of waiting time for transplantation, and the rules governing status on the waiting list should be carefully explained. Young people, especially, must be aware of the potential cosmetic impact of steroid requirements postoperatively. The likelihood of weight gain and the potential for diabetes mellitus, cataract formation, mood swings, irritability, impaired concentration, and tremor must be discussed. Potential complications must be presented with sensitivity. It may seem kind to withhold information, but patients who are uninformed and suffer adverse postoperative effects will expectedly feel that they were "led down the garden path."

Observation by the team in the course of teaching and informed consent provides important information about mental status and coping styles.

Teaching Venues

At the Massachusetts General Hospital (MGH), a "family meeting" format is used to interview kidney transplant patients prior to placing their names on the cadaveric organ list or proceeding with living donor evaluation. For other types of solid organ transplantation, the patient is admitted when feasible and a standard series of visits are arranged with surgery, nursing, psychiatry, social service, anesthesiology, and other medical and paramedical subspecialists as indicated. Some insurance plans require that this process occur on an outpatient basis.

Transplant teams may have a psychiatrist who is subspecialized in this area or they may rely on general hospital psychiatric consultation services. Some teams rely on a psychologist or social worker. The psychiatric interview compliments the process of informed consent and provides an excellent opportunity to instruct patients in relaxation techniques, to counsel them about mobilizing an effective support network, and to inform them about the potential for postoperative mental status change and how that is best managed. The psychiatrist or consulting psychologist and social worker are in an optimal position to reinforce adaptive skills and to assist in cognitive reframing and behavioral techniques for enhancement of perceived control and well-being (65–68). Several studies have demonstrated the favorable postoperative impact of preoperative psychological intervention (69–71).

Patient-to-patient interactions provide a valuable adjunct to preoperative teaching. Many successful transplant recipients enjoy this opportunity to "give something back" by sharing their experience with new transplant candidates. Patient groups are similarly effective. They may rely on lay leadership or on a skilled group therapist. The format may include teaching sessions to which members of the surgical team are invited. Some groups include both patients and family members. They may be specific to transplantation of one organ system or the group may encourage more diverse participation.

Printed materials are a useful educational supplement. Also, *Organ Transplants: A Patients' Guide*, coauthored by Hank Pizer and the Massachusetts General Hospital transplant team (72), is recommended.

Egbert et al (73) demonstrated that patients undergoing abdominal surgery had greater postoperative comfort and required less narcotics when they were taught prior to their operation about the normalcy of postoperative pain and encouraged to ask for pain medication as needed. Similarly, one can instruct patients about the risk of postoperative delirium while emphasizing that some degree of confusion or even hallucination is in the range of customary experience, that these are temporary phenomena, and that they respond to appropriate medication adjustments. (An example is a liver transplant recipient who imagined that one of her surgeons was having a party outside the window of her hospital room.)

One might think of the preoperative patient as a "cryptographer" in search of cues that will aid in the mastery of perioperative events. In an early study published in the experimental psychology literature, Schacter and Singer (74) found that healthy experimental participants responded differentially to injected adrenaline depending on their exposure to waiting room confederates who were either irritable or elated. In analogous fashion, one can teach preoperative transplant candidates how to cope within the range of experience that patients typically encounter. In the process, one must not deny pain or tell patients how to feel, and one's intention to provide long-term follow-up and support should be emphasized.

Psychotherapy

Indications

Patients with Axis I or Axis II psychiatric disorders should be encouraged to receive psychotherapy in preparation for transplantation. When compliance is a concern and when there are debilitating emotional symptoms, active treatment should be required as a condition of the patient's being listed as a waiting recipient.

Patients who are psychologically asymptomatic or who have mild adjustment disorders are best advised to mobilize whatever resources they find most beneficial. This may include supportive counseling for the patient and family, religious involvement, or community-based support. Patients should also be encouraged to give specific assignments to friends and family who wish to help.

The pretransplant psychiatric evaluation provides a format for brief therapy. I find it useful to tell patients that the purpose of the psychiatric interview is to teach, to form a basis for subsequent ad hoc psychiatric referral, and to ascertain whether there are any special needs that must be addressed for transplantation to be successful.

Goals

Even a one-time psychiatric interview may provide a unique opportunity for listening and debriefing. While underscoring the hope of transplantation, the therapeutic psychological encounter allows for a recognition of the patient's personal loss and attendant grief.

Guilt is eased by honoring the sick role. Patients who express feelings of guilt about the need for a cadaver organ are best reminded of the inevitability of death and of the relief that many bereaved families experience when informed of the opportunity for organ donation. Concern about identity and body image may also be responsible for negative feelings about cadaveric transplantation and can be addressed through psychotherapy.

The pretransplant psychiatric interview also provides an opportunity to help patients feel more accepting of the pretransplantation medical evaluation. Patients are best advised that the object is to see whether they can realistically benefit from a transplant and whether there are specific circumstances that need to be addressed before transplantation proceeds.

Above all, the pretransplant interview is an excellent opportunity to strengthen the therapeutic alliance and to inform patients that transplantation works best in the presence of a good working partnership between the transplant recipient and the surgical team.

The psychiatrist can also play an important role in shaping expectation, and the patient benefits from learning that adverse events can be managed successfully. Liver transplant candidates may benefit from learning that post-transplant pain has been shown to require less narcotic analgesic support than gallbladder surgery (75). This finding may be the result of denervation that occurs in the process of removing the native liver.

Techniques

Psychotherapy with pretransplant patients can be challenging because of their decreased autonomy and, in many instances, impairment of cognitive function. Brief sessions that are coordinated with the patient's schedule of other essential hospital visits are often most practical. Patients who are especially motivated and physically able may conform to a more traditional scheduling approach. Uncovering psychotherapeutic strategies may be unacceptably destabilizing. Generally, patients do best with types of psychotherapy that support coping abilities. Among these approaches are supportive, cognitive, behavioral, and interpersonal forms of therapy.

Hypnosis offers a practical means of teaching patients to relax and it can be an adjunct in the control of pain and pruritus for those who are hypnotically susceptible. Hypnotherapy and other cognitive strategies are especially beneficial for cardiac transplant candidates undergoing prolonged stays in the intensive care unit (ICU). Such approaches offer creative opportunity for distraction and may also be employed to help patients remain more in touch with meaningful aspects of their lives, thereby facilitating a "psychological bridge to transplantation" (76).

Substance abuse counseling and treatment is essential for those who are actively affected or recently abstinent. Family members should be actively included in the rehabilitation process.

Phobic disorders relevant to the surgical setting should be identified and behaviorally desensitized. A rehearsal technique, "postnoxious desensitization," encourages individuals to fantasize a favorable operative outcome, and then to work backward imaginally to gain mastery of events. One woman, for example, described a dread of endotracheal intubation. When asked to imagine under hypnosis that she had successfully completed heart transplantation, the patient pictured herself sitting in an enclosed porch that her husband had constructed. In subsequent scenes, she was guided in working backward imaginally through an expected sequence of perioperative events and encouraged to use her feelings of hope and renewal to favorably interpret the experience. Following a single therapy session, she was able to overcome her phobia and to use self hypnosis while undergoing pretransplant cardiac catheterization (76).

Skills

Referring physicians and surgeons can benefit their patients by becoming acquainted with the practice patterns of specific psychotherapists. Child psychiatrists should be selected for patients under age 18. Couples and family therapists may be especially effective in dealing with complex marital problems. Consultation psychiatrists have established psychopharmacologic knowledge that may be less available to the patient's customary mental health worker. Some psychiatrists excel with individuals suffering from specific disease categories, such as cystic fibrosis, diabetes mellitus, or cancer. Other psychiatrists may be very experienced and effective in treating specific immigrant groups, sensory-impaired patients, chronic pain sufferers, or substance abusers.

Psychopharmacologic Treatment

Psychopharmacologic care of the transplant patient has been reviewed in depth by Trezepacz et al (77,78). The judicious use of antidepressant, anxiolytic, and antipsychotic agents may improve function and facilitate other aspects of patient management. The choice and optimal dosage of specific medications are dictated to some extent by the type of organ failure. Treatment may be considered for outpatients or for the acute perioperative transplant recipient.

Among the antidepressants favored are the selective serotonin reuptake inhibitors or SSRIs because of their low incidence of problematic side effects and for their anxiety-reducing properties. This class of medication includes fluoxetine, sertraline, and paroxetine. Fluoxetine and sertraline differ in biologic half-life but are otherwise quite similar in their spectrum of action and side effect profiles. Dosing customarily begins with 5–10 mg daily of fluoxetine or 25–50 mg daily of sertraline. Weekly titration of dosage is advisable. Healthy outpatients tolerate up to 80 mg of fluoxetine or 200 mg of sertraline daily. These levels are not typically required in the transplant population. Paroxetine tends to be a more sedating agent and can be given in doses of 10–20 mg daily. The SSRIs variably inhibit cytochrome P450 2D6 and are weak 3A4 inhibitors. Appropriate caution should be taken to prevent toxicity with drugs that are metabolized through the 2D6 pathway.

Bupropion is also a safe and effective antidepressant. It tends to be more stimulating than other agents, but is less beneficial for treatment of concurrent anxiety states. Allergic reactions to fluoxetine and to bupropion occur in approximately 4% of patients.

Tricyclic antidepressants, such as desipramine, were formerly the first-line medications for depression and can be continued perioperatively in patients who have been successfully maintained on this class of drugs.

Monoamine oxidase inhibitors (MAOIs), such as phenelzine and tranylcypromine, are best avoided because of the risk of hypertensive crisis with sympathomimetic agents that may be required perioperatively. Meperidine must be avoided in combination with these agents because of the risk of hypotension. Other limiting factors are the dietary restriction imposed by the risk of hypertensive crisis when foods high in tyramine are combined with MAOIs. Nonetheless, there are rare instances in which these agents may be the only ones beneficial for treatment-resistant depression. In one instance, tranylcypromine was the only successful pharmacologic approach for a depressed heart transplant recipient.

Electroconvulsive therapy is an alternative approach to treatment-resistant depression and it may be preferred for those who are very severely depressed because of its relatively rapid action.

Anxiolytics vary in half-life. Among the benzodiazepines, alprazolam, oxazepam, and lorazepam are shorter-acting agents that are customarily given on a three or four times daily schedule. Diazepam and clonazepam are longer acting and are usually given twice daily. Alprazolam and clonazepam are most effective for panic attacks. Buspirone and tranxene are an alternative to benzodiazepines for treatment of generalized anxiety.

Bipolar mood disorders are typically managed with lithium carbonate, which must be monitored carefully in patients who are medically compromised. Lithium levels are generally maintained at 0.8 to 1.0 mEq/L. Serum levels are increased with diuresis and in renal failure. Valproate and carbamazepine are anticonvulsant agents that offer an alternative to lithium. Valproate is especially valuable for acute onset of mania.

Among the antipsychotic agents, there is an increasing array of new medications. Maintenance of an effective antipsychotic regimen, like maintenance of antidepressant medication, is very important to perioperative stabilization. For acute psychoses in the patient with end organ failure, haloperidol remains the agent of first choice. Extrapyramidal side effects are lessened with intravenous administration.

The pretransplant evaluation provides an excellent chance to learn which agents patients have best responded to in the past and to hear of any idiosyncratic drug reactions. Some patients give histories of medication intolerance, information which may prove invaluable in subsequent admissions if the patient's ability to communicate effectively is compromised.

In general, it is essential to tailor psychopharmacologic management to the demands of organ failure. Cassem's dictum to "start low and go slow" is a valuable way to avoid the pitfalls of oversedation and iatrogenesis (79).

Psychopharmacologic Intervention for Kidney Transplant Candidates Psychopharmacologic care of the patient with renal failure requires dosage adjustments of standard anxiolytic, antidepressant, and neuroleptic agents as described by Bennet (80). As an alternative to SSRIs and bupropion, psychostimulants, especially methylphenidate, may be chosen for their rapid onset of action in the treatment of depression (48). Short-acting antianxiety agents are generally preferable to avoid build-up of metabolites. Monitoring of anticonvulsant medications is complicated by spuriously low values that may result from changes in protein binding. Free levels of phenytoin and carbamazepine are more reliable than standard serum levels. Lithium carbonate is fully dialyzed and should therefore be administered after treatment on hemodialysis days. Some patients require continued administration on nondialysis days. Frequent initial monitoring is essential to avoid toxicity. Monthly levels prior to hemodialysis are advisable once a satisfactory dosing schedule has been established. When aluminum encephalopathy is suspect, deferoxamine, an iron- and aluminum-binding agent, may be administered (48).

Psychopharmacologic Intervention for Liver Transplant Candidates Psychopharmacologic limitations are imposed by the primary role of the liver in the metabolism of psychoactive medications. Preoperative anxiety and agitation can, however, be treated with low doses of short-acting benzodiazepines. In the presence of hepatic encephalopathy, oxazepam is preferred because of its relatively simple metabolism. A daily dose of 10 mg should not routinely be exceeded. Dyphenhydramine is a safe agent in low dosage for nocturnal sedation. Insomnia is very frequent in this patient population, but one must be gentle in striving to ameliorate it.

A full range of antidepressant agents can be used in liver transplantation. It is wise to use low doses at the outset and to monitor blood levels. We prefer bupropion because of its stimulating action. In one previously reported case, a patient with encephalopathy and severe pretransplant depression proved responsive to dosing at 37.5 mg daily.

Psychopharmacologic Intervention for Cardiopulmonary Patients Psychopharmacologic care for heart transplant candidates requires gentle use of anxiolytics to avoid exacerbation of cognitive impairment and secondary depression. Tricyclic antidepressants are especially disadvantageous in this population because of their potential for arrhythmogenicity and orthostatic hypotension. Constipation, another frequent tricyclic side effect, may increase cardiovascular risk related to Valsalva's maneuvers (81).

Delirium is common for patients who require intraaortic balloon pump management. Intravenous haloperidol should be administered for agitation by using escalating doses beginning with 0.5–1.0 mg every half hour. Supplementation with intravenous lorazepam may be necessary.

Oversedation must be scrupulously avoided for patients with pulmonary failure. This patient population is especially prone to panic-type anxiety attacks that can be optimally managed with alprazolam or clonazepam. The SSRIs provide a more delayed relief from panic, but they have an additional antidepressant benefit. Some clinicians believe that they favorably alter airway resistance in some individuals with obstructive pulmonary disease.

Social Service Intervention

It is most helpful to work with a medical social worker who is familiar with the demands of transplantation and who is available to attend work rounds on a weekly basis. The social worker is an invaluable source of patient and family support and plays a pivotal role in ensuring that the patient will have access to needed health care perioperatively.

Recreation Therapy

Patients who wait for weeks in a hospital require support and distraction. A recreational therapist or skilled volunteers may provide crafts and audiovisual materials or engage the patient in shared activities such as card play or board games. One heart transplant patient who enjoyed oil painting was able to overcome his depression by producing canvases that he offered for sale to the staff. At MGH, a series of relaxation videotapes play on the hospital's closed-circuit teaching channel. Teaching films are also available for kidney transplant patients and their potential donors.

POSTOPERATIVE PSYCHIATRIC CONSIDERATIONS

Postoperative Psychological Reactions

Improvement in Psychological Function

With reversal of end organ failure, neuropsychiatric function improves and patients experience improved well-being and, at times, a sense of rebirth. Psychological improvement generally occurs most rapidly after renal transplantation, where it is often evident within one to two postoperative days. Among heart transplant recipients, Riether et al (58) found marked improvement in depression and anxiety within the first three months after transplant. Neuropsychiatric recovery generally occurs more slowly for liver recipients, but improved psychological adjustment and quality of life have been well documented (61,82). Some patients undergo surprisingly rapid recovery and are ready for discharge from the hospital within two to three weeks. At the opposite end of the spectrum are those with prolonged postoperative encephalopathies, the majority of which slowly recover.

Organic Brain Syndromes

Metabolic impairment, infection, and medication effects are factors contributing to postoperative delirium (see Chapter 33). Anesthetic agents, analgesics, and antirejection medications should be considered in the etiology. Prednisone may cause sleep disturbance, emotional lability, and perceptual abnormality, but we do not typically see the affective psychoses that were relatively common in the earlier years of transplantation when rapid dose reduction was not yet in practice. Both cyclosporine and tacrolimus (FK506) may be associated with neurologic complications including seizures, delirium, and coma (83–86). Clues to cyclosporine toxicity are the concurrent development of hypertension, renal dysfunction, and tremor. Toxic levels of cyclosporine may follow from cytochrome P450 enzyme inhibitors such as erythromycin, ketoconazole, and diltiazem (87).

Among heart transplant recipients, intraoperative cerebral ischemia may occur as a result of decreased perfusion from hemorrhagic or embolic phenomena. Psychotic reactions may follow within the first two postoperative days. The etiology is more likely to be multifactorial when psychotic manifestations are delayed by two to five days and respond rapidly to neuroleptic treatment and environmental support (88).

Among liver transplant recipients, central pontine myelinolysis is a rare idiopathic demyelinating disorder that produces a locked-in syndrome (89,90).

Anxiety States

Anxiety often results in patients who experience failed post-transplant expectations. Rejection and infection are commonly associated with features of anxiety. Somewhat surprisingly, anxiety may occasionally follow from decreased medical dependence. Some lung transplant recipients, for example, have expressed worry about breathing on their own without oxygen support.

Intravenous pulses of methylprednisolone may give rise to mood swings or to anxiety that typically subsides within in a day or two once rescue therapy is completed. OKT-3, a monoclonal antibody used for acute rejection, may be associated with severe headache, joint pains, and other anxiety-generating systemic effects.

Post-transplant biopsy procedures are another source of stress. Renal and hepatic biopsies are typically performed with specific indications. Heart and lung transplant recipients undergo routine endocardial biopsy or bronchoscopy.

Anxiety is to be expected when there are delays in hospital discharge. Sometimes, however, psychiatric consultation may be required for the patient who complains that discharge is premature. These individuals may be fearful because of unresolved symptomatology or because of the transition from the close in-hospital observation.

Body Image Distortions

Cushingoid change from prednisone is especially distressing to young patients undergoing transplantation. Cyclosporine may also cause hirsutism. Common warts are another disfiguring complication that sometimes improves when immunosuppression is changed from azathioprine to cyclophosphamide.

Some consultation psychiatrists have focused on the psychological impact of the transplant recipient's incorporating a donor organ (91). A remarkable account was Harry Abrams' report about a Ku Klux Klan grand dragon who joined the NAACP on learning that his donor was an African American (92). Some patients wonder whether the donor's lifestyle may have contributed to changes in food choice that occur after transplant. One middle-aged heart–lung transplant recipient, who learned the adolescent age of her cadaver donor, spoke to a national daytime television audience about her subsequent youthful and energetic lifestyle.

Depression

Following transplantation, depression may be a recurrence of a prior affective disorder. Repeat episodes of major depression are common among even healthy individuals with a positive past history of similar mood impairment.

Corticosteroid-induced depression tends to be accompanied by irritability that is often less evident to the patient than to the family and attending surgical staff. Rejection is also a common cause of depression and may be related both to the attendant fear of graft loss and to cytokine production.

Most important for the transplant team is the link between depression and infection. Prodromal mood change often foreshadows a fever spike or evidence of systemic illness. We have found cytomegalovirus infection to be associated with a significant increase in first-time psychiatric consultation (93). Patients whose depressive symptoms are coincident with infection or with rejection do not usually express hopelessness or suicidal ideation. Appetite reduction, lethargy, and psychological withdrawal are common to these situations, along with evidence of systemic illness.

Psychological Rejection

Some psychiatrists have speculated about the possibility of psychologically induced allograft rejection (94). Rejection is clearly psychological in origin when noncompliance occurs as an outcome of depression, memory impairment, substance abuse, or a severe adjustment reaction. Noncompliance may follow loss of third-party funding or other adverse economic developments that make expensive immunosuppressants less attainable.

Sexual Concerns

Sexual function is a significant factor in perceived quality of life. It should be discussed routinely in the post-transplant period. Some clinicians may choose to employ a sexual history questionnaire (95). Among factors interfering with sexual potency in males and with sexual interest for people of both genders are medication effects, anxiety, depression, and perceptions about sexual participation by patients and significant others. Medications that affect sexual responsiveness include the commonly employed immunosuppressant medications, antihypertensives, anxiolytic agents, analgesics, and antidepressants. Strategies for assisting in this area include modification of medications, patient education and counseling, and urologic or gynecologic referral, when needed.

Pain Management Problems

Postoperative analgesic requirements are increased for those with routine preoperative use of narcotic agents that are either prescribed or illicitly acquired. Denarcotization for these individuals should be accomplished slowly, with the aid of a hospital pain service or with psychiatric consultation. Anxiety and depression can decrease pain thresholds and should be treated pharmacologically. Tricyclic antidepressants, typically at low dose, are helpful in migraine and in painful neuropathy. Relaxation techniques, including self hypnosis, can help reduce fear and increase the patient's perceived control.

Postoperative Psychiatric Intervention

Long-Term Care

Transplant patients are often told that they will end up with a new set of medical problems once end organ replacement has occurred. This is a function of rejection, medication side effects, and progression of systemic disease. The care of transplant patients is thus a long-term undertaking and the consulting psychiatrist may be reconsulted at intervals, especially for those who are most ill and/or least adaptive.

Patients who are at a high risk psychologically are best enlisted in follow-up plans prior to operative intervention. Patients with affective disorders, schizophrenia, substance abuse histories, and moderate mental retardation can be treated with a good management plan that includes supportive counseling, psychopharmacologic care, and social engineering, when appropriate.

Psychotherapeutic Intervention

Psychotherapeutic principles of postoperative care are similar to those discussed above. Some patients need help to reframe their expectations. For example, a patient undergoing prolonged intensive care may need help in interpreting the extent of progress signaled by absence of a monitor, reduction of intravenous lines, or moves toward mobilization. Guilt and shame may occur following an episode of delirium. Some may struggle with their preoperative wish for a donor organ. Patients can be helped to understand that these are usual aspects of the transplantation experience.

Behavioral interventions may assist the nursing staff to manage patients with excessive dependency, hostility, or resistance to routine care.

Group therapy offers an effective approach for patients and family members and may be conducted by the psychiatrist, social worker, psychologist, or psychiatric nurse clinician.

Psychopharmacologic Intervention

Antidepressant treatment and anxiolytics should be given as described for the pretransplant patient. Tricyclic antidepressants may be preferred for diabetics with peripheral neuropathy, or they may be used for depressed patients with insomnia who are not at cardiovascular risk from these agents. Serum levels should be followed carefully in the presence of hepatic dysfunction. For the most part, bupropion and SSRIs are better tolerated. Sertraline, fluoxetine, and paroxetine are equivalent SSRIs. As discussed earlier, these agents variably inhibit the cytochrome P450 2D6 system and weakly inhibit 3A4, but they are not known to interfere with the metabolism of cyclosporine or FK506. Strouse (96) has demonstrated that fluoxetine does not interfere with cyclosporine levels. Nonetheless, cyclosporine levels must be closely followed.

While it may be tempting for the surgical team to reduce the patient's burden of medication requirements, it is essential that appropriately prescribed psychopharmacologic agents not be casually discarded. Among those with prior depression, there is a risk that postoperative care will be compromised by recurrence of major depressive symptoms. The patient may suffer needlessly from precipitous benzodiazepine withdrawal or recurrence of debilitating anxiety and panic attacks. When it appears advantageous to modify benzodiazepine dosing postoperatively, intravenous or sublingual lorazepam may be substituted for longer-acting oral agents, and dosing can be gradually tapered.

Modification of immunosuppressant protocols, when feasible, is often beneficial to patients undergoing psychotic reactions. Correction of metabolic abnormality, treatment of bleeding, and identification of infection are also essential. Complex partial seizures are an uncommon but treatable cause of psychosis. When anticonvulsant medication is required, it is important to consider that a decrease in immunosuppressant medication levels may follow from inhibition of cytochrome P450 enzymes. Valproate is preferred in the management of post-transplantation seizures.

Acute psychotic disturbances usually respond rapidly to intravenously administered haloperidol. One should begin with 0.5–1.0 mg at half hourly to hourly intervals. Generally, low doses (under 5 mg daily) are sufficient. As discussed above, extrapyramidal side effects are less common with the intravenous route. Parenteral administration of lorazepam or morphine sulfate is an adjunctive or alternative approach to severe agitation.

Corticosteroid-related irritability and hypomania often improve with 0.5–2.0 mg of haloperidol at bedtime.

Lithium carbonate can be resumed postoperatively for those who require long-term maintenance. One must be aware of possible increase in the toxicity of both cyclosporine and lithium when both agents are used together. Frequent monitoring of serum levels is essential. Valproate is sometimes chosen as the first-line treatment for mania and has been found to have a more rapid onset of reduction in manic symptoms.

It is interesting to speculate about the theoretical effect of psychotropic medication on immunologic activity. Neuroleptics are known to increase prolactin levels but have had no discernible adverse impact on allograft function. Lithium carbonate has established immune-stimulant properties but has had no documented adverse effect on allograft function. Lithium is also interesting because of its inhibition of phosphatidyl inositase, a factor in T-cell signaling. Bromocriptine, a dopamine stimulant that is used by addictionologists to relieve cravings for cocaine, is known to have favorable immunosuppressant action levels (97).

CONCLUSION

Psychiatric consultation is an essential service for the perioperative and long-term care of transplant patients. In addition to the management requirements of specific psychiatric syndromes, transplantation poses challenging ethical issues related to patient selection and to the use of donor organs. Psychiatrists and allied mental health professionals who are familiar with the transplant setting offer a valuable perspective and resource for support. Optimally, a full range of psychiatric, social, and psychological services are available to the transplant team with initial patient evaluation. Routine preoperative exposure to psychiatric intervention assists adaptation to the demands of transplantation and facilitates postoperative psychiatric referral. When transplantation goes well, patients experience a wonderful improvement in longevity and life quality. When setbacks and adverse outcomes occur, there is often a specialized need for psychological intervention.

REFERENCES

1. Surman OS. The surgical patient. In: Cassem NH, ed. Massachusetts General Hospital Handbook of General Hospital Psychiatry. St. Louis: Mosby Yearbook, 1991.
2. Surman OS. Psychiatric aspects of organ transplantation. Am J Psychiatry 1989;146:972–982.
3. Taylor C. Sources of the self. The making of the modern identity. Cambridge, MA: Harvard University, 1989.
4. Surman OS, Purtilo R. Reevaluation of organ transplantation criteria: allocation of scarce resources to borderline candidates. Psychosomatics 1992;33:202–212.
5. Calabrese G, Bobbit P. Tragic choices. 1st ed. New York: Norton, 1978.
6. Surman OS, Cosimi AB. Ethical dichotomies in organ transplantation: a time for bridge building. Gen Hosp Psychiatry 1996;18(suppl 6):13S–19S.
7. Loewy EH. Drunks, livers and values: should social value judgments enter into liver transplant decisions? J Clin Gastroenterol 1987;9:436–441.

8. Freeman AM III, Folks DG, Sokol RS, et al. Cardiac transplantation: clinical correlates of psychiatric outcome. Psychosomatics 1988;29:47–54.
9. Olbrisch ME, Levenson JL. Psychosocial assessment of organ transplant candidates. Current status of methodological and philosophical issues. Psychosomatics 1995;36:236–243.
10. Olbrisch ME, Levenson JL, Hafner R. The PACT: a rating scale for the study of clinical decision making in psychosocial screening of organ transplant candidates. Clin Transplant 1989;3:164–169.
11. Robertson JA. Patient selection for organ transplantation: age, incarceration, family support, and other social factors. Transplant Proc 1989;21:3397–3402.
12. Didlake RH, Dreyfus K, Kerman RH, et al. Patient noncompliance: a major cause of late graft failure in cyclosporine-treated renal failure. Transplant Proc 1988;20(suppl 3):63–69.
13. Colon EA, Popkin MK, Matas AJ, et al. Overview of noncompliance in renal transplantation. Transplant Rev 1991;5:175–180.
14. Rodriguez A, Diaz M, Colon A, et al. Psychosocial profile of noncompliant transplant patients. Transplant Proc 1991;23:1807–1809.
15. Wilson P. Psychological risk factors. Presented at the First Working Conference on Psychological and Ethical Aspects of Organ Transplantation, Toronto, June, 1990.
16. Levenson JL, Olbrish ME. Psychosocial evaluation of organ transplant candidates: a comparative survey of process, criteria, and outcomes in heart, liver, and kidney transplantation. Psychosomatics 1993;34:314–323.
17. Moss AH, Siegler M. Should alcoholics compete equally for liver transplantation? JAMA 1991;265:1295–1298.
18. Surman OS. The morality of transplantation. JAMA 1991;266:213. Letter.
19. Merrican KJ, Overcast TD. Patient selection for heart transplantation: when is a discriminating choice discrimination? J Health Polit Policy Law 1985;10:7–32.
20. Beresford TP, Turcotte JG, Merion R, et al. A rational approach to liver transplantation for the alcoholic patient. Psychosomatics 1990;31:241–254.
21. Beresford TP, Turcotte JG, Merion R, et al. A rational approach to liver transplantation for the alcoholic patient. Psychosomatics 1990;31:241–254.
22. Knechtle SJ, Fleming F, Barry KL, et al. Liver transplantation for alcoholic liver disease. Surgery 1992;112:694–701.
23. Kumar S, Stauber RE, Gavaler JS, et al. Orthotopic liver transplantation for alcoholic liver disease. Hepatology 1990;11:159–164.
24. Gastfriend DR, Surman OS, Gaffey GK, et al. Preliminary outcome of liver transplantation in a matched sample of alcoholics and nonalcoholics. Presented at the Annual Meeting, American Psychiatric Association, New Orleans, 1991.
25. Berlakovich G, Rudolf S, Herbst F, et al. Efficacy of liver transplantation for alcoholic cirrhosis with respect to recidivism and compliance. Transplantation 1994;58:560–565.
26. Osorio RW, Ascher NL, Avery M, et al. Predicting recidivism after orthotopic liver transplantation for alcoholic liver disease. Hepatology 1994;20:105–110.
27. Arnold RM, Youngner SJ. Back to the future: obtaining organs from non-heart-beating cadavers. Kennedy Inst Ethics J 1993;3:103–111.
28. Surman OS. Toward greater donor organ availability for transplantation. N Engl J Med 1985;312:318. Letter.
29. Hanson MJ. The seductive sirens of medical progress: the case of xenotransplantation. Hastings Cent Rep 1995;25:5–6.
30. Miller M. A proposed solution to the present organ donation crisis based on a hard look at the past. Circulation 1987;75:20–28.
31. Burdick JF, Capron AM, Delmonico FL. Preferred status for organ donors: a report of the preferred status subcommittee of the UNOS Ethics Committee. UNOS Update 1994;10:15–16.
32. Cosimi AB. Update on liver transplantation. Transplant Proc 1991;23: 2083–2090.
33. Cosimi AB. The donor and donor nephrectomy. In: Morris PJ, ed. Renal transplantation—principle and practice. New York: Grunne and Stratton, 1979:69–87.
34. Fabro AJ. Legal aspects of organ transplantation. Strunk vs Strunk. Conn Med 1970;34:583.
35. Fellner CH, Marshall JR. Twelve kidney donors. JAMA 1968;206:2703–2707.
36. Simmons RG, Klein SD, Simmons RC. Gift of life: the social and psychological impact of organ transplantation. New York: Wiley, 1977.
37. Smith MD, Kappell DF, Province MA. Living-related kidney donors: a multicenter study of donor education, socioeconomic adjustment, and rehabilitation. Am J Kidney Dis 1986;8:223–233.
38. Gouge F, Moore J, Bremer CR. The quality of life of donors, potential donors, and recipients of living-related donor renal transplantation. Transplant Proc 1990;22:2409–2413.
39. Busuttil RW. Living-related liver donation. Transplant Proc 1991;23:43–45.
40. Morimoto T, Yamaoka Y, Tamaka K, et al. Quality of life among donors of liver transplants to relatives. N Engl J Med 1993;329:363–364. Letter.
41. Singer PA, Seigler M, Whitington PF, et al. Ethics of liver transplantation with living donors. N Engl J Med 1989;3211:620–622.
42. Habib NA, Higgs BD, Marwan I, et al. Living-related liver transplantation in Africa. Int Surg 1993;78:121–123.
43. Surman OS, Dienstag JL, Cosimi AB, et al. Liver transplantation: psychiatric considerations. Psychosomatics 1987;28:615–621.
44. Kimball CP. A predictive study of adjustment to cardiac surgery. J Thorac Cardiovasc Surg 1969;58:891.
45. Johnston M. Anxiety in surgical patients. Psychol Med 1980;10:145–152.
46. Craven J, Littlefiels C, Rodin G, Murray M. The endstage renal disease severity index (ESRD-SI). Psychol Med 1991;21:237–243.
47. Kimmel PL, Weihs K, Peterson RA. Survival in hemodialysis patients: the role of depression. J Am Soc Nephrol 1993;4:12–27.
48. Brown TM, Brown RLS. Neuropsychiatric consequences of renal failure. Psychosomatics 1995;36:244–253.
49. Tyler RH. Neurologic disorders in renal failure. Am J Med 1968;44:734–748.
50. Surman OS, Parker SW. Complex partial seizures and psychiatric disturbance in end stage renal disease. Psychosomatics 1981;22:1077–1080.
51. Evans RW, Manninen DL, Garrison LP, et al. The quality of life of patients with end-stage renal disease. N Engl J Med 1985;312:553–559.
52. Levy NB. Psychological aspects of renal transplantation. Psychosomatics 1994;35:427–433.
53. Blumenthal J, Burg MM, Barefoot J, et al. Social support, type A behavior and coronary artery disease. Psychosom Med 1987;49:331–340.
54. Hackett TP, Cassem NH. The psychological adaptation to convalescence of myocardial infarction. N Engl J Med 1984;311:552–559.
55. Ahern DK, Gorkin L, Anderson JL, et al. Biobehavioral variables and mortality for cardiac arrest in the cardiac arrhythmia pilot study (CAPS). Am J Cardiol 1990;66:59–62.
56. Ruberman W, Weinblatt E, Goldberg JD, et al. Psychosocial influences on mortality after myocardial infarction. N Engl J Med 1984;311:552–559.
57. Vlay SC, Olson LC, Fricchione GL, et al. Anxiety and anger in patients with ventricular tachyarrhythmias. Responses after automatic internal cardiovascular defibrillator implantation. PACE 1989;12:366–373.
58. Riether AM, Smith SL, Lewison BJ. Quality of life changes and psychiatric and neurocognitive outcome after heart and liver transplantation. Transplantation 1992;54:444–450.
59. Dimsdale JE. Research links between psychiatry and cardiology. Hypertension, type A behavior, sudden death and the physiology of emotional arousal. Gen Hosp Psychiatry 1988;10:328–338.
60. Parsons-Smith BG, Summerskill WHJ, Dawson AAM, et al. The electroencephalogram in liver disease. Lancet 1957;2:867–871.
61. Tarter RE, Switala J, Arria A, et al. Subclinical hepatic encephalopathy: comparison before and after orthotopic liver transplantation. Transplantation 1990;50:632–637.
62. Tarter RE, Switala J, Plail J, et al. Severity of hepatic encephalopathy before liver transplantation is associated with quality of life after transplantation. Arch Intern Med 1992;152:2097–2101.
63. Surman OS. Psychiatric aspects of liver transplantation. Psychosomatics 1994;35:297–307.
64. Pollack MH, Kradin R, Otto MW. Prevalence of panic in patients referred for pulmonary function testing at a major medical center. Am J Psychiatry 1996;153:110–113.
65. Ray C. The surgical patient: psychological stress and coping resources. In: Eiser JR, ed. Social and behavioral psychology. New York: Wiley, 1982.
66. Andrew JM. Recovery from surgery with and without preparatory instruction for three coping styles. J Pers Soc Psychol 1970;15:223–226.
67. Wilson JF. Behavioral preparation for surgery: benefit or harm? J Behav Med 1981;4:79–102.
68. Johnston M. Preoperative existential status and postoperative recovery. Adv Psychosomatic Med 1986;15:1–20.
69. Levitan SJ, Kornfeld DK. Clinical and cost benefits of liaison psychiatry. Am J Psychiatry 1981;138:790–793.
70. Mumford E, Schlesinger HJ, Glass GV. The effects of psychological intervention on recovery from surgery and heart attacks: an analysis of the literature. Am J Public Health 1982;72:144–151.
71. Rogers M, Reich P. Psychological intervention with surgical patients: evaluation outcome. Adv Psychosom Med 1986;15:23–50.
72. Pizer H and the Massachusetts General Hospital Transplant Unit. Organ Transplants: a patient's guide. Cambridge, MA: Harvard University, 1992.
73. Egbert LD, Battit GE, Welch GE, et al. Reduction of postoperative pain by encouragement and instruction of the patient. N Engl J Med 1964;270:825.
74. Schacter S, Singer JE. Cognitive, social and physiological determinants of emotional state. Psychol Rev 1962;69:379.

75. Eisenach JC, Plevak DJ, Van Dyke RA, et al. Comparison of analgesic requirements after liver transplantation and cholecystectomy. Mayo Clin Proc 1989;64:356–359.
76. Surman OS. Organ failure and transplant patients. In: Cassem NH, Stern T, Rosenbaum J, Jellinek M, eds. Massachusetts General Hospital handbook of general hospital psychiatry. 4th ed. St. Louis: Mosby, 1997:501–543.
77. Trzepacz PT, DiMartini A, Tringali R. Psychopharmacologic issues in organ transplantation, part I: pharmacokinetics in organ failure and psychiatric aspects of immunosuppressants and anti-infectious agents. Psychosomatics 1993;34: 199–207.
78. Trzepacz PT, DiMartini A, Tringali RD. Psychopharmacologic issues in organ transplantation, part 2: psychopharmacologic medications. Psychosomatics 1993;34:290–298.
79. Cassem NH. Depression. In: Hackett TP, Cassem NH, eds. Massachusetts General Hospital handbook for general hospital psychiatry. 2nd ed. Littleton, MA: PSG Publishing, 1986:227–260.
80. Bennett W, Singer I, Coggins CJ. A guide to drug therapy in renal failure. JAMA 1974;230:1544–1553.
81. Evans D. Antidepressant adverse effects and antidepressants in the medically ill. In: American Society of Clinical Psychopharmacology Progress Notes 1995–96;6:22–23.
82. Moore KA, Jones R, Hardy AK, et al. Psychosocial adjustment to illness: quality of life following liver transplantation. Transplant Proc 1992;24: 2257–2258.
83. de Groen PC, Aksamit AJ, Rakela J, et al. Central nervous system toxicity after live transplantation: the role of cyclosporine. N Engl J Med 1987;317:861–866.
84. Vogt DP, Lederman RJ, Carey WD, et al. Neurologic complications of liver transplantation. Transplantation 1988;45:1057–1061.
85. Craven JL. Cyclosporine-associated organic mental disorders in liver transplant recipients. Psychosomatics 1991;32:94–102.
86. Moreno E, Gomez SR, Gonzalez I, et al. Neurologic complications in liver transplantation. Acta Neurol Scand 1993;87:25–31.
87. Castelao AM, Sabate JM, Grino S, et al. Cyclosporine-drug interactions. Transplant Proc 1988;20(suppl 6):66–69.
88. Hotson JR, Enzmann DR. Neurologic complications of cardiac transplantation. Neurol Clin 1988;6:349–365.
89. Estol CJ, Faris AA, Martinez AJ, et al. Central pontine myelinolysis after liver transplantation. Neurology 1989;39:493–498.
90. Winnock S, Janvier G, Parmentier F, et al. Pontine myelinolysis following liver transplantation: a report of two cases. Transpl Int 1993;6:26–28.
91. Castelnuovo-Tedesco P. Transplantation: psychological implications of changes in body image. In: Levy NB, ed. Psychonephrology 1. Psychological factors in hemodialysis and transplantation. New York: Plenum Medical, 1981:218–225.
92. Abrams HS. Repetitive dialysis. In: Hackett TP, Cassem NH, eds. Massachusetts General Hospital handbook of general hospital psychiatry. St. Louis, Mosby, 1978:342–364.
93. Hibberd PL, Surman OS, Bass M, et al. Psychiatric disease and cytomegalovirus viremia in renal transplant recipients. Psychosomatics 1995;36:561–563.
94. Viederman M. Psychogenic factors in kidney transplant rejection: a case study. Am J Psychiatry 1975;132:957–959.
95. Tabler JB, Frierson R. Sexual concerns after heart transplantation. J Heart Transplant 1990;9:397–403.
96. Strouse TB, Fairbanks LA, Skotzko CE, et al. Fluoxetine and cyclosporine in organ transplantation: failure to detect significant drug interactions or adverse clinical events in depressed organ recipients. Psychosomatics 1996;37:23–30.
97. Surman OS. Possible immunology effects of psychotropic medication. Transplantation 1993;34:139–143.

Chapter

35

Renal Considerations of Organ Transplantation

NINA TOLKOFF-RUBIN ERIK LANGHOFF

ACUTE RENAL FAILURE

Although the success rate of organ transplantation has improved with new immunosuppressive agents, improved surgical technique, and better recognition and management of infectious disease complications, acute renal failure (ARF) nonetheless remains both a diagnostic and a therapeutic challenge in this setting. The major causes of acute renal failure in patients with organ transplantation are similar to those incurred in patients undergoing any major surgical procedure, and include: 1) prerenal azotemia due to volume contraction or congestive failure, 2) obstructive uropathy, 3) acute tubular necrosis (ATN) secondary to ischemic insults and sepsis, and 4) drug-induced renal dysfunction due to direct tubular toxicity or acute allergic interstitial nephritis. Technical complications, such as vascular occlusion, renal artery stenosis, and ureteral leaks, as well as acute and chronic allograft rejection, are of particular concern in the renal transplant recipient and are discussed in Chapters 17 and 18.

Prerenal Azotemia

As in nontransplant patients, prerenal azotemia occurring in the transplant setting is reversible if the underlying cause is corrected by appropriate fluid and electrolyte management. It can, however, progress to ischemic renal failure if not recognized or treated. In prerenal azotemia, the kidneys perceive a decrease in the "effective" intravascular volume and normal homeostatic mechanisms come into play in an effort to restore the perceived deficit. In this situation, the kidneys retain their ability to normally concentrate the urine and conserve sodium.

A number of laboratory parameters are helpful in differentiating prerenal azotemia from established ATN. Of particular interest are the urinary indices: the urine osmolality, urine sodium, and fractional excretion of sodium. Thus, in prerenal azotemia, at a time when the kidneys are attempting to maximally conserve salt and water, one generally sees a urine osmolality greater than 500 mOsm/kg, a urine sodium less than 20 mEq/L, and a fractional excretion of sodium less than 1%.

In contrast, in patients with ATN secondary to an ischemic insult, sepsis, or direct tubular toxins, the kidneys lose their concentrating ability and tubular damage leads to an inability to reabsorb sodium early in the course of the injury. Consequently, in this situation, the urine osmolality is generally less than 350 mOsm/kg, the urine sodium is greater than 20 mEq/L, and the fractional excretion of sodium is generally greater than 1%.

The urinary sediment can also be helpful in distinguishing prerenal azotemia from ATN. In patients with prerenal azotemia, the sediment is frequently devoid of cellular casts, cells, or protein. In contrast, in patients with tubular injury, pigmented "muddy brown" casts are frequently prominent.

Another frequent indicator of a prerenal state is the ration of blood urea nitrogen (BUN) to creatinine. Normally the BUN–creatinine ratio is 10:1. However, in prerenal azotemia secondary to significant gastrointestinal losses, overdiuresis, or poor cardiac function [congestive heart failure (CHF)], the BUN rises disproportionately to the creatinine because of increased urea reabsorption under low flow states. Frequently, BUN-to-creatinine ratios greater than 20:1 can be seen. This is in contrast to ATN, where the BUN and creatinine generally rise in parallel.

There are some caveats to keep in mind in the transplant setting:

1. Cyclosporine and tacrolimus (FK506) toxicity both can produce a picture of marked prerenal azotemia (with an elevated BUN relative to the serum

creatinine, as well as a low urine sodium concentration) secondary to arteriolar vasoconstriction.

2. Steroids alone, and particularly pulse dose steroids, are markedly catabolic and can increase the BUN out of proportion to the creatinine and mimic a prerenal picture.
3. Certain processes that lead to tubular damage, such as the use of radiocontrast agents, obstruction, hemoglobinuria, and myoglobulinuria due to rhabdomyolysis, can sometimes present with a low fractional excretion of sodium early in the course of the injury (1).

Thus, in the transplant setting, whether it be renal, heart, lung, pancreas, or liver, evaluation of the volume status of the patient is critical to help establish the diagnosis of prerenal azotemia. Accurate assessment of intake and output (urine and gastrointestinal losses) as well as measurement of daily weights is essential. Invasive monitoring may be required. One also needs to be aware of the potential impact of certain drugs in the setting of prerenal azotemia. For example, in patients with already diminished renal perfusion (such as those with severe volume contraction, CHF, liver failure, or nephrotic syndrome), nonsteroidal anti-inflammatory agents (NSAIDs) can exacerbate a prerenal picture and produce a hemodynamically mediated acute renal failure (1). In these settings, renal perfusion is maintained by efferent arteriolar constriction. The nonsteroidals inhibit cyclo-oxygenase, thereby decreasing the normal production of vasodilatory prostaglandins. This leaves unbalanced vasoconstrictive stimuli and sets the stage for hemodynamically mediated ARF.

Likewise, patients with significant renal artery stenosis may present with a prerenal picture, which may progress to acute oliguric renal failure in the face of angiotensin-converting enzyme inhibitors or angiotensin-2 receptor antagonists. This is of particular concern in the renal transplant patient, with a solitary kidney, or in other patients with solid organ transplants and bilateral renal vaso-ocular disease where renal perfusion is being maintained by efferent arteriolar vasoconstriction that will be blocked by these drugs (2). Renal function clearly has to be closely monitored in this setting if these agents are to be employed. Moreover, if a marked deterioration in renal function occurs with these drugs, further evaluation for renovascular disease should be undertaken. Thus, prerenal azotemia and ischemic renal failure (ATN) can be viewed as a continuum, with the former leading to the latter when the impairment in blood flow becomes severe enough to lead to tubular death (1).

Postrenal Causes

Acute renal failure occurs when both ureters are obstructed or if there is obstruction of a single functional kidney, such as a renal transplant. If a transplant patient is oliguric, a catheter should be inserted into the bladder to rule out prostatic obstruction. If this does not immediately relieve the problems, a renal ultrasound should be obtained. A renal ultrasound can be used to diagnose obstruction, although it should be recognized that the sensitivity of this test is 85% and may not exclude the possibility of obstruction if the condition is acute or if the patient is hypovolemic (1). Therefore, if there is a high index of clinical suspicion for obstruction, it may on occasion be necessary to proceed with an antegrade or retrograde contrast study to establish the site of obstruction and provide relief.

In addition to prostatic hypertrophy, obstruction can be due to retroperitoneal fibrosis, papillary necrosis, renal calculi, or malignant conditions leading to blockage of the ureters. Intratubular obstruction can also lead to acute oliguric renal failure. This can be seen with deposition of acyclovir crystals (3), calcium oxalate crystals, or uric acid crystals, as is seen in the tumor lysis syndrome (4,5). Tumor lysis syndrome has been observed in heart and liver transplant patients presenting with extensive post-transplant lymphoproliferative disorders [B-cell lymphomas related to Epstein-Barr virus (EBV)] and may occur spontaneously in untreated patients with a massive tumor burden, as well as in the setting of chemotherapy (4,5). Once recognized, patients at risk for tumor lysis syndrome should be premedicated with allopurinol prior to initiating chemotherapy to block the massive uricosuria seen in association with tumor breakdown. In addition, there must be appropriate attention to hydration and alkalinization of the urine to a pH greater than 7.5 in order to increase the solubility of the uric acid.

Postrenal causes are important to rule out as quickly as possible, since the potential for recovery of renal function is often related to the duration of obstruction.

Ischemic Renal Failure

Ischemic renal failure can be the end result of multiple insults in the transplant recipient. Clearly, hypotension, sepsis, and direct toxic injury due to drugs are the major culprits of ARF in transplant patients.

In the renal transplant patient, ischemic injury to a cadaver donor allograft can lead to delayed graft function (DGF). A number of investigators have clearly shown that the long-term outlook of those allografts experiencing DGF is significantly decreased compared to those with immediate function (6,7). The question that arises is whether the disparity between these groups merely reflects our inability to diagnose rejection in the face of ischemic injury, or whether, as has been recently demonstrated, ischemia caused by extensive local release of cytokines and by activation of the complement cascade, neutrophils, and adhesion molecules, as well as by upregulation of MHC class II molecules, sets the stage for rejection (8). If the latter is the case, then potentially any agent that can improve ischemia reperfusion injury might not only have a beneficial effect on short-term allograft results (i.e., decreasing the need for dialysis in those transplant patients with ATN, an incidence that now averages 20% to 30%), but also have the potential for decreasing the frequency of early rejection episodes.

ICAM, the intracellular adhesion molecule on endothelial cells, interacts with CD11A/CD18 and CD11B/CD18 on neutrophils, promoting the adhesion of neutrophils to endothelial cells (9,10). In the rat model of ischemic renal failure, the administration of a monoclonal antibody directed against ICAM protects animals from ischemic renal failure, even when given two hours after the ischemic event (10). Moreover, "knockout" mice with a deficiency of ICAM are protected against acute renal failure (11), supporting the role of activated neutrophils in the pathogenesis of this process.

While a pilot trial in humans using a monoclonal antibody against ICAM-1 has suggested the possible utility of this monoclonal antibody in the setting of cadaver recipients at high risk for DGF (highly sensitized patients, or allografts with a prolonged cold ischemic time) (12), the benefit of this monoclonal antibody has not been confirmed in a multicenter randomized, double-blind study using a cyclosporine-based immunosuppressive protocol from the outset. Possibly the potential benefit of this antibody is mitigated by the early addition of cyclosporine in the multicenter trial, which may exacerbate ischemic tubular injury. This has certainly been the rationale for induction protocols using OKT-3 and antithymocyte globulin (ATG), in which these agents are used not only for their antirejection properties but to avoid the need for cyclosporine in the early post-transplant period (13).

Preliminary studies with platelet-activating antagonists likewise suggest that platelet activation via its effect on the complement cascade and cytokine release, as well as on leukocyte endothelial cell interactions may be important in early post-transplant ARF and rejection in humans (14). These antagonists also have been demonstrated to be protective in animal studies of ARF (15). Clearly, any agent that can decrease ischemic injury in the renal transplant may also have important therapeutic potential in all forms of solid organ transplantation and organ preservation, as well as in nontransplant settings.

Other therapeutic approaches have been undertaken to prevent or treat ischemic renal failure. The structural injury in ATN results in intratubular obstruction due to necrotic cellular debris, transtubular back leakage of the glomerular filtrate across the damaged tubule, and reductions in glomerular ultrafiltration due to alterations in renal hemodynamics (intrarenal vasoconstriction) out of proportion to the decline in renal blood flow (1). A number of new therapies directed at these findings have been studied. Atrial natriuretic peptide (ANP), a hormone produced in the cardiac atria, is normally secreted into the circulation in response to atrial dilatation and produces systemic hypotension and diuresis (1,16). ANP promotes vasodilatation of the afferent arterioles and vasoconstriction of the efferent arterioles, resulting in an increase in the glomerular filtration rate that is independent of renal blood flow (16).

In experimental animals, ANP appears to attenuate the severity of renal failure and potentiates the recovery of renal function even when administered after an ischemic insult. This improvement is associated not only with favorable changes in hemodynamics, but also with protection of the tubular epithelial integrity (16). Although an initial clinical trial was encouraging (17) in that the treated group showed a reduced need for dialysis, other studies have not demonstrated a significant improvement in outcome (18,19). A recent multicenter randomized, double-blind, placebo-controlled study of anaritide (a 25-amino-acid synthetic form of ANP) in over 500 critically ill patients in the intensive care unit with ATN did not provide enthusiastic support for the agent (19). The overall mortality and dialysis-free interval was not affected by the administration of ANP, and in fact, the drug appeared to worsen the outcome in those patients without oliguria. On the other hand, the study suggested these agents may be useful in the subgroup of patients with oliguric ARF (19). Clearly, further clinical trials are necessary before the usefulness of this agent can be established (20,21).

Drug-Induced Renal Complications

Drugs are one of the major causes of renal failure in the transplant population. This can occur as a result of direct toxicity, drug interactions, or an acute allergic interstitial nephritis (Table 35.1). In each case, the recognition is critical, as removal of the offending agent or reduction of the dose of the drug may be crucial in reversing or ameliorating the process.

Cyclosporine and Tacrolimus Toxicity

The nephrotoxicity of cyclosporine and tacrolimus represent significant side effects of these immunosuppressive agents and are a problem not only in renal transplantation, but in all solid organ recipients (22–29) (see also Chapters 6 and 9).

Acute cyclosporine and tacrolimus toxicity present clinically with a decline in renal function of the native kidneys or impaired renal function of a renal allograft (22–29). The histologic appearance is frequently a diagnosis of exclusion (i.e., ruling out histopathologic signs of rejection) but may include the presence of giant mitochondria and vacuolization, sometimes in an isometric pattern in the renal tubular cells (22–29). This decline in renal function usually responds to lowering the dose of the drug.

The mechanism for acute nephrotoxicity with cyclosporine and tacrolimus is incompletely understood. The absence of tubular cell necrosis in most patients suggests that the toxicity is not due primarily to a tubular effect. Recent studies support the notion that the acute nephrotoxic effect of cyclosporine and tacrolimus is the result of acute vasoconstriction of the afferent glomerular arterioles followed by a reduction of glomerular blood flow and glomerular filtration (30–39). Endothelin and thromboxane are postulated to mediate this process (30–39). This glomerular arteriolar

Table 35.1. Drugs Associated with Acute Renal Failure in Transplant Recipients

Mechanism	Drug
Direct tubular toxicity	Aminoglycosides
	Cyclosporine, tacrolimus
	Amphotericin
	Foscarnet, pentamidine
	Radiocontrast agents
Decreased renal perfusion due to impaired intrarenal hemodynamics	NSAIDs
	Angiotensin-converting enzyme inhibitors or AII receptor antagonists
	Radiocontrast agents
	Cyclosporine, tacrolimus
Rhabdomyolysis	HMG co-reductase inhibitors gemfibrozil ± cyclosporine
Intratubular obstruction by agent or metabolic product	Acyclovir (IV)
	Sulfonamides
	Methotrexate
	Triamterene
	Tumor lysis syndrome (uric acid) with chemotherapy
Acute allergic interstitial nephritis	Penicillins
	Cephalosporins
	Sulfonamides, rifampin
	Diuretics
	Cimetidine
	Allopurinol
	NSAIDs ± nephrotic syndrome
	Any drug capable of causing this syndrome
Hemolytic uremic syndrome	Cyclosporine, tacrolimus
	Mitomycin

Source: Adapted from Thadhani R, Pascual M, Bonventre JV. Acute renal failure. N Engl J Med 1996;334:1448.

vasoconstriction is reversible with improvement in renal blood flow and filtration when cyclosporine or tacrolimus dosage is reduced (32,35). Some evidence suggests calcium antagonists may exert a protective effect against cyclosporine toxicity, presumably by reversing both thromboxane- and endothelin-mediated afferent arteriolar vasoconstriction (36,38).

Protracted ARF is most frequently reported in organ recipients of cadaveric renal grafts with preexisting ischemic damage to the donor kidney and reflects the ability of cyclosporine to potentiate the ischemic injury to such grafts (40–42). In approximately 25% of recipients of cadaveric renal allografts, recovery of renal function does not resume until cyclosporine is temporarily withdrawn (40–42). The protracted form of ARF is not restricted to renal allografts, as similar prolongation of acute failure of native kidneys has been reported in heart transplant recipients and bone marrow recipients (43,44). Histologic changes are more prominent in protracted cyclosporine nephropathy with development of vasculopathy (smooth muscle drop out in arterioles) in addition to the tubular and mitochondrial changes (22).

Chronic cyclosporine and tacrolimus toxicity are best characterized in liver, heart, and lung transplant recipients who have normal baseline native renal function and in whom the contribution of a concurrent chronic renal rejection is excluded. The histologic changes in the renal cortex include severe tubular atrophy, basement membrane thickening, interstitial fibrosis, and focal segmental sclerosis of glomeruli (22).

Despite the fact that long-term studies of renal transplant function (more than 10 years) have not revealed an adverse impact on the clinical outcome of renal transplantation (45,46), studies from several centers suggest that treatment with cyclosporine continuously for more than 12 months is associated with a progressive but slow decline in glomerular filtration rate indicating irreversible renal injury (22,25,47). Clearly, many patients with heart, lung, and liver transplants on cyclosporine or tacrolimus with previously normal renal function have developed evidence of chronic renal failure after transplant, with interstitial fibrosis and chronic vasculopathy on biopsy of their native kidneys. Increasingly these patients are requiring renal replacement therapy. A recent report suggests that 7% of adult cardiac allograft recipients exposed to cyclosporine for at least three years will develop cyclosporine-associated end-stage renal failure requiring dialysis therapy (47). Now that new immunosuppressive agents are emerging, the question that must be answered is whether we can alter our protocols to avoid or decrease the dose of the more nephrotoxic agents and substitute drugs such as mycophenolate mofetil or rapamycin (48).

A unique form of cyclosporine nephrotoxicity resembling the picture of hemolytic-uremic syndrome with fibrin thrombi in the glomeruli and arterioles also has been described (49) (see Chapter 32). This lesion appears to be idiosyncratic. Although most patients with this thrombotic microangiopathy tend to develop irreversible renal failure, some patients demonstrate partial recovery if cyclosporine is discontinued (49). Similar lesions have also been reported with tacrolimus (27,28). While patients may develop thrombocytopenia and evidence of microangiopathic hemolytic anemia with schistocytes on peripheral smear, at times these findings may be absent and the renal lesion may be the only manifestation of the process.

The side effects as well as the clinical manifestations of cyclosporine and tacrolimus toxicity are listed in Tables 35.2 and 35.3. Hypertension is a common side effect of cyclosporine treatment (50,51) and is presumed to be primarily a consequence of sodium retention secondary to a diminished fractional excretion of sodium as well as increased vascular resistance. Increased sympathetic tone has also been reported as a factor in hypertension after heart transplantation (34). Hypertension tends to be more common with cyclosporine than with tacrolimus (26,51).

Hyperkalemia associated with a hyperchloremic (nonanion gap) metabolic acidosis is another frequent manifestation of both cyclosporine and tacrolimus nephrotoxicity. The hyperkalemia is thought to be due to decreased renin-angiotensin system activity as well as tubular insensitivity to aldosterone, leading to decreased urinary potassium excretion (52). Clinical studies suggest that the inappropriate response to the hyperkalemia and tubular insensitivity to mineralocorticoid are in part due to an inability to generate a favorable electrical gradient in the distal cortical nephron (52).

Asymptomatic hyperuricemia associated with enhanced proximal reabsorption of uric acid is reported in approximately 50% of transplant patients on cyclosporine-based immunosuppression, and gout is reported in 10% of cyclosporine-treated patients (53–55). Care must be used in treating patients with allopurinol (i.e., by modifying dose) if azathioprine is used, to avoid potential life-threatening bone marrow toxicity. It appears that mycophenolate does not interact with allopurinol, and that the allopurinol dose does not need to be adjusted when mycophenolate mofetil is substituted for azathioprine (Roche, personal communication, 1998).

Table 35.2. Adverse Effects of Cyclosporine Versus Tacrolimus

	Cyclosporine	Tacrolimus
Hypertension	+++	++
Nephrotoxicity	+++	++
Hemolytic-uremic syndrome	+	+
Hyperglycemia	+	+++
Hepatotoxicity	+	+
Hirsutism	++	–
Gingival hyperplasia	+++	–
Fibroadenoma of breast	++	–
Hypertrophic cardiomyopathy (children)	–	+

Table 35.3. Tubular Effects of Cyclosporine Toxicity

Clinical Symptom	Proposed Mechanism
Hypertension	Increased sodium reabsorption, increased afferent arteriolar resistance, and increased sympathetic tone
Hyperkalemia	Pseudohypoaldosteronism (aldosterone insensitivity) and increased intracellular potassium efflux
Hyperchloremic acidosis	Pseudohypoaldosteronism
Hyperuricemia	Increased uric acid absorption
Hypomagnesemia	Urinary wasting
Hypophosphatemia	Urinary wasting

Renal Complications Due to Drug Interactions with Cyclosporine and Tacrolimus

Cyclosporine and tacrolimus are the most common offenders implicated in drug-induced renal dysfunction in the transplanted patient, either alone or in combination with other drugs. The renal implications of drug interactions with immunophilin-based immunosuppression vary from mild renal dysfunction reversible after dosage modification to severe renal failure, including graft rejection and nephrotoxicity (22,25,47). Table 35.4 summarizes the most common drug interactions with cyclosporine and tacrolimus, which may cause either elevated blood levels with deterioration of renal (native or graft) function or decreased blood levels with the potential risk of rejection (56).

Cyclosporine is metabolized by the hepatic cytochrome P450 system (56). Drugs that inhibit the P450 system (e.g., erythromycin, other macrolides, diltiazem, ketoconazole, itraconazole, and fluconazole) will slow cyclosporine metabolism and increase blood levels, which may lead to nephrotoxicity if the cyclosporine dose is not reduced. In some instances, ketoconazole, diltiazem, or erythromycin have

Table 35.4. Drug Interactions with Cyclosporine and Tacrolimus

Drugs That Inhibit P450 and Increase Blood Levels	Drugs That Upregulate P450 and Decrease Blood Levels	No Effect on Cyclosporine and Tacrolimus Levels	Drugs That May Have a Nephrotoxic Effect Without Affecting Blood Level
Erythromycin	Rifampin	Nifedipine	Aminoglycosides
Clarithromycin	Isoniazid	Amlodipine	Amphotericin
Azithromycin	Phenobarbital		Nonsteroidal anti-inflammatory agents
Ketoconazole	Phenytoin		ACE inhibitors
Itraconazole	Carbamazepine		HMG coreductase inhibitors
Fluconazole			
Trimethoprim sulfa (high dose)			
Verapamil			
Diltiazem			
Nicardipine			

been specifically utilized in conjunction with cyclosporine in an effort to markedly reduce the dose of the immunosuppressive agent and thereby decrease the cost. Components of grapefruit juice are capable of inhibiting the intestinal cytochrome P450 system. Consistent use of grapefruit juice has resulted in an average increase of 30% in cyclosporine levels (57). Neoral, the new microemulsion preparation of cyclosporine (57), does not appear to have this interaction with grapefruit juice.

Drugs that induce the P450 system will increase metabolism of cyclosporine or tacrolimus and decrease blood levels, potentially leaving the patient at increased risk of rejection (56). Phenytoin and other antiepileptics as well as rifampin are examples of such drugs (56).

In clinical practice, the interaction of cyclosporine or tacrolimus with antimicrobial agents constitutes the most common interaction that requires monitoring of the cyclosporine or tacrolimus level. The most commonly observed interactions are listed in Table 35.4. The interaction of calcium channel blockers with cyclosporine is of particular note. Generally, nifedipine and amlodipine are thought not to interfere with cyclosporine or tacrolimus levels, whereas verapamil, diltiazem, and nicardipine increase cyclosporine and tacrolimus levels (56). This is important to remember when prescribing antihypertensive or antianginal agents.

Lovastatin is reported to cause myositis with elevations of the serum creatinine phosphokinase level in fewer than 0.5% of treated individuals, but administered concomitantly with cyclosporine or other drugs metabolized by the cytochrome P450 system the incidence is reported as high as 30%. Clinically, myalgias with elevated creatinine phosphokinase levels and rhabdomyolysis have complicated treatment of patients with cyclosporine and HMG-CoA reductase inhibitors (58). Similarly, cases of rhabdomyolysis with myoglobulinuric acute renal failure have been reported with gemfibrozil and niacin, which are also metabolized by the cytochrome P450 system (58–61). A low-dose regimen (20 mg/day or less) of the statins has been reported to be safely used in cyclosporine-treated patients (62,63).

Other potential nephrotoxic agents should be avoided in the setting of ARF to prevent exacerbating renal injury. Of particular note are radiocontrast agents. The risk for contrast nephropathy is highest in patients with diabetes mellitus, multiple myeloma, renal insufficiency (creatinine >2.8 mg/dL), and advanced age. Nonionic contrast agents offer no definitive advantage except perhaps in the highest risk patients (64). Diuretics and mannitol prophylactically may be detrimental in patients receiving contrast agents. Instead, efforts should be made to use the lowest possible dose of contrast, combined with saline administration to avoid volume depletion, maintain urine output, and reduce contact time of the dye with the renal tubular epithelial cell (65).

Acute Allergic Interstitial Nephritis

While the direct effects of cyclosporine and tacrolimus and the interactions of these agents with other drugs account for much of the renal dysfunction that is encountered in the transplant patient, nonetheless one must be alert to the possibility of a superimposed drug-induced acute allergic interstitial nephritis. This diagnosis may be especially difficult in the face of immunosuppressive treatment that can modify the picture.

Any drug may be a culprit, although the syndrome of acute allergic interstitial nephritis is most frequently described with beta lactam antibiotics such as nafcillin, oxacillin, the cephalosporins, as well as sulfa-containing drugs such as diuretics and trimethoprim sulfamethoxazole. The latter is of particular importance in that trimethoprim sulfa is the cornerstone of urinary tract infection prophylaxis in the renal transplant patient, as well as of pneumocystitis (PCP) prophylaxis in all transplant recipients. Consequently, documented allergic reactions require a consideration of other substitute medications such as atovaquone or pentamidine for PCP prophylaxis and a quinolone for urinary tract infection prophylaxis.

In nonimmunocompromised patients, fever, rash, eosinophilia, and a rise in the BUN and creatinine may point to the diagnosis of acute allergic interstitial nephritis (66). The urine sediment may demonstrate white cells and white cell casts, as well as eosinophils by Wright stain or Hensel stain. Acute oliguric renal failure occurs in about one-third of patients with this diagnosis (66). In immunosuppressed patients, however, steroids can mask many of these findings. Therefore, a high index of suspicion is critically important in the face of an unexplained rise in the serum creatinine in the absence of obstruction, rejection, or ischemic injury. Stopping the potential offending agent will generally lead to improvement in the renal insufficiency. In certain cases, however, particularly those with oliguric renal failure, high-dose steroids at 60 mg/day for one week then tapered gradually have been beneficial in speeding renal recovery and restoring baseline renal function (67).

RECURRENT DISEASE IN THE RENAL ALLOGRAFT

Virtually all diseases affecting the native kidney can recur in the kidney transplant with the exception of polycystic kidney disease and Alport's syndrome (hereditary nephritis) (75). Although the effect of recurrent disease on renal allograft survival is increasingly recognized as graft survival results continue to improve, the recurrence of the original disease accounts for only approximately 5% of all renal graft losses in both child and adult recipients (67–74). Recurrent diseases can be categorized as follows:

- Recurrent *primary* glomerular diseases (Table 35.5)
- Recurrent *secondary* glomerular diseases (Table 35.6)
- Recurrent nonglomerular (systemic) diseases (Table 35.7)

As a group, the recurrent diseases account for approximately 25% of patients with post-transplant nephrotic syn-

Table 35.5. Recurrent Primary Glomerular Diseases

Recurrent Glomerulopathy	Approximate Recurrence Rate	Graft Failure	Transplant Considerations
Focal segmental glomerulonephritis	20–30%	10–20%	In high-risk group possibly avoid living-related graft
IgA nephropathy	50%	<10%	Higher recurrence rate in living-related/haploidentical transplants
Membranoproliferative glomerulonephritis type 1	20–30%	30–40%	Histologic picture resembles transplant glomerulopathy (chronic rejection)
Membranoproliferative glomerulonephritis type 2	50–100%	10–20%	In high-risk group possibly avoid living-related graft
Membranous glomerulonephritis	10%	Rare	Higher recurrence rate in living-related/haploidentical transplants
Anti-GBM disease	10–20%	Rare	Monitor pretransplantation: transplant in absence of anti-GBM antibodies

Table 35.6. Recurrent Secondary Glomerular Diseases

Recurrent Glomerulopathy	Approximate Recurrence Rate	Graft Failure	Transplant Considerations
Diabetes mellitus	100%	<5%	Living-related or cadaveric grafts
Henoch-Schönlein purpura (HSP)	20%	10–15%	Delayed transplantation recommended
Hemolytic-uremic syndrome (HUS)	15–35%	40–50%	Avoid living-related donor Identification of high-risk patients
Lupus nephritis	<1%	None	Transplant when disease is serologically inactive
Wegener's granulomatosis	10–20%	Rare	Disease should be inactive, with low ANCA titers
Amyloidosis	5–15%	<5%	High mortality due to cardiac amyloid and infections

Table 35.7. Recurrent Nonglomerular (Systemic) Diseases

Recurrent Glomerulopathy	Approximate Recurrence Rate	Graft Failure	Transplant Considerations
Oxalosis	>90%	Most	Combined liver and kidney transplant
Cystinosis	10%	No	Graft results encouraging, but systemic cystine accumulation continues
Fabry's disease	Rare	Rare	Recent graft results encouraging
Alport's syndrome	Rare	<5%	Risk of anti-GBM disease

drome, whereas transplant glomerulopathy accounts for more than 60% of such patients (75). Transplant glomerulopathy is thought to be a consequence of chronic rejection with histologic features similar to membranoproliferative glomerulonephritis type 1 (MPGN type 1) (76).

The most frequent diseases that recur in the allograft are primary glomerular diseases. Among the recurrent glomerulonephritides, focal segmental glomerulonephritis (FSGS), MPGN type 2, and IgA nephropathy have the highest rate of recurrence (see Table 35.5). The donor and recipient factors that lead to recurrence of glomerulonephritis are not well understood, but some factors that have been associated with an increased risk (73) include young age of the recipient, a history of recurrence in previous transplants, and a rapidly progressive course of the primary renal disease (67,71–80). Recurrent glomerulonephritis is also observed more frequently in well-matched living-related renal transplants, suggesting a possible genetic susceptibility (78,79). Recent work does not show any impact of native nephrectomy on the incidence of recurrent disease following renal transplantation for primary glomerulonephritis (81).

Focal Segmental Glomerulosclerosis (FSGS)

The overall recurrence rate of FSGS is 20% to 30% (69–75,77–80). Within that group, recurrence leading to graft loss is seen in 30% to 40% (69–80). The histologic findings are the same as those in the native kidney disease, with focal segmental glomerular sclerosis and hyalinosis. Although some patients may present with nephrotic-range proteinuria as early as 24 hours after transplantation, most patients do not manifest the syndrome until three months after transplantation (70–75,77–80).

A subgroup of patients with a recurrence rate of greater than 50% has been identified. Risk of recurrence of FSGS is significantly increased in patients younger than 15, in those with a rapidly progressive course of disease with evolution to end-stage renal failure in less than three years, in those with mesangial proliferation on biopsy, and in patients with recurrence of FSGS in a previous graft (70–73,77–80).

Strategies for the management of recurrent FSGS include use of nonsteroidal anti-inflammatory agents, angiotensin-converting enzyme (ACE) inhibitors, cyclosporine, plasma exchange, and protein A immunoadsorption columns (78,82–84). While ACE inhibitors and NSAIDs have been demonstrated to diminish protein excretion in a number of cases, frequently this occurs at the expense of impaired glomerular filtration rate. Cyclosporine has not been shown to affect the course of recurrent FSGS, nor has switching from cyclosporine to FK506 (78).

The rapid recurrence of primary FSGS suggests the presence of a circulating factor in this disease (82–85). Several lines of evidence appear to support this hypothesis. Serum from patients with FSGS increases the permeability of isolated glomeruli to albumin (82). Evaluation of serum from pretransplant patients with FSGS in this in vitro system can identify those patients at high risk of recurrence (86% incidence of recurrence when glomerular albumin permeability was increased compared to 7% with sera of no or lesser activity) (82).

Use of a regenerating protein adsorption column (83) and plasmapheresis (82,84) have been reported to reduce protein excretion in transplant patients with recurrent FSGS and even induce complete remission in some cases (84). The factor removed, which does not appear to be an immunoglobulin, has an apparent molecular weight of 50 kilodaltons and appears to increase protein excretion when injected into rats (85). The exact nature of the toxin has yet to be identified.

IgA Nephropathy

Immunoglobulin A nephropathy recurs in about 50% of patients, with a reported range between 20% and 80% (52–55,77–79). Histologic changes are characterized by mesangial expansion and mesangial IgA deposits. The clinical picture of recurrent IgA nephropathy is that of hematuria with or without proteinuria, but graft failure occurs in less than 10% of patients (73).

It has been reported that the rate of recurrence of IgA nephropathy is higher in allografts from living-related donors (83%) (73,86–89), as compared with 14% in cadaveric kidney grafts (73,87). Because of the low rate of graft loss due to recurrent disease, however, living-related transplantation is generally not discouraged.

Membranoproliferative Glomerulonephritis

MPGN Type 1

The overall recurrence rate of idiopathic type 1 MPGN is reported to be approximately 20% to 30%, and the rate of graft loss varies between 30% and 40% (73). The histologic appearance of type 1 MPGN is similar to transplant glomerulopathy seen with chronic rejection, with reduplication of the glomerular basement membrane, subendothelial deposits, and increased mesangial matrix. The presence of significant immune deposits (C3), subendothelial deposits, and glomerular crescents may differentiate type 1 MPGN from transplant glomerulopathy (33). Clinically, the patients present with proteinuria and hematuria (70–73,90).

MPGN Type 2

Although type 2 MPGN is not a common cause of end-stage renal failure as compared with type 1 MPGN, its recurrence rate is 50% to 100% (70–73). Despite the high recurrence rate, graft loss appears to occur in only 10% to 20% of the patients (70–73). Analogous to FSGS, graft loss is reported to be increased in high-risk patients, which include those with rapidly progressive previous disease and recurrent nephrotic syndrome (82,91). Histologically, the lesions are similar to those observed in native kidneys, with prominent basement membrane dense deposits on electron micrographs (83). Clinically, the patient generally presents with proteinuria and hematuria.

Membranous Glomerulonephritis

The risk of recurrence of membranous glomerulonephritis (MGN) ranges widely from 3% to 26% (70–73,92–99). Ascertaining the true incidence is complicated by the occurrence of de novo MGN in renal allografts (2% to 9% in most series) (96–98). The clinical presentation of recurrent membranous nephropathy is characterized by nephrotic syndrome, which generally occurs within the first three months after transplant, and in two case reports even within two weeks after transplant (73,93). In contrast, de novo graft MGN tends to occur later (4 months to 6 years; mean 22 months) and the histologic picture more likely resembles that of chronic rejection, with evidence of interstitial fibrosis and vascular changes in addition to thickening of the basement membrane and evidence of subendothelial deposits (96–98).

Although the absolute risk of recurrence of MGN remains relatively low, approximately 50% of grafts with recurrent MGN fail (72,73). Males and patients with an aggressive pretreatment course marked by significant proteinuria and rapid deterioriation in renal failure appear to be at greater risk for early recurrence.

As in IgA nephropathy, the risk of recurrence appears higher in grafts from living-related (HLA-identical) siblings, with recurrence arising earlier than in those who receive cadaver grafts (73,95–99,101). These observations raise a note of caution about using living-related donors for patients with membranous nephropathy. While a possible association between the TAP1 B allele and MGN has been demonstrated, the role of this genetic marker has not been clearly identified (100).

Antiglomerular Basement Membrane Disease

The clinical recurrence rate of antiglomerular basement membrane (anti-GBM) disease is low (10% to 15%), although a higher percentage may demonstrate linear capillary immunoglobulin G (IgG) by immunofluorescent staining (70–73). The recommendation is to delay transplantation until anti-GBM antibodies are undetectable, usually 6 to 12 months after presentation of the disease, to avoid the risk of recurrent disease (70–73).

Diabetes Mellitus

Diabetic nephropathy recurs in 100% of renal allografts, based on histologic changes of mesangial expansion, glomerular basement membrane thickening, and arteriolar hyalinization (70–72,102). These occur within two to four years, whereas nodular glomerulosclerosis is rare (73,102). The clinical picture is recurrence of nephrotic syndrome, but graft failure due to diabetic nephropathy is rare in the first decade following transplantation (102).

Several mechanisms for the pathophysiology of the diabetic nephropathy have been proposed, including a genetic predisposition. Notably, HLA-DR4, B8, B15 have been associated with diabetic nephropathy (73). Hemodynamic factors, including increased glomerular pressures and flows (hyperfiltration), are also thought to contribute to the pathogenesis of diabetic microangiopathy (103), just as they are implicated in the primary disease process. The impact of normalizing blood sugar has been well demonstrated (104–107). Successful pancreas transplantation performed simultaneously or after renal transplantation has been shown to prevent or retard recurrent diabetic nephropathy in the allograft (104,106). Isolated reports suggest that early diabetic nephropathy can be reversed if diabetic kidneys are transplanted into euglycemic nondiabetic recipients (105).

At five years following isolated pancreatic transplant, diabetic glomerular lesions have not appeared to regress in native kidneys of patients with insulin-dependent diabetes mellitus (106). However, in a 10-year follow-up of these patients, an improvement has been observed (Mauer SM, personal communication, 1998). Thus, in nontransplanted patients, as demonstrated in the Diabetes Control and Complications Trial (DCCT) (107), as well as in the transplant setting (104–107), euglycemic control slows the progression of diabetic nephropathy (see also Chapter 21).

Henoch-Schönlein Purpura

Henoch-Schönlein purpura (HSP) and IgA nephropathy are two ends of the spectrum of the same disease. Reports of recurrence of this disease in renal allografts are based on small numbers of patients with HSP who have undergone transplantation (70–73,108–110). Clinical graft recurrence generally presents with hematuria and proteinuria in approximately 20% of patients, and graft failure due to recurrence occurs in 10% to 15% (73).

Histologic recurrence with mesangial IgA deposits is found with a prevalence of approximately 50% (109,110). It is recommended that transplantation be delayed for one to two years after the disappearance of the purpura or other active evidence of the disease process.

Hemolytic-Uremic Syndrome

Hemolytic-uremic syndrome (HUS) has a recurrence rate of 15% to 35%, with an incidence of graft loss varying from 30% to 50% (73,111–115). Clinically, the patients present with microangiopathic hemolytic anemia, thrombocytopenia, and renal failure. The histologic picture is that of intravascular coagulation with fibrin thrombi within the glomeruli. Recurrent disease must be distinguished from HUS occurring in association with cyclosporine or tacrolimus or with acute vascular rejection, which can present a similar clinical picture (111,112,116,117).

Increased risk for recurrent HUS is reported in patients receiving antilymphocyte globulin (ALG), OKT-3, and cyclosporine (73). On the basis of the findings in some studies that tacrolimus has less propensity than cyclosporine to induce HUS, some researchers have recommended the use of tacrolimus in place of cyclosporine in patients with previous loss of renal function due to HUS (118). Recurrent HUS is not at present described with rapamicin or mycophenolate mofetil, but the experience available with these drugs is limited.

Prevention of recurrent HUS should include avoidance of oral contraceptives and possibly low-dose aspirin or dipyridamole (73). Because of the possibility of an inherited endothelial defect that may predispose to HUS, caution has been advised in recommending living-related transplantation (111).

Lupus Nephritis

Graft survival in patients with systemic lupus erythematosus (SLE) has generally been similar to that in patients with other diseases (73,119–124). A recent report suggests that patients with SLE receiving a living allograft do better than those receiving a cadaver kidney (89% compared with 41% with a cadaver allograft) (123). This cadaver allograft survival is significantly lower than that reported for patients with other forms of renal failure (41% compared with 71%) (123). This has led to the suggestion of a possible preference for living-related donors in patients with lupus erythematosus (123,124).

Recent data suggest a recurrence rate of 2.7% to 3.8% of lupus erythematosus in renal allograft recipients (73,123,124). The incidence of recurrent symptoms of SLE has also been low as long as the SLE is clinically and serologically quiescent prior to transplant. Patients who have lupus anticoagulant identified prior to transplant and have a history of thromboembolic events should remain on anticoagulation if antiphospholipid antibody activity is documented (123).

Wegener's Granulomatosis

The experience with Wegener's granulomatosis is limited. Relapses with recurrence of vasculitis in the graft have been reported in 10% to 20% of patients, but rapidly progressive and lethal recurrence of Wegener's disease is rare (73, 125–131). It is generally recommended that transplantation of patients with Wegener's disease be postponed until antinuclear cytotoxic antibodies (ANCA) titers, particularly proteinase 3 specificity, are low-negative (70–73,127,129) and there is no evidence of acute disease. While ANCA titers pretransplant may herald relapses of systemic vasculitis, it is of note that recurrent Wegener's has been seen five days after transplant without increased ANCA levels (69). Treatment of recurrent Wegener's may include a switch to cyclophosphamide or the use of plasma exchange or intravenous immunoglobulin (73).

Amyloidosis

In clinical studies, the recurrence rate of symptomatic amyloidosis (primary, secondary, multiple myeloma, or familial) in allografts is reported to be 20% to 30%, although the rate of recurrence varies with the etiology of the underlying disease (73,132–134). Histologic but asymptomatic recurrence with fibrillar deposits (Congo red positive) in the glomerular basement membrane is common (10% to 30%) (73,132–134). The patients generally present with proteinuria that may progress to nephrotic syndrome or graft loss. The clinical outcome often is determined by the high mortality rate due to infections and cardiac amyloid disease, and by the evolution of any underlying hematologic malignancy (73,132–134). Recurrent renal disease heralded by onset of nephrotic-range proteinuria has also been reported in allograft recipients with underlying multiple myeloma and light-chain deposit disease. Recurrence of light-chain was found in 6 of 12 patients, with eventual graft loss in two patients despite plasma exchange, melphalan, and steroids (135).

Oxalosis

The underlying metabolic defect in primary hyperoxaluria (type 1) is deficiency in the enzyme glyoxalate aminotransferase. Instead of undergoing recycling to glycine, the glyoxalate is metabolized to oxalate, which is a dead-end metabolic pathway, and oxalate is eliminated unchanged by the kidneys. The increased oxalate load results in stone formation and obstructive uropathy with infection, usually before age 20 (136). Recurrent oxalosis and graft loss have resulted after renal transplantation in these patients (70–72).

Because the liver provides the missing enzyme activity, combined liver and kidney transplantation has led to successful therapy in this condition (137–140). This is the present recommended therapeutic approach. Two-year graft survival of 78% is reported (138–140). To maximize engraftment results, transplantation should be undertaken before the glomerular filtration rate (GFR) falls below 20 to 25 mL/min in order to minimize oxalate retention and to maximize renal graft urine output. For patients on dialysis, maximizing preoperative dialysis to reduce body stores of oxalate is recommended (137–140). Medical therapy with pyridoxine, neutral phosphate, and magnesium should be given after transplantation to reduce oxalate deposition and recurrence (136).

Cystinosis

The metabolic disorder of cystinosis is due to a deficient transport system for lysosomal cystine, leading to cystine accumulation in the interstitium of the kidney and calcific degradation of the tubules. Transplantation is the preferred mode of therapy for children with end-stage renal disease due to cystinosis, with a reported three-year graft survival of 80% (70,71,141). A comparable graft survival rate for adult patients with the disease has been reported. Recurrence occurs in approximately 10% of patients but does not impair the renal function (70–72). Unfortunately, renal transplantation does not correct the underlying metabolic disorder, and cystine continues to accumulate and deposit in the eyes, endocrine organs, and central nervous system (70).

Fabry's Disease

Recent transplant experience with Fabry's disease (angiokeratoma corporis diffusum universale) has shown three-year graft survivals of up to 80% (142–146), with rare recurrence of the disease. The biochemical defect results from a deficiency of alpha-galactosidase, leading to a visceral accumulation of glycosphingolipids (144). Renal transplantation does provide a source of alpha-galactosidase activity, and, in the majority of recurrences, the glycosphingolipid deposits have only been in the vascular endothelium. The latter suggests an inability of graft endothelial cells to metabolize the substrate, replacement of donor endothelium with recipient endothelium, or production of antigalactosidase antibodies (70–72).

Alport's Syndrome

Patients with Alport's syndrome (hereditary nephritis) have a defect in the $\alpha3$ chain of type IV collagen of the basement membrane, leading to renal failure and deafness (147). The transplant experience with Alport's syndrome has been generally favorable, with no difference in five-year allograft survival between Alport's patients and a matched control group (148,149). However, some Alport's patients can develop anti-GBM disease de novo in the post-transplant setting due to exposure to a kidney containing normal GBM, leading to development of anti-$\alpha3$ or anti-$\alpha5$ (type IV collagen) antibodies that are deposited along the basement membrane and may cause crescent glomerulonephritis (149–152).

LIVER DISEASE AND RENAL COMPLICATIONS

While patients with liver disease can develop all the usual forms of acute renal dysfunction previously discussed (i.e., ATN secondary to sepsis, hemorrhage, aggressive paracentesis, prerenal azotemia due to over-diuresis, drug-induced acute allergic interstitial nephritis, or contrast-induced nephropathy), several unique forms of renal involvement have been identified in this patient population.

Hepatitus C Virus (HCV)-Associated Glomerulonephritis

Hepatitis C virus (HCV) infection is a major cause of end-stage liver failure that often necessitates liver transplantation. Increasingly, there is a subset of patients presenting for liver transplant due to HCV who are identified as having concomitant glomerular disease of varying severity (153–159). Several renal manifestations have been identified in association with chronic HCV infection. Most commonly, hepatitis C virus is associated with MPGN type 1 (153–157). The histologic picture is one of a proliferative lobular glomerulonephritis with IgM, IgG, and C3 deposition. Cryoglobulins are occasionally noted on kidney biopsy (154). HCV has also been reported with membranous nephropathy (153).

Patients may present with the picture of mixed cryoglobulinemia syndrome: purpura, arthralgias, neuropathy, weakness, and abnormal liver function tests (153, 154,158,159). Renal manifestations include proteinuria (frequently nephrotic range) and an active urinary sediment, with red cells and red cell casts, as well as mild to moderate renal insufficiency (153–155,158). Laboratory tests suggestive of this disorder include a positive anti-HCV antibody by EIA2 or RIBA assays, positive HCV RNA polymerase chain reaction (PCR), positive rheumatoid factor (approximately 70% of patients), low complement levels (CH50 decreased in 75%, C3 low in 50%), and a negative ANCA titer (153,158,159). Fifty to seventy percent of patients with HCV-associated glomerulonephritis have circulating cryoglobulins in their serum (154,155,158). These cryoglobulins (proteins that precipitate from cooled serum) are generally composed of a polyclonal IgG bound to another immunoglobulin that acts as an anti-IgG rheumatoid factor. This antiglobulin component, usually of the IgM class, is generally monoclonal (154,155,158).

While the pathogenesis of HCV-associated glomerulonephritis is still debated, it is thought to be due to in situ formation of immune complexes in the glomeruli containing HCV, anti-HCV, and rheumatoid factor (153,158). Recently, there have been reports of direct identification of HCV antigen in the immune complexes in the glomeruli in 8 of 12 patients with HCV-associated MPGN (160).

Treatment with interferon-α in patients with HCV glomerulonephritis (3 million units three times a week for 6 to 12 months) has been demonstrated to reduce HCV viremia and cryoglobulin levels in approximately 60% of nontransplant patients, as well as to decrease proteinuria and stabilize renal function (156,161). The impact of decreasing viral load further suggests an etiologic relationship between hepatitis C and renal disease. Good clinical response is correlated with the disappearance of HCV RNA during treatment; however, relapse is common after stopping therapy (156,161).

There are other specific concerns about HCV glomerulonephritis following liver transplantation. In patients with HCV-associated liver failure undergoing liver transplant, standard immunosuppression results in a significant increase in the HCV viral replication and demonstrable viremia as soon as one month after transplant (157,161–164). Therefore, in patients who present with both liver and kidney involvement prior to transplant, there is the potential of exacerbating the glomerular disease after transplantation (165). Likewise, several cases of the new onset of nephrotic syndrome after liver transplant have been reported in patients with recurrent hepatitis C infection (164).

As the number of liver transplants for hepatitis C increases, the potential for associated renal involvement before and after transplant needs to be closely examined and may be important in the management of these individuals. Further studies are required to determine who may benefit from simultaneous liver and kidney transplant. Clearly, there is a critical need for more effective antiviral therapy for this disease entity (see also Chapter 19).

Hepatitis C in the Renal Transplant Recipient

As an increasing number of patients with renal failure wait on the cadaver renal transplant list, efforts are being considered as to how to expand the pool of organ donors. One question that has been raised concerns the possible use of hepatitis C cadaver donors: What might the impact of hepatitis C transmission be on HCV-negative renal allograft recipients?

Some information comes from the retrospective analysis of patients who received HCV organs prior to routine HCV testing (157,166). While it has been demonstrated that HCV-positive donors will transfer infection to virtually all HCV-seronegative recipients (157,166), there does not appear to be any clinically significant impact of hepatitis C on early renal allograft loss or mortality (157,167–171). Likewise, although biochemical evidence of HCV hepatitis occurs in approximately 50% to 65% of previously seronegative renal transplant recipients who have received an organ from an HCV-positive donor (157), the short-term morbidity and mortality related to the liver disease have been generally low, with only a minority of patients developing liver disease or fulminant hepatitis three to five years following transplant (157,167–171).

Beyond this period, however, there are increasing reports of excess morbidity and mortality due to HCV and evidence of portal hypertension and death due to hepatic disease (157,167,171). Thus, over the long term, it appears renal transplant using HCV-infected donors is associated with an increased risk of liver disease and death for the recipient, when compared with uninfected donors (157,171).

Therefore, as one considers expanding the criteria for organ donor, it may be necessary to closely match donor and recipient if using a hepatitis C donor is contemplated. For example, while it may be reasonable with informed consent to accept a hepatitis C donor for an older patient, for someone who has no available access, or for someone who desperately wants to get off dialysis and is highly sensitized, in the case of a young person one would have to weigh the long-term consequences of HCV transmission against the potential benefit of getting off dialysis.

Other questions concern the long-term impact of HCV, acquired prior to renal transplant, on the subsequent transplant course. Not only has de novo MPGN (with and without cryoglobulinemia) been demonstrated (172) following renal transplant in patients with hepatitis C, as well as membranous nephropathy (172–174) and transplant glomerulopathy (175), but recently a new syndrome has been described: an association between the presence of anticardiolipin antibodies and de novo renal thrombotic microangiopathy in HCV-positive renal transplant recipients (176). Cryoglobulins, complement level, and rheumatoid factors have been negative in these patients. The time between transplantation and the diagnosis of the syndrome has ranged between 5 and 120 days (with a median of two weeks) (176). These patients have also demonstrated an increased incidence of thrombotic complications including renal artery thrombosis, infarcted bowel, acute myocardial infarction, and pulmonary embolus (176). These findings suggest that the anticardiolipin antibodies demonstrated in the serum of these patients may be implicated in the pathogenesis of this syndrome (176,177).

Hepatorenal Syndrome

Hepatorenal syndrome is the development of progressive oliguric renal failure in patients with severe advanced liver disease in the absence of any other cause of acute renal failure (see Chapter 19). This syndrome generally occurs in cirrhotics with portal hypertension but may occur with acute fulminant hepatitis and alcohol cirrhosis; it has also been reported with some forms of liver cancer (178,179). The renal failure is secondary to a functional abnormality marked by severe renal vasoconstriction in the face of splanchnic vasodilatation and increased cardiac output, with a fall in systemic vascular resistance (178,179). The kidneys remain structurally normal in hepatorenal syndrome. In fact, the kidneys may resume function if the liver recovers, if a successful liver transplant is performed (180), or if the kidneys are transplanted into a patient with a normal liver but chronic renal failure (181). This suggests some factor related to the liver is responsible for the renal dysfunction (186–190).

The potential role of splanchnic dilatation in the syndrome is suggested by the response to portasystemic shunting as well as the response to ornipressin, an analogue of antidiuretic hormone that preferentially acts as a splanchnic vasoconstrictor (182). Administration of this drug to patients with advanced hepatic cirrhosis leads to a decrease in plasma renin and norepinephrine; an increase in mean arterial pressure, renal blood flow, GFR, and urine sodium; and correction of many of the hemodynamic abnormalities associated with hepatorenal syndrome (182).

The mediators of hepatorenal syndrome have been a subject of great debate. It has been suggested that there is an imbalance between the vasoconstrictor thromboxane and vasodilator prostacyclins (178,179). A number of other vasoconstrictor substances, such as endothelin, false transmitters, and increased sympathetic tone, have been postulated to be responsible for the hemodynamic effects observed in this syndrome (178).

Clinically, hepatorenal syndrome is characterized by oliguria, a urine sodium less than 10 mEq/L, a benign urine sediment, a urine osmolality greater than plasma osmolality, and a progressive rise in creatinine as well as a lack of response to volume expansion (178,179). The onset of renal failure may be insidious and can be precipitated by insults such as GI bleeding, spontaneous bacterial peritonitis, or overdiuresis (178). However, it must be remembered that hepatorenal syndrome is a diagnosis of exclusion. The best treatment for the renal failure in this setting is resolution of the primary hepatic failure or successful hepatic transplantation (178–180,183). Occasionally improvement has been reported with peritoneovenous (Levine) shunting (179).

Renal Replacement Therapy in Patients with Liver Failure

The mortality of patients with acute renal failure in the setting of acute hepatic failure (before or after liver transplant) remains high, and the issues of which renal replacement modality to utilize and the mode of anticoagulation, replacement fluid, and/or dialysis composition are matters of concern (184).

Patients with liver failure are particularly prone to cardiovascular instability with increased risk of renal ischemia from sepsis, GI bleeding, and overdiuresis. Following liver transplant there is also the increased risk of acute renal failure associated with nephrotoxic doses of tacrolimus, cyclosporine, or aminoglycosides.

In addition to cardiovascular instability, however, patients with liver failure both before and after liver transplant are prone to increased intracranial pressure and hypoxia. In fact, the most common causes of death in patients with acute fulminant hepatic failure remain cerebral edema and cerebral hypoxia (184). These two factors, cardiovascular status and concern about cerebral edema, need to be considered when selecting a mode of renal replacement therapy for these patients.

Acute peritoneal dialysis has the theoretical advantage of providing the most gradual form for dialysis and fluid removal, with fewer shifts in cardiovascular status or intracranial pressures and the avoidance of heparin anticoagulation. However, the placement of a peritoneal dialysis catheter pretransplant or soon after liver transplant presents very real hazards including the possibility of exit site infection or peritonitis, leakage, loss of albumin with decreased oncotic pressure, and ineffective clearances if there has been disruption of the peritoneal membrane. In addition, there is the risk of orthostatic pneumonia or impaired oxygenation as the result of increased amounts of fluid within the abdomen.

Hemodialysis, on the other hand, while effective in terms of clearance of potentially toxic compounds and the ability to remove volume, can be associated with marked hemodynamic lability, GI bleeding associated with heparin anticoagulation, and dialysis disequilibrium despite the use of mannitol and sodium modeling. While certainly heparin-free dialysis using saline flushes and blood flows greater than 200 cc/min can be utilized to minimize the risk of bleeding, and biocompatible membranes can be employed to avoid activation of complement and white cells that might exacerbate acute ischemic injury, what has become clear is that the major risk of hemodialysis in the setting of acute fulminant hepatic failure is the increase in intracranial pressure (Figs. 35.1 and 35.2) that can precipitate brainstem herniation (184). Marked rises in intracranial pressure may occur during hemodialysis in patients with acute liver failure and are often observed within the first hour as compared to dialysis disequilibrium, where cerebral edema tends to develop toward the end of the hemodialysis procedure due to rapid osmotic shifts (184).

In contrast, the newer continuous forms of renal replacement therapy such as continuous arterial venous hemofiltration (CAVH) and continuous veno-venous hemofiltration (CVVH) provide greater cardiovascular and intracranial stability, thereby decreasing the risk of hemodynamic and neurologic sequelae. Continuous renal replacement therapies enable removal of large amounts of fluid, maintenance of metabolic balance and solute clearance, and adequate nutritional support even in patients on pressor support (185). The disadvantage of CAVH is that it requires arterial access and anticoagulation to avoid clotting of the filter. This frequently presents problems in patients with liver disease and an underlying coagulopathy. CVVH, on the other hand, is performed utilizing veno-venous access but does require a blood pump and close nursing supervision (185).

Standard replacement solutions for CVVH contain lactate as the buffer. Unfortunately, in hepatic failure the liver may not be able to metabolize the lactate to bicarbonate, leading to marked elevations in the serum lactate level. At the same time, bicarbonate may be lost into the ultrafiltrate, exacerbating the metabolic acidosis.

Citrate has been utilized as a buffer in CVVH to replace lactate and also as a replacement for heparin anticoagulation. When citrate is used as a regional anticoagulant, this requires a calcium-free replacement solution and a separate calcium infusion post filter to avoid hypocalcemia in the patient (185). While the citrate solutions have been effectively utilized in patients with acute renal failure requiring CVVH who are at high risk for bleeding, citrate may pose

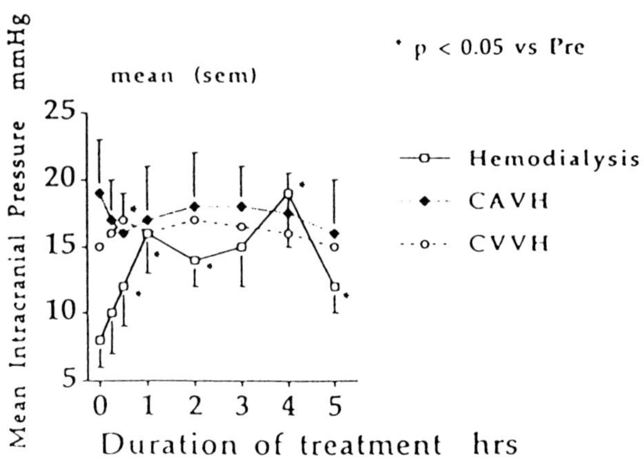

FIGURE 35.1. *The effect of treatment with intermittent hemodialysis (HD), continuous arteriovenous hemofiltration (CAVH), and continuous pumped veno-venous hemofiltration (CVVH) on the mean intracranial pressure in a group of patients with acute liver failure. (Reproduced with permission from Davenport A. Management of established renal failure in patients with liver failure. Semin Dial 1996;9:167.)*

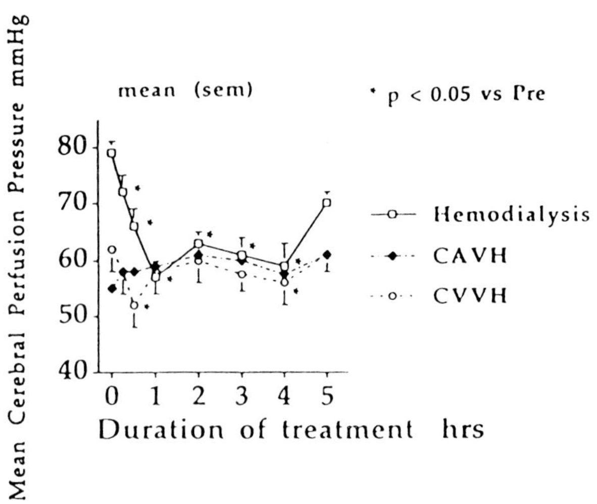

FIGURE 35.2. *The effect of treatment with intermittent hemodialysis (HD), continuous arteriovenous hemofiltration (CAVH), and continuous pumped veno-venous hemofiltration (CVVH) on the mean cerebral perfusion pressure (the difference between the mean arterial blood pressure measured at the level of the carotid syphon and the mean intracranial pressure) in a group of patients with acute liver failure. (Reproduced with permission from Davenport A. Management of established renal failure in patients with liver failure. Semin Dial 1996;9:168.)*

Table 35.8. Adjustment of Drug Dosages

Drug	Dosage for Normal Renal Function	Adjustment for Renal Failure GFR (mL/min)			Supplement for Dialysis
		>50	10–50	<10	
Amikacin	5 mg/kg q8h	70–100% q8–12h	30–70% q12h	20–30% q24–48h	Hemo: 2/3 normal dose after dialysis CAPD: 30% q24h CAVH: Dose for GFR 10–50 mL/min
Gentamicin	1 mg/kg q8h	70–100% q8–12h	30–70% q12h	20–30% q24–48h	Hemo: 2/3 normal dose after dialysis CAPD: 30% q24h CAVH: Dose for GFR 10–50 mL/min
Tobramycin	1 mg/kg q8h	70–100% q8–12h	30–70% q12h	20–30% q24–48h	Hemo: 2/3 normal dose after dialysis CAPD: 30% q24h CAVH: Dose for GFR 10–50 mL/min
Cefaclor	250 mg tid	100%	50–100%	50%	Hemo: Dose after dialysis CAPD: 250 mg q8–12h CAVH: Unknown
Cefazolin	0.5–1.5 g q6h	q6–8h	q12h	q24–48h	Hemo: Dose after dialysis CAPD: None CAVH: None
Cefotaxime	1 g q6h	q6h	q8–12h	q24h	Hemo: 1 g after dialysis CAPD: None CAVH: None
Cefoxitin	1–2 g q6–8h	q6–8h	q8–12h	q24–48h	Hemo: 1 g after dialysis CAPD: Dose for GFR 10–50 mL/min CAVH: Dose for GFR 10–50 mL/min
Ceftazidime	1 g q8–12h	q8–12h	q24–48h	q48–72h	Hemo: 1 g after dialysis CAPD: Dose for GFR 10–50 mL/min CAVH: Dose for GFR 10–50 mL/min
Ceftriaxone	1 g q12h	100%	100%	100%	Hemo: None CAPD: None CAVH: None
Cefuroxime	0.75–1.5 g q8h	q8h	q8–12h	q24h	Hemo: Dose after dialysis CAPD: None CAVH: Likely to be removed; dose for GFR 10–50 mL/min
Cephalexin	250–500 mg q6h	q6h	q6h	q8–12h	Hemo: 250 mg after dialysis CAPD: Dose for GFR 10–50 mL/min CAVH: Dose for GFR 10–50 mL/min
Cephalothin	0.5–2.0 g q6h	q6h	q6–8h	q12h	Hemo: Dose after dialysis CAPD: Dose for GFR 10–50 mL/min CAVH: Dose for GFR 10–50 mL/min
Clarithromycin	250–500 mg bid	100%	50–100%	50%	Hemo: Unlikely CAPD: Unlikely CAVH: Unlikely
Erythromycin	250–500 mg q6–12h	100%	100%	50–75%	Hemo: None CAPD: None CAVH: Unlikely
Amoxicillin	500 mg q8h	q8h	q8–12h	q12h	Hemo: Dose after dialysis CAPD: Dose for GFR 10–50 mL/min CAVH: Dose for GFR 10–50 mL/min
Azlocillin	2–3 g q4h	q4–6h	q6–8h	q6–8h	Hemo: Dose after dialysis CAPD: Dose for GFR <10 mL/min CAVH: Dose for GFR 10–50 mL/min
Dicloxacillin	250–500 mg q6h	100%	100%	100%	Hemo: None CAPD: None CAVH: None

Table 35.8. *Continued*

Drug	Dosage for Normal Renal Function	Adjustment for Renal Failure GFR (mL/min) >50	10–50	<10	Supplement for Dialysis
Methicillin	1–2 g q4h	q4–6h	q6–8h	q8–12h	Hemo: None CAPD: None CAVH: None
Mezlocillin	1.5–4.0 g q4–6h	q4–6h	q6–8h	q8h	Hemo: None CAPD: None CAVH: None
Nafcillin	1–2 g q4–6h	100%	100%	100%	Hemo: None CAPD: None CAVH: None
Penicillin G Potassium: 1.7 mEq/million U	0.5–4.0 million U q6h	100%	75%	25–50%	Hemo: Dose after dialysis CAPD: Dose for GFR <10 mL/min CAVH: Dose for GFR <10 mL/min
Piperacillin	3–4 g q4h	q4–6h	q6–8h	q8h	Hemo: Dose after dialysis CAPD: Dose for GFR <10 mL/min CAVH: Dose for GFR <10 mL/min
Ticarcillin Sodium: 5.2 mEq/g	3 g q4h	1–3 g q4h	1–2 g q8h	1 g q12h	Hemo: 3 g after dialysis CAPD: Dose for GFR <10 mL/min CAVH: Dose for GFR <10 mL/min
Ciprofloxacin	500–750 mg q12h	100%	50%	33%	Hemo: 250 mg CAPD: Dose for GFR 10–50 mL/min CAVH: Dose for GFR 10–50 mL/min
Norfloxacin	400 mg q12h	q12h	q12–24h	q24h	Hemo: None CAPD: Unlikely CAVH: Unlikely
Ofloxacin	400 mg/day	100%	50%	25%	Hemo: Dose after dialysis CAPD: None CAVH: Likely to be removed; dose for GFR 10–50 mL/min
Doxycycline	100–200 mg/day	100%	100%	100%	Hemo: None CAPD: None CAVH: Unlikely
Minocycline	100 mg q12h	100%	100%	100%	Hemo: None CAPD: None CAVH: Unlikely
Tetracycline	250–500 mg qid	q6–8h	q12–24h	Avoid	Hemo: None CAPD: Unlikely CAVH: Unlikely
Aztreonam	1–2 g q8–12h	100%	50–75%	25%	Hemo: 0.5 g after dialysis CAPD: Dose for GFR <10 mL/min CAVH: Dose for GFR 10–50 mL/min
Chloramphenicol	12.5 mg/kg q6h	100%	100%	100%	Hemo: None CAPD: Unlikely CAVH: Unlikely
Clindamycin	150–300 mg q6h	100%	100%	100%	Hemo: None CAPD: Unlikely CAVH: Unlikely
Imipenem	0.25–1.0 g q6h	100%	50%	25%	Hemo: Dose after dialysis CAPD: None CAVH: Dose for GFR 10–50 mL/min
Metronidazole	7.5 mg/kg q6h	100%	100%	50%	Hemo: Dose after dialysis CAPD: None CAVH: Likely to be removed; dose for GFR 10–50 mL/min

Table 35.8. *Continued*

Drug	Dosage for Normal Renal Function	Adjustment for Renal Failure GFR (mL/min)			Supplement for Dialysis
		>50	10–50	<10	
Teicoplanin	6 mg/kg/day	q24h	q48h	q72h	Hemo: None CAPD: None CAVH: None
Trimethoprimsulfamethoxazole	160 mg trimethoprim and 800 mg sulfamethoxazole q12h	100% q12h	100% q12–24 h	50% q24h	Hemo: 1/2 dose after dialysis CAPD: None CAVH: Likely to be removed; dose for GFR 10–50 mL/min
Vancomycin Monitor serum levels	1 g q12h	q12–24h	q2–7 days	q7–10 days	Hemo: Conventional—none; permeable membranes—dose for GFR 10–50 mL/min CAPD: Dose for GFR 10–50 mL/min CAVH: Dose for GFR 10–50 mL/min
Amphotericin B	0.3–0.5 mg/kg/day	100%	100%	100%	Hemo: None CAPD: Unlikely CAVH: Unlikely
Fluconazole	50–200 mg/day	100%	50%	25%	Hemo: Dose after dialysis CAPD: Dose for GFR <10 mL/min CAVH: Dose for GFR <10 mL/min
Flucytosine	150 mg/kg/day in 3–4 divided doses	25–50 mg/kg q12–24h	25–50 mg/kg q12–24h	50 mg/kg q24–48h	Hemo: Dose after dialysis CAPD: Dose for GFR 10–50 mL/min CAVH: Dose for GFR 10–50 mL/min
Itraconazole	100–200 mg q12h	100%	100%	100%	Hemo: None CAPD: None CAVH: Unlikely
Ketoconazole	200–400 mg/day	100%	100%	100%	Hemo: None CAPD: Unlikely CAVH: Unlikely
Chloroquine	1.5 g over 3 days	100%	100%	50%	Hemo: None CAPD: None CAVH: Unlikely
Pentamidine	4 mg/kg/day	q24h	q24–36h	q48h	Hemo: Unlikely CAPD: Unlikely CAVH: Unlikely
Praziquantel	Dose varies	100%	100%	100%	Hemo: None CAPD: Unlikely CAVH: Unlikely
Pyrimethamine	50–75 mg/day	100%	100%	100%	Hemo: Unknown CAPD: Unknown CAVH: Unknown
Quinine	10 mg/kg q8h	q8h	q8–12h	q24h	Hemo: Unlikely CAPD: None CAVH: Unlikely
Thiabendazole	Dose varies depending on infecting parasite	100%	50–100%	Avoid	Hemo: Unknown CAPD: Unknown CAVH: Unknown
Ethambutol	15 mg/kg q24h	100%	50–100%	25–50%	Hemo: Dose after dialysis CAPD: Dose for GFR 10–50 mL/min CAVH: Dose for GFR 10–50 mL/min
Isoniazid	5 mg/kg q24h	100%	75–100%	50%	Hemo: Dose after dialysis CAPD: Dose for GFR 10–50 mL/min CAVH: Dose for GFR 10–50 mL/min

Table 35.8. *Continued*

Drug	Dosage for Normal Renal Function	Adjustment for Renal Failure GFR (mL/min)			Supplement for Dialysis
		>50	10–50	<10	
Rifampin	600 mg q24h	100%	100%	100%	Hemo: None CAPD: None CAVH: None
Acyclovir	5 mg/kg q8h	5 mg/kg q8–12h	5 mg/kg q12–24h	2.5 mg/kg q24h	Hemo: Dose after dialysis CAPD: Same as for GFR <10 mL/min CAVH: 3.5 mg/kg/day
Amantadine	100 mg q12h	q12–24h	q48–72h	q16–8h	Hemo: None CAPD: Unlikely CAVH: Unlikely
Foscarnet Nephrotoxicity common	60–100 mg/kg q8–12h	50–100%	10–50%	Avoid	Hemo: Dose after dialysis CAPD: Unknown CAVH: Likely to be removed; dose for GFR 10–50 mL/min
Ganciclovir	2.5 mg/kg q8h	q8–12h	q24h	q48–96h	Hemo: Dose after dialysis CAPD: Unknown CAVH: 3.5 mg/kg/day
Ribavirin	200 mg q8h	100%	100%	50%	Hemo: None CAPD: Unlikely CAVH: Unlikely
Zidovudine (AZT)	200 mg q4h	100%	100%	50%	Hemo: Dose after dialysis CAPD: None CAVH: Likely to be removed; dose for GFR 10–50 mL/min
Quinidine	200–400 mg q4–6h	—	100%	75%	Hemo: None CAPD: None CAVH: Unlikely
Tocainide	400–600 mg q8h	—	100%	50%	Hemo: 200 mg CAPD: None CAVH: Unknown
Esmolol	50–150 μg/kg/min infusion	—	100%	100%	Hemo: None CAPD: None CAVH: Unknown
Labetalol	200–600 mg bid	—	100%	100%	Hemo: None CAPD: None CAVH: Unknown
Metoprolol	50–100 mg bid	—	100%	100%	Hemo: Dose after dialysis CAPD: Unknown CAVH: Likely to be removed; dose for GFR 10–50 mL/min
Nadolol	80–320 mg/day	—	50%	25%	Hemo: 40 mg CAPD: None CAVH: Likely to be removed; dose for GFR 10–50 mL/min
Pindolol	10–40 mg bid	—	100%	100%	Hemo: Unlikely CAPD: Unlikely CAVH: Unlikely
Propranolol	80–160 mg bid	—	100%	100%	Hemo: None CAPD: Unlikely CAVH: Unlikely
Sotalol	160–480 mg/day	—	30%	15–30%	Hemo: Dose after dialysis CAPD: None CAVH: Likely to be removed; dose for GFR 10–50 mL/min

Table 35.8. *Continued*

Drug	Dosage for Normal Renal Function	Adjustment for Renal Failure GFR (mL/min) >50	10–50	<10	Supplement for Dialysis
Timolol	10–20 mg bid	—	100%	100%	Hemo: None CAPD: None CAVH: Unlikely
Amlodipine	10 mg qd	—	100%	100%	Hemo: None CAPD: Unlikely CAVH: Unlikely
Diltiazem	30–90 mg q8h	—	100%	100%	Hemo: None CAPD: Unlikely CAVH: Unlikely
Felodipine	10 mg bid	—	100%	100%	Hemo: None CAPD: Unlikely CAVH: Unlikely
Nifedipine Nifedipine XL	10–30 mg q8h (XL: 30–120 mg qd)	—	100%	100%	Hemo: None CAPD: Unlikely CAVH: Unlikely
Verapamil Verapamil SR	80 mg q8h (SR: 180 mg qd–240 mg q12h)	—	100%	100%	Hemo: None CAPD: Unlikely CAVH: Unlikely
Digitoxin	0.1–0.2 mg/day	—	100%	100%	Hemo: None CAPD: None CAVH: None
Digoxin	1.0–1.5 mg load 0.25–0.5 mg/day	—	25–75% q24h	10–25% q48h	Hemo: None CAPD: None CAVH: Unlikely
Furosemide	40–80 mg bid	—	100%	100%	Hemo: None CAPD: None CAVH: NA
Omeprazole	20–40 mg/day	100%	100%	100%	Hemo: None CAPD: Unlikely CAVH: Unlikely
Sucralfate	1 g qid	50–100%	Avoid (contains aluminum)	Avoid (contains aluminum)	Avoid
Carbamazepine	200–1200 mg/day	—	100%	100%	Hemo: None CAPD: Unlikely CAVH: Unlikely
Phenytoin Protein binding decreased and distribution volume increased in renal failure; monitor free dilantin levels	1000 mg load, then 300–400 mg/day	—	100%	100%	Hemo: None CAPD: None CAVH: Unlikely

Source: Adapted from Swan SK, Bennett WM. Use of drugs in patients with renal failure. In: Schrier RW, Gottschalk CW, eds. Diseases of the kidney. Vol. III. 6th ed. Boston: Little, Brown, 1997: 2968.

problems in patients with liver failure who again may not be able to metabolize citrate to bicarbonate. Solutions containing sodium bicarbonate as the buffer are clearly the replacement fluids of choice. These are not commercially available in the United States at present, however, and must be individually prepared (184).

One factor in the treatment of all patients with renal failure requiring renal replacement therapies is the adjustment of drug dosages. Table 35.8 can be used to help estimate dosages of some frequently used classes of drugs according to each individual's degree of renal failure.

REFERENCES

1. Thadhani R, Pascual M, Bonventre J. Acute renal failure. N Engl J Med 1996;334:1448–1460.
2. Hricik DE, Browning PJ, Kopelman R, et al. Captopril-induced functional renal insufficiency in patients with bilateral renal artery stenosis or renal artery stenosis in a solitary kidney. N Engl J Med 1983;308:373–376.
3. Sawyer MH, Webb DE, Balow JE, Straus SE. Acyclovir-induced renal failure: clinical course and histology. Am J Med 1977;84:1067–1071.
4. Kjellstrand CM, Campbell DC, von Hartikch B, et al. Hyperuricemic acute renal failure. Arch Intern Med 1974;133:349–359.
5. Hande KR, Garrow GC. Acute tumor lysis syndrome in patients with high-grade non–Hodgkin's lymphoma. Am J Med 1993;94:133–138.
6. Troppman C, Gillingham KJ, Benedetti E, et al. Delayed graft function, acute rejection and outcome after cadaveric renal transplantation. Transplantation 1995;59:962–968.
7. Halloran PF, Aprile MA, Farrell V, et al. Early function as the principal correlate of graft survival. Transplantation 1988;46:223–228.
8. Goes N, Urmson J, Ramassar V, Halloran PF. Ischemic acute tubular necrosis induces an extensive local cytokine response: evidence for induction of interferon-gamma, transforming growth factor-beta 1, granulocyte-macrophage colony-stimulating factor, interleukin-2, and interleukin-10. Transplantation 1995;59:565–572.
9. Granger DN, Korthuis RJ. Physiologic mechanism of postischemic tissue injury. Ann Rev Physiol 1995;57:311–332.
10. Kelly KJ, Williams WW, Colvin RB, Bonventre JV. Antibody to intracellular adhesion molecule 1 protects the kidney against ischemic injury. Proc Natl Acad Sci USA 1994;91:812–816.
11. Kelly KJ, Williams WW, Colvin RB, et al. Intracellular adhesion molecule 1 deficit mice are protected against ischemic injury. J Clin Invest 1996;97:1056–1063.
12. Haug CE, Colvin RB, Delmonico FL, et al. A phase I trial of immunosuppression with anti-ICAM (CD54) mAb in renal allograft recipients. Transplantation 1993;55:766–772.
13. Norman DJ. Antilymphocyte antibodies in the treatment of allograft rejection: targets, mechanisms of action, monitoring and efficacy. Semin Nephrol 1992;12:315–324.
14. Grino JM. BN52021—a platelet activating factor antagonist for preventing post transplant renal failure: a double-blind randomized study. Ann Intern Med 1994;121:345–347.
15. Kelly KJ, Tolkoff-Rubin NE, Rubin RH, et al. An oral platelet-activating factor antagonist, Ro-24-4736, protects the rat kidney from ischemic injury. Am J Physiol 1996;271 (Renal Fluid and Electrolyte Physiology 40): F1061–F1067.
16. Shaw SG, Weidmann P, Hodler J, et al. Atrial natriuretic factor peptide protects against acute ischemic renal failure in the rat. J Clin Invest 1987;80:1232–1237.
17. Rahman SW, Kim GE, Mathews AS, et al. Effects of atrial natriuretic peptide in clinical acute renal failure. Kidney Int 1994;45:1731–1738.
18. Sands JM, Neylan JF, Olson RA, et al. Atrial natriuretic factor does not improve the outcome of cadaver renal transplantation. J Am Soc Nephrol 1991;I:1081–1084.
19. Allgren RL, Marbury TC, Rahman SN, et al. Anaritide in acute tubular necrosis. N Engl J Med 1997;336:828–834.
20. Humes HD. Acute renal failure: the promise of new therapies. N Engl J Med 1997;336:870–871.
21. Dubose TD, Warnock DG, Melita RL, et al. Acute renal failure in the 21st century: recommendations for management and outcomes assessment. Am J Kidney Dis 1977;29(5):793–799.
22. Myers BD. Cyclosporine nephrotoxicity. Kidney Int 1986;30:964–974.
23. Platz K-P, Mueller AR, Blumhardt G, et al. Nephrotoxicity following orthotopic liver transplantation. Transplantation 1994;58(2):170–178.
24. Porayko MK, Textor SC, Krom RA, et al. Nephrotoxic effects of primary immunosuppression with FK506 and cyclosporine regimens after liver transplantation. Mayo Clin Proc 1994;69(2):105–111.
25. Myers BD, Ross J, Newton L, et al. Cyclosporine associated chronic nephropathy. N Engl J Med 1984;311:699–705.
26. Textor SC, Wiesner R, Wilson DJ, et al. Systemic and renal hemodynamic differences between FK506 and cyclosporine in liver transplant recipients. Transplantation 1993;55:1332–1339.
27. Trimarchi HM, Truong LD, Brennam S, et al. FK506-associated thrombotic microangiopathy: report of two cases and review of the literature. Transplantation 1998;67:539–544.
28. Group TUMFLS. A comparison of Tacrolimus (FK506) and cyclosporine for immunosuppression in liver transplantation. N Engl J Med 1994;331(17):1110–1115.
29. Randhawa PS, Shapiro R, Jordan ML, et al. The histopathological changes associated with allograft rejection and drug toxicity in renal transplant recipients maintained on FK506. Am J Surg 1993;17:60–68.
30. Remuzzi G, Perico N. Cyclosporine-induced renal dysfunction in experimental animals and humans. Kidney Int 1995;52:S70–S74.
31. Lanese DM, Conger JD. Effects of endothelin receptor antagonist on cyclosporine-induced vasoconstriction in isolated rat renal arterioles. J Clin Invest 1993;91:2144–2149.
32. Kopp JB, Klotman PE. Cellular and molecular mechanisms of cyclosporine nephrotoxicity. J Am Soc Nephrol 1990;1:162–179.
33. Simonson MS, Dunn MJ. The molecular mechanisms of cardiovascular and renal regulation by endothelin peptides. J Lab Clin Med 1992;119(6):622–639.
34. Scherrer U, Vissing SF, Morgan BJ, et al. Cyclosporine-induced sympathetic activation and hypertension after heart transplantation. N Engl J Med 1990;323:693–699.
35. Curtis JJ, Luke RG, Dubrovsky E, et al. Cyclosporine in therapeutic doses increases renal allograft vascular resistance. Lancet 1986;2:477–479.
36. Epstein M. Calcium antagonists and renal protection. Current and future perspectives. Arch Intern Med 1992;152:1573–1584.
37. English J, Evan A, Houghton DC, Bennett WM. Cyclosporine-induced acute renal dysfunction in the rat. Transplantation 1987;44:135.
38. Loutzenhiser R, Epstein M, Horton C, Sonke P. Reversal of renal and smooth muscle actions of the thromboxane mimetic U-44069 by diltiazem. Am J Physiol 1986;250:F619–F626.
39. Kon V, Sugiura M, Inagami T, et al. Role of endothelin in cyclosporine induced glomerular dysfunction. Kidney Int 1990;37:1487–1491.
40. Hall BM, Tiller DJ, Duggin GG, et al. Post transplant acute renal failure in cadaver renal recipients treated with cyclosporine. Kidney Int 1985;28:178–186.
41. Group CMT. A randomized clinical trial of cyclosporine in cadaveric renal transplantation. N Engl J Med 1983;309:809–815.
42. Group EMT. Cyclosporine in cadaveric renal transplantation: one-year follow-up of a multicenter trial. Lancet 1983;2:986–989.
43. Copeland JG, Emery RW, Levinson MM, et al. Cyclosporine: an immunosuppressive panacea? J Thorac Cardiovasc Surg 1986;91:26–39.
44. Shulman H, Striker G, Deeg HJ, et al. Nephrotoxicity of cyclosporin A after allogeneic marrow transplantation. N Engl J Med 1981;305:1392–1395.
45. Lewis RM. Long-term use of cyclosporine A does not adversely impact on clinical outcomes following renal transplantation. Kidney Int 1995;S52:S75–S78.
46. Almond PS, Gillingham KJ, Sibley R, et al. Renal transplant function after ten years of cyclosporine. Transplantation 1992;53:316–323.
47. Goldstein DJ, Zuech N, Sehgal V, et al. Cyclosporine-associated end stage nephropathy after cardiac transplantation: incidence and progression. Transplantation 1997;63:664–668.
48. Halloran P, Mathew T, Tomlamovich S, et al. Mycophenolate mofetil in renal allograft recipients. Transplantation 1997;63:39–47.
49. Walfe JA, McCann RL, Sanfilippo F. Cyclosporine-associated microangiopathy on renal transplantation: a severe but potentially reversible form of early graft injury. Transplantation 1986;41:541.
50. Bennett WM, Porter GA. Cyclosporine-associated hypertension. Am J Med 1988;85:131–133.
51. First MR. An update on new immunosuppressive drugs undergoing preclinical and clinical trials: potential applications in organ transplantation. Am J Kidney Dis 1997;29:303–317.

52. Kamel KS, Ethier JH, Quaggin S, et al. Studies to determine the basis for hyperkalemia in recipients of a renal transplant who are treated with cyclosporine. J Am Soc Nephrol 1991;2:1279–1284.
53. West C, Carpenter BJ, Kakala TR. The incidence of gout in renal transplant recipients. Am J Kidney Dis 1987;10:369–322.
54. Noordzij TC, Leunissen KM, Van Hooff JP. Renal handling of urate and the incidence of gouty arthritis during cyclosporine and diuretic use. Transplantation 1991;52:64–67.
55. Lin HY, Rocher LL, McQuillan MA, et al. Cyclosporine-induced hyperuricemia and gout. N Engl J Med 1989;321:287–292.
56. Lake KD. Drug interactions in transplant patients. In: Emery RW, Miller LW, eds. Handbook of cardiac transplantation. Philadelphia: Hanley & Belfus, 1995.
57. Ducharme MP, Provenzano R, Dehoorne-Smith M, Edwards DJ. Trough concentrations of cyclosporine in blood following administration of grapefruit juice. Brit J Clin Pharmacol 1993;36:457–459.
58. Ballantyne CM, Radovancevic B, Farmer JA, et al. Hyperlipidemia after heart transplantation: report of a 6-year experience, with treatment recommendations. J Am Col Cardiol 1992;19:1315–1321.
59. Reaven P, Witztum JL. Lovastatin, nicotinic acid, and rhabdomyolysis. Ann Intern Med 1988;109:579–598.
60. Marais GE, Larson KK. Rhabdomyolysis and acute renal failure induced by combination lovastatin and gemfibrozil therapy. Ann Intern Med 1990;112:228–230.
61. Pierce LR, Wysowski DK, Gross TP. Myopathy and rhabdomyolysis associated with lovastatin–gemfibrozil combination therapy. J Am Med Assoc 1990;264:71–75.
62. Cheung AK, DeVault GA, Gregory MC. A prospective study of treatment of hypercholesterolemia with lovastatin in renal transplant patients receiving cyclosporine. J Am Soc Nephrol 1993;3(12):1484–1491.
63. Kobashigawa JA, Murphy FL, Stevenson LW, et al. Low-dose lovastatin lowers cholesterol after cardiac transplantation. Circulation 1990;82:281–283.
64. Rudnick MR, Goldfarb S, Wexler L, et al. for the Iohexol Cooperative Study. Nephrotoxicity of ionic and nonionic contrast media in 1196 patients: a randomized trial. Kidney Int 1995;47:254–261.
65. Solomon R, Werner C, Mann D, et al. Effects of saline, mannitol and furosemide on acute decreases in renal function induced by radiocontrast agents. N Engl J Med 1994;1331:1416–1420.
66. Cameron JS. Allergic interstitial nephritis: clinical features and pathogenesis. QJM 1988;66:97–115.
67. Galpin JE, Shinberger JH, Stanley TM, et al. Acute interstitial nephritis due to methicillin. Am J Med 1978;65:756–765.
68. Cameron JS. Recurrent primary disease and de novo nephritis following renal transplantation. Pediatr Nephrol 1991;5:412–421.
69. Dantal J, Giral M, Hoormant K, Soulillou JP. Glomerulonephritis recurrences after kidney transplantation. Curr Opin Nephrol Hypertens 1995;4(2): 146–154.
70. Cameron JS. Recurrent disease in renal allografts. Kidney Int 1993;44: S91–S94.
71. Ramos EL, Tisher CC. Recurrent diseases in the kidney transplant. Am J Kidney Dis 1994;24(1):142–154.
72. Haviharan S, Peddi VR, Savin VJ, et al. Recurrent and de novo renal diseases after renal transplantation: a report from the renal allograft disease registry. Am J Kidney Dis 1998;31:928–931.
73. Kotanko P, Pusey CD, Levy JB. Recurrent glomerulonephritis following renal transplantation. Transplantation 1997;63:1045–1052.
74. Schwarz A, Kraus PH, Offerman G, Keller F. Recurrent and de novo renal disease after kidney transplantation with or without cyclosporine A. Am J Kidney Dis 1991;17:524–531.
75. Cheigh JS, Mourandian J, Susin M, et al. Kidney transplant nephrotic syndrome: relationship between allograft histopathology and natural course. Kidney Int 1980;18:358–365.
76. Habib R, Broyer M. Clinical significance of allograft glomerulopathy. Kidney Int 1993;44(43):S95–S98.
77. Stephanian E, Matas AJ, Mauer SM, et al. Recurrence of disease in patients retransplanted for focal segmental glomerulosclerosis. Transplantation 1992;53(4):755–757.
78. Artero M, Biava C, Amend W, et al. Recurrent focal glomerulosclerosis: natural history and response to therapy. Am J Med 1992;92:375–383.
79. Senaqutuvan P, Cameron JS, Hartley BB, et al. Recurrence of focal sequential glomerulosclerosis in transplanted kidneys: analysis of incidence and risks factors in 59 allografts. Pediatr Nephrol 1990;4:21–30.
80. Tgani A, Stablein DH. Recurrence of focal sequential glomerulosclerosis post transplantation: a special report of the North American Pediatric Renal Transplant Cooperative Study. J Am Soc Nephrol 1992;2(suppl):S258–S265.
81. Odorico JS, Knechtle SJ, Rayhill SC, et al. The influence of native nephrectomy on the incidence of recurrent disease following renal transplantation for primary glomerulonephritis. Transplantation 1996;61(2):228–234.
82. Artero ML, Sharma R, Savin VJ, Vincent F. Plasmapheresis reduces proteinuria and serving capacity to injure glomeruli in patients with recurrent focal sequential glomerulosclerosis. Am J Kidney Dis 1994;23:574–585.
83. Dantal J, Bigo T, Bogers W, et al. Effect of protein adsorption on protein excretion in kidney transplant recipients with nephrotic syndrome. N Engl J Med 1994;330:7–12.
84. Dantal J, Baatard R, Hourmant M, et al. Recurrent nephrotic syndrome following renal transplantation in patients with focal glomerulosclerosis: a one center study of plasma exchange effects. Transplantation 1991;52:827–831.
85. Savin VJ, Sharma R, Sharma R, et al. Circulating factor associated with increased glomerular permeability to albumin in recurrent focal sequential glomerulosclerosis. N Engl J Med 1996;334(14):878–883.
86. Odum J, Peh CA, Clarkson AR, et al. Recurrent mesangial IgA nephritis following renal transplantation. Nephrol Dial Transplant 1994;9(3):309–312.
87. Bachman U, Biava C, Amend W, et al. The clinical course of IgA-nephropathy and Henoch-Schönlein purpura following renal transplantation. Transplantation 1986;42(5):511–515.
88. Berger J. Recurrence of IgA nephropathy in renal allografts. Am J Kidney Dis 1988;12:371–372.
89. Brensilver JM, Mallat S, Scholes J, McCabe R. Recurrent IgA nephropathy in living related donor transplantation: recurrence or transmission of familial disease? Am J Kidney Dis 1988;12:147–151.
90. Glicklich D, Mata AJ, Sablay LB, et al. Recurrent membranoproliferative glomerulonephritis type I in successive renal transplants. Am J Nephrol 1987;7:143–149.
91. Droz D, Nabarra B, Noel LH, et al. Recurrence of dense deposits in transplanted kidneys: I. Sequential survey of lesions. Kidney Int 1979;15:386–395.
92. Eddy A, Sibley R, Mauer SM, Kim Y. Renal allograft failure due to recurrent dense intramembranous deposit disease. Clin Nephrol 1984;21:305–313.
93. Montagnino G, Colturi C, Banfi G. Membranous nephropathy in cyclosporine treated renal transplant recipients. Transplantation 1989;47:725–727.
94. Rubin RJ, Barnes BA, Harrington JT. Recurrent idiopathic membranous glomerulonephritis. Transplantation 1977;24:4–9.
95. Couchoud C, Pouteil-Noble C, Colon S, et al. Recurrence of membranous nephropathy after renal transplantation: incidence and risk factors in 1614 patients. Transplantation 1995;59:1275.
96. Berger BE, Vincenti F, Biava C, et al. De novo and recurrent membranous glomerulopathy following kidney transplantation. Transplantation 1983;35:315–319.
97. Heidet L, Gagnadoux ME, Beziau A, et al. Recurrence of de novo membranous glomerulonephritis in renal grafts. Clin Nephrol 1994;41:314.
98. Schwartz A, Krause PH, Offerman G, et al. Impact of de novo membranous glomerulonephritis on the clinical course after kidney transplantation. Transplantation 1994;58:650.
99. Agarwal SK, Dash SC, Mehta SN, Bhuyan UN. Recurrence of idiopathic membranous nephropathy in HLA-identical allograft. Nephron 1992;60:366.
100. Chevrier D, Giral M, Braud V, et al. Membranous nephropathy and a TAP 1 gene polymorphism. N Engl J Med 1994;331:133–137.
101. Garcia RO, Espinoza RS, Silva GR, et al. Recurrent membranous glomerulonephritis in an HLA-identical allograft. Nephrol Dial Transplant 1991;20(6):647–649.
102. Najarian JS, Kaufman DB, Fryd DS, et al. Long-term survival of kidney transplantation in 100 type 1 diabetic patients. Transplantation 1990;47:106–113.
103. Aztz R, Brenner BM. Pathogenesis of diabetic microangiopathy: the hemodynamic view. Am J Med 1986;80:443–453.
104. Wilczek HE, Jaremko G, Tyden G, Groth CG. Evolution of diabetic nephropathy in kidney grafts. Evidence that a simultaneously transplanted pancreas exerts a protective effect. Transplantation 1995;59:51–57.
105. Abouna GM, Kremer GD, Daddah SK, et al. Reversal of diabetic nephropathy in human cadaver kidneys after transplantation into nondiabetic recipients. Lancet 1983;2:1274–1276.
106. Fioretto P, Mauer SM, Bilous RW, et al. Effects of pancreas transplantation on glomerular structure in insulin-dependent diabetic patients with their own kidneys. Lancet 1993;342:1193–1196.
107. The Diabetes Control and Complications Trial Research Group. The effect of intensive treatment of diabetes on the development and progression of long

term complications in insulin-dependent diabetes mellitus. N Engl J Med 1993;329:977–986.

108. Hasegawa A, Kawamura T, Ito H, et al. Fate of renal grafts with recurrent Henoch-Schönlein purpura nephritis in children. Transplant Proc 1989;21:2130–2133.
109. Meulders Q, Pirson Y, Cosyns J-P, et al. Course of Henoch-Schönlein nephritis after renal transplantation. Transplantation 1994;58(11):1186–1197.
110. Nast CC, Ward HJ, Koyle MA, Cohen AH. Recurrent Henoch-Schönlein purpura following renal transplantation. Am J Kidney Dis 1987;9:39–43.
111. Agerwal A, Mauer SM, Matas AJ, Nath KA. Recurrent hemolytic uremic syndrome in an adult renal allograft recipient: current concepts and management. J Am Soc Nephrol 1995;6:1160–1169.
112. Bonsib SM, Ercolani L, Ngheim D, Hamilton HE. Recurrent thrombotic microangiopathy in a renal allograft. Am Med J 1985;79:520–527.
113. Eijgenraam FJ, Donckerwolker RA, Monnens LAH, et al. Renal transplantation in 20 children with hemolytic-uremic syndrome. Clin Nephrol 1990;33:87–93.
114. Van den Berg-Wolf MG, Kootte AMM, Weening JJ, Paul LC. Recurrent hemolytic uremic syndrome in a renal transplant recipient and review of the Leiden experience. Transplantation 1988;45:248–251.
115. Hebert D, Kim EM, Silbley RK, Mauer SM. Post transplantation outcome of patients with hemolytic uremic syndrome: update. Pediatr Nephrol 1991;5:162–167.
116. Remuzzi G, Bertani T. Renal vascular and thrombocytopathic effects of cyclosporine. Am J Kidney Dis 1989;18:261–272.
117. Hebert D, Sibley RK, Mauer SM. Recurrence of hemolytic uremic syndrome in renal transplant recipients. Kidney Int 1986;30:S51–S58.
118. McCauley J, Shapiro R, Bronster O, et al. Renal transplantation under FK506 in patients with previous loss of renal function due to hemolytic uremic syndrome. Transplant Proc 1991;23:3068–3070.
119. Gross JA, Cole BR, Jendrisak MD, et al. Renal transplantation for systemic lupus erythematosus and recurrent lupus nephritis: a single center experience and review of the literature. Transplantation 1991;52:805–809.
120. Baumgardner GL, Mauer SM, Payne W, et al. Single-center 1–15-year results of renal transplantation in patients with systemic lupus erythematosus. Transplantation 1988;46:703–709.
121. Nossent HC, Swaak TJC, Berden JH, and the Dutch Working Party on Systemic Lupus Erythematosus. Systemic lupus erythematosus after renal transplantation: patient and graft survival and disease activity. Ann Intern Med 1991;111:183–188.
122. Cheigh JS, Stenzel KH. End-stage renal disease in systemic lupus erythematosus. Am J Kidney Dis 1993;21:2–12.
123. Lochhead KM, Pirsch JD, D'Allessandro AM, et al. Risk factors for renal allograft loss in patients with systemic lupus erythematosus. Kidney Int 1996;49:512–519.
124. Mojcik CF, Klippel JK. End-stage renal disease and systemic lupus erythematosus. Am J Med 1996;101:100–108.
125. Schmitt WH, Haubitz M, Mistry N, et al. Renal transplantation in Wegener's granulomatosis. Lancet 1993;342:860–862.
126. Tzardis PJ, Gruessner RWG, Matas AJ, et al. Long-term follow-up of renal transplantation for Wegener's disease. Clin Transplant 1990;4:108–111.
127. Oberhuber G, Prior C, Bosmuller C, et al. Early recurrence of Wegener's granulomatosis in a kidney allograft under cyclosporine treatment. Transplant Int 1988;1:49–50.
128. Clarke AE, Bitton A, Eappen R, et al. Treatment of Wegener's granulomatosis after renal transplantation. Is cyclosporine the preferred treatment? Transplantation 1990;50:1047–1051.
129. Curtis JJ, Deithelm AG, Herrera GA, et al. Recurrence of Wegener's granulomatosis in a cadaver renal allograft. Transplantation 1983;36:452–454.
130. Aunsholt NA, Ahlbom G. Recurrence of Wegener's granulomatosis after kidney transplantation involving the kidney graft. Clin Transplant 1989;3:159–161.
131. Steinman TI, Jaffe BF, Monaco AP. Recurrence of Wegener's granulomatosis after kidney transplantation. Am J Med 1980;68:458–460.
132. Harrison KL, Alpers CE, Davis CL. De novo amyloidosis in a renal allograft: a case report and a review of the literature. Am J Kidney Dis 1993;5:162–167.
133. Harmann A, Holdaas H, Fauchald P, et al. Fifteen year's experience with renal transplantation in systemic amyloidosis. Transplant Int 1992;5:15–18.
134. Pasternack A, Ahonen J, Kuhlback B. Renal transplantation in 45 patients with amyloidosis. Transplantation 1986;42:598–601.
135. Gerlag PG, Krenc RA, Berden JH. Renal transplantation in light chain nephropathy: case report and review of the literature. Clin Nephrol 1986;25:101–108.
136. Watts RWE. Treatment of primary hyperoxaluria type 1. J Nephrol 1994;7:208–214.
137. DePauw L, Gelin M, Danpure CJ, et al. Combined liver–kidney transplantation in primary hyperoxaluria type 1. Transplantation 1990;50:886–887.
138. Watts RWE, Morgan SH, Danpure CJ, et al. Combined hepatic and renal transplantation in primary hyperoxaluria type I: clinical report of nine cases. Am J Med 1991;90:179–188.
139. McDonald JC, Landdreneau MD, Rohr MS, DeVault GA. Reversal by liver–kidney transplantation in primary hyperoxaluria type 1. N Engl J Med 1989;321:1100–1103.
140. Jamieson NV. The European primary hyperoxaluria type 1 transplant registry report on the results of combined liver/kidney transplantation for primary hyperoxaluria 1984–1994. Nephrol Dial Transplant 1995;10(suppl 8):33–37.
141. Thedoropoulos DS, Kransnewich D, Kaiser-Kupfer MI, Gahl WA. Classic nephropathic cystinosis in adult disease. JAMA 1993;270(18):2200–2204.
142. Popli S, Molner ZV, Leehy DJ, et al. Involvement of renal allograft by Fabry's disease. Am J Nephrol 187;7:316–318.
143. Peces R, Aguado S, Renandez F, et al. Renal transplantation in Fabry's disease. Nephron 1989;51:294–295.
144. Donati D, Novario R, Gastaldi L. Natural history and treatment of uremia secondary to Fabry's disease: a European experience. Nephron 1987;46:353–359.
145. Gantenbein H, Bruder E, Burger HR, et al. Recurrence of Fabry's disease in a renal allograft 14 years after transplantation. Nephrol Dial Transplant 1995;10:287–289.
146. Mosnier JF, Degott C, Bedrossian J, et al. Recurrence of Fabry's disease in renal allograft eleven years after successful renal transplantation. Transplantation 1991;51:759–762.
147. Bodziak KA, Hammond WS, Molitoris BA. Inherited diseases of the glomerular basement membrane. Am J Kidney Dis 1994;23(4):605–618.
148. Peten E, Pirson Y, Cosyns J-P, et al. Outcome of thirty patients with Alport's syndrome after renal transplantation. Transplantation 1991;52:823–826.
149. Gobel J, Olbricht CJ, Offner G, et al. Kidney transplantation in Alport's syndrome: long-term outcome and allograft anti-GBV nephritis. Clin Nephrol 1992;38(6):299–304.
150. Kalluri R, Weber M, Netzer KO, et al. COL4A5 gene deletion and production of post-transplant anti-alpha 3(IV) collagen alloantibody in Alport's syndrome. Kidney Int 1994;45(3):721–726.
151. Rassoul J, al-Khadder AA, al-Sulaiman M, et al. Recurrent allograft antiglomerular basement membrane glomerulonephritis in a patient with Alport's syndrome. Am J Nephrol 1990;10(1):73–76.
152. Diaz JI, Valenzuela R, Gephardt G, et al. Anti-glomerular and anti-tubular basment membrane nephritis in a renal allograft recipient with Alport's syndrome. Arch Pathol Lab Med 1994;118(7):728–731.
153. Johnson R, Wilson R, Yamabe H, et al. Renal manifestations of hepatitis C virus infection. Kidney Int 1994;46:1255–1263.
154. Angedov V, Chung RT, Kaplan LM. A role for hepatitis C virus infection in type II cryoglobulinemia. N Engl J Med 1992;237:1490–1451.
155. Johnson RJ, Gretch DR, Yamabe H, et al. Membranoproliferative glomerulonephritis associated with hepatitis C virus infection. N Engl J Med 1993;328:465–470.
156. Johnson RH, Gretch DR, Couser WG, et al. Hepatitis C virus associated glomerulonephritis. Effect of alpha interferon therapy. Kidney Int 1994;46:1700–1704.
157. Fishman JA, Rubin RH, Koziel MJ, Periera BJ. Hepatitis C virus and organ transplantation. Transplantation 1996;62:147–154.
158. D'Amico G, Fornasier A. Cryoglobulinemic glomerulonephritis: a membranoproliferative glomerulonephritis induced by hepatitis C. Am J Kidney Dis 1995;25(3):361–369.
159. Bursetin DM, Rodby RA. Membranoproliferative glomerulonephritis associated with hepatis C virus infection. J Am Soc Nephrol 1993;4:1288–1293.
160. Sansonno D, Gesualdo L, Manno C, et al. Hepatitis C-related proteins in kidney tissue from hepatitis C virus infected patients with cryoglobulinemic membranoproliferative glomerulonephritis. Hepatology 1997;25:1237–1241.
161. Misiani R, Bellavita P, Fenili D, et al. Interferon alpha 2a therapy in cryoglobulinemia associated with hepatitis C virus. N Engl J Med 1994;330:751–756.
162. Gane EJ, Portimann BC, Naovmov NV, et al. Long-term outcome of hepatitis C infection after liver transplantation. N Engl J Med 1996;334:815–820.
163. Johnson M, Washburn W, Freeman R, et al. Hepatitis C viral infection in liver transplantation. Arch Surg 1996;131:284–291.
164. Rahamimon R, Ilan Y, Eid A, et al. Hepatitis C-associated cryoglobulinemia

after liver transplantation. Transplantatioon 1995;60:1050–1051.
165. Pascual M, Thadhani R, Chung RT, et al. Nephrotic syndrome after liver transplantation in a patient with hepatitis C virus associated glomerulonephritis. Transplantation 1997;64:1073–1076.
166. Pereira BJ, Wright TL, Schmid CH, Levey AS. A controlled study of hepatitis C transmission by organ transplantation. Lancet 1995;345:484–487.
167. Martin P, Friedman LS. Chronic viral hepatitis and the management of chronic renal failure. Kidney Int 1995;47:1231–1235.
168. Stemple CA, Lake J, Kuo G, Vincenti F. Hepatitis C—its prevalance in end stage renal failure and chronic course after kidney transplantation. Transplantation 1993;55:273–277.
169. Roth D, Zucher K, Cirocco R, et al. The impact of hepatitis C virus infection on renal allograft recipients. Kidney Int 1994;45:238–241.
170. Pereira BJ, Natov SN, Bouthot BA, et al. Effects of hepatitis C infection and renal transplantation on survival in end-stage renal disease. Kidney Int 1998;53:1374–1381.
171. Pereira BJ, Levey AS. Hepatitis C virus infection in dialysis and renal transplant. Kidney Int 1997;5:981–999.
172. Roth D, Cirocco R, Zucker K, et al. De novo membranoproliferative glomerulonephritis in hepatitis C virus infected renal allograft recipients. Transplantation 1995;59:1676–1682.
173. Gallay BJ, Alpers CE, Davis CL, et al. Glomerulonephritis in renal allograft associated with hepatitis C infection: a possible relationship with transplant glomerulopathy in 2 cases. Am J Kidney Dis 1995;26:662–667.
174. Cruzado JM, Gil-Vernet S, Ercilla G, et al. Hepatitis C-virus associated membranoproliferative glomerulonephritis in renal allografts. J Am Soc Nephrol 1996;7:2469–2475.
175. Cosio FG, Sedmak DD, Henry ML, et al. The high prevalence of severe early post transplant renal allograft pathology in hepatitis C positive recipients. Transplantation 1996;62:1054–1059.
176. Baid S, Pascual M, Williams WW, et al. Renal thrombotic microangiopathy associated with anticardiolipin antibodies in hepatitis C-positive renal allograft recipients. J Am Soc Nephrol 1999;10:146–153.
177. Prieto J, Yuste JR, Beloqui O, et al. Anticardiolipin antibodies in chronic hepatitis C: implication of hepatitis C virus as the cause of the antiphospholipid syndrome. Hepatology 1996;23:199–204.
178. Epstein M. Hepatorenal syndrome: emerging perspectives of pathophysiology and therapy. J Am Soc Nephrol 1994;4:1735.
179. Gines A, Escorsell A, Gines P, et al. Incidence, predictive factors, and treatment of the hepatorenal syndrome with ascites. Gastroenterology 1993;105:229–333.
180. Iwatsuki S, Popovtzer MM, Corman JL, et al. Recovery from hepatorenal syndrome after orthotopic liver transplantation. N Engl J Med 1973;289:1155–1159.
181. Koppel MH, Coburn JW, Mimes MD, et al. Transplantation of cadaveric kidneys from patients with hepatorenal syndrome: evidence of the functional nature of renal failure in advanced liver disease. N Engl J Med 1996;280:1367–1371.
182. Lenz K, Horthagl H, Druml W, et al. Ornipressin in the treatment of functional renal failure in decompensated liver cirrhosis. Effects on renal hemodynamics and atrial natriuretic factor. Gastroenterology 1991;101:1060–1064.
183. Gonwa TA, Klintmal GB, Levy M, et al. Impact of pretransplant renal function on survival after liver transplantation. Transplantation 1995;59(3):361–365.
184. Davenport A. Management of established renal failure in patients with liver failure. Semin Dial 1996;9(2):166–172.
185. Forni LG, Hilton PJ. Continuous hemofiltration in the treatment of acute renal failure. N Engl J Med 1997;336:1303–1309.

Chapter

36

Infection in the Organ Transplant Recipient

Robert H. Rubin Jay A. Fishman

The past decade has seen remarkable advances in organ transplantation, with one-year allograft survival rates of 85% to 90% being achieved at many transplant centers following cadaveric renal, heart, and liver transplantation. Indeed, the control of acute rejection processes has become so expert that attention has now turned to long-term allograft survival ("chronic rejection"), the complications of immunosuppressive therapy, and the development of new, even more challenging forms of transplantation–lung, small bowel, and pancreatic islet cell transplantation. At the same time, it should be recognized that post-transplant infection remains a major problem throughout the duration of immunosuppressive therapy, with evidence of possibly significant infection being found in more than 2 of 3 transplant patients. The impact of microbial invasion in transplant patients can go far beyond the *direct* causation of infectious disease syndromes such as pneumonia, hepatitis, or tissue abscess. In recent years, it has become apparent that cytokines, chemokines, and growth factors released in association with microbial replication and invasion (or as part of the rejection process) can have a variety of *indirect* effects as well (1,2):

1. The production of a global suppression of host defenses that leads to an increased risk of invasive superinfection with such opportunistic organisms as *Pneumocystis carinii*, *Candida* species, *Cryptococcus neoformans*, *Aspergillus* species, *Listeria monocytogenes*, and others
2. The modulation of the state of endothelial cell and leukocyte activation, as well as the display of major histocompatibility complex (MHC) antigens, thus affecting the recipient's response to the allograft and contributing to allograft injury
3. The participation in the pathogenesis of certain forms of malignancy, particularly those that occur at an increased rate in transplant recipients (post-transplant lymphoproliferative disease, squamous cell carcinoma of mucocutaneous surfaces, and Kaposi's sarcoma) following viral infection (see Chapter 37)

In addition, it is now clear that the indirect effects of infection are not unidirectional; that is, not only can cytokines liberated in the course of infection modulate the processes listed, but cytokines liberated in the course of such processes as rejection, trauma, and so forth can modulate the course of infection. The bidirectionality of these relationships is perhaps best illustrated by the answer to a question that has been a subject of intense controversy for the past two decades: "Which comes first, rejection or infection?" The answer is "Yes!"—the process can go in either direction (Fig. 36.1). It should be recognized, then, that infection and allograft rejection are inextricably intertwined, linked by the current requirement for lifetime immunosuppressive therapy after transplant. Any intervention that decreases the risk of rejection, thus permitting the use of lesser amounts of immunosuppression, will be translated into a lower risk of life-threatening infection; conversely, any intervention that decreases the risk of infection, thus permitting the safer use of more intense immunosuppression, will result in decreased allograft rejection. Thus, the *therapeutic prescription* for the transplant recipient should be recognized as having two components: an *immunosuppressive program* to prevent and treat rejection, and an *antimicrobial program* that is linked to the nature of the immunosuppression required in order to make the use of immunosuppression as safe as possible. Inherent in this view is the recognition that the goal of the infectious disease clinician in managing transplant patients is the *prevention* rather than the treatment of infection. The purpose of this chapter is to review the pathogenesis, clinical impact, and management of the most important infections affecting the organ transplant recipient (1–4).

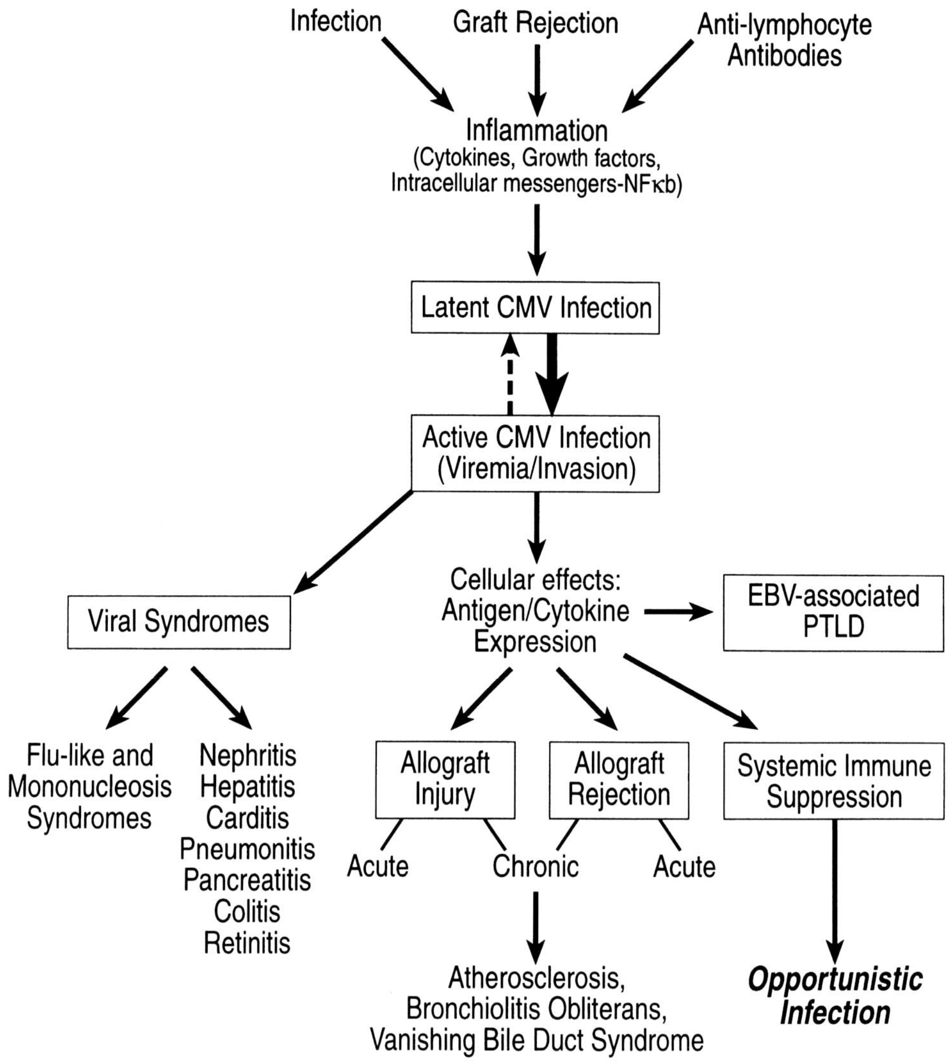

FIGURE 36.1. *Interactions among infection [particularly with cytomegalovirus (CMV) and Epstein-Barr virus (EBV)], allograft rejection, and post-transplant lymphoproliferative disease (PTLD). (Reproduced with permission from Fishman JA, Rubin RH. Infection in the organ transplant patient. N Engl J Med 1998;338:1741–1751.)*

RISK OF INFECTION

The microorganisms causing infection in the transplant patient can be divided into three general categories: 1) true pathogens (organisms capable of causing invasive disease in any individual through their ability to invade tissue planes or to produce a variety of toxins); 2) sometime pathogens (organisms usually found on the mucocutaneous surfaces of the body, causing no harm, but if damage to these surfaces or interference with their normal functioning occurs, then these organisms can cause life-threatening infection); and 3) nonpathogens (commensal organisms that are easily controlled by natural and acquired immunity such that even when inoculated into tissues they rarely produce disease). By convention, the term *opportunistic infection* is applied to infection caused by nonpathogens or to the occurrence of a clinical syndrome that is potentially life-threatening and that is caused by an organism usually incapable of producing such a syndrome (Table 36.1). The risk of infection, particularly opportunistic infection, in the transplant recipient is largely determined by the interaction of two factors: the environmental *exposures* that the patient encounters, and the patient's *net state of immunosuppression*. The relationship between these two factors is a semiquantitative one: if the exposure is great enough, even normal hosts will develop clinical disease; conversely, if the net state of immunosuppression is great enough, then minimal exposures to nonpathogens can have grave consequences. The clinician should keep this relationship constantly in mind as a clue to the presence either of excessive environmental hazards (when infection occurs in a patient whose net state of immunosuppression is not great) or of overimmunosuppres-

Table 36.1. Classification of Infections Occurring in Transplant Patients

Infections related to a technical complication[a]
Transplantation of a contaminated allograft
Anastomotic leak or stenosis
Wound hematoma
Intravenous line contamination
Iatrogenic damage to the skin
Mismanagement of endotracheal tube leading to aspiration
Infection related to biliary, urinary, and drainage catheters
Infections related to excessive nosocomial hazard
Aspergillus species[b]
Legionella species
Pseudomonas aeruginosa and other gram-negative bacilli
Vancomycin-resistant enterococci, methicillin-resistant *Staphyloccus aureus*
Infections related to particular exposures within the community
Systemic mycotic infection exposure in certain geographic areas[b]
Histoplasma capsulatum
Coccidioides immitis
Blastomyces dermatitidis
Strongyloides stercoralis[b]
Community-acquired opportunistic infection resulting from ubiquitous saprophytes in the environment[b]
Cryptococcus neoformans
Aspergillus species
Nocardia asteroides
Pneumocystis carinii
Respiratory infections circulating in the community[a]
Mycobacterium tuberculosis
Respiratory viruses (respiratory syncytial virus, influenza, etc.)
Infections acquired by the ingestion of contaminated food/water[a]
Salmonella species
Listeria monocytogenes
Viral infections of particular importance in transplant patients[a]
Herpes group viruses
Hepatitis viruses
Papillomavirus
Human immunodeficiency virus

[a] High probability of opportunistic infection, with the incidence and severity modulated by the nature and intensity of the immunosuppression being administered.

[b] Opportunistic infection (invasive infection of a nature and type not seen in nonimmunosuppressed individuals), again modulated by the nature and intensity of the immunosuppression being administered.

Source: Modified from Rubin RH. Infection in the organ transplant recipient. In: Rubin RH, Young LS, eds. Clinical approach to infection in the compromised host. 3rd ed. New York: Plenum, 1994:629–705.

sion (when infection occurs in the absence of an environmental hazard) (1,2,5).

The exposures of importance can be divided into two main categories: those occurring in the community and those occurring within the hospital. Within the community the most important issues are the geographically restricted, systemic mycoses (e.g., blastomycosis, coccidioidomycosis, and histoplasmosis), *Mycobacterium tuberculosis*, *Strongyloides stercoralis*, community-acquired respiratory viruses, salmonellosis, and *Campylobacter jejuni* infection. The types of infection observed with the mycoses and *M. tuberculosis* are very similar: reactivation of long-dormant infection due to attenuation of host immunity by post-transplant immunosuppression, with secondary dissemination; progressive primary infection, with primary dissemination; and, perhaps most interesting, superinfection, in which a transplant patient whose previous immunity has been diminished by immunosuppression develops invasive disease in association with a new exposure. The net result of all of these epidemiologic patterns is a high rate of progressive pulmonary infection (the portal of entry) and disseminated or metastatic infection. The resulting clinical syndromes include fever of unclear origin, pneumonia, or such manifestations of metastatic infection as meningitis, osteomyelitis, hepatic, renal, or mucocutaneous infection (1,2,5).

Strongyloides stercoralis is the parasitic infection with the greatest potential for affecting the transplant patient. Because of its unique autoinfection cycle, *S. stercoralis* can be maintained for decades asymptomatically in the gastrointestinal (GI) tract of individuals with normal host defenses. With the initiation of immunosuppression the organism is activated and two clinical syndromes can ensue: 1) a hyperinfestation syndrome, which is an exaggeration of the normal infection, resulting in hemorrhagic pneumonia and/or hemorrhagic entercolitis, or 2) disseminated infection, in which the organism actually invades tissues throughout the body, often accompanied by normal gut flora such as *Escherichia coli*, so that the clinical presentation is that of gram-negative bacteremia or meningitis unresponsive to apparently appropriate antimicrobial therapy. Effective treatment requires not only appropriate antibacterial therapy, but also anti-*Srongyloides* therapy with thiobendazole or ivermectin. After transplant these syndromes carry a mortality rate greater than 50%, and the emphasis should be on prevention with preemptive therapy prior to transplant. Routine examination of stool for this organism has a sensitivity of approximately 20%, which is clearly not adequate. Fortunately, an enzyme-linked immunosorbent assay (ELISA) for antibody to this organism is now available, and any transplant patient with a history of residence in endemic areas such as Latin America and Southeast Asia should be screened with this test, with seropositive individuals treated preemptively prior to transplant with thiabendazole or ivermectin (1,2,6–8).

Although cases of toxoplasmosis have been reported in other forms of organ transplantation, this parasitic infection is of major concern now only in heart transplant recipients. It is possible that the common use of trimethoprim-sulfamethoxazole prophylaxis is responsible in part for the low incidence of toxoplasmosis in noncardiac allograft recipients. Heart transplant recipients who are seronegative for *Toxoplasma gondii* and who receive an allograft from a seropositive donor are at high risk for developing life-threatening toxoplasmosis. In these patients, myocarditis (often mistaken for rejection), central nervous system and pulmonary infection, and disseminated infection can develop. Because of this concern, heart transplant recipients at risk for primary infection (donor seropositive, recipient seronegative) are treated with pyrimethamine and sulfasoxazole for four months (which also provides effective *Pneumocystis* prophylaxis) (1–3,9–12).

With the increasing success of transplantation and the return of patients to the community, such community-acquired infections as those due to respiratory viruses and gastrointestinal infections due to *Salmonella* species or *Campylobacter* are not uncommon. In particular, such viruses as influenza, parainfluenza, and respiratory syncytial virus have a significant impact on transplant patients, with an increased attack rate for both viral pneumonia and bacterial superinfection of the lungs. Influenza vaccination appears to be safe in transplant patients, but as with most vaccines given after transplant, has decreased efficacy (13,14). Respiratory syncytial virus, previously thought to be a pathogen only for young children, causes significant morbidity and occasional mortality in adult transplant patients. Strategies to prevent these infections are still evolving. At present, avoidance of exposure whenever possible appears to be primary. In the case of the gastrointestinal pathogens, more prolonged and severe disease, with a higher rate of bacteremia than in the nonimmunosuppressed host, is common and, again, avoidance of exposure is of importance. In this case, systemic antibiotics should be administered to prevent the consequences of invasive infection (1,2).

The most important points to be emphasized about community exposures are the following: a detailed recent and remote epidemiologic history regarding possible exposures to the pathogens listed is essential in the evaluation of a patient presenting with an infectious disease syndrome from the community; and patients should be advised regarding the avoidance of exposures (i.e., infected individuals, or travel to underdeveloped areas of the world where contamination of the water or food is not uncommon) (1–3).

Even more important than community exposures are those occurring within the hospital environment. Outbreaks of nosocomial infection due to contamination of the air or potable water with such pathogens as *Aspergillus* species, *Legionella* species, and gram-negative bacilli are well recognized to occur in transplant patients. Two epidemiologic patterns are observed: 1) domiciliary, in which exposures occur on the ward where the patient is housed, and 2) nondomiciliary, in which the exposure occurs in other parts of the hospital (e.g., radiology suite, operating room, catheterization laboratory) where the patient is taken for an essential procedure. Domiciliary exposures are relatively easy to detect because of clustering of cases in time and space. Nondomiciliary exposures are more common, however, though detection of the source of exposure may be difficult because of the lack of clustering. The best clue to the presence of a potentially important nosocomial hazard is the occurrence of a significant infection at a time when the net state of immunosuppression is not great enough for this to occur under normal circumstances (1–3,15,16). In recent years, person-to-person spread, often carried on the hands of medical personnel, of such organisms as methicillin-resistant *Staphylococcus aureus*, vancomycin-resistant *Enterococcus faecium*, and *Clostridium difficile* has become an increasing problem in transplant patients. Strict hand-washing precautions are essential in the management of all transplant patients, as is the institution of barrier nursing procedures when a patient is identified as being infected or colonized with one of these organisms.

Table 36.2. Factors Contributing to the Net State of Immunosuppression

Host defense defects engendered by the underlying disease process
Dose, duration, nature, and temporal sequence of immunosuppressive therapy
Technical factors that damage tissue, abridge the primary mucocutaneous barrier to infection, or result in the need for an indwelling foreign body
Neutropenia
Such metabolic factors as protein-calorie malnutrition, uremia, and perhaps diabetes mellitus
Infection with an immunomodulating virus (e.g., CMV, EBV, HBV, HCV, HIV)

The net state of immunosuppression is a complex function determined by a number of factors (Table 36.2). The major determinant of this function is clearly the nature of the immunosuppressive therapy being administered, but the importance of the other contributing factors is underlined by the following observations: Not only is infection virtually inevitable in the face of technical complications that lead to devitalized tissue or fluid collections, but the success of antimicrobial therapy is, to a significant degree, determined by the ability of the transplant team to correct this abnormality. The important contribution of protein-calorie malnutrition to the net state of immunosuppression is underlined by the finding at the Massachusetts General Hospital that patients with a serum albumin less than 2.8 g/dL have a ten-fold greater risk of life-threatening infection than those with higher levels of serum albumin; more than 90% of opportunistic infections occur in patients with immunomodulating viral infection, particularly that due to cytomegalovirus (indeed, the occurrence of opportunistic infection in the absence of such viral infection should trigger a search for a hitherto undetected environmental hazard) (1,2,5).

TIMETABLE OF POST-TRANSPLANT INFECTION

The immunosuppressive programs used in the management of all forms of organ transplantation are quite similar, with cyclosporine or tacrolimus being the cornerstones of these programs, usually accompanied by prednisone and either azathioprine or mycophenolate. In addition, induction courses of antilymphocyte antibody therapy are often utilized for the first 5 to 14 days after transplant to minimize the use of cyclosporine or tacrolimus if ischemia-reperfusion injury of the kidneys is occurring, or of prednisone if wound healing is a major concern (as in lung transplantation). Acute cellular rejection is usually managed with high-dose steroids, with antilymphocyte antibody therapy being employed for steroid-resistant rejection. With the standardization of immunosuppressive programs, it is apparent that there is a stereotyped pattern or "timetable" as to when different infections occur in the post-transplant period (Fig. 36.2); that is, although an infectious disease syndrome such as pneumonia can occur at any point in the post-transplant period, the microbial etiology (and hence treatment) is very different at different points in the post-transplant course. Such a timetable is useful to the clinician in three ways: in generating a differential diagnosis in the individual patient; as a tool for infection control, as exceptions to the timetable usually constitute unsuspected environmental exposures, especially within the hospital; and as the basis for designing targeted antimicrobial strategies that are cost effective (1,2,5).

The timetable for infection following organ transplantation is conveniently divided into three time periods (1,2,5):

1. *The First Month After Transplant.* There are three causes of clinical infection in the first month after transplant: 1) infection present in the recipient that was not eradicated prior to transplant, and which may be exacerbated by the surgery, anesthesia, and the need for immunosuppression; 2) infection conveyed via a contaminated allograft; and 3) the same bacterial and candidal infections of the wound, lungs, urine, vascular access device, and drainage catheters that occur in nonimmunosuppressed patients undergoing comparable forms of surgery (these last account for more than 95% of infections in this first month). The first rule of transplant infectious disease practice is to eradicate all treatable infection prior to transplant, with infections of the lung and bloodstream being particularly important—pulmonary tissue injured by infection, chemical aspiration, or infarction is at high risk of secondary infection with gram negatives and fungi after transplant. Ongoing bloodstream infection of donor or recipient carries a high risk for seeding vascular suture lines, resulting in mycotic aneurysms and catastrophic rupture. The key factor in determining the incidence of infection in the first month is the technical success of the transplant operation and the skill with which endotracheal tubes, vascular access devices, and drainage catheters are managed; a technical mishap almost invariably leads to infection. Indeed, the higher incidence of infection in liver, lung, and heart–lung allograft recipients is directly related to the technical complexity of these procedures (1,2,5).

   Notable by their absence during this time period are opportunistic infections despite the fact that the daily dose of immunosuppressive therapy is at its highest during this period. This observation has two implications: the major determinant of the net state of immunosuppression is not the daily dose of immunosuppression, but rather the sustained effect, the "area under the curve"; a single case of opportunistic infection occurring in this time period should be taken as prima facie evidence of an excessive environmental hazard that needs to be corrected (1,2).

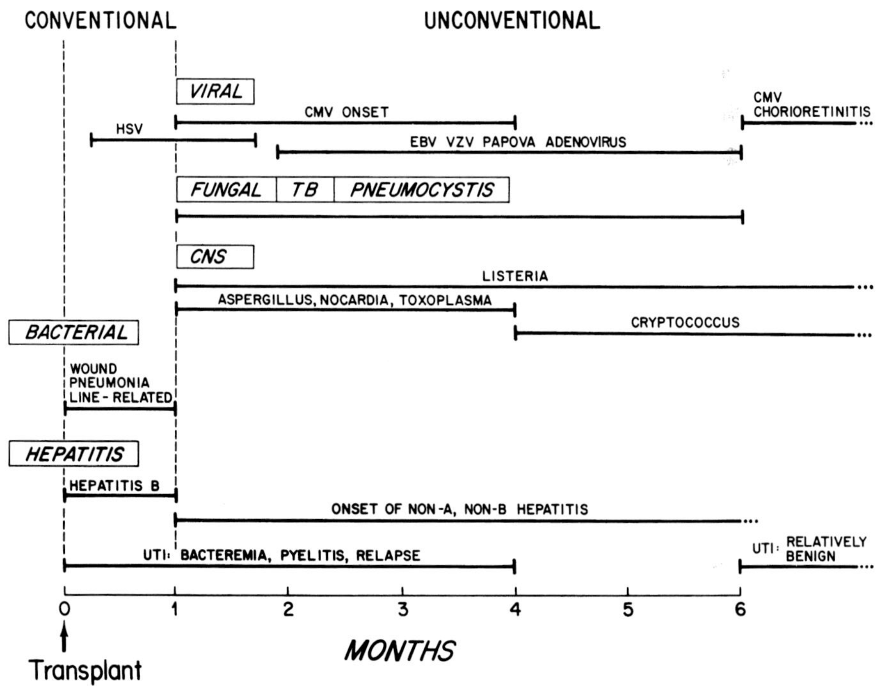

FIGURE 36.2. *Timetable for the occurrence of infection in the organ transplant patient. Exceptions to this timetable should initiate a search for an unusual hazard. CMV = cytomegalovirus; HSV = herpes simplex virus; EBV = Epstein-Barr virus; VZV = varicella-zoster virus; CNS = central nervous system; UTI = urinary tract infection; Papova = papillomavirus; TB = tubeculous. (Modified from Rubin RH, Wolfson JS, Cosimi AB, et al. Infection in the renal transplant recipient. Am J Med 1981;70:405–411.)*

2. *One to Six Months After Transplant.* During this time period, the etiology of infection changes markedly. In addition to residual or continuing effects of technically related infections that presented earlier, there are two major causes of infection in this time period: 1) the direct clinical effects of the immunomodulating viruses—cytomegalovirus (CMV), Epstein-Barr virus (EBV), hepatitis B and C (HBV and HCV), and the human immunodeficiency virus (HIV)—are manifested during this time period; and 2) the combined effects of sustained immunosuppression and often viral infection increases the risk of opportunistic infection due to such organisms as *P. carinii*, *Aspergillus* species, and *Nocardia asteroides* even in the absence of an unusual epidemiologic hazard (1,2,5).
3. *More than Six Months After Transplant.* In this late period, patients with surviving allografts can be divided into three groups: 1) 70% to 80% have had an excellent result from transplant, with satisfactory graft function maintained on baseline immunosuppression (their infection risks resemble those of the general community—respiratory viruses, urinary tract infection, etc.); 2) 5% to 15% have chronic viral infection, particularly with the hepatitis viruses (but also including HIV, papillomavirus, EBV, human herpesvirus-8, and others), which leads inexorably to severe organ dysfunction, AIDS, and/or malignancy; and 3) 5% to 15% (the "chronic ne'er-do-wells") have had a less than satisfactory result, with poor graft function, repeated courses of increased immunosuppression, and, often, chronic viral infection with one or more of the immmunomodulatory viruses. These last are at highest risk for opportunistic infection, particularly with *P. carinii*, *L. monocytogenes*, *C. neoformans*, and other pathogens, and should be maintained on long-term antimicrobial prophylaxis with trimethoprim-sulfamethoxazole and, possibly, fluconazole (1,2,5).

PRINCIPLES OF ANTIMICROBIAL THERAPY IN THE ORGAN TRANSPLANT RECIPIENT

There are three modes in which antimicrobial therapy can be prescribed for the transplant recipient: *therapeutic*, in which antimicrobial agents are utilized to treat established clinical infection; *prophylactic*, in which antimicrobial agents are administered to an entire population to prevent the occurrence of an infection common enough to justify this intervention; and *preemptive*, in which antimicrobial agents are prescribed to a portion of the population to prevent clinical disease on the basis of a laboratory marker or a clinical epidemiologic characteristic that defines a high risk for subsequent clinically important infections (1–3).

The most important factor in determining therapeutic success is how early a particular infection is diagnosed and effective therapy is initiated. This task is rendered particularly difficult in these immunosuppressed patients whose inflammatory response is muted, thus diminishing the signs and symptoms of infection often until late in the course of this process. In terms of therapeutic courses of antimicrobial drugs, rather than advocating fixed courses of therapy (e.g., two weeks or six weeks), our approach is based on the following principles:

- If clinical infection is associated with a technical/anatomic abnormality (e.g., devitalized tissue, fluid collection, anastomotic leak), then antibiotic therapy is ineffective without simultaneous correction of those factors that led to the infection in the first place.
- For those infections (e.g., fungal infection and tuberculous infection) with a high propensity for metastatic spread, initial diagnosis should then lead to a "metastatic work-up," as therapy should be directed at eradicating all sites of infection, not just the original site of discovery.
- Therapy should be designed to eliminate all evidence of the infection, with duration of therapy determined by clinical and microbial evaluation, with the addition of a "buffer period" of continued therapy since the objective evaluation of success of therapy is often quite insensitive.

The duration of the extra buffer period is determined by the seriousness of the infection and whether antimicrobial toxicity has occurred. Thus, the buffer period for systemic fungal infection may be several weeks, whereas for a urinary tract infection it is usually a few days. Implicit in these recommendations is the application of a major lesson from the HIV experience; that is, microbial burden is of critical importance in determining response to therapy and the needed duration of therapy. Cessation of therapy at a point when a significant microbial burden is present in these immunosuppressed individuals will have a high probability of inducing two undesirable events—relapsing infection and antimicrobial resistance (1–3).

Given both the impact of clinical infection and the difficulties in both recognizing and treating it, increasing emphasis is being placed on the prevention of clinical disease, with the use of both prophylactic and preemptive strategies. The two most successful prophylactic strategies are the use of perioperative prophylaxis at the time of surgery and the use of low-dose trimethoprim-sulfamethoxazole prophylaxis. The latter (i.e., one single-strength tablet at bedtime) should be utilized in every transplant patient who tolerates it, because it essentially eradicates urosepsis and urinary tract infection (indeed, breakthroughs should connote anatomic or functional abnormalities of the urinary tract), *P. carinii* pneumonia, nocardiosis, listeriosis, and probably toxoplasmosis. Whereas low-dose prophylaxis is well tolerated, the doses of trimethoprim-sulfamethoxazole required to treat clinical *Pneumocystis* infection are far greater and are associated with a more than 50% incidence of bone marrow, renal, and/or hepatic toxicity in this patient population (1–3).

There are two forms of preemptive therapy: one based on a laboratory assay, usually for evidence of presymptomatic infection; and one based on clinical/epidemiologic assessments of risk. Three examples of laboratory-based preemptive therapy are already being utilized at many transplant centers:

1. Asymptomatic CMV viremia, as determined by antigenemia or polymerase chain reaction (PCR) assay, is associated with a high risk of subsequent clinical disease, so many transplant centers are monitoring their patients and instituting ganciclovir therapy on the basis of this laboratory test.
2. Asymptomatic candiduria in the renal transplant patient, particularly one whose bladder function is less than optimal, is associated with the development of obstructing fungal balls at the ureterovesical junction, and subsequent ascending pyelonephritis. Thus, the finding of candiduris should trigger the initiation of systemic antifungal therapy preemptively to block this series of events.
3. Surgical removal of a pulmonary nodule that is found to be due to *Mycobacterium tuberculosis* or a fungus is associated with a 5% to 15% incidence of dissemination and subsequent central nervous system infection. This can be effectively preempted with two-week courses of systemic antifungal therapy (or with a six-month course of antituberculous therapy).

The prime example of the other category of preemptive therapy is with CMV infection. CMV-seronegative recipients of seropositive organs with conventional immunosuppression have a risk of clinical CMV disease of 15% or less; if antilymphocyte antibody therapy is required to treat rejection, the incidence of clinical CMV disease rises to approximately 65%. This excessive occurrence of CMV disease can be eliminated by a preemptive course of ganciclovir, initiated at the same time as the antilymphocyte antibody therapy (1–3,17–21).

Antimicrobial prescription in transplant patients is determined not only by consideration of the susceptibility of the pathogen(s) being treated, but also by the possibilities of interactions with the mainstays of immunosuppressive programs, cyclosporine and tacrolimus. There are three ways in which antimicrobial agents can interact with these immunosuppressive drugs; two of them have to do with the ability of a given antimicrobial agent to influence the key step in the metabolism of both these immunosuppressive agents, that mediated by hepatic cytochrome P450 enzymes. The third, synergistic nephrotoxicity, is due to unknown mechanisms. These three forms of drug interaction are as follows (1–3):

1. *Upregulation of Hepatic Cytochrome P450 Function.* Certain drugs, most notably rifampin, isoniazid, and nafcillin, increase the rate of cyclosporine and tacrolimus metabolism, thus decreasing blood levels and increasing the risk of allograft rejection.
2. *Downregulation of Hepatic Cytochrome P450 Function.* Certain drugs, most notably the macrolides (erythromycin, clarithromycin, and azithromycin) and the azoles (ketoconazole, itraconazole, and fluconazole) decrease the rate of cyclosporine and tacrolimus metabolism, thus increasing blood levels, causing nephrotoxicity and the possibility of overimmunosuppression with an increased risk of infection.
3. *Idiopathic Synergistic Nephrotoxicity.* Certain drugs, most notably aminoglycosides, amphotericin, vancomycin, high-dose trimethoprim-sulfamethoxazole and fluoroquinolones, cause synergistic nephrotoxicity in the face of therapeutic levels of the immunosuppressive agent. This is manifested in two ways: in some patients a single therapeutic dose of these agents can cause oliguric renal failure; more commonly, the toxicity seen with a drug such as amphotericin is greatly enhanced and accelerated.

The implications of these possible drug interactions are several. First, they provide even further impetus for attempts at preventing infection. Second, choices of antimicrobials are greatly influenced by these considerations, with a particular emphasis on the use of advanced-spectrum beta lactams, low-dose trimethoprim-sulfamethoxazole and fluoroquinolones, and fluconazole, with the particular avoidance of aminoglycosides and amphotericin. Third, the recognition that whenever antimicrobial therapy with azoles, macrolides, antituberculous agents, and nafcillin is required, readjustment of previously stable cyclosporine or tacrolimus doses is necessary, based on measurement of blood levels, *not only with the initiation of therapy with one of these antimicrobial agents, but also upon the termination of antimicrobial therapy* (1–3).

INFECTIONS OF PARTICULAR IMPORTANCE IN ORGAN TRANSPLANT RECIPIENTS

Cytomegalovirus

Cytomegalovirus (CMV) is the single most important infection observed in organ transplant patients, with at least 50% of transplant patients manifesting evidence of viral replication after transplant. The epidemiology, pathogenesis, and consequences of CMV infection are essentially identical in all forms of organ transplantation, with one notable exception: the organ transplanted is more affected by the virus than is the native organ. Thus, CMV hepatitis is a clinical problem almost exclusively in liver allograft recipients, CMV pancreatitis in pancreatic allograft recipients, CMV myocarditis in heart allograft recipients, and pneumonia in lung allograft recipients (although CMV pneumonia can occur in all forms of transplantation, both the attack rate and severity are greater in lung and heart–lung recipients) (1–5).

Three characteristics of herpes group viruses help explain why this group in general and CMV in particular are such effective pathogens in transplant patients: latency, cell association, and possible oncogenicity. The term *latency* refers to the fact that long after active viral replication has ceased, latent infection of a variety of cells and tissues remains and is capable of being reactivated under specific circumstances. The laboratory marker for latent infection is seropositivity in the absence of replicating virus. *Cell association* refers to the fact that this virus is transmitted through the exchange of infected cells between individuals (i.e., through intimate personal contact, transfusion, or transplantation) and is spread within individuals through the dissemination of cells with actively replicating virus. This means that humoral immunity is rendered inefficient and that the key host defense is mediated through the action of MHC-restricted, virus-specific, cytotoxic T cells—the arm of host defense most inhibited by presently employed immunosuppressive programs. Also, when there is MHC disparity between donor and recipient, it is likely that the allograft becomes a privileged site for viral replication, perhaps explaining the propensity for the virus to cause more severe disease in an allografted as opposed to a native organ. Finally, all herpes group viruses are considered potentially *oncogenic*, with EBV being clearly shown to play an important role in the pathogenesis of post-transplant lymphoproliferative disease (PTLD) (1,2). In addition, it is important to note that CMV disease increases the risk of PTLD by a factor of 7 to 10 (22).

There are three different patterns of CMV infection in the transplant patient, which depend on the past experience of donor and recipient with the virus, as revealed by serologic testing (1,2,4,5,23–26):

1. *Primary Infection.* When a seronegative recipient (R−) receives latently infected cells from a seropositive donor (D+), there is a 50% to 70% chance of the recipient developing symptomatic CMV disease. More than 90% of the time, the latently infected cells are within the allograft; in virtually all of the remaining cases the virus is obtained from latently infected, viable leukocytes present in red cell or platelet transfusions derived from seropositive donors. Studies performed in liver transplant recipients suggest that transfusion-derived CMV is milder than allograft-derived infection. Occasionally, a CMV-negative individual acquires primary CMV through intimate contact in the community. D+R− transplants account for 5% to 15% of organ transplants.
2. *Reactivation Infection.* When a seropositive recipient (R+) reactivates endogenous latent infection, there is a 10% to 20% chance of the recipient developing symptomatic CMV disease when routine immunosuppression (e.g., cyclosporine or tacrolimus, prednisone, with or without azathioprine or mycophenolate) is administered. Approximately 75% to 85% of organ transplant patients are at risk for reactivation CMV disease.
3. *Superinfection.* When a seropositive recipient (R+) receives an allograft from a seropositive donor (D+), in at least 50% of instances the virus that is activated is of donor rather than recipient origin. Although available data are incomplete, it appears that approximately twice as many D+R+ patients develop symptomatic CMV disease as do D−R+ patients. D+R+ transplants account for 25% to 40% of transplants performed.

CMV infection is initiated when latent virus is reactivated, a process requiring the action of such proinflammatory cytokines as tumor necrosis factor (TNF). These, in turn, stimulate a variety of intracellular messengers in latently infected cells (e.g., the nuclear transcription factor, NFκB) that trigger active viral replication. The key role of TNF and other proinflammatory cytokines explains the clinical and laboratory observations in which symptomatic CMV disease has been reported to follow such disparate processes as allograft rejection, urosepsis, antilymphocyte antibody treatment, and severe trauma. These disparate processes share in common the elaboration of proinflammatory cytokines, with the activation of CMV from latency representing a final common pathway (see Fig. 36.1) (2,27).

Other than the serologic status of donor and recipient, the most important determinant of the course of CMV infection is the nature of the immunosuppressive drugs being administered. Three categories of effects are observed in murine models and patients: 1) monoclonal and polyclonal antilymphocyte preparations cause systemic release of proinflammatory cytokines, which are extremely potent in terms of reactivating CMV; 2) cytotoxic drugs, such as azathioprine, cyclophosphamide, and mycophenolate, have moderate potency in terms of reactivating CMV; 3) cyclosporine, tacrolimus, prednisone, and rapamycin have no ability to reactivate CMV from latency (4,15). Since allograft rejection is also a potent stimulus for reactivating latent virus, one would expect that the use of antilymphocyte antibody therapy to treat rejection would be a particularly potent stimulus for reactivating virus and causing clinical disease. Indeed, when CMV-seropositive individuals receive such therapy, the incidence of clinical disease rises three-fold to four-fold (1,2,17,18).

Once there is active, replicating virus present, there is a marked change in the impact of the immunosuppressive drugs, with a reversal in the potency of their effects. Cyclosporine, tacrolimus, rapamycin, and prednisone amplify viral replication by inhibiting the cytotoxic T-cell antiviral response once CMV replication has been initiated by other factors such as alloimmune reactivity of cytokine release. Also, cytotoxic agents and antilymphocyte antibodies are only moderately active in terms of increasing the impact of replicating CMV. These observations have several implications. First, when assessing the impact of a given immunosuppressive program on the course of CMV, the entire program and the temporal sequence in which it is deployed need to be considered. Second, anti-CMV preventative strategies need to be linked to the nature of the immunosuppressive program that the patient requires. In particular, the use of antilymphocyte antibodies to treat rejection requires an escalation in the intensity of the antiviral program that is employed. Third, in the present era of cyclosporine- and tacrolimus-based immunosuppression, relapsing CMV disease (i.e., clinical symptoms returning after an initial response to antiviral therapy that has been completed) unrelated to the development of antimicrobial resistance is quite common. Such relapse is due to the amplifying effect of immunosuppression on small amounts of residual, replicating virus present after completion of a standard two- to three-week treatment course (1–3,17,18).

The direct effects of CMV replication are usually seen one to four months after transplant, although recent experience has shown that clinical CMV disease may recur or occur for the first time months after resolution of systemic inflammatory syndromes (particularly other forms of infection) in individuals who are highly immunosuppressed. As with most other viral processes, CMV usually begins insidiously with constitutional symptoms of anorexia, malaise, and fever, often accompanied by myalgia and arthralgias. In many patients, unexplained fever and constitutional symptoms, often with accompanying neutropenia and/or thrombocytopenia, subclinical hepatitis (symptomatic in liver allograft recipients), and a slight atypical lymphocytosis (a mononucleosis-like syndrome that differs from that caused by EBV in the normal host by the absence of pharyngitis, splenomegaly, and lymphadenopathy) are the only manifestations of this systemic infection. Other human herpes viruses (e.g., human herpes virus-6, -7, and -8, with HHV-8 being the putative cause of Kaposi's sarcoma) may be reactivated during the course of CMV infection. It has been difficult to sort out the contribution of these closely related viruses to clinical illness, but it would not be surprising if HHV-6 and -7 contributed to the pathogenesis of a mononucleosis syndrome or other illnesses that are now attributed solely to CMV (or EBV). This is particularly true of HHV-6 (1,2,28).

The two more serious manifestations of CMV are those involving the lung and the gut. In the lung, a bilateral interstitial pneumonia resembling that caused by other viruses, *Mycoplasma*, *Pneumocystis*, and other atypical pathogens occurs not uncommonly. Dual or sequential infection with *P. carinii*, fungi, and *N. asteroides*, as well as more conventional bacterial pathogens are not uncommon in this setting. The stomach appears to be the most frequent site of symptomatic CMV infection in the GI tract, not infrequently causing subjective complaints of nausea, a sense of abdominal fullness, and dysphagia, with poor gastric emptying. CMV infection at other sites in the upper GI tract is also common, with both esophagitis and duodenitis being well described. Colonic ulceration, often involving the right colon, presenting as GI hemorrhage, perforation, or even pseudomembranous colitis is also not uncommon. GI manifestations of CMV infection can occur in the absence of fever, leukopenia, or other manifestations of systemic disease, and assays for CMV viremia may be falsely negative in the face of active CMV gut involvement (2,29–34).

Because of the systemic nature of CMV disease, with the vasculitis component, CMV uncommonly can produce inflammatory states at other sites, including endometritis, encephalitis, hemorrhoiditis, transverse myelitis, and a cutaneous vasculitis. Chorioretinitis, typically appearing for the first time more than four months after transplant is the major late manifestation of CMV infection. Although chorioretinitis may present with only a single eye being involved, it invariably progresses to involve both eyes and to blindness unless prolonged antiviral therapy is instituted (1,2,35).

Thus far, only the direct effects of CMV have been discussed. Of the indirect effects, the one that has been most clearly delineated, in both humans and mice, is a rather global suppressant effect on host defenses that leads to a high rate of superinfection. Thus, preceding CMV disease has been clearly linked to an increased risk of *P. carinii* pneumonia, invasive fungal and nocardial infection, listeriosis, and even invasive bacterial infection. Indeed, there is a body of information to suggest that the successful prevention of CMV disease leads to a decrease in these infections as well. Traditionally, the risk of such superinfection has been correlated with the occurrence of symptomatic CMV disease. Since "asymptomatic" viral replication is a common event, an important unanswered question is whether all CMV replication, symptomatic or not, increases the patient's susceptibility to opportunistic superinfection (1,2,36–42).

An even more important issue is the relationship between CMV and acute and chronic allograft injury. As delineated in Figure 36.1, recent information about the roles of cytokines in inflammatory and immune responses suggests that the relationship between rejection and CMV is bidirectional, with CMV inducing rejection and the inflammation caused by rejection (and some antirejection therapies) increasing viral replication. Thus, both acute rejection and various forms of chronic allograft injury (e.g., bronchiolitis obliterans in lung allograft recipients, accelerated coronary atherosclerosis in cardiac allograft recipients, the disappearing bile duct syndrome in liver allograft recipients, and a particular form of glomerulopathy in renal allograft recipients) have been linked with CMV infection, both symptomatic and asymptomatic (1,2,4,43–55). The finding that 80% of renal allograft recipients with "biopsy-proven rejection" more than six months following transplantation responded to ganciclovir therapy without further immunosuppressive treatment, whereas others in the same group failed to respond to increased immunosuppression, is an important observation in this regard (56). However, what is also clear is that this is not a specific effect of CMV; rather, the operating hypothesis is that cytokines and growth factors elaborated in response to CMV replication *and other inflammatory states* can modulate the rejection process. [It is of interest in this regard that a glomerulopathy first linked with CMV has now been reported to be associated with hepatitis C as well (57).] CMV has been singled out because it is such a ubiquitous process in transplantation. Proof of this proposed link between CMV and allograft injury will come from studies of the effects of effective antiviral prophylaxis on the occurrence and rate of progression of allograft injury. Such studies have been initiated.

There are four approaches to the diagnosis of CMV infection: serologic, microbiologic, rapid nonculture assays, and analysis of biopsy specimens. Serologic assays, the measurement of circulating antibody levels, have their primary use in the assessment of donor and recipient prior to transplant to determine the risk of subsequent CMV disease and the type of preventative antiviral strategy that is indicated. Serial measurements of antibody level and the measurement of anti-CMV IgM levels are not sufficiently sensitive or timely to be worth measuring in this era when antiviral therapeutic decisions must be made. The gold standard for CMV diagnosis has long been tissue culture, with an end point of cytopathic effect. However, this often required up to six weeks for definitive results, which again is not adequate for therapeutic decision making. The first advance was the shell vial technique, in which the specimen to be tested was centrifuged against a fibroblast monolayer (which increases the yield approximately four-fold), with the monolayer then assayed 24 to 48 hours later with a fluorescein-labeled monoclonal antibody against the immediate early antigen of CMV. Although a very satisfactory technique for assaying respiratory secretions, biopsy specimens, or urine, the shell vial technique has a sensitivity of less than 50% in demonstrating viremia. Since the demonstration of viremia is the single most valuable diagnostic test for CMV, other techniques have been brought to bear. At present, the most valuable diagnostic techniques for CMV are the CMV antigenemia assay (which provides a semiquantitative assessment of the level of viremia) and quantitative PCR (which, unfortunately, is as yet only available at a few centers). Significant CMV disease requiring therapy is presently diagnosed either by the demonstration of viremia or by demonstrating the presence of virus in biopsy specimens taken from abnormal tissue (1–3,34,58–63).

The antiviral management of CMV can be divided into two general categories, *preventive* and *therapeutic*. In the preventive category, there are two approaches, prophylactic and preemptive. Prophylactic therapy is clearly indicated in those individuals at risk for primary infection (D+R–), since the attack rate for clinical disease is so high (50% to 70%). Although hyperimmune anti-CMV globulin and/or high-dose acyclovir have shown some protective effect in this setting, the most effective prophylactic strategy is prolonged ganciclovir therapy. Six months of intravenous therapy has been shown to be quite effective but is expensive and logistically difficult to deliver. Preliminary data suggest that for all of organ transplant patients except lung recipients, a prolonged course of oral ganciclovir (2–3 g/day for four months), particularly after a 10- to 14-day induction course of intravenous ganciclovir, is the most satisfactory approach to this problem (68). Whether hyperimmune globulin can add to the efficacy of this regimen remains to be determined (in mice, combination therapy is more effective than either by itself). It is clear that lung allograft recipients require more intensive and prolonged anti-CMV prophylaxis than do the other organ transplant patients. Currently, a minimum of six to eight weeks of intravenous ganciclovir is used, with or without hyperimmune globulin, with oral ganciclovir then continuing for several months thereafter (1–3,34,64–67).

For seropositive patients, prophylaxis with high-dose acyclovir and/or hyperimmune globulin have efficacy that is attenuated by the use of antilymphocyte antibody therapy. Oral ganciclovir is probably even more effective (1–3,68). However, since the risk of symptomatic CMV is relatively low (10% to 20%) if antilymphocyte antibody therapy is not used, the preferred approach is a preemptive one: intravenous ganciclovir at a dose of 5 mg/kg/day (with dosage modification for renal dysfunction) during the course of the antilymphocyte antibody therapy. This will decrease the incidence of CMV disease from approximately 65% to less than 20%. Recently, we have found that following the intravenous ganciclovir in this circumstance with three months of oral ganciclovir (2–3 g/day) will essentially eradicate infectious disease syndromes due to CMV in seropositive patients being treated with antirejection antilymphocyte therapy (17,18). Alternatively, one can monitor at frequent intervals for CMV viremia (which usually occurs one to seven days before the onset of symptoms), and then initiate intravenous therapy on the basis of these results (21).

Any consideration of anti-CMV prevention at present must recognize certain points:

1. All regimens that have been defined have been studied in terms of their ability to prevent the direct infectious disease syndromes caused by CMV. There is currently inadequate information available in terms of the efficacy of these regimens in preventing such indirect effects as allograft injury, oncogenesis, or prevention of secondary infection. Such trials are currently underway, and the results of these trials will likely modify significantly the recommendations listed above.
2. Anti-CMV therapies are most effective as the virus emerges from latency, when the multiplicity of virus is at its lowest level. In this circumstance, antiviral resistance has not occurred (1–3).
3. Any change in immunosuppressive programs will likely require a reevaluation of anti-CMV preventive strategies, as the success of any particular antiviral program is closely linked to the nature of the immunosuppressive program employed.
4. New anti-CMV drugs are critically needed, particularly ones that can be utilized orally.

The standard of care for treating CMV is two to three weeks of intravenous ganciclovir (5 mg/kg twice daily, with dosage adjustments in the face of renal dysfunction). In addition, it may be of interest that HHV-6 is also sensitive to ganciclovir, and should respond to anti-CMV courses of therapy. Many groups will combine intravenous ganciclovir with hyperimmune globulin in patients with tissue invasive disease, particularly pneumonia. However, the standard regimen of intravenous ganciclovir is associated with a relapse rate of approximately 20% in seropositive individuals and approximately 65% in those with primary infection. In this situation, relapse is defined as patients with virologically documented symptomatic disease that responds to the ganciclovir, but with recurrent symptoms within six weeks of therapy cessation. Antiviral resistance is not the issue in the great majority of individuals. Usually, relapse of this type can be prevented by treating with intravenous therapy until viremia is totally cleared (as assessed by antigenemia or PCR), and then continuing with oral ganciclovir (2–3 g/day for two months in seropositive individuals, and for three to four months in those with primary infection) (1–3). Ganciclovir resistance has now been documented in organ transplant patients, with the following factors seeming to play a role: a high burden of virus present (akin to the HIV experience); cessation of intravenous ganciclovir before viremia is cleared; and/or premature switch to oral therapy. The bioavailability of oral ganciclovir is less than 10%, so this therapy should be reserved for prophylaxis or "wrap-up therapy" once the viral burden has been essentially eliminated. The primary alternative to ganciclovir, foscarnet, has a prohibitive rate of nephrotoxicity in transplant patients and should be avoided if at all possible through the appropriate use of ganciclovir (2).

Epstein-Barr Virus

The effects of Epstein-Barr virus (EBV) in the organ transplant patient are quite diverse, ranging from a mononucleosis syndrome akin to that observed in normal hosts, to clinical hepatitis (most commonly in liver transplant recipients), to a variety of malignant states (see also Chapter 37). These last are by far the most important effects of EBV in this patient population. Although in other patient populations, nasopharyngeal carcinoma (endemic in young men from South China and in certain Native Americans), and Burkitt's lymphoma (in Ugandan children and in such other immunosuppressed hosts as those with AIDS and congenital immunodeficiency states) are more common, in transplant patients the most important effect of EBV is in the pathogenesis of common PTLD. This last has been reported to occur in 1% to 2% of renal transplant recipients, 2% to 5% of liver and heart transplant recipients, and as many as 10% of heart–lung recipients—these differences not reflecting the differences in organs but rather the intensity of immunosuppression utilized in the different transplant settings (1,2,22).

The epithelial cells of the upper respiratory tract are the natural reservoir for EBV, causing lytic infection of the pharynx as the first manifestation of such infection. Long-lived B lymphocytes become secondarily infected with EBV as they travel through the lymphoid tissues of the oropharynx where lytic, infectious virus is being produced. Infection of these B lymphocytes results in latent infection without replication or release of virus and, consequently in *transformation and immortalization.* Latently infected B lymphocytes harbor the virus in a circular episomal form (which is not susceptible to antiviral chemotherapy) in which only a few genes, those necessary for transformation, are expressed. Individuals who are seropositive for EBV (more than 90% of adults) harbor latently infected B lymphocytes that have the potential for unlimited growth. However, lymphoproliferation does not occur because of an active immunologic surveillance mechanism based primarily on MHC-restricted, EBV-specific, cytotoxic T cells. Suppression of this mechanism in vitro or in such in vivo situations as EBV infection in mice with severe combined immunodeficiency, AIDS patients, and transplant patients results in outgrowth of these immortalized B cells and evident lymphoproliferation (1,2,22).

Current concepts of the pathogenesis of PTLD suggest that the expanded pool of immortalized B cells that result from inhibition of the cytotoxic T-cell surveillance mechanism have the potential for producing a polyclonal lymphoproliferative process. If a second step occurs, such as certain forms of chromosomal rearrangement, then a monoclonal lymphoproliferative process—one that is likely to be far more malignant in character than the polyclonal process—can develop. Of interest, EBV-immortalized B cells produce growth factors including lactic acid and interleukin-6 that stimulate their own proliferation in an autocrine loop. It is likely that cytokines and growth factors produced in the course of such other processes as rejection, other infections, antilymphocyte antibody therapy, and so forth, can also promote this process. For example, the greater than seven-fold increase in PTLD in organ transplant patients with a history of symptomatic CMV disease is thought to be mediated primarily through such a mechanism (see Fig. 36.1) (1,2,22).

From the preceding description, it is clear that the occurrence of PTLD is determined primarily through the interaction of two processes: the level of EBV latently infected and transformed B lymphocytes (which, in turn, is a reflection of the level of EBV replication in the pharynx) and the activity of the virus-specific cytotoxic T-cell response. Thus, increased immunosuppression, particularly with regimens that include antilymphocyte antibody therapy, and primary EBV infection (as seen almost exclusively in pediatric organ transplant patients) are important risk factors for PTLD. The MHC restriction of the cytotoxic T-cell–controlling mechanism suggests that MHC-mismatched allografts would be privileged sites for PTLD development, a prediction that appears to be borne out clinically (1,22).

The clinical presentation of EBV-associated PTLD can be quite variable, with almost any organ capable of being involved. Usually, one or more of the following features ushers in the illness: unexplained fever; a mononucleosis-type syndrome with fever, malaise, and lymphadenopathy, with or without pharyngitis; tonsillitis; a GI presentation, which can include GI bleeding, abdominal pain, gut perforation or obstruction; hepatocellular dysfunction; and central nervous system dysfunction such as seizures, altered state of consciousness, and focal neurologic dysfunction. An important clinical point is that absence of adenopathy on radiologic imaging does not rule out PTLD, as this disease can be totally extranodal in nature (1).

Pathologically, PTLD represents a continuum, both in terms of histology (nonspecific reactive hyperplasia, polymorphic B-cell hyperplasia, polymorphic B-cell lymphoma, and immunoblastic sarcoma) and clonality (polyclonal, oligoclonal, and monoclonal), from the reactive to the frankly malignant. Although conceptually this classification system is helpful, it is often not helpful in the individual patient because all levels of clonality and histology can be found at different sites in the same patient. A useful staging system that has prognostic value is badly needed in developing therapy for this condition (1).

Optimal therapy for PTLD is still being defined. Approximately 20% of individuals will respond to marked diminution of immunosuppression with or without antiviral therapy (68). Whether antiviral therapy has a role is as controversial as any other aspect of treatment; that is, the episomal form of EBV is not susceptible to antiviral therapy, but unanswered is whether or not active viral replication "feeds" the process and is best aborted with acyclovir or ganciclovir. There are "testimonials" to the efficacy of antiviral therapy in individual patients, but, as with other forms of therapy for PTLD, the characteristics of patients who will best respond to this intervention with or without immunomodulating therapy using interferon or immunoglobulin are currently unknown. It is more likely, although currently unproven, that antiviral preventative strategies aimed at both CMV and EBV, by cutting down on the EBV burden, could decrease the incidence of PTLD, particularly in patients receiving intensive antirejection therapy (1,22,70,71).

The one aspect of treating PTLD that is noncontroversial is the absolute requirement for significant decrease or cessation of immunosuppressive therapy, particularly cyclosporine, tacrolimus, and antilymphocyte antibody. Debulking procedures appear to have merit in some patients with localized disease. However, most groups approach PTLD as a systemic disease requiring systemic therapy. Currently, cytotoxic chemotherapy similar to that utilized in the treatment of non-Hodgkin's lymphoma in the nontransplant setting is the most common form of treatment employed. However, experimental therapies with anti-B-cell monoclonal antibodies, adaptive immunotherapy with lymphocyte infusions, and immunomodulating therapy with interferon alpha plus immunoglobulin are all being explored. Unfortunately, the whole area of therapy for PTLD suffers from the lack of an adequate prognostic staging system that would allow precise prescription for the individual patient (1,2,22).

Hepatitis B

Hepatitis B virus (HBV) has long been known to be an important pathogen in transplant patients due to its high prevalence in dialysis patients, and hence in patients presenting for renal transplantation. The most complete information on the impact of HBV infection comes from studies of renal transplant recipients, but it is likely that the information acquired from these patients is applicable to cardiac and lung transplant patients as well. Renal transplantation of HBV carriers is associated with an increased risk of opportunistic infection in the first 12 to 24 months after transplant; that is, it contributes to the net state of immunosuppression. The level of replicating virus and the rate of progression of the disease are increased significantly by post-transplant immunosuppression. There has been great controversy regarding whether patients with end-stage renal disease who are carriers of HBV should be transplanted. By ten years after transplant, at least 50% of these individuals will have developed end-stage liver disease or hepatocellular cancer, with patients having circulating HBV DNA or HBeAg prior to transplant being particularly likely to progress. It is likely that the advent of lamivudine, and perhaps other antiviral drugs active against HBV, will improve this prognosis (72). At present, HBV infection should be regarded as a relative contraindication for transplantation of the nonhepatic organs, requiring careful assessment of the patient's condition (including liver biopsy) before proceeding (1,2,73).

Patients with end-stage liver disease due to HBV have traditionally done significantly worse than those with other causes of liver failure, with a one-year survival of around 50% as compared to an expected rate of more than 80% (see Chapter 19). The expected rate of recurrence approaches 100% after transplant, with accelerated liver disease, and an increased risk of life-threatening infection. Because of these discouraging results, even when large doses of hepatitis B immunoglobulin (HBIG) are given during transplant, many centers had stopped offering liver transplantation to patients with end-stage liver disease due to HBV. It has now been shown that administration of 10,000 units of HBIG during the anhepatic phase of the operation, followed by daily administration for six days, and then approximately monthly (to keep the anti-HBs titer >1 : 100 IU) provides sufficient protection so that the results now being achieved in these patients are similar to those achieved in patients undergoing hepatic transplantation for other indications. The optimal duration for this therapy is unknown. Lamivudine and other antivirals are increasingly being used prior to and after transplantation in these patients. The cost of HBIG therapy is quite high, exceeding $15,000 per year. It has been shown that patients receiving such therapy have replicative forms of HBV in their mononuclear cells, even when the liver is free of detectable virus, hence the reluctance to stop HBIG and allow late infection of the allograft. Mutants of HBV resistant to both

HBIG and lamivudine have been reported as emerging during these therapies in the liver transplant patient with HBV infection (1,2,73–80).

The efficiency of transmission of HBV by transfusion or transplantation of an allograft from an HBV carrier approaches 100%. Fortunately, the techniques available for testing for HBsAg (and hence the presence of infectious virus) are so sensitive and specific that the current incidence of post-transfusion HBV infection is estimated to be approximately 0.002% per transfusion, with a comparable figure for organ transplantation. Of greater concern than the sensitivity of the assay is ensuring that appropriate blood specimens from the prospective donor are being assayed. Thus, both HIV and HBV have been transmitted from a donor who had received more than 50 units of blood in a vain resuscitative attempt before initiating the work-up for organ donation. When the blood specimens were obtained for pretransplant testing, they were falsely negative (representing transfused and not native blood), and virus-laden organs were inappropriately transplanted, resulting in viral transmission (1,2).

The efficacy of serologic testing in prevention of HBV transmission by transplantation is fortunate, as there is a relatively high rate of rapidly progressive liver failure when such transmission occurs in the peritransplant period (1). Fulminant hepatitis has been reported following liver transplantation when hepatitis delta virus infection has occurred in the setting of replicating HBV (81). With present testing methods and more effective infection control measures, HBV accounts for a small fraction of the 5% to 15% of allograft recipients who have chronic, usually progressive, liver disease (1).

Hepatitis C

Hepatitis C virus (HCV) accounts for virtually all of the cases of chronic liver disease in organ transplant patients. The clinical course of post-transplant HCV is far more indolent than that of HBV infection, with some increased incidence of opportunistic infection in the first few years, but no major impact on mortality until more than five years after transplant. From this point on, progressive liver failure and hepatocellular carcinoma begin to develop. In addition, cryoglobulinemia, membranoproliferative glomerulonephritis, and possibly a glomerulopathy akin to that associated with CMV infection may occur as a consequence of HCV infection (1,82,83).

HCV is a member of the flaviviridae family of RNA viruses and as such has considerable genetic variation, both in isolates from different individuals as well as from the same individual. This heterogeneity probably explains the failure of previous infection (even when anti-HCV is produced) to protect against rechallenge, even with the homologous strain. Depending on the method of analysis, there are 6 to 12 major HCV genotypes; the genotype present in a given population appears to be dependent on geography, mode of acquisition of HCV, and the time at which HCV infection was acquired. Whether genotype differences translate into different clinical effects or response to interferon therapy is currently an area of active research. In particular, genotype 1b has been reported to have higher replication rates, higher tissue RNA levels, more rapid disease progression, and a lower response rate to interferon alpha (1,82,83).

Primary HCV infection may be acquired from blood products, through sharing of needles for illicit drug use, by transplantation of an organ from an infected donor, during dialysis (again, through exposure to virus laden blood), or from unspecified sources within the community. Intrafamilial spread occurs sporadically and at a very low rate. Following infection, viremia can be demonstrated by PCR assay within a week. A serologic response to the virus can be demonstrated as early as three to four weeks or as late as several months after acquisition of the infection. Although incompletely studied, it is likely that immunocompromised patients may have greatly delayed or even absent antibody responses to the virus. When both antibody and PCR testing are carried out in the same individuals, it is clear that approximately 50% of antibody positive individuals harbor transmissible virus, with an undefined percentage of individuals who are anti-HCV negative also harboring the virus (1,82,83).

In the normal host, acute HCV is usually quite mild (overwhelming hepatic failure being a rare complication of this infection); fewer than 30% having symptoms referable to this infection. However, over time the majority of those infected develop evidence of chronic infection, with up to 20% of chronically infected individuals developing progressive liver disease with cirrhosis, hepatic failure, and/or hepatocellular carcinoma. Indeed, at many liver transplant centers, hepatitis C is the leading cause of liver disease requiring transplantation (1,82,83).

Renal transplantation (and likely also cardiac and lung) in the HCV-infected individual is associated with an increased risk of liver disease and death when compared with uninfected individuals, as immunosuppression appears to amplify the extent and effects of viral replication (see Chapter 17). We advocate careful evaluation of liver function, including biopsy, of anti-HCV–positive individuals prior to transplant because of the accelerated course HCV can sometimes take in these patients. However, the pace and impact of HCV infection is significantly less than that for HBV (1,82,83).

HCV is the cause of at least 60% of histologically demonstrated post-transplant hepatitis. Two patterns of infection are noted: primary infection acquired at the time of transplant and reinfection of the donor liver with endogenous HCV, which occurs in virtually all patients who are viremic at the time of transplant. In both groups of patients, histologic evidence of hepatitis is found in at least 2 of 3 individuals, with abnormal liver function tests being observed in less than half of these. In a small minority of individuals (<10%), a rapid progression to hepatic failure and/or cirrhosis, with the clinical course often being further complicated by life-threatening superinfection, will be noted. Overall, however, the first five years after transplant are not associated with excessive morbidity or mortality (1,82,83).

Therapy of HCV infection with interferon alpha is unsatisfactory; sustained responses are observed in fewer than 20% of individuals. Because of the lack of therapy, a great deal of attention has been focused on the prevention of acquisition of HCV, with significant controversy being engendered. The issue is the shortage of donors. Because of the lack of a statistically significant effect over the first three to five years after transplant, some centers advocate the utilization of anti-HCV–positive donors, particularly for recipients who are already anti-HCV positive. It should be emphasized that anti-HCV–positive recipients are not protected from rechallenge, and this policy is probably creating an artificial distinction between these two groups of recipients. While more information is being gathered (and until an effective therapy is available), we advocate the following approach: The use of HCV-infected extrahepatic allografts is justifiable in patients awaiting liver or heart transplants who are in extremis on life supports, in highly sensitized dialysis patients who are unlikely to have access to other kidneys, in elderly patients whose expected life span is less than 10 years, and, perhaps, in patients such as diabetics, in whom the improved duration and quality of life following transplantation might outweigh the risks of HCV infection. By contrast, every effort should be made, for the present, to exclude the use of such donors for children or young adults who have the potential for more than 10 years of life following successful transplantation (1,82,83).

Fungal Infection

Fungal infection in the organ transplant patient can be divided into two general categories: 1) pulmonary and/or disseminated infection with one of the geographically restricted systemic mycoses that have been previously discussed, and 2) opportunistic infection with fungal species that rarely cause invasive infection in the normal host (*Candida* species, *P. carinii*, *Aspergillus* species, *C. neoformans*, the *Mucoraceae*, etc.). These last are the most important forms of fungal infection observed in transplant patients, with three patterns of infection observed: primary infection, usually of the lungs, occasionally of the nasal sinuses, most commonly by *P. carinii, C. neoformans*, or *Aspergillus* species; sequential or concurrent secondary infection, either of the lungs or via infected intravenous lines, by *Candida* species or *Aspergillus* species; and primary cutaneous infection following a breach of skin integrity due either to trauma, an intravenous line that infiltrates with a necrotizing solution delivered to the skin and subcutaneous tissues, or water immersion injury due to *Aspergillus* species, the *Mucoraceae*, *Paecelomyces*, *Pseudallescheria boydii*, and a variety of dermatophytes. Quantitatively, as well as qualitatively, the most important opportunistic fungal infections in organ transplant patients are those caused by *Candida* species, *P. carinii*, *Aspergillus* species, *C. neoformans*, and the *Mucoraceae*. With the exception of *Pneumocystis*, it should be emphasized that the opportunistic fungal infections that occur in this patient population are highly associated with systemic metastases, particularly to brain, skin, and bone. Indeed, the first presenting complaint may be related to the metastasis rather than the primary portal of entry (1,84,85).

Candidal Infection in the Organ Transplant Recipient

Mucocutaneous infection with *Candida* species is not uncommon in transplant patients, due to overgrowth of colonizing species. Such overgrowth occurs when the nutrient supply (particularly glucose and glycogen) is increased because of elimination of the competing bacterial flora with broad spectrum antibacterials or because of the metabolic effects of uncontrolled diabetes, high-dose steroids, or pregnancy. The end result is oropharyngeal thrush, candidal esophagitis, vaginitis, intertrigo, and/or onychomycosis. Topical therapy with nonabsorbable fungal agents such as clotrimazole or nystatin will prevent the development of mucocutaneous infection and is usually effective treatment. If a prompt therapeutic response is not achieved, then systemic therapy with fluconazole or low-dose amphotericin is quite effective (1,84,85).

Invasive candidal infection in organ transplant patients usually occurs in the setting of surgery or some form of procedure or device that bypasses the primary mucocutaneous barrier to infection. These include the following (1,84,85):

1. Intravenous access device-related candidemia. Even transient candidemia of this sort requires systemic therapy with fluconazole or an amphotericin preparation (conventional amphotericin B, or one of the lipid-associated preparations of amphotericin that have recently been developed in order to decrease the nephrotoxicity of the amphotericin). Untreated candidemia in transplant patients carries a risk of visceral seeding of greater than 50%. In addition, the access device must be removed.
2. Technical complications of the transplant operation are highly associated with the development of deep wound/invasive candidal infection. This is particularly true when the previously described overgrowth factors are operative as well. In liver transplant patients, intra-abdominal bleeding, the need for re-exploration, vascular compromise with resulting tissue infarction, and undrained fluid collections are associated with a high risk of candidal infection. In renal transplant patients, indwelling catheters, nephrostomy tubes, and undrained fluid collections are similarly associated with candidal infection. In heart transplant patients as well, technical complications that require

indwelling foreign bodies, devitalized tissue, or are associated with a risk of candidal invasion. In lung transplant recipients, the bronchial suture line is at particular risk for candidal infection, and most centers employ systemic antifungal therapy (usually with fluconazole, unless colonization with fluconazole-resistant species, e.g., *C. glabrata, C. krusei*, and so forth, is noted). Similar considerations are involved with pancreatic transplants but, in addition, because of the increased burden of mucocutaneous *Candida* colonization in these diabetic individuals, the risk of infection is high enough to recommend fluconazole prophylaxis to all pancreas allograft recipients.

3. Renal transplant patients with poorly functioning bladders who develop asymptomatic candiduria (usually these are diabetics who have had Foley catheters in place) are at risk for the development of obstructing fungal balls at the ureterovesical junction, which, in turn, is associated with ascending candidal pyelonephritis and systemic dissemination. Less commonly, in liver transplant patients a similar phenomenon can occur in the biliary tree. Because of the gravity of these syndromes when fully developed, we advocate preemptive antifungal therapy to eliminate asymptomatic candidal carriage at these sites.

The group of transplant patients in whom candidal infection has been most completely studied are the liver transplant patients, in whom rates of candidal infection as high as 40% have been reported (see Chapter 19). In addition to technically impeccable surgery, there has been great interest in developing preventive antimicrobial strategies. Some groups advocate selective bowel decontamination with nonabsorbable antibacterials plus oral amphotericin; others advocate systemic fluconazole therapy peritransplant; and still others employ systemic amphotericin, particularly one of the newer lipid preparations. What is optimal is as yet unclear. It is clear, however, that no antifungal regimen can take the place of technically perfect surgery. Our own approach is to try to decrease bowel colonization with oral clotrimazole or nystatin prior to and following the transplant operation, and when systemic antibacterials are utilized, to reserve fluconazole for those patients with choledochojejunostomy biliary anastomoses, those who have been receiving high-dose antibacterial therapy prior to transplant, and those in whom the bowel is entered during the operation (1,85,86).

Systemic antifungal therapy for candidal infection should be linked to an aggressive approach to correcting any metabolic and anatomic abnormalities that led to infection in the first place. The choice of which systemic agent should be employed is based on the degree of clinical illness and knowledge of the species isolated. Patients who are acutely ill ("a therapeutic emergency") should have therapy initiated with conventional amphotericin, with a switch made to either fluconazole or a lipid amphotericin preparation once clinical stability has been achieved. Patients more subacutely ill ("diagnostic dilemmas") can be treated primarily with fluconazole or, in the case of a fluconazole-resistant infection, with a lipid amphotericin preparation (1–3).

Pneumocystis carinii *Infection in the Organ Transplant Recipient*

Pneumocystis carinii, long considered a protozoan (in part because of its response to certain forms of antiprotozoan therapy), is now classified as a fungus on the basis of studies of its ribosomal mRNA. *P. carinii* pneumonia occurs commonly in two groups of organ transplant patients in whom anti-*Pneumocystis* prophylaxis is not administered: 1) most transplant centers note an incidence of *Pneumocystis* without prophylaxis in 10% or more of patients from one to six months after transplant that is particularly associated with the occurrence of CMV infection; and 2) the 5% to 15% of patients who have had a poor outcome from transplantation, as previously described ("the chronic ne'er-do-wells"), have an incidence of *Pneumocystis* of 15% to 25% per year without prophylaxis (1,87,88).

Pneumocystis infection in transplant patients is thought to be primarily due to reactivation of previously acquired dormant infection. However, a variety of animal experiments, as well as human epidemiologic studies, suggest that *Pneumocystis* infection can be transmitted between immunosuppressed individuals. It is our policy, therefore, to isolate *Pneumocystis* patients from other transplant patients, particularly those patients whose net state of immunosuppression is at its highest. In addition to immunosuppressive therapy, especially recent exposure to high-dose corticosteroids, the components of the net state of immunosuppression that appear to be the most important risk factors for *Pneumocystis* are CMV infection, especially if CMV pneumonia is present (dual infection in the lung with CMV and *P. carinii* is not uncommon), and protein-calorie malnutrition (1,87,88).

The usual clinical presentation of *Pneumocystis* pneumonia is subacute, characterized by fever, nonproductive cough, tachypnea, and progressive dyspnea without pleurisy over several days. Physical examination is usually not very revealing other than fever, a rapid respiratory rate, and, on occasion, signs of bronchospasm. The degree of hypoxia and the extent of infiltrate on chest x-ray are often out of proportion to the subjective complaints or physical findings of the patient. More than 80% of patients have an x-ray picture that resembles that of viral or *Mycoplasma* pneumonia—a diffuse, bilateral, symmetric interstitial and alveolar pattern. The other major differential diagnostic consideration is congestive heart failure. Occasionally, atypical radiologic pictures may be noted—unilateral consolidation or nodular disease. Pleural effusions, cavitation, and lymphadenopathy on x-ray are quite unusual and, when present, suggest a concomitant process (1,87,88).

Diagnosis of *Pneumocystis* requires the demonstration of organisms in respiratory secretions or lung tissue by means of staining with Giemsa stain, Gomori methenamine-silver stain, or, optimally, fluorescein-labeled monoclonal antibodies directed against the organism. Bronchoalveolar lavage in these patients has a diagnostic sensitivity of greater than 90% (1,87,88).

Ideally, *Pneumocystis* should not occur in transplant patients because of the efficacy of prophylaxis. Low-dose trimethoprim-sulfamethoxazole (e.g., one single-strength tablet at bedtime) is the regimen of choice because of its near 100% efficacy in preventing not only *Pneumocystis* but also listeriosis, nocardiosis, urinary tract infection and urosepsis, and, possibly, toxoplasmosis. At this dose there is no adverse interaction with cyclosporine or tacrolimus. Patients who cannot tolerate trimethoprim-sulfamethoxazole should be considered for desensitization or be provided with alternative anti-*Pneumocystis* prophylaxis—atovaquone, monthly pentamidine, or dapsone. Optimal duration of anti-*Pneumocystis* prophylaxis is a matter of controversy, with some groups advocating it for life while others restrict it to the first 6 to 12 months after transplant as well as for the chronic ne'er-do-wells (1,87,88).

Treatment of *P. carinii* pneumonia in transplant patients is far more difficult than preventing it, as both trimethoprim-sulfamethoxazole and pentamidine (the two first line therapies for this infection) at the doses required to treat this infection have a high rate of toxic side effects and adverse interactions with cyclosporine and tacrolimus. Typically, trimethoprim-sulfamethoxazole is given at a dose of 20 mg of trimethoprim and 100 mg of sulfamethoxazole per kg daily in three or four divided doses for 14 to 21 days (with dosage adjustments for renal dysfunction); pentamidine is administered at a dose of 4 mg/kg/day for a similar time period. The two drugs appear to be equally effective, with the combination of drugs offering no therapeutic advantage. Of note, the administration of folinic acid to prevent bone marrow toxicity from high-dose trimethoprim-sulfamethoxazole may result in an increased rate of therapeutic failure. Patients presenting with clinically significant hypoxemia will likely benefit from a brief course of high-dose steroids in conjunction with the anti-*Pneumocystis* drugs. A commonly employed regimen is 40 mg of prednisone twice daily for five days, followed by 40 mg a day for five days, 20 mg a day for five days, and then a return to the baseline prednisone dose (1,87,88).

Aspergillus *Infection in the Organ Transplant Recipient*

Aspergillus species are commonly found in the environment as saprophytes on decaying vegetation. *Aspergillus* infection in the organ transplant patient usually occurs in one of two ways. Most commonly, aerosolized spores are delivered to the lower respiratory tract (75% to 90% of infections), nasal sinuses (5% to 10%), palate, or epiglottis (occasional cases). Alternatively, direct implantation occurs into tissues injured by trauma or surgery (5% to 10% of infections). Another potential source of *Aspergillus* infection for these immunosuppressed patients is the smoking of marijuana, as marijuana samples are often heavily laden with *Aspergillus* spores. Person-to-person spread of this infection does not occur. The major effect of *Aspergillus* infection in transplant patients is invasive infection (unlike the nonimmunosuppressed host, in whom a variety of allergic and colonization syndromes are not uncommon consequences of the inhalation of these spores). *Aspergillus* species can colonize any abnormal mucocutaneous surface, which is most apparent in the lung, where areas of bronchiectasis or preexisting cavities may become colonized with these organisms. Transplant patients differ from nonimmunosuppressed patients in regard to such colonization in one important respect: tissue invasion will occur in 50% to 70% of individuals whose respiratory tracts are colonized (1,3,85).

A single *Aspergillus* species, *A. fumigatus*, accounts for 50% to 75% of cases of invasive aspergillosis, with *A. flavus* responsible for most of the remaining cases. There are three hallmarks of invasive aspergillosis whatever the portal of entry, all stemming from the ability of these organisms to invade blood vessels: 1) hemorrhage, 2) tissue infarction, and 3) metastatic spread. In approximately 50% of cases metastases, particularly to the brain and skin, have occurred at the time of initial diagnosis, and in a significant number of these patients, the presentation is due to the metastasis (e.g., a seizure or focal neurologic defect secondary to a brain metastasis or an unexplained skin lesion) rather than the primary infection at the portal of entry (1,3,85).

Patients with invasive aspergillosis may present with a fever of unclear origin (in addition to the previously mentioned metastatic disease). More commonly, however, the presentation reflects disease at the portal of entry. In the case of the lung, the presenting symptoms are dyspnea, tachypnea, nonproductive cough, pleuritic chest pain, and hemoptysis in addition to fever and chills. In the lung transplant recipient, a necrotizing process involving the bronchial suture line can occur following the inoculation of *Aspergillus* spores. In all transplant patients, the characteristic x-ray picture reveals one or more nodular infiltrates that progress rapidly, are often cavitating, and not infrequently cross lung fissures. However, early in the process the conventional chest x-ray may be negative, while the chest computerized tomographic (CT) scan can reveal the process in a timely fashion. Additionally, the full extent of the disease, as well as a guide to biopsy, is best defined by CT (1,3,85,89,90).

Definitive diagnosis of invasive aspergillosis is via biopsy for culture and pathology. Blood cultures are almost invariably negative; indeed, most blood cultures positive for *Aspergillus* species should be regarded as contaminants. A presumptive diagnosis of invasive pulmonary aspergillosis can be made in patients with a clinically compatible syndrome and x-ray, coupled with the isolation of *A. fumigatus* or *A. flavus* from respiratory secretions. This is sufficient to initiate systemic antifungal therapy; however, other agents may have a similar presentation (1,3,85,89).

Amphotericin B remains the gold standard for the treatment of invasive pulmonary aspergillosis. Whether one of the lipid preparations of amphotericin is as effective as conventional amphotericin as primary therapy remains to be demonstrated. At present, it would seem appropriate to initiate therapy with conventional amphotericin (0.6–1.5 mg/kg/day), switching to a lipid preparation (5.0–7.5 mg/kg/day) once renal toxicity intervenes, and utilizing oral itraconazole (200–400 mg/day) only as long-term wrap-up therapy. The concern with itraconazole is the reliability of absorption. In those patients in whom itraconazole is utilized earlier in the course, there is a need to monitor blood levels to ensure adequacy of therapy. In patients with focal disease of the lung, in those with invasion of the nasal sinuses, and in those with primary cutaneous invasion, surgical resection in combination with systemic amphotericin therapy is necessary (1–3).

Cryptococcal Infection in the Organ Transplant Recipient

Cryptococcosis is a systemic fungal disease caused by the yeast *Cryptococcus neoformans*. The organism is found throughout the world, with sites contaminated by pigeon and chicken excreta being particularly enriched. Aerosolized cryptococci are inhaled and primary infection is established in the lung, with subsequent spread to regional lymph nodes via draining lymphatics. This event is probably quite common in the general population, causing at most an influenza-like syndrome and, in the majority, asymptomatic infection. In a small number of patients, progressive primary infection of the lung and/or bloodstream dissemination occurs. Alternatively, reactivation of a dormant focus results in recognizable pulmonary disease with secondary dissemination (1,89).

Cryptococci in nature are often unencapsulated; after inhalation a polysaccharide capsule develops that is markedly antiphagocytic for both granulocytes and monocytes. The organism itself is quite bland, producing no toxins and causing subacute and chronic disease that is often quite subtle in clinical presentation. Person-to-person spread is not recognized to occur. Cell-mediated immunity is the key host defense against this process, and hence organ transplant patients are at high risk. Either primary or reactivation infection, particularly the latter, can occur in the transplant patient. For unclear reasons, cryptococcosis is rare in the first six months after transplant, occurring primarily in the late period. Asymptomatic pulmonary nodules can occur in any transplant patient, with the more serious disease (e.g., central nervous system disease and disseminated infection) occurring primarily in the "chronic ne'er-do-well" population (1,85,89).

The clinical effects of cryptococcal infection in the transplant patient can be divided into the following three general categories (1,85,89):

1. *Pulmonary Infection*. Pulmonary disease is the most common manifestation of cryptococcosis in the transplant patient. Asymptomatic nodules discovered on routine chest x-ray is the most common manifestation of such infection. Diagnosis and treatment of this "benign" disease is important because, if left untreated, there is a high risk of subsequent disseminated disease. In the most immunosuppressed of transplant patients, a progressive pneumonia, with enlarging mass lesions or segmental consolidation, often with cavitation, is observed on x-ray. As a general rule, unless the x-ray is taken for other reasons, the x-ray reveals far more extensive disease than the clinical presentation would suggest—a "flu-like syndrome," minimal nonproductive cough or dyspnea, and a low-grade fever or none at all.
2. *Central Nervous System Infection*. *C. neoformans* possesses a unique tropism for the central nervous system (CNS), with meningitis and meningoencephalitis being common manifestations of infection with this organism. In contrast, mass lesions of the brain and spinal cord are relatively unusual. The most common presentation is unexplained fever and headache of several days' to weeks' duration, occasionally accompanied by nausea, dizziness, ataxia, impaired mentation, and irritability. The major feature of this condition is a basilar meningitis, which can result in decreased visual acuity, diplopia, facial numbness and weakness, papilledema, and a variety of cranial nerve palsies (most commonly of the sixth cranial nerve). Although patients may complain of a stiff neck, true meningismus is seen in the minority of patients. As the disease progresses, hydrocephalus may develop. The key point to be emphasized is that unexplained headache may be the only presenting manifestation of CNS cryptococcosis.
3. *Disseminated/Metastatic Infection*. *C. neoformans* can metastasize to any site of the body, but most commonly does so to the skin, skeletal system, or urinary tract. In particular, the skin is involved in approximately 1 of 4 patients with invasive cryptococcal infection and may be the first clue to the presence of disseminated disease. Skin lesions most often appear as erythematous papules or acneiform lesions, but cellulitis closely mimicking bacterial cellulitis and vesicular lesions resembling herpetic vesicles may also occur. In approximately 10% of cases involvement of the skeletal system occurs, with slowly progressive osteolytic lesions unaccompanied by periosteal proliferation being the usual presentation. The kidney and other sites in the urinary tract are not uncommonly seeded during the course of bloodstream dissemination, and the prostate serves as a potential reservoir for recrudescent infection.

Diagnosis of cryptococcal infection is made by demonstration of the organism in tissue biopsies, isolation of the organism from bodily fluids, or the demonstration of the cryptococcal capsular polysaccharide in a body fluid. The capsular polysaccharide antigen may be found in the blood, cerebrospinal fluid (CSF), or bronchoalveolar lavage fluid of infected patients. Detection and titering of antigen levels is important not only for diagnosis and assessment of the microbial burden, but also to determine the response to therapy. An essential part of the diagnostic evaluation of any transplant patient with cryptococcosis is a "metastatic work-up"—bone scan, CT scan of the brain and chest, lumbar puncture, and blood and urine cultures—in order to assess the full extent of disease. Therapy is designed to cure infection at all sites of involvement, not just the site of initial diagnosis (1,85,89).

Treatment of cryptococcosis can be with either amphotericin (with or without flucytosine) or fluconazole. Available evidence suggests that at six months the two therapies are equally effective, although amphotericin may gain control earlier. Our approach is to use fluconazole (400 mg/day) as the sole treatment if the patient is subacutely ill, but to initiate therapy with amphotericin (0.6–1.0 mg/kg/day) if the patient has more advanced disease, switching to fluconazole once improvement has occurred. It is important to reemphasize that fluconazole therapy will almost invariably require a decrease in cyclosporine or tacrolimus dose in order to avoid toxic levels. Duration of therapy is controversial, with some groups advocating fixed courses of six to eight weeks. Our approach is to treat until all evidence of disease is gone, and then add an additional "buffer" of two to four weeks (1,85,89).

Mucoraceae Infection in the Organ Transplant Recipient

The term *mucormycosis* encompasses infection caused by fungi of the family Mucoraceae, the most important of which are *Rhizopus*, *Mucor*, and *Absidia* species. These organisms are ubiquitous saprophytes that grow on decaying vegetable matter or other organic materials. In the transplant patient, mucormycosis is most common in diabetics, those with acidosis (particularly ketoacidosis), those being treated with deferoxamine for iron-overload syndromes, and those whose skin has been damaged by adhesive or Elastoplast tape laden with fungal spores or a caustic, infiltrating intravenous line (1,85,89).

Mucormycosis is initiated when aerosolized spores are inoculated onto the paranasal sinuses, nasal mucosa, or lower respiratory tract, or are introduced directly onto traumatized skin. The pathologic hallmark of mucormycosis is the invasion of blood vessels by broad, nonseptate hyphae that branch at right angles, resulting in hemorrhage and tissue infarction. In many ways this process resembles invasive aspergillosis. Important differences exist, however; mucormycosis spreads contiguously much more aggressively than invasive aspergillosis, producing more tissue infarction and hemorrhage. As a result, treatment of mucormycosis with antifungal agents alone is unrewarding and surgical resection is the therapy of choice. Conversely, metastatic spread via the bloodstream is relatively uncommon with mucormycosis (1,85,89).

There are three major forms of mucormycosis in the transplant patient (1,85,89):

1. *Rhinocerebral Mucormycosis.* Rhinocerebral infection usually begins on the palate or in the nasal sinuses and spreads contiguously into the orbit, and then into the brain. Early in the process the patient becomes febrile, toxic, with headache, lethargy, and loss of vision. A black eschar on the palate or nasal mucosa may be the earliest sign of this process. As the process evolves, retinal artery invasion (producing blindness, proptosis, and cavernous sinus thrombosis) or internal carotid artery thrombosis, or both, commonly occurs. Very quickly, the second, third, fourth, and sixth cranial nerves are affected. The typical picture is that of a blind, proptotic eye draining black necrotic pus with ptosis, pupillary dilatation, and complete ophthalmoplegia.
2. *Pulmonary Mucormycosis.* Mucormycosis of the lungs is a rapidly progressive necrotizing process that presents with fever, toxicity, pleurisy, nonproductive cough, and hemoptysis. Chest x-ray reveals focal, usually nodular, infiltrates that cavitate rapidly. Diagnosis requires biopsy.
3. *Cutaneous Mucormycosis.* Cutaneous infection occurs when Mucoraceae are inoculated into skin that has been damaged by trauma, catheters for intravenous infusion, or, uncommonly, as a result of hematogenous dissemination. A common series of events is the application of Elastoplast or adhesive tape laden with fungal spores to surgical wounds or intravenous sites. The end result is skin lesions characterized by frank infarction with a black eschar or ecthyma gangrenosum-like abnormalities.

Diagnosis of mucormycosis is based on pathologic assessment of biopsy material. Culture, even of biopsy material, is relatively insensitive, with sputum, blood, and other bodily fluids rarely yielding the correct diagnosis. Mucormycosis should be considered a medical emergency, with the need for early diagnosis and therapy. Therapy is ablative surgery (a "cancer operation with clean margins"), with adjunctive high-dose amphotericin therapy (1.25–1.5 mg/kg/day) directed at treating microscopic foci that remain. Careful assessment of the surgical specimen, both by frozen section in the operating room and after processing of permanent slides, must be carried out to ensure that the total process has been removed. The usual error in patient management is the failure to resect sufficient tissue at first operation (1,85,89).

Mycobacterial Infection in the Organ Transplant Recipient

The incidence of tuberculosis and the rate of extrapulmonary disease are considerably higher in the transplant population than that observed in the general population. A variety of forms of disease have been observed, ranging from cavitary pulmonary disease to miliary disease, from bowel disease to skeletal disease, and from skin to CNS disease. There have been instances in which the graft carried the infection from donor to recipient or when the graft was secondarily infected in the recipient as part of hematogenous dissemination of the organisms. An unusually high rate of bone and joint involvement has been noted in transplant patients with tuberculosis. Also, it is important to emphasize that epidemic disease can occur on a transplant unit if prompt identification and isolation of infected individuals is not accomplished. If active disease is detected in a transplant patient, we advocate 9 to 12 months of therapy, preferably with three bactericidal drugs (e.g., isoniazid, rifampin, pyrazinamide and fluoroquinolone are commonly used) (1–3,91–104).

Given the nature of the immunosuppressive therapy being administered, it is not surprising that mycobacterial infection is an important issue in transplant patients. Routine tuberculin testing prior to transplant should be part of the evaluation of every transplant candidate, although, admittedly, uremic and debilitated individuals could be falsely negative. An important and controversial issue is the appropriate response to a positive tuberculin test. On the one hand, the guidelines of the American Thoracic Society have traditionally recommended one year of isoniazid prophylaxis for individuals with positive tuberculin tests who are being treated with prolonged courses of immunosuppression. On the other hand, because of drug interactions with cyclosporine, tacrolimus, and perhaps corticosteroids, and because of the common occurrence of viral hepatitis in transplant patients, some transplant centers have advocated watchful waiting unless other risk factors are present. We advocate that reliable patients with positive tuberculin tests and no other risk factors should be closely followed after therapy. Those with one or more of the following risk factors should receive one year of isoniazid prophylaxis: recent tuberculin conversion; Asian, African, or Native American heritage; the presence of other immunosuppressing conditions, including protein-calorie malnutrition; a history of active tuberculosis, particularly if it was inadequately treated; and the presence of significant abnormalities on chest x-ray (1–3,105,106).

In addition to typical mycobacterial infection, atypical mycobacterial infection has been observed in transplant patients. This can be divided into two general categories: 1) pulmonary, skin, skeletal, and disseminated infection related primarily to *M. kansasii*, but occasionally also to such other species as *M. chelonae* and *M. xenopi*; and 2) skin infection alone with a variety of relatively less virulent mycobacterial species, including *M. marinum*, *M. haemophilum*, *M. thermoresistibile*, and *M. chelonae*. Atypical mycobacterial infection is often superimposed on sites of previous tissue injury. Management of atypical infection is with surgical debridement and treatment with a multiple-drug regimen (isoniazid, rifampin, and other drugs) that is chosen on the basis of in vitro sensitivity testing (1).

CLINICAL SYNDROMES OF PARTICULAR IMPORTANCE IN THE ORGAN TRANSPLANT RECIPIENT

Pneumonia

Pneumonia is the most common form of life-threatening infection observed in organ transplant patients (see Chapter 28). In approaching this problem, the epidemiologic and timetable considerations previously discussed are of great importance in arriving at an appropriate diagnosis. As outlined in Table 36.3, the combination of the mode of presentation of the pneumonia and the type of radiologic abnormality seen is quite helpful in narrowing the diagnostic considerations. In addition, the following principles should be kept firmly in mind (1,90):

1. Early diagnosis is the cornerstone of effective therapy. Because the prognosis of transplant patients is quite good if the pneumonia is effectively treated, then an aggressive diagnostic approach is clearly indicated.
2. CT scanning of the chest is of great utility in evaluating the extent of the pulmonary process, in helping with differential diagnostic considerations, and in guiding invasive diagnostic procedures.

Table 36.3. Differential Diagnosis of Fever and Pulmonary Infiltrates in the Compromised Host According to Roentgenographic Abnormality and the Rate of Progression of the Symptoms

Chest X-ray Abnormality	Acute*	Subacute/Chronic
Consolidation	Bacterial, including *Legionella* Thromboembolic Hemorrhage (Pulmonary edema)	Fungal Nocardial Tuberculous Tumor (Viral, drug-induced, radiation, *Pneumocystis*)
Peribronchovascular	Pulmonary edema Leukoagglutinin reaction (Bacterial)	Viral *Pneumocystis* Drug-induced (Fungal, nocardial, tuberculous, tumor)
Nodular infiltrate	(Bacterial, pulmonary edema)	Tumor Fungal Nocardial Tuberculous (*Pneumocystis*)

* An acute process is one that develops and requires medical attention in a relatively few hours (<24). A subacute/chronic process develops over several days to weeks. Note that unusual causes of a process are in parentheses.

Source: Modified from Rubin RH, Greene R. Clinical approach to the compromised host with fever and pulmonary infiltrates. In: Rubin RH, Young LS, eds. Clinical approach to infection in the compromised host. 3rd ed. New York: Plenum, 1994:121–162.

3. Invasive diagnostic procedures are essential for evaluating transplant patients with pneumonia. Such diagnostic procedures are initiated if the etiology of the pneumonia is not immediately apparent on examination of an expectorated or induced sputum specimen. At the present time, there are three major diagnostic procedures to be considered in this context: open or thorascopic lung biopsy; percutaneous aspiration biopsy; and bronchoscopic evaluation by bronchoalveolar lavage with or without transbronchial biopsy. Choice among these procedures is determined by two factors: pace of the illness, and morphology and location of the infiltrate. If the patient is acutely ill, and is deteriorating rapidly, then immediate lung biopsy is indicated as it is likely that only one opportunity for diagnosis will exist and the definitive (or most invasive) procedure should be carried out without delay. If the patient is more subacutely ill, then one of the less invasive procedures should be performed, with lung biopsy available if such an attempt fails to yield the diagnosis. Patients with focal, pleural-based lesions, particularly if a cavity is present, should be approached via a percutaneous aspiration biopsy; those with diffuse disease should undergo bronchoscopy based procedures (see also Chapter 28).

Central Nervous Infection

CNS infection is a not uncommon cause of morbidity and mortality in the organ transplant patient, occurring in 1% to 5% of individuals (see Chapter 33). There are four distinct clinical CNS syndromes that occur in organ transplant patients, each with its own diagnostic considerations (1,107–109):

1. *Acute Meningitis.* The most important cause of acute meningitis in this patient population is *L. monocytogenes*. In addition, the more common causes of meningitis that affect the general population can occur in these patients (there being nothing protective about immunosuppressive therapy in preventing pneumococcal, meningococcal, or *Haemophilus influenzae* meningitis), but these are uncommon.
2. *Subacute to Chronic Meningitis.* The most important cause of meningitis that presents over several days to weeks is *C. neoformans*, although such organisms as *M. tuberculosis*, *Coccidioides immitis*, and *Histoplasma capsulatum* can cause an identical clinical syndrome (subacute onset of fever and headache, sometimes associated with a decreased state of consciousness, with a lymphocytic pleocytosis and hypoglycorrhachia on cerebrospinal fluid examination) in the proper epidemiologic setting.
3. *Focal Brain Infection Causing Focal Neurologic Disturbances.* The most important causes of focal brain infection are those processes that are metastatic from a pulmonary portal of entry—most commonly, *Aspergillus fumigatus*, but also *N. asteroides* and other less common processes such as other fungi and *M. tuberculosis*. In addition, *L. monocytogenes* and *T. gondii* can produce focal brain disease (in the case of *Listeria* there is a particular propensity for producing brainstem disease, either alone or in combination with a meningitis picture).
4. *Progressive Dementia.* Although the most common causes of dementia in the transplant patient are metabolic disturbances and cyclosporine or tacrolimus toxicity, progressive dementia caused by the polyomavirus, JC virus, can be an important part of the presentation of the CNS disease, progressive multifocal leukoencephalopathy.

If one then considers these entities in the context of the timetable of expected infection after transplant, the following observations can be made: In the first month after transplant CNS infection is uncommon, unless an unusual epidemiologic exposure has occurred or the infection was initiated pretransplant. Virtually all CNS syndromes in this time period are due to toxic (CNS effects of cyclosporine or tacrolimus or toxicity from OKT-3, which can include an aseptic meningitis) or metabolic abnormalities. In the period from one to six months after transplant, listeriosis, aspergillosis, toxoplasmosis, and nocardiosis occur in the absence of antimicrobial preventative strategies, particularly in patients with CMV infection. In the late period, cryptococcosis and other opportunistic infections occur, primarily in the chronic ne'er-do-wells (1).

The presentation of CNS infection in the organ transplant patient may be very different from that in the normal host. In particular, the anti-inflammatory effects of the immunosuppressive therapy being administered may obscure the signs of meningeal irritation usually associated with meningitis in the nonimmunosuppressed individual. Any transplant patient with an unexplained headache, especially if febrile, should undergo a neurologic evaluation, including CT scan and lumbar puncture. Magnetic resonance imaging (MRI) should be considered in the patient with spinal cord findings, the patient with unexplained focal neurologic finding, and the patient with an abnormal CSF examination that is unexplained even in the face of a negative CT scan. The MRI scan is more sensitive than the CT, although more nonspecific findings may be observed (1) (see also Chapter 33).

Dermatologic Infection

The skin is important in the consideration of infection in the organ transplant patient, serving as both a potential portal of entry for pathogens and as a site of common metastasis for disseminated disease, which is often the first such manifestation of this event ("an early warning system"). The rich blood supply of the skin makes dissemination of infection from the skin and to the skin quite possible, particularly in immunocompromised individuals. Normally, the skin is quite resistant to microbial invasion because of at least three nonspecific factors: 1) intact keratinized layers of the skin, which prevent penetration of microorganisms; 2) dryness of the skin, which retards the growth of such organisms as the Enterobacteriaceae, *Pseudomonas aeruginosa*, and *Candida* species; and 3) the suppressant effect of the normal skin flora, which appears to reduce colonization of pathogens, a phenomenon known as *bacterial interference*. Thus, the chances of significant infection of cutaneous origin are increased, particularly in the following circumstances (1,110,111).

1. Destruction by trauma or bypass by introduction of intravascular catheters of the previously intact keratinized layer of skin
2. Water immersion injury, including maceration that occurs under occlusive dressings
3. Alteration of the normal colonizing flora due to antibacterial therapy or metabolic disturbances such as diabetes mellitus

The effect of chronic steroid administration on the skin is another factor that may contribute to the susceptibility of the skin to microbial invasion. Steroid therapy appears to inhibit proliferation of fibroblasts, synthesis of mucopolysaccharides, and deposition of collagen. The net effect is thin and atrophic skin that heals poorly. Minor trauma generates lesions that tend to persist, providing potential portals of entry for pathogens (110).

It is useful to categorize cutaneous infections in transplant patients into four categories (1,110,111):

1. Infection originating in skin and being typical of that which occurs in immunocompetent persons, albeit with the potential for more serious illness (e.g., staphylococcal or streptococcal cellulitis)
2. Extensive cutaneous involvement with pathogens that normally produce trivial or well-localized disease in immunocompetent patients (e.g., extensive dermatophyte infection or warts)
3. Infection originating from a cutaneous source and caused by opportunistic pathogens that rarely cause disease in immunocompetent patients but that may cause localized or widespread disease in compromised persons (e.g., *Paecelomyces*, *Penicillium*, and atypical mycobacterial infection)
4. Cutaneous or subcutaneous infection that represents metastatic spread from a noncutaneous site (e.g., 15% to 25% of cases of disseminated cryptococcosis, aspergillosis, candidiasis, and nocardiosis will manifest skin lesions early in their clinical course)

Perhaps the most important point to be emphasized about cutaneous infection, other than the need to protect the skin and to prevent it, is the fact that the morphology of the skin lesion may be greatly altered by the exogenous immunosuppression. The general rule that bears emphasis is that any unexplained skin lesion, even if innocent in appearance, merits biopsy for histology and culture. The usual dermatologic differential diagnosis based on morphology does not apply in many transplant patients, and an aggressive diagnostic approach is mandatory (1,110,111).

SUMMARY AND CONCLUSIONS

Despite the advances over the past three decades that have transformed organ transplantation from an interesting experiment in human immunobiology to the most practical means of rehabilitating patients with a variety of diseases causing destruction of kidney, heart, liver, and lung function, infection remains a major consideration. The risk of infection, particularly opportunistic infection, is determined by the interaction of three factors: the technical skill with which the perioperative care of the patient is accomplished, the epidemiologic exposures encountered, and the net state of immunosuppression. This last is a complex function, the most important ingredients of which are the nature of the immunosuppressive therapy being administered and the occurrence of infection with one of the immunomodulating viruses (CMV, EBV, HBV, HCV, and HIV). All of these factors are integrated into a timetable that delineates when different infections occur in the post-transplant course.

The effects of infection in the transplant patient go beyond the causation of particular infectious disease clinical syndromes. It is now apparent that cytokines, chemokines, and growth factors elaborated in the course of one process will influence others. In particular, allograft rejection and CMV infection are closely linked in a bidirectional relationship between these two processes. It is also important to emphasize that the altered inflammatory response of transplant patients can change the morphology of skin lesions and x-ray findings and render the clinical presentation of most infections more occult. For this reason, and because the most important factor in successful therapy is early diagnosis, an aggressive diagnostic approach, including invasive biopsies, is a cornerstone of patient management in this clinical setting.

Antimicrobial therapy in transplant patients is rendered difficult by the possibility of drug interactions with cyclosporine or tacrolimus. Because of this and the potential effects of infection in these patients, a particular emphasis is placed on the prevention of infection. Three modes of antimicrobial therapy are employed: therapeutic, prophylactic, and preemptive. A particularly important theme is that the therapeutic prescription for the transplant patient includes both an immunosuppressive strategy to prevent and treat rejection and an antimicrobial one to make it safe. Changes in one should trigger changes in the other.

REFERENCES

1. Rubin RH. Infection in the organ transplant recipient. In Rubin RH, Young LS, eds. Clinical approach to infection in the compromised host. 3rd ed. New York: Plenum, 1994:629–705.

2. Fishman JA, Rubin RH. Infection in the organ transplant recipients. N Engl J Med 1998;338:1741–1751.
3. Rubin RH, Tolkoff-Rubin NE. Antimicrobial strategies in the care of organ transplant recipients. Antimicrob Agents Chemother 1993;37:619–624.
4. Rubin RH, Colvin RB. The impact of cytomegalovirus infection on renal transplantation. In: Racusen LC, Solez K, Burdick J, eds. Kidney transplant rejection. 3rd ed. New York: Marcel Dekker, 1998:605–626.
5. Rubin RH, Wolfson JS, Cosimi AB, et al. Infection in the renal transplant recipient. Am J Med 1981;70:405–411.
6. Scowden EB, Schaffner W, Stone WJ. Overwhelming strongyloidiasis: an unappreciated opportunistic infection. Medicine (Baltimore) 1978;57: 527–544.
7. Purtilo DT, Meyers WM, Connor DH. Fatal strongyloidiasis in immunosuppressed patients. Am J Med 1974;56:488–493.
8. DeVault Jr GA, King JW, Rohr MS, et al. Opportunistic infections with *Strongyloides stercoralis* in renal transplantation. Rev Infect Dis 1990;12:653–671.
9. Luft BJ, Naot Y, Araujo FG, et al. Primary and reactivated *Toxoplasma* infection in patients with cardiac transplants. Ann Intern Med 1983;99: 27–31.
10. McGregor CG, Fleck DG, Nogington J, et al. Disseminated toxoplasmosis in cardiac transplantation. J Clin Pathol 1984;37:74–77.
11. Hakim M, Esmore D, Wallwork J, et al. Toxoplasmosis in cardiac transplantation. Br Med J 1986;292:1108.
12. Michaels MG, Wald ER, Fricker FJ, et al. Toxoplasmosis in pediatric recipients of heart transplants. J Clin Infect Dis 1992;14:847–851.
13. Dengler TJ, Strand N, Buhring I, et al. Differential immune response to influenza and pneumococcal vaccination in immunosuppressed patients after heart transplantation. Transplantation 1998;66:1340–1347.
14. Huzly D, Neifer S, Reinke P, et al. Routine immunization in adult renal transplant recipients. Transplantation 1997;63:839–845.
15. Hopkins C, Weber DJ, Rubin RH. Invasive aspergillus infection: possible non-ward common source within the hospital environment. J Hosp Infect 1989;12:19–25.
16. Rubin RH. The compromised host as sentinel chicken. N Engl J Med 1987;317:1151–1153.
17. Hibberd PL, Tolkoff-Rubin NE, Cosimi AB, et al. Symptomatic cytomegalovirus disease in the cytomegalovirus antibody seropositive renal transplant recipient treated with OKT3. Transplantation 1992;53:68–72.
18. Hibberd PL, Tolkoff-Rubin NE, Conti D, et al. Preemptive ganciclovir therapy to prevent cytomegalovirus antibody positive renal transplant recipients: a randomized controlled trial. Ann Intern Med 1995;123:18–25.
19. Grossi P, Kusne S, Rinaldo C, et al. Guidance of ganciclovir therapy with pp65 antigenemia in cytomegalovirus-free recipients of livers from seropositive donors. Transplantation 1996;61:1659–1660.
20. Rubin RH. Preemptive therapy in immunocompromised hosts. N Engl J Med 1991;324:1057–1059.
21. Singh N, Yu VL, Mieles L, et al. High dose acyclovir compared with short course preemptive ganciclovir therapy to prevent cytomegalovirus disease in liver transplant recipients. Ann Intern Med 1994;120:375–381.
22. Basgoz N, Preiksaitis JK. Post-transplant lymphoproliferative disorder. Infect Dis Clin N Am 1995;9:901–923.
23. Betts RF, Freeman RB, Douglas Jr RH, et al. Transmission of cytomegalovirus infection with renal allograft. Kidney Int 1975;8:385–392.
24. Ho M, Suwansirikul S, Dowling JN, et al. The transplanted kidney as a source of cytomegalovirus infection. N Engl J Med 1975;293:1109–1112.
25. Fiala M, Payne JE, Berne TV, et al. Transmission of cytomegalovirus infection with renal allograft. Kidney Int 1975;8:385–392.
26. Suwansirikul S, Rao N, Dowling JN, et al. Primary and secondary cytomegalovirus infection: clinical manifestations after renal transplantation. Arch Intern Med 1977;137:1026–1029.
27. Fietze E, Prosch S, Reinke P, et al. Cytomegalovirus infection in transplant recipients. The role of tumor necrosis factor. Transplantation 1994;58: 675–680.
28. Ward KN, Sheldon MJ, Gray JJ. Primary and recurrent cytomegalovirus infections have different effects on human herpesvirus-6 antibodies in immunosuppressed organ graft recipients. Absence of virus cross-reactivity and evidence for virus interaction. J Med Virol 1991;34:258–267.
29. Rubin RH. Impact of cytomegalovirus infection on organ transplant recipients. Rev Infect Dis 1990;12(suppl 7):S754–S766.
30. Rubin RH, Cosimi AB, Tolkoff-Rubin NE, et al. Infectious disease syndromes attributable to cytomegalovirus and their significance among renal transplant recipients. Transplantation 1977;24:458–464.
31. Marker SC, Howard RJ, Simmons RL, et al. Cytomegalovirus infection: a quantitative prospective study of 320 consecutive renal transplants. Surgery 1981;89:660–671.
32. Simmons RL, Lopez C, Balfour Jr HH, et al. Cytomegalovirus: clinical virological correlations in renal transplant recipients. Ann Surg 1974;180:623–634.
33. Simmons RL, Matas AJ, Rattazzi LC, et al. Clinical characteristics of the lethal cytomegalovirus infection following renal transplantation. Surgery 1977;82:537–546.
34. Hibberd PL, Snydman DR. Cytomegalovirus infection in organ transplant recipients. Infect Dis Clin N Am 1995;9:863–877.
35. Grefte A, van der Giessen M, van Son W, et al. Circulating cytomegalovirus (CMV)—infected endothelial cells in patients with active CMV infection. J Infect Dis 1993;167:270–277.
36. Gilbert MJ, Riddell SR, Plachter B, Greenberg PD. Cytomegalovirus selectively blocks antigen processing and presentation of its immediate early gene products. Nature 1996;383:720–722.
37. Patel R, Portela D, Badley AD, et al. Risk factors of invasive *Candida* and non-*Candida* fungal infections after liver transplantation. Transplantation 1996;62:926–934.
38. Falagas ME, Snydman DR, Griffith J, Werner BG. Exposure to cytomegalovirus from the donated organ is a risk factor for bacteremia in orthotopic liver transplant recipients. Boston Center for Liver Transplantation CMVIg Study Group. Clin Infect Dis 1996;23:468–474.
39. Braun WE, Nankervis G. Cytomegalovirus viremia and bacteremia in renal allograft recipients. N Engl J Med 1978;299:1318–1319.
40. Rand KH, Pollard RB, Merigan TC. Increased pulmonary superinfections in cardiac-transplant patients undergoing primary cytomegalovirus infection. N Engl J Med 1978;298:951–953.
41. Chatterjee SN, Fiala M, Weiner J, et al. Primary cytomegalovirus and opportunistic infections; incidence in renal transplant recipients. JAMA 1978;240:2446–2449.
42. Mackowiak PA, Goggans M, Torres W, et al. Relationship between cytomegalovirus and colonization of the oropharynx by gram negative bacilli following renal transplantation. Epidemiol Infect 1991;107:411–420.
43. Simmons RL, Fallon RJ, Schulenberg WE, et al. Do mild infections trigger the rejection of renal allografts? Transplant Proc 1970;1:419–423.
44. Rubin RH. The indirect effects of cytomegalovirus infection on the outcome of organ transplantation. JAMA 1989;261:3607–3609.
45. Kooijmans-Coutinho MF, Hermans J, Schrama E, et al. Interstitial rejection, vascular rejection, and diffuse thrombosis of renal allografts. Predisposing factors, histology, immunohistochemistry and relation to outcome. Transplantation 1996;61:1338–1344.
46. Lewis RM, Johnson PC, Golden D, et al. The adverse impact of cytomegalovirus infection on clinical outcome in cyclosporine–prednisone treated renal allograft recipients. Transplantation 1988;45:353–359.
47. Fryd DS, Peterson PK, Ferguson RM, et al. Cytomegalovirus as a risk factor in renal transplantation. Transplantation 1980;30:436–439.
48. Smiley ML, Wlodaver CG, Grossman RA, et al. The role of pretransplant immunity in protection from cytomegalovirus disease following renal transplantation. Transplantation 1985;40:157–161.
49. Richardson WP, Colvin RB, Cheeseman SH, et al. Glomerulopathy associated with cytomegalovirus viremia in renal allografts. N Engl J Med 1981;305:57–63.
50. Schooley RT, Hirsch MS, Colvin RB, et al. Association of herpesvirus infections with T-lymphocyte-subset alterations, glomerulopathy, and opportunistic infections after renal transplantation. N Engl J Med 1983;308:307–313.
51. Grattan MT, Moreno-Cabral CE, Starnes VA, et al. Cytomegalovirus infection is associated with cardiac allograft rejection and atherosclerosis. JAMA 1989;261:3561–3566.
52. Koskinen PK, Nieminen MS, Krogerus LA, et al. Cytomegalovirus infection and accelerated cardiac allograft vasculopathy in human cardiac allografts. J Heart Lung Transplant 1993;12:724–729.
53. Koskinen P, Lemstrom K, Bruggeman C, et al. Acute cytomegalovirus infection induces a subendothelial inflammation (endothelialitis) in the allograft vascular wall. A possible linkage with enhanced allograft arteriosclerosis. Am J Pathol 1994;144:41–50.
54. Normann SJ, Salomon DR, Leelachaikul P, et al. Acute vascular rejection of the coronary arteries in human heart transplantation: pathology and correlations with immunosuppression and cytomegalovirus infection. J Heart Lung Transplant 1991;10:674–687.
55. O'Grady JG, Alexander GJ, Sutherland S, et al. Cytomegalovirus infection and donor/recipient HLA antigens: interdependent cofactors in pathogenesis of vanishing bile duct syndrome after liver transplantation. Lancet 1988;2:302–305.

56. Reinke P, Fietze E, Ode-Hakim S, et al. Late acute renal allograft rejection and symptomless cytomegalovirus infection. Lancet 1994;344:1737–1738.
57. Gallay BJ, Alpers CE, Davis CL, et al. Glomerulonephritis in renal allografts associated with hepatitis C infection: a possible relationship with transplant glomerulopathy in two cases. Am J Kidney Dis 1995;26:662–667.
58. Chou S. Newer methods for diagnosis of cytomegalovirus infection. Rev Infect Dis 1990;12(suppl 7):S727–S736, 1990.
59. Erice A, Holm MA, Gill PC, et al. Cytomegalovirus (CMV) antigenemia assay is more sensitive than shell vial cultures for rapid detection of CMV in polymorphonuclear blood leukocytes. J Clin Microbiol 1992;30:2822–2825.
60. Fox JC, Griffiths PD, Emery VC. Quantification of human cytomegalovirus DNA using the polymerase chain reaction. J Gen Virol 1992;73:2405–2408.
61. Manez R, Kusne S, Rinaldo C, et al. Time to detection of cytomegalovirus (CMV) DNA in blood leukocytes is a predictor for the development of CMV disease in CMV-seronegative recipients of allografts from CMV-seropositive donors following liver transplantation. J Infect Dis 1996;173: 1072–1076.
62. Niubo J, Perez JL, Martinez-Lacasa JT, et al. Association of quantitative cytomegalovirus antigenemia with symptomatic infection in solid organ transplant patients. Diagn Microbiol Infect Dis 1996;24:19–24.
63. Sinzger C, Plachter B, Stenglein S, et al. Immunohistochemical detection of viral antigens in smooth muscle, stromal, and epithelial cells from acute cytomegalovirus gastritis. J Infect Dis 1993;167:1427–1433.
64. Snydman DR, Werner BG, Dougherty NN, et al. A randomized, double-blind, placebo-controlled trial of cytomegalovirus immune globulin prophylaxis in liver transplantation. Ann Intern Med 1993;119:984–991.
65. Winston DJ, Wirin D, Shaked A, et al. Randomised comparison of ganciclovir and high-dose acyclovir for long-term cytomegalovirus prophylaxis in liver transplant recipients. Lancet 1995;346:69–74.
66. Duncan SR, Gugurich WF, Iacono AT, et al. A comparison of ganciclovir and acyclovir to prevent cytomegalovirus after lung transplantation. Am J Respir Crit Care Med 1994;150:146.
67. Sen P, Winston DJ, Holt CD, et al. Long-term ganciclovir prophylaxis for successful prevention of primary cytomegalovirus (CMV) disease in CMV-seronegative liver transplant recipients with CMV-seropositive donors. Transplantation 1997;64:1614–1617.
68. Turgeon N, Fishman JA, Basgoz N, et al. Effect of oral acyclovir or ganciclovir therapy after preemptive intravenous ganciclovir therapy to prevent cytomegalovirus disease in cytomegalovirus seropositive renal and liver transplant recipients receiving antilymphocyte antibody therapy. Transplantation 1998;66:1780–1786.
69. Starzl TE, Nalesnik MA, Porter KA, et al. Reversibility of lymphomas and lymphoproliferative lesions developing under cyclosporine–steroid therapy. Lancet 1984;2:584–587.
70. Straus SE, Cohen JI, Tosato G, et al. Epstein-Barr virus infections: biology, pathogenesis, and management. Ann Intern Med 1993;118:45–58.
71. Preiskaitis JK, Diaz-Mitoma F, Mirzayans F, et al. Quantitative oropharyngeal Epstein-Barr virus shedding in renal and cardiac transplant recipients: relationship to immunosuppressive therapy, serologic responses, and the risk of posttransplant lymphoproliferative disorder. J Infect Dis 1992;166:986–994.
72. Rostaing L, Henry S, Cisterne JM, et al. Efficacy and safety of lamivudine on replication of recurrent hepatitis B after cadaveric renal transplantation. Transplantation 1997;64:1624–1627.
73. Davis CL, Gretch DR, Carithers Jr RL. Hepatitis B and transplantation. Infect Dis Clin N Am 1995;9:925–942.
74. Stevenson WC, McCullough C, Pruett TL. Liver transplantation for hepatitis B cirrhosis: clinical sequela of passive immunization. Clin Transplant 1996;10:668–675.
75. Terrault NA, Zhou S, Combs C, et al. Prophylaxis in liver transplant recipients using a fixed dosing schedule of hepatitis B immunoglobulin. Hepatology 1996;24:1327–1333.
76. Grellier L, Mutimer D, Ahmed M, et al. Lamivudine prophylaxis against reinfection in liver transplantation for hepatitis B cirrhosis. Lancet 1996;348:1212–1215.
77. Tipples GA, Ma MM, Fischer KP, et al. Mutation in HBV RNA-dependent DNA polymerase confers resistance to lamivudine in vivo. Hepatology 1996;24:711–713.
78. Ling R, Mutimer D, Ahmed M, et al. Selections of mutations in the hepatitis B virus polymerase during therapy of transplant recipients with lamivudine. Hepatology 1996;24:711–713.
79. Carman WF, Trautwein C, van Deursen FJ, et al. Hepatitis B virus envelope variation after transplantation with and without hepatitis B immune globulin prophylaxis. Hepatology 1996;24:714–717.
80. Bartholomew MM, Jansen RW, Jeffers LJ, et al. Hepatitis B virus resistance to lamivudine given for recurrent infection after orthotopic liver transplantation. Lancet 1997;349:20–22.
81. Marsman MA, Wiesner RH, Batts KP, et al. Fulminant hepatitis B virus; recurrence after liver transplantation in two patients also infected with hepatitis delta virus. Hepatology 1997;25:434–438.
82. Terrault NA, Wright TL, Pereira BJG. Hepatitis C infection in the transplant recipient. Infect Dis Clin N Am 1995;9:943–964.
83. Fishman JA, Rubin RH, Koziel MJ, Pereira BJG. Hepatitis C virus and organ transplantation. Transplantation 1996;62(2):147–154.
84. Paya CV. Fungal infections in solid organ transplantation. Clin Infect Dis 1993;16:677–683.
85. Hadley S, Karchmer AW. Fungal infections in solid organ transplant recipients. Infect Dis Clin N Am 1995;9:1045–1074.
86. Arnow PM. Prevention of bacterial infection in the transplant recipient: the role of selective bowel decontamination. Infect Dis Clin N Am 1995;9: 849–862.
87. Fishman JA. Prevention and treatment of infection due to Pneumocystis carinii. Antimicrob Agents Chemother 1998;42:995–1004,1300–1314.
88. Fishman JA. *Pneumocystis carinii* and parasitic infections in transplantation. Infect Dis Clin N Am 1995;9:1005–1044.
89. Wheat LJ. Fungal infections in the immunocompromised host. In: Rubin RH, Young LS, eds. Clinical approach to infection in the compromised host. 3rd ed. New York: Plenum, 1994:211–238.
90. Rubin RH, Greene R. Clinical approach to the compromised host with fever and pulmonary infiltrates. In: Rubin RH, Young LS, eds. Clinical approach to infection in the compromised host. 3rd ed. New York: Plenum, 1994:121–162.
91. Rattazzi LC, Simmons RL, Spanos PK, et al. Successful management of miliary tuberculosis after renal transplantation. Am J Surg 1975;130:359–361.
92. Oliver WA. Tuberculosis in renal transplant patients. Med J Aust 1976;1: 828–829.
93. Bell TJ, Williams GB. Successful treatment of tuberculosis in renal transplant recipients. J Soc Med 1978;71:265–268.
94. Ascher NL, Simmons RL, Marker S, et al. Tuberculous joint disease in transplant patients. Am J Surg 1978;135:853–856.
95. Riska H, Kuhlback B. Tuberculosis and kidney transplantation. Acta Med Scand 1979;205:637–640.
96. Vaz AJ. Miliary tuberculosis and the adult respiratory distress syndrome in a renal transplant recipient. Chest 1979;75:412.
97. Lloveras J, Peterson PK, Simmons RL, et al. Mycobacterial infections in renal transplant recipients: seven cases and a review of the literature. Arch Intern Med 1982;142:888–892.
98. Coutts II, Jegarajah S, Starsk JE. Tuberculosis in renal transplant recipients. Br J Dis Chest 1979;73:141–148.
99. Spence RK, Dafoe DC, Rabin G, et al. Mycobacterial infections in renal allograft recipients. Arch Surg 1983;118:356–359.
100. Qumibi WY, al-Sibai MB, Taher S, et al. Mycobacterial infection after renal transplantation—report of 14 cases and review of the literature. QJM 1990;77:1039–1060.
101. Al-Sulaiman MH, Dhar JM, Al-Hasani MK, et al. Tuberculous interstitial nephritis after kidney transplantation. Transplantation 1990;50:162–164.
102. Higgins RM, Cahn AP, Porter D, et al. Mycobacterial infections after renal transplantation. QJM 1991;78:145–153.
103. Sterneck M, Ferrell L, Ascher N, et al. Mycobacterial infection after liver transplantation: a report of three cases and review of the literature. Clin Transplant 1992;6:55–61.
104. Sundberg R, Shapiro R, Darras F, et al. A tuberculosis outbreak in a renal transplant program. Transplant Proc 1991;23:3091–3092.
105. Thomas Jr PA, Mozes MF, Jonasson O. Hepatic dysfunction during isoniazid chemoprophylaxis in renal allograft recipients. Arch Surg 1979;114:597–599.
106. Higgins RSD, Kusne S, Reyes J, et al. Mycobacterium tuberculosis after liver transplantation: management and guidelines for prevention. Clin Transplant 1992;6:81–90.
107. Hooper DC, Pruitt AA, Rubin RH. Central nervous system infections in the chronically immunosuppressed. Medicine (Baltimore) 1982;61:166–188.
108. Rubin RH, Hooper DC. Central nervous system infection in the compromised host. Med Clin N Am 1985;69:281–296.
109. Hall WA, Martinez AJ, Dummer JS, et al. Central nervous system infections in heart and heart lung transplant recipients. Arch Neurol 1989;46:173–177.
110. Wolfson JS, Sober AJ, Rubin RH. Dermatologic manifestations of infections in immunocompromised patients. Medicine (Baltimore) 1985;64:115–133.
111. Haim S, Friedman-Birnbaum R, Better O, et al. Skin complications in immunosuppressed patients: follow-up of kidney recipients. Br J Dermatol 1973;89:169–173.

Chapter

37

Neoplastic Complications of Organ Transplantation

ISRAEL PENN

During the last 30 years numerous studies have shown that organ transplant recipients are prone to develop a variety of malignancies, many of which are rare in the general population. In this chapter we review the characteristics of these neoplasms and discuss the different patterns of tumors that are seen in nonrenal allograft recipients compared with renal transplant patients. We shall also discuss children compared with adults.

This chapter is based largely on data collected by the Cincinnati Transplant Tumor Registry (CTTR) (1–10), the only worldwide repository of data on this subject, but the observations of many investigators are included. Until March 1996 the CTTR accumulated data on 9120 types of cancer that arose in 8566 organ transplant recipients: 7116 kidney, 820 heart, 354 liver, 152 bone marrow, 60 pancreas, 30 lung, 29 combined heart and lung, 4 upper-abdominal organ "cluster" transplants, and 1 small bowel transplant.

AGE AND SEX OF PATIENTS

The tumors occurred in a relatively young group of patients whose average age at the time of transplantation was 42.5 years (range 8 days to 80 years) (1–3). Forty-two percent were younger than 40 years at the time of transplantation. The average age of the patients at the time of diagnosis of their neoplasms was 47 years. Sixty-seven percent of patients were male and 33% female, in keeping with the 2:1 ratio of male to female patients who undergo renal transplantation (1–3).

INCIDENCE OF POST-TRANSPLANT CANCERS

Overall the incidence of cancer is increased threefold to fourfold in organ allograft recipients compared with age-matched controls in the general population (11), but the incidence of some malignancies is increased even more (1–3). Many neoplasms that are frequently seen in the population at large (carcinomas of the lung, breast, prostate, and colon, and invasive uterine cervical carcinomas) showed no increase, or even a decrease, among transplant patients (Table 37.1) (1–3).

Only one type of cancer frequently seen in the general population was also encountered in significant numbers in transplant patients. Excluding lip cancers, the percentage of non-melanoma skin tumors (34%) was very similar to that observed in the general population (36% of all tumors) (12), but the proportion of squamous cell carcinomas (SCCs) was markedly increased (1–3,13). If non-melanoma skin cancers and in situ carcinomas of the cervix (2.4% of all tumors in transplant patients versus 1.4% in the general population) were excluded, as they are from most cancer statistics, a variety of tumors that occur infrequently in the general population were observed commonly in transplant patients (Table 37.2) (1–3).

These results are consistent with several epidemiologic studies that showed a 28- to 49-fold increased incidence of non-Hodgkin's lymphomas (11), a 29-fold increase in lip carcinomas (14), a 400- to 500-fold increase in Kaposi's sarcoma compared with controls of the same ethnic origin (15,16), a 100-fold increased incidence of vulvar and anal carcinomas (14), a 20- to 38-fold increased incidence of hepatocellular carcinomas (17), and a 4.3-fold increased risk of genitourinary cancers (13) (a rather broad definition including carcinomas of the kidney, ureter, bladder, cervix, vulva, and vagina).

The incidence of malignancy increases with the length of follow-up after transplantation. The actuarial probability of developing cancer among patients who received cardiac transplants during childhood was 7% at 1 and 2 years, 12% at 3 years, and 15% at 4 and 5 years (18). An Australasian study of 6596 recipients of cadaver renal transplants showed that the percent probability of developing neoplasia 24 years after transplantation was 66% for skin cancers, 27% for non-skin tumors, and 72% for any type of malignancy (13). These exceptional figures must be treated with some reserve, as most of the neoplasms were skin cancers (which are very common in Australia) and the number of 24-year survivors was small. Nevertheless, they stress the need to follow transplant patients indefinitely (1–3).

Table 37.1. General Population Versus Cincinnati Transplant Tumor Registry Patients (Percent of All Cancers)

Neoplasm	General Population	Transplant Recipients
Non-melanoma skin cancer	36%	34%
Carcinomas of prostate	23%	2%
Carcinomas of breast	14%	4%
Carcinomas of lung	13%	8%
Carcinomas of colon/rectum	10%	5%
Carcinomas of bladder	4%	3%
Invasive cancer of uterus	4%	2%
In situ cancer of cervix	1.4%	2.4%

Table 37.2. General Population Versus Cincinnati Transplant Tumor Registry Patients

Neoplasm	General Population[a]	Transplant Recipients[a]
Lymphomas	5%	24%
Carcinomas of lip	0.2%	6.7%[b]
Kaposi's sarcoma	Negligible	5.6%
Carcinomas of vulva/perineum	0.5%	3.5%
Carcinomas of kidney	2.3%	4.8%
Hepatobiliary cancers	1.5%	2.4%
Sarcomas (excluding Kaposi's)	0.5%	1.7%

[a] Percentage of all cancers, excluding non-melanoma skin cancer and in situ cervical cancers.
[b] Skin cancers also appeared in 49%.

INTERVAL BETWEEN TRANSPLANTATION AND DIAGNOSIS OF CANCER

Some cancers appeared at fairly distinct intervals after transplantation (1–3). In the general population, an interval of 5 to 20 years or even more elapses between exposure to many carcinogens and the development of overt tumors. In contrast, among transplant patients many neoplasms appeared a relatively short time after transplantation (Table 37.3).

VARIETIES OF DE NOVO MALIGNANCY

The CTTR data are shown in Table 37.4.

Cancers of the Skin and Lips

Cancers of the skin and lips were the most common neoplasms, comprising 3315 of the 9120 cancers (36%) (see Table 37.4). Cancers appeared on sun-exposed areas (Fig. 37.1 and Plate 39), particularly of the head and neck and

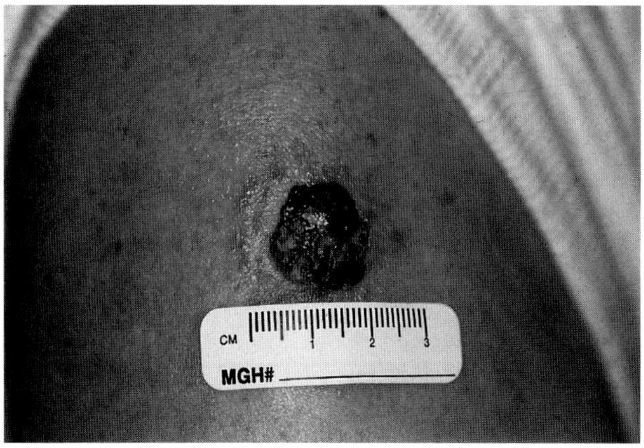

FIGURE 37.1. *Squamous cell carcinoma on the lateral upper arm in sun-damaged skin. This 52-year-old woman had undergone lung transplantation 7 years earlier and was being maintained on cyclosporine, azathioprine, and prednisone immunosuppression.*

Table 37.3. Time of Appearance of Neoplasms Following Transplantation and Initiation of Immunosuppression

Type of Cancer	Range in Months	Average in Months	Median in Months
Lymphomas	0.25–305.5	33	12
Kaposi's sarcoma	1–225.5	21	12.5
Carcinomas of kidney	1–213.5	55	41
Sarcomas (excluding Kaposi's)	2–239.5	70	43.5
Carcinomas of cervix	1.5–250	59	46
Hepatobiliary carcinomas	1–289.5	82	67.5
Skin cancers	1–313	83	69
Carcinomas of vulva/perineum	1.5–285.5	114	113.5
All cancers	0.25–324	62	46

Table 37.4. De Novo Cancers (n = 9120) in Organ Allograft Recipients

Type of Neoplasm	Number of Tumors*
Cancers of skin and lips	3315
Lymphomas	1560
Carcinomas of the lung	509
Kaposi's sarcoma	366
Carcinomas of uterus (309 cervix; 51 body; 3 unspecified)	363
Carcinomas of colon and rectum	320
Carcinomas of the kidney (273 host kidney; 30 allograft kidney; 12 unspecified)	315
Carcinomas of the breast	291
Carcinomas of the head and neck (excluding thyroid, parathyroid, and eye)	260
Carcinomas of the vulva, perineum, penis, and scrotum	229
Carcinomas of urinary bladder	202
Metastatic carcinoma (primary site unknown)	202
Leukemias	172
Hepatobiliary carcinomas	154
Carcinomas of prostate gland	154
Sarcomas (excluding Kaposi's sarcoma)	112
Carcinomas of thyroid gland	109
Cancers of stomach	107
Testicular carcinomas	74
Carcinomas of pancreas	72
Ovarian cancers	63
Miscellaneous tumors	171

* There were 8566 patients of whom 517 (6%) had two or more distinct tumor types involving different organ systems. Of these, 35 patients each had three separate types of cancer and 1 patient had four types.

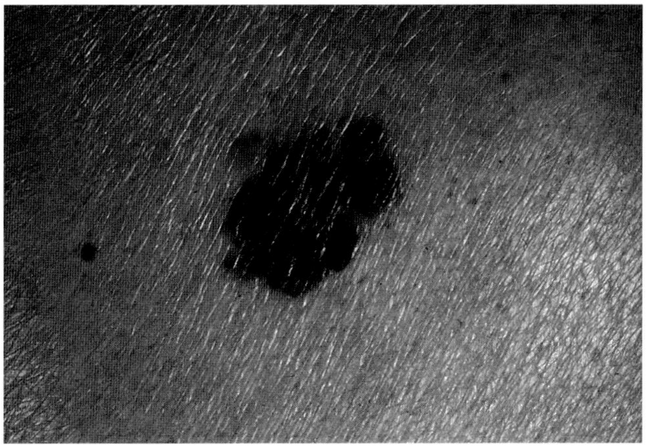

FIGURE 37.2. *Early superficial spreading melanoma on the back of a kidney transplant recipient receiving azathioprine and prednisone. Note the irregularly scalloped borders and central hypopigmentation that distinguish this lesion from a benign nevus.*

upper limbs (1–3,19). They occurred particularly in light-skinned individuals with blue eyes and blonde or red hair (19). The incidence of skin cancers frequently was related to the intensity of sunlight exposure (20–22). In geographic areas with limited exposure, there was a fourfold to sevenfold increase, but in localities with copious sunlight there was an almost 21-fold rise over the already high incidence expected in the local population. Almost all of the increase was in SCC (see below). However, exposure to sunlight was not the only factor involved. A surprisingly high incidence of SCC was reported from areas at higher latitudes, including Canada, Sweden, and Scotland, and may have been related to malignant change in papillomavirus-induced cutaneous warts, under the influence of immunosuppression, sunlight, and possibly other factors (1–3,11,21,23). For example, a British study of 291 renal allograft recipients showed that 59% had cutaneous warts and 22% had non-melanoma skin cancers (24).

As noted earlier, the incidence of skin cancer increases with the length of follow-up after transplantation. Australasian studies of 6596 recipients of cadaveric renal transplants showed a linear increase in the incidence of cutaneous neoplasms, reaching 66% to 70% at 20 years after transplantation (13,21). Similarly, a Dutch study showed a 10% incidence of non-melanoma skin cancers in renal transplant recipients at 10 years after transplantation, rising to 40% after 20 years (25).

The characteristics of skin cancer in transplant patients differed in several ways from those seen in the general population (1–3,13,19,21). Basal cell carcinoma (BCC) outnumbers SCC in the general population by 5 to 1, but the opposite occurred in transplant recipients in whom SCC outnumbered BCC by 1.8 to 1.0. SCC was calculated to occur at a frequency between 40 and 250 times higher than in the general population, BCC 10 times higher (25), and malignant melanoma 5 times higher (19). Malignant melanomas (Fig. 37.2 and Plate 40) comprised 5.4% of cutaneous neoplasms in the CTTR, in contrast with an incidence of 2.7% in the general population of the United States. In the general population SCC occurs mostly in persons over 60 years old; however, the average age among transplant patients was 30 years younger (22). In addition, the incidence of multiple skin cancers in the CTTR was remarkably high (at least 43%). Despite the CTTR representing a worldwide collection, the incidence of such skin cancers was similar to that seen only in nonimmunosuppressed individuals living in areas of copious sunlight (1–3). Some individual patients had more than 100 skin cancers. In some patients there apparently is a widespread skin abnormality with areas of unstable epithelium containing multifocal premalignant and malignant lesions (19).

The behavior of skin tumors in transplant patients also differed markedly from that seen in the general population, in whom skin tumors cause only 1% to 2% of all cancer deaths, the great majority from malignant melanoma. Squamous cell carcinoma was much more aggressive in transplant patients than in the general population, accounting for the majority of lymph node metastases and deaths from skin cancer (1–3). In the CTTR database, 5.8% of patients with skin cancers had lymph node metastases. In 195 patients with nodal metastases, 145 were from SCC, 35 from malignant melanoma, 14 from Merkel's cell tumor, and 1 from BCC. Similarly, 168 (5.1%) patients died of their skin cancers: 101 from SCC, 54 from malignant melanoma, 10 from Merkel's cell tumor, and 3 from BCC. Patients with skin cancer are also more likely to develop additional, more fulminant types of neoplasia than are allograft recipients without skin cancer (19).

Non-Hodgkin's Lymphomas

Of a total of 1560 lymphomas in the CTTR (see Table 37.4) only 42 (2.7%) were cases of Hodgkin's disease, which comprise 10% of lymphomas in the general population (12). Similarly, myeloma and plasmacytoma comprised only 58 cases (3.7%) compared with a 19% incidence among lymphomas in the general population (12). The bulk of post-transplant lymphomas (n = 1460) were non-Hodgkin's lymphomas (NHLs), which made up 93.6% of lymphomas compared with only 71% in the general population (1–3).

Morphologically, most NHLs were classified as immunoblastic sarcomas, reticulum cell sarcomas, microgliomas, or large cell lymphomas (1–3). Because many lesions straddle the ill-defined zone between infection and neoplasia, the term *post-transplant lymphoproliferative disorder* (PTLD) is frequently used to describe Epstein-Barr virus (EBV)-induced lymphoid proliferations (26). Although EBV infection occurs in most NHLs in transplant patients, some patients show no evidence of this virus despite a careful search for it (27). One author suggests that PTLD encompasses four disease groups: 1) uncomplicated post-transplant infectious mononucleosis, 2) benign polyclonal polymorphic B-cell hyperplasia, 3) early malignant transformation into polyclonal polymorphic B-cell lymphoma, and 4) monoclonal polymorphic B-cell lymphoma (28).

Of 608s NHLs in the CTTR that were studied immunologically, 86.3% arose from B lymphocytes, 13.3% were of T-cell origin, and 0.3% were of null cell origin (1–3). Fifty-three percent involved multiple organs or sites, while 47% were confined to a single organ or site. Post-transplant NHL differed from its counterpart in the general population in several ways (1–3,26,28,29). Whereas extranodal involvement occurs in from 24% to 48% of NHL patients in the community at large, it was present in 69% of NHLs in transplant patients. Surprisingly, one of the most common extranodal sites in transplant recipients was the central nervous system (CNS), which was involved in 296 of 1430 patients (21%) studied (1–3,9). (These figures excluded 11 patients with meningeal involvement only, and 8 patients whose cerebrospinal fluid showed lymphomatous cells without apparent CNS lesions.) Of this percentage, 9% included patients with systemic disease involving both the CNS and other organs, while 12% were confined to the CNS only. The 9% was similar to the 8% to 12% of CNS involvement

Table 37.5. Involvement of the Allograft by Non-Hodgkin's Lymphoma (1430 patients)

Renal	164
Hepatic	87
Pulmonary	33
Cardiac	27
Pancreatic	10
Bone marrow	8
Abdominal cluster organs	3
Small bowel	1
Total	**333 (23%)**

These figures include one patient with a combined kidney–pancreas transplant in whom both allografts were involved. Of 23 recipients of combined heart–lung transplants who developed NHL, in 15 (65%) it involved the heart and one lung allograft, in 1 (4%) it involved the heart and both lungs, and in 1 (4%) it involved the trachea. Almost all of the transplanted organs were affected in patients receiving abdominal cluster transplants.

by systemic NHL in the general population (9). However, most lesions in transplant patients occurred in the brain parenchyma, whereas in the general population they most often involved the leptomeninges, perivascular spaces, and nerve roots (9). The other 12% contrasted markedly with the percentage in the general population, in whom there is only a 1% to 2% incidence of primary CNS involvement by NHL (9). In both groups with primary CNS disease, the brain parenchyma was usually involved and meningeal involvement occurred infrequently (9). In the CTTR series, spinal cord lesions were most uncommon, resembling CNS lymphomas in the general population where the spinal cord was involved in only 0% to 5% in different series (9).

A remarkable finding in the CTTR data was the frequency of either macroscopic or microscopic allograft involvement, which occurred in 23% of patients with NHL (Table 37.5) (1–3). In some individuals with renal, cardiac, or hepatic allografts, the lymphomatous infiltrate was misdiagnosed as rejection when biopsies, performed because of allograft dysfunction, were studied microscopically.

The outcomes were studied in 999 patients with NHL (Table 37.6) (1–3). Of these, 178 patients (18%) had no treatment; in 88 of these patients (45%) the tumor was discovered only at autopsy. It is frustrating that 18% of patients with NHL died without treatment, because the diagnosis either was missed or was made too late for effective therapy to be instituted. No treatment data were available in 46 patients (5%). Treatment was given to 775 patients (78%), and of these, 307 (40%) had complete remissions. In 60 of these recipients (20%) the *only* treatment used was reduction or cessation of immunosuppressive therapy (1–3).

Kaposi's Sarcoma

The frequent occurrence of Kaposi's sarcoma (KS) in transplant recipients (see Table 37.4) was in marked contrast with

Table 37.6. Treatments Used in Non-Hodgkin's Lymphoma Patients Having Complete Remissions

Treatment	Multimodality Therapy[a] (Number of Patients)	Single Modality Therapy[b] (Number of Patients)
Decrease or cessation of immunosuppression	138	60
Excision	83	25
Acyclovir or ganciclovir	74	3
Chemotherapy	40	36
Radiotherapy	36	13
Immunotherapy		
Interferon	15	4[c]
Gamma-globulin	11	1[c]
Donor leukocytes/T cells	6	1[c]
Monoclonal anti-B-cell antibodies	3	—

[a] Used in 166 patients.
[b] Used in 141 patients.
[c] One patient received several types of immunotherapy (interferon, gamma-globulin, and donor T cells).

its incidence in the general population of the United States [prior to the acquired immunodeficiency syndrome (AIDS) epidemic] where it comprised only 0.02% to 0.07% of all neoplasms (1–3,10). The high incidence of KS in this worldwide collection of transplant patients is comparable to that seen in the general population only in tropical Africa, where it occurs with greatest frequency and comprises 3% to 9% of all neoplasms. It is remarkable that the number of transplant patients with KS in the CTTR (n = 366) exceeded those with carcinomas of the colorectum (n = 320), breast (n = 291), or prostate (n = 154) (see Table 37.4). Apart from individuals with AIDS, who frequently have KS, there is probably no other large series, except possibly in tropical Africa, in which the numbers of patients with KS exceed those who have these common tumors.

KS affected males more than females in a 3:1 ratio, a figure far less than the 9:1 to 15:1 ratio seen with KS in the general population (1–3,10,16). Transplant-related KS was rare in children (29). Nine of 116 patients (8%) who were tested for the human immunodeficiency virus (HIV) were positive (10). Three had acquired the infection from blood transfusions, one from homosexual activity, and one from the allograft, whose donor was HIV-positive.

KS was most common in transplant patients who were Arab, black, Italian, Jewish, or Greek (10,16). Two studies reinforce these findings. KS occurred in 1.6% of 820 Italian renal transplant recipients (30). Kaposi's sarcoma was the most common cancer in renal transplant recipients in Saudi Arabia, making up 76% of all neoplasms (31).

Fifty-nine percent of patients in the CTTR had nonvisceral KS confined to the skin, conjunctiva, or oropharyngolaryngeal mucosa. Forty-one percent had visceral disease, which involved mainly the gastrointestinal tract, lungs, and lymph nodes, but also affected other organs (1–3,10). Of 217 patients with nonvisceral disease, the lesions were confined to the skin in 212 patients (98%) and to the mouth or oropharynx in 5 (2%). The 148 patients with visceral disease had no skin involvement in 34 instances (23%), but 4 of them (3%) had oral involvement, which provided a readily accessible site for biopsy and diagnosis of the disease. Of those with nonvisceral disease, 117 (54%) had complete remissions following treatment. Interestingly, 38 (32%) of these remissions occurred when the *only* treatment was a drastic reduction of immunosuppressive therapy. In patients with visceral disease, only 40 of 148 patients (27%) had complete remissions. However, 25 of the 40 remissions (63%) occurred in response to reduction or cessation of immunosuppressive therapy only. Fifty-six percent of patients with visceral KS died. Of the deaths, 60 of the 83 patients (72%) died of the malignancy per se.

Of 39 kidney allograft recipients, in whom renal function was recorded following reduction or cessation of immunosuppressive therapy, 21 lost their allografts to rejection, 2 had impaired function, and 16 retained stable function (10).

Renal Carcinomas

There were 315 patients with carcinomas of the kidney (see Table 37.4). This figure excludes 273 patients who had lymphomatous involvement of the native or allograft kidneys and 3 patients who had renal sarcomas. Of the tumors, 249 (79%) were described as renal cell carcinomas, hypernephromas, clear cell carcinomas or adenocarcinomas; 38 (12%) as transitional cell carcinomas or urothelial carcinomas; and 28 (9%) as miscellaneous carcinomas.

An unusual feature was that 75 of the 315 patients (24%) had incidentally discovered renal malignancies, mostly renal cell carcinomas. These were discovered at the time of native nephrectomy for hypertension or other reasons, during work-up for other disorders, during operation for some other disease, or at autopsy examination.

Unlike most other neoplasms, which occurred as complications of immunosuppressive therapy, many renal carcinomas were related to the underlying kidney disease in renal allograft recipients (1–3,8). No explanation is available for the 16 carcinomas that occurred in cardiac transplant recipients and the 4 that occurred in liver allograft recipients. Most malignancies in renal allograft recipients arise in their own diseased kidneys, although 9% appeared in the renal allograft in the range of 2 to 213.5 (average 64) months after transplantation (8). Six of the 30 allograft tumors (20%) were diagnosed within 2 years of transplantation. It is possible that they may have been present in the allograft at the time of transplantation but were small enough to escape notice (8).

In various studies in the general population, 5% to 10% of renal neoplasms are carcinomas of the pelvis, whereas in the CTTR series, these accounted for 14% of malignancies (8). The increase is almost certainly due to the high incidence of analgesic nephropathy among renal allograft recipients, which occurred in 8% of CTTR patients with carcinomas of their native kidneys (8). This disorder is known to cause carcinomas in various parts of the urinary tract (32). This is borne out in the CTTR series in which 68% of patients with analgesia-related renal carcinomas have similar tumors elsewhere in the urinary tract (8). Another predisposing cause of cancers in renal transplant recipients is acquired cystic disease (ACD) of the native kidneys. It occurs in 30% to 95% of patients receiving long-term hemodialysis (33,34), and it is complicated by renal adenocarcinoma, which is increased 30- to 40-fold over its incidence in the general population (35). With a successfully functioning transplant, the ACD tends to regress (33), and presumably the risk of developing carcinoma also recedes. However, cases of persistent ACD and development of renal cell carcinoma have been reported in patients with successfully functioning renal allografts (9,36). The precise incidence of ACD-related carcinomas in renal transplant recipients is not known.

Carcinomas of the Vulva and Perineum

With the group of tumors that includes carcinomas of the vulva, perineum, scrotum, penis, perianal skin, or anus (see Table 37.4) (1–4), females outnumbered males by 2.5 : 1.0. This is in contrast with most other post-transplant cancers, where males outnumbered females by more than 2 : 1.

One-third of patients had in situ lesions (4). A disturbing feature is that patients with invasive lesions were much younger (average age 42 years) than their counterparts in the general population, whose average age is usually between 50 and 70 years. Of the 129 patients for whom information was available, 73 (57%) had a history of condyloma acuminatum (genital warts), which must be regarded as a premalignant lesion. In women, multicentric lesions were quite frequent; they not only involved several sites in the vulva, perianal area, or anus, but sometimes the cervix and/or vagina as well (1–4). Many patients with cancers of the vulva and perineum responded well to local or extensive excisions of their lesions, but 12% succumbed to the malignancy despite abdominoperineal resections or radical vulvectomies.

Carcinomas of the Uterus

Carcinomas of the cervix occurred in 11% of women with post-transplant cancers (see Table 37.4) (1–3). At least 72% of patients had in situ lesions. As mentioned above, the CTTR data showed only a small increase in the incidence of in situ uterine cervical carcinoma compared with the general population. This is surprising in view of two epidemiologic studies that showed a 14- to 16-fold increased incidence in transplant patients (37,38). This suggests that many cases are being missed. To avoid this error, every post-adolescent female transplant recipient should have regular pelvic examinations and cervical smears (1–4).

Hepatobiliary Tumors

Two epidemiologic studies showed a 20- to 38-fold increased incidence of hepatobiliary tumors, compared with controls (11,17). Most cases in the CTTR (see Table 37.4) were hepatomas. A substantial number of patients gave a preceding history of hepatitis B infection (1–3,39). A few cases with preceding hepatitis C virus infection have been encountered.

Sarcomas (Excluding Kaposi's Sarcoma)

The majority of non-Kaposi's sarcomas involved the soft tissues or visceral organs; cartilage or bone involvement was uncommon (1–3,10). Of the 112 sarcomas recorded in the CTTR database, the major types were fibrous histiocytoma (21 cases), leiomyosarcoma (19 cases), fibrosarcoma (12 cases), rhabdomyosarcoma (10 cases), hemangiosarcoma (9 cases), mesothelioma (6 cases), synovial sarcoma (4 cases), and miscellaneous sarcomas (31 cases).

Other Cancers

An increased incidence of other tumors was reported in some studies. For example, the Australia and New Zealand Dialysis and Transplant Registry noted a 289-fold increased incidence of endocrine cancers, a 5.6-fold increase of leukemia, a 2.5-fold increase in digestive organ cancers, a twofold increase in respiratory system tumors, and a 4.6-fold increase of miscellaneous cancers (13).

BIOLOGIC BEHAVIOR OF POST-TRANSPLANT NEOPLASMS

Neoplasms that occur in organ allograft recipients frequently demonstrate a more aggressive nature than do similar cancers in patients who have not undergone transplantation (39).

Tumors in Renal Versus Nonrenal Recipients

There were significant differences in tumor incidence in renal compared with nonrenal recipients (Table 37.7) (1–3,40). The striking incidence of lymphomas (45% versus 12%) in nonrenal transplant recipients is most likely related to the intensity of the immunosuppression given to this group. With renal transplant patients, severe rejection can be handled by returning the patient to dialysis treatment and discontinuing immunosuppressive therapy. With severe rejection of a cardiac, pulmonary, or hepatic allograft, death will result unless the patient's immunosuppressive therapy is substantially increased, except in rare instances when a new organ can be found to replace the failing allograft.

Table 37.7. Common Cancers in Renal Versus Nonrenal Recipients

Neoplasm	Renal (7630 tumors[a])	Nonrenal (1490 tumors[b])
Skin cancers	2965 (39%)	350 (23%)
Lymphomas	892 (12%)	668 (45%)
Kaposi's sarcoma	334 (4%)	32 (2%)
Carcinomas of cervix	297 (4%)	12 (<1%)
Renal tumors	295 (4%)	20 (1%)
Carcinomas of vulva/ perineum	217 (3%)	12 (<1%)

[a] In 7116 patients.
[b] In 1450 patients.

Table 37.8. Tumors in Pediatric Versus Adult Recipients (Percent of All Cancers)

Neoplasm	Pediatric: 447 Neoplasms[a]	Adult: 8673 Neoplasms[b]
Lymphoma	237 (53%)	1323 (15%)
Skin cancers	80 (18%)	3235 (37%)
Sarcomas	17 (4%)	95 (1%)
Carcinomas of vulva/anus	16 (4%)	213 (2%)
Kaposi's sarcoma	12 (3%)	354 (4%)
Hepatobiliary carcinomas	12 (3%)	142 (2%)

[a] In 434 patients.
[b] In 8132 patients.

Many renal recipients have been followed for 10 to 30 years after transplantation, whereas only a minority of nonrenal recipients have been followed for so long. This may account for the higher incidence of late-appearing malignancies of the skin, uterine cervix, vulva, and perineum in the renal recipients. The higher incidence of carcinomas of the kidney in renal recipients may reflect the influence of analgesic nephropathy and ACD of the kidney in predisposing patients to renal neoplasms (8).

Cancers in Pediatric Versus Adult Recipients

The types of cancers seen in pediatric organ allograft recipients (patients aged 18 years or less) were very different from those observed in the general childhood population and from those seen in adult organ allograft recipients (Table 37.8) (7). By far the most common malignancy was NHL. This is surprising as most NHLs occur in adults at a median age of 56 years; these lymphomas are relatively uncommon in children (7). However, children with congenital immunodeficiency disorders are prone to develop cancers, of which the most common (44%) is NHL (41).

One reason why NHL is more common in immunodeficient pediatric patients is because children have more lymphoid tissues than adults. These tissues become the sites of NHL when they are exposed to EBV infection or other stimuli (7). Primary EBV infections are more common in children than in adults, and, in immunosuppressed patients, EBV infection is more likely to lead to NHL (7). Even more striking is the high incidence of NHL in pediatric recipients of nonrenal organs, among whom NHL comprises the great majority of tumors (7) (see also Chapter 20).

As regards skin cancers among transplant recipients, children differ from adults in that melanomas comprised 14% of skin cancers among children compared with 5% among adults (7). In the general population malignant melanoma is rare during childhood, yet in the CTTR series 6 of 11 melanomas occurred in patients aged 9 to 18.5 years (average 12 years) at the time of their diagnosis. Four of the 11 patients (36%) were bone marrow transplant recipients.

Leiomyosarcoma is most uncommon in childhood, but 3 cases of smooth muscle tumors were recently reported in liver or liver and small bowel recipients (42). Of 19 leiomyosarcomas and smooth muscle tumors in the CTTR, 6 occurred in children. Another case, labeled as a fibrosarcoma, may possibly have been a myofibroblastic variant of leiomyosarcoma (10). Remarkably, in six of these seven cases the liver was involved, including four liver allografts. Smooth muscle tumors are also seen in AIDS patients, mainly children, with liver involvement in at least five cases (43).

Among patients who received transplants during childhood, carcinomas of the vulva and perineum subsequently occurred in 16 when they were between 20 and 39 years of age (7). It is disturbing to see these types of neoplasms, which typically occur among the elderly, in such young individuals (7). All cases occurred in renal allograft recipients. Fortunately, 50% of the lesions were "in situ" carcinomas and were readily treatable.

With increasingly prolonged follow-up times, we must be concerned about the types of cancer that may appear in patients who received transplants during childhood and thus were maintained on chronic immunosuppressive therapy for several decades (7).

DIAGNOSIS OF THE COMMON POST-TRANSPLANT CANCERS

Some cutaneous disorders that frequently occur in transplant patients may closely resemble skin cancers (1,2). They include warts, hyperkeratoses, and keratoacanthomas. If there is any question of malignancy one should biopsy suspicious lesions. Lip cancers may also pose diagnostic problems, as they are often atypical, appearing as superficial ulcers that do not have an indurated base or rolled everted edges. Occasionally multiple superficial lip carcinomas may occur simultaneously.

The clinical presentation of NHL is extremely variable (1,2). Some patients are completely asymptomatic or present with a syndrome resembling infectious mononucleosis. Other presenting features include fever, night sweats, upper respiratory infection, weight loss, diarrhea, abdominal pain, lymphadenopathy, and tonsillitis. Occasionally tonsillar enlargement may be so severe as to require emergency tracheostomy. As the gastrointestinal tract is often involved, a not infrequent presentation is acute perforation of an intestinal lesion causing peritonitis. Less commonly, gastrointestinal bleeding or intestinal obstruction is the major feature. At times patients present with a solitary lesion in the liver, lung, spleen, or other organ. Occasionally, allograft involvement imitates rejection and the diagnosis is made when an atypical lymphoblastic infiltrate is found in a biopsy specimen. Some patients with widespread disease present with a confusing picture of disseminated sepsis and multiple organ failure, and the diagnosis is made only at autopsy examination.

A possible CNS lymphoma should be suspected whenever an allograft recipient develops neurologic symptoms (1,2). A comprehensive work-up is necessary and may include examination of the cerebrospinal fluid, computerized axial tomography, electroencephalography, radionuclide brain scan, cerebral angiography, and magnetic resonance imaging. Such tests are useful in excluding other causes of neurologic symptoms such as hypertensive encephalopathy, meningitis, brain abscess, or intracranial bleeding (see also Chapter 33).

A clinician should suspect KS whenever a transplant patient, particularly one belonging to the ethnic groups mentioned above, presents with reddish blue macules (Fig. 37.3 and Plate 41) or plaques in the skin or oropharyngeal mucosa, or with apparently infected granulomas that fail to heal (1,2). If the diagnosis is confirmed, a thorough work-up, including CT scans of the chest and abdomen and upper and lower gastrointestinal endoscopy, is needed to exclude any internal visceral involvement.

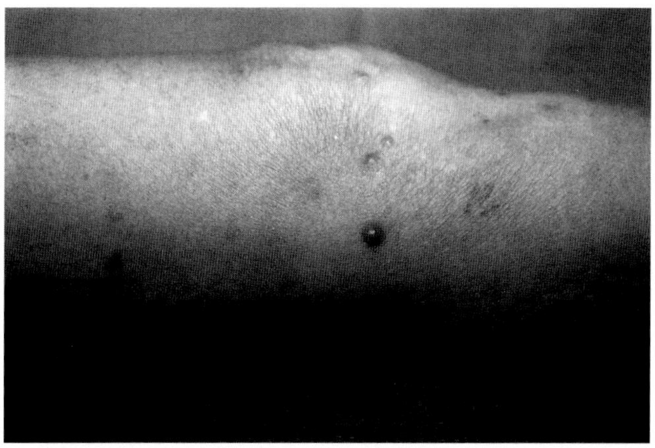

FIGURE 37.3. *Typical clinical appearance of reddish, elevated, nodular Kaposi's sarcoma lesion of the skin. This 57-year-old liver allograft recipient had received tacrolimus, azathioprine, and steroid induction therapy and was then maintained on tacrolimus–prednisone suppression.*

There is no evidence to support routine screening of the transplant population with serum tumor markers as a useful approach to the early diagnosis of neoplasia in these patients (44).

PREVENTION OF POST-TRANSPLANT MALIGNANCIES

Immunosuppression

The level of immunosuppressive therapy should be kept as low as is compatible with good allograft function (5). Renal transplant physicians and surgeons have learned by bitter experience that it is foolhardy to persist with intense immunosuppressive therapy in the face of repeated or persistent rejection; rather, they have found it safer to discontinue immunosuppression and return the patient to dialysis therapy until he or she has recovered sufficiently to attempt another transplant procedure.

In dealing with severe rejection of a nonrenal allograft, the transplant team does not have the means to provide long-term artificial support should the transplant fail. Consequently, high doses of immunosuppressive agents are often administered to salvage the graft. One may try to replace a failing liver or cardiac allograft before the patient develops complications of heavy immunosuppression, but the shortage of donors frequently precludes timely retransplantation.

Viral Infections

Whenever possible, one should attempt to prevent viral infections in immunosuppressed patients (5). As the incidence of hepatocellular tumors is increased mainly in renal transplant patients, and as this disease is frequently preceded by hepatitis B infection, inoculation of potential renal transplant candidates with hepatitis B vaccine may well prevent this type of tumor (5).

Many groups use prophylactic acyclovir or ganciclovir in the first few weeks after transplantation in patients who are at high risk for EBV infection, particularly when OKT-3 or ALG is used to treat rejection (45,46). Whether these prophylactic agents will truly reduce the incidence of EBV-related malignancies remains open to question, as both agents are virustatic rather than virucidal, and viral proliferation may resume once administration of these drugs is discontinued (5) (see also Chapter 36).

As papillomavirus infections (suspected as causes of carcinomas of the cervix, vulva, and perineum) are transmitted sexually, patients should be advised to practice barrier methods of contraception (condoms) (5,37). All postadolescent females should undergo regular pelvic examinations and cervical smears. All premalignant lesions, such as condyloma acuminatum or uterine cervical dysplasia, should be treated at an early stage to try to prevent progression to in situ or frankly invasive cancers (5).

Sunlight Exposure

As sunlight exposure is an important contributory factor to the development of skin cancers (1–3), patients should be advised to avoid excessive exposure; light-skinned individuals with blue eyes and blond or red hair are at particularly high risk for skin cancer (5).

Unfortunately, many patients, such as farmers, sailors, or construction workers, already had many years of sun exposure before becoming candidates for transplantation (5). If patients' occupations or hobbies make it necessary for them to spend much time in the sunlight, they should wear a wide-brimmed hat or a sun visor as well as long-sleeved shirts. Alternatively, they should protect their skin by regular use of sunscreens that filter out the harmful ultraviolet-B rays. After transplantation, those patients who spend prolonged periods of time in the sun must be examined on a regular basis, and any premalignant skin lesions must be carefully observed or treated.

Because metabolites of azathioprine, mainly methylnitrothioimidazole and related imidazole compounds (47), sensitize the skin to sunlight, some investigators have suggested that azathioprine therapy should be phased out and substituted by other immunosuppressive agents (5).

Ulcerative Colitis

Liver allograft recipients with chronic ulcerative colitis need regular colonoscopies to detect any dysplastic changes which may indicate the need for panproctocolectomy to prevent colon cancer (see also Chapters 19 and 29).

TREATMENT OF POST-TRANSPLANT MALIGNANCIES

In managing patients with premalignant skin lesions or early cancers, a useful treatment is topical use of 0.05% tretinoin cream (a retinoid). This is effective in treating warts and keratoses in organ allograft recipients, and it may perhaps inhibit cutaneous carcinogenesis (48). Treatment of skin cancers includes surgical excision, cryosurgery, chemosurgery, or radiotherapy (1–3).

In situ carcinomas of the uterine cervix respond well to simple hysterectomy, cervical conization, or cryotherapy (1–3). In situ carcinomas or small neoplasms of the vulva and perineum are treated by local excision. Large lesions require extensive operations such as total vulvectomy and inguinal node dissection, or abdominoperineal resection (4).

Other malignancies are treated by standard surgical, radiotherapeutic, or chemotherapeutic modalities.

The antiviral agents acyclovir or ganciclovir may be used to treat EBV-related NHL (1–3,28). Interferon alpha (IFN-α) has been used to treat some patients with KS, NHL, or other neoplasms (1–3). Interferon is a potent immune modulator that increases membrane expression of class I antigens of the major histocompatibility complex, T-cell–mediated cytotoxicity, and natural killer (NK) cell function (49,50). Thus, it may stimulate rejection, but conflicting findings have been reported in renal allograft recipients. Two studies showed an increased number of acute rejection episodes leading to graft failure when either high-dose or low-dose interferon was used immediately after transplantation, whereas two other studies showed no difference in the incidence of rejection or graft dysfunction using low-dose regimens (51).

Immunosuppression Strategies

In managing post-transplant malignancies, we must consider reduction or cessation of immunosuppressive therapy (1–3,10,29). The value of this approach is borne out by experience with inadvertently transplanted malignancies, some of which regressed completely following cessation of immunosuppressive therapy and removal of a renal allograft (1–3). Furthermore, cessation or reduction of immunosuppressive therapy when used by itself resulted in a substantial number of complete remissions of NHL (20%; 61 of 307 remissions) and KS (40%; 63 of 157 remissions) (24). Disappointingly, such treatment has rarely caused regression of epithelial tumors.

A limitation of the reduction or cessation of immunosuppressive therapy is that this may precipitate allograft rejection. Renal allograft recipients may be salvaged by return to dialysis therapy, but nonrenal allograft recipients may die of this complication. For example, this approach caused impaired function or allograft loss from rejection in 22 of 34 renal recipients treated for KS (10). Similarly, in a series of 14 renal recipients whose NHL was treated by reduction or cessation of immunosuppression (among other methods), 8 of 12 survivors lost their allografts (52). The CTTR does not routinely collect data on allograft function, but in 22 patients with NHL for whom such data are available and whose lymphomas underwent complete remission when the *only* treatment was reduction of immunosuppression, 16 (73%) had either acute or chronic rejection (6 of 9 kidney, 5 of 7 heart, 4 of 5 liver transplants, 1 combined kidney and pancreas allograft). More encouraging findings were noted in the Pittsburgh series of 131 cases of PTLD. Although histologic evidence of rejection of liver allografts was often seen, the graft could be salvaged in most cases (53). Similarly, although histologic rejection was observed in heart and heart–lung recipients, no grafts were lost as a result of this therapy (53).

Questions arise as to whether it is safe to resume immunosuppressive therapy without neoplastic recurrence in patients whose tumors regressed following reduction or cessation of immunosuppression. Two of eight renal allograft recipients who lost their kidneys following treatment of NHL were subsequently retransplanted 8 months and 4 years, respectively, after the original diagnosis of tumor without recurrence (52). Of eight liver allograft recipients with post-transplant NHL, six died despite reduction of immunosuppression, while two survived with complete remissions following cessation of immunosuppression except for a small maintenance dose of prednisone. Both eventually developed chronic rejection and underwent retransplantation 10 and 12 months after the initial transplantation. They were well 2 and 12 months, respectively, after their second transplants (54). Of 157 patients in the CTTR who had complete remissions of KS following reduction or cessation of immunosuppressive therapy, 7 had recurrent KS either when immunosuppressive therapy was resumed in the regular dosage or when they underwent second transplants. KS regressed once more when immunosuppression was again reduced or discontinued, but at least four patients lost their allografts to rejection (10).

In patients requiring cytotoxic therapy of widespread cancers, we must remember that most antineoplastic agents depress the bone marrow (1–3). Therefore, it is prudent to stop or reduce azathioprine dosage during such treatment to avoid severe bone marrow depression. As most cytotoxic drugs have immunosuppressive side effects, satisfactory allograft function may persist for prolonged periods. Treatment with prednisone may be continued, as it is an important component of many cancer chemotherapy protocols. Because many patients, particularly those with NHL, are already heavily immunosuppressed, chemotherapeutic agents should be used with caution. Some patients have died of overwhelming infections following intensive chemotherapy.

Non-Hodgkin's Lymphomas

As NHL is so important, special mention should be made of its management. In suitable patients with localized disease, excision or radiotherapy may suffice. In other patients with localized lesions or with widespread disease, immunosuppressive therapy should be reduced. In patients who are seriously ill, immunosuppressive therapy may even be stopped except for a small maintenance dose of prednisone. Theoretically, polyclonal lesions are more likely to respond to reduced immunosuppression than are lesions with clonal rearrangement involving a high proportion of cells. However, this distinction is not absolute, and a trial of reduced immunosuppression appears to be indicated regardless of clonal status (54).

Because most lesions are associated with EBV infection, the patients should be given acyclovir or ganciclovir. High doses of intravenous gamma globulin have been used as part of the treatment of NHL (55). Successful results have occurred in some patients with B-cell lymphomas treated with B-cell–specific monoclonal antibodies (56). In addition, infusions of allogeneic leukocytes containing cytotoxic T cells presensitized to EBV have been used successfully to treat a small number of lymphomas that occurred after solid organ or bone marrow transplantation (57,58).

In situations where no improvement occurred with the above measures, further attempts to boost antiviral immunity have included the administration of IFN-α and other forms of immunotherapy (59). Failure to cause complete regression is an indication for using chemotherapy.

ETIOLOGY OF POST-TRANSPLANT MALIGNANCIES

There is probably a complex interplay of multiple factors in the etiology of the various malignancies. Among these, oncogenic viruses and defective immunity probably are the major influences.

Oncogenic Viruses

Transplant recipients frequently are infected by viruses that are believed to cause a variety of neoplasms in animals and humans. The short induction time of KS and many types of NHL is in keeping with a viral etiology (1,6).

Epstein-Barr Virus

In the general population, nasopharyngeal carcinoma, Burkitt's lymphoma, Hodgkin's disease, rare T-cell lymphomas, and some thymomas have been linked to EBV. In immunodeficient patients, such as those with congenital defects, AIDS patients, and transplant recipients, there is a strong association between EBV infections and the development of lymphoproliferative disorders and lymphomas (1,6).

Infection of B lymphocytes usually results in latent infection without replication or release of virus (60). When EBV infects B cells, its linear genome circularizes to form an episome, an extrachromosomal element, in the cell nucleus (60). The result is transformation of B cells, which acquire the capacity to proliferate indefinitely. In vitro, latently infected B cells express only 10 of approximately 80 genes encoded by the virus: small RNAs called EBERS, six nuclear proteins called EBNAs, and one alert membrane protein (LMP) (60,61). Of these, two have known oncogenic potential: LMP and EBNA-2 (62).

Important in the process of the immortalization of B cells is the establishment of an autocrine loop whereby they produce growth factors, including interleukin 6 (IL-6) (60), that stimulate their proliferation. It is possible that large cyclosporine doses may foster development of EBV-transformed B-cell lymphomas by superinduction of the IL-6 gene (63). IL-6 may play an important role by limiting many immune responses or by directly promoting growth of EBV-infected B-cells (60,64).

Other cytokines (IL-4, IFN-α, and IFN-γ) play important regulatory roles in B-cell growth and development (65). IL-4 promotes B-cell proliferation, while IFN-α and IFN-γ inhibit this effect, resulting in a homeostatic balance of B-cell proliferation. It was hypothesized that uncontrolled B-cell proliferation, leading to lymphomas, was due to an imbalance caused by elevated levels of IL-4 and low levels of IFN-α (65).

When EBV infects B cells it is theorized that the following sequence of events occurs: it stimulates a polyclonal B-cell proliferation, which in normal individuals is controlled by EBV-specific cytotoxic T lymphocytes, by antibodies against virally determined antigens, and possibly by NK cells. However, these defenses are impaired in immunosuppressed patients, and the proliferation continues unabated. A cytogenetic event may then occur with the emergence of a monoclonal autonomous tumor bearing a chromosomal marker (26,28). This hypothesis is supported by findings of high EBV serum titers, by identification of EBV nuclear antigen in lymphoma cells, and by molecular hybridization studies showing EBV-DNA specific sequences in tumor specimens (26,28).

That all infected persons do not succumb to lymphomas points to the existence of potent durable restraints on EBV-transformed cells (61). Activated cytotoxic T cells that are neither EBV specific nor HLA restricted play a major role, but some cytotoxic T-cell clones are both specific for virus-infected cells and HLA restricted (60). In contrast, viral IL-10 may limit host responses by inhibiting T-cell growth and IFN-γ production (66). Another way that EBV may avoid T-cell recognition and clearance is by failure to express certain genes, such as those for LMP and EBNA-2, that transactivate other viral genes (60). Immunosuppressive agents such as OKT-3 may contribute to the development of EBV-related lymphomas by liberating IL-6, which favors the growth of EBV-infected cells, and IL-10, which impairs T-cell defenses against EBV (67).

Some investigators suggest that the presence of EBV genomes in tumor cells does not necessarily indicate that EBV is an oncogenic virus (68). Its presence may simply have stimulated cell division, which provided the substrate for malignant transformation.

It is unlikely that EBV alone is responsible for the development of lymphomas, as only a small minority of immunodeficient patients with EBV infections develop these tumors. It appears that some other factor(s) must also play a role. Furthermore, not all lymphomas in immunodeficient patients are associated with EBV. Careful search for EBV genomes has yielded negative results in several lymphomas in allograft recipients (27) and in numerous patients with AIDS-related lymphomas (69). It is possible that in some cases EBV may have no primary role in lymphomagenesis but may secondarily infect the neoplastic cells.

The view of EBV as a strictly B-lymphotrophic agent has been challenged by a series of studies suggesting that the virus infects T lymphocytes and, more speculatively, may be capable of deregulating T-cell growth and possibly cause T-cell lymphomas (70).

EBV has recently been found in a clonal form in several smooth muscle tumors in organ allograft recipients, suggesting that the virus may have a role in the development of these malignancies as well (71,72). EBV has also been linked to several leiomyosarcomas occurring in patients with AIDS (73).

Human T-Cell Lymphotrophic Virus-1

At least one T-cell lymphoma appears to have been caused by human T-cell lymphotrophic virus-1 (HTLV-1) in a renal transplant patient from the Caribbean, an area endemic for T-cell leukemia/lymphoma (74).

Viruses in Kaposi's Sarcoma

Many features of KS suggest a viral etiology: its short induction time after the onset of immunosuppression, the frequent history of relapses and remissions of individual lesions, the occasional history of apparently spontaneous cures in the "classic" variety of KS, and the regression of KS in transplant patients when immunosuppressive therapy is reduced or discontinued (1–3,6,10). In fact, some investigators do not regard KS as a true neoplasm but rather as a benign, potentially controllable and reversible hyperplasia (75). Atypical cells and mitotic figures are extremely rare histologic findings, and the multiple lesions, which are so frequently present, do not fit the classic understanding of metastases (76).

In addition, the occurrence of clusters of the disease in endemic areas of Africa and among AIDS patients favors an infectious etiology. Among viruses that have been linked with KS are hepatitis B virus, EBV, herpes simplex types 1 and 2, human herpes virus type 6, cytomegalovirus, and papillomavirus type 16 (10). The data in favor of any of them are not convincing. Recently, a new herpesvirus tentatively labeled HHV-8 has been isolated from AIDS-related KS, classic KS, and the KS that occurs in HIV-negative homosexual men (77,78). It is either an etiologic agent or a highly preferred passenger, but the available data do not permit discrimination between the two alternatives (78).

Papillomaviruses

More than 60 serotypes of human papillomaviruses have been identified in the general population. HPV-16 and HPV-18 are regarded as high-risk types for anogenital cancers and particularly cancers of the uterine cervix (79). In the dermatologic disorder epidermodysplasia verruciformis—which is characterized by impaired cellular immunity, disseminated warts, and the development of SCC in 30% of patients (mostly in skin areas exposed to sunlight)—HPV-5 and, less commonly, HPV-8 are the types most often associated with cancer (23).

The incidence of condyloma acuminatum in renal transplant recipients ranges from 2.4% to 4%. In a study of 48 renal transplant recipients, the prevalence of HPV DNA (predominantly HPV-16 and HPV-18) was 46% compared with 2% in controls (80). In three studies of female renal transplant recipients, the incidence of HPV lower genital infection showed a 5- to 17-fold increase, and the risk of carcinoma in situ showed an 11- to 14-fold increase (38,79,80). The genital infections and neoplasms were frequently multifocal in distribution, with varying combinations of involvement of the cervix, vagina, vulva, perineum, and anus (81).

As warts commonly develop in immunosuppressed renal transplant recipients, occurring in 77% of patients with graft function lasting more than 5 years (23), and as skin cancers are also common in these patients, the question arises as to whether or not warts in sun-exposed skin areas on immunosuppressed patients may undergo malignant change. The answer appears to be affirmative. In a study of 202 renal allograft recipients, 53 (77%) of 69 patients with graft survival of more than 5 years had warts, 26 (38%) had keratoses, and 8 (12%) had skin cancers. Of 133 recipients with graft survival of less than 5 years, 27 (20%) had keratoses and 2 (1.5%) had skin cancers (23). Fifteen of 24 SCC cases (60%) contained HPV-5/8 DNA, and one contained HPV-4 DNA. The authors emphasize that renal transplant recipients resemble patients with epidermodysplasia verruciformis in that they are immunosuppressed, have extensive viral warts, and develop SCC in sun-exposed skin areas. Another study demonstrated HPV-5 DNA in SCC of a renal allograft recipient (83). In a third study, SCC in a renal allograft recipient was found to contain HPV-2 and HPV-4 DNA (84). In addition, HPV-2 DNA was found in the BCC of two immunosuppressed patients (one a renal transplant recipient) (85), although it was questioned whether the HPV was a causative factor or merely a passenger in the BCC.

In the general population, HPV-2 DNA and HPV-16 DNA have been found in occasional oral cancers, but thus far no studies of HPV have been reported in 130 oral and lingual cancers reported to the CTTR.

Hepatitis Virus

The increased incidence of hepatocellular cancer in renal transplant recipients (1–3) may be related to the frequent occurrence of hepatitis B virus infections in dialysis and transplant patients (17). Hepatitis C–related hepatomas in transplant patients are increasingly being recognized.

Other Viruses

As several studies have shown that herpes simplex virus types 1 and 2 (HSV-1) and (HSV-2) may transform animal and human cells in culture, we may theorize that infections with HSV-1 could be related to the high incidence of lip cancers, and infections with HSV-2 to carcinomas of the uterine cervix in organ allograft recipients. However, there is little supporting evidence.

It is possible that oncogenic viruses may potentiate the effects of other carcinogens. For example, the high incidence of uterine cervical carcinomas in organ allograft recipients may be related partly to cervical dysplasia caused by azathioprine administration (1–3,6) and partly to infection by HPV. Nononcogenic viruses may also enhance the effects of known carcinogens. Experiments in mice subjected to various nononcogenic virus infections and treated with a chemical carcinogen showed an increased incidence of benign and malignant tumors (86).

Disturbances of Immunity

Deficient immune responses may contribute to the development of neoplasms in several ways.

Immune Surveillance

The immune surveillance hypothesis (87–89) suggests that a major function of the immune system is to control the development of malignancies. Daily wear and tear leads to replacement of millions of cells. Occasional mutations occur, some of which are potentially malignant. The immune system is believed to recognize these abnormal cells and destroy them. However, when a malignant cell escapes surveillance it gives rise to a neoplastic clone, which eventually presents as a clinical cancer.

The theory has stimulated considerable controversy (1,6). It is argued that if the concept is correct, there should be an increased incidence of all types of tumors, not only the disproportionately high incidence of the neoplasms described above. However, the counterpoint is made that if immunoincompetent patients were to live long enough, they eventually would develop more malignancies that usually have long latent periods of 15 or 20 years or more (such as carcinomas of the breast, bronchus, colon, and prostate). This does not occur because these patients tend to die at an earlier stage from intercurrent infections and lymphomas. Nevertheless, in the present state of our knowledge, the pattern of tumors encountered after transplantation fits more with a presumed viral etiology of many of the neoplasms, rather than with impaired immune surveillance.

Chronic Antigenic Stimulation

Chronic stimulation of lymphoid tissues may cause hyperplasia and eventually neoplasia. Experiments in animals involving repeated or continuous administration of foreign antigens have caused a high incidence of lymphomas (90–92). Chronic stimulation by foreign antigens of transplanted organs, repeated infections, transfusions of blood or blood products, or administration of polyclonal or monoclonal antilymphocyte preparations can overstimulate a partially depressed immune system and lead to NHL. Nonspecific B-cell activation with resultant expansion of B-cell clones increases the risk of chromosomal translocation and rearrangement of c-myc and Ig loci at the time of Ig gene rearrangement. Subsequently, external growth factors, possibly provided by EBV infection, could then cause neoplastic change of the cells. Supporting a role for this mechanism in the development of post-transplant malignancies is the observation that many are large cell lesions that have all the morphologic features of antigen-stimulated lymphocytes and are sometimes described as "immunoblastic sarcomas" (93).

Experiments with rejection of skin grafts in animals have shown that chronic antigenic stimulation may cause lymphomas by another mechanism, namely the immunologic activation of endogenous C-type oncornaviruses (94).

One model for producing lymphomas through chronic antigenic stimulation involves the establishment of chronic graft-versus-host disease (GVHD) in adult F_1 hybrid mice (90). Chronic GVHD may also activate C-type viruses, and continued viral replication in blastogenic lymphoid tissue may progress to malignant change (94). Similar mechanisms possibly could explain the development of lymphomas in organ transplant recipients, because donor lymphocytes or lymphoid tissues are transplanted with solid organs and may cause GVHD. However, if GVHD causes post-transplant lymphomas in humans, then it is surprising that these malignancies occur frequently after renal, hepatic, and cardiac transplantation in which the full-blown syndrome of GVHD is rare. Also, relatively few lymphomas have been described in many thousands of bone marrow transplant recipients, in whom GVHD is common.

KS is believed to arise from endothelial cells (95). There are structural and functional interactions between vascular and lymphatic endothelium and the immune system (95). Endothelial cells play an important role in lymphocyte traffic and participate in the immune response by acting as antigen-presenting cells. Theories that may explain the frequent occurrence of KS in transplant patients suggest that prolonged exposure to the foreign histocompatibility antigens of a transplanted organ; or repeated infections by viruses, fungi, bacteria, or protozoa; or a chronic immunologic reaction between antigenically altered lymphoid cells and normal lymphocytes may stimulate macrophages and lymphocytes to liberate the cytokines and growth factors (especially angiogenesis factors) that cause endothelial and mesenchymal cells to proliferate, resulting in KS (96,97). It is also possible that an oncogenic virus is either transferred to or induced in the cells responsive to the angiogenesis factor, causing their malignant change (97).

Impaired Immunoregulation

Because cellular and humoral feedback mechanisms limit the extent of immune reactions, defective control may allow unrestrained proliferation of lymphoid cells, ultimately resulting in the development of lymphomas. This may explain the unusually high incidence of these tumors in organ allograft recipients (1–3,6). One hypothesis is that thymic suppressor function, which normally restricts lymphoid proliferation, is impaired, thus permitting unregulated growth and lymphomagenesis (98). Another theory is based on observations that immunologic reactions may activate latent oncogenic viruses and that continuous antigenic stimulation of partially immunodeficient mice may lead to the development of lymphoreticular tumors (94,99,100). As many transplant patients are also only partially immunodeficient, it is postulated that defective antibody production fails to control lymphocyte proliferation and activation of oncogenic viruses in a milieu that favors their multiplication. The viruses shed from lymphoblasts attack cells in the microenvironment of the immunologic reaction and cause their malignant transformation (100).

Direct Carcinogenic Effects of Immunosuppressive or Chemotherapeutic Agents

Most experimental studies have demonstrated carcinogenicity only when these compounds were used in combination with physical or chemical agents, with foreign proteins, or with viral infections, or when they were used in animals such as NZB mice, which suffer from autoimmune diseases. For example, cyclosporine facilitated the development of transplanted, chemically induced, and virally induced tumors in several species, as well as the growth of human cancer xenografts in immunoincompetent mice or rats (1). Most immunosuppressive agents apparently did not cause "spontaneous" neoplasms when administered alone (1,101).

The International Agency for Research on Cancer found limited evidence for the carcinogenicity of azathioprine in mice and rats, and insufficient evidence that it is carcinogenic in humans (101). Cyclosporine markedly increased the induction of thymic lymphomas in AKR mice (which are known to have a high incidence of such malignancies), owing to its action as a tumor promoter (102). In addition, rats given dietary cyclosporine developed lymphoproliferative lesions similar to those in humans (103). In studies of peripheral blood lymphocytes of patients treated with azathioprine or cyclosporine for more than 1 year, 31 of 50 patients treated with azathioprine showed chromosome aberrations, and 17 of 25 cyclosporine patients had similar changes. These results suggest that both drugs could be regarded as teratogenic agents (104) (see also Chapters 6 and 7). In vitro studies of human cells showed that cyclosporine is mutagenic because it induced sister chromatid exchanges (105). However, the concentrations of cyclosporine (1 μg/mL) used in the experiments were much higher than those used clinically.

Synergistic Effects of Immunosuppressive Therapy with Other Carcinogens

It is possible that immunosuppressive agents may potentiate the effects of environmental carcinogens such as sunlight, tobacco, and other agents (1,6). Studies in mice treated with ultraviolet light and four commonly used agents—azathioprine, prednisolone, cyclophosphamide, and cyclosporine—showed that azathioprine and cyclophosphamide had strong tumor promoting effects, prednisolone had none, and cyclosporine caused a moderate reduction in the latent period for tumor induction (1,6). A possible mechanism to explain these differences is that metabolites of azathioprine, mainly methylnitrothioimidazole and related imidazole compounds, cause chemical photosensitization and thus promote skin carcinogenesis (47). If these results can be extrapolated to humans, they may help to explain the high incidence of skin cancers seen in organ allograft recipients.

Dysplasia of the uterine cervical epithelium follows therapy with a number of immunosuppressive agents including azathioprine (1,6). It is possible that this agent, in combination with HPV infection, may be responsible for the high incidence of in situ carcinomas of the cervix observed in transplant patients.

Other Potentially Carcinogenic Factors

Some transplant patients may have been exposed to other potentially carcinogenic drugs. These may have acted independently or synergistically with immunosuppressive agents. Several examples may be cited (1,6). Renal transplant recipients sometimes develop carcinomas in their own kidneys, some of which may have been caused by previous phenacetin abuse (1,6,8). Isoniazid, which is used in the prevention and treatment of tuberculosis in immunoincompetent patients, is a potential carcinogen (1,6). Diphenylhydantoin (Dilantin), which is used in some renal transplant patients to prevent seizure disorders, may cause pseudolymphomas or true lymphomas (106).

Variations in Susceptibility to Cancer

A puzzling feature is that only a small percentage of all immunosuppressed transplant patients develop malignancies. Perhaps these individuals may be genetically prone to develop neoplasms under certain circumstances.

Genetic factors control the individual's ability to activate or deactivate carcinogens, to produce interferon, which may affect their susceptibility to viral infections or malignancies, and to regulate the immune response via the major histocompatibility system (107–109).

HLA antigens also play an important role in host defenses against the development and spread of tumors, especially in virus-induced neoplasia (110,111). For example, in renal transplant recipients, HLA-A11 may protect against skin cancer, whereas HLA-B27 and HLA-DR7 are associated with an increased risk of this neoplasm (110). Allogeneic HLA antigens may also play a role in the development of skin cancer, as HLA-B mismatching is significantly associated with an increased risk of squamous cell carcinoma in renal transplant recipients (112).

Several authors reported altered frequencies of certain HLA phenotypes in patients with KS (113). These include an increased frequency of A-19, A-23 and B-49, B-18, and DR-5, as well as a decreased frequency of B-8 and DR-3. However, none of these studies specifically examined the transplant population. The HLA phenotype and ethnicity of patients reported to the CTTR were examined in 188 patients; HLA-A and HLA-B typing were available in 135 and HLA-DR typing in 67. When their ethnic background was considered (56% were Arab, Italian, Greek, or Jewish) (113), the expected HLA phenotype frequencies were almost exactly the same as in the KS patients. The quality of donor–recipient HLA match also was examined in 106 patients. Only 22% had four or more mismatches, and 59% had at least two antigens matched. This argues against poor donor–recipient matching as a risk factor for developing KS after transplantation.

ACKNOWLEDGMENTS

The author wishes to thank his many colleagues throughout the world who have generously contributed data concerning their patients to the CTTR. This study was supported in part by a grant from the Department of Veterans Affairs.

COMMENTARY

Darlene S. Johnson, Jessica L. Fewkes, and Arthur J. Sober

Renal transplants have been carried out extensively since the 1960s, and since the 1970s, an increased incidence of non-melanoma skin cancer has been reported in this population. With more transplantations, longer patient survival times, and more potent immunosuppressive agents, the problem of secondary malignancies has become an important issue in the complex management of transplant patients. As we continue to explore the possible role of immunologic mechanisms in the development of skin cancers in renal transplant patients, our current goals are the identification of patients at increased risk, preventive measures, and early aggressive treatment.

As Penn discusses in this chapter, the ratio of basal cell carcinoma (BCC) to squamous cell carcinoma (SCC) is reversed in the transplant population relative to the general population. Also, the incidence of skin cancer increases with the length of follow-up after transplantation. A key question is: Who among these already high-risk patients comprises our target population?

Cumulative sun exposure and the patient's age at the time of transplantation seem to be the most important risk factors (1). The incidence of SCC in renal transplant recipients decreases proportionately with an increase in latitude. Large multicenter studies in Australia, England, and Canada reported that the incidence of SCC at 10 years after renal transplantation was approximately 45% (2), 14% (3), and 10% (4), respectively. An increased incidence of premalignant and malignant lesions is seen in light-skinned patients with blue eyes and blond or red hair, and in patients who pursue outdoor occupations or hobbies.

Conflicting studies exist regarding increased rates of melanoma in the transplant population. If there is an increase in melanoma, it has not been dramatically evidenced by clinical experience. The finding of increased numbers of nevi in renal transplant patients and in HIV patients would suggest that longer follow-up times and monitoring for melanoma development would be reasonable (5).

Preventive measures for the non-melanoma skin cancers focus on minimizing sun exposure as early in life as possible. Physicians must inform patients about sun avoidance and protection: patients should minimize outdoor activities between 10 AM and 4 PM, wear physical sunblocks such as hats and long-sleeved shirts, and use sunscreens that block not only ultraviolet B rays but also ultraviolet A. Years before their patients undergo transplantation, nephrologists can begin educating those with an elevated BUN or creatinine about the dangers of sun exposure. Physicians can begin early ultraviolet exposure reduction programs in families prone to renal failure, such as those with polycystic kidneys.

The role of warts continues to be evaluated in transplant recipients. It is well documented that transplant recipients have an increased incidence of warts. Both oncogenic strains of human papillomavirus (HPV) and numerous other non-malignancy-associated strains have been isolated from multiple sites, including nonlesional skin, warts, and premalignant and malignant lesions (6). How HPV or other viral infections and the incidence of skin cancer in transplant recipients correlate is complex, and is currently under further investigation (7).

Also controversial is the role of individual immunosuppressive agents in facilitating the development of non-melanoma skin cancers. Early protocols of prednisone and azathioprine, and more recent triple therapies with prednisone, azathioprine, and cyclosporine, have been studied with inconclusive results regarding the increased risk associated with the use of any single immunosuppressive agent in many studies (8,9). Nevertheless, it is clear that the risk of post-transplant malignancy is directly related to the overall intensity of long-term immunosuppression (10).

We know that non-melanoma skin cancers are more anaplastic on biopsy, behave more aggressively, and lead to greater morbidity and mortality in transplant recipients as compared to immunocompetent patients. Therefore, early diagnosis and treatment are critical. Premalignant and malignant lesions may have a surprisingly benign clinical appearance, and multiple lesions may occur simultaneously. Aggressive treatment should begin with premalignant lesions, and can include liberal use of topical tretinoin, chemical peels, 5-fluorouracil, and cryotherapy. Once a skin cancer has been diagnosed, multiple treatment modalities may need to be combined to ensure clearance, including wide local excision, deep cryotherapy, or parenteral approaches such as systemic retinoids (11). Once we have a better understanding of the potential immunologic mechanisms leading to secondary malignancies in transplant recipients, we may develop more effective treatment modalities in the future.

CHAPTER REFERENCES

1. Penn I. Why do immunosuppressed patients develop cancer? In: Pimentel E, ed. CRC critical reviews in oncogenesis. Volume 1. Boca Raton: CRC, 1989:27–52.
2. Penn I. The problem of cancer in organ transplant recipients: an overview. Transplant Sci 1994;4:23–32.
3. Penn I. Malignancy after immunosuppressive therapy: how can the risk be reduced? Clin Immunotherapeut 1995;9:207–218.
4. Penn I. Cancers of the anogenital region in renal transplant recipients. Analysis of 65 cases. Cancer 1986;58:611–616.
5. Penn I. Post-transplant malignancies: clinical preventive measures. In: Schmähl D, Penn I, eds. Cancer in organ transplant recipients. Berlin: Springer-Verlag, 1991:157–160.
6. Penn I. Possible causes of cancer in transplant patients. In: Schmähl D, Penn I, eds. Cancer in organ transplant recipients. Berlin: Springer-Verlag, 1991:135–152.
7. Penn I. De novo malignancy in pediatric organ transplant recipients. J Ped Surg 1994;29:221–228.
8. Penn I. Primary kidney tumors before and after renal transplantation. Transplantation 1995;59:480–485.
9. Penn I, Porat G. Central nervous system lymphomas in organ allograft recipients. Transplantation 1995;59:240–244.
10. Penn I. Sarcomas in organ allograft recipients. Transplantation 1995;60: 1485–1491.
11. Kinlen LJ. Incidence of cancer in rheumatoid arthritis and other disorders after immunosuppressive treatment. Am J Med 1985;78:suppl 1A:44–49.
12. Parker SL, Tong T, Bolden S, Wingo PA. Cancer statistics, 1996. CA Cancer J Clin 1996;46:5–27.
13. Sheil AGR, Disney APS, Mathew TH, Amiss N. De novo malignancy emerges as a major cause of morbidity and late failure in renal transplantation. Transplant Proc 1993;25:1383–1384.
14. Blohme I, Brynger H. Malignant disease in renal transplant patients. Transplantation 1985;39:23–35.
15. Harwood AR, Osoba D, Hofstader SL, et al. Kaposi's sarcoma in recipients of renal transplants. Am J Med 1979;67:5:759–765.
16. Penn I. Kaposi's sarcoma in transplant recipients. Transplantation 1997;64: 669–673.
17. Schröter GPJ, Weil R III, Penn I, et al. Hepatocellular carcinoma associated with chronic hepatitis B virus infection after kidney transplantation (Letter to the editor). Lancet 1982;2:381–382.
18. Bernstein D, Baum D, Berry G, et al. Neoplastic disorders after pediatric heart transplantation. Circulation 1993;88:230–237.
19. Sheil AGR. Skin cancer in renal transplant recipients. Transplant Sci 1994;4:42–45.
20. Hoxtell EO, Mandel JS, Murray SS, et al. Incidence of skin carcinoma after renal transplantation. Arch Dermatol 1977;113:436–438.
21. Bouwes Bavinck JN, Hardie DR, Green A, et al. The risk of skin cancer in renal transplant recipients in Queensland, Australia. Transplantation 1996;61:715–721.
22. Mullen DL, Silberberg SG, Penn I, Hammond WS. Squamous cell carcinoma of the skin and lip in renal homograft recipients. Cancer 1976;37:729–734.
23. Barr BB, Benton EC, McLaren K, et al. Human papilloma virus infection and skin cancer in renal allograft recipients. Lancet 1989;1:124–129.
24. Glover MT, Niranjan N, Kwan JTC, Leigh IM. Non-melanoma skin cancer in renal transplant recipients: the extent of the problem and a strategy for management. Brit J Plastic Surg 1994;47:86–89.
25. Hartevelt MM, Bavinck JN, Koote AM, et al. Incidence of skin cancer after renal transplantation in the Netherlands. Transplantation 1990;49:506–509.
26. Nalesnik MA, Starzl TE. Epstein-Barr virus, infectious mononucleosis, and posttransplant lymphoproliferative disorders. Transplant Sci 1994;4:61–79.
27. Wilkinson AH, Smith JL, Hunsicker LG, et al. Increased frequency of posttransplant lymphomas in patients treated with cyclosporine, azathioprine, and prednisone. Transplantation 1989;47:293–296.
28. Hanto DW. Classification of Epstein-Barr virus-associated posttransplant lymphoproliferative diseases: implications for understanding their pathogenesis and developing rational treatment strategies. Ann Rev Med 1995;46:381–394.
29. Starzl TE, Nalesnik MA, Porter KA, et al. Reversibility of lymphomas and lymphoproliferative lesions developing under cyclosporine-steroid therapy. Lancet 1984;1:583–587.
30. Montagnino G, Bencini PL, Tarantino A, et al. Clinical features and course of Kaposi's sarcoma in kidney transplant patients: report of 13 cases. Am J Nephrol 1994;14:121–126.
31. Al-Sulaiman MH, Al-Khader AA. Kaposi's sarcoma in renal transplant recipients. Transplant Sci 1994;4:46–60.
32. Catalona WJ. Urothelial tumors of the urinary tract. In: Walsh PC, Retik AB, Stamey TA, Vaughn ER Jr, eds. Campbell's urology, 6th ed. Philadelphia: Saunders, 1992:1094–1158.
33. Ishikawa I. Acquired cysts and neoplasms of the kidneys in renal allograft recipients. Contrib Nephrol 1992;100:254–268.

34. Vaziri ND, Darwish R, Martin DC, Hostetler J. Acquired renal cystic disease in renal transplant recipients. Nephron 1984;37:203–205.
35. Kliem V, Kolditz M, Ehlerding G, et al. Risk of renal cell carcinoma after kidney transplantation. Clin Transplantation 1997;11:255–258.
36. Lien Y-H H, Kam I, Shanley PF, Schröter GPJ. Metastatic renal cell carcinoma associated with acquired cystic kidney disease 15 years after successful renal transplantation. Am J Kidney Dis 1991;18:711–715.
37. Sillman F, Stanek A, Sedlis A, et al. The relationship between human papillomavirus and lower genital intraepithelial neoplasia in immunosuppressed women. Am J Obstet Gynecol 1984;150:300–308.
38. Porreco R, Penn I, Droegemueller W, et al. Gynecologic malignancies in immunosuppressed organ homograft recipients. Obstet Gynecol 1975;45:359–364.
39. Barrett WL, First R, Aron BS, Penn I. Clinical course of malignancies in renal transplant recipients. Cancer 1993;72:2186–2189.
40. Ciancio G, Giguijor AP, Burke GW, et al. Post-transplant lymphoproliferative disease in kidney transplant patients in the new immunosuppressive era. Clin Transplantation 1997;11:243–249.
41. Kersey JH, Shapiro RS, Heinitz KJ, et al. Lymphoid malignancy in naturally occurring and post bone marrow transplantation immunodeficiency diseases. In: Good RA, Lindenlaub E, eds. The nature, cellular and biochemical basis and management of immunodeficiencies. Stuttgart: FK Shattaeur Verlag Symposia Medica Hoechst, 1987;21:289–294.
42. Doyle H, Tzakis AG, Yunis E, Starzl TE. Smooth muscle tumor arising de novo in a liver allograft: a case report. Clin Transplant 1991;5:60–62.
43. Van Hoeven KH, Factor SM, Kress Y, Woodruff JM. Visceral myogenic tumors: a manifestation of HIV infection in children. Am J Surg Pathol 1993;17:1176–1181.
44. Oberbauer R, Banyai S, Schmidt A, et al. Serum tumor markers after renal transplantation. Transplantation 1997;62:1506–1511.
45. Darenkov IA, Marcarelli MA, Basadonna GA, et al. Reduced incidence of Epstein-Barr virus-associated post-transplant lymphoproliferative disorder using preemptive antiviral therapy. Transplantation 1997;64:848–852.
46. McDiarmid SV, Jordan S, Lee GS. Prevention and preemptive therapy of post-transplant lymphoproliferative disease in pediatric liver recipients. Transplantation 1998;66:1604–1611.
47. Hemmens VJ, Moore DE. Photochemical sensitization by azathioprine and its metabolites: II. Azathioprine and nitroimidazole metabolites. Photochem Photobiol 1986;43:3:257–262.
48. Euvrard S, Verschoore M, Touraine JL, et al. Topical retinoids for warts and keratoses in transplant recipients. (Letter to editor.) Lancet 1992;340:48–49.
49. Peters M. Mechanisms of action of interferons. Semin Liver Dis 1989;9:235–239.
50. Faro A, Kurland G, Michaels MG, et al. Interferon alpha effects the immune response in post-transplant lymphoproliferative disorder. Am J Respir Crit Care Med 1996;153:1442–1448.
51. Min AD. Does interferon precipitate rejection of liver allografts?. Hepatology 1995;22:1333–1335.
52. Hickey DP, Nalesnik MA, Vivas CA, et al. Renal retransplantation in patients who lost their allografts during management of previous post-transplant lymphoproliferative disease. Clin Transplant 1990;4:187–190.
53. Nalesnik MA, Locker J, Jaffe R, et al. Experience with posttransplant lymphoproliferative disorders in solid organ transplant recipients. Clin Transplant 1992;6:249–252.
54. Klintmalm GB. De novo lymphoma after liver transplantation. Clin Transplant 1992;6:272–274.
55. Shapiro RS, Chauvenet A, McGuire W, et al. Treatment of B-cell lymphoproliferative disorders with interferon alpha and intravenous gamma globulin. N Engl J Med 1988;318:1334.
56. Benkerrou M, Durandy A, Fischer A. Therapy for transplant-related lymphoproliferative disease. Hematol Oncol Clin North Am 1993;7: 467–475.
57. Emanuel DJ, Lucas KG, Mallory GB, et al. Treatment of post-transplant lymphoproliferative disease in the central nervous system of a lung transplant recipient using allogeneic leukocytes. Transplantation 1997;63:1691–1694.
58. Rooney CM, Smith CA, Ng CY, et al. Use of gene-modified virus-specific T lymphocytes to control Epstein-Barr-virus-related lymphoproliferation. Lancet 1995;1:9–13.
59. Randhawa PS, Whiteside TL, Zeevia A, et al. Effects of immunotherapy on experimental immunodeficiency-related lymphoproliferative disease. Transplantation 1998;65:264–268.
60. Straus SE, Cohen JI, Tosato G, Mier J. Epstein-Barr virus infections: biology, pathogenesis, and management. Ann Int Med 1993;118:45–58.
61. Joab I. Biology of the Epstein-Barr virus. In: Dammacco F, ed. Advances in tumor immunology and allergic disorders. Milan: Edi-ermes, 1992:83–99.
62. MacMahon EME, Glass JD, Hayward SD, et al. Association of Epstein-Barr virus with primary central nervous system lymphomas in AIDS. AIDS Res Hum Retrovir 1992;8:5:740–742.
63. Walz G, Zanker B, Melton LB, et al. Possible association of the immunosuppressive and B cell lymphoma-promoting properties of cyclosporine. Transplantation 1990;49:191–194.
64. Emilie D, Coumbaras J, Raphael M, et al. Interleukin-6 production in high-grade B lymphomas: correlation with the presence of malignant immunoblasts in acquired immunodeficiency syndrome and in human immunodeficiency virus-seronegative patients. Blood 1992;80:498–504.
65. Mathur A, Kamat DM, Filipovich AH, et al. Immunoregulatory abnormalities in patients with EBV-associated B cell lymphoproliferative disorders. Transplantation 1994;57:1042–1045.
66. Vieira P, de Waal-Malefyt R, Dang MN, et al. Isolation and expression of human cytokine synthesis inhibitory factor cDNA clones: homology to Epstein-Barr open reading frame BCRF-1. Proc Natl Acad Sci USA 1991;88:1172–1176.
67. Goldman M, Gérard C, Abramowicz D, et al. Induction of interleukin-6 and interleukin-10 by the OKT3 monoclonal antibody: possible relevance to posttransplant lymphoproliferative disorders. Clin Transplant 1992;6:265–268.
68. Case records of the Massachusetts General Hospital. Weekly clinico-pathological exercises. Case 2-1987. A 30-year-old man with ataxia-telangiectasia and dysphagia. N Engl J Med 1987;316:91–100.
69. Subar M, Neri A, Inghirami G, et al. Frequent c-myc oncogene activation and infrequent presence of Epstein-Barr virus genome in AIDS-associated lymphoma. Blood 1988;72:667–671.
70. Editorial. Epstein-Barr virus and T-cell lymphoma. Lancet 1988;2:723–724.
71. Lee ES, Locker J, Nalesnik M, et al. The association of Epstein-Barr virus with smooth-muscle tumors occurring after organ transplantation. N Engl J Med 1995;332:19–25.
72. Timmons CF, Dawson DB, Richards S, et al. Epstein-Barr virus associated leiomyosarcomas in liver transplant recipients: origin from either donor or recipient tissue. Cancer 1995;76:1481–1489.
73. McLain KL, Leach CT, Jenson HB, et al. Association of Epstein-Barr virus with leiomyosarcomas in young people with AIDS. N Engl J Med 1995;332:12–18.
74. Zanke BW, Rush DN, Jeffery JR, Israels LG. HTLV-1 T cell lymphoma in a cyclosporine-treated renal transplant patient. Transplantation 1989;48: 695–697.
75. Brooks JJ. Kaposi's sarcoma: a reversible hyperplasia. Lancet 1986;2:1309–1311.
76. Dalgleish AG. Kaposi's sarcoma. Br J Cancer 1991;64:3–6.
77. Moore PS, Chang Y. Detection of herpesvirus-like DNA sequences in Kaposi's sarcoma in patients with and without HIV infection. N Engl J Med 1995;332:1181–1185.
78. Roizman B. New viral footprints in Kaposi's sarcoma. N Engl J Med 1995;332:1227–1228.
79. Zur Hausen H. Human papillomaviruses in the pathogenesis of anogenital cancer. Virology 1991;184:9–13.
80. Kelly GE, Sheil AGR, Rose BR, et al. HPV infection in the lower genital tract of women undergoing hemodialysis and women with renal allografts. Clin Transplant 1991;5:7–12.
81. Halpert R, Fruchter RG, Sedlis A, et al. Human papillomavirus and lower genital neoplasia in renal transplant patients. Obstet Gynecol 1986;68: 251–258.
82. Schneider V, Kay S, Lee HM. Immunosuppression as a high-risk factor in the development of condyloma acuminatum and squamous neoplasia of the cervix. Acta Cytol 1983;27:220–224.
83. Lutzner MA, Orth G, Dutronquay V, et al. Detection of human papilloma virus type 5 DNA in skin cancers of an immunosuppressed renal allograft recipient. Lancet 1983;2:422–424.
84. Van Der Leest RJ, Zachow KR, Ostrow RS, et al. Human papilloma virus heterogenecity in 36 renal transplant patients. Arch Dermatol 1987;123:354–357.
85. Obalek S, Favie M, Jablonska S, Szymanczyk J, Orth G. Human papillomavirus type 2-associated basal cell carcinoma in two immunosuppressed patients. Arch Dermatol 1988;124:930–934.
86. Southam CM, Tanaka S, Arata T, et al. Enhancement of responses to chemical carcinogens by nononcogenic viruses and antimetabolites. Prog Exp Tumor Res 1969;11:194–212.
87. Ehrlich P. Über den jetzigen Stand der Karzinomforschung. In: The Collected Papers of Paul Ehrlich. Vol 2. London: Pergamon Press, 1957:550.
88. Burnet FM. Immunological surveillance in neoplasia. Transplant Rev 1971;7:3–25.
89. Penn I. Immunosuppression—a contributory factor in lymphoma formation. Clin Transplant 1992;6:214–219.

90. Gleichmann E, Gleichmann H, Schwartz RS, et al. Immunologic induction of malignant lymphoma: identification of donor and host tumors in the graft-versus-host model. J Natl Cancer Inst 1975;54:107–116.
91. Metcalf D. Induction of reticular tumors in mice by repeated antigenic stimulation. Acta Int Cancer 1963;19:657–659.
92. Walford RL, Hildemann WH. Life span and lymphoma-incidence of mice injected at birth with spleen cells across a weak histocompatibility locus. Am J Pathol 1965;47:713–721.
93. Lukes RJ, Collins RD. Immunologic characterization of human malignant lymphomas. Cancer 1974;34(suppl 4):1488–1503.
94. Hirsch MS, Proffitt MR, Black PH. Autoimmunity, oncornaviruses, and lymphomagenesis. Contemp Top Immunobiol 1977;6:209–227.
95. Ziegler JL. Etiology angiogenesis. In: Ziegler JL, Dorfman RF, eds. Kaposi's sarcoma: pathophysiology and clinical management. New York: Dekker, 1988:151–168.
96. Ensoli B, Barillari G, Gallo RC. Cytokines and growth factors in the pathogenesis of AIDS-associated Kaposi's sarcoma. Immunol Rev 1992;127: 147–155.
97. Warner TF, O'Loughlin S. Kaposi's sarcoma. A byproduct of tumor rejection. Lancet 1975;2:687–689.
98. Gershwin ME, Steinberg AD. Loss of suppressor function as a cause of lymphoid malignancy. Lancet 1973;2:1174–1176.
99. Krueger G. The significance of immunosuppression and antigenic stimulation in the development of malignant lymphomas. In: Grundmann E, Gross R, eds. The ambivalence of cytostatic therapy, recent results in cancer research. Vol 52. Berlin: Springer-Verlag, 1975:88–95.
100. Schwartz RS. Another look at immunologic surveillance. N Engl J Med 1975;293:181–184.
101. IARC monographs on the evaluation of the carcinogenic risk of chemicals to humans: some antineoplastic and immunosuppressive agents. Lyon: World Health Organization. International Agency for Research on Cancer, 1981;26.
102. Hattori A, Perera MIR, Witkowski LA, et al. Accelerated development of spontaneous thymic lymphomas in male AKR mice receiving cyclosporine. Transplantation 1986;41:784–787.
103. Demetris AJ, Nalesnik MA, Kunz HW, et al. Sequential analyses of the development of lymphoproliferative disorders in rats receiving cyclosporine. Transplantation 1984;38:239–246.
104. Fukuda M, Aikawa I, Ohmori Y, et al. Chromosome aberrations in kidney transplant recipients. Transplant Proc 1987;19:2245–2247.
105. Yuzawa K, Kondo I, Fukao K, et al. Mutagenicity of cyclosporine. Induction of sister chromatid exchange in human cells. Transplantation 1986;42:61–63.
106. Li FP, Willard DR, Goodman R, Vawter G. Malignant lymphoma after diphenylhydantoin (Dilantin) therapy. Cancer 1975;36:1359–1362.
107. Grossberg SE. The interferons and their inducers. Molecular and therapeutic considerations. N Engl J Med 1972;287:13–19,79–85,122–128.
108. McDevitt HO. Regulation of the immune response by the major histocompatibility system. N Engl J Med 1980;303:1514–1517.
109. Miller DG. On the nature of susceptibility to cancer. Cancer 1980;46: 1307–1318.
110. Festenstein H, Garrido F. MHC antigens and malignancy. Nature 1986;322:502–503.
111. Dausset J, Colombani J, Hors J. Major histocompatibility complex and cancer, with special reference to human familial tumors (Hodgkin's disease and other malignancies). Cancer Surv 1982;1:119–147.
112. Bouwes Bavinck JN. Epidemiological aspects of immunosuppression: role of exposure to sunlight and human papillomavirus on the development of skin cancer. Hum Exp Toxicol 1995;14:98.
113. Brunson ME, Balakrishnan K, Penn I. HLA and Kaposi's sarcoma in solid organ transplantation. Hum Immunol 1990;29:56–63.

COMMENTARY REFERENCES

1. Fernandiz C, Fuente MJ, Rivera M, et al. Epidermal dysplasia and neoplasia in kidney transplant recipients. J Am Acad Dermatol 1995;33:590–596.
2. Leigh IM, Glover MT. Cutaneous warts and tumours in immunosuppressed patients. J R Soc Med 1995;88:61–62.
3. London NJ, Farmery SM, Will EJ, et al. Risk of neoplasia in renal transplant patients. Lancet 1995;346:403–406.
4. Dyall-Smith D, Ross JB. Cutaneous malignancies in renal transplant recipients from Nova Scotia, Canada. Aust J Dermatol 1995;36:79–82.
5. Grob JJ, Bastuji-Garin S, Vaillant L, et al. Excess of nevi related to immunodeficiency: a study in HIV-infected patients and renal transplant recipients. J Invest Dermatol 1996;107:694–697.
6. Chopra KF, Tyring SK. The impact of the human immunodeficiency virus on the human papillomavirus epidemic. Arch Dermatol 1997;133:629–633.
7. Ternesten-Bratel A, Kjellstrom C, Ricksten A. Specific expression of Epstein-Barr virus in cutaneous squamous cell carcinomas from heart transplant recipients. Transplantation 1998;66:1524–1529.
8. Kinlen LJ, Sheil AG, Peto J, Doll R. Collaborative United Kingdom–Australasian study of cancer in patients treated with immunosuppressive drugs. BMJ 1979;2:1461–1466.
9. Bergfelt L, Larko O, Blohme I. Skin disease in immunosuppressed patients in relation to epidermal Langerhans' cells. Acta Derm Venereol 1993;73:330–334.
10. Jensen P, Hansen S, Moller B, et al. Skin cancer in kidney and heart transplant recipients and different long-term immunosuppressive therapy regimens. J Am Acad Dermatol 1999;40:177–186.
11. Bavinck JN, Tieben LM, Van der Woude FJ, et al. Prevention of skin cancer and reduction of keratotic skin lesions during acitretin therapy in renal transplant recipients: a double-blind placebo controlled study. J Clin Oncol 1995;13:1933–1938.

Part VI

The Future of Transplantation

Chapter

38

Bone Marrow Conditioning

Douglas A. Hale Anthony P. Monaco

Within the context of this chapter, the use of donor-specific bone marrow (BM) to induce tolerance refers to the injection of donor BM into immunologically mature, adult allograft (or xenograft) recipients in association with transient or chronic immunosuppression to induce various degrees of specific immunologic unresponsiveness to the allograft (or xenograft). Such unresponsiveness can take the form of specifically augmented graft survival over that achieved with a finite amount of immunosuppression, reduced need for chronic immunosuppression to maintain prolonged survival, or (most desirably) indefinite specific tolerance without the requirement for any maintenance immunosuppression. The use of donor-specific BM or marrow components given before, during, or after the grafting process will be analyzed.

In their landmark study, Billingham, Brent, and Medawar (1) were the first to establish actively acquired immunologic (allograft) tolerance through the administration of fetal and (later) neonatal donor-specific antigen (such as lymph node cells and splenocytes, but not BM cells) followed by subsequent donor skin allografts when the animal reached maturity (2). Several years later, Billingham and Brent (3) demonstrated that BM also could be used as a source of donor-specific antigen in the induction of neonatal tolerance. The prevalent scientific interpretation at that time was that the neonatal immune system was not physiologically mature and was immunologically incompetent. Thus, the neonatal immunologic milieu provided an environment that was uniquely conducive to the induction of donor-specific tolerance. Currently these experiments are not particularly relevant to the prolongation of allograft survival in a clinical scenario, but recent evidence confirming that the immune system of the neonatal animal is quantitatively, though not qualitatively, different from that of the mature animal underscores the fact that they represent the foundation upon which most of the subsequent research on tolerance is based (4–6).

Subsequent experimental attempts to induce tolerance in adult, immunologically competent animals were based on the concept of inducing a transient state of immunologic incompetence (similar to the neonate) using peripheral immunologic ablation techniques followed by donor-specific antigen, usually in the form of replicating lymphoid cells (Fig. 38.1). In early studies beginning in the 1950s, the preparative, ablative regimens relied on the use of various forms of host irradiation (such as whole body and total lymphoid irradiation) prior to infusion of donor-specific BM, followed by tissue or whole organ grafting. In the majority of these studies the object was to accomplish complete donor BM engraftment and gross chimerism to facilitate allograft acceptance. In this chapter this model will be referred to as the irradiation/BM (rad-BM) model. In the latter part of the 1960s, conditioning for tolerance induction in immunologically competent animals focused on the use of peripheral lymphocyte ablation by various antilymphocyte preparations and/or chemical methods, followed by donor-specific BM infusion. In this regimen, the goal was not to achieve a permanent complete BM transplant engraftment (so-called gross chimerism). Nevertheless, the persistence of small numbers of donor BM cells (so-called microchimerism) was postulated and demonstrated (see below). In this type of tolerance model, the role of BM was to induce various types of immunomodulatory cells whose regulatory function facilitated tolerance. This general regimen will be referred to as the antilymphocyte serum/BM (ALS-BM) model.

Although both general regimens were conceived in simplistic terms of peripheral lymphocyte depletion, extensive studies by various groups have demonstrated that a complex series of tolerance facilitating and regulatory mechanisms are

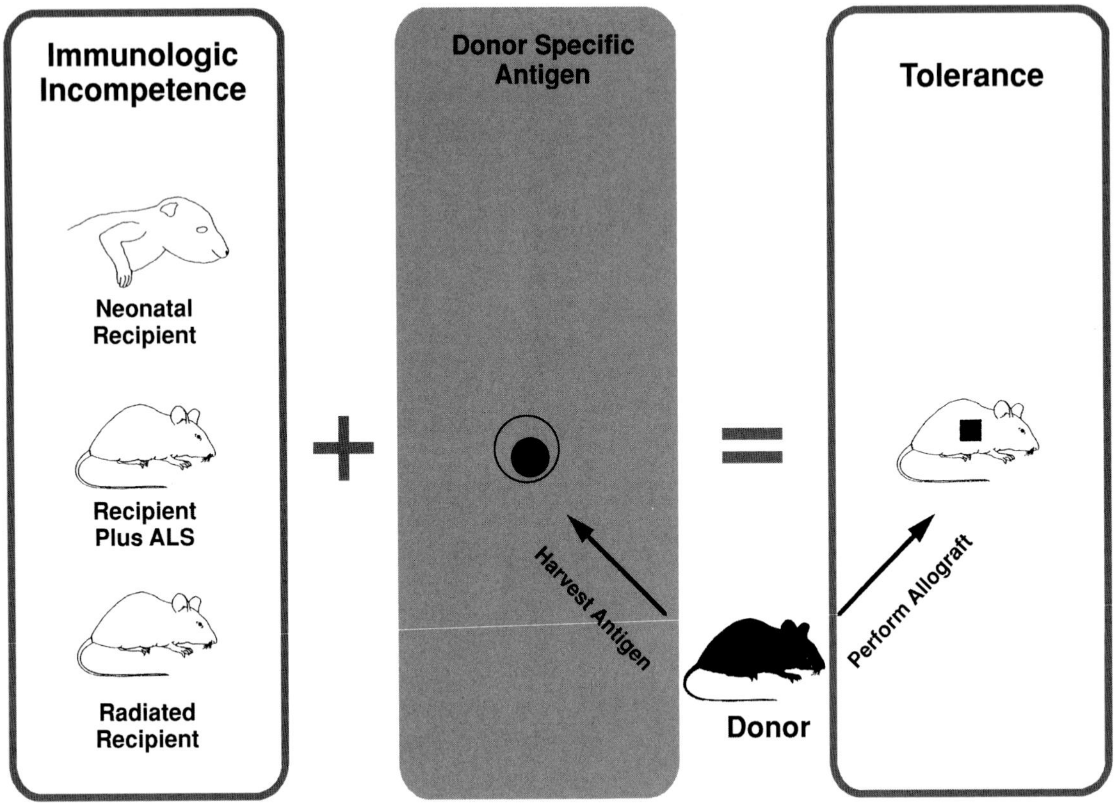

FIGURE 38.1. *Early theoretical basis for bone marrow conditioning was based on the landmark observations of Medawar regarding the active acquisition of tolerance. The administration of donor-specific antigen (in the form of cell suspensions) to animals with immature (neonatal tolerance) or incapacitated (through administration of ALS or radiation) immune systems would lead to tolerance.*

involved in both models. Furthermore, as will be seen later, these two approaches have recently converged as researchers ponder the benefits of combining elements of both these preparatory regimens in their protocols, especially in higher mammalian models.

This chapter is a comprehensive survey of relevant experimental and clinical data accumulated for each of the two classes of preparatory regimens that have developed in parallel over the past several decades. We hope to present the reader with the major developments in each of these two schools of BM conditioning as well as provide an appreciation of their similarities and differences. Finally we will conclude with a discussion regarding the future direction of research and clinical applications of this topic.

ANTILYMPHOCYTE SERUM PRECONDITIONING: THE ANTILYMPHOCYTE SERUM/BM TOLERANCE MODEL

Rodent Studies

The first comprehensive studies regarding the use of donor-specific BM infusion for tolerance induction using antilymphocyte serum (ALS)-based peripheral lymphocyte ablation were begun in 1970 by Monaco and colleagues in Boston. This work began as a logical extension of the observation that ALS produced dramatic tissue and peripheral lymphopenia in which the paracortical (circulating T-lymphocyte) areas of lymph nodes were profoundly depleted. Mouse skin allografts and rat skin xenografts enjoyed prolonged survival under ALS.

The impetus for the use of ALS to facilitate tolerance was the observation of the extraordinary effect that prior adult thymectomy had on the recovery of ALS-induced immunosuppression (7). Mice given a finite course of ALS showed profound tissue and blood lymphopenia that persisted for a month, during which time the animals showed depressed thymus-dependent humoral antibody responses and an inability to reject skin allografts. After one month, lymphocyte levels returned to normal and immune competence was restored. Adult thymectomy prior to ALS treatment resulted in peripheral blood and tissue lymphocyte depletion and depression of antibody formation that lasted twice as long as in normal (nonthymectomized) ALS-treated mice. This resulted in skin allograft survival many times longer than in adult nonthymectomized, ALS-treated recipients, with some grafts persisting over 100 days in perfect condition. It was known at the time that lethally irradiated mice rescued with syngeneic spleen cells recovered immune responses whether or not they were thymectomized as adults (8) but thymectomized irradiated recipients given bone marrow did not recover as readily as their nonthymectomized counterparts. These early ALS thymectomy studies were consistent with the concept that recovery from ALS peripheral depletion was affected by the bone marrow and was somehow thymus dependent or sensitive.

The prolonged state of immunosuppression associated with profound peripheral and tissue lymphopenia induced by ALS and adult thymectomy mimicked the immune incompetence and underdeveloped immune system of the neonate. Exploiting this observation, Monaco and colleagues (9) sought to reproduce in transiently immunosuppressed adults (ALS and thymectomy) the tolerance induction that had been achieved in neonates by Billingham, Brent, and Medawar (1). Normal or adult thymectomized mice were given ALS followed by donor-specific F_1 hybrid allogeneic spleen and lymph node cells (to avoid a graft-versus-host reaction) and donor skin grafts (9). The results were dramatic. Although ALS-treated, adult thymectomized mice not given donor cells showed prolonged skin graft survival, none exceeded 80 days. In contrast, the overwhelming majority of mice given donor cells survived over 100 days, and most survived indefinitely. These "tolerant" mice were chimeras by the gross chimera assay of Mitchison (10), and they accepted second donor-specific skin grafts but rejected third-party grafts. Furthermore, reinfusion of normal recipient strain isogeneic lymphoid cells terminated the tolerant state. These animals were therefore tolerant by all the criteria originally defined by Medawar.

The identification of bone marrow as the optimal replicating cellular antigen to induce tolerance resulted from the efforts of Monaco and colleagues to define a clinically applicable protocol. It was obvious that F_1 hybrid cells would never be available for clinical application. For eventual induction of tolerance in the ALS-prepared recipient, one would need easily available, nontoxic, highly effective antigen. When large doses of homozygous lymphoid cells were substituted for F_1 hybrid cells, severe graft-versus-host (GVH) reactions occurred in ALS-treated thymectomized mice. Attempts to avoid graft-versus-host disease (GVHD) used cell-free splenic antigens (11), haptenic forms of cell-free liver antigen (12), and nonreplicating living cells (i.e., kidney, epidermal) (13) in combination with ALS, but they were demonstrated to be ineffective. This necessitated further studies of lymphoid cells, which demonstrated that low doses of homozygous (non-F_1 hybrid) cells induced some tolerance without causing GVHD. Lance and Medawar subsequently showed that low doses of F_1 hybrid cells (blood, spleen, lymph nodes, thymocytes) all induced some degree of tolerance in ALS-treated mice (14,15), but they failed to examine BM. Further studies from Monaco's laboratory evaluated lymphocytes from lymph nodes, thymus, spleen, and BM over several dose ranges for tolerogenicity in ALS-treated mice (16). These studies were restricted to nonthymectomized mice, as adult thymectomy was not an attractive clinical option. They demonstrated that BM was superior in inducing specific unresponsiveness (tolerance) at each dose tested. Splenocytes were always second, and cells isolated from lymph nodes and the thymus had minimal effects and even caused sensitization at certain doses (Fig. 38.2).

The ability of BM to induce tolerance in ALS-treated mice without producing GVHD suggested that BM contains stem cells that are capable of inducing tolerance but are devoid of immune competence and the associated potential for GVH reactions. At this point it became apparent that appropriate fractionation studies might yield the optimal cellular antigen from BM for clinical tolerance

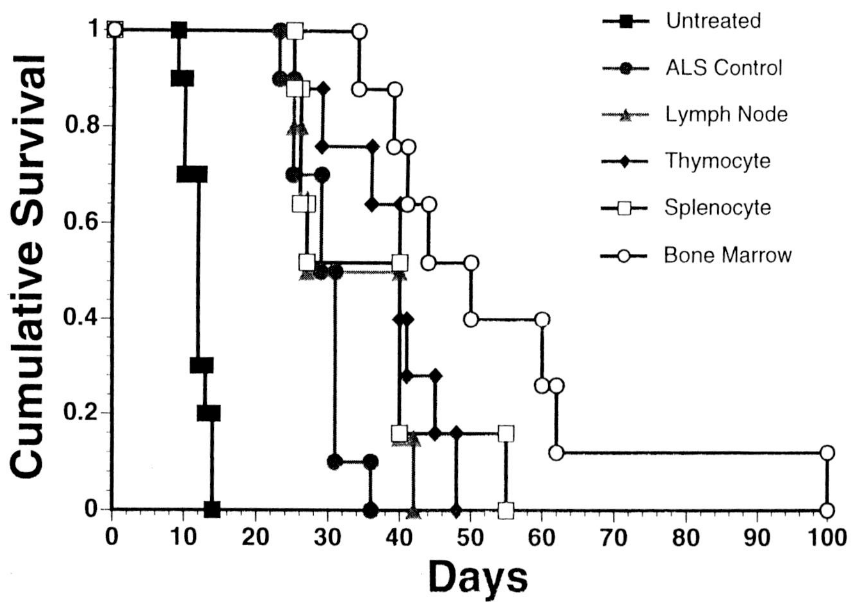

FIGURE 38.2. *Determination of optimal antigen for use with ALS. The 25 × 10^6 C3H/He cells of each listed type were administered intravenously to A/He recipients of C3H/He skin grafts on day +8. Rabbit anti-mouse ALS was administered on days −1 and +2.*

induction (16). In addition, it was postulated that various organs may contain variable numbers of mobilizable lymphoid cells, constituting a significant antigenic inoculation, and that treatment with ALS might facilitate induction of tolerance by these cells. Given the potentially important observation that long-term organ graft survivors may have persistent extratransplant donor cells in the periphery (17), this postulate was indeed prescient.

The unique tolerogenic effect of BM in ALS-treated recipients has been explored in detail. Dose was absolutely critical; at low doses (25×10^6 cells per mouse), BM was distinctly superior to all other lymphoid cell sources. As the dose was increased, spleen cells became more tolerogenic but lymph nodes and thymus became sensitized. This was consistent with the hypothesis (later verified) that tolerance was facilitated by a relatively nonimmunogenic stem cell and that the presence of mature lymphocytes (T cells) from lymph node and thymus was counterproductive. Additional studies using extremely low (0.01×10^6) to high (100×10^6) BM doses showed that, with a fixed amount of immunosuppression (ALS), the result could vary from sensitization, to no effect, to tolerance (Fig. 38.3) (13).

Timing of BM infusion was also critical. The optimal effect occurred only when BM was given 2 to 6 days after ALS treatment. BM given in proximity to ALS caused sensitization, and BM given 2 or 3 weeks after ALS had no effect (Fig. 38.4) (18). These studies clearly established that the recipient's state of immune competence (effect of ALS) and type of antigen (BM) were critical for tolerance induction. These original mouse studies, which underscored the necessity for delayed BM infusion after ALS, remain the basis for use of BM infusion clinically. It soon became clear that ALS-BM tolerance was not typical "Medawar" tolerance.

Studies evaluating various methods of delivering the BM inoculum demonstrated that the intravenous route of administration was not obligatory (19). Nevertheless, it was adopted by Monaco and Wood as part of the standard ALS-BM protocol (Fig. 38.5). Using this standard model (ALS days −1, +2; BM day 7), BM failed to induce tolerance when it was administered by the intraperitoneal, intrakidney, or subcutaneous routes—but sensitization was never induced. In contrast, BM given intrahepatically or intrasplenically (both by direct injection) was highly tolerogenic. Splenocytes were tolerogenic (but less so) using these unorthodox routes of administration while, again, lymph nodes and thymocytes failed. In a surprising series of experiments, it was demonstrated that BM administered into the spleen was even superior to intravenous BM in tolerance induction. Splenectomy 2 days after intrasplenic injection of BM reduced the tolerogenic effect, while splenectomy any time after intravenous BM injection had no effect (19,20). It is now known that exposure of donor BM to recipient antigens is critical for the tolerogenic effect (see below).

Whereas tolerance induction in ALS-treated, thymectomized mice using large doses of F_1 hybrid lymphoid cells induced a classic Medawar type of tolerance (9), it soon became apparent that the tolerance in the ALS-BM model was distinctly different and its etiology was multifactorial.

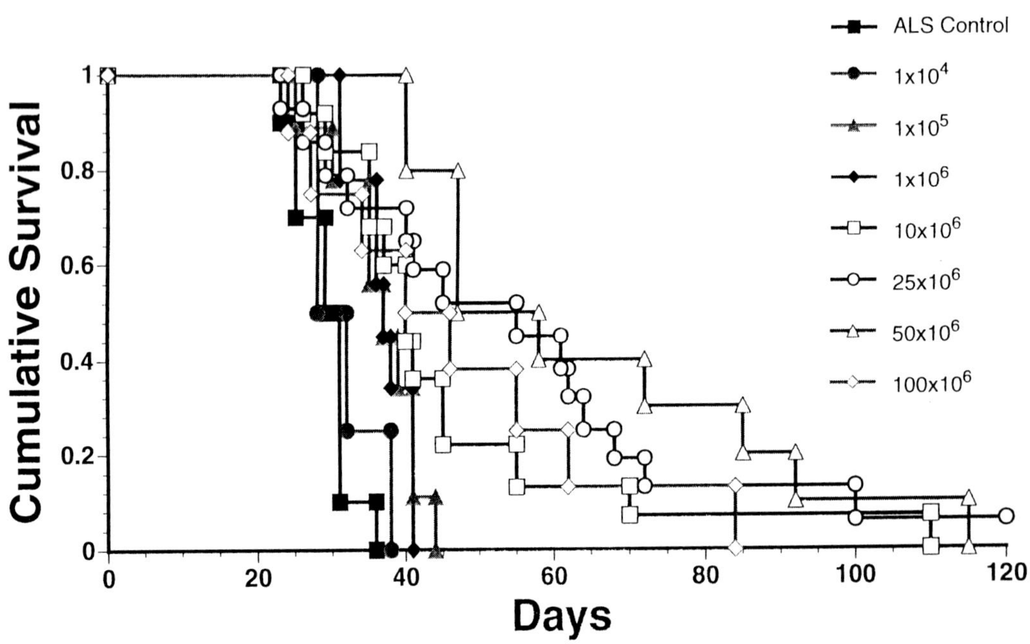

FIGURE 38.3. *Determination of optimal dose of donor-specific bone marrow to use with ALS. The specified number of viable C3H/He bone marrow cells were adminstered intravenously to A/He recipients of C3H/He skin grafts on day +8. Rabbit anti-mouse ALS was administered on days −1 and +2.*

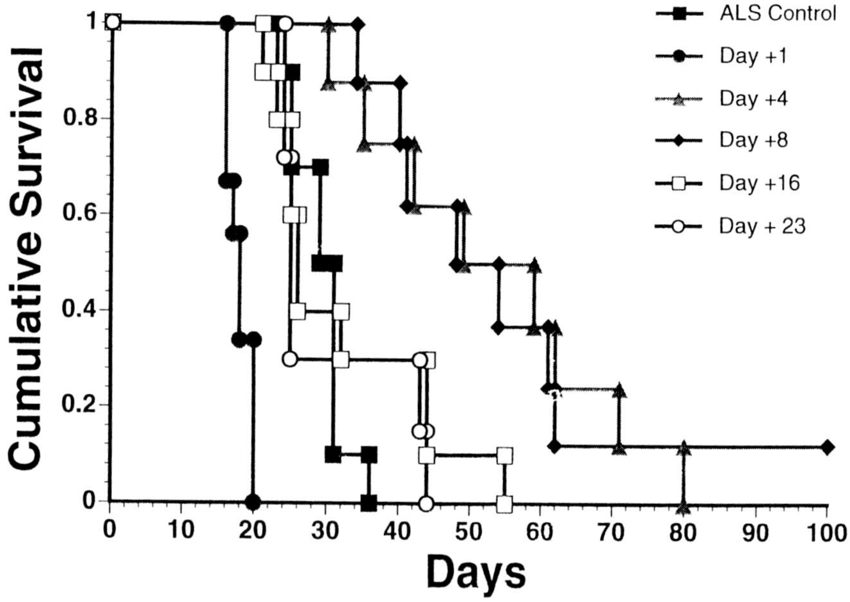

FIGURE 38.4. *Determination of optimal timing of administration of donor-specific bone marrow to use with ALS. The 25 $\times 10^6$ viable C3H/He bone marrow cells were adminstered intravenously to A/He recipients of C3H/He skin grafts on the days indicated. Rabbit anti-mouse ALS was administered on days −1 and +2.*

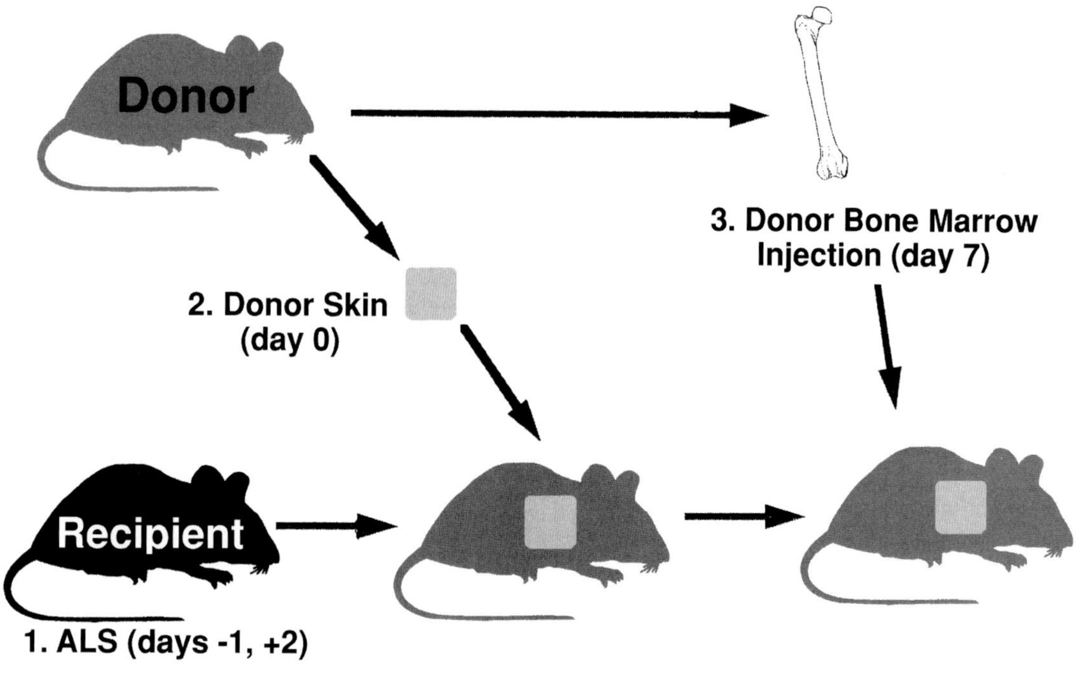

FIGURE 38.5. *Standard ALS-BM regimen developed by Monaco and Wood for application in murine models. The 0.5 mL of rabbit anti-mouse ALS are administered on days −1 and +2 relative to skin grafting on day 0. The 25 $\times 10^6$ viable donor-specific bone marrow cells are administered intravenously on day 7.*

The presence of gross chimerism was never demonstrated in the ALS-BM model, even in animals with long-surviving perfect grafts. However, the possibility that small levels of donor cells could persist in tolerant mice (microchimerism) was not excluded. Liegeois subsequently showed that donor BM persisted in certain animals under specific circumstances. Using a sensitive (at that time) T6 chromosome marker technique, he showed (21) that in ALS-treated mice given donor-specific BM and skin grafts in an ALS-BM protocol, intrasplenic proliferation of donor BM was identified up to 134 days after injection, but not in mice given just ALS or ALS and nonspecific BM. The conclusion was inescapable that exposure of donor BM to its own antigens (graft) in the recipient was critical for its proliferation and persistence; whether it caused tolerance could be inferred but not proven.

Another difference of ALS-BM "tolerant" mice was that second donor-specific grafts (applied while the first graft was 100 to 200 days old) were slowly rejected, whereas third-party grafts were rejected normally (20), and these "tolerant" mice seemed to have some level of donor-directed cell-mediated immunity by crude assays (22). The suggestion was that these apparently unresponsive animals had some type of active immune response that allowed acceptance of their well-tolerated grafts. Indeed some immunostimulants (adjuvants) could abrogate the tolerance, although *Bordetella pertussis*—known to cause lymphocytosis—could increase it when judiciously administered (23). This concept was reinforced by the finding that animals given BM on day +23 showed no tolerance and even evidence of sensitization (24). In essence, the use of ALS and BM generated an immune response that augmented the survival of early placed grafts and shortened the survival of late placed grafts. There was also evidence for humoral immunity in mice with well-tolerated grafts after ALS and BM (22,25), albeit with limited assays.

This active immune state in what appeared to be an unresponsive (tolerant) animal was confirmed in an additional study in which paired donor grafts were placed at various times simultaneously before BM injection in the standard ALS model and enjoyed prolonged survival (i.e., they were both tolerated) (26). In contrast, separate identical donor grafts placed before and several days after BM had different fates: the early graft was tolerated and the late graft was rejected. In addition, if a mouse was given ALS and BM but no donor graft on day 0, and then grafted on day +56, the graft was violently rejected, indicating that the previous marrow injection had sensitized the recipient. But if additional ALS was given with the day +56 graft, survival was indefinite. Tolerance was apparently induced in a sensitized animal.

It is of interest that cyclophosphamide given before BM injection abrogated the tolerogenic effect, possibly because cells facilitating tolerance were destroyed. Cyclophosphamide given after BM potentiated tolerance, perhaps by causing destruction of immunocompetent cells responding to the challenge of marrow (27). These studies and others in which the timing of donor skin graft placement was varied weekly from day 0 to day 56 led to the conclusion that BM (and other lymphoid cellular antigens) administered in proximity to ALS immunosuppression induced both a cytotoxic (sensitizing) and an enhancing (prolonged survival) response (28). If grafting was delayed for 14 days or more after ALS and cellular antigen, the sensitizing response was expressed as accelerated rejection. However, with additional ALS the enhancing response was expressed by prolonged survival.

Maki et al provided the first in vitro analysis of immune reactivity in ALS-BM–treated mice bearing long-term surviving grafts (29). Mice given ALS alone or ALS and a skin graft (but no BM) both showed prolonged nonspecific depression of T-cell and B-cell mitogen responses, which correlated with the persistence of the ALS effect. The ALS-grafted mice developed high direct lymphocyte-mediated cytotoxicity (DLMC), strong reactions in mixed lymphocyte reaction (MLR) cultures, and strong generation of cell-mediated lymphocytotoxicity in CML as immunosuppression from ALS wore off and graft rejection was imminent. Skin-grafted mice given ALS and BM showed prolonged suppression of DLMC and MLR to donor alloantigens, but they demonstrated high secondary type CML in association with prolonged skin graft survival. This indicated that spleen cells (used in the CML assay) from tolerant ALS-BM mice contained a population of precursor cells that were sensitized to skin donor alloantigens and were capable of differentiating into highly reactive cytotoxic cells upon reexposure to donor alloantigens. This observation argued against a classic clonal deletion mechanism of tolerance (see Chapter 5). It also suggested some type of immune regulatory phenomenon to explain the unresponsiveness present in vivo.

Although the mechanisms underlying tolerance in the ALS-BM model are multifactorial, the majority of experimental data suggest that donor-specific BM leads to a regulatory cell environment in the putatively tolerant recipient. Simpson et al showed that mice given skin allografts after ALS alone contained nonspecific suppressor cells (Fig. 38.6) (30). In the standard ALS-BM model using a standard suppressor cell transfer assay, Wood and colleagues showed that suppressor cells persisted in the spleens of BM–infused ALS-treated recipients with long-term grafts (31). They were specific for the donor strain (i.e., they did not transfer unresponsiveness to other donor strains) and were presumably T cells (anti-theta positive). Indeed, the ability of cytoxan given before BM injection to abrogate tolerance might be due to inhibition of a suppressor cell generation (32). Monaco and Wood subsequently evaluated the induction of unresponsiveness to skin allografts using adult congenic B10 mice disparate either at isolated K, I, or D regions of the H2 complex or at combined K/D and I regions (33). This series of studies demonstrated that unresponsiveness to antigens of the isolated K or D regions (class I) could not be induced, as shown by the inability of BM to prolong graft survival in these mice compared with ALS-treated controls. On the other hand, unresponsiveness to class I antigens could be induced when they were presented with antigens of the I region (class II). This indicated that the I region exerted a tolerogenic effect on the K and D regions. This requirement for the concomitant presentation of antigens of the K/D and I regions to achieve unresponsiveness was consistent with previous observations that active suppression is one possible mechanism for the induction of unresponsiveness in ALS-treated, marrow-injected mice.

Indeed, a follow-up study was conducted that involved analysis of the evolution and presence of suppressor cells in the various lymphoid compartments of ALS-BM tolerant mice (34). Suppressor cells appeared first in the spleens but then disappeared there and appeared later in the lymph

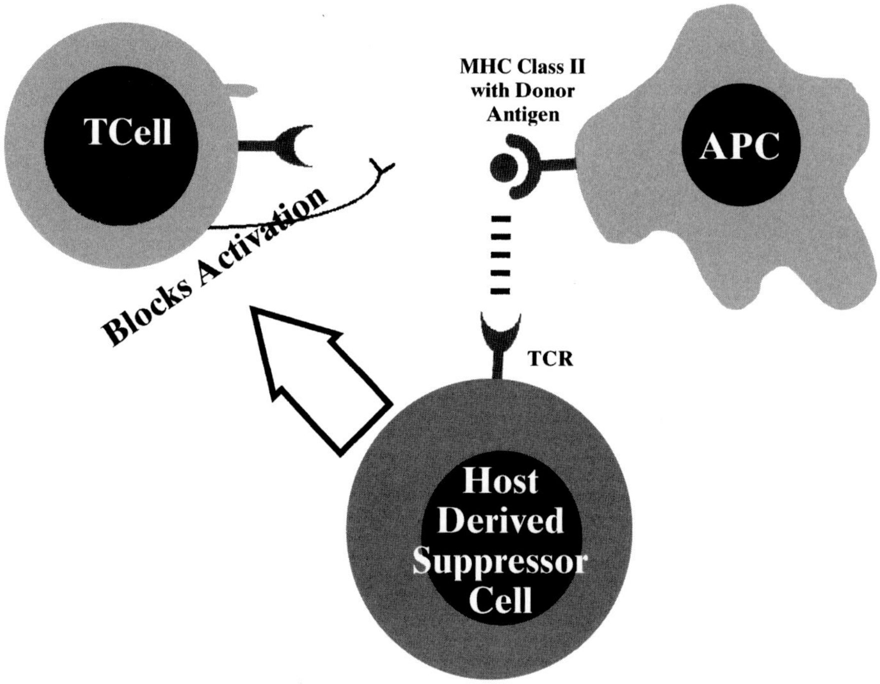

FIGURE 38.6. *Schematic depiction of the mechanism of action of putative suppressor cells in the ALS-BM model. Suppressor cells are cells of host origin that specifically inhibit T-cell activation in the presence of donor antigen.*

nodes, where they persisted for prolonged periods. Thymocytes and BM never showed suppressor cells. The identification of suppressor cells in this model depended on the time and lymphoid compartment studied. One should always keep this in mind when excluding the presence of suppressor cells (in any transplantation experiment) on the basis of a single assay at one given time point: multiple lymphoid compartments and times must be studied.

Maki et al extended this in vitro analysis of immune responses in ALS-BM tolerant mice (above) by showing the presence of suppressor cells using in vitro co-culture techniques (35,36). He showed that after ALS administration, nonspecific suppressor cells of recipient origin are generated; skin grafting of these animals resulted in or caused the appearance of recipient-origin anti-donor–specific suppressor cells. The most exciting finding was that when BM was infused into ALS grafted mice, specific suppressor cells of donor origin were generated and persisted during the late tolerant state. This work was clearly the forerunner of the idea that some type of veto cell is generated in ALS-BM tolerant models (Fig. 38.7) (37), a concept later reinforced by the non-human primate experiments of Thomas and colleagues (see below). A detailed description of this hypothesis relative to the interplay of the various suppressor cells in shifting the immune (cytotoxic) response to one of tolerance in the suppressed state has been presented (35–37). In a later study, Maki confirmed the important (and probably unique) effect of ALS treatment in generation of suppressor cells. He showed that animals given ALS alone possess antigen-nonspecific suppressor T cells that inhibit the proliferative response as well as the generation of cytotoxicity in MLC (38). The additional antigen stimulation provided by skin allografting shifts the specificity of suppressor cells from antigen nonspecific to specific for the donor skin antigen through an as yet unidentified mechanism. In some way this sets the stage for generation of a donor-specific, BM origin suppressor cell in the ALS-BM model.

How the putative regulatory cells (suppressor?, veto?, other?) work remains a subject of great speculation. Early studies suggested that suppressor-type cells are actively recruited to long-term grafts in ALS-treated mice (35).

Wood and Monaco next proceeded to study the effect of injection of donor-specific BM on the frequency of donor reactive cytotoxic lymphocytes in ALS-treated mice (39). This study utilized limiting dilution assay techniques that were modified so that only the population of cytotoxic T lymphocytes (CTLs) activated in vivo by alloantigens could be distinguished from the total CTL population. These quantitative determinations were made in spleens and lymph nodes of experimental and control mice on days 8, 14, 21, 58, and 365 after skin grafting. This study demonstrated that donor reactive CTLs in the BM–injected group remained suppressed as long as the animals maintained their grafts. The frequency of CTLs specific for third-party antigens was normal in mice bearing long-term donor-specific skin grafts. When the marrow-injected mice rejected their donor skin grafts, the total donor-specific reactive CTL frequency returned to normal. In contrast, in ALS-treated controls that did not receive BM, the total number of donor reactive CTLs returned to normal levels with recovery from the immunosuppressive effects of the ALS. The suggestion of this study was that donor marrow prevented the regeneration of donor reactive CTLs in the lymphoid tissues of ALS-treated mice.

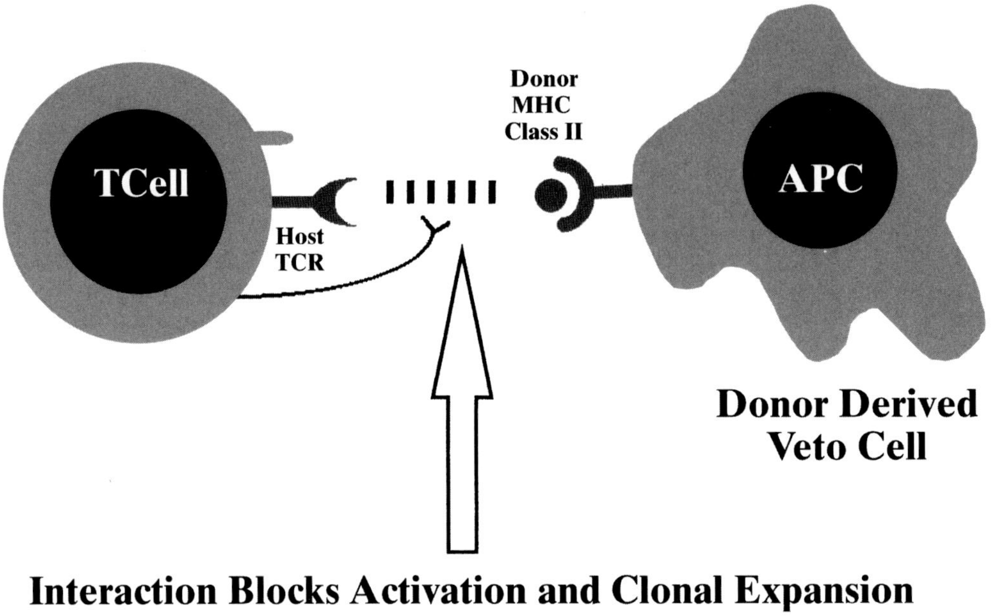

FIGURE 38.7. *Schematic depiction of the mechanism of action of putative veto cells in BM conditioning models. A veto cell is a cell of donor origin that acts as a fraudulent APC and specifically inhibits host T-cell activation in the presence of donor antigen.*

In a similar study, Pourshadi et al demonstrated that abrogation of secondary skin allograft rejection was accomplished by a veto-like mechanism provided by donor BM (40). In this study, mice received skin allografts and were injected on the following day with recipient strain spleen cells sensitized to the donor strain or with sensitized recipient strain spleen cells in combination with donor strain BM cells. When skin and BM cell donors from an F_1 strain were combined with a parental strain as recipient, donor BM abrogated the second set rejection observed in recipients of sensitized spleen cells alone. This occurred even though the F_1 BM cells were naturally tolerant of sensitized spleen cells. Thus, immunologic recognition of the sensitized spleen cells by the BM cells is not necessary for this abrogation. In this experimental system, the characteristics of the sensitized spleen cell suppressive activity of BM cells were consistent with a veto cell nature. These results suggested that the donor BM suppresses the regeneration of donor reactive CTLs in the lymphoid tissues of ALS-treated mice, possibly by veto cell activity.

De Fazio and colleagues have studied the tolerogenic efficacy of various BM cell fractions and demonstrated that for whole marrow to be effective the cells must be alive. Fresh marrow of adults and juvenile animals were equally effective (41). BM cells retain their effectiveness if stored at 4°C in 10% fetal calf serum for 18 hours but not if maintained at 37°C. Freezing the cells for 10 days in a cryoprotective medium preserved the ability of the cells to prolong graft survival (42).

The first fractionation study used velocity sedimentation on a bovine serum albumin gradient. Four fractions were obtained and one (fraction 3) containing predominantly small lymphocytes was very active in graft prolongation. Indeed 1–4 $\times 10^6$ fraction 3 cells were as effective as 25 $\times 10^6$ unfractionated cells in inducing unresponsiveness. A second fractionation method utilized Ficoll gradients (43). The 1 $\times 10^6$ lymphoid-like cells derived from donor BM that sedimented at a rate of 3 mm/hr in a 2% to 4% Ficoll gradient at unit gravity were as efficacious as 25 $\times 10^6$ whole BM cells. These allograft-prolonging lymphoid-like cells appeared not to be colony-forming unit (CFU) cells, had suppressive activity in vitro in MLR, and contained both nylon wool adherent and nonadherent cells. In the Ficoll separation, two major white cell fractions were obtained, the second of which (4 to 2 mm/hr fraction) was analogous to the fraction 3 achieved by BSA gradients.

Gozzo and De Fazio performed extensive additional studies using enrichment and depletion techniques (41) and fractionation by continuous density gradient centrifugation in Percoll (44). These studies showed the active cell in BM fractions displayed receptors for the Fc portion of IgG (FcR), but were negative for Thy-1, Ia, and Ig complement receptors, and for interleukin (IL)-2 receptors. The active Percoll fraction was 97% lymphoid cells. The cells had a density of 1.060 to 1.070 and represented 1% of total recovered cells. Using these highly purified Percoll fractions, they also showed that the active BM cells were positive for PNA (peanut agglutinin) and SBA (soybean agglutinin) receptors and positive for anti-asialo granulocyte-macrophage (GM) ganglioside, findings consistent with the concept that the active cells were stem cells or immature T cells (45).

Mature T cells have a negative effect in this model. It was found that peripheral blood lymphocytes (PBLs) could be substituted for BM in the ALS-BM model (46,47). This phenomenon resembled the effect of post-grafting BM infusion. The active PBLs were Thy-1$^-$ and had Percoll gradients similar to the active BM cells. However, if PBLs were mixed with BM, the tolerogenicity of BM was reduced. The cells associated with partial abrogation of the BM effect appeared to be mature T cells. This experiment suggested that, in the clinical application of BM, mature T cells in blood should be avoided—the reason vertebral BM is currently used in clinical applications of the ALS-BM model. Also, active cells could be obtained from blood PBLs using the Percoll fraction technique to eliminate the tolerance-abrogating mature T cells.

Since all the fractionation studies suggested that the active BM cells were some type of early stem cell, it was logical to see if the concept of expansion of the active cells could be achieved. Maki established suppressor cell clones from fresh adult BM that obviously contained a population of cells capable of specifically downregulating the immune response directed toward self major histocompatibility complex (MHC) antigens (48). C3H BM was cultured in various media containing IL-2 and/or IL-3, and the cultured cells were screened by limiting dilution for their capacity to suppress CTL generation against self MHC antigens. Several suppressor clones with strong suppression against self MHC antigens were produced. When administered with IL-3 in vivo, certain clones substituted for BM in the ALS-BM model prolonged specific skin allografts in mice. Northern blot analysis showed that these clones expressed full-length transcripts of the T-cell receptor (TCR) γ gene, but not those of TCR α, β, or δ genes. Flow cytometry showed that the BM suppressor clones were Thy-1 positive (in contrast to above) but negative for CD3, CD4 (L3T4), and CD8 (Lyt-2), and that they expressed only class I MHC antigens. The conclusion was that some type of suppressor cell from adult bone marrow may play an important role in extrathymic induction of self-tolerance.

Maki's studies on in vitro BM expansion suggested an in vivo approach to expand the active BM cell fractions. Monaco et al treated BM donors with granulocyte-macrophage colony-stimulating factor (GM-CSF) for two weeks, and their BM and other lymphoid tissues were harvested (49). The tolerogenicity of BM from GM-CSF–treated donors was significantly better in the ALS-BM model. The effect on spleen cells was variable—high doses of spleen cells from treated donors were not more tolerogenic but low doses were. Extensive fractionation studies showed that GM-CSF treatment activated a cell population in BM that promoted tolerance. This cell population was recovered in the 60% Percoll fraction. In contrast, GM-CSF treatment appeared to affect two cell populations in the spleen, one beneficial (tolerogenic) to graft survival, the other detrimental (decreased tolerance). The predominant effect depended on the dose used. The spleen cell(s) active in prolonging graft survival in ALS-treated mice was identified to be a non-T, non-B cell, as it lacked Thy-1, Ia, and Ig surface markers. Both FcγR$^+$ and FcγR$^-$ spleen cells were effective in prolonging grafts, but FcγR$^-$ cells were more effective (50). These findings explained the contradictory data on tolerance observed in attempting to use spleen cells in the ALS-BM model. They also showed the potential for using growth factors in conjunction with BM for tolerance induction.

In the usual ALS-BM protocol only a modest number of animals became tolerant indefinitely. In the standard (C3H/He to B6AF$_1$) class I–mismatched combination, all BM recipients enjoyed augmented survival of skin grafts, but only 15% to 25% were tolerant indefinitely. Clinical application of BM–induced tolerance would be more attractive if higher percentages of recipients became tolerant. Also, of concern has been the recognition that initial tolerance-inducing regimens will be introduced with standard immunosuppression therapies (cyclosporine) that might abrogate tolerance (recall that cyclophosphamide abrogated tolerance when given before BM) (27). Therefore, it was encouraging to find in mice that a short course of cyclosporine given after BM markedly increased the number of indefinite survivors to 50% to 60% (cyclosporine given before BM had marginal effects but did not abrogate tolerance) (51). More important, this improved tolerogenicity was accompanied by a powerful suppressor response.

Next, the effect of rapamycin (Sirolimus) in the ALS-BM model was studied. Using short courses of rapamycin in doses that had shown minimal effect on skin graft survival alone, investigators demonstrated that the drug had a dramatic effect in augmenting tolerance in ALS-BM–treated recipients. At 1.5 mg/kg, 100% of BM recipients became tolerant (over 200 days) (52). Using limiting dilution analysis, a dramatic reduction in CTL cells in tolerant animals was identified. Experiments using thymectomized, ALS-BM–treated mice suggested that the extraordinary effect of rapamycin might be mediated in part via its known property of decreasing the number of double positive (CD4/CD8) cells in the thymus. Hale et al compared the effects of cyclosporine versus rapamycin in augmenting tolerance in the ALS-BM model involving more severe histocompatibility differences. Rapamycin was superior in augmenting tolerance across combinations involving class I and II differences, complete mismatches, and nondiscordant xenografts (53). Of interest, the tolerance induced with rapamycin was multifactorial—skin allograft unresponsiveness was specific in vivo but in vitro analysis showed some nonspecificity. It had been previously shown that spleen cells from ALS-BM tolerant animals do not make IL-2 in vitro when challenged with donor-specific alloantigens. However, this study could not confirm the T_H1–T_H2 paradigm in rapamycin–ALS-BM tolerant animals; that is, there was not a preferential secretion of IL-4 and IL-10 in the tolerant mice. More recent work in Monaco's laboratory has demonstrated that permanent (>250 days) skin allograft survival could be achieved in a murine class I and II mismatch skin allograft model by combining a single dose of rapamycin with the standard ALS-BM protocol (ALS days −1, +2, and BM day 7). Again it was demonstrated that the recipient passed through a phase of nonspecific immunosuppression that evolved into a donor-specific state of tolerance after 60 to 90 days. Moreover, these animals demonstrated a clear state of stable donor-specific chimerism (approximately 5% to 10%) in the spleen, peripheral blood, and bone marrow.

These experiments with cyclosporine and rapamycin bode well for the clinical application of the ALS-BM model. The effects of tacrolimus and other new agents on the tolerance induced in the ALS-BM model have not been studied in detail to date, but these represent relevant experiments for eventual clinical application.

Further understanding of the processes underlying the beneficial effects of donor-specific BM administration was provided by a study conducted by Murase, Starzl, and colleagues (54). This study was designed to test the validity of the bidirectional paradigm of tolerance induction proposed by Starzl, but most of the findings bear direct relevance to other models of BM conditioning. In this rat model, leukocytes obtained from BM, spleen, lymph node, and thymus were used in conjunction with tacrolimus in an attempt to induce long-term donor-specific tolerance and chimerism. Some rats received heart, liver, intestine, or kidney allografts in conjunction with tacrolimus alone in order to compare their potential for inducing donor-specific tolerance with that of the cell suspensions. Without the concomitant administration of tacrolimus, all organs and cell suspensions were acutely rejected. Moreover, GVHD always ensued when intestinal grafts or cell suspensions of spleen or lymph nodes were administered in association with tacrolimus. In contrast, the administration of tacrolimus allowed engraftment of BM cells, liver, heart, and kidney without clinical evidence of GVHD. Administration of a thymus cell suspension and small doses of whole blood neither engrafted nor showed evidence of GVHD when administered in conjunction with tacrolimus. At 100 days, rats that had initially received heart, liver, or BM were tolerant in that they accepted a challenge heart or liver allograft for 100 more days in spite of persisting in vitro evidence of donor-specific reactivity. At this point, histopathologic studies of the challenge livers were normal, regardless of the nature of the priming graft. In contrast, the still-beating challenge hearts exhibited a range of changes from no evidence of acute or chronic rejection to severe rejection. The tolerogenicity of the priming grafts, from best to worst, was defined as liver, then bone marrow, then heart. After 30 days, the greatest degree of chimerism and a clear dominance of donor T cells were demonstrated in rats whose primary grafts had been liver. Animals whose primary graft was BM were less densely chimeric but demonstrated multilineage chimerism without a clear dominance of either donor or recipient cells. At 100 days after primary allografting, donor-specific class II cells had become sparse in both the liver and BM recipients; however, T-, B-, and dendritic cell lineages still could be detected. In animals receiving other primary grafts (kidney, heart, and other cell suspensions), no significant chimerism could be detected. The suggestion is that there may be a sufficient number of tolerogenic BM–derived cells within some organ grafts, so as to render unnecessary the administration of donor bone marrow. On the other hand, simultaneous administration of BM may facilitate tolerance induction to certain organs with low numbers of tolerogenic cells (i.e., heart, kidney, etc.).

Canine Studies

The concept of exploiting the unique properties of the neonatal immune system for the induction of donor-specific tolerance was extended to a higher phylogenetic model by Grosjean et al. In this study, they were able to demonstrate that dogs injected with donor BM in the neonatal phase of development were specifically tolerant to these same antigens when they were reexposed at maturity (55). In 1967, Grosjean and colleagues followed up on this work and reported on the use of ALS in conjunction with BM injection in order to augment the induction of tolerance in immature dogs (56). The rationale behind these experiments was that the administration of ALS would reconstruct the neonatal immunologic milieu in young dogs and facilitate the induction of tolerance. In this series of experiments, they found modest synergism of ALS and donor-specific BM in prolonging kidney allograft survival.

In 1970, Yamamoto attempted to create a more tolerogenic milieu in mature dogs by combining the effects of azathioprine and BM transplantation in a canine renal allograft model (57). These experiments found that donor BM administered alone 4 days prior to allografting sensitized the recipient, leading to a second set rejection pattern. Azathioprine administered alone at a dose of 5 mg/kg/day beginning 7 days prior to allografting resulted in a modest prolongation of kidney survival to 21 days (control = 9 days). The combination of donor-specific BM and azathioprine resulted in prolongation of graft survival to 37 days, whereas use of nondonor marrow afforded no survival benefit. Yamamoto then attempted the same experiment but this time combined the use of rabbit anti-dog ALS and azathioprine (58). These experiments demonstrated an additive effect of combining ALS with azathioprine [mean survival time (mst) = 39 days] and a further potentiating effect of BM (mst = 48 days).

Caridis and colleagues also demonstrated that the success of this model of tolerance induction was not limited to lower species. Their first dog experiments clearly showed an effect of ALS and BM (59). Dogs given ALS daily for a week before and after renal allografting received approximately 300×10^6/kg BM cells (from ribs of donors) on day 10. BM–infused dogs showed prolonged survival over those given ALS alone (Fig. 38.8). In a group given a second dose of BM (day +20) the survival was remarkable (100 to 200 days versus a control ALS group of 14 to 31 days). Most interesting was the observation that some dogs with long-term surviving renal allografts after ALS-BM had transient bouts of renal dysfunction from which they spontaneously recovered. Given the observations (above) of evidence in mice of sensitization and tolerance after ALS and BM, it was postulated that BM infusion may produce a transient host-versus-graft (HVG) reaction, which may in turn lead to the establishment of an enhancement-type phenomenon resulting in an augmented graft survival. These improved results over those achieved earlier by Grosjean were the result of the continuing studies designed to optimize the dosage and timing of each of the components of this therapy.

Hartner and colleagues (60) showed that BM Percoll fraction 3 (fraction 3 BM) was as effective or more effective than fresh whole BM and that frozen-thawed fraction 3 BM was also effective. This finding in dogs was obviously important for the eventual clinical application of BM or its fractions. In this study the dogs were treated with ALS from days −6 to +7 relative to kidney transplantation. Fresh unfractionated BM or fraction 3 BM (produced by centrifugation in a discontinuous Percoll density gradient) was intravenously infused into the recipients on post-graft day 13 or 14. As in the mouse model, use of the fractionated BM resulted in superior allograft prolongation compared to unfractionated BM (46 vs. 35 days, respectively). In this study it was also noted that frozen/thawed BM or fraction 3 BM was as effective in prolonging allograft survival as the fresh counterpart. In vitro analysis of the recipients at 30 to 45 days after transplant demonstrated a globally reduced MLR to donor as well as third-party antigens and reduced responses to ConA, PHA, and pokeweed mitogens, suggesting that the animals were nonspecifically suppressed. By 60 days after transplant, the MLR to third-party antigens and responsiveness to ConA, PHA, and pokeweed mitogens had returned to normal levels, whereas donor-specific unresponsiveness was maintained.

The effect of combining pharmacologic immunosuppression in combination with ALS-BM was then studied (61,62). This study demonstrated that the long-term renal allograft survival with specific unresponsiveness to the donor induced through the use of ALS and fractionated BM could be improved on with a limited course of cyclosporine in a canine model. ALS was administered daily from days −5 to +7 relative to grafting on day 0 with an MLR-mismatched donor renal allograft. Fractionated donor BM cells were infused 3 to 7 days following the last dose of ALS. The administration of adjuvant cyclosporine (20 mg/kg/day) was

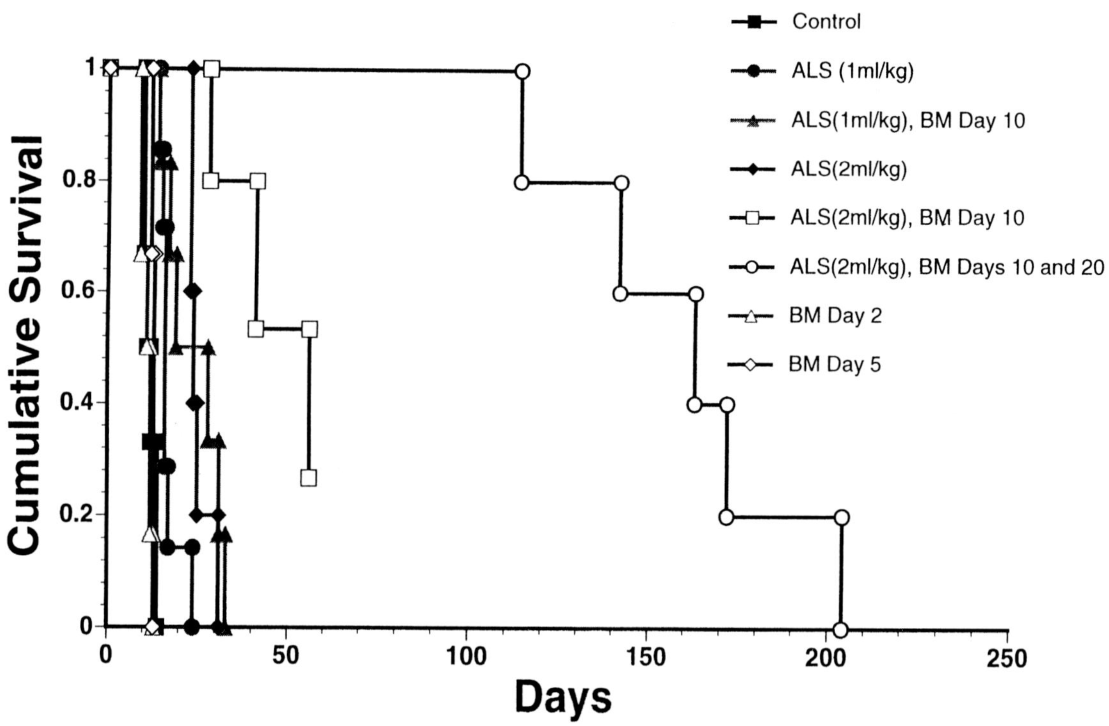

FIGURE 38.8. *Demonstration of efficacy of the ALS-BM regimen in the canine model. Rabbit anti-dog ALS was administered daily from day −7 to day +7 at the dosage indicated. The 2–4 × 10^6/kg viable donor-specific bone marrow cells were administered intravenously on the days indicated.*

begun 3 to 7 days following the BM infusion and continued for 60 days. Relevant median graft survivals were 19 days for animals treated with ALS alone, 23 days in animals treated with ALS plus cyclosporine, and 95 days for animals treated with ALS, cyclosporine, and fractionated BM. Follow-up studies including rapamycin demonstrated that when combined with a cyclosporine–ALS–BM regimen, rapamycin given at a dose of 0.3 mg/kg through day 39 after allografting significantly increased overall survival when compared to the use of cyclosporine–ALS–BM alone (63).

Nonhuman Primate Studies

Study of the ALS-BM model was first applied to a primate model by Smits et al when they demonstrated in 1971 that the administration of antilymphocyte globulin (ALG) for six days following transplantation followed by a single injection of 25 million BM cells into a baboon was superior to the continuous use of ALG and equal to or slightly superior to the standard immunotherapy at the time (azathioprine and prednisolone) (64). Control animal hepatic grafts survived 11 days, whereas continuous administration of ALG resulted in graft survival of 19 days, and ALG-BM administration resulted in a median graft survival of 31 days. In a follow-up study one year later, Myburgh et al further studied this ALG-BM model in baboons by studying the effects of other immunomodulatory agents (65). An intensified period of post-transplant immunosuppression was created via the addition of a single injection of 50 mg/kg of cyclophosphamide at the time of transplant. This was found to result in no improvement in median allograft survival (31 days vs. 35 days for ALG-BM alone), but it did result in a markedly increased animal mortality secondary to sepsis. The addition of whole body irradiation immediately preoperatively completely abrogated the beneficial effects of ALG and BM. The prolongation of donor antigen exposure through the use of multiple pulsed doses of BM (25 million cells given on day 7 and three times weekly thereafter) was inferior to a single dose given on postoperative day 7 (25 million cells) and frequently resulted in sensitization. This finding is at variance to results obtained with multiple doses of BM in the canine renal allograft model discussed previously.

This group then conducted experiments designed to elucidate the underlying mechanism of the ALS-BM regimen. They began by exploring the concept of passive and active enhancement in live allografting using a polyspecific cytotoxic serum (prepared in a pool of ten baboons by hyperimmunization with allogeneic lymphoid tissue) and donor-specific BM injection (Fig. 38.9) (66). Again using an outbred baboon population, control hepatic allograft survival was 12.9 ± 2.5 days. Administration of the polyspecific serum (passive enhancement) given in doses of 1 mg/kg for 2 weeks following transplantation significantly prolonged allograft survival to 32 days. This passive enhancement was felt to be the result of antibody binding the antigenic targets of the donor tissue, thereby inhibiting the cell-mediated response. The combination of passive and active enhancement was studied through the administration of the polyspecific serum in combination with 25 million donor-specific BM cells. This regimen resulted in significant further prolongation of allograft survival to a median of 51 days. Subsequent testing demonstrated circulating donor-specific alloantibodies in the serum of animals with long-term surviving hepatic allografts.

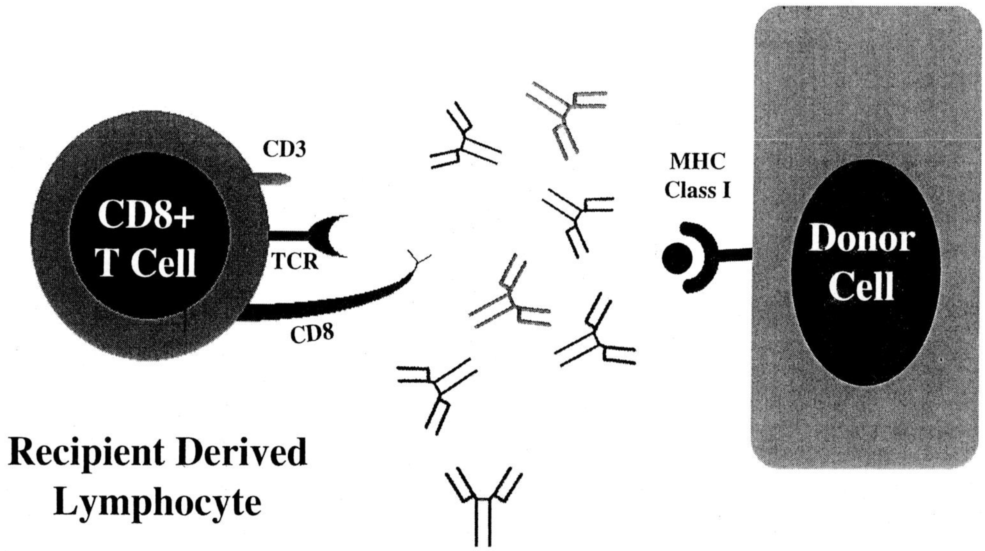

FIGURE 38.9. *Schematic depiction of the mechanism of action of humoral enhancement in BM conditioning models. Antibody specific for donor class I antigen competitively inhibits the recognition of this antigen by cytotoxic T cells, thereby preventing cell-mediated cytotoxicity.*

Smit et al expanded on this earlier work in a study in which outbred baboons were preimmunized with donor-specific BM fractions after having been conditioned with either cyclophosphamide or incomplete Freud's adjuvant. Both of these protocols resulted in a predominantly anti-donor B cell antibody response that significantly prolonged the survival of orthotopic liver allografts from the BM donors (67). They suggested that the beneficial effects of BM were the result of a relatively high concentration of MHC class II antigens in comparison with other sources of donor-specific antigen, which had been found to be inferior for the induction of tolerance (68).

The use of ALS in conjunction with the administration of donor-specific BM was then attempted in outbred rhesus monkeys by Thomas and colleagues. Among the first of their observations was that skin allograft survival could be significantly prolonged in an outbred primate model using this treatment regimen (69). Encouraged by these findings, they then set out to apply this treatment regimen to an outbred rhesus monkey kidney allograft model (70,71). Four groups were initially studied: control animals that received no immunosuppression, a second group that received only rabbit anti-thymocyte globulin (RATG) (50 mg/kg daily, days 0 to 5 after transplant), a third group that received RATG in conjunction with one intravenous dose of donor-specific BM (70 million cells/kg) on day 12, and a fourth group that received RATG and donor-specific BM (70 million cells/kg) on days 12 and 20. Standard renal allografts were performed on day 0. Control animals had a median graft survival of 9 days. Median graft survival in animals receiving only RATG was 35 days. Animals receiving two doses of donor-specific BM in conjunction with RATG had a median graft survival of 50 days, whereas all animals receiving a single dose of donor-specific BM experienced graft survivals in excess of 365 days. On histopathologic analysis, these long-term surviving kidneys demonstrated moderate mononuclear cell infiltration and minimal changes in extraglomerular vessels. These studies demonstrated an inverse relationship in the ratio of CD4 and CD8 cell subsets that occurred in all RATG-treated groups. The elevation in relative proportion of $CD8^+$ cells was greatest in animals receiving a single dose of donor-specific BM in conjunction with RATG, with these animals having a $CD4^+$-to-$CD8^+$ cell ratio of 0.18 (normal 1.1) for at least 4 months after transplant. It subsequently recovered (0.42–0.71) at 6 to 8 months after transplant, although it never achieved normal levels. They demonstrated that the lymphocytes of animals receiving RATG and a single dose of donor-specific BM on day 12 became nonspecifically unresponsive to polyclonal antigens and allogeneic cell stimulation in a one-way MLR in the first 4 months after transplant. Later in vitro studies demonstrated that the nonspecific unresponsiveness began to recover by 6 months after transplant and was normal by 8 months after transplant. The MLR to donor-specific antigen consistently remained negative. Thus the early state of nonspecific lymphocyte unresponsiveness appeared to evolve over time to a state of donor-specific antigen unresponsiveness.

Subsequent studies demonstrated that the regimen consisting of RATG administration followed by donor-specific BM on day 12 following allografting was associated with the presence of pan-lymphocyte reactive antibody in the recipient until the tenth post-transplant day (72). Pan-specific antilymphocyte antibody was no longer detectable after 11 days, but cytotoxic antibody specific for mature T cells remained in the recipient's serum. These findings may explain the critical time relationship between antilymphocyte therapy and BM infusion required for the induction of tolerance in rodents, noted previously by Monaco and Wood. This study also seemed to suggest that the tolerance-promoting cell present in BM was not a mature T cell, as cytotoxic antibodies specific for mature T cells were present at the time of BM administration. Rather, it might be a pre-T or non-T cell. Finally, this study demonstrated that the RATG-BM protocol resulted in the development of lymphoid nodules in the transplanted kidney that express a $CD8^+$, FcIγG-receptor–positive phenotype and appear to be of donor origin. This suggested the possibility of locally mediated immunosuppression via a veto cell type of mechanism, veto cells being donor-derived cells of BM origin that act as fraudulent antigen presentation cells.

Further studies have demonstrated that the adjunctive use of azathioprine did not have a beneficial effect and, in fact, resulted in decreased median graft survival and increased anti-donor lymphocyte-mediated cytotoxicity. In contrast, the adjunctive use of cyclosporine and low-dose prednisone exerted an additive immunosuppressive effect and resulted in a 50% increase in median renal allograft survival and no discernible anti-donor lymphocyte-mediated cytotoxicity (73). This study was notable in that cyclosporine and low-dose prednisone appeared to enhance the humoral alloimmune response, increasing the incidence of recipients with anti-donor antibody-dependent cell-mediated cytotoxicity.

The Thomases then extended their work on the ALS-BM model to include fractionated total lymphoid irradiation (TLI). TLI has been effective in promoting allograft tolerance without chronic immunosuppressive therapy in animal models but has not been widely accepted in clinical transplantation due to the logistical and practical limitations associated with pretransplant conditioning. The potential use of a more practical (for cadaveric transplants) post-transplant TLI protocol had not been critically evaluated. In the ATG-BM experiments the RATG was administered for 3 to 5 consecutive days beginning on day 0, and a total dose of 500–625 cGy of fractionated TLI was given in treatments of 125 cGy each beginning on day +1. Interestingly enough, either post-transplant TLI nor ATG monotherapy induced long-term graft acceptance, but the combination of the two treatments was remarkable in promoting long-term allograft acceptance (75% >100 days) without subsequent immunosuppressive therapy. The post-transplant TLI accentuated and prolonged the changes in peripheral blood lymphocyte subpopulations that were initially effected by RATG. For example, depressed levels of $CD3^+$ cells were present for 4 to 5 months, with large numbers of $CD4^+$ and $CD8^+$ $CD3^-$ cells. The infusion of DR^- $CD3^-$ donor-specific BM in recipients treated with post-transplant TLI and RATG appeared to further increase the incidence of stable long-term allograft acceptance (80% >100 days).

Simultaneously, further studies of the mechanisms underlying the beneficial effect of donor BM administration and the role of veto cells in this model were pursued (74). This series of studies began with the observation of the importance of carefully timing the donor BM cell infusion (59,71,75). Also important was the observation that no sensitization, GVH reactions, or serially detectable chimerism had been observed in these models (35,72,76). Also notable was the finding of specific anti-donor CTL activity detected in 90% and 85% of the nonimmunosuppressed and RATG-treated controls, respectively, at or before the time of rejection. However, the investigators were not able to detect anti-donor CTL activity in any of the recipients treated with ATG and donor BM cell infusion, even after most allografts eventually succumbed to a chronic type of rejection process late in the post-transplant period. Moreover, the suppression of donor CTL responses by donor BM appeared to be specific in that third-party CTL responses could be elicited in these animals. One hypothesis was that veto cells have a role in the induction of allograft tolerance and suppression of CTL responses following donor BM cell infusion in ATG-treated monkey renal allograft recipients. The authors set up a series of depletion experiments with donor BM cells depleted of particular subsets. This was accomplished through the use of monoclonal antibodies for CD2, CD3, CD8, CD16, CD38, and DR antigens. Bound cells were then removed with anti-IgG–coated magnetic beads. The depletion of DR- and CD38-positive cells from the inoculum did not affect the activation of cell-mediated lympholysis. The absence of any effect in spite of depletion of DR-positive cells suggests that the veto cell population in rhesus BM is not represented by mature dendritic cells or cells of the macrophage/monocyte lineage. Since CD38 is expressed on lymphoid progenitors, activated lymphocytes, natural killer (NK), and leukocyte-activated killer (LAK) cells, the lack of adverse effect associated with depleting these populations suggests that the veto cell population is not activated and is of a nonlymphoid, very early lymphoid, or non-NK/LAK cell lineage. In contrast, depletion of $CD2^+$ cells resulted in a complete loss of veto activity. In addition, depleting $CD3^+$ cells not only failed to diminish veto activity, but actually enhanced it somewhat. These results suggest that the veto cell population in fresh BM is not represented by mature T cells. Depletion of either $CD16^+$ or $CD8^+$ cells also eliminated in vitro veto activity. These in vitro findings were confirmed with in vivo applications.

Limiting dilution assays demonstrated the donor specificity of clonal inactivation of CTL precursors after in vitro or in vivo exposure to BM depleted of DR bright cells (77). In addition minimal bystander effects were seen on normal CTL precursor responses to third-party stimulator cells, while CTL responses to donor-specific cells were abrogated in the same cultures. Donor BM cells mediating the veto effect were resistent to L-leucyl-L-leucine methyl ester, which excluded BM cell–mediated cytotoxicity by NK cells, CTLs, or activated macrophages. In contrast, the veto activity was abolished if the marrow was pretreated with UV-B light irradiation, mitomycin, or gamma irradiation, indicating that BM cells contained a UV-B–sensitive precursor of the veto effector that required a proliferative step prior to having full veto capacity. Again, both the administration of cyclophosphamide and irradiation of BM depleted of DR bright cells were capable of abrogating its tolerogenic effect. Only recipients given nonirradiated donor BM depleted of DR bright cells demonstrated PBL chimerism, which was associated with the functional deletion of anti-donor CTL precursors and correlated with the duration of graft survival.

A subsequent study investigated the veto mechanism of CTL precursor suppression and the role of CD8 and transforming growth factor (TGF)-β in these events (78). These studies were based on the previous observation that depletion of $CD8^+$ subsets from the BM inoculum ablated the tolerogenic effect. A role of CD8 in the veto effect was also suggested by rhesus MLR-induced CML experiments in which pretreatment of normal responder cells with monoclonal antibody to MHC class I (the natural ligand of CD8) blocked the suppressive activity of allogeneic BM cells. In addition, pretreatment of the BM cells with anti-CD8 monoclonal antibody blocked strong veto activity, suggesting that CD8 functions as an accessory or adhesion ligand. Anti-CD8 treatment significantly enhanced weak BM-cell–mediated veto activity, suggesting that it may serve as a signal transducer to increase veto activity, perhaps by the induction of cytokine release. TGF-β was studied because it, like BM veto cells, inhibited MLR-induced CML reactions in a dose-dependent manner and anti-TGF-β immunoglobulin blocked the BM cell–mediated veto activity. In this series of studies, active TGF-β was found only in the supernatants of CML cultures containing BM cells. Pretreatment of the BM cells with L-leucyl-L-leucine methyl ester (which eliminates cytotoxic precursor and effector lymphocytes and monocytes) did not affect the level of active TGF-β. As noted in the previous study, the veto effect of BM cells was also noted to be L-leucyl-L-leucine methyl ester resistant. Also noted was that the treatment of isolated BM cell cultures with anti-CD8 antibody elicited TGF-β secretion, suggesting that CD8 functions as an immunoregulatory molecule in veto effects by BM and may act by inducing low-level secretion of TGF-β, which mediates or facilitates the veto mechanism of CTLp inactivation in a paracrine manner.

A recent study further investigated the immunologic basis for the heterogeneity in the duration of long-term graft acceptance following an ALS-BM regimen (79). This study examined the relationship between recipient–donor MHC class I and class II DR matching and the development of anti-donor antibody-dependent cellular cytotoxicity and renal allograft survival. The study demonstrated a requirement for sharing one DR allele to achieve long-term graft acceptance and that this was correlated with the early suppression of anti-donor antibody-dependent cellular cytotoxicity responses. The implication of this study is that the presentation of donor class I peptide by a shared DR allele allows a veto effect by donor BM cells and that this mechanism may be responsible for the tolerogenic effect. In this manner, DR sharing would allow specific donor BM veto cells to reduce clonal expansion elicited by both the direct and the indirect antigen presentation pathways.

Human Studies

The first clinical application of the ALS-BM model in human transplantation was made in the pre-cyclosporine era. Monaco et al suggested the efficacy of ALS and donor-specific BM administration in one human renal transplant case (80). In this case report they described the rejection-free post-transplantation course of a 38-year-old woman who received a zero-antigen match, crossmatch-negative cadaveric kidney in 1973. The patient received ALG for the first 14 days after transplantation and donor-specific BM (11×10^9 cells) on postoperative day 25 in addition to the standard prednisone-Imuran therapy available at that time. The graft functioned well and the patient experienced no episodes of rejection for 8 months, at which time she died of perforated sigmoid diverticulitis. At autopsy, the renal allograft appeared normal and histology showed minimal infiltration of the graft with mononuclear cells. A similar study was subsequently conducted in several patients receiving living-related kidney allografts (81). Again, the BM was well tolerated, there was no clinical or laboratory evidence of GVHD, and the patients did quite well from a rejection point of view.

Barber et al reported the first long-term results of a controlled prospective study involving the use of donor-specific BM in 57 cadaveric renal allograft recipients in the cyclosporine era (82). This study involved the administration of Minnesota antilymphocyte globulin (MALG) for 10 to 14 days following allograft placement. Cryopreserved donor-specific BM ($2–3 \times 10^8$ cells/kg) was transfused 7 days after the last dose of MALG. A group of 54 patients received the contralateral kidney and similar immunosuppression with the exception of BM. All patients received standard triple-agent immunosuppression (cyclogporine, steroids, azathioprine) with a median follow-up of 16 months. Sixteen grafts were lost in the control group (13 rejections, 3 deaths). Six grafts were lost in the BM group (3 rejections, 2 deaths, 1 recurrent disease). Interestingly enough, the graft survival rates for the BM group at 12 and 18 months were 90% and 85%, respectively. In the control group the 12 and 18 month allograft survival rates were 71% and 67%, respectively. While this difference was significant at the $P < 0.01$ level, the surprisingly low allograft survival rates in the control groups led to a less than enthusiastic acceptance of these findings. MLC analyses demonstrated a trend toward donor-specific hyporesponsiveness in the BM group. Examination of the differences in number of rejection episodes, estimated renal plasma flow, glomerular filtration rate, and urine protein between the control and treatment groups revealed no differences.

A subsequent report evaluated the incidence of chimerism and its association with rejection-free graft survival in these patients (83). Immediately after transplantation, 26.4% of patients in the BM treatment group and 18% of patients in the control group demonstrated low levels of chimerism even prior to BM infusion. Following donor-specific BM administration, the rate of chimerism in the treatment group was approximately 50% after 12 months of follow-up. The rate of chimerism in the control group was 10% to 20% over the same time period. Twenty-one of the 23 transfused patients (91.3%) who demonstrated detectable chimerism were rejection free over this 12-month period, whereas only 14.3% of the BM–transfused patients with no detectable chimerism were rejection free. The presence of chimerism in the control group was also correlated with a decreased incidence of rejection; however, it was statistically insignificant.

Other clinical studies using donor-specific BM conditioning have demonstrated mixed results. A brief report from England by Rolles et al examined the use of donor-specific BM transfused ($2–3 \times 10^8$ nucleated cells/kg) 5 days after a 10-day course of ATG in liver allograft patients in a prospective randomized study (84). Maintenance immunosuppression was provided by cyclosporine only. In this study there was no difference between the treatment and control group in terms of the number of rejection episodes per patient. Moreover, chimerism could not be demonstrated in the peripheral blood or BM of recipients utilizing PCR for donor MHC class II DNA.

There have been three reports of immunologic tolerance to renal allografts performed after the recipients had previously undergone myeloablation and BM transplantation as treatment for neoplasia and then received a renal allograft from the same donors (85–87). The four patients represented in these studies accepted their kidney allografts without the need for adjuvant immunosuppressive agents.

Finally, Ricordi and the Miami group have reported superior results in allograft survival and reduced rejection rates in liver allograft recipients given donor-specific BM, including the observation that multiple BM infusions gave the best results—a finding similar to those previously described by Monaco in a canine model (59,88).

TOLERANCE MODELS USING RADIATION PRECONDITIONING AND DONOR BM

Rodent Studies

The earliest studies using BM conditioning to affect prolongation of allograft survival were published in the mid-1950s and concerned the combined use of radiation and administration of donor-specific BM in mouse skin allograft models (see also chapter 5). It began with the observation that high doses of radiation given prior to grafting could significantly prolong the survival of skin allografts (89). It was noted, however, that increasing levels of radiation resulted in shortened animal survival. Two years later, Lorenz and colleagues discovered that animal survival could be restored by the injection of syngeneic, allogeneic, and (in some cases) xenogeneic BM immediately following exposure to the radiation (90). In 1955, Main and Prehn reported on skin allografts performed with the combination of high-dose irradiation of the recipient and BM rescue (91). In this study they described a novel phenomenon whereby skin allograft survival was for all intents and purposes permanent if the F_1 hybrid BM used for rescue therapy contained antigens identical to those of the allograft. This was subsequently confirmed by others (92). Similar results were demonstrated in later experiments extending this concept to the administration of homozygous donor-specific marrow as rescue therapy (93). While technological limitations prevented in-depth mechanistic studies regarding the role of BM in this model, it was noted via chromosomal markers that irradiated animals subsequently injected with allogeneic or xenogeneic BM were chimeras at least out to 49 days after injection (94). This series of experiments culminated in the report of a kidney allograft performed in a canine model using an irradiation and donor-specific BM injection protocol (95). The animal died of infectious complications 48 days following transplant, with the graft still functioning normally.

The exploration of various forms of host irradiation as a preparatory regimen for donor-specific BM injection began in earnest with a series of reports by Slavin et al that studied the induction of specific transplantation tolerance using various forms of fractionated TLI. The first study demonstrated that fractionated TLI was sufficient preparation for induction of long-term tolerance in conjunction with BM injection, resulting in a markedly decreased incidence of complications and mortality when compared to whole body irradiation (96). Slavin and colleagues were also successful in demonstrating that fractionated TLI prevented the onset of GVHD in animals subsequently treated with allogeneic BM injections, whereas whole body irradiation did not (97). In addition, they were able to demonstrate through in vitro microcytotoxicity assays that the mice rendered tolerant through this regimen were BM chimeras. This technique was later extended to rats with the findings that adult rats treated with fractionated TLI and donor-specific BM injection permanently accepted heterotopic placed heart or skin allografts from the donor. Furthermore, these animals were BM chimeras and were specifically tolerant to donor tissues. There was no evidence of GVHD present (98).

In much the same fashion as Monaco and Wood performed the first comprehensive and systematic evaluation of the ALS-BM model, Sachs and colleagues from NIH and later the Massachusetts General Hospital undertook a thorough and comprehensive evaluation of the immunologic mechanisms underlying the induction of tolerance in animals receiving donor-specific BM following a course of radiation conditioning. The first of these mechanistic studies was performed in mice. Induction of chimerism was accomplished through the administration of 750 cGy whole body irradiation followed by the intravenous injection of 20 million donor-specific BM cells 1 to 3 hours later (99). This study demonstrated that for about 2 months after reconstitution the chimeras had very weak anti-host cell-mediated lymphocytotoxicity reactivity and little third-party reactivity. During this period of time a cell population capable of suppressing CML reactivity against both host and third-party alloantigens was demonstrated in chimeric spleens by in vitro mixing experiments. These putative suppressor cells were Thy-1 negative and in most cases radiation sensitive. After 10 weeks, however, the mature chimeras demonstrated donor-specific tolerance and strong third-party alloreactivity, and at this point suppressor mechanisms could no longer be demonstrated via in vitro mixing experiments. Thus, in much the same way as it had been demonstrated that donor-specific unresponsiveness secondary to the administration of ALS and BM is a dynamic process involving changes in the recipient's immune responsiveness over time, so too did it appear that the same concept applied to radiation-based regimens.

A subsequent study looking at the suppression phenomenon more closely used recombinant strains of mice as a source of stimulator cells for in vitro analyses of suppressor cell function (100). These recombinant animals possessed both tolerated MHC antigens and nontolerated (third-party) MHC antigens on the same stimulator cells. These studies were performed to determine whether the tolerated antigens might elicit nonspecific suppression mechanisms affecting cell-mediated lymphocytotoxicity responses to nontolerated antigens. No evidence for such nonspecific suppression was observed in this study, and the conclusion was drawn that if suppressor mechanisms mediate such tolerance in mature allogeneic chimeras that they must be highly antigen specific.

Ildstad and Sachs then began to explore the therapeutic benefits of reconstituting the irradiated host with T-cell–depleted BM containing both host (syngeneic) and donor (allogeneic or xenogeneic) components in a mouse-to-mouse or mouse-to-rat model (101). The optimal number of syngeneic and allogeneic/xenogeneic BM cells needed to achieve consistent reconstitution and tolerance was determined to be 5 million and 15 million per 40 million cells, respectively. In this study, the recipient B10 mice were given a single dose of 950 cGy that resulted in 100% mortality within 2 weeks in otherwise untreated animals. These studies were stimulated by numerous previous observations that elimination of mature T cells from donor BM inocula can lead to long-term survival of fully allogeneic BM chimeras (99,102). The realization that the survival of such animals was generally not as good as those reconstituted with syngeneic BM and that the health of these animals was compromised led to the conclusion that this was the result of partial immunoincompetence (103,104). In an effort to circumvent this immunoincompetence, the use of mixed syngeneic and allogeneic BM was attempted. This study demonstrated that reconstitution with mixtures of syngeneic and allogeneic or syngeneic and xenogeneic BM led to long-term survival of recipients equivalent to that of animals reconstituted with syngeneic BM alone. Moreover, the animals remained healthy and demonstrated no evidence of infections or GVHD. Typing of mixed allogeneically reconstituted mice at 2 to 3 months following reconstitution demonstrated them to be mixed chimeras bearing variable percentages of syngeneic and allogeneic lymphoid cells in their peripheral circulation. These animals were immunocompetent and specifically tolerant to donor-specific skin grafts. In the mice reconstituted with mixed syngeneic and xenogeneic BM, there was little evidence of persistence of the xenogeneic lymphoid compartment; however, the animals did appear to be specifically hyporeactive to donor-specific (rat) skin grafts.

Next, Ildstad et al published a study dissecting the influence of T-cell depletion on either the syngeneic or the xenogeneic marrow component on prolongation of rat skin allografts in B10 mice (105). This study revealed that mice that received mixed marrow inocula in which the syngeneic component was T-cell depleted, whether or not the xenogeneic component was T-cell depleted, showed specific prolongation of donor skin grafts. In contrast, the rat skin grafts were promptly rejected by animals that were treated with mixed BM cell inocula that had not been T-cell depleted. In vitro analysis demonstrated that animals that had received untreated syngeneic BM demonstrated high levels of reactivity to donor-specific rat target cells, while animals reconstituted with mixed inocula in which the syngeneic component had been T-cell depleted exhibited low levels of serologic activity (if any) against donor-specific splenocytes.

Using these same techniques, Ildstad et al then studied the influence of T-cell depletion of host or donor BM on lymphopoietic repopulation in mixed allogeneic chimeras (106). In this series of studies when B10 recipients received mixed marrow inocula in which the syngeneic component had not been T-cell depleted, regardless of whether the allogeneic component was treated, they repopulated exclusively with host-type cells, promptly rejected donor-type skin grafts, and were reactive in vitro to the donor by CML and MLR assays. In contradistinction, T-cell depletion of the syngeneic component resulted in specific acceptance of donor skin grafts regardless of whether the allogeneic component had been T-cell depleted. Such animals were specifically unreactive to allogeneic donor lymphoid elements by CML and MLR assays, but were reactive to third-party antigens. When both the syngeneic and the allogeneic marrow components were T-cell depleted, variable percentages of host and donor lymphoid elements were detected in the reconstituted host. When only the syngeneic component was T-cell depleted, however, the animals repopulated exclusively with donor-type cells. Although these animals had detectable in vitro anti-host (B10) reactivity by CML and MLR, they exhibited excellent survival and demonstrated no in vivo evidence of GVHD.

Subsequent experiments noted that spleens from early mixed chimeras contained recipient strain cells capable of markedly suppressing in vitro cell-mediated lympholysis (107). Furthermore, they also realized that spleens from recipients of T-cell–depleted syngeneic marrow alone contained similar suppressor cells. This suppression was manifest 8 days following BM administration when spleen cell numbers were beginning to recover. Because of this, it was reasoned that if such suppression was involved in resistance to GVHD then allowing for an 8-day delay following the administration of T-cell–depleted syngeneic BM before injecting a T-cell–containing allogeneic inoculum may confer even further protection against GVHD. In a series of experiments using this approach in a murine model, they demonstrated that irradiation and infusion of syngeneic T-cell–depleted marrow allowed engraftment of allogeneic marrow given 8 days later with the development of complete, stable allochimerism. The 8-day delay, moreover, resulted in marked protection from GVHD induced by an otherwise unprotected large allogeneic BM inoculum.

Aksentijevich et al then reported on two studies with important ramifications for potential use of BM transplantation in a xenograft model. The first study demonstrated that normal murine serum contained natural antibodies (NAb)—IgM, IgG3—that bound with much higher affinity to rat BM cells than to rat splenocytes or thymocytes (108), despite the fact that the mouse–rat animal combination is considered concordant. The second study, using the adoptive transfer of rat BM cells into SCID mice with or without the concurrent adoptive transfer of normal BALB/c serum, demonstrated that the ability of the sera to inhibit the engraftment of rat BM cells correlated with their cytotoxic NAb content, and that the inhibitory effect of the sera could be overcome by the administration of large numbers of rat BM cells, ostensibly via adsorption of the naturally occurring antibody (109).

Further exploration into the veto-like mechanism underlying the beneficial effect of donor-specific BM transfusion (with sublethal radiation preparation) on allograft survival was conducted by Pierce et al. They noted that, in contrast to conventional suppression in which suppressor cells are syngeneic to the cells they suppress, tolerance in the models utilizing donor-specific transfusion could be transferred only by cells of the donor allotype (110–112). These studies were based on the observation that depletion of Thy-1–positive cells eliminated the capacity of the donor BM population to transfer tolerance and markedly reduced the capacity of the BM to induce tolerance (113). These studies also demonstrated that spleen cells from tolerant chimeras when co-injected in a 1:1 ratio reduced the high GVHD mortality induced by the injection of allogeneic spleen cells alone. When co-injected at a 5:1 ratio, spleen cells from mice rendered tolerant by BM injection and sublethal irradiation completely eliminated GVHD. Furthermore, depletion of the splenocytes specific for the MHC of the original BM donor in chimeric mice removed the capacity of the spleen cell inoculum to inhibit GVHD caused by normal mouse splenocytes. Thus, in contrast to conventional suppression, which required the continued presence of suppressor cells, the BALB/c cells isolated from the tolerant splenocyte injectate, although unable to inhibit GVHD disease induced by normal BALB/c splenocytes, remained nonreactive against the $H2^b$ allotype for a prolonged period following depletion of the B6 cells. This prolonged response reduction, dependent on some interaction with allogeneic donor cells (which are specifically nonreactive to host antigens), is compatible with a veto mechanism.

The mechanisms underlying the induction of tolerance via a BM–irradiation regimen were further delineated in a novel study by Tomita and colleagues (114). This study utilized the fact that B10 mice generate two endogenous superantigens that require I-E for their expression. These superantigens (Dvb11-1 and Dvb11-2) interact with Vβ11 of the T-cell receptor. Thus, in B10.A mice that possess an I-E antigen, and thus express the superantigens, T cells with the Vβ11 chain bind to the superantigens in the thymus and are deleted as self-reactive thymocytes. Conversely, B10 mice, which are I-E negative, do not express the superantigen and thus do not delete those T-cell clones bearing a Vβ11 chain. In this study, BM cells from I-E–positive B10.A mice were infused into I-E–negative B10 mice within the context of 3 Gy whole body irradiation, pretreatment with anti-CD4 and anti-CD8 monoclonal antibodies, and thymic irradiation. This study demonstrated the absence of detectable Vβ11 T cells in the splenocytes of long-term stable chimeras. The implication was that the presence of even very small numbers of donor-specific I-E–positive cells in the thymus of the recipient was responsible for the deletion of Vβ11-positive T cells in the recipient. In untreated B10 mice, an average of 5% of $CD4^+$ or $CD8^+$ PBLs expressed Vβ11, whereas only 0.3% of B10.A $CD4^+$ or $CD8^+$ PBLs expressed Vβ11. In chimeras created through the infusion of B10.A BM into B10 mice, Vβ11-positive PBLs were not detectable above the levels seen in B10.A mice when analyzed at 5, 6, 12, 20, and 73 weeks after BM transplantation. This occurred in spite of the fact that low levels of Vβ11 positive T cells were clearly detectable in the splenocytes of the chimeras at the earliest time points tested. In the splenocytes possessing Vβ11 positivity, attempts at stimulation of these lymphocytes through cross-linking of the Vβ11 T-cell receptor chains through the use of monoclonal antibodies resulted in a demonstration of anergy. Immunohistochemical staining with anti-I-E^k monoclonal antibody demonstrated rare I-E–positive cells in the chimeric thymus at day 10, with greater numbers detected on day 14 and large numbers detectable 6 weeks following BM transplantation. Taken together these results suggest that the T cells with receptors that recognize donor-specific antigen are not completely deleted in this model of tolerance induction and that those remaining donor-specific T cells may be tolerized via an anergy mechanism.

In an attempt to develop a more clinically relevant conditioning regimen with reduced potential for morbidity and mortality, non-myeloablative models for achieving multilineage mixed chimerism and tolerance across major histocompatibility barriers have been developed (115–117). These studies noted that the amount of chimerism demonstrated in animals receiving allogeneic BM directly correlated with the degree of disparity between the donor and the recipient and also correlated with the dose of total body irradiation administered. Treatment of the recipient with cyclophosphamide 2 days following allogeneic BM transplantation reduced the dose of total body irradiation necessary for reliable engraftment regardless of major and hematopoietic histocompatibility disparity. Allogeneic chimerism (BALB to B10 or B10.BR to B10) was stable and present in all cell lineages including lymphoid, NK, and myeloid cells. Moreover, these mixed chimeras exhibited donor-specific tolerance in vitro as assessed by MLC and cytotoxic assays, and in vivo to skin and primarily vascularized cardiac allografts. Ildstad then applied this tolerance induction regimen to a primarily vascularized rat cardiac model and studied its effect on the incidence of chronic rejection. In this study they found that donor-specific skin (mst ≥ 177 days) and primarily vascularized cardiac (mst ≥ 213 days) grafts were accepted without evidence of acute or chronic rejection. Moreover, the immunosuppression was specific in that MHC-disparate third-party skin (mst = 14 days) and cardiac grafts (mst = 13 days) were rapidly rejected. This tolerance was systemic since donor-specific tolerance was present in vitro as assessed by mixed lymphocyte proliferation assay.

This BM conditioning regimen has also been applied to the transplantation of allogeneic islets (118). In this series of studies, B10 ($H2^b$) mice rendered diabetic via streptozotocin were irradiated (950 cGy) and reconstituted with 5×10^6 T-cell-depleted syngeneic and 15×10^6 T-cell–depleted B10.Br ($H2^k$) BM cells. Islet allografts, genetically matched or disparate to the BM donor, were placed under the renal capsule within 24 hours following the infusion of BM cells. All donor-specific islet allografts were permanently accepted, while 7 of 9 MHC-disparate islet allografts were rejected. With the non-lethal conditioning regimen, diabetic mice received 500 cGy total body irradiation followed by an infusion of 15×10^6 untreated allogeneic B10.BR BM cells. A simultaneous islet allograft matched or MHC disparate to the BM donor was performed on the same day. Two days following BM transplantation a single dose of cyclophosphamide (200 mg/kg) was injected intraperitoneally. Once again, islet allografts matched to the BM donor demonstrated marked prolongation of survival (mst ≥ 226 days) and showed no evidence of chronic rejection, while MHC-disparate grafts were rejected (mst = 34 days). Animals receiving islet grafts without the concomitant administration of BM rejected their grafts over a similar time course as those receiving an MHC-disparate graft. The nonlethal conditioning regimen was then extended to an islet xenograft (rat-to-mouse) model (119). Here the diabetic recipients were conditioned with 700 cGy total body irradiation and transplanted with 4×10^7 donor-specific BM cells. All animals repopulated as mixed donor–host chimeras and demonstrated permanent acceptance of donor islet xenografts.

Canine and Swine Studies

In 1981 Howard and colleagues reported on renal allografts performed in 12 splenectomized dogs treated with fractionated TLI (total dose 1950–3000 rad) before their transplant (120). In eight dogs receiving BM from the kidney donor, two died immediately after transplantation, two rejected at 3 and 13 days, and one animal died with a functioning graft on day 13. Two animals experienced graft survivals in excess of 500 days. Chimerism was not detected in these long-term surviving animals. Control dogs had median graft survivals of 12 days. Four dogs treated with fractionated TLI without BM infusion had a median graft survival of 15 days.

At around the same time several studies were performed using skin allografts in pigs (121). In these experiments, various protocols of fractionated lymphoid irradiation were used in conjunction with 700 million donor-specific BM cells per kilogram. The BM was given one day following the cessation of radiation. Skin grafting was carried out 1 to 2 days following the administration of BM, with the exception of one protocol in which the skin grafts were delayed for approximately 2 weeks. Despite the use of various irradiation protocols, this study was able to achieve only moderate prolongation of median skin allograft survival (21.4 days compared to 10 days for control animals). Furthermore, as in the Howard study, no donor-specific chimerism was ever detected. In utilizing the same basic protocols extended to renal allografts, Vaiman et al demonstrated modest success in terms of achieving kidney allograft survivals of 6 to 7 months without additional immunosuppression (122). The regimen consisted of fractionated lymphoid irradiation followed 24 hours later by donor-specific BM injection. Renal allografting was performed 1 day following BM administration. Again, no permanent chimerism was obtained in this semi-incompatible SLA model.

Following previous demonstrations that permanent lymphopietic chimerism could be induced in MHC-disparate miniature swine by BM transplantation after lethal whole body irradiation, Sachs et al sought to determine whether such chimerism would lead to permanent tolerance to a donor-specific vascularized allograft without the requirement for exogenous immunosuppression (123). In this study, eight miniature swine that had received MHC-mismatched BM transplants more than 5 months previously underwent kidney transplantation from either an MHC-matched (to the BM donor) or an MHC-mismatched (to the BM donor) donor. All animals had regained in vitro responsiveness to third-party antigens by the time of transplantation. Animals that received kidney grafts mismatched for the BM donor rejected within 7 days. Of the animals that received kidneys matched to the BM allograft, 80% (4 of 5) had excellent renal function 200 days following kidney transplantation. This study demonstrated that BM transplantation can be an effective means for the induction of tolerance to an MHC-mismatched kidney transplant in a large animal model.

Nonhuman Primate Studies

The concept of using fractionated TLI as a preparatory regimen for donor-specific allogeneic BM conditioning was extended to primates in the early 1980s by Myburgh, Smit, and colleagues in a series of experiments that built on their previous work with the ALS-BM model. They first studied the extension of this concept to an orthotopic liver allograft in baboons (124). In this study, baboons were exposed to various fractionated TLI protocols prior to the administration of BM and allografting. Most of the irradiation protocols yielded no survival benefit when combined with donor BM injection. In one exception, the animals received eight separate doses of 200 cGy each, 3 times weekly ending 1 month prior to allografting, and 60 million donor-specific BM cells immediately following the last fraction of irradiation. Median graft survival was extended from 19 days in control animals to nearly 90 days. A small degree (<15%) of chimerism was found in some recipients via sex chromosome analysis and was documented in only half of the animals having long-term graft survival. Chimerism could not be demonstrated in any of the baboons exposed to alternative irradiation protocols. Despite the fact that only some of these animals experienced long-term graft survival, this study demonstrated that tolerogenesis induced by fractionated TLI and donor specific-BM injection is well tolerated and operative in a primate model.

In a second study, these researchers extended their newfound protocol to a baboon renal allograft model (125). This study demonstrated that fractionated TLI given in eight doses as outlined above, followed immediately by injection of approximately 200 million donor-specific BM cells, and followed 3 weeks later by kidney allografting, resulted in donor-specific tolerance in the recipients for donor kidney allografts and substantial BM chimerism without evidence of GVHD in this outbred baboon model. The levels of chimerism identified were significantly greater (i.e., between 30% and 50%) than those found in the liver allograft study previously discussed.

Smit et al then proceeded to follow these studies with in vitro assays of recipient lymphocyte proliferative responsiveness (126). In these studies they demonstrated the possible presence of both donor-specific and nonspecific lymphocytic suppression. These lymphocytes were recovered from animals following irradiation whether or not they had received a donor-specific BM infusion and organ transplantation. These preliminary studies demonstrated that like the ALS-BM model, the regimen of fractionated TLI and donor-specific BM injection is associated with prolonged periods of decreased donor-specific and nonspecific recipient lymphocyte responsiveness, which were perhaps mediated by suppressor cell activity. These findings were consistent with previous observations by Zan-Bar et al in which they reported the adoptive transfer of tolerance to bovine serum albumen in mice after fractionated TLI (127). The effect was mediated by a putative suppressor cell that was antigen specific when adoptively transferred in modest quantities.

In more recent studies, investigators at the Massachusetts General Hospital developed a regimen consisting of ATG, total body irradiation, thymic irradiation, and donor-specific BM infusion and applied it to a renal allograft model in cynomolgus monkeys (128,129). In these studies they looked at various manipulations of the ATG–irradiation preparative regimen and studied the effects of these manipulations on allograft survival and the induction of chimerism. The basic regimen consisted of horse anti-human ATG administered at a dose of 50 mg/kg intravenously on days −2, −1, and 0. Three hundred cGy of total body irradiation was administered as two fractions of 150 rad on days −6 and −5. Seven hundred cGy of local thymic irradiation was administered on day −1. Kidney transplantation and splenectomy were performed on day 0. Donor-specific BM cells at a dose of approximately 1×10^8 cells/kg were administered on day 0. Cyclosporine was administered for 28 days after transplant and then discontinued. This study was notable for the finding that monkeys treated with this regimen developed multilineage chimerism and accepted renal allografts for as long as 3 to 4 years with no further immunosuppression. Conversely, if total body irradiation was administered in a single dose of 300 cGy or a single dose of 150 cGy, chimerism could not be demonstrated and there was no long-term graft survival even with the addition of cyclosporine to the regimen. Similarly, monkeys treated with the basic regimen minus the infusion of donor-specific BM rejected the kidney allografts by day 52. This study suggests that, in this model, at least transient engraftment of donor BM appears to be essential for the induction of donor-specific tolerance.

Human Studies

In an early investigation into the induction of tolerance through the administration of lymphoid irradiation and BM, a clinical trial was attempted with six recipients of human cardiac allografts based on studies in dogs in which donor-specific tolerance was induced through the administration of BM after a conditioning regimen using TLI (130,131). Interestingly enough, in this study the patients received their TLI over a 39- to 49-day period. Heart transplantation was accomplished 7 to 13 days later. Donor-specific BM was administered (5 billion cells) intraperitoneally at the time of transplant. Four of these patients died within 2 months of transplant—one from uncontrolled and unmoritored rejection, two from sepsis, and one from hemodynamic compromise but with no evidence of rejection on autopsy. Two patients, both with heterotopic cardiac allografts, were long-term survivors with in vitro evidence of donor-specific unresponsiveness.

CONCLUSION AND FUTURE DIRECTIONS

Experimental donor-specific BM infusion as defined by the ALS-BM tolerance protocol has been effective in varying degrees in inducing some degree of specific unresponsiveness in every species tested (mouse, rat, dog, non-human primate) and with every tissue or organ tested (skin, heart, islets, liver, kidney). It seems reasonable to conclude that this will also apply to humans.

In the initial clinical applications of BM, expectations and criteria of efficacy should not be too high. It is unrealistic to expect that the complex immune system of humans will behave like that of an inbred rodent. Rather than seeing an immediate dramatic induction of donor-specific tolerance (without the need for maintenance immunosuppression), it is likely that the salutary effect of BM will become apparent in patients over time—much like histocompatibility matching. Eventually BM–infused patients should show improved survival, improved graft survival, and better function with less rejection episodes and reduced immunosuppressive requirements. Whether we will ever be able to remove all immunosuppression in all patients remains open to question. Since many experimental studies suggest that a major effect of BM (perhaps not the only effect) is production of a suppressor-regulatory cell environment, it might be necessary to keep a very low background of nonspecific immunosuppression to keep down the cytotoxic response and keep the suppressor cell response dominant. Indeed, suppressor activity is most demonstrable experimentally on a background of transient or minimal nonspecific immunosuppression; therefore, it seems reasonable to expect that this concept will also be applicable clinically.

Current methods of clinical BM application are limited by the amount of available BM. One donor can provide the BM for only one recipient—not for all six potential recipients of a multiorgan harvest. Also, the procurement of BM from multiple bones and vertebrae is tedious, time consuming, expensive, frequently disruptive to the retrieval process, and frankly aesthetically unappealing. It is essentially a research project beyond the capabilities of most organ transplant programs. In order for widespread application of

BM infusion to become a reality, a simple BM infusion protocol must be developed.

The authors believe that donor-specific BM will be used as a biologic reagent to facilitate the production of a suppressor-type immune response or state in essentially all recipients of solid organ transplants. For this to occur, one cannot expect to procure whole fresh BM in sufficient quantity for all potential organ recipients of a specific cadaver. Rather, we will have to obtain relatively small quantities of cadaver BM (taken relatively easily by routine aspiration) and expand it in culture to generate a sufficient quantity to provide BM for the recipients of two kidneys and a liver, heart, pancreas, and small bowel from the single cadaver. Similarly, one could imagine taking a small amount of BM from a living kidney or liver donor (perhaps even in the office or clinic), expanding it in culture, and subsequently infusing it after transplantation. Such expanded cultures maintained after transplantation could be the source for BM in repeated BM infusion protocols. Provision of expanded donor-specific BM cultures will be most likely the responsibility of regional organ banks. Small samples of BM will be harvested from each cadaver and expanded in culture and then supplied to the transplant centers that received the specific cadaver organs.

Widespread application of cultured BM will only take place when BM efficacy is demonstrated. This can really only occur when simple techniques of culture expansion are evolved and used in multicenter, carefully controlled trials involving different types of transplants. Well-controlled studies could be done in which small aliquots of BM could be removed from the recipient and the donor on the day of transplantation (and donor harvest). At 10 to 14 days after transplant, recipients could receive randomly either syngeneic or allogeneic BM with their usual immunosuppression. The experimental evidence presented herein would seem to suggest that the best results will be obtained when peripheral ablation by a finite course of ALS is included in the immunosuppression program because ALS fosters development of suppressor (natural regulatory) cells. All standard parameters of efficacy could be studied, but given the excellent current results with standard immunosuppression, efficacy will best be demonstrated most likely by absence of rejection, improved graft function, better histology, and most of all reduction of immunosuppression. Over time, improved graft survival should predominate.

When considering the fate of radiation-based regimens, we are faced with an interesting paradox. On one hand, these regimens have demonstrated clear superiority in terms of allograft survival and induction of stable chimerism in animal models. On the other hand, there is no compelling evidence that these measures will work in humans, and physicians are understandably reluctant to expose their patients to the potential risks of radiation without clear evidence that the patient stands a reasonable chance to benefit from it. Another limitation of this approach arises from the need for preoperative conditioning. As a result, radiation-based regimens, as they are currently defined, can only apply to living-donor allograft procedures. This limitation would not apply to a xenograft scenario, and as the science of xenotransplantation advances, interest in this model of BM conditioning will escalate.

COMMENTARY

Haval Shirwan and Suzanne T. Ildstad

Bone marrow transplantation (BMT) is a widely used and effective therapeutic regimen for the treatment of a steadily increasing number of life-threatening malignant, hereditary, hematologic, immunodeficiency, and autoimmune disorders. Additionally, it has recently become obvious that BMT resulting in hematopoietic stem cell (HSC) chimerism induces tolerance to allogeneic as well as xenogeneic cells, tissues, and organ grafts in a variety of species, including humans (1). Animals rendered chimeric exhibit donor-specific tolerance whether they engraft as 100% or only 1% donor (2). Moreover, HSC chimerism prevents chronic rejection in transplanted grafts, thereby offering the potential to overcome another major limitation to solid organ and cellular transplants (3).

The widespread clinical application of conventional BMT to induce tolerance in the clinic is limited by two major immunologic complications: 1) graft-versus-host (GVHD) disease, and 2) host-versus-graft (HVG) disease, a failure to engraft because of rejection by the host immune cells. Moreover, the morbidity and mortality associated with fully ablative conditioning could not be accepted in clinical attempts to induce tolerance to transplanted grafts. Depletion of mature T cells in the donor BM has been used to prevent GVHD, and treatment of the recipient with some form of immunosuppressive or myeloablative regimen has been used to prevent HVG reactions. Both of these approaches, however, are associated with complications, ranging from immunoincompetence to morbidity and mortality. Our ability to develop more effective transplantation tolerance protocols depends on a comprehensive understanding of the factors that play critical roles in the engraftment of allogeneic and xenogeneic BM grafts and the survival of the host. As we come to understand the mechanism for conditioning of the host as well as securing HSC chimerism without GVHD, new strategies to induce tolerance will become possible in the clinic.

In BMT, the HVG response that mediates HSC rejection differs mechanistically from that associated with rejection of solid organ allografts (see also Chapter 2). The rejection of solid organ allografts is primarily initiated by recipient T cells that recognize foreign histocompatibility (minor and MHC) antigens of the graft, either indirectly as peptides presented by the recipient MHC molecules or directly as intact MHC molecules on the surface of the cells of the graft (4). In contrast, the rejection of foreign BM grafts is believed to be mediated primarily by natural killer (NK) cells that fail to recognize allogeneic MHC molecules on the surface of cells of the graft (5).

The role of NK cells in the rejection of BM grafts has been demonstrated using both naturally occurring and genetically manipulated mutant rodents lacking selected populations of immune cells in their body (6). For example, beige mice that lack NK cells but have functional T and B cells accept allogeneic BM grafts. In marked contrast, SCID mice that have normal NK cells, but lack functional T and B cells, reject BM grafts in a normal tempo. Additionally, BM grafts from β_2-microglobulin knockout mice or knockout mice for transporters associated with antigen processing (TAP) molecules that lack class I expression on the cell surface are rejected by wild-type syngeneic recipients (7).

A series of recent investigations have provided direct evidence that NK cells use two distinct sets of receptors for their recognition of foreign antigens (8). These two distinct receptor families are represented by the Ly-49 and NKR-P1 molecules. The Ly-49 receptor recognizes MHC class I molecules on the surface of syngeneic cells and delivers a negative signal to inhibit the function of second receptor NKR-P1 molecules that recognize complex carbohydrate structures on the cell and deliver a positive signal for the killing function. This hypothesis is consistent with the hybrid resistance phenomenon observed in certain mouse strain combinations; that is, the rejection of BM grafts, but not solid organ grafts, occurs in the parent-to-F_1 hybrid, but not in the F_1 hybrid-to-parent combination. This is believed to be due to the presence of NK cells in the F_1 progeny that express Ly-49 molecule isotypes. These isotypes cannot recognize class I molecules on the surface of P cells and deliver a negative signal for killing function (5).

The two-signal hypothesis is further substantiated by the findings that BM cells that lack the expression of class I MHC molecules on the surface in class I, β_2-microglobulin, and TAP knockouts or tumors that express low levels of MHC molecules serve as targets for NK cells (7). A better understanding of NK receptors and the molecular nature of their recognition of self and foreign antigens and further knowledge of the events for effector function may allow for the development of novel molecular approaches for the prevention of rejection of foreign BM grafts.

In their chapter, Hale and Monaco have elegantly presented a historical perspective of approaches used to overcome complications of conventional BMT and to induce tolerance to solid organ allografts. These approaches are grouped into two categories: irradiation of the recipient with lethal or sublethal doses of radiation (the latter in conjunction with some forms of immunosuppression), and treatment of the recipient with antilymphocyte serum either alone or in combination with a variety of immunosuppressive regimens. Although these approaches have proven effective for fully allogeneic BM engraftment, they result in severe instances of GVHD and immune incompetence.

To overcome these complications, several groups have attempted to establish mixed allogeneic chimeras using T-cell–depleted allogeneic and syngeneic BM for transplantation. Although this approach proved successful for restoring immunocompetence and preventing GVHD, it is frequently associated with failure of engraftment. This complication has led to a series of studies that tested the effect of different cellular components of BM for the enhancement of engraftment and prevention of GVHD. These studies have demonstrated that purified stem cells can be transplanted over allogeneic barriers to establish engraftment, but they can only do so when given in significantly higher numbers as compared with those in unfractionated whole BM (6,9).

These observations suggested that there are other cell types in the BM that facilitate the engraftment of stem cells, which led to the concept of facilitating cells (9). The facilitating effect can be demonstrated by the use of several different cell types, including thymocytes, lymph node cells, and cells of BM origin. We have recently identified a $CD8^+$, $CD3^+$, TCR^- cell type in the BM that greatly facilitated the engraftment over allogeneic barriers when co-transplanted with stem cells into conditioned recipients (9).

The nature of facilitating cells and the molecular basis of their facilitation effect are currently unknown. It is also unknown whether the facilitating effect observed with other cell populations, such as thymocytes and lymph nodes, is mediated by the same cell type present in all these different populations and whether it uses the same mechanisms. This is a new area in BMT that holds a great promise for the future. Further study of the characterization of facilitating cells, the type of receptors they use to mediate facilitation, and their mechanisms of facilitation will be of particular utility for the routine clinical application of BMT without undesirable complications.

There are presently limitations for routine clinical application of BMT for the treatment of a variety of malignant, autoimmune, and hereditary disorders as well as the induction of tolerance to foreign grafts, but there has been tremendous progress in our knowledge of these limitations in recent years. Great promise for this area of transplantation has come of the recent advances in our understanding of T, NK, and stem cell immunobiology, the discovery of facilitating cells, and molecular manipulations at the level of whole organisms or cells. Furthermore, BMT presents great promise for the induction of tolerance across a xenogeneic barrier (see also Chapter 40). The use of xenografts for human transplantation has the potential to eliminate one of the greatest limitations of allotransplantation, the shortage of organ donors in clinics.

All these advances will, however, depend on a comprehensive understanding of cells and molecules that play critical roles in BM engraftment and elucidation of mechanisms that are needed for BM engraftment and the induction of tolerance to foreign organs across species and intraspecies barriers.

CHAPTER REFERENCES

1. Billingham RE, Brent L, Medawar PB. Actively acquired tolerance of foreign cells. Nature 1953;172:603.
2. Billingham RE, Brent L, Medawar PG. Quantitative studies on tissue transplantation immunity. III. Actively acquired tolerance. Philos Trans R Soc Lond 1995;239:357.
3. Billingham R, Brent L. Quantitative studies on transplantation immunity: IV. Induction of tolerance in newborn mice and studies on the phenomenon of runt disease. Philos Trans R Soc Lond B Biol Sci 1959;242:439.
4. Ridge JP, Fuchs EJ, Matzinger P. Neonatal tolerance revisited: turning on newborn T cells with dendritic cells. Science 1996;271:1723.
5. Sarzotti M, Robbins DS, Hoffman PM. Induction of protective CTL responses in newborn mice by a murine retrovirus. Science 1996;271:1726.
6. Forsthuber T, Yip HC, Lehmann PV. Induction of TH1 and TH2 immunity in neonatal mice. Science 1996;271:1728.
7. Monaco AP, Wood ML, Russell PS. Adult thymectomy: effect on recovery from immunologic depression in mice. Science 1965;149:432.
8. Cross AM, Leuchars E, Miller JFAP. Studies on the recovery of the immune response in irradiated mice thymectomized in adult life. J Exp Med 1964;119:837.
9. Monaco AP, Wood ML, Russell PS. Studies on heterologous antilymphocyte serum in mice. III. Immunologic tolerance and chimerism produced across the H-2 locus with adult thymectomy and antilymphocyte serum. Ann NY Acad Sci 1966;129:190.
10. Mitchison NA. The colonization of irradiated tissue by transplanted spleen cells. Br J Exp Pathol 1956;37:239.
11. Abbott WM, Monaco AP, Russell PS. Antilymphocyte serum and cell-free antigen loading. Transplantation 1969;7:291.
12. Mandel MA, Monaco AP, Russell PS. Destruction of splenic transplantation antigens by a factor present in liver. J Immunol 1965;95:673.
13. Monaco AP, Wood ML, Lytle B, Barrett I. Studies on heterologous antilymphocyte serum in mice. Colloques Internationaux C.N.R.S. 1971;190:361–373.
14. Lance EM, Medawar PB. Antilymphocyte serum and the induction of tolerance to transplantation antigens. Fed Proc 1970;29:151.
15. Lance EM, Medawar PB. Induction of tolerance with antilymphocyte serum. Proc Roy Soc (Biol) 1969;173:447.
16. Monaco AP, Wood ML. Studies on heterologous antilymphocyte serum in mice. VII. Optimal cellular antigen for induction of immunologic tolerance with antilymphocyte serum. Transplant Proc 1970;2:489.
17. Starzl TE, Demetris AJ, Murase N, et al. Donor dendritic cell repopulation in recipients after rat to mouse bone-marrow transplantation. Lancet 1992;339:1610.
18. Wood ML, Monaco AP, Gozzo JJ, Liegeois A. Use of homozygous allogeneic bone marrow for induction of tolerance with antilymphocyte serum: dose and timing. Transplant Proc 1971;3:676.
19. Monaco AP, Gozzo JJ, Wood ML, Liegeois A. Use of low doses of homozygous allogeneic bone marrow cells to induce tolerance with antilymphocyte serum (ALS): tolerance by intraorgan injection. Transplant Proc 1971;3:680.
20. Wood ML, Gozzo JJ, Monaco AP. Studies on tolerance/enhancement produced by antilymphocyte serum and bone marrow. Behring Inst Mitt 1972;51:220.
21. Monaco AP, Liegeois A, Wood ML, Clark AW. Active enhancement of tissue allografts with antilymphocyte serum and bone marrow. Adv Nephrol Necker Hosp 1975;5:135.
22. Wood ML, Gozzo JJ, Heppner G, Monaco AP. Cell-mediated immunity and serum blocking factor in tolerance produced in mice with antilymphocyte serum and bone marrow cell infusion. Transplant Proc 1972;4:383.
23. Clark AW, Monaco AP. The effect of bacterial adjuvants on allograft survival after anti-lymphocyte serum (ALS) and donor bone marrow in mice. Immunology 1974;27:887.
24. Wood ML, Gozzo JJ, Monaco AP. Use of antilymphocyte serum and bone marrow for production of immunological tolerance and enhancement: review and recent experience. Transplant Proc 1974;4:523.
25. Wood ML, Heppner G, Gozzo JJ, Monaco AP. Mechanism of augmented graft survival in mice after ALS and bone marrow infusion. Transplant Proc 1973;5:691.
26. Wood ML, Monaco AP. The effect of timing of skin grafts on subsequent survival in ALS-treated, marrow-infused mice. Transplantation 1977;23:78.
27. Wood ML, Monaco AP. The effect of cyclophosphamide on the splecific unresponsiveness to skin allografts induced in ALS-treated mice infused with donor bone marrow. J Immunol 1977;118:1456.
28. Wood ML, Monaco AP. Induction of cytotoxic (sensitization) and enhancing (prolonged survival) responses by injection of lymphoid cells in ALS-treated mice. Transplant Proc 1979;11:1456.
29. Maki T, Gottschalk R, Homsy FN, et al. In vitro analysis of immune reactivity in ALS-treated, bone marrow injected mice bearing enhanced skin allografts. Transplant Proc 1981;13:596.
30. Simpson MA, Maki T, Gozzo JJ, Monaco AP. Characterization of antilymphocyte serum induced suppressor cells. Transplant Proc 1983;15:740.
31. Wood ML, Monaco AP. Adoptive transfer of specific unresponsiveness to skin allografts by spleen cells from ALS-treated, marrow-injected mice. Transplant Proc 1979;11:1023.
32. Wood ML, Monaco AP. Differential effect of cyclophosphamide on states of specific allograft unresponsiveness in immunosuppressed mice. Transplantation 1979;27:186.
33. Wood ML, Monaco AP. Induction of unresponsiveness to skin allografts in adult mice disparate at defined regions of the H-2 complex. I. Effect of donor-specific bone marrow in ALS-treated mice. Transplantation 1984;37:35.
34. Wood ML, Monaco AP. Suppressor cells in specific unresponsiveness to skin allografts in ALS-treated, marrow-injected mice. Transplantation 1980;29:196.
35. Maki T, Gottschalk R, Wood ML, Monaco AP. Specific unresponsiveness to skin allografts in anti-lymphocyte serum-treated, marrow-injected mice: participation of donor marrow-derived suppressor T cells. J Immunol 1981;127:1433.
36. Maki T, Wood ML, Gozzo JJ, Monaco AP. Donor marrow derived suppressor cells in skin allograft unresponsiveness induced in antilymphocyte serum treated, marrow injected mice. Ann NY Acad Sci 1982:397.
37. Monaco AP. Studies in rodents on the use of polyclonal antilymphocyte serum and donor-specific bone marrow to induce specific unresponsiveness to skin allografts. Transplant Proc 1991;23:2061.
38. Maki T, Simpson M, Monaco AP. Development of suppressor T cells by antilymphocyte serum treatment in mice. Transplantation 1982;34:376.
39. Wood ML, Orosz CG, Gottschalk R, Monaco AP. The effect of injection of donor bone marrow on the frequency of donor reactive CTL in antilymphocyte serum treated, grafted mice. Transplantation 1992;54:665.
40. Pourshadi M, De Fazio SR, Gozzo JJ. Abrogation of secondary skin allograft rejection by veto-like cells in donor bone marrow. Transplantation 1993;56:385.
41. De Fazio S, Hartner WC, Monaco AP, Gozzo JJ. Mouse skin graft prolongation with donor strain bone marrow and anti-lymphocyte serum: surface markers of the active bone marrow cells. J Immunol 1985;135:3034.
42. De Fazio SR, Hartner WC, Monaco AP, Gozzo JJ. Mouse skin graft prolongation with donor-strain bone marrow and antilymphocyte serum. Effect of bone marrow cell storage. Transplantation 1986;41:26.
43. Gozzo JJ, Crowley M, Maki T, Monaco AP. Functional characteristics of a Ficoll-separated mouse bone marrow cell population involved in skin allograft prolongation. J Immunol 1982;129:1584.
44. De Fazio SR, Hartner WC, Monaco AP, Gozzo JJ. Prolongation of graft survival in ALS-treated mice by donor-specific bone marrow. Density gradient fractionation of the active bone marrow cells. Transplantation 1987;43:564.
45. De Fazio SR, Monaco AP, Gozzo JJ. Bone marrow cells that prolong graft survival in ALS-treated mice: characterization for markers related to lymphocyte ontogeny. Transplant Proc 1989;21:267.
46. De Fazio SR, Hartner WC, Monaco AP, Gozzo JJ. Effect of posttransplantation administration of peripheral blood lymphocytes in skin-grafted mice treated with antilymphocyte serum or antilymphocyte serum plus bone marrow. Transplantation 1987;44:70.
47. De Fazio SR, Monaco AP, Gozzo JJ. Prolongation of skin allograft survival in antilymphocyte serum-treated mice by posttransplant administration of peripheral blood lymphocytes. Transplantation 1989;48:163.

48. Takahashi T, Mafune K, Maki T. Cloning of self-major histocompatibility complex antigen-specific suppressor cells from adult bone marrow. J Exp Med 1990;172:901.
49. Monaco AP, Wood ML, Gottschalk R, Seiler FR. Effect of granulocyte-macrophage colony-stimulating factor on the induction of unresponsiveness by lymphoid cells. Transplantation 1991;51:213.
50. Wood ML, Monaco AP, Gottschalk R. Characterization of spleen cells capable of inducing unresponsiveness in ALS-treated mice. Transplantation 1991;51:208.
51. Wood ML, Gottschalk R, Monaco AP. The effect of cyclosporine on the induction of unresponsiveness in antilymphocyte serum-treated, marrow-injected mice. Transplantation 1988;46:449.
52. Bobbio SA, Wood ML, Monaco AP. Significant augmentation of specific unresponsiveness by rapamycin in ALS-treated, bone marrow injected mice. Transplant Sci 1993;3:51.
53. Hale DA, Gottschalk R, Fukuzaki T, et al. Superiority of sirolimus (rapamycin) over cyclosporine in augmenting allograft and xenograft survival in mice treated with antilymphocyte serum and donor-specific bone marrow. Transplantation 1997;63:359.
54. Murase N, Starzl TE, Tanabe M, et al. Variable chimerism, graft-versus-host disease, and tolerance after different kinds of cell and whole organ transplantation from Lewis to brown Norway rats. Transplantation 1995;60:158.
55. Grosjean O, Otte H. Immunologic tolerance induced in dogs by single or repeated neonatal injections of bone marrow from unrelated adult donors [in French]. C R Seances Soc Biol Fil 1966;160:216.
56. Otte H, Grosjean O. Anti-lymphocyte serum, bone marrow and immunological tolerance in the young dog [in French]. C R Seances Soc Biol Fil 1967;161:959.
57. Yamamoto M. Effect of donor bone marrow transplantation on canine renal allotransplants. Tohoku J Exp Med 1970;101:325.
58. Yamamoto M. Prolongation of canine renal allograft survival in combined therapy with rabbit-anti-dog antilymphocytic serum, azathioprine and the allotransplantation of the donor's bone marrow. Tohoku J Exp Med 1970;101:333.
59. Caridis DT, Liegeois A, Barrett I, Monaco AP. Enhanced survival of canine renal allografts of ALS-treated dogs given bone marrow. Transplant Proc 1973;5:671.
60. Hartner WC, De Fazio SR, Maki T, et al. Prolongation of renal allograft survival in antilymphocyte-serum-treated dogs by postoperative injection of density-gradient-fractionated donor bone marrow. Transplantation 1986;42:593.
61. Hartner WC, Markees TG, De Fazio SR, et al. The effect of antilymphocyte serum, fractionated donor bone marrow, and cyclosporine on renal allograft survival in mongrel dogs. Transplantation 1991;52:784.
62. Hartner WC, Markees TG, De Fazio SR, et al. Effect of early administration of donor bone marrow cells on renal allograft survival in dogs treated with antilymphocyte serum and cyclosporine. Transplantation 1995;59:131.
63. Hartner WC, Van der Werf WJ, Lodge JP, et al. Effect of rapamycin on renal allograft survival in canine recipients treated with antilymphocyte serum, donor bone marrow, and cyclosporine. Transplantation 1995;60:1347.
64. Myburgh JA, Smit JA, Mieny CJ, Mason JA. Hepatic allotransplantation in the baboon. 3. The effects of immunosuppression and administration of donor-specific antigen after transplantation. Transplantation 1971;12:202.
65. Myburgh JA, Smit JA. Hepatic allotransplantation in the baboon. IV. Further studies with the post-transplant administration of donor bone marrow and a soluble donor splenic antigen. Transplantation 1972;14:191.
66. Myburgh JA, Smit JA. Passive and active enhancement in baboon liver allografting. Transplantation 1972;14:227.
67. Myburgh JA, Smit JA. Active enhancement in the primate by bone marrow. II. B cell antibody, production and prolongation of liver allograft survival. Transplantation 1978;26:76.
68. Smit JA, Myburgh JA, Gaillard VJ. Active enhancement in the primate by bone marrow I. Ia-like determinants on nucleated bone marrow cells. Transplantation 1978;26:73.
69. Thomas JM, Carver FM, Burnett CM, Thomas FT. Enhanced allograft survival in rhesus monkeys treated with antihuman thymocyte globulin and donor lymphoid cells. Transplant Proc 1981;13:599.
70. Thomas JM, Carver FM, Foil MB, et al. Renal allograft tolerance induced with ATG and donor bone marrow in outbred rhesus monkeys. Transplantation 1983;36:104.
71. Thomas FT, Carver FM, Foil MB, et al. Long-term incompatible kidney survival in outbred higher primates without chronic immunosuppression. Ann Surg 1983;198:370.
72. Thomas J, Carver M, Cunningham P, et al. Promotion of incompatible allograft acceptance in rhesus monkeys given posttransplant antithymocyte globulin and donor bone marrow. I. In vivo parameters and immunohistologic evidence suggesting microchimerism. Transplantation 1987;43:332.
73. Thomas JM, Carver M, Cunningham P, et al. Promotion of incompatible allograft acceptance in rhesus monkeys given posttransplant antithymocyte globulin and donor bone marrow. II. Effects of adjuvant immunosuppressive drugs [published erratum appears in Transplantation 1989;47:928]. Transplantation 1989;47:209.
74. Thomas JM, Carver FM, Cunningham PR, et al. Kidney allograft tolerance in primates without chronic immunosuppression—the role of veto cells. Transplantation 1991;51:198.
75. Wood ML, Monaco AP. The effect of timing of skin grafts on subsequent survival in ALS-treated, marrow infused mice. Transplantation 1977;23:78.
76. Monaco AP, Wood ML, Maki T, Gozzo JJ. Future strategies for induction of unresponsiveness to organ allografts. Transplant Proc 1988;28:1207.
77. Thomas JM, Carver FM, Kasten-Jolly J, et al. Further studies of veto activity in rhesus monkey bone marrow in relation to allograft tolerance and chimerism. Transplantation 1994;57:101.
78. Verbanac KM, Carver FM, Haisch CE, Thomas JM. A role for transforming growth factor-beta in the veto mechanism in transplant tolerance. Transplantation 1994;57:893.
79. Thomas JM, Verbanac KM, Smith JP, et al. The facilitating effect of one-DR antigen sharing in renal allograft tolerance induced by donor bone marrow in rhesus monkeys. Transplantation 1995;59:245.
80. Monaco AP, Clark AW, Wood ML, et al. Possible active enhancement of a human cadaver renal allograft with antilymphocyte serum (ALS) and donor bone marrow: case report of an initial attempt. Surgery 1976;79:384.
81. Monaco AP, Wood ML, Maki T, et al. Attempt to induce unresponsiveness to human renal allografts with antilymphocyte globulin and donor specific bone marrow. Transplant Proc 1985;17:1312.
82. Barber WH, Mankin JA, Laskow DA, et al. Long-term results of a controlled prospective study with transfusion of donor-specific bone marrow in 57 cadaveric renal allograft recipients. Transplantation 1991;51:70.
83. McDaniel DO, Naftilan J, Hulvey K, et al. Peripheral blood chimerism in renal allograft recipients transfused with donor bone marrow. Transplantation 1994;57:852.
84. Rolles K, Burroughs AK, Davidson BR, et al. Donor-specific bone marrow infusion after orthotopic liver transplantation. Lancet 1994;343:263.
85. Sayegh MH, Fine NA, Smith JL, et al. Immunologic tolerance to renal allografts after bone marrow transplants from the same donors [see comments]. Ann Intern Med 1991;114:954.
86. Helg C, Chapuis B, Bolle JF, et al. Renal transplantation without immunosuppression in a host with tolerance induced by allogeneic bone marrow transplantation. Transplantation 1994;58:1420.
87. Jacobsen N, Taaning E, Ladefoged J, et al. Tolerance to an HLA-B,DR disparate kidney allograft after bone-marrow transplantation from same donor [letter]. Lancet 1994;343:800.
88. Ricordi C, Karatzas T, Nery J, et al. High-dose donor bone marrow infusions to enhance allograft survival: the effect of timing. Transplantation 1997;63:7–11.
89. Dempster W, Lennox B, Boag JW. Prolongation of survival of skin homotransplants in the rabbit by irradiation of the host. Br J Exp Pathol 1950;31:670.
90. Lorenz E, Congdon C, Uphoff D. Modification of acute radiation injury in mice and guinea-pigs by bone marrow injection. Radiology 1952:58:863.
91. Main JM, Prehn RT. Successful skin homografts after the administration of high dosage X radiation and homologous bone marrow. J Nat Cancer Inst 1955;15:1023.
92. Trentin JJ. Effect of x-ray dose on mortality and skin transplantability in mice receiving F1 hybrid marrow. Proc Soc Exp Biol Med 1956;93:98.
93. Main JM, Prehn RT. Fate of skin homografts in x-irradiated mice treated with homologous marrow. J Nat Cancer Inst 1957;19:1053.
94. Ford CE, Hamerton JL, Barnes DWH, Loutit JF. Cytological identification of radiation-chimeras. Nature 1956;177:452.
95. Mannick JA, Lochte HL, Ashley CA, et al. A functioning kidney homotransplant in the dog. Surgery 1959;46:821.
96. Slavin S, Strober S, Fuks Z, Kaplan HS. Induction of specific tissue transplantation tolerance using fractionated total lymphoid irradiation in adult mice: long-term survival of allogeneic bone marrow and skin grafts. J Exp Med 1977;146:34.
97. Slavin S, Fuks Z, Kaplan HS, Strober S. Transplantation of allogeneic bone marrow without graft-versus-host disease using total lymphoid irradiation. J Exp Med 1978;147:963.

98. Slavin S, Reitz B, Bieber CP, et al. Transplantation tolerance in adult rats using total lymphoid irradiation: permanent survival of skin, heart, and marrow allografts. J Exp Med 1978;147:700.
99. Auchincloss HJ, Sachs DH. Mechanisms of tolerance in murine radiation bone marrow chimeras. I. Nonspecific suppression of alloreactivity by spleen cells from early, but not late, chimeras. Transplantation 1983;36:436.
100. Auchincloss HJ, Sachs DH. Mechanisms of tolerance in murine radiation bone marrow chimeras. II. Absence of nonspecific suppression in mature chimeras. Transplantation 1983;36:442.
101. Ildstad ST, Sachs DH. Reconstitution with syngeneic plus allogeneic or xenogeneic bone marrow leads to specific acceptance of allografts or xenografts. Nature 1984;307:168.
102. Singer A, Hathcock KS, Hodes RJ. Self recognition in allogeneic radiation bone marrow chimeras. A radiation-resistant host element dictates the self specificity and immune response gene phenotype of T-helper cells. J Exp Med 1981;153:1286.
103. Zinkernagel RM, Althage A, Waterfield E, et al. Restriction specificities, alloreactivity, and allotolerance expressed by T cells from nude mice reconstituted with H-2 compatible or incompatible thymus grafts. J Exp Med 1980;151:376.
104. Rayfield LS, Brent L. Tolerance, immunocompetence, and secondary disease in fully allogeneic radiation chimeras. Transplantation 1983;36:183.
105. Ildstad ST, Wren SM, Stephany D, Sachs DH. Effect of selective T cell depletions in mixed xenogeneic reconstitution on specific hyporeactivity to transplantation across a species barrier. Transplantation 1986;41:372.
106. Ildstad ST, Wren SM, Bluestone JA, et al. Effect of selective T cell depletion of host and/or donor bone marrow on lymphopoietic repopulation, tolerance, and graft-vs-host disease in mixed allogeneic chimeras (B10 + B10.D2—B10). J Immunol 1986;136:28.
107. Sykes M, Chester CH, Sachs DH. Protection from graft versus host disease in fully allogeneic chimeras by prior administration of T cell depleted syngeneic bone marrow. Transplantation 1988;46:327.
108. Aksentijevich I, Sachs DH, Sykes M. Natural antibodies against bone marrow cells of a concordant xenogeneic species. J Immunol 1991;147:79.
109. Aksentijevich I, Sachs DH, Sykes M. Natural antibodies can inhibit bone marrow engraftment in the rat-mouse species combination. J Immunol 1991;147:4140.
110. Pierce GE, Watts LM, Clancy JJ. Sublethal fractionated total-body irradiation and donor bone marrow infusion for induction of allograft tolerance. Transplantation 1985;39:236.
111. Pierce GE, Watts LM. The role of donor lymphoid cells in the transfer of allograft tolerance. Transplantation 1985;40:702.
112. Pierce GE, Watts LM. Do donor cells function as veto cells in the induction and maintenance of tolerance across an MHC disparity in mixed lymphoid radiation chimeras? Transplantation 1993;55:882.
113. Pierce GE, Watts LM. Effects of Thy-1+ cell depletion on the capacity of donor lymphoid cells to induce tolerance across an entire MHC disparity in sublethally irradiated adult hosts. Transplantation 1989;48:289.
114. Tomita Y, Khan A, Sykes M. Role of intrathymic clonal deletion and peripheral anergy in transplantation tolerance induced by bone marrow transplantation in mice conditioned with a nonmyeloablative regimen. J Immunol 1994;153:1087.
115. Sharabi Y, Sachs DH. Mixed chimerism and permanent specific transplantation tolerance induced by a nonlethal preparative regimen. J Exp Med 1989;169:493.
116. Colson YL, Wren SM, Schuchert MJ, et al. A nonlethal conditioning approach to achieve durable multilineage mixed chimerism and tolerance across major, minor, and hematopoietic histocompatibility barriers. J Immunol 1995;155:4179.
117. Ildstad ST, Wren SM, Bluestone JA, et al. Characterization of mixed allogeneic chimeras: immunocompetence, invitro reactivity and genetic specificity of tolerance. J Exp Med 1985;162:23.
118. Li H, Colson YL, Ildstad ST. Mixed allogeneic chimerism achieved by lethal and nonlethal conditioning approaches induces donor-specific tolerance to simultaneous islet allografts. Transplantation 1995;60:523.
119. Li H, Abou el-Ezz AY, Gambrell BE, Ildstad ST. Mixed xenogeneic chimerism and tolerance III. A nonlethal approach to induce donor-specific transplantation tolerance to simultaneous islet xenografts. Transplantation 1995;60:59.
120. Howard RJ, Sutherland DE, Lum CT, et al. Kidney allograft survival in dogs treated with total lymphoid irradiation. Ann Surg 1981;193:196.
121. Vaiman M, Daburon F, Remy J, et al. Allograft tolerance in pigs after fractionated lymphoid irradiation. I. Skin grafts after partial lateral irradiation and bone marrow cell grafting. Transplantation 1981;31:358.
122. Fradelizi D, Mahouy G, de Riberolles C, et al. Allograft tolerance in pigs after fractionated lymphoid irradiation. II. Kidney graft after conventional total lymphoid irradiation and bone marrow cell grafting. Transplantation 1981;31:365.
123. Guzzetta PC, Sundt TM, Suzuki T, et al. Induction of kidney transplantation tolerance across major histocompatibility complex barriers by bone marrow transplantation in miniature swine. Transplantation 1991;51:862.
124. Myburgh JA, Smit JA, Browde S, Hill RR. Transplantation tolerance in primates following total lymphoid irradiation and allogeneic bone marrow injection. I. Orthotopic liver allografts. Transplantation 1980;29:401.
125. Myburgh JA, Smit JA, Hill RR, Browde S. Transplantation tolerance in primates following total lymphoid irradiation and allogeneic bone marrow injection. II. Renal allografts. Transplantation 1980;29:405.
126. Smit JA, Hill RR, Myburgh JA, Browde S. Transplantation tolerance in primates after total lymphoid irradiation and allogeneic bone marrow injection. III. Lymphocyte responsiveness and suppressor cell activity. Transplantation 1980;30:107.
127. Zan-Bar I, Slavin S, Strober S. Induction and mechanism of tolerance to bovine serum albumin in mice given total lymphoid irradiation (TLI). J Immunol 1978;121:1400.
128. Kawai T, Cosimi AB, Colvin RB, et al. Mixed allogeneic chimerism and renal allograft tolerance in cynomolgus monkeys. Transplantation 1995;59:256.
129. Kimikawa M, Sachs DH, Colvin RB, et al. Modifications of the conditioning regimen for achieving mixed chimerism and donor-specific tolerance in cynomolgus monkeys. Transplantation 1997;64:709.
130. Kahn DR, Dufek JH, Hong R, et al. Heart and kidney transplantation using total lymphoid irradiation and donor bone marrow in mongrel dogs. J Thorac Cardiovasc Surg 1980;80:125.
131. Kahn DR, Hong R, Greenberg AJ, et al. Total lymphatic irradiation and bone marrow in human heart transplantation. Ann Thorac Surg 1984;38:169.

COMMENTARY REFERENCES

1. Sayegh MH, Fine NA, Smith JL, et al. Immunologic tolerance to renal allografts after bone marrow transplants from the same donors. Exp Hematol 1991;13:581.
2. Ildstad ST, Sachs DH. Reconstitution with syngeneic plus allogeneic or xenogeneic bone marrow leads to specific acceptance of allografts or xenografts. Nature 1984;307:168.
3. Colson YL, Zadach K, Nalesnik M, Ildstad ST. Mixed allogeneic chimerism in the rat—donor-specific transplantation tolerance without chronic rejection for primarily vascularized cardiac allografts. Transplantation 1995;60:971.
4. Bradley JA, Mowat AM, Bolton EM. Processed MHC class I alloantigen as the stimulus for $CD4^+$ T cell-dependent antibody-mediated graft rejection. Immunol Today 1992;13:434.
5. George T, Yu YYL, Liu J, et al. Allorecognition by murine natural killer cells: lysis of T lymphoblasts and rejection of bone marrow grafts. Immunol Rev 1997;155:29.
6. Aguila H, Akashi K, Domen J, et al. From stem cells to lymphocytes: biology and transplantation. Immunol Rev 1997;157:13.
7. Lanier LL. The natural killer cells in transplantation. Curr Opin Immunol 1995;7:626.
8. Malanti MS, Peruzzi M, Parker KC, et al. Peptide specificity in the recognition of MHC class I by natural killer cell clones. Science 1995;267:1016.
9. Kaufman CL, Colson YL, Wren SM, et al. Phenotypic characterization of a novel bone marrow-derived cell that facilitates engraftment of allogeneic bone marrow stem cells. Blood 1994;84:2436.

Chapter

39

Gene Transfer

KATHRYN J. WOOD

The possibility that recombinant DNA technology might be used to transfer genes to mammalian cells for therapeutic purposes has stimulated enormous interest. Significant progress has been made in the last few years in the development of novel methods for gene delivery. Clinical trials exploiting the technology in a limited number of disease states have been approved and are already in progress. However, many more advances will be required before this approach will be accepted as commonplace in the clinic. Nevertheless, the scene has been set for the use of gene transfer as a therapeutic tool in the future. Importantly, although gene therapy was originally conceived as an intervention strategy to replace or correct defective genes in patients with inherited diseases, the realization that it may have much broader potential for the delivery of protein therapeutic agents such as cytokines, antibodies, and recombinant ligands has stimulated further interest. This chapter reviews the strategies that are currently being used for gene delivery and highlights some of the areas where this approach may be applicable for use in transplantation in the future.

Any strategy that results in the modification of the genetic repertoire of somatic cells for therapeutic purposes can be considered to fall under the general heading of gene therapy. In straightforward terms, gene transfer involves the delivery of one or more new genes and the sequences that regulate their expression to a target cell using an appropriate gene delivery system. The process of gene transfer can be carried out either ex vivo or in vivo, depending on the purpose for which it is intended. In the former case, cells are removed from the individual before manipulation. The new genes are then introduced into the cells in the laboratory before they are reintroduced into the recipient. For in vivo gene transfer, the genes are delivered directly to the cells in situ in the recipient. One can envisage different circumstances in transplantation where either of these approaches might be appropriate. In both situations, a delivery system is required to enable the new genes to be transferred efficiently to the target cells. Selection of the most appropriate gene transfer system for the situation where it is to be employed is obviously one of the factors that is critical for the success of the procedure. Numerous novel approaches for gene transfer have already been developed, although as yet the perfect transfer system is still elusive.

When gene transfer was first proposed as a possible therapeutic approach there was much skepticism. However, gene transfer is no longer just a hypothetical possibility. Over the past 15 or so years, it has progressed from experimental studies to a strategy that is being applied clinically. Gene transfer is certainly feasible clinically, and trials are already in progress for the treatment or investigation of certain diseases (1). Some might argue that progress to this stage has been slower than was originally predicted by the field's enthusiasts (2). Yet, progress has been made and will continue to be made as gene delivery systems are refined and improved, and gene transfer may be applicable to transplantation in the future (3).

GENE DELIVERY SYSTEMS

The selection of the gene transfer strategy to be used is determined by the clinical use to which this approach is being applied. All of the systems currently in use have both advantages and disadvantages, and it is fair to say that the perfect gene transfer system is certainly not available at present. The delivery system selected for use must therefore be chosen very carefully to ensure that the advantages are maximized for the application.

The gene transfer systems that have been used in clinical trials to date are replication-defective recombinant retroviruses, replication-defective recombinant adenoviruses, and plasmid liposome complexes. Many more are currently in development, and in the coming years there will undoubtedly be an explosion in the number of ways genes can be transferred to mammalian cells. Rather than describe each of the numerous delivery systems in turn, I will focus on the three that are currently approved for clinical use, highlighting the advantages and disadvantages of each system.

Replication-Defective Recombinant Retroviruses

Retroviruses have the advantage of transferring the genetic information they carry into the genome of the target cell (Fig. 39.1). In other words, the new genes that the recombinant vector carries will become integrated into the DNA of the target cell, thereby potentially modifying the genotype of the target cell permanently once the transfer has taken place. Moreover, as the target cell divides, the new gene will be transferred to the progeny (4,5). Integration of the transferred genes has both advantages and disadvantages. The potential of long-term expression of the transferred gene could be very advantageous, particularly if it was possible to regulate expression effectively. However, expression might also be a disadvantage if, for example, the transferred gene is toxic when overexpressed. In addition, because the site at which the gene integrates cannot be controlled, the possibility of insertional mutagenesis has to be considered. If integration were to result in activation of an oncogene or disruption of a tumor suppressor, this would be a major problem.

The use of retrovirus delivery systems has other potential limitations. The target cells must be proliferating for the retroviral vector to be integrated into the genome. Uptake of the retrovirus is receptor mediated; therefore, the target cells must express the appropriate viral receptor. Recombination and rearrangements are relatively common, and the vectors are sensitive to inactivation. In addition, the standard retrovirus constructs are only produced at relatively low titer, which also limits the efficiency of target cell transduction. These problems are being addressed by vector engineering and the development more efficient packaging cell lines (6–9).

One significant advance in the development of replication-defective retroviruses for gene transfer was the generation of specialized cell lines, referred to as packaging cells. Packaging cells permit the production of a "high" titer virus that is theoretically free from wild-type virus (see Fig. 39.1) (7). A wild-type retrovirus contains three genes—the gag,

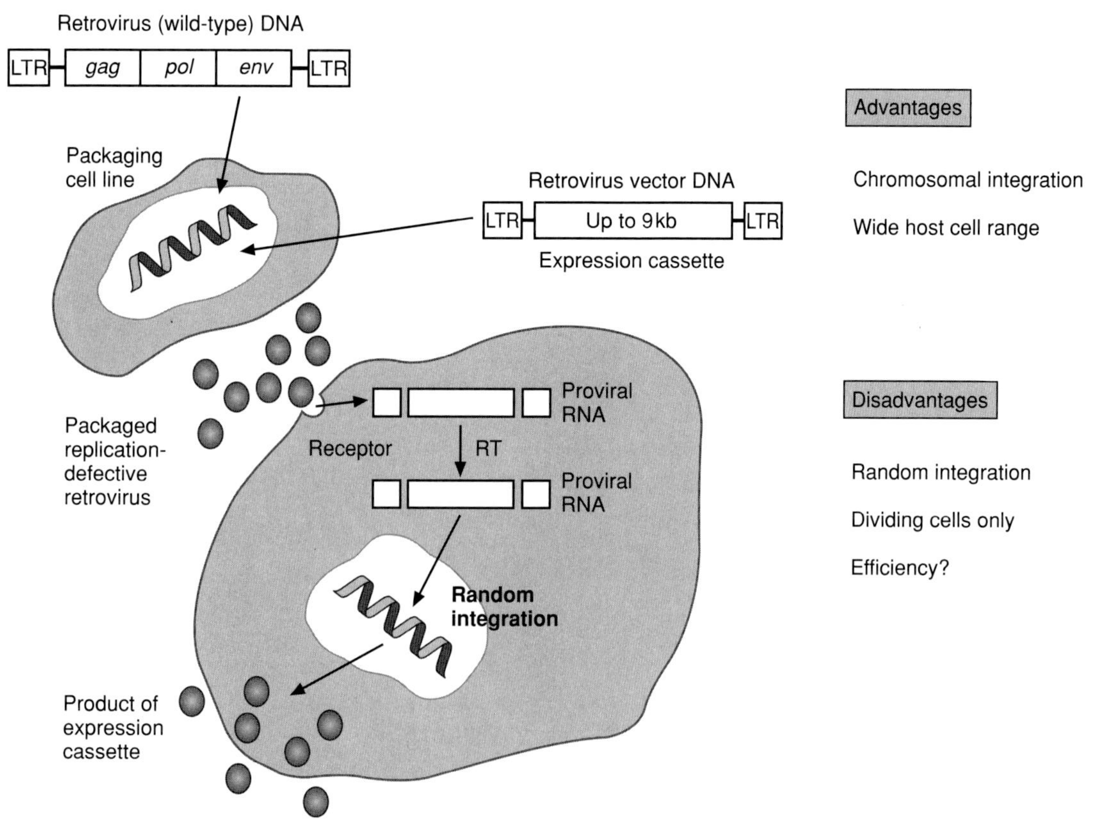

FIGURE 39.1. *Schematic illustration of gene transfer mediated by replication-defective retrovirus vectors. LTR, long terminal repeat; RT, reverse transcriptase.*

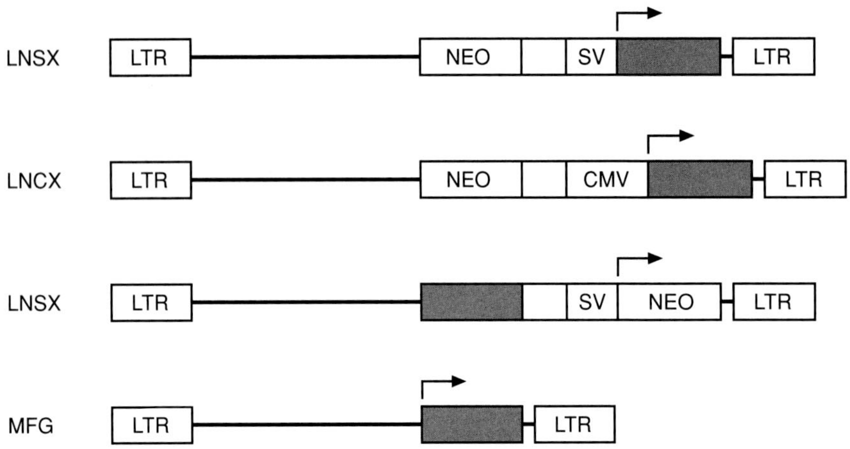

FIGURE 39.2. *Schematic representation of retroviral vectors to demonstrate alternative approaches for expressing novel genes. LN series of vectors were designed by Miller and colleagues (6), and MFG by Mulligan and colleagues (73). LTR, long terminal repeat; NEO, neomycin resistance gene; SV, early promoter from SV40; CMV, immediate early promoter from human cytomegalovirus.*

polymerase (pol), and envelope (env) genes—that are essential for viral replication. To ensure that a retrovirus is replication defective, these three genes must be deleted from the viral genome. In this state, once viral particles are formed they can undergo one round of infection but cannot replicate in the target cell. To produce viral particles that have the capacity to infect target cells, the replication-defective construct containing the gene of interest has to be processed through a packaging cell in which the gag, pol, and env genes have been introduced at different sites in the genome (see Fig. 39.1). These sequences provide the proteins necessary for packaging viral particles, and the cells that contain them are often referred to as virus-producer cells.

In principle, no genetic information for virus production should be transferred from the packaging cells to the target cells, thus no spread of the virus should be possible. This issue has been one of major concern as replication-defective retrovirus vectors have been approved for clinical use. Several reports have been made of the production of wild-type virus by replication-defective virus-producer cell lines in vitro. Moreover, in an experiment in which bone marrow stem cells were transduced with replication-defective retrovirus that was contaminated with wild-type virus, the animals receiving the transduced bone marrow developed lymphomas (10). It is clearly critical that this issue be resolved; packaging cell lines must be improved to ensure that escape of wild-type virus is impossible.

The choice of a specific retroviral vector for a particular protocol is empirical at present. There are three general classes of mouse Moloney leukemia virus-based retroviral vectors in current use. All contain the 5′ and 3′ long terminal repeats (LTRs), the packaging signal positioned just downstream from the 5′ LTR, and a portion of gag to increase the titer of the viral vector. The gene to be transferred can be expressed from the LTR, an internal heterologous promoter such as the SV40 or CMV promoters, or the gene's own promoter. In addition, a selectable marker may or may not be included in the construct (Fig. 39.2). The type of vector that gives the highest titer may vary depending on the precise conditions employed. A comparison of different constructs may therefore be productive if a high level of expression is required (11).

Adenovirus Vectors

Adenovirus gene delivery does not result in integration of the transferred genes into the genome of the target cell (Fig. 39.3). Instead, the transferred gene remains epichromosomal. Therefore, the risks of permanently altering the genotype of the targeted cell or of mutagenesis as a result of insertion do not exist when adenovirus vectors are used. Unfortunately, despite this potential advantage over retrovirus delivery systems, adenovirus vectors are not problem free.

First-generation adenovirus vectors were highly immunogenic, eliciting both innate and adaptive immune responses after delivery (12,13). Immune responses are triggered to both the vector and the transgene it contains, thereby limiting the duration of expression of the transferred gene and preventing readministration of the vector. The immune responses elicited by adenovirus vectors can be prevented effectively by co-administration of immunosuppressive agents, including drugs such as cyclosporine, cyclophosphamide, and tacrolimus (FK506) (14,15) as well as biological agents such as interleukin-1 (IL-1) receptor antagonist (16) and the cytokine IL-12 (17).

Immune response would not be a critical issue if adenovirus vectors were to be used only to deliver biologically active molecules to transplanted tissue or to a recipient at the time of transplantation who is receiving immunosuppressive agents. However, this is a severe limitation for the more general uses of these vectors as gene delivery systems for the administration of therapeutic genes to patients who are not receiving immunosuppressive therapy. Moreover, the majority of humans are already sensitized to adenovirus via environmental exposure. Thus, vector inactivation as a result of a secondary immune response may be even more of a problem in the clinical setting.

Ways of circumventing the immune response triggered by first-generation adenovirus vectors are being explored. Identifying and eliminating the targets of the response from

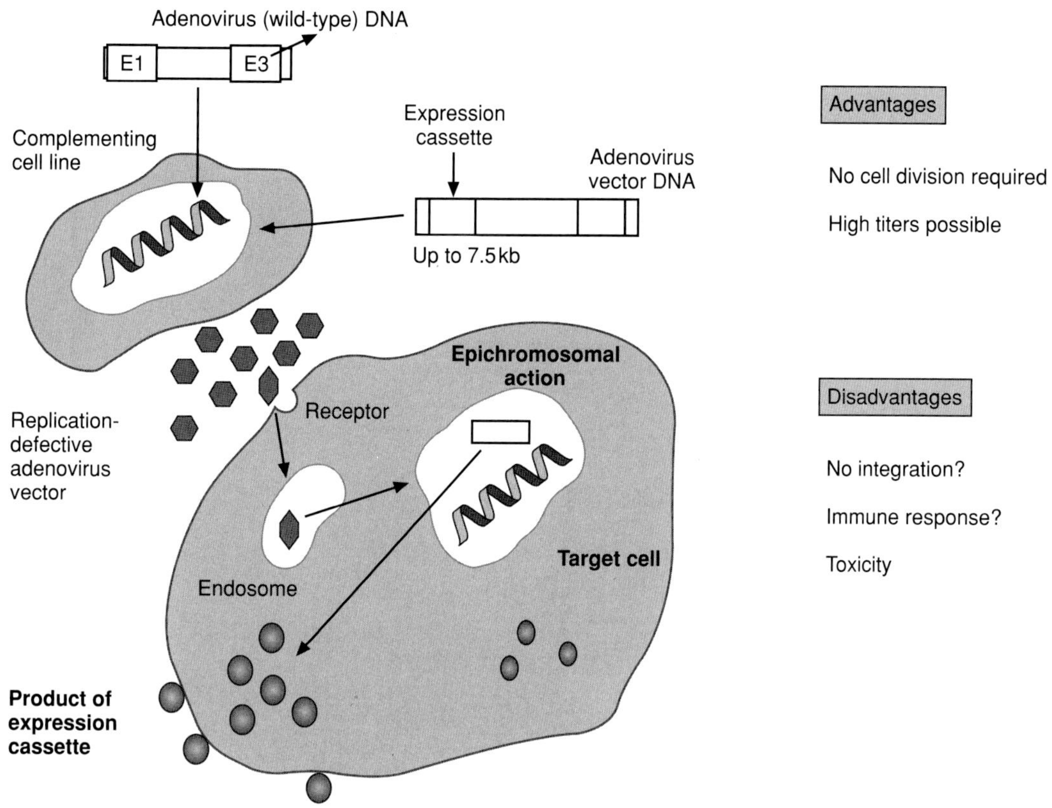

FIGURE 39.3. *Schematic illustration of gene transfer mediated by replication-defective adenovirus vectors.*

the vector would be one approach. The primary antigens that elicit the response to the intact virus are thought to be E1A and, to a lesser degree, E2 and the late antigens (18). The E1 and E3 regions were deleted from first-generation adenovirus constructs, but clearly this was insufficient to eliminate the immune response. Second-generation constructs (Ad2) have both E1 and E2A deleted from the adenovirus backbone. However, repeated administration of these vectors to primates has also resulted in the development of significant cellular and humoral immunity (19). If engineering the vectors is ultimately unsuccessful, another option would be to identify the components of the immune response that are most harmful and to target these specifically with more selective immunosuppression (20).

An alternative approach for repeated vector administration would be to use adenovirus expression vectors with different serotypes. In this situation, immune responses directed against the vector would not affect administration of the same gene in a vector prepared using a different adenovirus serotype (21). A further possibility would be to induce tolerance to the adenovirus vector. This has been achieved by delivering recombinant adenovirus to the thymus in combination with manipulation of the peripheral immune system using antilymphocyte serum (22,23).

The escape of replication-competent viruses after gene transfer is also of concern with adenovirus vectors. Although the vectors have been rendered incompetent for replication by deletion of the E1 genes, they are propagated by growth in cells engineered to express the E1 genes (see Fig. 39.3) (24). A low level of replication-competent virus may arise as a result either of recombination events in the packaging cells or of the ability of E1-defective adenovirus to replicate in some cells. The capacity of replication-defective adenoviruses to revert could be critically dependent on the properties of the target cell; it is unclear whether data from animal models will reflect accurately the situation that will arise once specific protocols are implemented clinically. If replication does occur, concerns about the safety of these vectors will have to be addressed.

Other Viral Vector Delivery Systems

Other viral vector delivery systems are also being developed, including adeno-associated virus, herpes simplex virus, vaccinia virus, and a number of other RNA viruses.

Adeno-Associated Vectors

Adeno-associated vectors are small, stable viruses that can infect human cells. Genes transferred using this approach will integrate into the genome of the target cell, but the integration process appears to be less efficient and less precise than that achieved using retrovirus vectors. However, a recent report suggests that adeno-associated vectors transduce muscle cells in situ with high frequency (25).

An interesting property of the intact virus is that insertion most commonly occurs with a small region of human chromosome 19. However, this region is associated with chromosomal rearrangements that occur in chronic B-cell leukemias, and therefore adeno-associated vectors that retained this property might not be suitable for exploitation as a site-specific integration strategy. Nevertheless, if the property of site-specific integration could be harnessed without adverse consequences, this would be very important (26). Another interesting property that has been attributed to these vectors is that they can integrate into nondividing cells. If substantiated, this property would offer a major advantage over retrovirus vectors (27).

Adeno-associated vector delivery has been reported to induce a humoral response against the viral capsid proteins that can prevent or limit the efficiency of gene transfer when repeat delivery is required. Moreover, most people have been exposed to adeno-associated virus, so resistance to different serotypes must be explored before clinical trials can be considered.

Herpes Simplex Vectors

Herpes simplex vectors may be highly effective for delivery of genes to the central nervous system (28,29). Unfortunately, a number of the viral genes are highly toxic. Much work is needed to produce a form of these vectors that will allow efficient gene delivery without excessive toxicity.

Nonviral Methods of Gene Transfer

In order to ensure effective entry and expression in the target cells, most nonviral methods of gene transfer rely on the normal mechanisms by which mammalian cells take up macromolecules. Nonviral delivery systems are thought to offer many advantages over viral vector systems:

1. The size of the DNA transferred can be much larger than with viral vectors.
2. The complexes used cannot replicate or recombine, so escape of replication-competent pathogens is not an issue.
3. The immune and inflammatory immune responses evoked as a consequence of gene delivery should be insignificant.

On the other hand, the disadvantage of nonviral delivery systems is that they are very inefficient.

The approaches that have been investigated include plasmid–liposome complexes (Fig. 39.4), receptor-mediated uptake pathways, and particle bombardment.

For plasmid liposome complexes and receptor-mediated uptake pathways, the DNA to be transferred has to be complexed with liposomes or the appropriate polypeptide or carbohydrate ligand to allow recognition by the receptor. One of the problems associated with the latter strategy is that endocytic vesicles formed as a result of uptake are usually targeted for fusion with lysosomes, which contain highly effective degradative enzymes. Thus, effective gene transfer using this approach requires escape of the DNA from this compartment. One strategy that may be effective is to use either whole adenovirus or fusion peptides from the influenza hemagglutinin gene to induce efficient uptake and disruption of DNA-containing endosomes. Whether these type of approaches will ultimately allow long-term, stable expression of the transferred genes remains to be determined.

For particle bombardment, DNA is absorbed onto submicron gold or tungsten particles and then accelerated to high velocity using a variety of different methods.

The Ideal Gene Transfer Strategy

As will have become clear from the preceding discussion, gene transfer methodology is still in the design stage. The perfect system does not exist at present, and much work is required before the perfect delivery system is available for clinical use. The ideal system would allow efficient delivery of the gene of interest to a specific target without any inflammation or immune recognition. Once expression has been initiated, it should be possible to regulate expression of the transferred gene effectively. Moreover, the vector should be stable and easy to produce and to purify to high titer. It seems unlikely that a single delivery system would be appropriate for every clinical situation. More likely is the development of designer delivery systems that are optimized for a particular use.

The debate as to the merits of viral versus nonviral delivery systems has been attracting attention. Proponents of viral delivery argue that replication-defective viral vectors are the best way to deliver genes to target cells efficiently. Those who support nonviral delivery systems believe that an inflammatory or immune response will always be initiated using a viral vector, however disabled the vector might be; thus, they feel that nonviral delivery is the only way to ensure long-term expression of the transferred gene. At present, the jury is still out. Only as new strategies for delivering genes both ex vivo and in vivo are developed will the best approach emerge.

POTENTIAL USES IN TRANSPLANTATION

Tolerance

Alloantigen pretreatment has long been used as a means of modulating immune response to an allograft (30,31). Although blood transfusions have been the most common source of alloantigen in clinical transplantation, there is increasing interest in using bone marrow as a vehicle for alloantigen delivery. Donor bone marrow can be given before, during, or after transplantation and still have a beneficial effect (32–38). The way in which the recipient is

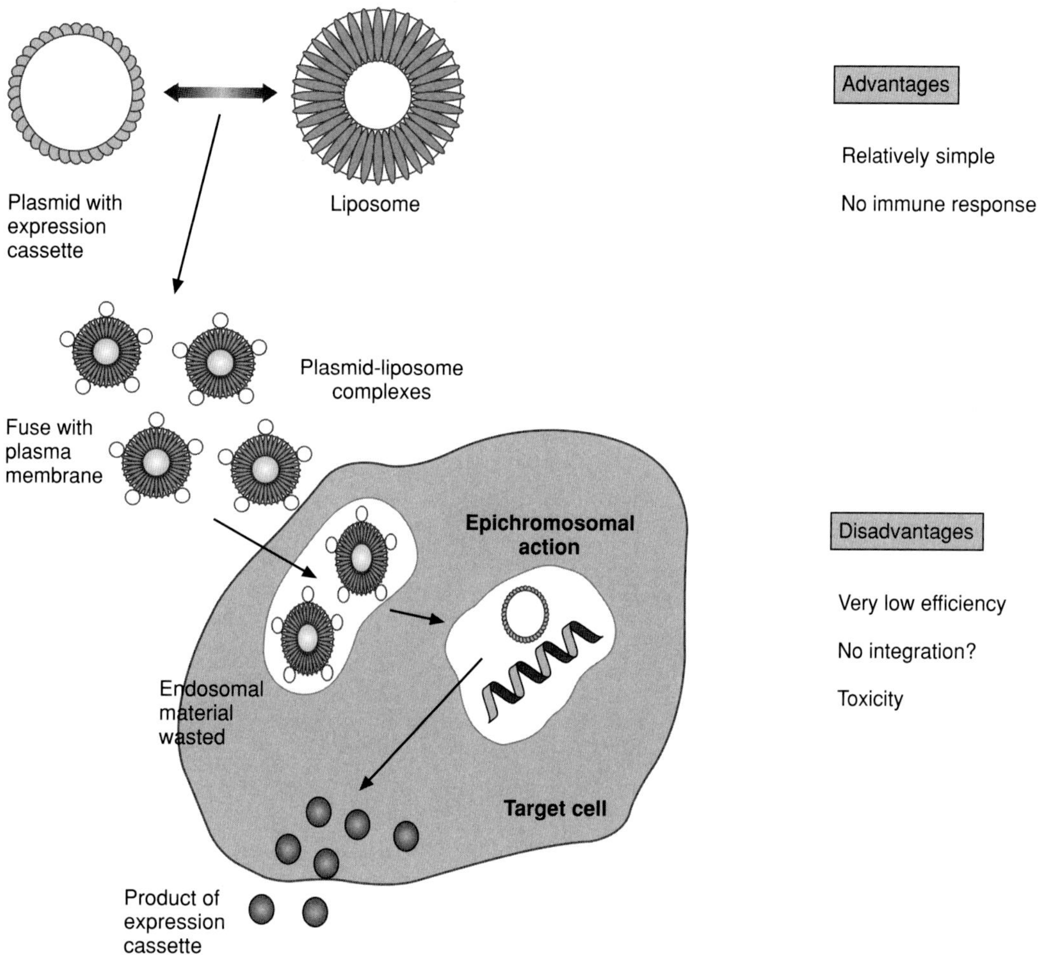

FIGURE 39.4. *Schematic illustration of gene transfer mediated by plasmid liposome complexes.*

manipulated before bone marrow infusion results in different mechanisms of tolerance being brought into play in the different systems (see Chapter 5).

Donor marrow originally was selected as the source of bone marrow for infusion because it was thought that the recipient would need to be exposed to every donor histocompatibility molecule in order to induce specific immunologic unresponsiveness. However, in certain circumstances this might not be the case, particularly for vascularized organ grafts. Indeed, exposure to cells expressing a single donor MHC molecule can be sufficient to prolong the survival of vascularized allografts (39). When bone marrow expressing a single donor MHC molecule is used, long-term survival and operational tolerance can be induced (38). For gene transfer strategies designed to induce specific unresponsiveness in vivo, this observation may be very important (see below).

The interests of my own group in using gene transfer as a strategy for inducing tolerance began with a series of experiments designed to unravel the requirements for the induction of specific unresponsiveness using alloantigen pretreatment. For these studies we introduced single or multiple MHC genes from the organ donor into fibroblasts of recipient origin in vitro using standard transfection methodology. The transfected cells were selected for cell surface expression of the allogeneic MHC molecule; we used them to treat recipient mice intravenously before transplantation of a vascularized cardiac allograft. This strategy demonstrated that exposure to a single donor MHC gene expressed by a cell of recipient origin was capable of prolonging the survival of fully allogeneic cardiac allografts (39). The addition of anti-CD4 monoclonal antibody therapy to this pretreatment protocol was able to promote the development of operational tolerance to the allografts (40).

As pointed out by Sundt and Sachs (41), this strategy had a number of limitations in the wider application of gene transfer for the induction of tolerance in transplantation. In particular, the use of a cell line for gene delivery was far from ideal. The advent of gene transfer strategies that allow genes to be transferred to cells immediately after isolation from the recipient (in particular, bone marrow cells) makes this approach much more attractive for the induction of tolerance.

Transduction of recipient bone marrow cells to express a donor MHC gene for use in a tolerance-induction protocol was first reported by Sykes and colleagues using a replication-defective retroviral delivery system (42). Recipient B10.AKM ($H2^k$) was transduced ex vivo to express a donor class I molecule $H2K^b$ using a recombinant retrovirus. The transduced bone marrow cells were shown to confer hypo responsiveness to K^b-mismatched skin grafts when they were used to treat recipient mice that had received nonlethal irradiation and monoclonal antibody therapy before bone marrow infusion. Sykes and colleagues are currently developing non-myeloablative conditioning regimens that will allow engraftment of the transduced bone marrow cells (43).

Transduction of bone marrow cells to express donor MHC genes might also facilitate the development of unresponsiveness to fully mismatched vascularized organ grafts. Wong and colleagues have also used a replication-defective retrovirus to transfer the $H2K^b$ gene to recipient CBA.Ca ($H2^k$) bone marrow cells ex vivo (44). The bone marrow cells were reinfused into recipient mice in combination with anti-CD4 monoclonal antibody therapy 28 days before transplantation of a fully allogeneic C57BL/10 ($H2^b$) vascularized cardiac allograft. Thus, the transplanted heart expresses the other alloantigens of the $H2^b$ haplotype as well as $H2K^b$, the gene transferred to the recipient bone marrow cells. In this experimental system, operational tolerance to the heart grafts was induced after pretreatment with recipient bone marrow cells expressing a single donor MHC antigen—a further example of linked unresponsiveness in vivo (45).

This approach has also been investigated in a pig kidney transplant model. Here, donor class II genes were transferred to bone marrow using a retroviral delivery system. As in the mouse, exposure to a single donor MHC molecule before transplantation was sufficient to induce prolonged survival of kidney grafts mismatched for multiple alloantigens (46). These observations are of key importance for the development of this approach for clinical application in the future.

The manipulation of bone marrow or cord blood by gene transfer is a strategy that has been considered for some time as a means of treating hematopoietic disorders (47,48). Indeed, gene therapy protocols using these cell populations as targets are already being investigated clinically (49). These strategies, combined with the considerable interest in identifying hematopoietic stem cells and developing strategies for mobilization of stem cells to the peripheral blood (50), provide a very solid basis for attempting to use this approach to manipulate bone marrow cells for the induction of tolerance to allografts and xenografts in the future.

Delivery of Biologically Active Molecules to the Graft

Gene transfer strategies offer the possibility of delivering molecules with immunomodulating activity to the graft itself or to defined sites in the recipient. Both of these options offer many advantages over the systemic delivery of immunosuppressive agents. Moreover, the former approach would allow molecules that could prevent or minimize ischemic damage or reperfusion injury to be expressed in situ at the time of transplantation.

Delivery of biologically active molecules to the graft can be achieved in two ways, by co-transplantation of genetically modified cells along with the graft or by modification of the graft itself.

The use of carrier cells that are transplanted alongside the graft could be an efficient way of delivering immunosuppressive molecules. To be useful, the carrier cells must be easy to transfect and expression of the transferred gene must be stable. In addition, the carrier cells must be able to survive when transplanted to the selected site in vivo, and they should not produce anything toxic that might compromise the function of the tissue transplanted alongside them. Very importantly, they must not have any tumorigenic potential. These requirements limit the number of potential applications of this approach, but, with cellular grafts such as islets of Langerhans, this strategy has been shown to prevent rejection (51–53).

Lau and colleagues transfected myoblasts of recipient origin ex vivo with expression plasmid(s) containing the cDNA for either CTLA4Ig or Fas ligand (FasL) together with a selection marker, such as the gene for neomycin resistance. Transfection was carried out using calcium phosphate precipitation, a standard technique. Transfected myoblasts were selected to ensure that colonies expressing the gene of interest were used for in vivo delivery. Myoblasts are relatively robust cells that will survive transfection using this fairly aggressive method of gene transfer. In this respect they are unlike many other populations of primary cells that might otherwise have been ideal vehicles for this type of application. To prepare the composite islet-muscle cell grafts, allogeneic islets and the transfected muscle cells were mixed before transplantation under the kidney capsule of recipient mice. In the case of co-transplantation of myoblasts expressing CTLA4Ig, islet grafts were prolonged from a mean of 11 days to 31 days (51). Expression of FasL by the myoblasts resulted in the long-term survival of the transplanted allogeneic islets (Fig. 39.5) (53). More recently, Li and colleagues have reported successful prolongation of FasL gene-transfected solid organ allografts (54).

Direct modification of the transplanted organ or tissue has also been shown to have potential as a strategy for modifying the response to allografts or xenografts. The strategy selected for gene transfer is clearly very important, and no clear favorite has emerged in the literature published to date. Indeed, the preferred strategy may vary among organs, depending on the susceptibility of the organ to transduction.

In one of the first studies of this type, Qin and colleagues compared the ability of the cytokines transforming growth factor beta (TGFβ) and viral IL-10 (vIL-10) to modulate the rejection response following their delivery directly to mouse myoblast and nonvascularized heart grafts (55,56).

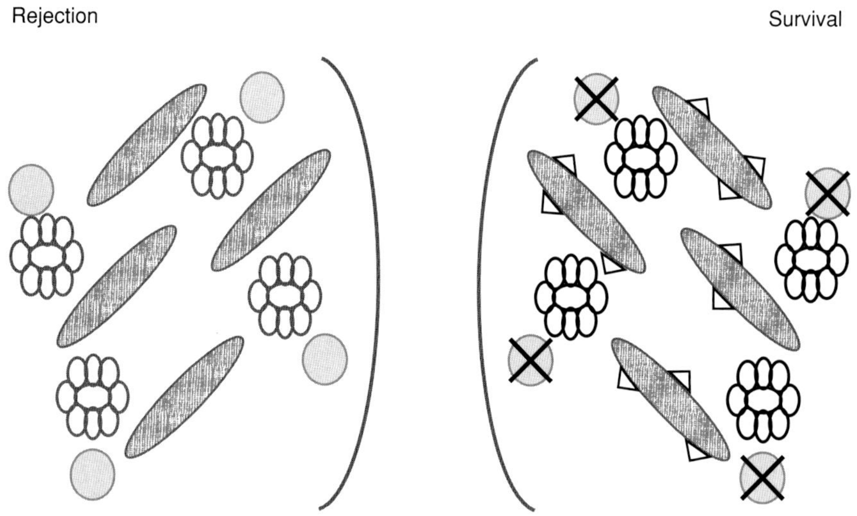

FIGURE 39.5. *Expression of Fas ligand in myoblasts can be used to protect allogeneic islets of Langerhans from rejection. (Based on data from Lau H, Yu M, Fontana A, Stoeckert C. Prevention of islet allograft rejection with engineered myoblasts expressing FasL in mice. Science 1996;273:109.)*

The efficiency of various viral and nonviral transfer strategies was compared, including retroviral, herpes simplex, and adenovirus vectors and naked DNA. (Unfortunately, in this study the same gene delivered by different vectors to the same tissue was not compared.) Not unexpectedly, Qin and colleagues found that the expression levels achieved varied according to the type of vector used. Interestingly, in their in vivo experiments, the retrovirus delivery of vIL-10 and the plasmid delivery of TGFβ directly to the graft resulted in prolongation of graft survival compared to the controls.

Viral IL-10 has also been expressed in human islets of Langerhans following their exposure to a replication-defective adenoviral construct incorporating the vIL-10 gene. The ability of the islets to stimulate a proliferative response was affected by the expression of vIL-10. At low concentrations, the response was augmented; at high concentrations (>5 ng/mL), the response was inhibited (57). The use of vIL-10 to manipulate immune responsiveness by direct modification of the allograft may be critically dependent on the level of expression achieved.

Adenovirus delivery systems have also been used to deliver biologically active molecules to liver and corneal grafts. In the former case, the efficiency of gene transfer to the liver during cold preservation, an attractive strategy for clinical use, was found to correlate with the ratio of the amount of vector to tissue mass as well as to the length of time the liver was exposed to the vector (58). Expression of a reporter gene was detectable within 12 hours of perfusion of the harvested organ and was produced at maximal levels by 48 hours. Further preliminary ex vivo perfusion experiments delivering TGFβ1 to the liver ex vivo using adenovirus have also been performed, with the rationale that this might downregulate both the inflammatory and immune response to the liver after transplantation. Given the additional ability of TGFβ to promote cell proliferation, this approach will need very careful evaluation (59).

The donor cornea is also amenable to manipulation by gene transfer to modulate the immune response or the function of endothelial cells before transplantation, as demonstrated in a feasibility study by Larkin and colleagues (60). Co-culture of isolated corneas with adenovirus constructs expressing the β-galactosidase reporter gene resulted in high levels of expression in the endothelial cells from 1 to 7 days after both ex vivo and in vivo exposure (60).

Data to support the idea that adenoviral strategies might be suitable for other types of endothelial cells are conflicting. For example, although primary cultures of human or pig vascular endothelial cells have shown efficient gene transfer, uptake by vascular endothelial cells in situ in pieces of aorta was found to be much less efficient, leading the researchers to conclude that this delivery system may be unsuitable for this type of manipulation (61). A study comparing direct injection of an adenovirus reporter construct into the coronary artery and the myocardium in vivo in minipigs produced similar findings. Delivery to the myocardium was found to be more efficient, resulting in expression in a localized area of the heart which peaked between days 3 and 6 after injection and returned to control levels within a month (62). Localized inflammatory responses were observed at the injection site, as had been reported by others (63).

Endothelial cells express a number of targets that might inhibit endothelial cell activation, prevent reperfusion injury, and promote graft acceptance; these are attractive targets for manipulation in the context of both allotransplantation and xenotransplantation (see below). For example, NF-κB is an inducible activator of transcription of a large array of genes, some of which are required for inflammatory and immune responses (64); inhibition of NF-κB may prevent endothelial cell activation. NF-κB exists in an inactive form in the cytoplasm of most cells, where it is bound to IκB. Activation of cells via a variety of different pathways, including IL-1, IL-6, and TNF-α, leads to the rapid release of IκB and the translocation of NF-κB to the nucleus. Genes regulated by NF-κB can be transcriptionally activated within minutes of exposure to an activating agent. Transfer of genes that encode molecules that inhibit the activity of NF-κB might prevent endothelial cell activation. One such approach used recombinant adenovirus to transfer the gene for an inhibitor known as A20. It was tested using aortic endothelial cells, and it has been shown to inhibit the upregulation of reporter genes and endothelial cell activation (65). If these and other related approaches are to be applied successfully in vivo, the development of gene transfer strategies that would lead to reliable uptake by endothelial cells is an important technical aim for the future.

If the aim of the gene therapy is to treat or prevent reperfusion injury to the graft, increased inflammation as a consequence of the gene transfer itself is highly undesirable. Nonviral strategies may overcome the adverse consequences of inflammation associated with the use of viral vector delivery systems, and plasmid-liposome complexes may have some advantages in this situation. As expression of bcl-2 in tissue can prevent apoptotic cell death, delivery of an expression cassette encoding bcl-2 might be useful in transplantation. In vivo transfection of the liver with plasmid-liposome complexes encoding the bcl-2 gene has been shown to prevent the death of hepatocytes induced by hypoxia (66). However, the efficiency of transfer and expression of bcl-2 was very low. Much higher levels must be achieved before this approach can be a practical option in the future.

Particle bombardment does not seem the most obvious choice as a method of gene delivery to an organ for preventing graft rejection, because one might expect that uniform expression throughout the transplanted tissue would be a prerequisite for success. However, biolistic transfection of islets with a cDNA encoding human CTLA4Ig has been shown to prolong the survival of cultured islet allografts in mice (67).

THE FUTURE

In the future gene therapy may have a much broader range of applications. In addition to introducing novel genes, it might also be used to inactivate genes by gene targeting. Its potential as a means of delivering protein therapeutic agents might also be realized. For the latter purpose, a delivery and gene expression system that would allow controlled delivery of the therapeutic molecule would be essential. The attributes of such a gene transfer system would include an ability to switch the delivery system on and off as necessary, as well as a means of controlling the amount of the substance produced. As the discussion at the beginning of this chapter highlighted, the perfect gene transfer system has yet to be invented. However, our increased understanding of the mechanisms that operate in the regulation of the expression patterns of endogenous genes have permitted the development of several approaches.

One strategy is to use a small molecule to modify the activity of a transcription factor that affects a particular promoter placed upstream of the gene of interest. This requires transfer of both the transgene and the regulatory sequences that are to be used to control expression. Some approaches have been tested using transgenic animals with varying degrees of success. For example, transcription factor–based glucocorticoid response elements have been explored, but the high level of basal expression and lack of specificity in the regulation achieved has dampened enthusiasm for this approach. Promoters that are regulated by prokaryotic transcription factors such as those controlled by tetracycline, where transcription requires binding of a tetracycline-dependent chimeric transactivator on a minimal tetracycline promoter, have also been investigated (68,69). More recently, an inducible system in which the transactivator protein requires tetracycline derivatives such as doxycycline has been described (70). This system has been demonstrated to allow long-term control of erythropoietin expression in vivo when primary myoblasts transduced using a retrovirus delivery system were transplanted in mice (71).

A novel strategy that uses the immunosuppressive drug rapamycin to regulate expression of the gene of interest has recently been described (72). Eukaryotic transcription factors usually consist of two domains, each with a discrete function: DNA binding or activation. If the two domains are separated, the transcription factor is rendered inactive. In this system, rapamycin is used as a bridge to bring the two domains of the transcription factor together (Fig. 39.6). Rapamycin binds to the immunophilin FKBP12 (see Chapter 11 for information about the mechanism of action of immunosuppressive drugs). The rapamycin–FKBP12

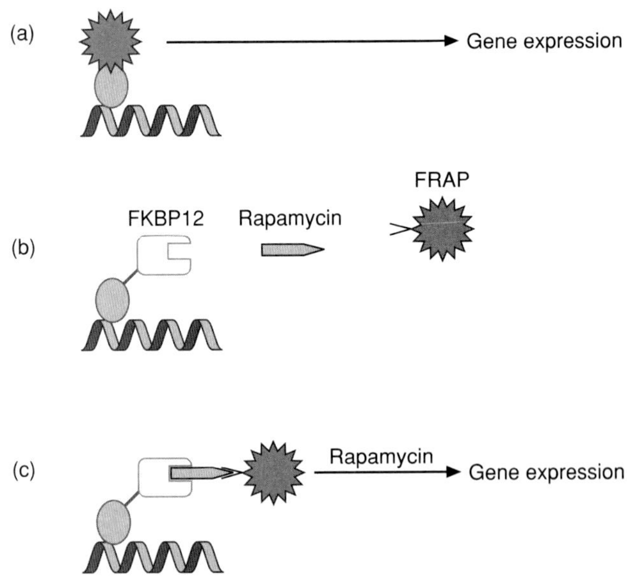

FIGURE 39.6. *A novel strategy for regulating gene expression after transfer in vivo using rapamycin. (Based on data from Rivera V, Clackson T, Natesan S, et al. A humanized system for pharmacologic control of gene expression. Nat Med 1996;2:1028–1032.)*

complex can then interact with another protein known as FRAP through the complexed rapamycin, and this leads to inhibition of the cell cycle. Rapamycin can therefore be thought of as acting as a small molecule bridge between FKBP12 and FRAP. Gilman and colleagues took advantage of this system by generating protein cassettes that produce the two domains of a transcription factor linked individually to FKBP12 and FRAP. Thus, only when rapamycin was added to the system would the two domains of the transcription factor be brought together by the bridge formed by rapamycin between FKBP12 and FRAP, and only then would the gene controlled by the transcription factor be turned on.

Conceptually, the rapamycin regulation approach is very elegant. However, implementation of this system is far from straightforward in its present configuration. To make it work, at least two and possibly three (as in this paper) different constructs must be generated. Both of the encoding chimeric proteins—the DNA-binding domain of the selected transcription factor and FKBP12, and the activation domain of the selected transcription factor and FRAP—must be under the control of constitutive promoters. The gene of interest is included in the third construct under the control of the transcription-factor–dependent promoter. Next, all three constructs have to be transferred and expressed in the cells of interest.

Despite its complexity, the utility of this system for regulating transgene expression in vivo was demonstrated by Rivera and colleagues (72), and the results were impressive. The group used replication-defective retroviruses as the backbones for each construct. Growth hormone was selected as the gene of interest. Once generated, the constructs were used sequentially to transduce the target cells in vitro. Selection was carried out at each stage. The selected clone of transduced cells was then transplanted to nude mice. The level of growth hormone produced in the presence or absence of rapamycin was then examined—only when rapamycin was administered was growth hormone detectable in the plasma.

One of the attractive properties of this type of approach is that the expression is only found when the drug is present. Thus, the effect of the transferred gene could be terminated by withdrawing the drug. However, as mentioned earlier, retroviral delivery systems may not be the ideal method of achieving gene transfer for clinical use. Clearly, in contexts other than transplantation and autoimmune disease, the immunosuppressive effects associated with rapamycin would be undesirable. Inactive analogues of rapamycin that retain FKBP12 and FRAP binding activity could be considered, but manipulation of the naturally occurring FKBP12 and FRAP could elicit an immune response that would reduce the efficacy of long-term therapy. The development of this type of strategy is only just beginning, and it offers an enormous number of possibilities for the future of gene therapy in the clinical setting.

CONCLUSION

Gene therapy is a rapidly developing field. New approaches for gene transfer will undoubtedly enable the technique to be used for the delivery of biologically active molecules at a particular site in vivo. It will be important to keep up with these developments to ensure that their potential application in transplantation is exploited in the future.

COMMENTARY

Stuart J. Knechtle

The innovative applications of gene therapy techniques to the field of organ transplantation are well summarized by Wood, who points out the great potential for this field, but also underscores how inadequate current gene transfer methods are for immediate clinical application. Furthermore, the immunomodulatory strategies employing gene therapy are, to date, inadequate to be considered for present clinical application.

One of the gene therapy strategies recently generating the greatest interest in the field of transplantation was that reported by Lau et al (1). This group found that syngeneic myoblasts expressing Fas ligand (FasL, CD95L) protected allogeneic islets of Langerhans for immunologic rejection when co-transplanted under the kidney capsule of mice. The immune privilege conferred on allogeneic tissue by FasL expression on host cells generated tremendous enthusiasm for generalizing this approach in organ transplantation. However, enthusiasm has been tempered by the inability of other expert groups to duplicate the results using the same general approaches. Kang et al reported that co-implantation of allogeneic C3H islets of Langerhans with congenic FasL-expressing myoblasts led to accelerated destruction of the islets by a granulocytic infiltrate (2). Others have also found that exogenous FasL expression, either by tumor cells or by islets, resulted in rapid destruction of the cells by neutrophils (3,4).

These more recent reports suggest that FasL may play a role along with other factors in the immune privilege of the eye and testis, but that exogenous FasL expression using currently practiced gene transfer strategies will not suffice for conferring immune privilege on other tissues. The findings of Lau et al suggest that FasL expression in the context of alloantigen or autoantigen may result in allospecific killing of T cells that are activated by coexpressed antigen; however, other factors must also be important in regulating the state of immune privilege. The nature of the immune privileged state with regard to FasL expression needs further clarification. The regulation of FasL expression by cells may turn out to be crucial in explaining the discrepant results reported.

Wood points out the limitations of cell lines modified by gene transfer for use in the induction of tolerance, and she indicates that the new methodologies for immediate gene transfer to harvested bone marrow cells are more attractive. The targeting of somatic stem cells would be particularly useful for transplantation if these cells could be grown and genetically modified without losing their multipotency and ability to self-renew. Unfortunately, our ability to identify, purify, and grow true somatic stem cells in culture is severely limited. Developments in stem cell biology and in our ability to target somatic stem cells for gene delivery are needed (5).

It may be the case that expression of allo-MHC directly in immunoregulatory tissues such as thymus will be a more feasible approach to tolerance using gene therapy than through genetic modification of bone marrow derived stem cells. For instance, we have found that direct injection of rat thymus by cDNA encoding allogeneic MHC class I was able to confer long-term unresponsiveness on fully MHC-mismatched liver allografts (6). Donor type MHC class I was expressed in the thymus and spleen of injected rats, perhaps in a manner similar to that achieved by the migration of injected bone marrow to these sites in other models. Direct in vivo cDNA transfer to thymus was used and was found to be effective despite its inefficiency. This experiment also points out the potential usefulness of linked recognition: unresponsiveness to a single alloantigen may confer unresponsiveness to additional alloantigens presented later along with it, because fully allogeneic liver transplants were accepted.

The view that gene therapy strategies to tolerance will require long-term, stable expression of donor antigen is difficult to substantiate, even though such expression would be useful. Rather, it may be that transient expression of donor antigen using genetic modification can adequately modify or deviate the host immune response, with the transplanted organ itself providing the continuous supply of alloantigen that has been found necessary for developing long-term unresponsiveness (7). This point remains controversial, and there are examples in experimental transplant models both of the utility of long-term stable bone marrow chimerism for tolerance and of tolerance existing in the absence of chimerism. In other words, gene therapy strategies relevant to tolerance do not necessarily require indefinite gene expression.

A potential problem with gene therapy approaches is the immune response that might be elicited by a newly expressed gene product, even in the context of autologous cells, because the host would not have acquired tolerance to such a product during development. Vilquin et al reported that normal muscle cells transplanted into dystrophin-deficient mdx mice elicited dystrophin-specific antibodies that did not harm the normal muscle cells, and a strong T-cell–mediated response did not develop (8). Tripathy et al found that mice injected intramuscularly with replication-defective adenoviruses expressing murine or human erythropoietin developed immune responses predominantly to the transgene-encoded products rather than to viral proteins (9).

In a dog model of myoblast transfer to dogs deficient in the lysosomal enzyme alpha-L-iduronidase, the reintroduction of transduced myoblasts expressing iduronidase resulted in IgG against iduronidase and cellular infiltration of the myoblast injection sites (10). Riddell reported that, in humans, five of six HIV subjects who received CD8 and HIV-specific T cells modified to express a combination gene encoding hygromycin and thymidine kinase permitting positive and negative selection developed cytotoxic T-cell responses to the novel proteins and eliminated the transduced cytotoxic T lymphocytes (11). These findings make it all the more important for immunologists to devise ways to avoid an immune response to a transgene product, because such strategies will be necessary for clinical gene therapy trials.

Given the limitations of viral and nonviral gene delivery methods, the application of gene therapy to organ transplantation will hinge on increasing the efficiency of gene transfer, developing inducible methods of in vivo gene transfer subject to nontoxic pharmacologic regulation, and finding nonimmunogenic vectors. Although adenoviral vectors have proven versatile (12), they have been disappointing from the standpoint of stability and immunogenicity. Gene delivery to a particular site in vivo using safer, more controlled parameters is likely to be developed by our colleagues in the gene therapy field. Somatic stem cell biology will hopefully develop means of targeting such cells for genetic modification.

In the meantime, as newer and better methods of gene transfer develop, it should be a major goal of transplant immunologists to learn more about how to achieve tolerance at a mechanistic level. Specifically, we must discern which cytokines or immunomodulatory proteins/peptides of the normal alloimmune response and normal tolerance mechanism could be used to change a host's alloimmune response to a tolerance response. How can we induce tolerance to a newly expressed gene product that the host did not see during immunologic development? I believe it would be honest to admit that, given the ideal gene transfer technique today (high levels of expression, indefinitely, with inducible expression), we do not yet know how to use the method to induce tolerance.

Of course, both fields will likely advance in parallel. Developments in our understanding of costimulation pathways using the CD40-CD40L and CD28-B7.1,B7.2 interactions as well as a better understanding of how lymphocytes kill (Fas-FasL, granzyme B, perforin pathways) have given us new and potentially more feasible approaches to gene therapy for the benefit of organ transplant patients.

CHAPTER REFERENCES

1. Crytal R. Transfer of genes to humans: early lessons and obstacles to success. Science 1995;270:404–410.
2. Friedmann T. Human gene therapy—an immature genie, but certainly out of the bottle. Nat Med 1996;2:144–147.
3. Prince HM. Gene transfer: a review of methods and applications. Pathology 1998;30:335–347.
4. Temin HM. Safety considerations in somatic gene therapy of human disease with retrovirus vectors. Hum Gene Ther 1990;1:111–123.
5. Boris-Lawrie K, Temin H. The retroviral vector. Replication cycle and safety considerations for retrovirus-mediated gene therapy. Ann NY Acad Sci 1994;716:59–70.
6. Miller A, Rosman G. Improved retroviral vectors for gene transfer and expression. Biotechniques 1989;7:980–990.
7. Miller A, Buttimore C. Redesign of retrovirus packaging cell lines to avoid recombination leading to helper virus production. Mol Cell Biol 1986;6:2895–2902.
8. Kasahara K, Dozy A, Kan Y. Tissue-specific targeting of retroviral vectors through ligand-receptor interactions. Science 1994;266:1373–1376.
9. Friedmann T, Yee J. Pseudotyped retroviral vectors for studies of human gene therapy. Nat Med 1995;1:275–277.
10. Donahue R, Kessler S, Bodine D, et al. Helper virus induced T cell lymphoma in nonhuman primates after retroviral mediated gene transfer. J Exp Med 1992;176:1125–1135.
11. Byun J, Kim S-H, Mook Kim J, et al. Analysis of the relative level of gene expression from different retroviral vectors used for gene therapy. Gene Ther 1996;3:780–788.
12. Yang Y, Nunes F, Berensci K, et al. Cellular immunity to viral antigens limits E1-deleted adenoviruses for gene therapy. Proc Natl Acad Sci USA 1994;91:4407–4411.
13. Yang Y, Ertl H, Wilson J. MHC class I-restricted cytotoxic lymphocytes to viral antigens destroy hepatocytes infected with E1-deleted recombinant adenoviruses. Immunity 1994;1:433–442.
14. Vilquin J, Guerette B, Kinoshita I, et al. FK506 immunosuppression to control the immune reactions triggered by first-generation adenovirus mediated gene transfer. Hum Gene Ther 1995;6:1391–1401.
15. Cassivi SD, Liu M, Boehler A, et al. Transgene expression after adenovirus-mediated retransfection of rat lungs is increased and prolonged by transplant immunosuppression. J Thorac Cardiovasc Surg 1999;117:1–7.
16. McCoy R, Davidson B, Roessler B, et al. Expression of human interleukin-1 receptor antagonist in mouse lungs using a recombinant adenovirus: effects on vector induced inflammation. Gene Ther 1995;2:437–442.
17. Yang Y, Trinchieri G, Wilson J. Recombinant IL-12 prevents formation of blocking IgA antibodies to recombinant adenovirus and allows repeated gene therapy to mouse lung. Nat Med 1995;1:890–893.
18. Mullbacher A, Bellet A, Hla R. The murine cellular immune response to adenovirus type 5. Immunol Cell Biol 1989;67:31–39.
19. Kaplan J, St George J, Pennington S, et al. Humoral and cellular immune responses of nonhuman primates to long-term repeated lung exposure to Ad2/CFTR-2. Gene Ther 1996;3:117–127.
20. Yang Y, Greenough K, Wilson J. Transient immune blockade prevents formation of neutralizing antibody to recombinant adenovirus and allows repeated gene transfer to mouse liver. Gene Ther 1996;3:412–420.
21. Kass-Eisler A, Leinwald L, Gall J, et al. Circumventing the immune response to adenovirus-mediated gene therapy. Gene Ther 1996;3:154–162.
22. de Matteo R, Raper S, Ahn M, et al. Gene transfer to the thymus. Annals of Surgery 1995;222:229–242.
23. Ilan Y, Attavar P, Takahashi M, et al. Induction of central tolerance by intrathymic inoculation of adenoviral antigens into the host thymus permits long-term gene therapy in Gunn rats. J Clin Invest 1996;98:2640–2647.
24. Jones N, Shenk T. Isolation of adenovirus type 5 host range deletion mutants defective for transformation of rat embryo cells. Cell 1979;16:683–689.
25. Fisher K, Jooss K, Alston J, et al. Recombinant adeno-associated virus for muscle directed gene therapy. Nat Med 1997;3:306–312.
26. Linden R, Burns K. Site specific integration by adeno-associated virus: a basis for a potential gene therapy vector. Gene Ther 1997;4:4–5.
27. Russell D, Miller D, Alexander I. Adeno-associated virus vectors preferentially transduce cells in S phase. Proc Natl Acad Sci USA 1994;91:8915–8919.
28. Kaplitt MG, Pfaus JG, Kleopoulos SP, et al. Expression of a functional foreign gene in adult mammalian brain following in vivo transfer via a herpes simplex virus type 1 defective viral vector. Mol Cell Neurosci 1991;2:320–330.
29. Fink D, Glorioso J. Engineering herpes simplex virus vectors for gene transfer to neurons. Nat Med 1997;3:357–359.
30. Fabre JW, Morris PJ. The effect of donor strain blood pretreatment on renal allograft rejection in rats. Transplantation 1972;14:608–617.
31. Opelz G, Sengar DPS, Mickey MR, Terasaki PI. Effect of blood transfusions on subsequent kidney transplants. Transplant Proc 1973;5:253–259.
32. Qin S, Cobbold S, Benjamin R, Waldmann H. Induction of classical transplantation tolerance in the adult. J Exp Med 1989;169:779–794.
33. Thomas FT, Carver FM, Foil MB. Long-term incompatible kidney survival in outbred higher primates without chronic immunosuppression. Ann Surg 1983;198:370.
34. Wood ML, Monaco AP. Induction of unresponsiveness to skin allografts in adult mice disparate at defined regions of the H-2 complex. II. Effect of donor-specific bone marrow in ALS-treated mice. Transplantation 1984;37:35–39.
35. Sharabi Y, Abraham V, Sykes M, Sachs D. Mixed allogeneic chimeras prepared by a non-myeloablative regimen: requirement for chimerism to maintain tolerance. Bone Marrow Transplant 1992;9:191–197.
36. Sharabi Y, Sachs DH. Mixed chimerism and permanent specific transplantation tolerance induced by a nonlethal preparative regimen. J Exp Med 1989;169:493–502.
37. Barber WH, Diethelm AG, Laskow DA, et al. Use of cryopreserved donor marrow in cadaver kidney allograft recipients. Transplantation 1989;47:66–71.
38. Wong W, Morris P, Wood K. Syngeneic bone marrow expressing a single donor class I MHC molecule permits acceptance of a fully allogeneic cardiac allograft. Transplantation 1996;62:1462–1468.
39. Madsen JC, Superina RA, Wood KJ, Morris PJ. Immunological unresponsiveness induced by recipient cells transfected with donor MHC genes. Nature 1988;332:161–164.
40. Saitovitch D, Morris P, Wood K. Recipient cells expressing single donor MHC locus products can substitute for donor specific transfusions in the induction of transplantation tolerance when pretreatment is combined with anti-Cd4 monoclonal antibody: evidence for a vital role of $Cd4^+$ T cells in the induction of tolerance to class I molecules. Transplantation 1996;61:1532–1538.
41. Sundt III TM, Sachs DH. Applications of molecular biology to transplantation tolerance. Immunol Today 1988;9:342–344.
42. Sykes M, Sachs DH, Nienhuis AW, et al. Specific prolongation of skin graft survival following retroviral transduction of bone marrow with an allogeneic major histocompatibility complex gene. Transplantation 1993;55:197–202.
43. Hayashi H, Le Guern C, Sachs D, Sykes M. Long-term engraftment of precultured post-5-fluorouracil allogeneic marrow in mice conditioned with a nonmyeloablative regimen: relevance for a gene therapy approach to tolerance induction. Transplant Immunol 1996;4:86–90.
44. Wong W, Stranford S, Morris P, Wood K. Retroviral gene transfer of a donor class I MHC gene to recipient bone marrow cells induces tolerances to alloantigens in vivo. Transplant Proc 1997;29:1130.
45. Wong W, Morris P, Wood K. Pretransplant administration of a single donor class I MHC molecule is sufficient for the indefinite survival of fully allogeneic cardiac allografts: evidence for linked epitope suppression. Transplantation 1997;63:1490–1494.
46. Yasamoto A, Yamada K, Sablinski, et al. Mechanisms of tolerance following class II gene transduction of autologous swine bone marrow. Transplant Proc 1997;29:1132.
47. Brenner M. Gene transfer to hematopoietic stem cells. N Engl J Med 1996;335:337–339.
48. Dunbar C. Gene transfer to hematopoietic stem cells: implications for gene therapy of human disease. Ann Rev Med 1996;47:11–20.
49. Rosenberg S, Blaese R, Brenner M, et al. Human gene marker/therapy clinical protocols. Hum Gene Ther 1996;7:1621–1647.
50. Eaves C. Peripheral blood stem cells reach new heights. Blood 1993;82:1957–1959.
51. Chahine A, Yu M, McKernan M, et al. Immunomodulation of pancreatic islet allografts in mice with CTLA4Ig secreting muscle cells. Transplantation 1995;59:1313–1318.
52. Benhamou PY, Moriscot C, Badet L, et al. Strategies for graft immunomodulation in islet transplantation. Diabetes Metab 1998;24:215–224.
53. Lau H, Yu M, Fontana A, Stoeckert C. Prevention of islet allograft rejection with engineered myoblasts expressing FasL in mice. Science 1996;273:109.
54. Li XK, Okuyama T, Tamura A, et al. Prolonged survival of rat liver allografts transfected with Fas ligand-expressing plasmid. Transplantation 1998;66:1416–1423.
55. Qin L, Chavin K, Ding Y, et al. Multiple vectors effectively achieve gene transfer in a murine cardiac transplantation model. Transplantation 1995;59:809–816.

56. Qin L, Chavin K, Ding Y, et al. Retrovirus mediated gene transfer of viral IL-10 gene prolongs murine cardiac allograft survival. J Immunol 1996;156:2316–2323.
57. Benhamou P, Mullen Y, Shaked A, et al. M. Decreased alloreactivity to human islets secreting viral interleukin 10. Transplantation 1996;62:1306–1312.
58. Drazan K, Wu L, Shen X, et al. Adenovirus-mediated gene transfer in the transplant setting. Transplantation 1995;59:670–673.
59. Wahl S. Transforming growth factor β: the good, the bad and the ugly. J Exp Med 1994;180:1587–1590.
60. Larkin D, Oral H, Ring C, et al. Adenovirus-mediated gene delivery to the corneal endothelium. Transplantation 1996;61:363–370.
61. Merrick A, Shewring L, Sawyer G, et al. Comparison of adenovirus gene transfer to vascular endothelial cells in cell culture, organ culture and in vivo. Transplantation 1996;62:1085–1089.
62. Muhlhauser J, Jones M, Yamada I, et al. Safety and efficacy of in vivo transfer into the porcine heart with replication-deficient, recombinant adenovirus vectors. Gene Ther 1996;3:145–153.
63. Kass-Eisler A, Falck-Pederson E, Alvira M, et al. Quantitative determination of adenovirus-mediated gene delivery to rat cardiac myocytes in vitro and in vivo. Proc Natl Acad Sci USA 1993;90:11498–11502.
64. Baldwin A. The NF-κB and IκB proteins: new discoveries and insights. Ann Rev Immunol 1996;14:649–683.
65. Cooper J, Stroka D, Brostjan C, et al. A20 blocks endothelial cell activation through an NF-KB-dependent mechanism. J Biol Chem 1996;271:18068–18073.
66. Yamabe K, Kamiike W, Shimizu S, et al. Prevention of hypoxic liver injury by in vivo transfection of the human bcl-2 gene. Transplant Proc 1997;29:384–385.
67. Gainer A, Korbutt G, Rajotte R, et al. Expression of CTLA4-Ig by biolistically transfected mouse islets promotes islet allograft survival. Transplantation 1997;63:1017–1021.
68. Gossen M, Bonin A, Freundlieb S, Bujard H. Inducible gene expression systems for higher eucaryotic cells. Curr Opin Biotechnol 1994;5:516–520.
69. Shockett P, Difilippantonio M, Hellman N, Schatz D. A modified tetracycline-regulated system provides autoregulatory, inducible gene expression in cultured cells and transgenic mice. Proc Natl Acad Sci 1995;92:6522–6526.
70. Gossen M. Transcriptional activation by tetracyclines in mammalian cells. Science 1995;268:1766–1769.
71. Bohl D, Naffakh N, Heard J. Long-term control of erythropoietin secretion by doxycycline in mice transplanted with engineered primary myoblasts. Nat Med 1997;3:299–305.
72. Rivera V, Clackson T, Natesan S, et al. A humanized system for pharmacologic control of gene expression. Nat Med 1996;2:1028–1032.
73. Guild B, Finer M, Housman D, Mulligan R. Development of retroviral vectors useful for expressing genes in cultured murine embryonal cells and hematopoietic cells in vivo. J Virol 1988;62:3795–3801.

COMMENTARY REFERENCES

1. Lau HT, Yu M, Fontana A, Stoeckert CJ Jr. Prevention of islet allograft rejection with engineered myoblasts expressing FasL in mice. Science 1996;273:109–112.
2. Kang S-M, Hoffmann A, Le D, et al. Immune response and myoblasts that express Fas ligand. Science 1997;278:1322–1324.
3. Allison J, Georgiou HM, Strasser A, Vaux DL. Transgenic expression of CD95 ligand on islet beta cells induces a granulocytic infiltration but does not confer immune privilege upon islet allografts. Proc Natl Acad Sci USA 1997;94:3943–3947.
4. Seino K, Kayagaki N, Okumura K, Yagita H. Antitumor effect of locally produced CD95 ligand. Nat Med 1997;3:165–170.
5. Porter ACG, Dallman MJ. Gene targeting. Techniques and applications to transplantation. Transplantation 1997;64:1227–1235.
6. Knechtle SJ, Wang J, Graeb C, et al. Direct MHC class I complementary DNA transfer to thymus induces donor-specific unresponsiveness, which involves multiple immunologic mechanisms. J Immunol 1997;159:152–158.
7. Mathew JM, Marsh JW, Susskind B, Mohanakumar T. Analysis of T cell responses in liver allograft recipients. Evidence for deletion of donor-specific cytotoxic T cells in the peripheral circulation. J Clin Invest 1993;91:900–906.
8. Vilquin J-T, Wagner E, Kinoshita I, et al. Successful histocompatible myoblast transplantation in dystrophin-deficient mdx mouse despite the production of antibodies against dystrophin. J Cell Biol 1995;131:975–988.
9. Tripathy SK, Black HB, Goldwasser E, Leiden JM. Immune responses to transgene-encoded proteins limit the stability of gene expression after injection of replication-defective adenovirus vectors. Nat Med 1996;2:545–550.
10. Shull RM, Lu X, McEntee MF, et al. Myoblast gene therapy in canine mucopolysaccharidosis. I: Abrogation by an immune response to alpha-L-iduronidase. Hum Gene Ther 1996;7:1595–1603.
11. Riddell SR, Elliott M, Lewinsohn DA, et al. T-cell mediated rejection of gene-modified HIV-specific cytotoxic T lymphocytes in HIV-infected patients. Nat Med 1996;2:216–223.
12. Wang J, Ma Y, Knechtle SJ. Adenovirus-mediated gene transfer into rat cardiac allografts. Comparison of direct injection and perfusion. Transplantation 1996;61:1726–1729.

Chapter

40

Xenotransplantation

IAN F. C. MCKENZIE BRUCE E. LOVELAND JAY A. FISHMAN
HUGH AUCHINCLOSS MAURO S. SANDRIN

INTRODUCTION

Xenotransplantation is the transplantation of tissue from one species to another. In the context of clinical transplantation, it includes nonhuman primate-to-human transplantation or pig-to-human transplants; in the experimental setting, many different models have been described (1). Although the concept of using animal organs to treat human disease has long been considered, there is now a renewed interest in xenotransplantation for several reasons. First, the advent of genetic engineering has led to the production of recombinant molecules and genetically modified or transgenic animals in which (at least theoretically) the targets of an immune response can be deleted or modified so that the subsequent immune reaction is decreased. Indeed, the ability of using such genetic engineering techniques in animals indicates that xenografts may ultimately take the place of allografts and the concept of using modified animal organs to transplant to the tolerant recipient may well come true. Second, there is a critical need for more organs for transplantation, due in part to the wider acceptance of transplantation and the improved survival of patients receiving liver and heart–lung allografts and other tissues. Moreover, fewer donors are available today due to the improvement in road traffic control and a diminishing interest in the community for organ donation, all of which adds up to an increasing demand and a diminishing supply. Data from the United Kingdom Transplant Support Service Authority (UKTSSA) clearly shows waiting lists are growing larger while transplants are being performed at the same rate (Fig. 40.1). Therefore, another source of organs for transplantation is required, and xenografts could provide the answer.

Will Patients Accept a Xenograft?

Before proceeding further with experimental studies, it is important to know whether patients would approve xenografting. Clearly, if patients would not accept a xenograft, then future experimental studies would be pointless. Several studies indicated a partial (but not total) acceptance of the use of animal organs for transplantation to humans. First, in the United States, the Partnership for Organ Donation used the Gallup Organization to survey approximately 6000 normal individuals and found that more than 50% supported the procedure (2). Second, in a survey of acute care nurses, most were opposed to xenotransplantation (3). Third, the Nuffield Council on BioEthics (UK) reported responses from many centers that varied from argument, to doubts, to acceptance (4). In our own study, 277 patients awaiting transplantation of either a heart or a kidney were asked various questions relating to the use of animal organs, including some regarding genetic engineering and whether they would accept a xenotransplant. Fifty percent found the procedure acceptable, 10% entirely unacceptable, and 40% wanted more information—presumably on the likelihood of success and possible dangers (5). The Nuffield Council has formulated the following practical guidelines:

1. Xenotransplantation may be able to supplement the inadequate supply of human organs.
2. The breeding of pigs (rather than higher primates) to supply organs would be ethically justified.
3. Advisory committees need to be established to set guidelines and, in particular, to monitor health risks from infection.
4. Once the necessary safeguards are in place, xenotransplantation may be offered to patients.

Problems with Xenotransplantation

It is currently held that the immune response to xenografts may be more vigorous than to allografts, and that increased immunosuppression would be required, which would be accompanied by severe side effects. Indeed, for the baboon-

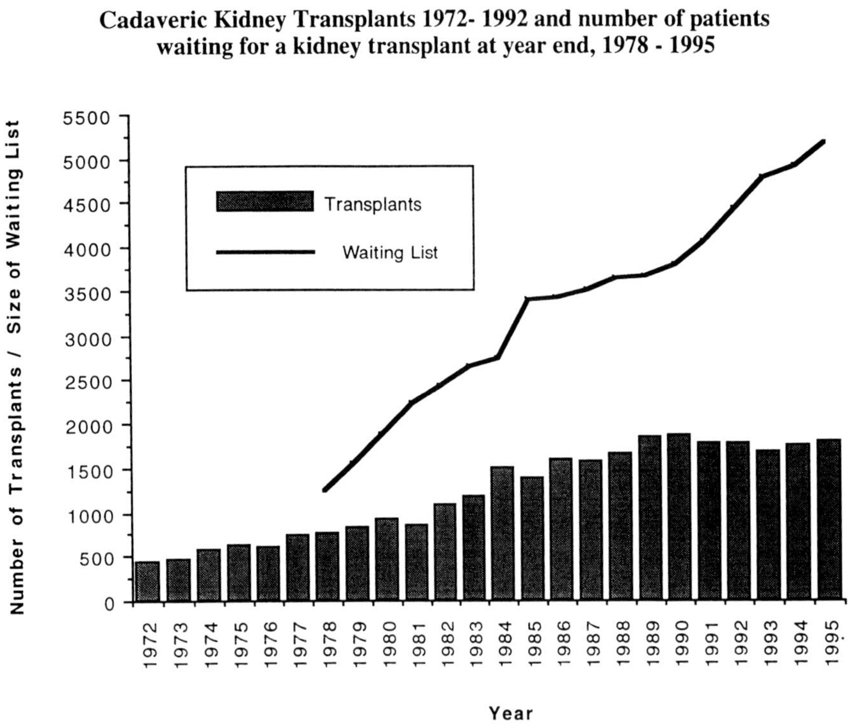

FIGURE 40.1. *Yearly transplant statistics for the UK and Republic of Ireland. (Reproduced with the permission of the United Kingdom Transplant Support Service Authority.)*

Table 40.1. Problems in Xenografting

Problem	Possible Solution	Predicted Time to Solve
Immunologic		
Hyperacute rejection	Antigen/antibody/C′ modification	2 years (2001)
Delayed rejection	? Antigen/antibody/C′ modification	5 years
Cellular rejection	Tolerance	5 years
Tolerance induction	Tolerance	5 years
Other		
Organ size	Selection	1 year
Species incompatibility of organs	? None	—
Inappropriate hormone secretion and regulation	Transgenic	5 years
Autoimmunity	Immunosuppression	5 years
Retroviral infection	Special breeding program	8 years
Patient acceptance/ethics	Explanation	None

to-human transplants done thus far, this seems to be the case. As will become apparent when the immune responses to xenografts are discussed, there appear to be three phases of rejection. The first major problem to be overcome in xenografting is hyperacute, antibody-mediated rejection (HAR) (Table 40.1), which, in pig-to-human transplantation, is likely to cause rejection of a vascularized organ within 10 to 60 minutes. This vigorous response is now not seen for allografts with crossmatching, where the presence of antigraft antibodies can be detected (see Chapter 4). However, unless HAR can be overcome, xenotransplantation cannot proceed. In the absence of HAR, a second phase of slower rejection [delayed xenograft rejection (DXR)] could occur, due to a number of immunologic and nonimmunologic factors. Third, there is a cellular immune response. At present, it is not clear whether the cellular response is greater or less for a xenograft than for an allograft.

Other than the immune system, there are additional potential problems associated with xenografting that cannot be readily identified until clinical xenografts are performed and survive for two to four weeks.

1. *Size.* It is not certain whether a transplanted xenograft will attain the size of the original donor or the appropriate size for the recipient.

2. *Compatibility.* Another potential problem is organ/tissue "incompatibility." This is difficult to define in spe-

cific terms but includes the endothelial cells and vessels of the donor organ being bathed in "foreign" blood components; pig endothelial cells may be adversely affected by some serum proteins, may not respond to the appropriate clotting factors, or indeed, any of the components differing in the species could lead to organ failure. Some experimental evidence suggests that tissue compatibility may not be a problem for all grafts. Nude mice can retain skin grafts of different species (e.g., chicken, lizard, human) for many months without obvious problems; whether this extends to vascularized organs is unknown.

3. *Hormones/Cytokines.* A further problem could be with hormone interactions; for example, in a pig kidney-to-human transplant, human interferon gamma (IFN-γ) does not react with pig tissue.

4. *Autoimmunity.* Autoimmunity can be induced in experimental animals by injecting tissue together with Freund's adjuvant. Perhaps a foreign organ could function in the same way; such autoimmune responses have recently been described in allografts (6).

5. *Infection.* The transfer of infection from donor to recipient is a potential risk and is considered in detail below.

None of the problems listed above are novel, and, indeed, they are similar to the problems presented to those performing the first allografts in the early 1960s. On a positive note, other than HAR, these problems have not appeared in the primate-to-human transplants done thus far, nor in the few pig-to-monkey transplants performed. Provided that there is careful planning (see the Nuffield Council's BioEthics recommendations above) and vigilance for the potential problems, they should not be an impediment to proceeding with xenotransplantation.

In this chapter we discuss the science and clinical studies in xenotransplantation with an emphasis on potential pig-to-human transplantation. The current lack of any significant clinical experience with xenotransplantation necessitates presentation of a more detailed review of the basic investigative approaches and consideration of potential applications than is presented for most other topics in this volume. Further descriptions of xenografting can be found in an excellent monograph (7), several reviews (8–11), and the journals *Xenotransplantation*, and *Transplantation*.

THE HISTORY OF XENOGRAFTING

The modern history of xenotransplantation began in 1963, when Reemtsma first reported a technically successful kidney transplant from a chimpanzee to a human patient (12,13). Over the next several years, Reemtsma, Starzl, and other investigators performed a series of kidney, liver, and heart transplants from chimpanzees, baboons, and even pigs (Table 40.2) (14–33). One of Reemtsma's patients survived with a chimpanzee kidney transplant for nine months with essentially normal renal function (14).

Table 40.2. Clinical Efforts at Xenogeneic Transplantation

Organ	Donor	Attempts	References
Kidney	Chimpanzee Monkey Baboon	14	14–17
Liver	Chimpanzee Baboon Pig	6 (plus many for perfusion)	18–27
Heart	Chimpanzee Baboon Sheep	5	28–31
Islets	Pig	10	32,33
Neural cells	Pig	4	
Bone marrow	Baboon	2	

These early efforts at clinical xenotransplantation were driven by the shortage of organs available for transplantation (the concept of brain death had not yet been accepted), and because there was no life-maintaining therapy, even for patients with renal failure (dialysis had yet to become widely available). Over the next seven years, however, both of these problems were solved, and the need for animal organs for human transplantation diminished. In addition, the immunologic barriers to xenotransplantation became more apparent. Recognition that hyperacute rejection of allogeneic transplants was due to preexisting antidonor antibodies was first achieved in the mid-1960s (34), and, as it was already known that there are natural antibodies in humans that react with antigens of most other species, it therefore became apparent that hyperacute rejection would be particularly important in xenogeneic transplantation in certain cases. Thus, the early clinical efforts at xenografting essentially ended as clinical allogeneic transplantation became more widespread.

While none of the early attempts at clinical xenografting were successful (in the sense of achieving long-term graft or patient survival), they demonstrated that humans can survive when dependent on the function of organs from an animal donor. In addition, survival for up to nine months, using the immunosuppression available in the 1960s, convinced many that it would be possible to achieve still longer survival of xenografts in human patients with newer and better tailored immunosuppressive strategies.

The early efforts at clinical xenografting had the additional effect of stimulating more research on xenogeneic transplantation during the next decade. Most of this research used experimental xenografts to study the mechanisms and possible therapies for hyperacute rejection (35,36). These studies provided valuable information on the contribution of complement and of inflammatory and thrombotic mediators in the rapid destruction of grafts by hyperacute rejection. However, they also generated the mistaken conclusion that all hyperacute rejection depends on the presence of preformed antibodies. More recent studies indicate that in some cases (such as the pig-to-dog combination often used in the early experiments) the alternative pathway of complement activation can initiate hyperacute rejection in the absence of preformed antibody. The assumption that natural antibodies were always involved, and the finding that hyperacute rejection occurred in all but the most closely related species combinations, gave rise to the widely held impression that natural antibodies occur in even greater number, along a continuum, related to the phylogenetic distance between species. Because of this view, it was surprising for many investigators to learn that hyperacute rejection of pig organs by primates is caused almost entirely by natural antibodies directed at a single antigenic determinant, Galα(1,3)Gal, whose immunogenicity was determined by a single discrete event in evolution (the loss of the α-galactosyl transferase gene in Old World primates and humans) (10,37). In some ways, therefore, the early research on hyperacute xenograft rejection generated important misconceptions. Only very recently has our understanding been modified such that the occurrence of hyperacute rejection in any given species combination is now thought to depend on at least three independent and discontinuous variables: 1) the presence of natural antibodies, 2) the ability to activate the alternative pathway of complement, and 3) the function of the complement regulatory proteins across that species barrier (38).

Although the growing success of clinical allogeneic transplantation was responsible for the diminished interest in xenografting during the 1970s, the continued growth of allografting eventually rekindled interest in xenogeneic transplantation. As organ transplantation became increasingly effective and more widely practiced, there were soon too few human organs available for the number of potential recipients who might benefit from receiving them. Since this disparity was most severe for very young recipients, it is not surprising that renewed efforts at clinical xenografting began with the desperate attempt in 1983 to transplant a baboon heart to the infant known as Baby Fae (31). While again not successful in saving the life of this child, the effort helped dramatize the growing shortage of organs for transplantation and certainly contributed to the subsequent rapid growth of interest and research in the field of xenogeneic transplantation. Despite the importance of this single clinical effort, the recent interest in xenografting has been driven, as it was originally, primarily by the disparity between the number of candidates for organ transplantation and the number of organs available for them (see Fig. 40.1). Despite vigorous efforts to increase the rate of cadaveric organ procurement, this disparity has been rapidly increasing (see Chapter 15).

The research achievements of the 15 years following the Baby Fae experiment are the subject of the remaining sections of this chapter. While this research has progressed there have continued to be sporadic efforts at clinical xenotransplantation. Two liver transplants from baboons to humans were performed in Pittsburgh (39), based on research in small animals showing that immunosuppression directed especially at B-cell responses can prevent the early antibody response and lead to prolonged survival of xenografts in concordant species combinations (40,41). One of these patients survived for several months before dying of infectious complications of the immunosuppression. In addition, baboon bone marrow has been transplanted to a patient with AIDS in the hope of reconstituting an immune system that would be resistant to HIV infection; however, engraftment apparently did not occur. Furthermore, there have been several efforts to use pig organs for human patients, including a temporary pig liver transplant as an effort to provide a "bridge" to allotransplantation (42), and several cases where ex vivo perfusion through a pig liver has been used to support patients with fulminant hepatic failure while they waited for a human liver transplant (27,43). Some of these patients have survived the entire process. Finally, two groups have used cellular transplants from pigs for human patients, including islets for the treatment of diabetes (33) and neural cells for the treatment of severe Parkinson's disease. There is evidence that some of these cell transplants have survived for long periods, although there was little substantial function of the transplanted tissues (44).

Further clinical efforts at xenografting will undoubtedly continue given the severe shortage of human tissue for clinical transplantation. However, the widespread clinical application of xenografting still appears likely to require a solution to many of the scientific issues described in this chapter.

ETHICAL PROBLEMS IN XENOGRAFTING

The ethical problems associated with xenotransplantation resolve into the following questions: 1) Should animal organs be used for human transplants? 2) Which species of animals could be used? 3) Should animals be specifically bred for transplantation, including the genetic engineering of donor animals? There are now internationally acceptable guidelines provided from a March 1996 meeting of the Nuffield Foundation Council on BioEthics (UK) (4), and there are national guidelines for the care and management of laboratory animals to which those in research must rigidly adhere (45).

As to the first question—whether it is ethically responsible to use animal organs—the Nuffield report (4) pointed out that our society accepts that animal parts be used for a variety of purposes: food, leather, tissues for transplantation (as has been done with skin and heart valves from pigs), a pituitary extract as a source of growth hormone (cattle, pigs), and insulin (extracted pig insulin was used prior to recombinant material being available). Thus, taking an organ for a transplant is no different in principle or in practice than what is currently happening today and is therefore acceptable.

The second question—concerning which animals could be used—resolves into a consideration of primates and domestic animals, of which the pig is the favored donor.

There are clear reasons why some primates should not be used—gorillas, orangutans, and chimpanzees are threatened species and while in Africa the baboon is not, establishing international baboon colonies is unlikely. Although some 30 primate grafts have been performed (see Table 40.2) with variable degrees of success (indeed, there are rare instances of a functioning graft lasting up to nine months in humans), the use of primates on a large scale to satisfy the transplantation needs of humans is not an attractive proposition. The domestic pig is therefore currently the favored donor.

The final question—whether it is acceptable to genetically engineer animals and use their organs—encompasses a number of possibilities beyond the ethical question, as such animals may express extraneous molecules that could ultimately be dangerous, for example, retroviruses (see below). However, is it morally responsible to modify an animal's genome by making transgenic animals or by "knocking out" genes by homologous recombination? In principle, genetic selection procedures have been conducted for centuries, wherein animals are selected for desirable characteristics such as breeding performance, quantity of lean meat (cattle, sheep, and pigs), wool production, and other characteristics in, for example, racehorses. While these procedures did not always involve laboratory experimentation, they are nonetheless the same as the early and subsequent genetic selection procedures that utilized random gene mutation. Today, with the advances in genetic engineering, such selection procedures can be controlled and performed rapidly, so that the result occurs within one generation rather than several. Thus, as genetic selection/engineering has been going on for decades, the recent advances are no different in principle and the ethical issues are therefore not new, but have been considered and resolved by the community. This is clearly a broad overview; opposing views on xenotransplantation are reviewed elsewhere (46). It should be noted here that the problems associated with xenografting (see Table 40.1) are not ethical issues. They are clinical or research problems to be dealt with by those working in that area.

THE CLASSIFICATION OF XENOGRAFT REJECTION

Some years ago Calne (47) proposed that xenografts performed between donor–recipient pairs be termed *concordant* or *discordant:* where early hyperacute rejection was noted (within minutes), this was discordant, whereas a later rejection, akin to that seen in allografts, was concordant. Examples of discordant grafts (Table 40.3) (1,47) were pig-to-monkey/human, guinea pig-to-rat, or dog-to-sheep. In all of these, large amounts of natural antibody in the recipient led to immediate antibody-mediated rejection (see below). By contrast, in other models such as primate-to-human or mouse- or hamster-to-rat, there were either no or lesser amounts of natural antibodies and graft rejection occurred more slowly. This classification is not absolute, however, and indeed nude mice bearing xenografts made considerable amounts of antibody but did not reject grafts. Adding an extraneous source of complement was required to destroy the graft (47–50). Furthermore, the rate of rejection depended on the tissue transplanted because some organs are more sensitive to antibody-mediated rejection than others. Thus, vascularized grafts are inordinately sensitive to antibody-mediated rejection as are single cell suspensions of bone marrow cells or lymphocytes. By contrast, islet cells, isolated liver cells, and skin appear to be more resistant to such mechanisms (see Table 40.3).

The endothelium of vessels is a critical target in vascularized xenotransplants, and it is clear that the starting point

Table 40.3. Classification of Xenograft Rejection

	Likely Immunologic Mechanisms		Nonimmunologic Participation	
Name	**Antibody**	**T Cell**	**Other Cellular (Neutrophils, Platelets, etc.)**	**Time**
Hyperacute rejection (HAR)	+	−	?	10 min–hours
Delayed acute XR (DXR)	+/−	?	+ → active endo cells	1 week
Late XR (LXR)	+ ?	+	+ ?	>1 week

Types
Discordant (Antibody, HAR): pig-to-monkey/human, guinea pig-to-rat, dog-to-sheep
Concordant (DXR?, LXR): primate-to-human, mouse-to-rat, hamster-to-rat

Tissue variability:
Sensitive to Ab: vascularized grafts, cell grafts (e.g., bone marrow, lymphocytes)
Relatively resistant to Ab: ?islet cells, liver cells, skin

Mediators of rejection:
Primary: antibody (C′, ADCC), T lymphocytes, ?NK
Secondary: NK, clotting factor, eosinophils, platelets, endothelial cells, serum proteins, neutrophils

for a classification involves consideration of the components that are both immunologic and nonimmunologic. The primary immunologic components are antibodies and lymphocytes, and these include NK cells, ADCC, and related phenomena. Nonimmunologic factors include tissue incompatibility and the activation of endothelial cells in vascularized grafts. Both the immunologic and the nonimmunologic factors induce an inflammatory response that involves, to a greater or lesser degree, all of the components involved in any acute or chronic inflammatory response and include neutrophils, eosinophils, macrophages, clotting factors, platelets, and the appropriate cytokines. Depending on the relative amounts of the immunologic and nonimmunologic components and the kinetics of the reaction, the xenograft response can vary from an acute Shwartzman-like reaction with an emphasis on intravascular clotting that occurs within a few minutes, to an antibody-mediated response occurring in 10 to 60 minutes and involving neutrophils—akin to an Arthus reaction (50,51). With the activation of endothelial cells and a lesser focus on antibody rather than on other components, the host response may then be more delayed and involve neutrophils, macrophages, and NK and other cells—the so-called delayed xenograft rejection (DXR). Later, the response also involves T cells, with a concomitant inflammatory response. In any particular model, one rejection mechanism may be dominant and the others may be absent or go unnoticed, but in clinical transplantation any one of these phenomena merges with the next. Other than for antibody-mediated effects, which can be studied in acute experiments with the transfer of antibody, it is difficult to study DXR or cellular responses in isolation (see section on cell-mediated xenograft rejection, below).

On the basis of all these interacting factors, a classification is possible based on the time of rejection rather than the components. Thus, the *hyperacute rejection* is most likely initiated entirely by antibody and complement and occurs within minutes to hours. This is succeeded by *delayed xenograft rejection*, perhaps involving a dominance of other mediators (but certainly not excluding antibody) and occurring in the first week. Finally, *cellular rejection* can be recognized (later) where T cells are the dominant initiating factors but where the role of the other mediators again cannot be excluded. There is also likely to be *chronic rejection* similar to that which occurs in allografts, wherein vascular occlusion and tissue atrophy can occur. This classification is not absolute but serves as a useful focus for description.

HYPERACUTE REJECTION

Definition

Hyperacute rejection (HAR) occurs when vascularized organs are transplanted into a recipient who has antibodies to the donor and consists of a series of events in which antibodies bind to the vascular endothelium of the grafted organ and the complement cascade is activated, leading to intravascular coagulation and loss of the organ. This reaction can occur within minutes, and in many aspects resembles a localized Shwartzman reaction. Polymorphonuclear leukocytes may also be involved in HAR, and in these cases the reaction is analogous to an Arthus reaction. The major mediators of hyperacute graft rejection are listed in Table 40.3 and will be discussed below.

History

Early animal models of transplantation, particularly in mice, used skin grafts to study graft rejection and demonstrated the importance of cellular mechanisms of graft rejection; there was difficulty in demonstrating that antibodies played any role in rejection. Thus, after allotransplantation, little antibody was formed, "second set" rejection could occur after adoptive transfer of cells but not antibody, and tolerance could be induced by the neonatal injection of cells but not antibody (52). In addition, rejecting grafts were infiltrated with cells and not antibody. These were all compelling reasons to consider that the cellular (lymphocyte) arm of the immune system caused rejection and that antibody did not. Furthermore, antibody administration to rodents bearing tumor, skin, or kidney grafts could lead to *graft prolongation* rather than rejection, a phenomenon known as *immunologic enhancement*, although in these early studies it was noted that grafts of leukemic tumors were destroyed by antibody and that sarcoma cells had to be used for enhancement studies (52–54). It was later realized that with a higher density of H-2 antigens, leukemic cells could bind more antibody and complement and be destroyed. Sarcoma cells, with a lower density of H-2 antigen, were resistant to the direct destructive effects of antibody (55). In later studies, the antibody-induced enhancement of vascularized kidney and heart allografts in rats was demonstrated by the passive administration of antibody. Nevertheless, in the 1960s, it was thought that antibodies played little role in rejection.

The rodent studies were misleading, however, for in the late 1960s HAR was described in kidney allografts (56,57) and IgM and IgG deposits were found in biopsies of rejecting allografts. Furthermore, the rejecting allografts in patients receiving immunosuppression did not have a cellular infiltration as the predominant feature of many biopsies; rather, they had vascular changes. The only examples of possible HAR in the rodent were the studies of Eichwald (58), wherein hyperimmunized mice would not accept a skin graft at all, but in these studies the role of active cellular immunity could not be excluded. The now classic studies of Winn and colleagues (48,49) established why rodents would not usually develop HAR. In these studies, the cellular rejection of rat-to-mouse skin was avoided by the use of immunosuppressive agents such as antilymphocyte serum (ALS), with which graft survival was extended to approximately 60 days, or nude mice could be used and had permanent graft survival. In these models, the role of antibodies could be studied in isolation in grafts that had "healed-in" and could be considered to be equivalent to vascularized organ grafts. In mice bearing healed-in rat skin grafts, the administration of mouse antirat antibodies led to skin graft damage within minutes and complete destruction within 24 to 48 hours (i.e., HAR) (48–50). The use of noncomplement-fixing antibodies or the depletion of complement prevented graft damage (49), and chicken antirat antibodies, which do not bind mammalian complement, prevented the mouse antirat antibody-mediated graft destruction. Of interest were subsequent studies showing that nude mice could reject grafts, provided that additional complement was given, as nude mice make T-cell–independent IgM antibody responses. Thus, provided that the right antibody is present (IgG2a in mice) with the appropriate complement, HAR of skin and other organs can occur in rodents in the absence of any lymphocyte component. The routine pretransplant assessment of human recipients for antidonor antibodies has virtually eliminated the hyperacute rejection of allografts (see Chapter 4), but HAR has re-emerged as the major barrier to xenotransplantation of nonprimate organs to humans.

Pathology of Hyperacute Rejection in Xenografts

The histologic examination of hyperacutely rejected vascularized organs (59–62) shows patterns that are characteristic of either an Arthus reaction or at times a Shwartzman reaction (Fig. 40.2 and Plate 42, Fig. 40.3), and includes features of a type II reaction in the classic Gell and Coombs classification—cytotoxic reactions that involve complement-

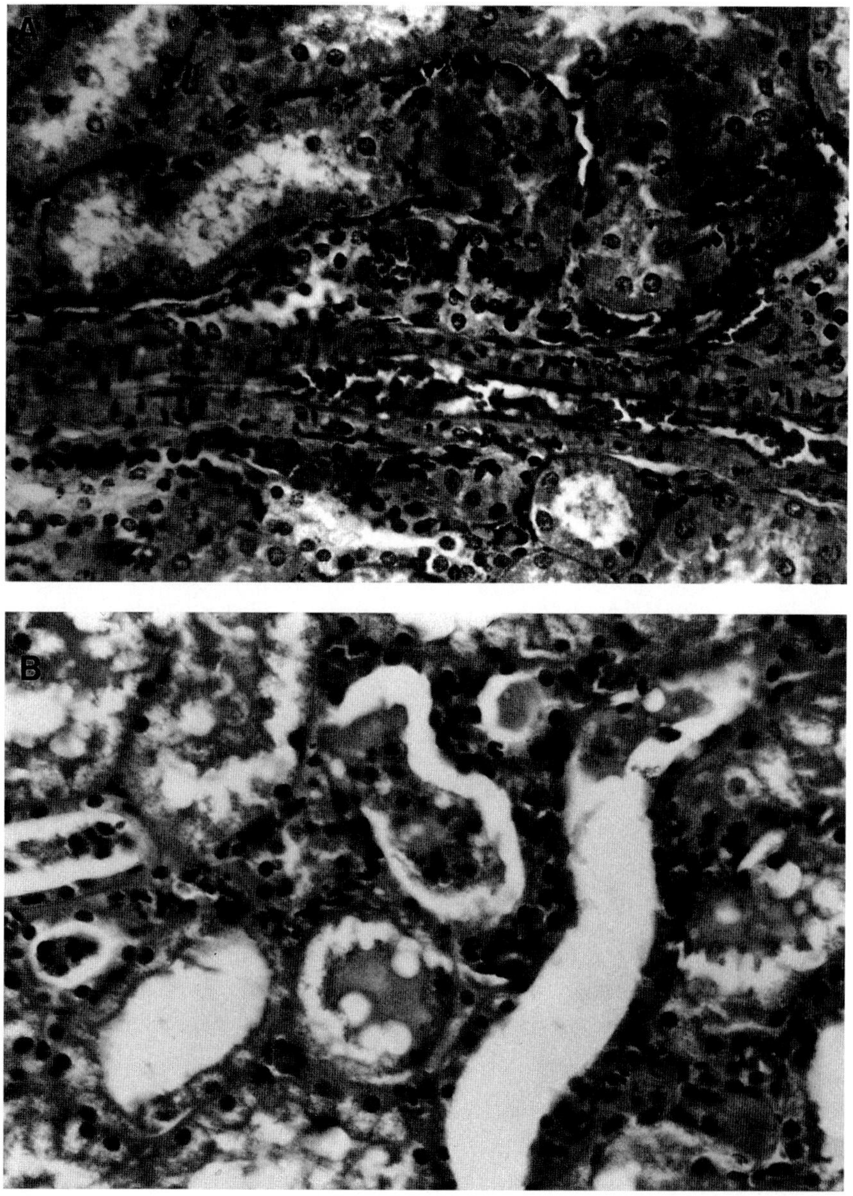

FIGURE 40.2. *Hyperacute xenograft rejection.* ***A.*** *Intravascular thrombosis and hemorrhage in a renal xenograft (sheep-to-dog). This has been likened to a Shwartzman-type reaction.* ***B.*** *Polymorphonuclear granulocyte accumulation in capillaries in the renal xenograft.*

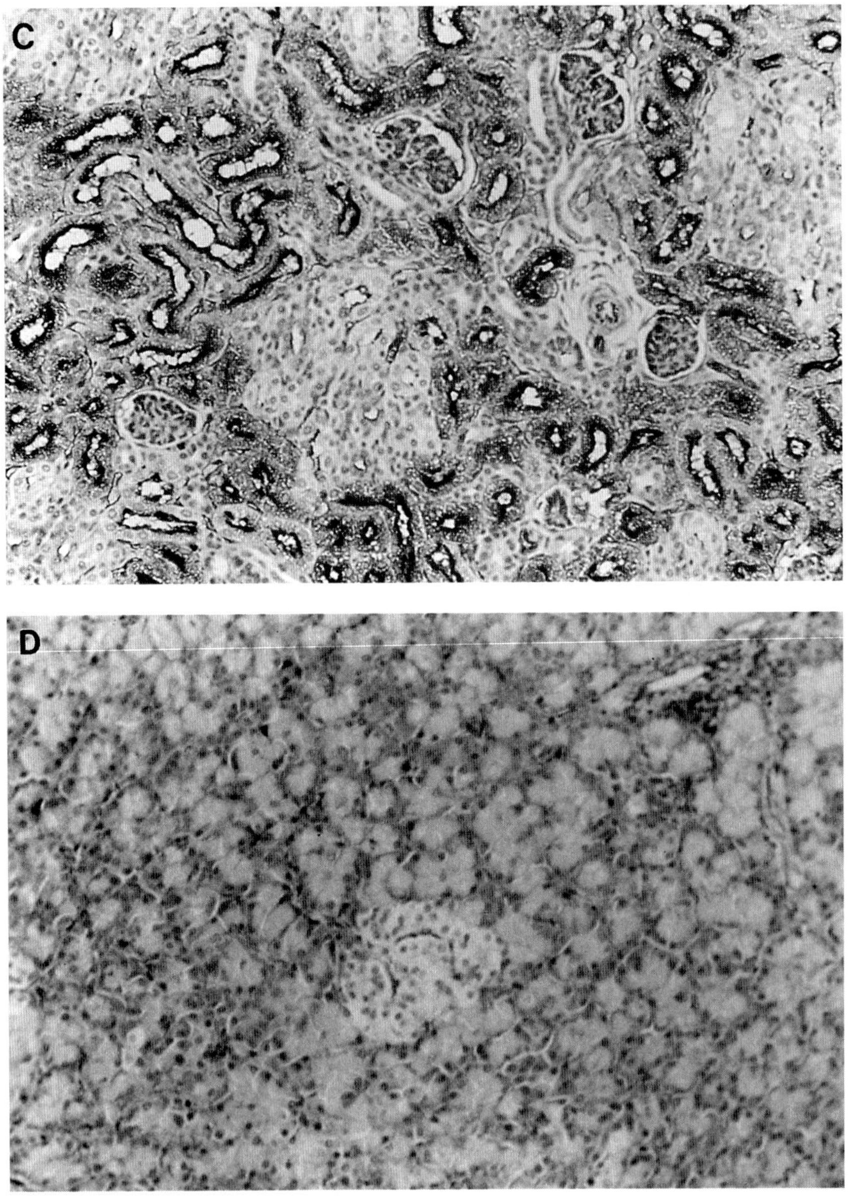

FIGURE 40.2. ***C.*** *Expression of Galα(1,3)Gal in pig kidney. Staining with the lectin IB4 and the immunoperoxidase method: dark staining [Galα(1,3)Gal] is lining tubules (proximal convoluted), collecting ducts, and capillary endothelium.* ***D.*** *Lack of expression of Galα(1,3)Gal in an adult pig islet cell (see* ***C*** *for details); the minimal staining is in capillary endothelium and in pancreatic ducts, but not in acini or islet cells.*

fixing antibodies binding to cell surface antigens, leading to cell destruction and usually involving polymorphic infiltration. Experimentally, the Arthus reaction can be induced by the intradermal injection of antigen into a sensitized animal that has circulating antibodies. Immune complexes form at the site of injection, deposit in the vessel wall, and complement is activated leading to the formation of chemotactic factors that attract polymorphonuclear granulocytes from the circulation. The recruitment of polymorphonuclear granulocytes is assisted by increased vascular permeability induced by the release of vasoactive amines from damaged platelets. Current dogma states that in an attempt to phagocytose the immune complexes, lysosomal enzymes are released, causing damage to the adjacent cells. Edema, erythema, and accumulation of polymorphonuclear granulocytes are seen approximately 30 minutes after injection, increasing to a maximum at three to six hours and leading to local tissue damage and necrosis.

The Shwartzman reaction can be caused by endotoxin, bacterial filtrates, or the injection of immune complexes or thrombin and results in immediate severe intravascular thrombosis, tissue hemorrhage, and ischemic necrosis. Of particular interest is endotoxic shock, in which endotoxin fixes complement, adheres to platelets, and triggers the coagulation system through the extrinsic pathway, leading to disseminated intravascular coagulation. HAR is dependent on antibody, but the end result of intravascular coagulation within xenotransplanted organs is very similar to the Shwartzman reaction. Recently, interleukin 12 (IL-12), interferon gamma (IFN-γ), and tumor necrosis factor alpha (TNFα) have been identified as key cytokines in the Shwartzman reaction (64).

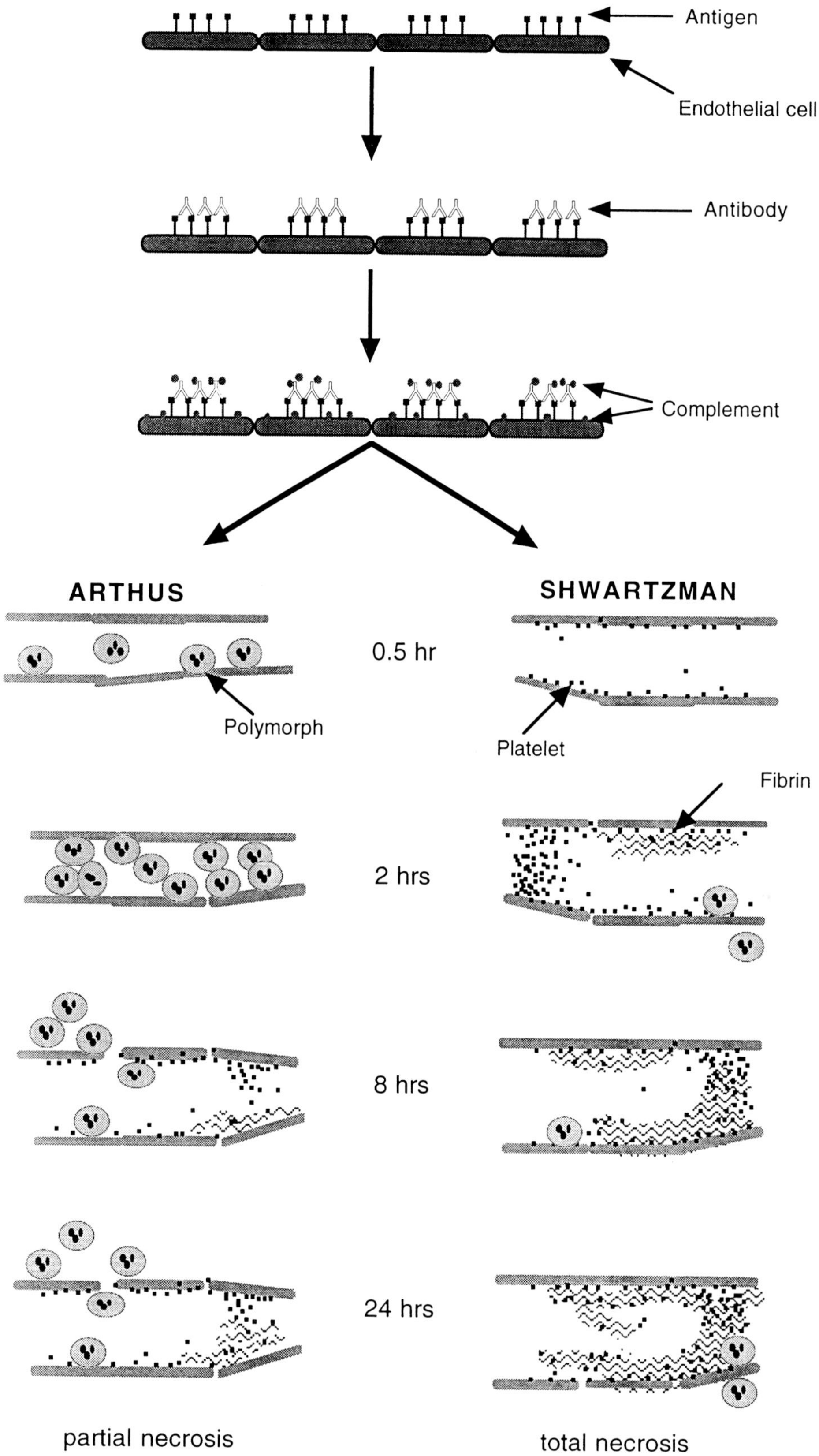

FIGURE 40.3. *Diagrammatic representation of hyperacute rejection. Events initiated by antibody binding to the endothelium and fixing complement, can proceed to either a Shwartzman-type reaction or an Arthus-type reaction (63). See Figure 40.2 for histology. (Adapted from Bogman MJJT. Hyperacute rejection as a model of antibody-induced vasculitis. Nijmegen: Stichting Studenenpers, 1983.)*

The characteristic pathology of hyperacute xenograft rejection includes interstitial hemorrhage, edema, thrombus formation, and, in some tissues and species combinations, the infiltration of polymorphonuclear granulocytes. Immunohistologic examination of rejected tissue shows linear deposition of immunoglobulin and complement along the endothelial lining of the vessels. Studies by Bogman et al (50,51) demonstrated that both the speed and the histologic outcomes of hyperacute rejection depend on the amount of antibody present: using a rat skin-to-mouse model similar to that used by Winn, these investigators showed that low doses of antibody gave rise to a slower Arthus-like reaction, whereas high doses of antibody rapidly induced a Shwartzman-like pattern. Furthermore, the partial depletion of complement changed the reaction from Shwartzman to Arthus and, conversely, administration of rabbit complement and greater antibody doses changed the Arthus reaction to the more violent Shwartzman histologic pattern (50,51). In pig-to-human transplants and in many other models, the literature refers extensively to polymorph accumulation, that is, an Arthus-type reaction. In our experience, however, HAR more closely resembles a Shwartzman reaction, particularly as intravascular coagulation and hemorrhage are more obvious features than polymorph adherence to vessels.

Components of Hyperacute Rejection: Antibody, Antigen, and Complement

The primary components in the hyperacute xenograft rejection are antibody and complement (Table 40.4), with coagulation and cellular inflammation being the secondary components.

Antibody

The crucial role of antibodies in HAR comes from several different lines of evidence: 1) hyperacute rejection occurs very rapidly, indicating a humoral factor; 2) antibody deposition on the donor endothelium is observed in rejected discordant xenografts; 3) ex vivo perfusion through xenogeneic organs or other modes of depletion of xenoreactive antibodies leads to a subsequent prolongation of graft survival in the antibody-depleted recipient; 4) reinfusion of antibody leads to hyperacute rejection of organs; 5) the transplantation of newborn primates, which have low titers of antipig antibodies, with pig hearts does not lead to hyperacute rejection; and 6) the time of onset and severity of hyperacute rejection is proportional to the titer of antibody.

Table 40.4. Evidence for Role of Antibodies and Complement in HAR

Antibody
Deposited on vascular endothelium in hyperacutely rejected organ
HAR occurs rapidly
HAR does not occur in recipient lacking antibody
Adoptive transfer with serum
Depletion of antibody (plasmapheresis, anti-Ig columns, immunoabsorbent columns) delays onset of HAR
Blocking antibody (neutralization) with antigen delays onset of HAR
Complement
Deposited on vascular endothelium in hyperacutely rejected organ
Depletion of complement (cobra venom factor, anticomplement antibodies) delays onset of HAR
HAR does not occur in complement-deficient animals

Antibodies of the IgM class, which are complement fixing, are considered to be the most important in HAR (65,66), although IgG antibodies can also play a role. Antibodies that cause xenogeneic HAR are "natural antibodies," which are present in the circulation of all individuals in the absence of an identified sensitizing antigen. Natural antibodies are not present at birth, but develop weeks to months later, presumably after colonization of the gut by microorganisms that sensitize the recipient. For example, chickens make a natural anti-B blood group–like antibody that appears within 30 days after hatching (67). However, if chicks are raised in a germ-free environment, these antibodies do not appear until normal gut bacteria are introduced into the feed (67). In the case of the long known human antipig antibodies (68), the majority recognize the carbohydrate Galα(1,3)Gal (see below) and are closely related to the natural anti-ABO blood group antibodies. In the pig-to-primate situation, a switch after transplantation in the anti-Galα(1,3)Gal from IgM to IgG is observed, accompanied by an increase in both the level (titer) (27,69) and the affinity of the antibody (69). It is likely that in other species combinations natural antibodies are also directed to carbohydrates, for example the anti-sialyl-Le^a antibodies in the hamster-to-rat model (70). As antibodies are a key component of HAR, it follows that their removal, blocking, or neutralization is an important strategy to avoid HAR.

Complement

The complement cascade is undoubtedly a major player in antibody-mediated hyperacute rejection: deposition of multiple complement components occurs in rejecting grafts, demonstrating that the cascade has been fully activated (71), but more importantly, grafts survive longer in complement-depleted animals (72–74) and in the absence of critical complement components, such as C6 in PVG (C-) rats (75,76) (Table 40.5).

The complement system involves more than 20 proteins, most of which are enzymes, that interact sequentially to amplify the initiating reaction and generate a variety of inflammatory sequelae. The initial reactions generate C3 convertases that cleave C3 into C3b, which can covalently attach to the targets of complement activation, and the anaphylatoxic fragment C3a (Fig. 40.4). Surface-bound C3b then becomes a focus for the generation of C5 convertases, which cleave C5 into C5b and the very potent C5a chemotactic peptide. C5b is the catalyst for resolution of the complement cascade, via the sequential activation and binding of the C6, C7, and C8 components, prior to polymerization of the multimolecular complex with C9 to form the pore-structure membrane attack complex (MAC), which is required for complement-mediated cell lysis. As summarized in Figure 40.4, the generation of chemokines in the early stages of the cascade (anaphylatoxins C3a, C4a, and C5a) enables other processes to occur, including increased vascular permeability by endothelial cell activation, mast and platelet cell degranulation, the clearance of antigen–antibody complexes, chemotaxis and activation of macrophages, neutrophils, and other cells, and development of the complex milieu of an inflammatory response, including coagulation.

The complement system can be activated either by antibody–antigen complexes that react with C1 and generate a sequence of events to utilize C4 in the "classic pathway" of complement activation, or by the cleaving of highly labile C3 protein by hydroxyl groups, zymogens, and free-radical ions in the "alternative pathway" of complement activation, a process that is constantly active (83). The two activation pathways converge at the cleavage of C5, resulting in

Table 40.5. Studies of Complement-Deficient Animals

Species	Deficiency	Study	Reference
Dog	C3	Effects of absence of C3a, C5a	77
Guinea pig	C3-low	Xenografts	78
	C2, C3, C4	Review of literature	79
Mouse	C3	Review of literature	80
Rabbit	C6	Dog heart xenograft	81
		Cat kidney xenograft	82
Rat	C6	Guinea pig heart xenograft	75, 76

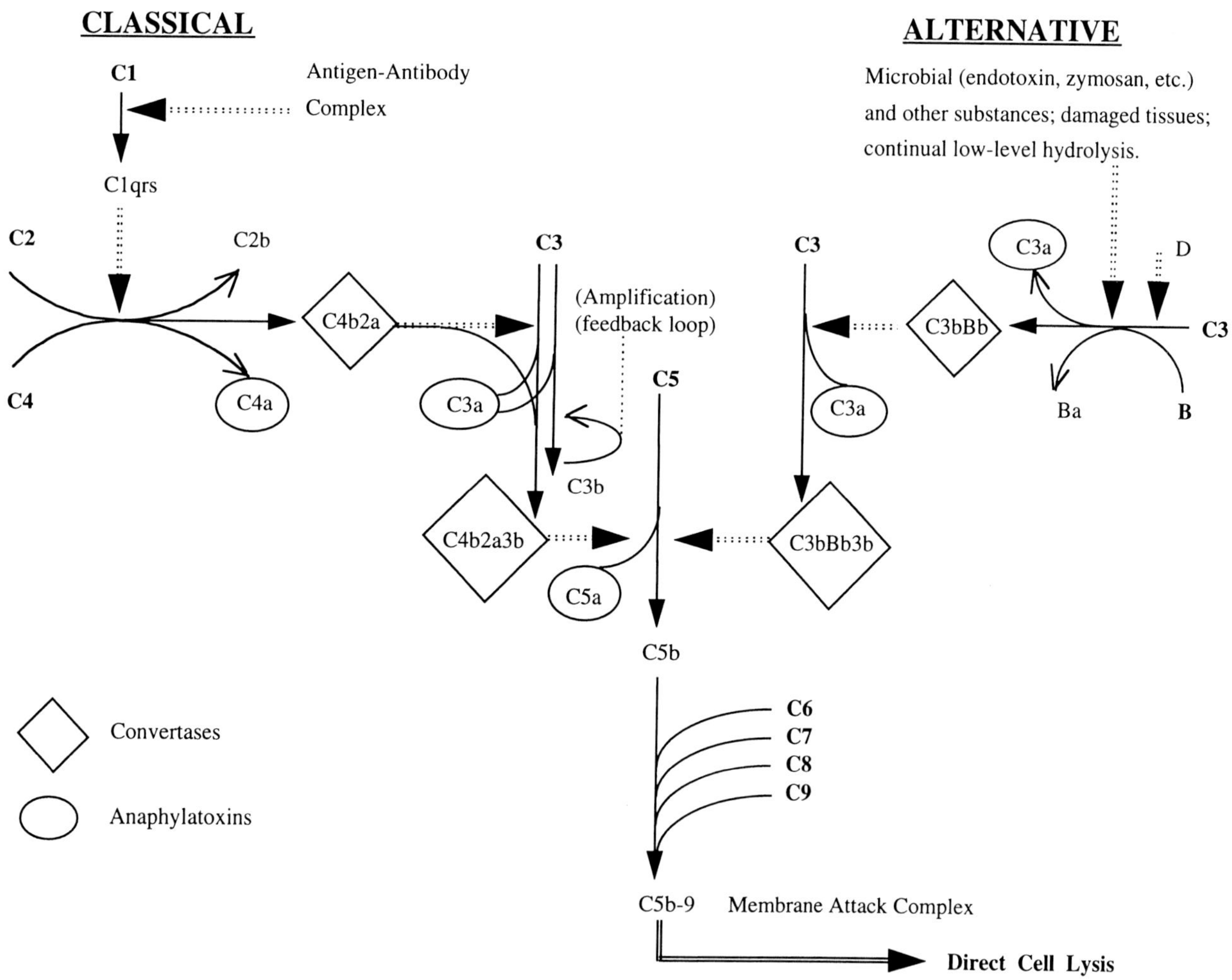

FIGURE 40.4. *The complement cascade: classic and alternative pathways of induction. Only the principal components are shown in order to demonstrate: 1) the production of the anaphylatoxins (circled) C3a, C4a, and C5a; 2) the generation and action of the convertases (outlined by diamonds); and 3) the convergence at the cleavage of C5. The classic pathway generates a C3 convertase (C4b2a) and a C5 convertase (C4b2a3b), whereas the alternative pathway utilizes C3bBb as the C3 convertase and C3bBb3b as the C5 convertase. Feedback amplification loops are established by the action of C3b on C3. The anaphylatoxins cause increased vascular permeability and the chemotactic migration of platelets, neutrophils, and macrophages, etc., and establish a procoagulant state.*

assembly of the terminal complex, MAC (see Figure 40.4). The interrelationship of the two pathways has been demonstrated by alternative pathway induction after C4b deposition (84) or IgG binding (85), thus they cannot be assumed to act in a mutually exclusive manner. This observation raises the possibility that in xenograft rejection not only is the classic pathway activated by natural antibodies reacting with the graft, but the alternative pathway may also be activated (83), depending on the donor–recipient combination. Furthermore, as indicated earlier, there is evidence that HAR can occur in the absence of antibody, deduced from the rejection of rabbit hearts by presuckled pigs (lacking immunoglobulin) after 92 minutes with the absence of Ig deposition in the graft but with C3 deposition, whereas hearts survived in pigs treated with cobra venom factor (CVF) (86).

Complement Regulation

The complement system can be viewed as a "hair-trigger" mechanism designed to react against microorganisms: there is no required instruction of the immune system and no memory, and once activated it provides a potent and damaging array of proteolytic reagents. In discordant xenogeneic combinations, the graft is the target for this reaction and can succumb within minutes. However, the complement system is normally held in check by a number of plasma and cell membrane proteins that limit the initiation of the cascade (87) and, at critical points, cascade amplification. Thus, they allow the complement system to "tick-over" rather than erupt. In particular, the "regulators of complement activation" (RCA) proteins [factor H, C4bp, CR2 (CD21), CR1 (CD35), membrane cofactor protein (MCP; CD46), and decay accelerating factor (DAF; CD55)] control the C3 and C4 amplification steps, and CD59 limits the polymerization of MAC (Table 40.6 and Fig. 40.5) (88–91). In proportion to the density of their expression, the complement regulators provide a threshold of protection against the *inappropriate* activation of complement both on cell surfaces and in the soluble phase. Once the threshold is surpassed, the catalytic effects of the complement enzymes overwhelm the regulators. In viewing the principal role of complement to be a rapid reaction against pathogens, this scenario is perfectly logical and eventually may be found to explain the variations in the tissue expression of complement regulators; for example, CD46 is at low density on PBLs but found at very high density on ductular cells in the salivary gland and kidney (92). In addition to purely regulatory functions, CR1 and CR2 are also involved, through receptor functions, in

Table 40.6. Molecules Regulating Complement Activity

Name(s)	CD No.	Ligands	Cofactor Activity	Decay Acceleration	Protein Size	Tissue Distribution	Therapeutic Potential
CR1	CD35	C3b, C4b	+	+	190–290 kd	RBC, monocytes, macrophages, neutrophils, most B and some $CD4^+$ T lymphocytes, follicular dendritic cells, Langerhans cells	rsCR1 for perfusion (in trials) [cell membrane CR1 has poor cell protection (intrinsic) function; it acts on C′ deposits on "adjacent" membranes]
MCP	CD46	C3b, C4b	+	−	56, 66, 74 kd	All tissues (?) except RBC	Transgenic MCP for cell protection Possibly rsMCP for perfusion
DAF	CD55	C3b, C4b	−	+	~70 kd	Most tissues, including RBC; not NK cells *GPI-anchored.*	Transgenic DAF for cell protection Possibly rsDAF for perfusion
CR2	CD21	C3dg	−	+	~145 kd	Most B lymphocytes, follicular dendritic cells, a T-cell subset, and some epithelial cells	Not tested? Role in signaling B lymphocytes may complicate potential therapeutic functions
Factor H		C3b	+	+	150 kd	Plasma	Possible; little data yet
C4bp		C4b	+	+	550 kd	Plasma (αβ heterodimer)	Not tested?
MACIF, HRF20, MIRL	CD59	C5b-8	Inhibition of C9 incorporation, thus blocking C5b-9 formation and MAC assembly		20 kd	Most tissues; not hepatocytes, glomerular epithelium, and oligodendrocytes *GPI-anchored.*	Transgenic CD59 for cell protection No likely use in soluble form

MCP = membrane cofactor protein; DAF = decay accelerating factor.

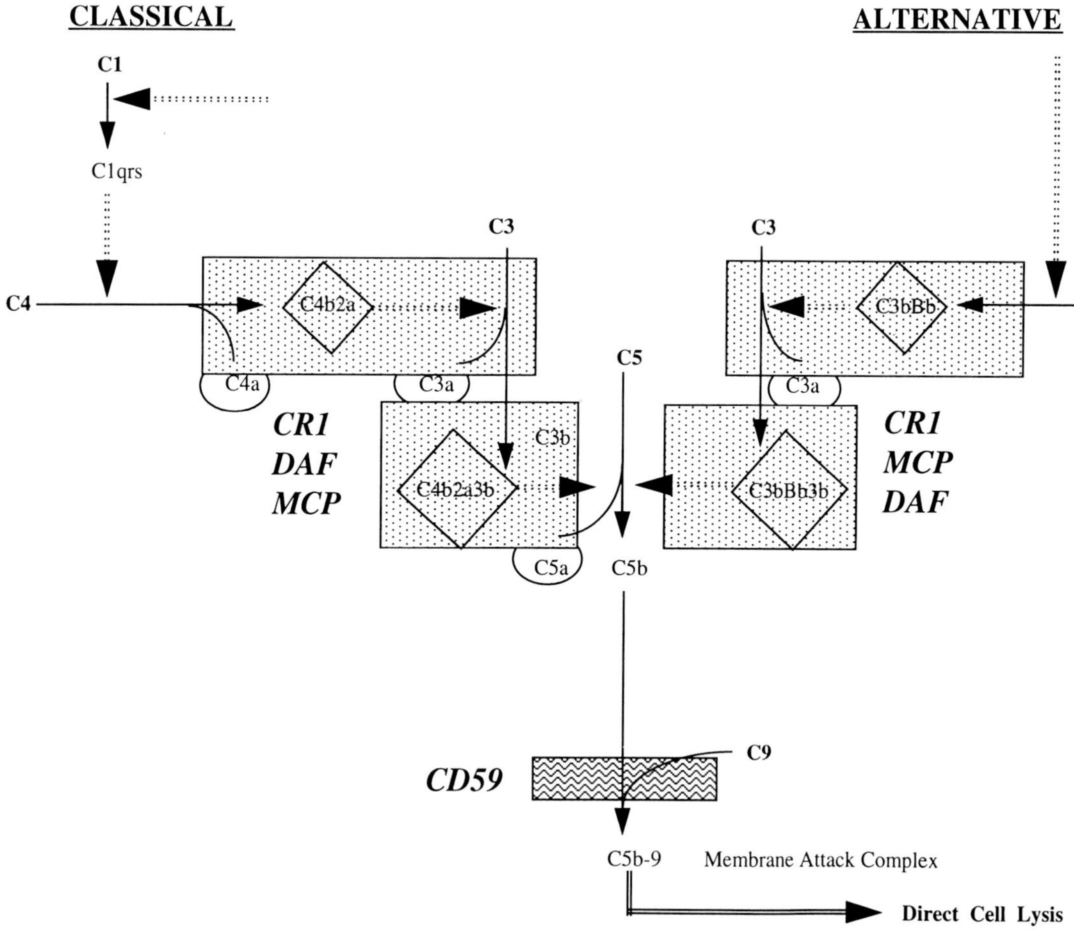

FIGURE 40.5. *Sites of action of complement regulators, focusing on the proteins used in transplantation studies. This figure should be compared with the detail of Figure 40.4. Two sites, shown as shaded boxes, are controlled: the activation of C3 and C4 (but also impinging on C5) by the RCA molecules CR1, DAF, and MCP; and the regulation of the terminal (MAC) complex by CD59. CR1 and DAF accelerate the decay of the convertases, and CR1 and MCP are cofactors for the serum protease, factor I, to cleave C3b and C4b. MCP and DAF differ in apparent regulatory efficiency for the two pathways, with CR1 probably most efficient. Note that in Table 40.6, both the CD nomenclature and the common descriptive acronyms for these molecules are shown: MCP (for membrane cofactor protein) is not a unique abbreviation, and should not be confused with the monocyte chemoattractant proteins (MCP-1, -2, etc.).*

immune complex clearance and activation of the immune system (89).

These regulatory proteins are relevant to xenotransplantation in two aspects. Because some of the complement regulators demonstrate species specificity, or at least species preference, in their interactions with complement (a characteristic called *homologous restriction* (93) and elaborated below), they may be impotent in mediating protection, thus providing a very low threshold for activation when exposed to nonhomologous complement components. Thus, the endogenous complement regulatory proteins of a xenografted tissue may be unable to prevent deposition of large quantities of the foreign (recipient) complement and amplification of the complement cascade. Perhaps this is a major reason why xenografts are so susceptible to antibody attack. Second, complement regulators that control the relevant complement proteins are tools for engineering donor organs. The human complement regulators that have been identified are listed in Table 40.6.

Complement and Xenograft Rejection

Complement Depletion by CVF Evidence of the causative role of complement in rejection has been obtained after its systemic depletion by treatment of the recipient with CVF, which binds factor B to form an unusually stable C3/C5 convertase, C5Bb, and "exhausts" serum C3 by rapidly activating it, thereby removing an essential component of the cascade (72,74). This is in itself sufficient to enable the extended survival of a pig-to-baboon cardiac xenograft (72); however, CVF treatment generates large amounts of the vasoactive and chemotactic C3a and C5a complement fragments and is associated with unacceptable morbidity (94). The complement components are continually synthesized and as C3 (largely from the liver) returns to normal levels, so can the capability of rejection, or at least of complement-mediated graft damage. Fortunately, the sensitivity of a graft to complement and antibody reduces with time after engraftment, a phenomenon called *accommodation* (see below).

Complement Depletion or Inhibition by Antibodies Antibodies directed to the C5 and C8 complement components have recently been tested with the prospect of developing a therapeutic reagent. The effect of the antibodies depends on which step in the complement cascade is targeted. Inhibition of MAC formation will limit cell lysis but will not limit the generation of chemotactic C3a and C5a peptides, and whether such a treatment is useful will depend on what mechanisms of rejection are critical to graft function and survival. Targeting C5 would appear to have strategic advantages. A likely limitation to their use is that antibody treatments in patients, except with "humanized" reagents, cannot be used repetitively because of the recipient's immune response to the foreign antibody (see also Chapter 13).

Complement Regulation by RCA Proteins The apparent, but not absolute, "homologous restriction" of some complement regulators to be species-matched to their complement components, in particular DAF (95) and CD59 (90), may be more than the failure to interact appropriately or efficiently with C3 and MAC fragments, respectively (93). Under certain circumstances, they may act as a focus for complement deposition and activation at the cell surface and thus cause increased sensitivity to complement. Recent data in our laboratory have suggested that MCP, when expressed on mouse cells at low to medium concentrations or introduced in soluble form for fluid-phase regulation, may sometimes increase cell sensitivity to rat or rabbit complement, presumably because of characteristics of the interaction with nonhomologous C3b or factor I. At higher MCP concentrations, these limitations with various complement sources have not been observed (96).

The immediate confrontation between graft cells and recipient blood in a vascularized tissue transplant poses the initial problem of xenotransplantation: any graft presents "damaged surfaces" to the recipient's blood because of the inevitable period of anoxia and ischemia during organ preparation. In particular, the graft's endothelial cells (EC), the immediate point of contact with the recipient, will have already responded to these insults and will have altered their shape and surface molecule composition, characteristics of "type I EC activation" (97) (see below). Therefore, complement deposition will occur immediately on reperfusion of the graft. For isografts and allografts, this is not recognized as a problem, probably because of the endogenous array of the protective molecules that regulate complement activation, in particular CR1, MCP, DAF, and CD59, and the lack of significant titers of reactive antibodies. This efficient function of endogenous RCA proteins to control the tick-over of C3 activation was imaginatively demonstrated by perfusion in vivo of rat kidneys with an antibody that blocked the function of rat 512Ag (rat Crry/p65), a homologue of DAF and MCP. C3 deposition and damage to autologous renal tubulointerstitial tissues occurred over the seven-day observation period (98).

For a xenograft, apart from the affected endothelial cells, there are additional stimuli for complement activation, principally the high density of surface carbohydrate moieties that are antigens for natural antibodies. Thus, whether it is the classic pathway and/or the alternative pathway of activation that initiates the complement cascade, a large quantity of complement can be deposited on each cell.

Structure and Function of Complement Regulators

Four of the complement-regulating proteins, whose characteristics are described in this section, are being tested as potential therapeutic molecules in xenotransplantation (see Table 40.6). Others, including C1INH, factor H, C4bp, and CR2, have not been widely tested as yet.

CR1 (CD35) The most effective complement regulator in molar terms may be complement receptor type 1 (CR1), a polymorphic cell surface protein of 190 to 290 kd that has two sites for binding C3b and one for C4b, and possesses multiple functions of complement regulation: decay acceleration of the C3 and C5 convertases, cofactor activity in factor I–mediated proteolysis of C3b and C4b through two stages of degradation, and immune complex clearance including enhanced phagocytosis (see Fig. 40.4) (99). CR1 has a restricted tissue distribution in humans, being found mainly on granulocytes, neutrophils, erythrocytes, monocytes, follicular dendritic cells, and most B and some T lymphocytes, and because of its long, rigid molecular structure predominantly regulates complement fragments on adjacent membranes (extrinsic activity) (89). The 290-kd isoform is a linear array of 30 disulphide-bonded tandem modules of 60 to 65 amino acids, referred to as short consensus repeats (SCR), which mediate the complement binding and regulatory functions. The SCR modules are also characteristic of several related regulatory proteins, including CR1, CR2, DAF, MCP, C4bp, and factor H (89), and nuclear magnetic resonance (NMR) studies have generated a putative 3-D structure (100).

MCP (CD46) MCP is the most widespread complement regulator (although it is not found on erythrocytes) and functions as a cofactor for the serum protease, factor I, to cleave C3b to C3bi and C3f. (Only CR1, with factor I, can mediate fragmentation of C3bi to C3d,g and C3c.) It is a highly efficient regulator of the alternative complement pathway (101–103) but also protects cells efficiently against classic pathway–mediated lysis (96,102,103). Human cells normally express four isoforms of MCP, glycoproteins of approximately 56 kd (C1 and C2 isoforms) and approximately 66 kd (BC1 and BC2 isoforms) that are generated by alternative splicing of a 14-exon transcript (92,104). Other isoforms are detectable, especially in tumor cells (105,106), which poses the question of which to choose in the context of transgenic organ donors. All isoforms have in common four SCR modules and differ in either the extracellular membrane-proximal glycosylated STP domains or in the cytoplasmic C-terminus.

Transfected cells expressing the common and another isoform have been compared for their resistance to complement-mediated lysis (96,107,108) and measles virus infection (109,110) (MCP is the measles virus receptor (111,112)); however, no distinct isoform-specific characteristics have been observed, and all isoforms appear to function equally. There is considerable diversity of total MCP protein expression between human tissues, with low to moderate densities found on lymphocytes, myocardium, hepatocytes, brain cells, and most interstitial cells, moderate quantities on endothelia, and very high densities found on syncytial trophoblasts of the placenta and on ductular cells in the salivary gland and kidney. There are also patterns to the expression of the isoforms identified by polymerase chain reaction (PCR) and Southern blot analyses, with preferences for BC2 in the kidney and C2 in the brain. However, since there are mendelian patterns of inherited isoform bias (best characterized in peripheral blood lymphocytes) observed as predominantly BC1 and BC2, predominantly C1 and C2, or having similar proportions of each (92), there is no functional explanation yet for the variation. It may be merely tissue-specific differences in the cells' splicing machinery, or there may be additional subtleties to MCP function yet to be identified.

DAF (CD55) The most widely tested cell-surface regulator in xenograft studies, DAF constructs have proven to be more amenable than MCP to expression as transgenes (113–119). DAF is an approximately 70-kd protein with a phospholipid [glycosyl-phosphatidylinositol (GPI)] plasma membrane attachment, is widely distributed on human cells, and is structurally very similar to MCP, having four SCR modules and a heavily O-glycosylated "STP" domain. However, it differs entirely in function, possessing decay acceleration activity for the classic (mainly) and alternative path C3 convertases, in particular inhibiting the formation of C4b2a and of C3bBb by competing with C2a and factor B, respectively, for binding to C4b or C3b, and enhancing the dissociation of C2a or Bb from C4b or C3b, respectively (see Table 40.6) (88,120).

CD59 Another cell-surface complement regulator that has been very extensively studied in xenotransplantation is CD59 (protectin, MIRL, MACIF, HRF20), an approximately 20-kd GPI-anchored protein that is widely expressed (121) and, at least in vitro, has been found to have a multitude of functions involving complement and coagulation regulation and T-cell signaling (90,91). CD59 inhibits cell lysis by competitively interfering with C9 incorporation into the C5b-C8 complement complex and thus blocking polymerization of the terminal MAC. It had originally been described as being homologously restricted to the regulation of human complement. However, more careful analyses of the molecular interactions have demonstrated that this was a misinterpretation (93). Although it acts at the final step of the complement cascade, it very effectively protects cells against lysis (120,122), and recent data confirm its ability to delay xenograft rejection.

Coagulation Pathways and Endothelial Cell Activation

Coagulation can be activated by: 1) an extrinsic pathway such as tissue damage, or 2) the intrinsic pathway, where clotting factors directly recognize foreign surfaces. In xenograft HAR, intravascular coagulation can be induced by several factors, including activation of the complement cascade, platelet adhesion and activation, tissue damage, and activation of endothelial cells. Bacterial toxins can directly activate the extrinsic pathway and give rise to the Shwartzman reaction and it has been suggested that the HAR seen in the rabbit-to-suckling pig model, which occurs in the complete absence of antibody, is due to the activation of the coagulation pathway rather than the alternative pathway of complement. Whether such mechanisms could also occur in pig-to-primate grafts is not known, although foreign carbohydrates can activate the coagulation pathway, which may be relevant in the pig-to-primate xenograft setting. Endothelial cell activation is also a part of the HAR process but is considered in detail below with DXR.

DELAYED XENOGRAFT REJECTION, ACCOMMODATION, AND MOLECULAR INCOMPATIBILITY

As described above, the subdivision of graft rejection into categories has been according to both the mediators and the time course of the rejection process, each defining particular roles for thrombosis, antibody, complement, T lymphocytes, granulocytes, and macrophages. Recently, the studies of antixenograft reactions occurring in the absence of hyperacute rejection have led Bach's group to introduce a new category: delayed acute xenograft rejection or discordant xenograft rejection (DXR). They have attempted to understand the factors involved in acute rejection occurring in the absence of antibody or complement activity, before T lymphocyte responses become apparent, and have suggested that endothelial cells are primarily responsible (97,123) and cause disordered thromboregulation.

In the absence of significant antibody titers, guinea pig hearts in rats are rejected hyperacutely in less than 10 minutes, presumably by the alternative activation pathway of complement because after complement depletion graft function can be extended to approximately 80 hours (123). In the absence of complement, however, leukocyte infiltration (particularly by macrophages and NK cells) was significant within four hours, IFN-γ was expressed by 48 hours, and tissue factor (TF), TNFα, and cytokines (including IL-1, IL-2, and IL-7) were detected. These mediators were thought to be involved in the development of fibrin deposits and platelet plugs in the rejected heart. Similar events are thought to occur in pig heart grafts in antibody-depleted monkeys (124).

Endothelial cells are the primary barrier between a vascularized graft and the host, and their susceptibility to activation by anoxia and temperature changes certainly presents difficulties in transplantation. Activated endothelial cells induce both thrombosis, resulting in coagulation and platelet aggregation, and inflammation. Therefore, it is essential that the molecular events of the activation process(es) are understood. They are likely to be the necessary targets of preoperative and postoperative treatments in the future. The immediate effects of endothelial activation occur without protein synthesis and are denoted *type I activation*: cell retraction allowing interstitial hemorrhage, P-selectin expression, loss of thrombomodulin, loss of tissue factor pathway inhibitor (TFPI), loss of heparan sulphate, or expression of von Willebrand factor (vWF) (Fig. 40.6) (97). E-selectin upregulation in graft endothelium has been suggested to be a predictor of activation and is detectable within four hours.

Type II endothelial activation is associated with a progressive induction of endothelial genes after several hours and over a period of days with novel protein synthesis of the adhesion molecules E-selectin, P-selectin, ICAM-1, and VCAM-1, and cytokines IL-1, IL-6, IL-8, MCP-1, TF, and so forth (97) (see Fig. 40.6). The cells are in a procoagulant state. Cellular infiltration is observed, with particular attention now being paid to NK cells with the implication that an antibody-dependent (Fc-receptor–mediated) direct cytolytic response (ADCC) may be occurring. The transcription factor NK-κB is essential for the genes that are upregulated during type II EC activation, therefore there is currently much interest in targeting NF-κB, for example, by the natural inhibitor IκB, to prevent activation or switch off the endothelial cells (125,126). This strategy requires imaginative targeting, as it would seem necessary to affect only particular EC (in the graft) and only for the limited time period necessary to enable the graft to "recover" and heal-

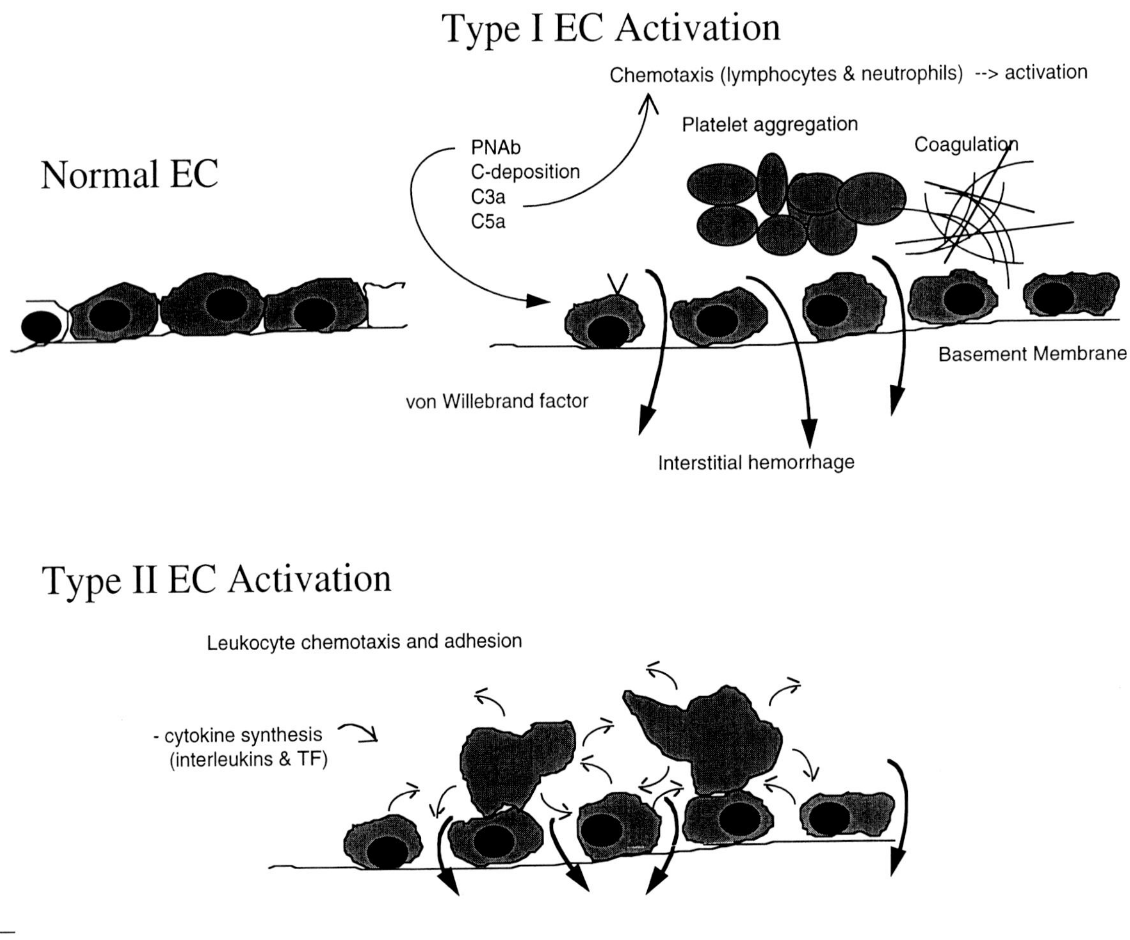

FIGURE 40.6. *Endothelial cell activation: type I and type II processes. Type I activation occurs without protein synthesis, driven by antibody and complement deposition on EC and the chemotactic and anaphylactic factors C3a and C5a. Platelet aggregation, coagulation, and interstitial hemorrhage are key features. As EC synthesize, express novel adhesion molecules and cytokines, and react to cytokines from infiltrating leukocytes, a procoagulant state is maintained and macrophages and NK cells adhere and are activated (123).*

in. Similarly, enhancing or preventing downregulation of thrombomodulin on the graft endothelium is expected to be beneficial after graft perfusion but is unlikely to be appropriate as a permanent alteration in the graft. Bach and colleagues are careful to point out that the initiation of any one component of DXR may lead to recruitment of other components; for example, platelet activation with vWF release can lead to adhesion and endothelial activation. Therefore, controlling one aspect may have little effect on the outcome of graft rejection.

Pig-to-primate cardiac transplantation models have presented conflicting evidence. CVF and immunosuppressive treatment of baboons prior to receiving heterotopic pig heart grafts prevented hyperacute rejection, and vascular changes were seen when rejection occurred—clear evidence of DXR—with unexpected T-lymphocyte involvement (127). In contrast, the DAF-transgenic pig hearts transplanted to monkeys were reported to have no signs of vascular rejection up to nine weeks after grafting, apparently due to the function of DAF on vascular endothelium. However, some of the normal pig hearts were not rejected as promptly as expected, and thus the mechanisms of rejection and role of DAF were not entirely clear, and DXR was not identified.

Accommodation

The unexpected survival of an incompatible graft under particular conditions has been noted for decades and termed either *adaptation* (128,129) or, more recently, *accommodation* (130,131). When systemic decomplementation or complement inhibition are combined with antibody depletion, pig heart xenografts into baboons are not hyperacutely rejected (132), neither are guinea pig heart xenografts into rats (123). Although the natural antibodies and complement reappear within a few days, and significant quantities of antibody (but not complement components) are deposited in the graft, the expected rejection does not necessarily occur immediately. In addition, in some human recipients of ABO-mismatched kidney allografts and a small number of patients with anti-HLA class I antibodies that were transplanted after plasmapheresis to temporarily deplete the antibodies, the grafts survived, the antibody returned, and yet the grafts appeared either to no longer bind the antibody (although by other measures they expressed the antigens) or to be unaffected by the bound antibody (130,133–135).

In some ways, this phenomenon resonates of immune tolerance, where a foreign graft can exist in the presence of a potentially reactive immune response; however, since a T-cell response is subsequently thought to be unaffected, it is likely to be entirely different. Necessary to this unusual state is the initial removal of antibody while the graft tissue is recovering from the major trauma of transplantation. If this state of coexistence of antibodies and antigen could be achieved consistently, it would simplify the strategies and procedures for undertaking xenografting.

Molecular Incompatibility

The concept of molecular incompatibility stems from the observation that certain molecules do not interact with the appropriate ligand or receptor from another species; that is, their interaction is "species specific." For example, a number of cytokines such as IL-1β and IFN-γ do not function across species. Molecular incompatibilities could clearly contribute to the hyperacute rejection of xenografts. The "partial dysfunction" of molecular interactions present more of a problem. For example, pig ECs produce a tissue factor inhibitor that regulates human TF-VIIa complex but is ineffective against human factor-Xa (136), and thus thromboregulation may be disturbed, at least within the microenvironments around the engrafted (pig) cells that synthesize the inhibitor. A different problem may arise from the interaction of vWF with the gpIb platelet receptor, which in humans requires shear stress to induce platelet aggregation. It has been observed that pig vWF can interact with human platelet gpIb receptor but aggregation occurs in the absence of shear stress (137). A greater incompatibility issue may arise for adhesion molecules, where cell recirculation, endothelial binding and release, or extravasation may function partially as normal and yet not entirely the same. Such effects would not necessarily be identified from in vitro models or short term survival studies, but they may contribute to chronic changes in a xenograft.

The evolutionary divergence between species is likely to include differences that will only be detected with the long-term function of a xenograft. It is likely that pig heart or kidney function in humans will be satisfactory; however, there is concern about liver function with the massive production of foreign proteins. At the cellular level, some compatibilities and incompatibilities have been tested, although the list is frighteningly short in comparison with the imagined total molecular load. It is already apparent that, for some proteins, partial function rather than total dysfunction occurs. The outcome may be innocuous (especially if other molecules can compensate) or a major problem. For example, of the cytokines, IL-2 functions perfectly across some species (the higher mammals; but mouse IL-2 will not stimulate human T cells), whereas human IL-1β and human IFN-γ do not act on pig ECs (138). Human IL-4 may also be less effective on pig cells.

CELL-MEDIATED XENOGRAFT REJECTION

As the sections above have indicated, the principal distinguishing feature of xenograft compared with allograft rejection lies in the humoral mechanisms of xenograft destruction. Because these mechanisms are so powerful and so rapid, it has been difficult to prolong xenograft survival long enough to examine the cell-mediated mechanisms that might subsequently play a role. As a result, our understanding of cellular xenograft rejection is poorly developed, allowing investigators to hold widely divergent views on its importance (139). Some investigators confidently predict that cellular immunity to xenografts is weaker, perhaps even trivial, when compared to allograft rejection, while others believe cellular immunity poses yet another severe immunologic barrier to successful xenotransplantation, and that it may include components that do not even participate in allograft rejection (140). This section reviews the data that are available on cell-mediated xenograft rejection, emphasizing especially the questions remaining to be answered.

Models for Studying Cell-Mediated Xenograft Rejection

Skin Grafts

Studies of T-cell–deficient "nude" mice have shown that these mutant animals can maintain healthy allogeneic and xenogeneic skin grafts without further immunosuppression (Fig. 40.7 and Plate 43) (141). Thus, it is clear that T cells can play a role in xenograft rejection and that they are an essential component for skin graft rejection by mice. A special feature of skin grafts is that their early survival does not depend on immediate revascularization, and only gradually, during the second week after transplantation, are anastomoses formed between donor and recipient blood vessels. This feature protects the donor endothelium from the immediate attack by preformed recipient antibodies, which is essential for hyperacute rejection. While studies have shown that once these vascular connections have been formed antidonor antibodies can cause rapid skin graft destruction, these studies have also indicated that large boluses of antibody are required for injury to occur (48). At least in rodents, either the level of endogenous, preformed antibodies is too low or their contact with donor endothelium too gradual for humoral mechanisms alone to cause xenogeneic skin graft rejection.

While the special feature of skin grafts allows their use for investigating cell-mediated rejection, the same feature may limit the conclusions that can be drawn from these studies. The mechanisms of skin graft rejection are probably not identical to those involved in the rejection of primarily vascularized organs, as suggested by the far greater difficulty in prolonging skin graft compared to heart or kidney graft survival in allogeneic combinations. On the other hand, the lack of endothelial exposure, which protects skin grafts from hyperacute rejection, may also protect them from potential cell-mediated responses directed at xenogeneic endothelium. Furthermore, the absence of hyperacute rejection for skin grafts does not mean that humoral mechanisms do not subsequently contribute to the rejection process. Thus, studies of xenogeneic skin graft rejection cannot be used as a perfect model of the cell-mediated mechanisms that are involved for more clinically relevant tissues.

Cellular Transplants

Transplants of xenogeneic cells, such as hepatocytes, do not include donor endothelium and are thus not subject to the ordinary processes of hyperacute rejection. However, many types of cells besides endothelial cells express the antigens that bind natural antibodies and it is not yet clear whether this binding causes destruction of xenogeneic cellular transplants (142). There is evidence that preformed antibodies can play a role in preventing xenogeneic bone marrow engraftment, although that effect can be overcome by sufficiently large doses of donor cells (143). Pancreatic islets, which are often thought of as cellular transplants, represent clusters of cells supplied by their own microvasculature including donor endothelium. The engraftment of islets is thus very similar to that of skin grafts in the time it takes to form anastomoses between donor and recipient vessels (144). The scant information available suggests that islets, like skin grafts, are most susceptible to humoral rejection after the first week (145,146), despite the finding in vitro that natural antibodies are toxic to xenogeneic islets. With the informa-

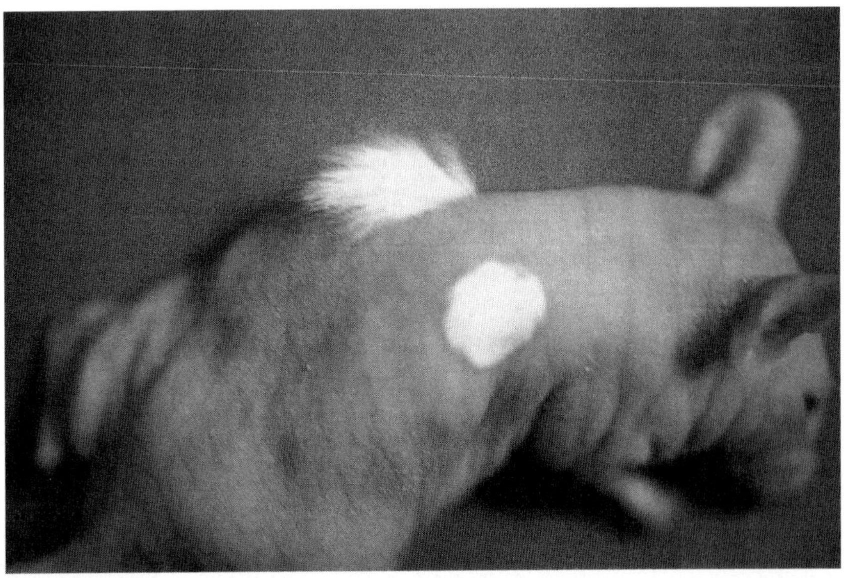

FIGURE 40.7. *Nude mouse with long-surviving allogeneic mouse and xenogeneic monkey skin grafts.*

tion currently available, it is not yet clear whether humoral mechanisms play a role in the rejection of xenogeneic cellular transplants and, therefore, to what extent the rejection of these transplants can be used to examine the cell-mediated response to xenografts.

Xenografts to Mutant Mice

The availability of mouse strains with natural or genetically engineered mutations has made it possible to test xenograft rejection by mice in the absence of selected components of the immune system. For example, B-cell–deficient mice rapidly reject xenogeneic skin grafts, demonstrating again that cell-mediated immunity is capable of causing xenograft rejection (147). Unfortunately, it is difficult to perform primarily vascularized organ transplants in mice from any but the most closely related species. Thus, even though such mutant recipient mice offer a way to examine component parts of the immune system, they cannot fully address the nature of cell-mediated rejection of primarily vascularized organs. In addition, the cell-mediated immunity of mice in response to pig tissues is not identical to the human antipig response (see below).

Concordant Species Combinations

Another approach to the investigation of cellular xenograft rejection has been to concentrate on concordant species combinations that, by definition, do not provoke hyperacute rejection (148). Many animal studies of this kind have been conducted, and most attempts at xenografting in human recipients have involved concordant donors. A striking feature of concordant xenografting, however, is the rapidity of the antibody response that occurs after transplantation and causes rapid graft destruction (40,41). Thus, humoral mechanisms can dominate even concordant xenograft rejection, and control of this humoral component has required the addition of immunosuppressive agents, such as methotrexate or cyclophosphamide, aimed at B-cell suppression. Therefore, transplantation in concordant species combinations is not a good experimental technique to analyze pure cell-mediated rejection mechanisms. Furthermore, the cell-mediated responses that are involved in concordant species combinations may not reflect the cell-mediated responses to more distantly related donors. Organs from transgenic pigs expressing complement regulatory proteins have survived in primate recipients for many weeks, but it is not yet clear whether the immune response in these modified discordant cases involves primarily T cells or a noncomplement-dependent humoral mechanism (38,149).

It is unfortunately true that none of the available models adequately isolates the clinically relevant, cell-mediated immune response of primates to primarily vascularized discordant xenografts. Either the humoral rejection of the graft obscures the cellular response of interest or the modifications of the recipient or of the donor tissue to avoid this response may alter the character of cellular rejection in significant ways. Although the conclusion has emerged that T cells can participate in xenograft rejection, it remains unknown whether this response is similar in strength and character to the allogeneic response. Under these circumstances, a great deal of the investigation of cell-mediated xenograft immunity has been performed in vitro, where cell-mediated immune responses can be isolated. This approach, however, is dangerous since many clear-cut conclusions from in vitro studies are not relevant to the in vivo mechanisms of graft destruction.

In Vitro Assays of Cell-Mediated Xenogeneic Responses

Cell-mediated xenogeneic immunity has been studied in vitro using the mixed lymphocyte reaction (MLR), measuring the proliferation of T cells stimulated by foreign cells, and the cell-mediated lympholysis (CML) assay, measuring the lysis of foreign cells by responding T cells. The striking feature of both assays in allogeneic combinations is the extraordinary strength of the T-cell response whenever there are differences in the major histocompatibility (MHC) antigens between the responder and stimulator populations. Not only can naive T cells respond to allogeneic stimulation in vitro without prior in vivo priming (a nearly unique feature of alloreactivity), but in addition, the precursor frequency of T cells responding to allogeneic MHC antigens is roughly 100-fold higher than the frequency of T cells that can respond to ordinary environmental pathogens (150).

The explanation for the extraordinary strength of alloreactivity in vitro is thought to involve two major components (Fig. 40.8). First, responder T cells, which have been selected in the thymus for their capacity to recognize peptides of foreign antigens presented by self MHC molecules, are able to recognize intact allogeneic MHC antigens "directly." This unusual feature of allogeneic MHC antigens occurs because of the similarity between allogeneic and self MHC molecules such that allogeneic MHC antigens appear to T-cell receptors like self MHC molecules presenting a foreign peptide (see Chapter 2). Second, the direct recognition of allogeneic MHC antigens gives rise to a high precursor frequency of responding T cells because of the high frequency of novel determinants generated by allo-MHC antigens. Whereas the peptides of environmental pathogens are presented by only a small fraction of the self MHC molecules on the responder's antigen presenting cells (APCs), all of the MHC antigens on allogeneic APCs are foreign to responding T cells (with numerous novel determinants produced by the endogenous peptides of the donor) (150).

The striking paradox stemming from these explanations for the strength of cell-mediated alloreactivity is that while the extreme polymorphism of MHC molecules within a species makes it unusual to find unrelated donors and recipients who are matched for their MHC antigens, and while MHC antigen disparities are primarily responsible for the

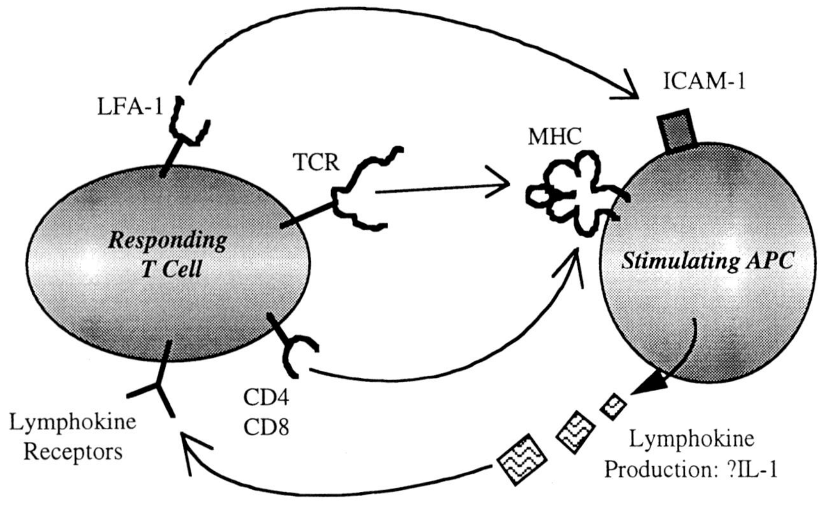

FIGURE 40.8. *Types of molecular interactions between T cells and APCs involved in T-cell activation. In addition to the interaction of T-cell receptors with MHC antigens and the peptides presented by these molecules, several other molecular interactions are involved in T-cell activation. The CD4 or CD8 molecules interact with monomorphic determinants on MHC class II and class I molecules, respectively. Lymphokines, produced by the stimulating cell, interact with lymphokine receptors of T cells. Several costimulatory and adhesion molecules also participate in T-cell activation. This diagram depicts only the interaction between ICAM-1 and LFA-1, but numerous other examples exist and are important in T-cell activation.*

strength of the T-cell response, it is the similarity of self and allogeneic MHC molecules that makes the in vitro immune response so strong. In addition, activation of T cells by allogeneic APCs also requires that the accessory molecules involved in T-cell stimulation (such as CD4 and CD8, the adhesion molecules, and the costimulatory molecules) can function effectively between different individuals of the same species. Therefore, direct T-cell activation by allogeneic MHC antigens expressed on allogeneic APCs is strong because of both the similarity within the species of the molecules involved in immune responses and the polymorphic differences in the MHC.

Based on this understanding of alloreactivity, many investigators have considered whether the cell-mediated response to xenogeneic stimulating cells is likely to be stronger, weaker, or the same as the allogeneic response. Since the strength of alloreactivity depends on the similarity of the molecular components of the immune system between members of the same species, cell-mediated xenoreactivity could be weaker if some of the molecular interactions required for T-cell activation do not function when donors and recipients come from different species. To examine this question, numerous MLR and CML experiments have been performed in different species combinations (151–154). The outcomes have varied, depending on the species combination involved, and the results can be grouped into one of the following three patterns.

1. Species combinations in which in vitro T cell responses are strong or that include unusual cell-mediated responses to xenogeneic antigens. The best example of this type of response is the clinically relevant, human antipig combination that shows a powerful direct response by human T cells but that also includes a response by NK cells not detected in allogeneic combinations (155).
2. Species combinations with T-cell responses that are similar to allogeneic reactions. Many concordant combinations fall into this category, including the human response to monkey stimulating cells (156).
3. Species combinations with strikingly weak direct recognition of xenogeneic antigens. In some species combinations it is difficult to detect any direct stimulation of T cells by discordant xenogeneic stimulating cells in either MLR or CML assays. Mouse responses to rabbit, pig, monkey, and human stimulators are examples of these combinations (157).

Human Antipig Cellular Immunity in Vitro

Because of its obvious clinical relevance, particular attention has been given to the human antipig cellular reaction in vitro. The magnitude and kinetics of cellular reactivity in both MLR and CML assays in this combination are similar to or stronger than human allogeneic reactions (158–164). The primary difference, however, is that when unseparated lymphocytes are used as responders, the reactivity is not inhibited by anti-T-cell reagents. This is because a substantial portion of the lymphocyte reaction is mediated by $CD16^{+}$ $CD56^{+}$ NK cells (138,155). This xenogeneic reactivity can often be detected when unprimed, unstimulated lymphocytes are used in lytic assays, especially if human antipig antibodies are present in the culture. Thus, some of this response is probably mediated by an ADCC mechanism (165). Even in the absence of antibodies, however, NK cells develop in vitro that lyse pig targets without apparent specificity for allelic MHC antigenic differences and the response is enhanced by IL-2 in the culture medium.

If NK cells are rigorously depleted from human lymphocyte responders, it is then possible to detect a direct T-cell response to pig stimulating cells that is very similar to an allogeneic T-cell response (155). Proliferation is largely by $CD4^{+}$ cells, stimulated by pig MHC class II antigens, and the cytotoxic T cells that develop after four to five days of in vitro stimulation are generally $CD8^{+}$ MHC class I–specific cytotoxic T lymphocytes (CTLs) that show allelic specificity for the xenogeneic MHC antigens of their targets (166).

Molecular Incompatibilities Responsible for Weaker Direct T-Cell Activation

Experiments have also been performed in species combinations with weak direct T-cell activation to determine which molecular incompatibilities are responsible for this "defect." As diagrammed in Figure 40.9, there are numerous possibilities. These possibilities have been examined by using genetically engineered APCs that are partly allogeneic and partly xenogeneic to correct some, but not all, of the potential defects responsible for weak T-cell activation (161,167–169). For example, mouse T cells have been stimulated by mouse APCs that express xenogeneic MHC antigens. This corrects potential defects of the cell surface accessory molecules, but not those of the interactions of CD4 or CD8 or of T-cell receptors with xenogeneic MHC

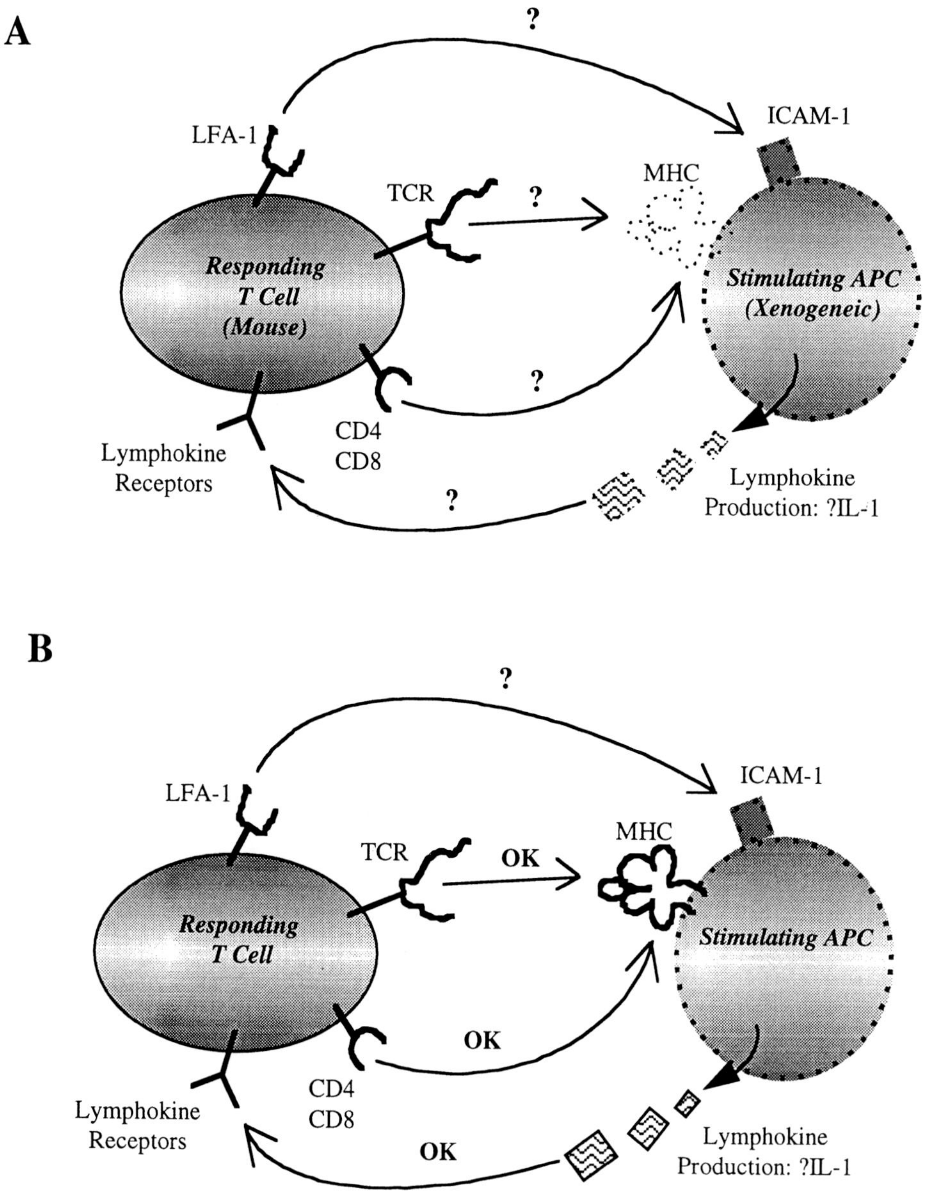

FIGURE 40.9. *Some of the molecular interactions required for T-cell activation may not function well when T cells and APCs come from different species.* ***A.*** *The xenogeneic APC is depicted in this diagram by dashed instead of solid lines. Failure of any of the molecular interactions between T cells and APCs might be responsible for diminished T-cell activation across species barriers.* ***B.*** *To determine which molecular interactions are defective in a particular combination, experiments can be performed using the techniques of molecular biology to create APCs that are partly xenogeneic and partly allogeneic. In the example depicted here, the APC remains xenogeneic but it expresses an allogeneic MHC molecule and stimulation can be tested in the presence of exogenous lymphokines derived from the same species as the responding T cell. Thus, this experiment will test whether the cell surface costimulatory and adhesion molecules are functional in this species combination.*

antigens. Alternatively, mouse T cells have been stimulated with human APCs that express allogeneic mouse MHC antigens. This corrects the opposite set of molecular interactions. With the molecular technology available today, numerous manipulations of APCs can be achieved to examine different combinations of potential defects.

The outcome of these types of studies have led to two general conclusions (151,170–173): 1) there are numerous "defects" in the molecular interactions that are responsible for weak T-cell activation, but the particular defects that exist depend on the species combination being studied; 2) the one potential defect that does *not* seem to be responsible is the interaction between T-cell receptors and the polymorphic regions of xenogeneic MHC antigens. Thus, it appears that xenogeneic MHC antigens with peptides in their cleft appear to T-cell receptors to be similar to self MHC molecules, as do allogeneic MHC antigens. These findings are consistent with studies of the amino acid sequence of the hypervariable regions of MHC molecules from different species, which have shown that there is as much homology in these regions between MHC molecules from different species as between molecules from different members of the same species (174).

Given the different outcomes in different species, it would be impossible to characterize the exact molecular interactions that are "defective" in every species combination. The important issue is which interactions are intact and which are defective in the clinically relevant combinations involving human responders. Although the human direct cell-mediated responses both to concordant primate and to discordant pig stimulating cells are intact, this does not prove that all of the molecular interactions involved in T-cell activation function normally in these species combinations. Therefore, recent experimental work has examined these molecular interactions individually, usually by attempting to inhibit T-cell responses in vitro by blocking particular accessory molecules (151,175–177). For example, the ability to prevent human T-cell lysis of pig cells by anti-CD8 antibody implies that the human CD8 interaction with its monomorphic binding site on pig class I MHC molecules is probably intact. Table 40.7 lists some of the molecular interactions of the human–pig combination that have been tested recently. This list is growing rapidly and it is likely to be modified substantially in coming years.

Table 40.7. Human T Cell-to-Pig Stimulating Cell Molecular Interactions That Have Been Tested

Human TCR	Pig SLA MHC class II	Intact
Human TCR	Pig SLA MHC class I	Intact
Human CD4	Pig SLA class II	May be less efficient than allo
Human CD8	Pig SLA class I	Intact
Human T cells	Pig B7	Intact [but not all individual molecules (e.g., B7.1, B7.2) have been tested]
Human LFA-1	Pig ICAM-1	Intact
Human CD2	Pig LFA-3	Intact (but unusual interactions may occur)

The search for molecular incompatibilities in the human antipig combination is based on the possibility that such incompatibilities might offer unique opportunities for immunosuppression in xenogeneic combinations. Since there appears to be significant overlap in the function of many of the accessory molecules involved in T-cell activation, therapies designed to inhibit only one of these interactions are often ineffective in allogeneic combinations. If there are molecular incompatibilities between human and pig cells that are compensated by other accessory molecules, then targeted therapy directed at these compensating molecular interactions might be more effective in xenogeneic than in allogeneic combinations.

Molecular Incompatibilities May Be Responsible for Stronger Cell-Mediated Xenogeneic Immunity

The idea that molecular incompatibilities between species are important in generating both the strength of hyperacute rejection and the weakness of in vitro T-cell responses in some species combinations has been well developed over the past 10 years. Only recently, however, has this concept been invoked to explain why cell-mediated immunity might be stronger in vitro in other species combinations (147). For example, molecular incompatibilities may be responsible for the ability of human NK cells to lyse pig but not allogeneic targets. Although NK cell activation remains poorly understood, it appears that these cells have two general types of receptors: 1) those that stimulate activation by recognition of carbohydrate determinants, and 2) those that inhibit activation by recognition of MHC class I molecules. Thus, it is possible (although not yet demonstrated) that human NK activation by pig cells is stimulated by unusual foreign carbohydrate determinants of the xenogeneic cells, and equally possible (but also not yet demonstrated) that human NK cells are activated because their inhibiting receptors fail to recognize pig MHC class I molecules.

Another example of molecular incompatibilities leading to stronger cell-mediated responses may involve the regulatory molecules of inflammation. For example, pig tissue factor pathway inhibitor does not inhibit human factor Xa (178–181). Thus, the inflammatory and procoagulant responses associated with even a routine transplant procedure may not be adequately controlled in this xenogeneic combination and may exacerbate the specific immunologic responses.

Finally, there is an emerging understanding in immunology that T-cell immunity may involve downregulating as well as upregulating signals, perhaps provided by molecular interactions between CTLA4 and B7.2 or between Fas and Fas ligand (160,182,183). While there is no clear example where failure of one of these interactions between species has been shown to be responsible for unusually strong T-cell responses, the search for such incompatibilities has now begun.

The Indirect Response to Xenoantigens in Vitro

The striking feature of allogeneic T cell responses in vitro is the ability to measure a response even without in vivo priming, a feature that depends fundamentally on the ability of T cells to recognize disparate MHC antigens "directly" (i.e., without the need to process peptides of these antigens for presentation by self MHC molecules). Nonetheless, peptides of foreign antigens of a donor graft (both from MHC and non-MHC proteins) can also stimulate recipient T cells by the more ordinary mechanisms of an immune response. This response has been called *indirect* T-cell activation, distinguishing it from the unusual but powerful activation of T cells by direct recognition of foreign MHC antigens (see Chapter 2). This terminology, however, fails to convey the important point that "indirect" T cell stimulation is the physiologic mechanism by which T cells respond to environmental pathogens (150). Because of their low precursor frequency, T cells stimulated by peptides of foreign antigens presented by self MHC molecules cannot usually be detected in primary in vitro cultures and can only be measured when the recipient has been previously immunized to these antigens in vivo. It would be expected, therefore, that after xenograft rejection, a secondary in vitro response to peptides of xenogeneic antigens (the indirect, but physiologic immune response) would be easily measured no matter what the species combination.

This expectation has been confirmed in all species combinations tested. Figure 40.10 shows an example of this

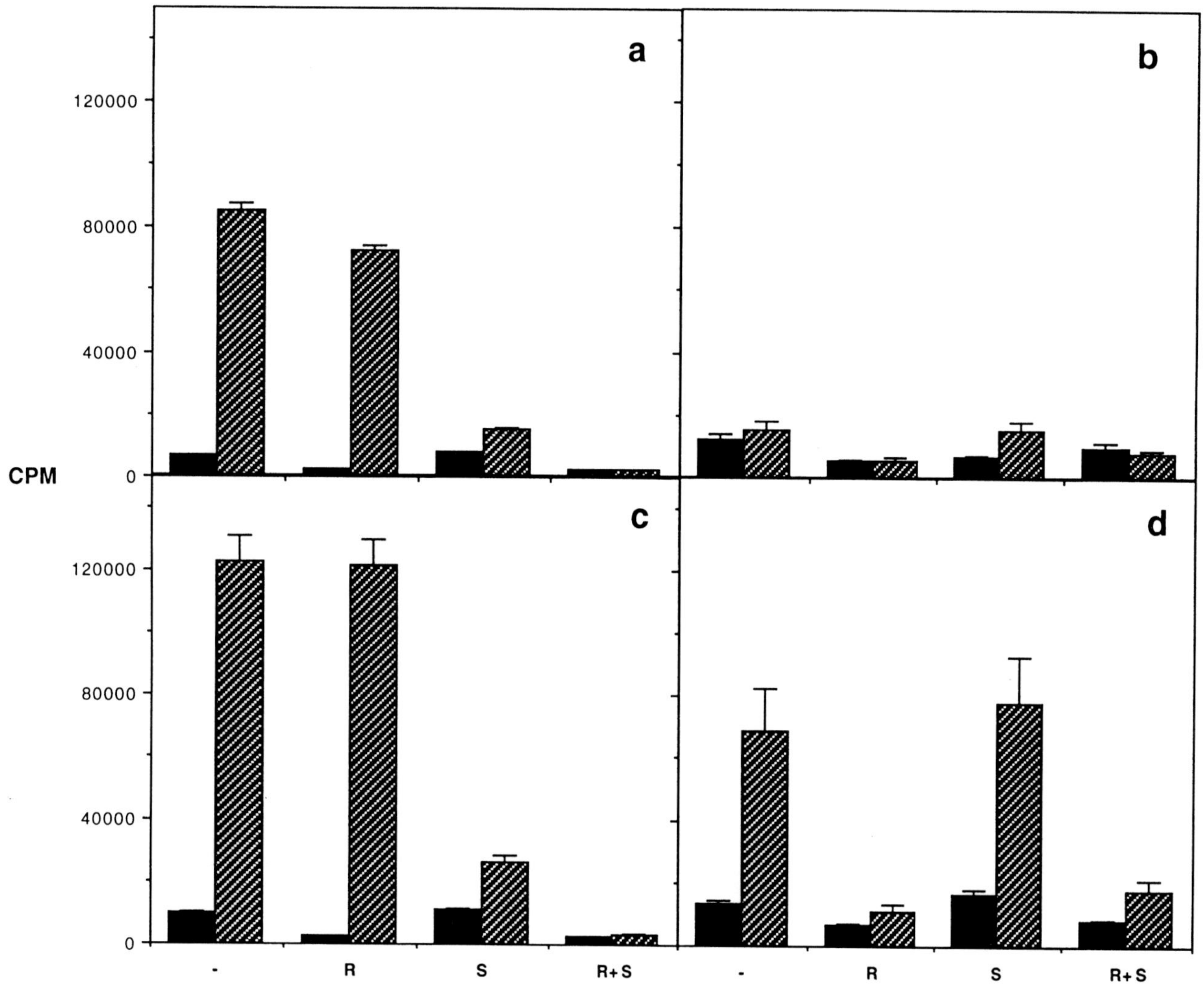

FIGURE 40.10. *Mixed lymphocyte responses of primed and unprimed mouse T cells with allogeneic and xenogeneic stimulators. In each panel, the APCs were depleted from either the responding T-cell population (R) the stimulating cell population (S) or both populations (R + S) together. The results in panel **a** show the strong in vitro response of unprimed mouse T cells to allogeneic stimulating cells when the stimulating antigens are expressed on the stimulator APCs. The results in panel **b** show the weak in vitro response of unprimed mouse T cells when stimulated with monkey (xeno) stimulating cells. However, the results in panels **c** and **d** show that after rejection of allo- or monkey skin grafts, respectively, mouse T cells have been sensitized to monkey antigens presented by mouse APCs. Filled columns represent antiself response, and hatched columns the antiallo or antixeno response, as CPM of ^{3}H-thymidine incorporation.*

result from the mouse antimonkey combination (in which direct T-cell activation in primary cultures is almost entirely absent) (156). Figure 40.10A shows the results of a mouse allogeneic MLR from an unprimed animal. There was a strong proliferative response that remained after the APCs of the responder population had been depleted (in keeping with the concept that direct T-cell stimulation is responsible for the powerful primary response to allogeneic MHC antigens). In contrast, Figure 40.10B shows little proliferation of unprimed mouse T cells stimulated by xenogeneic cells. Figure 40.10D, however, shows that after rejection of a xenogeneic skin graft, mouse T cells responded well in the presence of xenogeneic stimulators but that this response was eliminated by depletion of the responder APCs and not by depletion of the xenogeneic APCs. These results suggest that the mouse T cells were stimulated in vivo by the indirect pathway so that they could subsequently respond in vitro to peptides of xenogeneic antigens presented by mouse MHC molecules.

Sensitization of recipient T cells by the indirect pathway has been shown to occur in other species combinations as well, including those that demonstrate a direct response in primary in vitro cultures (166,184). Indeed, indirect sensitization of T cells to peptides of donor antigens also occurs during allograft rejection, which is not unexpected, since this is the normal mechanism by which T cells respond to any foreign protein. Nonetheless, the kind of results shown in Figure 40.10 have led to speculation that cell-mediated xenograft rejection might be distinguished from allograft rejection by the special importance of the indirect pathway for xenografts. This may be true in some cases, but the suggestion needs qualification in several ways. First, sensitization by the indirect pathway is not a unique feature of xenografting since it occurs during allograft rejection as well (185,186). The question has not yet been answered whether the indirect response stimulated by xenografts might be stronger than that stimulated by allografts because xenotransplants may have a larger number of disparate proteins to generate foreign peptides. Second, the weakness of the direct xenogeneic response in vitro is only a feature of some species combinations and not of the clinically relevant human response to other large animals. Third, the weakness of the direct response in mice has only been demonstrated in vitro and these assays may not reflect the actual mechanisms of graft rejection.

In Vivo Studies of Cell-Mediated Xenograft Destruction

The in vitro assays of cell-mediated xenogeneic responses described above are useful for examining the molecular compatibilities between the cells of the immune system of different species and for demonstrating the type of response occurring after graft rejection. Their value is much less clear, however, when they are used to describe the mechanisms of graft rejection. Substantial transplantation immunology data have shown the discordance between MLR or CTL activity measured in vitro and the survival or destruction of grafts in vivo. Even when T cells can be shown to have been sensitized in certain ways during graft rejection, it has not necessarily been clear that these responses were the ones that caused graft rejection. Thus, as in all areas of transplantation immunology, the study of the mechanisms of xenograft rejection in vivo are essential.

As described earlier, in vivo models of purely cell-mediated xenograft rejection are difficult to find and two approaches have been used: 1) to use small animals, especially mice, as recipients of xenogeneic tissues that are not primarily vascularized (such as skin grafts or pancreatic islets), an approach that avoids humoral rejection and allows extraordinary flexibility, or 2) to use large animals, or even human patients, as recipients of primarily vascularized organs, an approach that is more clinically relevant but that is complicated by the genetic diversity, the dominant humoral response, and by our diminished ability to characterize the cellular mechanisms. It is not surprising, given the limitations of both approaches, that fundamental issues in cell-mediated xenograft rejection have not yet been resolved.

Small Animal Studies of Cell-Mediated Xenograft Rejection

Skin grafts and pancreatic islets from xenogeneic donors are rapidly rejected by normal mice, usually faster than for allogeneic transplants. Rejection occurs at the same pace in B-cell–deficient mice, and the few studies performed indicated that the prolonged survival of xenogeneic transplants is more difficult to achieve using comparable doses of immunosuppressive agents such as cyclosporine (147). By contrast, prolonged xenograft survival occurs in nude mice and in mice depleted of both $CD4^+$ and $CD8^+$ T cells. Thus, despite the weak primary direct response in vitro of mouse T cells to xenogeneic stimulating cells, T-cell–mediated xenograft rejection is a powerful process in mice.

Additional studies have characterized the T-cell subsets involved in xenograft rejection by depleting either $CD4^+$ or $CD8^+$ T cells. Numerous experiments, using both skin grafts and islets, have indicated that xenograft rejection by mice is especially dependent on $CD4^+$ T cells in comparison to allograft rejection (187–190). For example, mice depleted of $CD4^+$ T cells allow longer survival of xenogeneic than allogeneic skin grafts. In addition, adoptive transfer experiments, in which immune deficient recipients have been reconstituted with purified T-cell subpopulations, have indicated that $CD4^+$ T cells can initiate xenograft destruction without the participation of B cells, $CD8^+$ T cells, or NK cells (191). By contrast, immunohistologic studies of rejecting xenografts have identified an unusually predominant macrophage component infiltrating the graft when compared to rejecting allografts (192), and other studies have suggested that NK cells are present in large numbers (193,194).

These results, especially when combined with the in vitro data, have led to a general impression that a principal mechanism of cell-mediated xenograft rejection involves powerful stimulation of $CD4^+$ T cells through the indirect pathway (because of the numerous foreign peptides of xenogeneic antigens) and that the resulting cytokines activate macrophages that destroy the xenograft through a delayed-type hypersensitivity (DTH) response (192,195). It has also been suggested that NK cells might play a role as the effector cells in this rejection (179).

As attractive as this model appears, there are experimental results that suggest that it is at least incomplete. First, while anti-CD4 treatment in mice can prolong skin graft survival, the combination of anti-CD4 and anti-CD8 treatment prolongs survival even more. Thus, $CD8^+$ cells can participate in murine xenograft rejection, with the suggestion that they are able to recognize xenogeneic target cells directly (196). Second, the survival of human islet transplants in mice has been prolonged by treatment with an anti-B7 antibody that reacts with human but not with mouse cells, indicating that a direct interaction between mouse T cells and human stimulating cells must be involved in the rejection mechanism (197). Finally, recipient mice that have $CD4^+$ cells but that lack class II MHC antigens (which therefore have no capacity for an indirect response) are still able to reject xenogeneic skin grafts (147). Thus, despite the in vitro data showing weak direct responses by mouse T cells to xenogeneic stimulating cells even after xenograft rejection, there is significant evidence that direct recognition of xenogeneic cells does occur in vivo and that it can lead to rapid graft destruction.

Clearly, the data generated by the in vitro assays in mice showing weak stimulation except through the indirect pathway do not provide an adequate picture of the in vivo events in xenograft rejection. This may be because the assays commonly used (such as proliferation, IL-2 production, and T-cell–mediated cytotoxicity) are measuring the wrong responses and that the actual mechanisms of xenograft rejection involve the other cytokines or other effector mechanisms. Alternatively, the in vitro assays may accurately reflect a weak initial response to xenogeneic stimulation, but one which is subsequently poorly regulated and controlled in vivo. As discussed above, it is also possible that molecular incompatibilities between species may weaken important downregulating interactions in vivo.

The studies of murine xenogeneic graft rejection have suggested that even when in vitro responses are weak, cell-mediated xenograft destruction is still a stronger process than is encountered in allogeneic transplantation. This conclusion suggests that when humans respond to pig organ transplants they may have multiple types of cell-mediated responses available:

- Those reflected in the normal T-cell responses in vitro that appear similar to allogeneic responses
- Those reflected in the unusual NK response detected in vitro to xenogeneic but not to allogeneic targets
- Those that are not measured at all in vitro, and are only detected in the murine experiments

Large Animal Studies of Cell-Mediated Rejection

Until recently, the only large animal studies of xenogeneic transplantation that permitted investigation of cell-mediated rejection were those involving concordant combinations. For example, some of the chimpanzee-to-human kidney transplants performed during the early 1960s survived for up to nine months (14). In addition, several groups have reported that very prolonged survival can be achieved in concordant combinations among the nonhuman primates (198,199). A striking finding in these examples was the limited evidence of cellular rejection present in biopsies of the xenogeneic transplants, indicating that within closely related species cell-mediated xenograft rejection can be controlled by nonspecific immunosuppressive agents. However, a consistent feature of these trials was the frequency of recipient death from complications of vigorous immunosuppression; no study has shown that comparable doses of immunosuppression can achieve as long a survival for xenografts as for allografts. While this may reflect the humoral elements of xenograft rejection even in concordant combinations, the results are consistent with the view that cell-mediated xenograft rejection is more powerful than allograft rejection.

More recently, large animal studies of cellular xenograft rejection have become possible using discordant combinations with genetic manipulations or targeted therapy to prevent hyperacute rejection. The results of these studies have been similar to those in the concordant species (38,149). For example, primarily vascularized organs from transgenic pigs expressing human complement regulatory proteins have survived for one to two months in primates, often with little evidence of rejection in the xenogeneic organ. However, the recipients of the longest-surviving transplants have always succumbed to the effects of the vigorous immunosuppression used to maintain the survival of their transplant. Other than to reaffirm the likelihood that the cellular rejection mechanisms for xenografts are powerful, these studies have not yet provided insight into the mechanisms of this rejection.

THE SPECIAL CASE OF PIG-TO-PRIMATE/HUMAN TRANSPLANTATION

As pigs are the most likely organ and tissue donors for xenotransplantation to humans (Table 40.8), the nature of natural human antipig antibodies–antigen interaction will be examined in some detail, particularly as the HAR of pig organs is currently the major obstacle to be overcome in xenotransplantation. The targets of these antibodies have been the subject of investigations for several years, as their identification would permit the development of strategies to overcome HAR. The evolutionary ancestors of pigs and primates diverged approximately 64 million years ago. Surprisingly

Table 40.8. Pigs as Xenotransplant Donors

Ethics
Less ethical problems than primates
Used now for pharmaceuticals (e.g., insulin) and heart surgery (valves)
Physiology
Choice of size, including minipigs
Breeding
Relatively short gestation period
Large litter size
Animal husbandry well established
Transgenesis available
Infection
Species trophism of pathogens (e.g., human hepatitis virus does not infect pigs)
Designated pathogen-free herds available

however, there is only one major epitope of pigs recognized by natural anti-pig antibodies, the carbohydrate Galα(1,3)Gal.

Galα(1,3)Gal Epitope

Many studies have concluded that Galα(1,3)Gal is the major xenoepitope of pigs that is recognized by natural human and primate antibodies (10,200–203). The observations that humans have substantial amounts of anti-Galα(1,3)Gal IgG antibodies were made by Landsteiner (204) and more recently by Galili (205–207); subsequently antibodies of the IgM and IgA classes have also been identified. The evidence that Galα(1,3)Gal is the major xenoepitope is summarized in Table 40.9.

Carbohydrate Inhibition

Carbohydrates had been implicated as determinants of xenoepitopes detected by naturally occurring antibodies, as monosaccharides (galactose, methyl-α-D-galactose), disaccharides (melibiose), and complex sugars can specifically inhibit the binding of natural human antibodies to pig cells (37,201–203); this was shown to be a terminal α-linked galactose, and in particular Galα(1,3)Gal (37,202,203).

Absorption Studies Complete absorption of cytotoxic antibodies was achieved using either melibiose (Galα(1,6)Glu) or Galα(1,3)Gal coupled to a matrix (208–211).

Transfection Studies COS cells [which are of Old World monkey origin and do not express Galα(1,3)Gal] could bind natural human antibodies after transfection with the mouse or pig α1,3galactosyltransferase cDNA (201,211). Human serum was able to lyse COS cells after transfection with the α1,3galactosyltransferase cDNA (210). Furthermore, these Galα(1,3)Gal$^+$ COS cells could remove all antipig antibodies in absorption experiments (212).

In Vivo Studies Cooper demonstrated that infusion of baboons with carbohydrates prevented hyperacute rejection (202). Furthermore, the ex vivo absorption of baboon blood over a melibiose or Galα(1,3)Gal column removed all cytotoxic antipig antibodies and prevented the subsequent HAR of a transplanted pig heart to a baboon (209).

Table 40.9. Evidence for Galα(1,3)Gal as the Major Xenoepitope in Pig-to-Human Xenografting

Enzymatic
Treatment with α-galactosidase leads to decreased antibody binding
Inhibition
Carbohydrates [Galα(1,3)Gal, melibiose] inhibit binding of natural antibodies and cytotoxicity
Transfection
Transfection with α1,3galactosyltransferase cDNA converts non-antibody-binding cell to antibody-reactive cell
Absorption
Galα(1,3)Gal columns remove all antipig antibodies
Galα(1,3)Gal$^+$ COS cells remove all antipig antibodies
Transplantation
Removal of anti-Galα(1,3)Gal antibodies prior to transplant prevents HAR
Infusion of Galα(1,3)Gal in vivo prevents HAR

Thus Galα(1,3)Gal is the major target of natural antibodies in humans to pigs. This does not exclude the presence of other antibodies, indeed, there are antibodies to subterminal carbohydrates such as *N*-acetyl lactosamine. These are nonfunctional in the presence of Galα(1,3)Gal as the terminal galactose masks the *N*-acetyl lactosamine epitope, but could be functional if the carbohydrate is exposed.

Tissue and Molecular Distribution of Galα(1,3)Gal

Absorption studies using different cell preparations have shown that the same epitope is found on erythrocytes, lymphocytes, and endothelial cells (201). More complete tissue distribution studies of Galα(1,3)Gal using both human antibodies (213) and the Galα(1,3)Gal specific IB4 lectin of *Griffonia simplicifolia* (214) have shown that all endothelial cells have very high expression of Galα(1,3)Gal, except the aorta, which showed weaker staining (213,214). As this would be the first cell type to interact with anti-Galα(1,3)Gal antibodies in a vascularized transplant, HAR ensues. Galα(1,3)Gal was found in most of the other tissue examined (liver, heart, kidney, and lung), with intracellular as well as cell membrane staining observed (see Fig. 40.2 and Plate 42). Adult pancreatic islets were of interest in that they were nonreactive (see Fig. 40.2 and Plate 42); however, fetal islets were slightly reactive and the level increased on in vitro culture (215). Yet, when the cultured islets were transplanted into nude mice and allowed to mature, Galα(1,3)Gal decreased to nondetectable levels, as in the adult (215).

Galα(1,3)Gal is expressed on many molecules as a normal component of glycosylation, including O-linked and N-linked oligosaccharide chains and glycolipids. On the cell surface, Galα(1,3)Gal is expressed on many molecules (216–219). For example, on platelets it is predominantly found on fibrinogen, von Willebrand's factor, α2 integrin, and β3 integrin (220). On endothelial cells, more than 20 glycoproteins carry Galα(1,3)Gal (216), some of which have been identified as von Willebrand's factor, DM-GRASP, and the α1, αv, α3/α5, β1, and β3 integrins (221).

α1,3galactosyltransferase

The Galα(1,3)Gal epitope (Fig. 40.11) is synthesised by the α1,3galactosyltransferase, which catalyzes the addition of a terminal α-linked galactose to *N*-acetyl lactosamine. cDNA clones encoding the α1,3galactosyltransferase have been isolated from the mouse (222,223), ox (224), pig (211,225), and New World monkeys (226), all encoding a type II integral membrane protein typical of all glycosyltransferases thus far isolated. Unlike these species, Old World monkeys and humans do not have a functional α1,3galactosyltransferase, as the gene has several nucleotide deletions and substitutions leading to a pseudogene (227,228). There are some pertinent similarities between the Galα(1,3)Gal epitope and human B blood group epitope: 1) B blood group epitope has an α1,2-linked fucose residue on the subterminal galactose (see Fig. 40.11); 2) the B blood group transferase [which is also an α1,3galactosyltransferase (229)] will only use fucosylated *N*-acetyl lactosamine (H substance) as substrate for the transfer of the terminal galactose, whereas the α1,3galactosyltransferase will only use *N*-acetyl lactosamine; and 3) the human α1,3galactosyltransferase pseudogene and the B blood group transferase are linked on chromosome 9, thus sharing a common evolutionary ancestor (10,227). These similarities and differences can be used in transgenic approaches to eliminate the Galα(1,3)Gal epitope (see below).

Anti-Galα(1,3)Gal Antibodies

Natural antibodies are IgM molecules encoded by germline genes (230), and for the most part their specificity is directed to carbohydrate epitopes: blood groups and galactose. For example, Wu et al characterized a rat antihamster IgM monoclonal antibody that could elicit HAR of hamster heart grafts in the rat and reacted with a carbohydrate epitope on the surface of hamster endothelial cells (70). It is of great interest that the antibody nucleotide sequences (for the heavy and light chains) indicated that no gene rearrangements occurred to produce the anticarbohydrate specificity and therefore were germline immunoglobulin genes (231). Most species also have natural IgG and IgA antibodies directed to the same epitopes as the natural IgM antibodies. The precise mechanism that induces an immunoglobulin class switch for these antibodies is unclear, although it appears that stimulation of the B cells with normal gut microorganisms may be involved.

Galili has shown a correlation between the distribution of Galα(1,3)Gal epitope and natural anti-Galα(1,3)Gal antibodies: species that do not express the Galα(1,3)Gal antigen were Old World monkeys and humans (i.e., those in which the α1,3galactosyltransferase is a pseudogene), and these produced natural anti-Galα(1,3)Gal antibodies (205,232,233). The anti-Galα(1,3)Gal antibodies may be induced in response to or as innate protection to infectious agents, as Galα(1,3)Gal is expressed on bacteria (e.g., *Escherichia coli*, *Klebsiella*, and *Salmonella*) and protozoa (e.g., *Plasmodium falciparum*, *Tryponosoma cruzi*, and *Leishmania mexicana*). It has been suggested that the selective pressure to

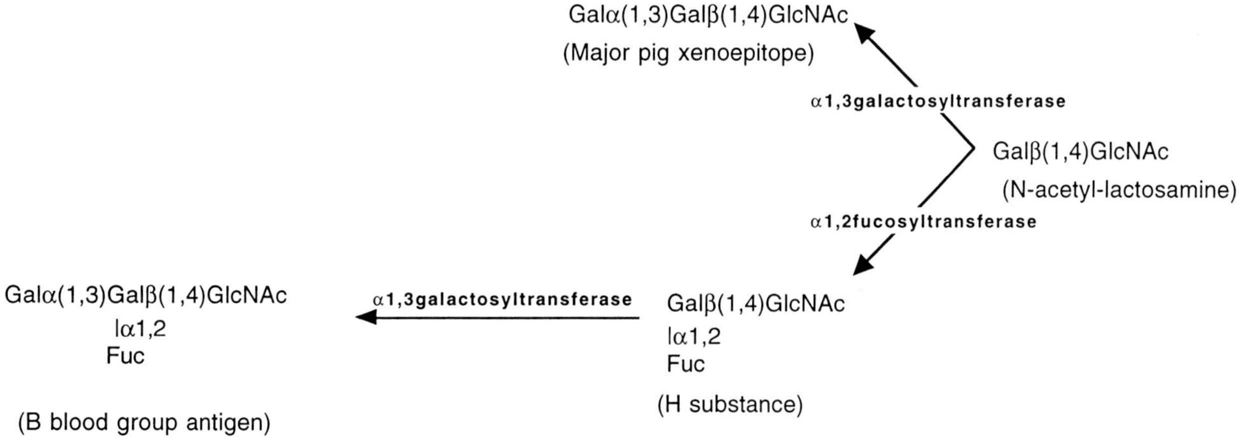

FIGURE 40.11. *Biosynthetic pathway for Galα(1,3)Gal and B blood group. The pathway begins with* N-acetyl-lactosamine *[Galβ(1,4)GlcNac] and the α1,3galactosyltransferase adds galactose to form Galα(1,3)Gal. To synthesize B blood group by the B blood group transferase (also an α1,3galactosyltransferase), Galβ(1,4)GlcNac must first be converted to H substance by the α1,2fucosyltransferase.*

produce anti-Galα(1,3)Gal antibodies was caused by *P. falciparum* (234). Individuals acquiring mutations within the α1,3galactosyltransferase and the subsequent loss of Galα(1,3)Gal would have a selective advantage over those expressing Galα(1,3)Gal, as they could produce anti-Galα(1,3)Gal antibodies to destroy the protozoan.

Anti-Galα(1,3)Gal antibodies constitute a large proportion of serum immunoglobulins, accounting for 1% to 2% of total IgG and 20 to 100 μg IgM (207,233,235). Moreover, antibodies from different individuals have similar properties: the specificity and affinity of the antibodies are similar.

As the major problem in pig-to-primate grafts is HAR due, predominantly, to the Galα(1,3)Gal antibody, major efforts are being directed to the reaction of these antibodies and to complement (see the section on therapeutic approaches, below). When this problem is overcome, DXR, cellular reactions, and other molecular problems will need to be addressed as they arise. The survival of pig tissue in tolerant monkeys (see Chapter 5) and of heterotopic pig heart transplants for 20 to 60 days indicates that, at least for these tissues, problems other than HAR may not be insurmountable.

FEATURES OF DIFFERENT ORGANS AND TISSUES FOR XENOTRANSPLANTATION

Vascularized Organs

Vascularized organs are highly susceptible to HAR, as the recipient antibodies bind to donor antigens of the vascular endothelium. Thus, it would be predicted that pig heart, liver, kidney, lung, or pancreas would all be rejected within minutes to hours of reperfusion. This may not always occur, however, and there are differences in the xenotransplant response to these organs.

Kidneys

Kidneys are particularly susceptible to antibody- and complement-mediated destruction, with coagulation in vessels that occurs within a few minutes. In two recent pig-to-human "grafts," pig kidneys were attached to the A–V fistula of patients undergoing hemodialysis and rejection occurred with the histologic features described earlier (236). In pig kidney-to-baboon grafts, rejection within 60 minutes has been described (208,237).

Lung

The lung may well be different. In a recent study (238), it was found that pig orthotopic lung grafts to primates were not hyperacutely rejected and indeed were functioning for up to 72 hours at the termination of the experiments. There was evidence of antibody and complement deposition in these grafts, and evidence of delayed rejection in that the grafts were hyperemic and there was fibrin and platelet deposition on the xenograft endothelium. Other studies, using ex vivo perfusion, do not support these findings (239).

Liver

The fate of liver xenografts in humans is not clear. Some 25 years ago, ex vivo perfusion of pig livers was performed as a possible treatment of liver failure (240). These studies appeared not to be accompanied by HAR, although at that time the phenomenon of HAR had barely been described. However, it is doubtful if the procedure benefitted the patients. Ex vivo pig liver perfusion is being re-examined and there is evidence of function of the liver and HAR being delayed. In the one pig-to-human liver transplant performed, anti-Galα(1,3)Gal antibodies were removed prior to grafting and HAR was delayed until a fresh plasma infusion was given (undoubtedly containing anti-Galα(1,3)Gal antibodies), at which point HAR occurred immediately (42). It is also known that for allograft HAR, which usually occurs in ABO-incompatible heart and kidney allografts, liver grafts appear to be relatively resistant.

Heart

No pig-to-human heart xenografts have been reported, but both orthotopic and heterotopic pig heart transplants have been performed in monkeys and baboons (241). Graft rejection is usually within minutes with a typical HAR response; that is, the pig heart behaves as expected.

Another feature of interest are the vascular changes that occur in xenografting. Among the difficulties with heart allografting are the arteriosclerotic changes that eventually occur in vessels in the transplanted heart. These consist of endothelial and submucosal hyperplasia and duplication of the elastic lamina that is a feature of chronic rejection, occurring many months or years after allograft transplantation and presumably due to the repeated insults of antibody and cellular immunity directed to the graft or other factors. The endothelial hyperplasia and intimal thickening has also been found in experimental heart transplant models in rodents. It was surprising, therefore, that when pig tissue was transplanted to baboons (242) vascular changes in the absence of HAR, particularly intimal thickening, occurred within days rather than months. This could be a major problem with heart xenotransplants.

Nonvascularized Tissue

Lymphoid cells, including bone marrow, appear to be particularly susceptible to antibody- and complement-mediated rejection as they are very accessible to circulating antibody and, in general, have a high density of cell surface antigens and a low density of complement-regulating proteins. Thus, xenogeneic bone marrow grafts performed in the presence of antibodies universally fail; but if the antibodies are removed, then successful transplantation may be obtained, which, in the case of mixed bone marrow chimerism (see Chapter 5), can lead to tolerance.

Islet Cell Transplants

Xenotransplantation has been considered thus far in the context of transplanting vital organs such as heart, lung, and liver, the justification being the long waiting list for allogeneic human organs. However, if pancreatic islet cell xenotransplantation is considered, there are enormous numbers of diabetic patients (almost 1 million in the United States) who could be eligible for an islet xenograft transplant. It is now considered that although insulin is useful to achieve a normoglycemic state, it does not avoid the long-term complications of diabetes with vascular disease affecting the kidneys, heart, eyes, and brain and that an intact islet is required for the correct control of blood sugar levels (see also Chapter 21 and commentary). Experimental studies clearly indicated that islet cell grafts can normalize the blood sugar and in this light xenografts are being examined. There is not a ready source of islets for allografts, and although islets have been isolated from human fetal tissue this is difficult because of the ethical issues and because of the supply of tissue. Xenografts, particularly from pig tissue, would provide an acceptable solution, particularly as the transplantation of islets is not a major procedure, pig insulin is very similar to that of humans (differing by only one amino acid), and pig insulin was used for many years to treat diabetics before recombinant human insulin became available.

The Source of Pig Islet Cells

The most obvious source of pig islets would be adult pigs; however, major difficulties have been found with the mechanical isolation of adult pig islet cells (243). The current procedures use mechanical disruption and collagenase, although a new enzyme "Liberase" has recently been used and has increased the yield of adult islet cells (244). Fetal pig islets could be another source. In particular, cultured islets could provide a relatively less immunogenic source of islet cells, although the logistics of obtaining and culturing sufficient islets for transplantation is a problem.

Islet Cell Rejection

While there have been many studies on islet allografts and xenografts into rodents, there have been few pig-to-primate studies. However, from the studies performed it appears that islets do not undergo acute antibody-mediated destruction, at least not within minutes, although rabbit islets transplanted underneath the kidney capsule of monkeys undergo rejection within six hours. It may be that this is equivalent to HAR, with six hours being the time for antibody to diffuse into the site. In this six-hour rejection model, heavy infiltration with neutrophils occurred, and it has been suggested that for islet grafts, neutrophils may be a primary component in the graft rejection procedure (245).

From another aspect, pig islets should be ideal for transplantation to humans in that the adult islet cells express little or no Galα(1,3)Gal antigen, although its expression appears to increase on culture and to decrease on subsequent transplantation (215,246). There certainly appears to be some Galα(1,3)Gal in islet cells, since in the clinical studies performed (see below), the patients have a dramatic increase in the amount and affinity of anti-Gal antibodies after receiving pig islet cells (69). Perhaps the endothelial expression of Galα(1,3)Gal could account for this, or there may be an increase as rejection proceeds.

Pig-to-Human Islet Cell Transplantation

The preferred site of islet transplantation is not yet clear—the peritoneal cavity, intraportal vein injection, or under the kidney capsule are possible sites. Thus far, 10 patients in Sweden have received pig xenograft islets, either under the kidney capsule or by the intraportal route, and immunosuppression was given, either as part of the suppression for a kidney transplant, or ALG or desoxyspergualin were given separately (33,247,248). There was evidence of survival with production of C-reactive protein in the urine and by biopsy of the kidney. All patients showed an increase in anti-Gal antibody by titer and affinity; however, there was no evidence of production of pig insulin.

THERAPEUTIC APPROACHES

The investigational approaches to xenotransplantation as a therapeutic measure naturally focus on how to overcome HAR in pig-to-human transplants and the subsequent DXR and cellular rejection. However, the research is likely to have repercussions in other areas where there is antibody-mediated damage of tissue, such as in autoimmunity. Clearly, as HAR is due to the interaction of antibody with antigen and complement fixation, therapeutic approaches should address: 1) antibody, 2) the Galα(1,3)Gal antigen, and 3) complement (Table 40.10). The strategies vary from simple antibody removal by plasmapheresis to sophisticated techniques of genetic engineering.

Table 40.10. Therapeutic Approaches to Prevent HAR

Antibody
Nonspecific
Plasmapheresis
Perfusion through anti-immunoglobulin columns
Splenectomy, deoxyspergualin
Specific
Ex vivo organ perfusion
Perfusion through Galα(1,3)Gal columns
Infusion with carbohydrate or peptide
Complement
Deplete complement: CVF, anticomplement antibodies
Inhibit complement: peptides, antibodies, soluble complement regulators
Transgenic expression of human complement regulators
Antigen
Prevent expression of Galα(1,3)Gal
Inactivate α1,3galactosyltransferase gene by homologous recombination
Antisense RNA/oligonucleotides
Remove Galα(1,3)Gal enzymatically
α-galactosidase transgene
Substrate competition
α1,2fucosyltransferase transgene

Antibody Removal or Neutralization

To overcome HAR in the pig-to-primate model, three basic approaches can be used: 1) reduce or deplete the natural antibody, 2) prevent the activation of complement, and 3) alter or remove the antigens recognized by the natural antibodies.

Antibody Removal by Plasmapheresis or Absorption Using Affinity Columns

Plasmapheresis has been successfully used to remove anti-donor antibodies prior to allotransplantation and to prolong xenotransplant survival in nonprimate species. For example, the survival of pig kidney-to-baboon transplants was extended to 22 days (249) and pig hearts to 2 days, or 17.5 days when used in conjunction with immunosuppression and complement depletion (250) (Table 40.11). Circulating antibodies are only depleted for one to two days unless the procedure is progressively repeated, or splenectomy performed, or immunosuppression used to achieve sustained antibody depletion. Splenectomy results in the long-term depletion of circulating natural antibodies and may ultimately be included as a routine step in the protocol for xenotransplantation. An alternative to plasmapheresis is to remove all immunoglobulin from the recipient prior to transplantation by the use of anti-human Ig (251).

A better approach would be to deplete only the xenoreactive antibodies by absorption, using ex vivo perfusion of isolated pig organs (e.g., livers or kidneys) or immunoabsorbent columns bearing Galα(1,3)Gal. The ex vivo perfusion of pig livers has been used as a treatment for fulminant hepatic failure in humans (23,240), as a bridge to human allotransplants (43), and for antibody removal prior to xenotransplantation to both primates (254,256,257) and humans (42). Like plasmapheresis, this is a short-term measure when used alone, as the xenoreactive antibodies reappear rapidly, unless splenectomy or immunosuppressive drugs such as cyclophosphamide or deoxyspergualin are administered. Using immunoabsorbent Galα(1,3)Gal columns, ex vivo perfusion of baboons on four consecutive days dramatically reduced the levels of circulating cytotoxic antipig antibodies (203,208). As IgM antibodies are an important class of antibodies that activate complement, anti-IgM antibodies have been used to deplete the natural antipig antibodies (258). However, HAR of a pig kidney still occurred, despite the reduction of the IgM level to 0.6% of the pretreatment level, presumably due to residual IgM and IgG antibodies.

Blocking of Anti-Galα(1,3)Gal Antibodies

Alternatively, antibodies could be neutralized or blocked. Antibody neutralization may be examined by infusing baboons with the oligosaccharides Galα(1,3)Gal or melibiose, where complete elimination of cytotoxic antibodies and prolonged cardiac xenograft survival has been achieved (202,209,259). Recently, peptides that mimic Galα(1,3)Gal and bind to anti-Galα(1,3)Gal antibodies have been described (260,261) and could prove to be of therapeutic value. HAR could also be prevented by blocking the natural anti-Galα(1,3)Gal antibodies with a noncomplement-fixing antibody or antibody fragment. Fab fragments of anti-Galα(1,3)Gal antibodies have been examined, but these are not of clinical use as their affinity is less than intact immunoglobulin molecules (262). However, high-affinity anti-Galα(1,3)Gal antibodies produced in chickens (263) could be of therapeutic value, since chicken antibodies do not fix mammalian complement and chickens naturally make anti-Galα(1,3)Gal antibodies.

Regulation of Complement by Cell Surface Molecules

Because complement activation is one of the critical barriers to immediate xenograft survival as well as to longer-term function (if the chemotactic C3a and C5a complement peptides prove to be significant mediators), many resources have been directed toward diminishing the effects of complement using the RCA molecules or other inhibitors.

Table 40.11. Pig Xenografts to Primates

Recipient	Organ	Treatment	Number	Survival	Reference
Baboon	Liver	−/±steroids ± azathioprine	7	6 hrs–3.5 days	252
Rhesus	Liver	ALS	3	<12 hr	253
Chimpanzee	Liver	—	1	8 hr	253
Baboon	Heart	—	4	<8 hr	254
Baboon	Heart	Splenectomy	3	<8 hr	254
Baboon	Heart	CsA + Methylprednisolone (MP)	5	<2 hr (×4), 5 days (×1)	254
Baboon	Heart	Ab absorption	7	<20 hr (×3), 4–5 days (×4)	254
Baboon	Heart	Ab absorption + CsA + MP	4	<24 hr (×3), 4 days (×1)	254
Baboon	Kidney	Plasmapheresis + ALG + CsA + MP	5	1–22 days	249

Source: Adapted from Ye Y, Cooper DKC. Experimental xenotransplantation in nonhuman primates using distantly related donor species. In: Cooper DKC, Kemp E, Reemtsma K, White DJG, eds. Xenotransplantation—the transplantation of organs and tissues between species. New York: Springer, 1991:389–393.

MCP

MCP (CD46) is a good candidate protein for a therapeutic role in controlling complement deposition in hyperacute xenograft rejection, and several research groups are trying to assess its suitability. It does regulate the classic pathway, it is highly efficient at controlling the alternative path "tick-over" (which may prove to be especially important in long-term xenograft survival and function), and it does not exhibit homologous restriction and thus (together with the endogenous regulators of the graft tissue) should control the activity of complement produced by cells of a graft. However, it does have multiple isoforms of unknown functional significance that may be relevant to the strategies of generating transgenic animals.

One way to avoid the limitation of selecting a particular MCP isoform in transgenic animals is to use genomic DNA; however, this has not yet been successful for YAC constructs containing the >40-kb MCP gene (113), apparently because of an inherent instability in the genomic DNA. Constructs using a cDNA sequence with a promoter of choice, or a minigene constructed from partial genomic and cDNA clones, have been used to make transgenic mice (119,264). The rodent xenotransplantation experiments have been disappointing, however. Hearts from a MCP-BC1 isoform transgenic mouse are hyperacutely rejected in rats (after administering rat-antimouse serum), chickens, and monkeys, with the rejection times being slightly delayed in comparison with normal mouse hearts (119). At best, the transgenic MCP had a minor effect in delaying the extremely powerful rejection reaction, although deposition of rat complement was initially prevented. A model of human plasma perfusion into transgenic mice followed by analysis of the liver showed that complement deposition was being controlled (264). In the absence of organ transplantation, however, it is not possible to predict whether the MCP expression would be sufficient to affect hyperacute graft rejection.

DAF

When transfected into cultured cell lines, DAF expression provides good protection against complement-mediated lysis (108,122), and both cDNA and genomic or minigene constructs have been used to make transgenic mice (113,115,116,264–266) and pigs (114,117,265,267). Indeed, the expression on transgenic pig tissues appears to have been much more effective in enabling xenografts to survive hyperacute rejection than could have been expected from the in vitro data. Recently, White and colleagues have reported the survival of beating transgenic pig hearts in immunosuppressed monkeys for weeks, with the absence of histologic features of antibody deposition or complement activation (268), which certainly augured well for the scheme of xenotransplantation. However, when the hearts were transplanted orthotopically, recipient survival was extended only to 9 days (269).

An interesting observation has been made with the GPI-linked DAF and CD59 molecules. For some time there has been discussion of the intermembrane transfer of GPI-linked proteins by mechanisms that have remained obscure; however, new evidence of transfer of DAF and CD59 from transgenic mouse erythrocytes to endothelial cells in vivo has been published (270). It was suggested that such transfer from a reservoir of protein on erythrocytes would act to maintain levels on endothelial cells. However, one interpretation not discussed is the role this may have in graft accommodation—namely, the gradual transfer of GPI-linked host complement regulators onto graft cells—which may not have been looked at in this context.

The initial transgene constructs utilized the mouse H-$2K^b$ promoter, which in general does not provide strong expression on endothelial and other critical cells. Data from other constructs that should generate much greater levels of expression should also begin to address the issue of "how much DAF is enough."

CD59

Transgenic mice and pigs expressing CD59 (115,117,265, 267,271–275), or CD59 and DAF (but with DAF expression and function not clearly apparent) (267), have been used as organ donors or in ex vivo perfusion models, and either a lack of MAC formation or an extension of organ function has been observed. It is unknown whether the levels of protein expression and the tissue distribution are comparable in the two models. It has generally been assumed that the combination of CD59 with DAF or MCP would provide better protection, and thus such experimental models are being pursued as discussed below.

Other Transgenic Approaches and Chimeric Molecules

Several studies use a multimolecular approach to complement regulation and three strategies are in progress: the construction of multigene DNA constructs for transgenesis, such as CD59 with DAF (and MCP) (267); the generation and crossing of transgenic animals independently expressing CD59, DAF, or MCP; and the construction of recombinant chimeric proteins with dual functions, such as CD59 and DAF (276) or DAF and MCP (277).

Initially tested in transfected cells, it was soon proven that coexpression of DAF and CD59 was more protective than single regulators (278,279). Similarly, once the transgenic animals were available, the data demonstrated that joint expression resulted in less complement deposition, including MAC (118). In particular, a problem posed for all these studies is whether the multiple proteins are each expressed sufficiently on the appropriate tissues, rather than one being high and another low and ineffective. The solution to good expression may depend on the choice of promoters or the site of transgene integration.

For the chimeric proteins, it remains to be seen whether or how the structural differences between them and the native molecules will affect their functions. Recent data have demonstrated that a DAF-CD59 but not a CD59-DAF chimera has functions of both parental molecules, as the

CD59-DAF lacks CD59 function (276). Thus, the exact protein structure and probably its positioning on the cell surface are, as expected, of great importance.

How Much Complement Regulation Is Enough?

Transfection data indicate that higher concentrations of regulators enable more effective protection of target cells, and the transgenic animal data revealed that low to moderate levels of expression have provided only marginal evidence of protection when tested against diluted human blood or plasma. Currently, therefore, the aim is to increase expression levels and combine graft protective strategies until a range of expression levels can be tested. It can be surmised from "normal" levels of expression for MCP, DAF, and CD59 that the range of densities on different tissues is large; thus, 5-fold to 10-fold increases of transgene expression over currently obtained levels may be useful and without detriment. It is not known whether, for instance, a 10-fold increase in the regulators on lymphocytes (which normally express near the lowest levels) may disturb their functions or increase their susceptibility to microbial infection. Thus, many basic questions remain unanswered.

Soluble Complement Regulators

Three molecules—CR1, DAF, and MCP—have been produced as recombinant soluble proteins and tested in a number of models to evaluate their therapeutic potential.

CR1

An approximately 230-kd recombinant soluble form of CR1 (rsCR1) (280) is being widely tested for its therapeutic potential, and experimental studies have been promising, leading to clinical trials in the adult respiratory distress syndrome (281). Because it does not demonstrate any homologous restriction, it has successfully been used to control complement activation in rats, mice, pigs, and monkeys. It has delayed (but not prevented) HAR of guinea pig hearts in rats (282,283) and pig hearts in monkeys (284). However, the effective concentrations have been 3 mg/kg or more and were most effective when given as continuous infusions or frequently repeated bolus injections. It has been widely tested for effective regulation of reperfusion injury in experimental models using rat heart (280,285), pig heart (286), rat liver (287), mouse skeletal muscle (288), and rat colon (289), and to limit vascular injury in the reversed passive Arthus reaction in rats (290) and rabbits (291).

Only one published in vitro comparison of rsCR1 with other recombinant soluble regulators (rsMCP and rsDAF) has been reported. At comparative protein concentrations, the rsCR1 was approximately 100 times more effective in protecting cells against lysis by the classic activation path (102,103) and was of similar potency to rsMCP in regulating the alternative pathway. At present, its most likely applications may be in protection against reperfusion injury, myocardial infarction ischemic damage, and respiratory distress syndrome, and as part of a combination therapy to prevent HAR.

MCP

Recombinant soluble forms of MCP (CD46) have been engineered and proven to effectively protect cells in vitro against lysis, both by classic and alternative pathway activation, to limit the reverse passive Arthus reaction in rats, to slightly delay the hyperacute rejection of mouse hearts in rats (102,103), and to inhibit measles virus infection of cells (292,293). These proteins require further testing to determine if they have therapeutic value; however, they are unlikely to be an improvement over rsCR1 (103).

DAF

The DAF (CD55) molecule has also been produced in recombinant soluble form and several observations suggest its potential. It has been reported to reduce the reverse passive Arthus reaction after intradermal administration (294), and in vitro it controls the classic pathway of activation quite effectively (103).

Other Regulators

Factor H, one of the endogenous fluid phase complement regulators with structural and functional similarities to CR1, MCP, and DAF, had not been considered to control cell surface deposition. Recent data, however, have demonstrated that this can occur. A human melanoma cell line was found to be protected against lysis by increasing the concentration of factor H in the solution (295). Whether such an observation has any significance for the xenograft system remains to be tested.

Cobra Venom Factor Treatment

Systemic depletion of complement by the intravenous infusion of CVF, which activates C3 and thus prevents the cascade from functioning, has been an extremely useful procedure to help define the roles of various mediators in the xenograft response (see section on hyperaccute rejection, above). It has allowed the effects of C3 and subsequent components to be distinguished from those of antibody alone and, since it prevents HAR, has enabled the activation of endothelial cells to be more closely observed in vivo. However, the side effects of the near-immediate C3 activation frequently risk the life of the subject, and thus CVF treatment cannot be envisaged as a clinical therapy. In addition, CVF has a high Galα(1,3)Gal content and therefore is a target for natural antibodies, and it is highly immunogenic, which would limit its use to a single treatment.

Transgenic Proteins as Microbial Receptors

Infecting microbes, both bacteria and viruses, have evolved with their hosts to accommodate their life cycles. Thus, it should not be surprising that cell surface proteins are found to be receptors for viruses and bacteria, although it is not clear whether the number of complement-binding proteins that are microbial receptors represents some adaptive drive. MCP is the receptor for measles virus, which binds via its hemagglutinin molecule to the N-terminal SCR modules of the protein. Some anti-MCP antibodies are able to block measles binding (and infection), and the transfection of MCP into animal cells generally enables measles infection (111,112). The identity of the isoform does not appear to be important (109,110). More recently, MCP was deduced to play an important role in the infection of keratinocytes by group A *Streptococci*, which cause suppurative diseases of the human skin (296). DAF has also been observed to bind bacteria (an adhesin of *E. coli*) (297), and two families of viruses, echoviruses (298,299) and coxsackieviruses types B1, B3, and B5 (300,301).

Are these observations of concern in xenotransplantation? It is possible that high expression of a particular receptor may make a cell more susceptible to infection. It could be argued, however, that most organs are bathed in the host's immune system and thus a vascularized organ graft should be well shielded from most pathogens.

Therapies Directed to C5 and C8

Because of the critical role of C5a peptide in inflammation, antibodies directed to C5 have recently been tested in xenogeneic models. Both monoclonal anti-C5 and a recombinant single-chain scFv fragment anti-C5 antibody have successfully blocked cell lysis. The monoclonal antibody was infused into pig hearts perfused with 6% human blood and extended function was observed (302). The Fv fragment has been successfully tested in the same model, preventing C5b-9 deposition, and a 100-mg bolus dose into rhesus monkeys inhibited the serum hemolytic activity for up to two hours (303). C8 has also been targeted with a monoclonal antibody, with dual effects being noted: prevention of C5b-9 deposition and cell lysis, and inhibition of the complement-induced prothrombinase activity (304). These novel approaches may have useful applications in reducing the immune assault on a reperfused xenograft, when given in combination with other pretransplant and posttransplant therapies.

Prevention of Synthesis or Elimination of Galα(1,3)Gal Epitopes

Perhaps the most likely approach to successful xenotransplantation in humans is to modify the donor in such a way that the targets for the antibodies are removed or masked. With the identification of Galα(1,3)Gal as the major xenoepitope, several strategies to remove or alter this carbohydrate structure have been investigated.

Homologous Recombination

The most direct approach to prevent the synthesis of Galα(1,3)Gal would be to inactivate the gene encoding the α1,3galactosyltransferase by a gene knockout. This has been achieved in mice that do not express Galα(1,3)Gal (305,306), and, like humans and Old World monkeys, produce natural anti-Galα(1,3)Gal antibodies. However, cells from these Gal-deficient mice still bind other natural human antibodies (306), most likely anti-*N*-acetyl lactosamine antibodies (262). Thus, gene inactivation of the α1,3galactosyltransferase alone is not the ultimate solution to the production of the universal donor pig. Furthermore, while gene inactivation by homologous recombination is the most direct approach, this technique is not yet available for the pig.

Transgenic Galactosidases

An alternative approach to eliminate Galα(1,3)Gal would be to use α-galactosidase, an enzyme that cleaves terminal α-linked galactosyl residues. Treatment of pig cells in vitro (using α-galactosidase of either bacterial or coffee bean origin) removes Galα(1,3)Gal and eliminates antibody binding (146,213,221). Expressing the cDNA clone encoding human α-galactosidase A within cells decreases Galα(1,3)Gal, resulting in decreased anti-Galα(1,3)Gal antibody binding and decreased lysis by antibodies and complement (307). Transgenic mice have been produced and this approach is feasible in pigs. However, α-galactosidase transgenic pigs, while having decreased Galα(1,3)Gal, would still express "uncapped" *N*-acetyl lactosamine residues that could bind human antibodies and lead to HAR.

H Transgenes

Competition for the α1,3-galactosyltransferase substrate by another glycosyltransferase utilizing the same substrate could lead to reduced expression of Galα(1,3)Gal. Such a transferase is the α1,2fucosyltransferase (H transferase), which catalyzes the production of the O blood group antigen or H substance (308). In H transgenic mice there is preferential expression of H substance and a marked decrease in Galα(1,3)Gal expression, a decrease in binding of anti-Galα(1,3)Gal antibody, and abrogation of complement-mediated lysis (308,309). The advantage of this approach is that the transgenic animals express O blood group antigen (the universal donor) and do not expose the "next" carbohydrate epitope, to which humans may have antibodies. The production of transgenic pigs is feasible, and the ideal transgenic pig that would be resistant to HAR could contain the α1,2fucosyltransferase, α-galactosidase, and one or more of the complement regulators.

Combined Strategies

An obvious and necessary extension of the therapeutic strategies is to combine the removal or masking of antigen with the provision or enhancement of resistance to complement and other inflammatory mediators. However, the problems inherent in creating and testing any one of the components has delayed examining the combined approach. If predictions are plausible, it is likely that the modulated tissues will survive long enough for further effects of species incompatibilities and lymphocyte-mediated responses to be more apparent. Then they will need to be addressed.

Immunosuppression for Cell-Mediated Xenograft Rejection

Although a number of nonspecific immunosuppressive agents have been found to be especially useful in xenogeneic transplantation, their value has probably been primarily in their ability to suppress B-cell responses. At this point, no study has suggested that any of the nonspecific immunosuppressive drugs that act primarily on T cells is more effective for xenografts than allografts. In fact, the available evidence indicates that more immunosuppression is required to prevent cell-mediated xenograft rejection. If this is true, then clinical application of xenogeneic transplantation is likely to represent an inferior alternative compared to allogeneic transplantation for most patients, until some way can be found to remove the immunologic disadvantage of animal donors for human patients. Even if manipulations of donor animals or new treatment strategies can effectively prevent humoral rejection of xenografts, the amount of immunosuppression required to clinically maintain allograft survival is still very close to the maximum that patients can tolerate. Therefore, adding more immunosuppression to maintain xenograft survival or attempting xenografting with our current levels of suppression is likely to cause the death of more recipients or the loss of more transplants to rejection. In addition, the biggest immunologic problem in clinical transplantation today is chronic rejection, for which no effective treatment is available (see Chapter 3). It is very likely that xenogeneic transplants will be even more susceptible to this form of rejection. With these considerations in mind, it seems likely that the clinical application of xenografting will require strategies that minimize the immunologic disadvantage of xenografts.

Genetic Manipulations of Donor Animals

The recent success of genetic engineering approaches in preventing hyperacute rejection (see section on therapeutic approaches, above) suggests that similar approaches might be used to prevent cell-mediated rejection. Potential genetic modifications that might be used for cellular rejection include the removal or modification of the target antigens or increases in the expression of potential regulatory molecules. While removing antigens is possible in mice through targeted gene disruption, this technology is currently not available for larger animals. Furthermore, even complete elimination of MHC antigens in mice has not prevented cell-mediated rejection (310). On the other hand, the production of transgenic pigs is possible today, although it is not yet clear what genes to insert to lessen the cellular mechanisms of xenograft rejection; possibly transgenic antisense DNA constructs could decrease pig class I and II MHC antigens.

Numerous suggestions for genetic manipulations have been offered. For example, if NK cells play a role in xenograft rejection, then perhaps transgenic pigs should be generated that express human MHC molecules (a counterintuitive suggestion from the point of view of those who seek better MHC matching in allogeneic transplantation). Perhaps transgenic pigs should be made that overexpress Fas ligand (making their tissues a privileged site like the testes) or that produce soluble receptors that would bind and inhibit T-cell ligands such as CD28. However, speculative solutions such as these are too easily generated in the absence of a better understanding of the cellular rejection mechanisms involved.

Tolerance Induction

The other approach to equalizing the immunologic response to xenografts and allografts is to eliminate the response altogether by inducing tolerance to donor antigens. However, achievement of this goal, even for allografts, has been the object of much transplantation research for over 40 years, suggesting that it is not simple to accomplish. Efforts to achieve transplantation tolerance for allografts have included either attempts to modify the responses of mature lymphocytes (peripheral tolerance) or attempts to eliminate the mature immune system and then allow subsequent reconstitution in the presence of donor antigens (deletional tolerance) (311). The ability to modify xenogeneic animals genetically may help to accomplish peripheral tolerance induction, although there is concern that the resulting donor-specific unresponsiveness may be unstable, especially in the face of the powerful immunologic stimulus of a xenograft. On the other hand, efforts to accomplish "deletional" tolerance through the induction of bone marrow chimerism will probably require modifications to support the engraftment and differentiation of xenogeneic bone marrow in a foreign environment (312–314). These strategies are described elsewhere in this book (see Chapter 5).

Despite the difficulties in achieving tolerance for xenogeneic donors, it is likely that widespread clinical application of xenogeneic transplantation will require some form of tolerance induction (140). Given the multiple additional immunologic barriers to xenogeneic transplants, the best approach for removing the immunologic disadvantage of animal organs will probably be to eliminate the immune response entirely.

INFECTIOUS DISEASE ISSUES IN XENOTRANSPLANTATION

A major concern with the use of nonhuman donor or "source" animals in clinical transplantation is uncertainty about the potential for the transfer of infection from animal species both to the recipient and to the general population. Particular concerns have been expressed regarding the inadvertent spread of novel or unidentified pathogens, particularly viruses, to the xenograft recipient. Detractors of primate donors cite herpesvirus B infections from macaque monkeys in humans, the proposed evolution of HIV-1 and HIV-2 from related simian immunodeficiency virus (SIV), and the high frequency of infection of baboons with foamy viruses and with other agents similar to those that cause disease in humans.

Pigs have been proposed as the main alternate source of organ donation for human xenotransplantation. Data on the nature, transmissability, and behavior of pathogens between nonhuman primates or pigs and humans are very limited. Thus, the risk of such transplanted, interspecies infection or "xenosis" or "xenozoonosis," cannot be accurately assessed at present (315–319). However, it is apparent that the "species specificity" of many pathogens, particularly viruses, may limit or prevent the transmissibility of animal-derived pathogens to humans and of human-derived pathogens to the xenograft. By contrast, the unique advantage of xenotransplantation to individuals with chronic viral infections (including hepatitis B and C, HIV, and cytomegalovirus) may prove to be one of the most valuable contributions of xenotransplantation, as pig tissue is not susceptible to these viruses.

The Risk of Opportunistic Infection in the Xenograft Recipient

The risk of opportunistic infection in the transplant recipient is a function of the epidemiologic exposures and the "net state of immune suppression" of the recipient; that is, the dose and duration of pharmacologic immune suppression and metabolic, technical, and infectious factors that predispose to the development of infection. Multiple factors *may* increase the likelihood of interspecies infections in addition to the common opportunistic infections seen in transplantation (Table 40.12). The combination of immune suppression, the use of organs across histocompatibility barriers, and the absence of preexisting immunity in the recipient to such animal-derived organisms render the host more susceptible to infection.

The term *xenosis* was coined to describe the transplantation of infection with xenogeneic transplants (315). In contrast with the natural spread of infection between species (termed *zoonosis*), xenosis poses unique epidemiologic hazards due to the efficiency of transmission of pathogens, particularly viruses, with viable, cellular grafts. A number of factors conspire to increase the risk of infection including: 1) the xenograft itself serves as a nidus or "culture plate" from which such organisms can spread in the human host, avoiding the need for a "vector" to achieve disease transmission; 2) the potential for infection with novel pathogens for which clinical laboratory testing is not available (either culture systems for species-specific organisms or serologic tests for human antibodies to animal pathogens); 3) the migration of cells from the graft to other sites in the host may carry cell-associated infection throughout the host; 4) the inability to recognize clinical syndromes caused by new pathogens (Table 40.13); 5) the lack of immunity to animal-derived pathogens in the xenograft recipient; and 6) the lack of knowledge about the behavior of potential pathogens from the donor species in immunosuppressed humans.

Assessing the Microbiologic Risks and Donor Selection

The theoretical risks of xenosis are dependent upon the presence of organisms in the graft tissue and the availability of the appropriate conditions for growth. Experience with allotransplantation suggests that virtually any organism can cause infection in the compromised host (see Chapter 36). While concern has focused on viruses, in the immediate post-transplant period common surgical complications (aspiration, wound infections, infected fluid collections, catheter-related processes) predominate, with the causative organisms being either bacterial or nosocomial yeasts and fungi. Many of these organisms are common to most species and easily identified: *Staphylococcus aureus*, streptococci, *Klebsiella* species, and *E. coli*. Some strains of organisms are thought to be species specific; for example, in studies of pigs, some *Mycoplasma* and *Streptococcus* strains could be speciated only by veterinary laboratories.

Recognition of the common pig-derived pathogens seen in humans may indicate those most likely to be of

Table 40.12. Factors Favoring the Development of Xenosis

No need for vector transmission; animal-derived pathogens implanted with the xenograft
Continuous exposure; species-specific organisms may replicate in the xenograft and spread to distant sites once adapted to the donor species
Animal-derived pathogens not previously associated with human disease
Failure to recognize clinical syndromes
Lack of appropriate microbiologic tests for animal-derived organisms in clinical laboratories
Rejection and immune suppression: stimuli for activation of latent infection
Recombination or coinfection: creation of new pathogens with altered biologic behaviors

Table 40.13. Nonrecognition of New Infectious Disease Syndromes

New human pathogens
New clinical syndrome or altered manifestations in humans
Suppression of host responses due to immune suppression
Low incidence or scattered or sporadic cases
Coinfection with other opportunistic pathogens
Absence of diagnostic tests for animal-derived organisms
High background rate of opportunistic infection
Common syndromes (respiratory, liver)
Latency
Carrier state

importance in the immediate post-transplantation period. Zoonotic infections have been observed in meat handlers, in farmers, and in individuals ingesting undercooked pork. Common bacterial and parasitic infections in these occupations include those due to *Salmonella* species, *Cholera suis, Brucella* and *Trichinella* species, rabies, anthrax, brucellosis, *Campylobacter* and *Cryptosporidia* gastroenteridities, *Streptococcus suis*, toxoplasmosis, leptospirosis, listeriosis, erysipeloid, and yersiniosis. An excess mortality, especially due to lung cancer, has been associated with the occupation of pork butchers over other meat handlers and the general population. No excess mortality due to infection has been described in these workers. Similarly, up to 20% of slaughterhouse workers and 25% of pigs have serologic evidence of exposure to swine influenza (generally H1N1 or H3N2 subtypes) (320,321). Recombinant strains of influenza (H1N2) have been observed in pig populations in which H1N1 strains are endemic and coinfection from humans with other strains (H3N2) occurs (322,323). There is no evidence of increased virulence of these "new" strains.

In the period from one to six months post-transplantation, the impact of postoperative complications is displaced by the opportunistic fungi, parasites, and immunomodulatory viruses. The fungi (including *Aspergillus, Candida*, and the geographic mycoses) and *Toxoplasma gondii* are not species specific and are easily identified, and standard therapies are available, although possible species specificity exists in *Pneumocystis carinii*.

The common cell-associated viruses that are activated in the first six months after transplantation are present in both pigs and in primates and are likely to be species specific. In humans, CMV, hepatitis B and C, herpes simplex virus, and Epstein-Barr virus cause systemic clinical syndromes, are globally immunosuppressive, and contribute to the development of cancer. These viruses also contribute to the development of other life-threatening opportunistic infections (e.g., *Pneumocystis* pneumonia) and to graft injury and rejection. In the xenograft, after activation by immune suppression, ischemic injury, and/or graft rejection, animal-derived viruses may be expressed, including herpes viruses (CMV, Papio, SA8, cercopithecine herpesvirus 1 or "B virus"), adenoviruses, hepatitis viruses, pseudorabies (e.g., Aujeszky's) or rabies viruses, reovirus, or papovavirus. These viruses are present in latent form in many if not most wild-caught animals, and have been associated with a variety of interspecies infections. Simian immunodeficiency virus and herpes B virus have been associated with human infection (324,325). Human Epstein-Barr virus can infect marmosets, while human CMV can infect chimpanzees.

Using this paradigm, some of the likely human pathogens derived from animals can be predicted, and general exclusion criteria developed, to guide the development of donor animal herds (Table 40.14). Those organisms thought to pose unacceptable microbiologic risks in the transplantation recipient will determine the approach to the microbiologic screening of donor animals or of xenograft tissues (Table 40.15). This list will vary depending on the donor species and the use intended for the xenograft. If microbiologic or serologic tests are available for these organisms, it is possible to exclude them from prospectively evaluated, closed, and microbiologically isolated donor animal herds. By contrast, wild-caught animals in open herds require individual screening for potential pathogens. Regardless of the donor species, screening will be limited by the nonavailability of appropriate tests. The transmissibility of human and animal pathogens can be assessed by periodic screening of animal handlers working with donor herds for exposure to potential pathogens. Excluded from this list are the retroviruses that form a component of the genomes of all species, and are discussed below.

Table 40.14. Microbiologic Screening of Xenograft

Donor Swine: Exclusion Criteria*
Known pathogens of humans (e.g. rabies, *Mycobacterium* tuberculosis)
Known pathogens of immunocompromised human hosts (e.g., *Toxoplasma gondii, Salmonella* species)
Similar to common pathogens of transplant recipients (e.g., porcine CMV, adenovirus)
Antibiotic-resistant organisms
Viruses at high risk for recombination (e.g., parvovirus, rotavirus)
Organ-specific exclusion list (e.g., *Mycoplasma* species in lung donors)

* The potential risks associated with retroviral agents merit separate consideration.

Table 40.15. Designated Pathogen-Free (DPF) Miniature Swine for Xenotransplantation

Exclude the presence of:	
Ascaris summ	*Cryptosporidium parvum*
Brucella suis	Neospora
Leptospira	*Sarcocystis suihominis*
Listeria monocytogenes	Trichinella spiralis
Mycobacterium bovis	Adenovirus (porcine)
Mycobacterium tuberculosis	Cytomegalovirus (porcine)
Mycobacterium avium—intracellular complex	Encephalomyocarditis virus
Mycoplasma hyopneumoniae (lung transplant)	Influenza virus (porcine and human)
Salmonella typhi	Porcine parvovirus
Salmonella typhimurium	Porcine reproductive and respiratory syndrome virus
Salmonella cholerasuis	Pseudorabies
Shigella	Rabies
*Aspergillus**	Rotavirus
*Candida**	
Histoplasma capsulatum	
Toxoplasma gondii	
Strongyloides ransomi	

* Exclude animals with lesions.

Organisms spread rapidly between closely quartered animals and also over long distances (326). Thus, the introduction of new animals into a herd or unregulated contact with other species (birds, rodents, farm animals, dogs, cats, ticks, fleas, humans) may be detrimental. Further, the spread of antibiotic-resistant organisms will be rapid, necessitating the limitation of the use of antibiotics in herd maintenance.

The manner in which the level of safety created by the exclusion criteria or lists of organisms is achieved need not be uniform as long as the transplanted tissues do not pose a microbiologic hazard to the recipient. For example, cellular transplants (e.g., bone marrow, microencapsulated tissues) pose a unique set of opportunities and challenges. Xenogeneic bone marrow transplants, used in immunologic tolerization procedures for example, spread throughout the body. These cells are exposed to graft rejection, host irradiation, immune suppression, and a variety of drugs and may cause graft-versus-host disease, all stimuli for the activation of latent, cell-associated viruses. By contrast, encapsulated cells or tissues do not spread through the body and may not elicit the level of host immune response observed in vascularized organ grafts. Compared with whole organs, each batch of cells can be cultured and examined, allowing for the exclusion of microbiologically contaminated lots of cells. In this case, the need to develop herds of designated pathogen free (DPF) animals may be reduced if the absence of potential pathogens can be demonstrated, or such organisms removed, during processing.

Unknown Pathogens: The Retroviruses and Prion Disease

Retroviruses

Public health concerns regarding xenotransplantation have grown out of the recent study of "emerging infections." These are newly described organisms, reemergent infections, or clinical syndromes that are recognized by virtue of clustering of unusual clinical syndromes (as with HIV and AIDS or hantavirus pneumonia) or a sudden change in the epidemiology of disease (antibiotic-resistant bacteria). Changes in the geographic distribution or manifestations of disease may render a previously unexposed and nonimmune population susceptible to infection. In general, this involves movement of people into an endemic area for the infectious agent (as with ebola virus), alteration of the pathogen (as with bacterial acquisition of plasmid-mediated antibiotic resistance or the evolution of SIV into HIV strains), or the movement of the natural hosts for a pathogen into new territories (as with the emergence of Lyme disease following conversion of many farms to forest in the eastern United States with the growth of deer, mice, and ticks carrying *Borrelia burgdorferi*). Xenotransplantation poses the challenge of novel (for the nonveterinarian) pathogens growing in graft tissues within an immunocompromised host. The ability of unknown pathogens to replicate and "adapt" to the human host is unknown, and altered behavior in humans or selective pressures favoring mutant or recombinant strains may occur.

The immunocompromised host is a "sentinal chicken" for new pathogens, particularly those of modest native virulence that cannot cause disease in the immunologically normal host. In AIDS, the clinical syndromes associated with HIV, microsporidia, *Cyclospora, Cryptosporidium, Rhodococcus equi*, JK virus, Kaposi's-associated herpes virus, and *Bartonella* species have been described. Thus attention must be paid to all types of potential pathogens. However, the risk of a pandemic on the scale of AIDS, which is derived from mutated or recombinant animal-derived viruses, has caused attention to be focused on the risks of retroviral infection.

What is the nature of this risk? Animal-derived, undescribed viruses capable of replicating in humans cannot be excluded. Xenotropic viruses or defective viruses may be undetectable in the native host species. The conditions most often associated with retroviral activation (e.g., immune suppression, graft-versus-host disease, graft rejection, viral coinfection, cytotoxic therapies) are present in the transplant recipient. The activation and behavior of the retroviruses in allotransplantation have not been well studied in vivo. However, the course of accidentally transmitted infection due to HIV-1 has been accelerated in transplant recipients, manifesting disease within six months (327,328). The activation of latent virus and the development of clinical manifestations, if any, may be delayed for over a decade. The manifestations of retroviral infection may be clinically inapparent or subtle: altered gene regulation, oncogenesis, or recombination with other viruses. Interspecies transmission of retroviruses has been identified in a number of models: seroconversion of humans to simian immunodeficiency virus (324); human foamy virus genes inducing encephalopathy in mice; pseudotyping of Rous sarcoma virus with avian and murine tumor viruses (329); pseudotyping of HIV with murine amphotropic retrovirus (330,331); simian Agent 8 in baboons (332); and HIV infection of cells of baboons, apes, and New and Old World monkeys by HIV-1 and -2. While productive infection was not always established in vivo, the ability of both known and unknown viruses to infect humans merits investigation.

By contrast, most intact endogenous proviruses (usually types B and C), once activated, are nonpathogenic and most are relatively restricted in host range. Coinfection and recombination with other viruses, mutation, or modification of viral behavior in the foreign human environment may alter the pathogenicity, organ specificity, or replication of the retroviruses or of other infectious agents (333–337). Viruses may gain *or* lose "virulence" following passage in other species or under environmental or antibiotic pressure. Thus, the main issue regarding retroviruses is the potential for infection of humans with animal-derived strains. It is likely that nonhuman primate-derived strains may be "better adapted" to the human milieu, but the risk of infection, regardless of source, is not known.

Some degree of assurance regarding the risk of xenosis requires, when possible, the exclusion of animal donors carrying known or potential human pathogens. Retroviruses of primates have been more thoroughly characterized than those of pigs. In part due to studies related to AIDS, up to 30 strains of lenteviruses have been described in primates. Only type C retroviruses have been characterized in pig-derived tissues. A virus from the PK15 cell line and another derived from a malignant lymphoma-derived cell line (Shimozuma cells) have been described (338–341). The latter isolate, Tsukuba-1, causes B- and T-cell lymphomas in wild boars (342). A large portion of this clone has now been sequenced and used to obtain the sequences of a naturally occurring porcine endogenous retrovirus of miniature swine and pigs. Limited studies have not demonstrated interactions between porcine retrovirus with proviruses of rat, mouse, or mink cells in vitro (342). However, a series of related porcine endogenous retroviruses (PERV) have now been isolated from pig-derived cell lines including PK-15. While the ability of these isolates to cause disease in human hosts is not known, at least one of these viruses is capable of causing productive infection of human cells in vitro (343). These observations have altered the "theoretical" risk of infection associated with xenotransplantation from swine donors, but no evidence of such infection has been found to date (344,345).

Of the baboon and other primate retroviruses, foamy (spuma-) viruses, endogenous retroviruses (e.g., baboon), STLV, SIV's and other type C, D, and endogenous viruses, infectivity for human cells has been demonstrated for SIV (human T cells) and baboon foamy virus (human fibroblasts) (Allen J, personal communication, 1997). The ubiquitous nature and genetic homologies of the primate immunodeficiency viruses (SIV, STLV, endogenous viruses), and the ability of these pathogens to infect other species, suggest a potential risk for human infection. Nevertheless, to date, none of the recipients of tissues from nonhuman primates have had nonhuman viral infection identified.

Prion Disease

Prion diseases are progressive neurodegenerative diseases associated with transmissible agents that contain protein and no apparent DNA or RNA. After prolonged latency (often over 30 years), disease is manifested with a typical astrocytosis and spongiform vacuolization of the neutrophil. Recent concerns regarding prion disease relate to the possible transmission of prion disease of cows ("mad cow disease" or bovine spongiform encephalopathy) to humans (Creutzfeldt-Jakob disease) via ingestion of beef contaminated by food containing infected sheep neural tissue (scrapie). Interspecies spread of prion disease has been demonstrated in animal models, and the spread of such diseases should be avoidable by the removal of any animal products from the feed of pig or primate donors. The presence of prion disease (or rabies) must be considered in any potential donor pool developing abnormal or degenerative neurologic function.

Risks Associated with Alterations of the Donor

Strategies developed to reduce the level of rejection occurring after xenotransplantation may also alter the risk of viral activation. Transgenic animals developed to minimize acute rejection of xenografts may change the expression of latent virus as a result of insertion or deletion of genes (267). These transgenes may also encode receptors for new pathogens, for example, MCP and measles virus and DAF and the echoviruses and coxsackie viruses (see section on therapeutic approaches, above). In humans, natural antibodies to Galα(1,3)Gal may be a part of an intrinsic defense mechanism against exogenous retroviral, bacterial, and parasitic infections (346–351). It is likely that such antibodies emerge as a result of chronic exposure to this epitope on the normal bacterial flora of the gastrointestinal tract. These same antibodies provide a major transplantation barrier to the use of vascularized organs from pigs carrying the endothelial Galα(1,3)Gal sugars. Techniques that remove the anti-Galα(1,3)Gal natural antibodies from the recipient (or remove the epitope from the transplanted organ) have prevented HAR in xenogeneic recipients of pig-derived organs (267,308,352). In Old World primates and in humans, the serum-mediated inactivation of retroviruses in vitro is probably due in part to the antibody-independent activation of complement on the retroviral surface (protein p15E) or to virally infected T cells (353–355). However, the anti-Galα(1,3)Gal antibodies present in human sera also bind to the gp70 of murine leukemia virus, which is infective for human cells, resulting in inactivation of this type C retrovirus (346,349,353,356). These natural antibodies have been proposed as a mechanism for the prevention of the transmission of retroviruses from species carrying the α-galactosyl epitope to humans. Viruses grown in human cells are generally less susceptible to serum-mediated inactivation than are viruses grown in the native host (350,357). Thus, removal of these natural antibodies may remove a barrier to retroviral transmission and, if infection is established in the human host, these viruses may be less susceptible to inactivation by serum-mediated mechanisms.

Microbiologic Advantages of Xenotransplantation

Despite the potential risks, clinical xenotransplantation may provide significant tangible benefits in the clinical care of patients with progressive organ failure (Table 40.16). In addition to unlimited supply, xenogenic organs may be resistant to infection with viral pathogens of humans including HIV (1 and 2), HTLV, hepatitis viruses, and herpes viruses including human CMV. In our laboratory, a variety of permissive cell lines from pigs and from humans have been shown to be resistant to infection with CMV across species' lines. It is not known whether in vitro data reflect the inability of animal-derived pathogens to infect human hosts or of human pathogens to infect the xenograft in vivo. However, human hepatitis B virus does not appear to infect

Table 40.16. Microbiologic Advantages of Xenotransplantation

Decreased recipient hospitalization time prior to surgery
Reduced nosocomial pathogen exposure
Decreased ischemic time (decreased rejection?)
Characterized microbial flora
Resistance to infection with human pathogens

baboon in vivo (358). This "species specificity" may reflect the absence of receptors and/or of cellular "machinery" necessary for viral replication in a novel host.

Most cadaver donor organs are derived from hospitalized patients potentially infected with nosocomial pathogens. The microbiologically characterized donor animal should be free of such increased infectious risk. Shortened graft ischemic times may also reduce the incidence of rejection, the need for prolonged antilymphocyte therapy, and the duration of hospitalization (e.g., less acute tubular necrosis). Many pancreatic cellular transplants have been performed without any apparent infections derived from the donor (344,359). Thus, the risks, while real, may have little impact over the short term.

Recipient Selection

The infectious risk posed to the individual and, in turn, to the community, is increased by preexisting immunodeficiency states or infections. Patients may be stratified, initially, based on life expectancy; those with limited life spans may not survive beyond the period of retroviral latency and may pose a reduced risk to the community. As candidates for xenografting, the increased infectious risks of common opportunistic infections in persons with HIV (1 or 2) or with hepatitis B or C may render these individuals poor choices for initial studies. It is equally apparent, however, that the urgency for transplantation may be greatest in persons with relatively short life expectancies and particularly in individuals with chronic viral infections. Informed consent is critical and should be obtained by individuals expert in the controversies (scientific, microbiologic, ethical) inherent to the proposed protocols. Because life-long surveillance may be needed to assess the incidence of opportunistic infections or of other complications of xenotransplantation, the recipient must be willing to participate in such an enduring experiment.

Strategies for the Future: Minimizing the Risks

Do the benefits of xenotransplantation justify the risks to the recipient and the community? Strategies have been proposed to eliminate infections due to known pathogens. The use of microbiologically closed and isolated herds screened for likely pathogens will minimize the chance of graft-derived infection. As was noted, not all xenografts need identical screening. For example, cellular transplants might be screened after isolation from the donor. Specific organs merit unique considerations, for example, for *Mycoplasma* species in lung xenografts or coxsackie viruses in heart xenografts (especially if DAF-transgenic pigs were used as donors).

How is the public health protected? Xenogeneic infections may be clinically inapparent, and silent trasmission of infection to medical workers or to family members might occur without symptomatic infection. Thus, initial studies might include a period of isolation of transplant recipients with routine screening (e.g., monthly blood cultures or imaging studies) for evidence of infections. Clinical trials must include careful archiving of sera and tissues from the donor, recipient, medical staff, and other patient contacts to aid in both prospective and retrospective microbiologic and epidemiologic studies of emerging infections in xenograft recipients. Changes, whether immunologic, infectious, or engineered, in either the donor or the recipient, may alter the risk of xenosis and must be evaluated in terms of need and benefit.

The risk of xenosis will never be zero. Significant dangers of infection exist for all transplant recipients given the relatively crude, though improving, immune suppressive regimens that are currently available. *Strategies that reduce the level of immune suppression needed to maintain graft function are the most important protection against emerging xenosis.* Careful donor animal selection may allow the risks to the recipient and to the community to be reduced and may confer substantial benefits when the potential of xenotransplantation is recognized. This risk must then be evaluated in terms of both the individual and the broader potential dangers to public health.

THE FUTURE OF XENOTRANSPLANTATION

The stage is now set to build on the clinical experience of the past using the recent advances to re-explore the clinical possibilities of xenografting—pig-to-human transplants of heart, kidney, liver, and pancreas as vascularized organs or pancreatic islets, bone marrow, and other cellular grafts. Genetically modified pigs are now being produced, expressing the complement-binding molecules (MCP, DAF, and CD59), and already improvements in survival have been reported using such donors. Further advances are developing now with the removal of antibody by plasmapheresis or affinity purification on anti-Galα(1,3)Gal columns, and expression of the Galα(1,3)Gal antigen is being modified in pigs by various transgenic approaches. Thus, as it is possible to define the critical components in HAR (see Table 40.3), it is also possible to describe and make the appropriate modifications to antigen, antibody, and complement, the three primary components causing HAR. Once HAR can be avoided, the stage will then be set to examine other procedures such as delayed graft rejection, chronic rejection, and the other problems alluded to in this chapter. Only when

HAR is solved can the other problems be clearly examined. We are optimistic that HAR can be solved in the not too distant future, and that appropriate immunosuppression could avert or delay DXR and the cellular modes of graft rejection. Whether this will suffice for permanent graft survival cannot be predicted at this stage; our optimism can extend only to short-term grafts of days or weeks utilized in life-threatening situations. However, in unrelated studies, tolerance induction across species is progressing and a Boston team (see Chapter 5) already has pig kidneys surviving in monkeys for some two to three weeks; the graft survival depends on the maintenance of chimerism. In these inordinately difficult experimental models tolerance can be achieved, and if the history of allografts is anything to go by, then xenotransplants to humans may well be simpler than in the primate models.

In time, other procedures can be examined, for example, the development of gene knockout technology for pigs (currently not available) leading to the inactivation of any or all genes involved in transplantation, such as the MHC class I and class II molecules, which from the mouse gene knockout data do not seem to be required for the survival of the animal. It is theoretically possible to produce a "universal donor." In addition, cytokines and immunomodulatory agents of both human and pig organ are now being produced by recombinant DNA methods, and these should be available to manipulate the immune response in the desired direction to promote prolonged graft survival. The remaining problems would then be the long-term acceptance of a foreign graft and its physiologic function and ability to adapt to the human environment (360).

COMMENTARY

David K. C. Cooper

"Clinical xenotransplantation is just around the corner, but it may be a very long corner."

These words, spoken by Sir Roy Calne, who has more experience than most with the rate of progress in organ transplantation, have haunted me since I first heard them in 1995. How long will the corner be? Will we feel confident enough to embark on a realistic clinical xenotransplantation program this year or next—or will we still be struggling to make sufficient progress in the experimental laboratory in 10 years' time?

The hurdles that nature has set before us are undoubtedly considerable. According to Claus Hammer, we are faced with no less a task than that of "outwitting evolution"(1), a goal that surely only surgeons and scientists with the very largest egos would even consider pursuing! I am in no position to cast an opinion on the sizes of the egos of Ian McKenzie and his colleagues, but in the foregoing chapter they have provided us with a valuable overview of the problems we face and of the many innovative therapeutic approaches being investigated. Those who wish to delve further into the details of present day research in this field are referred to a recent volume dedicated to this topic (2).

Successful therapy to enable xenotransplantation to become a clinical reality will almost certainly involve a combination of approaches. Just as in allografting, no single "magic bullet" has been discovered. Indeed, the complexity of the immune attack on a discordant xenograft, involving as it does both antibody-mediated mechanisms (some of which activate complement and some of which appear to induce ADCC) and cellular mechanisms, makes it even more likely that a combination of several different therapeutic approaches will prove necessary if we are to extend pig organ survival in human recipients for a clinically valuable period of time.

These approaches will almost certainly include genetic engineering of the donor and suppression of B-cell function in the host, as well as more standard therapy aimed at the host's T-cell response. Modification of the donor may not be confined only to the introduction of genes for human complement regulatory proteins and for such enzymes as H-fucosyltransferase, but may also necessitate techniques that downregulate the activation of the pig vascular endothelium that is believed to be a factor in the development of the various phases of xenograft rejection (3).

Even with successful donor modification, toward which a first step has already been taken by White and his colleagues with the breeding of pigs transgenic for human DAF (4), it is likely that, at least at times of rejection "crises," the recipient will require a combination of therapies directed toward inhibition of complement activation (e.g., CVF, SCR1), removal or inhibition of antipig (anti-Gal) antibody (e.g., extracorporeal immunoadsorption, intravenous oligosaccharide therapy), and suppression of antibody production (drug therapy aimed at B and plasma cells), as well as T-cell suppression.

Recent studies by several groups utilizing different approaches to inhibit the destructive effect of complement have indicated that very heavy pharmacologic immunosuppressive therapy can, at least temporarily, suppress some of the features associated with delayed xenograft rejection as well as cellular rejection (4,5). The morbidity and mortality associated with such therapy, however, strongly suggests that clinical xenotransplantation will require a more refined approach if it is to be truly successful. We therefore continue to search for new, more sophisticated, and more specific methods of interrupting the pathologic processes involved.

One such approach is the potential of anti-idiotypic antibodies (AIA) directed against anti-Gal antibodies (6). If AIA could transport a "toxin" to those B cells and plasma cells involved in the manufacture of anti-Gal antibodies, then we may be able to halt production of those specific antibodies without affecting the remainder of the immune system.

Indisputable proof that accommodation will indeed occur in relation to the presence of a discordant xenograft would be an encouraging step forward. The prospect for long-term survival of pig organs in humans in the absence of some form of accommodation appears to be poor unless genetic engineering techniques can be perfected to ensure the transplanted organ is totally protected from the host's antibody-mediated response.

The greatest hurdles may as yet be unknown to us and could be in the form of early and aggressive graft vasculopathy (chronic rejection), frustratingly reducing xenograft survival just when we thought the major problems had been resolved, or of nonimmunologic metabolic incompatibilities, preventing satisfactory long-term function of pig organs in the human environment. With time and persisting endeavor, however, these hurdles are also likely to be resolved.

The establishment of xenotransplantation as an accepted form of surgical therapy does not depend solely on resolution of the numerous immunologic hurdles it presents, although these are our first priority. Steps will be required to ensure that serious infection is not transferred with the donor organ and that the presence of pig endogenous retroviruses, possibly by some form of interaction with their human counterparts, will not lead to malignant change in the cells of the graft or host.

The logistics of supplying pig organs over wide geographic regions will require attention. Should a small number of centralized organ distribution centers be set up, or should the pigs be transported to the individual transplantation centers and the organs excised locally? Will a centrally controlled and regulated system for the allocation of organs serve us best, or will free market pressures dominate? Ethical and legal concerns will undoubtedly be raised (7). For example, does a "humanized" pig have any legal rights? As ridiculous as this question may appear to some, it is almost certain that others will raise it at some stage.

How close are we to successful clinical xenotransplantation? Although it is likely there will be sporadic attempts within the next few years—some of which may be deemed ill-judged—the inherent problems in "outwitting evolution" make it unlikely that this form of therapy will soon be established successfully on a *routine* basis. Indeed, a recent survey of those interested in xenotransplantation indicated that 2010 was the year by which most thought this would be achieved.

We are steadily and frustratingly learning the truth of Sir Roy's words—the corner is undoubtedly proving longer than we had hoped. Nevertheless, significant progress has taken place within the past ten years and we can remain cautiously optimistic that the outstanding problems will be resolved. Indeed, we are fortunate that we have both a vision and a task, for in the words of the unknown writer:

A vision without a task is a dream,
A task without a vision is drudgery,
A vision with a task is the hope of the world.

CHAPTER REFERENCES

1. Auchincloss H, Sachs DH. Xenogeneic transplantation. Ann Rev Immunol 1998;16:433–470.
2. Gallup. The American public attitudes towards organ donation and transplantation. Conducted for the Partnership for Organ Donations 1993.
3. Mohacsi PJ, Blumer CE, Quince S, Thompson JF. Correspondence. Nature 1995;378:434.
4. Nuffield Council on Bioethics. Animal-to-human transplants: the ethics of xenotransplantation. London: April, 1996.
5. Arundel M, McKenzie IFC. The acceptability of pig organ xenografts to patients awaiting a transplant. Xenotransplantation 1997;4:62–66.
6. Fedoseyeva EV, Tam RC, Popov IA, et al. Induction of T cell responses to a self-antigen following allotransplantation. Transplantation 1996;61:679–683.
7. Cooper DKC, Kemp E, Reemtsma K, White DJG. Xenotransplantation—the transplantation of organs and tissues between species. New York: Springer-Verlag, 1991.
8. Moller G. Xenotransplantation. Immunol Rev 1994;141:1–276.
9. Auchincloss H. Xenografting: a review. Transplant Rev 1990;4:14–27.
10. Sandrin MS, Vaughan HA, McKenzie IFC. Identification of Galα(1,3)Gal as the major epitope for pig-to-human vascularised xenografts. Transplant Rev 1994;8:134–149.
11. Kaufman CL, Gaines BA, Ildstad ST. Xenotransplantation. Annu Rev Immunol 1995;13:339–367.
12. Reemtsma K, McCracken BH, Schlegel JV, Pearl M. Heterotransplantation of the kidney: two clinical experiences. Science 1964;143:700–702.
13. Reemtsma K, McCracken BH, Schlegel JU, et al. Renal heterotransplantation in man. Ann Surg 1964;160:384–408.
14. Reemtsma K. Renal heterotransplantation from nonhuman primates to man. Ann N Y Acad Sci 1969;162:412–418.
15. Hitchcock CR, Kiser JC, Telander RL, Seljeskob EL. Baboon renal grafts. JAMA 1964;189:934.
16. Porter KA, Marchioro TL, Starzl TE. Pathological changes in six treated baboon to man renal heterotransplants. Br J Urol 1965;37:274.
17. Starzl TE, Marchioro TL, Peters GN, et al. Renal heterotransplantation from baboon to man: experience with six cases. Transplantation 1964;2:752.
18. Starzl TE, Ishikawa M, Putnam CW, et al. Progress in and deterrents to orthotopic liver transplantation, with special reference to survival, resistance to hyperacute rejection, and biliary duct reconstruction. Transplant Proc 1974;6;129.
19. Hollander D, Klebanoff G, Osteen RJ. Human baboon cross-circulation for treatment of hepatic coma. JAMA 1971;218:67.
20. Giles GR, Boehmig HJ, Ameniya H, et al. Clinical heterotransplantation of the liver. Transplant Proc 1970;2:506.
21. Hume DM, Gayle WEJ, Williams GM. Cross circulation of patients in hepatic coma with baboon partners having human blood. Surg Gynecol Obstet 1969;128:495.
22. Starzl TE. Experience in hepatic transplantation. Philadelphia: Saunders, 1969.
23. Ham JM, Pirola RC, Davidson GM, et al. Pig liver perfusion for the treatment of acute hepatic coma. Surg Gynecol Obstet 1968;127:453.
24. Eiseman B. Cross circulation in heterologous systems. Colston Papers 1967; The Liver: 279.
25. Abouna GM, Amemiya H, Andres G, et al. Immunological studies in patients receiving repeated allogeneic and xenogeneic liver hemoperfusions. Transplantation 1974;18:395–408.
26. Norman JC, Saravis CA, Brown ME, McDermott WVJ. Immunochemical observations in clinical heterologous (xenogeneic) liver perfusions. Surgery 1966;60:179.
27. Cotterell AH, Collins BH, Parker W, et al. The humoral immune response in humans following cross-perfusion of porcine organs. Transplantation 1995;60:861–868.
28. Hardy JD, Chavez CM. The first heart transplant in man. Am J Cardiol 1968;22:772.
29. Hardy JD, Chavez CM, Kurrus FD, et al. Heart transplantation in man: developmental studies and report of a case. JAMA 1964;188:1132.

30. Barnard CN, Wolpowitz A, Losman JG, et al. Heterotopic cardiac transplantation with a xenograft for assistance of the left heart in cardiogenic shock after cardiopulmonary bypass. S Afr Med J 1978;52:1035.
31. Bailey LL, Nehlsen-Cannarella SL, Concepcion W, Jolley WB. Baboon-to-human cardiac xenotransplantation in a neonate. JAMA 1985;254:3321.
32. Andersson A, Groth CG, Korsgren O, et al. Transplantation of porcine fetal islet-like cell clusters to three diabetic patients. Transplant Proc 1992;24:677–678.
33. Groth CG, Andersson A, Korsgren O, et al. Transplantation of porcine fetal islet-like cell clusters into eight diabetic patients. Transplant Proc 1993;25:970.
34. Williams GM, Hume DM, Hudson RP, et al. "Hyperacute" renal-homograft rejection in man. New Engl J Med 1968;279:611–618.
35. Perper RJ, Najarian JS. Experimental renal heterotransplantation: I. In widely divergent species. Transplantation 1966;4:377.
36. Shons AR, Moberg AW, Najarian JS. Xenotransplantation. In: Najarian JS, Simmons R, eds. Transplantation. Philadelphia: Lea and Febiger, 1972.
37. Good AH, Cooper DKC, Malcolm AJ, et al. Identification of carbohydrate structures that bind human antiporcine antibodies: implications for discordant xenografting in humans. Transplant Proc 1992;24:559–562.
38. Platt JL, Logan JS. Use of transgenic animals in xenotransplantation. Transplant Rev 1996;10:69–77.
39. Starzl TE, Fung J, Tzakis A, et al. Baboon-to-human liver transplantation. Lancet 1993;341:65–71.
40. Monden M, Valdivia LA, Gotoh M, et al. A crucial effect of splenectomy on prolonging cardiac xenograft survival in combination with cyclosporine. Surgery 1989;105:535–542.
41. Hasan R, Van den Bogaerde JB, Wallwork J, White DJG. Evidence that long-term survival of concordant xenografts is achieved by inhibition of antispecies antibody production. Transplantation 1992;54:408–413.
42. Makowka L, Cramer DV, Hoffman A, et al. The use of a pig liver xenograft for temporary support of a patient with fulminant hepatic failure. Transplantation 1995;59:1654–1659.
43. Chari RS, Collins BH, Magee JC, et al. Treatment of hepatic failure with ex vivo pig-liver perfusion followed by transplantation. New Engl J Med 1994;331:234–237.
44. Lanza RP, Cooper DK. Xenotransplantation of cells and tissues: application to a range of diseases, from diabetes to Alzheimer's. Mol Med Today 1998;4:39–48.
45. Institute of Medicine Committee on Xenograft Transplantation. Xenotransplant science, ethics, and public policy. Washington, DC: National Academy, 1996.
46. Hutchinson A, Singer P. Xenotransplantation: is it ethically defensible? Xeno 1995;3:58–60.
47. Calne RY. Organ transplantation between widely disparate species. Xeno 1994;2:80–83.
48. Baldamus CA, McKenzie IFC, Winn HJ, Russell PS. Acute destruction by humoral antibody of rat skin grafted to mice. J Immunol 1973;110:1532–1541.
49. Winn HJ, Baldmus CA, Jooste SV, Russell PS. Acute destruction by humoralantibody of rat skin grafted to mice—the role of complement and polymorphonuclear leukocytes. J Exp Med 1973;137:893–910.
50. Bogman MJJT, Berden JHM, Cornelissen IMHA, et al. The role of complement in the induction of acute antibody-mediated vasculitis of rat skin grafts in the mouse. Am J Pathol 1982;109:97–106.
51. Bogman MJJT, Berden JHM, Hagemann FHM, et al. Patterns of vascular damage in the antibody-mediated rejection of skin xenografts in the mouse. Am J Pathol 1980;100:727–738.
52. Najarian JS, Foker JE. The expression of immunity: the efferent arm. In: Nanjarian JS, Simmons RL, eds. Transplantation. Philadelphia: Lea and Febiger, 1972:94–122.
53. Gorer PA. Some recent work on tumor immunity. Adv Cancer Res 1956;4:149–186.
54. Gorer PA, Kaliss N. The effect of iso-antibodies in vivo on three different transplantable neoplasms in mice. Cancer Res 1959;19:824–830.
55. Boyse EA, Old LJ, Thomas G. A report on some observations with a simplified cytotoxic test. Transplant Bull 1962;29:435.
56. Kissmeyer-Neilsen F, Olsen S, Petersen VP, Fjeldborg O. Hyperacute rejection of kidney allografts associated with preexisting humoral antibodies against donor cells. Lancet 1966;2:662–665.
57. William GM, Hume DM, Hudson RPJ, Morris PJ. Hyperacute renal homograft rejection in man. New Engl J Med 1968;279:611.
58. Eichwald EJ, Wetzel B, Lustgraaf EC. Genetic aspects of second set skin grafts in mice. Transplantation 1966;4:260–273.
59. Larsen S, Starklint H. Histopathology of kidney xenograft rejection. In: Cooper DKC, Kemp E, Reemtsma K, White DJG, eds. Xenotransplantation—the transplantation of organs and tissues between species. New York: Springer-Verlag, 1991:181–205.
60. Rose AG. Histopathology of cardiac xenograft rejection. In: Cooper DKC, Kemp E, Reemtsma K, White DJG, eds. Xenotransplantation—the transplantation of organs and tissues between species. New York: Spinger-Verlag, 1991:231–242.
61. Wight DGD. Histopathology of liver xenograft rejection. In: Cooper DKC, Kemp E, Reemtsma K, White DJG, eds. Xenotransplantation—the transplantation of organs and tissues between species. New York: Springer-Verlag, 1991:253–272.
62. Starzl TE, Lerren RH, Dixon FJ, Groth CG. Shwartzman reaction after human renal homo-transplantation. New Engl J Med 1968;278:642–648.
63. Bogman MJJT. Hyperacute rejection as a model of antibody-induced vasculitis. Nijmegen: Stichting Studenenpers, 1983.
64. Ozman L, Pericin M, Hakimi J, et al. Interleukin 12, interferon γ, and tumor necrosis factor α are the key cytokines of the generalized Shwartzman reaction. J Exp Med 1994;180:907–915.
65. Platt JL, Vercellotti GM, Dalmasso AP, et al. Transplantation of discordant xenografts: a review of progress. Immunol Today 1990;11:450–456.
66. Gambiez L, Salame E, Chereau C, et al. The role of natural IgM in hyperacute rejection of discordant heart xenografts. Transplantation 1992;54:577–583.
67. Springer GF, Horton RE, Forbes M. Origin of anti-human blood group B agglutinins in white leghorn chicks. J Exp Med 1959;110:221–244.
68. McKenzie IF, Stocker J, Ting A, Morris PJ. Human lymphocytotoxic and haemagglutinating activity against sheep and pig cells. Lancet 1968;2:386–387.
69. Galili U, Tibell A, Samuelsson B, et al. Increased anti-Gal activity in diabetic patients transplanted with fetal porcine islet cell clusters. Transplantation 1995;59:1549–1556.
70. Wu G-D, Cramer DV, Chapman FA, et al. Genetic control of the humoral immune response to xenografts. Transplantation 1995;60:1497–1503.
71. Baldwin WMI, Pruitt SK, Brauer RB, et al. Complement in organ transplantation. Contributions to inflammation, injury and rejection. Transplantation 1995;59:797–808.
72. Leventhal JR, Dalmasso AP, Cromwell JW, et al. Prolongation of cardiac xenograft survival by depletion of complement. Transplantation 1993;55:857–866.
73. Miyagawa S, Hirose H, Shirakura R, et al. The mechanism of discordant xenograft rejection. Transplantation 1988;46:825–830.
74. Gewurz H, Clark DS, Cooper MD, et al. Effect of cobra venom-induced inhibition of complement activity on allograft and xengoraft rejection reactions. Transplantation 1967;5:1296–1303.
75. Brauer RB, Baldwin WMI, Daha MR, et al. Use of C6-deficient rats to evaluate the mechanism of hyperacute rejection of discordant cardiac xenografts. J Immunol 1993;151:7240–7248.
76. Leenaerts PL, Stad RK, Hall BM, et al. Hereditary C6 deficiency in a strain of PVG/c rats. Clin Exp Immunol 1994;97:478–482.
77. Winkelstein JA, Johnson JP, Swift AJ, et al. Genetically determined deficiency of the third component of complement in the dog: in vitro studies on the complement system and complement-mediated serum activities. J Immunol 1982;129:2598–2602.
78. Bitter-Suermann D, Burger R. Guinea pigs deficient in C2, C4, C3 or the C3a receptor. Prog Allergy 1986;39:134–158.
79. White DJ. Unos Update 1992;8:6–7.
80. Rosenberg LT, Tachibana DK. Mice deficient in C5. Prog Allergy 1986;39:169–191.
81. Zhow X-J, Niesen N, Pawloskwski I, et al. Prolongation of survival of discordant kidney xenografts by C6 deficiency. Transplantation 1990;50:896–898.
82. O'Regan CC, Robitaille P, Pinto-Blonde M, Chartrand C. Delayed rejection of cardiac xenografts in C6-deficient rabbits. Immunology 1979;38:245–248.
83. Weill BJ, Regimbeau J-M, Calmus Y, et al. The alternative complement pathway in hyperacute xenograft rejection. Xeno 1994;2:92–94.
84. Farries TC, Steuer KL, Atkinson JP. The mechanism of activation of the alternative pathway of complement by cell-bound C4b. Mol Immunol 1990;27:1155–1161.
85. Moore FD, Fearon DT, Austen KF. IgG on mouse erythrocytes augments activation of the human alternate pathway by enhancing deposition of C3b. J Immunol 1981;126:1805–1809.
86. Johnston PS, Lim SML, Wang MW, et al. Hyperacute rejection of xenografts in the complete absence of antibody. Transplant Proc 1991;23:877–879.

87. van den Berg RH, Faber Krol M, van Es LA, Daha MR. Regulation of the function of the first component of complement by human C1q receptor. Eur J Immunol 1995;25:2206–2210.
88. Lublin DM, Atkinson JP. Decay accelerating factor and membrane cofactor protein. Curr Top Microbiol Immunol 1989;153:123–145.
89. Liszewski MK, Post TW, Atkinson JPA. Membrane cofactor protein (MCP or CD46): newest member of the regulators of complement activation gene cluster. Annu Rev Immunol 1991;9:431–455.
90. Walsh LA, Tone M, Thiru S, Waldmann H. The CD59 antigen multifunctional molecule. Tissue Antigens 1992;40:213–220.
91. Davies A, Lachmann PJ. Membrane defence against complement lysis: the structure and biological properties of CD59. Immunol Res 1993;12:258–275.
92. Johnstone RW, Loveland BE, McKenzie IFC. Identification and quantitation of complement regulator CD46 on normal human tissues. Immunology 1993;79;341–347.
93. van den Berg CW, Morgan BP. Complement inhibiting activities of human CD59 and analogues from rat, sheep and pig are not homologously restricted. J Immunol 1994;152:4095–4101.
94. Brauer RB, Baldwin WMI, Sanfilippo F. Complement deficient animals in the study of hyperacute rejection. Xeno 1994;2:35–37.
95. Dalmasso AP, Vercellotti GM, Platt JL, Bach FH. Inhibition of complement mediated endothelial cell cytotoxicity by decay accelerating factor. Potential for prevention of xenograft hyperacute rejection. Transplantation 1991;52:530–533.
96. Loveland BE, Johnstone RW, Russell SM, et al. Different membrane cofactor protein (CD46) isoforms protect transfected cells against antibody and complement mediated lysis. Transpl Immunol 1993;1:101–108.
97. Bach FH, Robson SC, Winkler H, et al. Barriers to xenotransplantation. Nat Med 1995;1:869–873.
98. Nomura A, Nishikawa K, Yuzawa Y, et al. Tubulointerstitial injury induced in rats by a monoclonal antibody that inhibits the function of a membrane inhibitor of complement. J Clin Invest 1995;96:2348–2356.
99. Weiss L, Fischer E, Haeffner-Cavaillon N, et al. The human C3b receptor (CR1). Adv Nephrol 1989;18:249–270.
100. Barlow PN, Steinkasser A, Norman GD, et al. Solution structure of a pair of complement modules by nuclear magnetic resonance. J Mol Biol 1993;232:268–284.
101. Kojima A, Iwata K, Seya T, et al. Membrane cofactor protein (CD46) protects cells predominantly from alternative complement pathway-mediated C3-fragment deposition and cytolysis. J Immunol 1993;151:1519–1527.
102. Christiansen D, Milland J, Thorley BR, et al. Engineering of recombinant soluble CD46: an inhibitor of complement activation. Immunology 1996;87:348–354.
103. Christiansen D, Milland J, Thorley BR, et al. A functional analysis of recombinant soluble CD46 in vivo and a comparison with recombinant soluble forms of CD55 and CD35 in vitro. Eur J Immunol 1996;26:578–585.
104. Johnstone RW, Russell SM, Loveland BE, McKenzie IFC. Polymorphic expression of CD46 isoforms due to tissue-specific RNA splicing. Mol Immunol 1993;30:1231–1241.
105. Russell SM, Sparrow RL, McKenzie IFC, Purcell DFJ. Tissue-specific and allelic expression of CD46 is controlled at the level of alternative splicing. Eur J Immunol 1992;22:1513–1518.
106. Hara T, Suzuki Y, Semba T, et al. High expression of membrane cofactor protein of complement (CD46) in human leukaemia cell lines: implication of an alternatively spliced form containing the STA domain in CD46 up regulation. Scand J Immunol 1995;42:581–590.
107. Oglesby TJ, Allen CJ, Lizsewski MK, et al. Membrane cofactor protein (CD46) protects cells from complement-mediated attack by an intrinsic mechanism. J Exp Med 1992;175:1547–1551.
108. Lublin DM, Coyne KE. Phospholipid-anchored and transmembrane versions of either decay-accelerating factor or membrane cofactor protein show equal efficiency in protection from complement-mediated cell damage. J Exp Med 1991;174:35–44.
109. Gerlier D, Loveland B, Varior-Krishnan G, et al. Measles virus receptor properties are shared by several CD46 isoforms differing in extracellular regions and cytoplasmic tails. J Gen Virol 1994;75:2163–2171.
110. Manchester M, Liszewski MK, Atkinson JP, Oldstone MB. Multiple isoforms of CD46 (membrane cofactor protein) serve as receptors for measles virus. Proc Natl Acad Sci USA 1994;91:2161–2165.
111. Naniche D, Varior-Krishnan G, Cervoni F, et al. Human membrane cofactor protein (CD46) acts as a cellular receptor for measles virus. J Virol 1993;67:6025–6032.
112. Dorig RE, Marcil A, Chopra A, Richardson CD. The human CD46 molecule is a receptor for measles vrius (Edmonston strain). Cell 1993;75:295–305.
113. Platt JL, Logan JS. Use of transgenic animals in xenotransplantation. Transplant Rev 1966;10:69–77.
114. White DJG, Langford GA, Cozzi E, Young VJ. Protective effects of human DAF in transgenic pigs. Xeno 1995;3:48–51.
115. Byrne GW, McCurry KR, Kagan D, et al. Protection of xenogeneic cardiac endothelium from human complement by expression of CD59 or DAF in transgenic mice. Transplantation 1995;60:1149–1156.
116. van Denderen BJW, Pearse MJ, Katerelos M, et al. Expression of functional decay accelerating factor (CD55) in transgenic mice protects against human complement mediated attack. Transplantation 1996;61:582–588.
117. Cozzi E, White DJG. The generation of transgenic pigs as potential organ donors for humans. Nat Med 1995;1:964–966.
118. Mora M, Mulder LCF, Lazzeri M, et al. Protection from complement-mediated injury in livers and kidneys of transgenic mice expressing human complement regulators. Xenotransplantation 1996;3:63–68.
119. Thorley BR, Milland J, Christiansen D, et al. Transgenic expression of a CD46 (membrane cofactor protein) minigene: studies of xenotransplantation and measles virus infection. Eur J Immunol 1997;27:726–734.
120. Miyagawa S, Shirakura R, Matsumiya G, et al. Test for ability of decay-accelerating factor (DAF, CD55) and CD59 to alleviate complement-mediated damage of xeno-erythrocytes. Scand J Immunol 1993;38:37–44.
121. Meri S, Waldmann H, Lachmann PJ. Distribution of protectin (CD59), a complement membrane attack inhibitor, in normal human tissues. Lab Invest 1991;65:532–537.
122. Charreau B, Cassard A, Tesson L, et al. Protection of rat endothelial cells from primate complement-mediated lysis by expression of human CD59 and/or decay-accelerating factor. Transplantation 1994;58:1222–1229.
123. Hancock WW, Bach FH. The immunopathology of discordant xenograft rejection. Xeno 1994;2:68–74.
124. Lesnikoski BA, Shaffer DA, van der Werf WJ, et al. Endothelial and host mononuclear cell activation and cytokine expression during rejection of pig-to-baboon discordant xenografts. Transplant Proc 1995;27:290–291.
125. Baeuerle PA, Henkel T. Function and activation of NF-kB in the immune system. Annu Rev Immunol 1994;12:141–179.
126. Bach FH. Discordant xenotransplantation: a therapy whose time has come. Xeno 1994;2:57–59.
127. Kobayashi T, Taniguchi S, Ye Y, et al. Delayed xenograft rejection in C3-depleted discordant (pig-to-baboon) cardiac xenografts treated with cobra venom factor. Transplant Proc 1996;28:560.
128. Cannon JA. The question of host adaptation versus graft adaptation in sucessful homografts. Transplant Bull 1957;4:22–24.
129. Woodruff MFA, Simpson LO. Induction of tolerance to skin homografts in rats by injection of cells from the prospective donor soon after birth. Br J Exp Pathol 1955;36:494–499.
130. Bach FH, Platt JL, Cooper DKC. Accommodation—the role of natural antibody and complement in discordant xenograft rejection. In: Cooper DKC, Kemp E, Reemtsa K, White DJG, eds. Xenotransplantation: the transplantation of organs and tissues between species. New York: Springer Verlag, 1991:81–99.
131. Bach FH, Turman MA, Vercellotti GM, et al. Accommodation: a working paradigm for progressing toward clinical discordant xenografting. Transplant Proc 1991;23:205–207.
132. Fishel RJ, Platt JL, Matas AH, et al. Prolonged survival of a discordant cardiac xenograft in a rhesus monkey. Transplant Proc 1991;23:589–590.
133. Paul LC, van Es LA, de la Reviere GB, et al. Blood group B antigen on renal endothelium as the target for rejection in an ABO-incompatible recipient. Transplantation 1978;26:268–271.
134. Chopek MW. Simmons RL, Platt JL. ABO incompatible renal transplantation: initial immunopathologic evaluation. Transplant Proc 1987;19:4553.
135. Palmer A, Welsh K, Gjorsturp P, et al. Removal of anti-HLA antibodies by extracorporeal immunoadsorption to enable renal transplantation. Lancet 1989;1:10–12.
136. Kopp CW, Siegal JB, Hancock WW, et al. Effect of porcine endothelial tissue factor pathway inhibitor on human coagulation factors. Transplantation 1997;63:749–758.
137. Pareti FI, Mazzucoto M, Bottiri E, Marucci PM. Interaction of porcine von Willebrand factor with the platelet glycoproteins Ib and IIb/IIIa complex. Br J Haematol 1992;82:81–86.
138. Goodman DJ, von Albertini M, Willson A, et al. Direct activation of porcine endothelial cells by human natural killer cells. Transplantation 1996;61:763–771.

139. Auchincloss HJ. Cell-mediated xenoresponses: strong or weak? Clin. Transplantation 1994;8:155–159.
140. Dorling A, Lechler RI. T cell-mediated xenograft rejection: specific tolerance is probably required for long-term xenograft survival. Xenotransplantation 1998;5:234–245.
141. Manning DD, Reed ND, Shaffer CF. Maintenance of skin xenografts of widely divergent phylogenetic origin on congenitally athymic (nude) mice. J Exp Med 1973;138:488–494.
142. Hodgson RJ, Loudovaris T, Charlton B, Mandel TE. Destruction of transplanted β cells into diabetic mice is not mediated by antibody alone. Transplant Proc 1992;24:2300.
143. Aksentijevich I, Sachs DH, Sykes M. Normal mouse serum contains natural antibody angainst bone marrow cells of a concordant xenogenic species. J Immunol 1991;147:79–85.
144. Gill RG, Wolf L. Immunobiology of cellular transplantation. Cell Transplant 1995;4:361–370.
145. Simeonovic CJ, Wilson JD, Ceredig R. Antibody-induced rejection of pig proislet xenografts in CD4+ T cell-depleted diabetic mice. Transplantation 1990;50:657–662.
146. Satake M, Kawagishi N, Rydberg L, et al. Limited specificity of xenoantibodies in diabetic patients transplanted with fetal porcine islet cell clusters. Main antibody reactivity against α-linked galactose-containing epitopes. Xenotransplantation 1994;1:89–101.
147. Auchincloss HJ. Why is cell-mediated xenograft rejection so strong? Xeno 1995;3:19–22.
148. Calne RY. Organ transplantation between widely disparate species. Transplant Proc 1970;2:550.
149. Zaid A, Schmoeckel M, Bhatti F, et al. Life-supporting pig-to-primate renal xenotransplantation using genetically modified donors. Transplantation 1998;65:1584–1590.
150. Auchincloss HJ, Sachs DH. Transplantation and graft rejection. In: Paul WE, ed. Fundamental immunology. New York: Raven, 1993:1099–1141.
151. Moses RD, Auchincloss HJ. Mechanisms of cellular xenograft rejection. In: Cooper DKC, ed. Xeno-transplantation—the transplantation of organs between species. (2nd ed.) Berlin: Springer-Verlag, 1996.
152. Lindahl KF, Bach FH. Genetic and cellular aspects of xenogeneic mixed lymphocyte culture reaction. J Exp Med 1976;144:305–318.
153. Nielsen HE. Reactivity of lymphocytes from germfree rats in mixed leukocyte culture and in graft-versus-host reaction. J Exp Med 1972;136:417–425.
154. Shons AR, Kromrey C, Najarian JS. Xenogeneic mixed lymphocyte response. Cell Immunol 1973;6:420–428.
155. Chan DV, Yamada K, Auchincloss HJ. Human anti-pig cell-mediated cytotoxicity in vitro involves non-T as well as T-cell components. Xenotransplantation 1996;3:158–165.
156. Bach FH, Engstrom MA, Bach ML, Sell KW. Histocompatibility matching: VII mixed leukocyte cultures between chimpanzee and man. Transplant Proc 1972;4:97–100.
157. Moses RD, Pierson RNI, Winn HJ, Auchincloss HJ. Xenogeneic proliferation and lymphokine production are dependent on CD4+ helper T cells and self antigen-presenting cells in the mouse. J Exp Med 1990;172:567–575.
158. Murray AG, Khodadoust MM, Pober JS, Bothwell ALM. Porcine aortic endothelial cells activate human T cells: direct presentation of MHC antigens and costimulation by ligands for human CD2 and CD28. Immunity 1994;1:57–63.
159. Bravery CA, Batten P, Yacoub MH, Rose ML. Direct recognition of SLA- and HLA-like class II antigens on porcine endothelium by human T cells results in T cell activation and release of interleukin-2. Transplantation 1995;60:1024–1033.
160. Kirk AD, Li RA, Kinch MS, et al. The human antiporcine cellular repertoire: in vitro studies of acquired and innate cellular responsiveness. Transplantation 1993;55:924–931.
161. Kumagai-Braesch M, Satake M, Korsgren O, et al. Characterization of cellular human anti-porcine xenoreactivity. Clin Transplant 1993;7:273–280.
162. Rollins SA, Kennedy SP, Chodera AJ, et al. Evidence that activation of human T cells by porcine endothelium involves direct recognition of porcine SLA and costimulation by porcine ligands for LFA-1 and CD2. Transplantation 1994;57:1709–1716.
163. Vallee I, Watier H, Thibault G, et al. Evidence of noninvolvement of swine MHC class II in the in vitro proliferative response of human lymphocytes to porcine endothelial cells. Transplantation 1995;59:897–901.
164. Dorling A, Binns R, Lechler RI. Direct human T-cell anti-pig xenoresponses are vigorous but significantly weaker than direct alloresponses. Transplant Proc 1996;28:653.
165. Schaapherder AFM, Daha MR, te Bulte M-J, et al. Antibody-dependent cell-mediated cytotoxicity against porcine endothelium induced by a majority of human sera. Transplantation 1994;57:1376–1382.
166. Yamada K, Sachs DH, DerSimonian H. Human anti-porcine xenogeneic T cell response: evidence for allelic specificity of mixed leukocyte reaction and for both direct and indirect pathways of recognition. J Immunol 1995;155:5249–5256.
167. Moses RD, Winn HJ, Auchincloss HJ. Evidence that multiple defects in cell-surface molecule interactions across species differences are responsible for diminished xenogeneic T cell responses. Transplantation 1992;53:203–209.
168. Barzaga-Gilbert E, Grass D, Lawrance SK, et al. Species specificity and augmentation of responses to class II major histocompatibility complex molecules in human CD4 transgenic mice. J Exp Med 1992;175:1707–1715.
169. LaFace DM, Vestberg M, Yang Y, et al. Human CD8 transgene regulation of HLA recognition by murine T cells. J Exp Med 1995;182:1315–1325.
170. Alter B, Bach FH. Cellular basis of the proliferative response of human T cells to mouse xenoantigens. J Exp Med 1990;171:333–338.
171. Kalinke U, Arnold B, Hammerling GJ. Strong xenogeneic HLA response in transgenic mice after introducing an alpha-3 domain into HLA B27. Nature 1990;348:642–644.
172. Vignali DAA, Moreno J, Schiller D, Hammerling GJ. Species-specific binding of CD4 to the b2 domain of major histocompatibility complex class II molecules. J Exp Med 1992;175:925–932.
173. von Hoegen P, Miceli MC, Tourvieille B, et al. Equivalence of human and mouse CD4 in enhancing antigen responses by a mouse class II-restricted T cell hybridoma. J Exp Med 1989;170:1879–1886.
174. Gustafsson K, Germana S, Hirsch F, et al. Structure of miniature swine class II DRB genes: conservation of hypervariable amino acid residues between distantly related mammalian species. Proc Natl Acad Sci USA 1990;87:9798–9802.
175. Kumagai-Braesch M, Schachter B, Yan Z, et al. Identification of swine and primate cellular adhesion molecules (CAM) using mouse anti-human monoclonal antibodies. Xenotransplantation 1995;2:88–97.
176. Mueller JP, Evans MJ, Cofiell R, et al. Porcine vascular cell adhesion molecule (VCAM) mediates endothelial cell adhesion to human T cells. Transplantation 1995;60:1299–1306.
177. Herrlinger KR, Eckstein V, Muller-Ruchholtz W, Ulrichs K. Human T-cell activation is mediated predominantly by direct recognition of porcine SLA and involves accessory molecule interaction of ICAM1/LFA1 and CD2/LFA3. Transplant Proc 1996;28:650.
178. Grey ST, Hancock WW. A physiologic anti-inflammatory pathway based on thrombomodulin expression and generation of activated protein C by human mononuclear phagocytes. J Immunol 1996;156:2256–2263.
179. Bach FH. Xenotransplantation: problems and prospects. Annu Rev Med 1998;49:301–310.
180. Robson SC, Candinas D, Siegel JB, et al. Potential mechanism of abnormal thromboregulation in xenograft rejection: loss of ecto-ATPases upon endothelial cell activation. Transplant Proc 1996;28:536.
181. Robson SC, Young VK, Cook NS, et al. Thrombin inhibition in an ex vivo model of porcine heart xenograft hyperacute rejection. Transplantation 1996;61:862–868.
182. Tivol EA, Borriello F, Schweitzer AN, et al. Loss of CTLA-4 leads to massive lymphoproliferation and fatal multiorgan tissue destruction, revealing a critical negative regulatory role of CTLA-4. Immunity 1995;3:541–547.
183. Takahasbi T, Tanaka M, Inazawa J, et al. Human fas ligand: gene structure, chromosomal location and species compatibility. Int Immunol 1994;6:1567–1574.
184. Dorling A, Binns R, Lechler RI. Significant primary indirect human T-cell anti-pig xenoresponses observed using immature porcine dendritic cells and SLA-class II-negative endothelial cells. Transplant Proc 1996;28:654.
185. Sayegh MH, Watschinger B, Carpenter CB. Mechanisms of T cell recognition of alloantigen: the role of peptides. Transplantation 1994;57:1295–1302.
186. Auchincloss HJ, Lee R, Shea S, et al. The role of "indirect" recognition in initiating rejection of skin grafts from major histocompatibility complex class II-deficient mice. Proc Natl Acad Sci USA 1993;90:3373–3377.
187. Pierson RN, Winn HJ, Russell PS, Auchincloss AJ. Xenogeneic skin graft rejection is especially dependent on CD4+ T cells. J Exp Med 1989;170:991–996.
188. Kowalski L, Falqui L, Lacy PE, Scharp DW. Production of marked prolongation of survival of canine islet xenografts in mice by antilymphocyte sera and L3T4 antibody. Transplantation 1991;52:1094–1097.
189. Simeonovic CJ, Wilson JD. Role of CD4+ and CD8+ T cells in proislet allograft and xenograft rejection. Transplant Proc 1992;24:252–253.

190. Weber CJ, Zabinski S, Koschitzky T, et al. The role of CD4+ T cells in the destruction of microencapsulated islet xenografts in mice. Transplantation 1990;49:396–404.
191. Wecker H, Winn HJ, Auchincloss HJ. CD4+ T cells, without CD8+ or B lymphocytes, can reject xenogeneic skin grafts. Xenotransplantation 1994;1:8–16.
192. Wallgren AC, Karlsson-Parra A, Korsgren O. The main infiltrating cell in xenograft rejection is a CD4+ macrophage and not a T lymphocyte. Transplantation 1995;60:594–601.
193. Malyguine AM, Saadi S, Platt JL, Dawson JR. Human natural killer cells induce morphologic changes in porcine endothelial cell monolayers. Transplantation 1996;61:161–164.
194. Inverardi L, Samaja M, Motterlini R, et al. Early recognition of a discordant xenogeneic organ by human circulating lymphocytes. J Immunol 1992;149:1416–1423.
195. Markmann JF, Jacobson JD, Choti MA, et al. Modulation of major histocompatibility complex antigens and the immunogenicity of islet allografts. Transplantation 1989;48:478–486.
196. Bluestone JA, Pescovitz MD, Frels WI, et al. Cytotoxic T lymphocyte recognition of a xenogeneic major histocompatibility complex antigen expressed in transgenic mice. Eur J Immunol 1987;17:1035–1041.
197. Lenschow DJ, Zeng Y, Thistlethwaite JR, et al. Long-term survival of xenogeneic pancreatic islet grafts induced by CTLA4Ig. Science 1992;257:789–792.
198. Michler RE, McManus RP, Smith CR, et al. Prolongation of primate cardiac xenograft survival with cyclosporine. Transplantation 1987;44:632–636.
199. Ko DSC, Bartholomew A, Poncelet AJ, et al. Demonstration of multilineage chimerism in a nonhuman primate concordant xenograft model. Xenotransplantation 1998;5:298–304.
200. Sandrin MS, McKenzie IFC. Galα(1,3)Gal, the major xenoantigen(s) recognised in pigs by human natural antibodies. Immunol Rev 1994;141:169–190.
201. Sandrin MS, Vaughan HA, Dabkowski PL, McKenzie IFC. Anti-pig IgM antibodies in human serum reacts predominantly with Galα(1,3)Gal epitopes. Proc Natl Acad Sci USA 1993;90:11391–11395.
202. Cooper DK, Good AH, Koren E, et al. Identification of alpha-galactosyl and other carbohydrate epitopes that are bound by human anti-pig antibodies: relevance to discordant xenografting in man. Transpl Immunol 1993;1(3):198–205.
203. Cooper DK, Koren E, Oriol R. Oligosaccharides and discordant xenotransplantation. Immunol Rev 1994;141:31–58.
204. Landsteiner K. The specificity of serological reactions. Rev. ed. New York: Dover, 1962.
205. Galili U. Evolution and pathophysiology of the human natural anti-α-galactosyl IgG (anti-Gal) antibody. Springer Semin Immunopathol 1993;15:155–171.
206. Galili U, Macher BE, Buehler J, Shohet SB. Human natural anti-α-galactosyl IgG II. The specific recognition of α(1,3)-linked galactose residues. J Exp Med 1985;162:573–582.
207. Galili U, Rachmilewitz EA, Peleg A, Flechner I. A unique natural human IgG antibody with anti-α-galactosyl specificity. J Exp Med 1984;160:1519–1531.
208. Sablinski T, Gianello PR, Bailin M, et al. Pig-to-monkey bone marrow and kidney xenotransplantation. Surgery 1997;121:381–391.
209. Neethling FA, Koren E, Ye Y, et al. Protection of pig kidney (PK15) cells from the cytotoxic effect of anti-pig antibodies by α-galactosyl oligosaccharides. Transplantation 1994;57(6):959–963.
210. Vaughan HA, Loveland BE, Sandrin MS. Gal α(1,3)Gal is the major xenoepitope expressed on pig endothelial cells recognized by naturally occurring cytotoxic human antibodies. Transplantation 1994;58(8):879–882.
211. Sandrin MS, Dabkowski PL, Henning MM, et al. Characterization of cDNA clones for porcine α1,3 galactosyltransferase: the enzyme generating the Galα(1,3)Gal epitope. Xenotransplantation 1994;1:81–88.
212. McKenzie IFC, Vaughan HA, Sandrin MS. How important are anti-Galα(1,3)Gal antibodies in pig-to-human xenotransplants? Xeno 1994;2:107–110.
213. Oriol R, Ye Y, Koren E, Cooper DK. Carbohydrate antigens of pig tissues reacting with human natural antibodies as potential targets for hyperacute vascular rejection in pig-to-man organ xenotransplantation. Transplantation 1993;56(6):1433–1442.
214. McKenzie IF, Xing PX, Vaughan HA, et al. Distribution of the major xenoantigen (gal (α1–3)gal) for pig to human xenografts. Transpl Immunol 1994;2(2):81–86.
215. McKenzie IFC, Koulmanda M, Mandel TE, et al. Pig-to-human xenotransplantation: the expression of Galα(1,3)Gal epitopes on pig islet cells. Xenotransplantation 1995;2:1–7.
216. Vaughan HA, McKenzie IFC, Sandrin MS. Biochemical studies of pig xenoantigens detected by naturally occurring human antibodies and the galactoseα(1–3)galactose reactive lectin. Transplantation 1995;59(1):102–109.
217. Platt JL, Lindman BJ, Chen H, et al. Endothelial cell antigens recognized by xenoreactive human natural antibodies. Transplantation 1990;50:817–822.
218. Tuso PJ, Gramer DV, Middleton YD, et al. Pig aortic endothelial cell antigens recognized by human IgM natural antibodies. Transplantation 1993;56:651–655.
219. Thibaudeau K, Anegon I, Lemauff B, et al. Human natural antibodies to porcine platelets. Transplantation 1994;57:1110–1115.
220. Platt JL, Holzknecht ZE. Porcine platelet antigens recognized by human xenoreactive natural antibodies. Transplantation 1994;57:327–335.
221. Holzknecht ZE, Platt JL. Identification of porcine endothelial cell membrane antigens recognized by human xenoreactive natural antibodies. J Immunol 1995;154:4565–4575.
222. Larsen RD, Rajan VP, Ruff M, et al. Isolation of a cDNA encoding a murine UDPgalactose:β-D-galctosyl-1,4-N-acetyl-glucosaminide-α-1,3-galactosyltransferase: expression cloning by gene transfer. Proc Natl Acad Sci USA 1989;86:8227–8231.
223. Joziasse DH, Shaper NL, Kim D, et al. Murine α1,3 galactosyltransferase: a single gene locus specifies four isoforms of the enzyme by alternative spicing. J Biol Chem 1992;267:5534–5541.
224. Joziasse DH, Shaper JH, Van den Eijnden DH, et al. Bovine α1,3 galactosyltransferase: isolation and characterisation of a cDNA clone. Identification of homologous sequences in human genomic DNA. J Biol Chem 1989;264:14290–14297.
225. Strahan KM, Gu F, Preece AF, et al. cDNA sequence and chromosome localization of pig alpha 1,3 galactosyltransferase. Immunogenetics 1995;41:101–105.
226. Henion TR, Macher BA, Anaraki F, Galili U. Defining the minimal size of catalytically active primate α1,3galactosyltransferase: structure-function studies on the recombinant truncated enzyme. Glycobiology 1994;4:193–201.
227. Joziasse DH, Shaper JH, Jabs EW, Sharper NL. Characterisation of an α1,3-galactosyltransferase homologue on human chromosome 12 that is organised as a processed pseudogene. J Biol Chem 1991;266:6991–6998.
228. Larsen RD, Riverra-Marrero CA, Ernst LK, et al. Frameshift and non sense mutations in a human genomic sequence homologous to a murine UDP-Gal:β-D-Gal 1,4-D-GlcNAcα1,3-galactosyl-transferase cDNA. J Biol Chem 1990;265:7055–7061.
229. Yamamoto F, Clausen H, White T, et al. Molecular genetic basis of the histo-blood group ABO system. Nature 1990;345:229–233.
230. Coutinho A, Kazatchkine MD, Avrameas S. Natural autoantibodies. Curr Opin Immunol 1995;7:812–818.
231. Borie DC, Cramer DV, Shirwan H, et al. Genetic control of the humoral immune response to xenografts. II. Monoclonal antibodies that can cause rejection of heart xenografts are encoded by germline immunoglobulin genes. Transplantation 1995;60:1504–1510.
232. Galili U, Shohet SB, Korbin E, et al. Man, apes, and Old World mokeys differ from other mammals in the expression of α-galactosyl epitopes on nucleated cells. J Biol Chem 1988;263:17755–17762.
233. Galili U, Clark MR, Shohet SB, et al. Evolutionary relationship between the natural anti-Gal antibody and the Galα1–3Gal epitope in primates. Proc Natl Acad Sci USA 1987;84:1369–1373.
234. Ramasamy R. Is malaria linked to the adherence of α-galactosyl epitopes in Old World primates? Immunol Today 1994;15:140.
235. Parker W, Bruno D, Platt JL. Xenoreactive natural antibodies in the world of natural antibodies: typical or unique? Transplant Immunol 1995;3:181–191.
236. Aurell M, Samuelsson B, Breimer ME, et al. The first part of the goal of a project on xenotransplantation is achieved: porcine kidney in human circulation. LaKartidningen 1995;92:2655–2656.
237. Gianello PR, Latinne D, Alexandre GP. Pig-to-baboon renal xenografts. Xeno 1995;3:26–30.
238. Kaplon RJ, Platt JL, Kwiatkowski PA, et al. Absence of hyperacute rejection in pig-to-primate orthotopic pulmonary xenografts. Transplantation 1995;59:410–416.
239. Peirson III RN. Pig-to-primate lung xenografts: are they hyperacutely rejected? Xeno 1995;3:61–63.
240. Watts JM, Douglas MC, Dudley HAF, et al. Heterologous liver perfusion in acute liver failure. Br Med J 1967;2:341.
241. Lambrigts P, Sachs DH, Cooper DKC. Discordant organ xenotransplantation in primates. Transplantation 1998;66:547–561.

242. Fukushima N, Gundry SR, Matsumiya G, et al. Histological findings in heart grafts after orthotopic pig to baboon cardiac transplantation. Transplant Proc 1996;28:788–790.
243. Inverardi L, Ricordi C. Adult pigs as a source of insulin-producing tissue for xenotransplantation: islet separation technology. Xenotransplantation 1995;2:169–171.
244. Gores PF. New perspectives on islet transplantation. Xeno 1995;3:39–42.
245. Gray DWR, Song Z, Glover L, et al. Tissue culture prevents hyperacute rejection of islet xenografts. Xenotransplantation 1995;2:157–158.
246. McKenzie IFC, Koulmanda M, Sandrin MS, Mandel TE. Expression of Galα(1,3)Gal by porcine islet cells and its relevance to xenotransplantation. Xenotransplantation 1995;2:139–142.
247. Groth CG, Korsgren O, Tibell A, et al. Transplantation of porcine fetal pancreas to diabetic patients. Xeno 1994;2:102–106.
248. Groth CG, Korsgren O, Tibell A, et al. Transplantation of porcine fetal pancreas to diabetic patients. Lancet 1994;344:1402–1404.
249. Alexandre GPJ, Gianello P, Latinne D, et al. Plasmapheresis and splenectomy in experimantal renal xenotransplantation. In: Hardy MA, ed. Xenograft 25. New York: Elsevier, 1989:259–266.
250. Leventhal JR, Sakiyalak P, Witson J, et al. The synergistic effect of combined antibody and complement depletion on discordant cardiac xenograft survival in nonhuman primates. Transplantation 1994;57:974–978.
251. Leventhal JR, John R, Fryer JP, et al. Removal of baboon and human antiporcine IgG and IgM natural antibodies by immunoabsorption: results of in vitro and in vivo studies. Transplantation 1995;59:294–300.
252. Calne RY, White HJO, Herbertson BM, et al. Pig-to-baboon liver xenografts. Lancet 1968;1:1176.
253. Calne RY, Davis DR, Pena JR, et al. Hepatic allografts and xenografts in primates. Lancet 1970;1:103.
254. Cooper DKC, Human PA, Lexer G, et al. Effects of cyclosporine and antibody adsorption on pig cardiac xenograft survival in the baboon. J Heart Transplant 1988;7:238–246.
255. Ye Y, Cooper DKC. Experimental xenotransplantation in nonhuman primates using distantly related donor species. In: Cooper DKC, Kemp E, Reemtsma K, White DJG, eds. Xenotransplantation—the transplantation of organs and tissues between species. New York: Springer-Verlag, 1991:389–393.
256. Roslin MS, Zisbrod Z, Burack JH, et al. 15-day survival in pig-to-baboon heterotopic cardiac xenograft. Transplant Proc 1992;24:572–573.
257. Fukushima N, Bouchart F, Gundry SR, et al. The role of anti-pig antibody in pig-to-baboon cardiac xenotransplant rejection. Transplantation 1994;57:923–928.
258. Soares M, Havaux X, Latinne D, Bazin H. Depletion of xenoreactive natural antibodies by anti-μ monoclonal antibodies. Xeno 1994;2:88–92.
259. Ye Y, Neethling FA, Niekrasz M, et al. Evidence that intravenously administered alpha-galactosyl carbohydrates reduce baboon serum cytotoxicity to pig kidney cells (PK15) and transplanted pig hearts. Transplantation 1994;58(3):330–337.
260. Vaughan HA, Oldenburg KR, Gallop MA, et al. Recognition of an octapeptide sequence by multiple Galα(1,3)Gal-binding peptides. Xenotransplantation 1996;3:18–23.
261. Kooyman DL, McClellan SB, Parker W, et al. Identification and characterization of a galactosyl peptide mimetic. Implications for use in removing xenoreactive anti-A Gal antibodies. Transplantation 1996;61:851–855.
262. McKenzie IFC, Osman N, Cohney S, et al. Strategies to overcome the anti-Galα(1,3)Gal reaction in xenotransplantation. Transplant Proc 1996;28:567.
263. McKenzie IFC, Paton K, Smit JA, et al. Definition and characterisation of chicken anti-Galα(1,3)Gal antibodies. J Immunol 1996 (in press).
264. Mulder LCF, Ciccopiedi E, Mora M, et al. Livers of mice transgenic for human CD46 are protected from complement attack. Transgenics 1995;1:629–637.
265. McCurry KR, Kooyman DL, Diamond LE, et al. Transgenic expression of human complement regulatory proteins in mice results in diminished complement deposition during organ xenoperfusion. Transplantation 1995;59:1177–1182.
266. Somerville C, van Denderen B, Adam B, et al. Expression and function of human CD59 and human CD55 in transgenic mice. Transplant Proc 1995;27:3565–3566.
267. McCurry KR, Kooyman DL, Alvarado CG, et al. Human complement regulatory proteins protect swine-to-primate cardiac xenografts from humoral injury. Nat Med 1995;1:423–427.
268. Waterworth PD, Cozzi E, Tolan MJ, et al. Pig-to-primate cardiac xenotranslantation and cyclophosphamide therapy. Transplant Proc 1997;29:899–901.
269. Schmoeckel M, Bhatti FNK, Zaidi A, et al. Orthotopic heart transplantation in a transgenic pig-to-primate model. Transplantation 1998;65:1570–1577.
270. Kooyman DL, Byrne GW, McClellan Nielsen D, et al. In vivo transfer of GPI-linked complement restriction factors from erythrocytes to the endothelium. Science 1995;269:89–92.
271. Somerville CA, Kyriazis AG, McKenzie A, et al. Functional expression of human CD59 in transgenic mice. Transplantation 1994;58:1430–1435.
272. Diamond LE, McCurry KR, Oldham ER, et al. Human CD59 expressed in transgenic mouse hearts inhibits the activation of complement. Transpl Immunol 1995;3:305–312.
273. Kroshus TJ, Bolman RM, Dalmasso AP, et al. Expression of human CD59 in transgenic pig organs enhances organ survival in an ex vivo xenogeneic perfusion model. Transplantation 1996;61:1513–1521.
274. Fodor WL, Williams BL, Matis LA, et al. Expression of a functional human complement inhibitor in a transgenic pig as a model for the prevention of xenogeneic hyperacute organ rejection. Proc Natl Acad Sci USA 1994;91:11153–11157.
275. Fodor WL, Squinto SP. Engineering of transgenic pigs for xenogeneic organ transplantation. Xeno 1995;3:23–25.
276. Fodor WL, Rollins SA, Guilmette ER, et al. A novel bifunctional chimeric complement inhibitor that regulates C3 convertase and formation of the membrane attack complex. J Immunol 1995;155:4135–4138.
277. Iwata K, Seya T, Ariga H, Nagasawa S. Expression of a hybrid complement regulatory protein, membrane cofactor protein decay accelerating factor on Chinese hamster ovary cells. Comparison of its regulatory effect with those of decay accelerating factor and membrane cofactor protein. J Immunol 1994;152:3436–3444.
278. Hayashi S, Emi N, Isobe K, et al. Evidence that double transfection to endothelial cells using GPI-anchoring complement regulatory factor (DAF and HRF20) genes is useful for the inhibition of human complement-mediated cytolysis. Xenotransplantation 1995;2:298–294.
279. Hayashi S, Emi N, Isobe K, et al. Inhibitory effect of double transfection to xenoendothelial cells using both decay accelerating factor and homologous restriction factor 20 genes on complement dependent cytolysis. J Surg Res 1996;61:165–169.
280. Weisman HF, Bartow T, Leppo MK, et al. Soluble human complement receptor type 1: in vivo inhibitor of complement suppressing postischemic myocardial inflammation and necrosis. Science 1990;249:146–151.
281. Morgan BP. Complement regulatory molecules: application to therapy and transplantation. Immunol Today 1995;16:257–259.
282. Pruitt SK, Baldwin WM, Marsh HC, et al. The effect of soluble complement receptor type 1 on hyperacute xenograft rejection. Transplantation 1991;52:868–873.
283. Zehr KJ, Herskowitz A, Lee PC, et al. Neutrophil adhesion and complement inhibition prolongs survival of cardiac xenografts in discordant species. Transplantation 1994;57:900–906.
284. Pruitt SK, Kirk AD, Bollinger RR, et al. The effect of soluble complement receptor type 1 on hyperacute rejection of porcine xenografts. Transplantation 1994;57:363–370.
285. Shandelya SML, Kuppusamy P, Herskowitz A, et al. Soluble complement receptor type 1 inhibits the complement pathway and prevents contractile failure in the postischemic heart. Evidence that complement activation is required for neutrophil-mediated reperfusion injury. Circulation 1993;88:2812–2826.
286. Gillinov AM, de Valeria PA, Winkelstein JA, et al. Complement inhibition with soluble complement receptor type 1 in cardiopulmonary bypass. Ann Thorac Surg 1993;55:619–624.
287. Chavez-Cartaya R, de Sola GP, Wright L, et al. Regulation of the complement cascade by soluble complement receptor type 1. Protective effect in experimental liver ischemia and reperfusion. Transplantation 1995;59:1047–1052.
288. Pemberton M, Anderson G, Vetvicka V, et al. Microvascular effects of complement blockade with soluble recombinant CR1 in ischemia/reperfusion injury of skeletal muscle. J Immunol 1993;150:5104–5113.
289. Hill J, Lindsay TF, Ortiz F, et al. Soluble complement receptor type 1 ameliorates the local and remote organ injury after intestinal ischemia-reperfusion in the rat. J Immunol 1992;149:1732–1728.
290. Yeh CG, Marsh HC, Carson GR, et al. Recombinant soluble human complement receptor type 1 inhibits inflammation in the reversed passive Arthus reaction in rats. J Immunol 1991;146:250–256.
291. Rossi AG, Norman KE, Donigi-Gale D, et al. The role of complement, platelet-activating factor and leukotriene B4 in a reversed passive Arthus reaction. Br J Pharmacol 1992;107:44–49.

292. Seya T, Kurita M, Hara T, et al. Blocking measles virus infection with a recombinant soluble form of, or monoclonal antibodies against, membrane cofactor protein of complement (CD46). Immunology 1995;84:619–625.
293. Devaux P, Loveland B, Christiansen D, et al. Interactions between the ectodomains of haemagglutinin and CD46 as a primary step in measles virus entry. J Gen Virol 1996;77:1477–1481.
294. Moran P, Beasley H, Gorrell A, et al. Human recombinant soluble decay accelerating factor inhibits complement activation in vitro and in vivo. J Immunol 1992;149:1736–1743.
295. Ollert MW, David K, Bredehorst R, Vogel CW. Classical complement pathway activation on nucleated cells. Role of factor H in the control of deposited C3b. J Immunol 1995;155:4955–4962.
296. Okada N, Liszewski MK, Atkinson JP, Caparon M. Membrane cofactor protein (CD46) is a keratinocyte receptor for the M protein of the group A streptococcus. Proc Natl Acad Sci USA 1995;92:2489–2493.
297. Nowicki B, Hart A, Coyne KE, et al. Short consensus repeat-3 domain of recombinant decay-accelerating factor is recognized by *Escherichia coli* recombinant Dr adhesin in a model of a cell-cell interaction. J Exp Med 1993;178:2115–2121.
298. Ward T, Pipkin PA, Clarkson NA, et al. Decay-accelerating factor CD55 is identified as the receptor for echovirus 7 using CELICS, a rapid immuno-focal cloning method. EMBO J 1994;13:5070–5074.
299. Bergelson JM, Chan M, Solomon KR, et al. Decay-accelerating factor (CD55), a glycosylphosphatidylinositol-anchored complement regulatory protein, is a receptor for several echoviruses. Proc Natl Acad Sci USA 1994;91:6245–6249.
300. Bergelson JM, Mohanty JG, Crowell RL, et al. Coxsackievirus B3 adapted to growth in RD cells binds to decay-accelerating factor (CD55). J Virol 1995;69:1903–1906.
301. Shafren D, Bates RC, Agrez MV, et al. Coxsackieviruses B1, B3, and B5 use decay acceleration factor as a receptor for cell attachment. J Virol 1995;69:3873–3877.
302. Kroshus TJ, Rollins SA, Dalmasso AP, et al. Complement inhibition with an anti C5 monoclonal antibody prevents acute cardiac tissue injury in an ex vivo model of pig to human xenotransplantation. Transplantation 1995;60:1194–1202.
303. Evans MJ, Rollins SA, Wolff DW, et al. In vitro and in vivo inhibition of complement activity by a single chain Fv fragment recognizing human C5. Mol Immunol 1995;32:1183–1195.
304. Rollins SA, Matis LA, Springhorn JP, et al. Monoclonal antibodies directed against human C5 and C8 block complement mediated damage of xenogeneic cells and organs. Transplantation 1995;60:1284–1292.
305. Thall AD, Maly P, Lowe JB. Oocyte Galα1,3Gal Epitopes implicated in sperm adhesion to the zona pellucida glycoprotein ZP3 are not required for fertilization in the mouse. J Biol Chem 1995;270:21437–21440.
306. Tearle RG, Tange MJ, Zannettino ZL, et al. The α-1,3-galactosyltransferase knockout mouse: implications for xenotransplantation. Transplantation 1996;61:13–19.
307. Osman N, McKenzie IF, Ostenried K, et al. Combined transgenic expression of α-galactosidase and α-1,2-fucosyl transferase leads to optimal reduction in the major xenoepitope Galα(1,3)Gal. Proc Natl Acad Sci 1997;94:14677–14821.
308. Sandrin MS, Fodor WL, Mouhtouris E, et al. Enzymatic remodelling of the carbohydrate surface of a xenogenic cell substantially reduces human antibody binding and complement-mediated cytolysis. Nat Med 1995;1:1261–1267.
309. Cohney S, McKenzie IF, Patton K, et al. Downregulation of Galα(1,3)Gal expression by α1,2fucosyltransferase: Further characterization of α1,2-fucosyl transferase transgenic mice. Transplantation 1997;64:495–500.
310. Grusby MJ, Auchincloss HJ, Lee R, et al. Mice lacking major histocompatibility complex class I and class II molecules. Proc Natl Acad Sci USA 1993;90:3913–3917.
311. Charlton B, Auchincloss HJ, Fathman CG. Mechanisms of transplantation tolerance. Annu Rev Immunol 1994;12:707–734.
312. Ildstad ST, Wren SM, Sharrow SO, et al. In vivo and in vitro characterization of specific hyporeactivity to skin xenografts in mixed xenogeneically reconstituted mice (B10 + F344 rat to B10). J Exp Med 1984;160:1820.
313. Sharabi Y, Aksentijevich I, Sundt III TM, et al. Specific tolerance induction across a xenogeneic barrier: production of mixed rat/mouse lymphohematopoietic chimeras using a nonlethal preparative regimen. J Exp Med 1990;172:195–202.
314. Sachs DH, Sykes M, Greenstein JL, Cosimi AB. Tolerance as the key to long-term xenograft survival. Nat Med 1995;9:969.
315. Fishman JA. Miniature swine as organ donors for man: strategies for prevention of xenotransplant-associated infections. Xenotransplantation 1994;1:47–57.
316. Fishman JA. Preventing Infections in xenotransplantation: xenosis from miniature swine. Xeno 1995;3:72–77.
317. Michaels MG, Simmons RL. Xenotransplant-associated zoonoses: strategies for prevention. Transplantation 1994;57:1–7.
318. Michaels MG. Infectious concerns of cross-species transplantation. World J Surg 1997;21:968–974.
319. Ye Y, Niekrasz M, Kosanke S, et al. The pig as a potential organ donor for man. A study of potentially transferable disease from donor pig to recipient man. Transplantation 1994;57:694–703.
320. Pirtle EC. Incidence of antibody to swine influenza virus in Iowa breeder and butcher pigs correlated with signs of influenza-like illness. Am J Vet Res 1973;34:83–85.
321. Schnurrenberger PR, Woods GT, Martin RJ. Serologic evidence of human infection with swine influenza virus. Am Rev Respir Dis 1970;102:356–361.
322. Sugimura T, Yonemochi H, Ogawa T, et al. Isolation of a recombinant influenza virus (Hsw1N2) from swine in Japan. Arch Virol 1980;66:271–274.
323. Hinshaw VS, Bean WJJ, Webster RG, Easterday BC. The prevalence of influenza viruses in swine and the antigenic and genetic relatedness of influenza viruses from man and swine. Virology 1978;84:51–62.
324. Khabbaz RF, Heneine W, George JR, et al. Infection of a laboratory worker with simian immunodeficiency virus. New Engl J Med 1994;330:172–177.
325. Holmes GP, Chapman LE, Steward JA, et al. Guidelines for the prevention and treatment of B-virus in exposed persons. Clin Infect Dis 1995;20:421–439.
326. Gloster J, Sellers RF, Donaldson AI. Long distance transport of foot-and-mouth disease virus over sea. Vet Rec 1982;100:47–52.
327. Schwarz A, Offermann G, Keller F, et al. The effect of cyclosporine on the progression of human immunodeficiency virus type 1 infection transmitted by transplantation—data on four cases and review of the literature. Transplantation 1993;55:95–103.
328. Bowden RA, Coombs RW, Nikora BH, et al. Progression of human immunodefiency virus type-1 infection after allogeneic marrow transplantation. Am J Med 1990;88(5N):49N–52N.
329. Levy JA. Murine xenotropic type C Viruses. III. Phenotypic mixing with avian leukosis and sarcoma viruses. Virology 1977;77:811–825.
330. Spector DH, Wade E, Wright DA, et al. Human immunodeficiency virus pseudotypes with expanded cellular and species tropism. J Virol 1990;64:2298–2308.
331. Lusso P, Di Marzo Veronese F, Ensoli B, et al. Expanded HIV-1 cellular tropism by phenotypic mixing with murine endogenous retroviruses. Science 1990;247:848–852.
332. Levin JL, Hilliard JK, Lipper SL, et al. A naturally occurring epizootic of simian agent 8 in the baboon. Lab Anim Sci 1988;38:394–397.
333. Katz RA, Skalka AM. Generation of diversity in retroviruses. Annu Rev Genet 1990;24:409–445.
334. Javier RT, Sedarati F, Stevens JG. Two avirulent herpes simplex viruses generate lethal recombinants in vivo. Science 1986;234:746–748.
335. Isfort R, Jones D, Kost R, et al. Retrovirus insertion into herpesvirus in vitro and in vivo. Proc Natl Acad Sci USA 1992;89:991–995.
336. Rando RF, Srinivasan A, Feingold J, et al. Characterization of multiple molecular interactions between human cytomegalovirus (HCMV) and human immunodeficiency virus type 1 (HIV-1). Virology 1990;176:87–97.
337. Temin HM. Reverse transcription in the eukaryotic genome, retroviruses, pararetroviruses, retrotransposons, and retrotranscripts. Mol Biol Evol 1985;6:455–468.
338. Todaro GJ, Benveniste RE, Lieber MM, Sherr CJ. Characteristics of a type C virus released from the porcine cell line PK(15). Virology 1974;58:65–74.
339. Bouillant AMP, Grieg AS, Lieber MM, Todaro GJ. Type-C virus production by a continuous line of pig oviduct cells (PFT). J Gen Virol 1975;27:173–180.
340. Lieber MM, Sherr CH, Benveniste RE, Todaro GJ. Biologic and immunologic properties of porcine type C viruses. Virology 1975;66:616–619.
341. Suzuka I, Sekiguchi K, Kodama M. Some characteristics of a porcine retrovirus from a cell line derived from swine malignant lymphomas. FEBS Lett 1985;183:124–128.
342. Kaeffer B, Bottreau E, Thanh LP, et al. Histocompatible miniature boar model: selection of transformed cell lines of B and T lineages producing retrovirus. Int J Cancer 1990;46:481–488.

343. Patience C, Takeuchi Y, Weiss A. Infection of human cells by an endogenous retrovirus of pigs. Nature Med 1997;3:282–286.
344. Heneine W, Tibell A, Switzer WM, et al. No evidence of infection with porcine endogenous retrovirus in recipients of porcine islet-cell xenografts. Lancet 1998;352:695–699.
345. Patience C, Patton GS, Takeuchi Y, et al. No evidence of pig DNA or retroviral infection in patients with short-term extracorporeal connection to pig kidneys. Lancet 1998;352:699–701.
346. Rother RP, Fodor WL, Springhorn JP, et al. A novel mechanism of retrovirus inactivation in human serum mediated by anti-alpha-galactosyl natural antibody. J Exp Med 1995;182:1345–1355.
347. Welsh RM, Jensen FC, Cooper NR, Oldstone MBA. Inactivation and lysis of oncornaviruses by human serum. Virology 1976;74:432–440.
348. Almeida IC, Milani SR, Gorin AJ, Travoassos LR. Complement mediated lysis of *Trypanosoma cruzi* tryptomastigotes by human anti-αgalactosyl antibodies. J Immunol 1991;146:2394–2400.
349. Snyder HWJ, Fleissner E. Specificity of human antibodies to oncovirus glycoproteins: recognition of antigen by natural antibodies directed against carbohydrate structures. Proc Natl Acad Sci USA 1980;77:1622–1626.
350. Barbacid M, Bolognesi D, Aaronson SA. Humans have antibodies capable of recognizing oncoviral glycoproteins: demonstration that these antibodies are formed in response to cellular modification of glycoproteins rather than as consequence of exposure to virus. Proc Natl Acad Sci USA 1980;77:1617–1621.
351. Hamadeh RM, Jarvis GA, Galili U, et al. Human natural anti-Gal IgG regulates alternative complement pathway activation on bacterial surfaces. J Clin Invest 1992;89:1223–1235.
352. Platt JL, Parker W. Another step towards xenotransplantation. Nat Med 1995;1:1248–1250.
353. Welsh RM, Cooper NR, Jensen FC, Oldstone MBA. Human serum lyses RNA tumour viruses. Nature 1975;257:612–614.
354. Cooper NR, Jensen FC, Raymond MW, Oldstone MBA. Lysis of RNA tumor viruses by human serum: direct antibody-independent triggering of the classical complement pathway. J Exp Med 1976;144:970–984.
355. Bartholomew RM, Esser AF, Muller-Eberhard HJ. Lysis of oncornaviruses by human serum: isolation of the viral complement (C1) receptor and identification as p15E. J Exp Med 1978;147:844–853.
356. Cornetta K, Moen RC, Culver K, et al. Amphotropic murine leukemia retrovirus is not an acute pathogen for primates. Hum Gene Ther 1990;1:15–30.
357. Takeuchi Y, Cosset FC, Lachmann PJ, et al. Type C retrovirus inactivation by human complement is determined by both the viral genome and the producer cell. J Virol 1994;68:8001–8007.
358. Michaels MG, Lanford R, Demetris AJ, et al. Lack of susceptibility of baboons to infection with hepatitis B virus. Transplantation 1996;61:350–351.
359. Bjoersdorff A, Korsgren O, Feinstein R, et al. Microbiological characterization of porcine fetal ilset-like cell clusters for intended clinical xenografting. Xenotransplantation 1995;2:26–31.
360. Rogers NJ, Dorling A, Moore M. Xenotransplantation: steps toward a clinical reality. Immunol Today 1998;19:206–208.

COMMENTARY REFERENCES

1. Hammer C. Evolutionary obstacles to xenotransplantation. In: Cooper DKC, Kemp E, Platt JL, Wite DJG, eds. Xenotransplantation, 2nd ed. Heidelberg: Springer, 1997:716–725.
2. Cooper DKC, Kemp E, Platt JL, White DJG, eds. Xenotransplantation. 2nd ed. Heidelberg: Springer, 1997.
3. Bach FH, Robson SC, Winkler H, et al. Barriers to xenotransplantation. Nat Med 1995;1:869–873.
4. White DJG. hDAF transgenic pig organs: are they concordant for human transplantation? Xeno 1996;4:50–54.
5. Davis EA, Pruitt SK, Greene PS, et al. Inhibition of complement, evoked antibody, and cellular response prevents rejection of pig-to-primate cardiac xenografts. Transplantation 1996;62:1018–1023.
6. Koren E, Milotic F, Neethling FA, et al. Monoclonal antidiotypic antibodies neutralize cytotoxic effects of anti-αGal antibodies. Transplantation 1996;62:837–843.
7. Chae SJ, Cooper DKC. Legal implications of xenotransplantation. Xenotransplantation 1997;4:132–139.

Chapter 41

Understanding Organ Procurement and the Transplant Bureaucracy

JAMES F. BURDICK JOHAN DEMEESTER ISAMU KOYAMA

Transplantation, although a relatively recent area for federal consideration, has engendered a national bureaucracy in the United States that is in certain respects singular. How and why this is so may be understood at the organizational level and, more profoundly, at the level of the medical and historical forces responsible. This chapter considers both perspectives regarding transplantation in the United States and in other parts of the world. The fundamental issue in transplantation that distinguishes it from other aspects of medicine is that it involves transfer of a living portion of a human being from one person to another. This has had a powerful effect in every setting in which it has been practiced.

THE UNITED STATES

Historical and Legislative Background: Formation of the National System

When the US Congress passed the National Organ Transplant Act (NOTA) of 1984 (Pub. L. No. 98-507), it was partly the result of a few years of deliberation but was also an ad hoc response to recent publicized donor appeals and a directive from President Ronald Reagan. The remarkable improvement in transplantation outcomes provided by cyclosporine had produced a sense of urgency to make more organs available to respond to the increased demand relative to the supply. A series of hearings had been held by then Congressman Albert Gore that illuminated these issues and created fertile legislative soil. The bill was passed because of concerns that the field had succumbed to special interests, that its practices were not in the best interest of the public in general, and that there was no national impetus to maximize the possible public health benefits of the recently expanded capabilities of transplantation. In a detailed account of the sociologic background of this national movement, it was noted that a major influence on public thinking regarding oversight of medical resource allocation was the recent experience with choosing which patients would be funded to receive dialysis before there was general coverage for end-stage renal disease (1). Exclusively public control had been found unsatisfactory, but there was too much suspicion of professionals in the field, engendered in part by sensationalist press reports, to allow them to control it without public input.

The exact form support for transplantation should take represented an interesting tension between the Reagan administration and the Republican Senate, which wanted strong controls but a completely private process, and the Democratic House of Representatives (2). Some of the draft legislation provided for organ transplantation to be managed completely within the administration. Ultimately it was clearly stipulated that a private entity was to be responsible.

Among the ingredients of NOTA in 1984 were prohibition on the buying of organs, establishment of grants to organ procurement agencies, and recommendation of a national organ sharing system. In addition, the Act established a Task Force on Organ Transplantation. The Task Force was composed of 25 individuals from the areas of medicine, law, theology, ethics, allied health, the health insurance industry, and the general public. National Institutes of Health, Food and Drug Administration, and Health Care Financing Administration representation was included. Chaired by Dr. Olga Jonasson, the Task Force carried out extensive deliberations through focus groups, public meetings, and hearings.

The Report of the Task Force on Organ Transplantation (3) provided an extensive series of recommendations in all areas of transplantation. To facilitate organ and tissue donation, it was recommended that a Uniform Determination of Death Act be enacted by all states without one, hospital and medical examiner facilitation of donation be provided, hospital regulatory bodies make provision for donation efforts, public and professional education be extended, organ procurement agencies be centralized and certified, national data on organ retrieval and transplantation be collected, and tissue and organ recovery efforts be coordinated. The Task Force concluded that a unified national system of organ sharing was desirable, and recommended a network with broad governance and specific policy considerations. It also provided a detailed proposal for the structure and function of an Organ Procurement and Transplant Network (OPTN). Commercialization of the organ recovery and sharing process was rejected, and a restriction on the fraction of recipients that could be foreign nationals was specified. The Report of the Task Force also endorsed support for diffusion of technology and research. The foundation of the structures recommended was a balance of "procedural justice" and medical utility (1), which was echoed in a more recent national referendum on organ allocation by John Whelchel (4).

Many of the details in these national provisions were derived from less generalized practices underway at the time. For years transplant professionals had quietly been collaborating regionally on various aspects of the field that were dealt with on the national level by the Task Force. For instance, under the aegis of Paul Terasaki, the UCLA registry was studying characteristics and outcomes of large numbers of kidney transplants in its database, particularly with regard to the benefits of histocompatibility matching (5). The New England Organ Bank had been sharing kidneys on a regional basis from the late 1970s, with an emphasis on arranging for transplantation of the patient with high levels of panel reactive antibody (PRA) when possible. However, the structure and functions of the South Eastern Organ Procurement Foundation (SEOPF) were most generally in line with the Task Force recommendations.

Under pioneers such as David Hume and Bernard Amos, SEOPF had started as a complex of small centers in the southeast that had banded together to share organs because they were often unable to use a specific donor due to small numbers of medically suitable recipients. The process included networked collaboration on the still relatively primitive tissue typing techniques to optimize these and study their effects, a computerized listing and sharing system, and a stringent requirement that all transplants and their outcomes be reported centrally for analysis. By the mid-1980s, because of the advantage of the real-time computerized organ sharing system that it had pioneered and refined, membership in SEOPF had grown beyond the southeastern United States to encompass major portions of the country. SEOPF enabled nonmembers to participate in organ sharing via its computer matching system, which SEOPF called the *United Network for Organ Sharing*. In 1984, when SEOPF and American Society of Transplant Surgeons (ASTS) were forming a national organization and testifying in the hearings that led to NOTA (6), UNOS was a natural choice.

By 1985 a request for proposals (RFP) was published soliciting competitive proposals for the formation of the OPTN. Not surprisingly, UNOS won the OPTN and Scientific Registry contracts. The executive director and a principal architect of SEOPF, Gene Pierce, and a large number of other key SEOPF staff moved to the UNOS headquarters in Richmond. The transfer of personnel, equipment, and license for computer code was provided to UNOS by SEOPF for $1.00. UNOS began to construct the national process, based largely in all aspects from conceptual to computer code on the SEOPF system. During the first year, all existing patients awaiting transplant were incorporated into the national lists and the organ center began functioning 24 hours a day for national organ placement. The SEOPF matching code was used to generate a new point system based on Tom Starzl's proposal for renal and extrarenal allocation. The Policy Board and committees were formed, and membership criteria for transplant centers were developed.

A major organizational difference from the proposal by the Task Force was that the Scientific Registry was contracted separately from the Organ Center, where the responsibility lay for the day-to-day process of organ sharing. This has been rationalized as important to ensure appropriate competition in some way. However, since the data necessarily flow from the process, the distinction is conceptually inappropriate and potentially harmful insofar as completeness and validity are more accurately and efficiently ensured by a union of the two endeavors. The Scientific Registry contract was sole source, granted to UNOS, in 1987; since 1991, when this became a competitive contract, UNOS has won the bids. Because of the expertise available in the country, and in order to ensure the most broad-based support from the transplant community, established non-UNOS-based registries were appointed to subcontract the data collection and analysis effort. These "distributed registries" were the UCLA Terasaki database for kidneys; the Pittsburgh liver registry that had been developed largely by Robert Gordon; the Minnesota pancreas transplant database under Katherine Detre and David Sutherland; and the International Society of Heart Transplantation under Michael Kaye. Over time it has been necessary to incorporate data flow increasingly into UNOS, with special access for additional scientific studies retained by these registries.

The Social Security Act in 1987 was amended to require transplant centers and organ procurement organizations (OPOs) to belong to the OPTN in order to be deemed a Medicare provider. Reauthorization occurred in 1988 and 1991, and there has been no successful passage of reauthorization since. In 1994, bills passed both congressional houses but died in conference. In 1996, a version of NOTA reauthorization with important restrictive alterations cleared the House precipitously as part of the term wrap-up, but was not addressed in the Senate. Reauthorization is technically required only to authorize funding appropriations by Congress. For the fiscal years since reauthorization, implied funding has been carried through.

Federal funds have never supplied the majority of the budget. However, UNOS was already doing much of the work of the OPTN before the contract with its own funding. A registration fee is paid to UNOS for each patient put on the waiting list that supplements federal funds and, in fact, supplies the majority of the UNOS operating budget. However, in the cost-cutting environment of the new Republican Congress that came to Washington after the 1994 elections, even this degree of federal support is threatened, and it has become clear that UNOS must become financially self-sufficient. Legislative re-enactment will not be important for funding, although specifics about the contract, the flow of funds, control over policy, and enforcement could have major impacts if and when NOTA is reauthorized.

HCFA, HRSA, and DOT: The Organizational Relationships

To administer the federal transplant program, the Division of Transplantation (DOT—easily confused with the Department of Transportation, which does not seem to be a problem in acronymically sophisticated Washington), was authorized by NOTA. Figure 41.1 depicts how the DOT fits in the formal bureaucratic structure of the Department of Health and Human Services (DHHS). It is under the Bureau of Health Resources Development in the Health Resources and Services Administration (HRSA), an arm of the Public Health Service (PHS), along with the National Institutes of Health (NIH), the Food and Drug Administration (FDA), and the Centers for Disease Control (CDC). There is often confusion on the structural relationship to the Health Care Financing Administration (HCFA), which is another branch of the DHHS at the same level as the PHS. In general, the NIH, the HRSA, and other agencies are increasingly uninvolved with the intermediary of PHS involvement, in contrast to the formal structure depicted.

In addition to the OPTN, a major component of NOTA was the formation of the current OPO system, in which HCFA designates OPOs with exclusive service areas. The legislation mandates OPO responsibilities, including the requirement that each OPO have a system to allocate organs equitably. The goals of HRSA include several minority and rural health care initiatives, participating in the campaign against HIV and AIDS, and development of a comprehensive quality assurance program for health care, in addition to administering NOTA. Of a budget for fiscal year 1995 of just over \$3 billion for HRSA, \$7.7 million were assigned to the Bureau of Health Resources Development, which administers three other programs in addition to the DOT. In fiscal year 1995, UNOS received \$2,356,500. There is no improvement foreseeable in this paucity of federal funding. Within the administration the view has been expressed that, since the contract mandates patient registration fees, the government should

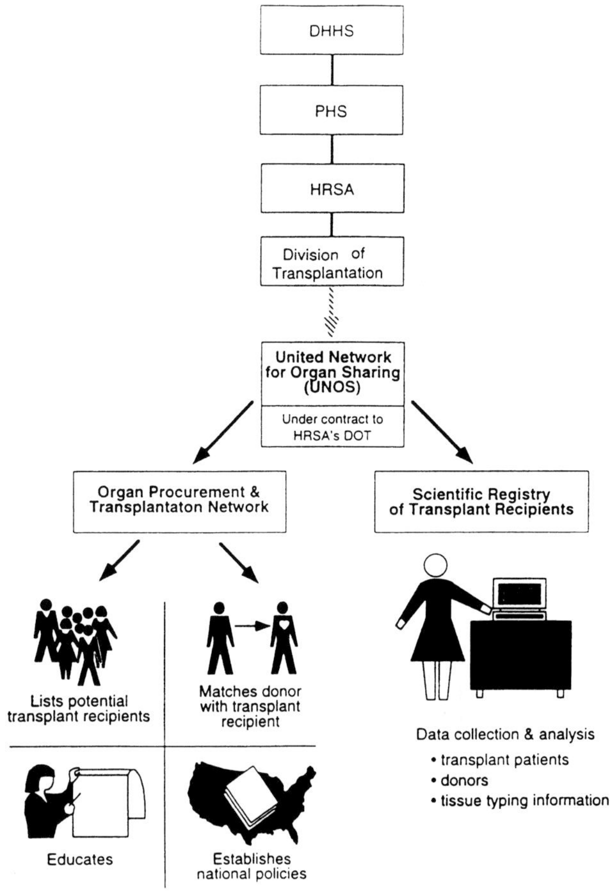

FIGURE 41.1. *UNOS within the administrative structure of DHHS.*

consider this income to fall under its control, but this idea is unlikely to be either publicly or legally supportable.

Although HCFA organizationally is a separate branch of HHS, a powerful potential tie with DOT exists. Effective in 1987, OBRA specified that if it was determined after due process that a center did not observe the rules of the OPTN, eligibility for HCFA reimbursement for all services could be withdrawn from that center. Since this would be a major financial issue for almost every hospital, it would seem to be a powerful enforcement tool. However, after a brief period beginning October 1987, during which this policy had the effect of law, the DHHS stated in 1991 that the OPTN rules are not binding until finalized as regulations, which has not yet occurred. Proposed regulations were published in 1994, but since these have never been finalized, they are not in force. Since there is nothing that formally details policy, and nothing vesting UNOS rules with this authority, OPTN policy remains voluntary in the sense that the threat of withdrawal of HCFA funding is moot.

The situation of DOT within the organizational structure of the DHHS may help to explain the difficulty with the OPTN dictating HCFA reimbursement policy, and this enforcement tool may never materialize. However, as a practical matter, the major policies that have been put in place after debate among the interested parties are probably disregarded no more than any other federal regulation or law. This general compliance, which has allowed the field to retain a relatively unsullied reputation, is a testimony to both the idealism and the realism of those involved. Another disagreement within the administration regarding the way UNOS is constituted, as opposed to its being a formal agency or entity within the executive structure of the DHHS, is found within HRSA, for instance in the Office of Planning, Evaluation and Legislation.

A source of difficulty in coordinating transplantation activities stems from the designation by NOTA of the OPOs to be overseen by Medicare, which is administered by HCFA. With the national OPTN under a different branch—namely, HRSA—problems can arise in communication, and potentially in substance, regarding policy.

Two other agencies that might have an impact on transplantation are the FDA and CDC. Recently, the CDC has become concerned about disease transmission by organs and tissues and issued a set of guidelines (7) that many transplant professionals felt represented an onerous lack of perspective based on the certain major risks of the diseases treated by transplantation versus the statistically demonstrable known minimal risk of transmission of disease (such as HIV) by transplantation ensured by the highly protective practices already in place. After further dialogue, a clarification indicating the importance of reasonable policies for organ use was issued.

The FDA has indicated an interest in two areas related to transplantation. It has been announced that any setting in which cells are removed from the body, processed in any way, and then replaced in a patient is subject to FDA regulation. This could affect islet cell transplantation and the use of treated cells for infusion to establish chimeric tolerance. Second, the FDA seems to be committed to regulation of the use of xenotransplantation should this technique become a reality. Since xenotransplant outcomes are likely to affect human allograft procedures for some time to come, interference with UNOS policies is foreseeable and may cause major problems if accommodation between UNOS and the FDA is not arranged well in advance. If it were to become reasonably successful, the medical possibilities of xenotransplantation would produce an irresistible tide that could quickly become difficult to control.

Given this administrative context, it is apparent that survival of UNOS has been critically dependent on its excellent service to the field of transplantation in all its complexity.

UNOS Structure

UNOS is a nonprofit entity incorporated in the state of Virginia. Its mission statement presently is: "We strive for continual improvement in transplantation through collective self-governance to benefit patients with organ failure." From the beginning, the description of work by HRSA was divided into two contracts, one for the Scientific Registry and one for the OPTN. This division was not in the original authorizing legislation and, as noted above, could be harmful. UNOS has been awarded these contracts on a three-year cycle since 1986. Funding for UNOS operations including the OPTN is derived, in addition, by fees from the membership in the form of a registration fee paid by the transplant program for each potential recipient listed on the computer. The UNOS Foundation is a not-for-profit subsidiary that is wholly owned by UNOS, and the Foundation owns Transplant Informatics, which is responsible for proprietary computer and other information activities underway within UNOS outside of contract deliverables.

When it was formed, UNOS divided the country into nine regions, based on established sharing patterns, for the purposes of representation. Subsequently, Region 9 split in two, and the large southeastern Region 3 was also divided in two, with northern West Virginia being annexed by Region 2. The present structure of UNOS is shown in Figure 41.2. Notably, in addition to not conforming to state boundaries in some cases, the UNOS map represents a distinct set of boundaries that do not much resemble other arbitrary national divisions, such as the HCFA regions or the End-Stage Renal Disease (ESRD) Network map. Each UNOS region elects a Councilor who serves for two years and generally was first elected two years previous to serve as Associate Councilor. The Councilor chairs the local regional meetings and serves as the regional representative on the Board.

An important ingredient in the way UNOS is constituted is the membership, which is composed of institutions, not individuals. This construction was inherited from the structure of SEOPF and allows generalized participation of the membership with a minimum of need for scrutiny of individuals during the application for membership. It also provides a direct connection with the institution as a whole for purposes of ensuring that policies are followed. The membership meets annually, mainly by a large proxy vote, and generally with the only usual business being to elect the Board and its officers.

The basic governing structure in UNOS is the Board of Directors. In 1994, it appeared that the next authorization of NOTA would specify categories of Board representation, and this structure was subsequently put in place in anticipation, although then NOTA was not passed. The Board consists of the Councilor from each region, representatives of certain national transplant societies, public members, and representatives of patients and patient families. It has the conventional responsibilities of governorship of a tax-exempt institution, plus the special responsibilities of determining public policy as represented by the activities of the OPTN and the Scientific Registry. At two regular meetings annually, the Board considers membership applications, policies regarding organ allocation, and other activities of the

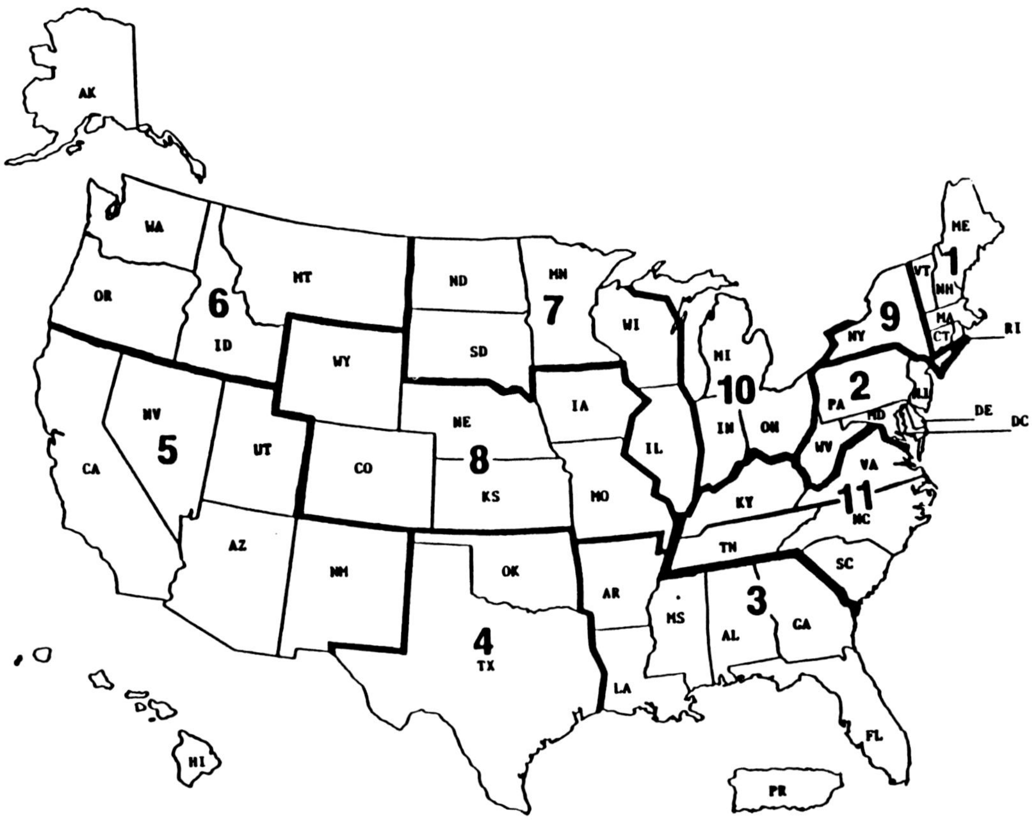

FIGURE 41.2. *UNOS regional map.*

organization, recently focusing more intensively on organ donation. The meetings are open to the public except for membership and contract items, which are considered in closed session.

The Executive Director of UNOS works closely with the Executive Committee and the Board regarding policy issues. The Executive Director is also in charge of administering the staff of the organization, which has grown to a total of over 150 persons in four major organizational areas, as shown in Figure 41.3. A major strength of the organization is that it has held both the Registry and OPTN contracts since they were first awarded in 1987, thus utilizing and deepening the experience of its staff.

Much of the detailed policy assessment is done by the UNOS committees, which generally each mirror the Board in a smaller way, being comprised of representatives from each region as well as members of the public and professionals who represent any particular interests. Committee members generally serve for two years. This two-year turnover at the Board and the committee level ensures a wide participation by the community over time. There are committees designed to deal with scientific issues, organ-specific issues, and topics of interest to patients and the general public Table 41.1. Recently the Council on Organ Availability was formed to oversee within UNOS the maximiza-

Table 41.1. UNOS Committees

UNOS Committees
Allocation Advisory
Communication
Ethics
Executive
Finance
Histocompatibility
Kidney/Pancreas Transplantation
Liver/Intestine Transplantation
Membership and Professional Standards
Minority Affairs
Organ Procurement Organization
OPTN Planning
Patient Affairs
Pediatric Transplantation
Scientific Advisory
Thoracic Organ Transplant
Ad Hoc Allocation Modeling Oversight
Ad Hoc Donations
Ad Hoc Foreign Relations
Ad Hoc Standardized Patient Listing Criteria
Ad Hoc Transplant Administrators

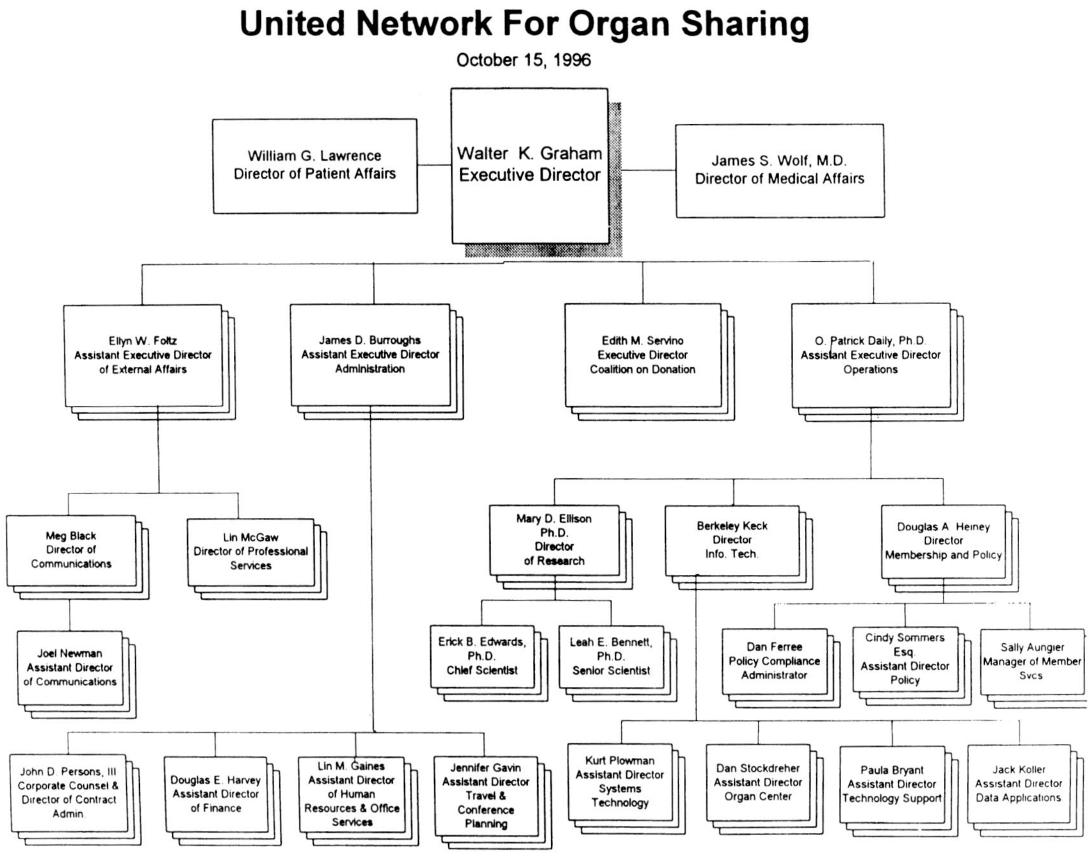

FIGURE 41.3. *Structure of the major offices within UNOS.*

tion of efforts to improve organ donation. The committees usually meet two to four times a year to take up issues as they see fit, or as referred by the Board or from other committees. For many issues two to four is an established group of committees that review them, with one or more bringing recommendations to the next Board meeting. In general, the committee members are not Board members, and the Board has not functioned by accepting subcommittee reports pro forma but has debated important issues as a committee representing the whole, using subcommittee input as one data source. This unorthodox approach to the corporation's business is gradually shifting for certain purposes. Some subcommittees of the Board are now in place, including the Allocation Advisory Committee.

A major element in the effectiveness of UNOS involves the large amount of time donated to committee and Board work by transplant professionals and private citizens. Since the great majority of the committees' members are not on the Board, the total number of individuals involved in a given year is over 200, working many thousands of hours without compensation, aside from reimbursement for expenses, mainly for travel. The result is a wealth of professional expertise and personal experience to deal with the issues under consideration. There is also a continuous, widely distributed availability of input and feedback, which provides the likelihood of conformity with the technically voluntary policies by the transplant community.

The extensive representation allowed by positions on the Board and also on committees, both regional and national, has worked well thus far. However, fair representation remains an issue, as it does with any governance structure. At present, each transplant institution, regardless of number of different programs or numbers of patients served, has one vote in the regional meetings and in the national elections. This was inherited from the SEOPF structure with its institutional, rather than individual, members. Such equality is a source of tension between the large and the smaller centers, and a proposal to allow voting, perhaps at the regional level, proportional to the number of patients listed or transplanted has been proposed. Difficulties in resolving the details of this proposal have prevented its enactment; meanwhile, the debate continues.

The number of transplant programs in the United States has grown from 466 in 1987 to 890 in 1995, and the total organs transplanted from 11,922 to 20,060. Although the majority of the day-to-day work of the UNOS staff is in fulfilling contract obligations, increasingly the transplant community is expecting more of UNOS in the form of services and donor awareness. Therefore, in addition to the increase in work from increased activity, the work has grown in variety over the years that UNOS has been in existence, and the staff has grown from 18 to 152 over that time. This development is simultaneous with a progressive decrease in federal funding, with the result that the member institutions are paying more of the bill for the organization. In the late 1980s, the fraction of UNOS budget obtained from the federal government was approximately 20%, while in 1995 it was 9.7%.

Additional funding has been sought that would allow UNOS to continue to expand services while decreasing its reliance on federal funds, and at the same time hold steady or even decrease the tax on members represented by the registration fee. The expertise in computer systems for transplant-related work and the potential for importing such services into other medical areas represent important capacities within Transplant Informatics, which will work toward developing these services in the market under the aegis of the Transplant Foundation.

DOT interacts with UNOS in the most formal sense as the director of the two contracts, for the OPTN and the Scientific Registry, held by UNOS. However, there has generally been interest in more extensive interaction to further goals of common interest in transplantation, partly through the grants that DOT is empowered to provide for work in improvement in transplantation. In addition, the tension between the usual executive branch structures and the special entity that UNOS represents results in a natural tendency for attempts at increased control of activities of UNOS, both those directed by the contract and those outside of the contract.

UNOS is an unusual bureaucratic structure because it is a private nonprofit corporation that theoretically is endowed by Congress with the power to enforce its policies as federal regulations. The tension between the executive bureaucracy that generally produces and enforces regulations and the power of the legislature to create laws and regulatory boards is finely and uniquely drawn in its situation. The analogy occasionally drawn between UNOS and a public utility is quite inaccurate. The public utility is essentially a corporation that works to make a profit for its shareholders but that has special restrictions, oversight, and advantages, by way of providing for sale a critical public service as a monopoly, which is very different from the activities of UNOS.

Another interesting quasi-governmental role with some analogy to UNOS is played by the National Association of Securities Dealers, Inc. (NASD), which was created by Congress as a self-regulatory organization for the securities industry in the Securities Exchange Act of 1934. NASD owns and operates the NASDAQ stock market exchange. Originally "National Association of Securities Dealers Automated Quotation System," now, like "UNOS," "NASDAQ" is a stand-alone noun. Also somewhat like UNOS, it has 11 regional district committees that do much of the local work of the corporation and have representation on a national Board, which also includes members from segments of the industry and at-large representatives. Structured to provide trading and monitoring in a highly sophisticated electronic environment, NASDAQ dealers must act according to the corporate rules. The structure of NASD includes, in addition to NASDAQ, a subsidiary called NASD Regulation, Inc., with arbitration and disciplinary arms. If monitoring or complaints indicate a violation by a member, a sequence of informal remedial actions and, those failing, disciplinary actions are specified. Penalties include censure, monetary sanctions, suspension, and expulsion. The Securities and Exchange Commission (SEC) may be petitioned for review of decisions, and aggrieved parties may proceed through the judicial system from there, beginning with an appeal to a US Court of Appeals.

Of course, organizations like NASDAQ do not have the same sort of relationship to the public as does UNOS, which has the responsibility of fostering a positive societal attitude toward organ donation throughout the country. It is often noted that the most important aspect of any activity related to transplantation is whether it will advance, or at least not hinder, organ donation. Unlike other situations, in which the public may have a different interest than industry representatives, it seems manifest that the industry (UNOS) and the public share fundamental goals and interests. Other characteristics that set transplantation and UNOS apart from other government activities are the rapidly developing technology, which cannot be dealt with effectively on the time scale required for conventional federal activity, and the fact that increasingly the transplant community is paying for the activities of UNOS as funds from HRSA diminish.

UNOS Activities

The principal activities of UNOS are derived from the original goals of SEOPF, which preceded it: organ sharing (from which evolved the modern entity, the OPTN) and the study of outcomes based on a listing of all transplants done (which has given rise to the Scientific Registry). As noted, these goals are best pursued when intertwined organizationally. In particular, if the Registry has current data on donors and transplants, it greatly improves timeliness and accuracy of the scientific effort. An important policy matter of SEOPF was that listing a transplant was not optional—all members were expected to include every operation, which ensured the integrity of the denominator and therefore the accuracy of any conclusions drawn from the data. This is another important way in which a seamless relationship between the OPTN and Scientific Registry is key.

The OPTN operates a computer-based allocation system with operators available around the clock. By law, all transplant recipient candidates, all donors, and all transplants must be reported. The allocation rules for each organ are used to generate a list of possible recipients, and the organ procurement organization (OPO) in charge of the donor is expected to offer the organ to transplant centers for patients in that order. A center must provide a reason for any patient it passes on the list. At present, the allocation system is based on a local priority, which is generally defined as a single list for all centers collaborating in an OPO. The next zone, moving outward, for the sharing of kidneys and livers is the UNOS Region. For hearts, it is a 500-nautical-mile radius around the donor. If after this offering the organ is not used, it is then offered out nationally.

The points that determine the patient's ranking on the list are different for each organ, but the time the patient has been waiting is the dominant ingredient for them all. Special considerations exist for pediatric and multiple organ transplant recipients. SEOPF has retained ownership of the general construction, plus any enhancements, of the computer code specifying the calculation of points, and this program is leased to the UNOS Foundation by SEOPF. The allocation algorithm undergoes periodic revision as the transplant community works to achieve the best system, incorporating the differing perceptions about the degree of sharing that is best.

For kidney allocation, the degree of HLA match is a factor in the points. A kidney must be offered to any possible recipient in the country who has no HLA antigens mismatched before it is offered to less ideal matches, which receive 3 to 7 points, with each year's waiting time providing 1 point. This policy has been the source of considerable controversy. One issue is the degree to which histocompatibility matching is important. It is questioned whether the particular advantage of no mismatch transplants is sufficient to balance the costs of the system required, and whether lesser matches provide sufficient benefit to balance the longer cold ischemic times that sharing requires. Another objection is the degree to which the antigen frequencies in blacks are different than Caucasians who, being in the majority, provide more donors. A given donor HLA pattern is more likely to match a Caucasian than a black recipient's antigens. The problem is exacerbated because end-stage renal disease is more likely to occur in blacks. This concern is partially balanced as each center receiving an obligatory share of perfect match kidneys has to put a kidney back into the system.

It is often observed that the emphasis given to HLA matching is too dominant, based on the absolute points values. However, this is not a valid criticism in view of the fact that the average kidney is transplanted for recipients that have about 3 points on the list. This means that, given the long waiting times in the country, most kidneys are transplanted predominately on the basis of waiting time rather than points for histocompatibility match. Because these issues continue to be studied and re-evaluated, however, the system is evolving.

The process of formation of UNOS policy starts with identification of an issue, either as a problem with the current mechanisms or as something that has not been addressed by the present policies. Typically, the issue will then be dealt with by organ- and topic-specific committees, often then by an integrating committee such as the Membership and Professional Standards Committee or the Allocation Advisory Committee, and then taken to the Board. Concurrently, the issue will be dealt with at each regional meeting, and an advisory vote on the regional sentiment is usually taken. These deliberations are summarized at the Board meeting, and the Board may ratify a resolution that would modify or add to existing policies. This language then is sent out for public comment to the several thousand addresses of known interested parties, the comments received back are collated for further committee review and comment, and the discussions are then reviewed at the next Board meeting. The Board can then vote to finalize the policy. If the issue is not controversial, the process can take less than six months. Not surprisingly, other issues require several iterations, or issues may be decided one way only to surface for a repeat of the process a year or two later. One of the strengths of UNOS is the rotation every year or two of officers, Board members, and committee members, which ensures broad contemporary input from the community. However, the lack of continuity can produce some redundancy in policy deliberations and decisions.

The Scientific Registry has been collecting data since October 1987. All patients registered, all transplants, and all donors are expected to be listed. It appears that compliance has been excellent overall. The database has become an unusual resource in American medicine, in view of the relatively inclusive and accurate data. It has allowed further analysis of the major questions in transplantation, including the interaction of points for histocompatibility, cold ischemia times, and use of new immunosuppressive agents. It has also allowed correction of each center's outcomes for case mix and factors that were found to be important nationally, and subsequently periodic publication of the data specific to each center. This "Center-Specific Report" has been notable for the degree to which the results clustered about the mean, providing reassurance that outcomes are similar among most centers. A major demand on the system is the contractual requirement for data provided in response to DOT and other federal inquiries. In recent years, a position of Director of Medical Affairs was established to provide a physician with substantial time onsite. This doctor's duties include reviewing the basis and perspective of data requests before the staff puts extensive and, in retrospect, unprofitable resources into processing an improperly framed request for information.

The Center-Specific Report also has served as the basis for internal quality control by the transplant community. The original contract language, incorporated into the bylaws, was that centers with results in the lowest 5% should be reviewed. Of course, this did not take into account the possibility that the absolute differences could be very small and clinically unimportant if the results were grouped tightly, or that the significance of the differences could be statistically dubious for some centers. A process for defining poor performance was devised with the aim of identifying those centers with the most important differences and with a calculated threshold degree of statistical certainty. For the Center-Specific Report, the patient and graft survivals for each organ were compared with those expected based on the correction for case mix and factors influencing outcome to yield a ratio for expected-to-observed results, so that, for example, if a center were to have outcomes exactly as predicted from their patient mix the value would be zero. It was decided that about −10% was an appropriate threshold for review; centers with values less than that, regardless of how significant statistically, were determined to not warrant further attention. A line was drawn, running from −10% at a P value of 0.05, to −30% at a P value of 0.40, on the graph of expected-observed, versus P value of the statistical significance of the value. Thus, a center with particularly poor results, and therefore a much larger deviation from expected than −10%, but with small numbers and therefore relative statistical uncertainty of the result, would nevertheless be selected for further evaluation. The centers selected are then reviewed with one iteration of their data for the subsequent two years. If this places their results above the line, they are removed from further consideration. Otherwise, they are asked to consider a site visit by professionals organized by UNOS to provide advice on improvement. During this process, programs commonly have closed or reorganized voluntarily. Those that remain have generally had site visits that were able to help the center identify and correct problems.

An attempt has been made to keep current the data collected, but here, in one telling instance, the relationship with the federal system has intruded. Forms were changed to reflect new technology in the detection of hepatitis. However, the pathway for approval through the Office of Management and Budget (OMB) required years, during which time UNOS could not institute the forms. By the time of approval, precious opportunity for real-time data collection had been lost, and the science had evolved so that the forms were out of date. Efforts to obviate such administrative problems are underway. UNOS has developed an online electronic data system that will permit addition of data collected as a nongovernmental initiative, which will eliminate the impact of such approval delays.

Privacy and protection of the data are a key area. UNOS has developed specific bylaws to ensure that there not be release of data by the organization that includes, or from which there could be derived, patient-specific information. Although it cannot theoretically control data requests by DOT that result in release through the Freedom of Information Act (FOIA), in practice the privacy upon which cooperation from centers is posited has been well protected. Invasion of the system by "hackers" has been repulsed repeatedly and there are extensive provisions for backup in the event of disruption of the UNOS OPTN computer system. In addition to onsite backup for data loss and power outage, one of the requirements of the contract is that there be offsite record storage. This is in place, and occasional simulation drills are held by which it is ensured that retrieval of data and restoration of the real-time operations of the Organ Center from the offsite location, and restoration of system integrity, will be prompt.

Recently, emphasis on efforts related to organ donation has intensified within UNOS. In 1994, the Coalition on Organ Donation was founded through UNOS as a vehicle for these efforts. Fueled largely by past president James Wolfe, the Coalition successfully competed for an award from the Advertising Council. This has provided pro bono generation of advertising material and help with effecting the distribution of this material. In addition, in 1996 an internal UNOS committee—the Council for Organ Availability—was formed to be the link between UNOS and all efforts toward organ donation.

The Future of the OPTN and UNOS

As the number of patients awaiting transplant continues to grow much faster than the number of organs available overall nationally, the transplant community has in turn been increasingly concerned with perceived inconsistencies in utilization of the organs that are available, which has fueled increased donor efforts, as described above. As another means of expanding the number of donors available, there has also been increasing analysis of the outcomes of using donors with medical criteria that have previously been felt to be relative contraindications. However, the major areas of debate are the use of specific listing criteria and the possibility of further evolution in the allocation algorithms.

In general, a patient is listed when the physicians and patient agree that it is indicated. There are criteria for defining the degree of illness for the most urgent heart and liver recipients, and some aspects regarding the status of the most severely ill patients, which have the highest priority for receiving a heart or liver, are monitored by UNOS because of perceived violations. Otherwise, the severity of the patient's illness at registration has not been addressed. As the concern about differences in waiting times around the country has increased, it has become clear that a uniform practice is needed if there is to be equitable allocation either at the local or at the national level. This is an issue for the present allocation policy, but even more critically important for any future policy that would use waiting time as a criterion in a system that extends allocation beyond the present boundaries. In 1997 and 1998, UNOS put in place medically defined criteria for listing and status upgrading for potential liver and heart recipients. Similar policies for potential kidney recipients have not achieved a consensus within the transplantation community.

The allocation system is another major issue that has become increasingly contentious. The debate deals, on one hand, with the perception by centers with long waiting lists that their potential recipients are disadvantaged in terms of timeliness of transplant and in terms of likelihood of survival to undergo transplant while still medically optimal. These centers tend to be larger and to attract patients from outside the local area, are often in urban areas with large disadvantaged local populations, and may be in competition with other local centers. On the other hand, the centers with shorter waiting lists that are typically smaller and serve primarily their local population express the concern that the long lists stem from unjustified early listings and inadequate organ retrieval in the locale of the long waiting list centers. In response to these general issues and to lobbying from centers wishing to have access to more organs for the patients on their large waiting list, there has historically been sentiment expressed in some federal circles in favor of an unvarnished single national list. This is intuitively an extraordinarily unrealistic and impractical idea in the view of some transplant professionals, and as the problems with this proposal became clear to others, the interest in it had waned. However, recently finalized regulations from HHS have advocated moving toward a single national list. Congress has put a moratorium on implementation pending a study by the Institute of Medicine.

A remarkably insightful and detailed approach to determining the effect of the just-mentioned and other theoretical alternatives to the allocation system has been developed (8) as a computer model by the Pritsker Corporation under a private contract with UNOS. The problems with a single national list were demonstrated by this modeling effort. It is unclear that a major change in the outcome of transplantation in the country can be produced by a change in the algorithms envisioned, which are based on variations on the "local to national" shells of distribution. Other systems are presently being modeled, including the "Pierce-Graham" Patient-Grouped Distribution System (PGDS) and the Optimized Single National List. These are based on the removal of allocation from geopolitical boundaries of states, OPOs, or UNOS regions, and use criteria of medical importance balanced against distance, as expressed either in fraction of the total list (PGDS) or as size of population in the radius of distance from the donor hospital to the recipient center (Optimized Single National List). It thus becomes possible to adjust all factors deemed relevant, in whatever relationship desired, and have them balanced against each other to arrive at the best compromise of characteristics for ranking patients. In the formulation of this compromise by the Optimized Single National List, it remains possible for recipients to have organs shipped from far away when there is particular justification, but the wholesale senseless transport around the country entailed by a simple single national list is avoided. Regardless of whether the ultimate system may be a seamless national construct, political and logistic realities may result in an intermediate stage of regional or extraregional rules and monitoring that could evolve toward national consensus.

A major issue remains regarding the extent and limits of power vested in UNOS. Public and professional opinion has proven to be a powerful force in generating adherence with UNOS policies, in spite of the ultimate absence of federal punishment for misbehavior. Whether other specific punishments should become legally mandated is not clear. In a related issue, constitutional law delegates to the states powers that are not specified as national in scope by federal legislation. By this, it might be argued that states have the ultimate power to determine what happens within their bounds regarding organ transplantation (9). Since this does not seem to be the intent of NOTA, it may be that the next NOTA should be explicit regarding what role, if any, states might play in allocation or other activities of the OPTN.

Finally, UNOS will need to exert the oversight vested in it through the OPTN contract in regard to xenografting. It seems increasingly possible that the breakthroughs that would allow selective application of this extraordinary concept may occur before too many years. However, it is likely that the use of human organs will continue to be advantageous, or mandatory, in some settings for the foreseeable future. In that case, the possible practices that centers doing xenotransplants might develop could affect the use of human organs. Since human organ donation and allocation would still require supervision to optimize fairness and utility, UNOS will need to develop policies for xenotransplantation that will provide the best facilitation of that field, as well as allow it to fit into the present picture in transplantation with the best benefit for recipients of all organs.

EUROPE, NORTHERN AFRICA, AND THE MIDDLE EAST

Within the region comprising Europe, Northern Africa, and the Middle East, remarkable heterogeneity is found concerning the organization of organ donation and transplantation, the availability of supportive legislative measures, and the involvement of governmental structures. The current national structures and territories are the consequence of many geographic and political changes over centuries, of religious segregation, and of national culture and character.

The most important regions for consideration are the countries of western Europe, especially in view of their participation in the European Union; the countries of eastern Europe, because of new developments after the demolition of the Berlin Wall; and, finally, the countries in northern Africa and the Middle East, cooperating politically in the Arab League.

Western Europe

Current Situation

All types of cadaveric organ transplantation—kidney, heart, lung, liver, pancreas, and combined organ transplants—are available in the different countries of western Europe. Table 41.2 gives an overview of the number of transplant programs, the waiting list numbers as of December 31, 1994, and the mean transplant activities during the last three to four years with regard to cadaveric kidney, heart, and liver transplantation (10). It is clear that the cadaveric renal and nonrenal transplant activity varies widely among the western European countries.

Living kidney donor transplants are most frequently performed in Norway, Sweden, and Denmark, and to a lesser

Table 41.2. Organ Transplants in Western European Countries

	Kidney (Cadaveric)			Heart			Liver		
	Centers[a]	Wait List[b]	Annual Procedures[c]	Centers[a]	Wait List[b]	Annual Procedures[c]	Centers[a]	Wait List[b]	Annual Procedures[c]
Austria	5	1000	330	3	120	100	3	48	95
Belgium	7	1093	350	6	72	115	5	102	140
Germany	42	9092	2040	25	639	485	17	164	585
Netherlands	7	1643	410	2	37	46	3	20	75
Greece	2	1439	65	2	56	11	2	59	9
Italy	28	7000	800	13	500	300	11	400	300
Portugal	7	1885	340	3	27	8	5	61	45
Spain	38	4621	1600	7	44	275	9	218	600
France	39	4516	1600	30	404	480	23	359	650
Denmark	4	280	135	2	8	27	2	12	43
Norway	1	120	73	1	4	23	1	10	15
Finland	1	400	160	1	8	30	1	5	29
Sweden	4	450	230	3	10	32	2	18	90
Switzerland	6	419	185	4	14	43	4	6	51
Ireland	1	140	133	1	—	14	1	—	19
United Kingdom	36	4849	1620	9	320	310	8	115	640

[a] Number of active programs in 1993–1995.
[b] Wait list: 1993 or 1994.
[c] Annual procedures: average 1992–1995.
No indicative annual wait list or transplant data found for Yugoslavia, Romania, Bulgaria, Lithuania, Latvia, Estonia, Ukraine, and USSR.
Since figures were retrieved from multiple sources, often covering different calendar years, the figures should be seen as indicative.

extent in Greece, the Netherlands, and Switzerland. "Domino" heart transplantation has been most markedly developed in the United Kingdom, while living liver donor transplantation is still a single-center expertise (e.g., Hamburg, Brussels St. Luc, Paris).

Bureaucracy

In contrast to the United States, transplant-related organization and legislation in Europe shows a remarkable heterogeneity—many differences exist among the various nations as to transplant and donation legislation, organization and allocation, and the structure of organ exchange organizations and their interaction with national health care authorities and governmental bodies.

Law

A milestone in the European transplant and donation legislation was a resolution on removal, grafting, and transplantation of human substances that was formulated by the Council of Europe in 1978 (11). In particular, this declaration accepted brain death as death of a patient. It also promoted the so-called presumed consent law, which holds that, in the absence of an already effected formal objection against donation, deceased persons can be assumed to be donors. Recommendations on legislation regarding living organ donation and organ trading were also made. Further, the Council of Europe established a select committee of experts on the organizational aspects of cooperation in organ transplantation (10) aiming to promote organ donation, harmonize policies, regulate multiple listing at different centers and countries, evaluate the possibility of a common European waiting list for certain patient groups, and pursue other joint interests.

Since 1978, several European countries have initiated (or added) laws addressing brain death, living and cadaveric donation, or commerce in human organs—France in 1978, Spain in 1979–1980, Austria in 1982, Finland in 1985, Belgium in 1986, and Denmark in 1990. These changes have been slow in coming, however, and often create greater differences among the countries as to policy. Two European countries, the Netherlands and Germany, are now drafting their donation and transplant law. In the United Kingdom, the Human Organ Transplants Act (1989), which prohibits commercial dealings in human organs intended for transplantation and restricts the transplanting of such organs between persons who are not genetically related, was enacted as an amendment to the law of 1961 in response to the practice of some physicians in London who used kidneys bought from foreigners in transplants.

The choice of the donation consent system has been dependent on governmental coalition, societal and personal rights, medical professional attitudes, and public attitude. It should always be remembered that the phrases *opting-in/informed consent* and *opting-out/presumed consent* are often an oversimplification of the real legislative measures (12); for example, presumed consent laws often differ on the legal

Table 41.3. Legislation on Donation in Western Europe (1996)

Country	Legislation/Practice	Population by Million Inhabitants	Average Annual Number of Donors per Million Inhabitants[a]	Average Annual Percentage of Multiorgan Donation[a]
Austria	Presumed consent	8	23.5	70%
Belgium	Presumed consent	10	21.0	75%
Finland	Presumed consent	5	19.0	30%
France	Presumed consent	58	16.5	75%
Norway	Presumed consent	4	16.6	35%
Switzerland	Presumed consent	7	14.9	70%
Portugal	Presumed consent	10	17.5	55%
Spain	Presumed consent/Informed consent	38	23.6[b]	75%
Italy	Presumed consent/Informed consent	57	7.0	80%
Greece	Presumed consent/Informed consent	10	6.9	75%
Denmark	Informed consent	5	14.0	55%
United Kingdom	Informed consent	60	15.4	65%
Ireland	Informed consent	4	20.0	36%
The Netherlands	No transplant law/Informed consent	15	15.0	55%
Germany	No transplant law/Informed consent	80	13.3	55%

[a] 1991–1995.
[b] In 1998, the number was increased to 31.5 donors per million.
Since figures were retrieved from multiple sources, often covering different calendar years, the figures should be seen as indicative.

obligation and/or circumstances to inform the family about the planned organ removal and the donor's consent. Table 41.3 illustrates the types of legislation on organ procurement in various western European countries. Meanwhile, it has become clear that "presumed consent" legislation alone is not sufficient for a high incidence of donor organ procurement, but that the final result depends on several factors unrelated to low number of potential donors, number of intensive care beds, collaboration of medical profession, organization of organ retrieval, and media attention.

Many countries have created (Belgium, United Kingdom, France) or are now developing (Austria, Sweden, the Netherlands) a national donor registry, in which the citizens can enter their decision to donate or oppose donation (or sometimes, give instruction to ask the family).

Organ Exchange Organizations

With the emergence of renal transplantation in the late 1960s, plans were made to coordinate cadaveric transplantation, based on the prediction that pooling of transplant candidates and organ exchange would contribute to the realization of optimally HLA-matched kidney transplants and optimum graft outcome (13). As a result, organ exchange organizations were formed intranationally, nationally, and internationally. As of the early 1980s, these organizations also became involved in the disposition of nonrenal donor organs (14). Table 41.4 surveys the European organ exchange organizations as of 1996.

Table 41.4. Western European Organ Exchange Organizations (1996)

	Participating Countries
Scandiatransplant	Denmark Finland Iceland Norway Sweden
United Kingdom Transplant Support Service Authority (UKTSSA)	United Kingdom Ireland
Eurotransplant	Austria Belgium Luxemburg Germany The Netherlands
Etablissement Français des Greffes (EFG)	France
Organización Nacional de Transplantes (ONT)	Spain
Lusotransplante	Portugal
Nord Italia Transplant (NITp)	Italy
Associazione InterRegionale Trapianti (AIRT)	Italy
Coordinamento Centro Sud per i Trapianti (CCST)	Italy
Sud Italia Transplant (SIT)	Italy
Hellenic Transplant	Greece
Swiss Transplant	Switzerland

Today, the tasks of the organ exchange organizations are more or less the same. In summary, they involve: 1) maximum usage of all cadaveric donor organs, and 2) objective allocation of the available cadaveric donor organs according to a consensus policy, based on the common principles of medical justice and utility. In addition, some organizations regularly voice their interest for scientific research [e.g., United Kingdom Transplant Support Service Authority (UKTSSA), Eurotransplant] and several have developed professional educational donation programs [e.g., European Donor Hospital Education Programme (EDHEP) by Eurotransplant, courses for Transplant Procurement Management Coordinator by ONT]. Others have established a reference tissue typing laboratory in order to achieve and maintain reliable HLA typing and crossmatch results (e.g., Etablissement Français des Greffes (EFG), Eurotransplant, Swisstransplant, UKTSSA). Sometimes donation and allocation of cadaveric tissues, such as corneas and heart valves, are also considered (e.g., Eurotransplant/Bio Implant Services, UKTSSA, EFG), and occasionally there is a registry of unrelated living bone marrow donors (Swisstransplant, EFG).

The organ exchange organizations were originally created by building on the work of already established figures in the field of transplant medicine, who ran the various private foundations or foundation-like institutions in a more or less paternalistic way. Nevertheless, as the voluntary cooperating transplant units agreed to abide by the shared rules, the organ exchange organization acted as the custodian and arbitrator of those rules (15).

Over time, the purely medical nature of transplantation has gradually been affected by societal issues, and thus several national organ donation and transplantation systems have been paid attention to by various governments and ministries of public health. The motive has been the increasing weight of organ transplantation on the organization of the health care system, the constitutional right of equal access to medical care, the shortfall of cadaveric donors to meet the demand, and also the allegations of organ trading, transplant tourism, and noncompliance with the allocation rules. As a result, in some countries the existing organ exchange organizations were attached to the department of health (EFG, UKTSSA). In other countries, the opportunity was taken by the government to create a formal national organ exchange organization closely linked to the government (ONT).

Simultaneously, there has also been a remarkable movement toward more democracy in the structure and/or decision making of organ exchange organizations (Eurotransplant). This probably relates to the increased attention paid to equity of (nationally and/or locally) procured organs, sharp increase of transplant centers, constantly rising waiting lists, and conviction of self-provisional capacities (16). As a consequence, several advisory committees (often organ specific) on allocation and procurement were established, and the governing Boards composed by election instead of invitation (17).

The financial structure of the organ exchange organizations is dependent on the legal entity of the organization and on the characteristics of the national health care system(s). Eurotransplant is financed by the health insurance authorities in the participating countries by means of the payment of a fee for each patient registration on the waiting list (18). The contribution is related to the type of transplant procedure and to the extra activities that Eurotransplant provides—for example, salary of transplant coordinators, and HLA typing of recipient and donor. The fee is adjusted annually in order to meet the Board-approved budget. The operational maintenance of the UKTSSA is the responsibility of the Department of Health. Adequate funding coming out of public funds raised through general taxation is provided as a cash-limited budget within which the Authority must exist (15).

In contrast to the United States, organization of the donor report and procurement is managed differently and rather independently of the organ exchange organization. The transplant centers themselves act as the donor reporting agency. The procurement area of a transplant center consists either of a clearly defined geographic area (Austria, EFG, the Netherlands, Spain, UKTSSA) or of a conglomerate of affiliated donor hospitals (Belgium, Germany, Italy). Authorization of transplant programs is most often a matter of the Ministry of Health rather than of the organ exchange organization itself. Transplant coordinators are the key persons between the transplant programs and organ exchange organization, and are responsible for administering the donor report and organ offer as well. The number of transplant coordinators per million inhabitants is not equally distributed among the diverse western European countries and there is no uniform European job description.

The western European countries do not share a common waiting list for any organ transplant or category of transplant candidates (including "high urgent"). Waiting lists are compiled by each European organ exchange organization. Strictly speaking, access to a waiting list is not restricted to residents of the country or countries served; however, excessive numbers of so-called nonresident transplant candidates at some transplant centers in Belgium and France, mainly coming from Italy, have been a topic of national debate questioning the proper usage of national donor organ resources and the issue of financial incentives. Being listed on multiple organ exchange organizations is disapproved by the Council of Europe.

Significant variation exists, both related to the type of donor organ and among different organ exchange organizations, regarding allocation policies and achievement of organ matching. Is organ allocation organized in a patient-oriented or program-oriented fashion? Is there an obligation or a recommended mandate that organs be offered to certain patient groups? Is the central allocation office involved in the allocation of all reported donor organs? Often, the allocation procedures incorporate (sequentially) the different possibilities. For example, with regard to heart allocation in Eurotransplant, mandatory offer and/or exchange of any available donor heart involves patients in the need of an early acute heart retransplant, coordinated by the central office; then, the local transplant program selects the best suitable patient; then, the donor heart is allocated in a patient-oriented way by the central allocation office. Conversely, kidney allocation has become entirely patient-oriented, with 100% placement by the central office (19). Several organ exchange organizations have opted for a matching and allocation procedure that is fully initiated and executed by the donor center (Scandiatransplant, ONT, EFG).

If donor organs cannot be used within a given organ exchange organization, they are usually offered to the other European organ exchange organizations. Most often this involves organs from pediatric donors, ABO blood group type AB donors, and "marginal" donors; however, the real extent of this "European" exchange is not exactly known.

In the larger organ exchange organizations, computer networks between the transplant programs enable the 24-hour-a-day listing of transplant candidates on the waiting list, donor report, transplant registration, and entry of transplant follow-up data.

Scientific Cooperation

Major European scientific organizations and registries are the European Society for Organ Transplantation (ESOT); the European Dialysis and Transplant Association-European Renal Association (EDTA-ERA), with a long-standing tradition of the European Registry on renal replacement therapy; and the European Liver Transplant Registry (coordinated by H. Bismuth of Paris).

Eastern European Countries

Current Situation

During the Communist era (until 1990), only kidney transplants were performed in the eastern European countries, usually infrequently and using non-heart-beating cadaveric donors. Since the political reformation, several countries have experienced an increased renal transplant activity and nonrenal transplant programs have been launched. Table 41.5 surveys transplant centers, waiting lists, and transplantation data for some Eastern European countries.

Bureaucracy

Brain death criteria have been accepted by law, but with considerable variation among the countries (Hungary in 1972, Bulgaria in 1976, USSR in 1987, Poland in 1990, Latvia in 1991). Often, the procedure of brain death declaration is explicitly described; for example, in the Czech Republic, brain death must be confirmed by two cerebral angiographic examinations performed 30 minutes apart.

For cadaveric donation, consent legislation generally follows the "presumed consent" principle. Prohibition on the sale of human donor organs and the removal of organs and/or tissues from a living donor for transplantation purposes are also covered in the law governing the transplantation of human organs and/or tissues.

In the years following 1972, international cooperation existed in the fields of kidney transplantation through an international agreement signed by Bulgaria, Czechoslovakia, Cuba, the former German Democratic Republic, Hungary, Poland, and the former Soviet Union. Exchange was only effective, to some extent, between Czechoslovakia, the German Democratic Republic, and Hungary. Following the demolition of the Berlin Wall and its political consequences, the Intertransplant cooperation stopped its activities. The German Democratic Republic officially joined the Eurotransplant International Foundation in July 1991, due to the unification of the two German countries, while the other eastern European countries and former Soviet states continued independently.

Some western European organ exchange organizations offered their help (20) to establish an efficient transplant infrastructure by drafting organizational guidelines, aiming at the foundation of a national transplant society, and permitting educational collaborations in the fields of organ procurement and transplantation and tissue typing. Several nonrenal transplant programs from the Eurotransplant organization have established such training programs, with centers in the Czech and Slovak Republics and, to a lesser

Table 41.5. Organ Transplants in Eastern European Countries

	Kidney (Cadaveric)			Heart			Liver		
	Centers[a]	Wait List[b]	Annual Procedures[c]	Centers[a]	Wait List[b]	Annual Procedures[c]	Centers[a]	Wait List[b]	Annual Procedures[c]
Poland	8	1732	320	2	—	50	6	—	35
Hungary	4	1400	220	1	—	3	1	—	7
Czech Republic	7	1000	400	2	—	70	3	—	35
Slovenia	1	200	10	1	—	1	1	—	—
Croatia	2	850	40	1	—	4	—	—	—
Slovak Republic	3	350	60	—	—	—	—	—	—

[a] Number of active programs in 1993–1995.
[b] Wait list: 1993 or 1994.
[c] Annual procedures: average 1992–1995.
No indicative annual wait list or transplant data found for Yugoslavia, Romania, Bulgaria, Lithuania, Latvia, Estonia, Ukraine, and USSR.
Since figures were retrieved from multiple sources, often covering different calendar years, the figures should be seen as indicative.

extent, in Hungary, Poland, and Romania. The so-called Baltic states—Estonia, Lithuania, and Latvia—have established a relationship with the Scandiatransplant Organization since 1994.

The political reorganization of eastern Europe may positively influence the socioeconomic climate, the health care policy, and the welfare system in such a way as to establish efficient national transplant programs, although it may take some time. Currently, regional reports do not indicate problems of political will, but rather those of the lack of medical and paramedical support to organ procurement and listing of patients as transplant candidates (21). The larger transplant programs from the former eastern European countries regularly present their basic scientific and clinical data at European and international symposia and congresses.

Countries of Northern Africa and the Middle East

Current Situation

Transplant activities in the Arab world began in the late 1970s and the 1980s, and mainly involve kidney transplants for which living-related donors are the main source (Table 41.6). Some countries (Saudi Arabia, Kuwait) have also established a cadaveric donor kidney transplant program. Nonrenal transplant programs (heart, liver) have been initiated in Saudi Arabia, Kuwait, and Turkey, but these programs are in general marginally developed in the Arab world.

It is not uncommon that Arab patients in need of an organ transplant seek such treatment abroad in European countries and in the United States (renal and nonrenal transplantation), as well as in neighboring countries where commercial living-nonrelated donor kidney transplant programs are available. Many countries in North Africa and the Middle East participate in the Middle East Society for Organ Transplantation biennial congress.

Bureaucracy

Many countries of the Arab world are Islamic. Since Islam as a religion provides a complete code of life, religious teaching influences the discussion of current and new laws (22). Consequently, progress in transplantation had to await study and rulings by Islamic religious scholars. Nowadays, the principle of donation of organs for transplantation from both living and cadaveric donors is generally accepted by Islam. The Third International Conference of Islamic Jurists, held in 1986 in Amman, Jordan, passed a resolution that equated brain death with cardiac and respiratory death (23). Following the Fourth International Conference of Islamic Jurists, held in Jeddah, Saudi Arabia, in 1988, the selling of body organs was deemed to be absolutely prohibited by Islam, and thus also the issue of paid organ donation.

Following the favorable Islamic opinion toward the transplantation of organs from both living and brain-dead donors, a Unified Arab Draft Law on Human Organ Transplants was outlined during the 1987 meeting of the Council of Arab Ministers of Health in Khartoum. This draft law has been adopted by several Middle Eastern countries.

In countries where cadaveric donation is legalized, donation is governed by a "required consent," either having been previously given by the deceased or given by the family. In those countries where the sale of organs is forbidden, the concept of compensated donation is usually accepted.

The most well-known organ exchange organization in the Arab world is the Saudi Center for Organ Transplantation (SCOT), which before 1993 was the National Kidney Foundation. It is the central coordinating body for renal care facilities and for all types of organ transplants in Saudi Arabia. Guidelines covering every detail concerning transplantation have been laid down, and must, by Ministerial Resolution, be strictly adhered to by all hospitals in the Saudi kingdom (24).

In Iran, a nonprofit society assists in the process of donor evaluation and functions, in case of the need to use unrelated living donors, to minimize commercialization and possible exploitation of donors (25,26). All volunteer donors have to present themselves to the National Association for the Support of End Stage Renal Disease Patients.

Some of the difficulties in establishing transplant programs in the Arab world are due to poor economic resources and inadequate health care budget allocations. For example, in some countries, the health care administration has made it easier to transfer patients abroad for transplantation through a medical collaboration paid for by the government instead of improving the countries' own facilities and level of health care.

Several regional reports plead for the institution of modest transplant programs so that the infrastructure necessary for donation and transplantation can remain in place until greater progress in transplantation is realized. Such progress depends on, among other things, a consensus on brain death as the legal definition of death, which should propagate nonrenal organ transplantation; improved economics; and appropriate health care policies leading to higher transplant activity in view of the expense of hemodialysis programs (27).

Table 41.6. Kidney Transplants in Northern Africa and the Middle East

	Centers	Cadaveric	Living
Saudi Arabia	10	95	145
Turkey	20	47	245
Iran	15	—	950 (approximately)

Note: Countries currently performing renal transplants include: Morocco, Algeria, Tunisia, Egypt, Sudan, Cyprus, Turkey, Lebanon, Jordan, Syria, Saudi Arabia, Kuwait, Yemen, Oman, Qatar, Bahrain, United Arab Emirates, Iran, and Iraq.

Future

European heterogeneity will probably continue, despite the political desire for European harmonization and unification. Each country has currently adapted a program of donation and transplantation that reflects its own historical experience and its own national character. Changes in health care policy and the expected drastic cuts in the national health care budget will have a major effect on the field of donation and transplantation.

The countries of northern Africa, the Middle East, and eastern Europe can be expected to increase their collaboration with neighboring countries, western Europe, and the United States, which should help establish a basic and adequate infrastructure for renal transplantation, renal replacement therapy in general, and perhaps also nonrenal transplantation. National transplant societies are likely to be founded, contributing to better assessment of local needs and national transplant activities and to mutual international understanding concerning practice and outcome.

ASIA

The History and Character of Asian Organ Transplantation

Organ transplantation in Asia began in 1964 with kidney and liver transplantations in Japan (Table 41.7). The first heart transplantation was performed in Japan in 1968; the surgeon was sued for the murder of the donor. Since then, no liver or heart transplantation using a brain-dead donor has been performed in Japan. Living-related kidney transplantation has been mainly practiced.

In other countries in Asia, kidney transplantation began at the end of the 1960s or in the 1970s. Heart and liver transplantation began in the 1980s, and the legislation for transplantation and brain death was established in the end of the 1980s or 1990s.

Each country in Asia has a different religion, culture, and level of medical practice, and the status of transplantation also varies. Therefore, it is hard to discuss organ procurement and allocation in Asia as a whole. We will begin with the current statistics of transplantation and then discuss the problems that Asian countries are facing in organ transplantation.

Table 41.7. History and Characteristics of Asian Organ Transplantation

1964	Japan	First liver transplantation (non-heart-beating)
	Japan	First kidney transplantation (living-related)
1968	Taiwan	First kidney transplantation (living-related)
	Japan	First heart transplant
1969	Korea	First kidney transplantation (living-related)
1970	Singapore	First kidney transplantation (cadaveric)
	Hong Kong	First kidney transplantation (cadaveric)
1972	Thailand	First kidney transplantation (living-related)
	Singapore	Legislation for "opt-in" system
1975	Malaysia	First kidney transplantation (living-related)
1976	Singapore	First kidney transplantation (living-related)
1977	Indonesia	First kidney transplantation (living-related)
1979	Saudi Arabia	First kidney transplantation (living-related)
	Pakistan	First kidney transplantation (living-related)
1981	Indonesia	Legislation for organ transplantation
1983	Taiwan	First liver transplantation
	Korea	Definition of brain death by Korean Medical Association
1987	Thailand	First heart transplant
	Singapore	"Opt-out" law
	Taiwan	Legislation for brain death and organ transplantation
	Taiwan	First heart transplant
	Philippines	Legislation for brain death
1988	Taiwan	Asian Transplantation Society established
	Korea	First liver transplantation
	Philippines	First liver and pancreas transplantation
	Philippines	Legislation for prohibiting organ commercialism
	Singapore	Legislation for organ transplantation
1989	Thailand	Legislation for brain death
	Indonesia	First Congress for Asian Transplantation Society
	Japan	First living-related partial liver transplantation
1991	Taiwan	Second Congress for Asian Transplantation Society
1992	Korea	First heart transplantation
1993	Thailand	Third Congress for Asian Transplantation Society
1994	India	Legislation for prohibiting organ commercialism

Current Status of Organ Transplantation in Asia

Kidney Transplantation

Almost all countries in Asia are practicing kidney transplantation, but the details vary remarkably (Table 41.8). China is completely dependent on cadaveric transplantation. On the other hand, India, Bangladesh, Indonesia, Oman, and Pakistan depend almost entirely on living donors. In other countries, both cadaveric and living donors are available to varying degrees. The ratio of cadaveric to living donors was 100% in China, 88% in Taiwan, 73% in Thailand, 67% in Singapore, 60% in Hong Kong, 35% in Japan, 28% in Saudi Arabia, 18% in Philippines, 3.3% in Korea, and 1.4% in Malaysia (28,29).

Cadaveric transplantation in Asia has included both brain-dead and non-heart-beating donors. In Taiwan (30), Thailand (31), Singapore (32), Saudi Arabia (33), Hong Kong (34), and the Philippines, which have legislation for brain death, almost all cadaveric transplants utilize heart-beating, brain-dead donors. Brain-dead donors are used sporadically even in the countries without legislation for brain death, but these cases have not been prosecuted so far. In Korea, where there is no law for brain death, the medical society recognizes the concept of brain death, and transplantation using both heart-beating and non-heart-beating donors has been practiced. On the other hand, in China and Japan only non-heart-beating donors are used for cadaveric

Table 41.8. Kidney Transplantation in Asian Countries (1991–1993)

		Living Donor			Cadaver Donor		
	Total Cases	Related	Spouse	Unrelated	Brain Death	Cardiac Arrest	Dialysis Patients
Bangladesh	26	26	0	0	0	0	204
China	5568	0	0	0	0	5568	63,998
Hong Kong	159	59	5	0	95	0	1598
India	7250	2350	400	4500	0	0	3200
Indonesia	72	72	0	0	0	0	600
Japan	1162	721	43	0	0	402	134,372
Korea	2312	1204	85	947	65	11	900
Malaysia	292	104	0	184	4	0	—
Oman	112	19	0	93	0	0	208
Pakistan	1215	700	10	500	—	—	700
The Philippines	334	266	1	6	61	0	—
Saudi Arabia	784	337	0	225	222	0	3780
Singapore	192	54	10	0	124	4	1213
Thailand	236	69	0	0	167	0	1119
Taiwan	461	55	0	0	406	0	11,567
United Arab Emirates	20	19	1	0	0	0	62

transplantation. China utilizes as many as 1500 donors a year for transplantation, and most of them seem to be executed criminals (35). Such donors have never been used in Japan, where the concept of brain death has now been legislated by the Diet. The shortage of cadaveric donors is a serious problem even in the countries that have a law for brain death. Less than 100 cases of cadaveric transplantation are practiced each year in all countries in Asia except China (28).

Transplantation using living donors is performed in all countries other than China. Living-related transplantation is the main approach in most countries. However, living-non-related transplants account for 83% in Oman, 68% in India, 68% in Malaysia, 42% in Pakistan, and 45% in Korea (28,29). In India, more than 4500 kidneys were transplanted in three years from nonrelated living donors other than spouses. These transplants may involve commercialism, since, unfortunately, a commercial trade for organs exists in some countries. There is strong sentiment within and outside of Asia that this commercial activity is unethical and should be stopped, and that selection of the donor for living-related and living-unrelated transplants ought to be evaluated and characterized by justice and fairness.

Extrarenal Transplantation

Taiwan (30), Thailand (31), and Singapore (32) began to practice heart transplantation by 1990, some time after the first case that was transplanted in Japan in 1968. Thereafter, China, Saudi Arabia (33), Hong Kong (34), and Korea began by 1993, and a total of more than 100 heart transplants have been done in Asia. About half of them were performed in Taiwan. The first heart–lung transplant was performed in Thailand in 1988 (31), and this program continues in Taiwan and Thailand.

Five to ten liver transplants are regularly performed in Taiwan and Thailand each year, and Singapore, the Philippines, Japan, Saudi Arabia, China, Korea, and Hong Kong also have done liver transplantation. Of these counties, all except China, Korea, and Japan have a law for brain death. Heart transplantation in Thailand and liver transplantation in Taiwan preceded the legislation, and in fact, these events were a driving impetus in the establishment of the law.

A special situation for liver transplantation exists in Japan. Since the first two cases of liver transplantation in the 1960s, no transplants have been done using brain-dead donors for 30 years. Legislation for brain death was only finalized in October of 1997. Living-related partial liver transplantation has been practiced and over 800 such procedures had been done in Japan by 1998.

Transplantation Facilities

There are 150 institutions for kidney transplantation in Japan, 95 in China, 52 in India, 33 in Korea, and 10 to 15 in other Asian countries (29). The average number transplanted in 1990 per institution was 50 in Pakistan, 46 in India, and 10 to 30 in most other Asian countries. Japan has the fewest number of transplants per institution—2.5 cases a year. Fewer than 10 institutions in each country perform extrarenal transplantation.

Dialysis Patients

In order to fully understand the status of kidney transplantation in each country in Asia, one must also understand the status of dialysis—the other therapeutic modality for end-stage renal disease. Japan has the largest number of dialysis patients, about 150,000. There are approximately 64,000 dialysis patients in China, 11,000 in Taiwan, 3700 in Saudi Arabia, and 3200 in India. The patients who are on waiting lists for transplantation account for 0.3% of dialysis patients in China, 12% in Bangladesh, 13% in Japan, and 16% in India, but 40% to 90% in most other Asian countries. The number of patients on dialysis is extraordinarily high for the population in Japan. New patients with end-stage renal disease in Japan, more than 8000 patients each year, are essentially able to receive dialysis treatments under the financial support from the government. The reported prevalence of end-stage renal disease per population does not seem to be different among the countries in Asia (33,36,37).

Although the governments provide some financial support for dialysis in most countries in Asia, very few patients throughout Asia with end-stage renal disease actually receive the renal replacement therapy. This means that a considerable number of patients with end-stage renal disease die without receiving any treatment.

Transplantation Offshore

At least 500 cases of kidney transplantation were performed abroad in 1992 on Asian patients (Table 41.9) (29). Fifty to 100 patients went abroad for transplantation from Taiwan, Malaysia, Saudi Arabia, United Arab Emirates (UAE), India, Hong Kong, Oman, and other countries. What kinds of transplantation, cadaveric or living, they were provided with is not clearly known. However, it appears that most transplantation performed in foreign countries is nonrelated-living donor kidney transplantation and is done on a commercial basis. Asians rarely undergo liver or heart transplantation abroad, with the exception of Japanese patients.

Legislation

Brain death is legally codified as the definition of death in Hong Kong, India, Oman, Indonesia, the Philippines, Saudi Arabia, Singapore, Thailand, Taiwan, and UAE. Brain death has not been legally accepted in Japan, Korea, China, Bangladesh, Malaysia, and Pakistan (see Table 41.9.). Of the 10 countries that have legislation for brain death, Thailand and Hong Kong have no laws for organ transplantation. However, both countries are practicing liver and heart transplantation using brain-dead donors. The other eight countries have laws for both brain death and organ transplantation, but India, Indonesia, and Oman have no experience with liver or heart transplantation. On the other hand, in China and Korea heart and liver transplantation have been done without any legislation for brain death and organ transplantation. In Japan there is no liver or heart transplantation using brain-dead donors because there is no legislation governing organ transplantation from such donors. In most countries that have laws for organ transplantation from brain-dead donors, the organ can be procured under an "opt-in" system. Singapore introduced legislation for an "opt-out" system in 1987, and it is only Singapore that retains an "opt-out" system now in Asia. It is interesting to note that this "opt-out" system has not been reconciled with Islamic religion in Singapore, and thus excludes the 17% of the Singapore population who are Muslims (37).

Table 41.9. Legislation and Economical Status in Asian Countries (1993)

	Legislation			Transplant Off Shore			Economical Support		
	Accept Brain Death	Law for Organ Transplant	Network System	Kidney	Heart	Liver	Dialysis	Recipients	Donors
Bangladesh	X	X	X	10	1				X
China	X	X	X	X	X	X			
Hong Kong	0 (1980)	X	0	46	X	X			X
India	0 (1994)	X	X	50	X	10		X	
Indonesia	0	0	X	50	X	X			
Japan	X	0	0	0	1	16	0	0	0
Korea	X	X	X	0			0	0	0
Malaysia	X	0	X	52			0	0	0
Oman	0 (1989)	0	X	49			0	0	X
Pakistan	X	X	X	8			0	0	X
The Philippines	0 (1983)	0	X				X	X	X
Saudi Arabia	0 (1982)	0	0	75					
Singapore	0 (1980)	0	X	16	X	X			
Thailand	0 (1972)	X	X	27			X	X	X
Taiwan	0 (1987)	0	0	91	X	X	0	0	0
United Arab Emirates	0 (1994)	0	X	53	X	X	0	0	0

0 = yes; X = no.

Networks and Organ Allocation

A few countries, such as Japan, Hong Kong, Taiwan, and Thailand, established a network system (see Table 41.9) for organ allocation and select the recipients on the basis of matching of histocompatibility antigens (HLA). Many other countries allocate the organs locally (i.e., in the area of each transplantation facility).

In Japan, a new national network system was introduced in April 1996 through which all kidneys are supposed to be allocated. This system includes seven blocks of districts, and within each block the kidneys are allocated to the recipients in order of HLA matching. The kidneys are shipped out to the other blocks in instances of full matching of HLA. This system is now in effect only for kidney transplantation but is expected to be applied to the extrarenal organs after establishment of legislation for organ transplantation from brain-dead donors.

Problems in Asian Organ Transplantation

Shortage of Donors, Especially Living-Nonrelated Donors

Although countries all over the world are facing the problem of a shortage of donors, it is especially serious in Asian countries. Transplantation medicine can exist only with donation of vital organs. From the technical point of view, most countries in Asia can achieve the same good results as western countries in organ transplantation despite the limited experiences (30,32,34). If more extensive donation is obtained, the distorted situation of transplantation medicine in Asia would be ameliorated. The religious differences do not seem to be a reason for this problem. Socioeconomic condition, education, and lack of understanding about medical realities appear to be important factors.

There has been no living-nonrelated kidney transplantation in Thailand and Saudi Arabia, where this type of transplantation is prohibited by law (31,33). Singapore, Taiwan, and Hong Kong also have had few cases of nonrelated transplantation, and it is of interest that these countries have a relatively higher ratio of cadaveric transplantation in Asia. On the other hand, many cases of nonrelated-living transplantation have been performed in India, Korea, Oman, Pakistan, and Malaysia (29).

There is an extensive living unrelated kidney transplant program in South Korea. It is reported that nonrelated transplantation accounts for 67.5% of all kidney transplantation at Severance Hospital, Yonsei University, in Korea (39). That center accepts kidneys from well-matched—that is, minimally 1-HLA-DR-antigen–matched or 2 HLA-A-B-antigen–matched—emotionally related, healthy individuals. Moreover, the motivation of potential donors is carefully evaluated by a hospital ethical committee that includes social workers and psychiatrists. Half of the potential unrelated donors are referred by the Korean Organ Program or Korean Kidney Foundation rather than by personal contact, and only 53% of the potential donors are actually accepted by the committee.

However, consensus is very rare in other countries on ethical and medical criteria for evaluation and selection of the living-unrelated donors. In Pakistan, living-unrelated transplants are mostly performed in the private sector, and many patients go to India to receive the organs from unrelated donors. The problems are not only commercialism but also faulty follow-ups and poor survival rate (40).

Socioeconomic Status and Commercialization of the Organs

The disparity among Asians regarding access to transplantation is due primarily to poverty. In Japan, about 100 persons per 1 million of the population develop end-stage renal disease each year and require dialysis treatment, and fortunately all patients can be provided with this treatment because it is economically supported by the government. Although the incidence of end-stage renal disease is similar in other Asian countries, 70 to 100 per million, very few patients have access to renal replacement therapy. Only 2% to 3% in Bangladesh (36) and 30% in Malaysia (37) are able to survive with either dialysis or transplantation. Unfortunately, other patients are doomed to death as a struggling economy limits the amount of equipment and the number of facilities for dialysis.

The commercialization of organs, primarily kidneys, exists in some Asian countries. The recipients are desperate to survive with transplantation, the living donors want to earn money essentially in order to survive, and the brokers make money by trading the organs. These three groups apparently form a substantial business. In commercially obtained kidneys, the recipients rarely pay the money directly to the donor. Instead, the brokers or hospitals charge the patients a single bill for all expenses including surgical fee, the cost of medicine, drugs, and examinations, doctors fee, acquisition fee, and rewarding. Therefore, the patients usually do not feel that they buy the organs. Most donors are very poor and deeply in debt.

Clearly this commercialism regarding transplant organs should be eradicated. Yet it is easy to condemn this commercialism as unethical without understanding that the related problems are too complex to solve easily. For example, legislation for prohibiting the commercial trade in organs was established in India in 1994, but this law is not applied across all states in India and its effectiveness does not seem to be perfect. One should keep in mind that the problem of the commercialization of organs is complicated by a multitude of other problems such as undeveloped medical care for end-stage renal disease, a lack of financial support by governments, the shortage of donors for transplantation, the poverty of the people, and public misunderstanding of transplantation medicine.

Donation from Executed Criminals

In China, over 5000 cases of cadaveric renal transplantation have been performed in the last three years (29). Of these, a number of donors seem to be executed criminals. No reports from China are available, but a few reports indirectly suggest this to be true (35). Transplant operations from nonliving donors may be scheduled a day or two in advance. Recipients are not necessarily informed of the source of the organs. Although cultural differences always underlie how medicine is practiced throughout the world, perhaps especially transplant medicine, the use of executed criminals as donors is nevertheless a matter of serious concern. What is known about this practice in China is mainly inferential and incomplete, and further reports detailing this topic are needed.

Perspectives in Asian Transplantation

Various religions, races, cultures, and social structures are mixed in Asian countries. Value judgments also differ among the countries. So does transplantation medicine. Understanding transplantation medicine in Asia requires that one consider each country's economy, system of medical care, and religious or cultural traditions of ethical teaching and practice. Most countries are facing many problems in the level of treatment for end-stage organ failure before transplantation. Legislation for organ transplantation and brain death has been recently established in many countries, but the shortage of donor organs remains a most serious problem, which might in fact be responsible for the commercialization of organs or transplantation using executed criminals. In order to improve the condition of Asian transplantation practice, it is required that there be extensive public education to promote donation, strict legislation for prohibiting unethical activities, and economic and financial support for end-stage organ failure or transplantation.

COMMENTARY

Jeremy Chapman

Why is there a transplantation bureaucracy that needs to be understood? If one can answer that question to one's own personal satisfaction, then it is possible to measure how well the current bureaucracies meet their responsibilities. There are four basic human concepts that provide both the foundation for transplantation and the origin of some of the problems that the bureaucracies must tackle.

First and foremost amongst the foundations of transplantation is the concept of brain death—its precise definition and the general community's understanding and acceptance of that definition. Transplantation therapy has required the definition of brain death and its embodiment in law in a way that the society served by that law can comprehend and trust. The way in which different countries have defined death of the individual has been surprisingly diverse, as noted in this chapter. Legislation, regulation, community-accepted practices, and religious authority approval have all played a part in each transplant bureaucracy's approach to brain death. The bureaucracy has failed the community that it serves in the countries that lack clarity in the definition of brain death.

The second concept is the technical capacity to remove an organ from one living individual and transplant it into a patient in need. While most readers may only think in terms of living kidney transplantation, current worldwide practice in living organ donation includes transplantation of the heart (domino procedure), and parts of the liver, lung, and pancreas. What relationship is required between the donor and the recipient? How is that relationship regulated, reviewed, and permitted? Some bureaucracies have been forced to respond to overt cash payments for human tissue, a process viewed by most societies as fundamentally unethical. Other bureaucrats in different circumstances have gone to the extreme of defining a grandparent as unrelated in law as a response to this issue. A bureaucracy that interprets a community's views, needs, and circumstances and then provides leadership in this very difficult and complex area of human endeavour is to be applauded. The applause is not deafening, and it is easy to find critics of those that carry these responsibilities.

An organ that is donated to the general community of people in need of a transplant, as a truly altruistic gift, must be seen as one of the most precious therapeutic resources available. The limitations on the number of such gifts and the almost unlimited number of potential recipients worldwide mean that allocation of that resource becomes a great responsibility to those empowered to make the choices. The process by which countries decide who receives and who is denied an individual organ is the third concept that the bureaucracies must confront. They are responsible for the manner in which comparative patient needs, professional opinion, scientific analysis, and lay opinion are melded to produce general allocative principles that can then be converted to actual allocative practices. Should donations be made available only to individuals who are nationals of the country where donation takes place? Should those donations be determined by geography, the science of tissue matching, or the distributive injustice of a wait list irrespective of medical need? The implementation of information technology has allowed some countries to make use of increasingly sophisticated allocation algorithms to move the decision to a depersonalized debate, rather than the pressing reality of snap decisions taken in the middle of the night over the telephone with imperfect information.

This chapter provides a detailed insight into the evolution of the approach taken in the United States. It is interesting to understand the problems that the United States appears to struggle with, notably the roles of governmental versus private organizations, individual involvement versus institutional representation, and the balance of power created by different sources of funding. The issues that have beset other countries are, by contrast, almost products of allowing an unfettered market economy access to organ donation. For example, the level of paid organ donation and subsequent response to that practice have overwhelmed other considerations in several countries during the past 10 years. The principles adopted in one country at one time, such as the use of organs from executed prisoners or voluntary donation of a prisoner's kidney in return for remission of sentence, have become abhorrent in subsequent years and sharply criticized when adopted elsewhere.

The fourth and final human concept that bureaucracies must tackle is the level to which a proactive rather than reactive stance is taken to espousing the issues of transplantation and educating the community. It is insufficient to note that most individual members of a given community do not understand brain death or organ donation. Just as health authorities and governments have to deal with lack of knowledge of vaccination or other health programs, so they must also deal with the ignorance that surrounds organ and tissue donation at all levels. Whether such processes have been established could be regarded as a yard stick by which to judge the effectiveness with which a bureaucracy has met its responsibilities. The failure of understanding begins, somewhat alarmingly, with the individuals who make the diagnosis of brain death and discuss consent to donation with the next of kin, and extends throughout the community. The intensive care physician who fails to understand the emotional implications of brain death and organ donation for the family; the nurse who witnesses spinal reflexes in the operating room and believes the cadaver is still alive; the recipient who fails the donor family's expectations of declared gratitude; and the surgeon who believes in an institutional ownership of a donated organ—all can be seen as the responsibility of a bureaucracy that has failed in its educational tasks.

To summarize, the answer to the question posed above—"Why is there a transplantation bureaucracy that needs to be understood?"—can thus be seen to rest on the real and present needs for both process and decision making in the following four areas:

- Definition of brain death
- Determination of the conditions for living organ donation
- Provision of a dynamic and interactive process for allocation of all transplantation therapy
- Education of the wider professional and general community

In conclusion, one might pessimistically, but perhaps reassuringly, conclude that by understanding their failings the transplantation bureaucracies are exposed as merely human.

REFERENCES

1. Dennis JM. Scarce medical resources: hemodialysis and kidney transplantation. In: Elster J, ed. Local Justice in America. New York: Russell Sage Foundation, 1995:109.
2. Iglehart JK. The politics of transplantation. N Engl J Med 1984;310:13:864–868.
3. US Department of Health & Human Services. Organ transplantation: issues and recommendations. Washington, DC: Government Printing Office, 1986.
4. Graham WK, Whelchel JD, McGraw L, et al. The UNOS statement of principles and objectives with equitable organ allocation. Richmond, VA: UNOS, 1994:1–19.
5. Mickey MR. HLA matching in transplants from cadaver donors. In: Terasaki PI, ed. Clinical kidney transplants. Los Angeles: UCLA Tissue Typing Laboratory, 1985:45.
6. Salvatierra Jr O. National organ transplant act. In: Salvatierra Jr O, Lum CT, eds. History of the American Society of Transplant Surgeons. Minneapolis MN: Stanton: 1994:360–374.
7. Center for Disease Control and Prevention. Guidelines for preventing transmission of human immunodeficiency virus through transplantation of human tissue and organs. MMWR 1994;43:RR-8:1–17.
8. Pritsker AAB, Martin DL, Reust JS, et al. Organ transplantation modeling and analysis. Proceedings of the WMC '96 Simulation in Medical Sciences Conference, San Diego, CA, January 14–17, 1996.
9. UNOS. In focus with Walter Graham. Richmond, VA: Sep./Oct. 1996:3.
10. Matesanz R, Miranda B. Preliminary data report organ donation and transplantation. Council of Europe, Transplant Newsletter, March 1996.
11. WHO. Legislative responses to organ transplantation. The Netherlands: Martinus Nijhoff, 1993.
12. Michielsen P. Effect of transplantation laws on organ procurement. Touraine JL, et al, eds. Organ Shortage: the solutions. The Netherlands: Kluwer Academic, 1995:33–39.
13. Van Rood JJ. A proposal for international cooperation in organ transplantation. Eurotransplant. Histocompatibility Testing 1967:451–452.
14. Persijn GG, Cohen B. Eurotransplant Part I, organizational aspects. Clin Transpl 1986:35–46.
15. Pudlo P. European transplant programs: What can the U.S. learn? J Transpl Coord 1993;3:138–140.
16. De Meester J, Persijn GG, Wujciak T, et al. The new Eurotransplant Kidney Allocation System: report one year after implementation. Eurotransplant International Foundation. Transplantation 1998;66:1154–1159.
17. Schippers HMA. New structure Eurotransplant organization. Eurotransplant Newsletter 1994;120:2–6.
18. Haase-Kromwijk B. Financing of Eurotransplant organization. Eurotransplant Newsletter 1994;112:69.
19. Van Renterghem Y, Persijn GG. The implementation of the new Eurotransplant kidney allocation system. Eurotransplant Newsletter 1996;131:4–7.
20. Cohen B. Cooperation between Eurotransplant and Eastern European countries. Eurotransplant Newsletter 1989;89:7–10.
21. Council of Europe. Transplant. Vol. 6. 1994.
22. Hassaballah AM. Definition of death, organ donation and interruption of treatment in Islam. Nephrol Dial Transplant 1996;11:964–965.
23. Daar AS. Organ donation—world experience—the Middle East. Transplant Proc 1991;23:2505–2507.
24. Shaheen FAR, Salim FH, Hamoud TA. Directory of the regulations of organ transplantation in the kingdom of Saudi Arabia. Saudi J Kidney Dis Transplant 1994;5:37–98.
25. Ahmed E, Malek Hosseini SA, Salahi H, et al. Experience with 300 renal transplants in Shiraz, Iran. Transplant Proc 1995;27:2767.
26. Fazel I. Renal transplantation from living related and unrelated donors. Transplant Proc 1995;27:2586–2587.
27. Rizvi SAH, Naqvi A. The need to increase transplantation activity in developing countries. Transplant Proc 1995;27:2739–2740.
28. Ota K, Teraoka S, Takahashi K, et al. Situation of organ transplantation in Asian countries (1989–1990). Transplant Proc 1994;26:40:2457–2460.
29. Ota K, Teraoka S, Kawai T. Donor difficulties in Japan and Asian countries. Transplant Proc 1995;27:1:83–86.
30. Chu S-H. Transplantation in Taiwan. Transplant Proc 1995;27:1476–1477.

31. Ongcharit C. The current status of organ transplantation in Thailand. Transplant Proc 1996;28:3.
32. Vathsala A, Lee WT, Li MK, et al. Transplantation in Singapore. Transplant Proc 1995;27:1472–1475.
33. Shaheeen FAM. Transplantation in Saudi Arabia. Transplant Proc 1995;27:1470–1471.
34. Hawkins BR. Current status of organ transplantation in Hong Kong. Transplant Proc 1996;28:1190–1192.
35. Cheng KP, Lai KN, Au CT, et al. Comparison of the mortality and morbidity rate between proper and unconventional renal transplantation using organs from executed prisoners. Transplant Proc 1991;23:2533–2536.
36. Rashid HU, Rahman M, Wahab MA, et al. Renal transplantation in Bangladesh. Transplant Proc 1995;27:1461–1462.
37. Fan KS, Lim TO, Morad Z, et al. Renal transplantation in Malaysia. Transplant Proc 1995;27:1466–1468.
38. Teik KO, Durai TT, Woods HF. Organization of national kidney foundation and organ sharing system in Singapore. Transplant Proc 1996;28:3.
39. Park K, Kim Y, Lee E, et al. Single-center experience of unrelated living donor renal transplantation in the cyclosporine era. In: Terasaki P, Cecka M, eds. Clinical kidney transplants. Los Angeles: UCLA Tissue Typing Laboratory, 1992:249–255.
40. Naqvi SAJ. Transplantation in Pakistan. Transplant Proc 1995;27:1469.

Chapter

42

Transplantation and Society

A. G. R. Sheil

DEMOGRAPHICS

For the provision of treatment by organ transplantation, nations may be divided into two categories. *Developed nations* with affluent societies, such as the United States, the countries of Western Europe, Japan, Australia, and New Zealand, have the expectation that their citizens with organ failure will receive the best treatment available. *Developing nations* presently fall into two groups. Some nations, such as South Africa, Korea and Southeast Asia, South America and Mexico, the Middle Eastern countries, Greece, and Russia, have established health programs and some first-rate facilities practicing organ transplantation; however, their economies preclude organ transplantation for most nationals. The second group of nations, including India, China, and countries of Central and Eastern Africa, have a few high-class health centers, where priorities for health care are directed toward basic public health requirements; in these situations, organ transplantation is either not practiced or has a low priority. The proportion of the world population living in the developing countries is approximately 85%.

RENAL REPLACEMENT THERAPY

The introduction of renal dialysis in the late 1950s and the first successful non-twin renal transplantation in 1961 were followed by the rapid spread of these technologies in developed countries throughout the world. Although the extent of the need was unknown and the new therapies were costly, clinicians and administrators in all major hospitals were quick to embrace them and be part of the dramatic breakthroughs. As a result, in most developed countries, the centers providing dialysis and kidney transplantation exceed by far the number required to meet actual demand.

Renal Replacement in Developed Countries

Variations in the numbers presenting for treatment in different countries depend on a number of factors. Genetic backgrounds of the peoples differ, as do the environments, infections, and other risk factors that determine the prevalence of conditions affecting the organs. For example, the incidence of renal failure differs among races and countries, as illustrated by the high rates of diabetes-induced renal failure in the United States and Canada. Hypertension contributes to renal failure among African Americans, New Zealand Maoris, Australian Aborigines, and Pacific Islanders, and analgesic abuse affects rates in Australia and Switzerland.

In a 1990 to 1992 review of renal replacement therapy in many developed countries (1), the number of facilities providing regular dialysis therapy per million of population varied from 1.5 to 4.2 (United Kingdom, New Zealand, Canada, Australia), to 4.6 to 6.7 in most European countries (Belgium/Netherlands/Luxembourg, France, Spain, Germany, Switzerland, Sweden, Norway, and Finland), to 10.8 in the United States, 13.8 in Italy, and 20.3 in Japan. The number of new patients beginning dialysis during the last full year before the review for the above countries were in the range 50 to 181 (mean 88) per million population. In all countries reviewed, there was an increasing rate of presentation due predominantly to the acceptance of older patients. Patients aged more than 65 years varied from 17% to 45% (mean 36%) of the new dialysis patients accepted.

Of the mean 88 patients per million population presenting each year with renal failure (but excluding the aged patients), around 50 patients per million population each year might be suitable for and would wish to have kidney transplantation. However, kidney transplantation rates in developed countries are in the range 10 to 41 per million population each year (2,3). The shortfall in donor organs contributes to enlarging dialysis programs and so to increasing costs, as well as to prolonged waiting times for patients on dialysis and a steady loss of patients who die while waiting for transplantation (about 6% per year). Doctors, health authorities, and governments continue their efforts to increase the number of organ donors.

Currently, in the developed countries, patients with kidney transplantation comprise 17% to 53% (mean 39%) of the renal failure population. Of the transplants performed, living donation contributes 20% to 25% of kidneys in the United States and Canada and 10% to 15% in Australia, New Zealand, and Europe. The remaining patients receive cadaveric donor grafts. In Japan, where cultural, religious, and legal factors result in an exceptionally low cadaver donor incidence, the dialysis rate is the highest in the world. What transplantation there is—4.1% of the renal failure population—is largely (65%) from living donors.

In each country, the socioeconomic, political, and legislative factors reflected in the health care system play roles in the availability of organ transplantation services. These influences determine not only the quantity and quality of the services, but the accessibility to them of all or part of the community served. The development of services is also responsive to financial considerations. For example, the cheaper forms of dialysis (home dialysis, limited care facilities, or continuous ambulatory peritoneal dialysis) and transplantation are encouraged wherever renal replacement therapy is concentrated in public hospitals and funded by governments through the public purse (e.g., European countries, Australia, Canada, New Zealand). When funding is through private, for-profit organizations, as it is in Japan and the United States, the number of dialysis facilities is high and the incentive to remove patients from dialysis via transplantation is low.

Because of the scarcity of donors and the high costs, a number of factors limit access to kidney transplantation. They include co-morbid conditions such as coronary artery disease, congestive cardiac failure, left ventricular hypertrophy, and malignancy (4). In the United States, advancing age, female sex, non-white race, and low income have also been shown to limit access (4). Variations in the kidney transplantation rates also depend on the public attitude to organ donation, the laws relating to brain death and consent for donation, the attitude of medical practitioners, and the efficiency of organizations involved in organ donation and retrieval. Kidney transplantation is being pursued aggressively in the United Kingdom, Australia, New Zealand, Scandinavia, and in European nations such as France, Belgium, the Netherlands, and Luxembourg, where transplantation patients constitute 30% to 58% of the total renal failure population. The proportions in the United States and Italy are 27% and 18%, respectively (1).

TRANSPLANTATION OF ORGANS OTHER THAN KIDNEYS IN DEVELOPED COUNTRIES

From kidney transplantation and research laboratories, the surgical methodologies and immunosuppressive therapies necessary for other organ transplants—the liver, heart, lung, pancreas, and intestine—developed. The majority of these clinical programs were superimposed on established kidney transplantation programs. Clinical other-organ transplants had begun during the 1960s in the United States; however, only heart transplantation had a brief, widespread popularity as a result of the first successful heart transplantation in South Africa. It was not until the advent of the immunosuppressive agent cyclosporine in the late 1970s that transplantation of all the other organs moved beyond a few dedicated centers in the United States and Europe. By the mid-1980s, other-organ transplants had become sufficiently successful to be recognized by doctors and the public as desirable.

At the time other-organ transplants became viable, the governments of most developed countries were in a position to restrict the number of centers approved and supported to provide other-organ transplants—thus preventing a recurrence of the proliferation of units as had occurred with kidney transplantation. In Australia, New Zealand, and England and several other European countries, selected centers are strategically located according to population demands and are financed with public funds to provide the services. Patients at these centers receive their treatment for free or for a low cost. The restriction of organ transplantation centers has prevented costly duplication of facilities and personnel, as well as increased their efficiency and skill by maintaining substantial workloads. Retrieval activity under this system has been rationalized, as the surgeons in each area of the country perform multi-organ retrieval from cadaver donors even when tissue matching or other factors dictate that grafts are to be sent to recipients in other areas.

In the United States, where a significant proportion of medical services are paid for through medical insurance or private funds, most large hospitals have established other-organ transplant programs for prestige and profit motives. The result is an oversupply of transplantation institutions, duplication of facilities, and keen competition for donor organs. In the last few years, state authorities and insurance agents have begun to regulate the situation by designating the centers to which transplant candidates are directed for treatment.

Just as for kidney transplantation, differing genetic and risk factors among the populations of different countries affect the demand for other-organ transplants. For example, in the United States and Canada the high rates of diabetes and hypertension contribute to an increased need for heart and pancreas transplantation. In Southeast Asia, viral hepatitis has contributed heavily to the need for liver transplantation. Overall, the demand varies widely, according to different estimates. The number of transplants required per million population each year for the various organs is 15 to

40 (median around 30) for heart (including heart–lung) (5) and liver (6,7). Pancreas and small bowel transplantation remain relatively infrequent treatments.

RENAL REPLACEMENT AND OTHER-ORGAN TRANSPLANTS IN DEVELOPING COUNTRIES

In the 1970s, the physicians and surgeons of developing countries who had trained in the developed countries began to introduce the methodologies for dialysis and kidney transplantation. By the 1980s, methods for other organs began to be introduced as well. However, widespread application of these treatments has been delayed. Sophisticated new treatments have a low priority in the face of existing requirements for preventative medicine, infection control, and dietary supervision. Also, social, cultural, religious, and legal factors have contributed to a low rate of organ donation, particularly from cadaver donors. Of the approximately 6 billion world population, the 5 billion people in developing countries have no access to treatment for organ failure.

The provision of transplantation services in several developing countries followed a common pattern (8). At first, patients received living-related donor kidney transplantation. Patients who had relatives or spouses judged to be suitable donors, and who had the necessary financial support, received grafts. The treatments often placed the donors (mothers and wives especially) under familial or financial duress.

The practice of the wealthy purchasing kidneys from the poor soon appeared, and living-unrelated donor kidney transplantation began to flourish. Donors became available under coercion or through ignorance, deception, or poverty. The development of a national and international black market for kidneys, subject to all the usual market dynamics, followed. As dealers, brokers, middlemen, advertising agencies, and tourist agencies from all over the world became involved, wealthy recipients and organ sellers were attracted from other countries. The price of a kidney escalated rapidly, and some organs were sold at auction. There was no legal redress for misadventure, including the transfer of diseased organs.

In the majority of developing countries, mainstream clinicians were appalled at the developing market for organs. They moved to eliminate the trade in organs by outlawing from each country's medical societies any doctors who participated in renal transplantation using living-unrelated donors. The actual and potential human rights abuses in the developing countries became the focus of a 1991 World Health Organization (WHO) study, which published principles to be applied worldwide in organ transplantation—including the prohibition of organ sales (9). Today, many of the countries where profiteering from kidney transplantation was rife (the Middle East, India, Southeast Asia, South America), as well as the developed countries where organ trafficking was more sporadic, have now outlawed profiteering in transplantation.

As a result, living donor programs in developing countries have undergone considerable change in recent years. In many countries, living-unrelated donor transplantation is restricted to spouses and others in a caring relationship with the recipient. In some countries such as India and Middle Eastern nations, other living-unrelated donor renal transplants are permitted when committees—usually composed of administrators, theologians, lay individuals, social workers, and doctors—approve each donation. The system works reasonably well in the public sector and in many key institutions, but it provides a widely recognized loop hole. Paid living-unrelated kidney donations continue to be the subject of a flourishing trade in the private sector in a number of countries, constituting 50% to 70% of kidney transplantations.

Because dialysis cannot be provided on a large scale for financial reasons, doctors needing organs for transplants find themselves in a persistent situation of "buy or let die" (10). In developing countries, the numbers of patients with renal failure who can be treated by dialysis and/or transplantation are only 0 to 10 per million population each year. Cadaver donor programs either do not exist or are struggling. Progress has been made in some areas of South America, Singapore, Hong Kong, South Africa, Turkey, and Greece. In the exceptional case of Saudi Arabia, an advanced cadaver donor program has been established (11).

For developing countries, the difficulties associated with other-organ transplants remain formidable. Liver and heart transplantation can be performed in many countries, but the cadaver donors are scarce. Organs from executed criminals have been used in several countries (e.g., Singapore, Korea, Taiwan, Hong Kong), but they have gradually phased out the practice. In mainland China, however, executed criminals remain virtually the only source of organs for transplantation; the number of transplants conducted from this source (mostly renal) is considerable.

The total number of liver or heart transplantations performed annually in Eastern Europe, Asia, and Southeast Asia is probably fewer than 200 of each type, with similar low numbers in Africa, China, India, and South America. A gradual increase in the rate of transplantation can be expected in the future, but it is inconceivable that the demand for transplants can ever be met. The future will provide severe difficulties for the ethics of organ allocation.

TRANSPLANTATION AND THE LAW

Until the 1940s, the disposal of cadavers was regulated by relatively straightforward laws such as Great Britain's Anatomy Act of 1932. However, by the late 1940s and early 1950s, the benefits of corneal transplantation were widely appreciated, resulting in increased usage of bodies and body parts. As a result, legislatures worldwide began to produce laws regulating the donation and use of dead bodies and body parts for scientific and medical purposes.

The transplantation of a kidney between identical twins in 1954 in Boston, Massachusetts, heralded not only the era of organ transplantation, but also the birth of another enterprise new in clinical practice, the removal of a normal organ from a healthy individual for implantation into another (needy) individual. With the advent of effective immunosuppression in 1961, the invasion of the bodies of the living and recently dead for kidneys for transplant became frequent.

As harvesting was subsequently extended to include a range of other organs, the "anatomical gift" and "corneal donation" laws often did not apply. New laws were required to define the limits of the developing practice. Inevitably, in the absence of law, errors and crimes occurred, and highly respected medical practitioners were prosecuted and sued for their roles in transplantation procedures. Some physicians were viewed by the public, and even by medical colleagues, as contributing to homicide or to organ theft. Many disapproved of the use of their nation's organs to treat foreigners. Prosecutions over these matters occurred in England, the United States, Japan, and Sweden (12).

In 1969 the United States enacted the Uniform Anatomical Gift Act. Upon an individual's death and in the absence of any prior objection by the deceased, gifts of bodies or body parts could be authorized by relatives in a stated order of priority. Similar laws were adopted by many countries. However, just as had happened previously, the practice of organ transplantation ran ahead of the law with developments in medicine. Transplantation surgeons had discovered that the best outlook for recipients (especially for heart and liver transplantation) was obtained when organs were removed from donors whose respiration and circulation were maintained after death had resulted from destruction of the brain.

Certifying Death: The Brain Death Criterion

During the 1950s and 1960s, it became possible to maintain patients with severe cerebral insults in a hemodynamically stable state by means of artificial respiration and intravenous therapy during the assessment and early treatment stages. Thus, many of those with fatal cerebral injuries continued in the stable condition, with the rest of the body organs functional, for periods of hours to weeks. It fell to the lot of doctors (usually intensive care physicians) to conclude that further treatment was useless, and to withdraw respiratory and other support. Death was certified by subsequent absence of respiration and heartbeat. During the 1960s, transplant surgeons were part of this routine. After the certification of death in the manner described (often in the operating room with the cadaver fully prepared for operation), the kidneys were removed rapidly for urgent transfer to waiting recipients. However, the futility of subjecting the organs to anoxia and failing circulation was apparent to all.

In 1967, Christiaan Barnard of South Africa transplanted the heart, beating at the time of its removal, from a brain-dead automobile accident victim to a man with terminal heart failure. The procedure and its potential stunned the world. Around the world, precipitate cardiac transplantation efforts followed, almost always involving heart-beating donors and without legal or uniform medical support for the procedure. The newly established concept of "death certified on cerebral grounds" (DOCG) had yet to gain widespread acceptance.

In many countries, under government or health authority direction, surgeons, physicians, lawyers, and others were constituted as committees with instructions to review transplantation practices and model new laws regulating them. The outstanding requirements were the definition of DOCG, the regulation of organ donation, and the control of commerce in body parts. Within one year of the Barnard transplantation, a group of Harvard Medical School specialists published a report whose primary purpose was "to define irreversible coma as a new criterion for death" (13). The committee listed a set of criteria or tests which, if fulfilled, would determine that death had occurred, even though (artificial) ventilation and circulation persisted.

The Harvard report was widely endorsed by the medical profession. Through the 1970s, it served as the keystone to criteria developed by institutions, health departments, and government organizations in the United States, Europe, Canada, Australia, and New Zealand. Legislation, including legal recognition of DOCG, followed. In most cases the laws depended on the concept of whole brain death, including the brainstem. However, in the United Kingdom irremediable loss of function of the brainstem is sufficient to determine death. The laws do not set out the criteria for brain death, leaving this to the codes of practice of the institutions and health authorities.

As well as making organ transplantation practicable, the diagnosis of DOCG permits discontinuation of medical treatment of the patient and frees medical and paramedical staff and the intensive care unit to help other sick individuals. A delay in the diagnosis of death was recognized as not in the best interests of the patient, the family, the doctors, or the health care institution.

Most experienced clinicians assert that irreversible destruction of the brain can be established with certainty by history, physical examination, and an apnea test. The diagnosis must be made independently by two experienced doctors unconnected with the transplantation team, and the procedures must be repeated after 24 hours. However, there are some circumstances where the results of ancillary tests may be sought—for example, when the blood levels of therapeutically or self-administered drugs indicate continued effect, when relatives or other doctors demand evidence of brain death, or when the 24-hour interval before the second examination must be curtailed (as in response to the request of relatives or when the donor becomes hemodynamically unstable). The ancillary tests used include electroencephalography, radionuclide brain scan, computed tomography, evoked brainstem responses, magnetic resonance imaging, positron emission tomography, Doppler sonography, intracranial pressure monitoring, cerebral angiography, and assays of endocrine functions of the brain. To be of value, the tests must be performed and interpreted by experienced specialists. With the exception of four-vessel cerebral angiography revealing absence of cerebral blood flow, no test provides an incontrovertible diagnosis of death and each can be used for confirmatory evidence only.

There has been considerable debate as to whether the brain death criteria can be applied in children. From time to time it has been proposed that young children be excluded from consideration (14). Most now agree that the same criteria apply to all full-term newborns older than 7 days and to other children. However, the criteria do not apply to immature pre-term newborns or the newly born; apart from anencephalic babies who might become organ donors, the need to test and establish the criteria of brain death in the newly born is rare (15).

In a 1990 review of worldwide legal statutes (16), brain death criteria were defined and DOCG was accepted medically in 35 of 39 nations. Laws certifying death on cerebral grounds had been passed in 13 nations and in 27 of the states in the United States. Since that review, similar legislation has been passed in other countries, and many others are moving in that direction. The concept of DOCG has been recognized by Roman Catholic, Protestant, and Jewish theologians.

Consent and Commerce

Throughout the 1970s, in developed countries, regulations of organ donation and of commerce in transplantation were discussed concurrently with laws concerning the diagnosis of DOCG. Again, the need was urgent, as removal of organs without proper informed consent, frank theft of organs, and profiteering from organ transplantation were occurring.

In 1975 a Council of Europe report and subsequent model legal code (in 1978) (17) dealt with the removal of tissues from both the living and the dead. It emphasized the requirement for informed consent (excepting children and the legally incompetent), drew a distinction between "regenerative" and "nonregenerative" body parts, and prohibited commerce in human tissues. It provided that tissues and organs may be removed from a dead body if there is no recorded objection by the deceased. This is *presumed consent* (or "opting out"), in which no inquiry of the relatives is needed, as distinct from *affirmative consent* ("opting in") in which the donor, relatives, or persons in lawful possession of the body are required to give consent. The code marks the first appearance of the recommendation that the state appropriate the dead body, as making tissues and organs available for the treatment of the sick is implicit.

The Council of Europe Code, with modifications, has been widely adopted throughout Europe and in some non-European nations. The countries that have enacted laws embodying presumed consent include Austria, Belgium, Czechoslovakia, Denmark, France, Hungary, Iceland, Israel, Jamaica, People's Republic of China, Poland, Portugal, Switzerland, Turkey, and the member countries of the former Soviet Union (16). Other countries have enacted the presumed consent laws but still seek affirmative consent for organ donation, including Cyprus, England, Finland, Greece, Italy, Norway, Philippines, Spain, and Yugoslavia. Countries where affirmative consent must be given include Argentina, Brazil, Bulgaria, Ecuador, Egypt, Hong Kong, Iraq, Japan, Kuwait, Lebanon, Luxembourg, Romania, South Korea, Sweden, Uruguay, and Venezuela (16). Countries where affirmative consent is required but the need is waived under certain conditions (for example, when relatives cannot be located after a thorough search) include Australia, Bolivia, Canada, Germany, India, Ireland, Kenya, Mexico, Netherlands, New Zealand, Panama, Peru, Puerto Rico, Singapore, South Africa, Syria, Tanzania, Thailand, and the United States. In all 160 countries with established legislation on tissue and organ donation, consent from an authorized entity is a requirement (16).

In developing countries, the legal regulation of organ transplantation activities trails far behind the developed countries. While many now have statutes (as detailed above), which are often based on those of the developed countries, the majority of the world's nations have not yet enacted legislation governing procurement of cadaver tissue, but instead rely on tradition or tribal law (16).

As organ transplantation continues to consume greater amounts of health budgets, and as transplantation poses increasing ethical dilemmas, it has become a preoccupation of health authorities, governments, and lawyers. In developed countries, and increasingly in developing countries, the established laws are updated and additional laws are passed with some frequency. Many of these updates relate to consent, with the objective of increasing the supply of donor organs.

ECONOMICS

Once transplantation is established in a country, any authority seeking to control the extent of its application becomes enmeshed in difficulties. At present, the brake on transplantation (and so costs) is the availability of organs, essentially from cadaver donors. Because of the costs of maintaining renal failure patients on dialysis (with kidney transplantation expected to decrease these costs) and the demands for treatment by patients, their relatives, their clinicians, and their community, governments and societies are constrained to relentlessly pursue methods to increase the availability of cadaver donors.

Reducing health care costs by increasing kidney transplantation is a largely illusory reduction, as the dialysis spaces freed by transplantation are filled at once by other patients as a result of widening indications and diminishing contraindications for dialysis. In fact, as the cadaver kidney donor may provide multiple organs, other-organ transplants and their associated costs increase accordingly.

The cost of a transplantation operation is frequently thought of as referring to the operation itself. However, the cost of the surgery is relatively minor. The expenditure on transplantation of a particular organ, summed over a year, must embrace the salaries of all those involved with the procedure—including surgeons, physicians, nurses, tissue typers, technicians, transplantation coordinators, dieticians, social workers, administrators, data managers, back-up staff, and research staff—as well as part of the costs of those providing back-up hematologic, biochemical, pathologic, and numerous other services. Also included are the costs of the recipient's accommodations before and after transplantation (including housekeeping and dietary components), diagnostic fees for all investigations, and the charges for tissue matching, blood and blood products, pharmacology (including expensive immunosuppressive agents), and organ retrieval.

The organ retrieval expenses in particular can be considerable. They will include either the organ procurement organization's (OPO) fees or transport of a surgical team and perfusionists to the donor hospital (often requiring a helicopter or jet aircraft charter). Other retrieval expenditures relate to the donor hospital expenses, such as intensive care and operating room costs, organ perfusion and preservation costs, and surgeon and physician fees.

The outlays for organ transplantation must also include the ongoing immunosuppression and treatment of patients following transplantation. The expense of the postoperative management of organ transplantation patients can vary enormously. Many recipients become patients of the transplantation center for life, so their continuing care, the treatment of their complications, and (when necessary) management of their graft failure and/or retransplantation become additional "transplant" expenses.

On the other hand, in nonprofit institutions, the expenditure on patients who would have died in the hospital were it not for transplantation (18) should be subtracted from the transplantation costs when assessing the overall financial impact on an institute. The calculation of organ transplantation expenditure is further complicated because it is debatable which outlays should be attributed to "organ transplantation" and which should not. For example, once patients are accepted onto waiting lists it might generally be acceded that pretransplantation costs are part of the organ transplantation responsibility, but how much of the expenditure on dialysis should be accepted as a transplant cost when patients may wait on dialysis for several years before transplantation?

The expenditure on transplantation must be differentiated from other institutional costs. Most programs are established in large hospitals that already have a full complement of staff (medical, paramedical, administrative, lay) with back-up investigative and therapeutic facilities; thus, the transplantation undertaking begins with surgeons and other staff who are already employed, and a significant proportion of the costs of the service are provided in previously established wages and infrastructure. As the transplantation activity increases, complementary additions to the staff of surgeons, physicians, nurses, anesthetists, technicians, and employees in the back-up facilities may be required. The institutions also have variable background costs. Rent for the land they occupy and charges for basic utilities (electricity, water, gas) can vary from almost nothing to substantial.

Given all these vagaries, the actual and/or estimated costs of transplantation of the various organs cover a broad range. Costs are also not equal to charges, as the latter may include profit and may vary according to market conditions and payer mix. Thus, the charges (*not* costs) for the procedures in developed countries are in the range US$70,000 to $350,000 (median $150,000) for liver transplantation, US$50,000 to $300,000 for heart, heart–lung, or lung transplantation (median $150,000 heart, $210,000 heart–lung), and US$25,000 to $130,000 for renal or pancreas transplantation (median $40,000 renal, $67,000 pancreas) (5,6,19,20).

The costs for the various transplants are much less in developing countries, mostly because the salaries of all those involved are but a fraction of those in developed countries. Most programs concentrate predominantly on living-related kidney transplantation, and do not involve the massive costs involved in full-fledged cadaver donor or other-organ transplant programs. For example, in India the charge for a living-unrelated kidney transplant for an Indian national is US$2000 (includes some profit), and US$8000 for a foreigner (Chugh KS, personal communication, 1996).

In the developed countries, the methods to finance organ transplantation differ among countries. In those nations with governmental control of funding and with strategic location of transplant facilities according to geographic population demands (England, other European countries, Australia, New Zealand, Saudi Arabia), there is reasonable control of costs. The approximate number of transplantations performed per year for each type of organ is known (predicated by donor numbers), together with the additional costs to the institutions of providing the services. These amounts (usually calculated on a per transplant basis) are provided to the designated institutions. The clinicians and administrators of the institutions vary their staffing, equipment, maintenance, and research needs as they see fit, within the allocation. Significant variations of transplantation numbers require a health authority review and potential variations in financial allocation.

As of 1988, the advent of managed care in the United States ushered in new methods of administration. In the United States, major insurers contract transplantation work to networks of designated transplantation hospitals, thus linking price competition to outcome. As a result, charges in the selected institutions have fallen appreciably from the maximum figures cited above (which probably were based on true costs) to approximately one-half the maximum (5).

In this competitive climate, transplant centers pursue economic efficiencies and reduced spending in the face of diminished returns for the transplantation procedures. These apparently worthy goals ultimately may impact adversely on patient care, and on the center's ability to stay abreast of advances in diagnostic or treatment methodologies and conduct clinical or basic research. Already, institutions have to weigh the costs and benefits of patient selection. The system now favors prudent choice, avoiding expensive ill or complex patients who otherwise could be saved. On the other hand, much of the cash "lost" through organ transplantation may be recouped through increased patient admissions in other areas due to the prestige and infrastructure associated with the transplantation program.

In all countries there is considerable debate as to the cost-effectiveness of organ transplantation. How comprehensive should the provision of transplantation services be, given their high cost and the myriad other requirements for financial support, both medical and nonmedical? While the general public is supportive of transplantation, public health officials and policy makers are less so (21). Those arguing in support of organ transplantation point out that it is uneconomic to allow patients with renal failure to become chronically ill and be maintained by dialysis, or to allow those with other-organ failure to become chronically ill and die. These patients could be "cured" (at least for a good number of years) by transplantation and contribute to the economic growth of the community. That patients do benefit from organ transplantation in terms of both survival and quality of life is now accepted (22). Greater proportions of kidney transplantation recipients are rehabilitated to work or household duties than are dialysis patients (23). A majority of patients with successful liver (24) and heart (5) transplantation return to the workforce, though employer concerns and patient choice reduce the total number who could work (5).

Whatever the total cost, it appears that in developed countries the drive for more donors will continue, and that there can be no financial limit to the number of transplantations performed until the entire demand is met. Donor numbers permitting, it is extremely difficult to offer limited transplantation procedures on financial grounds alone, because whenever an imposed quota of transplantation is reached, those patients who have not received grafts demand them. The plight of these needy individuals is carried dramatically and effectively in the media, resulting in public dismay and pressure on governments. Moreover, the imposition of a quota necessitates the selection of a fortunate group from the waiting patients, a requirement that poses severe ethical dilemmas.

Nor has the complete story of the cost of organ transplantation yet unfolded. The expenditure on continuing care for the multiplying numbers of transplantation recipients similarly multiplies. Because chronic rejection remains unsolved, it seems likely that all but a small proportion of recipients will be subjected to—and thus subject the health care system to—failure of their transplantation organ, with occasional retransplantations. Current estimates of "demand" include those on waiting lists, those who die waiting, and those who receive grafts; however, the total "need" may be almost twice the demand (6) when patients who could have benefited from transplantation but did not have the opportunity to achieve waiting-list status. A confounding uncertainty is that, as organ transplantation becomes more and more successful, so the indications broaden and age and other restrictions diminish.

EXTENDING THE DONOR ORGAN SUPPLY

For three decades it has been the hope and expectation of transplantation clinicians in developed countries that the clinical need could be met from cadaver donor sources. However, mitigating this outcome has been the steadily improving results of organ transplantation, which has led to progressively broadening indications and steadily increasing demand—thus, the plateau of available organs well below the need (3,23,25). The time patients spend on waiting lists and the number of deaths while waiting have both increased alarmingly (26). In England and the United States, waiting lists of recipients increase by 15% to 20% per year (2,25,27). The claim that there will never be sufficient cadaver donor organs to treat those in need is being heard more and more frequently.

Donor Shortage

Estimates of the number of kidney transplantations required to meet today's demand are around 50 per million population each year (25 to 30 donors per million population per year) in Europe (3) and America (2,28). Since around 70% of donors are now "multiorgan" donors (3), this number could provide other solid organs to meet the demands of many countries (3,5,28). In the United States, however, the demand for livers is estimated at 32 per million population per year (6). In the 1990s, in many European countries and the U.S. cadaver donor numbers have remained at 15 to 22 per million population per year, resulting in cadaver donor kidney transplant rates of the order of 30 per million population per year, liver transplants at 6 to 12, and heart transplants at 4 to 11 (3). Living-related donor kidney transplants contributed additional small percentages (0 to 15) in most countries; however, in Sweden and United States the additions were around 25%, bringing the overall kidney transplantation rates in these countries to 37 and 40 per million population per year. The renal transplant numbers are of the same order as for Spain, where this is achieved almost solely with cadaver donors, but still remain below the required 50 per million population per year to meet the demand.

As mentioned earlier, the need may be up to twice the demand (6). The plateauing of cadaver donor numbers reflects an increased drive to locate donors but also a decreased death rate of young individuals as a result of fewer automobile fatalities and better medical treatment.

The lack of donors is serious for adults awaiting transplantation, but the situation for wait-listed small children is extreme. Here, size of the donor organ is critical. Deaths of small children who might be donors are relatively rare. Surgical techniques allowing the implantation of adult kidneys and cut-down livers in children have helped, but overall the situation remains desperate, especially for potential cardiac recipients.

The need for more organs has stimulated increased usage of living donors, related and unrelated, as well as the consideration of anencephalic infants, vegetative individuals, executed criminals, and those contemplating suicide or euthanasia as possible donors. Suboptimal donor organs are used. The human fetus has joined the list of donors. Children have been conceived and born to provide bone-marrow transplantation for older siblings. Governments are pressed toward legislation to increase access to cadaver donors. The possibility of compensation or payment for organs is repeatedly examined. Trade in organs persists. Thus, need has been fueling the drive toward xenografting.

Living Donors

As waiting times for kidney transplantation progressively elongate, clinicians in developed countries are turning increasingly to living-related donor transplantation. The increasing use of kidneys from spouses and those in caring relationships with the recipient is a reversal of the 1980s trend away from living donors when cadaver donor results improved. There is now more general approval of the use of kidneys from living-unrelated donors who donate purely through altruism to unspecified recipients, although few centers in developed countries have used such donors. This latter finding is in accord with the WHO Guiding Principles on Human Organ Transplantation (9) that "in general such [living] donors should be genetically related to the recipients." In developing countries the situation remains quite different. Because cadaver donors remain infrequent (providing 0% to 15% of kidney transplantations in most countries), living donors, predominantly living unrelated, remain the dominant source of kidneys for transplantation.

In an effort to overcome the virtual absence of cadaver donors, some developing countries, notably South Korea, have instituted controlled programs of living-unrelated donors involving the "swapping" of kidneys between incompatible donor–recipient pairs such that the new pairings are compatible (29). This system is being extended to provide larger "living donor pools" made up of volunteers, either those involved with a recipient (as in the "swapping" programs) or individuals from the general population donating through altruism. This concept is gaining support in other countries, including developed countries.

Cadaveric Donors

The methods tried in the hope of increasing cadaver donors are legion. Most developed countries now have, or are developing, regional and national agencies (discussed further in the organ allocation section of this chapter) whose charters include the promotion of organ donation.

Public and Medical Education

Transplantation clinicians have endeavored to foster professional, public, and governmental support for cadaver donation through dedicated attempts at education, including media coverage of successful and/or interesting transplantation outcomes, public forums, donor awareness campaigns, donor recognition events, support groups, and direct addresses to minority groups (30). The major goals are to ensure that relatives are aware of each individual's wishes with regards to organ donation, and that all doctors recognize their responsibility to ensure that those who agree to organ donation (and who die in suitable circumstances) become organ donors.

Surveys in the majority of developed countries have demonstrated that the education efforts have been successful, as organ transplantation is supported by a significant majority of the public (31). However, the support has not translated into the granting of permission by relatives for donation—negative responses almost always exceed one-third of cases in all countries. Many studies have revealed that the proportion of in-hospital suitable potential donors who convert to actual donors is less than one-half (31).

The benefits of public and medical education programs are well illustrated in Spain (3), where concerted collaborative efforts of doctors, coordinators, the government, the public, and the media, in association with extensive professional coordination in hospitals, have resulted in cadaver donor numbers almost doubling in 5 years (to 25 per million population per year in 1994), approaching the number required to meet the demand for organ transplantation (7). Although similar strenuous efforts over the past decade have not proved demonstrably fruitful in other countries, it is widely believed that the Spanish experience confirms that, in developed countries, the potential to meet the total demand lies in cadaver donors.

Donor Cards, Licenses

The clinicians and health authorities in most developed countries have promoted the signing of intent on "donor cards" or motor driving licenses. Such cards would provide a signed record of each individual's wishes to donate or not donate, so helping relatives in their decision making. However, the surveys that recorded the public's approval of donation also revealed that few individuals had signed their intentions. Of those who had signed donor cards, even fewer carried them (32,33). Even so, most transplantation doctors believe that publicity drives for the carrying of cards or the signing of licenses are worthwhile as a means of promoting discussions within families.

The Intensive Care Unit

It has been reported in England that only approximately one-half of potentially suitable organ donors in intensive care units (ICU) actually donate. Some authors have concluded that, in addition to refusal by relatives (34), a significant limitation to increasing organ donor numbers is the hesitancy or unwillingness of ICU doctors to request organ donation (35).

The shortage of (expensive) ICU beds in almost every country undoubtedly mitigates decisions either to ventilate dead patients or to refer such patients for organ donation. Not only do physicians find requesting donation difficult, but they hesitate to explain brain death to relatives when the donor appears to be alive, and to explain that they cannot be with the patient when support is withdrawn. There is the added stress of maintaining cadaver donors for an additional time (as long as 36 hours) to allow completion of certification of death and arrangements for organ retrieval, with necessary continuing care for both the cadaver donor and the relatives. The extended time is a further burden for the relatives, who may request that the whole matter be ended. In addition, cadaver donors involve a great deal of hard work and organization for overextended ICU doctors. All these considerations simply disappear if the potential donor is never notified.

Each hospital should ensure that referral of potential donors is a required responsibility of doctors—a requirement taught to undergraduates and intensive care physicians in training. A hospital organization must include caring individuals who are trained for grief counseling to discuss donation with relatives. The institution and the transplantation clinicians, coordinators, and retrieval teams must never forget the distressed relatives and must work to minimize the stresses and disruption that organ donation causes in the ICU and the operating room. They must be sensitive, accommodating, and professional, and acknowledge the contribution of all involved.

Consent

As discussed earlier, many countries have "presumed consent" regulations which, when acted upon, have resulted in increased cadaver donation in some nations (36), although not in most. However, the affirmative consent of relatives is still widely sought. To eliminate professional reluctance to request donations (37), a number of states, countries, and institutions have enacted "required request" and/or "routine inquiry" regulations. Under required request rules, doctors are directed to raise the matter of possible organ donation with relatives before support is withdrawn from dead suitable organ donors. Under routine inquiry mandates, relatives must be asked if the deceased intended to be a donor.

It has also been suggested that all potential donors in ICUs should be referred to professional procurement personnel to enhance the likelihood of relatives agreeing to donation. To relieve entirely the burden of decision from relatives, it has been proposed that all persons should record in a registry during life whether they wish to be organ donors or not (mandated choice). Another suggestion is that those who enroll as future donors are awarded priority for subsequent need for organs (38) or even that all and only those who enroll themselves as potential donors are eligible to receive transplant organs if there is subsequent need (39).

Marginal Donors

To enhance cadaver donor numbers, some groups have explored the use of "marginal" or "suboptimal" donors. The practice has included kidneys (40), livers (41), and hearts (42). Such donors are those with features that might preclude use of the organs in normal circumstances, such as age, hemodynamic instability, advanced atherosclerosis, prolonged ICU stay, drug overdose, infection, insulin-dependent diabetes, uncontrolled hypertension, prior malignancy, morbid obesity, sustained hypotension, cardiac arrest, high-dose inotropic support, abnormal biochemical or organ function tests, and, for liver transplantation, severe hepatic steatosis and alcoholism. Organs with greatly prolonged cold ischemic intervals are considered. On occasion, previously transplanted organs (kidneys and livers) have been reused when the initial recipients died. To use kidneys from the very young (43) and old (44), the implantation en bloc of both kidneys in one recipient is being explored.

A further suggestion is that a "seniors pool" of consenting older recipients be established to receive grafts from older donors (45). With careful selection and with final gross and histologic assessment of the organ, results have been rewarding (40–42). Inherent dangers are acknowledged (46), as are the needs for informed consent from those waiting who agree to be recipients of such organs (27). A further extension of this premise has been the use by some groups of organs (kidneys, livers) from donors who test positive for hepatitis C (47) or hepatitis B (48) but have normal function tests (and, for livers, normal histology), because the incidence of progressive liver disease in recipients of such grafts, in the short term, has been low. The recommendation is that such organs be restricted to recipients already infected with the specific virus (47,48). The livers from hepatitis-infected donors are considered also for transplantation to serologically negative recipients with fulminant hepatic failure (48).

As might be expected, marginal donor organs have not been accepted for transplantation in 10% to 20% of cases, either following final assessment or because recipient teams decline to use them. Some such kidneys have been made available to teams in other countries and have been transplanted. For example, US kidneys have been implanted in Japan (49).

Non-Heart-Beating Donors

The use of organs from non-heart-beating donors (NHBD), the accepted practice throughout the 1960s and early 1970s, largely ceased with the advent of heart-beating donors. Today, some investigators are reexamining this source. Such donors are usually those who suffered cardiopulmonary arrest (inside or outside of the hospital) and failed to respond to resuscitation; others were ventilated in ICUs and have a hopeless prognosis, but do not meet brain death criteria ("controlled" NHBD).

For cardiopulmonary arrest, the proposal is that the resuscitation efforts continue, together with organ cooling by cold electrolyte infusion via a femoral arterial cannula (50), while consent for donation and arrangements for immediate organ retrieval are made. Increasingly, as part of the methodology for kidney transplantation, the excised kidneys are being machine perfused, as the results of several studies suggest that this offers a benefit in decreasing the otherwise high incidence (and expense) of delayed graft function and allowing assessment of the viability of the organs as evaluated by various tests (51). In skilled hands the results have been satisfactory for kidney transplantation, though less so for liver transplantation (46). Registry results of the method show modestly inferior results for kidney transplantation (Terasaki P, personal communication, 1996). Where this method has been actively pursued, the increase in donor kidneys has been 20% (52). Problem areas include difficulties in requesting donation almost at the same time as relatives are informed of the patient's death, the need to interfere with the body before consent is obtained (the groin operation to insert the intraarterial catheter), the need for constant availability of teams who can operate with speed and expertise, and the advisability of informed consent of waiting recipients who would accept these organs.

There are also legal concerns. In England, the opinion was that "elective ventilation" of patients—endotracheal intubation at the time of cardiac arrest in a medical ward to allow brain death certification and organ retrieval (53)—was outside the law because it involved nonconsented treatment of an incompetent person (the dead donor) when the treatment was not in the patient's best interest (54). It would seem that a similar consideration might apply to maintenance and cooling of an NHBD whose wishes concerning organ donation were unknown. To address this, legislation allowing hospitals to take the steps necessary to ensure the viability of organs for transplantation during the search for the cadaver's next of kin has already been passed in certain states in the United States (55).

For controlled NHBD the situation is much less difficult, as the issues of consent and preparation for organ retrieval can be dealt with before discontinuation of respiratory support.

Payment for Notification of Potential Donors and for Organ Retrieval

Systems of payments to individuals or organizations for notifying transplantation centers or OPOs of potential donors have the potential to increase cadaver donor numbers both in general and for specific transplantation centers. Although reimbursement of donor hospital and retrieval team expenses is important for maintaining their involvement in cadaver donor programs, it is also important that the "expenses" be regulated and uniform to prevent excess payments in the hope of attracting an unfair proportion of notifications or retrievals, and to prevent profiteering by doctors or agencies resulting from tissue and organ procurement or distribution (56).

Payment for Organs

Of all the methods to increase cadaver donor organ supplies, the place of payment to the (potential) donors or the relatives for the organs is the most hotly debated. The payments suggested vary from relatively small amounts, such as burial fees (57), to huge amounts as could be derived from national auction markets for organs (58). The proposals include "futures" markets whereby individuals pledge their organs against payment to relatives of rebates after their death (59).

An alternative is a "death benefit" (60). Those involved in obtaining consent would inform relatives at the time of donor death that organ donation has a monetary benefit. Payment to the relatives occurs subsequently. In both cases the hope is that the offer of payment will persuade individuals to allow their own, or their relative's, organs to be donated. Thus, the donation may occur for financial rather than humanitarian reasons.

With any method it is likely that the public focus on organ donation resulting from the availability of the reward would have a positive effect initially, by causing families to establish each individual's wishes regarding donation. However, all the schemes have negative aspects, and are shadowed by the possibility of failures accompanied by damaging publicity that would not only eliminate any gain, but critically impact the delicate balance that determines the current rate of organ donation. On the other hand, a government-approved death benefit scheme involving the availability to relatives of donors of approximately US$10,000 together with the payment of burial fees and transport of the donor and a relative is working effectively in Saudi Arabia (Shaheen FAM, personal communication, 1996).

In developed countries, the public has declared that organ transplantation should be available in all its forms to meet whatever demand exists. So far, it seems, money will be found. The public must now further decide whether its support extends to the provision of sufficient cadaver donor organs for the purpose. This is the key decision, as other forms of organs, either artificial or xenografts, will not be available in significant numbers in the foreseeable future.

ORGAN ALLOCATION

Living Donor

For the patients with organ failure who have a relative, spouse, or other caring individual who wishes to donate a kidney, or part organ, the allocation issues are reasonably straightforward once the putative donor is found to be healthy and not under duress, and the organ or part is shown to be anatomically suitable for transplantation. The blood group and tissue matching requirements are presented in other chapters in this book.

Cadaveric Donor

The allocation of scarce cadaver donor organs is fraught with difficulty. The central issue is that selection of a patient to receive an organ graft increases the risks of other waiting patients dying. For each graft implanted it is certain that an unspecified other patient, who could have been saved, will die.

Before patients are accepted to cadaver donor transplant waiting lists, the established scarcity of organs has already resulted in patient selection, with exclusion of many because of age restrictions, other organ system abnormalities, presence or history of malignancy, and so on. In developed countries, most patients who meet generally approved standards are placed on waiting lists, but this is not the case in developing countries where only tiny proportions of suitable recipients achieve waiting-list status.

Potential recipients who accept a listing must place their faith in a team of individuals, some known to them but others not, in a risky enterprise that is embroiled in variables and aimed ultimately at their restoration to good health. Subject to stringent ethical codes and consent, what has to be achieved is the removal of an organ from a dead patient, the organ's ex vivo preservation, and its proper allocation to, and implantation in, a blood-group and T-cell compatible, tissue-typed recipient. The organ transferred must be free of infection or malignancy, and it must be implanted in such a way that it can return to normal function in the immunosuppressed recipient. To achieve this goal, intensive care physicians, nurses, coordinators, tissue matchers, retrieval surgeons, perfusionists, physicians, anesthetists, and transplantation surgeons and their staffs must be available around the clock, prepared to move at the word of a potential donor. All these individuals (on average 40 for each transplant) carry heavy responsibilities, as a single error in any aspect of the undertaking can be critical.

To aid in the procurement and allocation of organs, most geographic areas, states, and countries have local, national, or multinational organizations whose purpose it is to ensure equity in allocation. This role is combined with effecting distribution, maintaining surveillance, and promoting efficiency and cadaver donations. Such bodies include the United Network for Organ Sharing (UNOS) of the United States, Eurotransplant, the United Kingdom Transplant Support Service Authority, the National Transplant Organization of Spain, and many others. Each has highly sophisticated, computer-based organ allocation systems.

With cadaver-donor renal transplants, results of the T-cell crossmatch and tissue matching are available within a few hours of donor death. As kidneys also can be preserved safely by simple cold storage for at least 24 hours, these rapid tests provide the basis for renal allocation, despite challenges to tissue matching on the grounds of efficacy and practicality, and a suggested adverse effect of long-distance transfer on donor kidneys (61).

Because of the large number of waiting patients, it is not uncommon for several patients to have equivalent tissue matching with one presenting donor. It is usual for one of the donor kidneys to be allocated within the geographic area in which the donor presented, while the other is made available on a wider, sometimes national, basis. To assist in the organ's allocation, a range of factors are incorporated into the selection format, with varying weightings. They include patient age, duration of time on dialysis, presensitization to HLA antigens, presence or absence of diabetes mellitus, primary or secondary grafts, ethnic group (not permitted in some countries), import–export imbalance, and so on. Most cooperative groups have an agreement that recipients closely matched to donors (0 or 1 HLA-A, B, DR mismatches) are allotted the kidneys. Computer selection via agreed selection criteria reduces physician competition for grafts. To ensure fairness in allocation, repeated reviews and adjustments of the selection criteria and weightings by personnel from all the institutions and organizations involved in the collaborative projects are required, together with studies to evaluate the impact of agreed policies.

A consequence of decision making involving tissue matching in societies that have minority ethnic and racial groups is that patients from these groups with renal failure will be discriminated against by the HLA determinants common to the general community (62). Compensatory weighting in the computer matching or a search for more equitable matching by considering "permissible" HLA mismatches (63) or key amino-acid residues (64) may be required. On the other hand, difficulties can arise because certain cultural groups may not favor organ donation, but patients with renal failure from these groups will accept donated kidneys.

With other-organ transplants, ABO blood group compatibility and size (for heart, heart–lung, lung, and liver) are important factors in recipient selection. Also, two other factors complicate allocation. First, the logistics of transplantation are such that the results of donor–recipient tissue matching are seldom available preoperatively because of the short time available, as most groups strive to keep ischemic intervals to a minimum. Second, because of absence of effective organ support systems, the waiting lists are comparatively short and the patients are more threatened. Approximately 25% of listed cardiac and liver candidates will die without receiving a transplant (65). This percentage may be artificially low, as some groups with many waiting patients will list additional patients only when another is removed from the list by transplantation or death.

Thus, for heart, heart–lung, lung, liver, and pancreas cadaver donor transplantation, the role of tissue matching in allocation is much reduced. The T-cell crossmatch is taken into consideration for heart, lung, and pancreas–kidney transplantation, but not always for liver. Many other factors come into consideration. They include the imminence of death ("transplant the sickest"); length of time on the waiting list; primary or secondary graft; whether patients are ICU-bound, hospitalized, or at home; the patient's prognosis following transplantation (sometimes determined by the cause of failure of the native organ); age; mental status; and compliance. More difficult psychosocial criteria such as "social worth" (e.g., a physician, politician, artist, or athlete versus a criminal or handicapped patient), psychological status (sound versus unstable, such as suicide candidates), financial status, ethnic origin, family situation (parents versus single persons), criminal record, addictive drug habit (including alcohol), and motivation. In general, patients close to death, younger patients, and those without complicating features such as malignancy or infection are favored. However, the question is frequently asked whether it is better to select the most threatened individual on the waiting list (whose results will be inferior) over a stable candidate (whose likelihood of success is high).

Because of the overwhelming importance of selection for transplantation, there is considerable support for committees to help in the allocation of organs, rather than leaving the matter in the hands of doctors. Such groups avoid any physician bias that might interfere with fair selection, because numerous non-medical matters may be involved. The committees often include theologians, social workers, and lay individuals as well as doctors who are involved and doctors who are not involved with transplantation. It is widely held that the donated organs belong to society, so society should be involved in their distribution (66).

Other concerns in allocation include the listing of one patient to receive more than one organ, as happens when a patient needing other-organ transplants also requires kidney transplantation. Here, it is acknowledged that there are important benefits to the recipient when both organs come from the one donor. However, not only is one patient treated when two could be (reducing cost-effectiveness), but the waiting time for other-organ transplants is comparatively short, so that by simultaneous renal allocation the recipient receives priority over all those waiting for kidney transplantation.

There is also the matter of foreign individuals obtaining grafts, usually with inflated charges for the transplantation. Because of the payment, the foreign patient may be given preference over national citizens. In the United States and England, this practice has resulted in public outrage and legal action against the doctors involved. Most countries now have written or unwritten laws forbidding or restricting such procedures (at 5% to 10% in the United States), unless the organ for transplantation cannot be used for the treatment of citizens of that country. Some donors, or their relatives, may have offered organs in the belief that they would be implanted into national citizens, so it is conceivable that some donors might not wish their organs transplanted into (certain) foreigners, or might not wish them transplanted for a profit unshared by their relatives. In a similar vein, certain religious groups have determined that their organs cannot be transplanted into individuals of another religious persuasion.

For all organs, those making the allocation decisions have an unenviable task. Not only do the above factors require consideration, but other influences obtrude. For example, added pressures may be brought to bear on those selecting because waiting potential recipients are relatives, friends, or friends of friends; they may be relatives or friends of influential individuals, including those whose influence impacts on the transplantation program, such as politicians or hospital administrators. Attempts by physicians to have a patient queue-jump or cut in the waiting line via a dishonest classification (such as an unwarranted admission to an ICU to gain an "urgent" rating) are not infrequent. Financial and other factors also come into play. As was previously mentioned, in the United States, being female or non-white can adversely affect a patient's access to kidney transplantation (4).

ETHICAL ISSUES AND TRANSPLANTATION

From the mid-1950s onward, medical advances in transplantation became matters of public fascination and concern: sustaining respiration and circulation after the brain had permanently ceased function, the first successful kidney transplantation from living and dead donors, and the first cardiac transplantation with an organ beating at the time it was taken from an individual. In addition, humans were subjects of pioneering transplantation experiments of uncertain ethical probity, including skin grafting in convicted prisoners (to test the immunosuppression agent antithymocyte globulin), use of kidneys for transplantation taken from convicted prisoners, removal of kidneys from cadavers without consent, the (unexpected) transplantation of malignancy with kidneys from individuals dying of cancer, and the implantation in humans of organs from animals.

In their rush to explore these advances, transplantation surgeons were venturing where none had gone before. New laws were required, and committees of doctors, scientists, lawyers, administrators, theologians, and philosophers came together to advise institutions, health authorities, grant-giving bodies, and governments on the moral correctness of the new endeavors, not only in transplantation but in all fields of medicine. Thus, the advent of organ transplantation accelerated, focused, and extended medical ethics in all its applications. The era of the ethics committee had arrived.

Living Donors

Before the first successful clinical organ transplantation between identical twins in 1954, the profound ethical concerns were addressed as comprehensively as possible (67). As living-related renal donor transplants became more frequent, ethicists placed emphasis on altruism as a prime requirement for donation, and urged an absence of pressures, either familial or medical, on the donors. The immensely superior results compared to those of cadaver-donor transplants, together with the low risks to the donor, justified the unnatural procedure. Most doctors and the public not only approve the practice, but accord the donors high praise, sanctified by virtually all religious groups.

The requirements of altruism and absence of coercion have also justified renal donations by those in a caring relationship with the recipient (such as spouses or foster parents). More recently, donations have been made, usually by relatives, of parts of the pancreas, liver, and lung. Moreover, the "swapping" of altruistically offered kidneys between incompatible donor–recipient pairs (29) has received broad approval.

The use of kidneys from individuals donating purely through altruism for the good of the community (i.e., those who have no direct connection with a potential recipient) is a more difficult matter which has not found wide appeal (68). However, the donations are generally viewed as ethically appropriate, with the caveat that a committee must review potential donors and that stringent psychological requirements must be met.

While the outcomes of living donor transplants are positive, it must be remembered that there can be mental and/or physical complications in both donors and recipients, despite the best efforts of transplantation clinicians to prevent them. Though breakdowns in donor–recipient relationships are relatively rare (69), on occasions donors have become unfriendly, jealous, abusive, and vindictive; they can become depressed and withdrawn; or they have demanded money or goods from recipients or return of the transplanted organ. Suicide, clearly related to the transplantation, has been recorded in both donors and recipients.

The operations for both parties are major and some complications must be expected, including surgical misadventure leading to failure of the transplantation. In developed countries, the published living-related renal donor mortality rate of 0.03% to 0.10% (69,70) translates to over 100 altruistic individuals who died because of organ donation. It is likely that substantially more have died in the developing countries.

Most physicians adhere to the original constraints on living donation, but two groups have emerged with divergent attitudes. One actively encourages living donation, citing the scarcity of cadaver donors as a major incentive. The other, including some respected transplantation surgeons, has ceased any involvement with the practice.

The initial high principles and ethics of organ transplantation were corrupted by the advent of profiteering. Today, the use of bought kidneys for transplantation is prohibited throughout all developed countries and many developing countries. Ethicists, theologians, and most doctors condemn the sale of any human organs. Even so, paid living-unrelated donor renal transplantation remains a frequent practice in some developing countries, where doctors request that donations be altruistic but profiteering is still rampant.

Cadaveric Donors

With cadaver donors, the rights, dignity, and respect that should be afforded the dying have to be weighed against the needs or rights of the living. Again, the key concerns involved are the care of the donor family, the declaration of the donor's death, consent by the donor or his or her relatives, the shortage of donor organs, organ allocation, and commerce.

In developed countries most issues are by no means resolved. Distressful errors and omissions concerning proper respect for and care of the donor or the donor family are frequently made by clinicians, coordinators, nurses, administrators, or others, often resulting in dramatic publicity that is damaging to the cause of organ donation. Even though the determination of DOCG is widely (but by no means universally) accepted throughout the medical profession, concerns and distrust remain for many of the general public. There is continuing concern regarding the consent laws and regulations of governments and other authorities that are aimed at increasing access to cadaveric organs. For example, with the widely applied "presumed consent" laws, ethicists argue that it is improper to assume consent simply because there is no recorded objection (39). Others consider that presumed consent carries a hint of coercion and "smacks of body snatching" (71). Further, required (or mandated) request is objectionable to ethicists (39).

The fatal consequences for waiting patients when organs are allocated to others present a recurring ethical dilemma. Also, while all ethicists argue that no individual should be excluded from a transplant program on the grounds of inability to pay, in practice this continues to occur even in some developed countries.

Ethics and Developing Countries

In the developing countries, in addition to the previously discussed ethical issues, there are added difficulties because of social, cultural, and religious attitudes relating to death and to the importance of the intact body for burial. However, the now-established ethical standards and regulations of the developed countries are a resource that the developing countries can consider and modify for their own circumstances. Ethical principles are being promoted in many developing countries by dedicated groups of transplantation clinicians, but the hurdles are formidable. The desperate need for organs encourages commerce and profiteering, difficulties in communication with the vast and scattered populations are extreme, and there is a lack of political will in the face of competing health requirements.

In developing countries, just as living donor transplants were complicated by financial trafficking, so too has this occurred with cadaver donor transplants. An agent may receive inflated payments for provision of cadaver donor organs. Even when the organs are obtained from a legitimate cadaver donor, they may be transferred abroad, rather than kept within the country where they are needed and should be used. The agent in such cases is sometimes a senior transplantation clinician, who is at best misguided, at worst corrupt.

In other countries, criminals condemned to capital punishment become cadaver donors, and their organs are removed immediately after execution. Most doctors in developed countries (and increasingly in developing countries) feel that medical practitioners should not be involved in any way with the execution of prisoners (72,73)—and it is not possible to achieve successful organ retrieval without involvement. There are also the uncertainties of consent and the manner in which the putative donation might influence the term and conditions of the prisoner. For all these reasons, the Transplantation Society has recommended that this source of organs not be used (74). Should executed prisoner organs be made available for profit, either to a citizen of a country or to foreigners, any claim that the practice could be ethically correct is lost.

In some developing countries, the matter of organ theft or murder for organs has also been raised. Public preoccupation with transplantation and with this possibility has led to repeated, poorly researched, and often irresponsible media proclamations of such crimes, including tales of baby farms and kidnappings for body parts. The stories have a severe negative impact on organ donation rates everywhere they disseminate. The media hype, fanned by professional and public perturbation, has led to formal investigations by governments, police agencies, and military authorities, as well as organizations including WHO, UNOS, and the Paris-based International Federation for the Rights of Man. To date, not a single incident in any country has been confirmed. Because organ transplantation is a complicated and sophisticated undertaking that must necessarily involve a large number of individuals, the likelihood of a successful organ transplantation from a murdered donor happening once without discovery is remote. For it to happen repeatedly, as would be necessary to generate a continued profit, would be impossible.

The Fetus

The ethics of the use of tissues and organs from fetuses have been the matter of much discussion (75). Fetal tissues such as the pancreas, brain, liver, thymus, bone marrow, and adrenal gland have all been used in clinical transplantation, despite widespread concern over the legality and ethical probity of the procedures. The use of fetal umbilical cord blood stem cells for a variety of bone marrow deficiencies is increasing (76). The collection and sale of fetal tissue by corporations is known to occur.

Legal regulations concerning the use or disposal of fetal tissues are lacking in most countries, but codes of practice have been laid down in many (77). The use of fetal tissues for research, including transplantation, remains largely under the supervision of institutional ethics committees. It seems likely that increased usage of tissues from this source will occur, as it appears that the current majority opinion (in the face of vigorous opposition) is that scientific and medical use of fetal tissues is permissible as long as tight controls are in force and defined requirements of donation are met. Such current requirements include legal abortions, informed consent obtained after the decision for abortion has been made, certified fetal death, no designated beneficiary, approved institutions for abortions, complete separation of the doctors performing the abortion from those performing research, and no commerce.

Anencephalic Infants

Further ethical debate concerns the possible use of the organs of anencephalic babies for transplants (78). Some have argued that, because of absence of the neocortex, these are "non-persons" or are "brain dead." Thus, such infants should be available for organ donation, if this is the wish of the parents. However, as brainstem function is present in these infants, the "whole of brain" or "brain stem" requirements for certification of DOCG preclude removal of organs until cardiorespiratory death occurs. Therefore, useful donation is a rare event.

Xenografts

Since the 1960s, the transplantation community has viewed the use of animal organs to treat needy humans as the solution to organ shortage. However, the use of xenografts for the treatment of humans is highly controversial (79). The essential arguments concern whether animals have the same rights to life as do humans, whether animal lives should be forfeited on behalf of humans, and whether xenotransplantation poses a danger to the human race by the addition of previously unknown viral pathogens (79).

The first xenografts to humans in the 1960s and 1970s were from chimpanzees and baboons (80,81). However, public objection to the use of xenografts in general, but especially to those from subhuman primates, climaxed with public demonstrations of outrage in 1992 to the Pittsburgh baboon-to-human liver transplantation (82). As a result, xenograft research has shifted emphasis away from chimpanzees, the great apes, and other endangered species, and toward other animals, particularly those bred for human usage such as pigs, sheep, goats, and cattle. A good deal of transplantation research, including problematical genetic manipulation to implant human genes in animals, is now directed to these animals, especially pigs (83).

All advanced societies and countries now have their own codes of ethics for xenotransplantation research, most of which are continuously updated. In addition, all institutions in which animal or human experimentation can take place are required to have formally appointed ethics committees with defined guidelines indicating the requirements that must be met. Even so, the desperate need for organs to treat dying patients leads not only to the stretching of established guidelines but to their swamping as new methodologies and treatments are developed.

COMMENTARY

Ronald D. Guttmann

A discussion of transplantation and society must encompass not a single subject, but rather a complex series of subjects whose processes are too multidirectional and too poorly understood to be fully explored in a short essay on organ transplantation. For example, what is the central focus of transplantation? Is it the organ to be grafted, the operation, the surgeon, the immunosuppressive drugs, rejection, complications, the patient's quality of life, cost-effectiveness, survival outcomes, organ shortage, or the public organ donation strategies? The answer to this question depends on one's particular point of view, and will represent one's well-meaning, but inherently biased, self-interest. Rarely would the critical issues of transplantation be dealt with or identified by "society," because society is, in itself, an ill-defined entity in relation to most human activities. Within the context of society, transplantation would be a minuscule health care activity were it not for two very essential issues.

First, transplantation and its associated technologies are traditionally reserved for patients who have had end-stage organ failure, so only a relative minority of patients with a terminal illness will receive an organ. The rest of the patients will continue to be treated by other means until their deaths, and these other methods of prolonging life and alleviating suffering represent a significant level of human affliction and societal cost. Thus, regarding transplantation in isolation is a conceptual error. Rather, it should be seen as a discipline that currently addresses only a small segment of those patients who might benefit.

Second, transplantations with organ grafts of the liver, heart, and lung cannot succeed without programs to convince the public to part with those organs after death. "Societal" approval and cooperation are not essential in the case of kidneys—a kidney can be removed from a living person, or an artificial kidney can offer equivalent life prolongation (albeit a more expensive and less desirable prolongation in some cases)—but with the other organs, social approval is inescapable. The need for organs from the dead has become a special feature of the transplantation field.

DEFINING DEATH

To get viable organs from the dead, a process had to be developed to redefine death, and this definition still remains a troubling issue three decades after its development. Whether death conceptually needs to be considered as an event, a process, or both, the arguments are too complex and theoretical to be detailed here. However, society views death in cultural, religious, spiritual, or biologic ways that disturb those who wish to say in logical, pragmatic, and scientific terms that brain death is death—and who expect society to accept the label objectively. As much as the transplant field wants and needs the public to routinely accept its redefinition of death, the unwillingness and distrust of society continue as a serious problem. Society hesitates to put the goodness and virtue of the outcomes promised to patients ahead of ingrained values and processes observed in death and the choice of dying unperturbed by medical technology.

DONOR SHORTAGE AND RATIONING

Because too few die in a manner that "brain death" can be declared, because many families resist giving consent for organ removal, and because individuals fail to provide living wills for organ donation, there is an organ shortage that disturbs the medical profession and is frustrating, if not lethal, for patients on waiting lists. As the organ shortage worsens at a rapid pace, it has given rise to a more critical look at how organs are rationed.

Who makes the rules of rationing? How is it decided who receives the next organ? Traditionally, and paternalistically, the rationing rules have been made by the medical professionals who carry out the medical, surgical, and immunologic transplant activities. Although transplant professionals believe that they know best, often they fail to recognize that they are not without self-interest or other conflicts of interest. Their non-medical rationing act has effects, at once positive and negative, on many other unseen patients. It is in this realm that society must intervene to ensure that, whatever the rationing scheme of precious organs, it will reflect the society's values and its willingness to provide those organs.

Organ Sales

Ironically, only in the case of kidneys, for which an artificial organ offers an alternative to transplantation, could a viable solution to the organ shortage be found in the form of regulated sales from willing kidney vendors. This scheme seems to be abhorrent to many transplant professionals, although it is much less so to the public at large. Even though the sale of kidneys is currently illegal in most countries, the debate about a regulated industry may well increase in intensity.

TECHNOLOGY

A few words need to be said about the technologies of transplantation. The field has succeeded to its current halfway state through the efforts of charismatic surgeons and their brilliance in the operating rooms, the dedication of scientists who have a cure always just around the corner, the struggles of industry "partners" to make good business decisions to ensure their share of the pie, and the control of those who decide what information society needs about this field to form a reasoned understanding. We assume that the advanced technologies and the marketing and promotion are all in the best interests of society, but our assumptions must be questioned in depth.

For example, in spite of press releases to the contrary, xenografts from animals to address the organ shortage are *not* just around the corner. The hoopla about its near-term successes and the claims that it will be without significant risk play more to the financial community than to the community grounded in medical reality.

Nor do improvements in graft survival necessarily equate to a good quality of life. Life prolongation has been remarkable with the therapies available to date, but equally remarkable are the plethora of long-term complications that patients suffer. This subject is too often glossed over when communicating with the public. At present, we urgently need more and safer drugs with a higher level of specificity.

In many situations transplants may be quite inappropriate from a medical as well as a cultural perspective. There is no a priori reason to accept the notion that a transplant is better than death in all instances. Many individuals see their death as a personal choice based on their personal values, regardless of how it might be viewed by others. Conversely, families pressured to "do something" often transfer that pressure to the doctor—and the referral to the transplant center invariably results in an accepted candidate. The gatekeeping role of physicians in the community needs to become an issue for society.

Finally, some suggest that perhaps the resources consumed by the transplantation enterprise are not worth the effort. It is true that transplantation is expensive, treats relatively few patients, and is only partially successful. These are all arguments used by those whose agenda involves controlling or deviating the resources consumed by our field to other presumed needs. This type of argument is specious, however, in that it has no real set of points of reference. For example, how much does it cost *not* to transplant? How much does it cost to provide other types of less effective therapy to patients with terminal illnesses such as cancer or in vegetative states? How much does it cost to insure elective procedures for nonfatal diseases? The answers to such questions are slowly emerging: when outcomes are measured over periods of sufficiently realistic length, transplantation looks relatively good.

CONCLUSION

Our failure to ask the important questions—and properly answer them with accurate information—has kept our field on the defensive and has kept society in the dark. Such analyses are an issue for society, because they must be done by those outside our discipline. Our methodologies must be given the same sort of scrutiny applied to other fields such as education, defense, and business. Although it may hurt a little initially, my guess is that analyzing "us" relative to "them" will not be so bad in the end. This is the ultimate challenge to the field in its search for a relationship to society.

REFERENCES

1. D'Amico G. Comparability of the different registries on renal replacement therapy. Am J Kidney Dis 1995;25:113–118.
2. First MR. Transplantation in the nineties. Transplantation 1992;53:1–11.
3. Matesanz R, Miranda B, Felipe C. Organ procurement in Spain: impact of transplant coordination. Clin Transplant 1994;8:281–286.
4. Gaylin DS, Held PJ, Port FK, et al. The impact of comorbid and sociodemographic factors on access to renal transplantation. JAMA 1993;269:603–608.
5. Evans RW. Socioeconomic aspects of heart transplantation. Curr Opin Cardiol 1995;10:169–179.
6. Evans RW, Manninen DL, Dong FB. An economic analysis of liver transplantation: costs, insurance coverage and reimbursement. Gastroenterol Clin North Am 1993;22:451–473.
7. Matesanz R, Miranda B. Need for liver transplantation. Lancet 1995;346:1168–1169.
8. Barsoum RS. The Egyptian transplant experience. Transplant Proc 1992;24:2417–2420.
9. World Health Organisation. Human organ transplantation—a report on developments under the auspices of WHO (1987–91). 1991.
10. Reddy KC. Should paid organ donation be banned in India? To buy or let die! Natl Med J India 1993;6:137–139.
11. Shaheen FAM. Transplantation in Saudi Arabia. Transplant Proc 1995;27:1470–1471.
12. Scott R. The body as property. London: Allen Lane, 1981:150–158.
13. A definition of irreversible coma. Report of the Ad Hoc Committee of the Harvard Medical School to examine the definition of brain death. JAMA 1968;205:337.
14. Farrell MM, Levin DL. Brain death in the pediatric patient: historical, sociological, medical, religious, cultural, legal, and ethical considerations. Crit Care Med 1993;21:1951–1965.
15. Ashwal S. Brain death in the newborn. Clin Perinatol 1989;16:501–518.
16. Lee PP, Yang JC, McDonnell PJ, et al. Worldwide legal requirements for obtaining corneas: 1990. Cornea 1992;11:102–107.
17. Committee of Ministers. Council of Europe, Resolution (78) 29 on harmonisation of legislations of member states relating to removal, grafting and transplantation of human substances. 1978.
18. Williams JW, Vera S, Evans LS. Socioeconomic aspects of hepatic transplantation. Am J Gastroenterol 1987;82:1115–1119.
19. Evans RW, Manninen DL, Dong FB. An economic analysis of pancreas transplantation: costs, insurance coverage, and reimbursement. Clin Transplant 1993;7:166–174.
20. Eggers PW, Kucken LE. Cost issues in transplantation. Horizons Organ Transplant 1994;74:1259–1267.
21. Dean M. Is your treatment economic, effective, efficient? Lancet 1991;337:480–481.
22. Michel BC, Van Hout BA, Bonsel GJ. Assessing the benefits of transplant services. Baillieres Clin Gastroenterol 1994;8:411–423.
23. Disney APS. Demography and survival of patients receiving treatment for chronic renal failure in Australia and New Zealand: Report on dialysis and renal transplantation treatment from the Australia and New Zealand Dialysis and Transplant Registry. Am J Kidney Dis 1995;25:165–175.
24. Levy MF, Jennings L, Abouljoud MS, et al. Quality of life improvements at one, two, and five years after liver transplantation. Transplantation 1995;59:515–518.
25. Pierce GA, Graham WK, Kauffman HM Jr, Wolf JS, United Network for Organ Sharing (UNOS). The united network for organ sharing: 1984 to 1994. Transplant Proc 1996;28:12–15.
26. Alexander JW, Zola JC. Expanding the donor pool: use of marginal donors for solid organ transplantation. Clin Transplant 1996;10:1–19.
27. Wing AJ, Chang RWS. Non-heart beating donors as a source of kidneys. BMJ 1994;308:549–550.

28. Nathan HM, Jarrell BE, Broznik B, et al. Estimation and characterization of the potential renal organ donor pool in Pennsylvania. Transplantation 1991;51:142–149.
29. Park K, Kim YS. Use of kidneys from living-related or unrelated donors: pro. Current opinions: living donors. In: Terasaki PI, ed. Clinical Transplants, 1994. Los Angeles: UCLA Tissue Typing Laboratory, 1994:374–375.
30. Callender CO, Bey AS, Miles PV, Yeager CL. A national minority organ/tissue transplant education program: the first step in the evaluation of a national strategy and minority transplant equity in the USA. Transplant Proc 1995;27:1441–1443.
31. Evans RW, Orians CE, Ascher NL. The potential supply of organ donors: an assessment of the efficiency of organ procurement efforts in the United States. JAMA 1992;267:239–246.
32. Prottas JM, Batten HL. Attitudes and incentives in organ procurement: the attitudes of the American public. Report to the Health Care Financing Administration, April 1986.
33. West R. Organ transplantation. London: Office of Health Economics, 1991:10.
34. Gore SM, Cable DJ, Holland AJ. Organ donation from intensive care units in England and Wales: two year confidential audit of deaths in intensive care. BMJ 1992;304:349–355.
35. Luce J. Ethical principles in critical care. JAMA 1990;263:696–700.
36. Michielsen P. Unlimited admission of patients to the waiting list for transplantation. In: Land W, Dossetor JB, eds. Organ replacement therapy: ethics, justice, commerce. New York: Springer, 1991:364–367.
37. Farge EJ, Silverman LM, Khan MM, Wilhelmus KR. The impact of state legislation on eye banking. Arch Ophthalmol 1994;112:180–185.
38. Kleinman I, Lowy FH. Cadaveric organ donation: ethical considerations for a new approach. Can Med Assoc J 1989;141:107–110.
39. Jarvis R. Join the club: a modest proposal to increase availability of donor organs. J Med Ethics 1995;21:199–204.
40. Alexander JW, Vaughn WK. The use of "marginal" donors for organ transplantation: the influence of donor age on outcome. Transplantation 1991;51:135–141.
41. Teperman L, Podesta L, Mieles L, Starzl TE. The successful use of older donors for liver transplantation. JAMA 1989;262:2837.
42. Livi U, Bortolotti U, Luciani GB, et al. Donor shortage in heart transplantation: is extension of donor age limits justified? J Thorac Cardiovasc Surg 1994;107:1346–1355.
43. Nghiem DD, Hsia S, Schlosser JD. Growth and function of en bloc infant kidney transplants: a preliminary study. J Urol 1995;153:326–329.
44. Johnson LB, Kuo P, Schweitzer EJ, et al. Double renal allografts successfully increase utilization of kidneys from older donors within a single organ procurement organization. Transplantation 1996;62:1581–1583.
45. Gjertson DW, Terasaki PI, Cecka JM, et al. Senior citizens pool for aged kidneys. Transplant Proc 1997;29:129.
46. Casavilla A, Ramirez C, Shapiro R, et al. Experience with liver and kidney allografts from non-heart-beating donors. Transplantation 1995;59:197–203.
47. Diethelm AG, Roth D, Ferguson RM, et al. Transmission of HCV by organ transplantation. N Engl J Med 1992;326:410–411.
48. Casavilla A, Mazariegos G, Fung JJ. Cadaveric liver donors: what are the limits? Transplant Proc 1996;28:21–23.
49. Ross C. Towards acceptance of organ transplantation? Lancet 1995;346:42.
50. Yokoyama I, Uchida K, Tominaga Y, et al. Ten-year experience in the use of double balloon catheter for kidney procurement from non-heart beating donors in cadaveric kidney transplantation. Clin Transplant 1993;7:258–262.
51. Tesi RJ, Elkhammas EI, Davies EA, et al. Pulsatile kidney perfusion for evaluation of high risk kidney donors safely expands the donor pool. Clin Transplant 1994;8:134–138.
52. Kootstra G, Wijnen RMH, van Hooff JP, van der Linden CJ. Twenty percent more kidneys through a non-heart beating donor program. Transplant Proc 1991;23:912–913.
53. Feest TG, Riad HN, Collins CH, et al. Protocol for increasing organ donation after cerebrovascular deaths in a district general hospital. Lancet 1990;335:1133–1135.
54. Jones MA. Elective ventilation of potential organ donors. The legal background. BMJ 1995;310:717–718.
55. Light JA, Kowalski AE, Ritchie WO, et al. New profile of cadaveric donors: what are the kidney donor limits? Transplant Proc 1996;28:17–20.
56. Cerilli J. Ethical guidelines for organ procurement. Transplantation 1988;46:171–172.
57. Peters TG. Life or death: the issue of payment in cadaveric organ donation. JAMA 1991;265:1302–1305.
58. Kevorkian J. A controlled auction market is a practical solution to the shortage of transplantable organs. Med Law 1992;11:47–55.
59. Schwindt R, Vining AR. Proposal for a future delivery market for transplant organs. J Health Polit Policy Law 1986;11:483–500.
60. McGaw JL, Wesley AJ, Dilip KS, et al. Incentives for organ donation? Lancet 1991;338:1441–1443.
61. Fryd DS, Canafax DM, Matas AJ, et al. In: Terasaki PI, ed. Clinical Transplants. Los Angeles: UCLA Tissue Typing Laboratory, 1988:79–90.
62. Gaston RS, Ayres I, Dooley LG, Diethelm AG. Racial equity in renal transplantation; the disparate impact of HLA-based allocation. JAMA 1993;270:1352–1356.
63. Maruya E, Takemoto S, Cecka JM, Terasaki PI. HLA matching identification of permissible HLA mismatches. In: Terasaki PI, Cecka JK, eds. Clinical Transplants. Los Angeles: UCLA Tissue Typing Laboratory, 1994:285–292.
64. Takemoto S, Terasaki PI, Gjertson DW, Cecka JM. Equitable allocation of HLA compatible kidneys for local pools and for minorities. N Engl J Med 1994;331:760–764.
65. Annual Report of the U.S. scientific registry for organ transplantation and the organ procurement and transplantation network. UNOS, 1992.
66. Land W. Accepted resolutions. Resolution 8. In: Land W, Dossetor JB, eds. Organ replacement therapy: ethics, justice, commerce. Part VII. New York: Springer, 1991:555.
67. Merrill JP, Murray JE, Harrison JH, Guild WR. Successful homotransplantation of the human kidney between identical twins. JAMA 1956;160: 277–282.
68. Spital A. Unrelated living kidney donors. Transplantation 1994;57:1722–1726.
69. Jones J, Payne WD, Matas AJ. The living donor—risks, benefits, and related concerns. Transplant Rev 1993;7:115–128.
70. Bay WH, Hebert LA. The living donor in kidney transplantation. Ann Intern Med 1987;106:719–727.
71. Mason J, McCall Smith R. Law and medical ethics. 3rd ed. London: Butterworths, 1991:312.
72. Current Opinions. Capital Punishment. Chicago, IL: The Council on Ethical & Judicial Affairs of the American Medical Association, 1989.
73. Editorial: Doctors and death row. Lancet 1993;341:209–210.
74. Policy Statement from the Ethics Committee of the Transplantation Society. Transplant Soc Bull 1995;3:3.
75. Fine A. Human fetal tissue research: practice, prospects and policy. Cell Transplant 1994;3:113–145.
76. Gale RP. Cord-blood-cell transplantation—a real sleeper? N Engl J Med 1995;332:392–394.
77. Coutts MC. Fetal Tissue Research. Kennedy Inst Ethics J 1993;3:81–100.
78. Medearis DN, Holmes LB. On the use of anencephalic infants as organ donors. N Engl J Med 1989;321:391–393.
79. Chapman LE, Folks TM, Salomon DR, et al. Xenotransplantation and xenogeneic infections. N Engl J Med 1995;333:1498–1501.
80. Reemtsma K, McCracken BH, Schlegel JU, et al. Renal heterotransplantation in man. Ann Surg 1964;160:384–410.
81. Starzl TE, Marchioro TL, Peters GN, et al. Renal heterotransplantation from baboon to man: experience with 6 cases. Transplantation 1964;2:752–776.
82. Starzl TE, Fung J, Tzakis A, et al. Baboon to human liver transplantation. Lancet 1993;341:65–71.
83. Geller RL, Turman MA, Dalmasso AP, Platt JL. The natural immune barrier to xenotransplantation. J Am Soc Nephrol 1992;3:1189–1200.

INDEX

Note: Page numbers followed by *f* indicate figures; those followed by *t* indicate tables.